DISEASES AND ICD-9-CM CODES *Continued*

Laryngitis	464.0
Lead poisoning	984
Legionnaires' disease	482.83
Leishmaniasis	085, 089
Leprosy	030
Lichen planus	697.0
Low back pain	724.2
Lyme disease	088.81
Lymphogranuloma venereum	099.1
Malabsorption	579
Malaria	084.6
Measles (rubeola)	055.9
Meconium aspiration	770.1
Melanoma	172
Meniere's disease	386.0
Meningitis	320–322
Menopause	627.2
Migraine headache	346
Mitral valve prolapse	424.0
Monilial vulvovaginitis	112.1
Multiple myeloma	203.0
Multiple sclerosis	340
Mumps	072.9
Myasthenia gravis	358.0
Mycoplasmal pneumonia	483.0
Mycosis fungoides	202.1
Nausea and vomiting	787.01
Necrotizing skin and soft tissue infections	785.4
Neoplasms of the vulva	239.5
Neutropenia	288.0
Nevi	216, 448.1
Newborn physiologic jaundice	774.6
Nongonococcal urethritis	099.4
Non-Hodgkin's lymphomas	202
Nonimmune hemolytic anemia	283.1
Normal delivery	650
Obesity	278.0
Obsessive-compulsive disorders	300.3
Onychomycosis	110.1
Optic neuritis	377.3
Osteoarthritis	715
Osteomyelitis	730
Osteoporosis	733.0
Otitis externa	380.10
Paget's disease of bone	731.0
Panic disorder	300.01
Pap smear	V72.3
Parkinsonism	332.0
Paronychia	681.0
Partial epilepsy	345.4
Patent ductus arteriosus	747.0
Pediculosis	132
Pelvic inflammatory disease	614
Peptic ulcer disease	533
Pericarditis	423.9
Peripheral arterial disease	443.9
Peripheral neuropathies	356
Pernicious anemia and other megaloblastic anemias	281
Personality disorders	301
Pheochromocytoma	227.0
Phobia	300.2
Pigmentary disorders—vitiligo	709.01
Pinworms	127.4
Pityriasis rosea	696.3
Placenta previa	641.0
Plague	020
Platelet-mediated bleeding disorders	287.1
Pleural effusion	511.9
Polycythemia vera	238.4
Polymyalgia rheumatica	725
Porphyria	277.1
Postpartum hemorrhage	666.1
Post-traumatic stress disorder	309.81
Pregnancy	V22.2
Pregnancy-induced hypertension	642
Premature beats	427.6
Premenstrual syndrome (PMS)	625.4
Prescribing oral contraceptive	V25.01
Pressure ulcers	707.0
Preterm labor	644.2
Primary glomerular disease	581–583
Primary lung abscess	513.0
Primary lung cancer	162.9
Prostate cancer	185
Prostatitis	601
Pruritus	698.9
Pruritus ani	698.0
Pruritus vulvae	198.1
Psittacosis (ornithosis)	073
Psoriasis	696.1
Pulmonary embolism	415.1
Pyelonephritis	590
Q fever	083.0
Rabies	071
Rat-bite fever	026
Relapsing fever	087
Renal calculi	592
Reye syndrome	331.81
Rheumatic fever	390
Rheumatoid arthritis	714.0
Rib fracture	807.0
Rocky Mountain spotted fever	082.0
Rosacea	695.3
Roseola	057.8
Rubella	056
Salmonellosis	003.0
Sarcoidosis	135
Scabies	133
Schizophrenia	295
Seborrheic dermatitis	690.1
Septicemia	038
Sézary's syndrome	202.2
Shoulder dislocation	831.0
Sickle cell anemia	282.6
Silicosis	502
Sinusitis	473
Skull fracture	800, 801, 803
Sleep apnea	780.57
Sleep disorders	780.5
Snakebite	989.5
Stasis ulcers	454.0
Status epilepticus	345.3
Stomach cancer	151
Streptococcal pharyngitis	034.0
Stroke	436
Strongyloides infection	127.2
Subdural or subarachnoid hemorrhage	852
Sunburn	692.71
Syphilis	090–097
Tachycardias	785.0
Tapeworm infections	123
Telogen effluvium	704.02
Temporomandibular joint syndrome	524.6
Tendinitis	726–727
Tetanus	037
Thalassemia	282.4
Therapeutic use of blood components	V59.0
Thrombotic thrombocytopenic purpura	446.6
Thyroid cancer	193
Thyroiditis	245
Tinea capitis	110.0
Tinnitus	388.3
Toe fracture	826.0
Toxic shock syndrome	040.89
Toxoplasmosis	130
Transient cerebral ischemia	435
Trauma to the genitourinary tract	958, 959
Trichinellosis	124
Trichomonal vaginitis	131.01
Trigeminal neuralgia	350.1
Tuberculosis	011
Tularemia	021
Typhoid fever	002.0
Typhus fevers	080, 081
Ulcerative colitis	556
Urethral stricture	598
Urinary incontinence	788.3
Urticaria	708
Uterine inertia	661.0
Uterine leiomyoma	218
Varicella (chickenpox)	052
Venous thrombosis	453.8
Viral pneumonia	480.0–480.9
Viral respiratory infections	465.0
Vitamin deficiency	264–269
Vitamin K deficiency	269.0
Warts (verrucae)	078.10
Wegener's granulomatosis	446.4
Whooping cough (pertussis)	033
Wrist fracture	814.0

Adapted from Jones MK, Castillo LA, Hopkins CA, Aaron WS (eds): St. Anthony's ICD-9-CM Code Book for Physician Payment, Vols 1 and 2, 5th ed. Reston, VA, St. Anthony Publishing, 1996.

LATEST APPROVED METHODS OF TREATMENT FOR THE PRACTICING PHYSICIAN

Edited by

ROBERT E. RAKEL, M.D.

Professor, Department of Family and Community Medicine
Baylor College of Medicine, Houston, Texas

and

EDWARD T. BOPE, M.D.

Family Practice Residency Director, Riverside Family Practice Residency Program
Clinical Professor, Department of Family Medicine
The Ohio State University, Columbus, Ohio

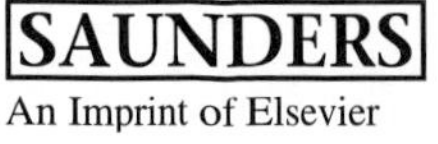

An Imprint of Elsevier

CONN'S CURRENT THERAPY 2004

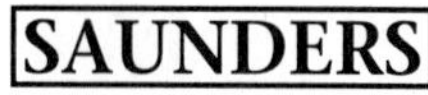
An Imprint of Elsevier

The Curtis Center
Independence Square West
Philadelphia, Pennsylvania 19106-3399

CONN'S CURRENT THERAPY 2004 ISBN 0-7216-0401-3

Notice

Medicine is an ever-changing field. Standard safety precautions must be followed but as new research and clinical experience broaden our knowledge, changes in treatment and drug therapy may become necessary or appropriate. Readers are advised to check the most current product information provided by the manufacturer of each drug to be administered to verify the recommended dose, the method and duration of administration, and contraindications. It is the responsibility of the treating physician, relying on experience and knowledge of the patient, to determine dosages and the best treatment for each individual patient. Neither the Publisher nor the author assume any liability for any injury and/or damage to persons or property arising from this publication.

The Publisher

Library of Congress Cataloging-in-Publication Data

Current therapy; latest approved methods of treatment for the practicing physician.
Editors: H. F. Conn and others
v. 28 cm. annual
ISBN 0-7216-0401-3
1. Therapeutics. 2. Therapeutics, Surgical. 3. Medicine—Practice.
I. Conn, Howard Franklin, 1908–1982 ed.

RM101.C87 616.058 49–8328 rev*

Publisher: Thomas H. Moore
Associate Editor: Tom Hartman
Senior Project Manager: Natalie Ware
Book Designer: Karen O'Keefe Owens

Printed in the United States of America.

Last digit is the print number: 9 8 7 6 5 4 3 2 1

Contributors

WALID ABUHAMMOUR, M.D.

Associate Professor of Pediatrics, Michigan State University College of Human Medicine, Lansing, Michigan; Director, Pediatric Infectious Disease, Hurley Medical Center, Flint, Michigan
Mumps

DAVID B. ADAMS, M.D.

Professor of Surgery and Head of General and Gastrointestinal Surgery, Medical University of South Carolina, Charleston, South Carolina
Chronic Pancreatitis

K. AFSHAR, M.D.

Fellow in Pediatric Urology, Hospital for Sick Children, Toronto, Ontario, Canada
Bacterial Infections of the Urinary Tract in Girls

SHARAREH AHMADI, M.D.

Specialist Registrar in Dermatology, Royal College of Surgeons in Ireland; Maier Hospital, Dublin, Ireland
Diseases of the Mouth

MICHAEL R. ALBERT, M.D.

Instructor, Department of Dermatology, Brown Medical School, Providence, Rhode Island
Smallpox

MARK S. ALLEN, M.D.

Associate Professor of Surgery, Mayo Medical School; Consultant in General Thoracic Surgery, Mayo Clinic; Chair, Division of General Thoracic Surgery, Mayo Clinic, Rochester, Minnesota
Pleural Effusion and Empyema Thoracis

OSCAR D. ALMEIDA, JR., M.D.

Clinical Associate Professor, University of South Alabama College of Medicine, Mobile, Alabama
Pelvic Inflammatory Disease

EZRA A. AMSTERDAM, M.D.

Professor, Internal Medicine (Cardiology), Director, CCU, University of California, Davis, Medical Center, Sacramento, California
Premature Beats

KELLEY P. ANDERSON, M.D.

Clinical Associate Professor of Medicine, Department of Cardiology, University of Wisconsin Medical School; Marshfield Clinic, Marshfield, Wisconsin
Heart Block

NANCY J. ANDERSON, M.D.

Professor, Division of Dermatology, Residency Director, Dermatology, Chief, Division of Dermatology, Loma Linda VA Hospital, Loma Linda, California
Granuloma Inguinale (Donovanosis)
Lymphogranuloma Venereum

WARREN A. ANDIMAN, M.D.

Professor of Pediatrics and Epidemiology and Public Health, Yale University School of Medicine; Attending Physician, Pediatric Infectious Diseases, Yale-New Haven Children's Hospital, New Haven, Connecticut
Infectious Mononucleosis

LOWELL B. ANTHONY, M.D.

Division of Gastroenterology and Neuroendocrine Oncology, Louisiana State University Medical Center, New Orleans, Louisiana
Nausea and Vomiting

CAROLINE M. APOVIAN, M.D.

Associate Professor of Medicine, Boston University School of Medicine; Director, Center for Nutrition and Weight Management, Co-Director, Nutrition Support Service, Boston Medical Center, Boston, Massachusetts
Obesity

GERARD V. ARANHA, M.D.

Loyola University School of Medicine, Maywood, Illinois
Acute Pancreatitis

DAVID J. ARATEN, M.D.

Instructor, Memorial Sloan-Kettering Cancer Center, New York, New York
Aplastic Anemia

JOSE R. ARIAS, JR., M.D.

Fellow, Allergy and Immunology, University of South Florida College of Medicine, The James A. Haley VA Hospital, Tampa, Florida
Nonallergic Rhinitis

OTTER Q. ASPEN

Harvard Medical School, Boston, Massachusetts
Acne Vulgaris and Rosacea

PAUL G. AUWAERTER, M.D., M.B.A.

Associate Professor of Medicine, Division of General Internal Medicine and Infectious Diseases, Johns Hopkins University, Baltimore, Maryland
Bacterial Pneumonia

TANDY AYE, M.D.

Fellow, Pediatric Endocrinology, Massachusetts General Hospital, Boston, Massachusetts
Diabetes Mellitus in Children and Adolescents

LEONARD B. BACHARIER, M.D.

Assistant Professor of Pediatrics, Washington University School of Medicine; Attending Physician, St. Louis Children's Hospital, St. Louis, Missouri
Asthma in Children

DAVID A. BAKER, M.D.

Professor, Obstetrics, Gynecology, and Reproductive Medicine, Health Sciences Center, State University of New York at Stony Brook, Stony Brook, New York
Vulvovaginitus

LAURA J. BALCER, M.D., M.S.C.E.
Associate Professor, University of Pennsylvania School of Medicine, Philadelphia, Pennsylvania
Optic Neuritis

JAMES F. BALE, Jr., M.D.
Professor and Vice-Chair, Department of Pediatrics, Division of Child Neurology, University of Utah School of Medicine; Medical Staff, Primary Children's Medical Center, Salt Lake City, Utah
Viral Meningitis and Encephalitis in Children and Adults

HENRY H. BALFOUR, M.D.
Professor, Department of Laboratory Medicine and Pathology, Professor, Department of Pediatrics, University of Minnesota Medical School, Minneapolis, Minnesota
Varicella (Chickenpox)

ROBERT A. BALK, M.D.
Professor of Medicine, J. Baily Center, Rush Medical College; Director of Pulmonary and Critical Care Medicine, St. Luke's Medical Center, Chicago, Illinois
Sepsis

JAMES N. BARANIUK, M.D.
Associate Professor of Medicine, Georgetown University, Washington, D.C.
Allergic Rhinitis Caused by Inhalant Factors

THEODORE D. BARBER, M.D.
Resident in Urology, Wayne State University School of Medicine, Detroit, Michigan
Trauma to the Genitourinary Tract

DEBORAH BARTHOLOMEW, M.D.
Clinical Associate Professor, Obstetrics and Gynecology, The Ohio State University College of Medicine and Public Health, The Ohio State University Hospitals and Clinics, Columbus, Ohio
Urinary Incontinence

NANCY L. BARTLETT, M.D.
Associate Professor, Washington University School of Medicine, St. Louis, Missouri
Hodgkin's Disease: Chemotherapy

JAMES C. BARTON, M.D.
Clinical Professor of Medicine, University of Alabama at Birmingham; Medical Director, Southern Iron Disorders Center, Birmingham, Alabama
Iron Deficiency

AHMET A. BASCHAT, M.D.
Clinical Instructor, Department of Obstetrics, Gynecology and Reproductive Sciences, University of Maryland School of Medicine, University of Maryland Medical Center, Baltimore, Maryland
Hemolytic Disease of the Fetus and Newborn

JOAN M. BATHON, M.D.
Johns Hopkins University School of Medicine; Active Staff, Johns Hopkins Hospital, Active Staff, Johns Hopkins Bayview Medical Center, Baltimore, Maryland
Osteoarthritis

NICHOLAS J. BEECHING, M.A., M.B.
Senior Lecturer, Liverpool School of Tropical Medicine, University of Liverpool; Honorary Consultant Physician, Tropical and Infectious Diseases Unit, Royal Liverpool University Hospital, Liverpool, United Kingdom
Salmonellosis

JEFFREY G. BELL, M.D.
Clinical Professor Obstetrics and Gynecology, Ohio State University; Director, Gynecologic Oncology, Riverside Methodist Hospitals, Columbus, Ohio
Cancer of the Uterine Cervix

GERALD C.J. BENNETT, M.B.*
The Royal London Hospital, Department of Health Care of the Elderly, London, United Kingdom
Pressure Ulcers

JOEL S. BENNETT, M.D.
Professor of Medicine and Pharmacology, University of Pennsylvania School of Medicine, Philadelphia, Pennsylvania
Platelet-Mediated Bleeding Disorders

BETHANY M. BERGAMO, M.D.
Assistant Professor of Dermatology, Department of Dermatology, University of Alabama, Birmingham, Alabama
Sunburn

BRIAN BERMAN, M.D., Ph.D.
Professor of Dermatology and Internal Medicine, University of Miami School of Medicine, Miami, Florida
Keloids
Cutaneous Warts

STANLEY J. BIRGE, Jr., M.D.
Associate Professor of Medicine, Washington University School of Medicine, Barnes-Jewish Hospital, St. Louis, Missouri
Osteoporosis

JACOB D. BITRAN, M.D.
Director, Hematology/Oncology, Lutheran General Hospital and Cancer Care Center, Park Ridge, Illinois
Primary Lung Cancer

ANTHONY J. BLEYER, M.D., M.S.
Associate Professor, Section of Nephrology, Wake Forest University School of Medicine, Winston-Salem, NC
Chronic Kidney Failure

CONRAD B. BLUM, M.D.
Professor of Clinical Medicine, Division of Preventive Medicine, Columbia University College of Physicians and Surgeons; Attending Physician, New York Presbyterian Hospital, New York, New York
Hyperlipoproteinemias

KRISTIE A. BLUM, M.D.
Fellow, Hematology/Oncology, Washington University School of Medicine, St. Louis, Missouri
Hodgkin's Disease: Chemotherapy

ANDREA K. BOGGILD, M.Sc., M.D.
Resident, Medical Microbiology, Department of Laboratory Medicine and Pathobiology, Faculty of Medicine, University of Toronto, Ontario, Canada
Amebiasis

JULIE A. BOOM, M.D.
Assistant Professor of Pediatrics, Baylor College of Medicine; Immunization Project Director, Texas Children's Hospital, Houston, Texas
Office-Based Immunization Practices

EDWARD T. BOPE, M.D.
Program Director, Riverside Family Practice Residency Program, Riverside Methodist Hospital, Columbus, Ohio; Clinical Professor, Department of Family Medicine, Ohio State University, Columbus, Ohio

*Deceased

WILLIAM Z. BORER, M.D.
Professor of Pathology, Jefferson Medical College, Thomas Jefferson University, Philadelphia, Pennsylvania
Reference Intervals for the Interpretation of Laboratory Tests

KAREN R. BORMAN, M.D.
Professor, Surgery, Vice-Chair for Surgical Education, Department of Surgery, University of Missisipi School of Medicine; Attending Staff, University Hospitals and Clinics, University of Mississippi Medical Center, Jackson, Mississippi
Thyroid Cancer

L. LUCY BOULANGER, M.D.
Medical Officer, Indian Health Service, United States Public Health Service, Crownpoint, New Mexico
Plague (Yersinia)

JAMES A. BOURGEOIS, O.D., M.D.
Director, Consultation-Liaison Service, Department of Psychiatry and Behavioral Sciences, University of California, Davis, Associate Professor of Clinical Psychiatry, University of California, Davis Medical Center, Sacramento, California
Delirium

PATRICK J. BOYLE M.D.
Professor of Medicine, University of New Mexico; Program Director, General Clinical Research Center, University of New Mexico, Albuquerque, New Mexico
Diabetic Ketoacidosis

CHAD M. BRAUN, M.D.
Clinical Assistant Professor; Associate Residing Director, Department of Family Medicine, The Ohio State University; Medical Director, Thomas E. Rardin Family Practice Center, Columbus, Ohio
Travel Medicine

JOEL G. BREMAN, M.D., D.T.P.H.
Senior Scientific Advisor, Fogarthy International Center, Bethesda, Maryland
Smallpox

DAVID C. BREWSTER, M.D.
Director, Endovascular Surgery, Division of Vascular Surgery, Massachusetts General Hospital, Boston, Massachusetts
Acquired Diseases of the Aorta

JOHN W. BRICE, M.D.
Associate Professor of Medicine, Medical College of Georgia; Chief of Medicine, Augusta VA Medical Center, Augusta, Georgia
Acute Respiratory Failure

S. LOUIS BRIDGES, JR., M.D., PH.D.
Associate Professor, Medicine and Microbiology, University of Alabama at Birmingham, Birmingham, Alabama
Polymyalgia Rheumatica and Giant Cell Arteritis

NICOLA BRINK, M.B., CHB., MMED.
Department of Virology (Bloomsbury) University College, London, United Kingdom
Rabies

ADAM BRODSKY, M.D.
Cardiology Fellow, Northwestern University Feinberg School of Medicine, Chicago, Illinois
Management of Angina Pectoris

PATRICIA D. BROWN, M.D.
Associate Professor of Medicine, Division of Infectious Diseases, Harper Grace Hospital, Detroit, Michigan
Bacterial Infections of the Urinary Tract in Women

CARLO BRUGNARA, M.D.
Professor of Pathology, Harvard Medical School; Director, Hematology Laboratory, Department of Laboratory Medicine, Children's Hospital Boston, Boston, Massachusetts
Nonimmune Hemolytic Anemia

LUCINDA S. BUESCHER, M.D.
Associate Professor of Dermatology, Southern Illinois University School of Medicine, Springfield, Illinois
Spider Bites and Scorpion Stings

SUPAWAN BURANAPIN, M.D.
Fellow in Nutrition, Section of Endocrinology, Diabetes and Nutrition, Boston University School of Medicine, Boston, Massachusetts
Obesity

JAMES J. BURKE, II, M.D.
Assistant Professor of Obstetrics and Gynecology, Mercer University School of Medicine; Attending Physician, Memorial Health University Medical Center, Savannah, Georgia
Endometrial Cancer

ROBERT L. BURNAUGH, M.D.
Fellow, Pulmonary and Critical Care, Medical College of Georgia, Augusta, Georgia
Acute Respiratory Failure

ANDREW BURROUGHS, M.B., CH.B., HONS.
Professor of Hepatology; Royal Free and University College Medical School, University of London; Consultant, Physician and Hepatologist, Royal Free Hospital, Hampstead, London, United Kingdom
Bleeding Esophageal Varices

DIEGO CADAVID, M.D.
Assistant Professor, Department of Neurology and Neuroscience, UMDNJ, New Jersey Medical School, Newark, New Jersey
Relapsing Fever

MARK P. CAIN, M.D.
Associate Professor of Urology, Indiana University; Staff Urologist, J.W. Riley Hospital for Children, Indianapolis, Indiana
Childhood Enuresis

JEFFREY P. CALLEN M.D.
Professor of Medicine (Dermatology), Chief, Division of Dermatology, University of Louisville, Louisville, Kentucky
Connective Tissue Diseases

THOMAS R. CARACCIO, PHARM.D.
Associate Professor of Emergency Medicine, State University of New York, Stony Brook, New York; Assistant Professor of Pharmacology/Toxicology, New York College of Osteopathic Medicine, Old Westbury, New York; Managing Director, Long Island Regional Poison Control Center, Winthrop University Hospital, Mineola, New York
Medical Toxicology: Ingestions, Inhalations, and Dermal and Ocular Absorptions

BRUCE R. CARR, M.D.
Holder, Paul C. MacDonald Chair in Obstetrics and Gynecology; Director, Division of Reproductive Endocrinology and Infertility, University of Texas Southwestern Medical Center at Dallas, Dallas, Texas
Leiomyomas

COLIN H. CHALK, M.D.
Associate Professor, Department of Neurology and Neurosurgery, McGill University Faculty of Medicine; Associate Physician, Department of Medicine, The Montreal General Hospital, Montreal, Quebec, Canada
Peripheral Neuropathies

MIRIAM M. CHAN, R.P.H., PHARM.D.
Clinical Assistant Professor of Pharmacy, The Ohio State University, Columbus, Ohio; Adjunct Assistant Professor of Pharmacology, Ohio Northern University, Ada, Ohio; Affiliate Faculty of Pharmacy Practice, Idaho State University, Pocatello, Idaho; Director of Pharmacy Education, Riverside Family Practice Residency Program, Riverside Methodist Hospital, Columbus, Ohio
Some Popular Herbs and Nutritional Supplements
New Drugs in 2002 and Agents Pending FDA Approval

ERNIE J. CHANEY, M.D.
Professor Emeritus, Department of Family and Community Medicine, University of Kansas School of Medicine-Wichita, Wichita, Kansas
Contraception

CHARLES CHAPPUIS, M.D.
Clinical Associate Professor of Surgery, Chief of Surgery, University Medical Center, Lafayette, Louisiana
Diverticula of the Alimentary Tract

CARLOS A. CHARLES, M.D.
Wound Healing Fellow, University of Miami School of Medicine, Dermatology and Cutaneous Surgery, Miami, Florida
Venous Ulcers

TSUNG O. CHENG, M.D.
Professor of Medicine, George Washington University Medical Center, Washington, D.C.
Mitral Valve Prolapse

ELISA I. CHOI, M.D.
Instructor in Medicine, Harvard Medical School; Instructor in Medicine, Beth Israel Deaconess Medical Center, Boston, Massachusetts
Q Fever

YOUNG K. CHOI, M.D.
Fellow, University of Iowa Hospital and Clinics, Carver College of Medicine, Iowa City, Iowa
Gaseousness and Indigestion

JOSEPHINE CHU, A.B.
Stanford University School of Medicine, Stanford, California
Bullous Diseases

MINA K. CHUNG, M.D.
Staff, Section of Cardiac Electrophysiology and Pacing Department of Cardiovascular Medicine; The Cleveland Clinic Foundation, Cleveland, Ohio
Atrial Fibrillation

THEODORE J. CIESLAK, M.D.
Chairman, San Antonio Military Pediatrics Center; Clinical Associate Professor of Pediatrics, University of Texas Health Science Center at San Antonio and Uniformed Services University of the Health Sciences, San Antonio, Texas
Anthrax

DAVID X. CIFU, M.D.
The Herman J. Flax, M.D. Professor and Chairman, Department of Physical Medicine and Rehabilitation, Virginia Commonwealth University/Medical College of Virginia; Chief, Rehabilitation Medicine Services, Medical College of Virginia Hospital, Virginia Commonwealth University Health System, Richmond, Virginia
Management and Rehabilitation of the Stroke Survivor

RICHARD D. CLOVER, M.D.
Department of Family Medicine and Clinical Epidemiology, University of Pittsburgh School of Medicine, Pittsburgh, Pennsylvania
Acute and Chronic Viral Hepatitis

DAVID E. COHN, M.D.
Assistant Professor, Division of Gynecologic Oncology, Department of Obstetrics and Gynecology, The Ohio State University College of Medicine and Public Health, Arthur G. James Center Hospital and Solove Research Institute, Columbus, Ohio
Neoplasms of the Vulva

NANCY ANDREWS COLLINS, M.D.
Associate Professor of Obstetrics and Gynecology, Director, Gynecology Division, Assistant Residency Director, University of Arkansas for Medical Sciences, Little Rock, Arkansas
Antepartum Care

DAVID E. COMINGS, M.D.
Director, Medical Genetics, Department of Medical Genetics, City of Hope National Medical Center, Duarte, California
Treatment of Tourette's Syndrome

COSTAS L. CONSTANTINOU, M.D.
Staff, Trinity Health System; Staff, Genesis Health System, Hematology Medical Oncology Consultants, Bettendorf, Iowa
Neutropenia

LARRY J. COPELAND, M.D.
Professor and Chair, Department of Obstetrics and Gynecology, The Ohio State University College of Medicine and Public Health; Chair, Obstetrics and Gynecology, The Ohio State Medical Center – James Cancer Hospital, Columbus, Ohio
Neoplasms of the Vulva

CHRISTINA M. COYLE, M.D.
Associate Professor of Medicine, Albert Einstein College of Medicine; Director of Clinical Infectious Disease, Jacobi Hospital, Bronx, New York
Malaria

BURKE A. CUNHA, M.D.
Professor of Medicine at the State University of New York School of Medicine, Stony Brook, New York; Chief, Infectious Disease Division, Winthrop-University Hospital, Mineola, New York
Prostatitis

CALHOUN D. CUNNINGHAM, III, M.D.
Clinical Fellow, House Ear Clinic, Los Angeles, California
Tinnitus

GUIDO DALBAGNI, M.D.
Associate Professor of Urology, Weill Medical College of Cornell University, New York, New York
Malignant Tumors of the Urogenital Tract

VICTORIA DALZELL, M.D.
Developmental and Behavioral Pediatrics, Barbara Bush Children's Hospital, Maine Medical Center, Portland, Maine
Attention Deficit Hyperactivity Disorder

ERNO S. DANIEL, M.D., PH.D.
Associate Clinical Professor of Medicine, University of Southern California School of Medicine, Los Angeles; Department of Internal Medicine and Geriatrics, Sansum-Santa Barbara Medical Foundation Clinic; Medical Director, Mission Terrace Convalescent Hospital and Vista Del Monte Retirement Community, Santa Barbara, California
Alzheimer's Disease

ANDRÉ DASCAL, M.D.
Associate Professor of Medicine and Microbiology and Immunology, McGill University; Associate Director, Division of Infectious Diseases, Sir Mortimer B. Davis–Jewish General Hospital, Montreal, Quebec, Canada
Toxic Shock Syndrome

JEFFREY B. DATTILO, M.D.
Assistant Professor of Surgery, Division of Vascular Surgery, Vanderbilt University Medical Center; Chief of Vascular Surgery, Veterans Affairs Medical Center, Nashville, Tennessee
Acquired Diseases of the Aorta

TERENCE M. DAVIDSON, M.D.
Professor of Surgery, University of California-San Diego School of Medicine, Veterans Affairs San Diego Healthcare System; Director, University of California-San Diego Nasal Dysfunction Clinic, Head and Neck Surgery, Sleep Clinic, San Diego, California
Snake Venom Poisoning

FAITH E. DAVIES, M.D.
Clinical Scientist, Department of Health, Academic Unit of Oncology and Haematology School of Medicine, University of Leeds, Leeds, United Kingdom
Multiple Myeloma

KATRINA R. DAVIS, M.D.
Assistant Professor of Obstetrics and Gynecology, Director, Junior/Senior Medical Student Internship Director, University of Arkansas for Medical Sciences, Little Rock, Arkansas
Antepartum Care

TAMI DE ARAUJO, M.D.
Research Fellow in Dermatology, Department of Dermatology and Cutaneous Surgery, University of Miami School of Medicine, Miami, Florida.
Cutaneous Warts

THOMAS G. DELOUGHERY, M.D.
Division of Hematology, Oregon Health and Science University, Portland, Oregon
Venous Thrombosis

JEAN-CHARLES DEYBACH, M.D.
Professor in Biochemistry and Molecular Biology; Faculté de Médicine Paris, Xavier Bichat Universités; Head of the Department of Biochemistry and Molecular Genetics and Centre Français des Porphyries, Paris, France
The Porphyrias

CAROL A. DIAMOND, M.D.
Assistant Professor, Pediatric Hematology/Oncology, University of Wisconsin Medical School, Madison, Wisconsin
Vitamin K Deficiency

H. ERHAND DINCER, M.D.
Senior Fellow in Pulmonary and Clinical Care Medicine, Medical College of Wisconsin, Milwaukee, Wisconsin
Silicosis

JEFFREY S. DOVER, M.D.
Adjunct Professor of Medicine (Dermatology), Dartmouth Medical School; Associate Clinical Professor of Dermatology, Section of Dermatologic Surgery and Oncology, Department of Dermatology, Yale University School of Medicine; Consultant Dermatologist, New England Baptist Hospital; Staff Physician, Dermatology, Beth Israel Deaconess Hospital; Consultant in Medicine (Dermatology), Dana Farber Cancer Institute, Boston, Massachusetts
Erythema Multiforme, Stevens-Johnson Syndrome, and Toxic Epidermal Necrolysis

CHARLES E. DRISCOLL, M.D., M.S.ED.
Clinical Professor of Family Medicine, University of Virginia, Charlottesville, Virginia; Director, Lynchburg Family Practice Residency, Lynchburg, Virginia
Postpartum Care

LAWRENCE M. DUBUSKE, M.D.
Instructor in Medicine, Department of Internal Medicine, Harvard Medical School, Consultant in Allergy, Brigham and Women's Hospital, Boston, Massachusetts
Asthma in Adolescents and Adults

WILLIAM DUCKWORTH, M.D.
Research Professor, Molecular and Cellular Biology Program, Arizona State University; Professor of Clinical Medicine, Department of Medicine; University of Arizona, Phoenix, Arizona
Diabetes Mellitus in Adults

JOHN D. EDWARDS, M.D.
Department of Surgery, University of Cincinnati Medical School, Cincinnati, Ohio
Peripheral Arterial Disease

GRAEME EISENHOFER, PH.D.
Laboratory Director and Staff Scientist, National Institutes of Health, Bethesda, Maryland
Pheochromocytoma

EDWARD M. EITZEN, JR., M.D., M.P.H.
Adjunct Associate Professor of Pediatrics; Adjunct Associate Professor of Military and Emergency Medicine, Uniformed Services University of the Health Sciences, Bethesda, Maryland; Senior Medical Advisor, Office of the Assistant Secretary for Public Health Emergency Preparedness, Department of Health and Human Services, Washington D.C.
Anthrax

NAYEF EL-DAHER, M.D., PH.D.
Clinical Associate Professor of Medicine, University of Rochester School of Medicine; Head, Infectious Diseases Unit, Department of Medicine, Park Ridge Hospital/Unity Health System, Rochester, New York
Pyelonephritis

WILLIAM J. ELLIOTT, M.D., PH.D.
Professor of Preventive Medicine, Internal Medicine, and Pharmacology, Rush Medical College of Rush University at Rush-Presbyterian-St. Luke's Medical Center; Attending Physician, Rush-Presbyterian-St. Luke's Medical Center, Chicago, Illinois
Hypertension

DIRK M. ELSTON, M.D.
Associate in Dermatology and Laboratory Medicine, Geisinger Medical Center, Danville, Pennsylvania
Hair Disorders

ELIHU ESTEY, M.D.
Professor, University of Texas, Professor of Medicine and Internist, Department of Leukemia, University of Texas M.D. Anderson Cancer Center, Houston, Texas
Acute Leukemia in Adults

GEOFFREY EUBANK, M.D.
Clinical Instructor, Ohio State University; Director, Neurology Education, Riverside Methodist Hospital; President, Neurological Associates, Inc., Columbus Ohio
Intracerebral Hemorrhage

ANNA F. FALABELLA, M.D.
Associate Professor, Dermatology and Cutaneous Surgery, Assistant Chief of Dermatology, VA Medical Center, University of Miami School of Medicine, Dermatology and Cutaneous Surgery; Director, Dermatology Wound Healing Clinic, Jackson Memorial Hospital, Miami, Florida
Venous Ulcers

RICHARD NEIL FEDORAK, M.D.
Professor of Medicine, Department of Medicine, University of Alberta; Director, Division of Gastroenterology, University of Alberta Hospital, Edmonton, Alberta, Canada
Malabsorption

ULLA FELDT-RASMUSSEN, M.D., D.M.S.C.
Associate Professor, Copenhagen University, Denmark; Chief of Department of Endocrinology PE2132, National University Hospital, Copenhagen, Denmark
Thyroiditis

CHRISTOPHER J. FINNEGAN, B.Sc., M.Sc.
Research Scientist, Veterinary Laboratories Agency, New Haw, Addlestone, Surrey, United Kingdom
Rabies

DAN FINTEL, M.D.
Associate Professor of Medicine; Director, Coronary Care Unit, Northwestern University Feinberg School of Medicine, Chicago, Illinois
Management of Angina Pectoris

STEPHANIE A. FISH, M.D.
Fellow, Division of Endocrinology, Diabetes, and Metabolism, University of Pennsylvania School of Medicine, Philadelphia, Pennsylvania
Hypothyroidism

ROBERT C. FLANIGAN, M.D.
Professor and Chairperson of Urology, Loyola University Medical Center, Department of Urology, Maywood, Illinois
Urethral Stricture

SCOTT E. FLETCHER, M.D.
Creighton/University of Nebraska, Children's Hospital, Omaha, Nebraska
Congenital Heart Disease

ANTHONY R. FOOKS, B.Sc., M.B.A., Ph.D.
Head, Rabies Research and Diagnostic Group, Veterinary Laboratories Agency, New Haw, Addlestone, Surrey, United Kingdom
Rabies

ANGELO FORMENTI, M.D.
Director of E.N.T. Videoendoscopy Center, E.N.T. Department, Fatebenefratelli e Oftalmico Hospital, Milano, Italy
Acute Facial Paralysis (Bell's Palsy)

JOSEPH F. FOWLER, Jr., M.D.
Clinical Professor of Dermatology, University of Louisville School of Medicine, Louisville, Kentucky
Contact Dermatitis

KATHLEEN FRANCHEK-ROA, M.D.
Baylor College of Medicine, Assistant Professor, Texas Children's Hospital, Preceptor Residents Primary Care Group, Houston, Texas
Parenteral Fluid Therapy for Infants and Children

JOHN P. FRANGIE, M.D.
Assistant Professor of Ophthalmology, Boston University School of Medicine, Boston, Massachusetts; Medical Director, Pioneer Valley Ophthalmic Consultants, Amherst, Massachusetts; Attending Surgeon, North East Laser Center, W. Springfield, Massachusetts, Franklin Medical Center, Amherst, Massachusetts
Conjunctivitis

CHAD I. FRIEDMAN, M.D.
Associate Professor, Department of Obstetrics and Gynecology, The Ohio State University College of Medicine, Columbus, Ohio
Dysfunctional Uterine Bleeding

MITCHELL FRIEDMAN, M.D.
Professor of Pulmonary Diseases, Chief, Section of Pulmonary Diseases, Critical Care, and Environmental Medicine, Tulane University of Medicine Medical Center, New Orleans, Louisiana
Management of Chronic Obstructive Pulmonary Disease

RICK A. FRIEDMAN, M.D., Ph.D.
Volunteer Clinical Faculty, University of Southern California, Department of Otolaryngology; Clinical Associate, House Ear Clinic, Los Angeles, California
Tinnitus

STEVEN M. FRUCHTMAN, M.D.
Clinical Director, Division of Hematology, Mount Sinai School of Medicine; Associate Attending Physician, Mount Sinai Hospital, New York, New York
Polycythemia Vera

JOSEPH M. FURMAN, M.D., Ph.D.
Professor, Department of Otolaryngology, University of Pittsburgh School of Medicine, Pittsburgh, Pennsylvania
Episodic Vertigo

GLENN FUSONIE, M.D.
Department of Surgery, University of Cincinnati Medical School, Cincinnati, Ohio
Peripheral Arterial Disease

JOHN N. GAITANIS, M.D.
Instructor in Neurology, Harvard Medical School; Assistant in Neurology, Children's Hospital of Boston, Boston, Massachusetts
Epilepsy in Infancy and Childhood

STEVEN L. GALETTA, M.D.
Van Meter Professor of Neurology and Ophthalmology, Director, Neuro-Ophthalmology, University of Pennsylvania Medical Center, Philadelphia, Pennsylvania
Optic Neuritis

DONALD B. GALLUP, M.D.
Professor and Chairperson, Department of Obstetrics and Gynecology, Mercer University School of Medicine; Attending Physician, Memorial Health University Medical Center, Savannah, Georgia
Endometrial Cancer

R. DON GAMBRELL, Jr., M.D.
Clinical Professor of Endocrinology and Obstetrics and Gynecology, Medical College of Georgia; Senior Staff, Department of Obstetrics and Gynecology, University Hospital, Augusta, Georgia
Menopause

JEAN-PIERRE GANGNEUX, M.D.
Faculté de Medicine de Rennes, Laboratoire de Parasitologie-Mycologie, Rennes, France
Leishmaniasis

NELSON M. GANTZ, M.D.
Clinical Professor of Medicine, Penn State School of Medicine, Hershey, Pennsylvania; Chief of Infectious Diseases, Boulder Community Hospital, Boulder, Colorado
Acute Bronchitis

STEVEN R. GARFINI, M.D.
Professor and Chair, University of California, San Diego, School of Medicine, San Diego, California
Low Back Pain

MITCHELL E. GEFFNER, M.D.
Professor of Pediatrics, Keck School of Medicine at University of Southern California; Fellowship Program Director, Children's Hospital of Los Angeles, Los Angeles, California
Hypopituitarism

KATHERINE G. GERGAS, M.S., L.N.P.
Certified Family Nurse Practitioner, Ohio State University Department of Family Medicine, Rardin Family Practice Center; Ohio State University, Columbus, Ohio
Travel Medicine

JAMSHID GHAJAR, M.D.
Clinical Associate Professor of Neurosurgery, New York-Presbyterian Hospital; Chief, Division of Neurosurgery, Jamaica Hospital, New York, New York
Acute Traumatic Brain Injury in Adults

HOSSEIN GHARIB, M.D.
Professor of Medicine, Mayo Medical School; Consultant, Mayo Clinic, Division of Endocrinology and Internal Medicine, Rochester, Minnesota
Hyperthyroidism

GEORGE J. GIANAKOPOULOS, M.D.
Clinical Assistant Professor of Medicine, The Ohio State University; Private Practice, Infectious Diseases, Riverside Methodist Hospital, Columbus, Ohio
Food-Borne Illness

PETER GIBSON, M.D.
Professor of Gastroenterology, Monash University; Director of Gastroenterology, Box Hill Hospital, Box Hill, Melbourne, Australia
Irritable Bowel Syndrome

GORDON G. GIESBRECHT, PH.D.
Professor, Faculty of Physical Education and Recreation Studies, University of Manitoba; Professor, Department of Anesthesia, University of Manitoba, Winnipeg, Manitoba, Canada
Disturbances Due to Cold

THOMAS P. GIORDANO, M.A., M.D.
Assistant Professor of Medicine, Section of Infectious Diseases and Health Services Research, Baylor College of Medicine; Staff Physician, The Thomas Street Clinic And Ben Taub General Hospital of the Harris County Hospital District, and the Houston VA Medical Center, Houston, Texas
Management of the HIV-Infected Patient

COL. STEPHEN M. GOLDEN, (M.D.), U.S.A.F., M.C.
Associate Professor of Pediatrics, Uniformed Services University of the Health Sciences, U.S.U.W.S., Bethesda, Maryland; Director, Newborn Services, Associate Chief of the Medical Staff; Chairman, Pediatric Research Committee; Travis A.F.B., California
Resuscitation of the Newborn

JOHN M. GOLDMAN, D.M.
Professor of Leukemia Biology; Chairman, Department of Hematology, Imperial College London at Hammersmith Hospital, London, United Kingdom
Chronic Leukemias

DAVID C. GORSULOWSKY, M.D.
Associate Clinical Professor, Department of Dermatology, University of California and San Francisco; Clinical Associate Professor, Department of Dermatology, Stanford University School of Medicine; Staff Physician, Veterans Affairs Medical Center, San Francisco, California
Papulosquamous Eruptions

MARY K. GOSPODAROWICZ, M.D.
Professor, Department of Radiation Oncology, University of Toronto; Chair, Department of Radiation Oncology, University of Toronto; Chief, Radiation Medicine Program, Princess Margaret Hospital, Toronto, Ontario, Canada
Hodgkin's Disease: Radiation Therapy

KIM R. GOTTSHALL, PH.D., P.T., A.T.C.
Assistant Professor, Department of Exercise and Nutrition Science, San Diego State University; Clinical Professor, Department of Biokinesiology, University of Southern California; Department of Defense Spatial Orientation Center, Naval Medical Center, San Diego, California
Ménière's Disease

MICHAEL B. GOTWAY, M.D.
Director, Radiology Residency Training Program, Assistant Professor-in-Residence, Diagnostic Radiology and Pulmonary/Critical Care Medicine, University of California, San Francisco; Director, Thoracic Imaging, Director, Body Imaging Protection Programs, San Francisco General Hospital, San Francisco, California
Atelectasis

DAVID F. GRAFT, M.D.
Clinical Professor of Pediatrics, University of Minnesota Medical School; Chairman, Asthma and Allergic Diseases, Park Nicollet Clinic, Minneapolis, Minnesota
Allergic Reactions to Insect Bites

LESLIE C. GRAMMER, M.D.
Professor of Medicine, Northwestern University, Chicago, Illinois
Hypersensitivity Pneumonitis

H.L. GREENBERG, M.D.
Dermatology Resident, University of Wisconsin, Madison, Wisconsin
Parasitic Diseases of the Skin

STEPHEN B. GREENBERG, M.D.
Herman Brown Teaching Professor, Baylor College of Medicine; Chief of Medicine, Ben Taub General Hospital, Houston, Texas
Influenza

JOSEPH GREENSHER, M.D.
Professor of Pediatrics, State University of New York, Stony Brook, New York; Medical Director and Associate Chair, Department of Pediatrics, Long Island Regional Poison and Drug Information Center, Winthrop-University Hospital Mineola, New York
Medical Toxicology: Ingestions, Inhalations, and Dermal and Ocular Absorptions

FRANK R. GREER, M.D.
Professor of Pediatrics, University of Wisconsin Medical School, Madison, Wisconsin
Vitamin K Deficiency

RICHARD M. GRIMES, B.B.A., M.B.A., PH.D.
Associate Professor, School of Public Health, Dental Branch, School of Nursing, University of Texas Health Science Center at Houston, Houston, Texas
Management of the HIV-Infected Patient

CELIA L. GROSSKREUTZ, M.D.
Instructor, Division of Hematology, Mount Sinai School of Medicine; Clinical Instructor, Mount Sinai Hospital, New York, New York
Polycythemia Vera

THERESA W. GYORKOS, PH.D.
Associate Professor, McGill University, Department of Epidemiology and Biostatistics; Associate Director, Division of Clinical Epidemiology, McGill University Health Centre (MUHC), Montreal General Hospital Site, Montreal, Quebec, Canada
Intestinal Parasites

DEREK A. HAAS, M.D.
Associate Instructor, Division of Reproductive Endocrinology and Infertility, University of Texas, Dallas, Texas
Leiomyomas

PETER H. HACKETT, M.D.
Associate Clinical Professor, Division of Emergency Medicine, University of Colorado Health Sciences Center; President, International Society for Mountain Medicine, Denver, Colorado
High Altitude Illness

DAVID N. HACKNEY, M.D.
Chief Resident, Department of Obstetrics and Gynecology, Ohio State University Medical Center, Columbus, Ohio
Hypertensive Disorders of Pregnancy

URIEL HALBREICH, M.D.
Professor of Psychiatry and Obstetrics and Gynecology, State University of New York at Buffalo; Director, Biobehavior Program, SUNY-AB, Buffalo, New York
Premenstrual Dysphoria

ROBERT E. HALES, M.D., M.B.A.
Joe P. Tupin Professor and Chair, University of California, Davis Medical Center, Department of Psychiatry and Behavioral Sciences, Sacramento, California
Delirium

ALLAN C. HALPERN, M.D.
Associate Member, Chief, Dermatology, Memorial Sloan-Kettering Cancer Center, New York, New York
Melanoma

M. BOWES HAMILL, M.D.
Associate Professor, Department of Ophthalmology, Baylor College of Medicine, Houston, Texas
Vision Correction Procedures

DOUGLAS H. HAMILTON, M.D., PH.D.
Adjunct Assistant Professor, Emory University Office of Public Health, Atlanta, Georgia
Cat-Scratch Disease

CHRISTINE M. HARDY, M.S., R.D., L.D.N.
Clinical Teaching Associate, Brown Medical School; Pediatric Nutrition Specialist, Department of Pediatric Gastroenterology and Nutrition, Rhode Island Hospital, Providence, Rhode Island
Normal Infant Feeding

MARY L. HARRIS, M.D.
Director, Fellowship Program, Associate Professor, Division of Gastroenterology, Johns Hopkins University, Baltimore, Maryland
Inflammatory Bowel Disease

ROGER HARTL, M.D.
Resident, Department of Neurosurgery, New York-Presbyterian Hospital, Weill College of Cornell University, New York, New York
Acute Traumatic Brain Injury in Adults

KATHRYN L. HASSELL, M.D.
Associate Professor of Medicine, Division of Hematology, Director, Colorado Sickle Cell Treatment and Research Center, University of Colorado Health Sciences Center; Director, Colorado Sickle Cell Treatment and Research Center, Denver, Colorado
Sickle Cell Disease

GABRIELLE M. HAWDON, M.D.
Department of Pharmacology, University of Melbourne, Melbourne, Australia
Hazardous Marine Creatures

J. OWEN HENDLEY, M.D.
Professor of Pediatrics, University of Virginia Health System, Charlottesville, Virginia
Viral Upper Respiratory Tract Infections

CHRISTIAN L. HERMANSEN, M.D.
Senior Resident, Lancaster General Hospital, Lancaster, Pennsylvania
Psittacosis (Ornithosis)

CHARLES B. HICKS, M.D.
Associate Professor of Medicine, Division of Infectious Diseases and International Health, Duke University School of Medicine, Durham, North Carolina
Syphilis

DARRYL T. HIYAMA, M.D.
Associate Professor of Surgery, David Geffen School of Medicine at University of California–Los Angeles, Los Angeles, California
Total Parenteral Nutrition in Adults

MICHAEL E. HOFFER, M.D.
Attending Professor, Uniformed Health Sciences University, Bethesda, Maryland; Director, Department of Defense Spatial Orientation Center, Department of Otolaryngology, Naval Medical Center–San Diego, San Diego, California
Ménière's Disease

DAVID HOSKING, M.D., M.B., CH.B.
Visiting Professor, University of Zagreb, Zagreb, Croatia; Consultant Physician, City Hospital, Nottingham, United Kingdom
Hyperparathyroidism and Hypoparathyroidism

JOSEPH M. HUGHES, M.D.
Clinical Associate Professor of Medicine, Columbia University School of Physicians and Surgeons, New York, New York; Attending Physician, Bassett Healthcare, Cooperstown, New York
Adrenocortical Insufficiency

TATYANA R. HUMPHREYS, M.D.
Clinical Associate Professor, Department of Dermatology, Thomas Jefferson University; Director, Division of Cutaneous Surgery, Jefferson Dermatology Associates, Philadelphia, Pennsylvania
Cancer of the Skin

SHAHID HUSSAIN, M.D.
Instructor, Department of Psychiatry and Behavioral Neurosciences, Wayne State University, Detroit, Michigan
Panic Disorder

THOMAS M. HYERS, M.D.
Clinical Professor of Internal Medicine, St. Louis University School of Medicine, St. Louis, Missouri
Pulmonary Embolism

NEIL H. HYMAN, M.D.
Associate Professor of Surgery, University of Vermont College of Medicine; Chief, Division of General Surgery, Department of Surgery, University of Vermont College of Medicine, Burlington, Vermont
Pruritus Ani and Vulvae

IGNACIO INGLESSIS, M.D.
Pericarditis

DAVID W. JACKSON, M.D.
Clinical Postdoctoral Fellow, Department of Ophthalmology, Baylor College of Medicine, Houston Texas
Vision Correction Procedures

JAMES J. JAMES, M.D., DR.P.H., M.H.A.
Director, Center for Disaster Preparedness and Emergency Response, American Medical Association, Chicago, Illinois
Toxic Chemical Agents Reference Chart: Clinical Considerations; Biologic Agents Reference Chart: Clinical Considerations

RASHID M. JANJUA, M.D.
Resident Neurosurgery, University of Louisville, Louisville, Kentucky
Acute Head Injuries in Children

JULIA V. JOHNSON, M.D.
Professor and Vice-Chair, Gynecology; Division Director, Reproductive Endocrinology and Infertility, Department of Obstetrics and Gynecology, University of Vermont College of Medicine, Burlington, Vermont
Endometriosis

ROYCE H. JOHNSON, M.D.
Professor of Medicine, David Geffen School of Medicine, University of California Los Angeles, Los Angeles, California; Chair, Department of Medicine, Chief, Infectious Disease, Kern Medical Center, Bakersfield, California
Coccidioidomycosis

M. PATRICIA JOYCE, M.D.
Director, Medical Services, National Hansen's Disease Programs, Baton Rouge, Louisiana; Adjunct Faculty, Tropical Medicine, Tulane University School of Public Health and Tropical Medicine, New Orleans, Louisiana
Leprosy (Hansen's Disease)

VERN C. JUEL, M.D.
Associate Professor of Neurology, University of Virginia School of Medicine, Charlottesville, Virginia
Myasthenia Gravis

KEVIN C. KAIN, M.D.
Professor of Medicine, University of Toronto; Canada Research Chair in Molecular Parasitology, Director, Centre for Travel and Tropical Medicine, Toronto General Hospital, Toronto, Ontario, Canada
Amebiasis

MATTHEW H. KANZLER
Clinical Professor, Stanford University School of Medicine; Chief, Division of Dermatology, Santa Clara Valley Medical Center, San Jose, California
Papulosquamous Eruptions

CAROL A. KAUFFMAN, M.D.
Professor of Internal Medicine, University of Michigan Medical School; Chief, Infectious Diseases Section, Ann Arbor Veterans Affairs Healthcare System, Ann Arbor, Michigan
Blastomycosis

ANDREW KEAT, M.D.
Consultant Rheumatologist, Northwick Park Hospital, Middlesex, United Kingdom
Ankylosing Spondylitis

JOHN KEFER, M.D., PH.D.
Resident, Urology, Cleveland Clinic, Cleveland, Ohio
Benign Prostatic Hyperplasia

DENNIS KELLAR, M.D.
Fellow, Pulmonary and Critical Care, St. Luke's Medical Center, Rush Medical College, Chicago, Illinois
Sepsis

ELIZABETH KENNARD, M.D.
Associate Professor, Clinical, Ohio State University; Division Director, Reproductive Endocrinology and Infertility, Department of Obstetrics and Gynecology, Ohio State University, Columbus, Ohio
Ectopic Pregnancy

SRIPATHI R. KETHU, M.D.
Assistant Professor of Medicine, Brown Medical School; Attending Physician, Rhode Island Hospital, Providence, Rhode Island
Gastritis and Peptic Ulcer Disease

ANTOINE E. KHOURY, M.D.
Professor, University of Toronto; Head, Division of Urology, The Hospital for Sick Children, Toronto, Ontario, Canada
Bacterial Infection of the Urinary Tract in Girls

EDWARD D. KIM, M.D.
Associate Professor, Department of Surgery/Urology, University of Tennessee Medical Center, Knoxville, Tennessee
Erectile Dysfunction

KAREN E. KING, M.D.
Assistant Professor, Pathology and Oncology, The Johns Hopkins School of Medicine; Medical Director, Hematopoietic and Therapeutic Support Service, Associate Medical Director, Transfusion Medicine Division, The Johns Hopkins Hospital, Baltimore, Maryland
Autoimmune Hemolytic Anemia

JEFFREY T. KIRCHNER, D.O., F.A.A.F.P.
Clinical Associate Professor, Temple University School of Medicine, Philadelphia, Pennsylvania; Medical Director, Comprehensive Care Clinic For HIV/AIDS, Lancaster, Pennsylvania
Psittacosis (Ornithosis)

DAVID C. KLONOFF, M.D.
Mills-Peninsula Health Services, San Mateo, California
Chronic Fatigue Syndrome

MICHAEL B. KNABLE, D.O.
Instructor in Psychiatry and Neurology, George Washington University Hospital, Washington, D.C.
Schizophrenia

RICHARD D. KOPKE, M.D.
Assistant Professor of Surgery, Uniformed Services, University of Health Sciences, Bethesda, Maryland; Staff Neurologist, Co-Director, Department of Defense Spatial Orientation Center, Department of Otolaryngology, Naval Medical Center–San Diego, San Diego, California.
Ménière's Disease

CHRIS G. KOUTURES, M.D.
Lecturer, Children's Hospital of Orange County, Orange, California
Common Sports Injuries

KRZYSZTOF KOWAL
Instructor in Medicine, Department of Allergology, University Medical School of Bialystok, Bialystok, Poland
Asthma in Adolescents and Adults

KRIS V. KOWDLEY, M.D.
Division of Gastroenterology, University of Washington School of Medicine, Seattle, Washington
Hemochromatosis

GRAHAM P. KRASAN, M.D.
Assistant Professor, Division of Infectious Disease, Department of Pediatrics, University of Michigan, Ann Arbor, Michigan
Streptococcal Pharyngitis

LESLEY A. KRESIE, M.D.
Co-Director, Core Laboratory, Director, Pathology Training Program, Baylor University Medical Center, Dallas Texas
Thrombotic Thrombocytopenic Purpura

STANFORD I. LAMBERG, M.D.
Associate Professor, Dermatology, The Johns Hopkins University, Baltimore Maryland
Cutaneous T-Cell Lymphoma

LENEE A. LANE, PHARM.D.

Clinical Assistant Professor, University of Oklahoma College of Pharmacy HSC, Oklahoma City, Oklahoma; Chief Pharmacist, Clinical Pharmacist, Norman Regional Hospital, Norman, Oklahoma; Eckerd Pharmacy, Oklahoma City, Oklahoma
Pernicious Anemia and Other Megaloblastic Anemias

DENNIS K. LEDFORD, M.D.

Professor of Medicine, University of South Florida College of Medicine and The James A. Haley VA Hospital; Chief of Allergy/Immunology, University Community Hospital, Tampa, Florida
Nonallergic Rhinitis
Anaphylaxis and Serum Sickness

WILLIAM M. LEE, M.D.

Meredith Mosle Distinguished Professor in Liver Diseases, University of Texas Southwestern Medical School; Attending Physician, Parkland Memorial Hospital, Dallas, Texas
Cirrhosis

GERTRUDE S. LEFAVOUR, M.D.

Associate Professor of Medicine, UMDNJ Robert Wood Johnson Medical School; Chief, Division of Nephrology, St. Peter's University Hospital, New Brunswick, New Jersey
Diabetes Insipidus

NEAL S. LELEIKO, M.D., PH.D.

Professor of Pediatrics, Brown University School of Medicine; Director, Division of Pediatric Gastroenterology, Nutrition and Liver Disease, Hasbro Children's Hospital of the Rhode Island Hospital, Providence, Rhode Island
Normal Infant Feeding

TOMMY LEONARD, JR., M.D.

Associate Professor of Pediatrics, Baylor College of Medicine, Houston, Texas
Care of the High-Risk Neonate

FRANCES R. LEVIN, M.D.

NYSPI; Q.J. Kennedy Associate Professor of Clinical Psychiatry, NYSPI, Columbia University; New York Presbyterian Hospital, New York, New York
Drug Abuse

MICHAEL J. LEVINSON, M.D.

Associate Professor of Medicine, University of Tennessee College of Health Sciences, Memphis, Tennessee
Constipation

MATTHEW E. LEVISON, M.D.

Professor of Medicine and Public Health, Medical College of Pennsylvania, Hahnemann University School of Medicine, Philadelphia, Pennsylvania
Infective Endocarditis

LYNNE L. LEVITSKY, M.D.

Associate Professor of Pediatrics, Harvard Medical School; Chief, Pediatric Endocrine Unit, Massachusetts General Hospital, Boston, Massachusetts
Diabetes Mellitus in Children and Adolescents

JAMES H. LEWIS, M.D.

Professor of Medicine, Division of Gastroenterology, Georgetown University School of Medicine; Georgetown University Hospital, Washington, D.C.
Hiccups

JAMES W. LEWIS, M.D.

Acute Renal Failure

NEIL R. LIEBOWITZ, M.D.

Assistant Clinical Professor, Psychiatry, University of Connecticut, School of Medicine; Medical Director, Connecticut Anxiety and Depression Treatment Center, Farmington, Connecticut
Anxiety Disorders

SHARI MIURA LING, M.D.

Assistant Professor, Johns Hopkins University School of Medicine; Staff Clinician, Clinical Research Branch, National Institute on Aging, Baltimore, Maryland
Osteoarthritis

ROBERT P. LISAK, M.D.

Parker Webber Chair in Neurology, Professor and Chair of Neurology, Professor of Immunology and Microbiology, Wayne State University School of Medicine; Neurologist-in-Chief, Detroit Medical Center; Chief of Neurology, Harper University Hospital, Detroit, Michigan
Multiple Sclerosis

GERALD L. LOGUE, M.D.

Professor of Medicine, State University of New York at Buffalo; Hematology Division Head, Erie County Medical Center, Buffalo, New York
Adverse Reactions to Blood Transfusions

NAOMI L.C. LUBAN, M.D.

Professor of Pediatrics and Pathology, George Washington University School of Medicine; Chief, Division of Laboratory Medicine and Pathology; Director, Transfusion Medicine/Donor Center, Children's Hospital National Medical Center, Washington, D.C.
Therapeutic Use of Blood Components

JAMES M. LYZNICKI, M.S., M.P.H.

Senior Scientist, Center for Disaster Preparedness and Emergency Response, American Medical Association, Chicago, Illinois
Toxic Chemical Agents Reference Chart: Clinical Considerations
Biologic Agents Reference Chart: Clinical Considerations

J. DICK MACLEAN, M.D.

Professor of Medicine, Director, McGill University Centre for Tropical Disease; Senior Physician, Director, Division of Tropical Medicine, Montreal General Hospital, Montreal, Quebec, Canada
Intestinal Parasites

KEN MADDEN, M.D., PH.D

Clinical Associate Professor of Neurology, University of Wisconsin Medical School, Madison, Wisconsin; Neurologist, Cerebrovascular Disease Subspecialist, Marshfield Clinic, Marshfield, Wisconsin
Ischemic Cerebrovascular Disease

DILIP MAHALANABIS, M.B.B.S.

Director, Society for Applied Studies, Kolkata, India
Cholera

MARK A. MALANGONI, M.D.

Professor of Surgery, Case Western Reserve University, Cleveland, Ohio; Chair, Department of Surgery, MetroHealth Medical Center, Cleveland, Ohio
Necrotizing Skin and Soft Tissue

YVONNE A. MALDONADO, M.D.

Associate Professor, Department of Pediatrics, Stanford University Medical Center, Stanford, California
Measles (Rubeola)

ANTHONY J. MANCINI, M.D.

Associate Professor of Pediatrics and Dermatology, Northwestern University Feinberg School of Medicine; Attending Physician, Children's Memorial Hospital, Chicago, Illinois
Atopic Dermatitis

SUSAN J. MANDEL, M.D.
Assistant Professor of Medicine and Radiology and Fellowship Program Director, Division of Endocrinology, Diabetes, and Metabolism, University of Pennsylvania School of Medicine; Associate Chief of Clinical Affairs, Hospital of the University of Pennsylvania, Philadelphia, Pennsylvania
Hypothyroidism

WILLIAM MUIR MANGER, M.D., PH.D.
Professor of Clinical Medicine, New York University Medical Center; Emeritus Lecturer in Medicine, Columbia College of Physicians and Surgeons; Attending Physician, Tisch Hospital; Attending Physician, Bellevue Hospital; Consultant, Southampton Hospital, New York, New York
Pheochromocytoma

LAUREN B. MARANGELL, M.D.
Brown Professor Psychopharmacology of Mood Disorders, Director of Mood Disorder Research, Baylor College of Medicine; Department of Veterans Affairs, Co-director, Psychopharmacology Research, Education, and Clinical Enhancement Program of the South Central Mental Illness Research, Education and Clinical Center, South Central MIRECC Department of Veterans Affairs, Houston, Texas
Mood Disorders

DAWN A. MARCUS, M.D.
Associate Professor, University of Pittsburgh Medical Center, Departments of Anesthesiology and Neurology, Pittsburgh, Pennsylvania
Headaches

M. PETER MARINKOVICH, M.D.
Department of Dermatology; Program in Epithelial Biology, Stanford University School of Medicine, Stanford, California
Bullous Diseases

JAMES M. MARTINEZ, M.D.
Assistant Professor of Psychiatry, Baylor College of Medicine, Houston, Texas
Mood Disorders

JOHN A. MATA, M.D.
Associate Professor of Urology, Louisiana State University Health Sciences Center, Shrevesport, Louisiana
Nongonococcal Urethritis

LAURA MAURI, M.D.
Instructor, Harvard Medical School; Staff Interventional Cardiologist, Brigham and Women's Hospital, Boston, Massachusetts
Acute Myocardial Infarction

ALEXANDER MAUSKOP, M.D.
Associate Professor, Clinical Neurology, State University of New York-Downstate Medical Center; Director, New York Headache Center, New York, New York
Pain

MICHAEL MCGUIGAN, M.D.
Medical Director, Long Island Regional Poison and Drug Information Center, Winthrop-University Hospital, Mineola, New York
Medical Toxicology: Ingestions, Inhalations, and Dermal and Ocular Absorptions

WILLIAM J. MCKENNA, M.D.
Professor of Cardiology, The Heart Hospital, University College, London, United Kingdom
Hypertrophic Cardiomyopathy

DANIEL MCNALLY, M.D.
Associate Professor, Department of Medicine, Chief, Pulmonary Division, University of Connecticut School of Medicine; Director, Pulmonary Laboratory, John Dempsey Hospital, Farmington, Connecticut
Cough

KATHERINE A. MCQUEEN, M.D.
Assistant Professor, Department of Internal Medicine, Baylor College of Medicine; Faculty, Section of General Internal Medicine, Ben Taub General Hospital, Houston, Texas
Alcoholism

BELLA H. MEHTA, PHARM.D.
Assistant Professor, Clinical, The Ohio State University, College of Pharmacy, Columbus, Ohio
New Drugs in 2002 and Agents Pending FDA Approval

MARIA MELA, M.D.
Clinical Research Fellow, Royal Free Hospital, Hampstead, London, United Kingdom
Bleeding Esophageal Varices

NICHOLAS A. MEYER, M.D.
Assistant Professor, University of Wisconsin; Director of Burn Center, University of Wisconsin, Madison, Wisconsin
Burns

LARRY E. MILLIKAN, M.D.
Professor, Tulane University Medical School, Department of Dermatology; Chairman, Tulane University Hospital and Clinic, New Orleans, Louisiana
Urticaria and Angioedema

GRACE Y. MINAMOTO, M.D.
Associate Professor of Clinical Medicine, Albert Einstein College of Medicine; Director, Fellowship Training Program in Infectious Diseases, Inpatient Medical Director, AIDS Center, Montefiore Medical Center, Bronx, New York
Rat-Bite Fever

EUGENE MINEVICH, M.D.
Assistant Professor, University of Cincinnati Department of Surgery, University of Cincinnati; Pediatric Urologist – Division of Pediatric Urology, Cincinnati Children's Hospital Medical Center, Cincinnati, Ohio
Epididymitis

HOWARD C. MOFENSON, M.D.
Professor of Pediatrics and Emergency Medicine, State University of New York, Stony Brook, New York; Professor of Pharmacological Toxicology, New York College of Osteopathic Medicine, Old Westbury, New York
Medical Toxicology: Ingestions, Inhalations, and Dermal and Ocular Absorptions

MARK E. MOLITCH, M.D.
Professor of Medicine, Northwestern University Feinberg School of Medicine; Attending Physician, Northwestern Memorial Hospital, Chicago, Illinois
Hyperprolactinemia

VICTOR M. MONTORI, M.D., MSC.
Assistant Professor of Medicine, Mayo Medical School; Senior Associate Consultant, Division of Endocrinology and Internal Medicine, Mayo Clinic, Rochester, Minnesota
Hyperthyroidism

ROSHANAK MONZAVI, M.D.
Fellow, Pediatric Endocrinology and Metabolism, Children's Hospital of Los Angeles, Los Angeles, California
Hypopituitarism

THOMAS M. MORIARTY, M.D., PH.D.
Director of Pediatric Neurosurgery; Kosair Children's Hospital, Norton Healthcare; Assistant Professor, Department of Neurological Surgery, University of Louisville, Louisville, Kentucky
Acute Head Injuries in Children

LYNNE H. MORRISON, M.D.
Assistant Professor of Dermatology, Department of Dermatology, Oregon Health Sciences University, Portland, Oregon
Skin Diseases of Pregnancy

STEVEN F. MOSS, M.D.
Associate Professor of Medicine, Brown Medical School; Attending Physician, Rhode Island Hospital, Providence, Rhode Island
Gastritis and Peptic Ulcer Disease

DEAN M. MOUTOS, M.D.
Associate Professor, Division of Reproductive Endocrinology, Department of Obstetrics and Gynecology, University of Arkansas for Medical Sciences, Little Rock, Arkansas
Amenorrhea

TARIQ I. MUGHAL, M.D.
Consultant, Haematology and Medical Oncology, Hammersmith Hospital at the Imperial College of Medicine, London, United Kingdom
Chronic Leukemias

KURT G. NABER, M.D., PH.D.
Apl. Professor, Technical University of Munich, Germany; Head of Urologic Clinic, Hospital St. Elisabeth, Straubing, Germany
Urinary Tract Infection in Males

AUAYPORN NADEMANEE, M.D.
Associate Clinical Director, Department of Hematology - Bone Marrow Transplantation; Director, Unrelated Donor Bone Marrow Transplantation Program, City of Hope National Medical Center, Duarte, California.
Non-Hodgkin's Lymphoma

SANJAY NANDURKAR, M.B.B.S.
Senior Lecturer, Department of Medicine, Monash University; Consultant Gastroenterologist, Box Hill Hospital, Box Hill, Melbourne, Australia
Irritable Bowel Syndrome

MAJOR JOHN NAPIERKOWSKI, M.D.
Instructor of Medicine, Uniformed Services University of the Health Sciences, Bethesda, Maryland; Gastroenterology Fellow, Walter Reed Army Medical Center, Washington, D.C.
Gastroesophageal Reflux Disease

DEAN K. NARITOKU, M.D.
Professor of Neurology and Pharmacology; Director, Center for Epilepsy; Director, Office for Therapeutics Research, Southern Illinois University School of Medicine; Director, Clinical Neurophysiology Laboratory, Memorial Medical Center, Springfield, Illinois
Epilepsy in Adolescents and Adults

THEODORE E. NASH, M.D.
Head, Gastrointestinal Parasites Section, Laboratory and Parasitic Disease, National Institutes of Allergy and Infectious Diseases, National Institutes of Health, Bethesda, Maryland
Giardiasis

VICTOR A. NEEL, M.D., PH.D.
Director, Division of Dermatologic Surgery, Dermatology Department, Massachusetts General Hospital, Harvard Medical School, Boston, MA
Premalignant Lesions

PAUL M. NESS, M.D.
Professor, Pathology, Medicine, and Oncology, The Johns Hopkins University School of Medicine; Director, Transition Medicine, Johns Hopkins Hospital, Baltimore, Maryland
Autoimmune Hemolytic Anemias

SHARON NESSIM, M.D.
Resident, Department of Microbiology, Infectious Diseases, Sir Mortimer B. Davis–Jewish General Hospital, Montreal, Quebec, Canada
Toxic Shock Syndrome

DAVID N. NEUBAUER, M.D.
Assistant Professor, Department of Psychiatry and Behavioral Sciences, Johns Hopkins University, School of Medicine; Associate Director, Johns Hopkins Sleep Center, Baltimore, Maryland
Insomnia

MIKHAIL V. NICKITA, M.D.
Research Fellow, Columbia University, College of Physicians and Surgeons; Fellow, Division of Substance Abuse, Columbia Presbyterian Medical Center, New York, New York
Drug Abuse

AGNIESZKA NIEMEYER, M.D.
Chief Resident, Department of Dermatology, Loma Linda University School of Medicine, Loma Linda, California
Granuloma Inguinale (Donovanosis)
Lymphogranuloma Venereum

STEPHEN D. NIMER, M.D.
Professor of Medicine, Cornell Medical College; Head, Division of Hematologic Oncology, Member, Sloan-Kettering Institute, Memorial Sloan-Kettering Cancer Center, New York, New York
Aplastic Anemia

JAMES J. NORDLUND, M.D.
Professor Emeritus, University of Cincinnati College of Medicine; Dermatologist, Group Health Associates, Cincinnati, Ohio
Pigmentary Disorders

KRISTIAN R. NOVAKOVIC, M.D.
Senior Resident, Loyola University Medical Center, Department of Urology, Maywood, Illinois
Urethral Stricture

PONSIANO OCAMA, M.D.
Research Fellow, Liver Division, University of Texas, Southwestern Medical Center at Dallas, Dallas, Texas
Cirrhosis

PATRICK T. O'GARA, M.D.
Associate Professor of Medicine, Harvard Medical School; Director, Clinical Cardiology, Vice Chairman, Clinical Affairs, Department of Medicine, Brigham and Women's Hospital, Boston, Massachusetts
Acute Myocardial Infarction

JEFFREY P. OKESON, D.M.D.
Professor, College of Dentistry, Director, Orofacial Pain Center, University of Kentucky, Lexington, Kentucky
Temporomandibular Disorders

MICHAEL OSBORNE, M.D.
Professor of Surgery, Weill Medical College of Cornell University; Chief, Breast Service, New York-Presbyterian Hospital, New York, New York; President, Strang Cancer Prevention Center, New York, New York.
Diseases of the Breast

JUDITH A. OWENS, M.D., M.P.H.
Associate Professor of Pediatrics, Brown Medical School; Director, Learning, Attention, and Behavior Program, Providence, Rhode Island
Attention Deficit Hyperactivity Disorder

BENZY J. PADANILAM, M.D.
Attending Cardiologist, St. Vincent Hospital, Indianapolis, India
Cardiac Arrest: Sudden Cardiac Death

TIKKI PANG, PH.D., F.R.C.PATH.
World Health Organization, Research Policy and Cooperation, Geneva, Switzerland
Typhoid Fever

DIANE E. PAPPAS, M.D., J.D.
Associate Professor of Pediatrics; Chief, Division of General Pediatrics, University of Virginia Health System, Charlottesville, Virginia
Viral Upper Respiratory Tract Infections

JAMES O. PARK, M.D.
Surgical Resident, Department of Surgery, The University of Chicago Hospitals and Health System, Chicago, Illinois
Tumors of the Stomach

CHRISTOPHER M. PARRY, M.B., BCHR.
Senior Lecturer, Department of Microbiology, University of Liverpool; Honorary Consultant Microbiologist, Department of Medical Microbiology, Royal Liverpool University Hospital, Liverpool, United Kingdom
Salmonellosis

ANAND C. PATEL, M.D.
Fellow, Pediatric Pulmonology, Washington University School of Medicine, Department of Pediatrics, Division of Allergy and Pulmonary Medicine, St. Louis Children's Hospital, St. Louis, Missouri
Asthma in Children

ARNOLD C. PAULINO, M.D.
Associate Professor, Departments of Radiation Oncology and Pediatrics, Emory University, Atlanta, Georgia
Brain Tumors

MASSIMILIANO PAZZAGLIA, M.D.
Fellow, Department of Dermatology, University of Bologna, Bologna, Italy
Diseases of the Nails

MARGARET S. PEARLE, M.D., PH.D.
Associate Professor of Urology, The University of Texas Southwestern Medical Center, Dallas, Texas
Renal Calculi

M.L. PEDRO-BOTET, M.D., PH.D.
Assistant Professor of Medicine, Universitat Autonoma de Barcelona; Staff Member of Infectious Disease Unit, Hospital Universitario Germans Trian i Pujol, Barcelona, Spain
Legionellosis

MICHELLE T. PELLE, M.D.
Assistant Professor, Boston University, Boston Medical Center, Boston, Massachusetts
Cutaneous Vasculitis

RONALD F. PFEIFFER, M.D.
Professor and Vice-Chair, Department of Neurology, University of Tennessee Health Science Center, Memphis, Tennessee
Parkinsonism

THEODORE PINCUS, M.D.
Division of Rheumatology and Immunology, Department of Rheumatology, Vanderbilt University School of Medicine, Nashville, Tennessee
Rheumatoid Arthritis

CHARLES A. POLNITSKY, M.D.
Adjunct Professor, Quinnipiac University, Hamden, Connecticut; Medical Director, Waterbury Hospital Regional Sleep Lab, Waterbury, Connecticut
Obstructive Sleep Apnea

VAREE POOCHAREON, B.S.
Medical Student and Clinical Research Fellow in Dermatology, Department of Dermatology, University of Miami School of Medicine, Miami, Florida
Keloids

MITCHELL C. POSNER, M.D.
Professor of Surgery, University of Chicago School of Medicine, Chief of Surgical Oncology, The University of Chicago Hospitals and Health System, Chicago, Illinois
Tumors of the Stomach

FABIO M. POTENTI, M.D.
Assistant Professor, Brown University; Division of Colorectal Surgery, Rhode Island Hospital, Providence, Rhode Island
Hemorrhoids, Anal Fissure, Anorectal Abscess, and Fistula in Ano

FRANK C. POWELL, M.D.
Lecturer in Dermatology, University College, Dublin, Ireland
Diseases of the Mouth

ERIC N. PRYSTOWSKY, M.D.
St. Vincent Hospital and Health Care, Indianapolis, Indiana
Cardiac Arrest: Sudden Cardiac Death

HERVÉ PUY, M.D.
Professor in Biochemistry and Molecular Biology; Faculté de Médicine Paris Ile de France Ouest; Assistance Publique des Hôpitaux de Paris, Paris, France
The Porphyrias

C. EGLA RABINOVICH, M.D., M.P.H.
Assistant Professor of Clinical Pediatrics, Duke University Medical Center, Durham, North Carolina
Juvenile Rheumatoid Arthritis

ROBERT E. RAKEL, M.D.
Professor, Department of Family and Community Medicine, Baylor College of Medicine, Houston, Texas

NATELLA RAKHMANINA, M.D.
Assistant Professor of Pediatrics, The George Washington University School of Medicine; Clinic Director, Special Immunology Service, Division of Hospitalist Services, Children's National Medical Center, Washington, D.C.
Fever

SATISH S.C. RAO, M.D., PH.D.
Professor of Medicine, Director, Neurogastroenterology and GI Motility, University of Iowa College of Medicine, Iowa City, Iowa
Gaseousness and Indigestion

AASE KROGH RASMUSSEN, M.D., M.SC.
Department of Medical Endocrinology PE2132, National University Hospital, Copenhagen, Denmark
Thyroiditis

K.P. RAVIKRISHNAM, M.D.
Clinical Assistant Professor, Department of Internal Medicine, University of Michigan, Ann Arbor, Michigan; Clinical Assistant Professor, Department of Internal Medicine, Wayne State University School of Medicine; Affiliate Assistant Professor, University of Detroit Mercy Hospital, Detroit, Michigan; Director, Pulmonary and Critical Care, William Beaumont Hospital, Royal Oak, Michigan
Tuberculosis and Other Mycobacterial Diseases

ROBERT V. REGE, M.D.
Professor and Chairman, Department of Surgery, University of Texas Southwestern Medical Center, Dallas, Texas
Cholelithiasis and Cholecystitis

GRAHAM D. REID, M.B., CH.B.
Clinical Associate Professor, Division of Rheumatology, Department of Medicine, University of British Columbia, Vancouver, Canada
Gout and Hyperuricemia

MICHAEL J. REITER, M.D., PH.D.
Professor of Medicine, Division of Cardiology, University of Colorado Health Sciences Center, Denver, Colorado
Tachycardias

JAMES P. RICHARDSON, M.D., M.P.H.
Clinical Professor, Department of Family Medicine, University of Maryland School of Medicine; Chief, Geriatric Medicine, Union Memorial Hospital, Baltimore, Maryland
Tetanus

MICHAEL J. RIEDER, M.D., PH.D.
Professor, Departments of Pediatrics, Physiology and Pharmacology, and Medicine, University of Western Ontario; Director, Division of Clinical Pharmacology, Children's Hospital of Western Ontario, University of Western Ontario, London, Ontario, Canada
Allergic Reactions to Drugs

EDWARD J. ROCKWOOD, M.D.
Staff, Glaucoma Department, Cole Eye Institute, Cleveland Clinic foundation, Cleveland, Ohio
Glaucoma

PETER S. ROLAND, M.D.
Professor and Chair of Otolaryngology, Head and Neck Surgery; Professor of Neurological Surgery, University of Texas Southwestern Medical Center, Dallas, Texas
Otitis Externa

KENNETH V.I. ROLSTON, M.D.
Professor of Medicine, The University of Texas, M.D. Anderson Cancer Center; Internist, M.D. Anderson Cancer Center, Houston, Texas
Primary Lung Abscess

ANNE ROMPALO, M.D., SC.M.
Professor, Division of Infectious Diseases, Department of Medicine; Professor, Division of Gynecology, Department of Obstetrics and Gynecology, The Johns Hopkins University School of Medicine; Professor, Division of Infectious Diseases, Department of Epidemiology, The Johns Hopkins School of Hygiene and Public Health; Medical Director, Centers for Disease Control and Prevention Sexually Transmitted Diseases/HIV Prevention Training Center, Baltimore City Health Department, Baltimore, Maryland
Gonorrhea

ROBIN D. ROTHSTEIN, M.D.
University of Pennsylvania Health System, Clinical Associate Professor of Medicine, University of Pennsylvania, Philadelphia, Pennsylvania
Dysphagia and Esophageal Obstruction

BRAD H. ROVIN, M.D.
Professor of Medicine and Pathology, Ohio State University College of Medicine and Public Health; Attending Physician, Ohio State University: University Hospitals, University Hospital East, James Cancer Hospital, Columbus, Ohio
Primary Glomerular Diseases

JEFFREY E. RUBNITZ, M.D., PH.D.
Associate Professor, University of Tennesee College of Medicine; Associate Member, St. Jude Children's Research Hospital, Memphia, Tennessee
Acute Leukemia in Children

LOUIS J. RUSIN, M.D.
Adjunct Assistant Professor, University of Minnesota, Department of Dermatology, Minneapolis, Minnesota; Staff Physician, Park Nicollet Clinic, Minnetonka, Minnesota
Pruritus (Itching)

CLODAGH RYAN, M.B.
Specialist Registrar in Haematology, National Centre for Hereditary Coagulation Disorders, St. James Hospital, Dublin, Ireland
Hemophilia and Related Disorders: A Practical Approach

DAVID A. SACK, M.D.
Director. Centre for Health and Population Research, International Centre for Diarrhoeal Disease, Dhaka, Bangladesh
Acute Infectious Diarrhea

THEODORE JOHN SACLARIDES, M.D.
Head, Section of Colon and Rectal Surgery, Professor of Surgery, Rush University Medical Center, Chicago, Illinois
Tumors of the Colon and Rectum

VENUSTO H. SAN JOAQUIN, M.D.
Professor of Pediatrics, University of Oklahoma Health Sciences Center; Chief, Section of Infectious Diseases, Department of Pediatrics, University of Oklahoma Health Sciences Center, Oklahoma City, Oklahoma
Whooping Cough (Pertussis)

RICHARD A. SANTUCCI, M.D.
Assistant Professor, Wayne State University School of Medicine; Chief of Urology, Detroit Receiving Hospital, Detroit, Michigan
Trauma to the Genitourinary Tract

ROBERT THAYER SATALOFF, M.D., D.M.A.
Professor, Otolaryngology–Head & Neck Surgery, Jefferson Medical College, Thomas Jefferson University, Philadelphia, Pennsylvania
Hoarseness and Laryngitis

RALPH M. SCHAPIRA, M.D.
Professor and Vice-Chair of Medicine, Medical College of Wisconsin, Milwaukee, Wisconsin
Silicosis

ROBERT T. SCHOEN, M.D.
Clinical Professor of Medicine, Yale University School of Medicine, New Haven, Connecticut
Bursitis, Tendonitis, Myofascial Pain, and Fibromyalgia

KATHRYN G. SCHUFF, M.D.
Assistant Professor of Medicine, Division of Endocrinology, Oregon Health Sciences University, Portland, Oregon
Cushing's Syndrome

DAVID M. SCOLLARD, M.D., PH.D.
Associate Professor, Pathology, Louisiana State University Medical Center; Chief, Research Pathology, National Hansen's Disease Programs, Baton Rouge, Louisiana
Leprosy (Hansen's Disease)

PETER J. SELBY, M.D.
Professor of Cancer Medicine, University of Leeds; Honorary Consultant Physician, St. James's University Hospital, Leeds, United Kingdom
Multiple Myeloma

KIMBERLY ANNE SELZMAN, M.D.
Assistant Professor of Medicine, Division of Cardiology and Cardiac Electrophysiology, University of North Carolina, Chapel Hill, North Carolina
Tachycardias

BRENT A. SENIOR, M.D.
Associate Professor, Otolaryngology–Head and Neck Surgery, University of North Carolina at Chapel Hill, Chapel Hill, North Carolina
Sinusitis

EDWARD J. SEPTIMUS, M.D.
Clinical Professor of Medicine, University of Texas Medical School; Associate Clinical Professor of Medicine, Baylor College of Medicine; Medical Director, Infectious Diseases and Occupational Health, Memorial Hermann Healthcare System, Houston, Texas
Osteomyelitis

DANIEL J. SEXTON, M.D.
Professor, Department of Medicine, Duke University Medical Center, Durham, North Carolina
Rickettsial and Ehrlichial Infections

HARRY SHARATA, M.D., PH.D.
Associate Professor of Dermatology, University of Wisconsin-Madison; Chief of Dermatology, VA Hospital, Madison, Wisconsin
Parasitic Diseases of the Skin

CURTIS A. SHELDON, M.D.
Professor, University of Cincinnati Department of Surgery, University of Cincinnati; Director, Division of Pediatric Urology, Cincinnati Children's Hospital Medical Center, Cincinnati, Ohio
Epididymitis

CHRISTOPHER E. SHIH, M.D.
Fellow, Division of Gastroenterology, Johns Hopkins School of Medicine, Baltimore, Maryland
Inflammatory Bowel Disease

PHILLIP J. SHUBERT, M.D.
Director of Perinatology, St. Ann's Hospital; Clinical Assistant Professor, Maternal-Fetal Medicine, The Ohio State University, Columbus, Ohio
Hypertensive Disorders of Pregnancy

LEONARD H. SIGAL, S.B., M.D.
Clinical Professor, Department of Medicine and Pediatrics, UMDNJ – Robert Wood Johnson Medical School, New Brunswick, New Jersey; Medical Director, Pharmaceutical Research Institute, Bristol-Meyers Squibb, Princeton, New Jersey
Lyme Disease

MARC A. SILVER, M.D.
Clinical Professor of Medicine and Associate Program Director, Cardiovascular Disease Fellowship, University of Illinois Medical Center, Chicago, Illinois; Chairman, Department of Medicine, and Director, Heart Failure Institute, Advocate Christ Medical Center, Oak Lawn, Illinois
Heart Failure

RACHE SIMMONS, M.D.
Associate Professor of Surgery, Weill-Cornell Medical School; Associate Attending Physician, The New York-Presbyterian Hospital, New York, New York
Diseases of the Breast

SYLVIA TITI SINGER, M.D.
Pediatric Hematologist/Oncologist, Children's Hospital and Research Center at Oakland, Oakland, California
Thalassemia

DANIEL A. SMITH, M.D.
Resident in Dermatology, Oregon Health and Science University, Portland, Oregon
Melanocytic Nevi

JACK D. SOBEL, M.D.
Professor of Medicine, Chief, Division of Infectious Diseases, Wayne State University, Detroit Medical Center, Detroit, Michigan
Bacterial Infections of the Urinary Tract in Women

ARTHUR J. SOBER, M.D.
Professor, Department of Dermatology, Harvard Medical School; Associate Chief of Dermatology, Massachusetts General Hospital, Boston, Massachusetts
Premalignant Lesions

TUULIKKI SOKKA, M.D., PH.D.
Research Assistant Professor, Division of Rheumatology and Immunology, Department of Rheumatology, Vanderbilt University School of Medicine, Nashville, Tennessee
Rheumatoid Arthritis

FREDERIC W. STEARNS, M.D.
Attending Staff, St. Francis Hospital; Attending Staff, South Crest Hospital, Tulsa, Oklahoma
Bacterial Diseases of the Skin

RICHARD STEEN, P.A., M.P.H.
Sexually Transmitted Infections Advisor, Family Health International, Geneva, Switzerland
Chancroid

ROBERT S. STERN, M.D.
Department of Dermatology, Beth Israel Deaconess Medical Center, Boston, Massachusetts
Acne Vulgaris and Rosacea

RACHEL E. STORY, M.D.
Fellow, Division of Allergy and Immunology, Department of Medicine, Northwestern University, Chicago, Illinois
Hypersensitivity Pneumonitis

MICHAEL STOWASSER, M.B.B.S., PH.D.
Senior Lecturer, Hypertension Unit, University of Queensland, Department of Medicine; Director, Hypertension Unit, Princess Alexandra Hospital, Brisbane, Queensland, Australia
Primary Aldosteronism

SHOBHA SWAMINATHAN, M.D.
Fellow, Infectious Diseases, Albert Einstein College of Medicine; Montefiore Medical Center, Bronx, New York
Rat-Bite Fever

CYRUS P. TAMBOLI, M.D.
Clinical Fellow, Division of Gastroenterology, University of Alberta; Clinical Associate, Grey Nuns Hospital; Clinical Associate, Royal Alexandria Hospital; Clinical Associate, Misericordia Hospital, Edmonton, Alberta, Canada
Malabsorption

MANUEL E. TANCER, M.D.
Associate Professor, Department of Psychiatry and Behavioral Neuroscience and Pharmacology, School of Medicine, Detroit, Michigan
Panic Disorder

RANDY A. TAPLITZ, M.D.
Assistant Professor of Medicine, Oregon Health and Sciences University, Portland, Oregon
Viral and Mycoplasmal Pneumonia

KAREN S. TARASZKA, M.D., PH.D.
Dermatology Resident, Yale University School of Medicine, Department of Dermatology, New Haven, Connecticut
Erythema Multiforme, Stevens-Johnson Syndrome, and Toxic Epidermal Necrolysis

STEPHANIE N. TAYLOR, M.D.
Assistant Professor of Medicine and Microbiology, Louisiana State University School of Medicine, New Orleans, Louisiana
Chlamydia Trachomatis

AYALEW TEFFERI, M.D.
Mayo Medical School; Professor of Medicine and Hematology, Mayo Medical Center, Rochester, New York
Neutropenia

RAJESH THAMAN, M.R.C.P.
Department of Cardiological Sciences, Cranmer Terrace, St George's Hospital Medical School, London, United Kingdom
Hypertrophic Cardiomyopathy

ANDREW E. THOMPSON, M.D., B.SC.
Chief Rheumatology Fellow, University of British Columbia, Vancouver, British Columbia, Canada
Gout and Hyperuricemia

CHENG HOCK TOH, M.D., M.B., CH.B.
Reader in Haematology, University of Liverpool; Royal Liverpool University Hospital, Liverpool, United Kingdom
Disseminated Intravascular Coagulation

M. TERESA TOME, M.D.
Department of Cardiological Sciences, St. George's Hospital Medical School, London, United Kingdom
Hypertrophic Cardiomyopathy

THAIS BROWN TONORE, M.D.
Assistant Professor, Family Medicine, Director of Student Programs, University of Mississippi Medical Center; Chief, Family Medicine, Mississippi Baptist Medical Center, Jackson, Mississippi
Dysmenorrhea

GISELA TORRES, M.D.
Dermatology Resident, Case Western Reserve University, Cleveland, Ohio; Clinical Research Fellow, University of Texas Medical Branch, Galveston, Texas
Viral Diseases of the Skin

ANTONELLA TOSTI, M.D.
Full Professor, Department of Dermatology, University of Bologna, Bologna, Italy
Diseases of the Nails

ISIDRO ZAVALA TRUJILLO, M.D.
Attending Physician, Head of Infectious Diseases Teaching Department, Universidad Autonoma de Guadalajara; Head, Internal Medicine Division, Head, Infectious Diseases Department, Hospital Angel Leano, Zapopan, Jalisco, Mexico
Brucellosis

RICHARD W. TSANG, M.D.
Associate Professor, Department of Radiation Oncology, University of Toronto; Radiation Oncologist, Princess Margaret Hospital, University Health Network, Toronto, Ontario, Canada
Hodgkin's Disease: Radiation Therapy

BRUCE Y. TUNG, M.D.
Associate Professor of Medicine, Riverside Nephrology Associates, Inc., Columbus, Ohio
Hemochromatosis

JAY H. TUREEN, M.D.
Clinical Professor of Pediatrics, University of California San Francisco, San Francisco, California
Bacterial Meningitis

STEPHEN K. TYRING, M.D., PH.D., M.B.A.
Professor, University of Texas Medical Branch; John Sealy Hospital, Galveston, Texas
Viral Diseases of the Skin

JOHN N. VAN DEN ANKER, M.D., PH.D.
Professor of Pediatrics and Pharmacology, The George Washington University School of Medicine; Executive Director, Pediatric Clinical Trials Unit, Chief, Division of Pediatric Clinical Pharmacology, Children's National Medical Center, Washington, D.C.
Fever

HARRY R. VAN LOVEREN, M.D.
Professor and Vice Chairman, University of South Florida, Tampa, Florida
Trigeminal Neuralgia

LAURIE VARLOTTA, M.D.
Associate Professor of Pediatrics, Department of Pediatrics, Drexel University College of Medicine; Director, Cystic Fibrosis Center; Attending Pediatric Pulmonology, St. Christopher's Hospital for Children, Philadelphia, Pennsylvania
Cystic Fibrosis

STEPHEN T. VERMILLION, M.D.
Assistant Professor, Division of Maternal-Fetal Medicine, Department of Obstetrics and Gynecology, Medical University of South Carolina, Charleston, South Carolina
Vaginal Bleeding in Late Pregnancy

MICHAEL J. VIVES, M.D.
University of Medicine and Dentistry of New Jersey, Newark, New Jersey
Low Back Pain

GEO VON KROGH, M.D., PH.D.
Associate Professor, School of Medicine, Department of Dermatovenereology, Karolinska Insititute; Associate Professor, Karolinska Hospital, Stockholm, Sweden
Anogenital Warts

MATTHEW D. VREES, M.D.
Chief Resident, Department of Surgery, Brown University; Chief Resident, Department of Surgery, Rhode Island Hospital, Providence, Rhode Island
Hemorrhoids, Anal Fissure, Anorectal Abscess, and Fistula in Ano

DAVID C. WAAGNER, M.D.
Associate Professor of Pediatrics and Chief, Division of Pediatric Infectious Diseases, Texas Tech School of Medicine; Attending Physician, University Medical Center, Lubbock, Texas
Rubella and Congenital Rubella

FLORIAN M.E. WAGENLEHNER, M.D., PH.D.
Urologic Clinic, Consultant Urologist, Hospital St. Elisabeth, Straubing, Germany
Urinary Tract Infection in Males

MICHAEL P. WAINSCOTT, M.D.
Professor, Division of Emergency Medicine, Department of Surgery, Univerity of Texas Southwestern Medical Center at Dallas; Program Director, Emergency Medicine Residency Program, Parkland Health and Hospital System, Dallas, Texas
Disturbances Due to Heat

STANLEY WALLACH, M.D.
Clinical Professor of Medicine, New York University School of Medicine; Executive Director, American College of Nutrition, Clearwater, Florida
Paget's Disease of Bone

THOMAS T. WARD, M.D.
Associate Professor of Medicine, Oregon Health Sciences University; Chief, Infectious Diseases, Portland Veterans Administration Medical Center, Portland, Oregon
Toxoplasmosis

CARL P. WEINER, M.D., M.B.A.
Professor, Obstetrics, Gynecology and Reproductive Sciences, Professor, Physiology, University of Maryland School of Medicine, Baltimore, Maryland
Hemolytic Disease of the Fetus and Newborn

LOUIS M. WEISS, M.D., M.P.H.
Professor of Medicine and Pathology, Albert Einstein College of Medicine; Attending Medicine (Infectious Diseases), Jack D. Weiler Hospital/Montefiore Medical Center/Albert Einstein College of Medicine; Attending Physician, Bronx Municipal Hospital (Jacobi Medical Center), Bronx, New York
Malaria

ATHOL WELLS, M.B.CH.B., M.D.
Consultant Physician, Royal Brompton Hospital, London, United Kingdom
Sarcoidosis

PAUL J. WENDEL, M.D.
Associate Professor of Obstetrics and Gynecology, Residency Program Director, University of Arkansas for Medical Sciences, Little Rock, Arkansas
Antepartum Care

JAY A. WERKHAVEN, M.D.
Associate Professor Department of Otolaryngology, Vanderbilt University, Nashville, Tennessee
Otitis Media

VICTORIA P. WERTH, M.D.
Professor, University of Pennsylvania, Hospital of the University of Pennsylvania VA Medical Center, Philadelphia, Pennsylvania
Cutaneous Vasculitis

L. JOSEPH WHEAT, M.D.
Mira Vista Diagnostics, Indianapolis, Indiana
Histoplasmosis

JOHN S. WHEELER, JR., M.D.
Professor of Urology, Loyola University Medical Center, Maywood, Illinois
Benign Prostatic Hyperplasia

BARRY WHITE, M.D. M.SC.
Lecturer in Haematology, Trinity College; Consultant Haematologist, National Centre for Hereditary Coagulation Disorders, St. James Hospital, Dublin, Ireland
Hemophilia and Related Disorders: A Practical Approach

CLIFTON R. WHITE, JR., M.D.
Professor of Dermatology and Pathology, Oregon Health and Science University School of Medicine; Associate Chairman, Department of Dermatology, Portland, Oregon
Melanocytic Nevi

THOMAS G. WIMMER, M.D.
Rheumatology Fellow, University of Alabama at Birmingham, Birmingham, Alabama
Polymyalgia Rheumatica and Giant Cell Arteritis

COLONEL ROY K.H. WONG, M.D.
Professor of Medicine, Director, Division of Digestive Diseases, Uniformed Services University of the Health Sciences, Bethesda, Maryland; Chief, Gastroenterology Service, Walter Reed Army Medical Center, Washington, D.C.
Gastroesophageal Reflux Disease

EDWARD C.C. WONG, M.D.
Assistant Professor, George Washington University School of Medicine and Health Sciences; Director of Hematology, Associate Director of Transfusion Medicine, Children's National Medical Center, Washington, D.C.
Therapeutic Use of Blood Components

JOEL YAGER, M.D.
Professor of Psychiatry, University of New Mexico School of Medicine, Albuquerque, New Mexico; Professor Emeritus, Department of Psychiatry and Biobehavioral Sciences, University of California at Los Angeles, Los Angeles, California
Bulimia Nervosa

OFER YOSSEPOWITCH, M.D.
Fellow, Urologic Oncology, Memorial Sloan-Kettering Cancer Center, New York, New York
Malignant Tumors of the Urogenital Tract

WILLIAM F. YOUNG, JR., M.D.
Professor of Medicine, Mayo Medical School; Vice-Chair, Division of Endocrinology and Metabolism, Mayo Clinic, Rochester, Minnesota
Acromegaly

VICTOR L. YU, M.D.
Chief of Infectious Diseases, VA Medical Center; Professor of Medicine, University of Pittsburgh, Pittsburgh, PA
Legionellosis

MARIA GUADALUPE ZAVALA, M.D.
Member of the Infectious Diseases Teaching Department, Universidad Autonoma de Guadalajara; Social Service and Research, Hospital General de Occidente, Zapopon, Jalisco, Mexico
Brucellosis

RICHARD KENT ZIMMERMAN, M.D., M.P.H.
Associate Professor with Tenure, Department of Family Medicine and Department of Behavioral and Community Health Sciences, University of Pittsburgh, Pittsburgh, Pennsylvania
Acute and Chronic Viral Hepatitis

BARRY S. ZINGMAN, M.D.
Associate Professor of Clinical Medicine, Albert Einstein College of Medicine; Medical Director, Infectious Diseases Clinic, Montefiore Medical Center, Bronx, New York
Fungal Diseases of the Skin

Preface

The goal for the 56th Edition of Conn's Current Therapy remains unchanged since Howard Conn published the first edition in 1949. That is to provide the practicing physician and other health professionals with the most up-to-date information on recent advances in therapy in an easy-to-read format. This year important tables of information are highlighted for you to provide quick-stop reading and reference. Specific information on the treatment of conditions the practicing physician commonly encounters in a clinical setting are presented by international authorities in the field who see these problems frequently and often have conducted research leading to changes in therapy.

Every year we turn to new authorities who provide their method for treating problems frequently encountered in practice and some less common problems that can be serious if not managed properly. Some diseases like smallpox were once excluded from the contents but have found their way back to medicine and so are reintroduced. Many of our authorities are outside the United States where English is their second language. The easy readability of their contribution is a tribute to their own skills and the excellent editorial staff at W.B. Saunders. This year 28 authors are from other countries such as Bangladesh (Acute Infectious Diarrhea), Switzerland (Typhoid Fever), India (Cholera), France (Leishmaniasis and Porphyria), Denmark (Thyroiditis), Italy (Bell's Palsy and Diseases of the Nails), Australia (Primary Aldosteronism and Irritable Bowel Syndrome), Ireland (Diseases of the Mouth and Hemophilia), as well as many authors from Canada and the United Kingdom.

Our greatest challenge each year is to meet the tight deadlines required in an annual publication to ensure that the information is correct. This year 85% of the authors are new from 2003 and the other 15% have thoroughly updated their material. Because each new authority presents his or her preferred method for managing the problem, the reader is encouraged to compare this with the previous editions that may provide alternative methods for consideration. The drugs recommended are the most effective according to their experience, even though some have not been FDA approved for that dosage or that indication. We have carefully marked them for your consideration.

Our special thanks to Norma Kessler, our editorial assistant, who organizes the manuscripts and galley proofs, and ensures that all the deadlines are met.

ROBERT E. RAKEL, M.D.
EDWARD T. BOPE, M.D.

Contents

SECTION 1. SYMPTOMATIC CARE PENDING DIAGNOSIS

SECTION 2. THE INFECTIOUS DISEASES

SECTION 3. DISEASES OF THE HEAD AND NECK

SECTION 4. THE RESPIRATORY SYSTEM

SECTION 5. THE CARDIOVASCULAR SYSTEM

SECTION 6. THE BLOOD AND SPLEEN

SECTION 7. THE DIGESTIVE SYSTEM

SECTION 8. METABOLIC DISEASE

SECTION 9. THE ENDOCRINE SYSTEM

SECTION 10. THE UROGENITAL TRACT

SECTION 11. THE SEXUALLY TRANSMITTED DISEASES

SECTION 12. DISEASES OF ALLERGY

SECTION 13. DISEASES OF THE SKIN

SECTION 14. THE NERVOUS SYSTEM

SECTION 15. THE LOCOMOTOR SYSTEM

SECTION 16. OBSTETRICS AND GYNECOLOGY

SECTION 17. PSYCHIATRIC DISORDERS

SECTION 18. PHYSICAL AND CHEMICAL INJURIES

SECTION 19. APPENDICES AND INDEX

Section 1

Symptomatic Care Pending Diagnosis

PAIN

method of
ALEXANDER MAUSKOP, M.D.
New York Headache Center
New York, New York

The significant progress in research on the basic science of pain over the past 10 years has thus far led to very few advances that can be applied in practice. However, most physicians do not use all the means of pain control now available to the fullest extent, mostly because of lack of knowledge and ingrained habits that have been shown to be hard to change despite educational efforts. Fear of legal complications is another obstacle. However, several successful lawsuits against physicians who failed to provide adequate pain relief may be the strongest incentive for physicians to change their habits. Ethical issues are an important aspect of pain management, not only in terminal cancer patients, where the distinction between euthanasia and pain relief is being debated, but also in opioid maintenance for nonmalignant pain.

The severity of pain can be measured only by the patient's report. Use of a verbal 1 to 10 scale allows the physician to monitor pain progression and treatment efficacy. Pain descriptions are inherently subjective, and the physician must trust these reports and take them at face value even if a particular condition "should not" result in severe pain. Malingering, especially in the presence of litigation and true drug abuse, is the exception to this rule.

PHARMACOTHERAPY

Pharmacologic management remains the mainstay of treatment for most pain syndromes. The major groups of drugs used in pain management are nonsteroidal anti-inflammatory drugs (NSAIDs), opioids, and adjuvant medications.

NSAIDs

Aspirin, ibuprofen (Advil, Motrin), naproxen (Aleve), and ketoprofen (Orudis) are sold over the counter, and many patients try them before seeking medical care. It is necessary to establish that the dosage and the frequency of self-administration were sufficient before giving up on this group of medications. Failure of one NSAID to relieve pain does not mean that another one will not be effective. Side effects can also be idiosyncratic. For example, naproxen (Naprosyn) and indomethacin (Indocin) can produce gastrointestinal side effects in a particular patient, whereas naproxen sodium (Anaprox) and diclofenac (Voltaren) do not. However, when pain is severe, it is inappropriate to keep trying various NSAIDs because they have a ceiling effect that makes them ineffective for more severe pain.

Opioids and NSAIDs have a different mechanism of action and together can have a synergistic effect. This combination may reduce the dose requirement of an opioid along with its side effects. Longer-acting NSAIDs such as naproxen (Naprelan), 750 to 1000 mg/d; piroxicam (Feldene), 20 mg once a day; meloxicam (Mobic), 7.5 to 15 mg/d; diflunisal (Dolobid), 500 mg twice a day; choline magnesium trisalicylate (Trilisate), 1500 mg twice a day; nabumetone (Relafen), 1000 mg once a day; and sustained-release indomethacin (Indocin SR), 75 mg once a day; are preferred in patients with continuous pain. Short-acting NSAIDs include ibuprofen, 400 to 600 mg every 4 hours; aspirin, 650 to 1000 mg every 3 to 4 hours; and ketoprofen, 50 mg four times a day. Ketorolac (Toradol) is the only NSAID that is available in parenteral form. The efficacy of a 30-mg intramuscular injection is comparable to that of a 10-mg morphine injection. Ketorolac (30 to 60 mg intravenously) is the author's second-line drug after injectable sumatriptan (Imitrex) for the office management of an acute migraine attack. The author occasionally injects ketorolac in the office to relieve acute low back or neck pain.

Selective cyclooxygenase 2 (COX-2) inhibitors such as celecoxib (Celebrex), rofecoxib (Vioxx), and valdecoxib (Bextra) have gained wide popularity, in part because of their reduced rates of gastrointestinal side effects, as well as the false impression of their superior efficacy. These important new drugs improve pain treatment in patients at high risk for gastrointestinal complications, such as the elderly; those with a history of peptic ulcers, cancer, or other serious conditions; or those with a risk of bleeding (COX-2 inhibitors do not affect platelets).

Opioids

Unlike NSAIDs, opioid drugs do not have a ceiling effect, which means that with the development of tolerance, the dose of an opioid can be escalated almost indefinitely to regain pain relief. Usually, the development of side effects limits such escalation, although some patients can tolerate an equivalent of up to several grams of morphine a day given parenterally. These patients remain functional because of a gradual escalation of the dose, which leads to the development of tolerance not only to pain relief but also to side effects. The development of tolerance to an opioid is usually manifested as a shorter duration of action. Because cross-tolerance between different opioids is incomplete, switching to a different opioid may forestall escalation of the dose. Using combinations of NSAIDs and adjuvant analgesics with opioids is another effective tactic. The development of tolerance and physical dependence is often mistakenly equated with addiction. In a tolerant patient receiving a high dose of an opioid drug, symptoms of withdrawal can appear within a few hours of the last dose. Addiction, on the other hand, is characterized by craving for the drug, taking the drug despite its harmful effects, and not following a physician's directions regarding proper use.

Both physicians and patients often have a fear of opioids because of their potential for addiction. A survey of 10,000 patients treated in burn units across the country looked at patients receiving large doses of opioid drugs on a daily basis for periods of up to several months. With the exception of those with a history of addiction, not a single patient became addicted. Sometimes the use of an opioid in a cancer patient is equated with imminent death. The author always brings this topic up because many patients do not verbalize their fears and, if not reassured, are reluctant to take sufficient amounts, if any, of the drug. Another obstacle to the proper use of opioids is an exaggerated concern about respiratory and central nervous system (CNS) depression. Tolerance to these side effects of opioids develops quickly. Patients do not become oversedated or stop breathing while in pain. When a patient taking a steady dose of an opioid suddenly becomes drowsy or experiences respiratory depression, the most likely cause is a new systemic problem, such as an infection or liver or kidney failure. When pain can be controlled only with some degree of sedation, a stimulant such as dextroamphetamine sulfate (Dexedrine),* 5 to 15 mg, dextroamphetamine with amphetamine (Adderall),* 5 to 30 mg, or methylphenidate (Ritalin),* 5 to 54 mg, all given once or twice a day, may not only improve alertness but can provide additional analgesia as well. These stimulants also have mild analgesic properties and are synergistic with opioid analgesics.

Meperidine (Demerol) is a popular drug, but it is the only opioid that should not be used with frequency for more than a few days. Meperidine is metabolized into normeperidine, which is a CNS stimulant. With chronic administration, meperidine can cause irritability, tremor, and generalized seizures.

The major side effect of opioids that must be anticipated is constipation. Senna concentrate (Senokot) is an anecdotal favorite to combat this problem because of its stimulating effect on peristalsis. Transdermal fentanyl (Duragesic) tends to produce less constipation than oral opioids do.

The author finds that transdermal fentanyl (Duragesic) has other advantages as well. This product provides a steady level of an opioid drug with practical and psychological benefits. Each patch lasts for about 3 days and comes in four strengths (25, 50, 75, and 100 μg/h). Because of the long half-life of the drug, the process of determining the optimal dose of the patch may take 1 to 2 weeks. While this adjustment is being made, patients should be given a short-acting opioid such as oxycodone (Percocet, Percodan, Tylox, Roxicet), morphine sulfate (Roxanol, MSIR), or hydromorphone (Dilaudid) as rescue medication for breakthrough pain. This practice also applies to the titration phase of other long-acting oral opioids, including sustained-release morphine (MS Contin, Oramorph SR, Kadian), sustained-release oxycodone (OxyContin), methadone (Dolophine), and levorphanol (Levo-Dromoran). Methadone is an excellent analgesic with good absorption and, in the author's experience, fewer side effects than other opioids. It is also one of the less expensive opioids.

Rectal suppositories of morphine (Roxanol, RMS), hydromorphone (Dilaudid), and oxymorphone (Numorphan) are useful for patients who cannot take oral preparations. The rectal route is not practical for long-term management and when high doses are needed.

Intranasal administration of butorphanol (Stadol NS) offers rapid onset of action. The limitation of this drug in its current formulation is that each spray contains a dose that is excessive for many patients and results in a high incidence of CNS side effects. Butorphanol is a partial agonist-antagonist drug that should result in a lower potential for addiction; however, the risk of addiction with this drug is still significant. It should not be given to patients who are maintained on opioids that are pure agonists because its antagonist properties can induce a withdrawal reaction. Patients undergoing chronic opioid maintenance become very sensitive to all opioid antagonists. Should a need arise to reverse the effect of an opioid in such a patient, naloxone (Narcan) must be diluted with saline and infused very gradually.

When a patient with continuous, severe pain cannot take oral medications, subcutaneous (SC) infusion of opioids is an alternative to the transdermal route and has many advantages over intravenous infusion. The patch should be tried first, but when it is ineffective at a high dose (e.g., two 100-μg Duragesic patches) or causes side effects, SC infusion is the method of choice. SC infusion is administered via a programmable, portable pump that can be filled with a solution

*Not FDA approved for this indication.

of any opioid, including morphine, hydromorphone, methadone, and levorphanol. The pump is connected to a 25-gauge "butterfly" needle that can be inserted subcutaneously by the patient or a family member. Intravenous infusion of an opioid may be necessary only if a patient requires a very large volume of an opioid or if other routes are not tolerated.

The use of opioid analgesics has been mostly limited to cancer patients, and their prolonged use in noncancer patients with pain remains controversial. A growing number of anecdotal reports and the author's personal experience suggest that under strict supervision, selected noncancer patients with pain can derive great benefit from chronic opioid therapy. Such patients are usually those in whom significant tolerance does not develop and who remain on a steady dose for long periods with few side effects. The author obtains a verbal or written informed consent from such patients in which they are warned about the risk of addiction, sees them at least once a month (for long-term, reliable patients, this requirement can be relaxed to once every 3 months), and tries to make opioids only a part of the pain management program.

Tramadol (Ultram) is an opioid drug that also has noradrenergic and serotoninergic effects. It is a relatively mild analgesic, but it lacks the potential for addiction and does not cause constipation.

Adjuvant Analgesics

This very diverse group of medications was not known to have analgesic properties when they were first introduced. One of the most effective groups of drugs for chronic pain and headache management is the tricyclic antidepressants (TCAs).

Among the TCAs, amitriptyline (Elavil)* has been studied most extensively, but nortriptyline (Pamelor),* imipramine (Tofranil), and desipramine (Norpramin)* are also effective and may produce fewer anticholinergic side effects. If one TCA is ineffective or produces unacceptable side effects, another TCA can be tried.

The starting dose of any TCA is 25 mg in young or middle-aged patients and 10 mg in elderly or debilitated persons. The average effective dose is 50 to 75 mg taken once a day in the evening. Some patients may require and tolerate antidepressant doses of up to 300 mg/d or more to achieve relief of pain or headache. Patients must be told that these medications are antidepressants but that they are also used for chronic painful conditions, even without any associated depression. If a patient discovers from another source that she was given an antidepressant drug, the patient may become angry and noncompliant and may think that her complaints were interpreted as depressive symptoms and not real pain. Warning patients about possible side effects such as dryness of the mouth, drowsiness, and constipation also improves compliance. Some contraindications to the use of TCAs include concomitant use of monoamine oxidase inhibitors, recent myocardial infarction, cardiac arrhythmias, glaucoma, and urinary retention. An electrocardiogram should be obtained before the initiation of treatment in all elderly patients.

*Not FDA approved for this indication.

Other antidepressants, including the selective serotonin reuptake inhibitors (SSRIs) fluoxetine (Prozac),* sertraline (Zoloft),* paroxetine (Paxil),* and citalopram (Celexa),* as well as the non-SSRI antidepressants bupropion (Wellbutrin SR)* and nefazodone (Serzone),* may have some utility in pain management. However, no large trials of these drugs for pain have shown any benefit beyond their antidepressant effect. The author frequently starts with these antidepressants before resorting to TCAs because of their favorable side effect profile. SSRIs do not cause weight gain, drowsiness, or anticholinergic side effects, all of which can occur with TCAs. Nefazodone and bupropion do not cause sexual dysfunction, which can occur with SSRIs.

It has been suggested that anticonvulsants are more effective for sharp, lancinating pain, whereas TCAs are better for burning, dysesthetic pain. However, this anecdotal observation has not been confirmed by a rigorous study, and it is worth trying this group of drugs for almost any pain syndrome, particularly neuropathic pain, neuralgias, and migraines. Anticonvulsants commonly used for pain relief are carbamazepine (Tegretol)* or its successors oxcarbazepine (Trileptal)* and gabapentin (Neurontin).* Carbamazepine, oxcarbazepine, and phenytoin (Dilantin)* are not effective for migraine headaches, whereas divalproex sodium (Depakote) is. Newer anticonvulsants such as lamotrigine (Lamictal),* topiramate (Topamax),* and levetiracetam (Keppra)* are being used and studied for their potential analgesic efficacy as well.

Dextromethorphan (Benylin),* which is in wide use as an antitussive agent, has been found to have analgesic properties and possibly delay the development of opioid tolerance. This drug produces analgesia through its blocking effect on the *N*-methyl-D-aspartate (NMDA) receptor. A gradual escalation of the dose up to 60 mg four times daily† or more is often necessary to achieve an analgesic effect.

Hydroxyzine (Vistaril, Atarax) may have some mild analgesic properties, but what makes it a useful adjuvant analgesic is its reduction of anxiety and nausea.

Caffeine has been shown to enhance the effect of other analgesics and to have mild analgesic properties of its own. It is useful in a variety of pain syndromes, but it is most commonly used for headaches. Overuse of caffeine in drinks (coffee, tea, colas) and medications (Excedrin, Anacin, Fiorinal, Esgic, Norgesic) can lead to severe withdrawal headaches and other symptoms. As few as 3 cups of coffee a day can induce a withdrawal rebound syndrome.

Corticosteroids can be very effective in relieving pain from various causes. Long-term side effects and loss of efficacy limit their use to the treatment of acute pain syndromes such as spinal cord, plexus, or nerve compression or severe migraine or back pain.

*Not FDA approved for this indication.
†Exceeds dosage recommended by the manufacturer.

Benzodiazepines usually have little utility in pain management, except for the acute pain of muscle spasm, such as in acute low back or neck pain or in a very anxious patient. A short course (up to a few weeks) of diazepam (Valium) or clonazepam (Klonopin)* in these circumstances carries little risk of addiction and may be of significant help.

Muscle relaxants can be effective not only for pain from muscle spasm but also for some neuropathic pain syndromes and neuralgias. Baclofen (Lioresal) and tizanidine (Zanaflex)* are generally used for chronic pain conditions, whereas metaxalone (Skelaxin), cyclobenzaprine (Flexeril), and carisoprodol (Soma) are more commonly used for pain caused by acute muscle spasm.

PSYCHOLOGICAL METHODS

Psychological methods are indispensable in the management of patients with chronic pain. Pain affects all aspects of chronic-pain patients' lives and the lives of people who surround them. For this reason, a psychologist is a crucial member of the pain management team. Chronic pain of long duration is very unlikely to respond to a single treatment modality, and patients should not be allowed to pick and choose their treatment. The author explains to such patients that pain control can be achieved only by attacking the problem with several methods at the same time. Psychological methods may include behavior modification, cognitive psychotherapy, biofeedback, and relaxation training. On occasion, in an anxious patient with acute or cancer pain, simple reassurance may reduce the need for opioid analgesics. In some patients, music therapy can have beneficial effects.

ANESTHETIC APPROACHES

Muscle spasm is a common primary cause of pain, and it often accompanies pain of other types. Trigger point injections are very effective in the management of acute pain from muscle spasm. These injections can be performed with a 1% lidocaine solution and must be combined with active physical therapy (by the word *active* the author implies an emphasis on strengthening exercises rather than passive modalities such as heat, ultrasound, and massage). Topical application of lidocaine (Lidoderm transdermal patch, ELA-Max cream) or lidocaine with prilocaine (EMLA cream) can be effective for postherpetic neuralgia, diabetic neuropathy, and other superficial pain.

For chronic pain of muscular origin (e.g., low back pain), botulinum toxin type A (Botox)* or type B (Myoblock)* can provide dramatic and sustained relief lasting an average of 3 months. The author finds that botulinum toxin type A is also highly effective for the prevention of migraine headaches. These biologic agents produce muscle relaxation by blocking the neuromuscular junction. Despite their origin, they are extremely safe products that, when used correctly, are virtually free of serious side effects.

Nerve blocks can provide temporary relief of pain in patients with local pain. Some use them to predict the possible efficacy of nerve ablation. Instead of a local anesthetic, which tends to have a very brief effect, the author usually injects a corticosteroid such as betamethasone (Celestone Soluspan) or methylprednisolone (Depo-Medrol) into an area around the nerve. Although such an injection cannot technically be considered a nerve block, similar techniques are used for both procedures. Examples of conditions that benefit from corticosteroid injections include carpal tunnel syndrome, meralgia paresthetica, and occipital neuralgia.

Sympathetic block is the most effective procedure for the treatment of reflex sympathetic dystrophy, especially when blocks are combined with vigorous physical therapy and, if necessary, pharmacotherapy and psychological methods. Such combined treatment works best if it is started early in the course of the disease.

Epidural and spinal infusions of opioids and local anesthetics are useful in some cancer patients and in a few selected patients with "failed back syndrome."

NEUROSURGICAL METHODS

In attempting to stop transmission of pain signals up along the nervous system, neurosurgeons have tried placing lesions anywhere from peripheral nerves all the way up to the frontal cortex. Nerve section can be effective in patients with meralgia paresthetica, occipital neuralgia, and some other focal neuropathic pain. It is not effective, however, in those with postherpetic neuralgia. Some patients with trigeminal neuralgia find temporary relief when the nerve leading to the trigger area is sectioned. A dorsal root entry zone (DREZ) lesion can sometimes relieve the pain caused by brachial plexus avulsion and anesthesia dolorosa. Sectioning of half the spinal cord (cordotomy) is very effective in patients with cancer who have unilateral pain below the waist. Bilateral cordotomy usually leads to loss of sphincter control and should be reserved for cancer patients who have already lost such control. Hypophysectomy should be considered in women with hormonal cancer (breast or ovarian) whose pain is resistant to other modalities.

PHYSICAL METHODS

Physical therapy is the main treatment modality for most patients with low back and neck pain. It is also essential in the management of complex regional pain syndrome (reflex sympathetic dystrophy). Patients with almost any pain syndrome can benefit from regular exercise. The improved cardiovascular and pulmonary function achieved with aerobic exercise is of significant benefit in itself, but it also provides important psychological benefit. Patients feel that they are regaining some control over their bodies and feel less helpless and hopeless. Regular exercise helps alleviate stress, which is a major contributing factor in chronic headache, back pain, and other pain syndromes.

Other physical methods include transcutaneous electrical nerve stimulation (TENS) and acupuncture.

*Not FDA approved for this indication.

Neither method has been scientifically proved to be effective; however, a large body of anecdotal evidence indicates that they can be very helpful in some patients. Results of experiments detailing opioid and nonopioid mechanisms of acupuncture analgesia in animals, as well as the successful use of acupuncture in veterinary medicine, suggest that the effect of acupuncture is superior to that of placebo. The author generally uses acupuncture in the elderly or other patients who do not tolerate any medications and in patients who have tried a variety of therapies without relief. In patients with chronic pain, acupuncture should be used as part of a multidisciplinary approach.

Chiropractic, osteopathic, and other methods of manipulation are in wide use for a variety of painful conditions. With the exception of vigorous neck manipulation, these methods are generally safe. These therapies can provide lasting relief for some acute pain syndromes such as low back pain, especially when they are used together with active physical therapy. Prolonged use of these methods should be avoided, however, because they divert patients from obtaining more effective treatment and because of the cost.

ETHICAL ISSUES

A fine line exists between euthanasia and pain relief in a terminally ill patient. Fortunately, this distinction is relatively easy to make in most cases, and the author believes that euthanasia almost never needs to be considered if relief of pain, anxiety, depression, and other symptoms is aggressively pursued. A patient who is clearly dying and is having severe pain must be relieved of this pain even though opioid drugs may hasten death by hours or days. When a patient with a painful terminal illness is not under imminent threat of death, pain relief should not result in death by overmedication. In rare patients, the only way that the pain is relieved is when the patient is asleep because of the sedative effects of opiates. Relief of severe anxiety with tranquilizers often reduces the need for opiates, although opiates are generally preferred because their action is easier to reverse if a patient is oversedated. Surgical and other invasive pain-relieving procedures should be considered earlier in terminally ill patients.

NAUSEA AND VOMITING

method of
LOWELL B. ANTHONY, M.D.
Louisiana State University Health Sciences Center
New Orleans, Louisiana

Nausea and vomiting are protective reflexes activated by a wide range of gastrointestinal (GI) and non-GI etiologies. Even though nausea is usually an accompanying symptom, emesis can occur with little or no warning. The general approach to the management of nausea and vomiting is to narrow the differential diagnosis by using subjective and objective data, followed by treating the most probable underlying cause. For the special circumstances of controlling iatrogenic causes of emesis, such as cancer chemotherapy–induced emesis, an effective antiemetic regimen should be administered before the emetogenic stimuli.

Nausea and vomiting are induced by efferent stimuli from the medullary vomiting center to striated muscles of the chest and abdomen and smooth muscles of the GI system. This final coordinating center in the medulla receives input not only from other areas within the brain (the medullary chemoreceptor trigger zone, the cerebrum, the limbic and vestibular systems) but also from visceral stimuli (cardiac and GI neuroreceptors). Central and peripheral neurotransmitters important in nausea and vomiting include dopamine, acetylcholine, serotonin, histamine, and endorphins.

INITIAL ASSESSMENT AND DIFFERENTIAL DIAGNOSIS

GI, central nervous system (CNS), iatrogenic, and systemic disorders may produce nausea and vomiting as an initial or late manifestation of an underlying disorder (Table 1). Iatrogenic causes may also be an unexpected warning of drug toxicity or an anticipated side effect of treatment. The patient's history provides crucial information regarding any relationship to

TABLE 1. **Some Causes of Nausea and Vomiting**

Gastrointestinal Disorders
Peptic ulcer disease/gastritis
Intestinal obstruction/ileus/perforation
Cholelithiasis/cholecystitis
Constipation/cecal impaction
Adhesions
Gastric cancer
Pancreatitis/pancreatic tumors
Motility disorders
Autonomic neuropathy
Central Nervous System Disorders
Migraine
Motion sickness
Vestibular dysfunction/Ménière's disease
Brain tumor/carcinomatous meningitis
Brain abscess
Hydrocephalus
Iatrogenic Causes
Medications
  Antineoplastic agents
  Morphine/analgesics
  Theophylline
  Digitalis/digoxin
  Anesthetic agents
  L-Dopa/bromocriptine
Radiation therapy
Postoperative
Systemic Causes
Pregnancy
Infections/food poisoning
Diabetic ketoacidosis
Uremia
Chromic hepatic disease
Adrenal insufficiency, paraneoplastic
Hypercalcemia
Drug overdose
Heavy metal poisoning
Psychogenic

meals, as well as the onset, character, frequency, and intensity of nausea and emesis. Pertinent historical data also include the presence of fever, pain (abdominal or cephalgic), changes in bowel habits, gallstones, kidney stones, jaundice, weight loss, medications, concomitant illnesses, previous operations, and personal habits.

Objective evaluation includes physical, laboratory, and radiologic examination. Physical examination allows one to not only observe signs accompanying the illness but also assess hydration and cardiovascular status so that supportive measures can be initiated before making the final diagnosis. Screening laboratory tests include (1) serum chemistries documenting acid-base–electrolyte status; levels of glucose, calcium, β-human chorionic hormone (if pregnancy is suspected), and amylase; urinary abnormalities; GI bleeding; drug levels (including urinary toxicologic screening if drug overdose is being evaluated); (2) peritoneal aspirate if ascites is present; and (3) evaluation of renal, cardiac, and hepatic function. Radiologic tests, including a chest radiograph, flat and upright abdominal films, and abdominal ultrasound, complete the initial evaluation and usually result in narrowing the diagnostic focus to one major organ system.

Assessment of Causes of Nausea and Vomiting in a Cancer Patient

Special consideration is required to determine whether the presence of these symptoms is iatrogenic or an indication of disease-related effects. Mechanical or nonmechanical bowel obstruction should be carefully excluded. Adhesions can develop from previous operations, but inactivity, metabolic effects, and drugs can also decrease bowel motility. Any constipation and fecal impaction accompanying the use of moderate to strong analgesics need to be considered as causes of nausea and vomiting in a cancer patient. Nausea and emesis can also be caused by CNS metastases as the initial indication of disease spread.

Cancer chemotherapy–induced nausea and emesis are usually temporally related to drug administration. The severity of nausea and vomiting depends on which drug or drugs are administered (Table 2). Nausea and emesis occurring in a cancer patient can also result from a conditioned response if antiemetic protection was not complete. These anticipatory symptoms develop in about 25% of patients and can affect compliance.

Delayed nausea and emesis occur more with cisplatin-based regimens and usually resolve within 4 to 14 days after treatment. Patients in whom pain, protracted nausea and emesis, fever, and metabolic effects develop and who do not respond to effective antiemetic measures should be evaluated for other causes of emesis.

TABLE 2. **Emetic Potency of Chemotherapeutic Agents**

Emetic Risk	Generic Agent	Brand Name
Severe (>30% Incidence)	Aldesleukin*	Proleukin
	Altretamine	Hexalen
	Carboplatin	Paraplatin
	BCNU	Carmustine
	Cisplatin	Platinol-AQ
	Cyclophosphamide	Cytoxan
	Cytarabine, ≥1 g/m^2	Cytosar-U DepoCyt
	Dacarbazine	DTIC-Dome
	Dactinomycin	Cosmegen
	Daunorubicin	DaunoXome Cerubidine
	Doxorubicin ≥20 mg/m^2	Adriamycin
	Epirubicin	Ellence
	Idarubicin	Idamycin
	Ifosfamide	Ifex
	Irinotecan	Camptosar
	Lomustine	CeeNu
	Mechlorethamine (nitrogen mustard)	Mustargen
	Melphalan	Alkeran
	Methotrexate, ≥250 mg/m^2	Methotrexate
	Mitoxantrone	Novantrone
	Pentostatin	Nipent
	Procarbazine	Matulane
	Streptozocin	Zanosar
Moderate (10–30% Incidence)	Asparaginase	Elspar
	Cytarabine, 100 mg/m^2 to <1 g/m^2	Cytosar-U DepoCyt
	Docetaxel	Taxotere
	Doxorubicin, <20 mg/m^2	Adriamycin
	Etoposide	VePesid Etopophos
	Fluorouracil	Fluorouracil
	Gemcitabine	Gemzar
	Methotrexate, >50 to <250 mg/m^2	Methotrexate
	Mitomycin	Mutamycin
	Paclitaxel	Taxol
	Pegaspargase	Oncaspar
	Teniposide	Vumon
	Thiotepa	Thioplex
	Topotecan	Hycamtin
Mild (<10% Incidence)	Bleomycin	Blenoxane
	Busulfan, oral, <4 mg/kg/d	Myleran
	Capecitabine	Xeloda
	Chlorambucil	Leukeran
	Cladribine	Leustatin
	Cytarabine, <100 mg/m^2	Cytosar-U DepoCyt
	Fludarabine	Fludara
	Hydroxyurea	Hydrea
	Isotretinoin	Accutane
	Melphalan, oral	Alkeran
	Mercaptopurine	Purinethol
	Methotrexate, ≤50 mg/m^2	Methotrexate
	Tamoxifen	Nolvadex
	Thioguanine	Tabloid
	Vinblastine	Velban
	Vincristine	Oncovin
	Vinorelbine	Navelbine

*Avoid corticosteroids as antiemetics.

TREATMENT

General Considerations

Successful control of nausea and vomiting depends on identifying the most likely cause of the patient's symptoms. Because antiemetics are routinely used empirically in many instances, except for pregnancy and drug overdose, initiating treatment with these agents alone or with intravenous (IV) fluids allows for patient comfort while evaluation is under way. If abdominal pain accompanies nausea and vomiting, surgical opinion may preclude early pharmacologic intervention.

Treatment of nausea and vomiting can be divided into pharmacologic and nonpharmacologic interventions. The latter encompasses dietary restrictions during pregnancy; behavioral techniques for conditioned behavior developing during cancer therapy; Alcoholics Anonymous for alcoholism; dialysis for uremia or drug overdose; radiation therapy, craniotomy, or both for CNS tumors; nasogastric tube for possible diagnostic and therapeutic interventions; lithotripsy for kidney stones; abdominal surgery for intestinal obstruction or refractory peptic ulcer disease; cholecystectomy for cholelithiasis or cholecystitis; and the use of mechanical or electrical stimuli.

Pharmacologic approaches include antiemetics and nonantiemetic agents, depending on the underlying cause. Reversing the underlying disease with antibiotics, insulin, nitrates, calcium channel blockers, steroids, anticonvulsants, and H_2 antagonists, among other agents indicated for specific diseases, may be accompanied by the empirical use of antiemetics for symptom control.

Antiemetics can be divided into eight major categories (Table 3). Classifying these drugs according to the mechanism of action allows one to select drugs from different classes when the emetic stimulus is strong and combination drug therapy is warranted. Avoiding combinations of two drugs within the same class decreases the likelihood of adverse drug reactions, such as acute dystonic reactions with dopamine antagonists.

Patient sensitivity, existing disease, and the severity of symptoms determine which specific antiemetic drug or antiemetic regimen is used. Antiemetics are effective in combination with regimens for the specific clinical circumstances shown in Table 4. In general, control of cancer chemotherapy–induced emesis includes a 5-HT_3 (serotonin) antagonist, a steroid, and a benzodiazepine. If cost is a primary consideration, oral formulations of the 5-HT_3 antagonist can be considered, or a dopamine antagonist such as metoclopramide (Reglan) can be substituted for the 5-HT_3 antagonist in the aforementioned regimen. However, 5-HT_3 antagonists are the antiemetic class of choice if the patient is younger than 30 years, has a history of motion sickness, or has had a previous dystonic reaction to dopamine antagonists.

Antiemetic Drugs

Serotonin Antagonists

A major development in antiemetic pharmacology has been the introduction of selective 5-HT_3 receptor antagonists such as ondansetron (Zofran), granisetron (Kytril), and dolasetron (Anzemet). This class of antiemetics is highly effective in controlling cisplatin-induced emesis and is well tolerated. Headache, which is mild and usually controlled with simple analgesics, occurs in about 15% of patients. Patients may also report lightheadedness, and serum transaminase elevations can occur transiently. Extrapyramidal symptoms occurring with dopamine antagonists are rarely seen after the administration of serotonin-inhibitory drugs. A single 32-mg IV dose has been shown to be equivalent to 32 mg in divided doses.

Dopamine Antagonists

Phenothiazines. These agents have been the most widely used in controlling non–cisplatin-based cancer chemotherapy–induced emesis. Prochlorperazine (Compazine) is usually given in doses ranging to 20 mg orally, rectally, or intramuscularly every 4 to 6 hours on an as-needed basis. Thiethylperazine (Torecan), chlorpromazine (Thorazine), perphenazine (Trilafon), and promethazine (Phenergan) are alternatives for other drugs in this class. Unfortunately, the activity of this class of drugs is modest at best, and dose escalation is associated with increased toxicity, including but not limited to hypotension, extrapyramidal effects, sedation, orthostasis, and anticholinergic effects, which restrict their use in controlling a strong emetic stimulus.

Butyrophenones. The limitations of these agents are similar to those of the phenothiazines. Droperidol (Inapsine) given as 0.5 to 10 mg IV every 2 hours can effectively control cisplatin-induced emesis. Sedation as well as diarrhea can occur at these dosages. Adverse effects are similar to those of the phenothiazines.

Substituted Benzamides. The most widely used agent in controlling cisplatin-induced emesis has been metoclopramide (Reglan). Successful dosage escalation to 2 mg/kg every 2 hours for five doses starting 30 minutes before the administration of cisplatin controls nausea and emesis effectively. Its action in these larger doses most likely involves nonselective serotonin blockade in addition to its dopamine antagonism.

A limitation to using metoclopramide is a relatively high incidence of extrapyramidal side effects, including acute dystonic reaction, which can be lessened somewhat with antihistamines or benztropine (Cogentin). Even though these side effects can be anticipated and controlled, they can be alarming to the patient, the family, and sometimes the hospital staff. Somnolence, anxiety, and diarrhea can also be observed.

Another drawback to the use of metoclopramide is the lack of a high-dose oral tablet. In the outpatient setting, patients take 5 to 15 of the 10-mg tablets every 2 hours if metoclopramide is to be used.

Steroids

Dexamethasone (Decadron)* and other steroids have moderate antiemetic activity when used as single agents (10 to 20 mg), with little, if any, toxicity. This class of drugs is generally used in combination with dopamine or serotonin antagonists. The mechanism by which steroids act as antiemetics is unknown. Lower doses of steroids have shown activity when used as single agents in low-dose cisplatin regimens. Because of transient rectal pain sometimes occurring with rapid dexamethasone infusion, slow infusion is recommended.

---

*Not FDA approved for this indication.

TABLE 3. **Antiemetic Classification and Recommended Dosage/Schedules**

Drug Category/Generic Name	Trade Name	Dosage/Administration
Serotonin Antagonists		
Ondansetron	Zofran	PO: 8–24 mg q24h IV: 0.15–0.36 mg/kg q4–8h or a single 32-mg dose
Granisetron	Kytril	PO: 2 mg IV: 1 mg or 10 μg/kg
Dolasetron	Anzemet	PO: 100 mg IV: 100 mg or 1.8 mg/kg
Dopamine Antagonists		
Phenothiazines		
Prochlorperazine	Compazine	PO: 5–20* mg q4–6h IV: 10–40* mg q3h IM: 5–20* mg q4–6h Rectally: 25 mg q4–6h
Thiethylperazine	Torecan	PO: 10 mg q6–8h IM: 10 mg q6–8h Rectally: 10 mg q6–8h
Promethazine	Phenergan	PO: 25 mg q4–6h IV: 12.5 mg q4–6h IM: 25 mg q4–6h Rectally: 25 mg q4–6h
Perphenazine	Trilafon	PO: 8–16 mg q4–6h
Chlorpromazine	Thorazine	PO: 10–25 mg q3–6h IV: 10–25 mg q3–6h Rectally: 50–100 mg q6–8h
Butyrophenones		
Droperidol	Inapsine	PO†: 1–2 mg q6–8h IV: 0.5–10 mg q2–4h IM: 1–2 mg q6–8h
Haloperidol‡	Haldol	IV: 1–3 mg q2–6h
Substituted† Benzamides		
Metoclopramide	Reglan	PO‡: 10 mg 30 min before meals IV: 1–3 mg/kg q2h
Steroids		
Dexamethasone‡	Decadron	PO: 10–20 mg q24h IV: 10–20 mg q24h
Methylprednisolone‡	Solu-Medrol	IV: 40–125 mg q4–6h
Antihistamines		
Diphenhydramine	Benadryl	PO: 25–100 mg q6–8h IV: 25–100 mg q6–8h IM: 25–100 mg q6–8h
Hydroxyzine	Vistaril	PO‡: 25–100 mg q6–8h IV: 25–100 mg q6–8h
Meclizine	Antivert	PO: 20–50 mg q24h
Dimenhydrinate	Dramamine	PO: 50mg q4–6h IV: 50 mg q4–6h
Benzodiazepines		
Lorazepam‡	Ativan	PO: 1–1.5 mg/m^2 IV: 1–1.5 mg/m^2 IM: 1–1.5 mg/m^2
Diazepam‡	Valium	PO: 5–10 mg q6–8h IV: 5–10 mg q6–8h
Cannabinoids		
Dronabinol	Marinol	PO: 5–10 mg/m^2 q4–6h
Nabilone†	Cesamet	PO: 1–2 mg q12h
Anticholinergics		
Scopolamine	Transderm Scōp	Dermal: 1 patch q3d behind ear
Miscellaneous		
Trimethobenzamide	Tigan	PO: 100 mg q4–6h IM: 100 mg q4–6h
Benzquinamide†	Emete-con	IV: 25 mg (1 mg/min) IM: 50 mg q3–4h

*Exceeds dosage recommended by the manufacturer.
†Not available in the United States.
‡Not FDA approved for this indication.

Antihistamines

Diphenhydramine (Benadryl), among others, has modest antiemetic activity and is generally used alone for weak emetic stimuli, for motion sickness, or in combination with metoclopramide for cisplatin-based chemotherapy. This class of drugs can potentially lessen the impact of the extrapyramidal symptoms induced by dopamine antagonists. Antihistamines may be

TABLE 4. **Antiemetic Regimens for Specific Emetic Conditions**

Clinical Situation	Agents	Dosage/Administration
Acute emesis from *severe* emetogenic agent	**5-HT$_3$ receptor antagonist**	
	Ondansetron (Zofran)	PO: 8–24 mg IV: 8 mg or 0.15 mg/kg
	or	
	Granisetron (Kytril)	PO: 2 mg IV: 1 mg or 10 μg/kg
	or	
	Dolasetron (Anzemet)	PO: 100 mg IV: 100 mg or 1.8 mg/kg
	and	
	Corticosteroid	
	Dexamethasone (Decadron)	IV: 10–20 mg
	or	
	Methylprednisolone (Solu-Medrol)	IV: 40–125 mg
	with or without	
	Lorazepam (Ativan)	IV: 1–1.5 mg/m^2
Acute emesis from *moderate* emetogenic agent	**Corticosteroid**	
	Dexamethasone (Decadron)	PO: 4–8 mg × 1 before chemotherapy *or* IV: 10–20 mg × 1 before chemotherapy
	or	
	Dopamine antagonist	
	Prochlorperazine (Compazine)	PO: 10–20 mg × 1 before chemotherapy *or* IV: 10–20 mg × 1 before chemotherapy
	or	
	Promethazine (Phenergan)	PO: 25–50 mg × 1 before chemotherapy *or* IV: 12.5 mg × 1 before chemotherapy
	or	
	Thiethylperazine (Torecan)	PO: 10–20 mg × 1 before chemotherapy *or* IV: 10–20 mg × 1 before chemotherapy
	or	
	Droperidol (Inapsine)	PO: 1–2 mg × 1 before chemotherapy *or* IV: 0.5–10 mg
Delayed *emesis* from *severe* emetogenic agent	**Corticosteroid**	
	Dexamethasone (Decadron)	PO: 8 mg bid for 2–3 or 3–4 d for high-dose cisplatin IV: 10 mg
	and	
	Substituted benzamide	
	Metoclopramide (Reglan)	PO: 30–40 mg bid–qid for 2–3 or 2–4 d for high-dose cisplatin
	or	
	5-HT$_3$ receptor antagonist	
	Ondansetron (Zofran)	PO: 8 mg bid for 2–3 d
Radiation-induced emesis		
Total-body irradiation	5-HT$_3$ receptor antagonist PO *and* Corticosteroid PO before each radiation fraction and 24 h afterwards	
Hemibody irradiation (upper abdominal, abdominal pelvic, mantle cranium, craniospinal)	5-HT$_3$ receptor antagonist PO *or* Dopamine antagonist PO before each radiation fraction	
Single-port irradiation (cranium, breast, head and neck, extremities, pelvis, thorax)	5-HT$_3$ receptor antagonist PO *or* Dopamine antagonist PO as needed	

administered orally, intramuscularly, or IV, with major side effects of sedation and anticholinergic symptoms.

Benzodiazepines

The antiemetic action of benzodiazepines is related to their effect on cortical pathways and possibly on the vomiting center. Amnesia accompanies the use of benzodiazepines, and this pharmacodynamic effect may be desired because it can lessen the conditioned behavior resulting from emetogenic therapy. This class of antiemetics may also assist in controlling the extrapyramidal side effects of the dopamine antagonists.

Lorazepam (Ativan),* a commonly used benzodiazepine because of its short half-life, is given in a dose of 1 to 1.5 mg/m^2 every 4 to 6 hours. Even though benzodiazepines have a wide therapeutic index, respiratory depression can occur.

Cannabinoids

In younger patients, particularly those with a history of marijuana use, cannabinoids may be an effective antiemetic. The antiemetic efficacy of this class of drugs is improved when used in combination with prochlorperazine. Present guidelines require that synthetic cannabinoids be used before initiating a request to the government for legal marijuana use. Dronabinol (Marinol) is representative of this class and is given in oral doses of 5 to 15 mg/m^2 every 4 to 6 hours starting an hour before chemotherapy. The high incidence of CNS side effects (including hallucinations, nightmares, and anxiety) severely limits their broader use, particularly in older patients.

Anticholinergics

This class of antiemetics is mostly used for motion sickness and is represented by scopolamine formulated as a patch (Transderm Scōp) placed behind the ear and changed every third day. Patients should be warned about the proper method of handling the scopolamine patch. After placing the patch, wearers should wash their hands to prevent inadvertent eye contact. Not doing so could result in an evaluation of the sudden onset of anisocoria. Even though the antiemetic activity of some of the other drug classes may in part be explained by anticholinergic mechanisms, this class of drugs is not generally used as a single agent in suppressing cancer chemotherapy–induced emesis.

Miscellaneous

Representative agents include trimethobenzamide (Tigan) and benzquinamide (Emete-con). These drugs are used more often with less serious emetic stimuli. They are well tolerated and have few side effects.

Special Circumstances in Controlling Nausea and Vomiting

Cancer Chemotherapy–Induced Nausea and Vomiting

Preventing nausea and vomiting from emetogenic therapy depends on giving antiemetics prophylactically and in combination (see Table 4). Using antiemetics as rescue agents is not as effective, but they are generally offered anyway. Avoiding rescue drugs in the same class as those given previously may lessen the likelihood of an adverse reaction.

Drug Overdose

Nausea and vomiting accompanying drug overdose may be a contraindication to antiemetic therapy until the risk for CNS and/or cardiac complications is lessened.

*Not FDA approved for this indication.

Parkinson's Disease/Pheochromocytoma

Managing nausea and emesis in patients with Parkinson's disease and pheochromocytoma represents two special situations in which dopamine antagonists can exacerbate the underlying disease. Carbidopa (Lodosyn) has fewer GI effects than L-dopa (Levodopa) does. Significant nausea and vomiting will develop in approximately 15% of patients treated with bromocriptine (Parlodel). The use of serotonin antagonists offers an additional treatment option.

Diabetes Mellitus

Promotility agents such as metoclopramide in low doses may be the antiemetic of choice for nausea and vomiting resulting from diabetic gastroparesis. Ten milligrams of metoclopramide taken 30 minutes before meals may improve these symptoms.

Carcinoid Tumor/Syndrome

Nausea and vomiting accompanying the hyperserotoninergic state, or carcinoid syndrome, are usually secondary to the effects of the tumor and not to serotonin stimulation of the chemoreceptor trigger zone or the vomiting center. Octreotide (Sandostatin) (50 to 150 μg subcutaneously every 8 to 12 hours), a somatostatin analogue, should be considered for managing nausea and vomiting in patients with hormonally active neoplasms.

Delayed Emesis After Cancer Chemotherapy

Prolonged nausea associated with anorexia and vomiting beginning 24 hours or more after cisplatin-based chemotherapy is referred to as delayed emesis. Continuation of effective antiemetics for at least 4 days after chemotherapy may be indicated. Because sustained use beyond 4 to 7 days may cause adverse effects, the administration of antiemetics as needed is preferred should nausea persist for longer than a week after cisplatin chemotherapy.

Anticipatory Emesis

Effectively controlling emesis is the best method to prevent the occurrence of a conditioned response. The amnestic effect of the benzodiazepines may also help reduce the incidence of anticipatory emesis if the antiemetic regimen is only partially effective. Behavioral methods using relaxation and imagery guided by an experienced clinician may offer an additional treatment option should conditioning interfere with compliance.

Nausea and Vomiting Accompanying Pregnancy

Morning or evening sickness is common during the first trimester of pregnancy, but these symptoms usually abate during the second trimester. More severe symptoms may be associated with multiple pregnancies or a hydatidiform mole.

Pharmacologic intervention is usually unnecessary. Reassurance, rest, frequent small meals, and dietary restrictions may be all that is required. For some patients, 50 to 100 mg pyridoxine (vitamin B_6)* per day is beneficial. If the symptoms are more persistent and protracted as in hyperemesis gravidarum, hospitalization and IV fluids may be required. No drugs have been approved for use in pregnancy. The selection of any pharmacologic agent should be based on the severity of symptoms and the potential risk to the fetus. The phenothiazines and metoclopramide* are effective in controlling pregnancy-related nausea and vomiting.

Postanesthesia Nausea and Vomiting

About 80% of patients will have nausea and vomiting during the perioperative or postoperative period. Using the 5-HT_3 antagonist class of antiemetics may avoid the sedation, hypotension, and extrapyramidal reactions associated with the phenothiazines and substituted benzamides.

Motion Sickness

Anticholinergics and antihistamines are commonly used in the management of motion sickness. Small, bland meals may be another effective measure. Scopolamine placed behind the ear may be convenient for those exposed to motion for long periods.

Radiation Therapy

The incidence of nausea and vomiting from radiation therapy is dependent on the dose and the region of the body receiving external beam treatment. With total-body and hemibody irradiation, combination regimens should be considered prophylactically (see Table 4). Single-port radiation treatments are associated with fewer GI side effects, and antiemetics can be used on an as-needed basis.

*Not FDA approved for this indication.

GASEOUSNESS AND INDIGESTION

method of
YOUNG K. CHOI, M.D., and
SATISH S. C. RAO, M.D., PH.D.
University of Iowa Carver College of Medicine
Iowa City, Iowa

"Doctor—I have gas" and "Doctor—I have indigestion" are common complaints. Mostly, they represent a benign illness, but they can cause significant morbidity, impair quality of life, and lead to loss of time at work. Here, we first discuss gas or bloating and thereafter indigestion.

GAS, FLATUS, AND BLOATING

Pathophysiology

Intestinal gas arises from four sources: (1) swallowed air; (2) CO_2 produced by chemical interaction among gastric acid, food, and alkaline secretions; (3) bacterial fermentation; and (4) diffusion of gas from blood supplying the gut. Mostly, intestinal gas consists of H_2, CH_4, CO_2, N_2, O_2, and other trace gases. Symptoms of gas and bloating may arise from an imbalance among production, transit, and expulsion of gas. Table 1 provides a list of common conditions that cause gas and bloating.

In some patients, excessive swallowing of air (aerophagia) may lead to frequent belching, eructation, or bloating. In others, there may be excessive gas production from fermentation of undigested food, malabsorption, or bacterial overgrowth. In patients with unexplained bloating, studies have shown impaired clearance (excess retention) of intestinal gas or hypersensitivity to bowel distention. In some, this may be due to high fat intake.

Etiology and Clinical Evaluation

The clinician's task is to determine whether the abdominal bloating is life threatening or a functional illness. If a patient presents with sudden onset of abdominal distention or inability to pass gas or stool, mechanical obstruction should be suspected. Sometimes, patients may not present with abdominal pain, especially if they are using narcotics or steroids or if they are mentally challenged or institutionalized.

Next, the clinician should consider the possibility of an infectious, inflammatory, or malabsorption disorder (see Table 1). The presence of alarm symptoms such as nausea, vomiting, diarrhea, blood in stool, weight loss, anemia, steatorrhea, or nocturnal pain may suggest an organic illness.

If alarm symptoms are absent, the possibility of carbohydrate intolerance must be explored. A detailed dietary history is useful. This is best assessed through a prospective 1-week food and symptom diary. If there is a temporal relationship between symptoms and ingestion of food containing lactose, fructose, or sorbitol, carbohydrate malabsorption is likely. Sometimes, malabsorption may be due to Crohn's disease, surgical resection, giardiasis, celiac disease, bacterial overgrowth, or eosinophilic gastroenteritis. If so, symptoms may resolve with treatment of the primary disease.

Motility dysfunction such as slow-transit constipation, dyssynergic or obstructive defecation, gastroparesis, or pseudo-obstruction syndromes can also cause gas and bloating. Rarely, functional disorders such as hepatic or splenic flexure syndrome, in which there is prolonged entrapment of colonic gas from anatomic aberrations, may be seen. Nissen fundoplication has become popular for treating gastroesophageal reflux disease. Following surgery, 10% to 20% of patients may experience severe postprandial bloating (gas-bloat syndrome) because of their inability to belch air. Finally, after excluding the aforementioned organic disorders, functional blasting or irritable bowel syndrome should be considered.

Physical Examination

The presence of abdominal tenderness, rebound, guarding, or absent or high-pitched bowel sounds suggests peritonitis or obstruction. In others, painless

TABLE 1. **A List of Common Conditions That Cause Gas and Bloating Together with Management Options**

Diagnosis	Cause(s)	Investigation(s)	Treatment(s)
Mechanical obstruction	Neoplasia, adhesion, stricture, volvulus, intussusception, or perforation	Plain abdominal films (erect/supine), barium study, endoscopy, colonoscopy, CT scan	Treatment of underlying disease Surgery
Aerophagia	Anxiety, GERD, smoking, chewing gum, sucking, drinking soda	History, plain abdominal film	Behavior modification: stop smoking, chewing gum, or drinking soda
Malabsorption	Lactose, fructose, sorbitol, beans, legumes, fat, gluten	History, food diary, breath test 3-day fecal fat	Withdrawal of the offending agent Enzyme supplements such as lactase, α-galactosidase (Beano), and pancreatic enzymes
Motility disorder	Gastroparesis, dumping syndrome, gas/bloat syndrome (after Nissen fundoplication), hepatic or splenic flexure syndrome, constipation	History, abdominal films, gastric emptying study, colon transit study, anorectal manometry	Prokinetics Laxatives Biofeedback
Bacterial overgrowth	Diabetes, chronic PPI usage, gastrectomy, Nissen fundoplication, scleroderma	Glucose breath test EGD + small-bowel aspirate culture	Antibiotics for 2 wk: ampicillin, metronidazole (Flagyl), or levofloxacin (Levaquin)
Cholecystitis	Gallstones	Ultrasound, CT scan, HIDA scan	Cholecystectomy, surgery
Functional gas or bloating	Irritable bowel syndrome, visceral hyperalgesia	History, ROME criteria, limited tests to exclude organic disease	Symptomatic, low-dose tricyclics, trazodone (Desyrel), tegaserod (Zelnorm)

CT, computed tomography; EGD, esophagogastroduodenoscopy; GERD, gastroesophageal reflux disease; HIDA, hydroxyiminodiacetic acid; PPI, proton pump inhibitor.

distention or the presence of excessive stool on abdominal or rectal examination suggests constipation with stool impaction or dyssynergia. Occasionally, particularly in young women, pseudocyesis or abnormal protrusion of the abdomen secondary to exaggerated lumbar lordosis may be seen.

Investigations

The workup should be focused, and one should avoid a fishing expedition. If obstruction is suspected, abdominal films, barium studies, or a computed tomographic scan should be obtained (see Table 1). If there is blood in the stool, colonoscopy should be performed, especially in older patients (>50 years). If celiac sprue is suspected, an upper endoscopy with small-bowel biopsy is helpful. If infection is suspected, stool examination for ova and parasites and stool culture should be obtained.

A diagnosis of carbohydrate malabsorption is made using breath tests. This noninvasive test has good specificity and sensitivity and can reproduce symptoms. Lactose intolerance is due to deficiency of lactase enzyme. Its prevalence varies from 10% to 30% in whites and 60% to 90% in Asians, Mexicans, and Africans.

Fructose intolerance is the inability to absorb fructose. Its absorption is limited, as there is no enzyme or active transport mechanism. Artificial sweeteners, fruits (pears, prunes), soft drinks, and juices contain fructose. An example of a fructose-positive breath test is shown in Figure 1. In tertiary care centers, 30% to 70% of patients with unexplained gastrointestinal symptoms may have fructose intolerance, and many fulfill ROME criteria for irritable bowel syndrome.

Excess intake of fiber, beans, or sorbitol-containing products (chewing gum, artificial sweeteners) can cause bloating through bacterial fermentation in the colon. Other sources include maldigestion of legumes from a deficiency of α-galactosidase.

Bacterial overgrowth is best identified by glucose hydrogen breath test or culture of small-bowel aspirate. Potential conditions that predispose to overgrowth are shown in Table 1.

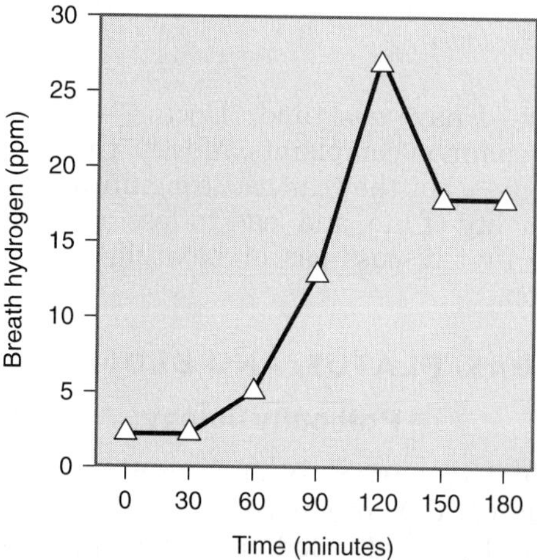

Figure 1. An example of a patient with fructose intolerance. After ingestion of fructose, there is a significant rise in breath hydrogen.

Management

The management depends upon the underlying etiology (see Table 1). If a life-threatening condition is suspected, the patient requires hospitalization.

The cornerstone for treating carbohydrate malabsorption is withdrawal of the offending agent. Fortunately, lactose-free milk and cheese are available and can be substituted. Also, lactase enzyme supplements may help. Fructose intolerance is best treated by withdrawal of the sugar. By modifying the diet, 70% of patients can improve. Adding dextrose powder to fructose products may also facilitate fructose absorption. Products such as α-D-galactosidase enzyme (Beano) or methylcellulose (Fiberase) can help patients with maldigestion of beans or legumes. Bacterial overgrowth is best treated with a 2-week course of antibiotics (see Table 1).

The management of functional bloating or irritable bowel syndrome is less satisfactory. Low-dose antidepressants such as amitriptyline (Elavil) or selective serotonin reuptake inhibitors or antispasmodics such as dicyclomine (Bentyl) or hyoscyamine (Levsin) may help. If a patient has constipation, osmotic laxatives such as milk of magnesia, polyethylene glycol (MiraLax), or bisacodyl may help. Fiber supplements and lactulose (Cephulac) must be avoided as they produce gas and can worsen symptoms. Tegaserod (Zelnorm), a serotonin partial agonist and a prokinetic, may help bloating with abdominal pain.

INDIGESTION

Indigestion or dyspepsia is defined as the occurrence of persistent or recurrent epigastric discomfort or pain, often after meals. Other associated features include nausea, fullness, vomiting, and heartburn. In the United States, the prevalence of dyspepsia is 5% to 20%. Most patients have acid reflux or peptic ulcer disease. Other common causes of indigestion, their workup, and treatment are summarized in Table 2.

Management

In younger patients with mild or occasional gastroesophageal reflux disease and no alarming symptoms, empirical treatment with H_2 blockers or proton pump inhibitors may be sufficient. In older patients (>50 years) or those with alarming symptoms such as dysphagia, nocturnal discomfort, weight loss, or atypical gastroesophageal reflux disease, a gastroenterologist should be consulted. Infection with *Helicobacter pylori* is associated with indigestion or peptic ulcer disease, and its eradication (see Table 2) may improve symptoms. Finally, there are patients with nonulcer or functional dyspepsia. Here, the underlying etiology is visceral hyperalgia (gastric hypersensitivity), although some patients may have decreased gastric accommodation or gastroparesis. These patients should be referred to a gastroenterologist for further workup and management.

TABLE 2. **A List of Common Conditions That Cause Indigestion Together with Management Options**

Diagnosis	Investigation	Treatment
Drug-induced dyspepsia (NSAID, theophylline, bisphosphonates, KCl)	History, endoscopy or biopsy	Withdrawal of drug PPIs (proton pump inhibitors) H_2 blockers Sucralfate (Carafate)
Helicobacter pylori gastritis	Serum antibody, breath test, stool antigen, and gastric biopsy	Triple therapy (metronidazole or amoxicillin, clarithromycin (Biaxin), and PPI)
Gastroesophageal reflux disease (GERD)	History, 24-h pH study, endoscopy	PPIs H_2 blockers, sucralfate
Peptic ulcer disease (PUD)	Endoscopy or biopsy, barium study	PPI, H_2 blockers, sucralfate
Functional or nonulcer dyspepsia	History, ROME criteria, EGD	PPI, low-dose antidepressants, prokinetics
Cholelithiasis	Ultrasonography, CT scan	Cholecystectomy

CT, computed tomography; EGD, esophagogastroduodenoscopy; NSAID, nonsteroidal anti-inflammatory drug.

HICCUPS

method of
JAMES H. LEWIS, M.D.
Georgetown University Medical Center
Washington, DC

Hiccups have long been considered a medical curiosity. Although most hiccups occur as brief, self-limited episodes lasting up to a few minutes, persistent hiccups that last longer than 48 hours or recur at frequent intervals often imply an underlying physical, structural, metabolic, or infectious cause. Occasionally, hiccups are intractable, occurring continuously for months or years, and can result in significant morbidity.

The term "hiccup" refers to the onomatopoeic attempt to vocalize the sound produced by the abrupt closure of the glottis after the sudden contraction of the inspiratory muscles. "Hiccough" was used in the older literature and likely represented the previously held belief that hiccups occur as a result of a respiratory reflex. The medical term for hiccups, singultus, is derived from the Latin root *singult,* meaning the act of catching one's breath during sobbing.

Hiccups do not appear to serve any particularly useful or protective function. However, because they may occur during fetal and neonatal life and are seen in other mammals, they may represent a primitive or vestigial reflex whose functional or behavioral significance has been lost. A relationship between hiccups and the phrenic nerve was recognized by an Edinburgh physician in 1833 who recommended blistering the skin over the course of the phrenic nerve in the neck as a means of treatment. In current theory, the afferent limb of the hiccup reflex is composed of the vagus and phrenic nerves and the sympathetic chain arising from T6-T12, with a hiccup center located in the upper spinal cord in C3-C5. The efferent limb remains primarily the phrenic nerve, although nerves to the glottis and accessory muscles of the respiration also are involved, as patients are reported to continue to hiccup even after transection of both phrenic nerves.

Conditions Associated with Hiccups

More than 100 conditions have been associated with hiccups, including a variety of structural, metabolic, inflammatory, neoplastic, infectious, and drug-related causes. For many, a relationship with one or more limbs of the reflex arc can be shown, whereas for others, the association is more obscure.

Overeating is a frequent cause of self-limited hiccups. The mechanism is presumed to be gastric distention leading to stimulation of the gastric branches of the vagus nerve or via direct irritation of the diaphragm by an overinflated stomach. Recently, sudden rapid stretch of mechanoreceptors in the proximal esophagus has been suggested as a cause.

Alcohol-induced hiccups may also be the result of gastric distention or the central effects of alcohol on the cerebral cortex, which remove inhibitions normally serving to dampen the hiccup reflex.

Intraoperative hiccups may occur from hyperextension of the neck, stretching the roots of the phrenic nerve, traction on the diaphragm or viscera, use of short-acting barbiturates, inadequate ventilation during anesthesia, or gastric distention or ileus that may continue into the postoperative period. A light plane of anesthesia may suppress inhibitory influences that normally function to prevent hiccups. As the neuromuscular blocking action muscle relaxant starts to diminish, a return of diaphragmatic activity may be associated with hiccups. Postoperative hiccups, which account for up to 25% of hiccups in men, usually appear within 4 days of surgery. A majority of these episodes follow intra-abdominal surgery, with the remainder resulting from urinary tract, central nervous system, and chest surgery.

Hiccups are frequently seen during endoscopy, relating to the use of opioids, midazolam (Versed), or gastric distention from insufflation.

HICCUP TREATMENT

Historical Cures

Many of the better-known hiccup "cures" can be traced back hundreds or thousands of years. Hippocrates wrote that in "the case of a person afflicted with hiccough, sneezing coming on removes the hiccough." Plato is credited with being the first to recommend a sudden slap on the back as a means of scaring away hiccups. This probably worked by inducing a sudden gasp in the person being struck, thereby breaking the hiccup cycle, giving rise to other therapies aimed at disrupting the respiratory rhythm. In ancient Greece, Aristophanes was told to hold his breath, gargle with water, and, if needed, tickle his nose to induce a sneeze. Plugging one's ears with one's fingers (in combination with breath holding) was advocated in London as early as 1627. Grandmothers going back several generations have recommended swallowing granulated sugar or eating peanut butter.

Physical and Mechanical Hiccup Cures

Some measures aimed at counteracting the diaphragmatic contractions that occur during hiccupping consist of pulling the knees up to the chest or leaning forward to compress the diaphragm (Table 1). Continuous positive airway pressure or other means to hyperinflate the lungs may stimulate the Hering-Breuer reflex, which disrupts not only the normal respiratory rhythm but also the abnormal hiccup pattern. Other means to reduce hiccup frequency include sneezing, performing a Valsalva maneuver, breath holding, hyperventilating, and involuntary gasping induced by inhaling smelling salts. Inhaling 5% carbon dioxide or breathing into a paper bag terminates hiccups through the effect of acute respiratory acidosis on diaphragmatic contractility.

Relief of gastric distention emetics, gastric lavage, or nasogastric aspiration may be effective when the stomach is overdistended by food, liquid, or air. Stimulation of the soft palate, uvula, and pharynx is often cited as a way to terminate a bout of hiccups. Forcible traction of the tongue (credited by William Osler), lifting the uvula with a spoon, and manipulating the pharynx with a catheter or cotton-tipped swab also have been used successfully. Intraoperative hiccups may be stopped with a rubber or plastic catheter–inserted spray of ethyl chloride. The success of these methods suggests that irritation of the soft palate or pharynx inhibits afferent impulses transmitted by the vagus nerve.

Stimulation of vagal afferents may also account for the success of swallowing dry granulated sugar, sipping ice water, or eating peanut butter. Although a few published reports on the use of sugar attest to its efficacy, as with nearly all other purported hiccup "cures," they are anecdotal and uncontrolled. Alcohol-related hiccups have been treated successfully with a lemon wedge soaked in angostura bitters. Drinking from the far side of the glass has been proposed as

TABLE 1. **Mechanical Methods Used to Treat Hiccups**

Stimulation of the uvula or nasopharynx
Forcible traction of the tongue
Lifting the uvula with a spoon
Catheter stimulation
Gargling with water
Sipping ice water
Sucking on hard candy
Swallowing dry granulated sugar
Swallowing hard bread or peanut butter
Noxious taste (vinegar, angostura bitters)
Interruption of respiratory rhythm
Valsalva maneuver
Gasping (noxious odor or sudden fright)
Sneezing
Continuous positive airway pressure
Holding the breath
Compressing the thyroid cartilage
Respiratory center stimulants
Breathing 5% carbon dioxide
Hyperventilating
Holding the breath
Rebreathing into a paper bag or dead space tubing
Counterirritation of the diaphragm
Pulling the knees up to the chest
Leaning forward to compress the chest
Applying pressure at points of diaphragmatic insertion
Relief of gastric distention
Gastric lavage
Nasogastric aspiration
Emetic-induced vomiting
Disruption of the phrenic nerve/glossopharyngeal nerve
Nerve block
Electric stimulation
Crush procedures
Transection
Counterirritation of the vagus nerve
Supraorbital pressure
Carotid sinus massage
Removal of hair or foreign body irritating tympanic membrane
Digital rectal massage
Acupuncture
Korean hand acupuncture
Acupuncture with electromagnetic stimulation
Psychiatric
Hypnosis
Behavior modification
Attempting to drink from the far side of a glass
Prayer

TABLE 2. **Pharmacotherapy of Hiccups**

Antispasticity agents
Baclofen (Lioresal),* 5-20 mg PO every 6-12 h
Major tranquilizers
Chlorpromazine (Thorazine), 25-50 mg, IV every 6 h; if successful, switch to oral use at the same dose
Haloperidol (Haldol),* 2-12 mg/d, PO
Anticonvulsants
Phenytoin (Dilantin),* 200 mg IV bolus, then 100 mg PO four times daily
Valproic acid (Depakene),* 15 mg/kg/d, PO or rectally
Carbamazepine (Tegretol),* 200 mg, PO four times daily
Magnesium sulfate,* 5 mL 25% solution IM
Central nervous system stimulants
Methylphenidate (Ritalin),* 6-20 mg, IV bolus***
Amphetamine sulfate combination (Adderall),* 10-20 mg, PO twice daily
Ephedrine,* 5 mg, IV bolus
Anesthetic stimulants
Ketamine (Ketalar),* 0.4-0.5 mg/kg, IV during anesthesia
Calcium channel blockers
Nifedipine (Procardia),* 10 mg, PO twice daily (increased to 20 mg three times daily)
Antidepressants
Amitriptyline (Elavil),* 10 mg, PO three times daily
Serotonin antagonists
Ondansetron (Zofran),* 4-32 mg, IV bolus or 8 mg, PO three times daily
Dopamine antagonists
Metoclopramide (Reglan),* 10 mg, PO every 6 h or 5-10 mg, IM or IV every 8 h
Dopamine agonists
Amantadine (Symmetrel),* 100 mg/d, PO
Parasympathomimetics
Edrophonium (Tensilon),* 5 mg, IV
Parasympatholytics
Atropine,* 1 mg, IV
Quinidine,* 10 grains, PO or IM every 3-4 h**
Antiarrhythmics
Lidocaine (Xylocaine),* 1 mg/kg IV loading dose followed by 2-4 mg/min continuous IV infusion

*Not FDA approved for this indication.
**Exceeds dosage recommended by the manufacturer.
***Does not come commercially in IV form.
Medications and doses listed are those with reported success in the literature.

a means of terminating hiccups through so-called "cerebral concentration" because it is nearly impossible to accomplish.

Miscellaneous Hiccup Cures

The successful use of hypnosis for hiccups has been reported for a variety of underlying causes. Acupuncture has been used for generations in Asia to treat hiccups, and its use is increasingly being reported for patients with intractable hiccups in the West. Korean hand acupuncture is a specialized form specifically reported to be successful.

Drug Therapy for Hiccups

Several pharmacologic agents have been used for persistent or intractable hiccups when mechanical or physical measures fail. As is the case with most reports on stopping hiccups, the results for nearly all medications remain anecdotal (Table 2). The following agents have been the most frequently employed for hiccups of various causes.

Baclofen

Baclofen (Lioresal)* is a derivative of the inhibitory neurotransmitter gamma-aminobutyric acid that was

*Not FDA approved for this indication.

initially developed for reducing the frequency and severity of spasticity in patients with multiple sclerosis and spinal cord disorders. It has been in use to treat hiccups for more than a decade and has emerged as the most successful general hiccup therapy, as noted by an increasing number of anecdotal reports and by randomized, controlled clinical trials. Baclofen is believed to reduce excitability and depress reflex hiccup activity, as demonstrated in animal studies in which its injection into the putative hiccup center in the nucleus raphe magnus of the cat medulla has terminated experimental hiccups. It blocks esophageal and gastric distention–induced relaxation of the lower esophageal sphincter and blocks inhibition of the crural diaphragm to end hiccups.

Baclofen is rapidly absorbed after oral administration, has a half-life of 3 to 4 hours, and is excreted largely unchanged by the kidneys. Side effects include drowsiness, insomnia, dizziness, weakness, ataxia, and confusion. Elderly patients may tolerate it poorly, and sudden withdrawal after long-term use may cause hallucinations, anxiety, and tachycardia. Respiratory depression, seizures, and coma have been reported after overdose; the drug should be used cautiously in patients with renal failure. Abrupt withdrawal (especially after intrathecal use) has led to a syndrome of high fever, altered mental status, seizures, rigidity, and rhabdomyolysis.

Chlorpromazine (Thorazine)

This major tranquilizer has been used to terminate hiccups since reports in the 1950s cited cure rates of 80% among patients with intractable hiccups from various causes. After successful intravenous therapy, oral chlorpromazine at the same dose can be maintained for 7 to 10 days. A related agent, haloperidol (Haldol),* also may be effective, perhaps relating to its dopamine antagonistic effects, although drowsiness, postural hypotension, and other side effects may limit their usefulness.

Anticonvulsants

Phenytoin (Dilantin),* administered as an initial intravenous bolus followed by oral therapy, has not been consistently effective in terminating hiccups. Valproic acid (Depakene),* given orally or rectally, has controlled hiccups for as long as 1 year, possibly by enhancing the inhibitory effects of gamma-aminobutyric acid. Carbamazepine (Tegretol)* also has successfully stopped hiccups when administered orally. Benzodiazepines, on the other hand, have not been useful in terminating hiccups and, in fact, may even be the cause of some hiccups.

Specific Hiccups Cures

A number of causes of chronic hiccups have been successfully treated by drugs or maneuvers specifically directed at the underlying condition (Table 3). For example, anesthesia-related hiccups have been stopped with methylphenidate (Ritalin),* ephedrine,* intranasal ethyl chloride spray,* and catheter stimulation of the pharynx. Postoperative hiccups have been terminated by amphetamine (Benzedrine)*/** and ketamine (Ketalar),* an anesthetic stimulant administered at 20% less than the usual anesthetic dose.

*Not FDA approved for this indication.

TABLE 3. **Some Successful Cause-Specific Hiccup Therapies**

Hiccup Cause	Successful Physical Maneuver/Drug Treatment
Addison's disease	Steroid replacement
Alcohol	Lemon wedge soaked in angostura bitters
Candida esophagitis	Antifungal treatment
Carcinomatosis with vomiting	Ondansetron
Cardiac arrhythmia (ventricular tachycardia)	Cardioversion
Coronary artery or valvular heart disease	Nifedipine
Esophageal obstruction or achalasia	Esophageal dilation
Foreign body in ear canal	Removal
Herpetic esophagitis	Acyclovir
Hyponatremia	Correct electrolyte imbalance
Intraoperative	Catheter stimulation of pharynx; instillation of ethyl chloride into nostrils
Parkinson's disease	Amantadine
Postoperative	Splanchnicectomy
Reflux esophagitis	Acid suppression or antireflux surgery
Renal failure requiring dialysis	Baclofen

Metoclopramide (Reglan)* has terminated hiccups of diverse causes and has a well-recognized effect on gastric distention caused by diabetic gastroparesis. Amantadine (Symmetrel),* a dopaminergic agonist, has had anecdotal success in treating hiccups relating to Parkinson's disease. Ondansetron (Zofran),* a specific 5-hydroxytryptamine-3 antagonist, has been used successfully to control hiccups in patients with metastatic adenocarcinoma who also may have uncontrolled vomiting. Baclofen (Lioresal)* has successfully managed hiccups associated with renal failure in dialysis patients, acquired immunodeficiency syndrome, and an interesting entity known as familial hiccups.

Chronic hiccups are sometimes associated with esophageal disorders. Achalasia-related hiccups have been eliminated after successful pneumatic dilation. Hiccups caused by herpetic esophagitis have been successfully treated with acyclovir, and patients with candida esophagitis–related hiccups may be cured by antifungal treatment. Gastroesophageal reflux disease has been considered a cause and a consequence of hiccups; therefore, treatment of acid reflux has not always brought relief.

Guidelines for Treating Transient Hiccups

Hiccup episodes that last only a few minutes may be annoying or embarrassing but rarely require treatment other than simple physical maneuvers. Holding

*Not FDA approved for this indication.
**Not available in the United States.

the breath, breathing into a paper bag, pulling on the tongue, sneezing, swallowing a tablespoon of granulated sugar or peanut butter, or sucking on hard candy are often effective, but in many instances, these hiccups would probably have spontaneously stopped without attempting these remedies. In patients in whom hiccups last longer than 30 to 60 minutes, manually stimulating the nasopharynx with the finger or rubber catheter, lifting the uvula with a spoon or other device, or inducing a gasp with smelling salts can be tried if simpler measures are ineffective. Not recommended as home measures are instilling ammonia or ether into the nasopharynx, performing carotid sinus massage, applying supraorbital pressure or digital compression to the root of the neck over the course of the phrenic nerve, or compressing the thyroid cartilage, all of which have been cited in the literature.

Women in their second or third trimester of pregnancy may note rhythmic fetal movements that are attributable to fetal hiccupping; these hiccups can be easily seen on sonography and can often be terminated when the mother leans forward or turns onto her side to change the fetal position.

Guidelines for Treating Persistent Hiccups

A thorough search shows an underlying organic cause in 90% of men with persistent hiccups. However, women are less likely to have an identifiable organic cause, according to reports. The extent of the evaluation varies, and at times unanticipated findings may be uncovered. One prospective evaluation of chronic hiccups lasting longer than 48 hours reported magnetic resonance imaging scans of the brain and upper spinal cord showing abnormalities in a number of patients who had a negative gastroesophageal evaluation that included endoscopy, pH monitoring, and manometry.

No studies have examined the percentage of patients in whom hiccups resolve when the underlying disorder is corrected. If hiccups remain refractory despite specific therapy and subsequent physical manipulations such as pharyngeal stimulation, pharmacologic agents may be required. Initially, baclofen (Lioresal)* can be tried, but should this fail, valproic acid (Depakene),* chlorpromazine (Thorazine),* or other agents can be used. Acupuncture or hypnotherapy is being increasingly attempted. Interestingly, persistent hiccups often spontaneously resolve during sleep, but return on awakening.

For hiccups that remain unresponsive to any or all of the measures previously mentioned, such as those by widespread intra-abdominal carcinomatosis or surgical adhesions, electrical stimulation or surgical or chemical disruption of the phrenic nerve needs to be considered, especially when the hiccups cause significant discomfort or morbidity. However, before phrenic nerve disruption is attempted, fluoroscopic examination of the diaphragm should be performed to determine whether one side of the diaphragm is dominant. Temporary phrenic nerve blocks and phrenic crush procedures have not been uniformly successful, even when both sides have been treated. Moreover, impaired pulmonary function and even respiratory failure have occurred as a result of bilateral diaphragmatic paralysis. This approach seems justified only in extreme instances, with ventilatory support services immediately available. Glossopharyngeal nerve blocks have been reported to stop chronic hiccups and are far less invasive than phrenic nerve disruption.

For hiccups that defy all treatment measures, unconventional approaches have been advocated, including praying to St. Jude, the patron saint of lost causes. The latter was said to be successful in one individual who had tried countless unsuccessful cures.

*Not FDA approved for this indication.

ACUTE INFECTIOUS DIARRHEA

method of
DAVID A. SACK, M.D.
Centre for Health and Population Research
Dhaka, Bangladesh

Acute diarrhea is defined as the passage of an increased number of loose or watery stools in association with other symptoms of intestinal illness, such as abdominal cramps or vomiting. As a general rule, diagnosis can be confirmed by at least three such stools in a day. In industrialized countries, diarrhea is a common inconvenience, affecting people one or two times per year, but it may become a serious condition in certain circumstances, such as when the diarrheal fluid loss is very high, when the symptoms persist and lead to electrolyte imbalance, when the symptoms are accompanied by signs of invasive disease, or when the symptoms represent signs of more serious underlying illness. In developing countries, diarrheal diseases are one of the leading causes of death because the dehydration, if not treated with appropriate rehydration therapy, can quickly lead to death. The number of deaths from diarrhea worldwide is estimated at 1 to 2 million, but this huge number actually represents a sizeable decrease from the mid-1990s, when it was about 5 million. The improvement in the number of deaths is believed to be the result of proper case management including the widespread use of oral rehydration therapy.

Because most cases of diarrhea are self-limited, the syndrome is divided into acute diarrhea, defined as lasting fewer than 14 days, and persistent diarrhea, in which the symptoms last more than 14 days. This cutoff of 14 days is somewhat arbitrary, but it is a helpful guide in identifying those patients who may require additional investigation. Either acute or persistent diarrhea may have blood (with or without mucus), and when this occurs the disease is called *dysentery* or *invasive diarrhea*. Diarrhea without blood in the stool is referred to as *watery* or *secretory diarrhea*. Some illnesses, especially those caused by *Shigella* or *Salmonella* species, may start as watery diarrhea and progress to dysentery.

Diarrhea may be caused by a wide variety of infectious agents, but it may also result from noninfectious causes such as laxatives, lactose intolerance, inflammatory bowel disease, pancreatic insufficiency, and irritable bowel syndrome. Among the infectious causes, certain viruses and bacteria are the most common, but parasites may also be considered. Among the viruses, rotavirus is by far the most common cause of diarrhea in infants, but other viruses (e.g., calicivirus) are more likely to cause diarrhea in older persons. Bacteria are much less likely to be the cause of diarrhea in industrialized countries but are common causes of diarrhea in developing countries that lack modern sanitation.

Evaluation of patients with acute diarrhea includes determining several key characteristics, such as age of the patient (because different pathogens tend to infect certain age groups), history of recent travel to developing countries (because bacterial pathogens are much more common in areas of poor sanitation), signs and symptoms of dehydration (because this will determine how aggressive to be with rehydration therapy), history of recent intake of risky foods or water, signs and symptoms of invasive diarrhea such as blood in the stool or fever, history of antibiotic use (because certain agents may infect the gut after use of antibiotics), and duration of symptoms (because chronic symptoms lead one to consider more chronic conditions). Key physical findings include evaluation for dehydration and evidence of systemic illness. Laboratory tests may be useful in the evaluation of some patients to confirm the presence of blood or pus cells in the stool or to evaluate patients suspected of having infection with *Shigella, Salmonella, Campylobacter, Vibrio, Clostridium difficile,* a parasite, or rotavirus. Although these tests may be useful in selected patients, a pathogen is found only rarely in patients in the United States; in developing countries, where bacterial pathogens are more common, the facilities and economic resources for such tests are limited. Thus, most mild cases of acute watery diarrhea can be managed without specific laboratory tests. During the search for pathogens, the fundamental management of fluids and electrolytes should not be overlooked.

CLINICAL SYNDROMES

Diarrhea may be classified into different clinical syndromes. These syndromes help to define the pathophysiologic mechanisms, the most likely infectious agents responsible, the treatment needed, and the clinical investigations that may help to define the illness further. These syndromes may further be refined depending on specific risk factors, epidemiologic factors, and age groups.

Acute Watery Diarrhea

By far the most common diarrheal syndrome is the sudden occurrence of loose or watery stools. This may be accompanied by nausea, vomiting, loss of appetite, abdominal cramps, and low-grade fever. However, fever greater than 102°F (38.9°C) generally suggests that the illness is not simply acute watery diarrhea but represents another invasive illness. The stools usually are very watery and of high volume but do not contain blood or mucus. A fecal leukocyte test, if performed, is negative for pus cells. Within the general category of acute watery diarrhea, a few types in specific groups of patients should be especially noted: infantile diarrhea, elderly diarrhea, traveler's diarrhea, seafood-associated diarrhea, outbreak-associated diarrhea, and cholera-like diarrhea.

Infantile Diarrhea

Infantile diarrhea occurs in nearly all infants during their first 15 months of life, but it usually does not occur during the first 3 months, when maternal antibody protects the infant. This condition continues to cause a large proportion of pediatric hospital admissions in the United States and is a major cause of pediatric admissions in the developing countries. The illness often starts with vomiting, but then diarrhea becomes the most prominent symptom, along with fussiness and resistance to feeding. Dehydration is the most dangerous complication of infantile diarrhea, which may result from the excess loss of diarrhea stool and vomiting. "Superabsorbent" disposable diapers may mask the large volumes of stool that are being lost and may also obscure the fact that urine output is decreasing. Thus, parents and providers must be alert to the signs of dehydration, including poor skin turgor, dry mucous membranes, increased thirst, depressed fontanelles, and low urine output.

Rotavirus is the most common cause of the infantile diarrhea syndrome in industrialized countries, where it usually occurs during a winter season. It is also the most common cause in developing countries, but bacterial pathogens, especially enterotoxigenic *Escherichia coli*, are also major causes. Regardless of the specific agent causing the diarrhea, the most important treatment is the restoration of fluids to correct dehydration and to maintain hydration until the diarrhea has resolved. Antibiotics and antidiarrheal drugs (e.g., diphenoxylate and atropine [Lomotil] or loperamide [Imodium]) should not be used in ordinary infantile diarrhea.

In the United States, few deaths are attributed to infantile diarrhea because it is readily managed with fluid and electrolyte replacement, but it does lead to many hospitalizations and much lost work for the parents and lost days from daycare. Globally, however, infantile diarrhea is estimated to kill about 1 to 2 million children each year.

Diarrhea frequently accompanies or follows the use of broad-spectrum antibiotics used to treat other illnesses, such as otitis or pneumonia in young children. These symptoms can usually be managed with oral rehydration solution (Table 1), as needed, to prevent dehydration.

Diarrhea In the Elderly

Just as dehydration is of great concern in infants, it is also a major problem in the elderly. The agents causing diarrhea in the geriatric age group are more

TABLE 1. **Composition of Rehydration Solutions Used to Treat Diarrheal Diseases**

Oral Rehydration Solution	Na^+	Cl^-	K^+	HCO_3	Carbohydrate	Osmolality (mmol/L)
Glucose-based oral rehydration solution (as recommended by World Health Organization)	75*	65	20	10†	13.5‡	245
Rice-based oral rehydration solution	70	60	20	10†	30-50§	~180
Intravenous fluids	—	—	—	—	—	—
Lactated Ringer's	130	109	4	28‖	—	271
Dhaka solution	133	154	13	48¶	—	292
Normal saline	154	154	0	0	—	308

*WHO and UNICEF lowered the preferred sodium concentration to 75 mEq. Previously it was 90 mEq/L.
†Base is given as trisodium citrate having 30 mEq (10 mmol)/L.
‡Glucose (13.5 g) containing 75 mmol/L.
§30 to 50 g of rice contains about 30 mmol/L, depending on the degree of hydrolysis.
‖Base in Ringer's is lactate.
¶Base in Dhaka solution is acetate.
Note: Commercial products in industrialized countries (e.g., Pedialyte in the United States contains 25 g of glucose and 45 g of sodium. CeraLyte contains 40 g of rice carbohydrate and 50 or 70 mEq of sodium (depending on the specific product).

varied. Calicivirus, *Salmonella, C. difficile,* and occasionally rotavirus are known to cause diarrhea in both endemic and epidemic forms. Although the diarrhea symptoms are similar to those in other age groups, the consequences may be much more severe because of the decreased ability of elderly patients to adapt to slightly decreased circulating blood volumes. The diarrhea episode, even with only mild dehydration, may result in cardiovascular complications, such as stroke, heart attack, and mesenteric artery thrombosis. Diarrhea in the elderly is also complicated by inconvenient nursing care, and the troublesome nursing care and cleaning may take precedence over the recognition that the patient is becoming dehydrated. Urine output and orthostatic blood pressure measurements should be monitored in such patients in addition to observing for other signs of dehydration, so that oral or intravenous fluids can be given as needed.

Because nursing homes house many elderly and disabled patients, and because enteric pathogens frequently spread in nursing homes, these institutionalized patients are especially at risk from outbreaks of diarrhea. *C. difficile* is of special concern in nursing home patients because these environments typically have exposure to antibiotics that select for *C. difficile,* and such patients can easily become infected with this bacterium.

Traveler's Diarrhea

Persons traveling from industrialized to developing countries are at high risk of developing acute diarrhea. As with other forms of watery diarrhea, it is usually accompanied by abdominal cramps and may also be accompanied by nausea, vomiting, anorexia, and inability to carry out planned activities. Thirty percent to 50% of travelers develop one or more episodes of diarrhea or loose stools during travel to developing countries, although illness sufficiently severe to lead to inability to function is much less common. Enterotoxigenic *E. coli* is the most common agent causing this syndrome, but other bacteria, and rarely viruses and parasites, may also cause these symptoms.

Symptoms of traveler's diarrhea are self-limited and usually last for 3 to 5 days in otherwise healthy people. Treatment includes maintenance of body fluids with oral rehydration solution and, in severe cases, use of an antibiotic such as ciprofloxacin (Cipro)* or norfloxacin (Noroxin).* Loperamide (Imodium) may be used along with the antibiotic. The antibiotic may be given for 1 to 3 days, but long courses of antibiotic are not needed. Such a course of antibiotic will decrease the duration of diarrhea significantly. Bismuth subsalicylate (Pepto-Bismol)* may be used to provide some symptomatic relief for mild cases.

The risk of traveler's diarrhea is less if one follows rules to ensure that food and water are hygienic (e.g., "cook it, peel it, or forget it"); however, even travelers who carefully follow such rules still frequently develop diarrhea. Prophylactic antibiotics can be given to persons who are at high risk if they are at such risk for a brief time (less than 3 weeks). Doxycycline (Vibramycin)* (100 mg/d with food) reduces the risk significantly; however, increasing numbers of enteric bacteria are resistant to this drug. Frequently, doxycycline is used to prevent malaria and, if given for this purpose, will also prevent most episodes of traveler's diarrhea. Prophylactic norfloxacin* (100 mg) or ciprofloxacin* (250 mg) daily will prevent nearly all episodes of diarrhea, and either agent is advised for persons who have a high risk of complications should they become dehydrated, such as elderly patients or those with cardiovascular disease. Use of such prophylactic antibiotics should be limited to less than 3 weeks; they are given only during days of actual travel, not before or after the travel.

Seafood-Associated Diarrhea

Certain diarrhea-causing bacteria are found in seafood, and these should be suspected when the history suggests an association with seafood such as shellfish, raw fish, or other fish that may not be fully cooked. Vibrios such as *Vibrio parahaemolyticus,*

*Not FDA approved for this indication.

Vibrio cholerae including both serogroup 01 and non-01, and other vibrios are especially common in seafood. The risk of *Vibrio* infection is much higher during the summer, when seawater temperatures are higher. Persons with immune deficiency who are more susceptible to *Vibrio* infection should avoid raw or undercooked seafood, especially during the summer months. Less commonly, caliciviruses and other enteric bacteria are associated with seafood. Other viruses (e.g., hepatitis A) may also be associated with seafood but do not commonly cause diarrhea. Travelers to cholera-endemic areas should avoid raw seafood or seafood served cold (e.g., shrimp salad). Even if once cooked, the cold seafood can be contaminated again with utensils or food juices from the kitchen.

Outbreak-Associated Diarrhea

Occasionally, the history will suggest that the patient may have been infected as part of a common-source outbreak. Such cases should be reported to the local health department immediately so that an outbreak investigation can be conducted. Illness after a "pot luck" meal should especially stimulate questions about whether others may have also become ill. The Centers for Disease Control and Prevention estimate that each year about 76 million persons experience food-borne illness in the United States, most of which is diarrheal disease. Many of these illnesses occur during common-source outbreaks. The most common bacterial agents causing these food-borne infections are *Salmonella, Campylobacter, Shigella,* and *E. coli.* Identification of such outbreaks can lead to preventive measures to stop the distribution of contaminated food.

Cholera Syndrome

Although rare in industrialized countries, cholera occurs in most developing countries. The occurrence of severe, rapidly progressing, dehydrating diarrhea with "rice-water stools" is the classic presentation for true "cholera gravis" caused by *V. cholerae* serotype 01 or 0139, but it may also be caused by enterotoxigenic *E. coli* and by other vibrios. This kind of illness is life threatening and requires aggressive rehydration.

Dysentery (Inflammatory Diarrhea)

The dysentery syndrome is characterized by frequent passage of loose stools containing blood (sometimes with mucus) and is the result of inflammation of the colon or lower small intestine. The patient tends to have the feeling of needing to pass stools frequently, but the volume is very small because the urgency is caused by inflammation of the rectum. Frequently, only small amounts of mucus or blood are passed. Because of the inflammation, patients with dysentery usually have severe abdominal cramps, they often have fever, body aches, and malaise, and they may have tenesmus (rectal pain that persists even after a stool has been passed). A fecal leukocyte test will reveal many polymorphonuclear leukocytes. In the case of shigellosis or salmonellosis, the illness may start as typical watery diarrhea and then progress to dysentery.

The most common causes of dysentery are *Shigella, Campylobacter,* and *Salmonella.* Amebic colitis may cause bloody stools but usually without inflammation, and stool microscopic examination is needed to identify the hematophagous trophozoites of *Entamoeba histolytica.*

Antibiotics are indicated for patients with shigellosis, but they are of questionable benefit in infections with *Campylobacter* and *Salmonella. Shigella* organisms are now commonly resistant to ampicillin and co-trimoxazole (Bactrim), and the newer quinolones have become the drugs of choice for most patients. In developing countries, where less expensive antibiotics may have an advantage, knowledge of the antibiotic sensitivities of local or endemic strains should guide immediate therapy. When possible, culture and sensitivity tests should be performed.

Proctocolitis is a syndrome involving inflammation of only the distal colon that leads to passage of small volumes of inflammatory exudates. Agents responsible for the syndrome include *Neisseria gonorrhoeae* and *Chlamydia,* often spread by anorectal intercourse.

DIAGNOSIS OF SPECIFIC AGENTS

Recognizing specific pathogens begins with suspecting their presence, based on history and physical examination.

Rotavirus

Rotavirus should be suspected in infants and young children, especially during the winter season (although in tropical climates rotavirus occurs year round). The illness often starts with vomiting and then progresses to watery diarrhea. Surveillance shows that nearly every infant is infected with rotavirus before he or she reaches 2 years of age, and 15% to 20% of infants develop diarrhea sufficiently severe to seek care from a provider each year. Pediatricians usually recognize the rotavirus season because many infants may be developing this illness during the same period of the year. There is some variability from year to year and in specific locations, but in the United States the "rotavirus season" usually starts in the southwestern states in late autumn and moves eastward, reaching the eastern states by mid-winter to late winter.

The infection is self-limiting, but children may be ill for several days, and total fluid losses during the illness can be life threatening unless they are corrected properly. The crucial treatment is the maintenance of fluids and electrolytes using oral rehydration solution, but occasionally children require intravenous fluid. Some infants may develop rotavirus infections more than once; however, the first one is usually the most severe, and subsequent infections tend to be mild or asymptomatic.

A stool enzyme-linked immunosorbent assay is available to confirm the diagnosis, but the results do not change the treatment of the patient. Patients who must be admitted to a hospital should be under contact precautions to prevent spread of the virus to other patients in the hospital because nosocomial spread is common.

A live, oral tetravalent vaccine (RotaShield)* for rotavirus was introduced to prevent this common infection. The vaccine consisted of a mixture of four reassortant, attenuated, virus vaccine strains. The parent virus for the vaccine originated from a rhesus monkey. Based on the extensive clinical trials, the vaccine was expected to greatly reduce rates of severe infantile diarrhea and reduce pediatric hospitalizations. Unfortunately, an unanticipated and serious adverse event, intussusception, occurred in a very small proportion of infants who received the vaccine, and the vaccine was withdrawn shortly after its introduction. Other vaccines, based on human and bovine strains, are still under development, and it is hoped that they will be protective without causing intussusception. Epidemiologic evidence suggests that natural infection with human rotavirus does not lead to intussusception, so there is an expectation that the other vaccines will be safe.

Rarely, rotavirus causes infection in the elderly, but it may cause mild diarrhea in family members of sick infants who handle the child's diapers. In immunosuppressed patients, rotavirus infection may cause persistent diarrhea. When diarrhea is persistent, in addition to fluids, a passive antibody transmitted through immune milk has proved helpful.

Calicivirus (Norwalk-like virus)

Norwalk-like virus may cause gastroenteritis in any age group. Generally, the illnesses occur in outbreaks and may affect people in camps and dormitories, who experience acute vomiting and diarrhea. The illness is usually short-lived, lasting a day or so, but outbreaks may involve many people. The role of these viruses as a cause of endemic diarrhea is still being investigated, but they may be relatively common causes.

Vibrio cholerae

Cholera is caused by *V. cholerae* serotype 01 or 0139. Currently, serotype 01 is found in nearly all developing countries, but serotype 0139 is only in South Asia, although it may be spreading to other areas. Cholera, sometimes referred to as epidemic cholera or cholera gravis, has major public health importance because of the ability to cause severe, life-threatening watery diarrhea. Deaths from dehydration may occur within a few hours of onset of symptoms, even in previously healthy persons. Contaminated seafood and water are common vehicles, but many foods have also been implicated. Travelers suspected of having cholera should have a stool culture performed using specific media for this organism, and positive cases should be reported to the authorities. In endemic countries, the number of cases are too great to culture all cases, and specimens from a sample of cases should be tested to confirm the type of organism and the antibiotic sensitivity patterns. Cases occurring in an area not previously infected should be confirmed and reported to the authorities.

Symptoms include severe watery diarrhea, and often the stool is so watery that it loses its fecal character and is like "rice water." Patients with severe cases usually also have severe vomiting, and with increasing dehydration they develop classic signs of acute dehydration proceeding to shock, coma, and death unless they are treated rapidly. The stools contain large amounts of bicarbonate and potassium, and patients may develop severe metabolic acidosis and potassium deficiency. Muscle cramps may be an especially painful occurrence during the illness.

The symptoms of cholera result from the protein toxin produced by *V. cholerae* that stimulates adenylate cyclase, resulting in increased levels of intracellular cyclic AMP, chloride secretion, and tremendous outpouring of fluids and electrolytes into the gut lumen. There is essentially no inflammation in the gut, and the intestinal mucosal cells remain healthy, but the cholera toxin maximally stimulates their cyclic AMP system. GM_1 ganglioside is the receptor for the toxin on the surface of the mucosal cells. High titers of antitoxin antibodies can neutralize the toxin by preventing the toxin from reaching its receptor.

V. cholerae organisms that are not serotype 01 or 0139, as well as other *Vibrio* species, may also cause diarrhea (as well as systemic infections) in individual patients, but they do not cause epidemic cholera.

The treatment of cholera includes rapid rehydration, correction of acidosis, replacement of potassium, and administration of antibiotics to shorten the illness and to decrease overall purging volumes. Patients with severe cholera become rapidly dehydrated, and most of the fluid deficit is from the circulating volume. Thus, intravenous fluids for these severely dehydrated patients need to be given rapidly (in less than 4 hours) in volumes of about 10% of the body weight to restore circulating volumes completely. Thus, a 50-kg patient will require 5 L in less than 4 hours. Slow or insufficient rehydration may lead to acute renal failure or other complications of shock. The most appropriate intravenous fluid is either lactated Ringer's or another polyelectrolyte solution (e.g., Dhaka solution) that includes a base to correct the acidosis as well as potassium to correct the potassium deficit.

Oral rehydration can be started as soon as the patient is able to drink, even while the intravenous fluids are being given. The best oral rehydration solution for cholera and other severely purging patients is one prepared with rice. Rice oral rehydration solution is available commercially (CeraLyte), or it can be prepared with homemade ingredients. The electrolytes should be those conforming to the standard oral rehydration solution of the World Health Organization, which contains 70 mEq of sodium, 20 mEq of potassium, and 30 mEq of citrate.

*Not available in the United States.

Doxycycline (Vibramycin) and tetracycline are the antibiotics of choice for adults, and co-trimoxazole (Bactrim)* is preferred for children. Other antibiotics can be used for resistant strains, including single-dose azithromycin (Zithromax).

Enterotoxigenic *Escherichia coli*

This group of *E. coli* causes illness through the production of a heat-labile enterotoxin (LT) that is similar to cholera toxin, a heat-stable enterotoxin (ST), or both. Either of these toxins leads to secretion of fluid from the small intestine. Frequently, these toxins also express specific colonization factor pili that allow them to colonize the small intestine. In general, the illness is less severe than cholera, but individual patients may have an illness that is indistinguishable from cholera. These organisms are among the most common causes of childhood and infant diarrhea in the world and are the leading cause of traveler's diarrhea, but they occur rarely in industrialized countries, usually in the context of a food-borne or water-borne outbreak.

Treatment is focused on rehydration using the same guidelines as for other watery diarrhea. Antibiotics are not recommended for most cases in endemic settings. However, the course of traveler's diarrhea caused by these organisms is shortened when effective antibiotics are used. The reason for recommending antibiotics for travelers and not for endemic disease in children is the high prevalence of the disease in children, and treatment with antibiotics is simply not practical and would lead to widespread antibiotic overuse.

Other Types of *Escherichia coli*

Other types of *E. coli* that may cause diarrheal illness include enteroaggregative *E. coli*, enteroinvasive *E. coli*, and enterohemorrhagic *E. coli*. The enteroaggregative *E. coli* organisms are likely to be common causes of illness in certain areas, but their true importance is still being determined. Other than rehydration, no specific treatment is needed for this illness. The enteroinvasive *E. coli* organisms are very similar to *Shigella* in terms of the virulence properties and clinical illness, and patients with this infection should be managed as if they had shigellosis. The enterohemorrhagic *E. coli* organisms, which produce a *Shiga*-like toxin, are fast becoming a major public health problem, with outbreaks of food-borne illness. They can cause severe, acute illness, often with severe bloody diarrhea, which may lead to hemolytic uremia syndrome. The strains appear to be primarily associated with beef and cattle; however, many foods have been vehicles for the transmission of organisms. The risk of enterohemorrhagic *E. coli* infection is a major reason to eat beef only if it is well cooked.

*Not FDA approved for this indication.

Shigella

The *Shigella* organisms are the ones that most commonly cause dysentery, or bloody diarrhea, although they may also cause a watery diarrhea syndrome. The genus is divided into four species and multiple serotypes. *Shigella sonnei* is the most common in industrialized countries, whereas *Shigella flexneri* is more common in developing countries. *Shigella dysenteriae* serotype 01 (*Shiga* bacillus) may occur in epidemics in developing countries, and these epidemics have become major public health emergencies because the disease is so severe, the strains are often resistant to usual antibiotics, and the disease spreads rapidly. *Shigella boydii* is generally less common, but the disease is similar to that caused by *S. flexneri.*

Patients with acute dysentery should be assumed to have shigellosis and should accordingly be treated with antibiotics based on the local sensitivity patterns. Unfortunately, *Shigella* species are becoming increasingly resistant to formerly effective antibiotics. For sensitive strains, ampicillin or co-trimoxazole is effective, but resistant strains will require other antibiotics, such as one of the newer quinolones or pivmecillinam (Selexid).* Nalidixic acid (NeGram)† is useful for many strains, but *S. dysenteriae* is now frequently resistant to this drug as well.

Campylobacter jejuni

Campylobacter jejuni, usually transmitted from poultry, is the most commonly isolated bacterial pathogen isolated in the United States from patients with diarrhea. It can cause either watery diarrhea or dysentery. A benefit from using antibiotics is not clear, especially if the start of treatment is delayed. Erythromycin is generally used if the treatment can begin within the first few days of the onset. Ten percent to 15% of healthy people in developing countries carry *Campylobacter* in their stools, so isolation of such a strain during illness does not necessarily mean that the bacterium is causing the illness in this setting. Occasionally, *Campylobacter* can lead to systemic illness with bacteremia, and these illnesses certainly require appropriate antibiotics according to sensitivity patterns.

Infection with *Campylobacter* has been associated with the subsequent development of Guillain-Barré syndrome. It is believed that certain strains express gangliosides that initiate an autoimmune disease through the process of molecular mimicry. Fortunately, this is a rare complication *of Campylobacter* infection.

Salmonella

Salmonella species are frequently associated with food-borne outbreaks and lead to acute diarrhea that is generally watery but may progress to dysentery. Treatment is with appropriate rehydration, and antibiotics are generally not needed except in

*Not available in the United States.
†Not FDA approved for this indication.

TABLE 2. **Recommended Antibiotics for Use in Patients With Common Diarrhea Pathogens**

Syndrome	Antimicrobial agent	Adults (amount per dose)	Children (amount per dose)
Acute diarrhea with no complications	No antibiotic recommended	No antibiotic recommended	No antibiotic recommended
Cholera	Doxycycline (Vibramycin), single dose	300 mg	Not recommended
	Tetracycline* qid for 3 days	500 mg	12.5 mg/kg
	Ciprofloxacin (Cipro)* bid for 3 days	500 mg	Not recommended
	Co-trimoxazole (Bactrim)* bid for 3 days	TMP 160 mg + SMX 800 mg	TMP 5 mg/kg + SMX 25 mg/kg
	Azithromycin (Zithromax),* single dose	1 g	20 mg/kg
Traveler's diarrhea	Ciprofloxacin* bid for up to 3 days	500 mg	Not recommended
	Co-trimoxazole bid for 3 days	TMP 160 mg + SMX 800 mg	TMP 5 mg/kg + SMX 25 mg/kg
Shigellosis	Ciprofloxacin* for 5 days	500 mg	Not recommended†
	Co-trimoxazole bid for 5 days	TMP 160 mg + SMX 800 mg	TMP 5 mg/kg + SMX 25 mg/kg
	Nalidixic acid (NeGram)*	1 g	15 mg/kg
	Pivmecillinam‡ qid for 5 days	400 mg	12.5 mg/kg
Giardiasis	Metronidazole (Flagyl)* tid for 5 days	250 mg	5 mg/kg
Cyclospora infection	Co-trimoxazole* bid for 3 days	TMP 160 mg + SMX 800 mg	TMP 5 mg/kg + SMX 25 mg/kg
Rotavirus infection	No antibiotic recommended	No antibiotic recommended	No antibiotic recommended

*Not FDA approved for this indication.
†When *Shigella* organism is resistant to other antibiotics, ciprofloxacin may be appropriate in severely ill children after the risks and benefits are weighed.
‡Not available in the United States.
SMX, sulfamethoxazole; TMP, trimethoprim.

complicated cases. Rarely, septicemia may occur that requires energetic treatment, including the use of an appropriate antibiotic.

Clostridium difficile

C. difficile is an anaerobic organism that can produce an enterotoxin leading to colitis. It most commonly occurs after the use of an antibiotic that selects for this organism. This can become a severe infection, especially in the elderly and otherwise compromised hosts. Detection of the toxin from stool specimens is important in diagnosing this infection. Treatment is with metronidazole (Flagyl),* or with vancomycin (Vancocin) for patients in whom treatment with metronidazole has failed.

REHYDRATION THERAPY

Patients with watery diarrhea lose excessive amounts of fluid. When the fluid loss is mild or moderate, the patient may feel weak, lethargic, and thirsty. When the fluid loss is severe, the condition becomes life threatening. Some illnesses start with mild fluid loss and mild dehydration, but as the illness continues, the dehydration worsens. Diarrheal stool is isotonic and contains large amounts of electrolytes. With severe purging, major losses of sodium, bicarbonate, and potassium occur, and these need to be corrected by a rehydration solution that has an electrolyte content similar to that of the lost fluid.

Most patients improve with oral solutions containing the proper mixture of salts and carbohydrate. Several studies have found complex carbohydrates (e.g., rice starch) to be more effective in severely purging patients and to reduce the purging rate. Although almost any fluid can be used with mild cases, the fluid loss from significant purging should be replaced with oral rehydration solution (e.g., CeraLyte, Pedialyte, Infalyte) that contains the proper concentrations of electrolytes and carbohydrates. Soft drinks, sports drinks, and many other commonly used fluids do not have the proper composition of salts, they may have excess sugars, or they may be hypertonic and are not acceptable for replacing significant loss from diarrhea.

Oral rehydration solution should be given in amounts sufficient to correct the fluid loss. A patient who is mildly dehydrated can be assumed to have lost about 5% of body weight, and this volume should be offered to correct the loss. Additional solution should then be given to make up for continuing losses until the illness subsides. If vomiting is a problem, the fluids can still generally be given in small but frequent volumes to replace the fluids needed. Additional water and other fluids should be given in addition to the oral rehydration solution to make up for normal physiologic fluid replacement.

With severe dehydration, more aggressive rehydration is needed with intravenous fluids, usually using lactated Ringer's solution. Normal or physiologic saline can be used in an emergency if lactated Ringer's

*Not FDA approved for this indication.

is not available, but saline will not correct the acidosis nor will it replace the needed potassium, and early introduction of oral rehydration solution is needed to correct for these deficiencies. Patients with severe dehydration can be assumed to have lost 10% or more of their body weight, and this loss needs to be corrected. Patients in shock need very rapid administration of fluids within 1 to 4 hours. Administration of oral rehydration solution can begin as soon as the patient is able to drink to make up for ongoing stool losses. The use of a "cholera cot" can ease assessment of ongoing stool losses and can thus guide the volumes of rehydration fluids that are needed.

SYMPTOMATIC MANAGEMENT

Bismuth subsalicylate (Pepto-Bismol) and loperamide (Imodium) are often used, especially in traveler's diarrhea, to relieve some of the symptoms of diarrhea, but they do not correct the fluid loss or restore electrolytes. A typical dose of bismuth subsalicylate is two tablets (or 1 tablespoon) every 6 to 8 hours. Patients should be warned that their stools will blacken and that they should avoid overdosing with salicylate. Loperamide is typically given as a 4-mg initial dose, followed by 2 mg every 6 hours until symptoms subside. Loperamide should not be given to children or to patients with dysentery.

ANTIMICROBIAL AGENTS

Antimicrobial agents are not needed for most cases of diarrhea but are indicated in a few conditions. These include cholera, shigellosis, severe traveler's diarrhea, *C. difficile* enterocolitis, amebiasis, giardiasis, and *Cyclospora* infection. Immunosuppressed patients may require specific antiviral agents depending on specific infections. A summary of the most common antimicrobial agents is found in Table 2.

CONSTIPATION

method of
MICHAEL J. LEVINSON, M.D.
University of Tennessee Medical School
Memphis, Tennessee

The symptom of constipation is very common. The aisles of any drugstore confirm the impact of this problem. The goal of this article is to provide a rational, efficacious, and ideally cost-effective approach to the patient with constipation.

Before we can approach the patient we must come up with a definition of what constitutes constipation. In a Western society it would be at least 12 weeks, which need not be consecutive, in the preceding 12 months of two or more episodes of straining in greater than one quarter of defecations, sensation of incomplete evacuation in greater than one quarter of defecations, sensation of anorectal obstruction or blockade in a quarter of defecations, manual maneuvers to facilitate greater than one quarter of defecations (e.g., digital evacuation, support of the pelvic floor), or less than three defecations per week. If these are present the patient is constipated. If accompanied by pain relieved by defecation then the patient has irritable colon "constipation type."

Simple constipation is seen in greater than 1% of the population and accounts for 2.5 million physician visits per year. Eighty-five percent of visits result in prescriptions for laxatives or cathartics, with an estimated $400 million spent on these products. Risk factors are being a woman and increasing age. Constipation is associated with inactivity, low caloric intake, number of medications being taken (which is actually independent of the profiles of their side effects), low income, and low education level. Constipation is also associated with depression and physical and sexual abuse.

CLINICAL FEATURES AND PATHOPHYSIOLOGY

Although physicians often focus mainly on the infrequency of bowel movements in the definition of constipation, patients have a broader set of complaints. The lower limit of normal stool frequency is three per week. In the ROME criteria it was two per week but included straining, hard stools, and a feeling of incomplete evacuation. After we answer what constitutes "constipation" in the view of the patient, the interview must also elicit a complete list of prescription and over-the-counter medications (Table 1).

Our definition of constipation comprises two parts—frequency and "evacuatory failure"—and herein is a significant conceptual advance in the understanding

TABLE 1. **Medications Associated With Constipation**

Class	Examples
Prescription drugs	
Opiates	Morphine
Anticholinergic agents	Clidinium/chlordiazepoxide (Librax), belladonna
Tricyclic antidepressants	Amitriptyline (Elavil) > nortriptyline (Pamelor)
Calcium channel blockers	Verapamil (Calan) hydrochloride
Antiparkinsonian drugs	Amantadine hydrochloride (Symmetrel)
Sympathomimetics	Ephedrine, terbutaline (Brethine)
Antipsychotics	Chlorpromazine (Thorazine)
Diuretics	Furosemide (Lasix)
Antihistamines	Diphenhydramine (Benadryl)
Nonprescription drugs	
Antacids, especially calcium-containing	Calcium carbonate (Tums)
Calcium supplements	
Iron supplements	
Antidiarrheal agents	Loperamide (Imodium), attapulgite (Parepectolin)
Nonsteroidal anti-inflammatory agents	Ibuprofen (Advil)

Adapted from *Gastroenterology*. Vol. 119, No. 6, p. 1768, Dec 2000. Copyright American Gastroenterology Association.

of constipation. Two major pathophysiologies can now be identified, with a third being the coexistence of both in the same patient. Slow transit colon (STC) ("colonic inertia") is thought to be a primary defect of slower-than-normal movement of contents from the proximal to the distal colon and rectum. In some individuals the basis for slow transit may be dietary or even cultural. In others, slow colonic transit probably has a true pathophysiologic basis in abnormal colonic motility. There are two subtypes of STC: (1) colonic inertia, possibly related to decreased numbers of high-amplitude propagated contractions; these peristaltic sequences are thought to be the mechanism for mass movement of contents, and their absence is expressed in a prolonged residence of fecal residues in the right colon; and (2) increased, uncoordinated motor activity in the distal colon that offers a functional barrier of resistance to normal transit. Most cases are idiopathic and separation of the types remains in the research setting.

The other major pathophysiology, pelvic floor dysfunction, features normal or slightly slowed colonic transit overall but a preferential storage of residue for prolonged periods in the rectum. In this instance, the primary failure is one of an inability to adequately evacuate contents from the rectum. The mechanisms can be subdivided into (1) examples of muscular hypertonicity (failure to relax, or "anismus"), incomplete relations or paradoxic contraction of the pelvic floor, and external anal sphincters during attempted defecation and (2) muscular hypertonicity. The role of excessive straining leading to or associated with excessive perineal descent, obstetric "trauma" to the perineal nerve, constipation, rectal intussusception, solitary rectal ulcer syndrome, and fecal incontinence is not entirely clear. Separation of STC from disorders of evacuation as the major cause of constipation is extremely important because the primary therapeutic approaches differ significantly. These patients should be referred to a gastroenterologist and has led to a new field of urogynecology.

Insight into the pathogenic mechanisms of intractable constipation can be gained from referral centers; 59% had normal colonic transit. These were likely irritable bowel syndrome (IBS) with constipation. Twenty-eight percent had pelvic floor dysfunction (with or without slow transit)—the hardest to treat—and 13% had slow transit only.

TABLE 2. **Common Medical Conditions Associated With Constipation**

Mechanical obstruction
Colon cancer
External compression from malignant tumor
Strictures: diverticular or postischemic
Rectocele (if large)
Postsurgical abnormalities
Megacolon
Anal fissure
Metabolic conditions
Diabetes mellitus
Hypothyroidism
Hypercalcemia
Hypokalemia
Hypomagnesemia
Uremia
Heavy metal poisoning
Myopathies
Amyloidosis
Scleroderma
Neuropathies
Parkinson's disease
Spinal cord injury or tumor
Cerebrovascular disease
Multiple sclerosis
Other conditions
Depression
Degenerative joint disease
Autonomic neuropathy
Cognitive impairment
Immobility
Cardiac disease

Adapted from *Gastroenterology*. Vol. 119, No. 6, p. 1770, Dec 2000. Copyright American Gastroenterology Association.

CLINICAL EVALUATION

Historical features are key, and the questioning must be specific when trying to separate the three types: slow transit, straining (evacuatory problems), or both. Women who have had multiple births and a hysterectomy must be asked about the evacuatory problem many times associated with urinary problems. A careful drug history must be obtained (see Table 1), and except for diabetes, hypothyroidism, and hypercalcemia, the many medical conditions associated with constipation are rare (Table 2).

Physical exam and screening tests, if deemed appropriate, should also eliminate diseases to which constipation is secondary. On physical, the findings of the perineal/rectal examination are key.

1. In the left lateral position with the buttocks separated, observe the descent/elevation of perineum and retention squeeze. Look for signs of soiling.
2. Rectal examiner should evaluate resting tone and its augmentation of a squeezing effort. The voluntary external sphincter will be tightened by squeezing the internal sphincter; the internal sphincter will not. Patient should be asked to "expel my finger."
3. An examination should be made for rectocele or consideration for good gynecologic exam. At conclusion of the initial clinical evaluation, it should be possible to classify tentatively the patient complaining of constipation into one of the following categories:
   a. IBS with constipation when pain, bloating, and incomplete defecation predominate.
   b. STC when the pelvic floor appears to be normal and symptoms of slow transit predominate.
   c. Rectal outlet obstruction.
   d. Items 2 and 3 combined, often in conjunction with IBS.
   e. Organic constipation (mechanical or drug side effect).
   f. Secondary constipation (metabolic disorders).

DIAGNOSTIC TESTS

The majority of patients presenting with constipation without warning signs (i.e., blood in stool, negative exam history and physical, normal complete blood count, sedimentation rate, calcium, thyroid, and diabetic studies) can be treated with diet (see Table 1). If there is no response, further testing may be necessary from the simple inexpensive "sitz" marker transit time to the costly colonoscopy to anorectal manometry and defecography at a tertiary care facility. There is no substitution for a good history and physical exam.

TREATMENT

An initial approach is to increase fiber gradually along with fluid intake. You must tell the patient it will take time and that they will have more bloating and gas at the beginning of therapy. Fiber supplements may facilitate fiber in the diet. There is a long list of fiber supplements. I start with methylcellulose (Citrucel), which causes less gas and bloating (not as soluble fiber). The cost is $0.50–$1.43 per use. I then advance to psyllium (Metamucil), which is soluble with bloating and gas. The cost is $0.10–$0.30 per use, increasing the dose every 7 to 10 days. They should begin with two daily doses (morning and evening) with fluids, usually 8 ounces of water. If more treatment is needed, an inexpensive saline agent such as Milk of Magnesia should be used at a cost of $0.11–$0.44 per use. In general, most STC should be controlled by one of these therapies. If the diagnosis is confirmed and if there is still no response, I add a polyethylene glycol drug (MiraLax), especially in elderly patients. Cost is significantly increased but highly effective for STC.

If not amenable to surgery, a glycerin suppository may help the patient evacuate if used nightly (cost, $0.20 per use). If not successful, I have had great success with Tegaserod (Zelnorm), a partial agonist of 5-HT_4 receptors. It thereby stimulates peristalsis and modulates gut motility. As a partial agonist, Tegaserod is less likely to induce receptor desensitization. The dose is 6 mg before breakfast and 6 mg before the evening meal. There are minimal side effects, but warn the patient that it may increase sensation of gas. It rarely causes diarrhea. The biggest drawback is the cost. I will not discuss surgical options. This should be left for gastroenterologists, especially urogynecologists and those interested in the subject.

Several big changes have occurred since the last review of this topic for this book. These are:

1. High incidence of inability to evacuate, which can be picked up on history and may need more extensive workup, leading to a new field of urogynecology.
2. There is no such thing as the laxative habit; since phenolphthalein has been removed from products, there is no longer nerve damage.
3. New medicines are starting to appear to specifically address the problem; these appear safe and very efficacious.
4. The majority of patients can be handled by the primary care physician if "they just listen to what the patient means by constipation."

FEVER

method of
NATELLA RAKHMANINA, M.D.
The George Washington University
Children's National Medical Center
Washington, D.C.

and

JOHN N. VAN DEN ANKER, M.D., PH.D.
Pediatric Clinical Trials Center
Division of Pediatric Clinical Pharmacology
Children's National Medical Center
Pediatrics and Pharmacology
The George Washington University
Washington, D.C.

Measurement of the body temperature is the most common clinical test performed, and the presence of fever is accepted as a reliable indicator of either acute or chronic disease. However, the question of fever as being convenient or harmful is not yet completely answered. Surprisingly, few studies have been performed to ascertain the physiologic consequences of fever and to validate the rationale behind antipyretic therapy.

DEFINITION OF FEVER

The upper limit of normal body temperature is 37.7°C (99.9°F) in adults and 37.9°C (100.2°F) in children. The normal daily temperature variation is typically 0.5°C (0.9°F), with the lowest occurring at 6 AM and the highest at 4 to 6 PM. Ovulatory cycle, pregnancy, heavy exercise, and metabolic dysfunction can affect body temperature.

Temperature can be measured from the skin, tympanic membrane, rectum, or mouth, or in the urine. Studies have indicated that a rectal temperature, obtained with the glass thermometer left in place for 3 minutes, is highly correlated with core body temperature. The rectal method is preferable for the measurement of temperature in infants, although not recommended in immunocompromised patients or patients with anorectal malformations. Oral temperatures are generally 0.6°C (1.0°F) lower than rectal readings as a result of mouth breathing. Devices that evaluate the temperature of the tympanic membrane are not considered to be sufficiently accurate because of a falsely low reading with a poor placement. Axillary temperatures have a sensitivity of only 50% to 70% compared with rectal thermometry.

In the clinical setting, fever is typically defined as a rise in body temperature above the normal range. During febrile illness, diurnal variation in temperatures are maintained but at elevated levels. Fever may not be present during infections in newborns, elderly, patients with chronic renal failure or septic shock, or those taking corticosteroids.

Questions about the risk-benefit quotient of fever have generated considerable controversy in recent years. Clinical data supporting an adaptive role for fever include evidence of beneficial effects of fever and adverse effects of antipyretics on the outcome of the infections. It has been reported that treatment with antipyretic drugs could increase mortality in severe infections, prolong viral shedding, and impair antibody response to viral infection. The potential of the febrile response for harm is reflected in a series of reports suggesting that pyrogenic cytokines might mediate some of the systemic and local manifestations of sepsis resulting from gram-positive bacteria, AIDS, meningitis, suppurative arthritis, and mycobacteriosis.

PATHOPHYSIOLOGY OF FEVER

An area of the brain located in and near the rostral hypothalamus seems to have a pivotal role in the complex process of thermoregulation. Several endogenous substances and drugs affect temperature regulation by altering the activity of hypothalamic neurons. Exogenous pyrogens are, for the most part, microbes, toxins, and other products of microbial origin, whereas endogenous pyrogens are the host cell–derived cytokines that are the principal central mediators of the febrile response. The list of currently recognized pyrogenic cytokines includes, among others, interleukin 1 (IL-1), tumor necrosis factor alpha (TNF-α), IL-6, and interferon gamma (INF-γ). The essential elements of the febrile physiologic pathway are release of pyrogenic cytokines by inflammatory cells in response to exogenous pyrogens, induction of cyclooxygenase (COX), activation of the arachidonic acid cascade, and enhanced biosynthesis of prostaglandin E_2 (PGE_2) by hypothalamic vascular endothelial cells. PGE_2 acts to raise the hypothalamic thermal setpoint and thereby induce peripheral and thermogenic mechanisms to increase core temperature.

During the febrile response the vasoconstriction redirects the blood flow from cutaneous to deep vascular beds to minimize heat loss. This leads to increased pulse and blood pressure, decreased sweating, and a noticeable cold sensation in the hands and feet. Shivering is initiated to increase muscular heat production. Endocrine and metabolic reactions include secretion of acute-phase proteins by the liver, increased production of glucocorticoids, and decreased secretion of vasopressin, which reduces the volume of body fluid to be warmed.

HYPERTHERMIA

Unlike fever, hyperthermia involves a failure of thermoregulation expressed by an uncontrolled heat production, inadequate heat dissipation, or defective hypothalamic homeostasis. These include heat stroke syndromes, certain metabolic diseases, central nervous system trauma, hemorrhage or tumor, intrinsic hypothalamic dysfunction, and the effects of pharmacologic agents. Exogenous heat exposure and endogenous heat production are two mechanisms by which hyperthermia can result in dangerously high internal temperatures.

Hyperthermia can be rapidly fatal and its treatment differs from that of fever. Antipyretics do not reduce the elevated temperature in hyperthermia. The treatment of hyperthermia is primarily targeted at rapid reduction of body temperature by physical means. This can be accomplished by cool and tepid (20°C) sponge bathing (without alcohol). Submersion should be avoided so that body heat loss by evaporation can occur. Cooling blankets are of potential danger because of excess vasoconstriction. Intravenous fluids can also be administered for dehydration, but cool fluids through a central line close to the heart are not advisable.

FEVER OF UNKNOWN ORIGIN

Fever of unknown origin (FUO) refers to a prolonged febrile illness (more than 3 weeks) without an established etiology despite intensive evaluation. Three general categories of illnesses account for the majority of "classic" FUO cases: infections, malignancies, and collagen-vascular diseases. Infections are the most common identified source of FUO in children (approximately 50%), followed by collagen-inflammatory and neoplastic disease. In contrast, multisystem diseases such as rheumatic diseases, vasculitis including giant cell arteritis, polymyalgia rheumatica, and sarcoidosis account for 30% of cases in patients older than age 65 with FUO. Geography and travel history have a significant impact on the etiology of FUO. Prolonged fevers in the developing world include infections of worldwide distribution such as tuberculosis, typhoid, amebic liver abscesses, and AIDS. Ease of travel has the potential to bring to developed countries more geographically restricted illnesses such as malaria, filariasis, and schistosomiasis. Many of these illnesses may have incubation periods that extend for months, with some remaining latent for years.

The degree of fever, nature of fever curve, and response to antipyretics do not provide enough specificity to guide the diagnosis of FUO. Therapeutic trials of antimicrobials and corticosteroids, although tempting in the effort to "do something," rarely establish a diagnosis. The use of empirical antimicrobials can delay the diagnosis of some occult infections and increase the number of drug fevers. The administration of corticosteroids for a presumed inflammatory process should not replace relevant biopsies for steroid-responsive disease.

FEVER IN CHILDREN

Fever is the most common presenting complaint in pediatric practice. The most challenging aspect of evaluating a febrile child without an apparent source of fever is to differentiate those who have a serious illness from those who do not. Occult bacteremia occurs most commonly in children younger than 36 months, and the most common serious illnesses are meningitis, bacteremia, urinary tract infection, soft-tissue infections, pneumonia, and bacterial enteric infections. In children older than 6 years of age infectious illnesses still predominate, but collagen vascular diseases and malignancy become more prominent. Important consideration in a child with persistent fever should be given to Kawasaki disease, especially in those who have an incomplete clinical picture with only three or four of six of the major diagnostic criteria.

Management of the infant with fever is related to age. For the febrile infant who is younger than 90 days of age, a full sepsis evaluation (including complete blood count with differential, urine analysis, lumbar puncture, and culture of all three body fluids) is indicated. Infants 30 days of age and younger should be admitted to the hospital for intravenous antibiotics while awaiting culture results. Children ages 31 to 89 days often are admitted to the hospital for observation, but recent studies indicate that they may be followed at home if the results of the screening laboratory tests are benign, the child appears well, and no findings on history or physical examination suggest serious illness. If infants are followed as outpatients, careful observation at home must be assured by physician follow-up.

TREATMENT OF FEVER

Acetaminophen is generally regarded as the safest antipyretic agent and is the preferred drug, especially in children with suspected varicella and influenza, because of the association of aspirin with the risk of Reye syndrome. Nevertheless, liver failure is a well-recognized consequence of acetaminophen overdose (>90 mg/kg/24 h) and should be taken into consideration with the chronic use of the drug. Recent reviews identified several factors associated with acetaminophen hepatotoxicity in children, including age less than 10 years old associated with cumulative toxicity from repeated doses, delays in onset of symptoms, and ingestion of acetaminophen along with another hepatotoxic drug. Children with a family history of hepatic toxicity resulting from acetaminophen have an increased risk of developing a toxic reaction. Aspirin, ibuprofen, and other nonsteroidal anti-inflammatory drugs may cause dyspepsia, gastrointestinal bleeding, nausea, and vomiting. Overdose of ibuprofen (>400 mg/kg/24 h) has been associated with renal toxicity, aseptic meningitis, and aplastic anemia.

Alternating acetaminophen with ibuprofen every 2 hours is sometimes recommended in cases of febrile seizures and refractory fever. Given the absence of published safety and efficacy data related to the practice of alternating acetaminophen and ibuprofen, it is prudent for health care providers to exercise discretion when considering this sequence of therapy. The use of cooling blankets or tepid water sponging facilitates the reduction of temperature, but physical methods should not be used without antipyretics. The common adverse effects of physical methods include shivering and discomfort.

Children with a previous febrile or nonfebrile seizure are aggressively treated to reduce fever. However, it is unclear what triggers the febrile seizure because there is no correlation between the absolute temperature elevation and onset of a febrile seizure in a susceptible child. Furthermore, treatment with antipyretics has not been demonstrated to reduce the risk of febrile convulsions.

The cytokines involved in the febrile response can induce discomfort, with sweats, anorexia, aches, somnolence, and irritability. Antipyretic agents are frequently used to alleviate these symptoms. Complete normalization of the body temperature is not an objective of antipyretic therapy.

COUGH

method of
DANIEL McNALLY, M.D.
University of Connecticut Health Center
Farmington, Connecticut

Cough is both a natural protective reflex, part of our body's host defense system covering the tracheal bronchial region, and a pathologic finding of disease. It is one of the most frequent patient complaints.

THE COUGH REFLEX

As a protective reflex, its afferent limbs arise in a variety of receptors throughout the respiratory tract. These receptors may respond to mechanical stimuli such as pressure or to chemical stimuli, including exposure to irritant gases or particles or to both. Depending upon the site of origin, the afferent signals take different pathways. The primary route from the larynx and the tracheobronchial tree is the vagus, which also may transfer signals from mediastinal structures such as the esophagus, from the abdomen, and even from the ears. The pericardial surfaces or the diaphragm may activate the phrenic nerve, whereas the posterior pharynx transmits signals through the glossal pharyngeal nerve and the nasal spaces by the trigeminal nerve. The centers that integrate and create the cough reflex are in the medulla. The efferent pathways for a cough include signals to the phrenic nerve regulating diaphragm function, the spinal motor tracts controlling the muscles of expiration, and again the vagus, which helps to form the pharyngeal musculature into an effective conduit for the cough process. Ultimately this chain of events leads to an inspiration followed by closure of the glottis and then an increase in pleural pressure with contraction of the muscles of the abdomen and the expiratory intercostals. When an adequate pressure has been generated in the airways, the glottis opens explosively, creating a sudden airflow that clears the airway. The anatomy of the airway plays a supporting role in this reflex—the posterior membranous portion of the trachea is forced inward during the expiratory effort, narrowing the airway. This reduced cross-sectional area dramatically increases the airflow velocity and, in turn, helps to clear the triggering material from the tracheobronchial tree.

Cough as a Sign of Disease

There is a transition from cough as a protective reflex to cough as a sign or symptom of disease.

Normal individuals with no airway disease raise and swallow small amounts of secretions brought to the larger airways by the mucociliary escalator. When that normal balance is disturbed by excess production of mucus or excess inhaled materials, a cough can result. However, cough may also occur when the defense mechanism is too easily stimulated, as in hyperreactive airway diseases such as asthma, or when the clearance is rendered ineffective by reduced airflow in obstructive lung diseases such as chronic bronchitis and emphysema. The cough may become a patient complaint when it becomes increasingly frequent or when it produces a noticeable quantity of mucus. Specific qualities of the material raised, such as hemoptysis or striking purulence, may bring a cough to attention, or secondary consequences of cough-like syncope, incontinence, or rib fractures may be what prompts the patient to seek help.

Cough can arise from some problems quite minor, in which the traditional advice not to make the cure worse than the disease is important, up to serious problems such as cancer or interstitial lung disease in which early identification and treatment may be important. An approach to diagnosis and treatment needs to take into account that the majority of patients will have one of several common problems that are often amenable to empirical therapy, and not all patients need a complete evaluation at their initial visit. Any such stepwise approach needs to have carefully planned checkpoints to gauge an adequate response or move the patient and practitioner to the next level of investigation.

THE INITIAL VISIT AND FOUR COMMON ETIOLOGIES

An understanding of the likely etiologies of cough greatly shapes the investigation and initial treatment. Fortunately, four problems, alone or in combination, account for the majority of coughs. Because they are benign, generally causing more morbidity than mortality, and because effective therapy with a relatively mild side effect profile is available, empiric therapy after a limited investigation may be appropriate. Further studies to confirm the mechanism of cough, or to search for other less common causes, can be deferred while this brief, initial trial is undertaken. The four most common causes are postnasal drip, airway hyperreactivity, gastroesophageal reflux, and bronchitis—the last concept including both acute sputum production after infection and chronic sputum production related to smoking.

At the initial visit, a thorough history and an appropriately focused physical exam remain important, with key elements indicated in Table 1. Specific questions focused on each of the four common items are important, even if more general questioning in review of systems has been negative. Physical examination focused on the respiratory system should be expanded to include observation of a forced expiratory effort. Although it lacks the quantitative precision of pulmonary function testing, it provides information about whether bronchospasm is present through a measurement of forced expiratory time and by auscultation for wheezes with or after the forced expiratory maneuver. It also provides a simple measure of bronchial hyperreactivity, because with the deeper breath and more forceful exhalation, some individuals who have no wheezing before will demonstrate wheezing or trigger a cough. These findings would be supportive of airway hyperreactivity as a process underlying the cough.

TABLE 1. **Initial Visit Evaluation for Cough**

History
What triggers the cough? Activity? Position? (suggesting reflux if worse supine)
Does the cough vary by season? By time of day? (nocturnal cough and reflux)
Does cold air trigger a cough? (suggesting airway hyperreactivity)
History of prior productive cough
Similar or preceding respiratory illness in family or coworkers
Medications in use: angiotensin converting enzyme inhibitors
Smoking history
Sputum: blood, purulence and volume
Systemic symptoms: fever, weight loss
Localized chest pain (suggesting more serious mechanism such as malignancy)
Dyspnea
Voice changes or stridor (suggesting laryngeal problem)
Examination
Crackles (suggesting interstitial disease)
Wheezing or prolonged forced expiratory effort (suggesting hyperreactivity)
Cough with forced expiratory effort (suggesting hyperreactivity)
Nasal mucosal erythema or increased secretions (suggesting postnasal drip)
Posterior pharyngeal "cobblestoning" (suggesting reflux)
Investigations (in some cases)
Chest radiograph (for pneumonia or malignancy)
Spirometry (to demonstrate obstructive changes in hyperreactive airway disease)
Lung volumes and diffusion (interstitial lung disease)

At that initial visit, a chest radiograph may often be included. Except for individuals who are smokers and manifest chronic productive cough, or individuals with an acute bronchitis where knowledge of whether or not a pneumonic infiltrate is present may be helpful in deciding the circumstances of follow-up later, the chest radiograph will often have relatively low yield. Obviously a history of smoking or increasing age, both of which increase the risk of carcinoma, would move for an earlier chest radiograph.

Postnasal Drip

Postnasal drip should be suspected in an individual who describes the sensation of materials coming from the nose into the posterior pharynx, when the appearance of cough symptoms coincides with the findings of increased nasal congestion or nasal secretions, or when the patient describes materials filling the posterior pharynx even if these are not perceived as dripping into the throat. On examination, swollen or inflamed nasal mucosa is suggestive, as are increased secretions seen at least in the nasal passages. Mottling or "cobblestoning" of the posterior pharynx is suggestive but may not be seen in all patients and should not be regarded as essential to the diagnosis. Cough that is prominent with changes of position, particularly changes of head position, is also suggestive, although it overlaps with cough triggered by gastroesophageal reflux occurring when patients are bent over. Initial therapy for postnasal drip should include an antihistamine decongestant combination and nasal steroids. An antihistamine would not be expected to be effective against all causes of postnasal drip, but the addition of the nasal steroid maximizes the likelihood that the inflammatory process will be controlled in a timely fashion. Most patients will require a 2-week period, and sometimes more, to determine if there is a response. Additional measures if needed include nasal ipratropium (Atrovent nasal spray). This is particularly effective in individuals who have thin, watery secretions rather than the more mucopurulent secretions for which a nasal steroid may be effective. Individuals who have signs of sinus infection will need antibiotic therapy. Patients in whom secretions are abundant or where obstruction of the sinus passages is suspected may benefit from nasal irrigation. This can be done in a simple fashion with nasal saline spray, but sometimes requires more dramatic irrigation with a 30 to 60 mL syringe or a "turkey baster" to reduce secretions and inflammation and allow healing.

Airway Hyperreactivity

Airway hyperreactivity as a source of cough is often referred to as cough-variant asthma. These individuals share the bronchial hyperreactivity of asthmatics, but may never have wheezing, even when they are symptomatic with their cough. However, the same mechanism of inflammatory mediator release in the mucosal and submucosal regions, and sometimes airflow obstruction below the level of perception, produce the same triggers that lead to a cough mechanism. These individuals frequently give a history of specific triggers that will elicit a cough—either materials in their environment or particular activities. Many of these share the quality of increased ventilatory demand or of sensitivity to cold or dry air. Cold air sensitivity is an inexpensive screening tool for bronchial hyperreactivity. Almost any environmental exposure that the patient relates to the onset of the cough should suggest this possibility. A trial of an inhaled β-agonist may be helpful and is quite specific for bronchial hyperreactivity. However, some individuals do not manifest bronchospasm, and the absence of a response to an inhaled bronchodilator when the remainder of the history is suggestive should not eliminate this mechanism. The more important portion of empirical therapy for airway hyperreactivity is inhaled corticosteroids. Use of systemic corticosteroids is also possible, but carries a greater potential for side effects, and for many patients awareness of the potential side effects may lead them to decline or be noncompliant with that therapy. Inhaled corticosteroids with metered-dose inhalers should always be used with a spacer to improve delivery to the airways and reduce the side effect from deposition in the posterior pharynx and mouth. Newer microscopic powdered, inhaled steroids, with their own unique delivery devices, eliminate the need for a spacer. The typical time for response to inhaled steroids is 2 weeks, although some patients respond somewhat more quickly.

Gastroesophageal Reflux

Gastroesophageal reflux is suggested when patients give a history of mid- and upper sternal burning or pain, or a sour, acid taste or partially digested food material in the mouth. This is often triggered by supine position or by bending, but the patient who does not experience this during waking hours may still have enough reflux during sleep to trigger cough. Although for some patients the acid does in fact reach the lungs, it may produce cough by activating receptors in the posterior pharynx without crossing the glottis or even receptors in the lower esophagus. Because gastroesophageal reflux relates to habits of eating, sleeping and position, careful inquiry about these items is important. Physical examination, even without indirect laryngoscopy, may show erythema in the posterior pharynx, but this is not unique to reflux and could arise from other causes including viral infection.

Therapy for reflux should include counseling of the patient to avoid foods likely to trigger symptoms. Weight reduction may also be important, but is unlikely to help quickly enough to establish a diagnosis. Late meals or assuming a supine position after an earlier meal may aggravate symptoms. The head of the bed should be elevated, without "bending" the patient in the middle and leading to increased abdominal force and pressure especially in obese patients. Because there may be a delay between when the reflux produces symptoms and when the cough is manifest, traditional use of antacid medications is not useful as part of empirical therapy. Many patients with reflux only at night will not awaken with symptoms that would lead them to use an antacid. Rather, empirical therapy should include an H2 blocker or, because of their superior consistency of effect, a proton pump inhibitor. At least initially, the dose used should be in the full antireflux range so that any response will be clear cut and helpful in making a diagnosis.

Bronchitis

A productive cough is the hallmark of bronchitis. Acute bronchitis may include other symptoms suggestive of an acute infection, such as fever or malaise. The history may include other family members or coworkers with similar symptoms. Likewise, many individuals who have an acute viral airway infection may develop hyperreactivity with cough as a manifestation. In the context of an acute cough with other findings suggestive of an infection, a chest radiograph may be appropriate to identify if pneumonia is present. Individuals with other signs of infection, with purulent sputum, and with cough may benefit from treatment with antibiotics, although some will not have specific pathogens identified on culture. Patients may benefit from measures that help to raise secretions more effectively. This includes inhaled bronchodilators, even in patients who do not have wheezing or detectable airflow obstruction. Inhaled bronchodilators may be used before exposure to increased humidity or steam, the latter readily available by standing in a hot shower for a few minutes. The bland aerosol from the steam may help to improve cough, with increased humidity mobilizing secretions, and prior treatment with the bronchodilator reduces any bronchospasm the bland aerosol might create.

In chronic bronchitis, daily sputum is the core definition of the disease. Often it is a change in the pattern of cough that prompts the patient to seek attention. Cough in this context may benefit from the same measures noted for an acute bronchitis, and in addition, therapy used for airway hyperreactivity may be helpful, because many individuals have a mixture of chronic sputum production and variable degrees of airway obstruction best labeled as asthmatic bronchitis. Because this population is often older, and many are smokers, they deserve a chest radiograph as part of the initial investigation out of concern for bronchogenic carcinoma.

In all these situations of initial evaluation and empirical therapy, it is important to involve the patient in the discussion. Patients who understand the possible mechanisms for their cough will be more compliant with therapy and better able to report changes in their status at the next visit. These therapies take some time to show a response, and it is important to provide these patients from the start with additional nonspecific therapies to try to reduce the cough.

NONSPECIFIC THERAPIES

These nonspecific therapies include medications that improve the efficiency of coughing, reduce the triggers of a cough, and suppress the reflex center in the brain that produces the cough (Table 2).

Nonspecific therapy may be aimed at making the cough more effective, thus reducing the work required to clear secretions. This would include measures to

TABLE 2. **Cough Therapy**

Classification	Drug	Dosage	Remarks/Precautions
To improve cough effectiveness			
Expectorant	Guaifenesin (Robitussin)	200-400 mg q 4 h PO	Effectiveness is not substantiated in clinical trials
Mucolytic	Acetylcysteine (Mucomyst)*	2-3 mL 10% solution NEB	May increase airway irritation and bronchospasm and should be administered with a bronchodilator
	Dornase alfa (Pulmozyme)*	2.5 mg q 12-24 h NEB	Useful in cystic fibrosis
Cough suppressing			
Afferent receptor	Benzonatate (Tessalon)	100 mg q 4-6 h PO	Must be swallowed whole to avoid oral and pharyngeal anesthesia; similarity to tetracaine causes toxicity in overdose
	Lidocaine (Xylocaine)*	3 mL of 4% solution NEB 3-4 times a day	Local anesthesia of pharynx and glottis can allow aspiration; system toxicity possible with overuse
Cough center	*Non-narcotic*		
	Dextromethorphan (Benylin)	10-30 mg q 4-8 h PO	Contraindicated in patients on MAOIs; reduced alertness in some cases
	Narcotic		
	Codeine	15-30 mg q 4-6 h PO	Sleepiness and constipation are occasional side effects
	Hydrocodone/homatropine (Hycodan)	5 mg q 4-6 h PO	Greater addiction potential than codeine
For postnasal drip			
Sympathomimetic decongestant	Pseudoephedrine (Sudafed)	60 mg q 4-6 h PO	Lower doses are less likely to produce hypertension
	Oxymetazoline (Afrin)	2-3 nasal sprays q 12 h	May cause rebound nasal congestion if used for >3 days
	Phenylephrine (Neo-Synephrine)	2-3 nasal sprays q 3-4 h	May cause rebound nasal congestion if used for >3 days
H_1 Antagonist			
First generation	Chlorpheniramine with pseudoephedrine (Chlor-Trimeton Allergy-D 4 hour)	4 mg /60 mg q 4-6 h PO not to exceed 4 per day	Caution in hypertensive patients. May produce sleepiness. Available in sustained-release (8 mg/120 mg) formulations
	Azatadine maleate with pseudoephedrine (Trinalin Repetabs)	1 mg /120 mg q 12 h PO	Caution in hypertensive patients. May produce sleepiness

Continued

TABLE 2. **Cough Therapy—Cont'd**

Classification	Drug	Dosage	Remarks/Precautions
Second generation	Fexofenadine* (Allegra)	60 mg q 12 h PO	Also available with pseudoephedrine for combined decongestant effect
	Loratadine (Claritin)	10 mg q 24 h PO	Also available with pseudoephedrine for combined decongestant effect
	Cetirizine (Zyrtec)	5-10 mg q 24 h PO	Also available with pseudoephedrine for combined decongestant effect
Nasal corticosteroids	Fluticasone (Flonase)	2 squirts each side twice a day	
For airway hyperreactivity			
Aerosol bronchodilator	Albuterol (Proventil)	2 puffs by MDI as needed up to 4 times a day	Tremor and tachycardia with overuse
Inhaled corticosteroids	Fluticasone (Flovent) 110 μg dose	2 puffs by MDI twice a day using spacer	Followed by oral rinsing to reduce risk of yeast pharyngitis
	Budesonide (Pulmicort)	2 inhalations twice a day	Followed by oral rinsing to reduce risk of yeast pharyngitis
For gastroesophageal reflux			
H2 antagonist	Ranitidine (Zantac)	150 mg 2 times a day PO	
Proton pump inhibitor	Lansoprazole (Prevacid)	15 mg PO once or twice daily	
	Metoclopramide (Reglan)	5-10 mg before meals and bedtime	
For bronchitis			
Aerosol bronchodilator	Albuterol (Proventil)	2 puffs by MDI as needed up to 4 times a day	Tremor and tachycardia with overuse. Albuterol may be followed by steam or other humidity source to improve secretion clearing
	Ipratropium (Atrovent)	2-4 puffs MDI up to 4 times a day	Tachycardia with overuse, but no tremor
Antibiotics	Biaxin (Clarithromycin)	1000 mg per day for 10 days PO	
	Amoxicillin/clavulanate (Augmentin)	875 mg q 12 h PO	Useful for bacterial sinorhinitis

* Not FDA approved for this indication.
MAOIs, monamine oxidase inhibitors; MDI, metered-dose inhaler; NEB, nebulizer; PO, orally.

provide additional humidity, either through increasing the ambient humidity that the patient inspires or providing adequate fluids and hydration for the patient, so the mucosal surfaces can produce adequate fluids. Therapy for underlying airway obstruction is also important, because an improved FEV1 will lead to a greater velocity of flow and better secretion clearing. Lesions of the chest bellows, such as kyphoscoliosis, obesity, or any process that causes pain related to respiratory effort may hinder cough and need to be addressed to improve the efficiency of the cough. Most ordinary over-the-counter cough syrups contain guaifenesin (Robitussin). This may produce some improvement in the liquefaction of secretions but in itself does not suppress the reflex center.

Suppression of a cough reflex itself can be attempted either centrally or peripherally. Central cough suppression includes noncontrolled prescription medications such as dextromethorphan (Benylin). Although it does produce some sleepiness, it provides a measure of cough suppression without as many side effects as a narcotic. More thorough suppression of cough by a central mechanism generally requires a narcotic. This can be particularly effective but will produce sleepiness, often constipation, and limits the patient's ability to drive and perform other attention-critical activities. Some patients will be controlled only when they are rendered nearly cough free for a sustained period of several days. Such an effort may require having the patient stay at home and minimize his or her activity, providing an environment of adequate humidification and treating any other airway disease present, and planning an adequate bowel regimen and a respite from dangerous or responsible activities so he or she can use the narcotic more frequently. These trials should have a defined period of a few days, with a clear understanding between the patient and the physician that narcotic cough suppression is a short-term tool.

Efforts to block the sites of triggering have met with mixed success. Aerosol lidocaine (Xylocaine)* can be administered and will reduce cough, but frequently produces enough systemic absorption that central nervous system toxicity can result, and commonly leads to sufficient numbing of the posterior pharynx that swallowing is compromised and aspiration can occur. Benzonatate (Tessalon Perles), a surface anesthetic, available in liquid form in small "pearls," can be swallowed whole, absorbed systemically, and then excreted through the lungs. Because the maximal

*Not FDA approved for this indication.

delivery of this medication is in the lower airways, the pharyngeal defenses are not as compromised and swallowing remains intact, whereas cough may be substantially reduced.

LESS COMMON ETIOLOGIES

Other mechanisms may be identified at the initial visit. The presence of stridor or changes in voice quality should prompt investigation by laryngoscopy looking for specific laryngeal abnormalities. When dyspnea is prominent, pulmonary function testing to look for unappreciated obstructive disease or concurrent restrictive disease should be undertaken. When there are systemic findings of weight loss or changes in appetite, clubbing, or focal pain, especially in the context of an individual who is a smoker and older, chest radiograph and further investigation for the possibility of bronchogenic carcinoma should not be delayed.

Cough related to angiotensin-converting enzyme (ACE) inhibitors is seen more frequently now because those medications are used in more patients. Estimates extend up to 20% of patients on these drugs, although the number who seek attention for it is probably less. The mechanism is believed to be activation of afferent nerve fibers by bradykinin accumulating in the tracheobronchial mucosa where ACE inhibitor has interfered with its normal degradation. Typically this occurs within the first 1 to 4 weeks after the start of therapy, but sometimes it is seen several months later. Spirometry may not reflect obstruction, because this is largely an irritant reflex mechanism, and it is not found with any greater frequency in patients with airway reactivity from other causes. Demonstrating the mechanism requires discontinuing the drug, with a response typically within 1 week, sometimes as short as 1 day, and occasionally as long as 1 month. Placing a patient back on another ACE inhibitor will generally cause a return of the symptoms, but angiotensin II receptor antagonists such as losartan (Cozaar) do not initiate this mechanism and may be an effective alternative.

Bronchiectasis is also a cause of cough. Unlike the patients of the preantibiotic era who presented with dramatically large sputum volumes, frequent episodes of hemoptysis, and systemic symptoms of infections, these patients may have subtle symptoms. Some may have a nonproductive cough, and others may show a measure of responsiveness to bronchodilator that, although not complete, still suggests asthma. Most, however, find that the cough is little improved with bronchodilators. Patients may localize their cough to a region of the lung, sometimes with localized pleuritic pain accompanying the cough, if the bronchiectasis is appropriately localized to a region near a pleural surface. Bronchograms are done infrequently now, and the diagnosis generally requires high-resolution computed tomography (CT) scans. Findings that are localized should raise a question of an obstructive lesion that may need further investigation by bronchoscopy. When this occurs, particularly in younger patients, investigation looking for immunodeficiency states such as combined variable hypogammaglobulinemia or cystic fibrosis is important. Patients with bronchiectasis require antibiotic therapy appropriate to any current infection and assistance in improving secretion clearing through airway humidification and positioning. Some patients may benefit from cyclic antibiotic therapy, such as doxycycline (Vibramycin) 100 mg daily for the first 10 days of each month, and rarely continuous antibiotics, in an effort to suppress bacterial flora and reduce the frequency of purulent exacerbation and cough.

Eosinophilic bronchitis generally produces a nonproductive cough and is often seen in patients who have multiple allergies. These patients may not demonstrate airway hyperreactivity on formal testing but will generally respond to corticosteroid therapy, either systemically or by inhaled steroid. Definitive diagnosis would require bronchial mucosal biopsy, but this will seldom be necessary if empirical therapy for airway hyperreactivity is given because the eosinophilic bronchitis will respond to that as well. Pathologically the specimen will show eosinophils in and surrounding the airways, but the biopsies usually lack the mast cells seen in asthmatics, explaining the reduced frequency of airway hyperreactivity in these patients.

Acute episodes of cough may follow with a fairly high frequency mycoplasma and chlamydial infections, upper respiratory viral infections, and infection with *Bordetella pertussis*. When the cough occurs concurrently with other symptoms of the infection, the acute effects of the organism are the likely cause, but frequently the cough will become more prominent as the other symptoms resolve, suggesting that the cough occurs because airway hyperreactivity has been initiated from the mucosal damage of the initial infection. Treatment for the acute cough related to these organisms involves antibiotic therapy for the organism itself when appropriate, whereas the later development of cough should be treated with the same measures noted previously for airway hyperreactivity.

Cough related to bronchogenic carcinoma remains a significant concern that many patients have when consulting a physician for cough. Most of the patients with cough as the presentation of their lung cancer will have lesions in the larger airways where the afferent trigger sites are most common. Cough in an older patient or a patient who has been a smoker should increase suspicion, particularly when physical examination or chest radiograph suggests a process that is localized to one side or one region of the lung.

Interstitial lung disease is another uncommon but serious cause of cough. Often these patients on examination will manifest their cough at full inspiration rather than when attempting a normal or forced expiration. It should also be suspected when cough is accompanied or overshadowed by shortness of breath at rest or with exertion. These patients describe little variability in their cough, dependent upon either climate or time of day, and will generally not report a response to an empirical trial of initial therapy. Identification of these patients comes with pulmonary function testing that shows restriction with combined diffusion and lung volume changes or, in the earliest cases, isolated reduced diffusion alone. It may also be recognized from a chest radiograph or a high-resolution CT scan that would show pulmonary fibrosis or the "ground glass" appearance suggestive of alveolar wall inflammation. Most of these patients will require a biopsy for confirmation of the nature of their interstitial lung disease, because the individual pathologic processes do provide a basis for choosing therapy and giving the patient important prognostic information.

Other uncommon causes of cough can include laryngeal disease, mild or early congestive heart failure, tracheomalacia, recurring episodes of aspiration, and even patients with cough on a psychogenic basis. This last phenomenon is often seen in patients who may have had in the past another reason for cough on a physical basis and who incorporated cough into their daily habits in an effort to clear secretions or reduce irritation. The habit may persist even after the initiating stimulus is removed.

LATER VISITS

Because the range of possible mechanisms is so broad, a stepwise approach to investigation is important. After the initial visit and an initial trial of therapy, a repeat office visit should follow in 2 to 4 weeks. At that point, if symptoms persist and a chest radiograph was not done initially, one is appropriate. The patient should have pulmonary function testing to look for more subtle evidence of airflow obstruction and to screen for restrictive lung disease. If there was a clinical suspicion of one of the four common causes, but there were inconsistent elements in the history or if the empirical trial was not successful, an escalation of the therapy may be appropriate. This might include addition of other agents to suppress nasal inflammation or secretion that were not used as part of the initial trial, such as nasal ipratropium (Atrovent), an extended course of antibiotic therapy if sinusitis was suspected but did not respond, or a higher dose of proton pump inhibitor if reflux was suspected but did not respond to the initial therapy. At this point it may also be appropriate to further investigate the upper airways with a sinus CT to demonstrate mucosal thickening or air fluid levels consistent with sinus inflammation as a source of postnasal drip, or nasopharyngolaryngoscopy to examine both the velopharynx region and the glottic region looking for evidence of inflammation or a structural lesion. Nasopharyngolaryngoscopy may be particularly helpful in identifying occult reflux, because localized erythema in the region of the arytenoids may be seen in refluxing patients who sleep supine.

The patients who show no response after this second visit and the subsequent studies and therapies will need further investigation. This would include 24-hour pH probe recordings to demonstrate acid reflux as a source of cough, particularly in patients who do not report the characteristic burning or sour taste. In patients in whom symptoms have not suggested airway hyperreactivity, methacholine change testing may be helpful. Last, a small subset of patients with persistent cough may require bronchoscopy looking for a mucosal or submucosal abnormality including polyps or bronchial adenomas that may be triggering cough but produce no lesion detectable by CT scanning or chest radiograph.

INSOMNIA

method of
DAVID N. NEUBAUER, M.D.
Department of Psychiatry and Behavioral Sciences
Johns Hopkins University School of Medicine
Associate Director
Johns Hopkins Sleep Disorders Center

Insomnia is the inability to sleep adequately when one is attempting to sleep. It is among the most common concerns encountered in clinical practice. Approximately one half of adults in our society occasionally experience insomnia within any year, and about 10% to 15% of the population has severe or chronic symptoms. The prevalence tends to be greater among women, and for both sexes it increases with age. Insomnia may be associated with nighttime distress and daytime fatigue, sleepiness, excessive arousal, anxiety, irritability, poor concentration, mistakes, and accidents. Persistent insomnia may increase the risk for the development of major depression. Acute insomnia, lasting no more than a week or two, often is associated with readily identifiable circumstances. Chronic and recurrent insomnia are more likely to result from multiple vulnerabilities and precipitants. The potential factors that may interfere with sleep are quite diverse and add to the challenge in evaluating and treating patients complaining of sleep disturbance.

NORMAL SLEEP

An appreciation of the two primary processes regulating the sleep-wake cycle under normal circumstances is important in understanding the context of a patient's sleep complaint. A *homeostatic process* represents the overall balance of sleep and wakefulness over time and promotes a total of about 8 hours of sleep during a 24-hour period. Sleep deprivation, whether acute or chronic, increases the sleepiness drive. The timing of the sleep propensity is strongly influenced by the *circadian process*, which synchronizes sleepiness with various other physiologic rhythms. Typically these two processes promote about 8 hours of nighttime sleep and 16 hours of daytime and evening alertness. A conceptual balance of factors that might contribute either to sleepiness or arousal at any point in the 24-hour cycle can be formulated. The influences of these intrinsic homeostatic and circadian processes, along with various factors (e.g., caffeine, distress, pain) that are extrinsic to the fundamental regulation of the sleep-wake cycle, together can aid in understanding a patient's sleep-related complaint at any particular time. A consideration of this broad context of insomnia is essential for a thorough evaluation.

CAUSES OF INSOMNIA

The potential causes of insomnia may be considered in several broad categories (Table 1) and are discussed below. However, it should be recognized that multiple simultaneous causes often are present and the negative influences on a person's sleep can shift over time. It is useful to consider those characteristics that might contribute to one's vulnerability or susceptibility to insomnia (e.g., circadian phase predisposition, personality features), specific triggers for an insomnia episode (e.g., major depression, jet lag, sleep apnea), and influences that can perpetuate insomnia symptoms (e.g., conditioned hyperarousal, napping, alcohol use).

Everyone is vulnerable to the experience of distress resulting from *situational disturbances* that may result from various personal or societal problems. Insomnia associated with acute distress usually is transient; however, it may initiate chronic insomnia symptoms that are reinforced by other perpetuating factors. Persistent distress from external stressors also may contribute to long-term insomnia.

Insomnia may result from exacerbations of any *psychiatric disorder* associated with emotional distress. With some psychiatric disorders, such as major depression, there likely is a direct negative physiologic influence on sleep architecture and perceived sleep quality. Mood and anxiety disorders are common among people with persistent insomnia. The majority of individuals diagnosed with major depression complain of insomnia, and in the course of recurrent major depression insomnia often is the first symptom to reappear.

Any *medical disorders*, whether acute or chronic, that are associated with nighttime pain or discomfort may undermine the experience of adequate sleep. Musculoskeletal problems are obvious examples; however, insomnia may result from various neurologic, endocrine, pulmonary, cardiovascular, gastrointestinal, genitourinary, and renal disorders, among others.

Although insomnia is a sleep complaint, it may be the presenting symptom of an underlying *sleep disorder*. For instance, sleep-disordered breathing may cause repeated nighttime arousals and awakenings, as well as a sense of unrefreshing sleep. Frequent, brief involuntary muscle contractions indicative of periodic limb movements of sleep similarly may promote sleep disruption. Restless leg syndrome often is associated with delayed sleep onset because of the uncomfortable sensations.

TABLE 1. **Causes of Insomnia**

Situational disturbances
Psychiatric disorders
Medical disorders
Sleep disorders
Circadian predisposition
Schedule abnormalities (jet lag, shift work)
Medication effects
Substance abuse
Psychologic conditioning
Poor sleep hygiene

Circadian rhythm disorders, a subset of sleep disorders, deserve special attention because they commonly contribute to insomnia and often are unrecognized. Although the circadian system typically promotes sleep from about 10 to 11 PM until about 6 to 7 AM, for some individuals the physiologic sleepiness drive occurs either earlier or later. At the extremes of this phase spectrum there often are significant clinical consequences. The history reflects a long-standing sleep-wake cycle trend. Severe "early birds" have a circadian sleepiness drive that is phase-advanced. The usual primary complaint is persistent early morning awakening or light and disrupted sleep during the later hours of the night. Early evening sleepiness and little difficulty with initial sleep onset are typical; however, people with this advanced predisposition often do not go to bed as early as when they might to be able to fall asleep. Significant clinical sleep problems resulting from a circadian phase advance are relatively rare among young adults; however, the potential sleep-disrupting effects increase progressively with age because of the general trend for the circadian cycle to shift earlier. A "night owl" tendency describes a delayed sleep phase pattern wherein people either stay up rather late before attempting sleep or complain of taking several hours to fall asleep after getting into bed at an earlier desired bedtime. Given the opportunity, they then are able to sleep well into daytime, perhaps to mid-afternoon. Awakening at a desired earlier morning hour, such as 7 to 8 AM, tends to be quite challenging and results in sleep deprivation. A complaint of daytime sleepiness commonly accompanies the sleep onset difficulty. This delayed circadian pattern occurs most commonly among adolescents and young adults.

The circadian system also is important in the insomnia commonly resulting from *schedule abnormalities*, as occurs with jet lag and shift work schedules. In these situations sleep is attempted at times outside the phase of the circadian sleepiness drive maximum. With jet lag the circadian system typically adjusts to the new time zone photoperiod, and the insomnia resolves within several days. Insomnia may be relapsing or chronic with continually changing shift work assignments or persistent work schedules that impinge on the individual's predisposed circadian sleep time.

The potential stimulating and sleep-disrupting effects of over-the-counter and prescribed *medications* always must be assessed in the evaluation of insomnia patients. A list of common substances and medication classes that may contribute to insomnia is listed in Table 2. *Substance abuse*, including alcohol and stimulant use, may lead to acute or chronic insomnia.

Psychologic conditioning can play a major role in chronic insomnia. The distress of sleeplessness from various precipitants can become associated with one's bedroom, bedtime routines, and the attempt to fall asleep. Over time the mental arousal and frustration can be reinforced and thereby increase the likelihood of further sleeplessness. In this manner the insomnia can become self-perpetuating, resulting in further

Table 2. **Common Medications and Substances That May Promote Insomnia**

Caffeine
Alcohol
Nicotine (inhaled and transdermal)
Selected herbal preparations
Selected over-the-counter diet, cold, and allergy preparations
Selective serotonin reuptake inhibitors and selected antidepressants
Selected antihypertensives
Corticosteroids
Nonsteroidal anti-inflammatory drugs
Theophylline
Diuretics
Stimulants

difficulty with sleep onset or exaggerated nighttime awakenings.

Assorted sleep-enhancing behaviors, routines, and habits may be described as promoting good sleep hygiene. In contrast, *poor sleep hygiene* can contribute to insomnia. Examples may involve irregular sleep-wake schedules (including napping), excessive or afternoon/evening caffeine, excessive evening physical exercise, excessive wakeful time in bed, the use of the bed and bedroom for activities unrelated to sleep or sex, and a bedroom environment that is not conducive to sleep (e.g., temperature extremes, disturbing noise or light).

ASSESSMENT

The history and physical examination are the foundations of the insomnia evaluation. These may provide evidence of suspected causative factors. In the primary care setting sleep issues routinely should be included in the history and review of systems. Patients do not necessarily volunteer sleep-related symptoms—those that do discuss it are just the tip of the iceberg. The insomnia history should detail the nighttime and daytime symptoms, duration, frequency, predictability, and any apparent associations with schedules and life events. Previous therapeutic trials by the patient or health care practitioners, along with the outcomes, also should be reviewed.

Having a patient maintain sleep log charts showing all sleep episodes (including naps) during sequential 24-hour episodes for at least several weeks can be quite helpful in documenting aspects of the insomnia symptoms, as well as any changes resulting from therapeutic interventions.

In a primary care setting the assessment of selected insomnia patients may include consultation with a sleep medicine specialist. This may be useful in complex cases or when other sleep disorders are suspected. In some cases sleep laboratory testing will provide valuable diagnostic information. The American Academy of Sleep Medicine (www.aasmnet.org) maintains a directory of accredited sleep disorder centers.

TREATMENT

The treatment of insomnia may include both specific and general strategies (Table 3). Specific approaches address underlying disorders contributing to the insomnia, as may occur with sleep apnea, major depression, chronic pain, and congestive heart failure. General approaches may be therapeutic in various clinical situations and may be combined with other treatments. *Education* is a cornerstone in insomnia treatment. An understanding of factors that can disturb sleep can help motivate patients to make necessary behavior changes. Sleep hygiene recommendations include various sleep-enhancing behaviors (Table 4). *Psychotherapy* may be beneficial for emotional distress, identifying and resolving conflicts, and changing attitudes about sleep. *Behavioral management* involves interventions designed to limit excessive time in bed and to reduce the conditioned excessive arousal that may be associated with attempts to sleep. A cognitive-behavioral therapy approach combines sleep and insomnia education, specific behavioral interventions, and a psychotherapeutic plan to diminish maladaptive assumptions and thought processes regarding sleep and insomnia. General pharmacologic approaches to insomnia typically involve the use of sedating medications.

Table 3. **General Approaches to Insomnia Treatment**

Education
Sleep hygiene
Psychotherapy
Behavioral management
Pharmacologic

The use of hypnotic medications should be part of an integrated approach to the insomnia that also has addressed appropriate specific underlying factors and sleep-enhancing behaviors. The benzodiazepine receptor agonists (Table 5) have been the primary hypnotic medications over the past three decades. The most recent generation includes zolpidem (Ambien) and zaleplon (Sonata). The elimination half-life and duration of action are short for zolpidem and ultrashort for zaleplon; therefore, there is little risk of residual sedation the following morning after bedtime use. Generally these medications are effective, safe, and well tolerated at the recommended doses, which for both is 10 mg for adults and 5 mg for elderly patients. The abuse potential is very small. Most insomnia patients treated with hypnotics do well and need the medication only for a few days or weeks. However, selected patients may continue to benefit from longer-term nightly or intermittent use.

Table 4. **Sleep Hygiene Recommendations**

Attempt to maintain regularity in the sleep-wake cycle timing
Avoid caffeine after lunchtime
Exercise regularly, but not within a few hours of bedtime
Avoid alcohol, especially within a few hours of bedtime
Avoid late heavy meals, but consider a small bedtime snack
Reserve the bedroom and bed for sleep and sexual activities
Develop a relaxing evening routine
Avoid excessive wakeful time in bed
Avoid bedroom temperature extremes
Avoid disruptive noises and consider a white-noise machine

TABLE 5. **Benzodiazepine Receptor Agonist Hypnotics**

Generic Name	Brand Name	Elimination Half-Life (H) (Including active metabolites)
Benzodiazepine		
Estazolam	ProSom	10–24
Flurazepam	Dalmane	40–250
Quazepam	Doral	40–250
Temazepam	Restoril	3.5–18
Triazolam	Halcion	1.5–5.5
Nonbenzodiazepine		
Zaleplon	Sonata	1
Zolpidem	Ambien	2.5

The traditional benzodiazepine-structure hypnotics may be effective, especially for short-term use. There should be greater concern for tolerance and withdrawal symptoms, which can be minimized with a tapered discontinuation. Several of these medications have long half-lives that can lead to residual daytime sleepiness and impairment.

Many other medications with some potential for sedation have been recommended for the primary goal of promoting sleep in insomnia patients. In these cases the consideration of potential adverse effects and drug interactions is important. All sedating substances, including alcohol, over-the-counter, and prescription medications, can have cumulative effects, with excessive central nervous system depression and residual daytime sedation. Antihistamines, such as diphenhydramine (Benadryl),* have a moderately long duration of action with increased potential for residual daytime effects, and they also can contribute to anticholinergic side effects, such as urinary retention and confusion. Trazodone (Desyrel)* also has a relatively long duration of action that can lead to residual daytime sleepiness. Because of the trazodone postsynaptic alpha antagonism there is increased risk of hypotension, especially among elderly patients. Priapism and serotonin syndrome are infrequent complications of trazodone use. Presently there is not sufficient data to support the efficacy or safety of the assorted dietary supplements that are promoted as sleep aids.

The majority of insomnia patients can be managed effectively in the primary care setting. The extent to which psychotherapeutic and behavioral interventions are provided in these practices depends upon the interest and skills of the health care professional. Additional resources may be available through a sleep medicine specialist.

Insomnia is a common problem that may have serious consequences, including quality of life deterioration and increased risk of depression. Insomnia has many potential causes, and several of these may be present simultaneously. Both specific and general treatment strategies may be necessary for sustained improvement in sleep. With chronic insomnia, effective treatment often requires a therapeutic alliance with the patient as different interventions are explored. The ultimate goal is helping the patient achieve an internal and external environment that allows the experience of adequate nighttime sleep and daytime alertness.

*Not FDA approved for this indication.

PRURITUS (ITCHING)

method of
LOUIS J. RUSIN, M.D.
Park Nicollet Clinic, University of Minnesota
Minnetonka, Minnesota

Pruritus, which is synonymous with itching, is the bane of the dermatologist and the patient. It is the sensation that provokes the desire to scratch. Although it is the most common patient symptom encountered by dermatologists, its pathophysiology is unclear, causes are numerous and varied, and the treatment is often difficult. Itching causes one to scratch, and the scratching often worsens and perpetuates the itching. The itching can become severe, causing discomfort, frustration, and loss of sleep for the patient (and the treating physician!).

ETIOLOGY

Itching is a complex psychoneurodermatologic phenomenon involving central nervous system processes and peripheral mediators but is complex and poorly understood. This sensation results from the activation of a network of free nerve endings at the dermal-epidermal junction. The cutaneous nerve stimulation is mediated by several substances including histamine and neuropeptides—including substance P, arachidonic acid transformation products, prostaglandin E, platelet activating factor, vasoactive peptides and proteases, and enkephalins. In the past, it was believed that itch sensation was transmitted by low-intensity stimulation of unmyelinated polymodal C nerve fibers. However, it has also been shown that there are two populations of fibers when unmyelinated C fibers are stimulated: the majority responds by causing pain, a small minority responds by causing itch. This sensation of itch is carried to specific areas of the brain that can respond through motor nerves with scratching. More recent studies have shown that enkephalins (opioid pentapeptides) exert a regulatory action on itch through the central nervous system.

CAUSES OF PRURITUS

Itching is a symptom, not a disease. It may be caused by a myriad of factors that may be classified as localized or generalized.

Localized Pruritus

Certain body areas are predisposed to external factors or disease processes that result in localized pruritus (Table 1).

TABLE 1. **Localized Pruritus**

Scalp—seborrheic dermatitis, psoriasis, acne necrotica, allergic contact dermatitis
Eyelids—irritant dermatitis, contact dermatitis, atopic dermatitis
Ears—psoriasis, seborrheic dermatitis, otitis externa
Hands—contact or irritant dermatitis, psoriasis, dyshidrotic eczema
Genitals—kraurosis vulvae, psoriasis, fungal or yeast infection
Anus—pruritus ani
Legs—asteatotic dermatitis, stasis dermatitis, lichen simplex chronicus
Feet—fungal infection, dyshidrotic eczema, psoriasis

Generalized Pruritus

Generalized itchiness may be caused by external factors or skin diseases or be a result of systemic factors.

External factors

a. environmental: low humidity, winter weather, electric blankets, heated mattress pads or heated water beds, frequent showering, high humidity with sweat retention
b. chemical: some detergents or additives to the wash, certain body soaps or washes, rubbing alcohol, witch hazel, some body lotions or bath additives, topical chemical irritants
c. particulate matter: foreign bodies such as fiberglass or hair
d. infestations, bites, or parasites: scabies, lice, black flies, no-see-ums, chiggers, sand fleas, swimmer's itch, animal mites or fleas, arthropod bites
e. aquagenic pruritus
f. radiation therapy

Skin Diseases

Innumerable diseases have been associated with itching. They are defined by history and presentation.

Systemic Factors

Estimates of generalized pruritus caused by systemic disease vary from 10% to 50%. These factors are many, varied, and include infections, drug eruptions, endocrine disease, hepatic disease, renal disease, hematologic disease, occult malignancy, allergies, psychogenic factors, and autoimmune disease.

a. infectious: viral disease such as HIV, varicella, rubella; fungal infection; trichinosis; intestinal parasites
b. drug eruptions: often associated with chemotherapy with antineoplastic drugs. May cause pruritus from cholestasis, renal impairment, allergic reaction, hypersensitivity, or chemical interference with neural pathways
c. endocrine: hyperthyroidism or hypothyroidism, parathyroidism, diabetes, carcinoid syndrome
d. hepatic disease: obstructive jaundice, primary biliary cirrhosis, intrahepatic or posthepatic biliary obstruction, hepatic cholestasis as seen in pregnancy
e. renal disease: occurs in 13% of all patients with chronic renal disease and about 70% to 90% of those on hemodialysis
f. hematologic disease: Hodgkin's disease (in 10% to 25% of patients), polycythemia vera, iron deficiency, paraproteinemia, mast cell disease, myelomatosis, leukemia, mycosis fungoides
g. occult malignancy: adenocarcinomas and squamous cell carcinomas of various organs
h. allergies: to ingestants, inhalants
i. psychogenic factors: neurotic excoriations, delusions of parasitosis, obsessive-compulsive disorder. Stress and psychologic trauma intensify all forms of pruritus. This is a diagnosis by exclusion and you must rule out all other causes first.
j. autoimmune disease: graft versus host disease

EVALUATION

Since pruritus is a symptom and not a disease, it may be especially difficult to evaluate if it is generalized and has been present for months to years. All evaluations should include a detailed history, physical exam, and appropriate laboratory studies.

History

The history is probably the most important part of the workup. It needs to be accurate and thorough, including the location, onset, duration, prescription and over-the-counter medications used, the time they were started, periodic or seasonal variation, current skin care practices, a thorough review of systems, and relationship to occupation. Answers to these questions may prompt more detailed questions regarding affected family members; exposures to plants, animals, or chemicals; history of recent travel; factors that make it worse or better; malignancy; chemotherapy; infection; and the patient's emotional state.

Physical Exam

The extent of the exam is based on the history and areas involved. If the onset is recent, the involved areas are localized or show a specific distribution, or any primary lesions are noted, the diagnosis will be easier.

Laboratory Testing

See Table 2.

TREATMENT

Treatment of pruritus is often difficult, exasperating, and frustrating for the patient and provider. Oftentimes the patient has had pruritus for quite some time, has been treated with several over-the-counter products that have aggravated and perpetuated the problem, and is caught up in the itch-scratch-itch cycle when initially seen. Treatment consists of trying to find and treat any underlying disease or external factor, topical therapy, and systemic therapy.

1. Treat the underlying disease and eliminate external factors. If the history, exam, and laboratory findings identify a specific cause, treat accordingly.

TABLE 2. **Laboratory Testing**

Routine chemistry profile including hepatic and renal function tests, fasting blood sugar, thyroid screening
Ferritin level
Complete blood count with differential
Stool for ova and parasites, chest radiograph, malignancy workup, and other appropriate tests if indicated by history and physical exam

2. Topical therapy

- Patient education: This is the *most* important part of the treatment. Spend time discussing the role of scratching in perpetuating pruritus, specific factors to avoid that aggravate the condition (excessive bathing; harsh soaps; liquid soaps; dry environment; electric blankets; hot environments; avoiding topical Benadryl, lidocaine [Xylocaine], and neomycin because many people develop contact dermatitis to them; extremely hot showers or baths), and preventive measures such as using mild soaps, applying emollients after bathing and drying, taking tepid baths or showers, wearing wicking clothing when exercising, using a humidifier, and avoiding botanical products, distraction, ice or cold compresses, and ultraviolet B light. Be as specific as possible.
- Pharmacologic therapy:
  a. Low-to-medium strength cortisone creams or ointments if the excoriations have created dermatitis. These work best with plastic wrap occlusion at night for 10 days. Not for facial use or moist skinfolds
  b. Menthol- or camphor-containing creams (Sarna Anti-Itch)
  c. Tacrolimus ointment (Protopic)* or pimecrolimus cream (Elidel)*
  d. Capsaicin cream (Zostrix)* and doxepin cream (Zonalon) have not been very effective.

3. Systemic therapy

a. Sedating antihistamines are helpful, especially when taken 1/2 to 1 hour before bedtime, when the itching is usually most intense. Diphenhydramine (Benadryl),* hydroxyzine (Atarax), cyproheptadine (Periactin),* and doxepin (Sinequan)* work well. The nonsedating antihistamines cetirizine (Zyrtec),* fexofenadine (Allegra),* loratadine (Claritin),* and desloratadine (Clarinex)* are relatively ineffective for itching unless caused by urticaria.
b. BuSpar or other antidepressants may help recalcitrant pruritus.
c. Sometimes a cortisone injection or short tapering course of oral cortisone is necessary to quiet the process down enough to treat with topical products and sedating antihistamines as needed.

Pruritus is a common, difficult, poorly understood, subjective sensation of itching that is always frustrating to have and often difficult to treat. There is relief for these patients, but the provider must *listen* to the patients, take a thorough and detailed history, do a physical exam, and order appropriate laboratory tests. Identifying a cause, eliminating external factors, and treating a skin disease or systemic disease are often curative. Symptomatic treatment or dealing with an underlying psychogenic etiology will still provide relief for these patients.

*Not FDA approved for this indication.

TINNITUS

method of
CALHOUN D. CUNNINGHAM III, M.D., and
RICK A. FRIEDMAN, M.D., PH.D.
House Ear Clinic, Inc.
Los Angeles, California

Tinnitus, or head noise, is a frequently presenting complaint estimated to affect up to 40 million Americans at some point in their lives. Although the majority of people are not bothered by its presence, tinnitus seriously affects an estimated 10 million people and it debilitates approximately 1 million. A basic understanding of this complex condition is necessary for all primary care physicians because most patients suffering from tinnitus can be helped.

Tinnitus is best defined as noise that is heard in the absence of external acoustic stimuli. It is typically classified as *subjective* (noise heard only by the patient) and *objective* (noise heard by the patient and observer). Subjective tinnitus is more common and is often seen in association with hearing loss. Objective tinnitus is less common and may reflect vascular abnormalities that facilitate turbulent blood flow in the region of the ear. Tinnitus is a symptom, not a disease, and an underlying etiology must first be sought.

In evaluating the patient with tinnitus, a few important points in the patient's history will steer the physician toward a diagnosis or further testing. Is the tinnitus unilateral, bilateral, or "inside the head"? What is the character of the tinnitus (and, of importance, is it pulsatile)? Is it acute or chronic (i.e., what is the onset)? Are there any exacerbating or relieving factors? Has there been a history of noise exposure? Ear infections? Hearing loss? Stress? What is the degree to which the head noise has affected or debilitated the patient's life (does it keep the patient awake at night; does it awaken him or her from sleep; can the patient focus, concentrate, and perform daily activities)? The physician must address and gain insight into the psychologic status of the patient; many affected patients are depressed, anxious, or "stressed out." Stress appears to play a large role in these patients and is discussed later.

Physical examination should include otoscopic examination; tuning fork testing; neurologic examination with special attention to the cranial nerves; and auscultation of the ears, mastoids, and carotid arteries if the tinnitus is pulsatile. Objective tinnitus necessitates a diagnostic workup different from that for subjective tinnitus.

The importance of audiometry cannot be overemphasized. Pure tone thresholds for air conduction, bone conduction, and speech testing are crucial in the evaluation of tinnitus; the answer often lies in the audiogram. If the audiogram is normal, reassurance of the patient is often all that is required.

After this information has been collected, the diagnosis is usually apparent. If the diagnosis is unclear, a differential diagnosis is generated, and further testing may be needed. We have found that classifying tinnitus as pulsatile or nonpulsatile aids in evaluating the patient. Table 1 lists some of the more common etiologies of pulsatile tinnitus; Table 2 displays common causes of nonpulsatile tinnitus.

The treatment of tinnitus is based on the underlying pathology, and diagnosis may require additional diagnostic testing. In the category of pulsatile tinnitus, temporal bone computerized tomography (CT) scanning is the imaging study of first choice to evaluate a middle ear mass (glomus tympanicum or jugulare; CT scanning also detects abnormalities of the jugular bulb or carotid artery). If identified, surgical removal of these tumors offers benefit. Carotid duplex scanning is indicated for patients with a carotid bruit. Benign intracranial hypertension is an often overlooked but frequent cause of pulsatile tinnitus. Affected patients tend to be obese females in their third to fifth decades of life. This idiopathic increase in intracranial pressure often presents with headaches, visual changes, and a venous hum heard by the patient. Gentle compression of the jugular vein in the neck often relieves the pulsatile tinnitus. Referral to a neurologist or neuro-ophthalmologist is appropriate for these patients. Magnetic resonance imaging (MRI) or magnetic resonance angiography is an excellent first-line study if there is a suspicion of increased intracranial pressure in the patient with pulsatile tinnitus and no mass behind the tympanic membrane. Myoclonus of either a middle ear muscle or the palate is generally described as an intermittent "clicking" sound, sometimes several times per second. Spasm of the soft palate can be observed when the patient is symptomatic. Muscle relaxants, botulinum toxin (Botox)* injection for the palate, or sectioning of the tensor tympani or stapedius muscles usually brings relief.

Eighty percent of patients with sensorineural hearing loss have subjective tinnitus at some point in their lives. This is the most common type of tinnitus. It is often described as high pitched (like the sound of crickets) or roaring (like a jet engine) and is most noticeable at night, when it is quiet. Although the precise pathophysiologic mechanism accounting for the generation of this tinnitus is not known, it appears to be related to changes in the auditory pathways as a result of loss of peripheral sensory cells or irritation to the inner ear or auditory nerve. Most often, the tinnitus is not particularly bothersome because most patients become used to it over time. An audiogram is helpful in diagnosing these cases because many of these patients will have a high-frequency sensorineural hearing loss related to aging (presbycusis) or previous noise exposure. Taking time to explain to these patients that their tinnitus is simply a manifestation of their hearing loss is often all that is needed to reassure them nothing serious is wrong. Exposure to loud noises—either brief, high-intensity sounds (acoustic trauma) or prolonged exposure to medium- to high-intensity sounds (noise-induced)—will cause tinnitus. Hearing protection and counseling are important for patients who are avid hunters or work in noisy environments.

*Not FDA approved for this indication.

TABLE 1. **Common Etiologies of Pulsatile Tinnitus**

Benign intracranial hypertension ("venous hum" tinnitus)
Atherosclerotic carotid artery disease
Glomus tumor (tympanicum or jugulare)
Vascular malformation (arteriovenous malformation)
Otosclerosis
Palatal myoclonus
Middle ear muscle (tensor tympani or stapedius) myoclonus
Hypertension

TABLE 2. **Common Etiologies of Nonpulsatile Tinnitus**

Hearing loss
Noise exposure/acoustic trauma
Acoustic neuroma
Otitis externa
Otitis media
Eustachian tube dysfunction
Labyrinthitis
Meniere's disease
Stress, depression, anxiety
Temporomandibular joint dysfunction
Tension headaches
Medications

Any patient with unilateral tinnitus or an asymmetric sensorineural hearing loss should undergo evaluation for a retrocochlear lesion such as an acoustic neuroma. MRI with *gadolinium contrast* is the study of choice for the diagnosis of acoustic neuroma.

Infections of the outer, middle, or inner ear are often accompanied by tinnitus; diagnosis is made on the basis of the history and physical examination. Treatment of the infection relieves the tinnitus.

Meniere's disease is characterized by the classic triad of fluctuating hearing loss, vertigo, and tinnitus. The diagnosis is a clinical one, usually based on the history and normal otologic examination. Meniere's disease can be difficult to manage and generally warrants referral to an otologist or neurotologist.

Stress is intimately related to tinnitus and may be the cause or a major contributing factor to its severity in certain patients. When taking the history the physician should carefully question the patients about current stresses in their lives at work and home. We use the mnemonic CAPPE (Table 3) to help identify these important stresses.

Chemical stresses include medications or other agents shown to cause or increase the severity of tinnitus (Table 4). Patients using such treatments are advised to seek alternative medications in consultation with their internists. Likewise, they are asked to

TABLE 3. **CAPPE Mnemonic for Tinnitus Evaluation**

Chemical
Acoustic
Pathologic
Physical
Emotional

monitor their caffeine intake (or switch to decaffeinated products) and alcohol consumption and to quit tobacco products.

Acoustic stresses include chronic noise exposure, acoustic trauma, sensorineural hearing loss (presbycusis, noise-induced), and conductive hearing loss. We strongly urge hearing protection for patients who are exposed to occupational noise, for people attending loud concerts, and for anyone exposed to loud noises.

Pathologic stresses include any infectious, inflammatory, vascular, or neoplastic process affecting the ear, including otitis externa, otitis media, labyrinthitis, acoustic neuroma, Meniere's disease, and glomus tumor. Diagnosis is usually made on the basis of the history and physical examination and further testing as indicated.

Physical stresses may be sequelae of natural events (you will hear your pulse in your ears after vigorous exercise) or nonotologic processes such as fever, upper respiratory tract infection, temporomandibular joint dysfunction (if you clench your teeth, you will hear noise in your ears), tension headaches, cervical muscle tension, or other major illness. Patients with normal or abnormal eustachian tube function describe a popping sound, the same sound you hear when you swallow. Treating these conditions will relieve the stress associated with these entities.

Finally, emotional stress can be a significant contributor to tinnitus. Screening questions for problems at home, in the office, or with the family often reveal such stresses. Stress reduction is very helpful for these patients, and we have recommended biofeedback or habituation (see below) to help control symptoms. When patients hear the tinnitus, their stress level increases; in other words, tinnitus itself causes stress. The increased stress serves only to make the tinnitus louder, further increasing the stress. Such a vicious cycle leads to insomnia, depression, inability to focus, and malaise. Breaking the cycle is important in the management of these patients. For most patients, simple reassurance is all that is required. Others more affected may need a short course of a low-dose tricyclic antidepressant to help, especially when sleep is affected. We occasionally use amitriptyline (Elavil),* 25 mg orally, at bedtime to help with symptoms of insomnia, stress, and depression. Consultation with the patient's internist is recommended. Stress management plays a large role in helping these patients.

TABLE 4. **Medications Causing Tinnitus**

Aminoglycosides
Erythromycin
Vancomycin
Furosemide (Lasix)
High-dose aspirin
Nonsteroidal anti-inflammatory drugs
Quinine/chloroquine (Aralen)
Antineoplastic drugs (platinum-based regimens)

For patients significantly distressed by their tinnitus, habituation has recently shown promising results in treatment. The goal of tinnitus habituation is to reach the stage at which, although patients may perceive tinnitus as unchanged when they focus on it, they are otherwise unaware of its presence. This is achieved by direct counseling combined with low-level, broadband noise generated by wearable devices that eventually help the patient become habituated to his or her tinnitus. Practitioners of this technique report successful of treatment in 75% of patients.

When no specific cause of tinnitus can be found, as is often the case, we find that a few conservative measures are often helpful. Patients are first instructed to eliminate excessive caffeine or tobacco from their diets. Home *masking* techniques are initiated that involve the use of background noise to overcome the sound of tinnitus. White noise generators or a radio tuned to low static will often help, especially at night, when it is quiet.

Tinnitus is a symptom, and an underlying disease process should be sought before simple reassurance of the patient. History, physical examination, and audiometry generally point to the correct diagnosis. Additional testing may be needed. Identification of various stresses in the patient's life helps physician and patient organize a differential diagnosis for head noise and helps sort out various possible causes. Most patients do well with education and reassurance, whereas others may require further testing and treatment.

*Not FDA approved for this indication.

LOW BACK PAIN

method of
STEVEN R. GARFIN, M.D.
Department of Orthopaedics
University of California, San Diego

and

MICHAEL J. VIVES, M.D.
Department of Orthopaedics
University of Medicine and Dentistry of New Jersey
Newark, New Jersey

Back pain is a ubiquitous complaint, second to only upper respiratory infection as a reason for physician office visits in the United States. Sixty to 80% of all people will experience a significant episode of disabling back pain at some point in their lives. Low back problems are the most common cause of disability in patients younger than 45 years of age. Although radiographic evidence of disc degeneration increases fairly linearly with age, the peak incidence of back pain is between the ages of 35 and 60. The symptoms of back pain will improve spontaneously in roughly 80% of the cases regardless of the treatment offered. Fifteen to

20% of patients, however, will have pain that may result in functional limitations for more than a year. Although not as common as back pain, sciatica, or radicular leg pain, may be experienced by up to 4.8% of men and 2.5% of women older than 35 years of age. The leg pain is preceded by an initial event of back pain in 76% of these patients, often up to a decade earlier. The prognosis for patients with leg-predominant symptoms is also favorable, with 75% improving within 30 days of the onset of their symptoms. In North America, back disorders generate direct and indirect costs of more than $100 billion per year in treatment and lost time from work. The majority of these costs are generated by the small subset of patients whose symptoms do not resolve spontaneously.

PATHOPHYSIOLOGY

Distinguishing radicular leg symptoms from axial back pain and referred pain is important, both for their differing etiologies and treatments. Axial and referred pain is caused by noxious stimuli affecting nerve endings in the annular outer portion of the discs, vertebral end plates, and facet joints. The pattern of referral is to the area designated the sclerotome, which has the same embryonic origin as the mesodermal tissues stimulated. This pain is often described as deep, aching, and diffuse. The intervertebral disc is the most common source of such axial somatic pain. Many independent investigators have reported that the outer layers of the annulus and the end plates have innervation from the sinuvertebral and sympathetic nerves. Nociceptive stimuli to these nerve endings may be biochemical byproducts of disc injury or abnormal stresses resulting from annular tears. A less common source of back and referred leg pain may be the facet joint. The postganglionic posterior primary ramus branch of the spinal nerve supplies afferent sensory input to the articular cartilage, synovium, and capsule of the facet joint. These findings are supported by the observation that injection of hypertonic saline into the joint produces pain, which subsequently can be blocked by lidocaine.

Radicular pain is caused by compression of a chemically sensitized nerve root, generating evoked ectopic responses in the dorsal root ganglion. Radicular pain is commonly described as lancinating or shooting with extension in a distinct band down the extremity. Although diffuse pain below the knee may be referred, distinct pain extending into the foot is more likely radicular. The most frequent cause of lumbar radiculopathy is disc herniation. An interaction of mechanical and inflammatory components is believed responsible. Nucleus pulposus within the epidural space results in an inflammatory response, and the specific role of various cytokines in symptom generation is an evolving field of study. Other sources of radiating lower extremity pain include foraminal or lateral recess stenosis caused by facet arthropathy and osteophyte formation, ligamentous hypertrophy, and spondylolisthesis (both degenerative and as a result of a defect in the pars interarticularis). Peripheral neuropathies may mimic or coexist with lumbar radiculopathies. Finally, although rare, spinal neoplasm or infection can present with complaints of axial pain or radicular symptoms.

EVALUATION AND TREATMENT

As physicians, our common practice is to encounter patients and generate a differential diagnosis based on the information gained by history taking and physical examination. Additional tests are frequently ordered to confirm or definitively establish a diagnosis before outlining a treatment plan. Given the favorable natural history of acute back and radicular pain and the difficulty in pinpointing the anatomic cause of the symptoms in many cases, such a conventional approach has proved costly and ineffective. A more useful approach is to exclude the rare conditions that require early aggressive intervention and adopt a symptom-directed approach to the remainder in an organized fashion.

Cauda equina syndrome and progressive muscle weakness are two conditions that should be ruled out at the initial presentation. If either of these is noted, then immediate magnetic resonance imaging (MRI) should be performed. If the study is positive, the patient should undergo a relatively urgent decompression, because bowel and bladder recovery is best accomplished with prompt surgery. If there is no history of cauda equina syndrome or progressive neurologic deficit, most patients can be treated with activity modification and nonsteroidal anti-inflammatory medications. Typically, opioids are reserved for selected cases of severe pain and for limited periods. If bed rest is recommended, it is usually for not more than a few days.

If the symptoms fail to resolve over the first few weeks, then physical therapy, focusing on range-of-motion and stabilization exercises, can be considered. Many different modality-based treatments and exercise programs have purported efficacy. Patients with continued symptoms should also have screening radiographs obtained that may demonstrate spondylolysis, spondylolisthesis, occult compression fractures, or, if present long enough, occult infection or malignancy. If any of these rare conditions are detected, then appropriate treatment can be initiated. In the majority of cases, however, nonspecific findings are present that do not clearly identify the pain generator. At this point, treatment recommendations differ based on the predominant complaint—sciatica or low back pain.

If leg pain is the predominant symptom and there is a positive tension sign or neurologic finding, then an MRI should be performed. If a lesion is demonstrated that correlates with the patient's complaints and physical findings, discectomy offers predictable relief with very little morbidity. Epidural steroid injection may be a consideration as an intermediate step before surgery in some cases, and selective nerve root injection may serve both diagnostic and therapeutic purposes. If the MRI is negative, electrical studies, glucose tolerance test, and so on are warranted to evaluate for a peripheral neuropathy.

Patients with primarily axial complaints that persist should have additional workup including a medical evaluation for gastrointestinal, genitourinary, hematologic, and biochemical abnormalities. In the past, bone scans were thought useful, but currently MRI may be most helpful at this stage because it is sensitive for pernicious sources of pain (occult tumor or infection) and allows a more detailed evaluation of common disc pathology. Although MRI can demonstrate disc derangement, it unfortunately cannot definitively confirm that these derangements are painful, as evidenced by similar findings in asymptomatic individuals. Although interest has arisen in minimally invasive approaches, such as intradiscal electrothermal therapy for treatment of painful annular lesions, additional data from independent investigators (with extended follow-up) are needed to clarify their role. Additionally, simple decompression alone is unlikely to improve predominantly axial symptoms. At this time, the main surgical option for treatment of mechanical back pain of discogenic origin is fusion. Because spinal fusion surgery carries more morbidity and less optimistic outcome than simple decompression, patient selection is critical to achieve success. Only a small percentage of patients with mechanical back pain are candidates for fusion. The authors favor additional nonoperative measures such as disease education or "low back school" programs to incorporate understanding of pertinent physiology with exercises and activity instruction to help patients maximize function with minimized back pain. More detailed psychosocial evaluation may be warranted to explore the possibility of confounding issues such as litigation, compensation, drug use, and untreated psychiatric disorders, which may potentiate the patient's dysfunction. If these measures have been exhausted and confounding issues have been excluded or addressed, fusion can be considered. Many favor additional provocative testing with discography to help isolate the painful levels to be fused with an interbody technique. One or, at most, two levels appear to have the most realistic chance for success. With such strict criteria, many patients will not be candidates for surgery. In these cases counseling on tolerance of symptoms, acceptance of functional limitations, and periodic (yearly) follow-up are the preferred routes.

Section 2

The Infectious Diseases

MANAGEMENT OF THE HIV-INFECTED PATIENT

method of
THOMAS P. GIORDANO, M.D.
Sections of Infectious Diseases and Health Services Research
Baylor College of Medicine
Houston, Texas

and

RICHARD M. GRIMES, PH.D.
Management and Policy Sciences
University of Texas Houston School of Public Health
Houston, Texas

EPIDEMIOLOGY, PATHOGENESIS, AND NATURAL HISTORY

Epidemiology of HIV Infection

Infection with the human immunodeficiency virus is a public health problem of enormous magnitude. The World Health Organization estimates that, as of December 2001, more than 60 million people have been infected with the virus, about 40 million of whom are still alive. About 28 million of the infections were in sub-Saharan Africa. Prevalence rates in some areas of Africa are estimated to be more than 30% in adults between the ages of 15 and 49. The epidemic is also rapidly expanding in South and Southeast Asia, where more than 6 million people are infected. Other rapidly growing epidemics are in Latin America (1.4 million infections) and Eastern Europe (1 million). The developed countries of Western Europe (560,000) and North America (940,000) have a large number of infected individuals but the rate of new infections has stabilized in these areas.

The major risk factor for disease acquisition also varies between developed and developing countries. In developing countries, the primary mode of transmission (>90%) is heterosexual and the ratio of male cases to female cases is 1:1. In developed countries, the epidemic was initially concentrated in white, gay males and IV drug users. Recently, there are increasing numbers of women and heterosexuals becoming infected. In the United States, 6% of the 1990 cases were due to heterosexual transmission, and the male:female ratio of AIDS cases was 8:1. In 2001, 16% of cases were due to heterosexual transmission and the male:female ratio was 3:1. In people who were found to be HIV infected in 2001 but who had not yet been defined as an AIDS case, the male:female ratio was 2:1. The U.S. epidemic is also concentrated in minorities. In males, 44% of the 2001 AIDS cases were among African Americans and 20% in Hispanics, although each of these groups constitutes about 10% of the U.S. population. Among women, 63% of the 2001 AIDS cases were in African Americans and 17% in Hispanics.

The potential for HIV infection should not be excluded because of age. The condition occurs at any age at which individuals are sexually active or may have shared needles. Although the bulk of AIDS cases have been found in people between 25 and 50 years of age, more than 10% of AIDS cases in the United States have occurred in people older than 50 years of age and 3% in people older than 60.

The Virus

There are two retroviruses that cause immunodeficiencies in humans, termed HIV-1 and HIV-2. The viruses infect and destroy CD4+ T lymphocytes, which are critical cells in the host immune system's cell-mediated immunity and memory responses. The two different viruses descended from viruses that infect different species of apes, and are only 60% homologous. HIV-1 is the more prevalent virus, causing more than 90% of the HIV infections in the world. HIV-1 has been divided into three groups, which are labeled M, N, and O. M is the most common of the groups, comprising as much as 95% of the world's HIV-1 infections. N and O groups have seldom been described outside of Africa. HIV-1 group M has been further subdivided into at least 11 subtypes, called "clades." These clades have been lettered A through K. These clades are likely to recombine, creating viruses that are mixtures of the clades. Recombinants are labeled by the letters of the clades that have combined (e.g., AG, AEF).

The predominant clade in North America and Western Europe has been clade B. However, non-B clades have been introduced into the United States. In a New York City study of individuals who were found to be HIV infected between 1993 and 1997, 68% of 517 HIV positive people born in Africa, 26 of 51 (52%) HIV positives from Asia, and 41% of 201 HIV positive immigrants from South America were infected with non-B clades. A surveillance system that has been established to determine prevalence of various clades in 10 U.S. cities showed that 64 of 271 (24%) newly diagnosed HIV patients were infected with non-B subtypes of HIV-1. Thus infection of U.S. patients, particularly immigrants, with non-B clades is not uncommon and may be becoming more frequent.

There is strong epidemiologic evidence that the non-B clades are more easily heterosexually transmitted. As the prevalence of non-B clades becomes better established in the developed world, there may be a larger number of heterosexually transmitted cases in those countries. In addition, the multiplicity of clades and recombinant forms of the virus will certainly make developing a vaccine to prevent HIV transmission more difficult. Furthermore, the effectiveness of antiretroviral drugs on non-B clade HIV infections is unclear because the clinical trials for these drugs have been conducted in areas where clade B predominates.

Among the outstanding characteristics of HIV-1 are its replication rate and its propensity to mutate. It has been estimated that more than 10 billion new virions per day are produced in an untreated person with HIV-1 infection and that more than 100,000 of these virions are mutants. Most of these mutants are not viable but those with replicative capacity and random mutations that confer resistance to antiretroviral drugs can potentially become the dominant species when the original form of the virus is suppressed with antiretroviral medication. Sub-lethal levels of antiretroviral drugs encourage the selection of resistant mutants, highlighting the importance of adherence to the drug regimens used for treatment of HIV infection.

Natural History of HIV Infection

HIV infection is a long-term infectious process that has characteristic stages. During the first few weeks of infection, there is enormous virus production and the amount of circulating virus, termed the HIV viral load, is quite high. After some weeks, the body mounts an incomplete immune response and the viral load drops to a level that is idiosyncratic to each individual. This level of viral load, called the "set point," is maintained until the patient becomes symptomatic, usually 3 to 15 years later. The set point has prognostic significance, with higher levels being associated with more rapid progression to disease (Table 1).

Clinically, the only early evidence of HIV infection is a self-limited syndrome that has been labeled primary HIV infection (PHIV) or acute retroviral syndrome, which occurs in 50% to 90% of infections. PHIV typically occurs a few weeks to a few months after infection. Symptoms of PHIV are common to many acute viral infections, including mononucleosis, so differentiating PHIV may be difficult (Table 2). It is not possible to diagnose PHIV clinically, and clinicians should consider PHIV in any patient with a prolonged viral syndrome or a constellation of conditions as described in Table 2. Suspicion is heightened by a sexual or substance use history that reveals recent behaviors associated with HIV transmission. Obtaining an accurate history and HIV testing are extremely important in patients suspected of having PHIV because this may be the only time that a patient appears for medical care for years after his or her infection, because of the prolonged asymptomatic phase following PHIV in most cases. Therefore, it is crucial that it be diagnosed to prevent transmission to others.

PHIV can be confirmed by detecting HIV nuclear material in the serum with an HIV viral load assay or a P24 antigen test. Conventional HIV antibody testing may not reveal the presence of HIV antibody because the body may not have yet mounted a sufficient immune response to the infection to produce antibodies, producing a false-negative result. However, in early infection, there will be a very elevated viral load. Any HIV infection that is diagnosed with a viral load should be confirmed at a later date with an antibody test.

After PHIV, most individuals have a long asymptomatic period, which typically lasts 8 to 12 years. During this period the primary impact of HIV infection is to gradually weaken the immune system through destruction of lymphocytes. Eventually the immune system is degraded to the point that the person experiences opportunistic infections that often become fulminant. In addition, HIV-related immunosuppression increases the risk for certain cancers, such as Kaposi's sarcoma and non-Hodgkin's lymphoma, which have viral pathogeneses. There are also systemic disease manifestations that have been linked to HIV infection. The appearance of these infections, cancers, and systemic manifestations generally corresponds to the level of immunosuppression as measured by the CD4+ T lymphocyte count.

TABLE 1. **Percentage of People Progressing to AIDS Within 3 Years (and 9 Years) Stratified by CD4+ Count and Viral Load**

	CD4+ <200	CD4+ 201-350	CD4+ >350
Viral load 1500-7000	*	0 (32.2)	2.2 (30.0)
Viral load 7001-20,000	14.3 (64.3)	6.9 (66.2)	6.8 (53.5)
Viral load 20,001-55,000	50.0 (90.0)	36.4 (84.5)	14.8 (73.5)
Viral load >55,000	85.5 (100.0)	64.4 (92.9)	39.6 (85.0)

*Insufficient data exist to provide an estimate for this category and for all CD4 categories with VL <1500 copies/mL. Data from the Multicenter AIDS Cohort Study: Guidelines for the Use of Antiretroviral Agents in HIV-Infected Adults and Adolescents, February 4, 2002. Available at http://www.aidsinfo.nih.gov.

TABLE 2. **Associated Signs and Symptoms of Primary HIV and Frequency of Their Appearance**

Sign or Symptom	Frequency of Appearance (%)
Fever	96
Lymphadenopathy	74
Pharyngitis	70
Rash*	70
Myalgia or arthralgia	54
Diarrhea	32
Headache	32
Nausea and vomiting	27
Hepatosplenomegaly	14
Weight loss	13
Thrush	12
Neurologic symptoms including:	12
Meningoencephalitis	
Aseptic meningitis	
Facial palsy	
Guillain-Barré syndrome	
Brachial neuritis	
Cognitive impairment or psychosis	

*The rash is usually erythematous and maculopapular with lesions on face and trunk and sometimes extremities, including palms and soles.

Adapted from Guidelines for the Use of Antiretroviral Agents in HIV Infected Adults and Adolescents, February 4, 2002. Available at http://www.aidsinfo.nih.gov.

The normal CD4+ count is approximately 1000 cells/mm^3. As long as this count stays above 500/mm^3 there is little likelihood of opportunistic disease, although the patient may complain of loss of energy, low-grade fever, or night sweats. The CD4+ count will decrease between 50 and 100 cells per year in the untreated state. With this decrease the host becomes susceptible to a wide range of opportunistic infectious and noninfectious conditions, as outlined in Table 3. These conditions are also important diagnostic clues for the presence of HIV, and any patient who has not been diagnosed with HIV infection who presents with one of these conditions should be offered an HIV antibody test. Testing for HIV infection should not be restricted to these diseases. Table 4 lists other conditions and situations for which testing should be considered. Testing should be particularly encouraged if the condition meets the criteria of the "3 R's"—recent onset, recurrent, and refractory to treatment.

Transmission of HIV

Transmission of HIV occurs when the potential host's mucous membranes or blood (in the case of percutaneous exposure) comes into contact with infected body fluids, especially blood, semen, and vaginal secretions. The most frequent modes of transmission are through heterosexual vaginal or anal sex, homosexual anal sex, sharing needles for injection drug use with an infected person, and maternal-to-fetus transmission, either in utero, at childbirth (most commonly), or through breast-feeding. The risk of acquisition through sex is increased by breakdown of the normal epithelial border such as occurs with ulcers or trauma, and is also increased by the presence of sexually transmitted diseases, whether ulcerative or not.

TABLE 3. **Correlation of CD4+ Count and HIV Complications**

CD4+ Count	Infectious Complications	Noninfectious Complications
>500/mm^3	Acute retroviral syndrome Candidal vaginitis	Persistent generalized lymphadenopathy Guillain-Barré syndrome Myopathy Aseptic meningitis
200-500/mm^3	Pneumococcal and other bacterial pneumonia Pulmonary tuberculosis Herpes zoster Thrush (oropharyngeal candidiasis) Kaposi's sarcoma Oral hairy leukoplakia	Cervical carcinoma (and CSIL) B-cell lymphoma Anemia Mononeuritis multiplex Idiopathic thrombocytopenic purpura Hodgkin's disease Wasting
<200/mm^3	*Pneumocystis carinii* pneumonia Disseminated histoplasmosis Coccidioidomycosis Miliary/extrapulmonary TB Progressive multifocal leukoencephalopathy	Peripheral neuropathy HIV-associated dementia Cardiomyopathy Vacuolar myelopathy Progressive polyradiculopathy Non-Hodgkin's lymphoma
<100/mm^3	Disseminated herpes simplex Toxoplasmosis Cryptococcosis Microsporidiosis *Candida* esophagitis	
<50/mm^3	Disseminated CMV Disseminated *Mycobacterium avium* complex	CNS lymphoma

Adapted from Hanson DL, Chu SY, Ferizo KM, Ward JW: Distributions of CD4 T lymphocytes at diagnosis of acquired immunodeficiency syndrome-defining and other human immunodeficiency virus-related illnesses. The Adult and Adolescent Spectrum of HIV Disease Project Group. Arch Intern Med 155:1537-1542, 1995. Copyright 1995, American Medical Association.

CMV, cytomegalovirus; CNS, central nervous system; CSIL, cervical squamous intraepithelial lesion; TB, tuberculosis.

TABLE 4. **Situations in Which HIV Testing Should Be Offered**

General Conditions
People with known risk factors for HIV
People who request testing
Pregnant women
Adults hospitalized in a hospital with a prevalence of HIV of >1% or AIDS of >0.1%
People with any condition listed in Table 3
Certain Infections
Severe herpetic lesions
Shingles, especially multidermatomal
Community acquired pneumonia
Recurrent bacterial infection or infection with unusual organisms
Atypical features of common infections
Other STDs
Oropharyngeal candidiasis
Recurrent vulvovaginal candidiasis
Tuberculosis
Symptoms
Weight loss
Chronic diarrhea
Unexplained fever
Generalized lymphadenopathy
Laboratory Tests
As part of work up for ITP, TTP, anemia, leukopenia, and unexplained renal insufficiency
Dermatologic Conditions
Severe psoriasis
Seborrheic dermatitis
Extensive HPV infection
Molluscum contagiosum
Oral leukoplakia
Neurologic Conditions
Neuropathies
Dementia
Guillain-Barré syndrome
Aseptic meningitis
Malignancies
Non-Hodgkin's lymphoma
Hodgkin's disease
Cervical carcinoma
Anal carcinoma

HPV, human papillomavirus; ITP, idiopathic thrombocytopenic purpura; STDs, sexually transmitted diseases; TTP, thrombotic thrombocytopenic purpura.

People at high risk for acquisition of HIV include people with a history of multiple sex partners, men who have sex with men, and users of illicit drugs, even if not intravenously used, because illicit drug use is often associated with multiple sexual partners and exchange of money for sex.

Oral sex carries a lower risk of transmission than does anal or vaginal sex. Condoms decrease the risk of infection but do not eliminate it. Exposure to nonbloody oral secretions, feces, urine, tears, and other nongenital fluids is very low risk, even when the exposure is via mucous membranes. There is no risk of acquisition through casual contact, including sharing eating utensils, toilet facilities, and contact with intact skin. The HIV viral load is directly related to the risk of that person transmitting HIV. Thus the use of highly active antiretroviral therapy (HAART), which can decrease viral load, decreases transmission risk. Circumcision also decreases acquisition risk in heterosexual men, likely because keratinization of the exposed epithelium fortifies it against trauma and infection. Though transmission of HIV through receipt of blood products can still occur, it occurs exceedingly rarely in developed countries but remains a high risk in places where blood is not screened.

MANAGEMENT OF PATIENTS INFECTED WITH HIV

The management of patients with HIV is complex and demanding. Recommendations on treatment of HIV, antiretrovirals available for use, knowledge about the toxicities of these agents, and tests available to help guide therapy are continually changing. Survival of patients with HIV has been shown to be better in people cared for by experienced providers, and all patients with HIV should be referred to experienced providers whenever feasible. When access to an experienced provider is limited, continual consultation with experts is strongly advised. Clinicians treating HIV infection should also be familiar with the latest guidelines for treatment, which can be found at www.aidsinfo.nih.gov. When patients are referred to other providers for chronic HIV treatment, the referring provider should not treat the patient hastily with antiretrovirals. Rather, acute opportunistic infections should be treated, appropriate opportunistic infection prophylaxis should be initiated, and timely referral made.

The Initial Evaluation

The History and Physical

Although the medical history is always important, it is crucial in the HIV-infected patient. A full history is necessary because immunosuppression can manifest itself in many ways, the success of treatment is determined by a complex interaction of social, biologic, psychologic, and medical factors, and polypharmacy is unavoidable in these patients. Table 5 lists the essential elements of the medical history. In addition to those items, the history should also include whether the person is sexually active and whether sexual or needle-sharing partners are aware of the person's HIV infection. In some states, physicians are obliged to inform such people of their possible exposure to HIV, but confidentiality laws require that this disclosure be handled in a careful way; providers are encouraged to avail themselves of expertise and resources particular to their practice setting. Consultation with the local health department will assist in these matters. The physical exam should include a thorough examination of all systems, with particular attention to the oropharynx, lymph nodes, lungs, and nervous system.

Laboratory and Other Tests

All patients should have a confirmatory HIV Western blot on record. Patients should also have a complete

TABLE 5. **Important Elements of the Medical History in People with Known HIV Infection**

History Item	Rationale
HIV risk factor	Certain illnesses are more common in injection drug users (e.g., hepatitis), whereas others are more common in men who have sex with men (e.g., Kaposi's sarcoma)
Presence of fevers, weight loss, night sweats, cough, pain, rash, diarrhea	Symptoms commonly associated with HIV and opportunistic infections
Nadir CD4+ count and peak viral load	Assess likely rate of disease progression and stage of disease
History of antiretroviral treatment, reasons for altering or discontinuing any therapy, response to therapy, and side effects from therapy	Determine likely drug resistance patterns and drug intolerances to assist in developing a plan for future treatment
Previous infectious disease history including chickenpox, tuberculosis, sexually transmitted diseases, pneumonia, and skin and soft-tissue infections	Determine the likelihood of recurrence of the conditions and stage of HIV disease
Comorbid conditions, such as coronary atherosclerosis, diabetes mellitus, and viral hepatitis	Determine the potential for these conditions to complicate antiretroviral treatment and drug selection
Current or past substance use and current or past psychiatric disorders	Referral for treatment, which may enhance ability to adhere to treatment regimen
Prescription, over-the-counter, and herbal medication	Avoid potentially harmful drug interactions
Social history that assesses social support system, housing stability, location of current and previous residences, travel history, occupational history, and exposure history (pets, chemicals, animals, etc.)	Determine risk for certain opportunistic infections (e.g., tuberculosis, histoplasmosis, toxoplasmosis). People who once lived in areas endemic for histoplasmosis and coccidioidomycosis may have reactivation of these infections regardless of where they presently live
Sexual history	Prevent transmission (see text)
Family history of diabetes mellitus, hypertension, and cancer	Determine the risk of developing these conditions secondary to immunosuppression or drug therapies

blood count to screen for cytopenias, chemistry panel to assess renal function and electrolytes, liver associated tests to assess for hepatitis, the rapid plasma reagin (RPR) test to screen for syphilis; hepatitis A, B, and C serologies; urinalysis; and fasting cholesterol fractions and triglycerides to establish a baseline cardiovascular risk. Toxoplasma IgG should be obtained to assess risk of toxoplasmosis, and all patients should undergo standard tuberculin skin testing for tuberculosis. All patients should also have a screening chest radiograph to serve as a baseline examination and to detect asymptomatic disease processes. Patients should also have a baseline CD4+ count and an HIV viral load performed. Prognosis of patients with HIV is related inversely to CD4+ count and directly to HIV viral load (see Table 1). CD4+ counts can fluctuate by as much as 30% with intercurrent illness or because of laboratory variability, and viral load can vary by as much as 0.5 $\log_{10}$, so these parameters should be assessed twice before decisions to initiate or change treatment are made. Whether to assess HIV resistance to antiretrovirals at baseline is somewhat controversial. However, many providers obtain a baseline resistance profile to determine if the patient has been infected with drug-resistant virus, a phenomenon that seems to be increasing in communities where many individuals are receiving HAART.

Immunizations

People with HIV are at increased risk for severe pneumococcal infections and should receive the pneumococcal vaccine. The vaccine is more effective when given at higher CD4+ cell counts, and people who are vaccinated with a low CD4+ count that subsequently rises to more than 200 cells/mm^3 in response to HAART should be offered revaccination. Patients who are not immune should be offered hepatitis B vaccine, and men who have sex with men should be offered hepatitis A vaccination. All patients should be offered influenza vaccine yearly, and tetanus vaccine should be kept up to date. Live vaccines should be avoided at all stages of HIV infection.

Subsequent Evaluations

Subsequent history and physical examinations should be tailored to the patient's current symptoms and drug therapy as well as history. The CD4+ count and viral load are the key parameters in determining whether HAART should be offered to patients and whether HAART is effective. Therefore, they should be measured every 3 or 4 months for patients stable on HAART or with early disease not yet on HAART. Patients newly started on HAART or with suboptimal responses to therapy should have these parameters followed more closely. The response to effective HAART should include between a one and two $\log_{10}$ drop in viral load at 4 weeks, a viral load below 500 copies/mL at 3 or 4 months, and a viral load below 50 copies/mL at 6 months. Symptomatology, physical examination, and complete cell counts, liver function, and renal function should be monitored to assess complications of therapy. In addition, an RPR should be performed annually in people with high risk of exposure to syphilis or a history of syphilis. For patients on HAART, fasting lipids should be assessed every 3 to 6 months because severe hyperlipidemia can complicate therapy. HIV resistance testing should be obtained before switching to a new regimen if that switch is made for virologic failure, though not if the switch is to be made because of drug intolerance or other reasons.

Antiretroviral Treatment

When to Start HAART

There is widespread agreement among experts that anyone with a CD4+ count lower than 200 cells/mm^3, a CD4 percent lower than 14%, or anyone with symptomatic HIV disease should be encouraged to initiate HAART (Table 6). Asymptomatic patients with CD4+ cell counts above 350 and viral loads below 55,000 copies/mL are generally not encouraged to take therapy. For patients who do not fit these categories, there is controversy about when to begin therapy. Patients with CD4+ cell counts above 350 and high viral loads (>55,000 copies/mL) are encouraged to take therapy by some, but not all, experts because of faster disease progression based on the higher viral load. Patients with CD4+ counts between 200 and 350 are encouraged to take therapy by most providers, especially if the viral load is high. Research on when to start therapy is ongoing, and providers are encouraged to seek timely expert advice in making this decision. Patient involvement in the decision to start therapy is critical, since the patient must embrace any therapy in order for it to be successful.

Antiretroviral Agents

There are three classes of antiretroviral agents, the protease inhibitors (PI), nucleoside reverse transcriptase inhibitors (NRTI), and non-nucleoside reverse transcriptase inhibitors (NNRTI). The nucleotide reverse transcriptase inhibitor tenofovir (Viread) can be thought of as an NRTI. These drugs and their most common side effects are described in Table 7A, 7B, and 7C. Most HAART regimens consist of a combination of either one to two PIs or an NNRTI together with two NRTIs. Alternative regimens that include only 3 NRTIs have also been used but are not currently recommended as first-line therapy. There is no indication to use single drug therapy except in pregnant women whose CD4+ count or viral load would not suggest a multidrug regimen. All two-drug therapies have been shown to be inferior to triple therapy. It should be noted that, because of drug interactions and overlapping resistance patterns, these drugs cannot be combined at will. Again, expert advice in constructing a regimen is essential. Current first-line recommended combinations are shown in Table 8.

Chronic Therapy and Salvage Therapy

Currently available therapy cannot eradicate HIV from an infected patient and so treatment will be lifelong. The goal of therapy is to achieve a sustained viral load less than 50 copies/mL. With a degree of sustained viral suppression, immune recovery, indicated by a rise in CD4+ cell count, will ensue in most patients. This immune reconstitution improves health and survival. Patients who achieve viral suppression may maintain that suppression for a brief time or for many years. Failure to achieve or sustain virologic suppression is associated with poor adherence to medications and development of resistance. When a regimen fails, as indicated by a persistent significant rise in the viral load (>0.5 $\log_{10}$ copies/mL), consideration should be made to switching to a new regimen provided that any problems with adherence can be addressed.

The selection of a salvage regimen should be guided by resistance testing, a knowledge of previously used antiretrovirals, the patient's tolerance of previous therapy, and the patient's comorbidities and concurrent medications. Resistance testing requires the patient to have a viral load of at least 1000 copies/mL and will only reliably test resistance to the drugs that the patient is currently receiving. Therefore, HIV resistance testing should be performed while the patient is on the failing regimen to maintain selective pressure on the virus. Cross-resistance within a class generally follows predictable patterns, and this knowledge should be used in selecting a salvage regimen. After resistance develops to a particular drug (and any cross-resistant drug), that resistance persists for the life of that patient, even if no longer detected on resistance testing. This persistence of resistance is due to the incorporation of mutant virus into host DNA, effectively archiving these mutant phenotypes and allowing them to resurface given the appropriate selective pressures. Thus resistance testing interpretation and salvage regimen design is complex and challenging and should be guided by an experienced provider.

Any salvage regimen should include at least two and preferably three drugs to which the patient's virus is reasonably expected to be sensitive. In general, a patient who has failed a first regimen that included an NNRTI without a PI should be placed on a PI-based regimen. A patient who is failing a first regimen based on a PI may be placed on a dual PI or ritonavir-boosted PI regimen, which provides very high drug levels that may overcome resistance. Alternatively, the patient may be switched to an NNRTI-based regimen. Two new NRTIs should be selected if possible. In the heavily treatment-experienced or resistant patient, inclusion of new agents that may be recently approved, such as enfuvirtide [T-20] (Fuzeon), or available through

TABLE 6. **Guidelines for Starting HAART in Asymptomatic Individuals**

Assess CD4+ and VL	CD4+ <200 cells/mm^3	CD4+ >200 and <350 cells/mm^3	CD4+ >350 cells/mm^3
VL <55,000 copies/mL	Recommend tx	Consider tx*	Defer tx
VL >55,000 copies/mL	Recommend tx	Recommend tx	Consider tx†

*Some experts would consider a delay in therapy given that <15% of patients in this category progress to AIDS at 3 years.

†Some experts would recommend starting therapy given that >30% of patients in this category progress to AIDS in 3 years, but others would observe patients with careful CD4 monitoring.

HAART, highly active antiretroviral therapy; tx, therapy; VL, viral load.

TABLE 7A. **Nucleoside Reverse Transcriptase Inhibitors**

NRTI*	Dose	Selected Side Effects
Zidovudine (AZT, Retrovir)	300 mg q12h	Gastrointestinal upset, headache, anemia, myopathy
Lamivudine (3TC, Epivir)	150 mg q12h	Minimal
Stavudine (d4T, Zerit)	40 mg q12h (if >60 kg), 30 mg q12h (if <60 kg)	Neuropathy, pancreatitis
Didanosine (ddI, Videx, Videx EC)	400 mg qd (if >60 kg); 125 mg q12h or 250 mg qd (if <60 kg or with TDF)	Neuropathy, gastrointestinal upset, pancreatitis†
Abacavir (ABC, Ziagen)	300 mg q12h	Hypersensitivity reaction‡
Tenofovir (TDF, Viread)	300 mg qd	GI upset, flatulence, headache
Dideoxycytidine (ddC, zalcitabine [Hivid])	0.75 mg tid	Peripheral neuropathy, pancreatitis, stomatitis§
Combivir (CBV, fixed combination AZT 300 mg and 3TC 150 mg)	1 pill q12h	As for individual drugs
Trizivir (TZV, fixed combination AZT 300 mg, 3TC 150 mg, and ABC 300 mg)	1 pill q12h	As for individual drugs

*All NRTIs can cause lactic acidosis and hepatic steatosis. Renal adjustments are available for all NRTIs except abacavir, tenofovir, and fixed combination formulations.

†Must be taken on an empty stomach. Doses are for tablets (chewed or dissolved), not powder. Videx EC is preferable because of improved tolerability.

‡The hypersensitivity reaction is characterized by abdominal pain, fever, rash, nausea, vomiting, and malaise. Do not rechallenge; the drug can be fatal if the patient discontinues and then restarts abacavir therapy if the patient has a history of hypersensitivity at any time. Most reactions occur within 6 weeks. Patients must be extensively educated about this side effect.

§ddC should be avoided because of its side effect profile and decreased efficacy.

TABLE 7B. **Non-Nucleoside Reverse Transcriptase Inhibitors**

NNRTI	Dose	Selected Side Effects
Efavirenz (EFV, Sustiva)	600 mg qhs	CNS effects,* rash
Nevirapine (NVP, Viramune)	200 mg qd × 14d, then 200 mg bid	Rash, hepatitis†
Delavirdine (DLV, Rescriptor)‡	400 mg q8h	Rash, headache

*CNS effects occur in 25% to 40% and consist of a feeling of dizziness, "disconnected" feeling, and strange dreams, all of which usually decrease within 2 weeks. It is recommended that efavirenz be given at bedtime, and the drug is contraindicated in pregnancy.

†The rash and hepatitis are more common in women. The hepatitis occurs within the first 4 weeks and can be fatal. Stevens-Johnson reaction is reported. Check liver function 2 to 4 weeks after starting therapy.

‡This regimen is used much less commonly because of q8h dosing and rash.

TABLE 7C. **Protease Inhibitors**

Protease Inhibitors	Dose	Selected Side Effects
Nelfinavir (NFV, Viracept)*	1250 mg q12h or 750 mg q8h	Diarrhea, gastrointestinal upset
Indinavir (IDV, Crixivan)†	800 mg q12h (with RTV, 100 or 200 mg q12h), or 800 mg q8h	Gastrointestinal upset, increased bilirubin, nephrolithiasis (take with 48 oz of water daily)
Saquinavir SGC (SQV-SGC, FTV, Fortovase)‡	1200 mg q8h, 400 mg q12h with RTV 400 mg q12h, or 1000 mg q12h with RTV 100 mg q12h	Gastrointestinal upset
Saquinavir HGC (SQV-HGC, INV, Invirase)‡	1000 mg q12h with RTV 100 mg q12h	Gastrointestinal upset but better tolerated than FTV; not recommended without RTV-boosting
Amprenavir (APV, Agenerase)§	1200 mg q12h, or 600-1200 mg q12h (with RTV, 100-200 mg q12h)	Rash, gastrointestinal intolerance
Lopinavir/ritonavir (LPV/r, Kaletra)	400/100 mg q12h (3 fixed-dose combination pills)	Gastrointestinal upset, diarrhea
Ritonavir (RTV, Norvir)‖	600 mg q12h	GI upset, hepatitis; not recommended as single PI

*Must be taken with food.

†An indinavir/ritonavir combination is preferred because of an improved dosing schedule and pharmacokinetic profile. Indinavir given alone must be taken on an empty stomach and separated from didanosine (ddI).

‡Saquinavir/ritonavir is preferred because of a smaller pill burden and an improved pharmacokinetic profile.

§Amprenavir alone is eight pills q12h. Administration with ritonavir decreases the pill burden.

#Increase the dose to 533/133 mg q12h when co-administrated with efavirenz and nevirapine.

‖Ritonavir is poorly tolerated at full dose and is primarily used to enhance serum levels of other protease inhibitors through cytochrome P-450 inhibition.

SGC, soft gel capsule; HGC, hard gel capsule.

TABLE 8. **Potential Choices for Initial HAART Regimens* (Choose a Dual NRTI Backbone and Either a PI, an NNRTI, or Abacavir†)**

Dual NRTI		PI
AZT + 3TC (Combivir)		Nelfinavir (Viracept)
d4T + 3TC		Lopinavir/ritonavir (Kaletra)
d4T + ddI‡	PLUS	Indinavir (Crixivan)/ritonavir (Norvir)
AZT + ddI§		Saquinavir (Invirase)/ritonavir (Norvir)
TDF + 3TC		**NNRTI**
		Efavirenz (Sustiva)‖
		Nevirapine (Viramune)¶
		Third NRTI
		ABC (with AZT + 3TC, as Trizivir)†

*This list does not contain all possible HAART regimens, but rather a list of those more commonly used in clinical practice.

†A triple NRTI regimen, AZT/3TC/ABC (Trizivir), can be considered in those with a viral load less than 100,000.

‡Higher risk of pancreatitis and neuropathy; risk of liver toxicity and lactic acidosis is higher in pregnant women; not commonly used because of its side effect profile.

§Not commonly used because of its side effect profile.

‖Contraindicated in pregnancy.

¶Nevirapine is less favorable because of a higher risk of hepatitis and rash, but has no CNS side effects compared with efavirenz.

HAART, highly active antiretroviral therapy; NRTI, nucleoside reverse transcriptase inhibitor; PI, protease inhibitor; NNRTI, non-nucleoside reverse transcriptase inhibitor; AZT, zidovudine (Retrovir); d4T, stavudine (Zerit); 3TC, lamivudine (Epivir); ddI, didanosine (Videx); TDF, tenofovir (Viread); ABC, abacavir (Ziagen).

expanded access programs or clinical trials, should be sought out. Even if a salvage regimen does not achieve ideal results based on viral load or CD4+ testing, it may have value. HAART is clinically beneficial to patients without optimal viral response or immune response and should be continued in patients with end-stage AIDS who have exhausted all therapeutic options unless a tolerable regimen cannot be constructed.

Adherence to Therapy

Although the previous section indicates that the decision to start and to change therapy is driven by laboratory values, it must be remembered that the only successful drug regimen is the one that a patient takes. Therefore, the most important factor in determining success of a regimen is patient adherence. The exceptional rate of mutation of HIV means that it can rapidly develop drug resistant forms of the virus when drug pressure is removed, even for a short while. Failing to take as few as 5% of the doses can greatly increase the probability of developing drug resistance. In concrete terms, a patient who is on a twice-a-day regimen who consistently misses a single dose in a 2-week period is at risk of developing drug resistance.

Therefore the only time to prescribe therapy is when the patient is ready to commit to meticulously following the therapeutic regimen. That being said, there is little to guide the determination of when a patient can be considered "ready" to start HAART. The patient is being asked to commit to treatment without first-hand knowledge of the consequences of therapy, which can include substantial alteration of one's lifestyle (e.g., eating at rigid times, fitting drug taking into already complex lives) and frequent or severe side effects. Because most patients will have some difficulty tolerating their drug regimens, a verbal commitment to start HAART needs to be reassessed after the patient has had some experience with the regimen. The primary guide to assess readiness is to make certain that the patient does not feel pressured by his or her physician to take therapy, as opposed to informed by the physician. If the patient is only starting to please the doctor, he or she is not ready and will likely fail to adhere to therapy. Negative consequences from poor adherence to therapy over time may be as severe as or more severe than the consequences of delaying therapy because of patient reluctance to initiate therapy. The physician must inform the patient of the risks and benefits of a starting versus delaying therapy. Patients must make the decision to initiate therapy freely and not simply in response to the physician's recommendation.

Numerous studies have been undertaken to identify predictors of adherence. None has identified a reliable way to predict adherence, nor can physicians reliably predict adherence. However, that does not mean that clinicians cannot assist patients in adhering. Regimens can be selected that minimally interfere with a patient's lifestyle. For example, one can avoid a regimen that is taken twice a day with meals for a patient who does not customarily eat breakfast. The patient should be fully informed of the likely side effects of drugs. Many antiretrovirals have side effects that moderate with time and patients are more likely to adhere if they know that the problems will subside in a few weeks. The clinician should anticipate common side effects and prescribe medication to manage those effects, which will both minimize side effects and increase the patient's trust in the physician. The physician should make the patient a full partner in selecting a regimen. Most patients should be seen 2 weeks after new antiretrovirals are started so side effects can be managed, adherence can be re-enforced, and modifications to therapy in response to severe side effects can be made early to minimize the development of resistance. Close monitoring and frank discussions with the patient are keys to success.

COMPLICATIONS OF ANTIRETROVIRAL THERAPY

As experience with antiretroviral therapy continues to accumulate, the toxicities of these drugs have been better recognized. Because therapy is prolonging survival, it has been particularly difficult to sort out the relative contribution of antiretrovirals to processes that occur with HIV and aging themselves, such as hyperlipidemias, fat redistribution, and coronary artery disease.

Neuropathy

Symptoms of peripheral neuropathy range from mild occasional pain or tingling in the feet to severe, constant, debilitating pain with numbness that results in inability to walk. Peripheral neuropathy can develop from HIV infection itself; however, dideoxycytidine (Hivid) (ddC), stavudine (Zerit) (d4T), and didanosine (Videx) (ddI) can all cause peripheral neuropathy, especially when used in combination in a patient with preexisting neuropathy. Dose reduction of the offending agents may relieve symptoms, and switching to other antiretrovirals should be considered. Nonsteroidal anti-inflammatory agents should be prescribed for mild symptoms and nortriptyline (Pamelor)* and gabapentin (Neurontin)* for moderate symptoms, with narcotics reserved for severe symptoms.

Lactic Acidosis

Symptoms of hyperlactatemia include abdominal pain, fatigue, nausea, and vomiting that can develop at any time while a patient is on chronic therapy. Although most cases of lactic acidosis have been associated with d4T, all NRTIs can cause the syndrome, which has a high fatality rate after the patient is frankly acidotic. Treatment is supportive and includes discontinuing NRTI therapy. Retreatment with HAART may be attempted after recovery, but NRTIs, especially d4T, should be avoided. Many patients on HAART develop asymptomatic hyperlactatemia, which generally should not be treated or prospectively ascertained.

Lipodystrophy and Metabolic Complications

Various lipodystrophy syndromes have been reported in patients with HIV, including central fat accumulation, visceral fat accumulation, facial and peripheral fat atrophy, lipomatosis, and hyperlipidemias. Management of hyperlipidemias in the HIV-infected patient is the same as in the uninfected patient, with attention to drug-drug interactions between HMG CoA reductase inhibitors and PIs and NRTIs. Treatment of the fat accumulation and atrophy disorders is uncertain, but may be helped by replacement of d4T with another antiretroviral if the patient is on that drug. Exercise and diet should be recommended. Hormonal therapies (growth hormone and testosterone) have been used to treat these conditions but are considered experimental.

Insulin resistance may develop in patients treated with PIs and occurs most often in those with central fat accumulation or a family history of diabetes. Switching to a PI-sparing regimen should be considered, and the use of metformin (Glucophage) or thiazolidinediones (such as rosiglitazone [Avandia] or pioglitazone [Actos]) may be beneficial in patients with both diabetes resulting from insulin resistance and central fat accumulation. Management of diabetes is the same as for the HIV-uninfected.

Osteonecrosis is a complication of HIV itself, but is more frequent in the HAART era, and most commonly involves the femoral or humeral heads, femoral condyles, proximal tibia, or bones of the hand and wrist. Osteoporosis and osteopenia may be increasing in HIV-infected populations. Treatment of these bone disorders is the same as for HIV-uninfected individuals.

Cardiovascular Disease

There is some evidence that HIV alone increases the risk of cardiovascular disease, and that treatment with PIs increases that risk further. Controversy exists, however, and more definitive studies are ongoing. In the meantime, many experts recommend aggressive management of cardiac risk factors in patients with HIV, including encouraging smoking cessation, weight loss, and exercise, and the treatment of hypertension, diabetes mellitus, and hyperlipidemias. HIV-specific guidelines for the management of cardiac risk factors and cardiac disease have not been developed, and providers should follow general population guidelines.

Drug-Drug Interactions

Drugs commonly used to treat HIV-infected people often interact with each other. This interaction can be exploited to benefit the patient. For example, low-dose ritonavir (Norvir) boosts levels of other PIs, allowing longer dosing intervals and fewer dietary restrictions. The antiretroviral drugs can also interact with literally dozens of different medications. These include calcium channel blockers, lipid lowering agents, antihistamines, gastrointestinal drugs, neuroleptics, psychotropics, oral contraceptives, anticonvulsants, methadone, antimycobacterials, antibiotics, antifungals, and antivirals, among others. Those who are treating an HIV-infected person should consult appropriate references, such as www.aidsinfo.nih.gov, when considering prescribing any medications, especially a medication metabolized through the cytochrome P450 system.

OPPORTUNISTIC INFECTIONS

Because immunosuppression can lead to the failure of the immune system to eliminate, contain, or suppress almost any new or commensal organism, HIV infection can lead to a wide variety of infectious processes. This review will cover the most common of these opportunistic infections. In addition, although syphilis and the forms of hepatitis are not strictly opportunistic infections, they are briefly discussed because of their frequency in HIV-infected patients.

Pneumocystis carinii Pneumonia (PCP)

Before the widespread use of prophylaxis for PCP and the development of HAART, PCP was the most common AIDS-defining condition and the leading cause of death in HIV-infected people. It is still regularly seen as a presenting condition in patients newly diagnosed with HIV infection or in those who have not adhered to their HAART regimen. *Pneumocystis* causes a subacute pneumonia that progresses to severe disease in people with HIV and low CD4 counts,

*Not FDA approved for this indication.

especially counts below 200 cells/mm^3. Patients commonly present with slowly progressive dyspnea on exertion and nonproductive cough with fever. Physical exam is usually unremarkable, although crackles may be heard on chest auscultation. Resting room air pulse oximetry may be normal, but should be checked with ambulation or stair-climbing, as desaturations with exertion suggest the diagnosis. Chest radiography typically shows bilateral interstitial infiltrates, although it may be normal in as many as one third of cases. Nodular infiltrates, focal infiltrates, and, especially in the person receiving aerosolized pentamidine PCP prophylaxis, lower lobe disease are not uncommon. Diagnosis rests on demonstrating the fungus in pulmonary specimens. A positive induced sputum can be diagnostic, although the sensitivity of the procedure is not high. In contrast, the sensitivity of bronchoalveolar lavage is more than 95%. Although it is not unreasonable to empirically treat at-risk patients with consistent signs and symptoms of PCP, failure to respond in 1 or 2 weeks or presence of severe disease should prompt an invasive diagnostic workup to establish a definitive diagnosis, because the differential diagnosis for fever and pulmonary infiltrates in a patient with HIV is long and includes tuberculosis, typical and atypical pneumonia, endemic fungi, pulmonary Kaposi's sarcoma, and many other diseases, both infectious and noninfectious. The treatment and prophylaxis choices for PCP are shown in Table 9.

Toxoplasmic Encephalitis

Toxoplasma gondii is an intracellular parasite transmitted by the ingestion of undercooked meat products or material contaminated by infected cat or dog feces. Most nonimmunocompromised hosts are

TABLE 9. **Treatment of *Pneumocystis carinii* Pneumonia (PCP)**

Regimens*	Side Effects
Acute Infection	
First Choice	
Trimethoprim/sulfamethoxazole (Bactrim, Septra), 15 mg/kg/d IV or PO trimethoprim and 75 mg/kg/d of sulfamethoxazole divided q6-8h × 21d†	Neutropenia, rash, GI upset, increased creatinine and potassium
Alternatives	
Pentamidine (Pentam), 4 mg/kg IV qd × 21‡	Pancreatitis, hypoglycemia, hyperglycemia, rash, neutropenia, decreased blood pressure, conduction abnormalities.
Clindamycin (Cleocin),*** 600 mg IV q8h or 300-450 mg PO q6h + primaquine,*** 15 mg base PO qd × 21d‡§	GI upset, neutropenia, diarrhea, *Clostridium difficile*
Trimethoprim (Primsol),*** 15 mg/kg PO divided q8 + dapsone,*** 100 mg PO qd × 21d§	Rash, pruritus, GI upset, hemolytic anemia (dapsone)
Trimetrexate (NeuTrexin), 45 mg/m^2 IV qd, and folinic acid (leucovorin), 20 mg/m^2 PO/IV q6h, ± dapsone, 100 mg PO qd × 21d	Neutropenia, rash, fever
Atovaquone (Mepron), 750 mg PO bid × 21d	GI upset, rash
Prophylaxis‖	
First Choice	
Trimethoprim/sulfamethoxazole (Bactrim, Septra) 1 DS or 1 SS tablet PO qd¶	Neutropenia, rash, GI upset, increased creatinine and potassium
Alternatives	
Dapsone,*** 100 mg PO qd	Rash, neutropenia, hemolytic anemia
Dapsone, 50 mg PO qd, pyrimethamine (Daraprim),*** 50 mg PO qwk, + leucovorin, 25 mg PO qwk	Rash, GI upset, hemolytic anemia, megaloblastic anemia, neutropenia
Dapsone, 200 mg PO qwk, pyrimethamine, 75 mg PO qwk, and leucovorin, 25 mg PO qwk**	Rash, GI upset, hemolytic anemia, megaloblastic anemia, neutropenia
Atovaquone (Mepron), 750 mg PO bid (liquid)	GI upset, rash
Aerosolized pentamidine (NebuPent), 300 mg aerosolized via Respirgard II Nebulizer monthly††	Cough (can give inhaled beta-agonist)
Trimethoprim/sulfamethoxazole, 1 DS PO three times weekly	Neutropenia, rash, GI upset, increased creatinine and potassium

*Check arterial blood gases before starting therapy. When Pa_{O_2} is less than 70 or the alveolar-arterial gradient is greater than 35, use prednisone, 40 mg PO bid for 5 days, then 40 mg qd for 5 days, then 20 mg qd for 11 days regardless of the regimen (administer 30 minutes before the first dose of antibiotic).

†This regimen has the most experience in the treatment of PCP and should be used if possible. Consider desensitization in patients with history of sulfa allergy.

‡This regimen can be used for patients who are allergic to sulfonamides with severe disease.

§Consider using these regimens for patients with mild to moderate PCP who are allergic to sulfonamides. These regimens are equally efficacious.

‖Secondary prophylaxis is required after treatment. Primary and secondary PCP prophylaxis can be stopped after the patient has started highly active antiretroviral therapy and is controlling viral replication with a CD4+ count >200 cells/mm^3 for >3 months.

¶Most efficacious PCP prophylaxis regimen.

**Only trimethoprim-sulfamethoxazole at a dose of 1 DS daily and dapsone/pyrimethamine/leucovorin protect against toxoplasmosis.

††Pneumocystis infection in the apices and extrapulmonary sites can develop in patients receiving this regimen, and it is less effective when the CD4+ count is less than 50.

***Not FDA approved for this indication.

GI, gastrointestinal; DS, double strength; SS, single strength.

asymptomatic, but with immunosuppression the disease can activate, manifesting in the central nervous system. Patients may present with headache, altered mental status, fever, focal neurologic signs, or seizures, and most will have a CD4 count below 100 cells/mm^3. Most patients will have multiple ring-enhancing lesions with mass effect on neuroimaging, typically involving the basal ganglia and corticomedullary junction. Cerebrospinal fluid (CSF) analysis will be unremarkable. An AIDS patient with symptoms or signs of meningoencephalitis should undergo brain imaging before lumbar puncture to rule out significant mass effect that would contraindicate the removal of CSF. More than 95% of patients diagnosed with toxoplasmic encephalitis will have serum IgG antibodies to *Toxoplasma*, although their absence does not rule out the disease, because some patients may have lost the antibody, and others may be presenting with acute toxoplasmosis rather than reactivation disease.

Treatment of toxoplasmosis is often presumptive because definitive diagnosis requires brain biopsy. The treatment and prophylaxis choices for toxoplasmosis are shown in Table 10. If a patient demonstrates clinical improvement after 1 week of empiric therapy, the diagnosis is established and treatment should be completed. Failure to improve clinically by 2 weeks should prompt consideration of other diagnoses, including central nervous system lymphoma, brain abscess, or progressive multifocal leukoencephalopathy, and single photon emission computed tomography imaging and brain biopsy may be necessary. Glucocorticoids may be needed to control edema, but make assessment of clinical improvement difficult. Radiographic improvement may lag behind clinical improvement. Anticonvulsants should be used if seizures are frequent. Secondary prophylaxis after treatment for acute disease is needed. Primary prophylaxis for toxoplasmosis should be offered to all patients with a CD4 count lower than

TABLE 10. **Treatment of *Toxoplasma gondii* Infection**

Regimens	Side Effects
Treatment*	
First Choice	
Pyrimethamine (Daraprim), 200 mg PO × 1, then 75-100 mg PO qd, + folinic acid (leucovorin), 10 mg PO qd, + sulfadiazine, 1-2 g PO q6h × 6 wk	Megaloblastic anemia, neutropenia, rash pruritus
Alternative	
Pyrimethamine + folinic acid (leucovorin) as above + Clindamycin (Cleocin),** 900 mg IV q6h or 600 mg PO q6h × 6 wk†	Megaloblastic anemia, neutropenia, diarrhea, *Clostridium difficile*
Pyrimethamine + folinic acid (leucovorin) as above and one of the following: azithromycin (Zithromax),** 1200-1500 mg qd, or clarithromycin (Biaxin),** 1 g PO bid or atovaquone (Mepron),** 750 mg PO qid	Megaloblastic anemia, neutropenia, GI upset, rash
Suppression‡	
First Choice	
Pyrimethamine, 25-75 mg qd + folinic acid 10 mg qd, + sulfadiazine, 0.5-1.0 g PO q6h§	Megaloblastic anemia, neutropenia, rash, pruritus
Alternative	
Pyrimethamine + folinic acid (leucovorin) 10 mg PO qd + clindamycin (Cleocin),** 300-450 mg PO q6h§	Megaloblastic anemia, neutropenia, diarrhea, Clostridium difficile
Prophylaxis‖	
Primary	
Trimethoprim/sulfamethoxazole, DS tablet PO qd	Neutropenia, rash, GI upset, increased creatinine and potassium
Alternative	
Dapsone,** 50 mg PO qd, + pyrimethamine 50 mg PO qwk, + folinic acid (leucovorin), 25 mg PO qwk	Rash, nausea/vomiting, hemolytic anemia (check G6PD level)
Dapsone, 200 mg PO qwk, pyrimethamine, 75 mg PO qwk, and folinic acid, 25 mg PO qwk	Rash, nausea/vomiting, hemolytic anemia (check G6PD level)
Trimethoprim/sulfamethoxazole, 1 SS tablet PO qd or 1 DS tablet PO three times weekly	Neutropenia, rash, GI upset, increased creatinine and potassium
Atovaquone (Mepron)** 1500 mg PO qd ± pyrimethamine 25 mg PO qd + folinic acid (leucovorin) 10 mg PO qd	GI upset, rash, megaloblastic anemia, neutropenia

*Dexamethasone (Decadron), 4 mg IV q6h for significant brain edema/mass effect.
†This is the preferred alternative.
‡Suppressive therapy is lifelong, but may be discontinued if all of the following have been achieved: successful completion of initial therapy, resolution of symptoms and radiographic evidence of edema, and a CD4 count of greater than 200 for 6 months with viral suppression.
§Clindamycin/pyrimethamine/leucovorin does not prevent *Pneumocystis carinii* pneumonia, while the sulfadiazine regimen does.
‖Primary prophylaxis may be discontinued after a CD4+ count of greater than 200 for 3 months and viral suppression have been achieved.
**Not FDA approved for this indication.
G6PD, glucose-6-phosphate dehydrogenase.

100 cells/mm^3, and people seronegative for *Toxoplasma* IgG should avoid cat litter and the consumption of undercooked meats.

Tuberculosis

After a person with HIV is infected with *Mycobacterium tuberculosis*, his or her risk of developing active tuberculosis disease is about 10% per year, in contrast to the risk of people without HIV, who have a 10% lifetime risk. Thus identification of people at high risk for tuberculosis disease is important, and all HIV-infected people should have baseline skin testing. People at high risk for exposure to tuberculosis (injection drug users, long-term residents of correctional facilities, and homeless individuals) should undergo yearly skin testing. Because a severely immunocompromised patient may fail to mount an immune response to the skin test, leading to a false negative result, some experts recommend retesting a previously negative individual after the CD4 cell count has been restored to more than 200 cells/mm^3. A positive test is induration of 5 mm or greater in the HIV-infected population but the absence of induration does not rule out tuberculosis. In addition, any HIV-infected person with prolonged contact with an infectious tuberculosis case should be treated with prophylaxis, regardless of the skin test result. People meeting these criteria should be evaluated for active disease and, if determined to have latent disease, offered treatment, regardless of their age. Preferred prophylaxis is with isoniazid (INH) for 9 months with supplemental pyridoxine (Vitamin B_6), although pyrazinamide combined with rifampin or rifabutin (Mycobutin)* for 2 months may be used, with attention to drug interactions and hepatotoxicity.

Patients with active tuberculosis will present with subacute or chronic symptoms, including cough, fever, weight loss, and fatigue, although some patients may be asymptomatic, detected only on screening skin testing and radiography. The radiographic findings include focal disease, cavitary disease, miliary disease, apical disease, or hilar adenopathy, and, in some cases, no abnormalities. Extrapulmonary disease may accompany pulmonary disease or may be the sole manifestation of tuberculosis. The prevalence of extrapulmonary disease increases as the CD4 cell count decreases. Treatment of tuberculosis is detailed elsewhere in this book, and guidance is also available at www.aidsinfo.nih.gov. All people with active tuberculosis and HIV should be treated with directly observed therapy containing either three or four drugs, depending on the local prevalence of isoniazid drug resistance. Paradoxic worsening of tuberculosis can occur in any person treated for tuberculosis, but appears to be more frequent in people with HIV who are also receiving HAART. This type of immune reconstitution phenomenon should not prompt discontinuation of HAART or antituberculosis therapy, and should be managed symptomatically or, in extreme cases, with corticosteroids. Rifampin and rifabutin have substantial interactions with PIs and NNRTIs, and expert consultation is advised when treating the HIV-infected person with active tuberculosis. Secondary prophylaxis after successful treatment of active or latent tuberculosis is not needed.

*Not FDA approved for this indication.

Disseminated *Mycobacterium avium* Complex (MAC) Infection

M. avium complex bacteria are commonly found in food and water. Disseminated infection is most common in patients with CD4 cell counts lower than 50 cells/mm^3. Patients present with fever, night sweats, weight loss, diffuse abdominal pain, and diarrhea. Examination may reveal diffuse lymphadenopathy, hepatosplenomegaly, and abdominal tenderness. Severe or acute abdominal signs, such as guarding or rebound, should suggest an alternative diagnosis. Laboratory analysis may reveal anemia or pancytopenia from marrow infiltration or elevated alkaline phosphatase from liver involvement. Diagnosis is established by mycobacterial blood cultures, which will be positive in most cases, bone marrow biopsy and culture, or lymph node biopsy and culture. The treatment and prophylaxis choices and their alternatives for MAC are shown in Table 11. Clarithromycin (Biaxin) is the most active agent against MAC, but resistance develops and another agent (ethambutol [Myambutol]* or rifabutin [Mycobutin]) must be given concomitantly, especially in the person who has failed macrolide prophylaxis. Fluoroquinolones* are also active against MAC. Prophylaxis should be offered to anyone with a CD4 cell count lower than 50 cells/mm^3. An immune reconstitution syndrome with MAC may develop as with tuberculosis, where symptoms and signs of the infection may worsen on initiation of HAART.

Candidiasis

Candida organisms are common on the skin and mucosal surfaces. In immunosuppressed people, these organisms can become pathogens of the oropharyngeal, esophageal, and vulvovaginal mucosa. Oropharyngeal candidiasis is described in Table 12. Primary treatment is with topical agents such as nystatin (Mycostatin) or clotrimazole (Lotrimin). Brief courses of fluconazole (Diflucan) may be needed for patients with severe or recurrent disease, but are discouraged because of the possibility of promoting azole resistance. Vaginal candidiasis will present as a typical yeast infection with thin discharge and vaginal irritation in women with any CD4 cell count. Topical therapy is preferred, although single-dose fluconazole (150 mg) is also effective. Esophageal candidiasis will be manifest as odynophagia, and 70% of patients with esophageal candidiasis will have concomitant oral thrush and most will have a CD4 count lower than 100 cells/mm^3. Treatment is with fluconazole 200 mg daily* for 2 to 3 weeks. Failure to respond indicates resistance or

*Not FDA approved for this indication.

TABLE 11. **Treatment of *Mycobacterium avium* Complex (MAC) infection**

Regimens	Side Effects
Treatment*	
First Choice	
Clarithromycin (Biaxin), 500 mg PO bid,† ethambutol (Myambutol),** 15 mg/kg/d PO, ± rifabutin‡ (Mycobutin), 300 mg qd PO	GI upset (Biaxin, Zithromax); optic neuritis, needs ophthalmologic follow-up (ethambutol); uveitis, GI upset and leukopenia (rifampin)
Alternative	
Can substitute azithromycin (Zithromax), 500-600 mg PO qd for clarithromycin	GI upset
Prophylaxis*	
First Choice	
Clarithromycin, 500 mg PO bid† or azithromycin, 1200 mg PO qwk	GI upset
Alternative	
Rifabutin, 300 mg PO qd‡	Leukopenia, GI upset, uveitis
Azithromycin, 1200 mg PO qwk, and rifabutin, 300 mg PO qd‡	Leukopenia, GI upset, uveitis

*Treatment for patients with disseminated MAC is lifelong. Primary prophylaxis for MAC may be discontinued if the CD4 cell count remains above 100 cells/mm^3 for >3 months. Secondary prophylaxis may be discontinued if the patient has completed 1 year of therapy, is asymptomatic and culture negative, and the CD4 cell count has been >100 cells/mm^3 for >6 months.

†Clarithromycin levels are altered in the presence of rifabutin, and rifabutin levels are significantly increased by clarithromycin.

‡Rifabutin interacts strongly with protease inhibitors and non-nucleoside reverse transcriptase inhibitors, so dose modification of both drugs is required; check the drug insert before concomitant use. For prophylaxis, rifabutin and azithromycin is less well tolerated than azithromycin alone, while rifabutin alone is less efficacious than a macrolide alone.

**Not FDA approved for this indication.

GI, gastrointestinal.

another etiology for the odynophagia. Retreatment with itraconazole (Sporanox) or amphotericin B (Fungizone)* can be considered in those with a history of recurrent exposure to fluconazole. Esophagoscopy is indicated to establish a diagnosis in those who fail to respond to empiric therapy, because the differential diagnosis of esophagitis in these patients also includes herpes, cytomegalovirus, aphthous ulcers, and other less common disorders. Suppressive therapy in patients with recurrent disease may be indicated until the immune system is restored, but should not be undertaken lightly because it may promote azole resistance. Primary prophylaxis works, but it is generally not recommended.

Cryptococcosis

Cryptococcus neoformans is a fungus commonly found in the environment. It can cause meningitis that presents with severe headache, fever, altered mental status, meningismus, and nausea and vomiting (from increased intracranial pressure) in a patient with a CD4 cell count lower than 100 cells/mm^3. A headache may be the only presenting sign or symptom. If focal signs, seizure, or altered mental status are present, the differential diagnosis includes mass lesions (such as toxoplasmosis and lymphoma), and imaging with contrast is recommended before lumbar puncture. Patients with cryptococcal meningitis will have no mass lesions on imaging but may have hydrocephalic changes. On lumbar puncture, the opening pressure will be elevated and should be recorded. Cell counts may show a mild monocytic leukocytosis, but may be entirely normal, as may be the glucose and protein levels. CSF cryptococcal antigen testing has a high sensitivity (95%) and the titer of the antigen can be followed to assess response to therapy; culture is nearly always positive as well. Therapy is with amphotericin B (Fungizone) (0.7-1.0 mg/kg/d IV) with flucytosine (Ancobon) (25 mg/kg every 6 hours PO) for 14 days of induction therapy, followed by fluconazole (Diflucan) 400 mg/d PO for 8 weeks, then fluconazole 200 mg/d as secondary prophylaxis. There is less experience with lipid amphotericin formulations (AmBisome and others), but they may be needed in people undergoing prolonged therapy or with pre-existing renal disease. In patients who have a normal mental status at diagnosis, a CSF white cell count higher than 20 cells/mm^3 (indicating a more robust immune response), and a CSF cryptococcal antigen titer less than 1:1024, oral fluconazole 400 to 800 mg/d PO for 6 to 8 weeks may be used initially, followed by suppressive therapy. In azotemic patients, flucytosine may cause cytopenias, nausea, vomiting, diarrhea, rash, hepatitis, and peripheral neuropathy, so serum levels of flucytosine should be monitored. Patients will often show symptomatic improvement after a diagnostic lumbar puncture because of the removal of fluid and resultant drop in intracranial pressure. Many patients will need daily therapeutic lumbar puncture to decrease intracranial pressure during the course of therapy, and with each tap the pressure should be lowered to less than 20 cm of H_2O or by 50%. After the induction phase of therapy a repeat lumbar puncture should be performed and if

*Not FDA approved for this indication.

TABLE 12. **Oral Manifestations of HIV Infection**

Condition	Location	Clinical Features	Diagnosis	Treatment
White or Yellowish–White Nonulcerative Lesions				
Pseudomembranous candidiasis—Thrush (common)	Palate, buccal and labial mucosa, and dorsal tongue	Curd-like raised painless lesions	Culture, biopsy or response to antifungals	Topical or systemic antifungals Recurrences common
Angular cheilitis caused by *Candida* infection (common)	Corners of the mouth	Macerated white radiating fissures, occasionally erythematous	Biopsy or response to antifungals	Topical or systemic antifungals Recurrences common
Candidal leukoplakia (less common)	Tongue	Painful, raised white lesion that does not rub off looks like oral hairy leukoplakia	Biopsy or response to antifungals	Topical or systemic antifungals Recurrences common
Oral hairy leukoplakia (common)	Lateral tongue, buccal mucosa	Painless raised white lesion that does not rub off; hairy "fingers" may lead from lesion	Biopsy or response to therapy	Acyclovir** Recurrences common
Human papillomavirus—warts (relatively rare)	Anywhere in the oral and perioral area	Spike-like projections, cauliflower masses or plaques that do not rub off	Biopsy	Podophyllin resin (Podocon-25), surgical excision, laser treatment
Red or Purplish–Red Nonulcerative Lesions				
Kaposi's sarcoma (common)	Hard palate or gingiva	Red or purple macules, papules, nodules that progress to bulky tumors	Biopsy. Kaposi's sarcoma may also be evident in skin or viscera	Surgical resection; radiotherapy; intralesional or systemic chemotherapy
Erythematous candidiasis (relatively rare)	Palate, buccal and labial mucosa and tongue	May be diffuse or discrete red lesion with painful or burning sensation	Biopsy or response to antifungals	Antifungal medications
Non-Hodgkin's lymphoma (rare)	Lymphoid tissue of gingiva, palate or tonsillar region	Firm, focal swelling or poorly defined alveolar masses	Biopsy	Systemic chemotherapy, surgical removal
Squamous cell carcinoma (rare)	Anywhere in oral cavity	Shiny violaceous lesions, variable	Biopsy	Surgical resection, radiotherapy or chemotherapy
Oral Ulcers				
Aphthous ulcers—Canker sores (idiopathic) (common)	Nonkeratinized (movable) surfaces	Painful well circumscribed shallow ulcers that deepen with time	Biopsy or visual appearance	Small ulcers respond to steroids; thalidomide (Thalmid)** for severe disease*
Herpes simplex ulcers—cold sores (common)	Hard palate, gingiva, lips and perioral area.	Begins as vesicular lesions that may coalesce into large erosive ulcerations	Biopsy or culture	Antiherpes drugs
Cytomegalovirus infections (rare)	Oral mucosa	Painful punched out lesions with non-indurated borders	Biopsy	Ganciclovir (Cytovene)** may be helpful
Herpes zoster (rare)	Appears along the trigeminal nerve.	Vesicular-erosive eruptions accompanied by severe pain	Viral culture	Antiviral medications may help reduce intensity of lesion
Structures with Abnormal Appearance				
Linear gingival erythema (common)	Gingiva	Bright red tissue at the margin of the teeth and gum; painless	Characteristic appearance	Aggressive plaque removal. Meticulous oral hygiene
Necrotizing gingivitis/periodontitis (less common)	Gingiva and underlying bone	Inflamed gums, pain, and loose teeth to the point of falling out	Appearance	Plaque removal, surgical débridement, antibiotics, oral hygiene
Other Conditions				
Xerostomia (less common)	Oral cavity	Poor salivary flow	Patient history, multiple caries	Saliva substitutes
Dental caries (very common)	Teeth	Multiple rapidly progressing caries which may be accompanied by pain, sensitivity to hot and cold	Visualization, dental exam	Fillings, meticulous oral hygiene, regular dental exams and oral hygiene education

*Thalidomide is contraindicated in pregnant women because it causes severe birth defects. It can only be used in people of child-bearing potential if strict contraception is insured.

**Not FDA approved for this indication.

Adapted from: Weinert M, Grimes RM, Lynch DP: Oral manifestations of HIV infection. Ann Intern Med 125:485-496, 1996; and Grimes RM, Stevenson GC: Oropharyngeal lesions in AIDS. Gastrointest Endosc Clin of North Am 8:783-809, 1998.

the CSF is still culture-positive, a longer induction phase may be needed. Serum cryptococcal antigens are positive in almost all cases of cryptococcal meningitis, but do not correlate with response to therapy. Primary prophylaxis with fluconazole is effective but does not improve overall survival, is expensive, and is associated with candidal azole resistance and drug-drug interactions, so is not recommended. Secondary prophylaxis may be discontinued after successful cryptococcal meningitis treatment if the patient has a sustained response to HAART with a CD4 cell count higher than 100 to 200 cells/mm^3 for more than 6 months.

Histoplasmosis and Coccidioidomycosis

Both of these endemic fungal infections can cause disseminated diseases in AIDS patients resembling tuberculosis. *Histoplasma capsulatum* is found in the environment in the Ohio and Mississippi river valleys and the Midwest, particularly in Indiana and Kansas City, as well as Puerto Rico. Diagnosis is by culture of sputum, blood, or bone marrow, or by urinary antigen detection. Treatment is with amphotericin (Fungizone) followed by itraconazole (Sporanox) maintenance therapy, and primary prophylaxis is not indicated but may be considered for those in hyperendemic areas or with significant occupational exposure to bird or bat droppings and CD4 cell counts lower than 100 cells/mm^3. *Coccidioides immitis* is endemic in the southwestern United States, and causes significant disseminated disease in patients with advanced immunosuppression. Diagnosis is by culture of pulmonary specimens, blood, bone marrow, or cerebrospinal fluid, or by serum IgG titer. Treatment is with amphotericin followed by fluconazole (Diflucan)* or itraconazole.* Patients with meningeal involvement should receive amphotericin with fluconazole initially. Maintenance therapy with an azole is required. Little data are available to recommend discontinuation of chronic suppressive treatment.

Cytomegalovirus (CMV)

CMV, a common herpes virus, can cause rapid blindness resulting from retinitis in people with CD4 cell counts lower than 50 cells/mm^3. Symptoms suggesting retinitis include increased "floaters," decreased visual acuity, and sudden loss of vision resulting from retinal detachment. All patients with a CD4 count lower than 50 cells/mm^3 should undergo a baseline ophthalmologic exam to detect and treat early disease. CMV infection is disseminated, and may also cause a periventricular encephalitis, pneumonitis, esophagitis, enteritis, colitis, proctitis, and rectal and oral ulcers. Therapeutic options include systemic ganciclovir (Cytovene) with or without intraocular ganciclovir implants (Vitrasert), foscarnet (Foscavir), cidofovir (Vistide), valganciclovir (Valcyte), and fomivirsen intravitreal injection (Vitravene). Acyclovir (Zovirax)* and valacyclovir (Valtrex)* are not useful. Therapy for CMV infection should be undertaken with expert assistance. Primary prophylaxis is generally not used because of the toxicity and cost of many of these agents. Secondary prophylaxis may be discontinued in patients with stable ocular disease, sustained increase in CD4 cell count to higher than 100 to 150 cells/mm^3 for more than 6 months, and ability to obtain regular ophthalmologic exams. A decision to discontinue secondary prophylaxis should be made in concert with the patient and the ophthalmologist.

Hepatitis C Virus (HCV) and Hepatitis B Virus (HBV) Infection

HCV can cause a progressive liver disease that may result in cirrhosis over decades. The course of HCV disease is accelerated by co-infection with HIV. HCV infection is common in HIV-infected intravenous drug users, with co-infection rates of 80%. HCV infection is suggested by IgG antibody positivity, though HCV RNA viral load should be assessed to confirm chronic active infection. People with HCV co-infection may be at higher risk of hepatic damage from PIs or NNRTIs, but HAART should not be withheld on that basis. All people with HCV should be counseled that alcohol consumption may dramatically increase the pace of the liver disease. Treatment of HCV is the same as in the HIV-uninfected population, though given the high prevalence of depression, substance abuse, and cytopenias in the co-infected population, interferon (Intron A) and ribavirin (Rebetol) are often contraindicated or poorly tolerated.

All people with HIV should be screened for active HBV, indicated by hepatitis B surface antigenemia. Patients without chronic active infection who are hepatitis surface antibody negative should be immunized against HBV. People chronically infected with HBV should be treated with an antiretroviral regimen that includes either lamivudine (3TC) (Epivir) or tenofovir (Viread), or perhaps both, if HIV treatment is indicated. If HIV treatment is not indicated, HBV-specific therapy should be considered on an individual basis, but mono or dual therapy with 3TC or tenofovir for HBV is not recommended because the patient's HIV will likely develop resistance to those agents.

Progressive Multifocal Leukoencephalopathy (PML) and HIV Dementia

PML is due to JC virus infection, and occurs in AIDS patients with CD4 cell counts lower than 100 cells/mm^3. Patients will present with chronically progressive cognitive and motor dysfunction. MRI reveals diffuse white matter disease. No specific therapy is available, although clinical improvements in this otherwise fatal disease have been noted with HAART. HIV dementia is a chronic progressive dementia resulting from HIV or other unidentified pathogens resulting in brain atrophy. Improvements have been noted in patients treated with HAART, and agents that penetrate into the central nervous system well, such as zidovudine (Retrovir) (AZT) and efavirenz (Sustiva), may be preferred.

*Not FDA approved for this indication.

Oral Manifestations of HIV Infection

More than 90% of HIV infected individuals who are not receiving HAART will experience at least one oral manifestation of HIV at some time in the course of their disease. Treatment of these lesions is crucial to patient comfort and to avoiding dehydration and the HIV wasting syndrome. Patients with oral pain are far less likely to eat and drink and may be less likely to adhere to a pill regimen and may have difficulty maintaining proper nutrition and hydration. Because oral diseases are located in a part of the body that can be visualized, they can be easily seen and diagnosis can be made by the characteristic appearance of the lesion or its location. Most oral manifestations are diagnosed by sight or by successful, empirical treatment. Excellent pictures of most oral manifestations of HIV infection can be found at www.hivdent.org/slides/index.htm. Common oral manifestations of HIV are outlined in Table 12. For most conditions there are curative treatments, and palliation can be achieved in all conditions. However, the successful management of these conditions requires a strong working arrangement between the treating physician and a dentist, and all HIV-infected people should be referred to a dentist, preferably one experienced in the care of HIV-infected patients. Because they are more prone to common dental disease such as caries and gingivitis, HIV-infected patients should be seen more frequently by a dentist than should the noninfected person.

Syphilis

Although not truly an opportunistic infection, syphilis is a concern among HIV-infected individuals because of an accelerated course in this population and because genital syphilitic lesions promote the transmission of HIV. Benzathine penicillin G (Bicillin L-A) 2.4 million units IM is the treatment of choice for primary, secondary, and early latent (<1 year) syphilis, whereas 3 weekly doses are required for late latent syphilis or syphilis of unknown duration. Patients with neurologic symptoms, late latent syphilis, latent syphilis of unknown duration, or inadequate serologic response to treatment of early disease (<4-fold drop in RPR titer at 6 months) should undergo lumbar puncture. If the CSF is positive by the Venereal Disease Research Laboratory test, then neurosyphilis is diagnosed and aqueous penicillin G 4 million units every 4 hours IV should be administered for 10 to 14 days, followed by 2.4 million units of benzathine penicillin IM given once. Patients with a history of penicillin allergy should undergo skin testing, and, if positive, should be desensitized. Ceftriaxone (Rocephin)* may be an acceptable alternative to penicillin, but data are limited, and penicillin is the treatment of choice for all stages of syphilis in HIV-infected people.

*Not FDA approved for this indication.

Malignancies

HHV-8 Infection (Kaposi's Sarcoma-Associated Herpesvirus)

Infection with HHV-8 causes Kaposi's sarcoma in people with AIDS, which can involve the skin and the mucosal surfaces of the respiratory or gastrointestinal tract. HHV-8 is most common in homosexual men, who are thus at greatest risk for Kaposi's sarcoma. The typical lesion is a violaceous plaque that may be raised, and could be confused with bacillary angiomatosis. Biopsy is necessary for diagnosis. Minor cutaneous lesions may be managed expectantly or with local therapy, but severe disease or visceral disease should be treated with chemotherapy or radiation. HAART has resulted in stabilization and even reversal of lesions, even without chemotherapy or radiation therapy. No antiviral prophylaxis is available to treat HHV-8.

Human Papillomavirus-Associated Malignancy

Women with HIV are at high risk of developing invasive cervical cancer if co-infected with certain strains of human papillomavirus. Initially, all women should undergo a pelvic examination with Papanicolaou smear, repeated at 6 months if results are negative, then yearly thereafter. Positive or indeterminate results should be handled as in the HIV-uninfected population. Human papillomavirus causes anal carcinoma in recipients of anal intercourse, and there is growing evidence that populations at risk should be screened with anal cytology smears as well, although there is of yet no recommendation.

Other Malignancies

Because survival for patients with HIV has increased, it has become apparent that HIV infection predisposes to other malignancies as well. Non-Hodgkin's lymphoma is now a relatively common AIDS-defining condition, and the risk in HIV-infected patients is many times higher than in noninfected people. Burkitt's lymphomas are aggressive lymphomas that respond poorly to treatment. Primary central nervous system lymphoma will present similarly to toxoplasmosis. All of these lymphomas are associated with Epstein-Barr virus (EBV), though the EBV is not active and anti-EBV therapy has no role in their management. Hodgkin's disease, although not AIDS-defining, is more common in HIV-infected patients than in HIV-uninfected people. Primary effusion lymphomas are associated with HHV-8. The treatment of all of these malignancies is improved if effective HAART is administered.

AMEBIASIS

method of
KEVIN C. KAIN, M.D.
University of Toronto and UHN-Toronto General Hospital
Toronto, Ontario, Canada

and

ANDREA K. BOGGILD, M.D.
University of Toronto
Toronto, Ontario, Canada

Amebiasis, caused by the protozoan parasite *Entamoeba histolytica*, accounts for an estimated 40 million to 50 million cases of colitis and liver abscess, resulting in 100,000 deaths annually. After malaria, amebiasis is the second leading cause of protozoan death in the world. While *E. histolytica* has a worldwide distribution, its prevalence is overrepresented in the developing world. In North America, *E. histolytica* infection is most commonly observed in immigrants from and travelers to developing countries. Amebiasis is typically acquired by ingesting food and water contaminated with fecal matter containing *E. histolytica* cysts. Control and prevention strategies are therefore similar to those for other food- and water-borne diarrheal organisms. Transmission in urban settings most frequently occurs in institutions such as daycares, nursing homes, residences for the developmentally challenged, and psychiatric facilities.

It has been recognized that *E. histolytica* (Eh) has a morphologically identical although genetically distinct sister species, *Entamoeba dispar* (Ed). Whereas Eh is the causative agent of invasive amebic colitis and amebic liver abscess (ALA), Ed is a gut commensal resulting in asymptomatic colonization of the large bowel. Antiamebic therapy to eradicate Ed infection is unnecessary. Enzyme immunoassays (EIAs) based on the galactose/*N*-acetylgalactosamine (Gal/GalNAc) adherence lectin differentiate the two species. These assays and molecular analyses have revealed that Ed accounts for more than 90% of infections previously attributed to Eh in nonendemic settings. Even in regions where invasive disease is common, Ed is considerably more prevalent.

PATHOPHYSIOLOGY

E. histolytica is an amitochondriate protozoan parasite. Its life cycle is direct, meaning that ingestion of the cyst, even just one, can lead to infection. In the small intestine, each cyst undergoes excystation to yield four trophozoites, at which time division occurs, and the eight organisms begin to colonize the large intestine. The mean incubation period for Eh is 7 days, although this can vary widely. The Gal/GalNAc lectin expressed on the surface of Eh trophozoites is a well-characterized virulence factor mediating the attachment of amebae to epithelial cells and contact-dependent cytolysis. Once lectin-mediated host-parasite adhesion occurs, Eh appears to kill target cells by activating host caspases, leading to host cell apoptosis. Apoptotic cells are then rapidly phagocytosed.

E. histolytica has developed a number of strategies to facilitate invasive disease, including adherence to colonic mucosa, cytolysis of epithelial and immune effector cells, and modification of host immunity. Risk factors for the development of invasive disease are summarized in Figure 1. A number of laboratories have described putative virulence factors contributing to invasion such as lectin-like adhesion molecules, cysteine proteases that can interfere with humoral immunity by degrading IgA and IgG antibodies, and cytolytic proteinaceous "amebapores." With these virulence systems intact, trophozoites penetrate the colonic epithelium and reach the lamina propria, where loose areolar tissue provides little resistance to the spread of amebae. Their movement within this compartment leads to the characteristic flask-shaped ulcer that is noted histologically with invasive disease. The majority of lesions occur in the cecum, appendix, or ascending colon, although ulceration can occur throughout. Chronic infection can lead to granulomatous inflammation and formation of "amebomas," often mistaken for malignancy and frequently occurring in the cecum and transverse and sigmoid colon.

Once the submucosa has been invaded, amebae can spread hematogenously to the liver, where amebic colonies coalesce to form ALAs containing variable amounts of necrotic debris and blood. ALAs are particularly dangerous as they have the potential to rupture into any adjacent cavity including the abdomen, pleural space, or pericardial sac. Rarely, abscesses can form at other metastatic foci such as the lungs, brain, spleen, and kidney.

CLINICAL FEATURES

Asymptomatic colonization may occur with *E. histolytica* but is 3 to 10 times more common with *E. dispar*. A proportion of those colonized with Eh progress to invasive disease characterized by amebic colitis or extraintestinal abscess formation.

Patients with invasive colitis typically present with an insidious onset of abdominal pain, weight loss, and dysentery. Fever is relatively uncommon (<50%), but the majority (>70%) have blood in the stool (macro- or

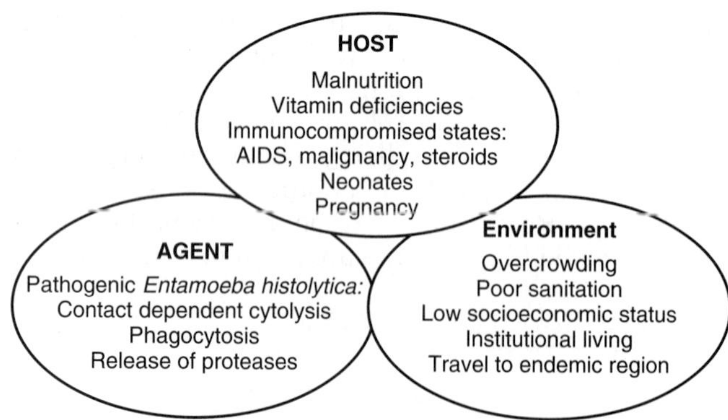

Figure 1. Predisposing risk factors for the development of invasive amebiasis.

microscopic). Involvement of the entire bowel may resemble ulcerative colitis, and it is important that all patients with a history of travel to or residence in endemic areas have Eh infection excluded before initiation of corticosteroid or other immunosuppressive therapy for presumed ulcerative colitis. Local sequelae of untreated amebiasis include hemorrhage, toxic megacolon and colonic perforation, distant metastases, stricture, chronic granulomatous inflammation (amebomas), cutaneous amebiasis, and rectovaginal fistulas.

ALA, the most common outcome of extraintestinal invasion by Eh trophozoites, may arise acutely with fever and right upper quadrant pain and tenderness or, in about 20% to 50% of cases, more insidiously with a several-week history of weight loss and more vague abdominal pain. Concomitant amebic dysentery is uncommon. ALAs are more common in young adult males, in whom they outnumber ALAs observed in adult females 10 to 1. In 80% of cases, ALAs are solitary and involve the right lobe of the liver, often with a concomitant elevation of the right hemidiaphragm on chest radiograph. Although abscesses of the left lobe account for less than 20% of ALAs, they have a predilection for rupture into the pericardium or left pleural cavity, which is associated with a higher mortality rate.

Routine laboratory investigations reveal a leukocytosis over 12,000/µL (~80%) and elevated alkaline phosphatase (~70%) in the majority of individuals with an ALA. Serum bilirubin and transaminases are less commonly elevated.

Several previous reports have revealed a high prevalence of amebiasis in men who have sex with men. These cases have been shown to be predominantly cases of nonpathogenic *E. dispar* infection. However, more recently invasive Eh disease including ALA has been reported in gay males.

ALAs may be complicated by secondary bacterial infection, pleural and pericardial effusions, and rupture. After successful therapy, the abscess cavity resolves slowly over many months, although in approximately 20% or more, patients have a persistent cystic defect on imaging studies.

DIAGNOSIS

Traditionally, the diagnosis of intestinal amebiasis has relied upon the microscopic examination of fecal samples. Any examination for parasites in fecal samples must include the use of a permanent stained smear and a micrometer. The identification of intestinal protozoa including *Entamoeba* species is based on unique characteristics of the trophozoite and cyst stages, including size and shape, nuclei number and structure, nuclear characteristics, motility (trophozoites), inclusions, and chromatoidal bodies. These features are most readily demonstrated using permanently stained fecal smears (trichrome or iron hematoxylin for amebae). However, microscopic diagnosis is laborious and cannot differentiate Eh from Ed. Isozyme pattern differences, serologic responses, detection of stool Eh antigen by EIA, and polymerase chain reaction (PCR) have all been reported to be useful in distinguishing Eh from Ed, although most remain research tools. Potential advantages of these molecular and immunologic techniques over microscopy include higher sensitivity and specificity, expedience of results, ease of use, and cost. Although antigen detection assays and PCR are reportedly sensitive and specific for Eh, the "gold standard" for discriminating Eh from Ed still remains isolation of trophozoites by stool culture combined with differentiation of the two species by zymodeme analysis. Using cultured trophozoites of Eh and Ed, comparisons revealed that PCR has greater sensitivity and specificity than EIA-based stool antigen detection in distinguishing the two organisms. However, field studies comparing PCR and antigen detection indicate that these methods perform equally well.

Patients with invasive Eh disease mount a systemic humoral response to the 170-kDa heavy lectin subunit. Serum antilectin IgG antibodies can be detected within 1 to 2 weeks of symptom onset in more than 70% of patients with amebic colitis and more than 90% of patients with ALA but may persist for years after infection. Thus, in endemic areas, long-term seropositivity rates limit the use of serum antilectin IgG for diagnosis. Fecal lectin antigen detection would appear to be more specific than serology for active intestinal infection and can provide quantitative differentiation of Eh and Ed. For ALAs, stool antigen is infrequently positive and the diagnosis in nonendemic areas is most commonly established through demonstration of a space-occupying lesion in the liver through abdominal ultrasonography, computed tomography, or magnetic resonance imaging combined with positive, and usually high, antiamebic serologic titers. An approach to the workup of patients with suspected ALA is outlined in Figure 2.

The differential diagnosis for ALA includes hepatocellular carcinoma, cystic hydatid disease, and pyogenic abscesses. In contrast to ALA, pyogenic abscesses occur primarily in older patients with underlying hepatobiliary disease, have an equal sex distribution, and are usually associated with positive bacterial cultures from blood and following aspiration of the abscess.

Occasionally, space-occupying lesions of the liver are aspirated for diagnostic purposes. Aspiration of pyogenic abscesses demonstrates bacteria by Gram stain and by culture. In ALAs, amebic trophozoites are rarely identified (usually found only in the periphery of the lesion) but Eh lectin antigen may be positive by EIA. The presence of bacteria in an ALA is indicative of secondary bacterial infection.

TREATMENT

The treatment objectives of amebiasis therapy should be to cure invasive disease at both intestinal and extraintestinal sites and eliminate the passage of cysts from the bowel lumen. As previously mentioned, most asymptomatic individuals diagnosed with "amebiasis," on the basis of stool microscopy, are infected with the harmless gut commensal *E. dispar*. However, until serology or new antigen or PCR-based assays

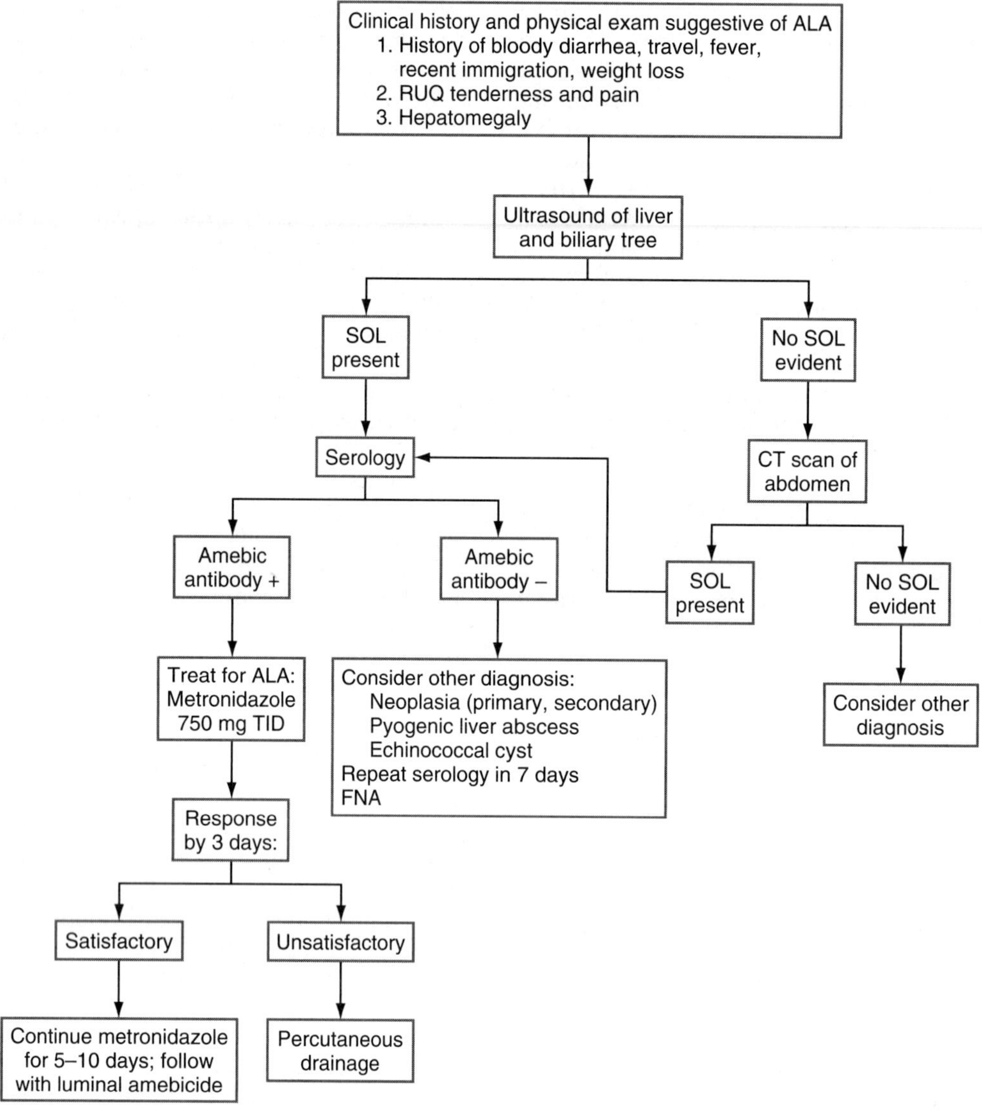

Figure 2. Approach to the patient with suspected amebic liver abscess (ALA). CT, computed tomography; FNA, fine-needle aspiration; RUQ, right upper quadrant; SOL, space-occupying lesion.

that differentiate Eh from Ed are readily available, all asymptomatic cyst passers should be treated with a lumen-active agent alone. A summary of current treatment recommendations for Eh infection is presented in Table 1.

Diloxanide furoate (Furamide) is a drug of choice in the management of asymptomatic cyst passage. It has a success rate of 85% in the elimination of Eh after a 10-day course of therapy. Treatment success is indicated by stools that remain free of Eh trophozoites and cysts 1 month after therapy. As there is great day-to-day variability in the excretion of organisms, several specimens should be examined for evidence of cure. Diloxanide is generally well tolerated, with reports of occasional gastrointestinal (GI) upset, diplopia, and urticaria. This drug is considered safe in pregnancy after the first trimester. Diloxanide can be obtained through the Centers for Disease Control and Prevention (CDC) in the United States and through the Bureau of Pharmaceutical Assessment, Health Protection Branch (HPB) in Canada. It is not otherwise available in North America.

Alternative intraluminal regimens include paromomycin (Humatin) and iodoquinol (Yodoxin), both of which are as effective as diloxanide in the eradication of cyst passage. Paromomycin is an aminoglycoside with poor GI absorption and is thus safe in pregnancy. Documented side effects include diarrhea and abdominal cramps. Iodoquinol necessitates a longer treatment course and may interfere with thyroid function in addition to its mild GI side effect profile. Rarely, dose-related neurotoxicity including optic neuritis has been reported with prolonged use of an inappropriately high dose. The failure rate of any of the aforementioned drugs is 10% to 15%; therefore, follow-up stool examinations are important for test of cure.

Metronidazole (Flagyl) is the recommended treatment for patients with any form of invasive amebiasis, including ameboma. Metronidazole, a 5-nitroimidazole derivative, has excellent oral bioavailability and is

TABLE 1. **Pharmacologic Treatment of Amebiasis**

Type of Infection	Drug	Adult Dose	Pediatric Dose
Asymptomatic cyst passage	Diloxanide furoate (Furamide)	500 mg tid × 10 d	20 mg/kg/d¶ × 10 d (max 1500 mg/d)
	Paromomycin (Humatin)	500 mg PO tid × 7 d or 25-35 mg/kg/d¶ × 7 d	25 mg/kg/d¶ × 7 d (max 1500 mg/d)
	Iodoquinol (Yodoxin)	650 mg tid × 20 d	30-40 mg/kg/d¶ × 20 d (max 2 g/d)
Amebic colitis*	Metronidazole (Flagyl)†	750 mg tid × 5-10 d	30-50 mg/kg/d¶ × 10 d (max 2250 mg/d)
	Tinidazole (Fasigyn)‡	2 g QD¶ × 3 d‖	50 mg/kg/d × 3 d (max 2 g/d)
Amebic liver abscess,* extrahepatic abscess,* ameboma*	Metronidazole (Flagyl)†	750 mg tid × 5-10 d	30-50 mg/kg/d¶ × 5-10 d

*Treatment of invasive amebiasis should always be combined with a luminal amebicide as for asymptomatic cyst passage.
†As an alternative, 2.5 g QD × 3 d may be used if short-course therapy is desired.
‡Not available in the United States.
‖Exceeds dosage recommended by manufacturer.
¶Total daily dose divided into 3 doses per day.

highly efficacious in the treatment of amebiasis, with a 90% cure rate. There is now evidence to suggest that 2.5 g of metronidazole daily for 3 days* is as effective as the standard 7-day course. As metronidazole fails to target luminal organisms, this regimen is best combined with a lumen-acting agent. Although the safety of metronidazole during pregnancy is controversial, treatment of invasive amebiasis during pregnancy is necessary. Most recently, a comparison of 1000 pregnant women who received metronidazole with those who did not demonstrated no teratogenicity or adverse effects on the fetus. Commonly reported side effects of metronidazole include headache, somnolence, nausea, abdominal discomfort, and metallic taste. Other side effects such as darkly pigmented urine, urticaria, and neutropenia are rarely documented. As metronidazole has disulfiram-like action, it is best for patients to avoid consuming alcohol while taking the drug. Tinidazole (Fasigyn)†, another 5-nitroimidazole, is the preferred first-line therapy for invasive amebiasis outside North America.

Medical therapy alone usually suffices in the management of ALA and metastatic disease. As with amebic colitis, metronidazole combined with a luminal agent is the treatment of choice. Most cases of ALA respond to metronidazole within 72 to 96 hours. Chloroquine (Aralen) or percutaneous drainage of ALA, or both, may be considered for nonresponders. Although chloroquine actively targets amebae in hepatic tissue, clinical trial data supporting its addition to metronidazole in the treatment of ALA are lacking. Potential indications for percutaneous drainage of ALA are outlined in Table 2.

*Exceeds dosage recommended by the manufacturer.
†Not available in the United States.

CONTROL AND PREVENTION

As *E. histolytica* has a fecal-oral route of transmission, interruption of its life cycle can be achieved through improved sanitation and access to clean drinking water. Treatment of those harboring parasites may also be an effective control strategy. Although these intervention strategies are straightforward, they are often unattainable in the developing world. As there are no known animal reservoirs of Eh, an effective vaccine could virtually eradicate this disease. Potential vaccine candidates include immunogens that generate antibodies that block lectin, incapacitate the amebapore, or inhibit receptor-mediated endocytosis of apoptosed cells. An oral vaccine that stimulates cellular and mucosal immunity has the potential to play a role in the global control of amebiasis.

TABLE 2. **Potential Indications for Aspiration of Amebic Liver Abscess**

Clinical	Radiographic	Diagnostic
Failure of medical therapy after 3 d of treatment	Abscess >10 cm	Rule out pyogenic abscess in context of multiple lesions
Increasing right upper quadrant pain or hepatic tenderness	Left lobe abscess with danger of rupture into pericardium	
Severe jaundice	Rapidly enlarging abscess	
Prerupture syndrome:	Thin rim of liver parenchyma around abscess cavity	
Abdominal wall distention		
Ileus		
Guarding		
Symptomatic relief		

GIARDIASIS

method of
THEODORE E. NASH, M.D.
National Institutes of Health
Bethesda, Maryland

Giardiasis is caused by infection with the protozoan parasite *Giardia lamblia* (*Giardia duodenalis, Giardia intestinalis*). It is among the most common parasitic infections of humans and causes both epidemic and endemic gastroenteritis manifested primarily as diarrhea although upper gastrointestinal symptoms may also be common. The parasite has two stages. An infectious cyst is excreted in the feces and is able to survive outside the host. When ingested by humans and other mammals, the cyst excysts in the upper small intestine liberating motile trophozoites that multiply within the small intestine. It is this form that is responsible for the manifestations of disease. As the trophozoites travel down the intestine, they develop into cysts. *Giardia* infections are common because very large numbers of cysts can be excreted in the feces, measured at 18 million cysts/mL of feces, and 100% of people become infected after ingestion of as few as 10 to 100 cysts. In addition cysts may remain infectious in cold water for months, which is why this parasite is one of the most common causes of defined waterborne outbreaks of gastroenteritis.

EPIDEMIOLOGY

The prevalence of *Giardia* infections varies but is consistently the most commonly diagnosed parasitic infection in the United States and most developed countries. It is the most common parasite detected in stools submitted to state health laboratories; prevalences average from 5.6% to 7.2%. Infections via person-to-person, water, or food are frequent whenever fecal contamination occurs. However, certain groups are more likely to become infected. Giardiasis is most common in the young and more frequent in the summer in temperate regions. In the United States hospitalizations are about as common as for shigellosis. In many developing countries infections are practically universal by the age of 2 and the proportion infected remains surprisingly high, although reduced, throughout adulthood. Because of the high level of endemic infections in these regions, travelers to these areas are at increased risk for infection. However, in reported series *Giardia* is a relatively uncommon cause of traveler's diarrhea. Giardiasis is particularly common in daycare settings—in which 40% or greater of the children can be infected. In this setting infections are commonly cryptic or not appreciated until the children infect their parents or other family members. Infected infants and toddlers contaminate recreational water supplies by indiscriminate defecation and are increasingly recognized as sources of epidemics in public swimming areas. Other groups more likely to be infected include homosexuals and backpackers. The latter become infected because lakes and streams become contaminated with cysts from people or animals such as beavers. Although contaminated foods have been vehicles in outbreaks, this has been recognized relatively infrequently.

Although most who become infected are immunocompetent, people with hypogammaglobulinemia, nodular follicular hyperplasia without hypogammaglobulinemia, or lymphoma of the small intestine commonly develop debilitating and sometimes life-threatening giardiasis. More recently, an increasing number of AIDS patients with severe and difficult to treat giardiasis have been recognized.

INFECTION

The hallmark of *Giardia* infections is variability. The incubation period is commonly between 1 and 2 weeks but can be considerably longer. Infections may be aborted, transient, or prolonged, sometimes lasting years. Because trophozoites inhabit the small intestine, signs and symptoms are related to alterations in the function of the small intestine and are to be distinguished from agents that cause colitis. Symptoms range from asymptomatic carriage, a relatively frequent occurrence, to fulminate diarrhea and vomiting resulting in dehydration and hospitalization. Diarrhea without blood or mucus, cramping, foul-smelling flatus, belching, nausea and vomiting, anorexia, and weight loss are the most common symptoms. Fever is unusual. Malabsorption and failure to thrive are particularly serious problems in infants, young children in developing regions of the world, and others with marginal nutrition such as in cystic fibrosis. One report correlated *Giardia* infections with decreased intellectual development. Compared with diarrheal illnesses resulting from bacteria, giardiasis has a longer incubation period, is associated with less systemic symptoms and therefore the patients are less frequently acutely ill, and has a more prolonged, intermittent course. Lactose deficiency may complicate giardiasis and contribute to continuing symptoms after therapy.

Extraintestinal manifestations such as uveitis, urticaria, and arthritis have been described. It is unclear if the concurrence of these represents two independent processes occurring at the same time or a casual relationship.

DIAGNOSIS

The diagnosis is established by detecting cysts and occasionally trophozoites in the feces, trophozoites in the small intestines, or by detection of specific *Giardia* antigen in the stool. A good practice is to perform standard ova and parasite examinations to rule out parasites other than *Giardia* and a stool *Giardia* antigen test. There are a number of commercially available antigen detection tests that have shown sensitivities and specificities of greater than 95%. The basis of these tests is detection of soluble cyst wall proteins that are likely released during the process of encystation so that antigen-based tests are positive even when cyst excretion is erratic or barely detectable, instances in which

TABLE 1. **Drugs Commonly Used to Treat Giardiasis**

Drug	Adult Dose	Pediatric Dose	Remarks
Metronidazole (Flagyl)	250 mg po tid × 7 d	5 mg/kg tid × 7 d	Gastrointestinal upset, disulfiram-like effect
Quinacrine (Atabrine)	100 mg qid × 5 d	2 mg/kg qid × 5 d	Not generally available. Gastrointestinal upset, yellow skin, urine, psychosis
Furazolidone (Furoxone)	100 mg qid × 7-10 d	6 mg/kg/d in 4 doses × 7-10 d	Best tolerated in children. Many potential side effects but usually well-tolerated
Paromomycin (Humatin)*	25-35 mg/kg tid × 5-10 d	—	Not absorbed. Likely less effective. Best use in pregnancy. GI upset.
Tinidazole	2 g single dose	50 mg/kg once with max 2 g	Similar but less frequent compared to metronidazole

*Not FDA approved for this indication.

the diagnosis would likely be missed by microscopic stool examinations. A positive stool antigen test is highly suggestive, if not indicative of the diagnosis. Previously, standard stool examinations for ova and parasites were unable to diagnose between 5% and 15% of *Giardia*-infected individuals after three stool examinations. Diagnosis required invasive techniques to detect trophozoites in small intestinal mucus and fluid. These included a string test, duodenal intubation, and examination of touch preps of small intestinal biopsies. However, in most cases, *Giardia* antigen detection tests should replace invasive techniques. Because both false-positive and false-negative results have been documented, more extensive evaluations are indicated in patients whose diagnosis is based solely on a positive *Giardia* antigen test and who fail to respond to repeated treatment courses. Similarly, in instances in which the diagnosis is clinically suspected, repeated antigen tests or invasive tests may be indicated.

Giardiasis is both overdiagnosed and underdiagnosed. The symptoms of giardiasis are nonspecific, intermittent, and frequently of mild-to-moderate intensity, leading to both a reluctance of the patient or parent to seek medical attention and a failure of the physician to consider the diagnosis. Sometimes, nausea and vomiting are the prominent manifestations of giardiasis and the diagnosis is not considered because diarrhea is not prominent. On the other hand because the symptoms and signs caused by other conditions mimic those of giardiasis, *Giardia* infections are also overdiagnosed and not uncommonly treatment offered without establishing the diagnosis. Not unexpectedly such patients frequently fail to respond to therapy. As mentioned previously, *Giardia* infections are relatively frequent, commonly asymptomatic, and long lasting, features that increase the possibility of two diseases coexisting. One should also keep in mind that *Giardia* infections come about after ingestion of feces and that more than one type of diarrhea-causing agent can be ingested at the same time or manner, causing confusion about which organism is actually responsible for the symptoms.

TREATMENT

The drugs commonly used for the treatment of giardiasis are listed in Table 1. All these drugs have significant side effects and drug interactions, and standard texts should be consulted before use. Metronidazole (Flagyl),* a nitroimidazole, is the most commonly used drug in the United States despite the fact that it has never been approved by the FDA for the treatment of giardiasis. Another nitroimidazole, tinidazole,** not marketed in the United States but commonly available elsewhere, is equal if not superior in efficacy to metronidazole and has fewer side effects. Metronidazole (Flagyl), although usually well-tolerated, can cause troubling upper gastrointestinal upset, which occasionally limits its use. Alcohol ingestion should be avoided because it causes a disulfiram-like reaction. For many years quinacrine (Atabrine)*** was the drug of choice to treat giardiasis but it is no longer manufactured in the United States and not readily available, although it can be obtained through a few pharmacies (Panorama Pharmacy, Panorama City, CA: 1-800-247-9767; Priority Pharmacy 1-800-487-7113). Major side effects include upper gastrointestinal symptoms, yellow discoloration of the skin and urine, and occasional psychosis or visual hallucinations. Furazolidone (Fluroxene), a broad-spectrum antibacterial nitrofuran, is less effective than either metronidazole or quinacrine. However, it is available as a liquid and therefore is more acceptable and effective than metronidazole or quinacrine for use in children. Although generally well-tolerated gastrointestinal upset is the most common side effect, but there is a large number of less common but nevertheless reported side effects such as hemolysis resulting from glucose 6-phosphate dehydrogenase deficiency, nitrofuran sensitivity reactions, and disulfiram-like reactions after ethanol ingestion. Furthermore, it is a monoamine oxidase (MAO) inhibitor, so that sympathomimetics and tyramine are contraindicated and drugs metabolized by MAO require dose adjustments. Paromomycin (Humatin)* is a nonabsorbable aminoglycoside less well-studied than the other antibiotics with anecdotal reports of effectiveness. Because it is not absorbed, it has been suggested as treatment for symptomatic infections in pregnancy. Other less

*Not FDA approved for this indication.
**Not available in the United States.
***May be compounded by pharmacists.

established drugs include albendazole (Albenza),* zinc bacitracin,* and neomycin.

With the exception of paromomycin (Humatin),* none of the commonly employed drugs should be used routinely in pregnancy. If the patient is able to clinically tolerate the infection and gains weight, he or she may not require treatment. Otherwise, in severe symptomatic giardiasis, metronidazole (Flagyl)* can probably be safely used in the second and third trimesters.

Treatment failures may be due to immunologic impairment, reinfection, or drug resistance. In immunocompetent people treatment failures are more frequent than commonly reported and may be due to biologic differences among isolates. However, organisms with proven drug resistance are unusual. In treatment failures, longer or increased dosing or a change to an alternate drug is usually effective. In immunologically impaired patients therapy with combined quinacrine and metronidazole has been extremely effective. Nitazoxanide (Alinia), recently approved for patients 1 to 11 years of age in the United States, appears to be effective in giardiasis and may be useful in the treatment of patients unresponsive to other drugs. Patients who fail to cure frequently respond transiently to treatment with lessening or abolition of symptoms but then relapse. Patients who continue to relapse should be questioned carefully about the possibility of reinfection including source of water, presence of infected household members, and sexual practices.

*Not FDA approved for this indication.

BACTEREMIA AND SEPSIS

method of
DENNIS KELLAR, M.D., and
ROBERT A. BALK, M.D.
Section of Pulmonary and Critical Care Medicine
Rush Medical College and
Rush-Presbyterian-St. Luke's Medical Center
Chicago, IL

Sepsis has been defined as the systemic inflammatory response to an infection. The true incidence of sepsis is unknown, in part because of the lack of a uniformly accepted definition. The Centers for Disease Control and Prevention (CDC) had previously reported a dramatic 139% increase in the septicemia discharge diagnosis over a decade of monitoring. Using discharge coding data from seven states, it has been recently suggested that there are more than 750,000 episodes of severe sepsis each year in the United States. Severe sepsis accounts for 1 of every 10 intensive care unit (ICU) admissions and represents 2% to 3% of all hospital admissions. Furthermore, the U.S. incidence of sepsis is projected to rise at a rate of 1.5% per year. Factors responsible for this increase include the continued growth in the number of elderly patients, an increased number of immunocompromised patients, the increased use of invasive procedures and devices to care for patients, the growing problem with resistant microorganisms, and a greater awareness and recognition of this disorder.

Sepsis is now reported to be the 10th most common cause of death in the United States and is one of the two most common causes of death in the noncoronary ICU. Using the extrapolated annual incidence of 750,000 episodes of sepsis in the United States and a relatively conservative mortality estimate of 28%, there would be an annual mortality of greater than 220,000. This surprisingly high mortality rate has been projected despite our enhanced understanding of the pathophysiologic alterations that occur in sepsis, our technologic improvements in monitoring and support of the critically ill patient, and our use of more potent antibiotic therapy. There have also been multiple attempts to improve the outcome of the septic patient using innovative therapeutic strategies that are designed to target selected aspects of the pathophysiologic response to the causative microorganism(s).

DEFINITIONS OF SIRS AND SEPSIS

The approach to management of patients with severe sepsis and septic shock begins with prompt recognition of the septic process (Table 1). As mentioned, in the past there has been difficulty in identifying septic patients, in part related to the lack of a uniformly accepted definition. In 1991, the American College of Chest Physicians and the Society of Critical Care Medicine convened a consensus conference that was charged with developing a set of definitions that would assist the medical community in communication about sepsis and would provide for the early recognition of the septic patient. The definition would incorporate predominantly readily available clinical criteria that would facilitate patient identification and enrollment in investigational trials of innovative therapeutic agents. The consensus conference recognized that there were patients with presumed sepsis based on their clinical presentation who lacked a positive culture or other evidence of a documented infection. These individuals were classified as having the systemic inflammatory response syndrome or SIRS. SIRS can result from a diverse group of insults, such as trauma, burns, or pancreatitis. Sepsis was defined as the SIRS response to a documented infection.

SIRS was defined as a widespread systemic inflammatory response to a variety of insults, including, but not limited to, infection. SIRS was operationally defined by the presence of two or more of the following:

- temperature >38°C or <36°C,
- heart rate >90 beats per minute,
- respiratory rate >20 breaths per minute or $Paco_2$ <32 mm Hg,
- white blood cell count >12,000 cells/mm^3, or <4000 cells/mm^3 or >10% immature band forms.

Sepsis is the systemic inflammatory response to a documented infection. The diagnosis of sepsis requires the presence of at least two of the these SIRS criteria,

TABLE 1. **SIRS and Sepsis Criteria***

ACCP & SCCM Consensus Conference Definitions—1992
Systemic Inflammatory Response Syndrome (SIRS): The systemic inflammatory response to a wide variety of severe clinical insults, manifested by two or more of the following conditions: 1. Temperature >38°C or <36°C 2. Heart rate >90 beats/min 3. Respiratory rate >20 breaths/min or $Paco_2$ <32 mm Hg 4. WBC count >12,000/mm^3, <4000/mm^3, or >10% immature (band) forms.
Sepsis: The systemic inflammatory response to infection. In association with infection, manifestations of sepsis are the same as those previously defined for SIRS. It should be determined whether they are a direct systemic response to the presence of an infectious process and represent an acute alteration from baseline in the absence of other known causes for such abnormalities.
Severe Sepsis/SIRS: Sepsis (SIRS) associated with organ dysfunction, hypoperfusion, or hypotension. Hypoperfusion and perfusion abnormalities may include, but are not limited to, lactic acidosis, oliguria, or an acute alteration in mental status.
Sepsis (SIRS)-Induced Hypotension: A systolic blood pressure <90 mm Hg or a reduction of ≥40 mm Hg from baseline in the absence of other causes for hypotension.
Septic Shock/SIRS Shock: A subset of severe sepsis (SIRS) and defined as sepsis (SIRS)-induced hypotension despite adequate fluid resuscitation along with the presence of perfusion abnormalities that may include, but are not limited to, lactic acidosis, oliguria, or an acute alteration in mental status. Patients receiving inotropic or vasopressor agents may no longer be hypotensive by the time they manifest hypoperfusion abnormalities or organ dysfunction, but nonetheless would be considered to have septic (SIRS) shock.
Multiple Organ Dysfunction Syndrome (MODS): Presence of altered organ function in an acutely ill patient, such that homeostasis cannot be maintained without intervention.

*Modified from Bone RC, Balk RA, Cerra FB, et al. American College of Chest Physicians/Society of Critical Care Medicine Consensus Conference: Definitions for sepsis and organ failure and guidelines for the use of innovative therapies in sepsis. *Chest.* 1992;101:1644-1655.

plus an infection. Signs of infection include an inflammatory response to the presence of microorganisms or the invasion of normally sterile host tissue by those organisms. There is a continuum of injury severity in SIRS and sepsis. Severe SIRS and severe sepsis are defined by the presence of organ dysfunction or hypoperfusion as a result of the inflammatory response. Hypoperfusion and perfusion abnormalities may include, but are not limited to, lactic acidosis, oliguria, or an acute alteration in mental status. Sepsis-induced hypotension occurs when systolic blood pressure falls to <90 mm Hg or there is a reduction of ≥40 mm Hg from baseline systolic pressure in the absence of other causes for hypotension.

Septic shock is a subset of severe sepsis with hypotension despite adequate fluid resuscitation, along with the presence of perfusion abnormalities. Patients receiving inotropic or vasopressor agents may no longer be hypotensive by the time they manifest hypoperfusion abnormalities or organ dysfunction, yet they would still be considered to have septic shock. When there is multiple dysfunction of organ systems present, it is termed multiple organ dysfunction syndrome, or MODS. The definition of MODS is the alteration of organ function such that normal homeostasis cannot be maintained without intervention. Unfortunately, there are no uniformly agreed-upon definitions to define the dysfunction or failure of specific organ systems. However, most would agree that the need for organ support or replacement therapy does signify the presence of specific organ failure.

Validation of these consensus conference definitions came from a prospective evaluation of University of Iowa patients who met the SIRS criteria, sepsis, severe sepsis, and septic shock definitions. They demonstrated an increase in mortality as patients moved down this continuum of injury severity.

PATHOGENESIS OF SEPSIS

The septic response begins as a normal physiologic response to an infection that attempts to wall off and eliminate the offending microbiologic organism(s). The pathologic process we clinically recognize as sepsis is the result of an excessive and uncontrolled physiologic response that may culminate in endothelial cell injury, MODS, or death. The normal response to infection involves a process that serves to localize and contain an invading organism usually resulting in the initiation of repair of injured host tissue. When this inflammatory response to infection becomes generalize and extends to healthy host tissue this becomes SIRS. With the onset of SIRS, normal host tissue, whether infected or not, becomes damaged. This results in the release of proinflammatory and anti-inflammatory molecules and mediators that are capable of producing injury or altering the host's immune response. These contrasting elements help facilitate host tissue repair in healing. However, when there is an imbalance in the complex and intricate septic cascade, either a SIRS or a compensatory anti-inflammatory response syndrome (CARS) can predominate. If the SIRS response predominates there is a predisposition for an exaggerated proinflammatory response that can culminate in the production of MODS. In contrast, when the anti-inflammatory CARS response predominates, there is a state of immune suppression that can result in secondary or nosocomial infections. These additional inflammatory insults may supply additional "hits" to the immune system and has been termed the "multiple hits hypothesis" for the production of multiple organ dysfunction or failure. The sepsis cascade has been categorized into five stages by Bone and colleagues, which are listed in Table 2.

Host factors responsible for important first-line of defense against the infectious insult include epithelial barriers, mucociliary flow, pH of body fluids, urine volume, and secretory immunoglobulins. Overall immune function of the host is also a key consideration. Chronic diseases such as diabetes mellitus, HIV infection, and chronic alcoholism commonly predispose the host to an infectious insult. The adaptive and innate immunity of the host also provide key defenses against infectious insults. The adaptive arm of host immunity is composed of specialized B cells and T cells. Receptors unique to each of these cell lines result in a proliferation of immune response when stimulated. The innate arm of the immune response uses receptors that recognize highly conserved antigenic regions in large groups of microorganisms. A group of cell surface receptors that have become of particular interest are the toll-like receptors (TLR). For example, activation of TLR-4 by circulating endotoxin from the gram-negative bacterial cell wall induces the transcription of a number of inflammatory and immune response genes. Gram-negative organisms contain a component of endotoxin within the cell wall that is responsible for many of the manifestations of sepsis. Gram-positive organisms produce exotoxins that may function as superantigens. The result is a massive activation of T-cells, with an overproduction of cytokines and an out-of-control immune response.

Mediators of the host inflammatory response are initially found in high concentrations locally, at the nidus of infection. In severe infections proinflammatory cytokines will produce systemic symptoms. This usually becomes the telltale sign that the infection is unable to be contained locally. Some of the more common primary pro- and anti-inflammatory molecules and mediators are listed in Table 3. Included in the list of proinflammatory cytokines are tumor necrosis factor (TNF-α), interleukin 1 (IL-1), interleukin 6 (IL-6), and interferon-γ.

An overwhelming systemic inflammatory response results when the host is unable to contain the proinflammatory response locally. The massive, uncontrolled production of proinflammatory molecules and cytokines produce SIRS. Endothelial dysfunction typically ensues from the inflammatory response coupled with the activation of the coagulation syndrome. The result is microvascular thrombi and upregulation of endothelial adhesion molecules, causing microvascular permeability, vasodilatation organ dysfunction, and shock.

The overwhelming response is then followed by CARS, which down-regulates the proinflammatory cascade. The balance that ensues during the mixed antagonistic response syndrome (MARS) will determine the clinical manifestations and outcome of the response to the infection. The principle mediators of the CARS response include; IL-4, IL-10, and transforming growth factor (TGF-β). In some cases the compensatory reaction can lead to excessive production of counterregulatory cytokines, leading to immune suppression. This can be recognized by a decreased production of IL-6 and TNF-α by monocytes. The final result may be immunomodulatory failure, progression of infection, or superinfection along with coagulation activation, abnormalities of fibrinolysis leading to MODS and death.

TABLE 2. **The Five Stages of Sepsis**

The infectious insult
Preliminary systemic response
Overwhelming systemic response
The compensatory anti-inflammatory reaction
Immunomodulatory failure

TABLE 3. **Potential Molecules Involved in the Pathogenesis of Sepsis and SIRS**

Proinflammatory Molecules and Cells
Polymorphonuclear leukocytes (PMNLs)
Tissue macrophages and monocytes
Platelets
Arachidonic acid metabolites
Prostaglandins, prostacyclin, thromboxane
Leukotrienes
Cytokines (interleukins 1, 2, 6, 8, 15, TNF, G-CSF)
Soluble adhesion molecules
Platelet activating factor (PAF)
Complement and activation of the complement cascade
Various kinins (i.e., Bradykinin)
Endorphins
Histamine and serotonin
Proteolytic enzymes
Elastase and lysosomal enzymes
Protein kinase, tyrosine kinase
Toxic oxygen metabolites
Superoxide, hydroxyl radical, hydrogen peroxide, peroxynitrite, etc.
Endotoxin and other bacterial and microbial toxins
Activation of the coagulation cascade
Neopterin
Plasminogen activator inhibitor-1 (PAI-1)
CD-14
Toll-like receptors 2 and 4
NfκB
Vasoactive neuropeptides
Monocyte chemoattractant protein (MCP)-1 and 2
Potential Anti-Inflammatory Molecules
Interleukin-1 receptor antagonist (Il-1ra)
Type II interleukin-1 receptor
IL-4
IL-10
IL-13
Transforming growth factor β (TGF-β)
IκB
Glucocorticoid receptors
Epinephrine
Soluble TNF receptor (sTNFr)
Leukotriene B_4 receptor antagonist
Soluble CD-14
Lipopolysaccharide (LPS) binding protein

MANAGEMENT OF SEVERE SEPSIS AND SEPTIC SHOCK

Management of sepsis and septic shock begins with prompt recognition of the process. Along with recognition and determination of a probable site of infection the initial management begins with an assessment of the physiologic derangements. In critically ill patients the general management involves source control, restoration, and maintenance of normal hemodynamic function, adequate oxygenation, ventilation, tissue oxygen delivery, and prevention of complications. Recently the assessment of adrenal function and detection of occult adrenal insufficiency in vasopressor-dependent patients with septic shock has been important for defining a potential role for physiologic adrenal replacement therapy. It is also important to evaluate for the presence of complications of critical illness and to administer preventive strategies where appropriate.

Source Control

Prompt, effective management of the source of the infection is the cornerstone of sepsis management. Early initiation of appropriate, effective, antimicrobial therapy is essential for a favorable outcome in the septic patient. Necessary specimens should be sent for culture and sensitivity testing as early as possible, because this information will guide subsequent antimicrobial therapy and allow for good antimicrobial stewardship. The initial antimicrobial therapy is empiric and should be directed toward the organisms that are likely to be causing the infection that has given rise to the septic response. A review of nosocomial infections suggests that the urinary tract, respiratory system, and bloodstream are the three most common sources of hospital-acquired infections. Clinical trials of new agents for the treatment of sepsis have observed that the respiratory tract and the abdomen are the most common sources of infection. After identification of the likely site and cause of the infection, the initial antibiotic selection should be made taking into account the antibiogram of the institution or specific unit where the infection was acquired. When the results of the various cultures and their sensitivity pattern are available, the antimicrobial therapy should then be appropriately tailored. It has been well-documented that the use of early effective antimicrobial therapy will decrease mortality, particularly in patients with gram-negative bacteremia, elderly patients with *Streptococcus pneumoniae* infection, and critically ill patients with bloodstream infections or hospital-acquired pneumonia. The use of early effective antibiotic therapy in critically ill patients has been associated with significant reductions in infection-related and all-cause mortality rates. This benefit was present despite the addition of effective antibiotics after the culture and sensitivity data was available. This observation underscores the importance of initiating the correct initial empiric therapy. Correct antibiotic decisions become even more important in this era of increasing antibiotic resistance. It is important to know the ecology of organisms in your institution along with the antibiogram for the institution. Several recent reviews have been published to assist with the initial empiric antibiotic selection.

Hemodynamic Management

Sepsis is characterized by vasodilatory or distributive shock, and there is an increase in vascular capacitance along with the decrease in the systemic vascular resistance. Septic patients are typically intravascularly volume depleted related to the presence of increased permeability as a result of endothelial cell injury along with an increase in fluid loss coupled with a decrease in fluid replacement. Early recognition of significant hemodynamic derangements and restoration of normal organ perfusion are vital in preventing organ dysfunction and failure. The goal of hemodynamic resuscitation should be to either raise the mean arterial pressure above 60–65 mm Hg or achieve a systolic blood pressure of ≥90 mm Hg. The resuscitative efforts and the adequacy of tissue perfusion can be assessed at the bedside by monitoring heart rate, blood pressure, orthostatic blood pressure changes, mental status, hourly urine output, and skin perfusion. The initial hemodynamic resuscitation should take the form of fluid volume replacement. The fluid resuscitation can be accomplished with a variety of fluids, including crystalloid, colloid, blood, synthetic starches, and hypertonic saline. Most clinicians accomplish the fluid resuscitation with intravenous infusion of either crystalloid or colloid. Bolus infusions are typically administered using the clinical response or measurements of central venous pressure or pulmonary capillary wedge pressure as a guide. In many instances adequate volume resuscitation may be sufficient to restore normal perfusion pressure. The choice of crystalloids versus colloids for fluid resuscitation has been the subject of numerous studies and reviews. Currently there is no clear benefit of one fluid over the other. Crystalloids tend to be cheaper and more readily available, but a larger volume is required. Generally it may take significant liters of fluid to adequately resuscitate patients with severe septic shock. Colloids are typically more expensive and may be associated with coagulation abnormalities, but smaller volumes are needed.

Invasive vascular monitoring may be used to aid in the determination of adequate hemodynamic resuscitation. If a central venous catheter is present, the central venous pressure can be measured to assess the adequacy of the intravascular volume status. In selected patients with hemodynamic insufficiency, the insertion of pulmonary artery catheters to measure the left- (and right-) sided filling pressures and the various hemodynamic parameters may be beneficial. A sphygmomanometer may not be reliable for blood pressure measurement in hypotensive septic patients. Insertion of an arterial line may be required, especially if the patient does not respond to volume resuscitation and requires the addition of vasopressor therapy for hemodynamic resuscitation.

Vasopressor Management

If adequate fluid resuscitation is not sufficient to restore adequate hemodynamic function, then vasopressor or inotropic therapy will be necessary. There is a wide variety of vasoactive medications that are useful in the hemodynamic resuscitation of septic shock. Table 4 lists some of the more commonly used agents. Despite a wide range of possible agents, dopamine (Intropin) and norepinephrine (Levophed) are typically used in most clinical units. Some centers

TABLE 4. **Vasoactive Agents Commonly Used in the Management of Severe Sepsis***

Drug	Receptor Activity	Dose	Effect	Notes
Norepinephrine (Levophed)	α_1: 3+, α_2: 2+, β_1: 2+	0.03–1.5 μg/kg/min	Vasoconstriction	Little change in heart rate or CI May decrease lactate
Epinephrine	α_1: 3+, α_2: 3+, β_1: 3+, β_2: 2+	0.1–0.5 μg/kg/min	Increase stroke volume and CI	Unpredictable dose-response Decrease splanchnic blood flow Increase oxygen consumption and delivery
Dopamine (Intropin)	α_1: 3+, α_2: 3+, β_1: 3+, β_2: 2+	<5 μg/kg/min	Vasodilation	Dopaminergic effects predominate Dilation of renal, mesenteric, and coronary arteries Increased glomerular filtration rate (GFR) Sodium excretion
Dopamine	α_1: 3+, α_2: 3+, β_1: 3+, β_2: 2+	5–10 μg/kg/min	↑ Inotropy and chronotropy	β-adrenergic effects predominate Increased CI due primarily to increased stroke volume
Dopamine	α_1: 3+, α_2: 3+, β_1: 3+, β_2: 2+	>10 μg/kg/min	Vasoconstriction	α-adrenergic effects predominate
Dobutamine (Dobutrex)	α_1: 1+, α_2: 1+, β_1: 3+, β_2: 2+	2–20 μg/kg/min	↑ Inotropy and chronotropy	25%–50% increase in CI Decreases PAOP
Phenylephrine (Neo-Synephrine)	α_1: 3+	0.5–8 μg/kg/min	Vasoconstriction	Increases MAP without change in heart rate CI may decrease
Vasopressin (Pitressin)	V_1	0.04 units/min	Vasoconstriction	"Hormone replacement therapy." May potentiate the vasoconstrictor effect of endogenous catecholamines or act directly on a V_1 receptor

*Modified From Steel A, Bihari D. Choice of catecholamine: does it matter? *Curr Opin Crit Care* 2000;6:347-53.

prefer to use phenylephrine (Neo-Synephrine) in patients with tachycardia or a history of arrhythmias because this pure alpha agent will cause less tachycardia and arrhythmias.

Unfortunately, there is a lack of large, prospective, randomized, protocol-controlled clinical trials that have compared dopamine with norepinephrine for the management of patients with septic shock. Therefore, until such data are available to guide the decision process, there is no clear benefit of one vasopressor strategy over the other. Therefore either agent is acceptable in the management of hypotensive patients. Dopamine has been the preferred agent in many units, in part related to its ease of use, the concept that it improves splanchnic and renal perfusion, and its safety record. Recent clinical trial results have revealed that there is no specific beneficial effect of so-called "renal dose dopamine" in preventing the development of renal failure or in decreasing the need for renal replacement therapy. In addition, the use of dopamine has been associated with an increased incidence of arrhythmias and a decrease in the gastric intramucosal pH (an indicator of splanchnic oxygen delivery and utilization). Norepinephrine is a potent vasoconstrictor that also has some increase in inotropic and chronotropic effect on the heart. There is no decrease in renal or splanchnic perfusion as was once thought and, in fact, there is an increase in the perfusion of these vascular beds as a result of the increased cardiac output and vasoconstriction. A large observational study of French septic shock patients who required high doses of vasopressor therapy demonstrated a significant improvement in survival with the use of norepinephrine as compared with high doses of dopamine with or without the addition of epinephrine.

Recently there has been renewed interest in the use of vasopressin* (Pitressin) in patients with vasodilatory shock. The initial release of stored vasopressin from the posterior pituitary during hypotension depletes the body's store of the hormone. As the shock state persists, there is a state of vasopressin deficiency, which some view as a hormone deficiency state that is amenable to replacement therapy. Some centers are now infusing vasopressin as a hormone replacement therapy in a constant, nonescalating dose to augment dopamine or norepinephrine's pressor effects. The importance of early goal-oriented hemodynamic resuscitation was emphasized in a recent trial comparing this technique with more traditional resuscitation efforts. The early goal-oriented protocol was associated with significant improvement in ICU and hospital survival and significantly less death from sudden hemodynamic collapse.

Some patients with severe sepsis and septic shock have a reversible biventricular myocardial dysfunction, which has been attributed to circulating TNF-α, IL-1, or nitric oxide that are elaborated as part of the SIRS response. Ventricular dilatation and a reduced

*Not FDA approved for this indication.

ejection fraction comprise this myocardial depression. Inotropic agents such as dobutamine (Dobutrex) or epinephrine can improve the myocardial contractility and hemodynamic function in these patients. By increasing stroke volume and heart rate, dobutamine increases the cardiac index. While epinephrine can also increase the cardiac index, its use should be limited in the septic patient because it can impair splanchnic blood flow and increase systemic and regional lactate concentrations.

Support Oxygenation and Ventilation

Abnormalities of the respiratory system are some of the most common evidence of organ systems involvement in sepsis. Septic patients should be assessed for adequacy of oxygenation, oxygen delivery, ventilation, and the ability to protect the airway. Septic patients commonly have abnormalities of oxygenation and increased work of breathing. Patients who are hypoxemic should be given supplemental oxygen with a goal of achieving arterial oxygen saturation ≥90%.

Another decision to make in caring for the septic patient is the need and timing for endotracheal intubation and ventilatory support. Acute lung injury and ARDS are relatively common manifestations of pulmonary dysfunction in the patient with severe sepsis and septic shock. Up to 35% of septic patients may manifest ARDS. The goal of mechanical ventilation is to maintain the PaO_2 in the 55 to 70 mm Hg range while keeping the FIO_2 below 60% (0.6). The traditional approach to mechanically ventilating patients with acute lung injury (ALI) and ARDS has been to employ tidal volumes in the 10 to 15 mL/kg range. The Acute Respiratory Distress Syndrome Network (ARDSNet) trial of low tidal volume ventilation of 6 mL/kg ideal body weight, coupled with maintaining an end-inspiratory plateau pressure ≤30 cm H_2O, and a nomogram for positive end-expiratory pressure (PEEP) titration based on FIO_2 and oxygenation goals demonstrated an overall decrease in hospital mortality along with an increase in ventilator-free and organ failure–free days.

The risk of infection and ventilator-associated complications increases with the duration of ventilatory support. Patients should be removed from the ventilator as soon as they no longer need mechanical ventilatory support. The use of weaning protocols implemented by trained ICU support staff have been shown to speed the weaning process and improve the overall process of extubating the critically ill patient. It is also important to use sedation and analgesia appropriately in this critically ill population. Excessive sedation and analgesia have been linked to prolonged stays on mechanical ventilatory support and increased complications.

In a large, multicenter controlled trial conducted in critically ill patients without ischemic cardiac disease or acute blood loss, the restrictive practice of packed red blood cell transfusions in the management of anemia and low hemoglobin levels (Hb levels between 7.0 and 9.0 g/dL) was shown to provide adequate oxygen delivery to the tissues and in a subgroup of younger patients and less ill patients was found to be associated with a lower mortality rate compared with a more liberal transfusion policy with Hb levels maintained in the 10.0–12.0 g/dL range. The use of weekly recombinant erythropoietin has also been shown to reduce the need for transfusions in critically ill patients. Aggressive use of packed red blood cell transfusions in an effort to achieve supernormal oxygen delivery states should be discouraged.

Supportive Care for the Critically Ill Patient

Patients with severe sepsis and septic shock are critically ill and susceptible to the multiple complications common in the critically ill population. These complications include deep vein thrombosis and pulmonary emboli, stress-related gastrointestinal bleeding, nosocomial infections, MODS, and critical illness polyneuropathy/myopathy. Patients in the ICU with sepsis or septic shock should receive prophylaxis for deep vein thrombosis with unfractionated or low-molecular-weight heparin or pneumatic compression devices if they have a coagulopathy or increased risk of bleeding. Prophylaxis for stress related gastrointestinal bleeding may be accomplished with H_2-receptor blockers, proton pump inhibitors,* sucralfate (Carafate),* or early enteral feeding.

Nutritional support of the patient with severe sepsis is important from multiple standpoints. Proper nutrition is important to maintain the necessary immune function during the catabolic septic metabolic process. Enteral administration of nutrition may prevent stress-related gastrointestinal bleeding and may prevent the translocation of bowel organisms or endotoxin by maintaining the integrity of the gastrointestinal tract's mucosal barrier function. Nutritional requirements during severe sepsis and septic shock have been addressed by numerous organizations and medical societies. Adequate nutrition is responsible for improved wound healing, decreasing susceptibility of critically ill patients to infection and optimizing immune function. The following nutritional guidelines have been recommended for patients with sepsis:

- daily caloric intake, 25–30 kcal/kg/usual body weight/day
- protein, 1.3–2.0 g/kg/day
- glucose, 30%–70% of total nonprotein calories to maintain serum glucose <225 mg/dL
- lipids, 15%–30% of total nonprotein calories
- Omega-6 polyunsaturated fatty acids should be reduced in septic patients, maintaining that level which avoids deficiency of essential fatty acids (7% of total calories-generally 1 g/kg/d).

Metabolic management also includes correction of electrolyte abnormalities as well as tight control of blood sugar, which may require constant insulin infusion. In a report of postsurgical predominantly ventilated patients, tight glucose control aimed at keeping the blood sugar between 90 and 110 mg/dL was associated with a significant improvement in ICU and hospital

*Not FDA approved for this indication.

survival. There were four times more deaths from multiple organ failure secondary to a proven septic focus in the group that did not receive the tight glucose control.

INNOVATIVE THERAPIES IN SEVERE SEPSIS AND SEPTIC SHOCK

Severe sepsis and septic shock have continued to be associated with a significant mortality rate despite the improvements in our understanding of the septic process, the use of powerful antibiotic agents, and the provision of basic sepsis management. Technologic advances have also brought forward antibodies, receptor blockers, and other innovative agents designed to interrupt or block aspects of the septic cascade. The majority of innovative experimental strategies were directed at various components of the proinflammatory response evident during the initial phases of SIRS and sepsis. Lack of success with the majority of these trials has led to a shift in the target for interruption toward a later stage aspect of the septic cascade. A number of these recent strategies have taken aim at the coagulation system in an effort to inhibit the generation of thrombin and fibrin, which may be instrumental in the disorder of the microcirculation that may be at least partially responsible for the organ system dysfunction and MODS seen in severe sepsis and SIRS.

Corticosteroid Therapy

Experimental studies in animal models of sepsis and septic shock have demonstrated improved survival with the pretreatment or early treatment with high doses of corticosteroids. The use of high doses of corticosteroids in humans with severe sepsis and septic shock has not been associated with significant improvements in survival except in one study. As a result of multiple trials of high-dose steroids in patients with severe sepsis showing no benefit and potential harm this practice has been abandoned. Recently, the observation that basal cortisol levels and the cortisol response to the administration of adrenocorticotrophic hormone (Corticotropin) (ACTH) could predict survival in patients with severe sepsis and septic shock has drawn attention back to the use of steroid therapy. A French study of patients with septic shock demonstrated that a basal cortisol level of ≤34 μg/dL along with the ability to increase the cortisol level by ≥9 μg/dL was associated with a 74% survival rate. In comparison, patients who had a basal cortisol level of >34 μg/dL and were unable to increase their cortisol level by ≥9 μg/dL had an 18% survival rate. The investigators proposed that some patients with septic shock have a state of relative adrenal insufficiency or problems with their glucocorticoid receptors that can be improved with the use of more physiologic corticosteroid replacement therapy. A recent multicenter, prospective, randomized, controlled trial of 300 patients with vasopressor-dependent septic shock who were all receiving mechanical ventilatory support and were resuscitated according to a defined protocol demonstrated an improved survival rate in those patients who failed to increase their basal cortisol level by >9 μg/dL and were given physiologic corticosteroid replacement therapy. For this trial the physiologic corticosteroid replacement therapy consisted of 50 mg of hydrocortisone (Solu-Cortef)* intravenously administered every 6 hours for 7 days combined with once daily fludrocortisone (Florinef)* given enterally at 50 μg/day. The authors of this trial concluded that physiologic corticosteroid therapy is beneficial and should be administered to vasopressor-dependent patients in septic shock who manifest relative adrenal insufficiency as defined by the failure to increase the cortisol level by more than 9 μg/dL after ACTH stimulation.

High-Volume Continuous Venovenous Hemofiltration Therapy

The use of high-volume, continuous hemofiltration (either continuous arteriovenous or venovenous) has been reported to benefit the hemodynamic course and outcome in patients with intractable circulatory failure resulting from septic shock. The use of this form of management is expensive, requires defined expertise, and may be associated with metabolic and coagulation abnormalities. Further studies are needed to determine if this mode of therapy improves outcome in septic patients. Its use should probably be limited to patients with renal indications for hemofiltration.

Antithrombotic Therapy

Newer therapies have been directed toward inhibitors of the coagulation system as a potential therapeutic strategy for patients with severe sepsis and septic shock. Earlier therapies targeting the proinflammatory stage have shown little benefit in reducing mortality. Among the therapies that have been used are antithrombin, tissue factor pathway inhibitor (TFPI), and activated protein C replacement therapy.

Antithrombin III (AT) is an endogenous serine protease that has antithrombotic and anti-inflammatory properties. In an early trial in a small number of patients the administration of AT* to patients with septic shock and disseminated intravascular coagulation demonstrated a trend toward improved survival. Subsequently a large multicenter, prospective, randomized, double-blind, placebo-controlled trial was conducted which unfortunately showed no difference in mortality compared to placebo at 30, 60, and 90 days.

Tissue factor pathway inhibitor (TFPI) inhibits Factor VIIa within the Factor VIIa/tissue factor complex, after first binding and inactivating Factor Xa. Recently, a Phase 3 multicenter, prospective, randomized, double-blind, placebo-controlled trial has been completed and reportedly failed to demonstrate a significant benefit in the primary endpoint, which was 28-day all-cause mortality.

As with antithrombin, the Protein C system is one of the endogenous antithrombotic agents. Drotrecogin alfa (activated) (Xigris) is recombinant human activated

*Not FDA approved for this indication.

protein C. A recent Phase 3 trial was stopped after the second interim analysis demonstrated a significant survival benefit associated with the use of activated protein C versus placebo in 1690 patients with severe sepsis and septic shock. Treatment with a 96-hour infusion of drotrecogin alfa (activated) produced a 6.1% absolute risk reduction and a 19.4% relative risk reduction in the 28-day all-cause mortality in patients with severe sepsis (P = .005). The use of drotrecogin alfa (activated) was accompanied by a significant reduction in D-dimer and IL-6 levels, supporting a beneficial effect on coagulation and inflammation, respectively. There was also restoration of the normal fibrinolytic pathway with the use of activated protein C. The drotrecogin alfa (activated)-treated population did experience more serious bleeding complications (3.5%) compared with the placebo group (2.0%), and this difference trended toward significance. These results suggest that for every 66 patients treated with drotrecogin alfa (activated), one additional serious bleeding event would occur. The number needed to treat to save an additional life was 16. A recent pharmacoeconomic analysis concluded that this agent is beneficial in patients with severe sepsis and septic shock who had a high risk of mortality and were young or had a high likelihood of surviving were it not for the complicating septic process.

The Food and Drug Administration (FDA) and 19 other regulatory bodies in other countries (including the European Union) have approved the use of drotrecogin alfa (activated) for the treatment of severe sepsis in adult patients with a high risk of mortality. The FDA gives the example of using the Acute Physiology and Chronic Health Evaluation (APACHE) II to estimate the risk of death (APACHE II score ≥25) and other means such as the number of dysfunctional organs to determine the target population of patients. Currently, the safety and efficacy of drotrecogin alfa (activated) in pediatric patients has not been determined. Contraindications for the use of drotrecogin alfa (activated) include patients with known sensitivity to drotrecogin alfa (activated) and those patients with a high risk of death from or significant morbidity associated with bleeding. This group would include patients with active internal bleeding, recent (within 3 months) hemorrhagic stroke, recent (within 2 months) intracranial or intraspinal surgery or severe head trauma, trauma with increased risk of life-threatening bleeding, the presence of an epidural catheter, an intracranial neoplasm, or mass lesion or evidence of cerebral herniation.

PROGNOSIS

Despite the tremendous advances in our appreciation of the pathophysiologic processes that comprise the septic response coupled with improved antibiotics and technologic support of the critically ill, the mortality rate for patients with severe sepsis and septic shock remains high. Clinical trials have reported placebo-group mortality rates attributable to severe sepsis and septic shock of 20% to 50%, with mortality rates up to 80% to 85% with septic shock and multiple organ failure. This high rate of morbidity and mortality demands an aggressive approach for early diagnosis and treatment in an attempt to improve the outcome of these critically ill patients. A number of factors have been found to impact survival including, age, comorbid condition, site and type of infection, severity of illness, the number, and specific organ system failures. In addition, a patient's genetic makeup or gender may have a dramatic impact on whether or not they develop sepsis, as well as the severity, clinical manifestations, and outcome of the sepsis. It has also been demonstrated that survivors of sepsis have increased 6- and 12-month mortality rates compared with matched nonseptic critically ill patients. There is also a reduced quality of life and more health-related issues in those patients who have survived an episode of sepsis. These observations underscore the importance of early aggressive management of the septic patient and suggest that our future focus should also be directed toward prevention of sepsis.

BRUCELLOSIS

method of
ISIDRO ZAVALA TRUJILLO, M.D., and
MARIA GUADALUPE ZAVALA, M.D.
Universidad Autónoma de Guadalajara
Guadalajara, Mexico

Brucellosis is distributed worldwide and remains endemic in many parts of the underdeveloped world. It affects mainly domestic animals. It continues to be one of the most widely distributed zoonoses, and humans are commonly infected.

Brucellae are small gram-negative coccobacillary, nonmotile microorganisms that possess great ability to survive within phagocytes. There are seven known species of brucellae (Table 1).

EPIDEMIOLOGY

The World Health Organization points out that cases of brucellosis are reported each year around the world. *Brucella abortus* is more prevalent in the United States and northern Europe, whereas *Brucella melitensis* is more common in Latin America, the Mediterranean, and the developing world.

TABLE 1. **Different Species of Brucella**

Microorganisms	Biovars	Infected Animals
B. melitensis	4	Goats, camels
B. abortus	8	Cows, camels, buffalo
B. suis	4	Domestic and feral swine
B. ovis		Sheep
B. neotomae		Desert rats
B. canis		Kennel-raised dogs
B. maris		Marine mammals and cetaceans

Brucellosis is transmitted from animals to humans by three main routes: through the digestive tract by eating contaminated meat and unpasteurized milk or milk products; by direct contact of conjunctiva or broken skin with infected tissues or blood; and by the respiratory system through inhalation by laboratory personnel of clinical isolates or the live vaccine. Other rare forms such as transmission through total blood transfusions and possible sexual transmission from person to person have been documented.

In the United States, after the implementation of effective programs for the eradication of this disease in animals, the incidence of brucellosis in humans has declined in a progressive and consistent manner. Nevertheless, in states bordering Mexico, such as Texas and California, the epidemiology of brucellosis is mainly linked to the ingestion of unpasteurized goat milk products imported from Mexico.

PATHOGENESIS

It is known that *B. abortus* is taken up by polymorphonuclear leukocytes and that 24 hours later brucellae are present in the Kupffer cells, followed by the formation of granulomas made up of epithelioid cells. Resolution starts by the sixth month, and the infection disappears completely by the end of a year. In contrast, an accumulation of neutrophils with tissue destruction was observed when *Brucella suis* and *B. melitensis* were used, resulting in abscess formation.

Infection by brucellae is obligatory intracellular infection, particularly within the cells of the reticuloendothelial system. This characteristic predisposes to future relapses because of the presence of brucellae within the blood causing the disease to be chronic.

IMMUNITY

Factors that affect the clinical presentation and evolution of the infection are nutrition, age, immune state, size of the inoculate, and route of acquisition of the infection.

In general, the infection induces both humoral and cellular immunity. In studies utilizing animal models, it has been found that immunity to brucellae is mediated by lymphocytes, which interact with the host's macrophages in an attempt to increase their ability to inactivate ingested bacteria. The serum antibody response to brucellosis in humans should be evaluated by agglutination methods complemented by the use of reducing agents (2-mercaptoethanol or dithiothreitol) to distinguish the class of immunoglobulin. This response is characterized by an initial rise in antibody titers of the class IgM, followed in several weeks by a predominance of IgG antibodies.

With the enzyme-linked immunosorbent assay (ELISA) technique, it was found that antibodies to brucellae were present 12 months after treatment in patients without relapse, and in patients with relapse a second peak of IgG and IgA antibodies was detected.

CLINICAL MANIFESTATIONS

Brucellosis manifests itself in a wide variety of clinical presentations and can be divided into three types (Table 2).

The bacteremic type has an acute evolution associated with signs and symptoms of systemic dissemination. Intermittent fever (temperature >38.5°C) is one of the most consistent signs. The headache tends to be intense and is accompanied by vomiting, simulating meningitis, profuse sweating, depression, anorexia, and significant weakness; also, muscular and articular pain often impedes walking. In this form the diagnosis is established by cultures and serology (Figure 1).

The chronic form classification should be reserved for those who have symptoms of the disease for over 1 year after the diagnosis of brucellosis is established.

The sites more frequently affected by localized brucellosis are bones, joints, central nervous system, liver, spleen, heart, prostate, kidney, bladder, testicles, eyes, and skin. This form is generally related to cases in which the organism is not present in blood, in which case the diagnosis is established by isolating *Brucella*, taking a biopsy of the affected area.

The osteoarticular manifestations can be present in less than 85%, including arthralgias, arthritis, spondylitis, osteomyelitis, tenosynovitis, bursitis, and sacroiliitis.

DIAGNOSIS

Blood cultures are generally accepted as the procedure of choice, processed using the Castaneda technique, and growth of brucella may require up to 6 weeks. In the localized forms, culture material should be taken from the affected zones.

Occasionally, the diagnosis is made serologically by several techniques such as the serum agglutination test (SAT) with standard tube dilution plus 2-mercaptoethanol; which inhibits the agglutinating activity of IgM but not IgG. The ELISA method has the characteristic of quantifying the total antibodies whether or not they are agglutinants (Table 3).

TREATMENT

Several antimicrobial agents are active against *Brucella* spp. Combination therapy with two active drugs is superior to monotherapy. It is important to use antibiotics that show excellent in vitro activity against brucellae and the ability to penetrate cells, reaching sufficient concentrations to inhibit growth of the organisms, or better to reach bactericidal concentrations.

TABLE 2. **Clinical Presentations of Brucellosis**

Clinical Form	Cultures	SAT, 2-ME
Acute (bacteremic)	Blood (positive)	≥1:160
	Bone marrow (positive)	≥1:160
Chronic	(Negative)	≥1:80
		≥1:80
Localized	Biopsy of tissue (positive)	≥1:160*
	Material from abscess (positive)	≥1:160

*In some cases serology test may be negative.

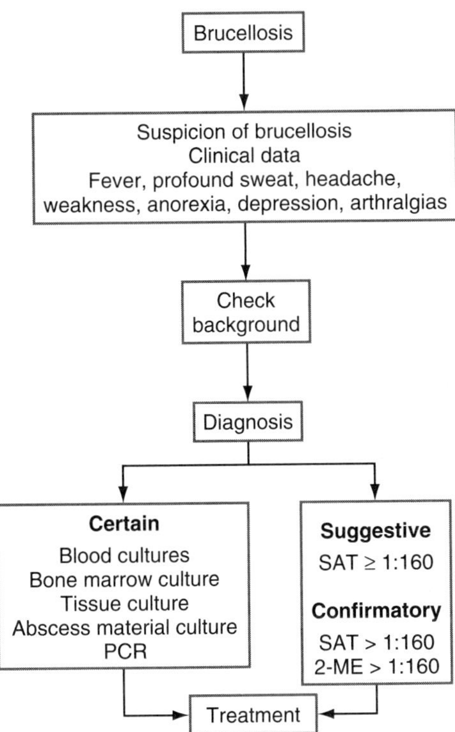

Figure 1. Essentials of the diagnosis of brucellosis.

Combinations such as doxycycline (Vibramycin) plus streptomycin, tetracycline plus streptomycin, doxycycline plus rifampin (Rifadin)*, and doxycycline plus ofloxacin (Floxin)* are considered appropriate treatments.

Rifampin plus trimethoprim-sulfamethoxazole (TMP-SMZ) (Bactrim)* is considered the drug combination of choice for the treatment of pregnant women. Combinations such as gentamicin (Garamycin) plus doxycycline, gentamicin plus rifampin, oxytetracycline (Terramycin) plus gentamicin, and TMP-SMZ with gentamicin have been used with no relapses. TMP-SMZ plus rifampin and gentamicin plus rifampin are an excellent combination for children older than 8 years.

PREVENTION

The prevention of brucellosis requires the eradication of the infection from domestic animals, the use of effective barriers by people at high risk, and pasteurization of milk.

*Not FDA approved for this indication.

TABLE 3. **Diagnosis of Brucellosis**

Blood culture (3)
Bone marrow culture
Tissue (biopsy) culture
Material abscess culture
CSF culture
PCR
Serology:
SAT* and 2-ME**, ELISA

*Serum agglutination test
**2-Mercaptoethanol

VARICELLA (CHICKENPOX)

method of
HENRY H. BALFOUR, JR., M.D.
Department of Laboratory Medicine and Pathology
Department of Pediatrics
University of Minnesota Medical School
Minneapolis, Minnesota

Chickenpox is both preventable *and* treatable. Like measles, mumps, and rubella, chickenpox is preventable by immunization with a live, attenuated vaccine. Unlike measles, mumps, and rubella, it can be successfully treated with specific antiviral therapy. Chickenpox is a mild disease for most children, but it can be serious and sometimes fatal for adults and immunocompromised patients of any age.

ETIOLOGY AND EPIDEMIOLOGY

Chickenpox (also called varicella) usually results from primary infection with varicella-zoster virus, a human herpesvirus. Shingles (also called herpes zoster) occurs when varicella-zoster virus, which has remained clinically latent in dorsal root ganglia after causing chickenpox, reactivates and travels down afferent sensory nerves to produce a painful dermatomal rash. Varicella-zoster virus is spread most readily by droplets aerosolized when an infected person talks, coughs or sneezes. This virus also may be contracted by direct contact with the skin lesions of a patient who has either chickenpox or shingles. Persons with chickenpox are most likely to transmit virus during the tail end of their incubation period and for the first 2 days of the rash. Chickenpox is quite contagious: when introduced into a household, 86% of susceptible children will contract it. In temperate climates, chickenpox is a seasonal illness that most commonly affects young children during the months of October through May. Children are infected less frequently in the tropics, leaving them susceptible to adult-onset chickenpox. Varicella-zoster virus is heat-labile, which may explain its apparent reduced infectivity among children in rural tropical settings. The incubation period of chickenpox is 14 days with a range of 10 to 21 days. Second cases are well documented but are uncommon. There were 4,000,000 cases of chickenpox annually in the United States until a live, attenuated vaccine was approved in 1995. Since then, the yearly incidence has steadily fallen.

CLINICAL COURSE

Otherwise Healthy Children

Children have a mild or unapparent prodrome of low grade fever, malaise and respiratory symptoms. A day or two later, a pruritic rash develops in the scalp and on the face. The rash quickly spreads to the trunk and then to the extremities. Skin lesions are usually most numerous on the trunk. The rash evolves rapidly from maculopapules to superficial vesicles and then more slowly to pustules which finally crust. I have actually seen papules turn into vesicles during the course of a physical examination. Vesicles form on mucosal surfaces as well as the skin but these rapidly rupture to become shallow ulcers. Lesions are frequently at different stages of development in the same area. New skin lesions continue to form for a median of 3 days after the onset of rash. The appearance of new lesions for more than 7 days suggests that the patient has an underlying immunocompromised condition. Children who are not treated with antiviral therapy average 350 to 400 skin lesions. Oral acyclovir (Zovirax) therapy results in 50 to 100 fewer lesions. A reduction in the total number of lesions is first appreciated on the fourth day after the onset of rash. The lesions usually crust within a week. When the crusts are shed, a small pit sometimes surrounded by hypopigmentation may remain. In controlled clinical treatment trials, children who received placebo averaged 33 of these residual lesions when examined 28 days after onset of illness as compared with 13 lesions among their acyclovir-treated counterparts. The vast majority of the residual lesions heal in several months without leaving a scar.

Adolescents and Adults

The prodrome in adults and adolescents is more pronounced than it is in children. The evolution and distribution of the rash is similar to that of younger patients, except that the lesions are more numerous and may be more pruritic. Patients are often systemically ill.

Pregnant Women and Newborn Infants

Pregnant women with chickenpox are prone to develop viral pneumonia. If chickenpox occurs during the first 20 weeks of pregnancy, there is a 1% to 2% risk of fetal damage resulting in ocular and central nervous system abnormalities, cicatricial skin lesions, and limb hypoplasia. If a mother develops chickenpox within 7 days before or after delivery, her infant may develop neonatal chickenpox. This disease resembles bacterial sepsis and can be fatal. Until the age of 28 days, neonates who contract chickenpox from any source are at some risk for a severe illness. In contrast, infants whose mothers have shingles during pregnancy rarely if ever sustain a clinically significant varicella-zoster virus infection.

Immunocompromised Hosts

Chickenpox in an immunocompromised patient is serious. Among 127 children with cancer not given prophylaxis or antiviral therapy, 28% developed chickenpox pneumonia and the overall mortality rate was 7%. Immunocompromised hosts have a prolonged course and may continue to form new skin lesions for several weeks unless treated with antiviral drugs. Rather than following its usual evolution, the rash often stalls at the vesicular or even papulovesicular stage. Vesicles may became bullous or hemorrhagic. The virus may substantially damage visceral organs, especially the lungs, liver, gastrointestinal tract, bone marrow, or central nervous system. Signs and symptoms of visceral involvement mean that the illness is potentially life-threatening.

COMPLICATIONS

In immunocompetent children, the most common complication is bacterial infection of skin lesions, which may progress to cellulitis or even necrotizing fasciitis. If patients become septic, suppurative arthritis, osteomyelitis, or bacterial pneumonia may result. Rare complications due to the virus itself include arthritis, carditis, cerebellar ataxia, encephalitis, glomerulonephritis, hepatitis, orchitis, pneumonia, thrombocytopenia, uveitis, and vascultis.

In the immunocompromised host, the virus has a predilection for the lungs, liver, gastrointestinal tract, central nervous system, and bone marrow. Any evidence of visceral involvement (such as dyspnea or abdominal pain) should prompt admission to the hospital for antiviral therapy as described below.

DIAGNOSIS

Chickenpox is almost always a clinical diagnosis. Most patients give a history of exposure to chickenpox 2 weeks before they present with characteristic skin lesions concentrated on the face and trunk. In atypical cases, the diagnosis may be confirmed by submitting lesion aspirates or swabs to a diagnostic virology laboratory for culture or antigen detection. Conditions most often confused with chickenpox are skin infections due to herpes simplex virus, streptococci, or staphylococci. If the central nervous system is involved and the diagnosis is uncertain, cerebrospinal fluid should be submitted for detection of varicella-zoster virus by a sensitive and specific diagnostic technique such as polymerase chain reaction.

PREVENTION

A live, attenuated vaccine (Varivax) is approved in the United States for prevention of chickenpox and should be part of routine childhood immunizations (Table 1). Chickenpox vaccine had a protective efficacy of 95% over a 7-year follow-up period in children who participated in a placebo-controlled research study. If vaccinees develop chickenpox after exposure to wild virus, their illness is usually mild. The United States has opted for a strategy of universal chickenpox immunization, whereas some other countries offer vaccine only to persons at high risk of exposure (as listed in Table 1). There are advantages and disadvantages to both approaches. Success of the universal immunization plan depends upon achieving herd immunity. If the velocity of transmission is slowed but not stopped, the result could be an increase in the age at which susceptible individuals contract chickenpox. Adults are sicker than children and are at greater risk for complications. Therefore, it is important that every

TABLE 1. **Prevention of Chickenpox**

Prophylaxis	Clinical Category	Dosage	Comments
Pre-exposure			
Chickenpox vaccine (Varivax)	Healthy child 1-12 years old	1 dose (0.5 mL SC)	Give after age 15 mo if possible
	Healthy susceptible person ≥13 years old*	2 doses, 4-8 weeks apart	It may be cost-effective to screen patients for antibody and only immunize the seronegatives, because ~80% of persons in this age group are seropositive
Post-exposure			
Varicella-zoster immune globulin (VZIG) MUST BE GIVEN WITHIN 96 HR OF EXPOSURE	Premature newborn	1 vial (1.25 mL) IM	Gestational age <28 wk: all hospital exposures; gestational age >28 wk: hospital exposures if mother is seronegative
	Term newborn	1 vial IM	If exposed in hospital when <28 days old
	Pregnant woman	5 vials IM	Or one large vial (6.25 mL)
	Infant with maternal chickenpox	1 vial IM	If mother develops chickenpox 7 days before or after delivery
	Immunocompromised host	1 vial/10 kg of body weight IM	
Acyclovir (Zovirax)**	Susceptible household member	20 mg/kg (maximum 800 mg) 4 times daily for 7 days	Best results when initiated 7-9 days post-exposure
	Pregnant woman Immunocompromised host	800 mg orally 5 times daily for 7-10 days	An option when the exposure is not recognized until the 5th day

*Susceptible persons to target for immunization include women of childbearing age (unless pregnant), workers in environments where transmission is likely (healthcare, day care, elementary and middle school), and residents in households with children who haven't had chickenpox.

**Not FDA approved for this indication.

effort be made to maximize acceptance and uptake of chickenpox vaccine in the United States.

Although chickenpox vaccine is approved only for otherwise healthy persons, certain immunocompromised patients may be safely and effectively immunized. They include children with acute leukemia in remission, transplant candidates, and HIV-infected individuals with CD4 cell counts >200/μL or CD4 percentages of at least 25%. Before immunizing such patients, it would be prudent to consult an infectious disease specialist.

Chickenpox vaccine can also provide post-exposure protection if given within 4 days of the exposure. If more than 4 days have elapsed and prophylaxis is deemed necessary, the best approach is to prescribe oral acyclovir. Post-exposure prophylaxis using varicella-zoster immune globulin (VZIG) or acyclovir (Zovirax)* is appropriate in certain settings as outlined in Table 1. VZIG is expensive and pain at injection site is a frequent complaint. Because VZIG is passive prophylaxis, it must be repeated after each exposure until the patient develops chickenpox or persistent antibodies to varicella-zoster virus indicating that a subclinical infection has stimulated active immunity.

TREATMENT

Antiviral Therapy

Acyclovir (Zovirax) is the mainstay of specific treatment (Table 2). Both valacyclovir (Valtrex)* and famciclovir (Famvir)* should be at least as effective as acyclovir, but they have not yet been studied appropriately in patients with chickenpox. Acyclovir shortens the clinical course by 25% to 30% in otherwise healthy persons. Many children and their parents find this desirable. My rationale for treating all children over the age of 24 months is that it is impossible to predict exactly which child is destined to have a severe case of chickenpox. Since oral acyclovir therapy is safe, the risk-benefit ratio favors treatment. Therapy is especially worthwhile in adolescents, adults, and children who represent secondary cases in their household, because patients in these categories tend to be sicker. Acyclovir is most effective when started within 24 hours of onset of rash, but recent data have shown a benefit if it is initiated on the second and perhaps even third day of the rash.

Immunocompromised patients with chickenpox should always be given antiviral therapy. The standard of care is acyclovir administered intravenously at a dose of 10 mg/kg every 8 hours (Table 2). There are data to support switching from intravenous to oral acyclovir once the patient has ceased forming new lesions and has no evidence of visceral disease. Antiviral therapy should be initiated as soon as possible, because it may not prevent spread to visceral organs if given more than 2 days after onset of rash. However, immunocompromised patients who present late in their clinical course should still be treated with intravenous acyclovir unless they have stopped forming new skin lesions and have no evidence of visceral disease.

Which immunocompromised patients are at risk for visceral chickenpox? Solid organ and bone marrow transplant recipients, patients receiving cytotoxic drugs or chronic corticosteroid therapy for malignancies or autoimmune diseases, and persons with AIDS who have <200 CD4 cells are at high risk. Patients who take aspirin regularly or use intermittent corticosteroids, as well as those with chronic cutaneous, cardiac or pulmonary disease are at some risk. Many

*Not FDA approved for this indication.

TABLE 2. **Antiviral Therapy for Chickenpox**

Clinical Category	Treatment of Choice	Alternative Treatment	Comments
Otherwise healthy child	Oral acyclovir (Zovirax), 20 mg/kg (maximum 800 mg) 4 times daily for 5 days	None	Treatment most effective when initiated within 24 hr of onset of rash; secondary household cases tend to be sicker than index case.
Otherwise healthy adolescent or adult	Oral acyclovir, 800 mg 4 times daily for 5 days	Valacyclovir (Valtrex),* 1000 mg 3 times daily for 5 days Famciclovir (Famvir),* 500 mg 3 times daily for 5 days	Both valacyclovir and famciclovir should be at least as effective as acyclovir but controlled trials have not been reported and these drugs are not approved for treatment of chickenpox
Pregnant woman	Oral acyclovir, 800 mg 4 times daily for 5 days	Intravenous acyclovir, 10 mg/kg every 8 hr for 7 days if there is evidence of visceral chickenpox	Acyclovir is not approved for use in pregnancy (Pregnancy Category B)
Neonatal chickenpox	Intravenous acyclovir,* 10 mg/kg every 8 hr for 7 days	None	
Immunocompromised host	Intravenous acyclovir,* 10 mg/kg every 8 hr for 10 days	Switch to oral acyclovir, 800 mg 5 times a day to complete 10-day course	The switch from intravenous to oral acyclovir should not be made until the patient is afebrile, has ceased forming new lesions, and has no evidence of visceral chickenpox

*Not FDA approved for this indication

clinicians elect to treat mildly immunocompromised patients with oral rather than intravenous acyclovir. If oral acyclovir is prescribed, these patients should be followed closely and admitted to the hospital for intravenous acyclovir if evidence of visceral disease develops.

Symptomatic Relief

Pruritus is the chief complaint, especially in adolescents and adults. Patients should avoid sunlight, especially in the summer, because it aggravates the rash, intensifying itching. Pruritus may be relieved with cold compresses applied periodically to the itchiest spots. Colloidal oatmeal baths (Aveeno) and oral diphenhydramine hydrochloride (Benadryl) may also be helpful. If fever is a problem, acetaminophen (Tylenol) is preferred. Aspirin should not be given to patients younger than 18 because its use in children with acute viral illnesses has been associated with Reye syndrome.

CHOLERA

method of
DILIP MAHALANABIS, M.B.B.S., F.R.C.P. (EDIN)
Society for Applied Studies
Kolkata, India

Cholera is characterized by severe uncontrolled purging of watery stools leading to life-threatening dehydration, hypovolemic shock, and acidosis. Although cholera carries a case fatality rate of 50% or more when left untreated, almost all patients recover fully and rapidly when they are treated adequately. With rapid rehydration, a seriously ill patient in profound shock with no detectable pulse or blood pressure is able to sit, talk, and eat within a few hours and can return to work or school within 2 to 3 days. This life-saving and dramatic treatment can be rendered at a low cost; this is important because cholera affects mainly poor people in developing countries.

Cholera is caused by the bacterium *Vibrio cholerae* serogroup O1 and O139, which colonizes the mucosal lining of the small intestinal lumen. The cholera toxin (CT) released is composed of one A (enzymatic) subunit and five B (binding) subunits. The B subunit binds the toxin molecule to the mucosal cell receptor GM_1 ganglioside; the A subunit is cleaved to produce fragments A1 and A2. The A1 subunit functions as an enzyme intracellularly to activate adenylate cyclase to produce increased levels of cyclic adenosine monophosphate, leading to increased secretion of salt and water. The net effect is the loss of copious amount of fluid and electrolytes manifesting as watery diarrhea. Other toxins produced by *V. cholerae* O1 or O139, such as the zona occludens toxin and accessory cholera toxins, are believed to contribute to the secretion of fluid, but their precise role is not fully defined.

TREATMENT

On examination, a typical cholera patient is extremely weak and thirsty, has a hoarse voice, and often complains of muscle cramps. Signs of dehydration include decreased skin turgor, sunken eyes, dry mucous membranes, and a weak or undetectable radial pulse. Patients often have severe metabolic acidosis. A remarkable aspect of the disease is how a healthy person can become so sick after only a few hours of diarrhea and vomiting. However, much less severe episodes of cholera are common, and mild cases cannot be distinguished clinically from other acute watery diarrheal diseases. Such an acute dehydrating diarrhea syndrome is sometimes caused by other etiologic agents, most notably the enterotoxigenic *Escherichia coli*.

Patients are assessed for signs of dehydration to estimate severity and fluid requirements. Rapid assessment is important because a severely dehydrated patient may literally be within minutes of death unless fluid therapy is started immediately. Clinical assessment is adequate for formulating a treatment plan for individual patients; laboratory tests (e.g., hematocrit, plasma specific gravity, total serum proteins) are used in research studies to compare groups of patients but are superfluous for clinical management. Clinical manifestations of severe cholera are mostly the result of loss of salts and water in the stool and vomitus. Complications arise only when appropriate rehydration is not accomplished rapidly.

Objectives of treatment are (1) rapid replacement of water and salts already lost; (2) maintenance of normal hydration until diarrhea stops, by replacing fluid losses as they occur; (3) reduction of the magnitude and duration of diarrhea with suitable antimicrobials; and (4) introduction of a normal diet as soon as the patient is able to eat without waiting for diarrhea to stop.

Until the early 1970s, fluid losses in cholera could be replaced only by intravenous therapy. Treatment has been revolutionized by the introduction of oral rehydration therapy (ORT), in which a solution containing glucose and three salts is used (Table 1). It has made cholera therapy practical, simple, inexpensive, and highly effective, particularly under field conditions. ORT is based on the fact that glucose-linked enhanced absorption of sodium and water from the small intestine remains largely intact during the massive secretory state of cholera. ORT is optimally employed by starting administration of the solution at the first sign of diarrhea in an amount equal to the losses that occur and continuing it until diarrhea stops. This may reduce the number of severe cases requiring intravenous therapy, conserving scarce medical resources. Research in the 1980s showed that replacing 20 g glucose with 50 g rice flour (which requires cooking; see Table 1) for 1 L oral rehydration salt solution increases absorption and reduces fluid stool losses by 35% to 40% in comparison with glucose oral rehydration salt (ORS) solution. Recently, the World Health Organization (WHO) recommended a universal ORS solution containing a reduced concentration of sodium (75 mmol/L), glucose (75 mmol/L) with a total osmolarity of 245 mOsm/L for use in diarrhea of any etiology and in all age groups. Although this ORS has shown improved effectiveness in children with acute noncholera diarrhea, its use is associated with an increased incidence of transient asymptomatic hyponatremia in adults with cholera. If it is used for treating adults with cholera, careful monitoring is advised for symptomatic hyponatremia.

Intravenous rehydration still plays a critical role in the treatment of cholera. In patients who present with severe dehydration and shock, infusion of appropriate intravenous fluids can be lifesaving. Intravenous fluids should replace the electrolyte losses via cholera stool, which in the severely affected patient range from 100 to 140 mmol/L of sodium, 30 to 50 mmol/L of bicarbonate, and 15 to 30 mmol/L of potassium with an osmolarity close to that of plasma (Table 2). Lactated Ringer's (Hartmann's) solution is commercially available and has a suitable composition (see Table 2). Normal saline with or without glucose should be used only if a more suitable polyelectrolyte solution is not available. In such a situation, a complete ORS solution should be given as early as possible to provide the base and potassium.

Patients with severe dehydration and signs of hypovolemia should be rehydrated intravenously to achieve complete rehydration in 2 to 4 hours. After initial complete rehydration, most patients can be maintained with ORT, although about 10% to 15% of hospitalized patients may need an additional short course of intravenous therapy because of high purging rates and

TABLE 1. **Oral Rehydration Salt Solution**

Amount of Oral Rehydration Salts Needed to Prepare 1 L of Solution	
Sodium chloride	3.5 g
Trisodium citrate dihydrate	2.9 g
OR	
Sodium hydrogen carbonate (sodium bicarbonate)	2.5 g
Potassium chloride	1.5 g
Glucose anhydrous*	20.0 g
(or rice powder)	(50 g)
Molar Concentration of Solution (mmol/L)	
Sodium	90
Potassium	20
Chloride	80
Citrate	10
Glucose	111
Estimated osmolarity (mOsmol/L)	311

*50 g rice powder can replace 20 g glucose. To prepare a rice-oral rehydration salt (ORS) solution, put 50 g rice flour in 1100 mL water and bring to a boil. Continue boiling for about 7-10 min. When the mixture is opalescent, cool, add the three salts. Serve warm and discard after 8 h. Rice-ORS can reduce purging by 30%-40% in comparison with glucose-ORS.

TABLE 2. **Electrolyte Composition of Cholera Stool and Some Intravenous Solutions***

Concentration (mmol/L)	Cholera Stool		Ringer's Lactate**	Normal Saline***
	Adults	*Children*		
Na^+	135	105	131	154
K^+	15	25	4	0
Cl^-	100	90	111	154
HCO_3^-	45	30	26	0

*Do not use 5% dextrose in water to treat dehydrating diarrheal diseases.

**The best commercially available solution. Lactate yields bicarbonate; low potassium concentration is made up by optimum use of oral rehydration therapy.

***Sodium concentration is high for children and solution does not contain a base or potassium. Prompt introduction of oral rehydration therapy may prevent potential problems.

recurrence of signs of dehydration. A single solution is adequate for all age groups in cholera.

Rehydration and Maintenance Therapy

The severity of dehydration must be assessed and the fluid requirement estimated quickly. A severely dehydrated patient with a deficit of about 10% of body weight is very weak with poor skin turgor, sunken eyes, and a barely perceptible or absent radial pulse. As an example, the estimated deficit in a 50-kg adult with severe dehydration is 5 L. A moderately dehydrated patient whose deficit is estimated at about 7.5% has obvious signs of dehydration with dry mucous membranes, sunken eyes, and poor skin turgor; the radial pulse is palpable but soft and rapid. In severely dehydrated patients, intravenous fluids are infused rapidly to quickly restore circulating volume. As a guide, half of the estimated volume of fluid required in a severely dehydrated patient should be given over the first hour, initially as fast as possible until the radial pulse is palpable. The patient should be fully hydrated in 2 to 4 hours, at which time intravenous therapy may be discontinued and oral rehydration therapy started and continued until diarrhea stops.

For most patients with mild and moderate dehydration, ORT can be given both for initial rehydration and for replacement of ongoing fecal losses. ORT can continue in spite of some vomiting, which is common; with persistence and with small frequent feedings, most patients retain enough fluid to become rehydrated.

Adequate replacement is signaled by the return of the radial pulse to normal strength and rate (the pulse rates in an adult are usually below 90 beats per minute), return of skin turgor to normal, and a feeling of well-being. Children who are drowsy or stuporous may not become fully alert for 12 to 18 hours despite adequate rehydration. In addition, weight gain of about 8% to 10% in a severely dehydrated patient is observed. Return of urine output usually occurs within 12 to 20 hours of initial rehydration.

Patients are most conveniently treated with a cholera cot, which allows efficient collection and measurement of stool. In its simplest configuration, a cholera cot consists of a foldable canvas camp cot covered by a plastic sheet with a suitable hole in the center. A sleeve fits into the hole and guides the diarrheal stool into a plastic bucket underneath the cot so that it can be measured periodically. A vomit basin should also be available. A simple input-output chart at the patient's bedside shows the amounts of intravenous and ORS solutions and the volume of stool. A few hospitalized cholera patients may show signs of dehydration while on ORT. If dehydration occurs, additional intravenous fluids are given rapidly as for initial rehydration, after which oral maintenance should be resumed.

Antimicrobial Therapy

The goal of antimicrobial therapy is to drastically reduce or eliminate *V. cholerae* from the intestinal lumen so that no more cholera toxin is produced and only the residual toxin already bound to the gut mucosa remains. The use of a suitable antibiotic such as tetracycline reduces the duration of diarrhea by about 50%, to an average of 2 days; reduces the volume of diarrhea after start of treatment by about 50%; and reduces the duration of *Vibrio* excretion to an average of 1 to 2 days. Therefore, the use of an appropriate antibiotic has a profound effect on the cost and convenience of treatment.

Antibiotics are usually given after completion of initial rehydration (i.e., about 4 to 6 hours after starting treatment). Tetracycline, the antibiotic of choice, is given to adults at 500 mg every 6 hours for 72 hours and to children at 50 mg/kg/d in four divided doses for 72 hours (tetracycline should be avoided in children younger than 8 years of age). Doxycycline (Vibramycin) can also be used in a single dose of 300 mg in adults and 6 mg per kg body weight for children younger than 15 years of age; doxycycline may cause nausea and should be given after the patient eats some food. Alternative antibiotics are furazolidone (Furoxone), 100 mg every 6 hours (for children, 5 mg/kg/d in four divided doses) for 72 hours; erythromycin,* 250 mg every 6 hours (for children, 30 mg/kg/d in three divided doses) for 72 hours; or trimethoprim-sulfamethoxazole (Bactrim)* (8 mg of trimethoprim and 40 mg of sulfamethoxazole per kg/day in two divided doses) for 72 hours. However, *V. cholerae* O139, isolated in 1992 and the recent strains of *V. cholerae* O1 isolated in certain cholera endemic areas, are resistant to trimethoprim/sulfamethoxazole. Chloramphenicol (Chloromycetin)* is also effective in the same dosage as tetracycline but is usually not used because of potential serious side effects. In view of the reported emergence of resistant strains of *V. cholerae* O1 and O139 to some of these drugs in some areas, norfloxacin (Noroxin)* (400 mg twice daily for 3 days) and ciprofloxacin (Cipro)* (500 mg twice daily for 3 days) have been shown to be effective alternatives. Ciprofloxacin and norfloxacin have been incriminated as causing cartilage toxicity in experimental animals and hence are not currently recommended for use in children and pregnant women. Prophylactic antibiotics are not recommended because of the risk of the emergence of antibiotic-resistant strains.

Diet

Patients should be offered normal food as soon as the dehydration and acidosis are corrected and they feel able to eat.

COMPLICATIONS

Complications of cholera are rare if correct treatment is provided quickly because most result from delay in therapy or provision of inappropriate fluid therapy. Risks of pyrogen reaction, excessive hydration, or too-rapid correction of hypernatremia or hyponatremia or acidosis are minimized by optimal

*Not FDA approved for this indication.

use of ORT and early resumption of a normal diet. Pneumonia, a not uncommon problem, may be due to aspiration of vomitus or altered tissue resistance secondary to shock and acidosis.

PREVENTION

The only effective means of preventing cholera is to ensure that healthy individuals are not infected with *V. cholerae* through food and drink. Therefore, washing hands with soap and water, using clean water for drinking and washing utensils and other activities, and appropriate excreta disposal are useful preventive measures. The injectable killed bacterial vaccines are not recommended because protection is inadequate, short-lived, and ineffective in children. Two new cholera vaccines—the inactivated oral whole cell recombinant B subunit vaccine* and the live oral CVD-103HgR vaccine*—are marketed in Sweden and Switzerland, respectively. A group of WHO experts observed that the killed whole cell B subunit oral vaccine (CHOLERIX)* could be considered for use in cholera prevention or control in emergencies. The recommendation for vaccination applies primarily to high-risk situations, such as refugee or displaced populations (either coming from or located in endemic areas) at risk or in natural disaster situations, when the crude death rates resulting from cholera are above 1 to 2 per 10,000 people per day. WHO discourages vaccination as a means of personal protection for foreign travelers.

*Not FDA approved for this indication.

FOOD-BORNE ILLNESS

method of
GEORGE J. GIANAKOPOULOS, M.D.
Clinical Assistant Professor of Medicine, Ohio State University
Private practice, General Infectious Diseases
Riverside Methodist Hospital
Columbus, Ohio

Food-borne illness remains an important and continually changing health problem in all countries of the world. In the United States over the last 20 years, several "new kids on the block" have emerged to take our attention, including E. coli 0157:H7, *Campylobacter jejuni*, *Listeria monocytogenes*, *Cyclospora*, and *Cryptosporidium*. The CDC recently reported that they estimate food-borne diseases will cause 76 million illnesses with 5000 associated deaths in the next year in the United States alone. There is a palpable paranoia in the United States when it comes to the perceived lack of safety in our food supply. This is because food-borne diseases are common and the notion that our food supply comes from places with less rigid sanitary standards than that of the United States. Technology and food science practices of the 21st century have not eradicated or reduced food-borne diseases because of the mass production and processing of meats, fruits and vegetables as well as the loss of smaller farmers and producers. Other contributing factors may include migrating and moving populations, more restaurants and "fast foods," and less emphasis on traditional home lifestyle and family meals.

Table 1 lists food-borne illnesses and their characteristics. The CDC web site at www.CDC.gov has an exhaustive list of articles on the subject and detailed chapters are available in the infectious disease textbooks in any medical library. The office physician will come into contact mostly with viral, bacterial and protozoal causes of food-borne illnesses. Included in this chapter's tables are toxin-associated syndromes from mushrooms and seafood.

Food-borne diseases cause the most morbidity-mortality in the very young and the very old. This reflects the immaturity of the infant's immune system and the waning immunity seen with aging that predisposes to other diseases. Also of note is the role of normal intestinal microflora and microenvironment or lack thereof in the susceptible host. The stomach's low pH is classically one of the "lines of first defense" of the alimentary canal and when altered by age, disease or antacids, may predispose to symptomatic infection with various organisms. This concept has been well documented with salmonellosis and it is even postulated that alteration of normal gut flora with antibiotics disrupts colonization resistance and creates an environment suitable for allowing symptomatic salmonellosis.

Salmonella will be handled extensively in a separate chapter. It, along with *Campylobacter*, is one of the most common bacterial causes of acute infectious colitis. Foods most commonly associated with salmonellosis include poultry and dairy products but also sources of *Salmonella* include reptiles and exotic pets, such as iguanas. Tens of thousands of these kinds of animals are being imported each year. There are many well-documented outbreaks of non-typhoidal *Salmonella* associated with pets. Classic typhoid fever is rare in the United States but can be seen in expatriates, travelers and migrant workers. *Salmonella* has a "tropism" for vascular endothelium and can cause mycotic aneurysm formation, particularly in patients with pre-existing atherosclerosis. Positive blood cultures for *Salmonella* should always be treated with at least two weeks of a susceptibility directed antimicrobial, typically ciprofloxacin (Cipro). Careful follow-up of patients with documented positive blood cultures for *Salmonella* species is prudent. If persistently positive blood cultures are noted, a search for an endovascular sanctuary site such as a pre-existing aneurysm should be undertaken.

Campylobacter is probably underappreciated by many primary care physicians as one of the most common causes of symptomatic and prolonged diarrhea syndromes. In adolescents and young adults, it is the most common cause of bacterial infectious colitis. This is essentially a zoonotic infection that can also contaminate food and water in a classic fecal-oral model. There also is an association between Guillain-Barré syndrome and *Campylobacter* infection. A high

TABLE 1. **Food-Borne Illnesses**

Etiologic Agent	Estimated U.S. Food-Borne Cases/Year*	Incubation	Signs and Symptoms	Associated Foods	Treatment
Viral Agents					
Calicivirus (Norwalk-like agents)	~9,200,000	24–48 h	Nausea, vomiting, watery diarrhea; may be fever	Fecally contaminated foods, ready-to-eat foods touched by infected food workers, shellfish	Fluids, antimotility agents
Rotavirus, astrovirus	~39,000 each	1–3 d	Vomiting, watery diarrhea, low-grade fever	Same	Same
Hepatitis A	~4200	30 d (range, 15–50 d)	Dark urine, jaundice, flulike symptoms, diarrhea	Same	Same
Bacterial Agents					
Campylobacter jejuni	~2,000,000	2–5 d	Diarrhea, cramps, fever, vomiting; may be bloody diarrhea Sequela: Guillain-Barré syndrome	Raw and undercooked poultry, unpasteurized milk, contaminated water	Fluids; antibiotics (ciprofloxacin [Cipro], 500 mg PO bid × 3 d, or azithromycin 500 mg PO qd × 3d
Salmonella (nontyphoidal)	~1,300,000	1–3 d	Diarrhea, fever, abdominal cramps, vomiting; occasional bloody diarrhea Sequela: septicemia	Raw or undercooked poultry, contaminated eggs *(Salmonella enteritidis)*, unpasteurized milk or juice, contaminated raw fruits or vegetables	Fluids; antibiotics *not* indicated unless extraintestinal spread (or immunocompromised host at risk for extraintestinal spread); for invasive/extraintestinal disease, ciprofloxacin, 500 mg PO bid × 5–7 d
Clostridium perfringens	~250,000	8–16 h	Watery diarrhea, nausea, abdominal cramps; fever rare	Meats, poultry, gravy; often precooked	Fluids, supportive care
Staphylococcal food poisoning	~190,000	1–6 h	Sudden onset of severe nausea and vomiting; may be diarrhea	Unrefrigerated or improperly refrigerated meat, potato and egg salad, cream pastries	Fluids, supportive care
Escherichia coli O157:H7 and STEC	~94,000	1–8 d	Diarrhea, often bloody; abdominal pain and vomiting; little or no fever Sequela: hemolytic-uremic syndrome	Undercooked beef (esp. hamburger), unpasteurized milk and juice, raw fruits and vegetables (sprouts)	Fluids, supportive care; *antibiotics contraindicated*
Shigella	~90,000	24–48 h	Abdominal cramps, fever, diarrhea; stool may contain blood and mucus	Fecally contaminated food or water, ready-to-eat foods touched by infected food workers	Fluids, supportive care. Treat with ciprofloxacin, 500 mg PO bid × 3 d, or TMP/SMZ (Bactrim), DS PO bid × 3 d
Yersinia enterocolitica	~87,000	24–48 h	Diarrhea and vomiting, fever, abdominal pain; may cause pseudoappendicitis syndrome	Undercooked pork, unpasteurized milk	Fluids, supportive care; antibiotics if suggestion of invasive disease (ciprofloxacin, 500 mg PO bid × 3 d, TMP/SMZ, DS PO bid × 3 d, or ceftriaxone [Rocephin], 2.0 g IV qd)
Food-borne streptococcus	~51,000	24–48 h	Pharyngitis	Contamination of foods by infected food workers	Pen V PO × 10 d, or azithromycin, 500 mg PO qd × 5 d
Bacillus cereus	~27,000	Emetic toxin: 1–6 h Diarrheal toxin: 10–16 h	Sudden onset of nausea and vomiting; diarrhea may be present Abdominal cramps, watery diarrhea, nausea	Improperly refrigerated/rewarmed cooked and fried rice Meats, stews, gravies; often precooked	Fluids, supportive care

E. coli, enterotoxigenic	~24,000	1–3 d	Watery diarrhea, abdominal cramps, some vomiting	Water or food contaminated with human feces	Fluids; antibiotics in severe cases (ciprofloxacin, 500 mg PO bid × 3 d; TMP/SMZ)
Vibrio cholerae (nonepidemic/non-O1/O139), *Vibrio parahaemolyticus*	~5200	6–72 h	Watery diarrhea; occasionally bloody diarrhea	Raw or undercooked shellfish, seafood	Fluids; doxycycline, 100 mg PO bid × 3 d in severe cases
Vibrio vulnificus		1–4 d	Sepsis in patients with liver disease or those who are immunocompromised; possible diarrhea	Same	Minocycline (Minocin), 100 mg PO q12 h, and cefotaxime (Claforan), 2.0 g IV q8h
Listeria	~2500	GI: 9–48 h; invasive disease: 2–6 wk	Fever, muscle aches, and nausea or diarrhea. Preganant women may have mild flulike illness, with infection leading to premature delivery or still birth. Elderly or immunocompromised patients may have bacteremia or meningitis	Fresh soft cheese, unpasteurized milk, ready-to-eat deli meats, hot dogs	Fluids for gastroenteritis; for invasive disease, ampicillin, 2 g IV q4–6h, or TMP/SMZ
Botulism	~60	12–72 h	Blurred vision, dysphagia, descending muscle weakness; may be vomiting, diarrhea	Home-canned foods with low acid content; foods where anaerobic growth possible	Supportive care. Botulinum antitoxin helpful if given early in course of illness. Call (404) 639-2206 or (404) 639-3753 workdays or (404) 639-2888 nights and weekends
Parasitic Agents					
Giardia lamblia	~200,000	1–4 wk	Acute or chronic diarrhea, flatulence, bloating	Untreated surface water, contamination of foods by water or infected food worker	Metronidazole (Flagyl), 250 mg PO tid × 5 d
Toxoplasma gondii	~110,000	6–10 d	Generally asymptomatic; cervical lymphadenopathy and/or flulike illness may develop in 20% Immunocompromised patients: CNS disease Preganant women: fetal CNS infection	Undercooked meats, including pork, lamb, venison; contact with cat fecal material	Asymptomatic infections: no treatment Pregnant women (first 18 weeks' gestation): spiramycin,[†] 3g qd, obtained from FDA, (301) 827-2335 Immunocompromised hosts: pyrimethamine (Daraprim) plus sulfadiazine, folinic acid
Cryptosporidium parvum	~30,000	2–28 d	Cramping, abdominal pain, watery diarrhea; fever and vomiting may be present and may be relapsing	Contaminated water, vegetables, fruits, unpasteurized milk	Supportive care
Cyclospora cayetanensis	~15,000	1–11 d	Fatigue, protracted diarrhea; often relapsing	Imported berries, contaminated water, lettuce	TMP/SMZ, DS PO bid × 7 d
Natural Toxins					
Ciguatera fish poisioning		GI: 2–12 h	Abdominal pain, nausea, vomiting, diarrhea; in severe cases, may be hypotension and bradycardia	Large predacious tropical reef fish: barracuda, grouper, red snapper, amberjack	Supportive care, atropine and blood pressure support; IV mannitol (20% solution, 1 g/kg piggybacked over 30 min) reported to be lifesaving in severe cases
		Neurologic: 12 h–5 d	Paresthesias, pain and weakness in legs, temperature reversal		In chronic cases, amitriptyline[‡] (Elavil) may be beneficial

Continued

TABLE 1. **Food-Borne Illnesses—Cont'd**

Etiologic Agent	Estimated U.S. Food-Borne Cases/Year*	Incubation	Signs and Symptoms	Associated Foods	Treatment
Scombroid (histamine toxicity)		1 min–3 h	Flushing, rash; burning sensation of skin mouth	Improperly refrigerated "scombroid" fish, including tuna, mahi-mahi	
Paralytic shellfish poisoning		30 min–3 h	Paresthesias, ataxia, dysphagia, mental status changes, hypotension; respiratory paralysis in severe cases	Scallops, mussels, clams, cockles harvested from beds exposed to blooms of the dinoflagellate *Alexandrium*; occurs primarily in Alaska, Pacific Northwest, California, and Maine	Supportive care

*Estimates of disease incidence (rounded to two significant figures) from Mead PS, Slutsker L, Dietz V, et al: Food-related illness and death in the United States. Emerg Infect Dis 5:607–625, 1999.
†Investigational drug in the United States
‡Not FDA approved for this indication.
Abbreviations: CNS = central nervous system; DS = double-strength tablet; FDA = Food and Drug Administration; STEC = Shiga toxin–producing *E. coli;* TMP/SMZ = trimethoprim/sulfamethoxazole.
Adapted from Diagnosis and management of foodborne illnesses: A primer for physicians. MMWR Morb Mortal Wkly Rep 50 (RR02):1–69, 2001.

percentage of individuals who have Guillain-Barré syndrome have either serologic or historical evidence of a recent *Campylobacter* infection. *Campylobacter* are commonly found as commensals in the gut flora of cows, sheep, fowl, as well as dogs and cats. A higher percentage of poultry probably are contaminated with *Campylobacter* than compared with *Salmonella*.

DIAGNOSIS

When first evaluating a patient with possible food-borne disease, historical factors will help narrow the differential diagnosis. The most common bacterial causes, *Campylobacter, Salmonella, E. coli* and *Shigella* do have a summer/fall seasonality and are most commonly seen among children. There is a second peak in the incidence of disease seen in young adults, particularly with *Campylobacter* associated illnesses. Staph aureus toxin mediated food poisoning syndromes occur typically in the summer months. Water conditions supportive for *Vibrio* infections are seen at the end of the summer. As far as chemical food poisoning syndromes are concerned, ciguatera is most commonly a spring/summer disease; paralytic seafood poisoning is often associated with summer/fall red tide and mushroom hunters are out in the warm months. The office clinician has little means at his or her disposal, other than the history and stool studies upon which to make a diagnosis. Health departments utilize powerful molecular typing methods allowing the tracking of food-associated illnesses and it is not unusual to see sporadic emergence of illnesses from a single source of contaminated food, that is, single individuals can become ill even when multiple individuals have eaten from the same source.

The presence of the following should prompt stool cultures, ova, and parasitic screenings:

1. crampy abdominal pain with tenesmus and fever,
2. bloody diarrhea,
3. prolonged diarrhea greater than seven days,
4. neurologic symptoms such as paresthesia, weakness or cranial nerve palsies,
5. the above symptoms in an immunocompromised patient,
6. pertinent travel history.

Blood cultures can be valuable and the physician should have a low threshold to order when any of the above symptoms are present in the immunocompromised host or when the degree of toxicity so dictates. Typhoid fever is associated with greater than 95% positive blood culture rate. It is not unusual to see positive blood cultures in older patients with *Campylobacter* colitis.

Evaluation of patients in whom food-borne illness is suspected must include a differential diagnosis of non-infectious, non-food-borne illnesses, such as inflammatory bowel disease, irritable bowel syndrome, malignancies and importantly a history of previous antibiotic administration since the diagnosis of *Clostridium difficile* colitis is so common. The use of antibiotics in the patient with *C. difficile* may precede the diarrheal illness and the seeking of medical attention by many weeks. The presentation of *C. difficile* can be subtle particularly in nursing home patients and a high index of suspicion is required. Occasionally in the elderly debilitated patient, the presentation of antibiotic associated colitis is characterized by paralytic ileus, toxic megacolon or perforation but minimal or no diarrhea. Any suspicion of this condition warrants a baseline CBC, electrolytes, renal function testing and close follow-up. *Clostridium difficile* is just one consequence of the overuse of our once-thought-invincible arsenal of antibiotics. Sadly, vancomycin-resistant enterococci, methicillin-resitant staphylococci and penicillin-resistant pneumococci are terms that have entered the day-to-day conversations in virtually all hospitals and nursing homes across the country. Strategy for long term control of these problems must first and foremost begin by emphasizing judicious antibiotic prescription and not by assuming the major pharmaceutical companies will be able to solve the problem with new antibiotics.

Other important historical issues to help define the pathogen in food-associated illnesses include the specific symptoms themselves. As outlined below and as seen in Table 1, vomiting, nausea, abdominal pain, diarrhea, bloody diarrhea, neurologic symptoms, and systemic inflammatory response syndrome due to bacteremia may help define the etiology in addition to laboratory testing. Recent travel suggests an enterotoxigenic *E. coli* (traveler's diarrhea), amebiasis, or giardiasis. Ingestion of seafood with neurologic symptoms and/or rapid onset symptoms suggests natural toxin ingestion associated with various shellfish and seafood (see Table 1). *Vibrio vulnificus* infection in patients with underlying liver disease is usually not subtle and is also associated with raw shellfish and undercooked seafood. *Campylobacter* and *Salmonella* exposures may be suspected with exposure to poultry, eggs and not uncommonly seen in epidemic settings in extended care facilities and subacute nursing facilities. Livestock handlers and participants in state fair livestock exhibitions have been infected with *E. coli* 0157:H7 outbreaks. Deli meats, soft cheeses and unpasteurized dairy products can transmit *Listeria monocytogenes*. *Listeria* can cause severe sepsis syndromes and meningitis in pregnant women, as well as groups more classically at risk such as the elderly and immunocompromised.

When a practitioner makes the diagnosis of a diarrhea-associated syndrome based upon a positive stool culture, the lab usually notifies the local health department. This may happen as a routine from the laboratory testing facility. If the lab is not automatically reporting the positive culture, then a call to the local or State Health Department is appropriate. Local and State Health officials will then report to the CDC who compile the data nationally. Patients recovering from a food-borne illness should be educated regarding hand washing and may be allowed back to work or school once the symptoms have abated and/or stool surveillance cultures are negative. There may be local health regulations with more specific requirements.

TREATMENT

Once the diagnosis is made, specific treatment regimens are outlined in Table 1. However, in the office setting, a clear diagnosis is initially often not apparent. A simple approach in this initial setting is to categorize patients into groups that cause (1) short incubation nausea and vomiting, (2) "classic" gastroenteritis with diarrhea, (3) gastroenteritis with a neurologic syndrome, (4) and the patient systemically ill with infectious colitis.

Short Incubation Vomiting Syndrome/ "Classic" Gastroenteritis with Diarrhea

Most food-borne illnesses in this category are self-limited and antibiotic administration is not indicated. Supportive care is the mainstay of treatment in most viral and toxin mediated food-borne illness syndromes. Enteral or parenteral rehydration with a solution that contains both sugar and salt in physiologic proportions is the key component of treatment. The World Health Organization suggests an enteral rehydration solution containing 3.5 g NaCl, 1.5 KCl, 2.5 g $NaCHO_3$ and 20 g glucose/liter boiled water. In the U.S., "clear liquids" or Pedialyte are reasonable alternatives. Care must be taken when giving parenteral hypotonic fluid resuscitation in the dehydrated patient in order to avoid rapid shifts in serum sodium. Bismuth subsalicylate (Pepto-Bismol)* is a time-honored over-the-counter medicine that is very useful in treating symptoms of viral gastroenteritis. Diarrhea symptoms can be ameliorated with over-the-counter medications such as loperamide (Imodium); see package insert for instructions. For intractable nausea and vomiting promethazine (Phenegran) or prochlorperazine (Compazine) can be taken by mouth or per rectum.

The self-limited nature of many causes of infectious colitis and food-borne diseases in the healthy host is testament to the robust nature of the immune system. The over-prescription of antibiotics and possibly the heavy use of antibiotics in food animals contributes to the continued escalation of resistance to common antibiotics and there is no end in sight. *Salmonella* testing routinely shows multi-resistance patterns and some strains were even resistant to previously thought first line drugs such as ciprofloxacin and Bactrim. *Salmonella* DT104 is one of the most notorious of these resistant strains with very high mortality rates associated with its infections in the United Kingdom. The CDC surveys resistance patterns and *Shigella* also routinely exhibits a multi-resistant pattern to commonly prescribed antimicrobials, including tetracycline, ampicillin, and in up to 10% of the strains, sulfamethoxazole (Bactrim). *Shigella* isolates from foreign countries sometimes can show the most extensive resistance patterns and sensitivity testing should direct care in these situations.

Gastroenteritis with a Neurologic Syndrome

One of the most feared toxin-associated illnesses remains botulinum toxin poisoning. Fatalities are still seen with botulism as well as with some mushroom ingestion syndromes. *Clostridium botulinum* toxin ingestion produces descending paralysis characterized initially by diplopia, dysphasia, and sometimes neurologic respiratory failure. Botulinal spore germination in improperly preserved foods remains the most common vehicle for disease. Treatment includes supportive care and antitoxin administration. The antitoxin is available through the CDC at 404-329-2888.

Ciguatera fish poisoning is caused when a toxin produced by tiny dinoflagellates is concentrated as it moves up the food chain in larger tropical reef fish such as barracuda and grouper. The larger fish are then eaten and a disease occurs characterized by gastroenteritis as well as paresthesia and weakness. When symptoms are severe, hospitalization with mannitol administration may be indicated (see Table 1). Similar toxin-associated syndromes have been described and include paralytic shellfish poisoning (clams and mussels), neurotoxic shellfish poisoning, amnesic shellfish poisoning, and histamine toxicity seen with improper storage of fish after being caught.

Table 2 lists food-borne illnesses associated with mushroom consumption. These also produce gastroenteritis with associated neurologic symptoms. In these scenarios, treatment includes gastric lavage with activated charcoal administration to aid removal of

TABLE 2. **Mushroom Syndromes**

Syndrome (Toxin)	Incubation	Symptoms	Mushrooms
Anticholinergic symdrome (muscarine)	30 min–2 h	Sweating, salivation, lacrimation, bradycardia, hypotension	*Inocybe* species
Delirium (ibotenic acid, muscimol isoxazole)	20–90 min	Dizziness, ataxia, incoordination, hyperactivity	*Clitocybe* species *Amanita* species
Hallucination (psilocin, psilocybin)	30–60 min	Mood elevation, hallucination	*Psilocybe* species *Panaeolus* species
Disulfiram-like (coprine)	30 min after alcohol	Headache, nausea, vomiting	*Coprinus* species
Hepatic failure (gyromitrin)	2–12 h	Nausea, vomiting, hemolysis, hepatic failure, seizures	*Gyromitra* species
Hepatorenal (amatoxins and phallotoxins)	6–24 h	Abdominal pain, vomiting, diarrhea, renal and hepatic failure	*Amanita phalloides*
Nephritis (orellanine)	3–5 d	Thirst, nausea, headache, abdominal pain, renal failure	*Corinarius* species

toxin and cathartics (e.g., magnesium citrate) to speed gut transit time. Ingestion of *Amantia phalloides* ("death-cap" mushrooms) can result in death and intensive support including hemodialysis and liver transplantation has been described. *A. phalloides* is endemic along the West Coast and Mid-Atlantic Coast.

The Systemically Ill Patient with Infectious Colitis

Antimicrobial chemotherapy is indicated for systemic syndromes, even before a specific diagnosis can be made. The initial antibiotic prescription should be directed against the most common pathogens and the quinolone class of antimicrobials is often first prescribed. However, depending on the severity of the illness and risk factors of the host, a broader spectrum "cocktail" may be appropriate. The risk of death from bacterial disease is highest with infections from *E. coli* 0157:H7, *Listeria* (in immunocompromised hosts), and *V. vulnificus* (in hosts with chronic liver disease). Antiperistaltics are probably contraindicated in patients acutely ill with high fever, bloody diarrhea, fecal leukocytes, or evidence of a systemic inflammatory response syndrome. Non-typhoidal, non-systemic salmonellosis syndromes classically are not treated with antimicrobials. Antibiotic intervention in *E. coli* 0157:H7 infection is yet unsettled. It is thought they have minimal use in these cases and generally these are followed carefully for the development of hemolytic uremic syndrome. These cases can be severe with extended ICU stays and hemodialysis.

ORGANISMS AND FOODS

The two classic preformed toxin mediated food poisoning syndromes are associated with outbreaks of *Staphylococcus aureus* and of *Bacillus cereus* food poisoning. The mechanisms are slightly different. Staphylococcal food poisonings are associated with contamination of food during preparation by a food handler. The food handler presumably contaminates the food from a cutaneous source such as an infected boil, the organism then replicates under suboptimal storage conditions and the toxin is produced. Individuals become ill almost immediately after ingesting the preformed enterotoxin. Symptom onset is within 6 hrs and includes nausea, vomiting, and occasional diarrhea. In contrast, *B. cereus* short incubation food poisoning syndromes are often associated with foods contaminated by the organism such as fried rice that has been cooked and then held for extended periods. Illnesses from both organisms are of short duration and spontaneously abate within 12-18 hours.

C. perfringens outbreaks and long incubation *B. cereus* food poisoning are associated with in-vivo toxin production from the consumed organism. Since the toxin is not preformed in these syndromes, abdominal cramping and diarrhea predominate the clinical picture as opposed to vomiting. Both of these organisms have been isolated from raw meat, poultry and fish and so it is not uncommon to see outbreaks when large quantities of food are prepared in institutional settings, including nursing facilities. *B.cereus* has also been isolated from dried foods including beans, cereals, spices and mixes.

E. coli 0157:H7 outbreaks have classically been associated with undercooked ground beef, raw milk, and foods that are associated with meat production. However, increasingly outbreaks have been seen with many other food groups. Often fertilizer or manure is contaminated with *E. coli* 0157:H7, which then contaminates food or water and in this way foods not associated with cattle production have been implicated in outbreaks. Raw eggs have been implicated and considered a major source of salmonellosis in the United States as well as unpasteurized orange juice products, milk, and other fresh produce. *Shigella* outbreaks are less common but associated with pre-prepared potato and egg salads, as well as fresh produce, including salad bars at restaurants. *Campylobacter* infections most often follow ingestion of undercooked poultry but are also considered a zoonotic infection associated with many domesticated animals.

Yersiniosis, although rare, can be seen with contaminated tofu, raw pork, and contaminated dairy products. Traveler's diarrhea from enterotoxigenic *E. coli* is a notorious condition with well-known risk factors. "If it is not cooked or you cannot peel it, do not eat it!" Well-documented outbreaks in foreign countries make salads less glamorous while dining at the seaside resort.

Botulism outbreaks continue and are associated with home canning of various foods. Honey can be the source of *Clostridium botulinum* in cases of infant infections and this natural food should be avoided in very small children. Other distasteful documented scenarios include Norwalk virus and Snow Mountain agent associated with shellfish and salad foods that have been contaminated by a fecal/oral mechanism possibly by a food handler. Norwalk-like agents are thought responsible for recent cruise ship outbreaks and a food handler or passenger source is thought responsible as opposed to contaminated food. Investigations of viral gastroenteritis outbreaks have implicated the fisherman who harvested the foods while ill from the same virus, which caused the outbreak. They contaminated the water where they were working because of lack of toilet facilities on the boat. There have been well-publicized *Cyclospora* outbreaks following imported raspberry consumption. They were imported from a Central American farm and the contamination occurred when sewage contaminated runoff went into the fields where the raspberries were grown.

PREVENTION

Proper processing and preparation most directly impacts the incidence of food-borne disease. Usually as consumers, we cannot control whether a food product is contaminated. Therefore most of the effort to prevent disease for an individual will revolve around food choices, preparation, storage, as well as careful attention to the food preparation area. If a meat product is contaminated with a pathogen such as *E. coli* 0157:H7, proper food handling and preparation can mitigate the risk of becoming ill after consumption. The same can be said for cooked vegetables. However, contaminated fruits that are not cooked essentially cannot be sterilized regardless of how much they are washed or rinsed; if contaminated, they will still transmit the organism. Food-borne disease from the common bacterial pathogens is usually transmitted as a result of contaminated food of animal origin as opposed to contamination from a food handler or a person harvesting seafood, that is, an outbreak of salmonellosis or campylobacter is likely related to food contaminated with its own indigenous flora during processing. This could not be said of staphylococcal food poisoning, viral gastroenteritis outbreaks, hepatitis A, or *Shigella* infections which are often a result of contamination by the food handler.

Our role as primary care givers includes diagnosis; treatment and education particularly to the high-risk hosts above discussed. A laundry list of foods to be avoided given to the HIV patient, the elderly, the pregnant, and those with severe chronic medical conditions may cause undue paranoia, but a few guidelines such as careful food preparation, avoiding unpasturized dairy products and raw shellfish is prudent and practical. Also, the clinician can play a role in detection of outbreaks and assist in reporting institutional illness that may reflect breakdown in the efforts to avoid food-borne disease.

NECROTIZING SKIN AND SOFT TISSUE

method of
MARK A. MALANGONI, M.D.
Case Western Reserve University
Department of Surgery, MetroHealth Medical Center
Cleveland, Ohio

DEFINITION AND CLASSIFICATION

Necrotizing skin and soft tissue infections comprise a spectrum of diseases characterized by rapidly progressive, extensive soft tissue inflammation and necrosis. These infections usually involve the subcutaneous tissue and muscular fascia but also can involve the skin and muscles. Although the course of disease is unpredictable, necrotizing soft tissue infections are often fulminant and mortality is high, particularly when the early manifestations are not recognized. These infections can involve any part of the body; however the lower extremities, perineum, and abdomen are the most common sites.

Various eponyms and terms have been used to describe these infections according to the affected area (Fournier's gangrene), the tissue involved (necrotizing fasciitis), or the causative bacteria (Streptococcal gangrene). Recently, there appears to be an increase in infections due to *Streptococcus pyogenes*, which has been dubbed "flesh-eating bacteria" to emphasize its rapidly progressive nature.

PREDISPOSING FACTORS

Necrotizing soft tissue infections can be either primary or secondary in origin. Primary or "idiopathic" infections are uncommon (10-15% of cases) and occur when there is no obvious portal of entry for bacteria. These infections result either from hematogenous bacterial spread or direct invasion through minuscule epidermal lesions. Secondary infections are much more common and occur in patients who have had some compromise of the skin, subcutaneous tissue, or muscle that increases their susceptibility to infection.

Secondary necrotizing skin and soft tissue infections generally occur as a complication of inadequately treated or unrecognized infections, but can occur after an operation or injury. Diseases or conditions that predispose to the development of infection include diabetes mellitus, immunocompromised states, obesity, chronic alcoholism, peripheral vascular diseases, and illicit drug injections. Neglected or inadequately treated cutaneous infections, decubitus ulcers, ischemic leg ulcers, perirectal or Bartholin's cyst abscesses, and strangulated hernias can also predispose to necrotizing infections. Blunt or penetrating injury to soft tissues, burns, skin closure after contaminated or dirty operations, the use of un-sterilized needles, and human, animal, or insect bites, when accompanied by bacterial inoculation, can result in infection in susceptible patients.

DIAGNOSIS

The diagnosis is primarily a clinical one and should be based on the history and physical examination. Establishing an early diagnosis depends on a high index of suspicion. Early in the course of infection, patients frequently complain of *localized pain that is disproportionately severe compared with the physical findings*. Early features on examination include edema and tenderness. As the infection progresses, cutaneous erythema, woody induration, crepitus, skin vesicles, bullae, cutaneous hypesthesia, and necrosis develop. Tachycardia is usually present early; however fever, changes in mental status, metabolic acidosis, and shock are late findings.

Associated laboratory findings usually include leukocytosis, hyponatremia, and hypocalcemia. The presence of anemia, disseminated intravascular coagulation, and rhabdomyolysis are later findings. An elevated serum creatine phosphokinase (CPK) is useful to determine muscular involvement. A normal CPK generally excludes muscle necrosis. Myoglobinuria can occur when muscular necrosis is present.

Radiographs of the associated soft tissues should be obtained when the diagnosis is unclear. These studies may demonstrate gas in the subcutaneous tissues, even in patients without crepitus. Magnetic resonance imaging (MRI) is sensitive for the detection of soft tissue necrosis and gas. MRI often can distinguish necrotizing from non-necrotizing infections, which usually do not require débridement. Computed tomography (CT) is a very sensitive test to demonstrate soft tissue gas and may be useful when an MRI scan is not feasible. These studies are not necessary when the diagnosis is obvious.

Fine-needle aspiration cytology can demonstrate the presence of microorganisms and is useful when findings are equivocal. Incisional biopsy with frozen section examination can identify necrosis and vascular thrombosis, as well as microorganisms.

MICROBIOLOGY

Necrotizing infections of the skin and soft tissues can be due to either single or multiple organisms. Idiopathic infections are most commonly monomicrobic and are caused principally by *S. pyogenes*, *Staphylococcus aureus*, or *Clostridium perfringens*. Group A streptococcal infections occur more commonly in younger patients, involve the extremities, and are associated with toxic shock syndrome. These infections tend to have a fulminant course in contrast to a more insidious presentation for polymicrobic infections. The rapid onset and progression of monomicrobic infections is related to the production of bacterial exotoxins, which cause extensive local tissue damage and necrosis. Monomicrobic infections occur in approximately 10-20% of all cases.

Polymicrobic infections are caused most often by facultative aerobic and anaerobic bacteria, which act in synergy to produce conditions that promote the progression of infection. The exact microbiology varies depending on the site of involvement but generally includes both Gram-positive and Gram-negative organisms (Table 1). Extensive necrosis is a common feature of this heterogenous group of infections and occurs as a result of vascular thrombosis of the dermal vessels. Bacterial toxins and tissue ischemia contribute to further injury. Soft tissue gas results from the production of insoluble gases such as hydrogen, nitrogen, and methane, but is highly variable. Soft tissue gas is characteristically absent in infections caused by *S. pyogenes*.

TABLE 1. **Causative Organisms for 45 Polymicrobic Necrotizing Soft-Tissue Infections (n = 127)**

Aerobes (Gram-Positive)	51 (40%)
Enterococci	21
Streptococcal species	11
Coagulase-negative staphylococci	10
Staphylococcus aureus	6
Bacillus species	3
Aerobes (Gram-Negative)	54 (43%)
Escherichia coli	15
Pseudomonas aeruginosa	13
Enterobacter cloacae	5
Klebsiella species	5
Proteus species	4
Serratia species	4
Acinetobacter calcoaceticus	3
Other	4
Anaerobes	19 (15%)
Bacteroides species	12
Clostridium species	4
Others	5
Fungi	3 (2%)

From McHenry CR, Piotrowski JJ, Petrinic D, Malangoni MA: Determinants of mortality for necrotizing soft tissue infections. Ann Surg 221:560, 1995.

TREATMENT

The early recognition and urgent treatment of necrotizing soft tissue infections is critical to obtain a successful outcome. There are three major components of treatment: fluid resuscitation, antimicrobial therapy, and operative débridement.

Fluid resuscitation is best done using an isotonic electrolyte solution such as lactated Ringer's solution. Large volumes are often required. Associated electrolyte abnormalities, particularly hyponatremia and hypocalcemia, should be corrected. Red blood cell transfusions may be required to correct anemia related to intravascular hemolysis.

Because of the wide range of microorganisms that cause these infections, empiric antibiotic therapy should be directed against a broad spectrum of pathogens. Useful antibiotics include carbapenems, extended spectrum penicillins with a beta-lactamase inhibitor, or a combination of antibiotics (Table 2). Clindamycin (Cleocin), 900 mg q8h, should always be given whenever infection due to *S. pyogenes* or *S. aureus* is suspected, since this drug is more effective against toxic shock syndrome. Patients with traumatic wounds should receive tetanus toxoid (Td) or human tetanus immune globulin (TIG), based on their immunization status.

Prompt operative débridement is essential. Débridement should remove all apparently necrotic and infected tissue. The underlying tissue necrosis typically extends beyond the obvious limits of cutaneous involvement; therefore, appropriate exposure and exploration are critical. Débridement should be continued until viable tissue is reached. Exudates and tissue specimens should be submitted for Gram stain and culture with antimicrobial susceptibility testing. Patients who have extensive loss of the abdominal wall may need prosthetic mesh for reconstruction and to prevent evisceration. Associated muscle compartments should be inspected for involvement and fasciotomies done as needed. Amputation can be lifesaving in extensive soft tissue infections of the extremities. A colostomy can prevent contamination from defecation and helps control wound sepsis when infection involves the perineum.

Following débridement, the affected area should be irrigated and packed lightly with gauze moistened with 0.9% normal saline. The use of topical antiseptic

TABLE 2. **Recommended Antimicrobial Therapy**

Agents	Dose
Single Agents	
Imipenem-cilastatin (Primaxin)	750 mg q6h
Meropenem (Merrem)	1 gm q8h
Piperacillin—tazobactam (Zosyn)	3.375 gm q6h
Combinations	
Penicillin plus	3-4 million units q4h
Gentamicin or tobramycin *plus*	1.7 mg/kg q8h
Clindamycin (Cleocin)	900 mg q8h

and antibacterial solutions usually does little to inhibit bacterial growth. Routine re-exploration should be performed in the operating room within 24-48 hours in all but the most minor cases. Repeated débridement should continue in the operating room until the infection is controlled.

Postoperatively, the patient should be monitored in the intensive care unit until stable. Intravenous antibiotics should be continued until signs of local wound sepsis and systemic toxicity have resolved. This includes eradication of fever and return of the white blood cell count to normal. Early nutritional support should be initiated, preferably by an enteral route. Strict control of hyperglycemia is important and vasopressors should be used as needed.

Once the infection has resolved, soft tissue coverage with split-thickness skin grafts or reconstructive flaps is recommended. The use of a vacuum-assisted closure device can help reduce the area requiring coverage. Premature closure of contaminated or persistently infected sites, however, will likely lead to recurrence of infection and increased mortality.

Hyperbaric oxygen (HBO) has been advocated as an adjunctive treatment for necrotizing infections, particularly those due to clostridia. There are no data, however, to support improved survival or earlier resolution of infection with the use of HBO. Its use should not delay or substitute for complete and adequate débridement of infected non-viable tissues.

Although the treatment outlined above has improved the outcomes for necrotizing, skin and soft tissue infections, recent large series demonstrate that mortality is between 25-35%. Delays in presentation and débridement are major factors contributing to a higher mortality rate. Patient age, the extent of body surface area involvement, underlying risk factors, and the degree of organ system dysfunction also have been shown to be predictors of outcome. Delays in recognition and treatment must be avoided in order to achieve optimal survival for this disease process.

TOXIC SHOCK SYNDROME*

method of
SHARON NESSIM, M.D., and
ANDRE DASCAL, M.D., F.R.C.P.C.
McGill University
Montreal, Quebec, Canada

Toxic shock syndrome (TSS) is a rapidly progressive, potentially lethal syndrome caused by toxin released from *Staphylococcus aureus* (SA) and group A β-hemolytic streptococci (GAS). Recently, TSS has also been described in association with infections caused by group B, C, and G β-hemolytic streptococci. In this article we will compare the epidemiology, pathogenesis, clinical manifestations, diagnosis, and management of group A β-hemolytic streptococcal toxic shock syndrome or "toxic strep" (GAS-TSS) and staphylococcal toxic shock syndrome (SA-TSS).

*This article is unchanged from *Conn's Current Therapy 2003*.

EPIDEMIOLOGY

Syndromes consistent with toxic shock caused by both SA and GAS were first described in the early part of the 20th century. Formal reporting of both syndromes, however, did not occur until more recently, 1978 for SA-TSS and the mid-1980s for GAS-TSS.

SA-TSS

Cases of SA-TSS have classically been categorized as either menstrual or nonmenstrual. Nonmenstrual cases have occurred in association with both surgical and nonsurgical wound infections, foreign bodies (including intrauterine devices and diaphragms), burns, bone and joint infections, and postinfluenza SA superinfection. SA-TSS has also followed colonization without infection by toxin-producing strains, with menstrual cases serving as the primary example. In 1999, 113 cases of SA-TSS were reported in the United States, a major decline from the 1264 cases reported from 1979 to 1980. Although menstrual cases accounted for nearly all the early reported cases of SA-TSS, their incidence has steadily declined over time to the extent that from 1987 to 1996, only 58% of cases were linked with menses. The reason for this decline probably relates to the withdrawal of highly absorbent tampons from the market. The case-fatality rate for menstrual SA-TSS has declined since its emergence approximately 20 years ago from 5.5% to 1.8% more recently. For nonmenstrual cases, the case-fatality rate is reported to be between 5.3% and 8.5% and has not changed significantly over time.

GAS-TSS

Unlike SA-TSS, cases of GAS-TSS have been reported with increasing frequency. Recent estimates of GAS-TSS suggest an incidence of approximately 1 per 100,000. As with SA-TSS, most of those in whom GAS-TSS develops do not have predisposing underlying disease, although diabetes, alcoholism, varicella, the use of nonsteroidal anti-inflammatory agents, and a history of trauma (including surgery) are risk factors. GAS-TSS usually occurs sporadically, but clusters among family members, health care workers, and nursing home residents have been reported. Although the mortality rate in SA-TSS is under 5%, GAS-TSS carries a more ominous prognosis, with appreciable morbidity and a mortality rate of 30% to 70%.

CLINICAL MANIFESTATIONS

The case definitions of SA-TSS and GAS-TSS (Tables 1 and 2, respectively) illustrate the hallmark of hypotension and multiorgan dysfunction present in both. Rapid onset of symptoms in otherwise healthy individuals should raise suspicion regarding the possibility of TSS.

TABLE 1. **Case Definition for *Staphylococcus aureus* Toxic Shock Syndrome**

Criteria*	Definition
1 Fever	Temperature >38.9°C
2 Hypotension	Systolic blood pressure <90 mm Hg
	Orthostatic drop in diastolic blood pressure >15 mm Hg
	Orthostatic syncope or dizziness
3 Rash	Diffuse macular erythroderma
4 Desquamation	1–2 wk after onset, particularly on the palms and soles
5 Multisystem organ involvement (≥3)	GI (vomiting or diarrhea at onset of illness)
	Muscular (severe myalgia or CK >2× the upper limit of normal)
	Mucous membranes (vaginal, oropharyngeal, or conjunctival hyperemia)
	Renal (BUN or creatinine >2× the upper limit of normal or pyuria in the absence of UTI)
	Hepatic (total bilirubin, AST, or ALT >2× the upper limit of normal)
	Hematologic (platelet count <100,000/mm^3)
	CNS (disorientation or altered level of consciousness without focal neurologic signs when fever and hypotension are absent)
6 Negative results of	Blood, throat, or CSF cultures (blood culture may be positive for *S. aureus*)
	Serologic tests for Rocky Mountain spotted fever, leptospirosis, or measles

*A definite case is an illness that meets six of six criteria, whereas a probable case is an illness that meets five of six criteria.
Abbreviations: ALT = alanine aminotransferase; AST = aspartate aminotransferase; BUN = blood urea nitrogen; CK = creatine phosphokinase; CNS = central nervous system; CSF = cerebrospinal fluid; GI = gastrointestinal; UTI = urinary tract infection.
Reingold, AL et al: Toxic shock syndrome surveillance in the United States, 1980 to 1981. Ann Intern Med 96:875-880, 1982.

SA-TSS

In menstrual cases, the median interval between the onset of menstruation and SA-TSS is 2 to 3 days. Similarly, the median onset after surgery is 2 days. A variety of skin manifestations can be seen in SA-TSS. Early in the course of disease, one may note a diffuse, red macular rash that also traditionally involves the palms and soles. In addition, patients may have mucosal involvement, and in severe cases, petechiae, ulcerations, vesicles, and bullae may be seen. One to 2 weeks after onset of the illness, a maculopapular rash may develop, and one may also observe desquamation of the palms and soles. Hypocalcemia and hypomagnesemia are frequently noted.

After recovery from SA-TSS, recurrences have been reported, mostly related to the absence of antibody response to SA toxins or inappropriate or inadequate antimicrobial regimens.

GAS-TSS

In contrast to SA-TSS, soft tissue infections occur in up to 80% of patients with GAS-TSS. Necrotizing fasciitis with or without myonecrosis is present in 50%. Infection usually begins within 1 to 3 days at a site of minor local trauma, which often does not result in a visible break in skin. The most common initial symptom of GAS-TSS is severe diffuse or localized pain of a relatively sudden onset that may precede objective evidence of local infection. The appearance of purple bullae or dusky-looking skin is an ominous sign. Approximately 20% of patients have an influenza-like syndrome that precedes the hypotension.

PATHOGENESIS

The search for a unifying hypothesis that would explain the common clinical features in SA-TSS and GAS-TSS has led to the emergence of the present superantigen (SAG) theory. SAGs are capable of activating large numbers of T cells at once, and such activation results in sudden, massive cytokine release. SAGs do not require processing by antigen-presenting cells and instead interact directly with the invariant region of the major histocompatibility complex (MHC) class II molecule. Furthermore, binding of the SAG-MHC

TABLE 2. **Case Definition for Group A Streptococcal Toxic Shock Syndrome**

Criteria*	Definition
I Isolation of group A streptococci	A: From a normally sterile site
	B: From a nonsterile site
II Clinical signs of severity	A: Systolic blood pressure <90 mm Hg
	B: Multisystem organ involvement (2 of the following):
	Renal impairment (creatinine >177 μmol/L or a >2-fold elevation over baseline)
	Coagulopathy (platelets <100,000/mm^3 or disseminated intravascular coagulation
	Liver involvement (total bilirubin, ALT, AST >2-fold elevation or >2× the upper limit of normal)
	Adult respiratory distress syndrome
	Generalized, erythematous, macular rash that may desquamate
	Soft tissue necrosis, including necrotizing fasciitis, myositis, or gangrene

*A definite case is an illness that meets criteria IA and IIA, whereas a probable case is an illness that meets criteria for IB and IIB.
Abbreviations: ALT = alanine aminotransferase; AST = aspartate aminotransferase.
Adapted from the Working Group on Severe GAS Infections: Defining the group A streptococcal toxic shock syndrome. JAMA 269:390-391, 1993.

complex to the T-cell receptor at one of its five variable regions (the β region) results in the stimulation of 5% to 20% of the total T-cell population. Such stimulation leads to cytokine release (interleukin-1 [IL-1] and tumor necrosis factor-α [TNF-α] from macrophages and IL-2, TNF-β, and interferon-γ from TH_1 cells) that is several orders of magnitude greater than that in response to antigen-specific activation. The hypotension and multisystem organ failure are related both directly to these cytokines and indirectly via cytokine-induced vasodilation, capillary leak, and myocardial suppression. Several of the toxins elaborated by SA and GAS belong to the SAG superfamily and are thus able to trigger the massive cytokine response just described.

SA-TSS

Staphylococcal enterotoxins (SE) A, B, C, D, E, G, H, I, J, K, L, and P and toxic shock syndrome toxin-1 (TSST-1) have been identified as belonging to the SAG superfamily. The primary toxin implicated is TSST-1, and this toxin is elaborated by 90% to 100% of menstrual SA-TSS–associated strains but only by approximately half of nonmenstrual SA-TSS–associated strains. Strains that are TSST-1–negative are frequently positive for enterotoxins SEB and SEC. Individuals in whom SA-TSS develops appear to lack antibodies to TSST-1 and/or the SEs that have developed in most others by the third decade.

GAS-TSS

The toxins produced by GAS, which are part of the SAG superfamily, include streptococcal pyrogenic exotoxins (SPE) A, C, G, H, and J, as well as streptococcal SAG and streptococcal mitogenic exotoxin Z. Of these toxins, SPE-A and SPE-C have been present in most cases of streptococcal TSS. Another virulence factor is the M protein, which is a filamentous protein anchored to the cell membrane that possesses antiphagocytic properties. Over 80 different serotypes of M protein have been differentiated, with types 1, 3, 12, and 28 accounting for most of the isolates from patients in whom GAS-TSS developed.

DIAGNOSIS AND DIFFERENTIAL DIAGNOSIS

The differential diagnosis of both SA-TSS and GAS-TSS includes septic shock and febrile mucocutaneous syndromes such as Rocky Mountain spotted fever, meningococcemia, leptospirosis, dengue fever, ehrlichiosis, measles, and Kawasaki's disease.

SA-TSS

Although SA is isolated from mucosal or wound sites in 80% to 90% of cases of SA-TSS, its isolation is not required for diagnosis. In addition, evidence of SA bacteremia is present in only approximately 5% of cases. Seroconversion of antibodies to any of the SA-elaborated products may be helpful in making a retrospective diagnosis.

GAS-TSS

Given the frequent soft tissue involvement in GAS-TSS, meticulous physical examination is mandatory. Unlike the situation in SA-TSS, in which only 5% of blood cultures are positive, 60% of blood cultures in GAS-TSS demonstrate the presence of streptococci. Seroconversion to GAS products such as DNase B and antistreptolysin O can be used as evidence of recent GAS infection.

MANAGEMENT

Management of both SA-TSS and GAS-TSS begins with resuscitation and supportive care by a team experienced in the management of these entities. These interventions should be combined with an effort to eradicate the causative organism and minimize its toxin-mediated effects. In GAS-TSS, surgery is often vital because of the frequency of soft tissue infection. However, surgical intervention should not be forgotten in SA-TSS, in which removal of foreign material, drainage of any identified infectious focus, or débridement of wounds may be required. Adjunctive hyperbaric oxygen for necrotizing fasciitis–associated GAS-TSS has been of benefit in some reports. Appropriate antibiotic therapy can help in management not only by reducing the number of infecting organisms (β-lactams or vancomycin [Vancocin]), but also by direct inhibition of toxin production (clindamycin [Cleocin]).

If allergy to β-lactams precludes the use of penicillins or cephalosporins, vancomycin should be substituted. Penicillin and vancomycin doses should be adjusted for the degree of renal dysfunction. Continued use of clindamycin beyond the initial period should be based on available susceptibility data. The macrolides have been shown to be superior to penicillin in in vitro and animal studies; however, increasing resistance precludes their routine use in severe GAS disease. Linezolid (Zyvox), quinupristin/dalfopristin (Synercid), and the newer fluoroquinolones have shown in vitro activity against both SA and GAS. Although they are used for gram-positive disease successfully, their use in TSS to date has been limited.

SA-TSS

Current recommendations for the treatment of SA-TSS include the combination of a penicillinase-resistant penicillin such as oxacillin (Bactocill), nafcillin (Unipen), or cloxacillin (Cloxapen) (2 g intravenously [IV] q4h) and high-dose clindamycin (900 mg IV q8h). In areas with a high prevalence of community-acquired methicillin-resistant SA, the addition of vancomycin (2 g IV per day in divided doses) is advised until sensitivity to penicillinase-resistant penicillins is confirmed.

GAS-TSS

Current recommendations for the treatment of GAS-TSS include the use of a combination of penicillin (4 million U q4h) and clindamycin (900 mg IV q8h).

Although GAS is exquisitely sensitive to penicillin, the use of penicillin alone is limited by its reduced efficacy when large numbers of organisms are present (Eagle effect), as is often the case in severe GAS disease. The reason for this reduced efficacy is diminished expression, during the stationary phase of growth, of the penicillin-binding proteins (PBPs) that act as targets for penicillin. Importantly, in vitro and animal studies have demonstrated greater bactericidal activity for ceftriaxone (Rocephin) than for penicillin at any given inoculum size. This difference probably relates to the relatively higher expression of PBPs targeted by ceftriaxone during the stationary phase of growth than PBPs targeted by penicillin. Based on these limited data, we believe that the addition of ceftriaxone (2 g IV q12h) to penicillin and clindamycin should be considered in severe GAS infections.

Intravenous Immune Globulins and Other Immunomodulators

The SAG theory described earlier has led to a limited number of case reports and one observational study reporting benefit with the use of intravenous immune globulin (IVIG, Gamimune N)* in GAS-TSS. The routine use of IVIG in the management of TSS, however, cannot be an evidence-based recommendation at this time for several reasons. First, reports on IVIG suffer from the classic methodologic problems inherent in any retrospective, nonrandomized, noncontrolled trial. Second, the composition of any given batch of IVIG is variable, and its effectiveness is dependent on the presence of the desired antibodies. Third, no consensus has been reached regarding the dose, and the effects of high-dose IVIG may be rather difficult to predict in such a complex pathogenesis. If the use of IVIG is to be based on the SAG hypothesis, it should be administered very early in the evolution of TSS. It is clear that appropriate trials on the benefit of IVIG in TSS are required.

Recently, several in vitro and animal studies have tested the ability of specific immunomodulating agents to inhibit the major cytokine mediators of toxic shock. These agents include the TNF-α inhibitor pentoxifylline (Trental),* IL-6 and IL-11 (which inhibit the synthesis of TNF-α and IL-1), and a newly designed peptide antagonist that inhibits the SAG-induced expression of TH_1 cytokines. Although these immunomodulators are promising, further studies demonstrating safety and efficacy in humans are needed. Other therapies that have been tried but for which the evidence is inadequate include TSST-1–specific monoclonal antibodies and corticosteroids.

Chemoprophylaxis

Because data on chemoprophylaxis for close contacts of patients with GAS-TSS is limited, the Centers for Disease Control and Prevention advised in 1998 that no clear recommendation could be made and that decisions should be individualized. In Canada, most public health authorities recommend chemoprophylaxis with a first-generation cephalosporin for close contacts (defined as persons spending more than 4 h/d or more than 20 h/wk together, sharing sleeping arrangements, or having direct mucous membrane contact) within 7 days of illness of the index patient.

*Not FDA approved for this indication.

INFLUENZA

method of
STEPHEN B. GREENBERG, M.D.
Department of Medicine
Baylor College of Medicine
Houston, Texas

Influenza is an acute respiratory illness occurring in yearly outbreaks and epidemics throughout the world. Epidemics typically occur in the winter season and are associated with increased morbidity and mortality. People are infected by aerosol or close contact. After an incubation period of 1 to 3 days, upper and lower respiratory tract signs and symptoms develop. These include sore throat and cough as well as systemic complaints of fever, headache, and myalgias. Although school-aged children have the highest attack rates, mortality is highest in people older than age 65.

Influenzavirus is an RNA virus from the orthomyxovirus family. Influenza types A and B are responsible for epidemic and pandemic disease. Influenza C is an uncommon cause of respiratory illness. The two surface glycoproteins, hemagglutinin (HA) and neuraminidase (NA), are important in the pathogenesis of this infection. Changes or mutations in one or both of these proteins are the major reasons for the repeated epidemics of influenza. Minor changes in HA or NA, or "antigenic drift," occur in both influenza A and B viruses. A major change in HA or "antigenic shift" is associated with a worldwide epidemic or pandemic. These pandemic strains are thought to occur when exchange (reassortment) of genes between human and avian influenza A viruses occurs during a dual infection and results in a new strain that can replicate in people who are susceptible.

Excess mortality from epidemic influenza has ranged between 10,000 and 40,000 deaths annually in the United States. Far greater numbers of deaths have been documented in those worldwide outbreaks that were recorded in 1918 (H1N1), 1957 (H2N2), 1968 (H3N2), and 1977 (H1N1). In 1918, it is estimated that more than 500,000 deaths occurred in the U.S. secondary to pandemic influenza.

Influenza is monitored each year by the Centers for Disease Control and Prevention (CDC) and the World Health Organization. Information can be found through the CDC at (888)232-3228 or at its web site: *http://www.cdc.gov/ncidod/diseases/flu/weekly.htm*. An epidemic of influenza is heralded by an increase in school absenteeism and visits to health care facilities.

Increases are also recorded in industrial absenteeism, hospitalization for pneumonia and influenza, and total deaths.

CLINICAL MANIFESTATIONS

Influenza-associated illness usually begins with the abrupt onset of fever, headache, myalgias, sore throat, and cough. Other presentations can include a "common cold" syndrome or systemic signs and symptoms without much respiratory tract involvement. Other signs and symptoms can include hoarseness and tracheal pain. Typically, the acute illness lasts 3 to 5 days with cough and malaise persisting for several weeks.

There are few physical findings in influenza. Hyperemia in the oropharynx is common. Mild cervical lymphadenopathy is seen most frequently in children. The chest examination is usually normal in uncomplicated influenza, even though ventilatory defects have been described in patients undergoing pulmonary function testing.

Common complications of influenza include otitis media, sinusitis, bronchitis, and pneumonia. The major serious complication of influenza is pneumonia that occurs in patients with underlying cardiovascular or pulmonary problems, patients with diabetes mellitus, renal diseases or immunosuppression, patients in nursing homes or chronic care facilities, and in individuals older than age 65. Three patterns of pneumonia have been reported: (1) primary viral; (2) secondary bacterial; or (3) mixed viral and bacterial. In primary influenza pneumonia, symptoms persist in a patient with acute influenza and include fever, tachypnea, and dyspnea. Primary viral pneumonia is the most severe but least common pneumonia complication of influenza. Because the influenza virus affects the integrity of the tracheobronchial epithelium, there is a predisposition for bacterial superinfections of the lungs. Although the most frequently detected bacterial cause is *Streptococcus pneumoniae*, *Staphylococcus aureus* is second in frequency (approximately 20% of cases). With secondary bacterial pneumonia, there is an exacerbation of fever and respiratory symptoms after an initial improvement in what appears to be acute influenza. Many patients have features of both viral and bacterial pneumonia. One can recover both influenza virus and bacterial pathogens from the sputum of such patients.

Other complications of influenza include myositis, rhabdomyolysis, Reye syndrome, central nervous system involvement, myocarditis, and exacerbations of asthma and chronic obstructive pulmonary disease. Acute myositis presents with tenderness of the affected muscles with marked elevation of serum creatine phosphokinase levels. Myoglobinuria and acute renal failure have been reported in such cases. Reye syndrome is reported in children with influenza B, and less frequently with influenza A. It presents with nausea and vomiting followed by change in mental status. Hepatomegaly and elevated blood ammonia levels are noted. An association with the use of aspirin has been noted in Reye syndrome cases. Central nervous system diseases associated with influenza also include encephalitis, transverse myelitis, and Guillain-Barré syndrome (GBS). Cases of toxic shock syndrome have also been reported in association with *S. aureus* infection and acute influenza.

DIAGNOSIS

Other respiratory viruses and infectious agents can give a clinical syndrome similar to influenza virus. Where influenza virus is known to be circulating in a community, influenza illness is likely to be caused by influenza virus in approximately 60% to 70% of cases. To make a specific diagnosis, one of several virus specific assays would be necessary.

Laboratory diagnosis requires detection of virus or viral antigen from throat swabs, nasal washes, or sputum. Virus isolation using embryonated eggs or cell culture monolayers is the gold standard for detecting influenza virus. After a respiratory sample is obtained, it should be placed in viral transport medium and taken immediately to the laboratory. Influenza viruses are usually isolated within 3 to 7 days of tissue culture inoculation.

Rapid viral diagnostic tests are becoming available in many laboratories. Some tests will distinguish between type A and B viruses and others do not. Immunofluorescence tests require expensive equipment, technical expertise, and take longer than enzyme immunoassays to perform. Enzyme immunoassay techniques can provide results within 30 minutes of collection and can be performed in physician offices. Although the specificity of these rapid tests is high, the sensitivity has ranged between 60% and 90%, with better results being observed in specimens from children.

Nucleic acid detection methods such as reverse transcriptase polymerase chain reaction (RT-PCR) assays are sensitive and specific but not available except in research laboratories. The use of RT-PCR may allow for the detection of influenza infection more quickly and aid in the use of specific antiviral treatment.

Influenza can be diagnosed retrospectively using serologic methods. Paired sera collected 2 to 4 weeks apart can demonstrate a more than fourfold antibody rise demonstrating that an acute illness has occurred. Serologic methods include hemagglutination-inhibition, complement fixation, and enzyme immunoabsorbent assay.

PREVENTION AND TREATMENT

Vaccine

The primary method of preventing influenza and its severe complications is influenza vaccination. The target groups recommended for annual vaccination include (1) people older than 65 years of age, (2) people of any age with certain chronic medical conditions, and (3) people who live with or care for people at high risk. Vaccination has led to fewer influenza-related respiratory illnesses and physician visits, hospitalizations, and deaths among high-risk individuals, otitis media among children, and lower work absenteeism among adults. Although the optimal time to receive influenza vaccine is during October and November, vaccination efforts in October should be for high-risk people and health care workers. Depending on supply of vaccine, other groups should receive vaccine in November. For as long as vaccine supplies are available, all targeted groups should receive vaccine into December and later. Influenza vaccination of healthy children ages 6 to 23 months is supported by the Advisory Committee on Immunization Practices.

Special populations should receive consideration for influenza vaccination. Because of the documented influenza-associated excess deaths among pregnant women, women who will be beyond the first trimester of pregnancy during the influenza season should be vaccinated. Regardless of the stage of pregnancy, pregnant women with medical conditions that increase the risk for complications from influenza should be vaccinated before the influenza season. There is limited information on the frequency and severity of influenza illness as well as the benefits of influenza vaccination among people with HIV infection. However, vaccine should be offered to HIV-infected people, including HIV-infected pregnant women. Breast-feeding mothers can receive influenza vaccine. Persons at high risk for complications of influenza should consider influenza vaccine if they were not vaccinated in the preceding fall or winter and plan to travel to the tropics, or with an organized tourist group at any time of year, or plan to travel to the Southern Hemisphere during April through September. People providing essential community services should also consider vaccination. Students or people in closed institutional settings should be encouraged to be vaccinated.

Certain individuals should not be vaccinated. Those known to have anaphylactic hypersensitivity to eggs or to other components of the vaccine should not receive the influenza vaccine. Those with an acute febrile illness should not be vaccinated until symptoms have lessened.

Dosage recommendations depend on the age of the person. Children younger than 9 years of age who are previously unvaccinated should receive two doses more than 1 month apart. All other individuals should receive one dose. Only FDA-approved influenza vaccine should be used in children ages 6 months to 3 years. The intramuscular route is recommended. Adults and older children should be vaccinated in the deltoid muscle; infants and young children should be vaccinated in the anterolateral area of the thigh.

The inactivated influenza virus vaccine is composed of virus antigens from three influenza virus strains: A/H1N1, A/H3N2, and B. Based on worldwide surveillance of new strains, the virus strains for vaccine development are selected to be those most likely to circulate in the upcoming season. Each vaccine strain is grown in embryonated chicken eggs, inactivated with a chemical agent, and partially purified. Vaccines are made from whole virus, disrupted virus particles (subvirion), or purified surface HA or NA antigens. Whole virus vaccine is not available in the United States. Split-virus vaccines contain subvirion or purified surface antigens. The vaccine contains 15 μg of HA antigen from each of the candidate strains in a 0.50 mL dose. Table 1 contains the recommended doses of vaccine to be used for different age groups (2002-2003 season).*

TABLE 1. **Influenza Vaccine Dose by Age Group**

Age Group	Dose*	Number of Doses†
6-35 months	0.25 mL	1 or 2
3-8 years	0.50 mL	1 or 2
≥9 years	0.50 mL	1

*Intramuscular administration in deltoid muscle for adults and older children and anterolateral thigh for infants and young children.

†Two doses given 1 month apart for children younger than 9 years of age who are receiving influenza vaccine for the first time.

People receiving vaccine should be told that the vaccine contains noninfectious killed viruses and cannot cause influenza and that incubating or coincidental respiratory illness unrelated to influenza vaccination can occur around the time of vaccination. The most frequent side effect is soreness at the vaccination site lasting less than 2 days. Systemic reactions including fever, malaise, and myalgia can begin 6 to 12 hours after vaccination, especially in individuals who have no prior exposure to the influenza virus antigens in the vaccine. Immediate reactions such as hives, angioedema, or anaphylaxis are rare. Recent studies have suggested no substantial increase in GBS associated with influenza vaccination. Most authorities believe the potential benefit of influenza vaccination, significantly outweighs the possible but low risks for vaccine associated GBS. Although there are no studies evaluating the simultaneous administration of influenza vaccine and other childhood vaccines, it is recommended that children at high risk for influenza-related complications receive influenza vaccine when receiving other routine vaccinations.

Intranasally administered cold-adapted, attenuated, influenza virus vaccines (LAIVs) are under development in the United States. Potential advantages of LAIVs include broad mucosal and systemic immune responses, ease, and acceptability of administration. Application for licensure of a LAIV is under review by the FDA.

Antivirals

Four licensed influenza antiviral agents are an adjunct to influenza vaccine for controlling and preventing influenza and are not substitutes for vaccination. The four drugs have different pharmacokinetics, side effects, routes of administration, approved age groups, dosages, and costs. When administered within 2 days of illness onset, both amantadine (Symmetrel) and rimantadine (Flumadine) reduce the duration of influenza A illness, and zanamivir (Relenza) and oseltamivir (Tamiflu) reduce the duration of influenza A and B illness by 1 day. No studies have demonstrated

*Not FDA approved for this indication.

the effectiveness of any of these four antiviral agents in preventing serious complications of influenza. There are only limited data on the effectiveness of these four antiviral agents for treatment of influenza among persons at high risk for serious complications of influenza. Few studies have been published on the efficacy of influenza antivirals in pediatric patients.

Amantadine (Symmetrel) and rimantadine (Flumadine) are M2 inhibitors that block proton ion channels in the virus membrane and prevent uncoating of virus and initiation of viral replication. Zanamivir (Relenza) and oseltamivir (Tamiflu) are neuraminidase inhibitors that block the activity of the viral NA or sialidase. Neuraminidase removes sialic acid residues from the surface of the infected cell and also helps virus pass through the overlying mucus layer to the respiratory epithelium.

Amantadine and rimantadine are approved for the chemoprophylaxis of influenza A but not B infections. Both drugs are effective in preventing illness from influenza A infections in approximately 70% to 90% of individuals. Amantadine and rimantadine do not inhibit the antibody response to vaccines. Only oseltamivir, among the neuraminidase inhibitors, has been approved for prophylaxis. However, oseltamivir and zanamivir have been shown to prevent influenza illness when given to people as chemoprophylaxis after a household member was diagnosed with influenza. No studies have demonstrated the effectiveness of these four antiviral agents in preventing influenza in severely immunocompromised persons. When any of these drugs are taken as chemoprophylaxis, it must be taken each day for the duration of influenza activity or at least during the period of peak activity in the community.

Chemoprophylaxis should be considered (1) for people at high risk who are vaccinated after influenza activity has begun, (2) for people who provide care to those at high risk, (3) for people who are expected to have an inadequate antibody response to influenza vaccine, and (4) for people who should not be vaccinated. Use of these drugs for treatment and prophylaxis of influenza is important in institutional outbreak control. Table 2 lists the FDA's approved indications for each drug and recommended drug doses by age group.

All four drugs are administered orally. Amantadine and rimantadine are available in tablet or syrup form. Oseltamivir is available in capsule or oral suspension. Zanamivir is available as a drug powder given by oral inhalation using a plastic device. Amantadine is excreted unchanged in the urine (90%) and thus dosages need to be reduced with renal insufficiency. Rimantadine is metabolized by the liver (approximately 75%) and therefore should be used with caution in patients with liver disease. Most of the orally inhaled zanamivir is deposited in the oropharynx with less than 20% being systemically absorbed. Approximately 80% of oseltamivir is absorbed systemically.

Amantadine and rimantadine can cause central nervous system (CNS) and gastrointestinal side effects. The CNS side effects include nervousness, anxiety, insomnia, difficulty concentrating, and lightheadedness and are more frequent with amantadine than with rimantadine. Gastrointestinal side effects are usually nausea and anorexia and occur in 1% to 3% of people taking either drug. Lowering the dosage of amantadine in those with renal insufficiency, seizure disorders, or certain psychiatric disorders can reduce the incidence and severity of side effects.

Zanamivir is currently not recommended for treating patients with chronic airway disease because of the potential for decline in respiratory function. Oseltamivir was associated with nausea (10%) and vomiting (9%), although only a small number of patients discontinued the drug because of these side effects. Oseltamivir is recommended to be taken with food to decrease these side effects.

No studies have been completed on the safety or efficacy of these antiviral drugs in pregnant women. There is limited information on drug-drug interactions with these drugs. Amantadine should be given cautiously to patients receiving drugs that also affect the CNS. No published data are available that address the safety and efficacy of combination therapy with any of these antiviral drugs.

Drug-resistant viruses have been reported in patients given either amantadine or rimantadine for

TABLE 2. **Approved Indications for Influenza Antiviral Medications**

		Age Group (y)				
Indication	**Antiviral Agent**	**1-6**	**7-9**	**10-12**	**13-64**	**≥ 65**
Treatment						
	Amantadine (Symmetrel)	5 mg/kg/d†	5 mg/kg/d†	100 mg bid	100 mg bid	≤100 mg/d
	Rimantadine (Flumadine)	Not approved	Not approved	Not approved	100 mg bid	100 mg/d
	Zanamivir (Relenza)	Not approved	Not approved	10 mg bid	10 mg bid	10 mg bid
	Oseltamivir (Tamiflu)	Varies by weight	Varies by weight	Varies by weight	75 mg bid	75 mg bid
Prophylaxis						
	Amantadine	5 mg/kg/d†	5 mg/kg/d†	100 mg bid	100 mg bid	≤100 mg/d
	Rimantadine	5 mg/kg/d†	5 mg/kg/d†	100 mg bid	100 mg bid	100 mg/d
	Zanamivir	Not approved	Not approved	Not approved	Not approved	Not approved
	Oseltamivir	Not approved	Not approved	Not approved	75 mg/d	75 mg/d

†Up to 150 mg per day.

therapy. Resistant strains have been recovered from patients within 2 to 3 days of starting therapy. The frequency of transmission of resistant viruses is unknown but already reported. In vitro resistance to zanamivir and oseltamivir has been demonstrated, and clinical isolates with demonstrated resistance have appeared but are infrequent. Surveillance for neuraminidase inhibitor-resistant influenza virus is ongoing.

Other Measures

Symptom management of influenza should include oral hydration, acetaminophen for fever and headache, nasal decongestant, and cough suppressant. Antibiotics should be given only for secondary bacterial infections.

LEISHMANIASIS

method of
JEAN-PIERRE GANGNEUX, M.D., PH.D.
Laboratoire de Parasitologie-Mycologie
Rennes Cedex, France

Leishmania parasites are kinetoplastid protozoa members of the family Trypanosomatidae. They are transmitted by phlebotomine sandflies and are responsible for a broad spectrum of human diseases: localized and disseminated cutaneous leishmaniasis (LCL and DCL), mucocutaneous leishmaniasis (MCL), and visceral leishmaniasis (VL). Variability of the disease outcome results from a complex host-parasite relationship. The host's genetic background and immunologic status and the parasite's intrinsic pathogenicity represent three main components that determine the clinical expression but also the therapeutic response.

Out of 350 million people at risk in 88 endemic countries, there is an estimated prevalence of 12 million cases with an incidence of 1.5 million cases annually of dermal and mucosal infections and 0.5 million cases annually of visceral infections. Difficulties remain for the control and treatment of leishmaniasis and new strategies are needed. Evaluation of optimal chemotherapeutic protocols or identification of new vaccine candidates is of prime interest but we should also take into account the host diversity, the parasite polymorphism, and the vector and reservoir controls.

LIFE CYCLE AND PATHOPHYSIOLOGY

Leishmania are dimorphic parasites. The flagellated promastigotes multiply in the female sandfly's intestinal tract and are transmitted during blood-sucking. More than 20 species of the *Leishmania* genus are transmitted to humans by sandfly vectors, members of the *Phlebotomus* genus (in the Old World) and of the *Lutzomyia* genus (in the New World). In the mammalian host, promastigotes are engulfed by phagocytic cells, and proliferate as nonflagellated obligate intracellular amastigotes. Experimental and clinical data suggest that an efficient host immune response involves a CD4+ T helper 1 cell-mediated response, leading to macrophage activation and elimination of intracellular amastigotes through nitrogen oxidation products. It has been shown that the course of *Leishmania* infection is under genetic control, in particular with the NRAMP1, TNF-α, TNF-β, and MHC genes implicated.

Besides, the clinical expression of *Leishmania* infection also depends on the causing species and on the strain's intrinsic virulence. Anthropophilic species belong to both *Leishmania* and *Viannia* sub-genus. It is convenient to classify species upon their geographical distribution and their tropism (dermal, mucosal, or visceral) (Table 1). However, this schematic view does not reflect the role of host factors on the outcome as mentioned previously, and for example, visceralizing diseases have been observed with typical dermotropic species such as *L. major* or *L. amazonensis* in immunosuppressed patients. Because microscopic examination does not allow for the differentiation between *Leishmania* species, identification of isolates mainly relies on the reference method of isoenzymatic characterization. More recently, molecular tools

TABLE 1. **Geographic Distributions, Vectors, and Clinical Forms of Major Anthropophilic Species of the *Leishmania* Genus**

	Old World Leishmaniasis	New World Leishmaniasis
Vectors	*Phlebotomus* genus	*Lutzomyia* genus
Parasites	***Leishmania* sub-genus**	***Leishmania* sub-genus**
	—*L. donovani:* VL, rarely LCL, PKDL and oronasal leishmaniasis	—*L. chagasi:* VL, rarely LCL
	—*L. infantum:* VL, rarely LCL and oronasal leishmaniasis	—*L. venezuelensis:* LCL
	—*L. major, L. tropica, L. killicki, L. arabica:* LCL	—*L. mexicana, L. amazonensis:* LCL, DCL
	—*L. aethiopica*: LCL, DCL	***Viannia* sub-genus**
		—*L. braziliensis:* LCL, MCL
		—*L. braziliensis panamensis, L. guyanensis:* LCL, rarely MCL
		—*L. peruviana, L. naiffi, L. lainsoni, L. shawi, L. colombiensis:* LCL

DCL, diffuse cutaneous leishmaniasis; LCL, localized cutaneous leishmaniasis; MCL, mucocutaneous leishmaniasis; PKDL, post-kala-azar dermal leishmaniasis; VL, visceral leishmaniasis.

proved to be relevant in distinguishing closely related strains in epidemiological studies.

CLINICAL MANIFESTATIONS AND DIAGNOSIS

Visceral Leishmaniasis

This life-threatening form corresponds to the generalized involvement of the reticuloendothelial system. After an incubation period of 2 to 12 months, VL presents itself with chronic fever (Kala Azar = "black fever" in Hindi), hepatosplenomegaly, and weight loss. Biologic signs are pancytopenia and hypergammaglobulinemia. If untreated, the infection evolves to a fatal form with cachexia and secondary complications, such as bacterial and viral infections, epistaxis, gingival bleeding, or petechiae. Nodules and hypo- or hyperpigmented macules named post-kala-azar dermal leishmaniasis (PKDL) may occur after treatment in the Indian and African forms of VL. India, Bangladesh, Nepal, and Sudan in the Old World (*L. donovani* and *L. infantum*) and Brazil (*L. chagasi*) in the New World are the major epidemic and endemic foci of VL. In the Mediterranean basin, VL resulting from *L. infantum* occurs sporadically in children and immunosuppressed patients (HIV infected patients, and patients undergoing organ transplantation). Atypical presentation of VL, gastrointestinal involvement, and concurrent opportunistic infection are usual in immunosuppressed patients. The diagnosis is based mainly on the demonstration of the parasite in blood buffy coat or bone marrow, lymph nodes, spleen, or liver aspirates. Two complementary methods are used: a Giemsa colored smear showing intracellular amastigotes or a promastigote growth in an axenic culture medium (Novy-Mac Neal-Nicolle, or various liquid media such as Schneider's Drosophila medium or RPMI medium supplemented with fetal calf serum). A positive culture allows a species identification by enzymatic characterization. Reference laboratories also use polymerase chain reaction for the diagnosis and a molecular identification. In case of negative parasitologic diagnosis, serology may contribute to help the decision to treat. Detection of anti-*Leishmania* antibodies is mainly performed using direct/indirect agglutination or indirect immunofluorescence assays, and detection of specific antibodies against recombinant K39 antigen are mainly performed using strip-test or ELISA assays.

Cutaneous and Mucocutaneous Leishmaniasis

LCL is the most common clinical expression of *Leishmania* infection. The lesion generally heals spontaneously within 1 month to 3 years. Except the nations of the Pacific region, including Australia and New Zealand, CL is found in all tropical and subtropical regions of the World. The incubation period varies from 1 week to several months after the infected insect bite. The localized lesions progressively evolve from erythematous papules to nodules and noduloulcerative lesions. Less typical lesions may include verrucous, eczematous, psoriasiform, varicelliform, keloidal, erysipeloid, and sporotrichoid morphologies. Inflammatory satellite papules and regional lymphadenopathy may be present during New World CL. Four major complicated cutaneous forms are described, depending on the causative species:

- *Leishmaniasis recidivans* (LR) is an oligoparasitic and recurrent localized form resembling lupus vulgaris. It corresponds to the development of new lesions within the scar of a healed acute lesion. *L. tropica* is the most causative species.
- DCL is an anergic polyparasitic form of CL resembling lepromatous leprosy. *L. aethiopica* in the Old World and *L. mexicana* and *L. amazonensis* in the New World are the principal causative species.
- PKDL manifests itself by skin lesions after resolution of VL or during relapses. This form is frequently disfiguring mainly due to *L. donovani* in India and East Africa.
- MCL, also known as Espundia, is a rare but severe event after *L. braziliensis* (more rarely *L. panamensis* and *L. guyanensis*) infection. It corresponds to oronasal mucosa tropism of the parasite after hematogenous or lymphatic dissemination from the skin, abutting on chronic disease with a risk of facial mutilation. Without treatment, no spontaneous healing is observed and relapses are observed even under treatment.

The diagnosis is based on the demonstration of the parasite in Giemsa-stained tissue smears or biopsies or on the identification of promastigotes in culture, thus allowing a species identification. PCR may improve the sensibility of the diagnosis.

CHEMOTHERAPEUTIC TREATMENTS

Pentavalent Antimony Derivatives (SB^v)

Organic pentavalent antimonials have been the first-line therapy for VL since their introduction in 1937. Sodium stibogluconate (Pentostam—100 mg SB^v/mL)* and meglumine antimonate (Glucantime—85 mg SB^v/mL)* are administered intravenously or intramuscularly, in doses of 20 mg SB^v/kg per day for 28 d for the treatment of VL. However, response rates have been decreasing, particularly in India, but also in East Africa and in the Mediterranean basin. In HIV-co-infected patients, relapses after initial treatment are almost ineluctable. These trends incite to lengthen duration of therapy or to increase doses, with a higher risk of reversible side effects (nausea, vomiting, myalgias, arthralgias, raised hepatic transaminase levels, subclinical pancreatitis, and minor electrocardiographic changes) and of severe cardiotoxicity (concave ST segment, prolongation of the QT, arrhythmia, and sudden death). Old World CL with multiple lesions at risk of disfiguring scars and New World CL at risk of mucosal metastasis should be treated with parenteral

*Not FDA approved for this indication.

TABLE 2. **Recommendations on Drug Regimens to Be Used in the Treatment of Mediterranean Zoonotic Visceral Leishmaniasis (WHO Conference, Roma, Italy, 1995)**

Drug	Posology
Pentavalent derivative antimony (SB^v)	20 mg SB^v/kg/d during 20–28 d
• meglumine antimonate = Glucantime* • sodium stibogluconate = Pentostam*	
Pentavalent derivative antimony + Allopurinol**	20 mg sbV/kg/d + 15 mg/kg/d during 20–28 d
Liposomal amphotericin B = AmBisome	3 mg/kg/d on d 0, 1, 2, 3, 4 and 10 (total dose: 18 mg/kg)
Aminosidine = paromomycin (Humatin)**	12–16 mg/kg/d during 14–63 d

*Investigational drug in the United States.
**Not FDA approved for this indication.

SB^v in doses of 20 mg SB^v/kg per day for 20 d. Localized CL is easy to treat with well-tolerated intralesional injections of 0.2-1 mL SB^v per lesion per week for 4 or 5 weeks, particularly during *L. tropica* infections.

Amphotericin B (AmB) and Lipid Formulations of AmB

During the past decade, deoxycholate AmB (Fungizone) has been considered to be an efficient alternative in the treatment of Old and New World VL (0.5 mg/kg daily for 28 d or 1 mg/kg daily for 15–20 d). However, its use is limited because of infusion-related reactions and nephrotoxicity. Liposomal AmB (AmBisome) in a simplified therapeutic protocol (Table 2) proved effective and much better tolerated than the deoxycholate formulation. Although it is costly, liposomal AmB is now a first-line treatment recommended for children as well as for adults and is a candidate of special interest for secondary prophylaxis in immunosuppressed patients because of its tolerance and long tissue half-life. Low-dose or single high-dose regimens with liposomal AmB were recently assessed and proved effective and more affordable. AmB lipid Complex (Abelcet), another lipid formulation of AmB, has been less evaluated but also proved effective. During CL and MCL, deoxycholate Amb is considered by some authors as a valuable alternative in case of resistance to first-line therapy with antimonials. Available data are insufficient to draw conclusions on lipid formulations of AmB for CL and MCL treatment.

Miltefosine*

Since 1997, only hexadecylphosphocholine (miltefosine, Miltex) has emerged as a new anti-*Leishmania* drug. Miltefosine, originally developed as an oral antineoplastic agent, is the first orally administered treatment that proved effective for VL including those with antimony-resistant infections. In multiple clinical trials, dose regimen of 100 mg/d for 4 weeks was well-tolerated in adults and allowed high rates (96%) of definitive cures (approximately 2.5 mg/kg of body weight for children). Even shorter courses of treatment (100 mg/d for 3 weeks) allowed high-level efficacy in preliminary series of patients. Since 2002, miltefosine (Impavido) is registered in India for the treatment of Kala Azar. Unfortunately, this promising treatment for the 21st century did not prevent relapses in the first few HIV-coinfected patients treated with it. This phospholipid derivative also proved effective for the treatment of New World CL at the dose of 2.25 mg/kg/d for 3–4 weeks. Little is known on the interest of a topical formulation of miltefosine.

*Not FDA approved for this indication.

Pentamidine Isethionate

Discovered in 1939, pentamidine isethionate (Pentacarinat) has been used for a long time as an alternative of choice for patients intolerant to or presenting with a refractory VL to antimonials. High cure rates were reported using a classical regimen (15 parenteral injections of 4 mg/kg on alternate day), but its efficacy has diminished over the years, particularly in India. This declining activity with an estimated cure rate lower than 70%, together with the drug toxicity (from reversible hypoglycemia to definitive insulin-dependent diabetes mellitus and cardiac toxicity), have led to its decreased use. Treatment regimens based on 3 to 4 intramuscular injections of 3–4 mg/kg on alternate days allow a cure rate of more than 80% either during Old World or New World CL. Similar cure rates are obtained only after at least eight injections during the treatment of MCL, DCL, or LR.

Aminosidine

Aminosidine sulfate[†] is an aminoglycoside antibiotic, with an identical chemical structure to paromomycin (Humatin)* and erythromycin (Monomycin). In VL, several studies reported a favorable outcome after administration of aminosidine alone or combined with pentavalent derivatives of antimony in African and Indian Kala Azar. It is considered as a valuable alternative drug in case of unresponsiveness to antimonials or can be used in combination with antimonials to reduce the duration of therapy (see Table 2). However, the parenteral formulation is not currently produced. Limited documented cases and experimental data

*Not FDA approved for this indication.
[†]Available as an orphan drug only.

are not in favor of using aminosidine for the treatment of Mediterranean *L. infantum* VL. Against *Leishmania major,* it has good in vitro activity and clinical trials have been performed with various formulations containing 15% aminosidine for the topical treatment of Old World and New World CL. Results are ranging from more than 85% cure rate to same rate as obtained with placebo, depending on the design of the study, the causing species, and the ointment formulation (methyl benzethonium chloride, urea or urea + 0.5% gentamicin).

Other Medications

Allopurinol (Zyloprim),* metronidazole (Flagyl),* ergosterol biosynthesis inhibitors (ketoconazole [Nizoral],* itraconazole [Sporanox],* fluconazole [Diflucan],* terbinafine [Lamisil])* or dapsone* have been used either for the treatment of VL or CL in monotherapy or combined with antimonials. However, only limited data are available with these drugs that proved inconsistently effective, mainly depending on the causal species. Recent studies suggest that fluconazole could be a treatment of prime interest for LCL resulting from *L. major*. Clinical trials are in prospect with the primaquine analogue WR6026 (Sitamaquine). This compound previously developed in the field of malaria showed antileishmanial activity and has the advantage of being taken orally.

STRATEGIES FOR OPTIMAL TREATMENT AND CONTROL OF LEISHMANIASIS

The declining activity and the toxicity of traditional leishmanicidal drugs, and the high rates of relapses in immunosuppressed patients stress the need for alternative compounds screening and for the optimization of therapeutic protocols.

- Drug adaptation to the presumed causative *species* of the parasite and drug monitoring resistance are relevant strategies because it's now admitted that the therapeutic response varies with the *Leishmania* species.
- A powerful drug delivery system can optimize tolerance and action of traditional drugs. For example, liposomes loaded with amphotericin B proved particularly effective in targeting the infected macrophages, permitting drug delivery into the parasitophorous vacuole.
- Multitherapy is an interesting approach to increase efficacy and tolerance, and to avoid the emergence of drug resistance. Principal protocols used in patients with refractory VL included antimonials combined with aminosidine, allopurinol, or immunotherapy. Other drug combinations were also experimentally evaluated.
- In immunosuppressed patients, mainly HIV-coinfected patients, a partial or complete restoration of immune functions remains the only warrant against relapses. Secondary prophylaxis proved inconsistently effective and no consensus has still been adopted.

Although "historical" immunization with parasites from active human lesions to produce self-cure CL and induce lifelong protection against reinfection have been reported, the development of a *Leishmania* vaccine will not be an easy task. First-generation vaccines with killed *Leishmania* showed no evidence of significant protection against VL during the past 50 years. More recently, native and recombinant antigens were screened and tested for second-generation vaccines. Their interest will depend on their potentiality to protect against all clinical forms of leishmaniasis, independently to the causative species.

Before disposing of an effective vaccine, the vector and reservoir controls remain of prime interest. To decrease the risk of being bitten, long pants and long-sleeved shirts should be worn; insect repellents containing DEET on uncovered skin and fine-mesh insecticide-impregnated bed-nets should be used. Besides, a better knowledge on the ecology of reservoir host species and of phlebotomine sandflies can direct towards new strategies of control of leishmaniasis.

*Not FDA approved for this indication.

LEPROSY (HANSEN'S DISEASE)

method of
M. PATRICIA JOYCE, M.D., and
DAVID M. SCOLLARD, M.D., PH.D.
National Hansen's Disease Programs
Baton Rouge, LA

Leprosy is a curable infectious disease. The causative agent, *Mycobacterium leprae*, primarily infects skin and peripheral nerve, although deep infections (e.g., liver and bone marrow) may be transient occurrences in heavily infected, untreated individuals. The organism is weakly acid-fast, noncultivatable, very slow growing (as determined in mouse foot-pad studies), and, in the laboratory, appears to be highly susceptible to freezing and probably to drying.

Infection is acquired through close contact with an infected person. Although the route of transmission has not been clearly determined, both aerosol transmission and skin-to-skin transmission are considered probable modes of transmission. Heavily infected patients have abundant organisms in the nasal mucosa and mucous secretions. *M. leprae* infection is enzootic among nine-banded armadillos in the U.S. Gulf States and areas of Central and South America, and is a potential, if unusual, source of human infection in these areas.

The information available suggests that more than 95% of adults are not susceptible to infection even after substantial exposure to large doses of bacilli. In susceptible persons, the infection has a median incubation time of 2 to 7 years, but may be as long as 20 years.

Because of this long incubation period and gradual, insidious onset, it is often difficult or impossible to identify the source of contact. The long incubation, together with the potential for deformity (greatly exaggerated in the minds of many laypersons), has resulted in an extraordinary stigma and fear of social ostracism that deter many patients from seeking treatment early in the course of the disease. If the disease is not recognized and treated at an early stage, however, some neuropathy and resultant deformity may persist even after antimicrobial treatment has successfully eliminated the pathogen.

As a result of widespread implementation of multidrug treatment programs and policy changes that remove individuals from the roster of patients to be followed (both promulgated by the World Health Organization [WHO]), the available figures indicate a sharp decline in the prevalence of Hansen's disease (HD) globally over the last two decades. The number of new cases of HD identified annually has not changed significantly during the same period, and continues to number approximately 800,000 worldwide. The U.S. experiences approximately 150 new cases per year, the majority of whom are immigrants from endemic countries, although native-born cases are reported from Texas and Louisiana in particular.

LABORATORY TESTS

A full-thickness skin biopsy from the active (advancing) margin of the most active lesion, stained with hematoxylin-eosin and Fite-Faraco stains, is the primary laboratory basis for the diagnosis and classification of HD. If another mycobacterial infection is suspected, a culture should be performed, and growth will exclude *M. leprae*. If fixed in formalin for less than 24 hours, paraffin-embedded tissue may also be satisfactory for polymerase chain reaction analysis for *M. leprae* DNA, should that be indicated.

The other laboratory test useful in the diagnosis and follow up in HD is the "slit-skin smear," which should be performed only by trained, experienced individuals. A shallow incision is made in the skin at six standard sites, as well as from other sites, including selected lesions. A small drop of dermal interstitial fluid is smeared onto a glass slide, and the number of acid-bacilli is determined and expressed as a "bacteriologic index." This may be used to assess the bacterial load before and during therapy.

In the absence of tissue confirmation, an empiric diagnosis of HD, with estimated 70% certainty, may be made for a patient from an endemic area with a typical anesthetic lesion. Although the WHO advocates this approach in resource-poor settings, in the United States and wherever resources are available patients with questionable skin lesions should be evaluated by trained specialists.

No serologic tests are available for the routine diagnosis of HD. Some serologic assays have been described, but these are used for research purposes. Similarly, no diagnostic skin test is available. (The lepromin test reflects the host's capability of producing a granulomatous response to *M. leprae* antigens, but does not measure prior exposure to the organism and is of no diagnostic value in individual patients.)

After the diagnosis of HD has been confirmed and treatment is being planned, tests for glucose-6-phosphate dehydrogenase deficiency are recommended, as are baseline erythrocyte and leukocyte counts and liver function studies.

Lepromatous patients (see the following section) have a polyclonal increase in antibody production, including antibodies that may produce several false-positive serologic tests, including those for syphilis and HIV.

CLASSIFICATION

M. leprae elicits a uniquely broad spectrum of immunopathologic responses in man. These many manifestations reflect the patients' differing capabilities to develop a cellular immune response to *M. leprae*, and this is the basis of the clinical and pathologic "Ridley-Jopling" classification system. This five-part classification identifies, at one extreme, patients with a high degree of cell-mediated immunity and delayed hypersensitivity, presenting with a single, well-demarcated lesion with central hypopigmentation and hypesthesia. Biopsies of these reveal well-developed granulomatous inflammation and rare acid-fast bacilli demonstrable in the tissues; this is termed polar tuberculoid (TT). Unlike tuberculosis, caseous necrosis is rare in tuberculoid HD. At the other extreme, patients have no apparent resistance to *M. leprae*; these patients present with numerous, poorly demarcated raised or nodular lesions on all parts of the body, biopsies of which reveal sheets of foamy macrophages in the dermis, containing very large numbers of bacilli and microcolonies called "globi." This nonresistant, highly infected form of the disease is termed polar lepromatous (LL). The majority of patients, however, fall into a broad "borderline" category between these two polar forms; this is subdivided into borderline lepromatous (BL), mid-borderline (BB), and borderline tuberculoid (BT).

Very early lesions may be manifested as relatively nonspecific perineural infiltrates in which rare acid-fast bacilli can be demonstrated, but without sufficient infiltrates to classify them—these are called "indeterminate." Care should be taken to use this term only when the biopsy shows diagnostic evidence of leprosy (nerve involvement and acid-fast bacilli) because a diagnosis of HD may often have significant impact on a patient's family, employment, and psychologic and social status.

The Ridley-Jopling classification has been used worldwide and enables comparisons of the distribution of different types of HD in different countries and racial groups. This classification system is the basis of almost all clinical immunologic studies of HD, is of considerable value in advising patients and their physicians regarding the risks of acute complications of HD (see the following section), and provides the basis for recommendations of the different MDT treatment regimens.

Recently, the WHO has recommended a simplified clinical classification scheme, identifying TT and BT types as "paucibacillary" (PB), and LL, BL, and BB types as "multibacillary" (MB). In many countries where histopathologic evaluation of biopsies is costly or not available, the WHO now advocates the use of this classification system, with skin smear results and the number of skin lesions to designate a patient as PB or MB.

TREATMENT

Dapsone, rifampin (Rifadin),* and clofazimine (Lamprene) remain the mainstay drugs of choice (Table 1), used in combined MDT regimens depending on the disease classification. Alternate agents can be used in these combinations (see Table 1) if there is evidence of drug intolerance or resistance.

*Not FDA approved for this indication.

Treatment recommendations of the U.S. National Hansen's Disease Programs (NHDP) (http://bphc.hrsa.gov/nhdp) and the WHO are based on the distinction between paucibacillary and multibacillary disease (Table 2), but differ in the length of minimal therapy and the use of monthly witnessed doses of rifampin* and clofazimine. The NHDP recommends daily rifampin* and only suggests monthly use in the setting of concomitant corticosteroid use for neuritis or control of immune reactions.

*Not FDA approved for this indication.

TABLE 1. **Antileprosy Drugs**

Agent	Routine Dose	Side Effects	Antibacterial Mechanism	Drug Effects and Drug Interactions
Dapsone	100 mg/d	Anemia, hemolysis (G6PD) Methemoglobinemia Agranulocytosis Liver toxicity Sulfone syndrome Peripheral neuropathy	Weakly bactericidal; competitive PABA antagonist	Substrate of CYP2C9, 2E1, and 3A4; increases marrow toxicity of zidovudine (Retrovir) and pyrimethamine (Daraprim); increases serum trimethoprim
Clofazimine (Lamprene)	50 mg/d	Nausea Skin pigmentation and xerosis Bowel motility/ileus Possible cardiac arrhythmias	Weakly bactericidal; binds mycobacterial DNA	None confirmed
Rifampin (Rifadin)*	600 mg/d (given as monthly dose if concurrent steroids used)	Nausea Hepatotoxicity Marrow suppression Interstitial nephritis Flulike syndrome Discolored body fluids Drug interactions	Bactericidal; inhibits DNA-dependent RNA polymerase	Strong inducer of CYP3A4; especially decreases levels of corticosteroids, estrogens, protease inhibitors, carbamazepine (Tegretol), macrolides, methadone (Dolophine), and others
Minocycline (Minocin)*	100 mg/d	Nausea Deposits in bone and teeth Photosensitivity Hyperpigmentation CNS toxicity Hypersensitivity	Bactericidal; inhibits ribosomal protein synthesis	Decreased absorption with cation preparations; decreases effect of estrogens; increases effect of warfarin (Coumadin)
Ofloxacin (Floxin)*	400 mg/d	Nausea CNS toxicity Phototoxicity Hypersensitivity Drug interactions	Bactericidal; inhibits DNA gyrase	Increases effect of theophylline (Uniphyl), caffeine, warfarin (Coumadin), antiarrhythmics; absorption decreased by didanosine (Videx) and cationic preparations
Levofloxacin (Levaquin)*	500 mg/d	Nausea CNS toxicity Phototoxicity Hypersensitivity Drug interactions	Bactericidal; inhibits DNA gyrase	Increases effect of theophylline (Uniphyl), caffeine, warfarin (Coumadin), antiarrhythmics; absorption decreased by didanosine (Videx) and cationic preparations
Ethionamide (Trecator-Sc)*	250 mg/d (Note: 500–750 mg/d for TB)	Nausea Hepatotoxicity Hypersensitivity Metallic taste Peripheral neuropathy	Bactericidal; inhibits peptide synthesis	None confirmed but use with caution if hepatic dysfunction, diabetes, or cycloserine use
Clarithromycin (Biaxin)*	500 mg twice/d	Nausea Motility disorder Cardiac arrhythmias Hypersensitivity Drug interactions	Bactericidal; inhibits ribosomal protein synthesis	CYP3A4 substrate, also inhibits CYP1A2 and 3A3/4; increases levels of theophylline (Uniphyl), cyclosporine (Neoral), carbamazepine (Tegretol), cisapride (Propulsid), astemizole (Hismanal),** others

*Not FDA-approved for this indication.
**Not available in the United States.
CNS, central nervous system; CYP, cytochrome P450; G6PD, glucose-6-phosphate dehydrogenase deficiency; PABA, para-aminobenzoic acid; TB, tuberculosis.

TABLE 2. **Treatment Regimens**

Multibacillary		
Agent	*U.S. NHDP*	*WHO*
Dapsone	100 mg/d for 24 mo	100 mg/d for 12 mo
Rifampin (Rifadin)*	600 mg/d for 24 mo	600 mg monthly given under supervision for 12 mo
Clofazimine (Lamprene)	50 mg/d for 24 mo (If refused, may substitute daily minocycline*)	50 mg/d, plus 300 mg each mo given under supervision for 12 mo
Paucibacillary		
Agent	*U.S. NHDP*	*WHO*
Dapsone	100 mg/d for 12 mo	100 mg/d for 6 mo
Rifampin (Rifadin)*	600 mg/d for 12 mo	600 mg monthly under supervision for 6 mo

*Not FDA-approved for this indication
NHDP, National Hansen's Disease Programs; WHO, World Health Organization.

Most recently a single-dose regimen of rifampin,* 400 mg, ofloxacin, (Floxin),* 400 mg, and minocycline (Minocin),* 100 mg (ROM therapy) has been recommended by WHO for use in patients with paucibacillary disease limited to a single lesion. The NHDP continues to recommend 12 months of daily therapy for all patients with PB disease, but a third drug (usually clofazimine) may be added if active neuritis develops.

Treatment of Acute Complications of HD

"Reactions" are acute inflammatory complications often manifesting as medical emergencies during the course of treated or untreated HD. Two major clinical types of leprosy reactions occur; together they may affect 30% to 50% of all leprosy patients. Because *M. leprae* infects peripheral nerves, the inflammation associated with reactions often leads to severe nerve injury with subsequent paralysis and deformity. These reactions appear to have different underlying immunologic mechanisms, but both are poorly understood and the factors which initiate them are unknown. Multidrug treatment of HD should be continued during the management of reactions.

TYPE 1 REACTIONS. Type 1 reactions, also known as "reversal" reactions, occur in patients in the borderline portion of the spectrum (i.e., BL, BB, and BT). They are manifested as induration and erythema of pre-existing lesions, frequently with prominent acral edema, and often with progressive neuritis causing sensory and motor neuropathy. These reactions develop gradually and their natural course may last for many weeks. Type 1 reactions are the result of spontaneous enhancement of cellular immunity and delayed hypersensitivity to *M. leprae* antigens, but the causes and mechanisms of this enhancement are poorly understood. Aggressive initial treatment with prednisone is indicated to protect nerve function, starting at 60 to 80 mg per day (1 mg/kg/d). Prolonged low-dose corticosteroids, over 4 to 6 months, have been shown more effective than very high dosage or very brief courses in the treatment of active neuropathy. Tapering should proceed slowly as the patient's condition permits.

TYPE 2 REACTIONS. Type 2 reactions, also known as erythema nodosum leprosum, occur in multibacillary patients (LL and BL). These patients experience abrupt onset of crops of very tender, erythematous nodules that may develop on various parts of the body, without predilection for pre-existing lesions. Systemically, these patients usually also experience fever, malaise, and some degree of neuritis with sensory and motor neuropathy. Iridocyclitis and episcleritis, orchitis, arthritis, and myositis may also accompany this reaction, and in severe type 2 reactions, cutaneous lesions may ulcerate. The natural course of type 2 reactions is 1 to 2 weeks, but many patients experience multiple recurrences over several months. Several features of these reactions suggest that antigen-antibody complexes may play a role, but such a relationship is not clearly established.

Treatment with corticosteroids is indicated if type 2 reactions do not quickly respond to nonsteroidal anti-inflammatory agents. These reactions may respond only poorly to prednisone even in doses of 60 to 80 mg daily. Thalidomide (Thalomid) is indicated for patients with multiple reactions that are poorly controlled with corticosteroids; 100 mg/d is usually sufficient, although higher doses (up to 400 mg/d in divided doses) may be used in the initial days of treatment of severe reactions. Thalidomide should be limited to bedtime dosing as soon as possible as it may be severely sedating. Its remarkable anti-inflammatory effect in treating type 2 reactions was the major reason that thalidomide was retained in the pharmacopoeia for several decades when it was otherwise generally proscribed due to its teratogenic properties. Multiple methods of birth control should be implemented before using thalidomide in women of childbearing age. To avoid nonprescribed self-medication, some programs restrict its use to inpatients or direct administration in outpatient clinics for both men and women. Clofazimine also has anti-inflammatory effects on type 2 reactions by still unexplained mechanisms and is given in doses of 100 to 200 mg/d as part of the antibiotic regimen in lepromatous (MB) disease.

THE LUCIO PHENOMENON. The Lucio phenomenon is an acute, severe, necrotizing vasculitis described originally in patients of Mexican ancestry and is associated with polar forms of lepromatous disease with longstanding and heavy infection. This complication is rare but has a high morbidity and mortality; its underlying mechanisms are unknown. Lucio reactions are often accompanied by a profound anemia, and they require intensive wound care and débridement comparable with the management of severe burns, and aggressive use of corticosteroids. These reactions require inpatient management, and consultation with the NHDP is highly recommended.

PROGRESSIVE NEURITIS. Progressive neuritis may develop slowly in patients with any type of leprosy, and rapid progression with pain and neuropathy may be seen in some patients who do not have systemic or cutaneous symptoms of typical type 1 or type 2 reactions. The possibility of neuritis should be carefully

*Not FDA approved for this indication.

evaluated at each clinic visit, and if observed, treatment with corticosteroids is indicated to prevent anesthesia and paralysis. Abrupt worsening of neurologic function is a medical emergency and requires aggressive use of corticosteroids and close monitoring by medical staff. Thalidomide is not effective for type 1 reactions and is not used for neuritis unless there is clear evidence of concurrent type 2 reaction.

OPHTHALMIC COMPLICATIONS. Ophthalmic complications in HD are serious and, without treatment, may lead to blindness. Iritis caused by infection by *M. leprae* may be identified by slit-lamp examination. It usually responds well to multidrug therapy, although killed bacilli are removed slowly, in the same manner that they are cleared from the skin and other tissues. As noted earlier, iridocyclitis and episcleritis may also complicate the course of type 2 reactions. Secondary glaucoma may result unless ophthalmologic steroids are prescribed. Severe keratoconjunctivitis is a serious complication of neuritis in branches of the trigeminal nerve, causing corneal and conjunctival insensitivity. Keratoconjunctivitis in HD is treated by prompt and regular application of conjunctival lubricating and moistening agents combined with oral corticosteroids to alleviate the neuropathy. Neuritis in branches of the facial nerve may cause weakness or paralysis of the orbicularis oculi muscles and lagophthalmos; it may develop during the course of type 1 reactions. If the nerve injury and muscle weakness are not reversible, tarsorrhaphy may be necessary to protect the eye.

Antileprosy Therapy in Special Circumstances

Multidrug Therapy During Leprosy Reactions

During leprosy reactions or active neuritis, the composition and length of multidrug therapy should be individually determined. Monotherapy of any type should never be used initially, but it may be used as maintenance therapy after multidrug therapy during corticosteroid use.

Treatment in Children, Pregnancy, and Lactation

Standard multidrug therapy is used for children with both PB and MB disease. Dapsone is given at 1 mg/kg/d, rifampin* at 1 mg/kg/d, and clofazimine at 1 mg/kg/d. Minocycline* and fluoroquinolones* are generally avoided (as they are also in pregnant women). Standard multidrug therapy may be used during pregnancy and lactation, with only minimal risk of significant transfer of medication to the child.

Treatment of persons with HIV Disease or Tuberculosis

Although the concurrence of leprosy and HIV disease has been associated with a shortened life expectancy in some studies, the two infections generally appear to be independent in incidence and severity, unlike the combined influence of HIV and tuberculosis. Standard multidrug therapy can be used in the HIV patient with leprosy, using conventional duration of therapy with close monitoring of clinical response. Special care must be given to the potential interactions of rifampin with antiretroviral medications, protease inhibitors in particular. Use of rifampin in antileprosy therapy has a prophylactic benefit against latent tuberculosis; however active tuberculosis should be identified before initiating rifampin, especially in persons with HIV disease, as standard multidrug therapy would represent rifampin monotherapy in tuberculosis.

*Not FDA approved for this indication.

Drug Intolerance or Microbial Resistance

If drug intolerance develops, or if resistant bacilli are suspected, the patient should be evaluated by a referral center for alternate combinations of medications. Minocycline* or a fluoroquinolone* can be substituted in multidrug therapy, but no set guidelines have been established for length of therapy.

PREVENTION AND MANAGEMENT OF DISABILITIES

The prognosis and well-being of leprosy patients have radically improved in the last half-century because of the use of effective antimicrobial treatment. Prompt, aggressive treatment of reactions has also reduced the severity of disabilities. Patient education remains essential for compliance, and for injury prevention in patients with insensate hands and feet. Protective footwear and ophthalmologic support are essential even after completion of multidrug therapy, because the leprosy patient may have lifelong neuropathic disabilities. Conservative management of plantar ulcers by casting and pressure reduction should be employed to avoid the need for amputation.

Prevention and Control Measures

Early clinical diagnosis, prompt initiation of multidrug treatment, and vigilant follow-up of contacts are the bedrock of HD leprosy prevention and control. Although no infectious disease is likely to be eradicated by treatment alone, the evidence clearly indicates that good treatment and follow-up will substantially reduce the number of highly infectious individuals and, in time, this will lead to a decline in transmission and in the number of new patients infected. Evaluation and treatment of infected household contacts remains the mainstay of infection control.

Patient compliance with treatment is a major issue because treatment regimens require several months or years of medication. Patient education to encourage compliance when the patient may feel no rapid benefit and to provide support if a reaction complicates the course of the disease is thus a critical part of the overall prevention strategy. Even highly infected patients become noninfectious to others almost immediately upon receiving multidrug therapy; education should

*Not FDA approved for this indication.

emphasize that compliance with treatment is thus also beneficial to family and other close contacts.

Prophylactic treatment is not recommended. No vaccine is available, although such research is being actively conducted. Similarly, although improving methods for early detection is a high priority in leprosy research, no current laboratory techniques can achieve better results than are obtained by careful, thorough skin examination by an experienced physician or paramedical worker.

MALARIA

method of
CHRISTINA M. COYLE, M.D., and
LOUIS M. WEISS, M.D., M.P.H.
Albert Einstein College of Medicine
Bronx, New York

Malaria, one of the most common infectious diseases in the world, infects about 500 million people, with a resultant mortality of 3 million people per year. Most of these infections occur in the developing world, where malaria is a leading cause of morbidity and mortality; it has a profound effect on the economy of endemic countries. Imported malaria is a common problem in nonendemic countries. For example, in the United States, about 1200 cases of malaria are reported to the Centers for Disease Control and Prevention (CDC), and more than 99% of these cases are in travelers who have visited or are from endemic countries. Rare cases of transmission within the United States have been reported. These cases have been caused by the presence of mosquito species capable of transmitting malaria that fed on patients with imported cases of malaria, with resulting microfoci of malaria transmission in the United States. Such microfoci have been reported in New Jersey, California, Texas, and Florida. Other sources of infection in patients without a history of travel include blood transfusion; the use of contaminated needles, and, rarely, imported insects (transmission at or near international airports). Congenital infection is uncommon, but it has been reported in nonimmune pregnant women.

Malaria is more severe in children, pregnant women, and travelers from nonendemic countries (e.g., patients with no immunity resulting from previous infection). In addition, within a few years after leaving an endemic country, a person loses the immune response that modulates infection and can develop severe malaria on return to an endemic country. *Plasmodium falciparum* is more likely to cause severe disease than the other malaria species that infect human beings. About half of the infections reported to the CDC are with *P. falciparum,* and most of these are acquired from travel to Africa or in immigrants arriving from Africa. The greatest burden of *P. falciparum* is in sub-Saharan Africa, where more than 90% of the deaths from malaria occur, mostly among children younger than 5 years of age. *Plasmodium vivax* infections have been reported from travelers to many parts of the world, but they are often seen in travelers to the Indian subcontinent.

ETIOLOGY

Obligate intracellular protozoa of the genus *Plasmodium* cause malaria. The four species of protozoa that cause malaria, in order of decreasing world prevalence, are *P. falciparum, P. vivax, Plasmodium malariae,* and *Plasmodium ovale.* Transmission occurs when sporozoites are inoculated into human beings from the salivary glands of a female *Anopheles* species mosquito during a blood meal. Within a half-hour, these sporozoites are cleared from the blood and enter hepatocytes, where they multiply asexually in a process called *exoerytocytic schizogony.* This process results in the formation of thousands of merozoites in each infected hepatocyte. In infections with *Plasmodium falciparum* and *Plasmodium malariae,* rupture of all the infected hepatocytes occurs at about the same time; however, in *P. vivax* and *P. ovale,* some of the hepatocytes become infected but do not rupture. These infected hepatocytes develop into latent tissue schizonts called *hypnozoites* that can cause a relapse of the malaria infection for up to 5 years after the original infection. Seven to 10 days after infection by a sporozoite, when the hepatocyte ruptures, merozoites enter the circulation, where they infect red blood cells. In red blood cells, the parasite undergoes further division and development (erythrocytic life cycle). Newly formed merozoites are released from erythrocytes and can then invade and multiply as merozoites in red blood cells or can invade and develop into mature sexual forms (gametes). These sexual forms (macrogametes and microgametes) can be transmitted to a feeding *Anopheles* mosquito to complete the life cycle. The cycle of rupture and infection of erythrocytes results in the classic fever pattern seen in malaria infection. The time it takes to compete the life cycle is associated with the classic periodicity of the fevers seen with each *Plasmodium* species.

The incubation period for *P. falciparum* is 9 to 14 days, that for *P. vivax* is 12 to 17 days (although primary attack can occur up to 1 year after initial infection), that for *P. ovale* is 16 to 18 days, and that for *P. malariae* is 18 to 40 days. The incubation period can be prolonged in patients taking chemoprophylaxis and in those who have developed partial immunity from repeated malarial infections. The development of immunity is slow, and it takes years of repeated exposures for immunity to malaria to become established.

EPIDEMIOLOGY

Malaria transmission occurs in Africa, Asia, Oceania, Latin America, and South America, with additional foci in Haiti, the Dominican Republic, Greece, Turkey, and the Middle East. Historically, indigenous malaria has been reported as far north as Russia and as far south as Argentina; however, North America, Europe, Australia, New Zealand, Japan,

Argentina, Russia, and the Caribbean currently have no malaria. Within malaria-endemic countries are large areas that are malaria free because transmission depends on local environmental and other conditions. *P. falciparum* is the most common malaria in the developing world, but *P. vivax* has the broadest geographic range and does occur in temperate zones. *P. ovale* is mostly limited to tropical Africa (where the Duffy blood group is found). The risk of acquiring malaria varies greatly from one region of a country to another; variables such as altitude, season, and the amount of rural travel by a traveler influence the density of the vector mosquito population. Because mosquito vectors feed from dusk to dawn, evening and nighttime exposure increases risk. In the United States, more than 60% of the cases of imported malaria are acquired in Africa. Travel risk data can be obtained from the CDC (*http://www.cdc.gov/travel/*), the World Health Organization (*http://www.who.int/ith/english/index.htm*), or the United Kingdom Health Department (*http://www.calaib.co.uk/launc-it/ travel.htm*).

The development of resistance to antimalarial drugs has complicated malaria therapy and prophylaxis. Chloroquine-resistant strains of *P. falciparum* have spread throughout most of the malarious regions of the world, leaving only Latin America west of the Panama Canal, Haiti, the Dominican Republic, Egypt, and parts of the Middle East (choloroquine resistance has been reported in Yemen, Oman, Saudi Arabia, and Iran) unaffected. Resistance to the combination of pyrimethamine and sulfadoxine (Fansidar) is prevalent in some areas of Southeast Asia, the Amazon Basin of South America, and many foci in sub-Saharan Africa. In areas of Southeast Asia, *P. falciparum* malaria has shown a reduced susceptibility to the standard 3-day course of quinine used for therapy in other parts of the world. Mefloquine (Lariam) and halofantrine (Halfan) resistance is important along the Thai-Kampuchean and Myanmar borders and in parts of Vietnam. Studies of isolates of *P. falciparum* suggest that, in West Africa and South America, some strains of malaria have an inherently decreased sensitivity to mefloquine. In addition to chloroquine-resistant *P. falciparum,* there are reports of chloroquine-resistant *P. vivax* in Brazil, New Guinea, and Indonesia. Primaquine resistance is well established in Southeast Asia and Oceania, where up to one-third of patients with *P. vivax* malaria will have a relapse after a standard 14-day course of therapy. Resistance to primaquine is uncommon in other areas of the world where *P. vivax* is endemic.

CLINICAL MANIFESTATIONS

In its early stages, malaria typically manifests as a flulike prodrome that includes headache, malaise, and myalgias, then fever. A travel history is therefore important in suggesting this infection. In a traveler with these symptoms, the differential diagnosis should include typhoid fever, early meningococcal disease and rickettsiosis (e.g., typhus), arboviral infections (e.g., Dengue fever), and leptospirosis. The presence of a rash is suggestive of these other infections. Malaria paroxysms usually develop with a few days of the prodromal period and correspond to the rupture of infected erythrocytes. When most of the parasites within infected erythrocytes undergo schizogony (maturation) at the same time, paroxysms will occur at 48-hour intervals (the length of the developmental life cycle) for all malaria species, except *P. malariae,* in which the developmental life is 72 hours long. Such synchronization is rare in *P. falciparum,* and in this infection, a hectic pattern of paroxysms and fever is what is most commonly seen. During paroxysms, fever can rise to 104°F to 105°F with associated rigors, severe heachaches, abdominal pain, and nausea. Splenomegaly and hepatomegaly may be present without peripheral lymphadenopathy. Blood tests are likely to reveal anemia, thrombocytopenia, neutropenia, hyponatremia, and mildly elevated transaminase levels.

In its early stages, falciparum malaria is clinically indistinguishable from infection with other species. Life-threatening complications can develop rapidly in *P. falciparum* infection, but they are rarely seen with other species. This is in part related to the ability of *P. falciparum* to infect erythrocytes of all ages, unlike the other species of malaria. *P. vivax* and *P. ovale* infect reticulocytes, and *P. malariae* is restricted to a subpopulation of older erythrocytes. It is also the result of cytoadherence of erythrocytes infected with *P. falciparum* to postcapillary venules and uninfected erythrocytes. The high levels of parasitemia and severe anemia that can develop in *P. falciparum* infection along with the cytoadherence of the infected erythrocytes can cause tissue hypoxia and organ dysfunction. As a result, symmetrical encephalopathy (termed *cerebral malaria*), acute tubular necrosis, and adult respiratory distress syndrome can occur in the setting of *P. falciparum* infection. The clinical and laboratory features of severe falciparum malaria are: depressed consciousness, convulsions, respiratory distress, shock, spontaneous bleeding, jaundice, acute renal failure, hematuria, parasite density greater than 2%, schizonts in the peripheral blood smear, acidosis, hypoglycemia, prolonged clotting time, thrombocytopenia, and hemoglobin lower than 7.5 g/dL.

DIAGNOSIS

For diagnosis, it is important that several sequential blood smears (finger stick or capillary blood) be examined for the presence of parasitized erythrocytes. The initial smear may be negative because symptoms of malaria can occur a few days before the appearance of infected erythrocytes at detectable levels. Ideally, both thick and thin smears should be obtained and examined on multiple occasions over a 72-hour period before the diagnosis of malaria is excluded. Some newer tests that can detect parasites at low concentrations are useful when there is a high clinical suspicion of malaria, but negative smears. The reported sensitivity of these tests is greater than 90%, and the specificity is greater than 95%. The *quantitative buffy coat* detects parasite nuclei using fluorescence microscopy and acridine orange. Specific identification of species is difficult with this method. *Rapid diagnostic tests,* which are immunochromatographic tests, are based on the capture of parasite antigen from peripheral blood using monoclonal antibodies prepared against a malaria antigen target. Malaria antigens currently targeted by rapid diagnostic tests are *P. falciparum* histidine-rich proteins (HRP-2), parasite lactate dehydrogenase, and *Plasmodium* aldolase. Parasight *F* and *ICT* Malaria *pf* detect *P. falciparum* (HRP-2) and thus detect only this malarial species. The OptiMAL test detects parasite lactate dehydrogenase and can distinguish between *P. falciparum* and *P. vivax* infection. *Polymerase chain reaction* techniques have also been developed, but they are used primarily for research purposes. Serologic testing can demonstrate prior infection, but it is not useful during most acute infections. The exception is chronic *P. malariae* infection, in which serologic testing may be used as proof of infection in the appropriate clinical setting.

Thick blood smears are prepared with Giemsa stain in a manner that optimizes the chance of detecting the parasites, but such smears are unreliable for species identification. Thin blood smears are examined for the latter purpose and are prepared in the same manner as routine hematologic smears. In addition to species identification, the degree of parasitemia should be estimated because it has prognostic value in severe *P. falciparum* infections. At low levels of parasitemia, this can be done on thick smears, but at higher levels, thin smears examined at several oil immersion fields can provide an adequate estimate of percent parasitemia. During treatment, the examination and quantification of parasitemia in sequential smears are useful for monitoring the effectiveness of antiparasitic treatment and for detecting the emergence of drug resistance during treatment.

Initial evaluation of newly diagnosed cases of malaria should include: percentage parasitemia, blood cell count, platelet count, electrolytes, creatinine, urea, calcium, glucose, liver function tests, and coagulation tests. Blood cultures should be obtained because of the presence of coincidental bacterial infection (e.g., typhoid) in some patients with malaria. In patients with severe malaria or respiratory symptoms, lactate and blood gas analysis should be obtained. After the treatment of malaria or before travel, glucose-6-phosphate dehydrogenase (G6PD) levels should be determined.

ANTIMALARIAL DRUGS

Chloroquine phosphate (Aralen Phosphate) and *chloroquine sulfate (Nivaquine)** are 4-aminoquinolones that act on the erythrocytic stage of all species of *Plasmodium.* Chloroquine is the drug of choice for the treatment of susceptible strains of *P. falciparum* as well as for the treatment of infection with *P. vivax, P. ovale,* or *P. malariae.* Chloroquine does not affect liver schizonts and thus does not prevent relapse in *P. vivax* or *P. ovale* infections. Subsequent treatment with *primaquine* is recommended to avoid relapses. Primaquine should not be administered, however, to patients with G6PD deficiency. Side effects of chloroquine occur in about 25% of users and include gastrointestinal upset, visual disturbances, headache, and nonallergic pruritus. With intravenous therapy, hypotension and heart block may occur, especially if the drug is administered rapidly.

Mefloquine (Lariam) is a 4-quinolinemethanol that acts on the erythrocytic stage of all species of *Plasmodium*, but like chloroquine, it does not affect liver schizonts. It is active against all four species of malaria including most chloroquine-resistant *P. falciparum* isolates. In the United States, mefloquine is generally recommended only for prophylaxis because, in the doses required for treatment, unacceptable central nervous system effects, such as seizures and psychosis, have been reported. These central nervous system effects can be confused with cerebral malaria. It is estimated that these side effects occur in 1 in 10,000 to 1 in 20,000 travelers who use 250 mg per week for prophylaxis or in 0.5% to 1.0% of patients given 1250 mg for treatment. Using a smaller divided dose for treatment can reduce the incidence of neurotoxicity. Mefloquine dosage is not standardized for children weighing less than 15 kg.

Mefloquine is contraindicated in patients with epilepsy or psychiatric disorders. It should be avoided in patients with cardiac conduction disorders because it prolongs QTc. In theory, quinine or quinidine may exacerbate the cardiodepressant effects of mefloquine, and thus loading doses of these drugs should not be given in patients who have received mefloquine recently. It should be used in caution with patients taking β-blockers. Although teratogenic in rodents, mefloquine has been taken by women during the second and third trimester of pregnancy, and no fetal malformations have been associated with its use. It is not known whether first-trimester exposure is harmful, and in general this drug should not be taken during pregnancy. Because of its long half-life, pregnancy should probably be avoided for at least 3 months after a woman takes mefloquine.

Cinchona alkaloids such as *quinine sulfate* (oral) or *quinidine gluconate* (intravenous) are very effective antimalarial agents. Both quinine and quinidine are effective against the erythrocytic stages of all four malarial species and are also active against the gametocytes of *P. vivax, P. ovale,* and *P. malariae.* Quinine sulfate (650 mg three times a day for 3 or 7 days), combined with pyrimethamine-sulfamdoxine, tetracycline, or clindamycin (Cleocin), is the first-line treatment (oral) of chloroquine-resistant malaria and should be used as empirical treatment in all patients in whom the malaria species is unknown. For severe cases, intravenous quinidine gluconate should be used, combined with tetracycline or clindamycin.

Quinine sulfate has a bitter taste and is associated with syndrome of cinchonism: headache, nausea, abdominal pain, tinnitus, and transient loss of hearing. This syndrome is associated with high serum levels of quinine or quinidine. These symptoms usually begin 48 hours after starting treatment and subside quickly

*Not available in the United States.

when the treatment is stopped. Both quinine and quinidine can cause insulin release from the pancreas and have been associated with hypoglycemia. For this reason, intravenous glucose is indicated in pregnant women undergoing therapy with these drugs. Potential cardiovascular effects include QRS widening and arrhythmias. Parental quinidine administration should be done with electrocardiographic monitoring.

Primaquine phosphate is an 8-aminoquinoline active against tissue schizonts and gametocytes that is used to prevent relapses from infection with *P. vivax* or *P. ovale*. Because primaquine can cause hemolysis in patients who are G6PD deficient, it should not be given to patients with this deficiency. Primaquine is contraindicated during pregnancy, because the G6PD status of the fetus cannot be ascertained.

Pyrimethamine-sulfadoxine (Fansidar) has been used for the treatment of chloroquine-resistant falciparum malaria. Because of drug resistance and the occurrence of allergic reactions to sulfadoxine, this agent is no longer used for prophylaxis. Fatalities from serious cutaneous allergy (Stevens-Johnson syndrome) occurred in 1 in 11,000 to 1 in 26,000 patients within the first 5 weeks of starting prophylactic therapy. No fatal reactions have been reported in patients with no history of sulfa allergy who were taking pyrimethamine-sulfadoxine (three tablets once) for the empirical treatment of chloroquine-resistant falciparum malaria. Patients with G6PD deficiency can develop hemolysis when they take this drug.

Tetracyclines are active against erythrocytic schizonts of all four species of malaria including chloroquine-resistant falciparum malaria. These drugs possess some activity against extraerythrocytic schizonts, but they are not active enough to be used to prevent relapses. Doxycycline (Vibramycin) is used for prophylaxis in patients unable to take mefloquine or in areas of mefloquine resistance (Vietnam and the Thai-Kampuchean border). Side effects of importance include gastrointestinal intolerance, photosensitivity reactions (SPF-15 or higher sunscreen should be used in patients taking this drug), and vaginal candidiasis (women can take fluconazole [Diflucan], 150 mg once, as empirical treatment for this complication).

Macrolides and *lincomycins* are active against erythrocytic schizonts of all four species of malaria. Clindamycin (Cleocin)* is used in combination with quinine for the treatment of chloroquine-resistant falciparum malaria. *Clostridium difficile* enterocolitis is the main side effect and can be managed with metronidazole treatment. Azithromycin (Zithromax)* has been effective for prophylaxis in a small trial.

Proguanil-atovaquone (Malarone) is active against both erythrocytic and extraerythrocytic schizonts. Atovaquone inhibits mitochondrial electron transport. It is highly effective against *P. falciparum*, but has a high recrudescent rate with the development of resistance when it is used as monotherapy. In combination with proguanil, it is highly effective and well tolerated. Side effects include: abdominal pain, diarrhea, nausea, and coughing. Malarone is a fixed-dose combination of 250 mg atovaquone and 100 mg of proguanil hydrochloride per adult tablet and 62.5 mg of atovaquone and 25 mg of proguanil hydrochloride per pediatric tablet.

Artemisinin, derived from the Chinese medicinal plant qinghao (*Artemisia annua*), is a rapidly acting antimalarial that has been established as an effective treatment in multidrug-resistant falciparum malaria found on the Thai-Kampuchean and Thai-Myanmar borders. The compound can be given parenterally, orally, or by suppository and is cidal for the asexual blood stages of *P. falciparum*. Currently, these drugs (artesunate and artemether) are not available in the United States.

Halofantrine (Halfan), 8 mg/kg (maximum dose is 500 mg) orally at 0, 6, and 12 hours and a course repeated in 7 days, is a phenthrenemethanol derivative of an amine alcohol that requires fat for optimal absorption. Recrudescence is a reported problem after single-dose treatment. Side effects have limited the use of this compound and include: cough, pruritus, hemolytic anemia, QTc prolongation, and PR prolongation. Torsades de pointes have been described with administration of this drug, and cardiotoxicity has limited this drug's usefulness.

Fluoroquinolones have antimalarial activity in vitro, but they have not proven effective in clinical trials.

TREATMENT

During the initial evaluation of a patient with suspected malaria, certain factors must be considered. These include the species of malaria, the parasite density, the geographic area of potential acquisition of infection, coexisting medical complications, and the ability of the patient to take oral medication. The geographic area of acquisition must be considered in evaluating the possibility of chloroquine-resistant *P. falciparum* or chloroquine-resistant *P. vivax* infection. Patients with *P. falciparum* infection, mixed infections with *P. falciparum* and other species, or infections in which the species cannot immediately be identified should be hospitalized.

Patients with malaria caused by organisms other than *P. falciparum* should receive a course of chloroquine phosphate by mouth (Table 1). When this treatment is completed, primaquine phosphate should always be administered to patients with *P. vivax* or *P. ovale* infections after screening for G6PD-related infection. Patients who acquired *P. falciparum* in Central America west of the Panama Canal, in Mexico, or in most of the Middle East can be treated with chloroquine unless they are unable to take medications by mouth or have complications that require parenteral therapy. *P. falciparum* from all other regions of the world should be considered resistant to chloroquine. For patients with chloroquine-resistant malaria, quinine is the drug of choice. Patients who can tolerate oral treatment should be given quinine sulfate for 3 days (or 7 days if the infection was acquired in Southeast Asia or Oceania, where reduced

*Not available in the United States.

TABLE 1. **Drug Treatment of Malaria**

Drug	Adult Dosage	Pediatric Dosage
All *Plasmodium* Species Except Chloroquine-Resistant *P. Falciparum* and Choroquine-Resistant *P. Vivax*		
Oral		
Chloroquine phosphate (Aralen)	600 mg base (1 g salt), then 300 mg base (500 mg salt) at 6, 24, and 48 h	10 mg base/kg then 5 mg base/kg at 6, 24, and 48 h
Parenteral		
Quinidine gluconate	10 mg/kg loading dose (max 600 mg) over 1 h, followed by continuous infusion of 0.02 mg/kg/min × 3 d (or until taking PO)	Same as adult dose
Chloroquine-Resistant *P. falciparum*		
Oral		
Quinine sulfate	650 mg tid × 3 d (7 d if acquired in Southeast Asia or Oceania)	25 mg/kg/d in three doses × 3 d (7 d if acquired in Southeast Asia or Oceania)
Plus Tetracycline	250 mg qid × 7 d (doxycycline 100 mg bid)	For children ≥7 y; 4 mg/kg/d qid × 7 d
or Clindamycin* (Cleocin)	450 mg qid (PO) × 7 d	20-40 mg/kg/d in three doses × 7 d
or Pyrimethamine-sulfadoxine (Fansidar)	Three tablets once on last day of quinine	<1 y old: 1/4 tablet[†] 1-3 y: 1/2 table 4-8 y: one tablet 9-14 y: two tablets >14 y: three tablets on last day of quinine
Alternatives		
Mefloquine (Larium)	15 mg base/kg followed by 10 mg/kg in 12 h	Same as adult dose
Atovaquone/Proguanil (Malarone)	4 tablets/d × 3 d	11-20 kg: one tablet/d 21-30 kg: two tablets/d 31-40 kg: three tablets/d >40 kg: four tablets/d × 3 d
Halofantrine (Halfan)	8 mg/kg q6h × 3 doses repeat in 1 wk (maximum adult dose 500 mg)	Same as adult dose
Parenteral		
Quinidine gluconate plus	10 mg/kg loading dose (max 600 mg) over 1 h, followed by continuous infusion of 0.02 mg/kg/min × 3 days (or until taking PO)	Same as adult dose
Clindamycin*	900 mg tid × 7 d	10 mg/kg first dose followed by 5 mg/kg tid × 7 d
Exchange transfusion in patients with high parasitemia		
Multidrug-Resistant *P. falciparum* With Failure of Standard Treatment		
Artemether*[‡] plus	4 mg/kg/d × 3-7 d	
Doxycycline	100 mg bid × 7 d	
Artemether[‡] plus	4 mg/kg/d × 3 d	
Atovaquone/Proguanil (Malarone)	Two adult tablets bid × 3 d	11-20 kg: one adult tablet/d × 3 d 21-30 kg: two adult tablets/d × 3 d 31-40 kg: three adult tablets/d × 3 d >40 kg: two adult tablets bid × 3 d
Artemether[‡] plus	4 mg/kg/d × 3 d	
Mefloquine (Lariam)	750 mg followed by 500 mg	15 mg/kg followed 8-12 h later by 10 mg/kg
Chloroquine-Resistant *P. vivax*		
Quinine sulfate plus	650 mg q8h × 3-7 d	25 mg/kg/d in three doses × 3-7 d
Doxycycline	100 mg bid × 7 d	For children 2 mg/kg/d in three doses × 3-7 d
Alternatives		
Mefloquine	750 mg followed by 500 mg 12 h later	15 mg/kg followed 8-12 h later by 10 mg/kg
Halofantrine	500 mg q6h × three doses	8 mg/kg q6h × three doses
Chloroquine plus	25 mg base/kg in three doses over 48 h	
Primaquine	2.5 mg base/kg in three doses over 48 h	
Prevention of Relapses in *P. vivax* or *P. ovale* Infection		
Primaquine phosphate	15 mg base (26.3 mg salt)/d × 14 d	0.3 mg base/kg/d × 14 d

*Not FDA approved for this indication.
[†]Do not give to infants <2 months old.
[‡]Not available in the United States.

sensitivity to quinine has been demonstrated). This regimen should be supplemented with tetracycline, clindamycin, or pyrimethamine-sulfadoxine to avoid recrudescence.

Patients with falciparum malaria who are unable to take oral medications because of depressed sensorium, vomiting, or other reasons, or those in whom more than 3% of erythrocytes are parasitized, or who have organ dysfunction resulting from infection (renal failure, cerebral malaria, adult respiratory distress syndrome) should be treated with parenteral quinidine gluconate (10 mg/kg loading dose to a maximum dose of 600 mg, followed by 0.02 mg/kg/minute for 3 days). Quinidine should be administered in 5% glucose while one monitors QTc, vital signs, and the electrocardiogram. This treatment should be accompanied by tetracycline or clindamycin. When stable, the patient can be switched to oral quinine to finish the course of treatment (as described earlier).

Adjuncts to antimicrobial therapy are often needed in cases of complicated falciparum malaria. Careful monitoring of blood glucose is needed because of the common complication of hypoglycemia. This complication is very common in pregnant women and children with malaria and in all patients with severe malaria. Severe anemia requires transfusion with packed erythrocytes. In nonimmune patients with falciparum malaria, the mortality rises to more than 60% with parasitemia greater than 10%. Exchange transfusion can be used to remove infected erythrocytes in cases of hyperparasitemia. Renal failure is associated with severe malaria and is usually secondary to hydration status. Peritoneal dialysis can be lifesaving for patients with acute renal failure. Severe malaria can be complicated by noncardiogenic pulmonary edema (adult respiratory distress syndrome), and this complication is associated with a poor prognosis.

Cerebral malaria is a life-threatening complication of *P. falciparum* infection. Coma or impairment in mental status during malaria infection needs to be distinguished from other causes of neurologic symptoms such as hyperpyrexia, hypoglycemia, and concurrent infection. Seizures are common in the early stages, followed by coma or a decreased level of consciousness often associated with hyperpyrexia. Neck rigidity and photophobia do not occur, but patients can develop neck retraction, opisthotonos, gaze disorders, and posturing. Corticosteroids are not indicated, because they are associated with increased mortality in this setting. Antipyretics, antiemetics, and anticonvulsants can all be used.

Malaria in pregnancy can compromise fetal development and can induce premature labor or spontaneous abortion. Chloroquine is safe for the fetus. Despite concerns about an oxytocic effect, quinine and quinidine have been used successfully and safely in malaria during pregnancy. The risks from malaria to the mother and child outweigh any concerns about the use of these drugs in this setting. There is a theoretical risk of hyperbilirubinemia and subsequent kernicterus with sulfonamide use late in pregnancy. Tetracycline is contraindicated during pregnancy. For this reason, quinine and clindamycin are used to treat malaria during pregnancy. Because primaquine is also contraindicated during pregnancy, patients with *P. vivax* and *P. ovale* disease should be treated with chloroquine alone and should be monitored for relapse, which should be treated. Once delivery has occurred, primaquine should be given to the mother. Congenital transmission has been reported, so all babies born to mothers with active malaria should be closely followed, and diagnostic testing should be performed.

PREVENTION

The combination of personal protection measures and prophylaxis (Table 2) can be highly effective in preventing malaria, but no chemoprophylactic regimen guarantees protection against the disease. Because the *Anopheles* mosquito bites from dusk to dawn, during this time, people should wear clothing that minimizes the amount of exposed skin and should remain in well-screened areas. Those in high-exposure areas should sleep in screened rooms and should use permethrin-impregnated bed nets. Pyrethrium insect

TABLE 2. **Malaria Prophylaxis Regimens**

Drug	Adult Dosage	Pediatric Dosage
Chloroquine-Resistant Areas		
Mefloquine (Lariam)	250 mg once/wk starting 1 wk before departure and for 4 wk after leaving endemic area	15-19 kg: 1/4 tablet 20-30 kg: 1/2 tablet 31-45 kg: 3/4 tablet >45 kg: one tablet
Doxycycline	100 mg/d starting 1 d before departure and for 4 wk on leaving endemic area	If >7 y old: 2 mg/kg/d (maximum dose 100 mg/d)
Atovaquone-proguanil (Malarone)	1 adult tablet daily starting 1 d before departure and for 7 d after leaving endemic area	11-20 kg: one pediatric tablet 21-30 kg: two pediatric tablets 31-40 kg: three pediatric tablets >40 kg: one adult tablet
Chloroquine-Sensitive Areas		
Chloroquine phosphate	300 mg base (500 mg salt) starting 1 wk before departure and for 4 wk on leaving endemic area	5 mg base/kg (8.3 mg salt/kg)
For Terminal Prophylaxis (Required With All Prophylaxis Except Atovaquone-Proguanil)		
Primaquine phosphate	15 mg base/d (26.3 mg salt/d) × 14 d	0.3 mg base/kg/d (0.5 mg salt/kg/d) × 14 d

sprays are also useful. Insect repellent containing N,N-diethyl-*m*-toluamide (DEET) is effective. Exposure to high concentrations for prolonged periods may be neurotoxic; this has been of particular concern for young children. DEET-related seizures have been reported in very young children using highly concentrated DEET; for this reason, no more than 35% DEET is recommended for skin application in children.

With the exception of the few areas where chloroquine-resistant malaria has not been described, travelers should take mefloquine or atovaquone-proguanil for prophylaxis. Doxycycline is an alternative for patients who cannot take either of these drugs. Chloroquine phosphate taken once weekly is appropriate for travel to Central America west of the Panama Canal, to Mexico, to Haiti, and to most of the Middle East (chloroquine resistance has been reported in Yemen, Oman, Saudi Arabia, and Iran). Travelers to areas of multidrug-resistant malaria on the Thai-Myanmar border, the Thai-Kampuchean border, and parts of Vietnam should take doxycycline.

Pregnant women should be discouraged from traveling to malarious areas. Mefloquine and doxycycline are both contraindicated in pregnancy. If travel is necessary, atovaquone-proguanil should be used.

Prophylactic drugs should be started before departure to ensure optimal blood levels and tolerance. Mefloquine and doxycycline do not prevent the exoerythrocytic life cycle and thus need to be continued for 4 weeks after leaving an endemic region. Atovaquone-proguanil is effective for the exoerythrocytic life cycle and thus needs to be continued for only 1 week after leaving an endemic region. All patients should be tested for G6PD before departure. After prolonged exposure in endemic regions, all patients taking either mefloquine or doxycycline should be given primaquine phosphate, 15 mg base (26.3 mg salt) daily for 14 days on leaving an endemic region. Regardless of the prophylaxis taken, travelers should be advised that malaria could be responsible for unexplained febrile illness occurring within a year of the trip. There is currently no commercial vaccine for malaria prevention.

Drug resistance is increasing in *P. falciparum*, and has spread to *P. vivax*. In addition, there is resistance among the anophelines to insecticide. For these reasons, malaria is recognized as a reemerging disease. Physicians should be familiar with diagnosis, management, and potential complications of malaria because it is likely that the number of cases of imported malaria seen annually will rise.

BACTERIAL MENINGITIS

method of
JAY H. TUREEN, M.D.
University of California San Francisco
San Francisco, California

Bacterial meningitis is an acute infection of the leptomeninges and subarachnoid space caused by a variety of pyogenic bacteria. It is a very serious disorder with a high incidence of death and neurologic sequelae. Bacterial meningitis is a medical emergency with urgent need for rapid diagnosis and institution of appropriate empiric antibiotic therapy and supportive measures.

Etiology of bacterial meningitis is influenced by several factors: age of the patient, underlying illness, and any potential communication between the external environment and the central nervous system. The pathogenesis of meningitis occurs by three possible mechanisms: hematogenous seeding of the choroid plexus during bacteremia; local extension from an infected contiguous site (paranasal sinus, cranial bone); and acquired breach of normal anatomic barriers or congenital defects (basilar skull fracture, neurosurgical procedures, congenital dermal sinuses communicating with the subarachnoid space). Hematogenous meningitis is by far the most common cause.

Age is the primary determinant of etiology in hematogenous meningitis. The period of greatest incidence of disease is the neonatal period, where meningitis occurs in approximately 1 in 300 infants. The principal pathogens are *Streptococcus agalactiae* (Group B streptococcus), gram-negative enteric organisms, principally K-1–positive strains of *Escherichia coli, Klebsiella pneumoniae*, and other Enterobacteriaceae, and *Listeria monocytogenes*. Meningitis occurs next most commonly in infants and toddlers, although the introduction of conjugate vaccines for *Haemophilus influenzae,* type b, has reduced the incidence dramatically. Currently, *Streptococcus pneumoniae* and *Neisseria meningitidis* are the most common pathogens from childhood through adulthood in normal hosts. In the elderly or in hosts with impaired immunity, there has been an increase in reports of meningitis due to Group B streptococcus, *Listeria,* and *Haemophilus influenzae*. These epidemiologic trends and changes in antimicrobial sensitivity must be considered when selecting empiric antibiotic therapy. Meningitis occurring as a postoperative complication is frequently caused by skin flora such as staphylococcal species and gram-negative enteric organisms, whereas basilar skull fracture involving the paranasal sinuses typically involves respiratory organisms such as *S. pneumoniae* or *Haemophilus* species.

CLINICAL PRESENTATION

Signs and symptoms of meningitis are age-dependent. The classic clinical triad of meningitis includes fever, stiff neck, and headache, often with symptoms of antecedent upper respiratory infection. However, in children younger than 2 years of age, meningeal signs are not reliably present, but abnormal thermoregulation (fever or hypothermia) and alteration in level of consciousness occur >90% of the time. Elderly patients may present with confusion, lethargy, or disorientation.

Meningitis may have a subacute presentation over a few days, with fever, malaise, nausea, vomiting, and other nonspecific signs and symptoms that then progress to more classic symptoms. Alternatively, meningitis can have a fulminant presentation, with a nonlocalized high fever and onset of altered consciousness that occurs over a few hours. Physical findings specific to meningitis are those of meningeal irritation. Stiff neck is diagnosed when the patient resists or reports pain on neck flexion, sometimes occurring only with the last 15 degrees of flexion. Brudzinski's sign is elicited with the patient in the supine position and is present when there is involuntary flexion at the hip when the neck is flexed; Kernig's sign is performed with the patient supine and the knee flexed at 90 degrees. Straightening of the leg causes stretching of nerves and is positive when patients report pain in the lower back on this maneuver. The presence of any of these signs is evidence of meningeal irritation; not all are necessarily present simultaneously. These signs are not reliably present in neonates and toddlers with meningitis; however, opisthotonic posturing may be noted. Fullness or bulging of the anterior fontanelle may be detected in infants and is evidence of intracranial hypertension.

Systemic signs may also be present in meningitis. Meningococcal meningitis is often accompanied by a rash, which can be erythematous and maculopapular, petechial, or purpuric. Abnormalities of vital signs are also common, though nonspecific. Tachycardia out of proportion to fever is frequently evidence of a serious infection. Blood pressure abnormalities are frequent: elevation may be evidence of intracranial hypertension or anxiety and shock may accompany the sepsis syndrome that can exist concurrently with meningitis.

Seizures occur in approximately 25% of patients with meningitis. They may be generalized or focal, and seizures that are difficult to control with anticonvulsants have poor prognostic implications. Focal seizures may be caused by vasculitis or stroke. Intracranial hypertension is almost universal in meningitis and may result in global cerebral ischemia or tentorial herniation. In spite of the frequency of intracranial hypertension, papilledema is a rare finding in bacterial meningitis, perhaps because of the rapidity with which intracranial hypertension occurs in this disease.

DIAGNOSIS

Bacterial meningitis is diagnosed by lumbar puncture with cerebrospinal fluid (CSF) examination and culture. Blood cultures should also be obtained and are positive in 50%–80% of cases. If the patient has received antibiotic therapy in advance of the spinal tap, CSF can be tested with latex particle agglutination to look specifically for the presence of bacterial antigens for *S. pneumoniae, N. meningitidis, H. influenzae,* and Group B streptococcus.

CSF should be sent stat for cell count and differential, protein and glucose measurement, and Gram stain and culture. Concomitant with the spinal tap, blood should be sent for serum glucose measurement and blood culture.

Opening pressure should be measured by manometer with the patient in the lateral recumbent position after free flow of CSF is established. Normal range of opening pressure varies with age: normal upper limit for newborns is 60 mm H_2O, for toddlers 80 mm, for school-age 90 mm, and for adolescents and adults 180 mm.

Typical CSF findings in bacterial meningitis are polymorphonuclear pleocytosis with CSF white blood cell (WBC) count ranging from several hundred to several thousand. In the neonatal period, up to 35 WBC/mm^3 can be present; however, no more than 60% should be polymorphonuclear cells with the remainder mononuclear cells and lymphocytes. Beyond the neonatal period, 6 WBC/mm^3 is the upper limit of normal with no polymorphonuclear cells.

CSF glucose concentration is depressed in bacterial meningitis. Normal CSF glucose concentration is 50–80 mg/dL and concentration less than 40 mg/dL is common in bacterial meningitis. The CSF/serum glucose ratio also is decreased in meningitis and is usually less than 0.5. Measurement of serum glucose and calculation of the CSF/serum glucose ratio is important in proper interpretation of the CSF glucose concentration. Hyperglycemia, whether the result of stress or diabetes may increase CSF glucose sufficient that it is in the normal range, yet the CSF/serum glucose ratio will still be depressed in the setting of bacterial meningitis. The mechanism of hypoglycorrhachia is still incompletely understood. Increased consumption of glucose by bacteria in the subarachnoid space and WBC utilization were proposed in the past; however, these explanations have been largely refuted by more recent work in animal models. Increased utilization of glucose by the brain through anaerobic metabolism and impaired transport of glucose across the blood-brain-CSF barrier are now considered to be more likely explanations.

CSF protein concentration in bacterial meningitis is increased, with values ranging from 50 to 500 mg/dL. Increased CSF protein occurs because of disruption of the blood-brain barrier. CSF lactate is increased in bacterial meningitis and is typically >3.0 mg/dL; however, is not routinely done in all labs. If available, it may be a useful test for differentiating bacterial meningitis from other causes of central nervous system (CNS) disease.

Gram stain is positive in approximately 90% of cases of bacterial meningitis. Interpretation of the Gram stain should be by a trained microbiologist because there are pitfalls in interpretation. *L. monocytogenes* are small, gram-positive rods and are often difficult to identify as organisms. Overdecolorized pneumococci often appear to be gram-negative diplococci and can be mistaken for meningococci, potentially leading to inappropriate narrowing of empiric antibiotic choice. In general, initial empiric antibiotic selection should not be narrowed until definitive identification of the causative organism and susceptibility data are reported by the laboratory.

Other diagnostic tests include latex particle agglutination (LPA), which detects bacterial antigen. Specific tests are available for *S. pneumoniae, N. meningitidis, H. influenzae,* K-1 positive *E. coli* and Group B streptococcus. These tests are highly specific and may be valuable in the setting of partially treated meningitis that may have negative Gram stain and culture. For *S. pneumoniae,* Group B streptococcus, and *H. influenzae,* the LPA test is >90% sensitive and specific; for *N. meningitidis* meningitis the LPA is highly specific but has sensitivity of only 50%. Similarly, the limulus lysate amoebacyte assay detects gram-negative bacterial endotoxin and is both sensitive and specific; however, it is not routinely available in all hospital labs.

DIFFERENTIAL DIAGNOSIS

Differential diagnosis of bacterial meningitis is broad when symptoms are nonspecific and clear signs are not present. When present, the combination of fever, meningeal signs, altered consciousness, and headache will suggest an infectious CNS process. The most common alternative diagnoses include viral meningitis, viral encephalitis, meningitis resulting from fungi or *Mycobacterium tuberculosis,* or space-occupying lesions such as brain abscess, epidural abscess, or subdural empyema.

Viral meningitis often presents with fever, stiff neck, and headache. Viral meningitis is usually distinguished from bacterial meningitis based on normal level of consciousness, although infants and children may show extreme irritability. CSF exam is critical in differentiating the two. In viral meningitis, pleocytosis is generally moderate, typically with a few hundred WBCs. In addition, protein is only moderately elevated and CSF glucose and the CSF/serum glucose ratio is normal. Exceptions to this are rare cases of enteroviral meningitis, typically caused by ECHO virus 11 and 3 and lymphocytic choriomeningitis virus meningitis, where CSF pleocytosis can be >1000 cells/mm^3. Early in viral meningitis, polymorphonuclear cells in CSF can predominate; however, lumbar puncture repeated 6–8 hours after initial lumbar puncture will show a conversion to mononuclear and lymphocytic cells. This diagnostic strategy can be used in the emergency department as a tool to differentiate aseptic from bacterial meningitis. Specific diagnosis may be made by viral culture or by RT-PCR for enteroviral RNA.

Viral encephalitis can be caused by *Herpes simplex* virus (HSV) and by arthropod-borne (ARBO) viruses. In the United States, St. Louis encephalitis and La Cross virus encephalitis are the most common causes; Eastern Equine and Western Equine virus encephalitis occur less commonly. Patients with a history of recent travel to Asia may present with Japanese B virus encephalitis.

Patients with viral encephalitis present with a prodromal, influenza-like illness with fever, malaise, and myalgia. This is followed by CNS symptoms of confusion, decreased level of consciousness, abnormal mentation, and seizures. CSF exam shows pleocytosis of several hundred cells with a mononuclear predominance. Protein is mildly elevated and glucose is normal. Diagnosis is made by PCR, viral culture, typically in public health department laboratories or by serologic testing demonstrating rise in specific antibody titer. HSV encephalitis can be suspected based on several characteristic features: the CSF typically has several hundred to thousands of red blood cells; there is a characteristic electroencephalogram (EEG) pattern and neuroimaging typically shows temporal lobe involvement. PCR testing is available for HSV-1 and HSV-2 and is both highly sensitive and specific.

Fungal and mycobacterial meningitis generally have a more prolonged prodromal phase than bacterial meningitis, with evolution over several days to a few weeks. Patients present with altered level of consciousness, headache, and stiff neck. CSF exam shows moderate mononuclear pleocytosis in the range of 100–500 WBC/mm^3. CSF pressure is usually elevated to the range seen in bacterial meningitis and CSF glucose may be low and protein elevated as seen in bacterial meningitis. Features differentiating the diseases can be epidemiologic of host risk factors, particularly the association of meningitis resulting from *Cryptococcus neoformans* in patients with HIV infection or other cause of immune suppression, meningitis resulting from *Coccidiodes imitis* with residence or travel to the Southwest or Central Valley of California, and tuberculous meningitis in patients known to be tuberculin positive of from tuberculosis (TB)-endemic areas. Clinical features that differentiate the diseases are the frequent occurrence of papilledema in fungal and mycobacterial meningitis and cranial nerve palsies in TB meningitis. Diagnosis is confirmed by specific KOH and acid-fast stains of CSF and culture.

Space-occupying lesions of the CNS should be considered in the differential diagnosis because they may present with headache and fever; however, there are often important differentiating features. These conditions usually present with focal features, either a focal seizure or with specific focal neurologic signs. When a mass lesion is suspected, lumbar puncture should be avoided until cranial computed tomography (CT) or magnetic resonance imaging scanning excludes a mass lesion with midline shift or evidence of severe intracranial hypertension.

Other conditions which share features with bacterial meningitis include noninfectious diseases as well. Subarachnoid hemorrhage is heralded by acute headache, decreased level of consciousness, and stiff neck. Fever is usually absent. Diagnosis is usually made by CT scanning demonstrating blood in the basal cisterns. If CT scanning is negative, lumbar puncture is performed and frankly bloody or microscopically detected red blood cells may be detected in CSF. Infants who have accidental or nonaccidental head trauma may develop subdural effusions that can cause low-grade fever, intracranial hypertension, decreased level of responsiveness and bulging fontanelle. Diagnosis is made based on suspicion of non-accidental trauma from other physical signs and cranial CT.

TREATMENT

Empiric Therapy

Treatment of bacterial meningitis includes selection of age- and host-appropriate antimicrobials, supportive care, and use of adjunctive therapy. Antibiotics are chosen empirically for the treatment of bacterial meningitis based on age of the patient, specific risk factors, and patterns of bacterial resistance. Empiric therapy is initiated when the diagnosis is strongly suspected based on history and physical exam findings and lumbar puncture findings that support the diagnosis, such as cloudy CSF and elevated CSF pressure. In this setting, it is not necessary to await laboratory confirmation of the diagnosis before therapy is initiated.

Empiric antibiotic therapy is principally determined based on age-specific pathogens, known bacterial resistance patterns in a given area, and specific risk factors for the patient. Organisms of neonatal meningitis include Group B streptococcus, gram-negative enteric bacteria, and *L. monocytogenes*. Accordingly, for the neonate, treatment with ampicillin (50 mg/kg/dose q 6-12 h) and gentamicin 2.5 mg/kg/dose q 8–12 h or cefotaxime (Claforan) 50 mg/kg/dose q 6-12 h based on gestational age and postnatal age, is used.

For infants beyond the neonatal period and all other patients, the major pathogens are *S. pneumoniae* and *N. meningitidis*. Because of the emergence of penicillin- and cephalosporin-resistant pneumococci, empiric regimens for treatment of meningitis should include vancomycin (Vancocin), until identification and sensitivity data are known. Suggested treatment is to initiate therapy with a third-generation cephalosporin, either ceftraixone (Rocephin) (pediatric dose 100 mg/kg/day divided q 12 h; adult dose 2 gm q 12 h) or cefotaxime (Claforan) (pediatric dose 200 mg/kg/day divided q 6 h; adult dose 2 gm q 6 h) *plus* vancomycin (pediatric dose 60 mg/kg/day divided q 6 h; adult dose 500 mg q 6 h). Ampicillin should be added for patients with impaired cell-mediated immunity (AIDS, cancer chemotherapy, organ transplant with immunosuppression, congenital immune deficiency, pregnancy) to cover the possibility of infection with *L. monocytogenes*. Patients with cirrhosis or ascites from alcoholism or chronic renal disease and patients with diabetes are at increased risk of infection with gram-negative enteric bacilli and pneumococcus and should be treated with a third-generation cephalosporin and vancomycin. Patients who have recently undergone neurosurgical procedures are at risk of infection with gram-negative enteric bacteria and staphylococci and should be treated with a third-generation cephalosporin and vancomycin or nafcillin (Unipen). Patients who are neutropenic may be at increased risk of infection with *Pseudomonas aeruginosa* and should receive ceftazidime (Fortaz) as the third-generation cephalosporin.

Specific Therapy

When definitive identification of the organism and antimicrobial susceptibility test results are known, antibiotic treatment should be modified. Table 1 lists recommended drugs and doses for neonates, infants, and children, and adults with bacterial meningitis.

Pneumococcal Meningitis

Therapy of pneumococcal meningitis will be determined by susceptibility testing. In recent years, pneumococci with reduced sensitivity to penicillin and the third-generation cephalosporins have increased in frequency, although they remain sensitive to vancomycin. Pneumococci are considered penicillin sensitive if the

TABLE 1. **Empiric Therapy of Bacterial Meningitis**

Age	Antibiotic	Total daily dose (frequency)
<1 wk	Ampicillin plus	100 mg/kg/d (q 12 h)
	Gentamicin or	5 mg/kg/d (q 12 h)
	Cefotaxime (Claforan)	100 mg/kg/d (q 12 h)
1–4 wk	Ampicillin plus	200 mg/kg/d (q 6 h)
	Gentamicin or	7.5 mg/kg/d (q 8 h)
	Cefotaxime	200 mg/kg/d (q 6 h)
1–3 mo	Ampicillin plus	300 mg/kg/d (q 6 h)
	Cefotaxime or	200 mg/kg/d (q 6 h)
	Ceftriaxone (Rocephin) plus	100 mg/kg/d (q 12 h)
	Vancomycin (Vancocin)	60 mg/kg/d (q 6 h)
3 mo–18 yr*	Cefotaxime or	200 mg/kg/d (q 6 h)
	Ceftriaxone plus	100 mg/kg/d (q 12 h)
	Vancomycin	60 mg/kg/d (q 6 h)
>18 yr	Cefotaxime or	8 gm/d (q 6 h)
	Ceftriaxone plus	4 gm/d (q 12 h)
	Vancomycin	2 gm/d (q 6 h)
Immune compromised	Cefotaxime or	Dose appropriate to age
	Ceftriaxone plus	
	Vancomycin plus	
	Ampicillin	
Postneurosurgery	Cefotaxime or	Dose appropriate to age
	Ceftriaxone plus	
	Vancomycin or	
	Nafcillin (Unipen)	200 mg/kg/d (q 6 h) (children) 12 gm/d (q 6 h) (adult)

*For larger children, maximal adult dose should be used.

MIC is <0.1 mcg/mL, moderately resistant if the MIC is 0.1–1.0 mcg/mL, and resistant if the MIC is >1.0 mcg/mL. For cefotaxime and ceftriaxone, organisms are considered sensitive if the MIC <0.5 mcg/mL, moderately resistant if MIC is 0.5–2.0 mcg/mL, and resistant if MIC is >2.0 mcg/mL. Pneumococci with reduced sensitivity to both penicillin and cephalosporins should be treated with vancomycin. Meropenem (Merrem) a newer carbapenem antibiotic has good in vitro activity against resistant pneumococci and may be a suitable alternative; however, clinical experience is limited. Patients with pneumococcal meningitis should be treated for 10–14 days.

Meningococcal Meningitis

Treatment of meningococcal meningitis should be with penicillin or ampicillin. Antimicrobial sensitivity testing should be performed, because meningococci with reduced sensitivity to penicillin have been reported in Spain, the United Kingdom, and South Africa. These isolates remain susceptible to third-generation cephalosporins. Antibiotic prophylaxis should be given to the index case (unless treated with ceftriaxone) and to close contacts and health care providers who have had mucous membrane contact with oropharyngeal secretions. Treatment for uncomplicated meningococcal meningitis should be for 7 days.

Gram-Negative Bacillary Meningitis

Treatment of gram-negative meningitis should be directed by antimicrobial sensitivity testing, usually with a third-generation cephalosporin, ampicillin or an extended-spectrum penicillin. Meningitis due to *Pseudomonas aeruginosa* should be with ceftazidime or an extended-spectrum penicillin. Treatment should be for 21 days.

Listeria Monocytogenes Meningitis

Listeria meningitis should be treated with penicillin or ampicillin plus an aminoglycoside or with trimethoprim-sulfamethoxazole (Bactrim). Treatment should be for 14–21 days.

Group B Streptococcal Meningitis

Treatment of group B streptococcal meningitis should be with penicillin or ampicillin. Treatment should be for 14–21 days.

Staphylococcal Meningitis

Meningitis resulting from staphylococcal species rarely occurs in the absence of a foreign body, usually a ventricular shunt device. Therapy must include removal of the device, usually with temporary external ventricular drainage, and treatment with an antistaphylococcal antibiotic, either intravenous nafcillin or vancomycin, depending on sensitivity testing. Rarely, staphylococcal meningitis occurs in premature infants, patients with cutaneous fistulas to the subarachnoid space, patients with immune deficiencies, and patients with occult hamartomas in the CNS.

Adjunctive Therapy

Bacterial meningitis has a high incidence of death and neurologic sequelae even with rapid diagnosis and institution of appropriate therapy. This is thought to be due to release of proinflammatory cytokines that is potentiated by lysis of bacteria in the subarachnoid

TABLE 2. **Antimicrobial Therapy for Specific Pathogens in Bacterial Meningitis**

Organism	Antibiotic	Total Daily Dose (Frequency)	Duration
S. pneumoniae			10–14 days
Penicillin sensitive	Penicillin G or	200,000 U/kg/d (q 4 h) (children) 24 million U/d (q 4 h) (adult)	
	Ampicillin	See Table 1	
	Cefotaxime or	See Table 1	
Intermediate penicillin sensitive	Ceftriaxone	See Table 1	
Penicillin resistant	Vancomycin or 3rd generation cephalosporin if sensitive		
N. meningitidis	Penicillin G or Ampicillin	See Table 1	7 days
Enterobacteriaciae (*E. coli, Klebsiella, Enterobacter, Citrobacter*)	3rd generation cephalosporin	See Table 1	21 days
S. agalactiae	Penicillin G or Ampicillin	See above and Table 1	14–21 days
Pseudomonas aeruginosa	Ceftazidime (Fortaz)	200 mg/kg/d (q 6 h) (children) 8 gm/d (q 6 h) (adult)	21 days
Staphylococci			14 days
Methicillin-sensitive	Nafcillin	200 mg/kg/d (q 6 h) (children) 12 gm/d (q 6 h) (adult)	
Methicillin-resistant	Vancomycin	See Table 1	
Listeria monocytogenes	Penicillin or ampicillin plus gentamicin or Trimethoprim-sulfamethoxazole (Bactrim)	See Table 1 20 mg/kg/d TMP-100 mg/kg/d SMX (q 6 h) (children) 1.2 g TMP-6 g SMX/d (q 6 h) (adult)	14–21 days

space. For that reason, there has been interest in modulating the host inflammatory response, in 1988, the first randomized, controlled trial of dexamethasone* (Decadron) as adjunctive therapy in meningitis demonstrated reduction of hearing loss in children with *H. influenzae* meningitis. This was followed by additional prospective studies that confirmed reduction in hearing loss and other neurologic sequelae in children given dexamethasone concurrent with or just before antibiotics were given. In 2002, a prospective, randomized, blinded controlled trial of dexamethasone in adults with bacterial meningitis showed reduction in death and neurologic impairment in patients given dexamethasone 15–20 minutes before antibiotics were started. This was particularly notable in adults with *S. pneumoniae* meningitis when subgroup analysis was performed. Results from other trials in which dexamethasone was given up to several hours after antibiotics were started have not shown benefit. Because reduction in CNS inflammation may reduce antibiotic penetration into the subarachnoid space, there is some concern that bacteria that are highly resistant to penicillins and cephalosporins may not be effectively treated with these drugs when dexamethasone is given.

Current recommendations for adjunctive use of dexamethasone are to initiate dexamethasone (0.15 mg/kg IV q 6 h × 4 days in children; 10 mg IV q 6 h × 4 days in adults) 15–20 minutes before or concurrent with antibiotic administration. In adults, if meningitis is not due to *S. pneumoniae,* dexamethasone should be stopped. If the organism is found to be highly resistant to penicillins and cephalosporins, the patient should be carefully monitored and have repeat CSF exam to assure CSF sterilization.

SUPPORTIVE CARE

General supportive measures for patients with meningitis are critically important. Patients with decreased level of consciousness or impaired gag reflex should have stomach contents emptied and be placed on nasogastric suction. Patients should be NPO until mental status improves and gag reflex is present. Hypoxia should be treated with supplemental oxygen. Patients with hypoventilation should be intubated and mechanically ventilated, because hypercarbia leads to cerebral vasodilation and can potentiate intracranial hypertension.

Passive measures to treat intracranial hypertension include elevation of the head of the bed to 30 degrees and positioning of the patient with the head in the midline position. Active measures to treat intracranial hypertension are hyperventilation and careful use of mannitol (0.25 g/kg IV) for signs of impending cerebral herniation.

*Not available in the United States.

Shock in meningitis has been shown in a number of studies to be a poor prognostic factor. Fluid therapy should initially be directed at repairing fluid and electrolyte deficits by intravenous fluid administration. When euvolemia is established, maintenance fluids should be calculated according to ongoing urine and insensible fluid loss. Serum electrolytes should be measured. Hyponatremia may indicate SIADH (syndrome of antidiuretic hormone secretion), which is defined by the constellation of hyponatremia, decreased urine output, increased urine specific gravity, and increased urine sodium. SIADH occurs in approximately 30% of children with meningitis; if present, fluids should be restricted to insensible water loss plus urine output after deficits are replenished. If SIADH is not present, routine fluid restriction is not indicated. Inotropic agents to treat shock in patients with meningitis should be administered with extreme care and with continuous monitoring of intracranial pressure by subarachnoid bolt or intraventricular catheter. Patients with meningitis have been shown to have impaired cerebrovascular autoregulation and rapid increases in blood pressure can lead to spikes in intracranial pressure and cerebral herniation.

PREVENTION

Two strategies are available for prevention of meningitis: active immunization and antibiotic chemoprophylaxis. Immunization with conjugate vaccines for *H. influenzae* have reduced incidence of meningitis resulting from this pathogen by 90%. Similarly, immunization with heptavalent conjugate vaccine for *S. pneumoniae* has been shown to reduce bacteremic disease from that organism and may reduce the incidence of meningitis resulting from vaccine strains. This vaccine is recommended for infants; individuals with humoral immune deficiency, asplenia, chronic disease (cardiopulmonary, diabetes mellitus, hepatic, renal) or AIDS; and adults >65 years. Tetravalent meningococcal vaccine (containing antigens for MenA, C, W135, and Y) (Menomune-A/C/Y/W-135) or MenC vaccine* (Meningitis Conjugate vac) is recommended for first-year college students in dormitories. Meningococcal vaccination may also be indicated for travelers to the "meningitis belt" of sub-Saharan Africa, Saudi Arabia, and Nepal.

Antibiotic chemoprophylaxis is recommended for close contacts (family members, day care and school contacts) of the index case of invasive meningococcal disease. In children, rifampin (Rifadin) (10 mg/kg PO divided q 12 h × 2 d) or ceftriaxone (125 mg IM < 12 yr, 250 mg IM > 12 yr) is recommended. For adults, rifampin (600 mg PO divided q 12 h × 2 d) or ciprofloxacin*† (Cipro) (750 mg PO × 1) is recommended.

*Not available in the United States.
†Not FDA approved for this indication.

INFECTIOUS MONONUCLEOSIS

method of
WARREN A. ANDIMAN, M.D.
Yale University School of Medicine
New Haven, Connecticut

Infectious mononucleosis (IM) is a clinical syndrome most often caused by the Epstein-Barr virus (EBV) and, in its most classical form, comprises fever, exudative tonsillitis, diffuse lymphadenopathy, and absolute lymphocytosis with many atypical forms. Other pathogens (e.g., cytomegalovirus, *Toxoplasma gondii*, the adenoviruses) may cause atypical or less full-blown expressions of this syndrome. Our discussion will be limited to EBV-associated IM, the most commonly encountered form of the disease. Although EBV is a ubiquitous pathogen, causing infection throughout the world and in all populations studied, the occurrence of classic IM is limited to the more economically advantaged countries of the world where primary infection with EBV is delayed until adolescence and young adulthood. In such populations primary EBV infection takes the form of heterophile-positive IM and significant numbers of persons become ill during high school, college, or in the years following. When primary infection occurs in early childhood, full expression of the mononucleosis syndrome is rarely seen; infections are much more likely to be subclinical or to take the form of minor illnesses or incomplete forms of IM.

LABORATORY DIAGNOSIS

The diagnosis of EBV-associated IM is supported by three pieces of laboratory evidence: the presence of many atypical lymphocytes in the peripheral blood, the elaboration of heterophile antibodies, and the production of virus-specific antibodies of various types which rise and fall according to a well-defined pattern. In persons with the classic disease, the diagnosis is supported when one finds that 10% to 30% of the total white blood cell count is comprised of atypical lymphocytes (Downey cells); the proliferation of such cells contributes to a relative and sometimes an absolute lymphocytosis.

Heterophile antibodies (human agglutinins directed against red blood cell antigens of another species) are commonly produced in the course of IM, usually reach significant levels by the end of the first week of illness, and peak within 2 to 3 weeks. There is great variation in the height of the titer and the duration of the response, neither of which correlates with the severity of the disease. Many labs perform qualitative assays only, using a latex agglutination technique. In some patients, the heterophile response is very brief and may be missed if the serum is taken too late; in others, there may be a 3- to 4-week delay before a rise in antibody occurs. Children do not commonly produce significant amounts of heterophile antibody.

EBV-specific antibody tests (or panels of such tests) should be ordered only in those unusual instances in which the diagnosis is still unclear following review of other more traditional test results. Patients with acute EBV-associated IM will normally have both IgM and IgG antibodies to the viral capsid antigens (VCA) of EBV in their blood at the time they present with their first clinical symptoms. Antibodies to the early antigens (EA) of the virus usually appear a few weeks to a few months later, whereas the appearance of antibodies to the EB nuclear antigens (EBNA) are normally delayed for 2 to 4 or more months. Therefore, in patients with acute IM, clinicians should expect IgM and IgG antibodies to VCA to be present and antibodies to EBNA to be absent in acute blood specimens; antibodies to EA may or may not be present in such acute specimens. Different laboratories use widely varying test procedures and apply different diagnostic standards when performing these tests. Test results from commercial labs should be viewed with some degree of circumspection, especially when they fail to correlate with clinical findings and the results of complete blood counts and heterophile antibody tests. Large commercial labs usually perform enzyme-linked immunosorbent assays (ELISA), but many university and research laboratories continue to use more traditional immunofluorescence assays because, although more labor-intensive, they are believed to be more sensitive and specific.

TREATMENT/MANAGEMENT

Care of Uncomplicated Cases

The great majority of patients with IM recover uneventfully, although the period of convalescence may be lengthy (weeks to months). Patients usually require additional sleep and bed rest, and either acetaminophen or ibuprofen (Motrin) to alleviate symptoms associated with fever and malaise. Most afflicted individuals return to full activity within 4 weeks' time, but some high school or college students may need their physicians to intercede on their behalf to request reduction in workload or revision of examination schedules. No treatment is required for those patients who develop subclinical or mildly symptomatic episodes of hepatitis.

Patients with sore throat may benefit from a soft or liquid diet. For the 10% to 30% of individuals who are discovered to have group A beta-hemolytic streptococci in their throat cultures, orally administered penicillin or erythromycin should be prescribed; if the patient cannot swallow pills, an intramuscular injection of long-acting penicillin (Bicillin-LA) can be administered. Because ampicillin has a strong propensity for inducing a widespread skin rash in patients with IM, it should *not* be used to treat concurrent strep infections.

Splenomegaly

Although splenic enlargement is a frequent accompaniment of IM, splenic rupture is extremely rare, occurring in only 0.1% to 0.2% of patients with clinically apparent disease. Rupture most often occurs during the first 3 weeks following onset of symptoms; such individuals have splenic volumes 2 to 3 times their normal size. Patients with splenomegaly should be advised to avoid contact sports (e.g., football) and heavy lifting for the 2 to 4 weeks when the spleen is likely to remain enlarged. For those athletes in whom palpation of the left upper quadrant may be an inaccurate measure of continuing splenomegaly, ultrasound examination may provide guidance as to when they may safely return to full athletic schedules.

Splenic rupture is now frequently managed conservatively, with intravenous fluids, blood transfusions (if needed), bed rest, and pressure applied to the left upper quadrant. Although surgical intervention for splenic rupture is less common now than in previous years, surgeons should always be consulted in cases of suspected or actual splenic rupture and should be actively involved in comanaging the patient.

Corticosteroids

The use of steroids to treat various complications of IM remains a matter of controversy and debate. The literature on this subject provides little clear guidance, as much of it is based on anecdotal or uncontrolled studies or on more well-constructed studies in which the results have varied. One can reasonably conclude from these reports that steroids will likely reduce the fever, ablate some of the constitutional symptoms, and reduce the discomfort associated with the cervical lymphadenitis and tonsillitis. In contrast, steroids have *not* been shown to reduce lymph node swelling or splenomegaly.

Cumulative clinical experience suggests that steroids are likely to prove beneficial in reducing the degree of airway obstruction (stridor, suprasternal retractions) caused by severe tonsillar enlargement and parapharyngeal suppuration. Extreme signs of impending airway obstruction may require the intervention of an otolaryngologist and subsequent intubation or tracheotomy.

IM is sometimes complicated by antibody-mediated thrombocytopenia or hemolytic anemia; encephalitis or other neurologic complications of EB virus infection (e.g., Guillain-Barré syndrome, Bell's palsy, transverse myelitis); and myocarditis or pericarditis, among others. Severe cytopenias are rare, but may last a month or more, and in such cases a short course of steroids may help correct the hematologic abnormality. Some experts also recommend brief courses of steroids to ameliorate the cardiac and neurologic complications of IM, as well as severe constitutional symptoms, such as prolonged hectic fevers and malaise. The benefit of such treatments has not been subjected to scrupulous analysis.

The use of steroids to treat complications of IM should not be taken lightly. Concerns have been expressed regarding the possible deleterious effects of steroids on the proper evolution of the complex cell-mediated immune responses to EBV, which must be evoked so as to result in long-term immunosurveillance of the virus. In most instances, when steroids are used, a few days or a week of therapy should suffice; they should then be tapered quickly. Steroids should *never* be used in routine cases of IM nor to merely hasten return to full-time school activity or athletic pursuits.

Antivirals

Although a number of antiviral agents are active against EBV in vitro, only acyclovir (Zovirax)* has been subjected to controlled analysis as to its effects on uncomplicated IM. Some such studies have shown that acyclovir treatment results in reduced shedding of EBV in the throat; however, viral excretion resumes when the drug is withdrawn. Acyclovir has no significant effect on either the clinical symptoms or signs of the uncomplicated disease. Furthermore, there are only scant data suggesting that acyclovir may benefit patients with fulminant or progressive disease resulting from EBV (e.g., severe hepatitis, pneumonitis, granulocytopenia). Because relatively high concentrations of acyclovir are needed to inhibit replication of the virus *in vitro*, similarly high doses are employed by those clinicians who use acyclovir (Zovirax) to treat patients with severe and progressive disease (1500 mg/m²/d or 30 mg/kg/d, divided q8h, intravenously).

---

*Not FDA approved for this indication.

CHRONIC FATIGUE SYNDROME

method of
DAVID C. KLONOFF, M.D.
Mills-Peninsula Health Services
San Mateo, California

Chronic fatigue syndrome (CFS) is a real illness. Many patients with this illness can be helped. In CFS, symptoms occur out of proportion to currently identifiable pathology. To work effectively with CFS patients, health care professionals must be comfortable with making a diagnosis based solely on history without abnormal physical findings or abnormal test results. The absence of objective measures of illness severity, functional limitations, and response to therapy is a challenge for CFS caregivers.

DEFINITION

Chronic fatigue syndrome is a new name for an old disorder characterized by fatigue and multiple somatic symptoms. Over the past 100 years the symptoms, now labeled as CFS, have been known as neurasthenia, chronic brucellosis, hypoglycemia, candidiasis, and environmental illness (also known as the "20th century syndrome"). In the 1980s, because of reports linking fatigue, somatic complaints, and a positive Epstein-Barr virus (EBV) serology, the illness became known as chronic EBV syndrome or chronic mononucleosis.

The U.S. Centers for Disease Control and Prevention (CDC) devised a case definition for CFS in 1988 and modified the definition slightly in 1994. The 1994 case definition of CFS is known as the International Chronic Fatigue Syndrome Study Group (ICFSG) case definition

TABLE 1. **International Chronic Fatigue Syndrome (CFS) Study Group Case Definition of CSF**

In a patient with severe fatigue that persists or relapses for 6 months, classify as CFS if fatigue is severe and accompanied by at least 4 symptom criteria

Fatigue severity: Fatigue of new or definite onset (not lifelong) and not substantially alleviated by rest, resulting in substantial reduction in previous levels of occupational, educational, or personal activities

Symptom Criteria: Beginning at or after onset of fatigue and concurrently present after 6 months:

1. Impaired memory or concentration
2. Sore throat
3. Tender cervical or axillary lymph nodes
4. Muscle pain
5. Multijoint pain
6. New headaches
7. Unrefreshing sleep
8. Postexertional malaise

(Table 1). According to this definition, CFS is excluded when fatigue can be explained by known medical or psychologic diagnoses (Table 2). Within the report that redefined CFS, the ICFSG also coined the term "idiopathic chronic fatigue" to mean a case of severe prolonged fatigue without sufficient associated symptom criteria to qualify as CFS. Future modifications of the case definition are likely.

DEMOGRAPHICS

Fatigue is usually caused by one of three types of disorders. These disorders, along with their approximate relative frequencies, are psychiatric diseases (usually anxiety, depression, or somatoform disorders), 60%; chronic fatigue syndrome, 30%; and medical diseases, 10%. The gender breakdown for CFS patients is approximately 70% female and 30% male. The mean age of onset is 38 years. The prevalence has been measured from 2 to 400 per 100,000. CFS usually occurs sporadically, but several apparent CFS epidemics have also been reported. An unanswered question about these epidemics is whether the symptom outbreak was due to mass exposure to a triggering agent or mass hysteria.

OTHER NAMES FOR CHRONIC FATIGUE SYNDROME

A variety of poorly understood illnesses characterized by fatigue and somatic complaints are probably closely related to CFS. These illnesses appear to represent extreme forms of the same underlying disorder known as the "affective spectrum disorder." This disorder is associated with a neurochemical imbalance and dysfunction of the central nervous system. Affective spectrum disorder is characterized by a spectrum of presenting symptoms. Whichever symptom predominates determines the name of the illness. Examples of illnesses that constitute the affective spectrum disorder include CFS, fibromyalgia, premenstrual syndrome, irritable bowel syndrome, chronic hypoglycemia, and chronic muscle tension headaches.

TABLE 2. **International Chronic Fatigue Syndrome (CFS) Study Group Criteria for Exclusion from a Diagnosis of CFS**

1. A documented fatiguing medical disease
2. A previously diagnosed fatiguing medical disease that has not fully resolved
3. A prior or current major depressive disorder with psychiatric features such as bipolar disease, schizophrenia, dementia, anorexia nervosa, or bulimia nervosa
4. Substance abuse within 2 years of the onset of fatigue

Other illnesses that are probably closely related to or identical with CFS include multiple chemical sensitivities, the yeast connection, environmental illnesses, seronegative Lyme disease, silicone breast implant syndrome, and Gulf War syndrome. In these illnesses, there is often a conflict between patients who ascribe their symptoms to an organic cause (which may not be evident even after extensive investigation) and the medical establishment, which tends to affix a psychiatric diagnosis to these symptoms.

Many patients with CFS and these other illnesses have founded activist organizations to lobby for increased funding for research to demonstrate an organic cause for their illness. These patients believe that they are being unfairly stigmatized as having a psychiatric illness. A psychiatric diagnosis, compared with a medical diagnosis, may also confer lesser disability payments by insurance payers.

ETIOLOGY

The exact cause of CFS is not known. The illness is often triggered by an acute physical stress such as an infraction, trauma, surgery, or even a long vacation. EBV is one of the possible triggers; however, the final pathways of symptoms for all acute-onset cases are similar. There is no reason to obtain EBV serology tests in the work-up for CFS. These tests are not specific enough to distinguish patients with CFS from the approximately 90% of adults with serologic evidence of a prior EBV infection.

Minor perturbations of the immune system have been reported in CFS. They are mostly not severe, not consistent, and not apparently mechanistically linked to the symptoms of CFS. Abnormal hypothalamic-pituitary adrenal axis functioning, including hypocortisolemia may occur in CFS, but it is unclear whether the changes are primary or are secondary to abnormal sleep or exercise. Impaired autonomic responses to extreme tilt-table orthostasis have been reported. The acronym CFIDS (chronic fatigue syndrome and immune dysfunction syndrome) is a less accurate description of the illness and is usually not used by mainstream CFS researchers or clinicians.

Patients with CFS often report a hyperactive, "high-powered" lifestyle before developing the illness. They were often managing many projects and were disinclined to refuse taking on additional tasks. In this overcommitted, overworked state, an acute physical stress that would usually produce days or weeks of debility resulted in a prolonged state of physical decompensation. Much research has been conducted on organic changes that occur in patients after they develop CFS, but additional studies are needed on the premorbid physical and psychologic health of these patients to identify attitudes or behaviors that predispose to or perpetuate the illness.

WORK-UP FOR THE FATIGUED PATIENT

CFS is a diagnosis of exclusion. When a patient presents with fatigue, every medical and psychiatric diagnosis must be excluded before CFS is diagnosed. If CFS is incorrectly diagnosed, then the patient will not receive treatment for the actual disease. That condition might irreversibly worsen while CFS is being inappropriately treated.

The diagnostic workup of fatigue consists of four parts: (1) a history; (2) a complete physical examination; (3) laboratory tests; and (4) psychologic testing. The history should include an estimate of the percentage of premorbid energy remaining. Most CFS patients estimate <50%. They also complain of symptoms from the eight CDC or four ICSFG criteria.

The physical examination should include measurement of temperature (which is usually normal and always <101.5°F) and a search for exudative pharyngitis or palpable lymph nodes (which are usually not found). Laboratory tests in a fatigue workup need to consist of only five tests: (1) a chemistry panel, (2) a complete blood count, (3) a sedimentation rate, (4) a thyroid-stimulating hormone level, and (5) a urinalysis. No other studies are needed unless the fatigue is accompanied by significant symptoms that require testing in their own right. Serologies for EBV, human herpesvirus 6, cytomegalovirus, *Borrelia burgdorferi*, *Candida* species, and magnetic resonance imaging of the brain are examples of tests that should not be routinely performed in the workup for fatigue, but are appropriate for selected patients. Psychologic testing can consist of a simple mental status examination to exclude a thought disorder.

TREATMENT

CFS is a chronic illness. The goal is not a "cure," which would be a return to the prior level of functioning. Instead, the goal is to accommodate the illness, minimize symptoms, and maximize performance. The premorbid lifestyle was generally unhealthy and should not be the target for rehabilitation. CFS patients need to recognize which activities increase symptoms and then modify their lifestyles to minimize symptoms.

The three principles of treatment for physicians who treat CFS are to (1) be optimistic, (2) aim for gradual improvement, and (3) recognize the mind-body connection. CFS treatment is directed at both the medical and psychologic aspects of the illness. No matter what psychologic problems may have preceded the onset of CFS, a patient with CFS expresses symptoms referable to multiple organ systems and requires the same symptom relief as any patient with a recognized medical disease. Symptom relief alone, however, will provide only temporary benefit if underlying psychological problems are perpetuating the illness. Most CFS patients achieve the best results when a medical approach to relieve current symptoms is combined with a psychologic approach to prevent future symptoms. CFS treatments can be divided into two categories: nonpharmacologic (Table 3) and pharmacologic (Table 4).

TABLE 3. **Nonpharmacologic Treatment of Chronic Fatigue Syndrome**

Exercise	Support group
Relaxation methods	Individual psychotherapy
Diet	

Nonpharmacologic Treatment

Exercise is the most important treatment for CFS. Exercise has three purposes in CFS: (1) reversing muscle atrophy, (2) relieving anxiety and depression, and (3) providing a metaphor for success when fatigued patients cannot perform simple tasks. Patients with CFS are usually too fatigued to exercise. They typically end up in a negative cycle consisting of rest, muscle atrophy, decreased cardiac performance, decreased exercise capacity, pessimism, disinterest in exercise, and more rest. Daily exercise can replace that cycle with a positive cycle consisting of exercise, muscle hypertrophy, increased cardiac performance, increased exercise capacity, optimism, interest in exercise, and more exercise.

Daily aerobic exercise such as walking, bicycling, or swimming is best. The duration can be as little as 5 minutes per day. The duration should be graded or increased each week by 3 to 5 minutes up to 60 to 120 minutes daily. The patient should not exceed the prescribed amount of exercise. CFS patients tend to incorrectly estimate exercise performance. They may overdo their exercise and then develop muscle pain the next day that will limit future performance.

Relaxation methods such as biofeedback, yoga, and hypnosis can decrease CFS symptoms. If patients want to read about CFS, they should be advised that printed material from the U.S. National Institutes of Health and the CDC are factual, but many books, magazines, and Internet web sites contain material that is incorrect or dangerous. The physician should approve materials about CFS before patients read them. The amount of reading by CFS patients has actually been shown to be inversely correlated with improvement.

*Not FDA approved for this indication.

TABLE 4. **Pharmacologic Treatment of Chronic Fatigue Syndrome**

One or more agents:
Nonsteroidal anti-inflammatory drugs (NSAIDs)*
Symptomatic medications
Tricyclic antidepressants*
Selective serotonin reuptake inhibitors (SSRIs)*

*Not FDA approved for this indication.

A hypoglycemia-avoidance diet is helpful because it prevents the autonomic hyperactivity response that is similar in CFS and reactive hypoglycemia. Patients should avoid five types of foods: simple sugars, fruit juice, large meals, caffeine, and alcohol. There is evidence that evening primrose oil,* 500 mg twice daily, decreases muscle and joint pains in CFS. Salt has been claimed to cure CFS symptoms by correcting neurally mediated hypotension provoked by tilt table testing, but this controversial recommendation is unproven and should not be routinely followed.

A professionally led support group is very helpful for stress reduction. External stresses such as family, job, finances, or transportation problems affect everyone and generally exacerbate symptoms in CFS patients. Stress reduction improves CFS symptoms and requires preparation. A CFS support group can help patients to avoid certain stressful situations and to manage other stressful situations. Behavior patterns can be modified to create a healthier lifestyle. This process of identifying and modifying self-destructive behavior is known as cognitive-behavioral therapy.

Ongoing internal stresses such as conflicting goals, unmet expectations, low self-esteem, and childhood sexual abuse can perpetuate symptoms of CFS. These problems are not appropriate topics for a support group but may respond to individual psychotherapy.

CFS is not the same as depression. Many CFS patients feel demeaned by a referral to a psychiatrist because they believe they have a medical disorder that will be overlooked after they begin psychotherapy. The physician should not say, "There's nothing wrong with you," "The problem is in your head," or "You are depressed" because the patient will hear, "You are crazy" and further communication will be blocked. Individual psychotherapy can help CFS patients cope with the frustration of developing a chronic illness. Often this treatment is essential to recovery.

Pharmacologic Treatment

Nonsteroidal anti-inflammatory drugs are useful for the muscle and joint pains of CFS. Long-acting medications are preferable because CFS patients might forget to take short-acting medications that require several daily doses. Symptomatic medications that are not habit-forming can reduce pain, muscle spasm, and bowel spasm in CFS. For pain, acetaminophen does not, and tramadol (Ultram) does require a prescription. For muscle spasms, cyclobenzaprine (Flexeril) is effective. It should be taken after dinner or several hours before bedtime because of its sedating properties. Nonsedating muscle relaxers such as carisoprodol (Soma) and metaxalone (Skelaxin) can be used in the daytime. For severe occipital and posterior cervical muscle tension headaches, patients may use stretching exercises, heat, massage, relaxation, or, in selected cases, home cervical traction if pretreatment cervical spine x-rays are negative.

For bowel spasm, antispasmodics plus insoluble dietary fiber are effective. Low-dose hydrocortisone therapy to correct hypocortisolemia has been associated with some improvement in symptoms of CFS, but adrenal suppression and decreased bone mineral density preclude its practical use for CFS. Fludrocortisone (Florinef) as monotherapy for hypothesized neurally mediated hypotension in CFS has been demonstrated to be no more efficacious than placebo for improving either symptoms or orthostatic hypotension.

Tricyclic antidepressants are effective for the insomnia of CFS. The dosage used in this setting is far lower than for depression. Amitriptyline (Elavil)* is the first choice among tricyclic antidepressants because of its sedating, pain-relieving, and mood-elevating properties. Doxepin (Sinequan)* is even more sedating. Imipramine (Tofranil) and nortriptyline (Pamelor)* are each less sedating and desipramine (Norpramin)* much less sedating than amitriptyline. Dosages of these medications should begin with 5 to 10 mg 1 hour after dinner (and not at bedtime) daily with weekly dosage increases in 5 to 10 mg increments until either sleep is restored or side effects occur. The most common side effects with these medications include excessive sleep if the dose is too high, dry mouth, and postural light-headedness. To minimize or prevent nocturnal orthostatic hypotension, patients on amitriptyline should be instructed how to arise from a sitting or lying position. They should arise slowly, sit on the edge of the bed for 1 minute, walk slowly, and hold onto the wall for support. Trazodone (Desyrel)* and nefazodone (Serzone)* are also effective sedatives but are not tricyclic antidepressants.

Selective serotonin reuptake inhibitors (SSRIs)* are effective for the hypersomnia that is common in CFS. Many patients with CFS report excessive sleep both at night (more than 8 hours) and during the day (a nap of more than 15 minutes), as well as fatigue.

SSRIs are very effective for these complaints and they also provide mood elevation. These medications are activating or stimulating and ameliorate obsessive-compulsive traits. Protriptyline (Vivactil),* bupropion (Wellbutrin),* and venlafaxine (Effexor)* are also effective stimulants for selected patients, but are not SSRIs. Other pharmacologic treatments, including drugs, vitamins, herbs, and biologic agents have been advocated but not demonstrated to be effective, for CFS. Such treatments may be dangerous and are not recommended.

PROGNOSIS

Whether the goal of treatment is rehabilitation from work disability or a less constricted lifestyle, adherence to treatment is the best prognosis factor. Patients who are unwilling or unable to comply with treatment do not generally improve. When CFS results in work disability, the most favorable prognostic factors include disability duration of up to 4 months, age onset of treatment of up to 30 years, not receiving disability payments, and an illness duration of up to 40 months. As is the case with other chronic illnesses, after 1 year of work disability because of CFS, rehabilitation is rare.

---

*Not FDA approved for this indication.

When the patient with CFS is motivated to improve and the physician uses a combined medical and psychologic treatment approach, then great improvement is possible.

MUMPS

method of
WALID ABUHAMMOUR, M.D., F.A.A.P.
Michigan State University
Hurley Medical Center
Flint, Michigan

Mumps is an acute, contagious viral infection of childhood with typical presentation of painful swelling of one or both parotid glands and fever. As a result of universal childhood immunization, mumps is an uncommon disease in the United States today.

Mumps virus is a single-stranded RNA virus and a member of the family *Paramyxoviridae*, genus paramyxovirus. It has two major surface proteins: the hemagglutinin neuraminidase and the fusion proteins. Mumps virus is sensitive to heat and ultraviolet light. The origin of the name mumps is not known. It may be from the English verb mumps "to be sulky or to grimace," or the noun mump, which means "a lump."

The growth of mumps virus in embryonated eggs was reported in 1945. Mumps vaccine was licensed in the United States in December 1967, and the Advisory Committee on Immunization Practices (ACIP) recommended that its use be considered for children approaching puberty, for adolescents, and for adults. In 1977, ACIP recommended the routine vaccination of all children aged 12 months or older.

The 666 cases of mumps reported for 1998 reflected a 99% decrease from the 152,209 cases reported in 1968. However, because the virus is present throughout the world, risk of exposure to mumps outside the United States may be high. Few countries use mumps vaccine, so mumps remains a common disease in many countries of the world.

The clinical manifestations of mumps are variable. One-third of mumps infections have subclinical or mild respiratory disease. The incubation period is usually from 16 to 18 days, but cases may occur from 12 to 25 days after exposure. After the onset of prodromal symptoms of low-grade fever, malaise, anorexia, abdominal pain, and headache, swelling and tenderness of the parotid glands (i.e. parotids, parotiditis) develop within a day. Acid-containing foods may aggravate discomfort of the parotid gland. Ordinarily the parotid gland is not palpable, but in patients with mumps, it rapidly progresses to maximum swelling over several days. Unilateral swelling usually occurs first, followed by bilateral parotid involvement.

Occasionally, simultaneous involvement of both parotid glands occurs. Unilateral parotid disease occurs in fewer than 25% of patients. Patients may complain of earache exacerbated by chewing or elicited by palpation of the gland. Fever subsides within 1 week and disappears before swelling of parotid gland resolves, which may require as long as 10 days. Other salivary glands may be involved, and orifices of the ducts may be erythematous and edematous.

Epididymo-orchitis and oophoritis are rare in the prepubertal child. Approximately one third of postpubertal male patients develop unilateral orchitis. Bilateral orchitis occurs much less frequently and, although gonadal atrophy may follow orchitis, sterility is rare even with bilateral involvement. Central nervous system involvement with mumps is not uncommon, and it more often occurs as meningitis rather than true encephalitis. Headache, fever, nausea, vomiting, and meningismus are common. Mumps meningoencephalitis carries a good prognosis and usually is associated with uneventful recovery. Other clinical manifestations of mumps include pancreatitis accompanied by severe abdominal pain, chills, fever, and persistent vomiting. Thyroiditis, oophoritis, and mastitis occasionally occur. Hearing loss, especially unilateral, has been rarely noted after mumps. Less common complications include arthritis, myocarditis, and hematologic complications.

In addition to mumps virus infection, a parotid swelling can be caused by other viruses (Parainfluenza virus type 3, cytomegalovirus, and Epstein-Barr virus), bacteria (staphylococcus, pneumococcus, and gram-negative bacilli), drug reaction (iodides, propylthiouracil, and phenothiazines), obstruction resulting from stones (sialolithiasis), stricture, or tumors, and a wide variety of other diseases. Bacterial (suppurative) parotitis is associated with high fever and unilateral symptoms involving a single salivary gland. It should be strongly suspected in a patient who is toxic or who has a purulent discharge from the Stensen duct. Cervical lymphadenitis is differentiated from parotitis by its well-defined borders and characteristic location.

Mumps is a clinical diagnosis and laboratory tests are unnecessary. Virus can be isolated from saliva, mouth washings, urine, and cerebrospinal fluid in primary monkey kidney tissue culture.

Serology can be used to confirm cases. Serum amylase is elevated in mumps parotitis but is produced from either salivary glands or pancreas. In mumps infection the white blood cell and differential counts are generally normal to mildly elevated with lymphocyte predominance. Droplet precautions are recommended until 9 days after the onset of parotid gland swelling. Children should be excluded from the onset of parotid gland swelling from going to school and child care centers.

The treatment of mumps infections consists of symptomatic relief and supportive measures. Adequate hydration is important. Foods and liquids containing acid may cause swallowing difficulty and gastric irritation. Analgesics (acetaminophen [Tylenol] or ibuprofen [Advil]) can be used for severe headache, pain, and fever. Bed rest is recommended for a faster recovery particularly in complicated cases. No specific treatment is available for mumps infections. Prevention of mumps through immunization cannot be overemphasized. Live attenuated mumps vaccine is recommended for children older than 1 year of age and is included with measles and rubella vaccine as MMR. The vaccine is safe and induces protective immunity in greater than 95% of recipients. Mumps immunoglobulin has not been shown to be protective and is no longer available or licensed for use in the United States.

PLAGUE (*YERSINIA PESTIS*)

method of
L. LUCY BOULANGER, M.D.
Indian Health Service
United States Public Health Service
Crownpoint, New Mexico

Yersinia pestis, a gram-negative bacillus that causes plague, has been responsible for at least three pandemics of disease. The first documented pandemic in 541 AD took 100 million lives in Europe and Africa, or one half the population. Europe's population had just recovered when the second pandemic, also known as "The Black Death" began in 1346.

The last global outbreak began in 1894 in China, and in that year, Dr. Alexandre Yersin first identified the organism, *Y. pestis*. This pandemic spread to America by rats aboard ships. This last outbreak likely infected wild rodents in the southwestern United States where plague is now endemic.

EPIDEMIOLOGY

Plague continues to remain endemic in many countries around the world including Myanmar, Vietnam, Peru, Brazil, Zaire, Tanzania, and Madagascar where the enzootic cycle of infection involves more than 200 species of rodents and small mammals including rats, mice, squirrels, prairie dogs, and rabbits. Humans frequently intrude into the natural foci of infection, and an average of 1700 cases of human plague has been reported each year worldwide for the past 50 years. More than 400 cases of human plague have been reported in the United States since 1950, the majority of which were contracted in New Mexico, Arizona, Colorado, and California. In areas where plague is endemic human outbreaks occur approximately every 5 years and typically last for 1 to 2 years.

MODES OF TRANSMISSION

Y. pestis is transferred from animal to animal through the blood meals of fleas. Humans are incidental hosts and acquire the infection through one of three modes of transmission. First, and predominantly, through flea bites from fleas of wild animals or domestic animals that have contact with wild animals. Second, through direct inoculation while handling the bodily fluids or tissues of infected animals (i.e., skinning a rabbit or draining a cat's bubo) or, last, and only very rarely, through inhalation of infectious droplets (i.e., the cough of an animal or another human with pneumonic plague or the aerosolization of a bioterrorist weapon).

Although historically human plague has been transmitted from fleas originating from infected rats in overcrowded urban settings, the majority of modern cases now occur sporadically in rural settings where wild rodents and their fleas are infected endemically.

BIOTERRORIST THREAT

Along with smallpox and anthrax, plague is considered one of the most significant bioterrorist threats. *Y. pestis* is considered a category A critical biologic agent of terrorism because it has high potential for morbidity and mortality, can be mass-produced, and can be easily disseminated through aerosolization among a large population. There also is efficient person-to-person transmission of the organism, and a very high fatality rate of primary pneumonic infection. In simulated bioterrorist attacks with plague, the World Health Organization estimated that 36,000 people would die after an attack on a city of 5 million people.

PATHOGENESIS AND CLINICAL SYNDROMES

There are three clinical syndromes associated with *Y. pestis* infection: bubonic, septicemic, and pneumonic plague. Bubonic plague occurs when the bacillus is acquired through a blood-borne route and travels to a regional lymph node where a painful suppurative lymphadenitis ensues. Buboes are most commonly found in the groin, axilla, or neck and are from 1 to 10 cm in size. They are typically tender, erythematous, and even necrotic and gangrenous, from which the name "Black Death" originated. Septicemic plague occurs in a subset of patients where the bacillus disseminates causing bacteremia.

Inhalation of *Y. pestis* leads to pneumonic plague. Patients present with signs and symptoms of pneumonia and frequently have hemoptysis. Because the bacillus is aerosolized with coughing, there is efficient person-to-person transmission.

The incubation period for plague is from 2 to 8 days, and common presenting symptoms include abrupt onset of fever, malaise, myalgias, abdominal symptoms (in more than 50% of patients), headache, and pharyngitis (in 10%–20% of patients).

Human-to-human transmission does not typically occur in bubonic and septicemic plague unless secondary pneumonia develops. The last reported case of person-to-person transmission of pneumonic plague in the United States occurred in 1924 in Los Angeles.

With the use of appropriate antibiotics the mortality rates for bubonic and septicemic plague have dropped from 50% to 5%–10%. Most fatalities in the United States are related to delay in seeking treatment or delay in proper diagnosis, and it is imperative that patients presenting with sepsis of unclear etiology in endemic areas be treated empirically for plague. Primary pneumonic plague has nearly a 100% fatality if not treated within 24 hours of symptom onset.

Complications of plague include meningitis and secondary pneumonia, which arise from hematogenous spread of infection. Plague meningitis typically presents several days after the initiation of antibiotic treatment for bubonic or septicemic plague.

DIAGNOSIS

Y. pestis is a nonmotile, gram-negative bacillus that has a bipolar, safety pin appearance with Gram or Wayson stains. *Y. pestis* grows on blood or MacConkey agar optimally at 28°C.

Clinical specimens are typically obtained from blood, sputum, or the aspirate of a bubo. Firm buboes can be injected with nonbacteriostatic saline and then aspirated. Clinicians should take respiratory precautions, and all specimens should be prepared and examined under a biosafety level 2 hood with a Gram stain and culture. Rapid diagnostic tests include direct fluorescent-antibody stain (available through public health reference laboratories), polymerase chain reaction, and immunoassay (available at some state health departments, the Centers for Disease Control and Prevention, and military laboratories). Acute and convalescent serum should be tested for antibody titers against *Y. pestis*.

TREATMENT

Since 1948, streptomycin has been considered the drug of choice for plague. It is given intramuscularly (IM) to adults and children at a dose of 15 mg/kg twice daily with a maximum daily dose of 2 grams. However, streptomycin is manufactured by only one pharmaceutical company, is available in modest supplies, and only by request.

Recently there has been increased interest in the use of gentamicin (Garamycin),* doxycycline (Vibramycin),* and ciprofloxacin (Cipro)* against plague, particularly for treatment or prophylaxis in response to a bioterrorist event. The Working Group on Civilian Biodefense has recommended each of these three antimicrobials in the event of plague bioterrorism.

Based upon expert consensus and a recent retrospective study, gentamicin is now recommended as a first-line treatment for plague. Gentamicin can be used as a single daily dose of 5–7 mg/kg intravenous (IV) or IM.

Doxycycline also is labeled for use in plague and is considered an alternative treatment. Doxycycline has rapid and reliable gastrointestinal absorption. It is easily administered at a dose of 100 mg IV twice daily. Doxycycline can be given orally and is therefore useful in the setting of mass casualties or for postexposure prophylaxis.

Ciprofloxacin has bactericidal and intracellular actions against plague and is considered an alternative treatment based on in vitro and animal studies. It can be given to adults in doses of 400 mg IV or 500 mg by mouth twice daily.

Trimethoprim-sulfamethoxazole (Bactrim)* is recommended for prophylaxis of plague in a nonbioterrorist setting when tetracyclines are contraindicated. It is given at a dose of two double-strength tablets twice a day. However, no sulfonamide is Food and Drug Administration–approved for the treatment of plague.

*Not FDA approved for this indication.

Chloramphenicol (Chloromycetin)* is recommended for use in plague meningitis because of its ability to cross the blood-brain barrier. It is administered at 25 mg/kg IV 4 times daily.

Both penicillins and cephalosporins are considered ineffective by expert consensus and are not currently recommended for plague treatment.

Length of treatment should be based on clinical response and 10-day course minimum should be completed to avoid relapse of infection. Oral treatment can be used to complete the 10-day course after an initial response to parental treatment is observed.

To date there have been no cases of drug-resistant *Y. pestis* in the United States. Some isolates from Madagascar, however, have been found to be multidrug resistant with resistance mediated by a transferable plasmid. Multidrug resistant plague is of concern in a bioterrorist event and should be considered should any patient fail to respond to treatment.

PREVENTION AND CONTROL

People living in areas with endemic plague should avoid contact with dead rodents, eliminate burrowing areas of rodents found near living areas including woodpiles and open trash receptacles, and use insecticides to control flea populations.

Patients who are admitted to hospitals with suspicion of plague should be placed in respiratory isolation until bacteremia has resolved. Contacts with patients with bubonic and septicemic plague should be evaluated if a febrile illness occurs but do not require antibiotic prophylaxis. Prophylaxis is recommended, however, for contacts with patients with pneumonic plague. A vaccine for plague was discontinued in 1999 after being found ineffective, and there is currently no vaccine available.

All suspect plague cases should be reported to state public health officials. Information and consultation is available at state health departments and at the National Center for Infectious Diseases, Centers for Disease Control and Prevention, Fort Collins, Colorado.

*Not FDA approved for this indication.

ANTHRAX

method of
THEODORE J. CIESLAK, M.D.
San Antonio Military Pediatric Center
San Antonio, Texas

and

EDWARD M. EITZEN, Jr., M.D., M.P.H.
Department of Health and Human Services
Washington, D.C.

Anthrax is one of the great diseases of antiquity. Considered by some scholars as the cause of the fifth and sixth plagues of Exodus, anthrax, in 1876, was the first disease to fulfill Koch's postulates; in other words, the first disease proven to be the result of an infectious microorganism. Five years later, in 1881, Pasteur developed a veterinary vaccine effective against anthrax, the world's first antibacterial vaccine. Anthrax was likely responsible for the "black bane," a 16th-century human plague that swept across Europe. Today, in parts of Asia and Africa, anthrax remains a relatively common enzootic affliction of grazing animals, such as cattle, camels, sheep, and goats. Large epizootics occur sporadically—an outbreak in Iran in 1945 resulted in the deaths of 1 million sheep. Naturally occurring human anthrax results from contact with infected animal products such as wool, hair, hides, meat, bone, and bonemeal. A 1979 outbreak in Zimbabwe originated in cattle, but ultimately resulted in more than 10,000 human cases.

Classically, three forms of endemic human anthrax were known. Cutaneous anthrax, or malignant pustule, had long been an occupational hazard of ranchers and textile workers. Gastrointestinal anthrax, contracted via the consumption of infected meat, still occasionally occurs in the developing world, but has always been extraordinarily rare in the West. Inhalational anthrax, or "woolsorter's disease," was a rare but fatal affliction of textile mill workers in the preimmunization era.

Changes in animal husbandry practices, a declining market for goat hair products (goat hair was the animal product most closely linked with the transmission of anthrax), improved workplace controls, and vaccination of textile workers and select animal herds rendered anthrax to a medical curiosity in much of the Western world in the latter half of the 20th century. In fact, only 224 cases of cutaneous anthrax in humans were reported in the United States between 1944 and 1992, and none were noted during the period from 1992 to 2000. Similarly, only 18 cases of inhalational anthrax were reported from 1900 to 2000, with the last of these occurring in 1976. More recently, myriad threats and hoaxes, as well as the intentional release of anthrax spores via contaminated mail (which resulted in 11 inhalational and 12 cutaneous cases), have resurrected the specter of human anthrax in the United States.

Anthrax is caused by infection with *Bacillus anthracis*, a large, aerobic, gram-positive, spore-forming rod that grows readily on standard media, including blood agar. Because other species of *Bacillus* are common culture contaminants, however, some clinical laboratories may discard such cultures without identifying organisms to the species level. Clinicians entertaining a diagnosis of anthrax should thus alert their laboratory promptly regarding this suspicion. *B. anthracis,* as a gram-positive organism, produces no endotoxin. Rather, its virulence depends in large part on two protein toxins: edema toxin (a combination of edema factor and protective antigen) and lethal toxin (lethal factor + protective antigen). These virulence factors figure prominently in the design of prophylactic and therapeutic strategies against anthrax. In this review, we discuss the management of anthrax in light of this knowledge, of recent events, and of improvements in therapy and prophylaxis that have occurred since anthrax last posed a significant endemic threat 50 years ago.

INHALATIONAL ANTHRAX

Inhalational anthrax typically begins as a nonspecific febrile illness after an incubation period that averages 1 to 6 days, but may occasionally be much longer. The disease often follows a biphasic course; in addition to fever, early symptoms include myalgias, headache, nonproductive cough, and chest discomfort. These symptoms typically persist for a few days, and a brief period of improvement follows in some patients. In the absence of prompt therapy, a second phase quickly ensues and deterioration is rapid. High fever, cyanosis, stridor, dyspnea, and shock characterize this second phase. Hemorrhagic meningitis develops in 50% of patients. During this phase, patients often have a very high-grade bacteremia. Bacteria are readily cultured from blood and, in fact, can often be seen on gram-stained specimens of peripheral blood.

Much of what we know today regarding the pathology of inhalational anthrax in humans derives from the Sverdlovsk incident of 1979. In that instance, an inadvertent release of spores from a Soviet bioweapons production facility in the city of Sverdlovsk resulted in at least 66 human fatalities, along with hundreds of animal deaths. Subsequently, the result of autopsies conducted on 42 of the victims were made public. All 42 of these victims had hemorrhagic involvement of the mediastinum; 21 had the classic "cardinal's cap" of hemorrhagic meningitis. These findings highlight that, although inhalational anthrax is acquired via the lungs, it is not a disease of pulmonary tissue per se. Rather, inhaled bacteria reaching the lungs are taken up by pulmonary macrophages and transported to regional lymph nodes in the mediastinum. It is within these lymph nodes that anthrax bacteria proliferate and release their two protein toxins. These toxins lead to enlargement and necrosis of mediastinal lymphatic tissue, giving rise to a hemorrhagic mediastinitis with its characteristic radiographic findings of a widened mediastinum.

Because mediastinal widening in an acutely ill, febrile patient presents a very limited differential diagnosis, fully developed inhalational anthrax should actually be relatively easy to diagnose. Unfortunately, because patients at this stage of illness are unlikely to survive, the challenge for the clinician is to make a diagnosis early in the course of illness, before mediastinal pathology is obvious radiographically. Such early diagnoses may be made on epidemiologic grounds; various rapid diagnostic assays are in development. Culture of blood, cerebrospinal fluid, or pleural fluid should yield the organism in symptomatic cases. Culture of the anterior nares may be useful epidemiologically in the event of an inhalational attack, but a negative culture from the nares does not preclude the possibility of anthrax exposure. Computed tomography or magnetic resonance imaging may detect swollen mediastinal lymph nodes or minimal pleural effusions before conventional radiographs are diagnostic.

Treatment

Endemic strains of *B. anthracis* are virtually always susceptible to penicillin G, which remains, in the opinion of some, a viable option for the treatment of naturally occurring woolsorter's disease (2 million units IV q 2 h or 4 million units IV q 4 h). Because resistant strains are readily selected for, however, anthrax in the setting of a potential terrorist attack should be treated with alternative antibiotics until sensitivity test results are available. Moreover, the discovery of constitutive and inducible beta-lactamases among *B. anthracis* strains has led to cautions against the use of penicillin or ampicillin as single-agent therapy. Fluoroquinolones and tetracyclines, on the other hand, appear to be reasonable choices, based on in vitro and animal data. An isolated report of a tetracycline-resistant *B. anthracis* strain has led some experts to call for the empiric use of ciprofloxacin (Cipro) (400 mg IV q 12 h) as initial therapy of presumed inhalational anthrax. Doxycycline (Vibramycin) (100 mg IV q 12 h) remains a reasonable alternative. Furthermore, because anthrax relies on its protein toxins for virulence, some have advocated the addition of antibiotic(s) targeting protein synthesis at the level of the bacterial ribosome. Rifampin* (Rifadin), clindamycin* (Cleocin), clarithromycin* (Biaxin), and chloramphenicol* (Chloromycetin) fall into this category and are usually effective in vitro. The cell-wall–active agents vancomycin, ampicillin, imipenem* (Primaxin) and meropenem* (Merrem) are likewise typically effective in vitro. Given the propensity of *B. anthracis* to invade the meninges, we advocate inclusion in the regimen of an agent with favorable cerebrospinal fluid penetration. Penicillin, ampicillin, imipenem, meropenem, or chloramphenicol would appear reasonable choices in this regard. Levofloxacin* (Levaguin) and ofloxacin* (Floxin) may be acceptable substitutes for ciprofloxacin (Cipro), and other quinolones are effective *in vitro* as well. Owing to the presence of a cephalosporinase in many strains of *B. anthracis,* cephalosporins should not be used to treat anthrax. Whenever possible, we advocate that therapeutic agents be given parenterally until the patient is clearly on the road to recovery. In the case of a mass casualty event, however, where parenteral therapy may not be possible on a large scale, oral therapy may be necessary. Ciprofloxacin (500 mg PO q 12 h) or doxycycline (100 mg PO q 12 h) would represent logical empiric oral options, combined with oral forms of other drugs as mentioned previously. Duration of therapy is somewhat controversial. Classically, endemic woolsorter's desease was treated for 7 to 10 days. More recently, information gleaned from the Sverdlovsk incident, as well as limited data from primate studies, has led some experts to recommend treatment courses as long as 60 days. We concur with these recommendations (our methods are summarized in Table 1) in the setting of a terrorist incident when resources and drug tolerance permit.

*Not FDA approved for this indication.

Postexposure Prophylaxis

In the setting of a terrorist attack, early involvement of public health authorities and epidemiologists is

TABLE 1. **Recommended Therapy and Prophylaxis of Anthrax**

Condition	Adults	Children
Inhalational, therapy† (patients who are clinically stable after 14 days can be switched to a single oral agent [ciprofloxacin or doxycycline] to complete a 60-day course‡)	Ciprofloxacin (Cipro)§ 400 mg intravenously (IV) q 12 h OR	Ciprofloxacin§ 10–15 mg/kg IV q 12 h OR
	Doxycycline (Vibromycin) 100 mg IV q 12 h	Doxycycline 2.2 mg/kg IV q 12 h
	and	and
	Clindamycin*‖ 900 mg IV q 8 h	Clindamycin*‖ 10–15 mg/kg IV q 8 h
	and	and
	Penicillin G 4 mil U IV q 4 h	Penicillin G 400–600,000 U/kg/d IV ÷ q 4 h
Inhalational, postexposure prophylaxis (60-days course‡)	Ciprofloxacin 500 mg by mouth (PO) q 12 h OR	Ciprofloxacin 10–15 mg/kg PO q 12 h OR
	Doxycycline 100 mg PO q 12 h	Doxycycline 2.2 mg/kg PO q 12 h
Endemic cutaneous, therapy¶	Penicillin V 500 mg PO q 6 h OR	Penicillin V 40–80 mg/kg/d PO ÷ q 6 h OR
	Amoxacillin 500 mg PO q 8 h OR	Amoxacillin 40–80 mg/kg/d PO ÷ q 8 h OR
	Ciprofloxacin 500 mg PO q 12 h OR	Ciprofloxacin 10–15 mg/kg PO q 12 h OR
	Doxycycline 100 mg PO q 12 h	Doxycycline 2.2 mg/kg PO q 12 h
Cutaneous in setting of terrorism, therapy¶	Ciprofloxacin 500 mg PO q 12 h OR	Ciprofloxacin 10–15 mg/kg PO q 12 h OR
	Doxycycline 100 mg PO q 12 h	Doxycycline 2.2 mg/kg PO q 12 h
Gastrointestinal	Same as for inhalational	Same as for inhalational

*Not FDA approved for this indication.
†In a mass casualty setting, where resources are severely constrained, oral therapy may need to be substituted for the preferred parenteral option.
‡Assuming the organism is sensitive, children may be switched to oral Amoxacillin (80 mg/kg/d ÷ q 8 h) to complete a 60-day course. We recommend that the first 14 days of therapy or postexposure prophylaxis, however, include ciprofloxacin or doxycycline regardless of age. A three-dose series of AVA may permit shortening of the antibiotic course to 30 days (see text).
§Levofloxacin* (Levaquin) or Ofloxacin* (Floxin) may be acceptable alternatives to Ciprofloxacin.
‖Rifampin* (Rifadin) or Clarithromycin (Biaxin)* may be acceptable alternatives to Clindamycin* (Cleocin) as drugs that target bacterial protein synthesis. If ciprofloxacin or another quinolone is employed, doxycycline may be used as a second agent, as it also targets protein synthesis.
¶Ten days of therapy may be adequate for endemic cutaneous disease. We recommend a full 60-day course in the setting of terrorism, however, because of the possibility of a concomitant inhalational exposure.

paramount. An aggressive and rapid attempt must be undertaken to delineate the limits of contamination and identify those persons likely to have been exposed. After such persons are identified, early institution of antimicrobial prophylaxis is critical. Based on limited data from nonhuman primate studies, a single-agent administered orally is probably adequate. Ciprofloxacin (500 mg PO q 12 h) or doxycycline (100 mg PO q 12 h) would be reasonable choices. The duration of postexposure chemoprophylaxis remains somewhat controversial and, again, no controlled human trials have evaluated various options. Many experts, however, currently recommend courses as long as 60 to 100 days. Similarly, the role of postexposure immunoprophylaxis remains unsettled. We feel that three doses of the licensed anthrax vaccine (anthrax vaccine adsorbed, AVA)* given in conjunction with antibiotics, may enhance protection or enable the clinician to shorten the postexposure antibiotic course. Based on very limited animal data, we allow that, when available, a three-dose series of AVA (given at time zero and at 2 and 4 weeks after the initial dose), combined with 30 days of antibiotics, may be an acceptable alternative to longer antibiotic courses alone.

Pre-Exposure Prophylaxis

AVA consists of a purified preparation of protective antigen (a potent immunogen, protective antigen is critical for entry of lethal and edema factors into mammalian cells; it is nonpathogenic when given alone). AVA was licensed by the Food and Drug Administration FDA in 1970 and, in a large controlled trial, has been shown effective at preventing cutaneous anthrax among textile workers. Based on an increasing amount of animal data, there is every reason to believe that this vaccine is quite effective at preventing inhalational anthrax as well. Moreover, 18 studies now attest to the safety of AVA. Nonetheless, logistical and other considerations make large-scale civilian employment of AVA impractical at present. The vaccine is licensed as a six-dose series, given at 0, 2, and 4 weeks, and again at 6, 12, and 18 months. Yearly boosters are recommended for those at ongoing risk. At present, we recommend pre-exposure AVA only in select military and occupational settings.

Gastrointestinal Anthrax

This infection, never reported in the United States, is said to have a mortality rate as high as 50%. It would seem prudent to treat cases in a manner similar to that used in inhalational anthrax.

*Currently not available for the general public.

Cutaneous Anthrax

Naturally occurring cutaneous anthrax, such as woolsorter's disease, is an occupational hazard of ranchers, textile workers, and others having contact with sheep, goats, and cattle. The characteristic lesion begins as a pruritic papule, which progresses to a necrotic ulcer. A black eschar forms, giving rise to the coal-like lesion for which the disease is named (anthrax derives from the Greek *anthrakos*, coal). The differential diagnosis of cutaneous anthrax is limited and includes brown recluse spider bites, ulceroglandular tularemia, pyoderma gangrenosa, and a few other rare conditions. In the preantibiotic era, cutaneous anthrax had a mortality rate of approximately 20%. Although likely the result to dissemination and secondary bacteremia, at least some of this mortality could be attributed to the massive edema associated with some cutaneous lesions. Such edema, when involving the head or neck, may result in airway compromise. Consideration must be given to aggressive airway protection in such cases. Because the disease is relatively easy to recognize, especially by those familiar with it in endemic areas, and because therapy is straightforward, few patients today, however, should succumb to cutaneous anthrax. In fact, in the 1979 anthrax outbreak in Zimbabwe, only 182 of 10,738 (mostly cutaneous) victims succumbed to the disease, despite the constrained resources in the setting of civil war in this African nation.

The therapy of naturally occurring cutaneous anthrax is likewise straightforward. A 7 to 10-day course of single-agent therapy (with penicillin or ampicillin) is probably adequate in most cases. Cutaneous anthrax in the setting of terrorism, however, poses additional considerations. Because a presumption can be made that the victim of cutaneous disease, in such instances, may also have been exposed to a significant inhalational inoculum, we advocate treating such patients in a manner analogous to that used in victims of inhalational anthrax. Thus we would use double or triple therapy for 2 weeks, followed by an additional month-and-a-half of ciprofloxacin or doxycycline. If the organism were known to be sensitive, amoxacillin could be substituted for these drugs in children so as to avoid long-term quinolone or tetracycline exposure. We strongly recommend, however, that the first 2 weeks of therapy consist of ciprofloxacin or doxycycline in even the youngest children.

Although naturally occurring strains of *B. anthracis* are normally sensitive to a wide range of antibiotics, including penicillin, recent bioterrorism considerations have added a great deal of complexity to the management of anthrax victims. Most of the current recommendations are based on animal studies or very scant human data. It is our hope that no further opportunities to acquire human data will ever present themselves.

PSITTACOSIS (ORNITHOSIS)

method of
JEFFREY T. KIRCHNER, D.O.
Temple University School of Medicine
Philadelphia, Pennsylvania

and

CHRISTIAN L. HERMANSEN, M.D.
Department of Family and Community Medicine
Lancaster General Hospital
Lancaster, Pennsylvania

Psittacosis is a zoonotic infection of humans. It is caused by the organism *Chlamydia psittaci,* which is one of the four described species of *Chlamydia* and an obligate intracellular parasite. The infection is usually acquired in humans by contact with infected birds. This feature led investigators to originally believe that only psittacine birds (e.g., parakeets, parrots, cockatoos, cockatiels, macaws) were responsible for transmission to humans. Ritter described an outbreak of the disease in 1879 and referred to it as *pneumotyphus.* However, it was Morange in 1892 who is credited with the term "psittacosis" (from the Greek for parrot). It has subsequently been determined that more than 100 bird species, including domestic types such as turkeys and chickens, are capable of transmitting *C. psittaci* to humans. The term psittacosis has persisted, although ornithosis more aptly describes the potential for any bird to spread the infection. Moreover, the infection has been described in a large number of domestic animals, including cows, goats, and sheep. Bird fanciers are considered the highest risk group but others at risk include pigeon fanciers, veterinarians, and employees of pet shops. Psittacosis is considered an occupational hazard among employees in poultry slaughtering and processing plants.

TRANSMISSION

Transmission of *C. psittaci* is through respiratory inhalation of the organism that has been aerosolized in bird feces, fecal dust, or respiratory secretions of infected birds. The agent then travels to the reticuloendothelial cells of the liver and spleen where it replicates. This is followed by hematogenous invasion of the lungs and other organs. It is during this period of early infection that the organism may be isolated from the sputum or blood.

CLINICAL MANIFESTATIONS

In humans, psittacosis usually presents as a respiratory illness. However, the systemic nature of the disease accounts for its diverse clinical manifestations (Table 1). Initial signs and symptoms are variable, often described as "influenza-like." After an incubation period that ranges from 7 to 21 days, infected individuals will have a gradual onset of fever, malaise, cough, and headache. The later symptom is often quite severe. The patient's cough will become more prominent and progresses from dry and hacking early on to productive of blood-tinged sputum in severe cases. A more abrupt onset of symptoms that includes shaking chills and high fever has also been described but occurs much less frequently.

TABLE 1. **Signs and Symptoms of Psittacosis in 1136 Patients***

Fever	72%
Cough	44%
Headache	38%
Chills	33%
Weakness/fatigue	33%
Myalgias	25%
Nausea/vomiting	14%
Anorexia	13%
Chest pain	11%
Diaphoresis	11%

*Adapted from CDC: Psittacosis Surveillance: Annual Summary 1975-1984. Bethesda, MD, DHHS, 1987.

Gastrointestinal symptoms such as nausea, vomiting, abdominal pain, and diarrhea are seen, but usually when psittacosis is contracted from turkeys. Dermatologic manifestations include urticaria, subungual splinter hemorrhages, erythema marginatum, and superficial thrombophlebitis. Often described but uncommonly seen is a pink macular rash (known as Horder spots) that resembles the rose spots of typhoid fever. Cardiac involvement may be manifest by a relative bradycardia, similar to what is seen with brucellosis, typhus, or Legionnaire's disease. Cases of pericarditis, myocarditis, and culture-negative endocarditis resulting from *C. psittaci* have been reported. Hepatic enlargement is common but splenic enlargement is found only in about 10% of patients. The presence of hepatosplenomegaly with pneumonia is highly suggestive of psittacosis. A reactive arthritis may occur 2 to 3 weeks after the onset of respiratory symptoms. It is usually polyarticular but may involve a single joint. Neurologic abnormalities are diverse and may include meningitis, encephalitis, cranial nerve palsies, transverse myelitis, and seizures. If a lumbar puncture is performed, the cerebrospinal fluid is usually normal but may exhibit a low-level pleocytosis.

LABORATORY FINDINGS

Similar to the clinical findings, lab findings with psittacosis are typically nonspecific. The total leukocyte count is normal or just mildly elevated with a left shift. Mild anemia secondary to hemolysis or hemocytophagia is often found. Liver involvement is manifested by elevations in serum transaminase levels along with bilirubin and alkaline phosphatase. In rare cases of renal involvement, such as with acute tubular necrosis or glomerulonephritis, an elevated creatinine level will be found. Chest radiographs are abnormal in the majority of instances with single lobar consolidation. Less commonly, multilobar, atelectatic, or miliary patterns may be seen. Radiographic appearance is often worse than the patient's clinical symptoms would suggest.

DIAGNOSIS

The diagnosis of psittacosis is suggested by the clinical presentation of fever, cough, and headache accompanied

TABLE 2. **Considerations in the Differential Diagnosis of Psittacosis**

1. Bacterial pneumonia
2. "Atypical" pneumonia (*Legionella, Mycoplasma*, or *Chlamydia*)
3. Viral pneumonia
4. Fungal pneumonia
5. Tuberculosis
6. Q fever
7. Influenza

by a history of exposure to birds. However, the clinical manifestations are myriad leading to an extensive differential diagnosis (Table 2). Therefore, a definitive diagnosis can never be made on clinical grounds alone.

Laboratory diagnosis of psittacosis can be challenging in that the organism is rarely isolated from culture specimens. It is possible to culture *C. psittaci* from blood or sputum but this is typically discouraged due to the risk it places on laboratory personnel. The current test of choice is serologic analysis for chlamydial antibodies. An acute-phase sample should be obtained as soon as the infection is suspected. However, standard lab testing via complement fixation (CF) is not species specific and cross-reactivity with *C. pneumoniae* and *C. trachomatis* can occur as a result of common antigens. A convalescent-phase specimen should always be obtained about 2 weeks after onset of symptoms. Because antibiotic therapy may affect the early immunologic response, some recommend a third serum specimen for diagnostic confirmation.

Most authorities recognize a single antibody titer of at least 1:64 and a clinical scenario consistent with psittacosis as diagnostic of recent infection. However, the Centers for Disease Control and Prevention (CDC) considers a *confirmed* case of psittacosis to include a clinical picture compatible with the disease *plus* one of the three following criteria: (1) A positive sputum culture for *C. psittaci*, (2) a fourfold or greater increase in antibody titer to at least 1:32 or greater via a CF assay on specimens drawn at least 2 weeks apart, or (3) a species-specific single IgM titer of at least 1:16 done by micro-immunofluorescence (MIF). Although more specific than CF testing, MIF is not as readily available. The CDC definition for a *probable* case of psittacosis includes presence of the clinical illness plus a single antibody titer of 1:32 or greater by CF or MIF.

Collectively, serologic testing for psittacosis remains problematic because of the low specificity of most current assays. Testing on sputum for *C. psittaci* with polymerase chain reaction should improve diagnostic accuracy when this becomes more readily available.

TREATMENT

Appropriate treatment of a patient with psittacosis should include eradication of active infection with antimicrobials. Tetracyclines represent first-line therapy. Recommended doses are 100 mg twice a day for doxycycline (Vibramycin) or 500 mg four times a day for tetracycline (Sumycin). For initial therapy in severely ill patients, intravenous doxycycline hyclate may be given at a dose of 4.4 mg/kg (2 mg/lb) divided into twice-daily infusions. Macrolides can be used in those with contraindications to tetracycline, such as pregnant patients, children younger than 9 years old, and those with tetracycline allergy. The recommended dose of erythromycin (E-Mycin)* is 333 mg three times a day. Clarithromycin (Biaxin)* and azithromycin (Zithromax)* also provide antimicrobial function. However, macrolides may be less affective than tetracycline and clinical data with these agents are lacking. Unlike *Chlamydia trachomatis*, *C. psittaci* is often not susceptible to sulfonamides and these agents should not be used.

After initiation of therapy, clinical improvement is often seen within the first 24 to 72 hours. However, appropriate antibiotics must be administered for a minimum of 10 to 14 days to prevent relapse of infection. In the pre-antibiotic era, mortality from psittacosis was 20% to 40%. Presently the case fatality rate is less than 1%.

Prevention and infection control measures are important to consider. Birds, classically parrots and parakeets, can also manifest symptoms of acute infection referred to as avian chlamydiosis. They often have ocular or nasal discharge and diarrhea and should be isolated while receiving chlortetracycline** for a minimum of 30 days. People handling infected birds should exercise specific precautions including wearing gloves, gowns, and respirators. Disinfection of contaminated cages should be performed with 1:1000 quaternary ammonium, or 70% isopropyl alcohol. Cleaning cages should also involve limitation of feather, dust, and fecal matter circulation. Prevention of further infection also includes reporting cases to the state health authorities and the CDC. No vaccine is available to prevent disease either in birds or humans and immunity also is not gained by previous infection.

*Not FDA approved for this indication.
**Not available in the United States.

Q FEVER

method of
ELISA I. CHOI, M.D.
Beth Israel Deaconess Medical Center
Harvard Medical School
Boston, Massachusetts

EPIDEMIOLOGY

Q fever is a wordwide zoonotic infection that can manifest as both an acute illness and a chronic disease. The etiologic agent of Q fever, *Coxiella burnetii* (historically classified in the order Rickettsiales, now more recently considered as belonging to Proteobacteria), is found among many different wildlife species and has many different reservoirs, including arthropods (mainly ticks), birds, and mammals. However, human beings are the only hosts known to develop disease from infection with this organism. The source of human infection is usually cattle, sheep, goats, and farm animals, and, less commonly, dogs, cats, rabbits, pigeons, and rats. The true prevalence of Q fever may be underestimated, owing to underrecognition, because disease can be asymptomatic in infected persons. Human disease can result from inhalation of contaminated aerosol (thus making it a possible agent of bioterrorism), contact with body fluids of infected livestock, or exposure to skins or placentas of infected animals. Sexual transmission of *Coxiella burnetii* has also been reported, and infection believed to be acquired through the consumption of raw milk has been noted. Congenital infections have been reported to occur transplacentally, through blood transfusions, and through intradermal inoculations. Q fever has been reported predominantly in Nova Scotia (Canada), Israel, southern France, Spain, Switzerland, Great Britain, and Germany.

CLINICAL FEATURES

Clinical manifestations of Q fever can be broadly divided into acute (infection of less than 6 months' duration) and chronic (infection of more than 6 months' duration) forms. Acute infection typically manifests as a self-limited febrile or flulike illness, pneumonia, hepatitis, or, more rarely, meningoencephalitis, myocarditis, pericarditis, maculopapular or purpuric rashes, and granulomatous lymphadenitis. Other clinical presentations include seizures, polyradiculoneuritis, optic neuritis, gastroenteritis, pancreatitis, erythema nodosum, lymphadenopathy, hemolytic anemia, hypoplastic anemia, thyroiditis, syndrome of inappropriate antidiuretic hormone, glomerulonephritis, and splenic rupture. The incubation period is 2 to 5 weeks, with an average incubation time of 20 days. When infection occurs during pregnancy, spontaneous abortion may result, with subsequent chronic uterine infection and recurrent miscarriages. Infected persons can present with clinically asymptomatic hepatitis with transaminase elevations and fever or with prominent hepatomegaly and abdominal discomfort, usually without significant jaundice. A third variation of hepatic manifestation is fever without any other localizing signs, with characteristic "doughnut-like" granulomas on liver biopsy examination (granulomatous hepatitis).

Chronic Q fever (occurring in about 1% to 5% infected persons) most commonly presents as culture-negative endocarditis, a particularly severe and fatal form of chronic Q fever infection. Persons with preexisting valvular heart disease are at greatest risk of this particular manifestation, and diagnosis is often difficult, because conventional blood cultures are not usually able to detect growth of the causative organism, and vegetations are infrequently seen on echocardiography. The most frequently affected organs are the heart, arteries, bones, and liver. Other less common manifestations of chronic Q fever infection include infection of aneurysms or vascular grafts, hepatic fibrosis or cirrhosis (complicating hepatitis), and osteomyelitis or osteoarthritis, with much rarer reports of pericardial effusions, pulmonary interstitial fibrosis, amyloidosis, mixed cryoglobulinemia, malignancy-like presentations (pseudotumor of the lung, mimicking lymphoma), and central nervous system manifestations. These presentations occur months or years after the acute disease, and they represent long-term sequelae of untreated (and possibly undiagnosed) acute Q fever infection. Older persons and immunocompromised patients are at greater risk of acquiring the chronic form of Q fever.

DIAGNOSIS

Diagnosis often rests on serologic confirmation of infection with *Coxiella burnetii*, because the organism is difficult to culture. Nonspecific laboratory findings include leukocytosis, elevated erythrocyte sedimentation rate, elevated creatine kinase, thrombocytopenia, moderate hepatic transaminase elevations (2 to 10 times normal values), and autoantibodies (antiphospholipid antibodies, anti–smooth muscle antibodies, antimitochondrial antibodies). Seroconversion usually is detected within 1 to 2 weeks after onset of clinical disease, and approximately 90% of patients with *Coxiella burnetii* infection have detectable antibodies by the third week after onset of symptoms. Antibody titers higher than 1:200 for anti–phase II IgG and higher than 1:50 for anti–phase II IgM indicate acute infection. A single anti–phase I IgG antibody titer higher than 1:800 and an IgA titer of more than 1:100 indicate evidence of chronic infection. IgM titers can be variable, and they may not be as diagnostically useful. In chronic Q fever endocarditis, there is a high titer antibody response to both phase I and phase II antigens of the organism. Antibody titers reach their highest levels approximately 4 to 8 weeks after the onset of acute Q fever, with gradually decreasing levels over the subsequent 12 months. A persistence of high levels of anti–phase I antibodies despite therapy, or the reappearance of antibodies in high titer after previously being undetectable or only present in low titers, may herald the development of chronic Q fever infection. If acute Q fever has been diagnosed, recommendations are for repeat serologic testing, monthly, for at least 6 months. Some more recent investigations, of the use of polymerase chain reaction technology to diagnose Q fever, have resulted in some promising results, with successful detection of the organism in cell cultures and clinical isolates. However, diagnostic approaches based on polymerase chain reaction have not become widely available in many parts of the world, and serologic testing currently remains the most widely used diagnostic method.

TREATMENT

For acute Q fever infection, in general, a 2-week course of doxycycline (Vibramycin) is currently the recommended first-line therapy. Fluoroquinolones may be an alternative regimen, particularly in the case of more unusual manifestations of acute Q fever infection, such as meningitis or encephalitis, because of the unreliable penetration of the tetracyclines into the cerebrospinal fluid. Recommendations for pediatric or pregnant patients remains problematic, because clinical data are insufficient to recommend alternative agents such as macrolides or co-trimoxazole conclusively.

In general, combination therapy is the most optimal means of attempting medical cure of Q fever endocarditis. Combination regimens include doxycycline plus rifampin (Rifadin), or ciprofloxacin (Cipro) or ofloxacin (Floxin), plus doxycycline. The optimal duration of therapy for Q fever endocarditis is controversial, but long-term therapy appears to be the rule. The doxycycline and hydroxychloroquine treatment regimen is recommended for at least 18 months of therapy, and other regimens may need to be continued for variable durations, from 3 years to lifetime therapy. Serologic testing is recommended during therapy for Q fever endocarditis, with repeat testing on a monthly basis for up to 1 year of therapy and decreased-interval testing (every 3 months for several more years, then decreasing to every 6 months indefinitely) thereafter to ensure adequate success of therapy and to survey for possible relapse. In patients who are at particularly high risk of developing chronic infection with *Coxiella burnetii* (those with valvular heart disease, immunodeficiencies, or vascular abnormalities), repeated serologic testing should be undertaken, especially in the setting of previously documented or diagnosed acute Q fever infection or unexplained recurrent febrile episodes. In patients with Q fever hepatitis, there are some anecdotal reports of successful therapy with a combination of prednisone and an antibiotic. Adjunctive prednisone therapy may be considered in patients with Q fever hepatitis who have persistent fevers, persistent high elevations of erythrocyte sedimentation rate, and high titers of autoantibodies, especially when these occur despite antibiotic therapy. A short, tapering, 1-week course of prednisone therapy may be indicated if patients with Q fever hepatitis have not started to defervesce after several days of antibiotic therapy.

RABIES

method of
CHRISTOPHER J. FINNEGAN, B.Sc., M.Sc.,
NICOLA BRINK, M.B.ChB. MMed., M.RCPath., and
ANTHONY R. FOOKS, BSC., M.B.A., PhD.
Rabies Research and Diagnostics Group, WHO Collaborating Centre for the Characterization of Rabies and Rabies-Related Viruses
Veterinary Laboratories Agency
Addlestone, United Kingdom

and

University College London
London, United Kingdom

Rabies, a fatal zoonotic disease that infects all warm-blooded mammals, including human beings, is caused by a viral infection affecting the brain, and for which there is no known cure. Classic rabies virus (RABV) is the archetype virus within the Lyssavirus genus, (family Rhabdoviridae) and is mainly transmitted via saliva, after a bite from an infected animal. The virus enters the central nervous system of the host and causes encephalomyelitis. As a result, rabies has been responsible for causing thousands of human deaths for as many years. RABV is endemic in all continents, with the exception of several islands and peninsulas including Australia and New Zealand, a few European countries, and Antarctica, which remain free of rabies. This is, however, at considerable cost and with a continual risk of reimportation. Global estimates from the World Health Organization are that rabies deaths account for up to 50,000 human deaths each year. The highest number of cases is reported in Africa and Asia, particularly the Indian subcontinent. These figures are still considered to be conservative estimates, however, because under-reporting of rabies is considered to be widespread in developing countries. This is largely the result of a poor health care infrastructure, as well as insufficient control measures and the huge reservoir present in domestic animals and wildlife species.

RABIES VIRUS STRUCTURE

RABV is one of seven lyssaviruses. Possibly all lyssaviruses (genotypes 1 to 7 [Table 1]) are capable of causing clinically indistinguishable fatal human disease. Lagos bat virus (LBV; genotype 2), Mokola virus (MOKV; genotype 3), and Duvenhage virus (DUVV; genotype 4) are restricted geographically to Africa. LBV is the only lyssavirus that has never been reported to infect human beings. Human fatalities caused by the MOKV, DUVV, and Australian bat lyssavirus (ABLV; genotype 7) are relatively rare. Two additional viruses, isolated from bats (Aravan and Khujand virus), were isolated in Central Asia in 1991 and have been proposed as members of a new Lyssavirus genus. In Europe, two bat lyssaviruses referred to as European bat lyssaviruses (EBLVs) types 1 and 2 (genotypes 5 and 6, respectively), pose a threat to any animal or person who may come into contact with an infected insectivorous bat.

The members of this family Rhabdoviridae display similarities with respect to their genomic structures. The genome is single-stranded, negative-sense, nonsegmented RNA encoding for five separate proteins. The genes are ordered from 5′ to 3′ end of the genome as follows: nucleoprotein (N), phosphoprotein (NS or M1), matrix protein (M or M2), glycoprotein (G), and polymerase (L). A pseudogene exists between the G and L cistrons. The seven genotypes fall into two distinct phylogroups: genotypes 1 (RABV), 4 (DUVV), 5 (EBLV-1), 6 (EBLV-2), and 7 (ABLV) comprise phylogroup 1, whereas phylogroup II contains the divergent African genotypes 2 (LBV) and 3 (MOKV).

RABIES EPIDEMIOLOGY IN NORTH AMERICA

In North America, in the early 1940s, there were approximately 40 cases of human rabies each year. This figure increased to a total of 99 in the 1950s and then dropped to 15 in the 1960s, 23 in the 1970s, 10 in the 1980s, and 22 from 1990 to 1996. Widespread

TABLE 1. **Lyssavirus Taxonomy**

Genotype	Strain	Distribution	Source
1	Classic Rabies (RABV)	Worldwide	Dogs, wild carnivores, livestock, man; bats in the Americas
2	Lagos bat (LBV)	Nigeria, Central Africa	Fruit bats, cats, and dogs
3	Mokola (MOKV)	Nigeria	Shrews, rodents, cats, dogs, human beings
4	Duvenhage (DUVV)	South Africa, Zimbabwe	Insectivorous bats, human beings
5	European bat lyssavirus 1 (EBLV-1)	Western, Central, and Eastern Europe	Insectivorous (*Serotine* sp.) bats, human beings
6	European bat lyssavirus 2 (EBLV-2)	Northern Europe	Insectivorous (*Myotis* sp.) bats, human beings
7	Australian bat lyssavirus (ABLV)	Australia	Insectivorous and frugiverous bats, human beings
Proposed	Aravan and Khujand virus	Central Asia	Insectivorous bats

vaccination of companion animals in the 1950s was partly responsible for the decrease in human cases. Vaccination campaigns were implemented in the 1940s and all but eliminated canine variants of the rabies virus by the 1960s in canids. However, the late 1970s and early 1980s witnessed the reemergence of a variant, well adapted to dogs, in south Texas. Rabies has been reported more frequently in wild animals than in domestic animals in the United States since the 1960s. In 2001, wild animals accounted for more than 93% of all reported cases, whereas domestic species accounted for 6.7%. Raccoons were the most commonly reported wildlife species to harbor the disease (37.2%), followed by skunks and bats (30.7% and 17.2%, respectively).

It appears that three variants of rabies virus cause disease in skunks in the north and south central states and in California. The disease spread in the 1950s affected foxes throughout Canada and New England. Although rabid foxes have diminished in Canada because of successful baiting tactics, Alaska still harbors the virus in the fox population. Outbreaks of rabies infections in terrestrial mammals inclusive of skunks, foxes, raccoons, and coyotes are found in broad geographic regions across the United States.

Currently, with the availability of molecular diagnostic tools such as nucleotide analysis, it is possible to suggest the source of exposure. It is apparent from present findings that bats are a significant epidemiologic factor and may account for a large proportion of human rabies incidents in the United States.

RABIES VIRUS VARIANTS IN NORTH AMERICAN BATS

In North America, bat rabies is caused by a variant of genotype 1 (RABV). The main species involved are: *Eptesicus fuscus*, the big brown bat; *Tadarida brasiliensis*, the Brazilian (Mexican) free-tailed bat; *Myotis lucifugus*, the little brown bat; *Lasiurus cinereus*, the hoary bat; *Lasionycteris noctivagans*, the silver-haired bat, *Lasiurus borealis*, the red bat; and *Pipistrellus hesperus*, the Western pipistrelle.

HUMAN CASES OF RABIES IN NORTH AMERICA

Since the 1900s, the number of deaths caused by rabies has decreased from 100 or more each year to less than 10. These data are mainly the result of increased awareness, vaccination, and animal control programs, which were formulated in the 1940s. California reported the only human case of human rabies in 2001 and was the result of infection with a canine variant, imported to the United States, most probably from the Philippines. In 2002, two cases of rabies in humans were reported caused by bat variants of RABV. The first occurred in California and was the Brazilian free-tailed bat (*Tadarida brasiliensis*) virus variant. The second case, caused by a silver-haired and eastern pipistrelle bat (*Lasionycteris noctivagans* and *Pipistrellus subflavus*) virus variant, was reported from Tennessee.

GLOBAL RABIES SITUATION

Rabies in the Americas is characterized by genotype 1 variants, in both terrestrial mammals and in species of bat. In Latin America, rabies in vampire bats causes a significant economic problem. In contrast, canine rabies is problematic in countries in Africa and Asia. In Australia, a bat variant, Australian bat lyssavirus, has been detected from indigenous colonies of fruit bats.

PATHOGENESIS

The usual entry route of infection is the exposure of underlying tissues to virus-contaminated saliva across punctured or damaged skin or mucous membranes. Under normal environmental conditions, the virus does not persist significantly outside an infected animal. Experimental studies in mice have shown that the virus persists at the inoculation site, where it seems to remain latent for most of the incubation period of the disease, before advancing rapidly to the central nervous system along the peripheral nerves. It is hypothesized that limited viral replication at the site of infection occurs (usually myocytes) before the virus enters local nerve cells. Only later are peripheral nerves of the limb infected. At the entry site, the virus appears to be taken up into local muscle cells, where it becomes sequestered without activating the host's immune system. After a delay, the virus may replicate in the muscle fibers to yield sufficient virus to invade peripheral nerves through the neuromuscular junction by attachment to acetylcholinesterase receptors. Uptake of virus into cells is mediated by attachment of the viral G protein to cell surface receptors, which are expressed on various nerve and muscle tissues as well as cells in the immune system. The virus travels up the peripheral nerve axons by retrograde axoplasmic flow to reach the spinal cord and brain as the principal focus of infection, where it replicates and spreads widely to coincide with the onset of clinical signs and symptoms. These are attributable to brain cell damage and inflammation (nonsuppurative), with initial lesions most commonly in the cervical spinal cord, hindbrain, and hypothalamus. After these initial lesions, the virus spreads centrifugally to peripheral organs along nerve axons, with resulting infection in most tissues. By using quantitative molecular techniques for measuring viral loads, it is clear that the highest levels of virus are located in the salivary glands, adrenals, cornea, and regions of the brain, especially the cerebellum, hippocampus, and medulla, before death ensues. Within the central nervous system, the virus infects neurons and dendrites, with virus budding occurring from neuronal cell surfaces and synapses. The incubation period between the entry of the infection and the onset of clinical disease signs and symptoms is highly variable, depending on the infective dose amount, the virus strain, the host species, and the entry site of infection.

There is currently no explanation of how the virus persists in the site of inoculation without stimulating the host's immune response. It is not certain whether the saliva of the rabid animal plays an immunomodulating or suppressive role. Studies have shown that pathogenic strains of rabies virus cause antigen-specific suppression of B- and T-cell–mediated immune responses compared with nonpathogenic or inactivated pathogenic strains.

CLINICAL FEATURES OF HUMAN RABIES

Although the incubation period from exposure to the development of clinical rabies is highly variable, ranging from 7 days to more than a year, in most cases it is 30 to 90 days. The onset of clinical rabies is characterized by nonspecific prodromal features consisting of headache, fever, anorexia, nausea, vomiting, and diarrhea. This may be associated with symptoms such as anxiety, aggression, insomnia, hallucinations, and nightmares. These symptoms include pain and pruritus at the site of virus entry. The patient may also complain of an intolerance to tactile, auditory, and visual stimuli. Paresthesia or pain at the bite site, observed in about 45% of cases, may be followed by progressive pain or numbness in the limbs. Usually within 4 to 7 days, from the onset of symptoms, pain from the neck is reported, and it increases in intensity before becoming a permanent headache. The two basic clinical patterns of human rabies are: furious rabies and dumb rabies. Hyperexcitability and hydrophobia are characteristic of the furious (encephalitic) form of rabies. Clinical symptoms progress rapidly, especially as the virus spreads through the central nervous system and the neurologic impairment increases. The sight or mention of water or the word *rabies* usually exacerbates hydrophobia and aerophobia, with hyperventilation and laryngeal and diaphragmatic spasms. Symptoms often fluctuate with paroxysms of hyperventilation and dysphagia, usually provoked by sight or sound of water, that are punctuated by periods of relative lucidity. Other symptoms include hypersalivation and altered perception. A fear of death is often continually expressed; then, confusion, urinary incontinence, and atrial fibrillation are followed by respiratory spasms, breathing difficulties, convulsions, profuse salivation, and, ultimately, cardiorespiratory arrest. In contrast, ascending paralysis with sphincter involvement is characteristic of the paralytic or dumb form of the disease. Paralysis usually involves the bitten limb initially. The paralysis then spreads rapidly and symmetrically, with a loss of sphincter control and paralysis of the muscles of deglutination and respiration. The latter usually occurs as a terminal event.

DIAGNOSTIC METHODS

Diagnosis can usually be made on clinical grounds in the first instance, especially if there is a history of travel to a rabies-endemic country or evidence of a bite wound. In general, rabies is diagnosed in many laboratories after positive histologic examination of brain tissue by the direct fluorescent antibody test (FAT), which employs the detection of the nucleocapsid protein. The FAT is a rapid test (2 to 3 hours) with high specificity. Histopathologic preparation on formalin fixed brain preparations, stained with hematoxylin and eosin, can be performed within 2 hours of sample receipt. Aggregates of viral protein (Negri bodies) often accumulate within certain brain cells (particularly the hippocampus) and can be seen under the light microscope. Although the method is rapid, it has a low specificity and sensitivity compared with other methods. Virus isolation is performed by a homogenized suspension of suspect tissue (normally brain tissue) by the mouse inoculation test, administered to mice by intracranial injection. The mice are monitored for up to 28 days after infection. The rabies tissue culture inoculation test is comparable to the mouse inoculation test, and the results are obtained within 4 days. Laboratories with access to highly specific monoclonal antibodies can use immunohistochemical techniques in detecting antigen in fixed tissues. Molecular techniques including the reverse transcriptase polymerase chain reaction provide the ability to investigate antemortem diagnosis and thus can be used to identify the presence of viral RNA. An advantage of molecular diagnostic techniques, especially reverse transcriptase polymerase chain reaction, is the ability to amplify template in preparation for sequencing.

The G and N gene products are the major stimuli involved in eliciting an immune response in vaccinated animals and therefore have been the focus of many studies including molecular epidemiology. In general, the highly variable regions of the genome are more likely to represent the natural evolution of the virus outside any external selective pressure and the most suitable for differentiating closely related isolates. In contrast, the conserved regions are suitable for typing distantly related lyssaviruses.

The effective use of antemortem testing was demonstrated in a human case of rabies imported to the

United Kingdom. The patient had recently returned from the Philippines, where he reported being bitten on the palm of the hand by a stray dog. Saliva, cerebrospinal fluid, and skin biopsies (from the wound site and nape of the neck) were submitted for conventional antemortem diagnostic techniques. Established diagnostic techniques, including the mouse inoculation test and the rabies tissue culture inoculation test, failed to detect the virus. In contrast, a hemi-nested reverse transcriptase polymerase chain reaction followed by automated sequencing confirmed the presence of a canine variant of RABV (genotype 1) in both the saliva and skin specimens within 36 hours of sample submission. Subsequent phylogenetic analysis demonstrated that this isolate was closely related to that of a currently circulating dog strain in the Philippines.

TREATMENT

Persons who are bitten in a rabies-endemic country by a wild or domestic animal are encouraged first to wash the bite site with soap and to seek immediate medical attention.

Rabies is preventable by correct postexposure treatment employing conventional (modern, cell culture–based) human rabies vaccines in combination with other therapies, particularly with rabies immunoglobulin (RIG). Postexposure treatment is also available to anyone seeking medical attention after a bite from a rabies-suspect animal, especially if the animal has tested positive for rabies at an established diagnostic laboratory.

In low-risk exposures, postexposure treatment incorporating a full course of vaccination with five intramuscular injections is used. This regimen elicits a slow but detectable rabies-specific neutralizing antibody response within a few weeks. In contrast, elicitation of a rapid immune response can be achieved using an accelerated regimen, normally with multiple (four or eight) sites.

Current data show that vaccination with RIG provides the best protection against rabies. In all human rabies exposures, immunoglobulin should be considered for use in combination with vaccine, administered on day 0 (20 IU/kg), except when a previous full course of prophylaxis has been completed. In countries where human RIG is not available, equine RIG is an alternative source of immunoglobulin.

RAT-BITE FEVER

method of
GRACE Y. MINAMOTO, M.D., and
SHOBHA SWAMINATHAN, M.D.
Albert Einstein College of Medicine
Bronx, New York

Rat-bite fever refers to similar acute febrile illnesses caused by two different gram-negative organisms: *Streptobacillus moniliformis*, responsible for the majority of the cases in the United States; and *Spirillum minus*, more commonly associated with cases seen in Asia. Accurate data about the true incidence in the United States are not available because the disease is not reportable in any state. Although most cases are acquired through the bites or scratches of infected rats, some cases have also been reported with the bites of mice, gerbils, and squirrels. Nasopharyngeal carriage rates in healthy laboratory rats range from 10% to 100%, as compared with wild rats, with an estimated carriage rate of 50% to 100%. The low incidence of reported cases may result from a true low incidence of disease, a low index of suspicion and reporting of rat bites, and the fastidious growth requirements of the organism. Although most cases involve laboratory personnel, sporadic cases involving children living in unsanitary conditions with possible exposure to food or water potentially contaminated with rat feces have been reported. Haverhill fever is a clinically similar disease occurring in epidemic form, caused by *S. moniliformis* via ingestion of contaminated food or water rather than by direct rodent contact. Two large outbreaks of Haverhill fever were reported in which the implicated sources were raw milk and contaminated drinking water. Human-to-human transmission has not been documented.

BACTERIOLOGY

S. moniliformis is a pleomorphic, anaerobic gram-negative filamentous rod. Its tendency to form long chains with intermittent beadlike swellings gives it the name *moniliformis*. It is a nonmotile, nonencapsulated, microaerophilic organism requiring a carbon dioxide pressure between 8% and 10 %. Culture media supplementation with 10% to 20% serum, blood, or ascitic fluid is required for optimal growth of the organism.

On blood agar plates, growth of colonies resembling cotton balls can be detected between 3 and 5 days. Growth can be inhibited by the presence of sodium polyanethol sulfonate, which is used as an anticoagulant in blood culture bottles. Hence, when this organism is suspected, cultures should be obtained using polyanethol sulfonate–free or resin-containing bottles. The organism is oxidase-, catalase-, indole-, and urease-negative; additional carbohydrate utilization tests may be performed (although these tests should be incubated for 3 weeks before the results are read). Rapid identification is possible using gas-liquid chromatography to identify its characteristic fatty acid profile or by enzyme strip assay for the detection of its various aminopeptidases and glycosidases. This organism is capable of forming cell wall–deficient L forms, thereby rendering itself resistant to penicillin both in vivo and in vitro.

S. minus is a short gram-negative spiral rod that cannot be cultured on artificial media. It may be visualized by Giemsa or Wright staining of specimens, by darkfield microscopic examination, and by examination of mice and guinea pigs intraperitoneally inoculated with specimens.

CLINICAL MANIFESTATIONS

Rat-bite fever caused by *S. moniliformis* presents with an abrupt onset of fever, chills, headache, severe myalgias, and migratory arthralgias, usually within 10 days (range, 2 to 22 days) of exposure. The bite or exposure may not be recalled by the patient; the wound may have healed, or the bite may have occurred during sleep. The disease is often accompanied by an erythematous maculopapular or petechial rash involving the distal extremities and at times the palms and soles. Although asymmetric migratory polyarthritis is often present, monoarthritis involving the hip, knees, ankle, and wrist joints has also been reported in the literature. Other focal septic complications that have been reported include endocarditis, pneumonia, pericarditis, myocarditis, meningitis, chorioamnionitis (with an intact membrane), and abscesses in most organs. Regional lymphadenopathy is minimal to absent. The peripheral white blood cell count may be as high as $30,000/mm^3$. Up to 25% of patients may have false-positive results of non-treponemal tests for syphilis. Typically, fever subsides spontaneously within 3 to 5 days, and the other symptoms usually resolve within 2 weeks even without specific therapy.

Haverhill fever, caused by *S. moniliformis* by ingestion of contaminated water or food, derives its name from the town in Massachusetts where it was first described in 1926. Generally similar to disease caused by direct inoculation, it differs by the prominence of vomiting and pharyngitis among patients.

Disease caused by *S. minus*, also called sodoku in Japan, is characterized by a more prolonged incubation period (1 to 6 weeks) and more pronounced local symptoms. The site of the bite can often become painful and ulcerated, and it is associated with localized lymphadenopathy. The local inflammation stage is followed by fever, chills, headache, malaise, and an erythematous maculopapular rash involving the extremities. It may present as intermittent febrile episodes lasting for 3 to 4 days at each occurrence before complete resolution of symptoms. The range of complications reported includes endocarditis, meningitis, pleural effusions, hepatitis, and splenomegaly.

DIAGNOSIS

The first step toward the diagnosis is the recognition of a compatible clinical picture in a patient with a history of a rodent bite or exposure. In the absence of such a history, the diagnosis can become challenging. The differential diagnosis may include meningococcemia, enteric fever, syphilis, Lyme disease, viral exanthem, rickettsial infection, septic arthritis, endocarditis, and acute rheumatic fever. Because disease caused by both organisms can resolve spontaneously without treatment and then relapse over subsequent months, the clinical presentation may be one of relapsing fever or fever of unknown origin. Additionally, the difficulty in isolation of the organism and the occasional occurrence of L forms of *S. moniliformis* that do not grow on artificial media contribute further to the difficulties in diagnosis. *S. moniliformis* can be cultured from blood, joint fluid, and other body fluid specimens, but the laboratory must be notified that a case is suspected, so enriched media can be used to increase the diagnostic yield. Serologic tests for *S. moniliformis* include detection of specific agglutinins with a documented fourfold rise in titer and an enzyme-linked immunosorbent assay for the detection of specific antibody. A polymerase chain reaction assay for the detection of specific deoxyribonucleic acid has also become available at research laboratories.

S. minus can be seen in tissue by Giemsa or Wright stain or darkfield microscopy. Xenodiagnosis by examination of peritoneal fluid from inoculated mice or guinea pigs is currently the only means of recovering the organism.

TREATMENT

Penicillin remains the drug of choice for the treatment of this disease, regardless of the causative organism. Initial therapy with intravenous penicillin G at a total of 12 to 24 million U/day for 1 week, followed by completion with oral penicillin or ampicillin therapy for an additional week, is recommended. Longer courses with higher-dose (up to 24 million U/day of penicillin) intravenous therapy may be needed for complicated cases such as in patients with endocarditis or other deep-seated infections. Patients should be alerted to the possibility of the Jarisch-Herxheimer reaction that may occasionally occur with treatment of *S. minus* infection. In patients allergic to penicillin, effective alternatives include tetracycline* (500 mg every 6 hours) or streptomycin* (7.5 mg/kg every 12 hours; limited by ototoxicity). There is limited information on the use of erythromycin (E-Mycin),* chloramphenicol (Chloromycetin),* clindamycin (Cleocin),* and cephalosporins for the treatment of this disease; however, cephalosporins have been reported to have significant in vitro activity against *S. moniliformis*. Mortality from untreated rat-bite fever can be up to 10%, especially among infants and the elderly.

PREVENTION

The most effective means of prevention include the minimization of exposure to rats by effective pest control measures, avoidance of potentially contaminated water and raw milk, and use of gloves by laboratory personnel during the handling of rodents. After a rodent bite, the wound should be cleansed thoroughly. The role of prophylactic antibiotics, such as a course of oral penicillin, although seemingly reasonable, is unclear. Tetanus prophylaxis should be administered as indicated by the patient's immunization history.

---

*Not FDA approved for this indication.

RELAPSING FEVER

method of
DIEGO CADAVID, M.D.
University of Medicine and Dentistry of New Jersey–New Jersey Medical School
Newark, New Jersey

Relapsing fever is one of several diseases caused by spirochetes. Other human spirochetal diseases are syphilis, Lyme disease, and leptospirosis. Notable features of spirochetes are wavy and helical shapes, length-diameter ratios of as much as 100:1, and flagella that lie between the inner and outer cell membranes. The spirochetes that cause relapsing fever are in the genus *Borrelia*. Other *Borrelia* species cause Lyme disease, avian spirochetosis, and epidemic bovine abortion. Table 1 shows the main species of relapsing fever *Borrelia* species, their vectors, and an estimate of their geographic ranges. In the United States, relapsing fever has been considered a disease endemic only in the West. However, the more recent finding of relapsing fever–like *Borrelia* species in ticks and dogs in the Eastern United States suggests that the risk of relapsing fever may extend into the East.

EPIDEMIOLOGY

There are two forms of relapsing fever: epidemic, transmitted to humans by the body louse *Pediculus humanus* (louse-borne relapsing fever [LBRF]), and endemic, transmitted to humans by soft-bodied ticks of the genus *Ornithodoros* (tick-borne relapsing fever [TBRF]). In LBRF, itching caused by skin infestation with lice leads to scratching, which may result in crushing of lice and release of infected hemolymph into areas of skin abrasion. Louse infestation is associated with cold weather and a lack of hygiene. Migrant workers and soldiers at war are particularly susceptible to this infection. Historically, massive outbreaks of LBRF have occurred in Eurasia, Africa, and Latin America, but currently the disease is found only in Ethiopia and neighboring countries.

The main risk factor for TBRF is exposure to endemic areas (see Table 1). The risk of infection increases with outdoor activities in areas where rodents nest, such as entering caves or sleeping in rustic cabins. *Ornithodoros* are soft-bodied ticks that feed for short periods (minutes), usually at night. They can live many years between blood meals and may transmit spirochetes to their offspring transovarially. Infection is produced by regurgitation of infected tick saliva into the skin wound during tick feeding. There are several natural vertebrate reservoirs for TBRF *Borrelia* species, but the most common are rodents (deer mice, chipmunks, squirrels, and rats). In contrast, the body louse *P. humanus* is a strict human parasite, living and multiplying in clothing.

CLINICAL DIAGNOSIS

Relapsing fever should be suspected in any patient presenting with two or more episodes of high fever and constitutional symptoms spaced by periods of relative well-being. The index of suspicion increases if the patient has been exposed to endemic areas for TBRF or to countries where LBRF still occurs (see Table 1). Whereas LBRF is usually associated with a single relapse, TBRF usually has multiple relapses (up to 13). In LBRF, the second episode of fever is typically milder than the first; in TBRF, the multiple febrile periods are usually of equal severity. The febrile periods last 1 to 3 days, and the intervals between fevers are 3 to 10 days. During the febrile periods, numerous spirochetes are circulating in the blood. This is called *spirochetemia* and is sometimes unexpectedly detected during routine blood smear examinations. Between fevers, spirochetemia is not observed. The fever pattern and recurrent spirochetemia are the consequences of antigenic variation of the relapsing fever *Borrelia* species, specifically of the variable outer membrane proteins that confer serotype identity.

The latency between exposure to ticks in the endemic form or to lice in the epidemic form and the onset of symptoms is around 6 days (range, 3 to 18). Because *Ornithodoros* ticks feed briefly and painlessly at night, patients with TBRF may not be able to recall having been bitten by a tick. The clinical manifestations of TBRF and LBRF are similar, although some differences do exist. Table 2 lists the frequency of the most common manifestations of TBRF. The usual initial presentation is sudden onset of chills, followed

TABLE 1. **Relapsing Fever *Borrelia* Species Pathogenic to Human Beings**

Relapsing Fever	*Borrelia* Species	Arthropod Vector	Distribution of Disease
Endemic	*B. hermsii*	*Ornithodoros hermsi*	Western North America
	B. turicatae	*Ornithodoros turicata*	Southwestern North America and Northern Mexico
	B. venezuelensis	*Ornithodoros rudis*	Central America and Northern South America
	B. hispanica	*Ornithodoros marocanus*	Iberian peninsula and Northwestern Africa
	B. crocidurae	*Ornithodoros erraticus*	North and East Africa, Middle East, Southern Europe
	B. duttoni	*Ornithodoros moubata*	Sub-Saharan Africa
	B. persica	*Ornithodoros tholozani*	Middle East, Greece, Central Asia
	B. uzbekistana	*Ornithodoros papillipes*	Tajikistan, Uzbekistan
Epidemic	*B. recurrentis*	*Pediculus humanus*	Worldwide (recently only in East Africa)

TABLE 2. **Frequent Clinical Manifestations of Tick-Borne Relapsing Fever**

Sign or Symptom	Frequency (%)
Headache	94
Myalgia	92
Chills	88
Nausea	76
Arthralgia	73
Vomiting	71
Abdominal pain	44
Confusion	38
Dry cough	27
Ocular pain	26
Diarrhea	25
Dizziness	25
Photophobia	25
Neck pain	24
Rash	18
Dysuria	13
Jaundice	10
Hepatomegaly	10
Splenomegaly	6

by high fever, tachycardia, severe headache, vomiting, myalgia and arthralgia, and often delirium. In the early stages, a reddish rash may be seen over the trunk, arms, or legs. The fever remains high for 3 to 5 days, and then it clears abruptly. After an asymptomatic period of 7 to 10 days, the fever and other constitutional symptoms can reappear suddenly. The febrile episodes gradually become less severe, and the person eventually recovers completely. As the disease progresses, fever, jaundice, hepatosplenomegaly, cardiac arrhythmias, and cardiac failure may occur, especially with LBRF. Jaundice is more common at times of relapses. Patients with LBRF are also more likely to develop petechiae on the trunk, extremities, and mucous membranes, epistaxis, and blood-tinged sputum. Rupture of the spleen rarely occurs. Multiple neurologic complications can occur in LBRF as a result of disseminated intravascular coagulation and in TBRF as a result of infection of the meninges and cranial and spinal nerve roots by spirochetes. The most common neurologic complications of TBRF are aseptic meningitis and facial palsy. Relapsing fever in pregnant women can cause abortion, premature birth, and neonatal death. Sometimes patients can have nonfebrile relapses, consisting of periods of severe headache, backache, weakness, and other constitutional symptoms without fever that occur at the time of expected relapses. Delirium may persist for weeks after the fever resolves.

Relapsing fever may be confused with many diseases that are relapsing or cause high fevers. These include thyphoid fever, yellow fever, dengue, African hemorrhagic fevers, African trypanosomiasis, brucellosis, malaria, leptospirosis, rat-bite fever, intermittent cholangitis, cat-scratch disease, and echovirus 9 infection, among others. TBRF *Borrelia* species have antigens that are cross-reactive with Lyme disease *Borrelia* species, and inasmuch as the endemic areas of relapsing fever and Lyme disease overlap to some extent, confusion between the two infections can be expected. Although the pattern of recurring fever is the clue to diagnosing relapsing fever, confirmation of the diagnosis requires demonstration of spirochetes in peripheral blood taken during an episode of fever.

LABORATORY DIAGNOSIS

The comparatively large number of spirochetes in the blood during relapsing fever provides the opportunity for the simplest method for laboratory diagnosis of the infection, light-microscopy of Wright- or Giemsa-stained thin blood smears or darkfield or phase-contrast microscopy of a wet mount of plasma. The blood should be obtained during or just before the peaks of body temperature. Between fever peaks, spirochetes often can be demonstrated by inoculations of blood or cerebrospinal fluid into special culture medium or experimental animals. Enrichment for spirochetes is achieved by using the platelet-rich fraction of plasma or the buffy coat of sedimented blood. In the United States, the most common causes of relapsing fever are *Borrelia hermsii* and *Borrelia turicatae*; both will grow in BSK-H medium (commercially available from Sigma) and in young mice or rats. Whereas direct visual detection of organisms in the blood or cerebrospinal fluid is the most common method for laboratory confirmation of relapsing fever, immunoassays for antibodies are the most common means of laboratory confirmation for Lyme disease. Although serologic assays have been developed for the agents of relapsing fever, these are not widely available and are of dubious utility. The antigenic variation displayed by the relapsing fever species means that there may be hundreds of different "serotypes." If a different serotype or species is used for preparing the antigen, only antibodies to conserved antigens may be detected. For this reason, a standardized enzyme-linked immunosorbent assay (ELISA) with Lyme disease *Borrelia* species as antigen may be the best available serologic assay for relapsing fever. ELISA for anti-*Borrelia burgdorferi* antibodies is routinely done across the United States and Europe. If a positive result for IgM or IgG antibodies is obtained, the Western blot for antibodies to *B. burgdorferi* antigens would be expected to discriminate current or past Lyme disease from relapsing fever, as well as from syphilis, another cause of the positive Lyme disease ELISA result. Other frequent laboratory abnormalities can occur in relapsing fever but are not diagnostic. These include elevated white blood cell count with increased neutrophils, thrombocytopenia, increased serum bilirubin, proteinuria, microhematuria, prolongation of the prothrombin time and partial thromboplastin time, and elevation of fibrin degradation products.

TREATMENT

Relapsing fever *Borrelia* species are very sensitive to several antibiotics, and antimicrobial resistance is rare. Treatment options for adults and children younger than 8 years old are summarized in Table 3. Children older than 8 years old can be treated with the same antibiotics as adults, but the doses should be adjusted by weight. Before antibiotics are given, the possibility of causing the Jarisch-Herxheimer reaction (JHR) should be considered (see later). The tetracycline antibiotics are most commonly used for treatment of LBRF and TBRF. The first antibiotic of choice in adults and children older than 8 years old is doxycycline (Vibramycin). In general, shorter treatments are needed for LBRF than for TBRF. Single-dose therapy is usually recommended for LBRF. In TBRF, sometimes multiple doses of tetracyclines for up to 10 days cannot prevent relapses, and re-treatment may be necessary. Alternative oral antibiotics to the tetracyclines are erythromycin, penicillin, and chloramphenicol (see Table 3). Erythromycin and penicillin do not appear to be as effective as the tetracyclines; however, they are the drugs of choice for children younger than 8 years old and for pregnant women.

Although treatment with antibiotics is usually given orally, these drugs may need to be given intravenously if severe vomiting makes swallowing impractical. If the patient has symptoms and signs of meningitis or encephalitis without clinical and/or radiologic signs of increased intracranial pressure, the cerebrospinal fluid should be examined to rule out central nervous system infection. The finding of elevation of cerebrospinal fluid cells and protein demands the use of parenteral antibiotics, such as penicillin G or ceftriaxone (Rocephin). Optimally, antibiotic treatment should be started during afebrile periods when spirochetemia is low. Starting therapy near the peak of a febrile period may induce the JHR, in which high fever and a rise and subsequent fall sometimes to dangerous low levels in blood pressure may occur. Dehydration should be treated with fluids given intravenously. Severe headache can be treated with pain relievers such as codeine, and nausea or vomiting can be treated with prochlorperazine.

TABLE 3. **Treatment Options for Tick-Borne Relapsing Fever***

Adults

Nonsevere Forms

1. Doxycycline 100 mg PO bid for 1-2 wk†
2. Tetracycline 500 mg PO qid for 1-2 wk
3. Erythromycin 500 mg PO tid for 1-2 wk
4. Chloramphenicol 500 mg PO qid for 1-2 wk

Severe Forms

1. Ceftriaxone 2 g IV qd for 1-2 wk
2. Penicillin G 4 million U IV q4h for 1-2 wk

Children ≤8 years old

Nonsevere Forms

1. Erythromycin 30-50 mg/kg/d divided tid for 1-2 wk
2. Penicillin V 25-50 mg/kg/d divided qid for 1-2 wk

Severe Forms

1. Ceftriaxone 75-100 mg/kg/d IV for 1-2 wk
2. Penicillin G 300,000 U/kg/d, IV divided q4h for 1-2 wk

*Single doses of oral agents are used for treatment of all forms of louse-borne relapsing fever.

†In general, treatment for 1 week is recommended in early/milder cases and for up to 2 weeks for more severe cases.

JARISCH-HERXHEIMER REACTION

Antibiotic treatment of relapsing fever causes JHR in as many as 60% of cases. The JHR is more common in LBRF than in TBRF. It is characterized by the sudden onset of tachycardia, hypotension, chills, rigors, diaphoresis, and high fever. Patients with the JHR have been known to say that they felt as if they were going to die. It is caused by the rapid killing of circulating spirochetes 1 to 4 hours after the first dose of antibiotic that results in the release of large amounts of *Borrelia* lipoproteins in the circulation, followed by massive release of tumor necrosis factor and other cytokines. If possible, patients with the JHR should be transferred to an intensive care unit for close monitoring and treatment. During several hours, the temperature declines and the patient feels better. Large amounts of intravenous fluids (0.9% sodium chloride solution) may be required to treat hypotension. Steroids and nonsteroidal anti-inflammatory agents have no effect on the frequency or severity of the JHR. One study found that pretreatment with sheep anti–tumor necrosis factor-α monoclonal antibody (Fab fragment) suppressed JHR after penicillin treatment for LBRF and reduced the associated increases in plasma cytokines. Death can occur as a result of the JHR secondary to cardiovascular collapse in up to 5% of patients with treated LBRF and much less frequently in TBRF.

OUTCOME

Complete recovery occurs in 95% or more of adequately treated patients. The prognosis varies for untreated cases or when treatment is delayed. Mortality as high as 40% has been reported in untreated epidemics of LBRF. Relapsing fever also has a high mortality in neonates. Some neurologic sequelae can occur in patients with TBRF complicated with neuroborreliosis.

PREVENTION

Prevention of TBRF involves avoidance of rodent- and tick-infested dwellings such as animal burrows, caves, and abandoned cabins. Wearing clothing that protects skin from tick access (e.g., long pants and long-sleeved shirts) is also helpful. Repellents and acaricides provide additional protection. DEET, N,N-diethyl-*m*-toluamide, repels ticks when it is applied to clothing or skin, but it must be used with caution: it loses its effectiveness within one to several hours when applied to skin and must be reapplied; it is absorbed through the skin and may cause central nervous system toxicity if used excessively. Permethrin, an acaricide, is safer and more effective. Applied to clothing, it provides protection for 24 hours or more, and it is poorly absorbed cutaneously and causes no adverse systemic effects. In LBRF, prevention can be achieved by promoting personal hygiene and by dusting undergarments and the inside of clothing with malathion or lindane powder when available. Widespread antibiotic use may be necessary to control epidemics of LBRF, using one or two doses of 100 mg doxycycline given within 1 week.

LYME DISEASE

method of
LEONARD H. SIGAL, M.D.
Pharmaceutical Research Institute
Bristol-Myers Squibb
Princeton, New Jersey

and

Department of Medicine and Pediatrics
UMDNJ-Robert Wood Johnson Medical School
New Brunswick, New Jersey

What is Lyme disease? Infection with *Borrelia burgdorferi* is the quick answer, but there is a swirl of controversy and debate about the correct answer. To simplify this issue I propose using terms to describe the various manifestations seen in the complex illness known as "Lyme disease."

Lyme borreliosis: active infection with *B. burgdorferi;* may persist for long periods in the absence of antibiotic therapy. Can be divided into three overlapping clinical groups:

- Early localized infection
- Early disseminated infection
- Late infection

Resolving Lyme disease: self-limited complaints that linger after antibiotic therapy

Post–Lyme disease syndromes: complaints that continue after cessation of antibiotics; a variety of underlying causes of debility include:

- Permanent damage from previous Lyme disease
- Intercurrent illness, unrelated to prior Lyme disease
- Problems that follow *B. burgdorferi* infection but are not due to ongoing infection, e.g.,
  - patellofemoral joint dysfunction due to quadriceps atrophy
  - fibromyalgia related to sleep disorder

Understanding the precise causes of a patient's debility is pivotal in developing appropriate therapies. Confusion about Lyme disease results in many incorrect and unfortunate therapeutic choices. Thus it may be quite helpful to discuss therapeutic interventions for each of the clinical entities described previously. Before beginning, however, it is important to note that Lyme borreliosis occurs in Europe but differs somewhat from the disease in the United States. In Europe Lyme borreliosis is often the result of other organisms within the species *B. burgdorferi* sensu lato and occurs in a patient population that differs from that seen in the United States. Thus it may not be wise to extrapolate from the European experience to practice in the United States, especially when it comes to recommended antibiotic regimens. As a general principle, appropriate antibiotic therapy usually rapidly cures and prevents progression of *B. burgdorferi* infection to later features of Lyme disease, although nonspecific symptoms may persist for many months before they, too, resolve without further antibiotic therapy.

LYME BORRELIOSIS

B. burgdorferi is introduced by the bite of an infected ixodid tick. In the unfed, infected tick *B. burgdorferi* is found on the inner aspect of the midgut. Many hours after the tick introduces its mouth parts into the skin of its unwitting host blood arrives in the tick's midgut, causing *B. burgdorferi* to proliferate and alter its repertoire of surface proteins, ultimately allowing the organism to escape the midgut and enter the rest of the tick, notably the salivary glands. This process takes 36 or more hours after initiation of feeding. After removing the nutrients from blood the tick is left with a large volume of water to dispose of—this is done by making and excreting saliva into the wound from which the blood was removed. If the organism is present in the salivary glands, it can pass into the mammalian host in the secreted saliva. Thus there is a long period between attachment of the tick and passage of the organism during which one can abort the infection. A tick check after outdoor activities may reveal an attached but nonengorged tick; removal of the tick prevents infection because the organism has not yet been passed. Especially useful during "Lyme disease season" is a daily shower—an unattached tick will be dislodged by the light abrasion of a washcloth. Thus inexpensive and nontoxic personal strategies can be quite useful in the prevention of Lyme disease.

We know much about the ecology of Lyme disease that can allow us to minimize the risk of becoming infected: (1) much Lyme disease is acquired peridomestically; (2) the tick is usually found in the leaf clutter at the floor of the forest; and (3) the tick desiccates in direct sun and cannot survive on exposed lawns and other surfaces. There are methods of modifying one's own property to minimize the likelihood of Lyme disease near one's house, including, but not limited to: (1) cleaning shrubs, grass, and clutter between the property and surrounding forest; (2) placing a yard's width of wood chips at the boundary; and (3) if deemed *absolutely* necessary, chemically treating the wood chips, not the entire lawn, with acaricides. In hyperendemic areas many people took advantage of the outer surface A protein (OspA) vaccine, but this product was removed from the market earlier this year. Other candidate vaccines are under consideration but none is yet in clinical trials.

Lyme borreliosis can be divided into three overlapping and nonexclusive clinical groupings (Table 1).

Early Localized Disease

Erythema migrans (EM; the virtually pathognomonic expanding erythematous skin lesion) develops in up to 90% of patients with Lyme disease 1 to 30 days after the tick bite (mean is 7 to 10 days). The tick seeks out warm and moist places and climbs against gravity to feed; the tick that causes Lyme disease in the northeast, middle Atlantic states and Midwest is named *Ixodes scapularis* because it climbs up to the deer's scapula (shoulder) for its preferred residence. EM is most common in the groin and under the

TABLE 1. **Clinical Manifestations of Lyme Disease**

Early localized disease: occurs days to a month after the tick bite
Erythema migrans (in up to 90% of patients; bull's eye rash in about 1/3 of these—multiple in 10% of patients with EM)
Non-specific "virus-like symptoms": Fatigue/malaise/lethargy; myalgia; arthralgia; headache
Sleep disorder
Arthralgias
Regional/Generalized lymphadenopathy
Early disseminated disease[1]***:*** occurs days to 10 months after the tick bite
Carditis—in 5% to 10% of **untreated** patients
  Conduction defects
  Mild cardiomyopathy
Neurologic—in 10% to 15% of **untreated** patients
  Meningitis
  Encephalitis
  Cranial neuropathy (most often facial, which can be bilateral)
  Peripheral neuropathy/radiculopathy
  Myelitis
Musculoskeletal—approximately 50% of **untreated** patients
  Migratory polyarthritis and/or polyarthralgias
Cutaneous: Lymphadenosis benigna cutis (Lymphocytoma)—Europe, rare in US
Ophthalmologic: Conjunctivitis, Iritis, Choroiditis—all uncommon
Late disease[1]***:*** occurs months to years after the tick bite
Musculoskeletal—about 50% of **untreated** patients develop migratory polyarthritis
  about 10% of **untreated** patients develop chronic monoarthritis, usually of the knee
Neurologic disease—Chronic, often subtle, encephalopathy
  Chronic, often subtle, axonal neuropathy
Cutaneous—Acrodermatitis chronica atrophicans—Europe, rare in US

[1]May occur in the absence of any prior features of Lyme disease, i.e., may be the first feature of *Borrelia burgdorferi* infection.

buttocks, in the popliteal fossa, at the midriff, under the arms, and on the scalp (especially in children). The serologic immune response to *B. burgdorferi* may not be measurable for up to 6 or 8 weeks after the infected tick bite—thus some patients develop EM but are still seronegative. For this reason, we do not obtain a blood sample from a patient with EM; if a lesion appears to be a classic EM we treat, but do not test.

There can be an asymptomatic period between tick feeding/organism passage and the development of a syndrome of *B. burgdorferi* infection, during which time the infection is developing. Nadelman and colleagues have shown a single dose of 200 mg of doxycycline (Vibramycin)* can interrupt the infection and prevent progression to clinical Lyme borreliosis. There is debate about the use of this approach; the 87% protection was from a rate of 8 of 247 (3.2%) placebo-treated to 1 of 235 (0.4%) antibiotic-treated subjects; although significant at $P < .04$, the 95% confidence intervals are 25% to 98%. Many people are bitten repeatedly, which would lead to multiple treatments. If clinicians cannot differentiate *I. scapularis* from other ticks these patients will be retreated repeatedly for no reason. Selective use of prophylaxis in people with known engorged *I. scapularis* bites might be more reasonable.

Some patients have nonspecific symptoms resembling a viral infection in the days preceding the EM. Others have "virus-like symptoms" and no observed EM: this may be because there never was an EM or because the EM may have occurred on a part of the body that is hard to see (EM may be best seen using daylight). We have been impressed with the frequency with which sleep disturbances occur in early disease; this often resolves with antibiotics, but may persist for months or years.

EM must be differentiated from a cutaneous reaction to tick saliva. Such a reaction produces an erythema about 1 cm in diameter without further expansion, lasting for less than 36 hours. The other arthropod bite mentioned in discussions of EM is that of the brown recluse spider. These bites cause an immediate rapidly expanding painful erythema that can have central necrosis. The spider is encountered only upon invading its domain, so the bite is found on hands and feet after a person reaches into the spider's territory (e.g., an old shed, a wood pile, the corner of a garage). Thus there should be no difficulty in deciding if an erythema is EM or a spider bite. Treatment for EM is oral antibiotics, regardless of severity of associated symptoms (Table 2). With all features of Lyme borreliosis, nonspecific symptoms may persist after adequate antibiotics for 6 months or more. There is no reason to repeat antibiotic therapy—as long as there is no worsening of the symptoms and no objective evidence of new loci of inflammation the correct approach is support and symptomatic therapy only.

Early Disseminated Disease

Early disseminated disease occurs weeks to months after the EM; if no EM was observed, these may be the first noted manifestations of *B. burgdorferi* infection. Timing of the onset of the infection is important; if a feature of early disseminated disease occurs within a few weeks to a month of the infecting tick bite the patient may be seronegative despite having *B. burgdorferi* infection. Objective evidence of inflammation and organ dysfunction is crucial in supporting the diagnosis. Neurologic features occur in up to 15% of untreated patients. If meningitis is suspected, spinal fluid analysis (glucose, protein, Gram stain, and specific anti–*B. burgdorferi* antibody levels in fluid and blood) should be obtained. Lyme meningitis resembles and occurs in the same season as enterovirus meningitis. Many neurologists suggest patients with Lyme disease–related facial palsy have spinal fluid analysis, because therapy for isolated facial palsy is oral, whereas meningitis should be treated intravenously. A detailed neurologic exam should seek evidence of other cranial or peripheral neuropathies. Most facial palsies resolve entirely, although weakness may take months to clear. Meningitis also has a good prognosis, with symptoms decreasing quickly after therapy is started. Intravenous antibiotics for meningitis or peripheral neuropathies can be given at home with close follow-up. Swedish studies have shown that 28 days of oral doxycycline* can cure meningitis, but, as noted,

*Not FDA approved for this indication.

*Not FDA approved for this indication.

TABLE 2. **Current Recommendations for Therapy in Lyme Disease**

Early localized disease	Oral	2 weeks
EARLY DISSEMINATED DISEASE		
Isolated facial palsy	Oral	2 to 3 weeks
Meningitis, peripheral neuropathy, multiple cranial neuropathies, other CNS disorders	Intravenous	2 to 4 weeks
Mild carditis	Oral	2 to 3 weeks
Severe carditis	Intravenous	2 to 4 weeks May add prednisone 40 to 60 mg PO qd if severe and/or does not respond within 4 days of starting antibiotic therapy. Temporary pacemaker occasionally required.
LATE DISEASE		
Arthritis—initial treatment	Oral	6 to 8 weeks
Arthritis—if refractory to oral therapy	Intravenous	4 weeks
Tertiary neuroborreliosis	Intravenous	4 weeks
Drug regimens		
Oral therapy		
ADULTS		
Doxycycline* (Vibramycin)	100 mg. p.o. b.i.d.	
Amoxicillin[1,2]*	250 to 500 mg. p.o. q.i.d.	
If intolerant/allergic to the above		
Cefuroxime axetil (Ceftin)	500 mg p.o. b.i.d.	3 weeks[3]
Azithromycin* (Zithromax)	500 mg q.d.	7 to 10 days[3]
CHILDREN		
Amoxicillin*	50 mg/kg/day, divided dose	
Doxycycline**	100 mg. p.o. b.i.d.	
Erythromycin*	30 mg/kg/day, divided dose	
Penicillin G*	25 to 50 mg/kg/day, divided dose	
Intravenous Therapy		
ADULTS		
Third generation cephalosporins		
Ceftriaxone (Rocephin)	2 G q.d. or 1 G b.i.d.	
Cefotaxime* (Claforan)	3 G b.i.d.***	
Penicillin		
Penicillin G*	20 million units in 6 divided doses	
Chloramphenicol* (Chloromycetin)	50 mg/kg/day in 4 divided doses	
CHILDREN		
Third generation cephalosporins		
Ceftriaxone*	75 to 100 mg/kg/day	
Cefotaxime*	90 to 180 mg/kg/day, in 2 or 3 divided doses	
Penicillin		
Penicillin G*	300,000 U/kg/day in 6 divided doses	

[1]Dosage determined by size of patient
[2]No studies comparing amoxicillin with amoxicillin plus probenecid have been done; there is probably no reason to use probenecid.
[3]Duration recommendation for early localized disease.
*Not FDA approved for this application.
**Not recommended for children <8 yrs of age.
***Exceeds dosage recommended by the manufacturer.

extrapolation to U.S. practice from European experience may not be warranted.

An electrocardiogram (ECG) should be done to identify carditis, which can occur as an isolated finding in early disseminated disease. Lyme carditis occurs in 5% to 10% of untreated patients and typically causes bradycardia resulting from second- or third-degree heart block or can manifest as asymptomatic first degree or fascicular block. Multiple levels of damage occur, and the ECG may change patterns of block, representing the dominant lesion in the conducting system at that time. Lightheadedness, near syncope or syncope, palpitations, or chest discomfort is often associated with higher degrees of heart block. Cardiomyopathy and pericarditis are rare features of Lyme carditis. Oral therapy with careful monitoring should be given for first-degree block. Patients with more severe degrees of AV block should be hospitalized and treated with intravenous antibiotics; prednisone can be added in severe and refractory cases. Rarely, temporary pacing is needed. The outcome is usually favorable—conduction defects often begin to resolve before antibiotics are initiated.

Later Disease

Late features of Lyme borreliosis occur months to many years after inoculation with *B. burgdorferi* and may be the first identified features of the infection. Nearly all patients with late disease are strongly seropositive. Arthritis is a relatively common feature of untreated late borreliosis; 60% or more of untreated patients will have migratory arthralgias and some develop true inflammation. Up to 10% of untreated patients develop a chronic usually mono-arthritis, most often of the knee. Initial therapy of Lyme arthritis should be oral antibiotics for 6 weeks; intravenous therapy is reserved for refractory arthritis. Some will not respond to oral and intravenous therapy. Many of these patients are of the genetic type HLA-DRB10401, but there is *no* reason to test patients with arthritis or refractory arthritis in clinical practice; the test is expensive, the commercial serologic tests do not identify the specific types that actually impart risk of chronicity, and positivity merely represents a risk, it does not *assure*, chronicity. Treatment decisions do not rest on the results and it is imperfect as a prognostic tool—thus it should not be done. Testing that *is* useful is synovial fluid analysis; moderate leukocytosis with the presence of antibodies to *B. burgdorferi* within the fluid is expected. The value of this specific test is to assure that the arthritis is in fact Lyme arthritis. Lyme arthritis patients are almost always seropositive, but people with arthritis of another source can be seropositive because of prior Lyme borreliosis; the finding of concentration of specific antibodies within the fluid assures the diagnosis of Lyme arthritis. Polymerase chain reaction (PCR) studies of synovial fluid are often negative (more often positive on synovial tissue), and a negative PCR does not rule out the diagnosis of Lyme arthritis. Although a positive PCR from a reputable lab goes a long way to make the diagnosis, PCR should be a research tool and has not yet found a place in clinical medicine. Autoimmunity has not been proven as the cause of refractory Lyme arthritis and there is *no* role for immunomodulatory therapy in such cases.

Tertiary neuroborreliosis (TNB), the late neurologic features of Lyme borreliosis, includes cognitive dysfunction ("Lyme encephalopathy") or axonal polyneuropathy. TNB is estimated to occur in 5% or less of untreated patients; it can also be the first feature of *B. burgdorferi* infection. Formal cognitive studies should be done; although not specific, results of neuropsychologic studies can help support the diagnosis or suggest other causes of cognitive impairment and can be useful to formulate a rehabilitation strategy and as objective evidence of improvement. Spinal fluid should be studied for concentration of specific immunity. The fluid does not contain inflammatory cells; the only abnormality may be an elevated protein and specific antibodies. Abnormalities on single photon emission computed tomography and magnetic resonance imaging scans are common but not specific. Intravenous therapy is warranted, but response is typically quite slow, often taking 18 to 24 months for significant improvement to become apparent.

Lyme disease complicating pregnancy should be treated as is appropriate for the features of disease and there is no proof of risk to the fetus. Lyme disease is common in children; the good news is they typically have less severe disease and respond more rapidly and completely to appropriate regimens.

RESOLVING LYME DISEASE

In many of the features of *B. burgdorferi* infection reviewed previously, total resolution of findings and complaints may take weeks or months. EM usually resolves during therapy, but associated symptoms may last for up to 6 months; the patient ultimately improves without further therapy. Conduction block often begins to reverse even before therapy is complete, although there may be residual lower level block; there are rare examples of persisting block requiring permanent pacemaker. Meningitis usually resolves rapidly, but facial palsy may dissipate slowly and there are rare examples of significant residual weakness. Both Lyme arthritis and TNB may take months to years to disappear. In all examples, absent new foci of Lyme borreliosis–related damage or demonstrable worsening of the initial features of the disease, there is no proven reason to re-treat. If a new joint becomes inflamed or there is worsening of heart block, neuropathy or encephalopathy it is important to re-evaluate the patient carefully to make sure that no intercurrent disease has occurred and that the new or worsening problems are *B. burgdorferi* related; if they are, re-treatment is warranted. However, a slow and progressive improvement (often unrecognizable by the patient) is expected and does not represent a cause for alarm. Persistent features (e.g., facial palsy or heart block) may relate to the severity of initial damage or delay in therapy; human tissues have only a certain potential to heal. It is crucial not to treat "until symptoms resolve"; such a plan results in false expectations and overtreatment and may have unforeseen psychologic consequences (e.g., a patient who then becomes convinced that he or she has "chronic Lyme disease" forever and will never improve). Without an attempt at rehabilitation such a patient may become emotionally crippled by a nondisease.

POST–LYME DISEASE SYNDROMES

Emotional problems are not the only difficulties that can follow real *B. burgdorferi* infection. Three common examples deserve specific mention. The first is patellofemoral joint dysfunction, developing in people with prior true Lyme arthritis. Quadriceps atrophy resulting from prior knee inflammation causes mild instability in the patellofemoral joint, leading to knee pain (usually with minimal if any swelling), often misinterpreted as being a recurrence of the initial Lyme arthritis.

Sleep disturbances seem quite common after Lyme disease and may persist long after antibiotics are given;

sleep deprivation can cause cognitive and emotional problems and fatigue and do not respond to antibiotics. Fibromyalgia is commonly misidentified as TNB, because both can be associated with fatigue and cognitive dysfunction. In fibromyalgia both are usually related to an underlying sleep disorder. We have seen many patients with fibromyalgia seemingly resulting from a sleep disorder acquired during preceding Lyme borreliosis. The fibromyalgia does not respond to further antibiotics, suggesting that it is not the result of ongoing infection. Often patients with idiopathic fibromyalgia are misdiagnosed with Lyme borreliosis based on misinterpretation of a serology or despite negative serologies. Patients with fibromyalgia should be treated for their fibromyalgia, not for *B. burgdorferi* infection. Finally, patients with depression, anxiety, chronic fatigue, or other psychologic dysfunction can be misdiagnosed as having active Lyme borreliosis in much the same way. Especially in patients who have come under the influence of doctors who believe in "chronic Lyme disease," emotional trauma related to the assumption of a chronic and permanent sick role can be devastating and can be emphasized by participation in support groups, chat rooms, and by ongoing interaction with the practitioner. Such patients are best treated by disabusing them of the incorrect diagnosis, evaluating, and treating for sleep or psychologic disorders, and starting a personalized rehabilitation strategy.

The evidence in favor of "chronic Lyme disease" is flimsy at best, based on extrapolation from individual case reports, often from the European literature. There has never been an isolate of *B. burgdorferi* resistant to doxycycline or amoxicillin, so there is no reason to believe that many (or any) patients will fail therapy with appropriate agent, duration, and route of administration. There is no evidence that the organism becomes dormant or hides from the immune system and antibiotics. Long-term infection resistant to antibiotics probably does not exist. A recent study gave patients with "post–Lyme disease syndrome" 30 days of ceftriaxone (Rocephin)* followed by 60 days of doxycycline; the study was cut short by an impartial monitoring board because there was no evidence that any benefit would accrue to participants. Believers in "chronic Lyme disease" have criticized the study design, but even so there is *no* evidence that long-term therapy is of any value.

Lyme borreliosis is an infection with *B. burgdorferi* an organism that is killed efficiently by doxycycline* and amoxicillin*; there are no oral agents superior to these. Intravenous therapy with third-generation cephalosporins is effective for many features of the infection, but should only be used prudently. Other antibiotics, long-term oral therapy after parenteral therapy, 1-day-a-week parenteral therapy, combination regimens, different agents in rotation, and hydroxychloroquine (Plaquenil)* to enhance potency of agents have no scientific basis and should be avoided. Even more disturbing is the use of novel remedies such as colloidal silver, hyperbaric oxygen, malariotherapy, and nutritional supplements. Ongoing ineffective treatments and reinforcement of the belief that the infection persists and cannot be cured produces a psychologic burden that may be the most damage done by "Lyme disease." By understanding the pathogenesis of the various features of "Lyme disease," one can treat appropriately, safely, and effectively. By understanding the natural history of untreated and treated Lyme borreliosis and syndromes following treated infection a rational physician can educate his or her patient and together they can craft a proper therapeutic and rehabilitation strategy. The mythology and anxiety surrounding "chronic Lyme disease" can be overcome by a rational therapeutic partnership to the betterment of our patients' and society's health.

*Not FDA approved for this indication.

RUBELLA AND CONGENITAL RUBELLA

method of
DAVID C. WAAGNER, M.D.
Texas Tech School of Medicine
Lubbock, Texas

Postnatal infection with rubella virus typically results in an acute self-limited disease characterized by a discrete maculopapular exanthem, fever, and lymphadenopathy. Conversely, intrauterine infection with rubella virus can cause fetal demise or result in a syndrome of diverse congenital anomalies. Rubella (Latin for "little red") has historically been known by many names, including third disease, German measles, and 3-day measles, an allusion to the similarity of the exanthem to measles.

BACKGROUND AND EPIDEMIOLOGY

Rubella is a spherical, enveloped, single-stranded RNA virus, the sole member of the genus *Rubivirus* in the Togaviridae family. Infection with rubella virus is confined to humans and is worldwide in distribution. In the Northern Hemisphere, postnatal rubella infection is most prevalent in March, April, and May. Before routine vaccination, rubella outbreaks occurred regularly in 6- to 9-year intervals, with major pandemics developing every 10 to 30 years. After the mass vaccination of children against rubella, widespread rubella outbreaks have not occurred in the United States. Since 1969, the number of rubella cases in the United States has decreased by more than 99%. Despite widespread vaccination, approximately 10% to 20% of the U.S. population remains susceptible to rubella because of suboptimal vaccination rates. The highest rates of susceptibility (approximately 22%) are in persons born from 1970 to 1974. This observation is of particular concern in that many women remain susceptible to rubella during their reproductive years. In susceptible populations, rubella attack rates range from 50% to 90% in community outbreaks, with almost 100% attack rates in closed population such as military bases and institutions for the disabled.

During the 1990s, notable shifts occurred in the epidemiology of rubella in the United States with regard to age distribution, ethnicity, country of origin, and outbreak settings. Before the mid-1990s, most reported cases of rubella developed in persons younger than 15 years. Since that time, the majority of U.S. rubella cases have occurred in persons older than 15 years, with 86% of the cases reported in 1999 occurring in adults. In 1991, only 4% of persons with rubella in the United States were Hispanic, in contrast to 73% in 2000. Most U.S. rubella outbreaks since the mid-1990s have occurred in persons who were non-U.S. born, predominantly from Mexico and Central America. Outbreak settings have likewise shifted from schools, jails, and other closed environments to workplaces and communities, particularly meat and poultry processing centers employing large concentrations of foreign-born laborers.

Transmission of postnatal rubella from infected persons occurs through direct exposure to respiratory droplets by inhalation or contact with droplet-contaminated environmental surfaces. Transmission is more likely to occur after prolonged repeated contact than after a single brief contact. The incubation period for postnatal rubella is typically 16 to 18 days, but it can range from 12 to 23 days. In volunteer studies, the period of maximal communicability occurs 5 days before to 7 days after onset of the rash, although virus can be detected in respiratory secretions 7 days before to 14 days after the rash appears. Persons with subclinical postnatal rubella are also potentially contagious during the same interval. Hospitalized patients with postnatal rubella should remain in isolation for droplet precautions until 7 days after appearance of the rash. Similarly, nonhospitalized patients with postnatal rubella should be excluded from work, school, or daycare for 7 days after onset of the rash.

Clinical Features

In young children, appearance of the rash is typically the first sign of infection. However, in 65% to 95% of adolescents and adults, the rash is preceded by 1 to 5 days of prodromal complaints such as sore throat, headache, fever, anorexia, malaise, cough, and lymphadenopathy, typically of the posterior auricular, suboccipital, and cervical nodes. Fever is usually low grade (<38.5°C) or absent and seldom occurs after the first day of the rash. Subclinical infections without rash are common and estimated to occur in 25% to 50% of cases.

The rubella exanthem begins on the face and rapidly spreads centrifugally to involve the entire torso within 24 hours of onset. The characteristic rubella rash is a pink to reddish maculopapular eruption, less erythematous than the rash of measles. Moreover, in contrast to measles, the rubella exanthem is seldom confluent, usually resolves within 3 to 5 days, and thus gives rise to the description "3-day measles." In adolescents and adults, the rash is often pruritic. Coryza and conjunctivitis may accompany the exanthem but are much milder than with measles. Soft palate petechiae (Forschheimer's spots) have been described as an enanthem of rubella, but they are not pathognomonic.

Complications of Postnatal Rubella

Arthralgia and arthritis occur in up to 70% of adult women with postnatal rubella infection but are less common in adult men and rare in children. The arthritis usually begins within 1 to 6 days after onset of the rash and most frequently involves the fingers, wrists, and knees. The joint manifestations can require up to 1 month for resolution. Hematologic complications, predominantly thrombocytopenic purpura, occur in approximately 1 in 3000 cases. Children are affected more often than adults. The thrombocytopenia generally resolves within several months. Encephalitis is an infrequent complication of postnatal rubella; it affects approximately 1 in 5000 cases and occurs predominantly in adults. Although the mortality associated with postnatal rubella encephalitis ranges from 20% to 50%, survivors usually have no sequelae. An extremely rare and fatal progressive panencephalitis similar to the subacute sclerosing panencephalitis associated with measles has been described. Other rare complications of postnatal rubella include myocarditis, hepatitis, and peripheral neuritis. Despite a frequent transient leukopenia associated with postnatal rubella, bacterial superinfections seldom occur. Immunocompromised patients with postnatal rubella do not appear to be at an increased risk for complications.

Congenital Rubella

The devastating effects of intrauterine rubella infection are in sharp contrast to the typical self-limited course of postnatal rubella infection. The epidemiologic changes of congenital rubella have paralleled those of postnatal rubella. From 1997 to 1999, only 26 cases of congenital rubella were reported in the United States. Of these infants, 81% were Hispanic and 92% were delivered to non–U.S.-born mothers. Gestational age at the time of maternal infection is the single most important determinant in the frequency of fetal infection and risk of defects. The risk of fetal infection has been determined to be 90% at less than 11 weeks' gestation, 68% between 11 and 12 weeks' gestation, 39% between 13 and 26 weeks' gestation, and 53% after 26 weeks' gestation. The risk of congenital defects is approximately 90% at less than 11 weeks' gestation, 11% to 33% between 11 and 14 weeks' gestation, and 24% between 15 and 16 weeks' gestation. The overall risk for congenital defects in the first trimester is approximately 61%. Although fetal infection can develop after 20 weeks' gestation, congenital defects seldom occur.

Rubella virus can infect virtually every organ system in the fetus. Up to 68% of infants with congenital rubella infection are asymptomatic at birth, but manifestations of infection develop in most by 5 years of age. Congenital rubella syndrome, a syndrome of diverse anomalies including ophthalmologic, cardiac, neurologic, and audiologic defects, occurs primarily in infants infected within the first 12 weeks of gestation. Infants infected in the third or fourth month of gestation are usually at risk for only a single defect. Sensorineural deafness is the most common sole manifestation of congenital rubella infection. Transient manifestations of congenital rubella infection include intrauterine growth retardation, hepatosplenomegaly, radiolucent bone lesions, thrombocytopenia, bluish red ("blueberry muffin") purpuric lesions, and interstitial pneumonitis. Permanent manifestations include ophthalmologic defects (cataracts, retinopathy), cardiac defects, sensorineural deafness, and neurologic defects (microcephaly, meningoencephalitis, mental retardation). Children with congenital rubella infection can shed rubella virus for up to a year of age and should be kept in contact isolation until nasopharyngeal and urine viral cultures are negative.

Congenital rubella infection should be considered a progressive disease with many manifestations worsening over time or not appearing until later in life. Hearing deficits can progressively worsen or develop despite normal hearing early in life. Behavioral disorders, mental retardation, and autism can be delayed in appearance. Insulin-dependent diabetes mellitus develops in approximately 20% of cases by adulthood. During the second decade of life, a progressive panencephalitis can occur.

DIAGNOSIS

Postnatal Rubella

Laboratory confirmation of suspected rubella infection should always be obtained because of the variable clinical manifestations. The most commonly used method for diagnosis is serologic determination of the presence of rubella-specific IgM antibody. Rubella IgM antibody may not always be detectable within the first 5 days of rash, thus necessitating repeat testing if negative serologic results are obtained during this interval. False-positive rubella IgM test results have been reported in persons with Epstein-Barr virus, cytomegalovirus, and human parvovirus B19 infection and in the presence of rheumatoid factor. Serologic confirmation can also be made by a fourfold or greater rise in rubella IgG antibody levels on acute and convalescent base titers by enzyme-linked immunosorbent assay (ELISA). Rubella virus can be isolated in tissue cultures from nasal, throat, blood, urine, and cerebrospinal fluid samples. Though highly sensitive, viral cultures are time consuming and expensive. Ideally, specimens for culture should be obtained within 4 days of the onset of rash. Rapid detection of rubella virus in tissue culture by reverse transcriptase polymerase chain reaction is currently under investigation.

Congenital Rubella

The clinical findings of congenital rubella infection can be associated with other intrauterine infections requiring laboratory testing for confirmation. Demonstration of rubella-specific IgM antibody in cord blood or infant sera is considered a reliable indicator of congenital infection. However, approximately 20% of infected infants may have no measurable rubella-specific IgM antibody titers before 1 month of age. False-positives have been reported after incomplete removal of maternal IgG from the assay or because of the presence of rheumatoid factor. Virus isolation should be attempted from culture of the nares, throat, urine, buffy coat of blood, and cerebrospinal fluid. The presence of passively acquired maternal antibody in the infant may confound a diagnosis made by measurement of infant rubella-specific IgG antibody titers. Maternally derived rubella IgG antibody titers decrease at an approximate rate of a twofold dilution per month of age and should not be detectable within 6 to 8 months of age. The presence of stable or increasing serum concentrations of rubella-specific IgG antibody on serial samples by 6 months of age is indicative of congenital infection.

Prenatal diagnosis of congenital rubella infection after maternal infection is possible through reverse transcriptase nested polymerase chain reaction (RT-nPCR) testing of amniotic fluid and chorionic villus sampling. The sensitivity of RT-nPCR has been reported to be as high as 100% in relation to the timing of specimen collection with regard to maternal infection. Rubella virus can also be cultured from chorionic villus specimens. Measurement of rubella-specific IgM antibody in fetal blood is a highly specific, but insensitive indicator of fetal infection.

TREATMENT

Currently available antiviral medications are not effective in the treatment of postnatal or congenital rubella. Uncomplicated postnatal rubella infection usually requires minimal supportive care. Arthritis and arthralgias respond rapidly to aspirin therapy. Patients with thrombocytopenic purpura after postnatal rubella should be monitored for hemorrhage and treated symptomatically with platelet and blood transfusions as needed. Splenectomy is not beneficial. The efficacy of corticosteroids has not been established. Intravenous immune globulin should be considered in patients with prolonged thrombocytopenia.

Investigational trials of amantadine hydrochloride (Symmetrel),* interferon,* and exchange transfusion have not been shown to significantly alter the course of congenital rubella infection. Management of infants with congenital rubella infection must be individualized, with supportive care and intervention directed at the specific defects present. Ideally, children with congenital rubella infection should be monitored by a multidisciplinary team with long-term surveillance for late manifestations such as insulin-dependent diabetes mellitus.

MANAGEMENT OF RUBELLA EXPOSURE IN PREGNANCY

Rubella antibody determination should be performed early in prenatal care in all pregnant women to identify susceptible individuals. Susceptible pregnant women should be monitored for signs of rubella during pregnancy and advised to avoid contact with persons with any rash illness. If rubella exposure is suspected, serologic confirmation should be sought

*Not FDA approved for this indication.

in the contact case. If exposure is confirmed in a susceptible pregnant woman, rubella-specific antibody should be measured 2 to 3 weeks after exposure. If negative, the test should be repeated 6 weeks after exposure. Negative serology 6 weeks after exposure indicates that no infection occurred. Clinical diagnosis is unreliable because of the frequent subclinical manifestation of rubella and should not be considered as a means of excluding maternal infection.

Management of confirmed rubella exposure in susceptible pregnant women is controversial. Administration of live rubella vaccine after exposure is contraindicated in pregnancy and does not prevent fetal infection. The use of immune globulin after rubella exposure can modify or suppress maternal symptoms but may not prevent maternal or fetal infection. The administration of immune globulin (20 mL of IgG intramuscularly) should be reserved for confirmed rubella exposure in susceptible pregnant women within 72 hours of exposure for whom termination of pregnancy is not an option.

If rubella antibody conversion is confirmed in pregnancy, the family must be counseled in regard to the risk of fetal infection and congenital defects based on the gestational age at which infection occurred. Termination of pregnancy should be considered for rubella infections occurring early in gestation.

RUBELLA VACCINE

The only currently available rubella vaccine in the United States is RA 27/3, a live attenuated vaccine, in combination with measles and mumps vaccine (MMR) or as a single preparation (Meruvax II). The RA 27/3 vaccine does not contain egg protein. A protective serum antibody response occurs in more than 95% of recipients after a single dose administered after 1 year of age. Over 90% of recipients have vaccine-induced immunity for at least 15 years. Long-term studies suggest that one dose of vaccine conveys lifelong protection with no evidence of waning immunity.

The first dose of rubella vaccine, in combination with measles and mumps vaccine, should be administered between 12 and 15 months of age. A second dose is given routinely as MMR vaccine at school entry (4 to 6 years of age) because of the two-dose recommendation for measles vaccine. Adults born after 1957 and older children who have not received at least one dose should be immunized with MMR vaccine. Birth before 1957 does not guarantee rubella immunity, so women born before 1957 who might become pregnant should be vaccinated. A previous clinical diagnosis of rubella must not be considered evidence of rubella immunity. Pregnant women identified as being rubella susceptible during prenatal screening should be vaccinated after delivery and before hospital discharge. Special effort should be made to vaccinate all susceptible individuals in settings with high potential for rubella exposure, such as educational institutions, military bases, child care centers, workplaces, and health care facilities.

Rubella vaccination is contraindicated in pregnant women and those attempting to become pregnant. Women receiving rubella vaccine are advised to avoid pregnancy for 3 months after immunization. Data accumulated on 226 susceptible women inadvertently given rubella vaccine during pregnancy revealed only 24% of offspring with asymptomatic infection and none with congenital defects. Rubella vaccination during pregnancy should not be a reason for termination of pregnancy. Although attenuated rubella virus can be shed in the nasopharynx of the vaccinee, it is not considered communicable. Children of rubella-susceptible pregnant women may safely receive rubella vaccine. Breast-feeding is not a contraindication to postpartum vaccination. Although attenuated rubella virus can be shed in human milk, infants remain asymptomatic. Administration of human anti-Rho(D) immune globulin (RhoGAM) after delivery is not a contraindication to postpartum vaccination, although documentation of seroconversion at 6 to 8 months is advised.

Patients with immunodeficiency should not receive live rubella virus vaccine. However, persons with symptomatic HIV infection who are not severely immunocompromised should be vaccinated, as well as their susceptible close contacts. Patients receiving high doses of corticosteroid therapy for longer than 14 days should wait 1 month before rubella immunization. Recent recipients of immune globulin preparations should delay vaccination for an interval dependent on the dosing of immune globulin. Infants receiving palivizumab (Synagis) for respiratory syncytial viral prophylaxis can receive rubella vaccine at the normal dosing schedule. Minor respiratory illness and fever are not contraindications to vaccination.

Although RA 27/3 vaccine is considered to be a very safe vaccine, adverse reactions have been reported. Mild lymphadenopathy, fever, and rash can develop in 5% to 15% of recipients within 5 to 12 days of immunization. Acute arthralgia of the small joints occurs in approximately 25% of postpubertal females, with acute arthritis developing in 10%. Joint involvement appears 7 to 21 days after vaccination and can persist for 3 weeks. No relationship between RA 27/3 vaccine and persistent arthritis has been confirmed. Other rare adverse reactions include thrombocytopenia and transient peripheral neuritic complaints.

MEASLES (RUBEOLA)

method of
YVONNE MALDONADO, M.D.
Stanford University School of Medicine
Stanford, California

Measles (rubeola) is an acute exanthematous illness of childhood. It is infrequent in the United States, although it is a major cause of childhood mortality in developing countries.

ETIOLOGY

Measles is an RNA virus of the genus *Morbillivirus* in the family Paramyxoviridae.

EPIDEMIOLOGY

Measles is endemic throughout the world. In the past, epidemics occurred in the spring at 2- to 4-year intervals as susceptible children were exposed. In the prevaccine era, the age at peak incidence was 5 to 10 years. Individuals born before 1957 are considered immune to measles. Infants acquire passive immunity transplacentally from mothers who have measles antibody. Passive immunity persists variably in the first year of life and may interfere with immunization administered to infants younger than 12 months. Most women of childbearing age in the United States have measles immunity by means of immunization rather than contraction of the disease, and their infants lose passive antibody at a younger age than do infants of mothers who had measles infection.

In the United States, the incidence of measles rose in the 1980s because of inadequate vaccination, as well as vaccine failure. Reported measles cases dropped by more than 99%, from almost 900,000 cases in 1941 to an all-time low of 80 cases in 2000 as a result of intensified immunization efforts. Measles now occurs most often in unimmunized preschool-aged children, as epidemics in high schools and colleges, and as imported cases. More than half of the 108 cases reported in 2001 in the United States were associated with imported measles.

The Pan American Health Organization had established a goal of eliminating measles from the Western Hemisphere by the year 2000. Although that goal was not met, effort has been directed at interrupting indigenous measles transmission. From 1990 to 2000, measles cases in the Western Hemisphere declined by more than 99%, from approximately 250,000 to 1754 (Figure 1). Achievement of greater than 90% immunization rates in infants has been shown to produce disease-free zones.

Transmission. Measles is very contagious, with a 90% attack rate. Aerosol transmission occurs during the early clinical stage.

CLINICAL MANIFESTATIONS

Measles has three clinical stages: an incubation (catarrhal) stage, a prodromal (enanthem) stage with Koplik spots, and a final (exanthem) stage with a maculopapular rash accompanied by high fever. The incubation period lasts 10 to 12 days to the first prodromal symptoms and another 2 to 4 days to appearance of the rash. The virus may be transmitted by the 9th to 10th day after exposure and before clinical symptoms have occurred.

The prodromal phase usually lasts 3 to 5 days and is manifested as a low-grade to moderate fever, a dry cough, coryza, and conjunctivitis. These symptoms nearly always precede the enanthem phase by 2 to 3 days, which is characterized by the appearance of Koplik spots, the pathognomonic sign of measles. An enanthem or red mottling is usually present on the hard and soft palates. Koplik spots are small grayish white dots with a red base. They are generally found opposite the lower molars but may spread over the buccal mucosa. The spots are evanescent and wane within 12 to 18 hours. Conjunctival inflammation and photophobia may precede the Koplik spots.

The exanthem phase is associated with evolution of a rash accompanied by an abrupt rise in temperature, which may reach 40°C (104°F) or higher. When the rash appears on the lower extremities, the symptoms and fever subside within about 2 days.

The rash proceeds in a cephalocaudal direction, with faint macules on the head and neck. The rash progresses to become maculopapular and spreads rapidly over the entire face, neck, upper part of the arms, and upper part of the chest within 24 hours. It continues to spread throughout the body, and by the time it reaches the feet on the second or third day, it begins to fade on the face. The rash fades downward. The severity of the disease is directly related to the extent and confluence of the rash. In mild measles, the rash tends to not be confluent, and in very mild cases, few, if any lesions are present on the legs. In severe cases the rash is confluent, the skin is completely covered, including the palms and soles, and the face is swollen and disfigured.

The rash is often slightly hemorrhagic. Itching is generally mild. As the rash fades, brawny desquamation and brownish discoloration occur and then disappear within 7 to 10 days.

Mild cervical lymphadenopathy and splenomegaly may be noted. Mesenteric lymphadenopathy may cause

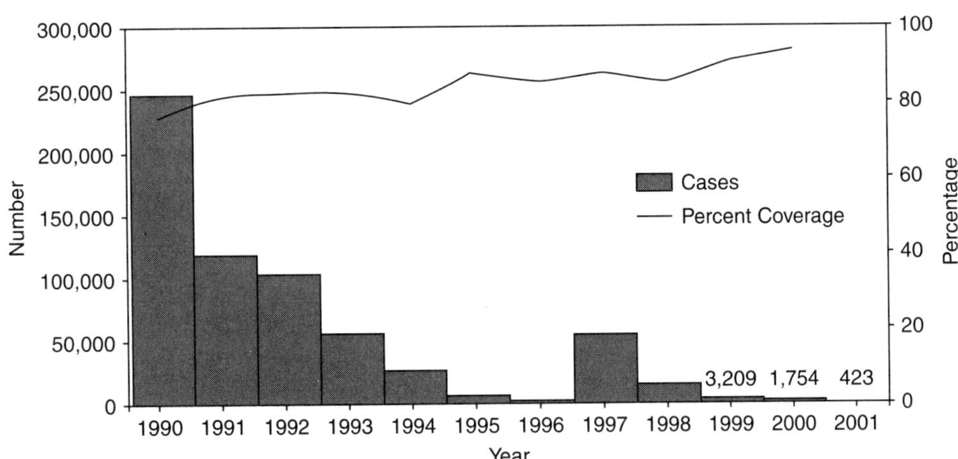

Figure 1. Number of reported and confirmed measles cases (1990 to 1994, total number of reported cases; 1995 to 2001, total number of confirmed cases) and percentage of routine measles vaccination coverage in infants by year in the region of the Americas. As of November 26, 2001, 423 confirmed cases were reported from nine countries. (From Centers for Disease Control and Prevention, 2001.)

abdominal pain. The characteristic pathologic changes of measles in the mucosa of the appendix may cause obliteration of the lumen and symptoms of appendicitis. Otitis media, bronchopneumonia, and gastrointestinal symptoms such as diarrhea and vomiting are more common in infants and small children (especially if they are malnourished) than in older children.

Atypical Measles. Atypical measles occurs in recipients of killed measles vaccine, which was used from 1963 to 1967, after exposure to wild-type measles. The hallmark of atypical measles is lack of a prodrome except for fever, the presence of severe headache, severe abdominal pain and vomiting, myalgias, respiratory symptoms, pneumonia with pleural effusion, and a distinct exanthem. The atypical measles rash first appears on the palms, wrists, soles, and ankles and progresses in a centripetal direction. The lesions are initially maculopapular but become vesicular and may become purpuric or hemorrhagic. Koplik spots rarely appear in patients with atypical measles.

DIAGNOSIS

Clinical diagnosis is based on the triad of cough, coryza, and conjunctivitis along with the typical rash and high fever. However, because indigenous measles rarely occurs in the United States, it is useful to serologically document infections to aid in disease surveillance. Detection of measles IgM is recommended and can be done by the state health department or the Centers for Disease Control and Prevention. IgM levels may be undetectable in the first 72 hours of the rash illness, so testing should be repeated in early cases of presumed measles. Isolation of measles virus from clinical samples is also useful in identifying the genotype of the strain to track transmission patterns. During infection, the virus can be isolated from nasopharyngeal secretions, blood, and urine. All suspected measles cases should be reported immediately to local or state health departments.

The white blood cell count tends to be low with a relative lymphocytosis. Cerebrospinal fluid in patients with measles encephalitis usually shows an increase in protein and a small increase in lymphocytes. The glucose level is normal.

Differential Diagnosis. The rash of measles must be differentiated from that of rubella; roseola infantum (human herpesvirus-6); infections by echovirus, coxsackievirus, and adenovirus; infectious mononucleosis; toxoplasmosis; meningococcemia; scarlet fever; rickettsial diseases; Kawasaki disease; serum sickness; and drug rashes.

TREATMENT

No specific antiviral therapy is available, and treatment is supportive. Antipyretics (acetaminophen or ibuprofen) for fever, bed rest, and maintenance of adequate fluid intake are indicated. Patients with photophobia should be protected from exposure to strong light. The complications of otitis media and pneumonia require appropriate antimicrobial therapy.

Complications such as encephalitis, subacute sclerosing panencephalitis, giant cell pneumonia, and disseminated intravascular coagulation must be assessed individually. Immune globulin and corticosteroids are of limited value.

Vitamin A. Treatment with oral vitamin A* reduces morbidity and mortality in children with severe measles in the developing world. Vitamin A supplementation is suggested for children 6 months to 2 years of age who are hospitalized for measles and its complications and for children older than 6 months with measles and immunodeficiency or evidence of vitamin A deficiency.

COMPLICATIONS

The primary complications of measles are otitis media, interstitial pneumonia, and encephalitis. Measles pneumonia in HIV-infected patients is often fatal and is not always accompanied by rash. Bacterial superinfection and bronchopneumonia are more frequent, however, and usually occur with pneumococci, group A streptococci, *Staphylococcus aureus,* and *Haemophilus influenzae* type b. Laryngitis, tracheitis, and bronchitis are common.

Measles may exacerbate *Mycobacterium tuberculosis* infection. Temporary loss of the hypersensitivity reaction to tuberculin skin testing may occur.

Myocarditis is an infrequent serious complication, although transient electrocardiographic changes may be relatively common.

Neurologic complications are more common in measles than in any of the other rash illnesses of childhood. The incidence of encephalomyelitis is estimated to be 1 to 2 per 1000 cases of measles. Its onset occurs 2 to 5 days after appearance of the rash. Other central nervous system complications, including Guillain-Barré syndrome, hemiplegia, cerebral thrombophlebitis, and retrobulbar neuritis, occur rarely. Subacute sclerosing panencephalitis is a chronic encephalitis caused by persistent measles virus infection of the central nervous system. It is extremely rare in the era of immunization.

PROGNOSIS

Case-fatality rates in the United States have decreased for all age groups, largely because of improved socioeconomic conditions, but also because of treatment of secondary bacterial infections. Despite this decline, the case-fatality rate is still 1 to 3 per 1000 cases. Deaths are primarily due to pneumonia or secondary bacterial infections. In developing countries, measles often occurs in infants, possibly because of malnutrition; the illness is severe and has high mortality.

PREVENTION

Institutional isolation precautions should be maintained from the seventh day after exposure until 5 days after the rash has appeared.

*Not FDA approved for this indication.

Vaccine. The initial measles immunization, usually as measles-mumps-rubella (MMR) vaccine, is recommended at 12 to 15 months of age, but it may be given after exposure to measles and for outbreak prophylaxis as early as 6 months of age. A second immunization, also as MMR, is recommended routinely at 4 to 6 years of age; it may be administered at any time during childhood, but at least 4 weeks after the first dose. Children who have not previously received the second dose should be immunized by 11 to 12 years of age. Adolescents entering college or the workforce should have received two measles immunizations.

Immune globulin will interfere with the immune response to measles vaccine. Anergy to tuberculin skin testing may develop and can persist for more than a month after measles vaccination. Children with active tuberculosis should be receiving antituberculosis treatment when measles vaccine is administered. A tuberculin test should be performed before or concurrent with measles immunization.

Measles vaccine is not recommended for pregnant women; children with primary immunodeficiency, untreated tuberculosis, cancer, or organ transplantation; those receiving long-term immunosuppressive therapy; or severely immunocompromised HIV-infected children.

Postexposure Prophylaxis. Passive immunization with immune globulin is effective for prevention and attenuation of measles within 6 days of exposure. Immunocompromised persons should receive immune globulin intramuscularly regardless of their immunization status.

TETANUS

method of
JAMES P. RICHARDSON, M.D., M.P.H.
Union Memorial Hospital
Baltimore, Maryland

Tetanus, one of the oldest afflictions of humankind, results from infection with the anaerobic gram-positive bacillus *Clostridium tetani.* The manifestations of the disease are caused by the neurotoxin elaborated by the organism, not by the infection itself. Tetanus usually presents as increased tone of the masseter muscles, or trismus, hence the former name of lockjaw.

ETIOLOGY

The causative organism of tetanus, *C. tetani,* exists as spores that are resistant to heating and disinfectants and thus is nearly ubiquitous. Spores have been found in animal and human feces and in soil, dust, human dwellings, and hospitals.

EPIDEMIOLOGY

Tetanus is a rare disease in the United States, with an annual incidence of about 0.02 per 100,000. Fewer than 50 cases are reported to the Centers for Disease Control and Prevention (CDC) each year. Probably many cases of tetanus go unreported, however. Sixty percent of recent cases reported to the CDC were 20 to 59 years old; 35% were age 60 years and older. There is a slightly higher incidence of tetanus in men, older adults, recent immigrants, and intravenous drug users. Serologic surveys document lower levels of protective antibodies in older adults, women, Mexican Americans, and those with lower incomes and educational levels. One-fifth of children 10 to 16 years of age do not have protective antibody levels. Untreated, tetanus is usually fatal. Even with treatment, the overall case-fatality rate is greater than 10%, increasing with increasing age to nearly 20% in those older than 60 years. Importantly, however, since 1989 no deaths have occurred in individuals in the United States who have received primary immunization.

Worldwide, the disease is much more common because of lower levels of immunization. About half a million infants succumb to neonatal tetanus every year.

PATHOGENESIS

Tetanus spores gain entrance to the body through injuries to the skin. These injuries are often so minor that they do not result in any medical attention (e.g., a prick from a thorn bush, a minor puncture wound). Because *C. tetani* is an obligate anaerobe, the spores will grow only in areas of low oxygen tensions, such as occurs with pressure sores, puncture wounds, or gangrene. Reports of tetanus after abortion, animal bites and stings, splinters, and body piercing are documented. Growing, or vegetative, *C. tetani* elaborate, tetanospasmin, one of the most potent neurotoxins known, which then spreads via axons to the central nervous system (CNS).

Tetanospasmin becomes bound to gangliosides within the CNS, suppressing inhibitory influences at the motor neurons by inhibiting gamma aminobutyric acid (GABA) and glycine release at the motor end-plate. This results in reflex irritability, rigidity, and disinhibition of spinal cord reflex arcs. Autonomic hyperactivity is common, resulting from direct stimulation by tetanospasmin. Hypertension and tachycardia, alternating with periods of hypotension and bradycardia, may occur.

CLINICAL PRESENTATION

The incubation period of tetanus is usually from 3 days to 3 weeks, but tetanus can occur several months after an injury. Cases with shorter incubation periods tend to be the most severe.

Generalized disease is the most common presentation of tetanus (Table 1). Common presenting complaints include trismus, neck rigidity, stiffness, dysphagia, restlessness, and reflex spasms. Tetanus patients may display risus sardonicus (a characteristic grimace manifested as raised eyebrows and a wrinkled forehead with the corners of the mouth pulled up). Muscle rigidity usually starts with the jaw and facial muscles

TABLE 1. **Presentation of Tetanus**

Generalized Disease
Trismus
Risus sardonicus
Dysphagia
Opisthotonus
Isolated cranial nerve palsies
Rigidity or stiffness in an extremity
Neck stiffness
Restlessness
Tetanic seizures
Poor sucking (newborns)
Localized Disease
Rigidity or stiffness in an extremity
Cephalic Disease
Single or multiple cranial nerve palsies

and then spreads to the trunk (opisthotonos) and extensor muscles of the limbs. Neonatal tetanus presents as an inability to suck 3 to 10 days after birth. Tetanic seizures, manifested by tonic muscle contractions, may occur in generalized tetanus. Tetanic seizures differ from major seizures in that patients with tetanic seizures remain conscious. Noise, light, or examination of the patient may provoke this activity. These seizures are extremely painful and portend a poor prognosis if frequent.

As the disease progresses, hypoxia may result from involvement of the respiratory muscles. Airway control is very important because laryngospasm may cause further compromise (see later).

Two less common types of tetanus are localized tetanus and cephalic tetanus. Localized tetanus is characterized by painful spasms of muscles near the site of injury. This disorder is usually self-limiting and lasts less than 2 weeks, but progression to generalized disease can occur if untreated. Cephalic tetanus is a frequently severe form of localized tetanus. The bacillus enters through minor head trauma or chronic otitis media. Cephalic tetanus may present as single or multiple cranial nerve palsies or trismus and will often progress to generalized tetanus if not treated.

DIAGNOSIS

Tetanus is a clinical diagnosis; there are no laboratory tests specific for the disease. A history of a predisposing injury and the development of the usual clinical features make the diagnosis clear in most cases. However, as noted previously, a history of injury is not always present. Laboratory tests such as complete blood counts and routine blood chemistry tests are not helpful. Cultures are positive in only 32% to 50% of patients, and in any event treatment cannot wait for their completion. Tetanus antitoxin antibody levels are not usually available quickly and are not reliable after the administration of human tetanus immune globulin (HTIG). Absence of any sensory deficits and a clear sensorium support the diagnosis of tetanus. It has been suggested that patients with tetanus will involuntarily bite a tongue blade before a gag reflex can be elicited (resulting from trismus). A well-documented history of primary immunization and a booster immunization within the last 10 years makes the diagnosis of tetanus much less likely.

Whereas established generalized tetanus is easily recognized, the diagnosis of early tetanus can present some difficulty. Cranial nerve involvement is common and may confuse the physician. Trismus may result from intraoral disease or an acute reaction to phenothiazines or metoclopramide (Reglan). Muscular stiffness can also be a manifestation of strychnine poisoning, meningitis, hepatic encephalopathy, rabies, and conversion reaction. A delay in the diagnosis of tetanus has occurred in patients presenting with dysphagia. Rigid abdominal muscles may simulate an acute abdomen.

TREATMENT

Whenever possible, patients with suspected tetanus should be transferred to a facility with experience with this disease. Patients should be kept in a quiet, dark environment. Treatment has the following goals: (1) neutralization of circulating toxin, (2) elimination of the source toxin by careful surgical excision, (3) prevention of respiratory and metabolic complications, and (4) prevention of muscle spasms.

Tetanus antitoxin should be given to prevent further fixation of the toxin to the central nervous system, although it will not reduce manifestations already present. Three thousand to 6000 units of human tetanus immune globulin (HTIG or Bay-Tet) should be given intramuscularly as soon as possible. Doses as small as 500 units may be as effective. Some authorities recommend giving some of this near the site of the wound. Immunization with tetanus-diphtheria toxoid (Td) or diphtheria toxoid-pertussis vaccine-tetanus toxoid (DPT or DTaP), as appropriate, also should be given, at a site different from that for TIG (Table 2).

Débridement is important for several reasons. Débridement removes live organisms, creates an aerobic environment unfavorable for further growth, and secures specimens for culture. Débridement should be delayed until several hours after the administration of antitoxin because tetanospasmin may be released into the bloodstream. Antibiotic therapy is essential to sterilize the wound and reduce bacteremia.

TABLE 2. **Routine Diphtheria and Tetanus Immunization Schedule for Persons 7 Years and Older**

Dose	Interval	Product
Primary 1	First dose	Td
Primary 2	4–8 weeks after first dose*	Td
Primary 3	6–12 months after second dose*	Td
Boosters	Every 10 years after last dose	Td

From: Immunization Practices Advisory Committee. Diphtheria, Tetanus, and Pertussis: Recommendations for Vaccine Use and Other Preventive Measures—Recommendations of the Immunization Practices Advisory Committee (ACIP). MMWR 1991;40(No. RR-10).

*Prolonging the interval does not require restarting series.

The antibiotic of choice is metronidazole (Flagyl) given at a dose of 7.5 mg per kg every 6 hours up to a maximum of 1000 mg. Acceptable alternatives are doxycycline (Vibramycin) and imipenem cilastatin (Primaxin). Penicillin, once the drug of choice, should not be used because it may worsen GABA-induced hypertonia.

Oxygenation is assured by protecting the airway. In all but the mildest of cases, prophylactic intubation should be initiated early. Intubation will usually require sedation with a benzodiazepine (e.g., lorazepam [Ativan], 2 mg intravenously) and neuromuscular blockade (e.g., vecuronium [Norcuron], 0.08 to 0.1 mg/kg). Patients requiring more than 10 days of intubation or who have generalized seizures should undergo elective tracheostomy. An oropharyngeal airway will allow removal of secretions and prevent biting in mild cases that do not require intubation.

Control of tonic spasms and tetanic seizures is best achieved with the benzodiazepines. Additional benefits are that these drugs produce sedation and amnesia. Diazepam (Valium) can be given at a dose of 0.5 mg/kg to 15 mg/kg per day intravenously. Alternatively, continuous infusions of lorazepam (Ativan) at a dose of 0.1 to 2.0 mg/kg per hour or midazolam (Versed) at a dose of 0.01 to 0.10 mg/kg per hour can be given. The goal is to control muscle rigidity and inhibition of spasm as well as produce the desired level of sedation.

In those patients whose muscle spasms do not respond to sedation, neuromuscular blocking agents, such as vecuronium (Norcuron), are often necessary. These patients will require assisted ventilation, often for several days or weeks. Because neuromuscular blocking agents prevent skeletal muscle movements only and do not reduce pain or provide sedation, it is essential that these patients be monitored very closely for adequate pain relief.

Later in the course of the disease cardiovascular instability may develop through effects on the autonomic nervous system. Both α-adrenergic and β-adrenergic blockade may be necessary with phentolamine (Regitine) and metoprolol (Lopressor) for treatment of hypertension and tachycardia (not Food and Drug Administration approved). Bradycardia may develop as well, at times requiring placement of a pacemaker. Hypotension may require monitoring of cardiac output and intravenous fluids or pressor agents.

COMPLICATIONS

Supportive care is critical to the prevention of complications. Most of these complications are those common to immobile patients. Attention to nutritional status and frequent turning of the patient will prevent pressure sores. Low-dose heparin or enoxaparin (Lovenox) should be administered to prevent deep venous thromboses and pulmonary emboli. Physical therapy should be begun as soon as possible to prevent contractures. Orthopedic management may be required for fractures and dislocations resulting from tetanic seizures.

Most patients will eventually make a full recovery, but some patients remain hypertonic. It is important that recovering patients complete a primary series of immunizations because having had the disease does not confer immunity (Table 3).

PREVENTION

Prevention of tetanus through immunization is the key to the elimination of tetanus. It is important to distinguish between primary and booster immunization, however. A never-immunized patient 7 years old or older requires two additional doses of Td beyond the dose given when wound is treated (see Table 3). Wounded patients who have never been immunized may require tetanus immunoglobulin (HTIG) (see Table 2). The elderly population is particularly susceptible, because so many have never been immunized or because their immunity has lapsed. The shortage of tetanus toxoid that occurred from 2000 to 2002 is now over and physicians should not hesitate to immunize adults as appropriate.

Physicians should use a case-finding approach to increase tetanus immunization rates. System changes (such as clinical pathways that allow immunization without a physician's order) are the most effective means to increase immunization rates. Reminders placed at physicians' desks or computer-generated reminders attached to charts or patients' bills also have increased rates. Tetanus-diphtheria toxoid should be given whenever tetanus immunization is necessary, to ensure immunity to diphtheria as well as tetanus.

Td is a safe vaccine. Adverse reactions consist primarily of local edema, tenderness, and fever. Anaphylactoid reactions are rare. Most adverse reactions occur in persons with evidence of hyperimmunization. The only

TABLE 3. **Guide to Tetanus Prophylaxis in Routine Wound Management**

History of Adsorbed Tetanus Toxoid (Doses)	Clean, Minor Wounds		All Other Wounds*	
	Td[†]	TIG[†]	Td[†]	TIG[†]
Unknown or				
<3	Yes	No	Yes	Yes
≥3[‡]	No[§]	No	No[‖]	No

From: Immunization Practices Advisory Committee. Diphtheria, Tetanus, and Pertussis: Recommendations for Vaccine Use and Other Preventive Measures—Recommendations of the Immunization Practices Advisory Committee (ACIP). MMWR 1991;40(No. RR-10)

*Such as, but not limited to, wounds contaminated from dirt, feces, soil, saliva; puncture wounds; avulsions; and wounds resulting from missiles, crushing, burns, or frostbite.

†For children younger than age 7, the diphtheria and tetanus toxoids and acellular pertussis vaccines (DTaP) or the diphtheria and tetanus toxoids and whole-cell pertussis vaccines (DTP)—or pediatric diphtheria and tetanus toxoids (DT) if pertussis vaccine is contraindicated—is preferred to tetanus toxoid (TT) alone. For those ages 7 years and older, the tetanus and diphtheria toxoids (Td) is preferred to TT alone.

‡If only three doses of fluid toxoid have been received, a fourth dose of toxoid, preferably an adsorbed dose, should be given.

§Yes, if more than 10 years since last dose.

‖Yes, if more than 5 years since last dose. (More frequent boosters are not needed and can accentuate side effects).

TIG, tetanus immune globulin.

contraindications of Td toxoid are a history of a neurologic sequela or a severe hypersensitivity reaction following a previous dose.

To reduce neonatal tetanus and protect the mother, pregnant women who are due for a booster should receive Td, preferable during the last two trimesters. HTIG should be given to pregnant women only when clearly indicated.

WHOOPING COUGH (PERTUSSIS)

method of
VENUSTO H. SAN JOAQUIN, M.D.
Section of Infectious Diseases
University of Oklahoma Health Science Center
Pediatric Infectious Diseases
Oklahoma City, Oklahoma

Pertussis is a Latin-derived word meaning intense cough. The commonly used name "whooping cough," however, is more descriptive of the disease. In the typical case, a series of hacking coughs during a single expiration ends in a forceful inspiratory whoop. Pertussis is a highly contagious respiratory infection caused by *Bordetella pertussis* or *Bordetella parapertussis*. Complications and mortality from the disease are highest in infants younger than 4 months old. After the introduction of the pertussis vaccine in the late 1940s, the number of cases in the United States decreased dramatically. Still, a cyclical increase in cases to epidemic degree occurs every 3 to 4 years.

EPIDEMIOLOGY

The worldwide burden of pertussis remains high, and is estimated at 50 to 60 million cases and half a million deaths each year. In the United States during the prevaccine era, the calculated attack rate was 872 per 100,000 population, causing an average of 7,300 deaths per year. Subsequent to widespread pertussis immunization (Figure 1), the reported incidence of pertussis declined to a historic low of 1,010 cases in 1976. Starting in the early 1980s, the incidence has increased cyclically with peaks every 3 to 4 years. The Centers for Disease Control and Prevention data for 1997 through 2000 showed an average annual incidence of 7,300 cases (2.7 per 100,000 population) and 16 deaths. The increased incidence involved three age groups: infants too young to receive three doses of pertussis-containing vaccine, adolescents, and adults. The low efficacy (70% to 90%) of the available pertussis vaccines and the short duration of the immunity after either vaccination or natural infection contribute significantly to the persistence of pertussis in this country.

Man is the only known host of *B. pertussis*. It is transmitted through contact with droplets of respiratory tract secretions generated by coughing. Up to 100% of nonimmune close contacts of the patient acquire the infection. Infants and young children often get pertussis from older siblings or adults in the household who have mild or atypical illness and are not suspected of having pertussis. Infected persons are most contagious during the catarrhal phase of the disease when symptoms are indistinguishable from that of viral respiratory infection.

PATHOGEN, PATHOGENESIS, PATHOPHYSIOLOGY

The genus *Bordetella* comprises six species: *B. pertussis, B. parapertussis, B. bronchiseptica, B. avium, B. hinzii,* and *B. holmesii. B. pertussis* accounts for 95% of cases of whooping cough, and *B. parapertussis* for most of the other cases. *B. bronchiseptica* is an animal pathogen that is a rare cause of pertussis-like illness in man. *B. pertussis* and *B. parapertussis* have 98.5% genetic homology; the most significant difference is the lack of production of pertussis toxin by *B. parapertussis*. The other *Bordetella* species have not been associated with respiratory infection in humans. *B. pertussis* produces several biologically active substances that are related to its pathogenicity and immunogenicity (Table 1). After inoculation onto the respiratory tract, *B. pertussis* adheres to the cilia of

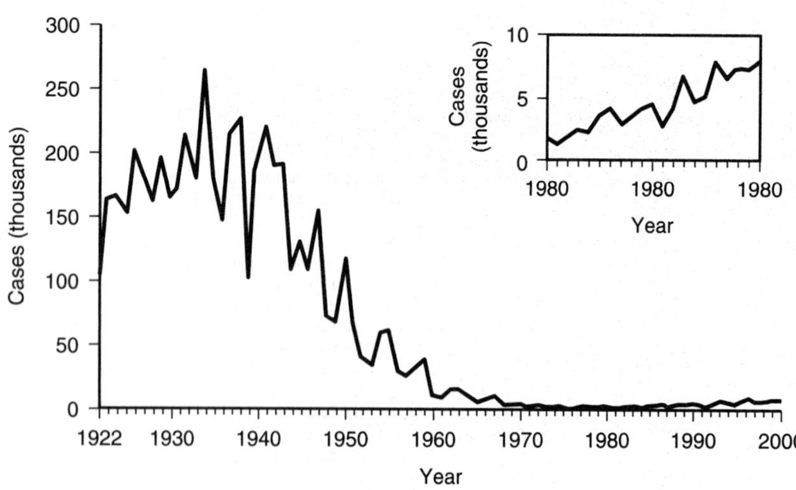

Figure 1. Number of reported pertussis cases, by year—United States, 1922-2000 (Adapted from Centers for Disease Control and Prevention; MMWR 51[04]: 73-76, 2002.)

TABLE 1. **Bacterial Components Related to Pathogenicity and Immunogenicity of *Bordetella pertussis***

Component	Biologic Activity
Pertussis toxin	Promotes lymphocytosis; induces histamine sensitization; stimulates insulin secretion; promotes adhesion to respiratory epithelium; stimulates IL-4 and IgE production; inhibits phagocytic function
Filamentous hemagglutinin	Promotes adhesion to respiratory epithelium; agglutinates erythrocytes
Fimbriae (pili), types 2 and 3	Promotes adhesion to respiratory epithelium
Adenylate cyclase	Inhibits phagocytic function; contributes to respiratory epithelial injury; causes hemolysis
Tracheal cytotoxin	Causes ciliary stasis and necrosis of respiratory epithelium; may impair neutrophil function
Pertactin	Promotes adhesion to respiratory epithelium
Dermonecrotic toxin	May contribute to epithelial injury
Endotoxin	Causes reaction to the whole-cell pertussis vaccine

the ciliated cells of the respiratory epithelium. The adhesion is mediated by the filamentous hemagglutinin, pertussis toxin, and pertactin. The fimbriae also function as adhesin but are probably not involved in primary attachment but serve to sustain the attachment. The organisms multiply in the ciliated epithelium and release components that cause lymphocytic and polymorphonuclear infiltration of the mucosa, and necrosis of the midzonal and basilar layers of the bronchial epithelium. In hamster organ cultures, the tracheal cytotoxin selectively destroys ciliated cells and is responsible for most of the respiratory epithelial damage. Other bacterial components that contribute to the epithelial injury include the dermonecrotic toxin and adenyl cyclase. The pertussis toxin and adenyl cyclase also impair leukocyte migration and phagocytosis, allowing the establishment of the infection. The pertussis toxin causes absolute lymphocytosis; both T and B lymphocytes are increased. *B. parapertussis* does not produce pertussis toxin; therefore, whooping cough caused by this species is usually not associated with lymphocytosis.

CLINICAL PRESENTATION

The incubation period ranges from 6 to 20 days; in most cases, the onset of illness occurs 7 to 10 days after exposure. The typical pertussis has three stages—catarrhal, paroxysmal, and convalescent—each lasting approximately 2 weeks. In the catarrhal stage, the child develops coryza, lacrimation, and occasional dry cough. The patient is usually afebrile, otherwise clinically well, and is difficult to differentiate from a child with common cold or viral respiratory infection. The occasional cough becomes hacking and progressively more frequent and severe, culminating in bouts of paroxysmal coughing. Between paroxysms, the patient appears well. Suddenly, the child develops a series of intense coughing during expiration, followed by a high-pitched inspiratory sound, the whoop, created by a forceful inspiration through a narrowed glottis. Severe paroxysms are associated with cyanosis, plethoric facies, bulging of the eyes, protrusion of the tongue, and distention of neck veins. Post-tussive vomiting is common. The child is exhausted and apathetic after a paroxysmal bout. The convalescent stage is characterized with gradual decline in the severity and frequency of the paroxysms.

Pertussis in the neonate and the very young is notable for the absence of the whoop, but the coughing spell is more likely to cause apnea, bradycardia, cyanosis, and seizures. The majority of infected infants require hospitalization. Complications are common and may include feeding problems, otitis media, pneumonia, encephalopathy, interstitial and subcutaneous emphysema, and pulmonary hypertension. The mortality rate is highest, at 1.3%, among neonates. In 2000, there were 17 pertussis-related deaths in the United States; all were infants younger than 4 months old.

The mild form of pertussis is seen in older children and adults who have prior exposure to *B. pertussis* antigens, either from immunization or natural infection. They may develop a protracted hacking cough without paroxysms, and are often misdiagnosed as cases of upper respiratory infection or bronchitis.

DIAGNOSIS

Paroxysmal coughing may be caused by a variety of bacterial, viral, fungal, and parasitic agents. The whoop and absolute lymphocytosis, however, are hallmarks of pertussis and their presence should facilitate making the diagnosis. The infant with a staccato cough and afebrile pneumonitis caused by *Chlamydia trachomatis* is probably the most difficult to differentiate clinically from the very young infant with pertussis. In older children and adolescents, the protracted brassy cough in *Mycoplasma pneumoniae* pneumonia is suggestive of pertussis. The clinical and radiographic findings of pneumonia favor *Mycoplasma* infection.

The laboratory diagnosis of pertussis rests on the isolation of *B. pertussis* and *B. parapertussis* in nasopharyngeal wash or swab specimens. Direct fluorescent antibody assay of the nasopharyngeal specimens will identify *B. pertussis* and *B. parapertussis* within 12 hours of performing the test, but is less sensitive and specific than culture, which may take up to 7 days to grow. *B. pertussis* is most likely to be isolated in the nasopharynx during the catarrhal stage; it is less likely to be found by the second week of the paroxysmal stage. Other diagnostic tests include immunoassays, polymerase chain reaction, and serology. They are not available in most clinical and commercial laboratories at this time but are done in research laboratories.

TREATMENT

The principal management of children with pertussis is supportive and symptomatic in nature. Infants younger than 6 months often require hospitalization. Paroxysms of cough associated with apnea, cyanosis, feeding difficulties, and seizures are common in these age groups and may require intensive care. The neonate and the premature infant with bronchopulmonary dysplasia are particularly at high risk of severe disease and should automatically be admitted.

Antibiotics do not have a notable effect on the paroxysmal stage, the stage that carries the brunt of the morbidity and mortality from pertussis. Treatment during the catarrhal stage attenuates the disease. However, it is rare for pertussis to be suspected or diagnosed during the catarrhal stage, except in a patient with known exposure but not given chemoprophylaxis. Notwithstanding the marginal effect on the clinical illness, antibiotic therapy eradicates *B. pertussis* from the respiratory tract. The patient is rendered noncontagious after 5 days of antibiotic therapy; therefore, every patient should receive antibiotic treatment. A major role of antibiotics in pertussis is chemoprophylaxis for all household members and close contacts of the patient, regardless of age, immunization status, or history of previous infection with *B. pertussis*. The antibiotics shown to induce bacteriologic cure in clinical studies are all macrolides: azithromycin (Zithromax), clarithromycin (Biaxin),* and erythromycin (E-Mycin) (Table 2). Erythromycin is the traditional drug of choice for pertussis. In vitro, azithromycin is the most active against *B. pertussis*. Recent data show azithromycin given for 5 days is at least as effective as erythromycin given for 10 days. It is better tolerated than erythromycin because of fewer gastrointestinal side effects and shorter duration of treatment. Because of better bioavailability and long half-life, it is administered once daily compared to three times daily for erythromycin. Azithromycin should probably be considered the antibiotic of choice for pertussis. A causal association between the development of pyloric stenosis and administration of erythromycin in neonates for pertussis prophylaxis has been reported. This association should be considered when deciding the management of pertussis in the very young infant. Other antimicrobial agents that are active against *B. pertussis* include trimethoprim-sulfamethoxazole (Bactrim)* and the quinolones. However, their efficacy has not been investigated.

Empiric use and small clinical trials of corticosteroids, albuterol (Proventil),* and pertussis immune globulin** in the treatment of whooping cough suggest possible effectiveness of these agents in reducing severity of the coughing spells. Well-designed clinical studies are needed. At present, the use of any of these drugs is not recommended.

PREVENTION

The effective control of pertussis by universal immunization of children with pertussis vaccine has been clearly demonstrated. From the 1940s to the 1990s, killed whole-cell (inactivated *B. pertussis*) vaccine combined with diphtheria and tetanus toxoids (DTP) was used in the United States. The less reactogenic acellular pertussis (aP) vaccines were first licensed and recommended for routine use in 1996. These vaccines all contain pertussis toxin but differ in the inclusion of the other pertussis immunogens (i.e., filamentous hemagglutinin, fimbriae 2 and 3, and pertactin). As of May 14, 2000, six aP-containing vaccines (DTaP) are licensed for use, but only three (Tripedia, Infanrix, and DAPTACEL) are distributed in the United States. Administration of DTaP is recommended at ages 2, 4, 6, and 15 to 18 months and the fifth dose at 4 to 6 years. Ideally, the same DTaP vaccine should be used throughout the entire vaccination series. However, if the previous vaccine received by the child is not known or not available, any of the licensed vaccines may be used to complete the vaccination series.

*Not FDA approved for this indication.
**Not available in the United States.

TABLE 2. **Antibacterial Drugs for Treatment and Chemoprophylaxis of Pertussis**

Drug*	Dosage
Azithromycin (Zithromax)**	10 mg/kg, single dose on day 1 5 mg/kg, single daily dose on days 2-5
Erythromycin	15 mg/kg, three times a day for 10 days
Clarithromycin (Biaxin)**	7.5 mg/kg, twice a day for 7 days

*Possible alternative drugs for children who are allergic or unable to tolerate the macrolides include trimethoprim-sulfamethoxazole (Bactrim)** and the quinolones.
**Not FDA approved for this indication.

OFFICE-BASED IMMUNIZATION PRACTICES

method of
JULIE A. BOOM, M.D.
Pediatrics
Baylor College of Medicine
Houston, Texas

The rates of most vaccine-preventable diseases in the United States are at record low levels. In 2001, there were only 2 cases of diphtheria, 27 cases of tetanus, and 108 cases of measles. However, pertussis incidence has been on a gradual increase since the 1980s. Of the 10,650 children ages 3 months to 14 years of age diagnosed with pertussis between 1990 and 1996, 54% were not appropriately immunized against diphtheria, tetanus toxoids, and pertussis (DTP). This recent increase in pertussis disease rates is of great concern as disease levels are often a late indicator of the soundness of the immunization system. In 2001, the National Immunization Survey conducted by the Centers for Disease Control and Prevention found that nationally, only 78.6% of children between age 19 and 35 months have been vaccinated with four doses of diphtheria, tetanus, acellular pertussis vaccine (DTaP), three doses of polio vaccine, and one dose of measles containing vaccine. The reasons for low immunization coverage levels are multifactorial: fragmentation of medical records, missed opportunities for vaccination, lack of reminder and recall systems, lack of provider education, and growing complacency regarding the need for immunization. Therefore, improving immunization coverage levels for all children is important for providers caring for children.

DIPHTHERIA, TETANUS AND ACELLULAR PERTUSSIS VACCINE

Since the early 1990s, new outbreaks of diphtheria have occurred in the newly independent states of the former Soviet Union due to low immunization coverage levels. Diphtheria is a toxin-mediated disease caused by *Corynebacterium diphtheriae*. The aerobic gram-positive bacillus, *C. diphtheriae*, produces toxin when the bacillus is infected by a bacteriophage that carries the genetic information for the toxin. Susceptible persons who live in crowded conditions may acquire the disease through colonization of the nasopharynx. The bacillus toxin causes local tissue destruction and membrane formation. The toxin then may be hematologically spread and result in severe complications including myocarditis, neuritis, otitis media, and respiratory insufficiency due to membrane formation and airway obstruction. The case fatality rate is 5% to 10% with rates up to 20% in children <5 years and adults >40 years. Case fatality rates in epidemics may range from 3% to 23%.

Tetanus is a toxin-mediated disease caused by *Clostridium tetani*. This gram-positive anaerobic rod can produce spores. The organism is sensitive to heat and oxygen, whereas the spores are very heat resistant and antiseptic resistant. Susceptible persons may acquire the disease through an open wound. If an anaerobic environment exists, such as in a deep puncture wound, *C. tetani* spores may germinate and produce toxins. Tetanus toxin binds within the central nervous system (CNS) and interferes with the release of neurotransmitters.

Symptoms are progressive and usually follow a descending pattern including trismus (lockjaw), neck stiffness, difficulty swallowing, muscle rigidity, and spasms. Complications include laryngospasm, spinal and long bone fractures, autonomic nervous system hyperactivity, and nosocomial infections resulting from prolonged hospitalization. This disease is fatal in 11% of reported cases, and most fatal in persons older than 60 years of age.

Pertussis, or whooping cough, is caused by the bacterium *Bordetella pertussis*. *B. pertussis* is an aerobic gram-negative rod, which produces many biologically harmful products including the following: pertussis toxin, filamentous hemagglutinin, agglutinogens, adenylate cyclase, pertactin, and tracheal toxin. The organism attaches to respiratory cilia. The disease is characterized by three classic stages. The catarrhal stage is characterized by mild upper respiratory symptoms. After 1 to 2 weeks, the paroxysmal stage begins. This stage is characterized by episodes of continuous, rapid coughs followed by a long inspiratory effort, which produces the high-pitched whoop. These attacks may be accompanied by cyanosis, vomiting, and exhaustion. The paroxysmal stage is followed by the convalescent stage. Complications are worst in young infants and include secondary bacterial pneumonia, seizures, and encephalopathy. Apnea is common in infants less than six months of age. The case fatality rate is 0.2%, with most deaths occurring in children <6 months of age.

Since 1996, the DTaP has been recommended for all doses of the primary pediatric series. The whole-cell vaccine (DTP) is no longer recommended for use in the United States because studies have shown that the acellular pertussis vaccine is significantly more effective with fewer mild and serious adverse events. The primary series of DTaP consists of four doses of vaccine beginning at 6 weeks to 2 months of age. The first three doses are given at 4- to 8-week intervals, with the fourth dose given at 15 to 18 months of age (Figure 1). The fourth dose may be given earlier if the following three criteria are met: the child is at least 12 months of age, at least 6 months have elapsed since the third dose, and the child is unlikely to return for vaccination at 15 to 18 months of age. A fifth dose is recommended after 4 years of age before school entry. The fifth dose is not necessary if the fourth dose was given on or after the fourth birthday. DTaP is not recommended for children >7 years of age because vaccine reactions are thought to be greater in older age groups. DTaP may cause local reactions including pain, redness, or swelling, especially after the fourth or fifth doses. Moderate to severe illness is a precaution to vaccination. Precautions to future doses of pertussis vaccine include: temperature >40.5°C within 48 hours with no other identifiable cause; collapse or shocklike state (also known as a hypotonic-hyporesponsive episode) within 48 hours; persistent, inconsolable crying lasting >3 hours within 48 hours; and seizures with or without fever occurring within 3 days. Contraindications to further vaccinations with DTaP include severe allergic reaction (anaphylaxis) and encephalopathy with no other identifiable causes occurring within 7 days of vaccination.

POLIO VACCINE

Polio virus is an enterovirus that is spread via the fecal-oral and respiratory routes. It enters the mouth and multiplies in the pharynx and gastrointestinal tract. The virus then spreads through the local lymphoid tissue to the bloodstream and may spread to the CNS. In less than 1% of cases, the virus then replicates and destroys neurons in the anterior horn and brainstem resulting in flaccid paralysis. Ninety-five percent of persons with polio infection will actually be asymptomatic. Approximately 4% to 8% of persons will have a minor, nonspecific illness characterized by upper respiratory symptoms, gastrointestinal symptoms, or an influenza-like illness. Nonparalytic aseptic meningitis occurs in 1% to 2% of infections. The death-to-case rate is 2% to 5% for persons with paralytic polio; the rates are higher in adults and those with bulbar involvement.

Since July 1999, inactivated polio vaccine (IPV) has been exclusively recommended by the Advisory Committee on Immunization Practices (ACIP). Oral polio vaccine (OPV) is no longer routinely available in

RECOMMENDED CHILDHOOD IMMUNIZATION SCHEDULE
UNITED STATES, 2003

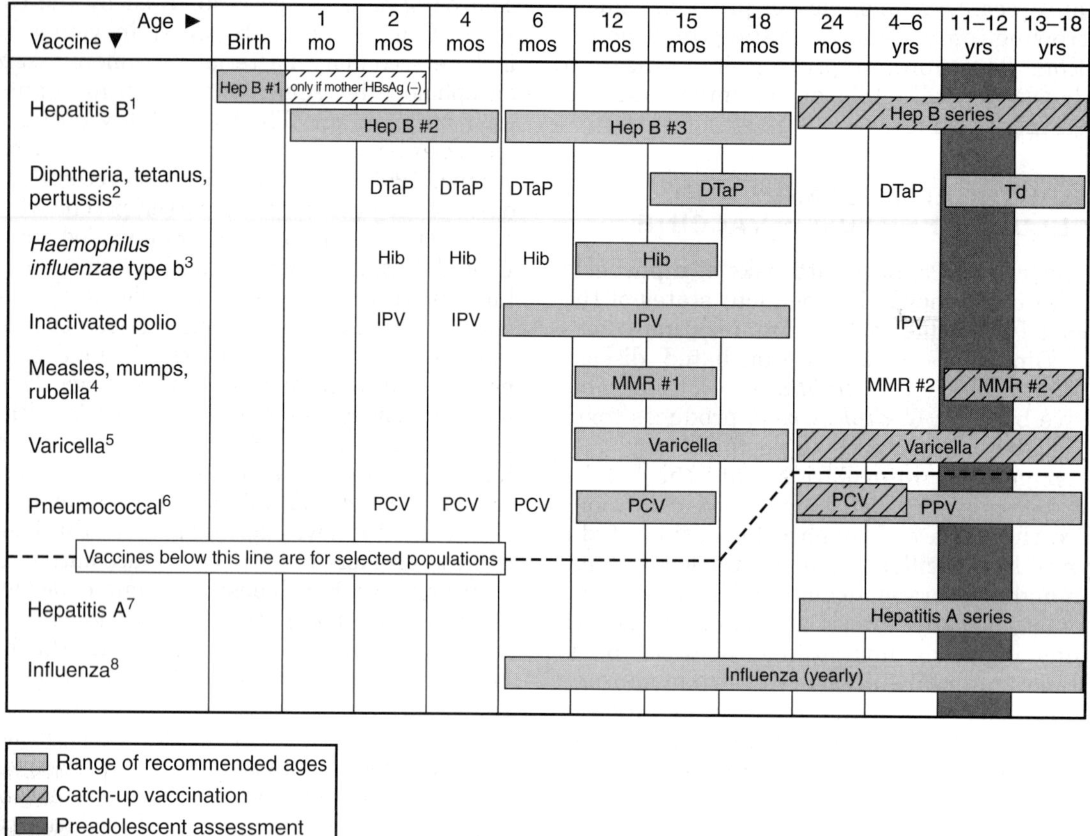

Age ►
Vaccine ▼
Birth
1 mo
2 mos
4 mos
6 mos
12 mos
15 mos
18 mos
24 mos
4–6 yrs
11–12 yrs
13–18 yrs
Hepatitis B1
Hep B #1
only if mother HBsAg (–)
Hep B #2
Hep B #3
Hep B series
Diphtheria, tetanus, pertussis2
DTaP
DTaP
DTaP
DTaP
DTaP
Td
Haemophilus influenzae type b3
Hib
Hib
Hib
Hib
Inactivated polio
IPV
IPV
IPV
IPV
Measles, mumps, rubella4
MMR #1
MMR #2
MMR #2
Varicella5
Varicella
Varicella
Pneumococcal6
PCV
PCV
PCV
PCV
PCV
PPV
Vaccines below this line are for selected populations
Hepatitis A7
Hepatitis A series
Influenza8
Influenza (yearly)
Range of recommended ages
Catch-up vaccination
Preadolescent assessment

Figure 1. Recommended Childhood and Adolescent Immunization Schedule, United States 2003.
Approved by the Advisory Committee on Immunization Practices (www.cdc.gov/nip/acip), the American Academy of Pediatrics (www aap.org), and the American Academy of Family Physicians (www.aafp.org).

This schedule indicates the recommended ages for routine administration of currently licensed childhood vaccines, as of December 1, 2002, for children through age 18 years. Any dose not given at the recommended age should be given at any subsequent visit when indicated and feasible. (■) Indicates age groups that warrant special effort to administer those vaccines not previously given. Additional vaccines may be licensed and recommended during the year. Licensed combination vaccines may be used whenever any components of the combination are indicated and the vaccine's other components are not contraindicated. Providers should consult the manufacturers' package inserts for detailed recommendations.

1. Hepatitis B vaccine (Hep B). All infants should receive the first dose of hepatitis B vaccine soon after birth and before hospital discharge; the first dose may also be given by age 2 months if the infant's mother is HBsAg-negative. Only monovalent hepatitis B vaccine can be used for the birth dose. Monovalent or combination vaccine containing Hep B may be used to complete the series. Four doses of vaccine may be administered when a birth dose is given. The second dose should be given at least 4 weeks after the first dose, except for combination vaccines which cannot be administered before age 6 weeks. The third dose should be given at least 16 weeks after the first dose and at least 8 weeks after the second dose. The last dose in the vaccination series (third or fourth dose) should not be administered before age 6 months.

Infants born to HBsAg-positive mothers should receive hepatitis B vaccine and 0.5 ml, Hepatitis B Immune Globulin (HBIG) within 12 hours of birth at separate sites. The second dose is recommended at age 1-2 months. The last dose in the vaccination series should not be administered before age 6 months. These infants should be tested for HBsAg and anti-HBs at 9-15 months of age.

Infants born to mothers whose HbsAg status is unknown should receive the first dose of the hepatitis B vaccine series within 12 hours of birth. Maternal blood should be drawn as soon as possible to determine the mother's HBsAg status; if the HBsAg test is positive, the infant should receive HBIG as soon as possible (no later than age 1 week). The second dose is recommended at age 1-2 months. The last dose in the vaccination series should not be administred before age 6 months.

2. Diphtheria and tetanus toxoids and acellular pertussis vaccine (DTaP). The fourth dose of DTaP may be administered as early as age 12 months, provided 6 months have elapsed since the third dose and the child is unlikely to return at age 15-18 months. **Tetanus and diphtheria toxoids (Td)** is recommended at age 11-12 years if at least 5 years have elapsed since the last dose of tetanus and diphtheria toxoid-containing vaccine. Subsequent routine Td boosters are recommended every 10 years.

3. *Haemophilus influenzae* type b (Hib) conjugate vaccine. Three Hib conjugate vaccines are licensed for infant use. If PRP-OMP (PedvaxHib® or ComVax® [Merck]) is administered at ages 2 and 4 months, a dose at age 6 months is not required. DTaP/Hib combination products should not be used for primary immunization in infants at ages 2, 4 or 6 months, but can be used as boosters following any Hib vaccine.

4. Measles, mumps, and rubella vaccine (MMR). The second dose of MMR is recommended routinely at age 4-6 years but may be administered during any visit, provided at least 4 weeks have elapsed since the first dose and that both doses are administered beginning at or after age 12 months. Those who have not previously received the second dose should complete the schedule by the 11-12 year old visit

5. Varicella vaccine. Varicella vaccine is recommended at any visit at or after age 12 months for susceptible children, i.e., those who lack a reliable history of chickenpox. Susceptible persons aged ≥13 years should receive two doses, given at least 4 weeks apart.

6. Pneumococcal vaccine. The heptavalent **pneumococcal conjugate vaccine (PCV)** is recommended for all children age 2-23 months. It is also recommended for certain children age 24-59 months. **Pneumococcal polysaccharide vaccine (PPV)** is recommended in addition to PCV for certain high-risk groups. See *MMWR* 2000;49(RR-9):1-38.

Continued

the United States as its use was associated with 8 to 10 cases of vaccine associated paralytic polio (VAPP) each year in the United States.

The primary series of IPV consists of three doses beginning at 6 to 8 weeks of age. The second dose is usually given at 4 months, and the third dose between 6 and 18 months of age (see Figure 1). A fourth dose is recommended on or after the fourth birthday before school entry. A fourth dose is not necessary if the third dose was given on or after the fourth birthday. A minimum interval of 4 weeks should separate all doses of the series. Minor local reactions including pain or redness may occur. Allergic reactions may occur in persons sensitive to streptomycin, polymyxin B, and neomycin because IPV may contain trace amounts of these antibiotics.

HAEMOPHILUS INFLUENZAE TYPE B VACCINES

Haemophilus influenzae type b (Hib) is a gram-negative coccobacillus which has six capsular subtypes (*a* through *f*). It enters the nasopharynx where it may colonize. In younger persons, the organism (especially types b and f) may then cause invasive disease. Hib disease peak attack rates in unvaccinated children are at 6 to 7 months of age; the disease is uncommon after 5 years of age. The most common types of invasive disease include meningitis, epiglottitis, septic arthritis, cellulitis, pneumonia, osteomyelitis, purulent pericarditis, endocarditis, and neonatal sepsis.

Since 1990, three polysaccharide-protein conjugate vaccines have been licensed for use in infants. All infants should receive a primary series of conjugate Hib vaccine (see Figure 1); the number of doses depends on the type of vaccine used and the age that the Hib series is initiated (Table 1). Regardless of the type of Hib protein conjugate vaccine used, a booster dose is recommended at 12 to 15 months. The minimum interval between doses is 4 weeks, with the optimal interval being 8 weeks. Children who initiate the Hib series after 7 months of age may not require the full series. Only one dose is needed between 15 and 59 months of age (see Table 1). Hib vaccine should not be given before 6 weeks of age because early doses may induce immunologic tolerance to additional doses of Hib vaccine.

Adverse events are uncommon after Hib vaccination. Five to thirty percent of vaccines report swelling, redness, or pain. Fever and irritability are infrequent. Precautions include moderate to severe illness. Contraindications include anaphylaxis to a prior dose and age <6 weeks because of the risk of immunologic tolerance.

MEASLES VACCINE

Between 1989 and 1991, a dramatic resurgence of measles recurred because of low immunization coverage levels in urban areas. The measles virus is a paramyxovirus that results in an acute viral systemic infection. The virus enters the nasopharynx and subsequently causes a primary viremia and infection of the reticuloendothelial system. The incubation period ranges from 7 to 18 days. The prodrome of measles classically includes a stepwise increase in fever (≥ 38.3°C), followed by cough, coryza, conjunctivitis, and Koplik spots on the mucous membranes. The classic measles rash begins at the hairline and proceeds with a downward, distal spread. Complications include diarrhea,

Table 1. **Detailed Vaccination Schedule for *Haemophilus influenzae* Type b Conjugate Vaccines**

Vaccine	Age at 1st Dose (Months)	Primary Series	Booster
HbOC (Hibtiter)/PRP-T (ActHIB)	2–6	3 doses, 2 months apart	12–15 months*
	7–11	2 doses, 2 months apart	12–15 months*
	12–14	1 dose	2 months later
	15–59	1 dose	—
PRP-OMP (PedvaxHIB)	2–6	2 doses, 2 months apart	12–15 months*
	7–11	2 doses, 2 months apart	12–15 months*
	12–14	1 dose	2 months later
	15–59	1 dose	—
PRP-D (*Connaught)	15–59	1 dose	—

*At least 2 months after previous dose.

Figure 1. ***Legend Continued***

7. Hepatitis A vaccine. Hepatitis A vaccine is recommended for use in selected states and regions, and for certain high-risk groups; consult your local public health authority. Children and adolescents in these states, regions, and high risk groups who have not been immunized against hepatitis A can begin the hepatitis A vaccination series during any visit. The two doses in the series should be administered at least 6 months apart. See *MMWR* 1999;48(RR-12):1-37.

8. Influenza vaccine. Influenza vaccine is recommended annually for children age ≥6 months with certain risk factors (including but not limited to asthma, cardiac disease, sickle cell disease, HIV, diabetes, and household members of persons in groups at high risk; see *MMWR* 2002;51(RR-3):1-31), and can be administered to all others wishing to obtain immunity. In addition, healthy children age 6-23 months are encouraged to receive influenza vaccine if feasible because children in this age group are at substantially increased risk for influenza-related hospitalizations. Children aged ≤12 years should receive vaccine in a dosage appropriate for their age (0.25 mL if age 6-35 months or 0.5 mL if aged ≥ 3 years). Children aged ≤8 years who are receiving influenza vaccine for the first time should receive two doses separated by at least 4 weeks.

For additional information about vaccines, including precautions and contraindications for immunization and vaccine shortages, please visit the National Immunization Program Website at www.cdc.gov/nip or call the National Immunization Hotline at 800-232-2522 (English) or 800-232-0233 (Spanish).

otitis media, laryngotracheobronchitis, pneumonia, encephalitis, and death. Death is usually secondary to neurologic and respiratory complications.

Currently, the first dose of measles-containing vaccine (MMR) should be given on or after the first birthday (see Figure 1). Ninety-nine percent of children respond to the first dose. A second dose is recommended at ages 4 to 6 years to produce immunity in children who failed to respond to the first dose (primary vaccine failure). The second dose may be given a minimum of 4 weeks after the first dose, as long as the first dose was given on or after 1 year of age. Adverse reactions may include fever (≥39.4°C or higher) or rash 6 to 12 days after vaccination. Rarely, thrombocytopenia, lymphadenopathy, or allergic reactions may occur.

Contraindications include the following: allergy to gelatin or neomycin, a severe allergic reaction after a prior dose, pregnancy, immunosuppression, moderate to severe illness, persons receiving large daily doses of steroids (>2 mg/kg/day or >20 mg/d) for 14 days or more, HIV infection with severe immunosuppression, or recipients of antibody-containing blood products. Egg allergy is not a contraindication to MMR vaccination, and skin testing to eggs is not indicated. If a tuberculin skin test (TST) is needed at the time of MMR vaccination, it should be placed simultaneously or separated by >4 weeks to eliminate any theoretical concern of the suppression of the TST reactivity after vaccination.

VARICELLA VACCINE

Varicella zoster is a herpesvirus that results in the disease commonly known as chicken pox. The virus enters through the respiratory tract and conjunctiva followed by a primary and secondary viremia. Clinical features begin after an incubation period ranging from 10 to 21 days. A mild prodrome of fever and malaise is followed by a generalized, pruritic rash. Classically, the rash follows a centripetal distribution with skin lesions in multiple stages of development (papules, vesicles, and crusts). Complications of varicella include secondary bacterial infection of skin lesions, arthritis, hepatitis, thrombocytopenia, pneumonia, and CNS involvement (ranging from aseptic meningitis to encephalitis). Death occurs in approximately 1 per 60,000 cases. Complications are highest in persons >15 years and infants <1 year of age.

The varicella zoster vaccine is a live attenuated viral vaccine. Routine vaccination is recommended at 12 to 18 months of age (see Figure 1). The vaccine is highly recommended by the 13th birthday, because severe complications from varicella disease are more frequent after this age. Children >13 years, who have not been immunized or had natural disease, should receive two doses of varicella vaccine separated by 4 to 8 weeks, as seroconversion rates in children >13 years after a single dose are lower than those in younger children. Contraindications and precautions are similar to those for MMR vaccine and include the following: severe allergy to a prior dose, allergy to neomycin or gelatin, immunosuppression, pregnancy, moderate to severe illness, or receipt of an antibody containing blood product. Salicylates should be avoided for 6 weeks after the varicella vaccine because of an association between aspirin use and Reye syndrome after chickenpox. If a child is due for both MMR and varicella vaccine, they either should be given simultaneously or separated by ≥28 days.

HEPATITIS A VACCINE

Hepatitis A is a picornavirus that is spread by the fecal-oral route. A long incubation period of 15 to 50 days may be followed by the abrupt onset of fever, malaise, anorexia, nausea, and jaundice. Children <6 years of age are symptomatic in 30% of cases, compared with older children and adults who are symptomatic in >70% of cases. Fulminant hepatitis A is rare, but may occur in those with underlying liver disease.

Hepatitis A vaccine is an inactivated whole virus vaccine. Currently, it is not licensed for children <2 years of age. Routine hepatitis A vaccination is recommended for children >2 years of age who live in states, counties, or communities where the annual hepatitis A disease rate between 1987 and 1997 was >20 per 100,000 persons (twice the national average). Children ages 2 to 18 years should receive an initial dose followed by a booster dose 6 to 12 months later (see Figure 1). Adverse reactions are mild and may include pain, erythema, or swelling at the injection site. Low-grade fever, fatigue, and malaise are even less common. Contraindications and precautions include severe allergic reaction after a previous dose, allergy to alum, or in the case of Havrix, allergy to 2-phenoxyethanol.

HEPATITIS B VACCINE

Hepatitis B virus (HBV) is a hepadnavirus. This virus is transmitted by parenteral or mucosal exposure from infected bodily fluids. After a prolonged incubation period ranging from 6 weeks to 6 months, the typical illness is characterized by a 3- to 10-day prodromal phase (i.e., malaise, anorexia, nausea, and abdominal pains) followed by a 1- to 3-week icteric period and a convalescent period in which malaise and fatigue may persist for weeks to months. Young children may be asymptomatic. Complications may include chronic HBV infection, which may result in chronic liver disease. Fulminant hepatitis may occur in 1% to 2% of persons.

Hepatitis B vaccination is recommended for all infants before hospital discharge. The primary dose may be given at 2 months of age if the infant's mother is HBsAg-negative. The second dose is recommended 1 to 4 months after the first dose with a 1-month minimum interval between doses 1 and 2. The third dose is recommended at age 6 to 18 months with a 2-month minimum interval between the second and third doses (see Figure 1). The minimum interval between doses 1 and 3 is 4 months. The third dose should not be given to infants before they are 6 months of age. Children not vaccinated during infancy should be vaccinated at 11 to 12 years of age. Adult hepatitis B vaccine candidates are many and include the following: men who have sex with men, heterosexuals with multiple partners, prostitutes, persons with other sexually transmitted diseases, intravenous drug users, prison inmates, persons on hemodialysis, health care workers, institutionalized individuals, Alaskan natives, Pacific Islanders, immigrants from HBV-endemic areas, household members of HBV carriers, and blood product recipients.

Contraindications to hepatitis B vaccine include serious allergic reaction to a previous dose or vaccine component or moderate to severe illness. Adverse events after vaccination include pain at the injection site and fever. Of note, no causal link between demyelinating disease, rheumatologic illnesses, or autoimmune diseases and hepatitis B vaccination has been found.

INFLUENZA VACCINE

Influenza is a RNA virus with three antigenic strains: A, B, and C. Influenza type A affects all age groups and results in moderate to severe illness. Influenza type B primarily affects children and causes milder disease than type A. Influenza type C is rarely associated with human illness.

Influenza type A has subtypes that are determined by surface antigens: hemagglutinin (H_1, H_2, and H_3) and neuraminidase (N_1 and N_2). The hemagglutinin and neuraminidase antigens periodically change. When major changes occur in one or both surface antigens (antigenic shift), worldwide pandemics may result from the large number of individuals with no prior immunologic experience to the new antigens. When minor changes occur in the surface antigens (antigenic drift), persons who are incompletely protected may transmit or develop disease. Antigenic drift occurs annually, however antigenic shift occurs at intervals of ≥ 10 years.

Influenza virus is spread by respiratory transmission. The virus attaches and penetrates respiratory epithelial cells. After an incubation period of 1 to 5 days (average 2 days), infected persons may develop the abrupt onset of fever, sore throat, myalgia and nonproductive cough. Symptoms usually last from 2 to 3 days and rarely longer than 5 days. Attack rates are highest among school-age children. Complications of influenza include secondary bacterial pneumonia, myocarditis, worsening of chronic bronchitis, myositis, Reye syndrome, and possibly death.

The influenza vaccine is an inactivated split-virus vaccine. Immunity after inactivated influenza vaccination rarely exceeds 1 year. Optimally, the vaccine is administered annually between early October and mid November. Influenza vaccine is recommended for the following at-risk individuals: persons >50 years of age, residents of long-term care facilities, pregnant women, persons 6 months to 18 years receiving chronic aspirin therapy, health care workers, and persons older than 6 months of age with chronic illness. Chronic illness includes the following: chronic pulmonary disease such as asthma, emphysema, bronchopulmonary dysplasia or chronic bronchitis, cardiovascular disease such as congenital heart disease or congestive heart failure, metabolic disease including diabetes mellitus, renal dysfunction, hemoglobinopathies, and immunosuppression. In 2002, the ACIP began encouraging influenza immunization of healthy children ages 6 to 23 months and their household contacts as these young children are at increased risk of influenza-related hospitalizations. Please see Table 2 regarding influenza dosages.

Following influenza vaccination, local reactions such as soreness, erythema, and induration may occur. The vaccine only contains inactivated products and cannot cause influenza disease. Fever, malaise, and myalgias occur in <1% of vaccine recipients. Allergic reactions are rare; however, egg allergy and thimerosal sensitivity are contraindications to immunization.

PNEUMOCOCCAL VACCINES

Streptococcus pneumoniae is a gram-positive organism that may result in serious invasive diseases such as pneumonia, bacteremia, and meningitis. Although many different serotypes exist, 10 of the most common serotypes produce about 62% of the invasive diseases. Pneumococci are commonly found in the respiratory tract. Asymptomatic carriage rates vary depending on age, environment, and presence of upper respiratory tract infections. The highest rates of invasive disease are in the following persons: children <2 years of age, persons with functional or anatomic asplenia such as in sickle cell disease, and persons with HIV. Children of certain ethnic groups (Alaskan native, Native American, and African American) and children in daycare are also at increased risk.

Two pneumococcal vaccines are available in the United States: 23-valent polysaccharide vaccine and the 7-valent polysaccharide conjugate vaccine. The 23-valent polysaccharide vaccine may be given to individuals older than 2 years of age and protects against 60% to 70% of invasive forms of pneumococcal disease. The 23-valent vaccine is recommended for all adults >65 years and persons >2 years who are immunocompromised or who have chronic diseases such as heart disease, lung disease, diabetes, liver disease, or cerebrospinal fluid leaks. The most common adverse events are local reactions occurring in 30% to 50% of recipients. Fever and myalgias occur in fewer than 1% of recipients. Severe systemic adverse events are rare.

A series of four 7-valent polysaccharide conjugate vaccines are recommended for infants. This vaccine has been shown to reduce invasive pneumococcal disease by 89%. Primary series doses are given at 2, 4, and 6 months of age (see Figure 1). Children who begin vaccination at >7 months of age require fewer doses

TABLE 2. **Influenza Vaccine Dosage, by Age Group—United States**

Age Group	Dosage	Number of Doses	Route
6-35 months	0.25 mL	1* or 2	IM
3-8 years	0.50 mL	1* or 2	IM
>9 years	0.50 mL	1	IM

*Only one dose is needed if the child received influenza vaccine during a previous influenza season.

TABLE 3. **Recommended Schedule of Doses for PCV7, Including Primary Series and Catch-Up Immunizations, in Previously Unvaccinated Children***

Age at First Dose	Primary Series	Booster Dose[†]
2-6 mo	3 doses, 6-8 wk apart	1 dose at 12-15 mo of age
7-11 mo	2 doses, 6-8 wk apart	1 dose at 12-15 mo of age
12-23 mo	2 doses, 6-8 wk apart	
≥24 mo	1 dose	

*Recommendations for high-risk groups are given in Table 3.
[†]Booster doses to be given at least 6 to 8 weeks after the final dose of the primary series.

(Table 3). After vaccination, local reactions occur in 10% to 20% of recipients with fever and myalgias occurring in 15% to 24% of recipients. For both types of pneumococcal vaccine, serious allergic reaction to a prior dose is a contraindication. Moderate to severe illness is a temporary contraindication to immunization.

TRAVEL MEDICINE

method of
CHAD M. BRAUN, M.D., and
KATHERINE G. GERGAS, M.S., CNP
Rardin Family Practice Center
Columbus, Ohio

Travel medicine is a subspecialty dedicated to the promotion of health and disease prevention in the traveling populace. With the advent of commercial air travel, our continental borders no longer restrict us. This freedom to travel throughout the world has exposed travelers to conditions not found commonly in the western world. According to the World Travel Association, international tourist arrivals amounted to 693 million in 2001. These numbers are expected to increase to 1.5 billion travelers by the year 2020. Many travelers do not seek pretravel advice from their primary care providers, and as a result face a higher risk of returning home ill.

Recent data compiled by GeoSentinel (2001), a global provider-based surveillance system that tracks infections in travelers, immigrants, and refugees, demonstrated acute diarrhea as the most common cause of morbidity among travelers. The exception to this was in sub-Saharan Africa, where the most common cause of morbidity was malaria. Other frequent causes of morbidity included skin conditions, viral syndromes, acute respiratory infections, helminths, and chronic diarrhea.

With this in mind, providers of primary care must know where resources are for current information regarding regional and country-specific disease risks, emerging infectious diseases, and anti-microbial resistance. The Centers for Disease Control and Prevention web site (www.cdc.gov/travelershealth) provides excellent up-to-date information for providers and patients. This web site also can direct patients and providers to local travel medicine specialists.

Ideally, the traveler should seek pre-travel care at least 4 to 6 weeks before departure. This allows time for routine medical and dental examinations, pretravel counseling and pretravel immunization.

TRAVEL COUNSELING

The consultation before travel is designed primarily to review the travel itinerary and then customize treatment accordingly. It is important to determine the destinations, length of stay, and activities planned. This history helps to determine potential risk as well as needs. A travel questionnaire can be quite helpful to obtain this information, especially when the patient is not well-known to the provider. This should assess medication allergies and allergies to vaccine components. Other areas of assessment should include immune system competency and presence of chronic disease. An accurate vaccination history should also be obtained. Further, the consultation should also focus on prevention and treatment of food, water, and insect-borne illnesses. Appropriate vaccines should also be administered.

PREVENTION OF FOOD AND WATER-BORNE ILLNESS

Prevention of food- and water-borne illnesses should be discussed with the patient planning international travel. In most circumstances, tap water should be avoided for drinking or even brushing teeth. In general water should be bottled or boiled. Water that is boiled should be boiled for 5 to 10 minutes at a rolling boil. Carbonated beverages are generally safe, as are pasteurized juices. All food should be well-cooked and served hot. Salads and precut fruit should be avoided. Fruits that can be peeled are generally safe. Meat should be well-done only. Unpasteurized milk, cheese, and other milk products should be avoided as well. Travelers should refrain from patronizing street vendors selling food.

Traveler's diarrhea is one of the most common ailments suffered by travelers. The best advice for the traveler is to replace the fluids lost during an episode of diarrhea. When an oral rehydration solution cannot be found, fluids should be replaced with reliable bottled water or caffeine free carbonated beverages. Bismuth subsalicylate (Pepto-Bismol) can be given to adults for whom there are no contraindications. Two tablets before meals and at bedtime can be used as prevention for traveler's diarrhea. Antimotility agents such as loperamide (Imodium) can be used with caution in adults. Antibiotic prophylaxis is no longer recommended for traveler's diarrhea. However, individuals may need a broad-spectrum antibiotic prescribed, especially when traveling to remote areas with limited access. For adults ciprofloxacin (Cipro) is an excellent choice. A dosage of 500 mg twice daily for 3 days is usually adequate. For children or allergic adults, azithromycin (Zithromax)* is an excellent alternative.

*Not FDA approved for this indication.

VACCINE PREVENTABLE ILLNESS

There are several vaccines recommended for international travelers. Many countries only require yellow fever vaccination. Cholera is no longer required, and there is no commercially available cholera vaccine for use in the United States. There are two recently developed vaccines available and licensed in other countries; however, neither of these is recommended for travelers. Infrequently some countries may still want to see proof of a cholera vaccine. In this case a stamp can be placed in the International Certificate of Vaccination (vaccine record recognized by the World Health Organization that can be purchased online from the U.S. government printing office).

Yellow Fever Vaccine

Yellow fever is a mosquito-borne viral illness occurring in tropical Africa and South America. The vaccine (YF-Vax) is live and produced from chick embryos. It should be avoided for individuals with a known hypersensitivity to eggs. The vaccine can cause fever and myalgias for 5 to 10 days after administration. It can be administered to children as young as 9 months. Evidence suggests that individuals age 65 or older are at an increased risk for adverse systemic events after administration of the vaccine. In this case, risks and benefits should be weighed carefully by the elderly patient and the health care provider. Yellow fever vaccine is contraindicated in pregnancy and conception should not be attempted for 3 months after administration. Yellow fever vaccine should not be given to those with immunosuppression. Low-dose steroid therapy (less than 10 mg per day), short-term corticosteroid therapy (less than 2 weeks), and bursal, tendon, or intra-articular steroid injections do not pose a risk to those receiving yellow fever vaccine. The individual who has received this vaccine poses no risk to household contacts that may be immunosuppressed. For those unable to receive vaccination because of contraindications, an exemption letter can be written. This should be on letterhead and bear an official stamp.

Hepatitis A

Hepatitis A is an enterically transmitted viral disease highly endemic in the developing world. It is the most common vaccine-preventable illness in travelers. Hepatitis A vaccine or immune globulin (IG IM) is highly recommended for all susceptible travelers planning on spending time in areas with high endemicity. The United States, Canada, Western Europe, Japan, Australia, and New Zealand have low rates. The rest of the world has intermediate to high risk. Two commercially available vaccines (Havrix, Vaqta) exist for use in the United States and they may be used interchangeably. Immunity can be expected by 4 weeks. Children older than age 2 may receive hepatitis A vaccines. It is recommended that individuals follow up with a second vaccine 6 to 12 months after the first. This is expected to provide the patient with at least 20 years of immunity. A combined Hepatitis A and Hepatitis B vaccine is now also available (Twinrix). Twinrix is not for use in children. Side effects are minimal, generally pain at the injection site for 24 to 48 hours. The safety of Hepatitis A vaccine in pregnancy has not been determined. Theoretically, there is little risk because Hepatitis A vaccine is produced from inactivated virus.

Hepatitis B

Hepatitis B is a viral illness transmitted through exposure to blood or blood-derived fluids. Risk to travelers is generally low except in areas with high endemicity. A risk assessment should be done to determine if a traveler is in need of hepatitis B protection. Factors to consider are activities planned, prevalence of chronic Hepatitis B in the general population, duration of stay, and any international adoptions. Two commercially available vaccines (Recombivax HB) exist in the United States. The vaccine is administered in a series of three doses at 0, 1 and 6 months. One of the vaccines, Energix-B, can be administered on an accelerated schedule at 0, 1, 2, and 12 months. Most individuals have 80% of their immunity after two doses. The final dose makes the immunity long-term. Hepatitis B vaccine is now recommended as a routine immunization for all children in the United States. Side effects are minimal, with the most common being pain at the injection site for 24 to 48 hours. Safety data in pregnant women is not known, but there is little theoretical risk because it is an inactivated vaccine.

Influenza

Respiratory disease caused by influenza A and B viruses can be a risk to travelers depending on time of year and destination. Influenza season is year round in the tropics, April through September in the temperate zones of the Southern Hemisphere and December through March in the temperate zones of the Northern Hemisphere. Vaccination is recommended for all international travelers. The vaccine is inactivated. Side effects include pain at the injection site for 24 to 48 hours and possible low-grade fever and myalgias for the same period, especially in those who have never received the vaccine before. Vaccine can be administered to children as young as 6 months. Children age 6 months to 9 years will require two doses at least 1 month apart to maximize antibody response. It is recommended that women who will be in at least their 14th week of pregnancy should be vaccinated.

Japanese Encephalitis

Japanese encephalitis is mosquito-borne viral encephalitis found mainly in Asia and the Pacific. Those who have the misfortune of developing clinical illness have a moderate rate (50%) of neuropsychiatric sequelae and case fatality rates can approach 30%.

Fortunately most cases are asymptomatic. Risk to short-term (less than 4 weeks' duration) travelers and those visiting urban areas is very low. Travelers residing for long periods of time in rural areas and expatriates are at highest risk. Travelers visiting risk areas are advised to take personal protective measures such as staying indoors from dusk to dawn and the utilization of repellents.

There is one vaccine licensed for use in the United States. The vaccine (JE-VAX) should be offered only to higher risk travelers. The vaccine is delivered in a series on days 0, 7, and 30. An accelerated schedule can be given on days 0, 7, and 14 but short-term immunity will only occur in 80% of vaccinees. Those receiving vaccination must not depart for 10 days after the last administration of vaccine to ensure adequate immune response and access to health care in the event of delayed adverse/allergic responses. Less than 1% of vaccinees may have delayed urticaria, angioedema, respiratory distress, and anaphylaxis. Nearly 20% of vaccinees experience pain at the injection site along with mild systemic complaints. Individuals with a known hypersensitivity to the vaccine or vaccine components (bee venom) should not be vaccinated. The vaccine is not recommended for those younger than age of 1 or for pregnant women.

Measles

Measles is an acute, highly communicable viral disease characterized by prodromal fever, coryza, conjunctivitis, cough, and Koplik spots on the buccal mucosa. Fewer than 1000 cases have been reported each year since 1993. Half of the cases reported each year come from people returning from visits overseas. Risk outside of the United States is high and can occur within developed Asian and European countries.

It is recommended that measles, mumps, rubella vaccine (MMR) be given if protection against any of the three viruses is needed. Individuals born before 1957, individuals with a known history of disease, individuals with proof of two live doses of measles vaccine on or after their first birthday, or those with laboratory evidence of immunity need not be vaccinated. MMR vaccine is recommended as part of the childhood immunization schedule for children in the United States. Adults never immunized or children behind on their immunization should be sure to receive two doses separated by at least 28 days. There is no contraindication to receiving two live vaccines simultaneously. But if two live vaccines are to be administered separately a period of at least 28 days must transpire between them. Pregnant women and immunosuppressed patients should not receive MMR vaccine.

Meningococcal Disease

Meningococcal disease occurs throughout the world. Symptoms include high fever, headache, stiff neck, nausea and vomiting, and a petechial rash. Due to early recognition and antibiotic therapy case fatality rates are 5% to 15%. Epidemics are known to occur frequently in sub-Saharan Africa especially during the dry season (December to June). Although the disease is rare in Americans who have visited that part of the world, the vaccine is still recommended. Individuals going to Mecca for an Islamic pilgrimage (Hajj or Umra) are required to have had the meningococcal vaccine.

There is one commercially available meningococcal vaccine (Menomune—A/C/Y/W-135) for use in the United States. The vaccine provides protection for 3 to 5 years. It is an inactivated polysaccharide vaccine and side effects are minimal, generally just pain at the injection site for 24 to 48 hours. The vaccine is not recommended for those younger than 2 years of age. Studies in pregnant women have not documented any adverse effects on the women or neonates.

Polio

Poliomyelitis transmission is via the oral-fecal route. Worldwide polio eradication projects have decreased the number of infected countries. There still are two large endemic areas in south Asia and sub-Saharan Africa. Travelers going to these areas should be fully immunized. Inactivated polio vaccine (IPOL) is the only vaccine available in the United States now. Side effects are minimal. Adults who have not received a primary series before visiting a polio endemic area should be vaccinated prior to travel. Three doses are given at presentation, 4 to 8 weeks later and in 6 to 12 months. If time before travel is less than 8 weeks, two doses should be given 4 weeks apart. If less than 4 weeks remain before travel, a single dose should be given and the series completed post travel. Children receive polio vaccine as part of the routine immunization schedule. The vaccine is avoided in pregnant women. Immunodeficient individuals may receive inactivated polio vaccine only.

Rabies

Rabies is almost always transmitted via animal bite. Travelers should be advised not to pet or feed animals, especially dogs. If bitten, travelers should wash the wound with soap and water, apply an antiseptic, and seek medical care immediately. Travelers with extensive outdoor or long-term travel to highly endemic areas should consider preexposure vaccination. Rabies vaccine (Imovax) is given intramuscularly at presentation and on days 7, 21, and 28. Side effects include pain, erythema, and pruritus at the injection site. Mild systemic side effects can also occur. The vaccine can be given to children. Preexposure vaccination is generally not recommended in pregnant women. Postexposure prophylaxis is not contraindicated in pregnancy.

Diphtheria, Tetanus, and Pertussis

An effort should be made to update the tetanus-diphtheria booster for traveling adults. It should also be stressed that this should be updated every 10 years as a matter of routine preventive care. If an adult or child older than age 7 has never received a primary series, three doses of tetanus-diphtheria (Td) should be given at presentation, 4 weeks later, and in 12 months. Diphtheria, tetanus, and acellular pertussis vaccines (DTaP) are given to children as a part of their routine childhood immunization schedule in the United States. The doses are given at 2, 4, 6, and 15 to 18 months. A booster is given at age 4 to 6 years. Side effects are generally minimal. It is preferred that Td be given as needed to pregnant women in the second or third trimesters.

Typhoid

Travelers are exposed to typhoid via contaminated food and drink. The risk of the disease is greatest on the Indian subcontinent and other developing countries in Asia, Central and South America, and Africa. Vaccination is especially recommended for those individuals traveling to remote areas or those who will have prolonged stays. There are two available vaccines with efficacy rates around 80%. The live oral vaccine (Vivotif Berna) provides some protection for up to 5 years. Four capsules must be taken each separated by 1 day. These must be taken on an empty stomach and there is potential for nausea, vomiting, and diarrhea. The vaccine should be avoided in those with impaired gastric defenses, children younger than 8 years of age and in pregnant women.

The polysaccharide-inactivated vaccine (Typhim Vi) offers protection for 2 years. It can be used in children at least 2 years of age. There are no safety data available about use of Typhim Vi in pregnancy; therefore, based on theoretical grounds the vaccine should be avoided in pregnant women. The oral vaccine (Vivotif Berna) should not be administered simultaneously with antibiotics or antimalarial medications as decreased immune response may occur. There should be at least 1 week between the last dose of the oral typhoid vaccine and the beginning of these medications. After the completion of antibiotics or antimalarials the oral typhoid vaccine cannot be started for at least 24 hours.

PREVENTION OF INSECT-BORNE ILLNESSES

There are a number of parasitic or viral diseases that travelers can be exposed to via the bite of an insect or mosquito. Travelers need to take personal protective measures when they are in areas at risk for exposure to such diseases. The following are some recommendations:

- Use unscented beauty products
- Cover up as much as you can with tightly woven fabrics that are light in color
- Avoid sheer fabrics and tight clothing
- Tuck pant legs into socks and tuck shirttails into pants
- Avoid sandals
- Check skin daily for insects
- Avoid walking in tall grass
- Do not lie directly on the ground
- Never dry clothing on the ground
- Check inside footwear and sleeping bags for insects
- Stay indoors at twilight or from dusk to dawn
- Use air conditioning when available and keep windows closed
- Choose camping areas that are high, dry, and away from food or rotting wood

Repellents

Travelers at risk for exposure to insect-borne illness should take the aforementioned precautions and use repellents. Permethrin (Insect Repellent Spray) is effective and can be sprayed on clothing, knapsacks, tents, and netting ahead of time. Its repelling effect lasts up to 20 launderings. Rooms can also be sprayed 1 hour before bedtime. Individuals should stay out of the room for 30 minutes after spraying. DEET is still recommended for repelling insects that may cause disease. It is applied to exposed skin. It is recommended that adults use a 30% to 35% concentration. DEET in a lower concentration (10%) can be used on children. In children 2 to 6 years of age, DEET should be used sparingly. It should not be used on children younger than 2 years of age. Pregnant women should use DEET sparingly in a low concentration.

Malaria Prophylaxis

Malaria is a mammoth international public health problem. Transmission of the disease occurs in Central and South America, Hispaniola, sub-Saharan Africa, the Indian subcontinent, Southeast Asia, the Middle East, and Oceania. Risk and need for prophylaxis depends on itinerary, length of stay, and activities planned. Health care providers advising international travelers should consult a reputable resource prior to prescribing an antimalarial medication for prophylaxis as there is an increasing amount of chloroquine-resistant *Plasmodium falciparum* worldwide. The Centers for Disease Control and Prevention web site is an excellent resource (*www.cdc.gov/travel*).

It should be stressed to all travelers that despite the use of personal protective measures, repellents, and chemoprophylaxis they still could develop the disease. Travelers should be advised the symptoms generally occur 10 to 14 days after an exposure and include high fever, severe myalgias, and nausea and vomiting. The symptoms may abate and then return. If these symptoms are experienced the traveler should proceed to his or her health care provider at once.

Malaria can be severe in pregnant women. Travel to endemic areas should be avoided or postponed until after delivery. Adverse outcomes include prematurity, abortion, and stillbirth. No chemoprophylactic regimen is 100% effective. If women cannot be dissuaded from traveling to endemic areas then they should at least postpone travel until the second trimester (18 to 24 weeks). At this point, an antimalarial can be prescribed and there is less risk. Pregnant women considering travel should consult their family doctor prior to international departures as a number of individual risk factors must be discussed.

Chloroquine (Aralen)

When traveling to areas without resistance, chloroquine should be prescribed if not contraindicated. The medication is generally tolerated very well. Side effects are mild and include stomach upset, dizziness, or headache. The regimen is 500 mg salt (300 mg base) weekly. This should begin 2 weeks before arrival, continue throughout the trip, and for 4 weeks after the traveler has returned home. Chloroquine should not be prescribed to travelers with a history of psoriasis as it may cause an exacerbation. This medication can be prescribed for children. The dosage is 5 mg/kg base (8.3 mg/kg of salt) weekly up to maximum adult dose. Chemoprophylaxis with chloroquine can be prescribed during pregnancy.

Presently, chloroquine-resistant malaria has been reported in Southeast Asia, Indonesia, and Latin America. When traveling to areas of resistance, other prophylactic options must be considered.

Mefloquine (Lariam)

This is the drug of choice for travelers going to areas with chloroquine-resistant *P. falciparum*. It is generally tolerated well. Side effects include stomach upset, loss of appetite, diarrhea, dizziness, fatigue, and insomnia. Rare individuals (1 in 10,000) develop severe reactions to this medication. These include reports of confusion, memory loss, nightmares, hallucinations, depression, paranoia, and agitation. The prophylactic regimen is 250 mg of salt weekly. This should begin 1 week before arrival, continue for the duration of the trip, and for 4 weeks after the traveler has returned home. Mefloquine (Lariam) should not be prescribed to individuals with a history of heart conduction problems, epilepsy, depression, or anxiety. Individuals on calcium channel blockers, β-blockers, or quinidine should not be prescribed this medication.

Mefloquine can be prescribed for children based on body weight. It cannot be made into suspension. Parents are advised to crush the medication and place it into a very sweet juice or food. Parents should be reminded to keep medications away from children because overdoses of antimalarials can be fatal. Clinical trials and reports of inadvertent use of mefloquine during pregnancy suggest that its use during the second and third trimesters pose no threat of adverse outcomes. It can be considered for women in their second or third trimesters when exposure to chloroquine resistant *P. falciparum* is unavoidable.

Doxycycline (Vibramycin)

This medication is tolerated well by most individuals. Potential side effects include nausea, vomiting, and diarrhea. Individuals should be advised to take this with food. Antacids should be avoided because they interfere with medication absorption. Photosensitivity also occurs and individuals on this medication should use a sunscreen with an SPF of 15 or greater. The dosage is 100 mg per day. This should begin 5 days before travel, continue through the duration of the trip and for 4 weeks after returning home. This medication cannot be used in children under the age of 8 and is contraindicated in pregnancy.

Atovaquone and Proguanil (Malarone)

This medication is generally tolerated very well. There is potential for stomach upset, so it should be taken with food. Malarone should not be given to individuals taking tetracycline, metoclopramide (Reglan), rifampin (Rifadin), or rifabutin (Mycobutin). The dosage is 1 tablet daily (250 mg atovaquone and 100 mg proguanil). This should begin 1 to 2 days before arrival, continue daily throughout the trip, and for 1 week after arriving home. This medication can be prescribed for children. It is not recommended in pregnancy.

MISCELLANEOUS CONSIDERATIONS

Acute Mountain Sickness

Travelers planning high-altitude excursions must ascend gradually. If climbers begin to experience nausea, vomiting, or headache they should descend. Travelers hiking or climbing should be sure to stay well hydrated. Those planning excursions above 7000 feet should consider acetazolamide (Diamox) before ascent. The dosage is 250 mg twice daily. This is to begin 1 day before ascent and continue twice daily for 3 days. Diamox should not be given to those with an allergy to sulfa or those with renal impairment.

Fresh Water Exposure

Travelers should be advised not to do any fresh water swimming. Schistosomiasis is a concern in many parts of the world including Africa and South America. Travelers should only swim in well-maintained chlorinated pools or ocean water known to be free from pollution.

Issues Related to Flying

Many individuals seeking pretravel advice may ask what are the best treatments for jet lag, barotrauma, and motion sickness. There is no easy solution for the problem of jet lag. Often the best advice is for the travelers to adopt local time as soon as possible. Over-the-counter diphenhydramine (Benadryl)* can often provide enough assistance to the traveler trying to get to sleep. Chewing or swallowing during ascent and descent can prevent barotrauma. Infants should be fed during these times. Diphenhydramine (Benadryl),* meclizine (Antivert), or scopolamine transdermal patches (Transderm-Scop) can help ease motion sickness.

Venous stasis caused by prolonged periods of sitting during flights has led to the development of deep vein thrombosis and pulmonary emboli. To help avoid this, alcohol consumption should be limited and hydration

*Not FDA approved for this indication.

should be maintained. Travelers should also move about the cabin during flight.

AFTER-TRAVEL CARE

Providers in a travel medicine clinic should have the capability to recognize, diagnose, and treat unusual conditions acquired during travel. Not all persons who travel need a post-trip evaluation. This is especially true for healthy persons and short-term travelers. Those returning from long trips and expatriates from the developing world should undergo evaluation even if asymptomatic. This should consist of a history and physical examination, complete blood count, chemistry profile, tuberculin skin test, and stool examination. Both travelers and physicians must consider previous travel in the evaluation of symptoms that appear months or even years later. Significant symptoms include fever, chills, sweats, fatigue, or persistent diarrhea.

TOXOPLASMOSIS

method of
THOMAS T. WARD, M.D.
Oregon Health Sciences University
Portland VA Medical Center
Portland, Oregon

Toxoplasmosis is the disease caused by infection with the obligate intracellular protozoan *Toxoplasma gondii*. Toxoplasmosis is a worldwide zoonosis and causes infection in both birds and mammals. Cats, the definitive hosts for *T. gondii*, are the animals in which the parasite maintains an enteroepithelial sexual cycle. Human beings and domestic animals are secondary hosts and are important in maintaining an extraintestinal asexual cycle of transmission. Although most human infection is asymptomatic, self-limited clinical disease can infrequently occur after primary infection in immunocompetent persons. Because of the persistence of dormant cyst forms, all infection becomes chronic and latent. Primary infection during pregnancy can result in transplacental transmission of infection to the fetus; resultant congenital toxoplasmosis has varied clinical manifestations. Reactivation of dormant cysts is an important cause of infection in immunocompromised patients with defective T-cell–mediated immunity, including those patients with advanced HIV infection, hematologic malignancies, and bone marrow and solid organ transplants.

T. gondii exists in three forms: the oocyst, the tissue cyst, and the tachyzoite. Oocysts are formed only in infected felines; these cats excrete large numbers of cysts for approximately 2 weeks after infection. Oocysts may remain viable in the soil for months and are an important environmental reservoir for infection of incidental hosts. Tachyzoites occur with acute infection in incidental hosts; their presence is required for the histologic confirmation of active disease. Tissue cysts occur after replication of tachyzoites and likely persist for the life of the incidental host. Dormant cysts are most commonly located in skeletal and smooth muscle, heart, brain, and eye. The presence of tissue cysts in histologic sections is indicative of past infection, but by itself it does not signify active infection.

The human incidence of seropositivity for *T. gondii* antibody varies greatly throughout the world. Within the United States, seropositivity increases with age, and the overall seroprevalence is approximately 15%. Within Western Europe, seroprevalence ranges between 50% and 70%. Human transmission occurs by oral exposure to oocysts that have contaminated water sources, vegetables, or other food products or, even more commonly, by ingesting poorly cooked or raw meat that contains tissue cysts. As many as 25% of lamb or pork samples have been shown to contain tissue cysts.

After human ingestion of either oocysts or tissue cysts, specialized forms of *T. gondii* emerge that penetrate the intestinal mucosa, establish intracellular infection within white blood cells, and enter the blood and lymphatic circulations to result in widespread dissemination throughout the body. Intact cell-mediated immunity leads to clearance of intracellular tachyzoites and the formation of dormant tissue cysts. Impaired cell-mediated immunity leads to either uncontrolled, primary infection (as in the fetus) or reactivation of infection later in life (as in AIDS and other immunosuppressed conditions).

DIAGNOSIS

The diagnosis of *T. gondii* infection can be established by serologic tests, amplification of specific nucleic acid sequences, or histologic demonstration of the parasite or its antigens. Rarely employed reference or research methods for diagnosis include isolation of the organism, specific IgG avidity tests, various antigen detection tests, and lymphocyte transformation tests.

IgG antibodies appear in immunocompetent individuals within 2 to 3 weeks after infection. A negative IgG test essentially excludes previous or past infection with *T. gondii*. IgG antibody may persist in high titers for years after infection; therefore, a single positive IgG titer does not differentiate whether infection is recently acquired, chronic and latent, or chronic and reactivated. Sequential IgG antibody tests that increase by more than two tube dilutions are consistent with recent infection. Specific IgM and IgA antibody tests are usually positive during the first 6 months after acquisition of infection, and negative tests have a high predictive value for excluding recent infection. A positive IgM test can indicate recent onset of infection; however both false-positive results and persistently positive IgM antibody test results in chronically infected individuals can occur. When therapeutic decisions will be based on the interpretation of a positive IgM antibody test, confirmatory testing by a reference laboratory should be performed if feasible. Serologic tests can be more difficult to interpret in immunocompromised patients.

Polymerase chain reaction (PCR) for detection of specific *T. gondii* nucleic acid sequences has been successfully employed using vitreous and aqueous humor, bronchoalveolar lavage fluid, peripheral blood buffy coat preparations, cerebrospinal fluid, and amniotic fluid after 18 weeks of gestation. False-positive brain tissue PCR tests may occur in patients with HIV infection and suspected toxoplasmic encephalitis.

Specific histopathologic findings on resected lymph nodes can be strongly suggestive of the diagnosis of toxoplasmosis in immunocompetent patients. Demonstration of tachyzoites in tissue is invariably diagnostic of active infection. Although the presence of a single cyst does not differentiate between active and chronic or latent infection, multiple cysts present on cytopathologic examination suggest the presence of active disease. Staining for specific antigens (e.g., immunoperoxidase techniques) is highly specific for active infection when positive, and it is much more sensitive than hematoxylin and eosin or Wright-Giemsa staining alone. Tests employing direct fluorescent antibody tests can be nonspecific and are best avoided.

CLINICAL MANIFESTATIONS

Most patients with acute *T. gondii* infection do not have symptomatic disease. Clinical manifestations of acute infection occasionally occur in immunocompetent adults, as does reactivation of infection within the retina of the eye. Infection during pregnancy results in congenital toxoplasmosis at an incidence of approximately 1 in 8000 live births in the United States; the frequency in which *T. gondii* causes spontaneous abortion is unknown. Reactivation infection from dormant cysts is the cause of toxoplasmic infections in patients with AIDS, patients with bone marrow or solid organ transplantations, and other immunosuppressed hosts. The clinical syndromes in each of the foregoing settings are sufficiently distinct to warrant separate comment.

Acute Infection in Immunocompetent Patients

Approximately 15% of immunocompetent patients who become infected have either regional lymphadenopathy or a mononucleosis-like syndrome characterized by generalized adenopathy and constitutional symptoms. Toxoplasmic lymphadenopathy is largely a self-limited disease in immunocompetent patients, and it rarely requires therapy. Epstein-Barr virus and cytomegalovirus infections are much more common causes of the mononucleosis syndrome. Other causes of lymphadenopathy that need to be considered include cat-scratch disease, lymphoma or metastatic malignancy, sarcoidosis, and tuberculosis and the deep mycoses. Serologic testing and lymph node biopsy are most beneficial in establishing a diagnosis. Infections acquired by blood transfusion or through a laboratory accident may be severe and should be treated.

Ocular Toxoplasmosis in Immunocompetent Patients

Approximately one third of all cases of chorioretinitis within the Unites States are caused by *T. gondii.* Most cases are believed to result from unrecognized congenital infection that reactivates, most commonly during the second and third decades of life. Retinal clinical findings are highly suggestive of *T. gondii* infection when evaluated by ophthalmologists experienced in managing this infection. Serologic testing is usually positive for prior exposure to toxoplasmosis, but in difficult cases, PCR testing may be performed on samples of aqueous or vitreous humor to confirm the diagnosis. Control of the host inflammatory response by the concomitant use of corticosteroids may be required in some patients receiving therapy for toxoplasmosis. Relapse of infection requiring repeated treatment is not uncommon.

Congenital Toxoplasmosis

Congenital toxoplasmosis results from transplacental spread of *T. gondii* infection that is asymptomatically acquired either during pregnancy or shortly before the onset of gestation. The risk of fetal infection varies with the stage of trimester; it is highest during the second and third trimesters. Approximately 60% of maternal infections acquired during the third trimester will result in fetal infection. Fetal infection occurring during the first trimester is believed to result frequently in spontaneous abortion. Clinical manifestations of congenital toxoplasmosis are varied. There may be no sequelae, or clinical disease may become manifest at birth or at various times after birth. Children may be born with the nonspecific manifestations of the TORCH syndrome, including chorioretinitis, hydrocephalus, intracranial calcifications, hepatosplenomegaly, rash, anemia, and/or jaundice. Other infectious causes such as herpes simplex, cytomegalovirus, rubella, and syphilis should be considered and excluded. In those infants born with subclinical congenital infection, studies suggest that most will eventually demonstrate evidence of clinical disease even though they appear normal at birth. Years or decades later, previously subclinically infected children may develop chorioretinitis, seizure disorders, or psychomotor and mental retardation. Early recognition and treatment of congenital infection reduce the likelihood of subsequent sequelae; therefore, congenital *T. gondii* infection should always be treated regardless of whether there are symptoms at birth. Treatment of acute maternal infection diagnosed during pregnancy reduces the risk of fetal infection by approximately 60%.

Because congenital toxoplasmosis occurs almost exclusively in women infected during pregnancy, it is important that such infection be recognized and treated aggressively. In some countries where there is a higher seroprevalence of *T. gondii* infection (e.g., France), routine screening for acquisition of infection during pregnancy is performed. Routine pregnancy screening is not currently advocated in the United States. Women who have IgG antibody but who lack specific IgM antibody are believed to have evidence of past, chronic infection and are not at risk of transmitting congenital infection. A positive IgM test requires further confirmatory testing through a reference laboratory to determine whether infection is recently acquired. Confirmation of acutely acquired maternal infection during pregnancy mandates testing during and after pregnancy to determine whether fetal or congenital infection has occurred. PCR testing of amniotic fluid at 18 weeks of gestation and beyond is approximately 60% sensitive and 100% specific in diagnosing fetal infection. Diagnosis of congenital toxoplasmosis at birth is usually confirmed by the presence of specific IgA (or IgM) in fetal serum, with careful attention to exclusion of maternal contamination of fetal blood. In children with suspected congenital toxoplasmosis, it is important to perform ophthalmologic evaluation and neuroimaging studies and to examine the cerebrospinal fluid for pleocystosis or elevated protein concentrations.

Toxoplasmosis in AIDS and Immunocompromised Patients

In immunocompromised patients, toxoplasmosis almost always occurs as reactivation infection. One exception is infection after heart transplantation, in which primary infection can occur when a seronegative host receives a donor heart from a seropositive donor. The central nervous system is the most commonly affected site, resulting in necrotizing focal or multifocal encephalitis and, less frequently, focal spinal cord involvement. Other forms of infection include chorioretinitis, myocarditis, and pneumonia. Active toxoplasmosis in immunodeficient patients can cause significant morbidity and mortality and always requires therapy. The duration of therapy is largely dependent on the degree of chronic immunosuppression, and, on occasion, lifelong maintenance therapy is indicated.

In natural history studies of HIV infection performed before effective antiretroviral therapy, it was observed that approximately one third of toxoplasmosis seropositive patients with AIDS developed toxoplasmic encephalitis before death. Daily receipt of one tablet of double-strength trimethoprim (160 mg)-sulfamethoxazole (800 mg) (Bactrim DS) largely eliminates the risk of disease. Most episodes of toxoplasmic encephalitis complicating AIDS occur in patients with CD4 counts less than 100 cell/mm^3, and infection is uncommon if the CD4 count exceeds 200 cell/mm^3. Patients with toxoplasmic encephalitis most commonly present with focal neurologic abnormalities of subacute (weeks) onset, often with fevers, headache, or subtle mental status or memory changes. Motor palsies are the most common focal abnormality, although cranial nerve abnormalities, visual field defects, and seizure disorders can be the major presenting symptoms. Neuroradiologic imaging is best performed using magnetic resonance imaging, with the most common finding being multiple, ring-enhancing cerebral lesions. Involvement of the basal ganglion area is common. Computed tomography is in general less sensitive in defining disease and its extent. Single lesions on magnetic resonance imaging are unusual in toxoplasmic encephalitis and suggest possible central nervous system lymphoma. Multifocal leukoencephalopathy resulting from JC virus can also cause neuroradiologic findings that resemble toxoplasmosis. PCR can be performed on cerebrospinal fluid for Epstein-Barr virus, JC virus, and toxoplasmosis.

A definitive diagnosis of toxoplasmic encephalitis is made by brain biopsy and by the histologic demonstration of tachyzoites. However, to avoid the morbidity associated with brain biopsy, in patients with HIV infection who are toxoplasmosis seropositive and who have consistent neuroradiologic findings, it is now standard practice to treat these patients for toxoplasmosis empirically and to observe the clinical response. Although neuroradiologic resolution is delayed, most patients with toxoplasmic encephalitis demonstrate clinical improvement within 7 days of initiating therapy. Failure to respond clinically to empirical therapy, seronegativity to *T. gondii* antibody, and the presence of a single lesion on magnetic resonance imaging all are findings that suggest the possibility of an alternative diagnosis and warrant consideration of performing a brain biopsy.

Tissue biopsies with histologic examination are usually necessary for diagnosing toxoplasmosis at other sites in immunocompromised patients. PCR testing on bronchoalveolar lavage fluid can be positive in cases of pneumonitis. Endomyocardial biopsy should be performed if toxoplasmosis is a consideration in the seronegative heart recipient of a seropositive donor.

THERAPY

Treatment of toxoplasmosis is summarized in Table 1. Most infections in immunologically normal adults are self-limited and do not require therapy. In ocular, central nervous system, and congenital toxoplasmosis, first-line therapy is the combination of pyrimethamine (Daraprim), and sulfadiazine, with folinic acid (leucovorin, not folic acid). Treatment duration is based on time of clinical resolution, but it is usually approximately 6 weeks in ocular and central nervous system infection and 12 months in congenital infection. In patients with AIDS who have persistently low CD4 counts (less than 200 cells/mm^3) and in other patients with continued profound immunosuppression, long-term maintenance therapy with pyrimethamine-sulfadiazine–folinic acid should be continued at the same doses used for primary therapy. Spiramycin* (not FDA-approved for this indication, 3 g/day, obtainable in the United States from the Food and Drug Administration; call 301-827-2335) is the drug of choice for pregnant women with acquired primary *T. gondii* infection. Spiramycin should be continued until term if there is no evidence of fetal infection. Spiramycin does not cross the placenta and will not treat infection in the fetus. If fetal infection is demonstrated to be present by amniotic fluid PCR, pyrimethamine–sulfadiazine–folinic acid should be administered during the second and third trimesters. Pyrimethamine is potentially teratogenic and should not administered during the first 16 weeks of pregnancy.

*Not available in the United States except from the FDA.

TABLE 1. **Therapy of Toxoplasmic Infection**

	Adult Doses	Pediatric Doses
Immunologically Normal		
Acute lymphadenopathy	No treatment	No treatment
Acute chorioretinitis	Pyrimethamine (Daraprim) 100 mg PO bid on day 1, then 25 mg PO qd + Sulfadiazine 1 g PO qid + Folinic acid (leucovorin) 5 mg PO qd	
Pregnancy	Spiramycin* 1.0 g PO q8h (see text)	
Congenital toxoplasmosis		Pyrimethamine 2 mg/k for 2 d, then 1 mg/kg PO qd + Sulfadiazine 50 mg/kg PO bid + Folinic acid 10 mg 3 × wk PO
AIDS and Immunologically Impaired		
Encephalitis and other tissue sites of infection	Pyrimethamine 200 mg PO × one dose, then 75 mg PO qd + Sulfadiazine 1 g PO qid + Folinic acid 5-10 mg PO qd	

*Not available in the United States except from the FDA.

Allergic reactions to sulfonamides are common in patients with HIV infection. Alternative drugs to sulfadiazine that may be employed in combination therapy include clindamycin (Cleocin)** 600 to 1200 mg every 6 hours intravenously or orally, clarithromycin (Biaxin)** 1 g every 12 hours orally, atovaquone (Mepron)** 750 mg every 6 hours orally, azithromycin (Zithromax)** 1200 to 1500 mg/d orally, and dapsone** 100 mg/d orally. Alternatively, increasing experience suggests that trimethoprim-sulfamethoxazole (Bactrim, Septra)** 5 mg/kg trimethoprim component every 6 hours orally or intravenously (20 mg/kg/ day total) is equally effective as the pyrimethamine-containing combination regimens in those patients who are not allergic to sulfa agents.

Corticosteroids can be administered to patients with ocular toxoplasmosis in whom a brisk inflammatory response is believed to be contributing to ocular pathology. Similarly, in toxoplasmic encephalitis with cerebral edema or significant mass effect, short-duration corticosteroids may be concomitantly employed with antitoxoplasmic antimicrobial therapy.

PREVENTION

Prevention of *T. gondii* infection is of major importance in pregnant women and immunodeficient patients who have not been previously exposed. Risk of primary infection can be reduced by not eating undercooked meat and by taking proper precautions when disposing of or cleaning cat litter material. Cysts in meat are killed at 60°C or higher. Hands should be thoroughly washed after soil contamination, and all fruits and vegetables should be washed before they are eaten.

Primary prophylaxis should be administered in patients with AIDS who have CD4 counts less than 100 cells/mm^3 and who are seropositive for toxoplasmosis antibody. Trimethoprim (160 mg)–sulfamethoxazole (800 mg)** as one double-strength tablet daily is highly effective for prevention of toxoplasmosis infection. Alternative prophylactic regimens include either (1) pyrimethamine 50 to 75 mg orally/week plus dapsone** 50 mg/d or 200 mg/week; or (2) pyrimethamine-sulfadoxine (Fansidar)** at three tablets every 2 weeks. Dapsone alone is not effective at preventing toxoplasmosis.

**Not FDA-approved for this indication.

**Not FDA approved for this indication.

CAT-SCRATCH DISEASE

method of
DOUGLAS H. HAMILTON, M.D., PH.D.
Centers for Disease Control and Prevention
Atlanta, Georgia

Cat-scratch disease (CSD) was first identified in 1930 by Robert Debré in Paris, who described a self-limited, regional lymphadenopathy occurring after a cat scratch or bite distal to the affected node. In 1983, researchers, using a Warthin-Starry silver impregnation stain, identified small, pleomorphic, gram-negative, non–acid-fast bacteria in the lymph nodes of patients with clinical CSD. Similar bacteria were later seen at the site of primary cat-scratch lesions, cultured from the tissues of patients with CSD, and these bacteria were subsequently identified as *Bartonella* (formerly *Rochalimaea*) *henselae*.

EPIDEMIOLOGY

Analyses of large national databases documented that: (1) 55% of persons with CSD are aged 18 years or younger, (2) 60% of cases occur in male patients, and (3) most cases occur in the fall and winter. An estimated 22,000 cases are diagnosed annually in the United States; more than 2000 of these patients require hospitalization, 90% have a history of contact with cats, and 57% to 83% have a history of a scratch from a cat. A case-control study of risk factors for CSD indicated that patients with CSD were more likely than controls to own a kitten aged 12 months or less, to have been scratched by a kitten, or to have had at least one kitten with fleas. A study of *B. henselae* infection of cats revealed that 72% of the kittens tested were bacteremic, whereas the adult cats tested had serologic evidence of past infection but had negative blood cultures. Fleas, implicated in the case-control studies, have been shown to harbor *B. henselae* and to be capable of transmitting the infection from cat to cat.

CLINICAL MANIFESTATIONS

Infection with *B. henselae* results in different clinical presentations depending on the immune status of the patient. Infection of an immunocompetent patient is likely to result in a classic CSD presentation (i.e., 3 to 5 days after exposure to a cat, most patients develop a small, round, red-brown papule). This lesion progresses through a vesicular and crusty stage within 2 to 3 days, and it may persist for up to 2 or 3 weeks. Within 1 to 2 weeks after appearance of skin lesions, patients develop gradual enlargement of the regional lymph nodes that drain the site of the primary lesion. Eighty-five percent of patients present with a solitary enlarged lymph node. Multiple nodes are usually found in a regional distribution, and only 2% of patients present with noncontiguous bilateral lymphadenopathy. The sites of lymph node involvement are most commonly: upper extremity (46%), neck and jaw (26%), groin (18%), preauricular (7%), and clavicular (2%). Additional constitutional symptoms noted in more than 50% of patients include: fever (28% to 39%), malaise or fatigue (29% to 34%), pharyngitis (7% to 13%), and headache (6% to 13%).

Unusual manifestations of CSD have been reported in 5% to 25% of patients. The most common complication is Parinaud's oculoglandular syndrome, which occurs in 6% of patients. Parinaud's oculoglandular syndrome presents as a unilateral granulomatous conjunctivitis with an ipsilateral preauricular lymphadenopathy. Ocular lesions are 2 to 10 mm or larger and are usually located on the palpebral conjunctiva. These lesions resolve in weeks to months and do not result in permanent scarring. Parinaud's oculoglandular syndrome may also be caused by other infectious agents (e.g., tuberculosis, tularemia, syphilis, and lymphogranuloma venereum), but CSD is believed to be the most common cause.

Neurologic manifestations may be evident in 1% to 7% of patients with CSD. In one case-series of 76 patients with neurologic symptoms, 80% had encephalopathy, and 20% had cranial or peripheral nerve involvement. Encephalopathy occurred 1 to 6 weeks after the onset of CSD and typically began with a headache that rapidly progressed to a change in mental status, delirium, and unresponsiveness. Convulsions occurred in 46% of these patients, and transient combative behavior occurred in 39%. In patients without a prior diagnosis of CSD, convulsions were often the initial symptom. Patients may become comatose for 1 to 4 days, but recovery is fairly rapid and complete without neurologic sequelae. Less common neurologic manifestations of CSD include persistent ataxia, transient hemiplegia, hearing loss, bilateral sixth cranial nerve palsy, and neuroretinitis with transient blindness.

Other rare complications of CSD in the immunocompetent host include hepatic and splenic abscesses (presenting as abdominal pain of unknown origin), osteolytic lesions, erythema nodosum, pneumonia or pleural effusions, and thrombocytopenic and nonthrombocytopenic purpura.

Infection of an immunocompromised person by *B. henselae* may result in a dramatically different clinical presentation called *bacillary angiomatosis* (BA). BA is a vasoproliferative disorder characterized by brown to violaceus or clear cutaneous and subcutaneous lesions. The BA lesions may be solitary but are usually multiple and tender; they can involve essentially all organ systems of the body, including lymph nodes, bone, brain, liver, and spleen. In HIV-infected patients, these lesions are often mistaken for Kaposi's sarcoma. Histologically, BA lesions consist of proliferating small vessels with prominent endothelial cells and varying numbers of neutrophils and neutrophil debris. The epithelial cells of BA lesions are protuberant and do not appear spindle-shaped or form the slitlike spaces seen in Kaposi's sarcoma. Morphologically, three distinct types of BA lesions have been described. The most common type is a pyogenic granuloma, followed by subcutaneous nodules and indurated hyperpigmented plaques. Warthin-Starry staining of BA lesions revealed clumps of the characteristic small, pleomorphic, gram-negative bacteria seen in classic CSD lesions. Subsequent investigators isolated *B. henselae* from the BA lesions of HIV-infected patients and demonstrated high levels of antibodies to *B. henselae* in patients with BA. Laboratory studies revealed that BA may also be caused by *Bartonella quintana*, a related bacterium and the agent of trench fever.

B. henselae infection in the immunocompromised host may also present as *bacillary peliosis*, which is an extracutaneous presentation of BA found in solid organs with reticuloendothelial elements (e.g., liver [peliosis hepatis], spleen, abdominal lymph nodes, and bone marrow.) Symptoms include fever, nausea, vomiting, diarrhea, and abdominal distention. Patients often present with hepatosplenomegaly.

B. henselae infection may also present as persistent or relapsing fever with bacteremia in the absence of lymphadenopathy or skin lesions. This condition has been observed in both immunocompetent and immunocompromised patients, although more commonly in the latter. These patients usually present with fatigue, fever, and anorexia without an obvious source of infection.

DIAGNOSIS

Diagnosis of CSD has traditionally required the presence of three of four criteria: (1) history of animal contact (usually a cat) and an abrasion, scratch, or ocular lesion; (2) a positive CSD skin antigen test; (3) regional lymphadenopathy for which other causes have been excluded; and (4) characteristic histopathologic changes consistent with CSD in a lymph node biopsy. The lack of an effective means of standardization and lingering doubts about the safety of the CSD skin test antigen led to the development and adoption of newer diagnostic tools. The most commonly used test is an indirect immunofluorescence assay for detection of anti–*B. henselae* IgG. Published studies examining the performance of the immunofluorescence assay test in a population of patients with CSD who met the classic case definition showed the test to be 98% sensitive and 98% specific. However, the ability to differentiate among *Bartonella* species using this test was not well established.

Enzyme immunoassays for either IgM or IgG antibodies to *B. henselae* have also been developed. Compared with the immunofluorescence assay, the enzyme immunoassay seems to have a lower sensitivity (71% to 85%) and a higher specificity (98% to 100%).

Polymerase chain reaction–based tests for detection of *B. henselae* DNA are available in a limited number of commercial laboratories. These tests have been helpful in identifying the causative agent of CSD as *B. henselae* and not as *Afipia felis,* as previously suspected.

Histologic findings on lymph node biopsy vary depending on the stage of the disease. Early CSD lesions show lymphoid hyperplasia, arteriolar proliferation, and reticular cell hyperplasia. This stage is followed by the development of granulomas with central necrosis and multinucleate giant cells. Late-stage lesions often show multiple stellate microabscesses. Rarely seen with routine tissue stains, bacteria may be seen as clumps in samples stained with the Warthin-Starry technique. The characteristic findings of BA are described earlier.

TREATMENT

In most immunocompetent patients with classic CSD, the disease is self-limiting, and antibiotic therapy has not proved beneficial. The lymphadenopathy usually regresses spontaneously within 2 to 6 months, but it may last up to 2 years. Patients with severe symptoms or unusual manifestations may benefit from a trial of antibiotics. Several proposed treatment regimens, based on small sample sizes, have been published (Table 1). The only randomized, double-blind clinical trial of antibiotic therapy of CSD involved azithromycin (Zithromax).* Incision and drainage of fluctuant lymph nodes are not recommended because of the tendency for these lesions to form chronic sinus tracts when they are managed surgically. If necessary, repeated aspiration of purulent material with a 16- or 18-gauge needle may provide symptomatic relief.

Managing patients with BA or as bacillary peliosis, both of which can be fatal if left untreated, is different from managing immunocompetent patients with classic CSD. Unlike patients with CSD, for whom treatment with antibiotics is of questionable efficacy, immunocompromised patients with BA have shown a dramatic response to antibiotic therapy. The current antibiotics of choice are erythromycin (E-Mycin)** or doxycycline (Vibramycin), although other regimens have been published (see Table 1). The reasons for the observed differences in clinical presentation and response to therapy after *B. henselae* infection in immunocompromised and immunocompetent hosts are not known.

*Not FDA approved for this indication.
**Not available in the United States.

TABLE 1. **Antibiotic Therapy for *Bartonella henselae* Infection**

Cat-Scratch Disease		
Antibiotic	*Dose/Route*	*Notes*
Axithromycin (Zithromax)*	Children (<45 kg): 10 mg/kg PO on day 1 and 5 mg/kg PO on days 2-5 Adults: 500 mg PO on day 1 and 250 mg PO on days 2-5	
Ciprofloxacin (Cipro)*	20-30 mg/kg/d PO divided into 2 doses for 7-14 d Adults: 500-750 mg PO bid for 7-14 d	For children aged ≥12 years
Rifampin (Rifandin, Rimactane, Rifocin)*	10-20 mg/kg/d PO divided into 2 or 3 doses for 7-14 d	600 mg is the maximum dose
Trimethoprim-sulfamethoxazole (Bactrim)*	10 mg/kg of the trimethoprim dose PO bid for 7 d	
Gentamycin (Garamycin)*	5 mg/kg/d IV or IM in divided doses q 8 h	For severely ill patients
Bacillary Angiomatosis/Bacillary Peliosis		
Antibiotic	*Dose/Route*	*Notes*
Erythromycin	500 mg PO qid for 6-8 wk	Duration of therapy depends on clinical response; some HIV-positive patients may require long-term, even lifelong disease suppression
Doxycycline (Vibramycin, Doryx, Monodox)	100 mg PO bid for 6-8 wk	
Clarithromycin (Biaxin)	500 mg PO bid for 6-8 wk	
Azithromycin (Zithromax)	250 mg PO qd for 6-8 wk	
Ciprofloxacin (Cipro)	500-750 mg PO bid for 6-8 wk	

* Not FDA approved for this indication.

SALMONELLOSIS

method of
CHRISTOPHER M. PARRY, FRCPath, MRCP
University Department of Medical Microbiology and Genitourinary Medicine
Royal Liverpool University Hospital
Liverpool, United Kingdom

and

NICHOLAS J. BEECHING, FRCP, FRACP, DCH, DTM&H
University Department of Tropical Medicine and Infectious Diseases
Royal Liverpool University Hospital
Liverpool, United Kingdom

Salmonellae are found widely in nature and in the gastrointestinal tracts of domesticated and wild mammals, reptiles, birds and insects, and they are a common cause of food poisoning. The majority of *Salmonella* isolates are classified as a single species, *Salmonella enterica*, with almost 2500 serotypes. *Salmonella enterica* serotype *Typhi* (abbreviated to *Salmonella typhi*) and *Salmonella paratyphi* are highly adapted to humans and cause the syndrome of enteric fever. The other non-typhi *Salmonellae* (NTS) are responsible for a variety of clinical syndromes in humans and animals. *S. typhimurium* and *S. enteritidis* are the most common serotypes worldwide. Identification of the infecting NTS serotype enables public health officials to identify the link between cases and source in a food-borne outbreak. Further subdivision of the serotypes can be achieved by bacteriophage typing and molecular methods.

EPIDEMIOLOGY

In industrialized countries there has been a pronounced increase in the incidence of infections due to NTS in humans in the last half-century. Much of this increase has been attributed to the widespread contamination of foods of animal origin, such as meat, poultry, eggs, and dairy products, leading to food poisoning. Uncooked or inadequately cooked food can be a source of infection. Furthermore, uncooked food can cross-contaminate cooked food. Although 95% of salmonellosis is related to food, occasional water-borne outbreaks have been described, and infections linked to exotic pets, particularly reptiles, are an increasing problem in some areas.

There are estimated to be 1.4 million cases of *Salmonella* infection in the United States each year, with 16,400 admitted to hospital and 580 deaths. Salmonellosis has a considerable economic impact in terms of days lost from work and use of health care resources. Manufactured foods, such as ice cream, powdered milk products and infant formula, and ready-to-eat snacks, may be a source of widespread outbreaks. New *Salmonella* serotypes have appeared linked to the increasing international trade of fresh fruit and vegetables and tourists returning from exotic locations with gastroenteritis. Fecal carriers can be important sources of *Salmonella* transmission in hospitals and other institutions. Person-to-person transmission can occur on the hands of patients, residents, or health care staff, particularly in elderly care nursing homes and infant daycare facilities. There has been increasing recognition of serious invasive infection resulting from NTS in humans in developing countries. In many sub-Saharan African countries NTS is a leading cause of bacteremia in children younger than age 5 years. In developing and developed countries it has also become an important cause of severe disease and death in children and adults infected with HIV.

During the 1980s, infection from *S. enteritidis* associated with eggs was a major problem. Many egg-laying and broiler flocks of chicken were colonized or infected with *S. enteritidis*. This problem has now declined because flocks have been vaccinated, pasteurization of eggs has become widespread, and stock control has improved. Multidrug resistant *S. typhimurium* DT104 has in turn become a significant problem in the United Kingdom, Europe, and the United States. This serotype is associated with a wide variety of animals and meat products and is invariably resistant to ampicillin, chloramphenicol (Chloromycetin), streptomycin, sulfonamides, and tetracyclines, and, in some instances, to trimethoprim (Proloprim) and fluoroquinolones.

Antimicrobials are widely used in the livestock industry as treatment for febrile illnesses and as growth promoters. This is considered one of the major factors in the emergence and dissemination of antimicrobial drug resistance in food-borne pathogens such as NTS. Resistance to ampicillin, chloramphenicol, and trimethoprim-sulfamethoxazole has led to the use of fluoroquinolones and extended-spectrum cephalosporins for treating invasive NTS infections in humans. The emergence of resistance to these drugs is therefore of considerable concern, particularly because they appear to be associated with a higher mortality. The emergence of fluoroquinolone resistance in animal and human isolates is likely to be related to the introduction of fluoroquinolones for veterinary use, particularly in poultry. Resistance to the third-generation cephalosporins has emerged in selected countries in North and South America, North Africa, Turkey, Eastern Europe, Russia, and India. *S. typhimurium*, Hadar, Virchow, and *S. infantis* are the serotypes commonly affected. Occasional carbapenem resistance has also been reported.

The infective dose varies according to the *Salmonella* serotype and the presence of host risk factors, but can be less than 10^3 organisms. Alterations in the gastrointestinal tract such as decreased gastrointestinal acidity, change in the normal gastrointestinal flora resulting from prior antibiotics, and gastrointestinal surgery all reduce host resistance. Those at the extremes of age often have relative achlorhydria, and this contributes to increased susceptibility to *Salmonella* infections. The risk of invasive salmonellosis is increased in patients in whom the intracellular killing of *Salmonella* by monocytes and macrophages is impaired. Some of the recognized conditions in which this occurs are listed in Table 1.

TABLE 1. **Host Factors Associated with Severe Gastroenteritis and Extra-intestinal Salmonellosis**

Age
<3 mo
>60 y
Immunosuppression
HIV/AIDS
Sickle cell disease
Malignancy
Lymphoproliferative disease
Organ transplantation
Diabetes mellitus
Renal failure
Primary hypogammaglobulinemia
Steroids
Chemotherapy
Radiotherapy
Transplant-related immunosuppressive medication
Decreased gastric acidity
Gastric surgery
Anti-acid medications
Disrupted host intestinal flora
Recent antimicrobial therapy
Bowel surgery
Endovascular abnormalities
Atheroma
Aneurysm
Valve abnormalities
Vascular graft
Other infections
Malaria (malarial anemia)
Histoplasmosis
Schistosomiasis
Bartonellosis
Relapsing fever

CLINICAL FEATURES

Salmonella infections result in several recognizable clinical syndromes with considerable overlap.

Gastroenteritis

The commonest manifestation in children and adults infected with NTS is acute diarrhea that is usually self-limited and indistinguishable from gastroenteritis caused by other pathogens. An incubation period of 6 to 72 hours is followed by the onset of diarrhea occurring several times a day, of moderate volume and without blood. Fever (38–39°C), abdominal cramps, nausea, vomiting, chills, headache, and myalgia may accompany this. Occasionally the diarrhea may be watery and of large volume, or small volume with tenesmus and blood. In the latter case the disease must be carefully distinguished from other bacterial causes of dysentery and inflammatory bowel disease. Rarely abdominal pain may be the main presenting feature and the infection may mimic appendicitis. Fecal cultures are not routinely required, as the diagnosis is clinical, but are useful for public health surveillance.

The illness is self-limiting, usually lasting for 3 to 7 days, rarely longer than 10 days, with the fever resolving within 2 to 3 days. The main complication, and reason for hospitalization, is dehydration requiring intensive oral or intravenous fluid replacement therapy. Associated mortality is low, less than 0.5%, but the risk is increased in the very young and elderly. Occasional serious complications, such as bacteremia and focal infections at other sites, may be associated with a higher mortality. After the symptoms have resolved, the mean duration of carriage of NTS in the stool is 4 to 5 weeks and varies according to *Salmonella* serotype and age.

Bacteremia

Any *Salmonella* serotype can cause bacteremia, but some serotypes, such as Choleraesuis, Dublin, and Virchow, are more commonly associated with bacteremia than others. Bacteremia may be secondary to an episode of gastroenteritis or may be primary without any associated gastrointestinal symptoms. In individuals admitted to hospital with gastroenteritis, between 5% and 10% will have an accompanying bacteremia, frequently unrecognized because blood cultures may not be taken. The prognosis is good, unless there is underlying immunosuppression or the patient is very young or elderly. Primary bacteremia, without gastroenteritis, occurs in people with severe underlying disease, immunosuppression, or AIDS. It is more common in adults than in children and can be associated with a high mortality, often because of the severity of the underlying condition.

Focal infections

Salmonella bacteremia leads to focal infections in a variety of sites in approximately 5 to 10% of cases (Table 2). Salmonellae have a predilection for vascular sites leading to infections that are difficult to treat. Endovascular infections are commonest in the elderly and those with atherosclerotic plaques or aneurysms.

TABLE 2. **Complications and Extra-intestinal Infections in Nontyphoidal Salmonellosis**

Urinary tract	Renal failure second to dehydration Urinary tract infection Pyelonephritis
Vascular	Arteritis (aorta) Prosthetic graft infection Endocarditis
Joints	Septic Reactive
Bones	Osteomyelitis
Central nervous system	Meningitis Brain abscess Ventriculitis
Hepatobiliary	Liver abscess Cholecystitis
Pulmonary	Pneumonia
Genital	Prostatitis Epididymitis Ovarian or testicular abscess
Gastrointestinal tract	Ileus Toxic megacolon Perforation Appendicitis
Soft tissue	Subcutaneous abscess Wound infection
Spleen	Splenic abscess

In one study it was estimated that the risk of endovascular infection complicating *Salmonella* bacteriemia was 25% in people older than 50 years. Meningitis usually occurs in children younger than 2 years of age and particularly in those below the age of 3 months and carries a high mortality. Osteomyelitis is a particular problem in those with sickle cell disease.

Chronic carriage

Convalescent carriage is commoner in neonates and infants and may sometimes last for up to 6 months. In some studies, antimicrobial therapy has increased the duration of carriage. Permanent carriage, defined as carriage in feces or urine for longer than a year, usually only occurs in adults. This occurs in approximately 0.2% of patients with nontyphoidal salmonellosis. Long-term carriage, as in enteric fever, may be associated with biliary abnormalities or concurrent bladder infections with *Schistosoma*.

HIV and Salmonella

The risk of salmonellosis in patients infected with HIV is estimated to be 20- to 100-fold greater than that of the general population. Furthermore, *Salmonella* is more likely to cause severe invasive disease such as fulminant diarrhea, recurrent bacteremia, meningitis, and death. Invasive infections occur at a late stage of the disease when the CD4 count is typically less than 100/mm^3. Recurrent *Salmonella* bacteremia is now included in the CDC diagnostic criteria for AIDS.

Treatment

Gastroenteritis caused by *Salmonella* is a self-limiting disease. The most important therapy is the replacement of fluid and electrolyte losses usually by oral rehydration solutions. Severe cases may require intravenous fluids. Antimotility drugs should be restricted to very mild cases and should be avoided if there is fever, mucus or blood in the stools and in children and the elderly. Antimicrobial therapy is not routinely required. Short-course or single-dose regimens with oral amoxicillin,* trimethoprim-sulfamethoxazole (Bactrim),* or fluoroquinolones* have not consistently decreased the duration of symptoms or eliminated stool carriage. Some studies have noted higher rates of bacteriological relapse in those treated with antimicrobials.

Empirical antimicrobial therapy should be considered for those who require hospitalization, who are severely ill, who have signs of systemic sepsis, or who have risk factors for severe or complicated disease (see Table 1). An oral or intravenous antimicrobial should be administered for 3 to 5 days or until the patient becomes afebrile. Longer courses of treatment may lead to an increased risk of relapse or chronic carriage. In adults, an oral fluoroquinolone is the treatment of choice. Ampicillin, ceftriaxone (Rocephin),* or cefotaxime (Claforan)* are suitable alternatives depending on the severity of the illness. In children the choice includes trimethoprim-sulfamethoxazole (Bactrim), ampicillin, ceftriaxone or cefotaxime. Fluoroquinolones are not usually recommended for pediatric use because of worries about possible joint or tendon damage, based on evidence from experimental animals. However, there is now a large body of evidence concerning the use of prolonged courses of fluoroquinolones in children with cystic fibrosis and short courses in children with dysentery and enteric fever that suggests that they are safe to use. In the face of increasing multiresistance in salmonellosis, fluoroquinolones have an important role in the treatment of salmonellosis in children when alternatives are unavailable.

In patients with bacteremia or focal infections, initial empiric therapy is with a fluoroquinolone or third generation cephalosporin until susceptibility patterns are known. The duration of treatment depends on the clinical problem, with focal infections often requiring tailored therapy. Failure adequately to drain the collection may lead to the emergence of resistance because of poor penetration of the antimicrobial into the site of infection. In general, simple bacteremia should be treated for 7 to 10 days; patients with pulmonary, biliary, and soft-tissue infection require 2 weeks of therapy; central nervous system infections should be treated for 3 weeks; bone and joint infections for 4 to 6 weeks; and endocarditis for 6 weeks. Infected aneurysms and other endovascular infections usually require surgical resection, including prosthetic grafts when possible, bypassing the infected area, as well as at least 6 weeks of antimicrobial therapy. Patients with an infected prosthetic graft that cannot be resected require suppressive oral therapy for life.

In patients with HIV infection and invasive salmonellosis treatment is needed to eradicate the infection and to prevent recurrence. One to two weeks of intravenous antimicrobial therapy should be followed by four weeks of oral fluoroquinolone therapy. Those who relapse require long-term suppressive therapy with a fluoroquinolone or trimethoprim-sulfamethoxazole.

Antimicrobial therapy with a fluoroquinolone has been found to be valuable in the control of outbreaks in institutions. Long-term carriage, as with typhoid, requires prolonged therapy with a fluoroquinolone, amoxicillin or trimethoprim-sulfamethoxazole, according to the susceptibility of the isolate. This may be ineffective in the face of biliary or urinary tract abnormalities.

CONTROL

Individuals can reduce their chance of exposure to NTS by care in food handling and preparation. This is particularly important in those with risk factors for severe disease. Avoidance of undercooked meat, poultry, eggs, and fish, the use of pasteurized milk, careful kitchen hygiene, and hand washing after contact with farm animals and pets (particularly reptiles) are simple steps. Tourists should stick to properly cooked foods and avoid ice creams and fruits that have already been peeled. Control of food-borne salmonellosis

*Not FDA approved for this indication.

requires attention to each stage in the process from farm to food manufacturers and food handlers to kitchen hygiene. Recognition of outbreaks requires a high index of suspicion by clinicians, microbiologists, and public health officials and national and international surveillance.

Food handlers need to play close attention to personal hygiene and the basic principles of good kitchen practice. Routine surveillance for asymptomatic *Salmonella* stool carriage, or for carriage of *Salmonella* after gastroenteritis, is not required. Patients may return to work when the diarrhea has resolved. Food handlers whose work involves touching unwrapped foods that are consumed raw or without further cooking, however, need two negative consecutive stools before returning to work. Health care workers with *Salmonella* gastroenteritis can also return to work after their diarrhea has resolved provided careful hand hygiene is observed. However, if they are caring for patients at high risk of complicated *Salmonella* infections, some authorities require two negative stool samples at least 24 hours apart.

TYPHOID FEVER

method of
TIKKI PANG, PH.D., FRCPATH
Research Policy & Cooperation
World Health Organization
Geneva, Switzerland

DEFINITION

Typhoid fever is an acute systemic illness caused by the Gram-negative bacterium *Salmonella typhi*. It is characterized by prolonged fever, disturbances of bowel function (constipation in adults or diarrhea in children), headache, malaise, and anorexia. Bronchitic cough is common in the early stage of illness. During the period of fever, up to 25% of patients show exanthem (rose spots), on the chest, abdomen, and back. The clinical presentation of typhoid fever varies from a mild illness with low-grade fever, malaise, and slight dry cough to a severe clinical picture, abdominal discomfort, and multiple complications. A very similar but often less severe disease is caused by *Salmonella paratyphi* A. One to five percent of patients become chronic carriers who harbor *S. typhi* in their gall bladder.

EPIDEMIOLOGY

It has been estimated that approximately 17 million cases of typhoid fever and 600,000 deaths occur annually. Incidence of typhoid fever in endemic areas varies between 45/100,000 per year to >1,000/100,000 per year. Studies in Bangladesh showed an incidence of typhoid of around 2,000/100,000 per year. Humans are the only natural hosts and reservoirs of *S. typhi,* and the infection is transmitted by ingestion of fecally contaminated food or water. Tainted ice cream, shellfish from contaminated waters, and raw fruit and vegetables fertilized by sewage are recognized sources of past outbreaks. The highest incidence occurs where water supplies serving a large population are fecally contaminated.

COMPLICATIONS

Approximately 5% to 10% of typhoid patients may develop serious complications. Occult blood is found in the stool of 10% to 20% of patients. Intestinal perforation is seen in around 3% of hospitalized cases. Altered mental status in typhoid patients has been associated with a high case fatality rate. Such patients generally have delirium or obtundation, although rarely with coma. Typhoid meningitis, encephalomyelitis, Guillain-Barré syndrome, cranial or peripheral neuritis, and psychotic symptoms, although rare, have been reported. Other serious complications include hemorrhages, hepatitis, myocarditis, pneumonia, disseminated intravascular coagulation, and thrombocytopenia.

DIAGNOSIS

Definitive diagnosis of typhoid fever depends on isolation of *S. typhi* from the blood, stool, bone marrow, urine, or specific anatomic lesion of a patient. Blood culture is likely to be positive in the first 7 to 10 days of illness, with stool isolation more common in the second or third week. Culture of bone marrow aspirate is the gold standard for diagnosis and is particularly valuable for patients who have been previously treated. Culture of duodenal aspirate has also been shown to be a good diagnostic test. Antimicrobial susceptibility testing is crucial to guide clinical management as many isolates are now multidrug resistant (MDR).

The low-cost Widal test, which measures agglutinating antibody levels against O and H antigens of *S. typhi*, is still widely used as a serodiagnostic aid in developing countries, despite its many limitations. The test has only moderate sensitivity and specificity and interpretation of results is complicated by background levels of antibodies in the normal population in endemic areas. Newer tests include the IDL Tubex test that detects IgM O9 antibodies from patients within minutes. Another rapid (3 hours) serologic test (Typhi dot) detects specific IgM and IgG antibodies to a 50 kD antigen specific to *S. typhi*. A newer version of the test, Typhi dot-M, was recently developed to detect specific IgM antibodies only. A dipstick test has also been developed based on the binding of *S. typhi*–specific IgM antibodies to lipopolysaccharide (LPS) antigen and the staining of bound antibodies by an anti-human IgM antibody conjugated to colloidal dye particles. The dipstick test, in particular, provides a rapid and simple serodiagnostic method in situations where culture facilities are not available.

THERAPY

Rapid treatment is imperative to avoid complications. Although standard first-line drugs, chloramphenicol

(Chloromycetin),* ampicillin or amoxicillin (Amoxil),* and trimethoprim-sulfamethoxazole (TMP-SMX) (Bactrim)* are effective, the fluoroquinolones are now widely regarded as the optimal choice for treatment of typhoid fever in both adults and children (Table 1). Fluoroquinolones are relatively inexpensive, are well tolerated, attain excellent tissue penetration, and achieve higher active drug levels in the gallbladder than other drugs. They produce a rapid therapeutic response with clearance of fever and symptoms in 3 to 5 days and very low rates of posttreatment carriage. However, treatment must take into consideration the emergence of MDR strains. Two types of drug resistance have been identified: resistance to chloramphenicol, ampicillin, and TMP-SMX (MDR strains); and resistance to the fluoroquinolone drugs.

In severe typhoid, the fluoroquinolones are also preferred but should be given for a minimum of 10 days (Table 2). If typhoid meningitis is suspected, patients should be immediately treated, in addition to antimicrobials, with high-dose intravenous dexamethasone (Decadron)* in an initial dose of 3 mg/kg by slow intravenous infusion over 30 minutes followed 6 hours later by 1 mg/kg every 6 hours for a total of eight times. This regimen can reduce mortality by 80% to 90% in these high-risk patients. In cases with intestinal perforation, surgical repair should not be delayed longer than 6 hours. Relapse of acute illness occurs in 5% to 20% of typhoid fever cases that have been apparently successfully treated. It is heralded by the return of fever after completion of antibiotics. Frequently the clinical manifestation is milder than the initial illness.

*Subcutaneous route not recommended by the manufacturer.

PREVENTION

The mainstays of prevention are health education, good sanitation, and vaccination. Typhoid is transmitted via the fecal-oral route through contaminated food and drinking water. Health education, clean water, food inspection, proper food handling, and proper sewage disposal have allowed developed countries to virtually eliminate typhoid fever. Health care providers can educate susceptible populations about the importance of personal hygiene and avoiding foods and drinks that may harbor bacteria, such as improperly cooked foods, snacks prepared by street vendors,

TABLE 1. **Treatment of Typhoid Fever: Uncomplicated Typhoid**

	OPTIMAL THERAPY			ALTERNATIVE EFFECTIVE DRUGS		
Susceptibility	**Antibiotic**	**Daily dose mg/kg**	**Days**	**Antibiotic**	**Daily dose mg/kg**	**Days**
Fully sensitive	Fluoroquinolone† (e.g., ofloxacin [Floxin]* or ciprofloxacin [Cipro])	15	5–7‡	Chloramphenicol Amoxicillin TMP-SMX	50–75 75–100 8–40	14–21 14 14
Multidrug resistant	Fluoroquinolone or cefixime (Suprax)*	15 15–20	5–7 7–14	Azithromycin or cefixime	8–10 15–20	7 7–14
Quinolone resistant§	Azithromycin (Zithromax)* or ceftriaxone (Rocephin)*	8–10 75	7 10–14	Cefixime	20	7–14

*Not FDA approved for this indication.
†The available fluoroquinolones (Ofloxacin,* Ciprofloxacin, Fleroxacin, Pefloxacin) are all highly active and equivalent in efficacy (with the exception of norfloxacin [Noroxin],* which has inadequate oral bioavailability and should not be used in typhoid fever).
‡Three-day courses are also effective, and are particularly effective in epidemic containment
The optimum treatment for quinolone-resistant typhoid fever has not been determined. Azithromycin, the §third-generation cephalosporins, or a 10–14 day course of high-dose fluoroquinolones are effective. Combinations of these are now being evaluated.

TABLE 2. **Treatment of Typhoid Fever: Severe Typhoid**

	OPTIMAL PARENTERAL DRUG			ALTERNATIVE EFFECTIVE PARENTERAL DRUG		
Susceptibility	**Antibiotic**	**Daily dose (mg/kg)**	**Days**	**Antibiotic**	**Daily dose (mg/kg)**	**Days**
Fully sensitive	Fluoroquinolone (e.g., ofloxacin [Floxin])*	15	10–14	Chloramphenicol (Chloromycetin) Ampicillin TMP-SMX (Bactrim)*	100 100 8–40	14–21 14 14
Multidrug resistant	Fluoroquinolone	15	10–14	Ceftriaxone or cefotaxime*	60 80	10–14
Quinolone resistant	Ceftriaxone (Rocephin)* or cefotaxime (Claforan)*	60 80	10–14	Fluoroquinolone	20	14

*Not FDA approved for this indication.

salads, ice, and tap water. Effective communication, adapted to local language, customs, and beliefs, together with close community participation, is important. Identification of carriers, and preventing their employment in food handling occupations, is another important preventive strategy.

VACCINES

Two safe and effective vaccines are currently available. One is composed of the Vi polysaccharide (Typhim Vi) given in one single dose subcutaneously* or intramuscularly. Protective efficacy is approximately 70% and revaccination is recommended every 2 to 3 years* for travelers. A second option is a live oral vaccine (Ty2la) (Vivotif Berna) available in enteric-coated capsules or as a liquid formulation** and normally administered in three to four doses* 2 days apart. This vaccine has a protective efficacy of 60% to 70%. The World Health Organization currently recommends vaccination for school children living in endemic areas, persons traveling to high-risk endemic areas, people in refugee camps, microbiologists, and sewage workers. Vaccination should also be considered as a tool to limit the spread of typhoid fever in a community facing an outbreak.

---

*Subcutaneous route not recommended by the manufacturer.
**Not available in the United States.

RICKETTSIAL AND EHRLICHIAL INFECTIONS

method of
DANIEL J. SEXTON, M.D.
Duke University Medical Center
Durham, North Carolina

ROCKY MOUNTAIN SPOTTED FEVER

Rocky Mountain spotted fever (RMSF) is caused by an obligate intracellular bacterium called *Rickettsia rickettsii*. RMSF occurs in western Canada, much of the United States, Mexico, Central America, Brazil, and Columbia. This disease occurs predominately between April and September but in southern areas of the United States or in Mexico or Central America, illness may occur during autumn and occasionally even in mid-winter.

In the eastern United States RMSF is transmitted by *Dermacentor variabilis* (the American dog tick), and in the western United States *Dermacentor andersoni* (the wood tick) is the principal vector. RMSF may occur after contact with ticks in rural, suburban, and even highly urbanized areas such as New York City. Rarely transmission may occur from crushing or removing infected ticks from humans or animals. Infection can be experimentally induced with aerosols of infected tick tissues or by mucosal contact. Most tick bites are painless and frequently tick bites are unnoticed or undetected. Thus many patients with RMSF have no knowledge of a tick bite before the onset of their illness.

After inoculation, *R. rickettsii* proliferates intracellularly and then subsequently spreads throughout the body via the bloodstream or lymphatics. *R. rickettsii* has a tropism for endothelial cells that ultimately results in widespread rickettsia-induced vasculitis that may in turn lead to innumerable minute foci of hemorrhage, increased vascular permeability, edema, and the activation of the humoral inflammatory and coagulation mechanisms. Vascular thrombosis and hemorrhage may occur in severe cases, resulting in widespread organ dysfunction often with hypovolemia and shock.

Host factors associated with increased severity of fatal outcome of RMSF include increasing age, male gender, and the presence of glucose-6-phosphate dehydrogenase deficiency. Black race and alcohol use have also been associated with a more severe disease and a higher fatality rate, but it is difficult to exclude the role of delay in seeking or receiving antimicrobial therapy in these patients. Delay in effective therapy has been associated with a significantly worse outcome—particularly if a delay in therapy exceeds 6 days.

The incubation period for RMSF ranges from 2 to 14 days. In the early phases of illness, symptoms are nonspecific. Most adult patients initially complain of headache, myalgias, malaise, and anorexia. Children may have prominent abdominal pain in the early phase of illness. Prominent gastrointestinal symptoms in children and adults with RMSF may lead to erroneous diagnoses such as acute appendicitis, cholecystitis, and even bowel obstruction.

Most patients with RMSF develop a rash between the third and fifth days of illness. However, rash is often absent when patients first contact a physician. In one study, 14% of patients had a rash on the first day of illness and less than half of all patients developed a rash during the first 3 days of illness. In a small percentage of patients, rash is delayed in onset for more than 5 days, and it may be atypical (e.g., confined to only one body region). Rash never occurs in up to 10% of patients. These cases of "spotless RMSF" may be severe and then fatal.

Most adult patients with RMSF complain of intense headache. Cough, abdominal pain, bleeding, edema (especially in children), confusion, and focal neurologic findings (including seizures) may occur in severe cases. Gangrene of the ears, digits, and scrotum may also develop in severe cases.

Most patients with RMSF have a normal white count at presentation but the white count in individual patients may be low, normal or elevated; thus it is not diagnostically useful. As illness progresses, most patients develop thrombocytopenia that may be severe. Low platelet counts may be accompanied by reduced fibrinogen concentrations and elevated fibrin split products. However, true disseminated intravascular coagulation is rare. Other laboratory abnormalities in severe cases include hyponatremia and elevated levels of amino transferases (transaminases), bilirubin, and creatinine. Jaundice and renal failure may occasionally be severe and confuse the clinical presentation.

Misdiagnosis is common. In early phases RMSF may be mistaken for undifferentiated viral illnesses. If oral antibiotics or other drugs are administered empirically during this phase of illness, subsequent skin rash may be incorrectly diagnosed as a drug eruption. RMSF has been confused with measles, meningococcemia, infectious mononucleosis, hepatitis, leptospirosis, streptococcal infections and viral meningitis. In addition the clinical features of RMSF overlap with those of monocytic and granulocytic ehrlichiosis.

There is no completely reliable diagnostic test for RMSF in the early phase of illness when therapy should begin. Thus it is imperative that therapy be based on individual clinical features and the epidemiologic setting. Any patient with suggestive symptoms in an endemic area who presents with a compatible illness in the spring or early summer warrants empirical therapy.

Diagnosis can be confirmed by biopsy of a skin lesion and use of direct immunofluorescent or immunoenzymatic staining methods. The sensitivity of detecting *R. rickettsii* in skin biopsy by direct immunofluorescent staining is approximately 70% with a specificity of 100%. However, sensitivity rapidly declines after antirickettsial therapy is begun. Moreover, such testing is available only in specialized medical centers. Rickettsia can be recovered from blood inoculated into tissue cultures or laboratory animals, but these techniques are available only in a small number of research facilities.

The mainstay of diagnosis of RMSF remains serologic testing. Indirect fluorescent antibody (IFA) testing is available through all state health departments and through several large reference laboratories. The minimum diagnostic titer in most laboratories is 1:64. Antibodies typically appear 10 to 12 days after the onset of illness but the optimal time to obtain a convalescent antibody titer is 14 to 21 days after onset of symptoms.

The preferred treatment for RMSF is doxycycline (Vibramycin), 100 mg intravenously or orally every 12 hours for adults. The dose for children older than 8 years of age is 3 mg/kg body weight in two divided doses for children under 45 kg (maximum dose 200 mg/d). Adjunctive measures such as oxygen therapy, mechanical ventilation, and hemodialysis are useful in severe cases. Although there are no published studies on the optimal duration of therapy for RMSF, doxycycline therapy is usually continued for 5 to 10 days or until the patient has been afebrile for at least 48 hours. Doxycycline is also the treatment of choice for children with RMSF as the risk of dental staining is minimal when short doses of therapy are given. Doxycycline should not be used in pregnant women (who should be treated with chloramphenicol [Chloromycetin] 500 mg intravenously every 6 hours).

Prevention of RMSF is difficult because of the ubiquity of ticks. However, persons exposed to tick-infested habitats should periodically inspect their body and clothes for ticks and remove any crawling or attached ticks. Fingers should be shielded with a cloth, tissue or paper towels, or gloves during tick removal when possible.

EHRLICHIOSIS

Ehrlichia are obligate intracellular bacteria that grow within membrane-bound vacuoles in human and animal leukocytes. Ehrlichia replicate within phagosomes in the host cell to produce intracellular colonies called morula. These morula are visible by light microscopy and can be stained with gram, Giemsa, Wright, or silver stains. Ehrlichia belonged to the family Rickettsiaceae. The Ehrlichia genus is complex and includes both human and animal pathogens. There are four genogroups of Ehrlichia that cause human disease: *E. chaffeensis* (the agent of human monocytic ehrlichiosis), *E. ewingii*, the Anaplasma *phagocytophilia* genogroup (which includes the human granulocytic Ehrlichia agent [HGE]), and the *E. sennetsu* genogroup.

As yet there is no clear understanding of the mechanism by which Ehrlichia produces human disease. Current knowledge about the pathogenic lesions of human monocytic ehrlichiosis is based on a small number of autopsies and bone marrow or liver biopsies. Humans infected with Ehrlichia do not show cell or tissue necrosis, abscess formation, or a severe inflammatory response. Ehrlichia do not produce vasculitis, thrombosis, or acute or chronic endothelial injury as seen in rickettsial infections. The major cellular target of *E. chaffeensis* is the mononuclear cell and macrophages; the major targets of the HGE agent are granulocytes. Patients with HGE infection may develop secondary opportunistic infections such as cryptococcal pneumonia or invasive aspergillus pneumonia.

Cases of HME have been recognized in the southeastern, south-central, and mid-Atlantic region of the United States. Since *E. chaffeensis* was first isolated from a soldier at Fort Chaffee, Arkansas, in 1990, a few cases of HME have been recognized in New England and the Pacific Northwest and isolated cases have recently been reported in Europe, Africa, and Mexico. In some locations, HME is more common than RMSF.

HGE was first described in 1994; since then, cases have been described in Wisconsin, Minnesota, New England, California, Florida, North Carolina, and Western Europe. *E. ewingii* infection was first described in 1999 in patients from Missouri and Oklahoma.

The principal vector of *E. chaffeensis* is the Lone Star tick (*Amblyomma americanum*). HGE is primarily transmitted by *Ixodes scapularis* (the tick that also is the vector of Lyme disease and babesiosis). *I. pacificus*, the black-legged tick, is the primary infector of HGE in the western United States. White tail deer are the principal animal reservoirs for *E. chaffeensis* infection; deer and the white-footed mouse are the principal animal hosts for HGE.

Most ehrlichial diseases have an incubation period of 7 to 14 days but shorter incubation periods occasionally occur. Most patients are febrile but self-limiting mild or unapparent infections probably occur. Nonspecific symptoms such as malaise, myalgias, headaches, and chills are present in most cases. Nausea, vomiting, joint pain, and cough may occur in some patients. Rash is uncommon in ehrlichiosis but a faint rash may occur in a small number of patients. When rash is striking, co-infection with another rickettsial or other tick-borne pathogens should be suspected. Neurologic symptoms may occur in patients with ehrlichiosis and include mental status changes, stiff neck and focal neurologic findings.

The most common laboratory abnormality in patients with HME is leukopenia. Thrombocytopenia and elevated plasma levels of amino-transferases (transaminases), lactate dehydrogenase, and alkaline phosphatase are commonly present. Anemia and an elevated plasma creatinine concentration may also occur. Leukopenia in patients with HGE can be caused by lymphopenia or neutropenia. Lymphopenia tends to occur in early stages of infection followed by lymphocytosis with atypical lymphocytes in the later phases of illness. The initial neutrophil count in patients with HGE is inversely related to the duration of symptoms before treatment is given.

Thrombocytopenia is present in many patients with HGE and HME and is a useful diagnostic clue. Patients with both HME and HGE may develop pleocytosis and cerebral spinal fluid abnormalities may mimic the changes of viral or aseptic meningitis.

Rarely subacute or chronic infection with *E. chaffeensis* may occur. Such patients may present subacutely with unexplained fever that may last for up to 6 to 8 weeks in untreated cases.

Complications of severe ehrlichiosis include seizures, comas, renal and respiratory failure, and congestive heart failure. Patients with ehrlichiosis who are co-infected with HIV may have an unusually severe course that ends fatally and patients with HGE may develop fungal superinfections late in the course of illness.

Differential diagnosis of ehrlichiosis is similar to that of RMSF. Both diseases may mimic an array of common viral illnesses such as mononucleosis as well as thrombotic thrombocytopenia purpura, hematologic malignancy, cholangitis and even community-acquired pneumonia. Diagnosis of ehrlichiosis is based primarily on serologic testing as culture of Ehrlichia is extremely difficult even in research laboratories. There are four primary methods to diagnose both HME and HGE: (1) examination of the peripheral blood or buffy coat for the presence of characteristic morulae in lymphocytes or granulocytes; (2) indirect fluorescent antibody testing; (3) polymerase chain reaction testing of bone marrow, spinal fluid or tissue samples; and (4) the synthesis of the history, clinical and laboratory, and epidemiologic features of an individual case.

All patients who present with a nonspecific febrile illness in the spring or summer months and have a recent history of tick bite or tick exposure should be evaluated for the possibility of ehrlichiosis. Although only a minority of patients with HME have morulae detectable in smears of their blood, a blood film should be examined on all patients with suspected infection. Morulae are more frequently seen in patients with HGE. In some studies more than two thirds of such patients have detectable morulae after careful microscopic examination. Serologic testing for ehrlichiosis is available in most state health departments. The minimum diagnostic IFA titer in most laboratories is 1:64; a fourfold-antibody rise is considered confirmatory of recent infection.

Although there are no controled trials that examined the efficacy of antimicrobial therapy for ehrlichiosis, tetracycline and chloramphenicol (Chloromycetin) both appear to be effective agents in treatment. Of these, doxycycline (Vibramycin) is preferred. Most patients treated with doxycycline defervesce within 48 hours of initiation of therapy. Doxycycline can be administered either orally or intravenously at a dose of 200 mg a day in two divided doses in adults. The dose of doxycycline for children older than 8 years of age is 3 mg/kg body weight in two divided doses for children under 45 kg. Children weighting more than 45 kg should receive the adult dose of doxycycline (maximum dose 200 mg/d). Therapy should be continued for at least 7 days or from 3 to 5 days after defervescence has occurred. Although all tetracyclines can cause dental staining in children, the risk of such staining after the use of doxycycline is minimal if a short course of therapy is administered. Because chloramphenicol (Chloromycetin) is not readily available in many parts of the United States and because of its risk of hematologic toxicity, doxycycline should be administered to all patients with noted or suspected infection except for women who are pregnant. Patients who are intolerant or allergic to tetracyclines and pregnant women can be treated with rifampin (Rifadin)* for 7 to 10 days, but the efficacy of such therapy is currently based on only anecdotal information. The possibility of perinatal transmission in HGE should be considered when HGE occurs in women near delivery.

---

*Not FDA approved for this indication.

SMALLPOX

method of
MICHAEL R. ALBERT, M.D.
Brown Medical School,
Providence, Rhode Island

and

JOEL G. BREMAN, M.D., D.T.P.H.
Fogarty International Center
National Institutes of Health,
Bethesda, Maryland

Smallpox is caused by variola virus and infects only humans. Historically, the more severe form of smallpox (variola major) had a mortality rate of 20% to 30% in unvaccinated individuals. Although occurrences of smallpox date back to antiquity in China, India, and Egypt, the disease ceased to be a natural threat after the success of the Global Smallpox Eradication Program of the 1960s and 1970s. This international campaign was based on immunization, surveillance, and containment of disease. The last endemic case of smallpox occurred in Somalia in 1977, and the disease was declared eradicated by the World Health Organization (WHO) in 1980. Since 1984, the virus is known to be retained in two laboratories, one each in the United States and Russia. However, there has been increasing concern over the possibility that the virus may exist outside these known locations and could be deliberately released as a bioterrorism agent.

ETIOLOGY

Variola virus is a member of the Poxviridae family. The genus orthopoxvirus includes variola virus, vaccina virus, and a number of animal viruses, such as monkeypox, cowpox, and camelpox, that cross-react serologically. The virions are large (approximately 300 × 250 × 200 nm), appear brick-shaped by electron microscopy, and contain single, linear, double-stranded DNA. The complete genomic sequences have been determined for numerous isolates of variola virus.

Human-to-human transmission of variola virus normally occurs via virus-laden droplets expelled from the oropharynx, with infection of the upper respiratory tract and subsequent passage to the draining lymph nodes. This is followed by a primary viremia in which the virus migrates to the reticuloendothelial system, where it replicates during a clinically latent period. A secondary viremia follows, with invasion of the oral mucous membranes and skin resulting in the onset of cutaneous manifestations. The patient is most infectious during the first 2 weeks after disease onset, when sloughing of oropharyngeal lesions is most prominent. Transmission less commonly may occur from contact with skin lesions, as well as infected clothing or bedding. Aerosol transmission without face-to-face contact has occasionally been reported, as in hospitals with shared ventilation systems.

CLINICAL MANIFESTATIONS

After infection, there is an approximately 7- to 17-day incubation period (mean 10 to 14 days) before the onset of signs and symptoms. Clinical onset begins with a 1- to 4-day pre-eruptive stage that commonly includes fever up to 40.5°C, malaise, chills, nausea, vomiting, headache, and backache. The enanthem of smallpox begins next with minute erythematous macules that evolve over a few days into papules and then vesicles, which erode. Upper respiratory tract involvement may include the mouth, tongue, pharynx, and larynx, and may be more extensive in severe cases. The characteristic skin eruption generally follows the start of the enanthem by a day, beginning on the face and spreading over the body in a centrifugal distribution, with greater involvement of the face and distal extremities than the trunk and proximal extremities. A hallmark of the smallpox rash is its monomorphic appearance, with lesions appearing essentially as a single "crop" and evolving together through different stages as erythematous macules, papules, vesicles, and pustules. Pustules often display a central umbilication or dimpling and dry into crusts by the end of the second week. The rash resolves during the third week, with lesions of the palms and soles persisting longest. The most common sequela is pitted scars, which have a predilection for the face and occur in more than half of severe cases. Complications of smallpox may include encephalitis, arthritis, pneumonitis, pneumonia, orchitis, and, occasionally, secondary cutaneous infection. Rarely, keratitis with corneal ulceration and scarring can lead to blindness. The cause of death from smallpox has not been completely elucidated but may be the cytopathic effects of the virus in the lungs, kidneys and other organs.

The classification system listed by the WHO divided smallpox (variola major) into five clinical types, based on patients studied in India. "Ordinary" smallpox constituted almost 90% of cases in unvaccinated individuals. The "modified" type occurred mainly in vaccinated individuals and was characterized by a milder course with fewer and smaller lesions, a more rapid disease resolution, and low mortality. In the "flat" type, the skin often had a cobblestone-like or leathery appearance, with lesions remaining flat and not progressing to pustules. Thought to reflect a deficient immune response to variola virus, this rare type occurred primarily in children and was usually fatal. "Hemorrhagic" smallpox was marked by petechiae and mucosal and conjunctival bleeding. This form of smallpox also held a grave prognosis and was more prevalent in pregnant women. Finally, "variola sine eruptione" occurred in immunologically protected individuals who developed constitutional symptoms but not a rash. Variola minor is a mild variety of smallpox that accounted for more than 95% of reported cases in the United States during the 20th century. Patients with variola minor often have fewer and smaller lesions that evolve more rapidly, they do not usually become seriously ill, and their mortality rate is less than 1%.

DIAGNOSIS

Clinically, the differential diagnosis of smallpox includes other eruptive skin diseases, such as viral exanthems and drug hypersensitivity reactions. In particular, varicella (chickenpox) may be misdiagnosed as smallpox. Distinguishing features of varicella include a history of exposure to an individual with chickenpox, a shortened and milder prodrome, the presence of lesions in different stages of development (polymorphic), lack of umbilication of pustules, concentration of lesions on the trunk, and infrequent involvement of the palms and soles. A human monkeypox, a zoonotic disease clinically resembling smallpox, has very limited ability to spread between humans. To aid in the clinical diagnosis of smallpox, the Centers for Disease Control and Prevention (CDC) has developed a rash illness assessment algorithm which is available online: (http://www.bt.cdc.gov/agent/smallpox/diagnosis/index.asp#poster).

Laboratory confirmation of smallpox has traditionally employed the isolation of virus on the chorioallantoic membrane of the chick embryo. Today, polymerase chain reaction methods are available for the rapid identification of variola virus. Electron microscopy can detect orthopoxviruses, although without speciation. Other techniques include immunofluorescence and immunohistochemical staining. Material should be taken from vesicles, pustules or scabs; handling and transport of clinical specimens must be coordinated with state and federal health agencies in accordance with CDC guidelines.

VACCINATION

Vaccination using live vaccinia virus induces protective immunity in more than 95% of recipients with a successful "take." The smallpox vaccine available for limited use in the United States is Dryvax,* which consists of lyophilized (freeze-dried) calf lymph containing vaccinia virus (New York Board of Health strain). Vaccination is administered using the tip of a sterile bifurcated needle that has been dipped into reconstituted vaccine. Perpendicular strokes are rapidly made, puncturing the skin overlying a 5-mm diameter area of the outer aspect of the upper arm. A trace of blood should appear to indicate that the strokes have been sufficiently vigorous. If successful, a primary reaction will occur, with erythema and pruritus developing after several days. This is followed by the formation of a central vesicle by day 5 or 6, which evolves into a pustule that crusts and heals with a scar after the third week. Vaccination may be associated with fever and regional lymphadenitis. Accelerated or modified reactions may occur in persons who have been previously vaccinated.

Vaccinia elicits both a humoral and cellular immune response. Neutralizing antibodies are detected in the majority of individuals following primary vaccination, and vaccinia virus–specific CD8+ cytotoxic T lymphocyte and interferon-γ–producing T lymphocyte responses have been demonstrated in vaccine recipients. Protective immunity acquired from smallpox vaccine is not lifelong, but generally wanes over a period of 5 to 10 years after the primary vaccination. However, patients with a history of vaccination who develop smallpox are more likely to develop mild disease with increased survival. Because vaccinia inoculated in the arm has a shorter incubation period than variola acquired via a respiratory route, vaccination is capable of ameliorating or even aborting smallpox if given early after exposure, particularly within the first four days.

*Available only from the CDC.

Routine smallpox vaccination of children was discontinued in 1972 in the United States, because potential adverse effects from vaccination outweighed the risk of contracting disease. Complications following vaccination include autoinoculation at other sites, generalized vaccinia, erythema multiforme, eczema vaccinatum, postvaccinial encephalitis, progressive vaccinia, and ocular vaccinia. Children younger than age 5 and those receiving primary vaccination are at the highest risk for developing complications. Sixty-eight deaths from complications of smallpox vaccination were reported in the United States in the nine years from 1959 to 1968; the risk of death was estimated to be approximately 1 per 1,000,000 primary vaccinations. A 10-state survey of complications of smallpox vaccination in 1968 determined that adverse reactions occurred in approximately 1250 persons per million receiving primary vaccination (Table 1). Accidental inoculation accounted for 42% of all complications, followed by generalized vaccinia (19%), erythema multiforme (13%), eczema vaccinatum (3%) and postvaccinial encephalitis (1%). Fifty-three persons per million need hospitalization for these complications. Other complications, such as severe reactions to vaccine that were uncomfortable or became superinfected, accounted for 21% of adverse reactions.

Unless there has been exposure to variola, smallpox vaccination is contraindicated in persons with immunodeficiency from any cause, a history of atopic dermatitis, acute or chronic dermatologic conditions causing a loss of skin integrity, or pregnant women. These individuals should also avoid close contact with recently vaccinated persons. Smallpox vaccine is also contraindicated in those who are allergic to the vaccine or its components, are less than 12 months of age, are currently breastfeeding, or have moderate or severe acute illness. Recent reports of myocarditis, pericarditis, and ischemic cardiac events following vaccination have added heart disease to the list of contraindications. In addition, vaccination should be avoided in patients with three or more of the following cardiac risk factors: hypertension, hypercholesterolemia, diabetes, a first-degree relative with onset of heart disease under age 50, or cigarette smoking. Currently, smallpox vaccination is not recommended in persons less than 18 years old or above 65 years old, or

TABLE 1. **Rates of Complications from Primary Vaccinia Vaccination and Indications for Vaccinia Immune Globulin (VIG)**

Complication	No. of Events/ 1 Million*	VIG Treatment†
Accidental infection	529	May be indicated in ocular inoculation without vaccinial keratitis
Generalized vaccinia	242	May be indicated in patients who are severely ill or have serious underlying illness
Erythema multiforme	165	Not indicated
Eczema vaccinatum	39	Indicated in severe cases
Postvaccinial encephalitis	12	Not indicated
Progressive vaccinia	2	May be effective, depending on immune defect
Other	266	Not indicated

*Data adapted from: Lane JM, Ruben FL, Neff JM, Millar JD: Complications of smallpox vaccination, 1968: Results of ten statewide surveys. J Infect Dis 122:303-309, 1970.

†Recommendations from: Vaccinia (Smallpox) Vaccine Recommendations of the Advisory Committee on Immunization Practices (ACIP), 2001.

those who have inflammatory eye diseases requiring corticosteroid eyedrops. However, there are no absolute contraindications to vaccination if confirmed exposure to smallpox virus has occurred.

Vaccinia immune globulin (VIG),** derived from the serum of individuals vaccinated with vaccinia, is available under an investigative new-drug protocol from the CDC for treating certain severe complications. Historically, the recommended dosage was 0.6 mL/kg of body weight administered intramuscularly in divided doses over 24 to 36 hours, which was repeated at 2- to 3-day intervals until the onset of recovery. VIG is effective for treating eczema vaccinatum, and may be indicated for certain cases of progressive vaccinia, generalized vaccinia, and autoinoculation of the eye or eyelid without vaccinial keratitis (see Table 1). Vaccinia immune globulin is not effective for postvaccinial encephalitis and is contraindicated in vaccinial keratitis because it may worsen corneal scarring.

Pre-exposure mass vaccination is not currently recommended in the United States because the threat of the deliberate release of smallpox is considered low and it would expose millions of individuals to potential adverse effects. However, because of smallpox's high mortality, and the fact that most of the population is now susceptible to the disease, political and scientific debate continues over vaccination policy; this includes discussion of the appropriate number of emergency and hospital personnel to vaccinate as well as whether voluntary vaccination should be made available in the future. The CDC has issued guidelines for smallpox vaccination; in the event of a confirmed smallpox outbreak, current strategy recommendations give priority to the initial vaccination of household and other close contacts of patients as well as medical, public health, laboratory, and disaster response personnel. Large-scale voluntary vaccination would be considered in such an emergency to supplement control in areas with smallpox cases as well as to decrease the number of individuals susceptible to further deliberate releases of smallpox virus. Although vaccine was removed from the commercial market in 1983, 15.4 million doses of Dryvax are held in stock, and a study of 680 previously unvaccinated adults suggests it is efficacious at dilutions of 1:5 or 1:10. In addition, the CDC has recently contracted for the manufacture of two different cell culture–grown vaccinia vaccines which will be stockpiled in large amounts for emergency use. The goal is to ensure that there is sufficient vaccine to protect the entire US population. Modified Vaccinia virus Ankara (MVA) is an alternative vaccinia undergoing clinical evaluation, and hopefully it will have fewer adverse events and be useful for immunosuppressed patients.

MANAGEMENT

Because of the importance of surveillance and containment in controlling smallpox, local and state health officers should be notified immediately if there is a patient with suspected infection. If diagnostic tests are deemed necessary, the CDC Rash Illness Evaluation Team should be contacted (telephone: 770-488-7100 or 404-639-2888). Patients with suspected or confirmed smallpox should be cared for in a facility meeting prescribed guidelines for airborne and contact isolation precautions. Treatment of clinical smallpox is largely supportive. Fluid and electrolyte balance, as well as nutritional needs, should be maintained. This is particularly important in patients with high fever, poor oral intake, vomiting, or widespread skin breakdown. Symptomatic care may be necessary for nausea, vomiting or diarrhea. Complications from secondary bacterial infection include impetiginization of cutaneous lesions or skin abscesses, pneumonia, osteomyelitis, joint infections and septicemia. Systemic antibiotic therapy should be guided by culture confirmation of the causative organism. In patients with respiratory complications, supplemental oxygen and, in severe cases, intubation and ventilation may be required. Topical idoxuridine (Herplex)† may be considered in cases of corneal ulceration and keratitis, although it is of unproven efficacy for smallpox.

Potential antiviral drugs for the treatment of smallpox are currently under intensive investigation. Cidofovir (Vistide),* a cytosine nucleotide analog licensed for the treatment of cytomegalovirus retinitis in patients with acquired immune deficiency syndrome AIDS, has broad-spectrum activity against DNA viruses including poxviruses. Cidofovir for the treatment of smallpox infection and complications of vaccinia vaccine is available from the CDC under an investigational new-drug protocol. Variola has been demonstrated to be sensitive to cidofovir in *in vitro* studies. In addition, cidofovir administered by either an intraperitoneal or intranasal route protected mice from fatal infection with vaccinia or cowpox. In humans, there are anecdotal reports of the efficacy of topical or systemic cidofovir to treat molluscum contagiosum and for skin diseases caused by poxviruses. Cidofovir has poor bioavailability when taken orally, and intravenous administration is associated with renal and ocular toxicity. Co-administration with probenecid as well as hydration before and after cidofovir therapy may lessen renal toxicity. Cidofovir modified with the lipid adduct hexadecyloxypropyl, to allow for oral absorption, was active against variola *in vitro* and protective against lethal cowpox infection in mice. Numerous other antiviral compounds, including cidofovir analogs, have potent *in vitro* efficacy against vaccinia virus and some have also been reported to inhibit vaccinia virus in *in vivo* animal studies. The safety and efficacy of these compounds for treating orthopoxvirus infections in humans remains unknown. Another potential treatment for smallpox that is under investigation is immunotherapy with neutralizing monoclonal antibodies directed against viral proteins. Treatment with a neutralizing monoclonal antibody has been reported to be effective prophylactically and therapeutically against vaccinia virus infection in mice.

**Investigational drug in the United States.

*Not FDA approved for this indication.

†Not FDA approved for this indication.

Section 3

Diseases of the Head and Neck

VISION CORRECTION PROCEDURES

method of
DAVID W. JACKSON, M.D., and
M. BOWES HAMILL, M.D.
Baylor College of Medicine
Houston, Texas

In an emmetropic patient (one who sees well at a distance without glasses), light from distant objects forms parallel light rays that enter the eye and are focused by the cornea and crystalline lens on the retina. When parallel light rays are not focused on the retinal photoreceptors, a refractive error exists.

REFRACTIVE ERRORS

In the United States, approximately 45% of people age 14 to 44 years wear spectacles for the correction of refractive errors. The proportion increases to 89% in people age 45 to 64 years because of the increasing prevalence of presbyopia (the loss of near vision with age). Myopia (nearsightedness), hyperopia (farsightedness), and astigmatism are types of refractive errors. In myopia, parallel light rays are brought into focus in front of the retina, and objects in the distance seem blurry. In hyperopia, objects are brought into focus behind the retina. However, distant objects are focused closer to the retina than near objects are. For this reason, distant objects are seen more clearly than near objects. In addition, our accommodative ability (the ability to focus incoming light with the crystalline lens of the eye on the retina) allows distant objects to be clearly refocused on the retina, but near objects remain focused behind the retina and continue to appear blurry. In patients with an astigmatic error, neither distant nor near objects are focused clearly on the retina.

The degree of refractive error is measured in diopters. A diopter is a measure of lens power and is the inverse of the focal length (in meters) of the lens. For example, a 2-diopter (D) lens focuses light to a point at half a meter. The cornea and crystalline lens together have a refractive power of approximately 63 D. The cornea alone is responsible for 43 D of refracting power and is the main refractive element of the eye. The average human lens has a power of 20 D. Because of the significant contribution of the cornea to the overall focusing power of the eye, alterations in corneal curvature can profoundly affect the patient's vision. In modern refractive surgery, most techniques involve reshaping the anterior corneal curvature by flattening it to correct myopia or steepening it to correct hyperopia.

The adult cornea measures approximately 12mm in diameter horizontally by 11 mm vertically and is composed of five layers. The corneal epithelium is the outermost layer. It is composed of nonkeratinizing, stratified squamous epithelium and is approximately 40 μm (10^{-6} m) thick. Bowman's layer lies beneath the epithelium. It consists of randomly dispersed collagen fibrils and is 14 μm thick. The underlying corneal stroma is made of uniform and regularly arranged collagen fibrils with a thickness of approximately 500 μm. Descemet's membrane lies beneath the corneal stroma. In the adult cornea it is 10 to 12 μm thick and is continuously laid down by corneal endothelial cells throughout life.

PHOTOREFRACTIVE KERATECTOMY AND LASER-ASSISTED IN SITU KERATOMILEUSIS

Most current surgical options for refractive vision correction use an excimer laser. The excimer laser emits ultraviolet radiation at a wavelength of 193 nm (10^{-9} m). The organic molecular bonds making up the corneal tissue absorb this wavelength. As the laser energy is absorbed, the bonds are disrupted, thereby resulting in non-thermal ablation of the corneal stroma. It is important to appreciate that the excimer laser is a non-thermal laser and thus tissue removal is exquisitely precise and without the collateral tissue damage that would be expected with a thermal laser. Both photorefractive keratectomy (PRK) and laser-assisted in situ keratomileusis (LASIK) techniques use the excimer laser for correction of refractive errors.

All patients should undergo rigorous screening before any refractive surgery. Contraindications and relative contraindications to refractive surgery include a history of herpes simplex or herpes zoster involving the eye, glaucoma, pupils larger than 8 or 9 mm in diameter, thin corneas, pregnancy or nursing, and dry eyes. Additionally, patients with poorly controlled diabetes or autoimmune disease should not undergo refractive surgery. Regular participation in contact sports where blows to the face and eyes are a normal occurrence is a relative contraindication to LASIK, but not PRK surgery.

During the preoperative examination, the patient's current glasses prescription and vision are determined. The refractive power of the glasses is compared with the patient's current refraction because it is important to have stable refraction before laser vision correction. In addition, patients with significant cataractous lens changes are not good candidates for the procedure. The patient's pupil size is checked in ambient and dim light. Pupil sizes larger than the available ablation diameters are at greater risk for the development of halos and glare at night. Current ablation diameters are up to 8 or 9 mm. Corneal curvature and thickness are also evaluated before refractive surgery. Any abnormal thinning or curvature anomalies are contraindications to refractive surgery.

Before the procedure, either PRK or LASIK, the periocular area is prepared with povidone-iodine (Betadine). An anxiolytic such as diazepam (Valium) and a topical anesthetic are given for comfort. Although both techniques use the excimer laser for refractive correction, the approach to each is different. PRK involves application of the laser directly to the cornea after removal of the epithelial surface. In this procedure, Bowman's membrane is ablated along with the underlying stroma to achieve recontouring of the corneal surface. After laser application in PRK, the epithelium is allowed to heal over the ablation site (healing generally takes 2 to 3 days). Advantages of PRK include the avoidance of a corneal flap and its applicability to patients with corneas too thin for LASIK. Disadvantages include patient discomfort, occasional corneal haze, scarring, and regression (loss of the desired correction from the healing response of the corneal tissue).

LASIK, on the other hand, involves the creation of a thin hinged corneal flap (140 to 180 μm thick) containing all the surface elements of the cornea. The flap is lifted and the laser is applied to the stromal bed. The flap is repositioned after laser application. Advantages of LASIK include significantly less regression (especially with higher corrections) than noted with PRK, along with less patient discomfort and more rapid visual recovery and stabilization. Disadvantages include a more complex procedure with the possibility of postoperative flap complications (rare).

Postoperative complications can include inflammation at the flap interface, infection, striae in the flap, decentered or irregular ablations, dry eyes, epithelial growth under the flap, and residual refractive error. Few complications cause loss of best-corrected acuity. However, many patients continue to require some spectacle correction after the procedure. For example, patients older than 40 years can expect to need reading glasses if they have been corrected for distance vision.

Currently, LASIK is available to correct spherical refractive errors of −14 to +6 D but performs best from −12 to +4 D. Astigmatic correction of up to 6 D is also possible. PRK is indicated for correcting small to moderate refractive errors or for treating corneas too thin for LASIK. Last year, over 1 million LASIK procedures were performed in the United States, and this number is expected to rise.

LASER-ASSISTED SUBEPITHELIAL KERATECTOMY

Laser-assisted subepithelial keratectomy (LASEK) is an attempt to combine the best features of LASIK and PRK. In LASEK, the corneal epithelium is first loosened with 20% ethyl alcohol and then gently moved aside. Excimer ablation then takes place exactly as in PRK. Unlike PRK, at the conclusion of LASEK the epithelium is repositioned. The discomfort experienced after LASEK is reportedly less than that after PRK, and visual recovery is faster. The primary advantage of LASEK over LASIK is that no stromal flap is cut, thus reducing the risk of the procedure. This technique is a recently developed procedure whose position in the refractive armamentarium has yet to be determined.

LASER THERMAL KERATOPLASTY AND CONDUCTIVE KERATOPLASTY

Both procedures are approved for the temporary correction of mild hyperopia in persons 40 years or older. These procedures can also temporarily give presbyopic patients better near vision. Spots of radio frequency energy (conductive keratoplasty [CK]) or laser energy (laser thermal keratoplasty [LTK]) are applied to the cornea to produce controlled shrinkage of collagen lamellae. The treatment spots are applied in an annular pattern in the periphery and result in steepening of the central portion of the cornea. The central corneal steepening increases the dioptric power of the cornea to correct hyperopia or produce myopia in an emmetropic presbyope.

CLEAR LENS EXTRACTION

Clear lens extraction is cataract surgery without the patient having a cataract and involves removal of the patient's clear crystalline lens with placement of a correctly powered intraocular lens (IOL). Although the surgical technique is identical, the goal of cataract surgery is to remove a lens opaque from cataract, whereas clear lens extraction is solely for refractive correction. This technique is best used for the correction of presbyopic hyperopes. Myopic patients have a significantly increased risk of retinal detachment over time after clear lens extraction, and for this reason, myopic patients should carefully consider alternative treatments of their refractive error.

PHAKIC INTRAOCULAR LENSES

This procedure entails the implantation of an IOL without previous removal of the patient's crystalline lens. By selecting the correct IOL power, the refractive error can be neutralized. The phakic IOL can be placed in front of the iris (colored part of the eye) or in back of the iris, or it can be clipped to the iris. Though not currently approved for use in the United States, phakic IOLs can be used to correct moderate to high myopia. The main risk of this procedure is subsequent cataract formation.

PERIPHERAL CORNEAL RELAXING INCISIONS

Peripheral corneal relaxing incisions (PCRIs) are arcuate incisions made just inside the limbus (junction of the cornea and sclera) to correct an isolated astigmatic error. Single or paired PCRIs are placed along the steep meridian of the cornea. The incisions flatten the steep meridian and slightly steepen the flat meridian, thereby causing the cornea to be more spherical and reducing astigmatic error.

It should be appreciated that although refractive surgery has benefited millions of people, no surgical procedure is appropriate for every patient. Different techniques have different applications, and every patient's needs are unique. Patients considering refractive surgery should meet with their refractive surgeon to discuss their individual goals and get a realistic estimation of the benefits in their individual case. As in all surgery, complications are possible and should be discussed thoroughly with the surgeon performing the procedure before surgery.

CONJUNCTIVITIS

method of
JOHN P. FRANGIE, M.D.
Pioneer Valley Ophthalmic Consultants
Amherst, Massachusetts

The conjunctiva is a mucous membrane that lines the posterior aspect of the lids and then sweeps around the anterior surface of the globe, ultimately fusing with the corneal epithelium at the limbus. Conjunctivitis connotes an inflammatory process of the conjunctiva that may be infectious or noninfectious. Noninfectious causes of conjunctivitis include exposure, allergy, and toxicity. Infectious conjunctivitis may result from bacterial, viral, or chlamydial agents. Although any age group may be affected by conjunctivitis, the implications of possible systemic sequelae in the neonatal population dictates that conjunctivitis in this age group be discussed separately.

NEONATAL CONJUNCTIVITIS

Neonatal conjunctivitis, or ophthalmia neonatorum, is conjunctival inflammation that occurs during the first 30 days postpartum. A complete workup of neonatal conjunctivitis requires a clinical examination including fluorescein staining, Gram and Giemsa stains, culture and sensitivity, and conjunctival scrapings. The physical signs of neonatal conjunctivitis tend to be nonspecific and include lid edema, discharge, conjunctival injection, and edema. Additionally, determination of an etiologic agent on the basis of onset with relation to birth has been proved to be an unreliable index. Meticulous workup is critical because isolation of an infectious agent may provide the clinician with information that has relevance on a systemic level. Although the pathogens in the neonatal population are not very different from those seen in adults, the immature neonatal immune system is more susceptible to systemic dissemination, occasionally with catastrophic results. Almost without exception, microbes responsible for ophthalmia neonatorum are encountered in the birth canal (unless premature membrane rupture allows *in utero* infection).

Buffered 1% silver nitrate solution is the most common ophthalmic agent instilled at birth. This agent tends to destroy *Neisseria* organisms with little effect on other pathogens, notably *Chlamydia* and viruses. The clinician should be aware that the silver nitrate compound is intrinsically toxic and has the potential to cause chemical conjunctivitis. Indeed, the most common form of neonatal conjunctivitis is secondary to the prophylactic agent. Chemical conjunctivitis secondary to silver nitrate is characterized by the nonspecific signs of conjunctivitis listed earlier; however, this entity is self-limited and typically resolves within 36 hours.

A wide spectrum of bacteria may cause ophthalmia neonatorum (Table 1). Staphylococci and streptococci represent the majority of gram-positive isolates. Gram-positive infections may be treated with topical erythromycin (0.5% ointment, 4 to 6 times per day) for 2 weeks. Gram-negative infections may be caused by a number of coliform bacteria including *Escherichia coli, Enterobacter* spp., *Proteus* spp., and *Serratia marcescens*. Additionally, *Klebsiella pneumoniae* and *Haemophilus* spp. have been isolated. Tobramycin (Tobrex), 0.3% ointment, four to six times per day for 2 weeks, is the drug of choice. With few exceptions, we recommend the use of ointments rather than solutions; instillation of solutions in crying neonates may result in a dilution or total washout of the antimicrobial agents. The one exception is *Haemophilus* spp., which tend to be resistant to tobramycin. The use of a polymyxin B/trimethoprim compound (Polytrim), four to six times per day, is indicated. If *Pseudomonas* spp. are isolated, one should instill tobramycin hourly.

Before the introduction of Credé prophylaxis (2% silver nitrate) in 1881, *Neisseria gonorrhoeae* was a major source of ophthalmic morbidity in the neonatal population. Although the occurrence of neonatal gonococcal conjunctivitis has decreased considerably, the significant morbidity associated with this condition mandates that this infection be diagnosed and treated promptly. *N. gonorrhoeae* has the ability to penetrate an intact corneal epithelium, and, therefore, is capable of causing corneal perforation. Gonococci appear as gram-negative diplococci. Thayer-Martin medium provides the best medium for growth of this agent.

TABLE 1. **Neonatal Conjunctivitis**

Organism	Topical Therapy	Systemic Therapy
Gram-positive	Erythromycin 0.5% 4–6 times daily	Not indicated
Gram-negative (except *Haemophilus* sp. and *Neisseria* sp.)	Tobramycin 0.3% (Tobrex) 4–6 times daily*	Not indicated
Haemophilus sp.	Polymyxin B compound (Polytrim) 10,000 U per ml 4–6 times daily	May be indicated if associated with cellulitis
Neisseria sp.	Penicillin G** 20,000 U per mL every half hour	Penicillin G** 50,000 U/kg/day in 4 divided doses
Neisseria sp. (resistant to penicillin	Bacitracin 500 units/g 8 times daily	Ceftriaxone (Rocephin) 50 mg/kg/day
Chlamydia	Erythromycin 0.5% 4–6 times daily	Erythromycin 40 mg/kg/day orally in 4 divided doses
Herpes simplex virus	Trifluorothymidine (Viroptic) 1.0% every 2 hours	If associated with signs of systemic dissemination

*Hourly instillation should be used for *Pseudomonas* sp.
**Not FDA approved for this indication.

Isolation of gonococci should prompt the physician to rule out other associated venereal pathogens including *Chlamydia*, syphilis, herpes simplex virus (HSV), and human immunodeficiency virus (HIV). Appropriate treatment of the mother and her sexual partner(s) should also be undertaken. It should be noted that owing to the chelating properties of tetracycline, this drug should not be used systemically in pediatric patients (up to age 8 years) or nursing or pregnant mothers. Lifelong discoloration of deciduous teeth has been reported in children after the administration of tetracycline.

Initial therapy of gonococcal conjunctivitis should include ceftriaxone (Rocephin), 50 mg/kg intramuscularly or intravenously every 24 hours for 1 week. Should culture sensitivity to penicillin G* exist, the suggested regimen is 50,000 U/kg per day intravenously, divided into four doses. Gonococcal conjunctivitis also requires simultaneous topical therapy. Penicillin G mixed* in a concentration of 20,000 U/mL may be applied every 30 minutes when the pathogen is susceptible. Alternative agents include bacitracin 500 units per gram or gentamicin (Garamycin)* 0.3%. Frequent lavage is also indicated to remove the typically copious exudate.

Chlamydia is the most frequent cause of infectious neonatal conjunctivitis, reflecting the prominence of this agent as a venereal pathogen. *Chlamydia* also is responsible for infectious neonatal pneumonitis, and this condition may be present in up to 20% of neonates with conjunctivitis. Chlamydial conjunctivitis has a spectrum of effects; although the condition is typically mild, corneal opacification and conjunctival scarring have been reported. The use of Giemsa stain may demonstrate chlamydial inclusion bodies in involved epithelial cells. The development of an enzyme-linked immunoassay permits rapid and accurate diagnosis. Systemic therapy is indicated in chlamydial conjunctivitis and consists of oral erythromycin, 40 mg/kg/day in four divided doses for 2 to 4 weeks. In addition, topical erythromycin ointment 0.5% may be used four times daily. Again, the clinician should suspect and rule out the presence of concurrent venereal pathogens.

*Not FDA approved for this indication.

VIRAL NEONATAL CONJUNCTIVITIS

HSV conjunctivitis in the neonatal period typically is caused by Type II virus encountered in the birth canal. HSV conjunctivitis may present unilaterally or bilaterally and has no defining characteristics unless there is coexistent HSV keratitis. Disseminated disease with significant morbidity may occur in up to two thirds of cases of HSV conjunctivitis and keratoconjunctivitis.

Ocular diagnosis has been aided by the development of monoclonal antibody immunologic techniques. Additionally, cell culture from associated skin lesions may be diagnostic. Ocular treatment consists of topical trifluorothymidine 1% (Viroptic) given every 2 hours while the patient is awake. Follow-up of HSV conjunctivitis should be undertaken by an ophthalmologist, whereas the pediatrician must monitor the patient for possible dissemination of the HSV agent, including encephalitis. As HSV conjunctivitis in the neonate has a nonspecific presentation, among the most important preventive tools is a high degree of clinical suspicion, a detailed maternal history of genital HSV infection, and close follow-up of these mothers. The presence of active genital lesions in these patients has been used as a criterion for proceeding with cesarean section. As in other cases in which a sexually transmitted disease is detected, workup for other agents in both the patient and mother is appropriate.

ADULT CONJUNCTIVITIS

Infectious or noninfectious agents may also cause conjunctivitis in the adult. Physical findings include lid edema, conjunctival edema and injection, and an associated discharge. The patient may complain of minimal irritation or foreign body sensation and, possibly, mild photophobia. Severe pain or photophobia suggests corneal involvement or anterior uveitis. Referral to an ophthalmologist is indicated.

Common noninfectious causes of conjunctivitis include toxicity and allergy. Toxic conjunctivitis typically is exhibited with conjunctival injection, mild to moderate ocular discomfort, and occasionally a serous discharge. The diagnosis is made on the basis of the patient's history of exposure to an inciting agent. The treatment of toxic conjunctivitis is primarily supportive; artificial tears may be used for comfort, and avoidance of exposure to the agent is curative.

The prominent component of allergic conjunctivitis is a subjective complaint of bilateral (or, less frequently, unilateral) ocular itching. If a discharge is present, it may be serous, or in advanced cases, tenuous ropelike deposits of matter may be removed from the eyes. It is not unusual for the patient to give a history of hay fever or similar atopic phenomena with associated seasonal occurrence.

The clinician's armamentarium against allergic conjunctivitis has been enhanced significantly over the course of the past decade. The treatment protocol should be administered in a "stepped" format. Initial treatment of uncomplicated seasonal allergic conjunctivitis should be supportive. Primary therapy should include using cold compresses and artificial tears four to six times daily (Table 2). The artificial tears appear to serve a dual purpose—serving as both a soothing lubricant in addition to providing the eyes with additional fluid to remove deposited allergens from the ocular surface.

Topical antihistamine agents such as pheniramine combined with decongestant such as naphazoline (Naphcon A) have been traditionally used to provide symptomatic relief. Levocabastine (Livostin) is a newer topical histamine blocker that displays a rapid onset and longer duration of action. Levocabastine has been shown to be some 15,000 times more potent than pheniramine. The topical histamine antagonist that has been found to have the greatest potency is emedastine (Emadine). Emedastine has an onset of action of less than 10 minutes.

Mast cell inhibiting agents prevent the allergic response by inhibiting the release of inflammatory mediators. It is believed that these agents bind to mast cell receptors and prevent IgE cross-linking by an inciting allergen. The initial members of this drug class, disodium cromoglycate (Cromolyn) and lodoxamide 0.1% (Alomide) have no intrinsic anti-inflammatory capabilities and do not relieve symptoms if mast cell degranulation has already occurred. Accordingly, a period of 1 to 3 weeks after instillation is not unusual before the patient appreciates the effect of these agents. Nedocromil 2% (Alocril) is a mast cell stabilizing agent that also seems to inhibit inflammatory cell chemotaxis. Two of the newer agents in this family, olopatadine (Patanol) and ketotifen 0.025% (Zaditor) have been shown to have direct antihistamine activity in addition to their membrane-stabilizing effects.

Topical corticosteroid preparations (loteprednol [Alrex, Lotemax], fluorometholone [FML],* prednisolone, and dexamethasone) tend to provide the greatest relief from allergic conditions. Unfortunately, steroid-induced adverse effects including elevation of intraocular pressure, potentiation of microbial proliferation, and cataractogenesis provide a significant risk factor given the usually self-limited course of allergic conjunctivitis. Because of the potential for sight-threatening complications, topical ophthalmic steroid use should be instituted and monitored by an ophthalmologist.

*Not FDA approved for this indication.

TABLE 2. **Conjunctivitis in Other Age Groups**

Etiology	Signs/Symptoms*	Treatment
Bacterial	Discharge with lids sealed shut in A.M., conjunctival injection	Erythromycin 0.5% or polymyxin B/trimethoprim compound (Polytrim) four times daily
Gonococcal	Hyperpurulent conjunctivitis Beefy-red conjunctival injection	Topical bacitracin 500 U/g 8 times daily *plus* Ceftriaxone 1 g intramuscularly every 24 hours for 5 days**
Chlamydial	Chronic unilateral or bilateral mucopurulent conjunctivitis	Tetracycline 500 mg or erythromycin stearate 500 mg orally four times daily for 3 weeks.
Viral	Serous discharge starting unilaterally, then spreading bilaterally, mild itching, conjunctival injection. Ipsilateral preauricular lymphadenopathy	Artificial tears Cold compresses Fomite precautions
Allergy	Bilateral itching, increased lacrimation, conjunctival injection, associated systemic allergy	Artificial tears 4–6 times/day Topical antihistamine 4 times/day Consider prophylactic treatment with a mast cell stabilizing agent in patients with documented seasonal allergic conjunctivitis
Toxic	Unilateral/bilateral irritation with conjunctival injection	Artificial tears Removal of inciting agent

*Corneal fluorescein staining and/or severe foreign body sensation suggest corneal involvement and should be managed with an ophthalmologist.
**Exceeds dosage recommended by the manufacturer.

Bacteria, viruses or chlamydial agents may cause adult infectious conjunctivitis. In contrast to the neonatal conjunctivitis, there are no data supporting the necessity to perform extensive laboratory work in the vast majority of cases. Obtaining a complete history generally gives a clinician insight about the etiologic agent. Viral conjunctivitis often causes symptoms of tearing and mild to moderate itching accompanying a serous discharge. The process typically starts in one eye with subsequent bilateral involvement within a matter of days. Viral conjunctivitis may be caused by a number of agents including picornavirus and adenovirus. Adenovirus subtypes are responsible for the highly contagious epidemic keratoconjunctivitis known as pink eye, which may be spread by fomites or person-to-person contact. An adenovirus subtype is also responsible for a symptom complex known as pharyngoconjunctival fever, in which the patient with conjunctivitis also is febrile and exhibits upper respiratory infection symptoms. The physical findings in viral conjunctivitis also may include a prominent ipsilateral preauricular lymph node.

HSV conjunctivitis in the adult is often a nonspecific conjunctival inflammation in the absence of associated corneal lesions. HSV conjunctivitis typically represents primary ocular infection and is difficult to differentiate from other forms of viral conjunctivitis. The primary importance of HSV infection in the eye is the subsequent recurrence with corneal involvement.

There are no specific cures for viral conjunctivitis. Treatment is primarily supportive with cold compresses and artificial tears. Occasionally, topical antibiotic preparations are prescribed as prophylaxis against secondary bacterial infections. Although steroids are known to provide symptomatic improvement for some types of viral conjunctivitis, these drugs potentiate HSV replication. Therefore, administration of corticosteroids for the treatment of viral conjunctivitis should be under the direction of an ophthalmologist.

The patient with bacterial conjunctivitis typically reports a unilateral, red, irritated eye, associated with a mucopurulent discharge that causes the eyelids to be sealed shut on waking. Culture and sensitivity testing of these cases has not been cost efficient. Indeed, sensitivity testing is somewhat useless because drug sensitivity is reported for drug levels obtained in the blood and soft tissues. These levels are easily surpassed on the ocular surface by topical application of antibiotics. Typically, conjunctivitis may be treated effectively with a polymyxin B/trimethoprim compound (Polytrim) or, in the more severe cases, a 0.3% aminoglycoside drop (gentamicin, tobramycin) four times daily for a 7- to 10-day course.

The presence of hyperpurulent conjunctivitis with a beefy red appearance to the conjunctiva in a sexually active adult should cause the clinician to consider gonococcal conjunctivitis. Unlike most other forms of adult conjunctivitis, gonococcal conjunctivitis requires concurrent parenteral therapy with ceftriaxone (Rocephin), 1 g intramuscularly every 24 hours for 5 days,** in addition to topical ophthalmic application of bacitracin 500 U per gram, eight times daily. Inadequate treatment may lead to rapid corneal perforation resulting in loss of the eye. Because of the virulent nature of this condition, gonococcal conjunctivitis should be managed with the aid of an ophthalmologist. Gonococcal conjunctivitis is typically an oculogenital condition; appropriate workup of the patient and his or her sexual partner(s) is indicated.

Adult inclusion conjunctivitis is another oculogenital process. The mucopurulent conjunctivitis is caused by *Chlamydia* and tends to have a chronic, remittent course. Adult chlamydial conjunctivitis typically results from sexual encounter with an infected partner. The infection is most commonly diagnosed in young (15 to 30 years of age) adults who have recently acquired a new sexual partner. Because this disease has a urogenital component, systemic therapy is indicated. Oral tetracycline 500 mg may be used in males or nonpregnant females who are not nursing; otherwise, erythromycin stearate 500 mg orally four times daily for 3 weeks is recommended.

An ophthalmologist should be consulted promptly to evaluate conjunctivitis that persists following the recommended treatment schedules or worsens significantly during the course of treatment.

ACKNOWLEDGMENT

The author wishes to acknowledge the contributions of Howard Leibowitz, M.D.

**Exceeds dosage recommended by the manufacturer.

OPTIC NEURITIS

method of
LAURA J. BALCER, M.D., M.S.C.E., and
STEVEN L. GALETTA, M.D.
Division of Neuro-Ophthalmology
Departments of Neurology and Ophthalmology
University of Pennsylvania School of Medicine, Philadelphia, Pennsylvania

Optic neuritis refers to an inflammatory disorder of the optic nerve. Most cases are related to multiple sclerosis (MS). Occasionally, optic neuritis may be caused by systemic disorders such as sarcoidosis or syphilis. This chapter will focus on diagnosis and treatment of the most common form of optic neuritis, *acute demyelinating optic neuritis.*

Acute demyelinating optic neuritis often represents the first clinical manifestation of MS. When signs or symptoms of MS are not present at the time of diagnosis, acute optic neuritis is referred to as idiopathic or *monosymptomatic*. Acute demyelinating optic neuritis affects primarily young patients (20 to

50 years of age), and is more common in women. Among populations at high risk for MS, acute monosymptomatic demyelinating optic neuritis has an incidence of approximately 3 per 100,000 per year (compared with 1 per 100,000 per year in lower risk populations).

CLINICAL FEATURES

The two most characteristic features of optic neuritis are subacute visual loss and pain upon eye movements. Many of the clinical features of this disorder were firmly established by the Optic Neuritis Treatment Trial (ONTT). The ONTT was a multicenter randomized trial of 457 patients that examined the effect of corticosteroid treatment on visual recovery in acute optic neuritis by comparing intravenous methylprednisolone* with oral prednisone* alone and with placebo (see Treatment). In the ONTT, loss of central visual acuity was reported in more than 90% of patients. Such loss of vision is usually subacute, progressing over hours to days. In fact, worsening or progression of visual loss beyond 2 weeks, or failure of visual recovery to begin within a 2- to 4-week period, should be considered atypical for acute demyelinating optic neuritis. Alternative etiologies for visual loss should be sought in such cases. Visual loss in optic neuritis is typically monocular, although involvement of both eyes may occur, particularly in children.

Pain in or around the eye is also a common presenting symptom of acute demyelinating optic neuritis. Reported by 92% of patients in the ONTT, ocular/periorbital pain is frequently worsened by eye movement (87% in ONTT), and may precede or occur concomitantly with visual loss. In typical cases, pain persists for no longer than a few days. During and even beyond the recovery of vision, patients with acute optic neuritis frequently experience temporary worsening of symptoms with exposure to heat (hot shower or exercise); this is referred to as Uhthoff's symptom. Positive visual phenomena, described as flashing bright lights or photopsias precipitated by eye movement, are also frequently reported by patients with optic neuritis (30% of ONTT participants).

The neuro-ophthalmologic examination reveals findings typical of optic nerve dysfunction. Visual function tests, performed at baseline within 8 days of symptom onset in the ONTT, revealed abnormalities of visual acuity, visual fields, contrast sensitivity, and color vision in both affected and fellow eyes. The degree of visual loss in the ONTT varied from mild field defects to marked loss of visual acuity (no light perception vision was noted in 3% of ONTT participants). In almost all cases, an afferent pupillary defect (APD) is present. Two-thirds of patients with acute demyelinating optic neuritis have a normal optic disc appearance at presentation *(retrobulbar optic neuritis)*. When optic disc swelling *(papillitis)* occurs, peripapillary hemorrhages are uncommon (6% in ONTT), and should suggest an alternative diagnosis such as anterior ischemic optic neuropathy. Visual recovery in the ONTT was generally favorable in all treatment groups; 95% of patients achieved visual acuities of at least 20/40. However, persistent symptoms may be reported months to years following acute optic neuritis.

*Not FDA approved for this indication.

DIAGNOSIS

The diagnosis of acute demyelinating optic neuritis is based upon the clinical history (typical vs. atypical course) and clinical features as outlined. In patients with monosymptomatic optic neuritis, magnetic resonance imaging (MRI) of the brain (T2-weighted and T1-weighted gadolinium enhanced images) should be performed. MRI is recommended, even in typical cases, to determine the presence of brain white matter lesions that would indicate that the patient is at high risk for the development of MS. In the ONTT, follow-up of patients at 5 years and beyond has shown that the number of white matter lesions, specifically the presence of two or more lesions, is highly predictive of the development of clinically definite MS (CDMS—defined as occurrence of a second clinical demyelinating event) in monosymptomatic patients (51% for ≥3 lesions vs. 16% for normal MRI).

MRI of the orbits with gadolinium and fat saturation is also useful in patients whose clinical course is not typical for acute demyelinating optic neuritis. In patients for whom MRI findings are abnormal but not classic for demyelinating disease, the detection of oligoclonal banding in the cerebrospinal fluid (CSF) may be helpful in guiding treatment decisions. Serologic studies and evoked potentials are generally not necessary for diagnosis of typical acute demyelinating optic neuritis.

TREATMENT

The most definitive investigation to date on the treatment of acute demyelinating optic neuritis has been the ONTT. The ONTT and its subsequent follow-up study (Longitudinal Optic Neuritis Study [LONS]) have had a significant impact on the practice patterns of ophthalmologists and neurologists, and have provided important data regarding clinical features, long-term visual outcome, and the role of brain MRI in determining prognosis for development of CDMS in monosymptomatic patients.

The ONTT enrolled 457 patients with acute unilateral optic neuritis, ages 18 to 46 years. The primary aim of the ONTT was to examine the effect of intravenous (IV) and oral corticosteroid therapy on visual outcome in acute demyelinating optic neuritis; the potential role for corticosteroid therapy in the development of CDMS (defined as a second demyelinating event) was a secondary outcome. Major findings of the ONTT are as follows: (1) IV methylprednisolone (250 mg every 6 hours for 3 days, followed by an oral prednisone taper) *hastened visual recovery* in acute optic neuritis, but *did not affect long-term visual outcome* at 6 months and beyond (5+ years) compared with oral placebo or oral prednisone alone (1 mg/kg/day for 11 days followed by 4-day taper); (2) treatment with oral prednisone alone was unexpectedly associated with an *increased rate of recurrent optic neuritis* in both affected and fellow eyes (30% at 2 years vs. 16% and 13% for placebo and IV steroids) that has persisted throughout follow-up of the ONTT cohort (5+ years); (3) patients with monosymptomatic optic neuritis in the IV methylprednisolone group had a reduced rate of CDMS during the first 2 years, but this benefit did not persist beyond 2 years' follow-up and was seen only in patients with high-risk brain MRI scans for CDMS (≥2 white matter lesions).

Data from the ONTT and similar trials demonstrate that there is no treatment for acute demyelinating optic neuritis that affects long-term visual outcome or visual prognosis compared with placebo. The most commonly used treatment, IV methylprednisolone (1 g/day for 3 days) followed by oral prednisone (1 mg/kg/day for 11 days followed by a 4-day taper), may hasten visual recovery by 2 to 3 weeks when started within 1 to 2 weeks of symptom onset. Oral prednisone alone, associated with an increased risk of recurrent optic neuritis in the ONTT, *should be avoided* in patients with typical acute demyelinating optic neuritis. If oral corticosteroids need to be used (e.g., because of difficulties with insurance coverage), we would recommend high-dose oral methylprednisolone (500 mg/d for 3 days followed by a taper).

As an alternative to the dosing regimen used in the ONTT (250 mg every 6 hours), the 3-day course of IV methylprednisolone may be given in single doses of 1 g/day. Although patients in the ONTT were hospitalized for IV methylprednisolone treatment, this therapy is now frequently provided in the outpatient setting by home care nursing and IV infusion companies. Short-term corticosteroid therapy is relatively safe when administered to young, healthy adults as in the ONTT. One patient in the ONTT who received IV methylprednisolone developed acute depression and another developed acute pancreatitis; both recovered without sequelae. Minor side effects of corticosteroid therapy in the ONTT included mild mood changes, sleep disturbances, facial flushing, stomach upset, and weight gain. Treatment with IV methylprednisolone (Solu-Medrol) was initiated within 8 days after symptom onset in the ONTT; however, such timing is frequently not realistic in the clinical setting. Beyond this time period, a decision to treat must be based upon the potential benefits vs. risks of therapy.

Among patients at high risk for the development of CDMS based on brain MRI criteria established by the ONTT (two or more white matter lesions, 3 mm or larger in diameter, at least one lesion periventricular or ovoid), the Controlled High-Risk Avonex MS Prevention Study (CHAMPS), a recent randomized trial of 383 patients with first demyelinating events (including optic neuritis, brainstem syndrome, or incomplete transverse myelopathy), demonstrated that treatment with interferon β-1a (Avonex, 30 μg intramuscularly [IM] weekly) significantly reduced the 3-year cumulative probability of CDMS vs. placebo by 44%.

All patients in CHAMPS received IV methylprednisolone (1 g/day for 3 days) followed by an oral prednisone taper as per the ONTT protocol (see above); steroid treatment was initiated within 14 days of symptom onset. After the steroid therapy, patients were then randomized to placebo or interferon β-1a (Avonex). To minimize the potential influenza-like side effects of interferon β-1a (reported by 54% who received active treatment), patients in both treatment and placebo groups were given 650 mg acetaminophen before each injection and then every 6 hours for 24 hours. In addition to flu-like side effects, depression was the only other adverse event whose incidence was at least 5 percentage points higher in the interferon β-1a group (20% vs. 13%, $P = .05$). Because anemia has been noted in previous trials of interferon β-1a (Avonex), patients should undergo laboratory testing before initiation and after 3 and 6 months of therapy (complete blood count with differential white cell count, platelet count, blood chemistries, liver function tests). The recommended duration of therapy has not yet been determined; follow-up in CHAMPS, with all patients now receiving active drug, will continue over 5 years to assess the long-term effects of interferon β-1a on clinical and MRI parameters (Controlled High-Risk Avonex MS Prevention Surveillance—CHAMPIONS Study).

Although the potential for long-term benefit of interferon β-1a in high-risk patients with acute monosymptomatic demyelinating optic neuritis or other first demyelinating event is not known, data from CHAMPS provide rationale for early therapy. Results from a randomized trial in Europe, the Early Treatment of Multiple Sclerosis Study (ETOMS), also provide evidence in favor of early interferon β-1a treatment. Patients in ETOMS ($n = 308$) received interferon β-1a (Rebif, 22 μg subcutaneously [SQ] weekly) or placebo; treatments were initiated within 3 months after a first demyelinating event. Similar to CHAMPS, a significantly lower proportion of patients in ETOMS who received interferon β-1a developed CDMS during the 2-year follow-up (24% reduction).

Before initiation of interferon β-1a, 70% of patients in ETOMS received corticosteroids (variable dose and route of administration), and 40% had multifocal neurologic deficits. As suggested by the ETOMS Study Group, differences between ETOMS and CHAMPS with respect to interferon β-1a dosage (22 μg vs. 30 μg), timing of initiation of therapy (3 months vs. 14 days following first demyelinating event), and patient population/disease severity (multi- vs. unifocal neurologic deficits at presentation) may account for the greater effect on delay of CDMS observed in CHAMPS.

SUMMARY

Based on data from the ONTT, CHAMPS, and ETOMS, patients with signs and symptoms consistent with acute monosymptomatic demyelinating optic neuritis should undergo evaluation and consideration of treatment, as outlined in Figure 1.

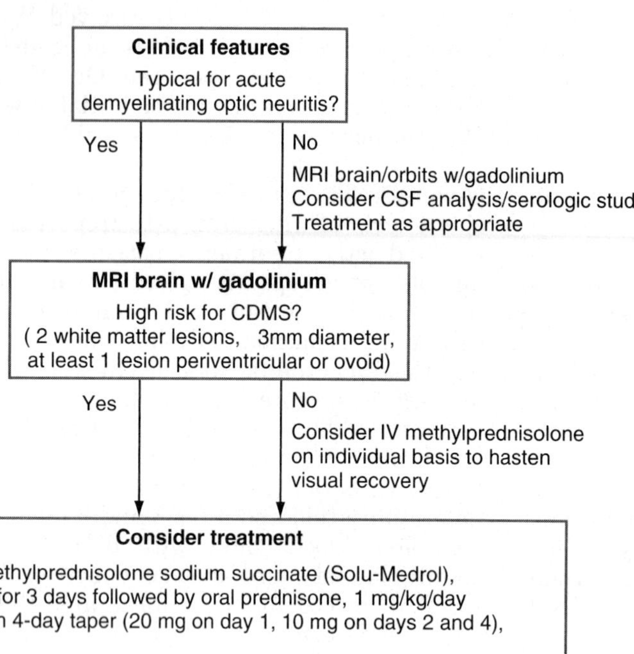
Clinical features
Typical for acute demyelinating optic neuritis?
Yes
No
MRI brain/orbits w/gadolinium
Consider CSF analysis/serologic studies
Treatment as appropriate
MRI brain w/ gadolinium
High risk for CDMS?
(2 white matter lesions, 3mm diameter, at least 1 lesion periventricular or ovoid)
Yes
No
Consider IV methylprednisolone on individual basis to hasten visual recovery
Consider treatment
Intravenous methylprednisolone sodium succinate (Solu-Medrol), 1 gram IV/day for 3 days followed by oral prednisone, 1 mg/kg/day for 11 days with 4-day taper (20 mg on day 1, 10 mg on days 2 and 4), followed by:
Interferon beta 1-a (Avonex 30 µg intramuscularly [IM] weekly, or Rebif 22 mg subcutaneously [SQ] weekly)–demonstrated to significantly reduce the risk of CDMS and the development of clinically silent MRI lesions in high-risk patients within 2–3 years follow-up.

Figure 1. Management of acute monosymptomatic optic neuritis.

GLAUCOMA

method of
EDWARD J. ROCKWOOD, M.D.
Cole Eye Institute, Cleveland Clinic Foundation
Cleveland, Ohio

Glaucoma is an ocular disorder characterized by optic nerve damage, seen as progressive enlargement of the optic disk cup with corresponding visual field loss, eventually leading to total and permanent blindness if untreated. Early visual loss tends to occur in the peripheral field of vision, with central visual acuity typically preserved until late in the disease process.

Elevated intraocular pressure is the most important risk factor for glaucoma. Normal intraocular pressure is about 16 mm Hg, with a range from about 10 to 21 mm Hg, and it tends to increase with increasing age. The higher the intraocular pressure, the greater both the risk and the rate of glaucomatous visual loss will be. However, different optic disks have different susceptibilities to intraocular pressure. Some patients have glaucomatous optic nerve damage despite normal or high-normal intraocular pressure (normal pressure glaucoma), and others have normal optic disk and no visual field loss despite elevated intraocular pressure (ocular hypertension).

Ciliary body epithelium produces aqueous humor, which circulates from the posterior to the anterior chamber of the eye, nourishes intraocular structures, and exits through the trabecular meshwork in the angle of the eye. In glaucoma, there is an abnormality of trabecular meshwork outflow.

The incidence of glaucoma increases with age in all races, but it is more common in African Americans and tends to be seen at an earlier age and with greater visual loss at presentation in this group. Angle-closure glaucoma is very common in Asians but seen in all races. Individuals with a family history of glaucoma have an increased risk of glaucoma. Diabetes mellitus and myopia (nearsightedness) are weaker risk factors.

TYPES

There are three major groups of glaucoma: open-angle glaucoma, angle-closure glaucoma, and developmental, or congenital, glaucoma. Primary open-angle glaucoma, the most common form, is genetically inherited. In primary open-angle glaucoma, the ocular examination is usually normal except for elevated intraocular pressure and glaucomatous visual field loss and optic nerve damage. Pigment dispersion from the posterior surface of the iris causes pigmentary glaucoma, more common in young myopic male patients, and in a condition of older adults, pseudoexfoliation glaucoma, an amyloid-like protein is released from intraocular epithelial cells into the anterior chamber and the trabecular meshwork. Other less common causes of secondary open-angle glaucoma include intraocular inflammation (iritis or uveitis), intracranial vascular shunts, blunt ocular trauma, chemical ocular burns (especially lye), and previous intraocular surgery.

Primary angle-closure glaucoma is less common than primary open-angle glaucoma and tends to occur in far-sighted persons with short axial length and eyes that are smaller than average. In these patients, the angle between the peripheral cornea and peripheral iris is narrow and may close acutely (acute primary angle-closure glaucoma) or, more commonly, may close gradually over months or years (chronic primary angle-closure glaucoma). Secondary angle-closure glaucoma occurs after processes that cause the development of adhesions between the peripheral iris and trabecular meshwork, such as iritis, ocular trauma, or infection, and after intraocular surgery. Patients with severe diabetic retinopathy may develop neovascular glaucoma with rapid angle closure, pain, and severe intraocular pressure elevation.

Primary infantile glaucoma is a rare inherited disorder usually diagnosed at, or shortly after, birth. Childhood glaucoma may also occur in association with congenital anomalies (cataract, aniridia, Marfan's syndrome, Lowe's syndrome, Rieger's anomaly) or as a result of blunt ocular trauma or iritis. Iritis, cataract, and glaucoma are frequent complications of juvenile rheumatoid arthritis in children.

SYMPTOMS

Glaucoma is usually asymptomatic until late in the disease, when the patient may notice limited vision in one or both eyes. Visual blurring and ocular pain are uncommon in glaucoma, except with severe intraocular pressure elevation. Acute primary angle-closure glaucoma may cause ocular pain, headache, blurred vision, haloes around lights, and nausea and vomiting. Pain from increased intraocular pressure is often felt in the globe, behind the eye, or in the brow area. Infants with glaucoma may demonstrate photophobia, tearing, and blepharospasm.

OPHTHALMOLOGIC EXAMINATION

Ophthalmologists test visual acuity, and intraocular pressure, usually with the Goldmann applanation tonometer. Manual (Goldmann) or automated visual field testing determines the extent of peripheral visual field loss, and gonioscopy is performed to detect angle closure or other angle abnormalities. A dilated retinal examination is performed to evaluate the optic disk and retina and to determine whether other ocular disorders (e.g., cataract, macular degeneration, diabetic retinopathy) are present. Optic disk examination is critical because glaucomatous optic nerve damage usually precedes detectable visual field loss, and changes in optic nerve appearance are the most reliable sign of glaucoma progression. Documentation of optic disk appearance is usually performed either with stereophotography or computerized optic disk image analyzers.

GENERAL ASPECTS OF THERAPY

The goal of glaucoma treatment is to reduce intraocular pressure with medication, laser, surgery, or a combination of these. Lowering intraocular pressure has been proven to reduce the incidence of glaucoma progression in large, prospective, multicenter clinical trials for both high-pressure and normal-pressure glaucoma. The Ocular Hypertension Treatment Study funded by the National Institutes of Health showed a reduction of the development of glaucoma from 9.5% (untreated) to 4.4% (medically treated) over 5 years in patients with ocular hypertension. Patients with ocular hypertension with large optic nerves and thin corneas were found to be at greatest risk of developing glaucoma. However, most patients with ocular hypertension do not require glaucoma treatment, and many can be observed, untreated, every 6 to 12 months, with treatment initiated once glaucoma damage is detected or if there is significant risk of developing glaucoma. Future glaucoma therapy may also focus on strengthening the optic nerve's resistance to intraocular pressure-induced damage, but at this time, there is no good clinical evidence of purported neuroprotective properties in any currently available glaucoma medication.

Traditionally in the United States, medication has been used first to treat open-angle glaucoma, with laser and then surgery reserved for patients whose disease is not controlled with the maximum tolerated medical therapy. However, laser and especially surgery provide lower mean intraocular pressures than glaucoma medication in many patients, and this approach reduces the likelihood of glaucoma progression. Clinical trials have demonstrated that early laser or surgical treatment can be beneficial for some patients with glaucoma. In the early 1990s medication was the least expensive option for managing glaucoma. However, with Medicare reimbursement reductions for ophthalmologic procedures, out-of-pocket costs to Medicare patients have commensurately declined such that laser or surgical treatment can cost less than a few months of glaucoma medical therapy and can provide long-term intraocular pressure reduction. The retail cost of some glaucoma medications can top $100 for a single bottle.

Variable compliance and noncompliance are frequent problems in glaucoma medical therapy. The high cost of glaucoma medication is an increasingly important reason. Glaucoma is usually an asymptomatic disorder, and medical agents may cause local and systemic side effects. Some patients are forgetful, and others may have difficulty incorporating eyedrop use into a busy daily schedule. Patients with arthritis may not be able to self-administer eyedrops. Patient education is helpful for reducing noncompliance. Other therapeutic options can be offered to patients who demonstrate repeated noncompliance.

All primary, and some secondary, angle-closure glaucomas require early laser peripheral iridotomy to relieve pupillary block. In some patients, laser iridotomy may be curative; however, additional medical or surgical therapy may be required to control intraocular pressure adequately. Early panretinal laser photocoagulation is required in the patient with neovascular glaucoma secondary to diabetic retinopathy and retinal venous occlusion. The glaucomas of early childhood usually require surgical management; medications are used only to temporize. Two groups of glaucoma medication (β-adrenergic antagonists and α_2-adrenergic agonists) may cause apnea in the neonate.

Medical Therapy

There are seven categories of U.S. FDA-approved glaucoma medications (Table 1). Most lower intraocular pressure by reducing aqueous production from the ciliary body, by increasing trabecular or nontrabecular outflow, or by a combination of both mechanisms. Hyperosmotics lower intraocular pressure by causing osmotic reduction of intraocular fluid.

β-Adrenergic Antagonists

Carteolol (Ocupress), levobunolol (Betagan), metipranolol (OptiPranolol), and timolol (Betimol, Timoptic) are nonselective β-adrenergic antagonists. Betaxolol (Betoptic) a selective β_1-adrenergic antagonist, has a reduced efficacy compared with nonselective agents, but it is preferred for patients with mild asthma. All five agents reduce aqueous production, can be administered once or twice daily, and, because

TABLE 1. **Glaucoma Medications**

Medication Class	Generic Name	Brand Name	Strength	Dosage
β_2-adrenergic antagonists				
Nonselective	Carteolol hydrochloride	Ocupress	1%	qd, bid
	Levobunolol hydrochloride	Betagan	0.25%, 0.5%	qd, bid
	Metipranolol	OptiPranolol	0.3%	qd, bid
	Timolol hemihydrate	Betimol	0.25%, 0.5%	qd, bid
	Timolol maleate	Timoptic	0.25%, 0.5%	qd, bid
	Timolol maleate gel	Timoptic XE	0.25%, 0.5%	qd, bid
Selective β_1	Betaxolol hydrochloride	Betoptic-S	0.25%	qd, bid
	Betaxolol hydrochloride	(generic)	0.5%	qd, bid
Nonselective adrenergic agonists				
	Dipivefrin hydrochloride	Propine	0.1%	qd, bid
	Epinephryl borate	Epinal	0.5%, 1%	qd, bid
	Epinephryl borate	Eppy/N	1%	qd, bid
	Epinephrine hydrochloride	Epifrin	0.5%, 1%, 2%	qd, bid
	Epinephrine hydrochloride	Glaucon	1%, 2%	qd, bid
α_2-Adrenergic agonists				
	Apraclonidine	Lopidine	0.5%	bid, tid
	Apraclonidine	Lopidine	1%	Prelaser
	Brimonidine	Alphagan P	0.15%	bid, tid
Parasympathomimetic agents				
Cholinergic agents	Carbachol	Isopto Carbachol	0.75%, 1.5%, 3%	bid, tid
	Pilocarpine	Ocuserts	20, 40 μg	Once weekly
	Pilocarpine hydrochloride	Akarpine	1%, 2%, 4%	
	Pilocarpine hydrochloride	Pilopine-HS gel	4%	qt bedtime
	Pilocarpine hydrochloride	Isopto Carpine	0.25%, 0.5%, 1%, 2%, 3%, 4%, 6%, 8%, 10%	bid to kid
	Pilocarpine hydrochloride	Pilocar	0.5%, 1%, 2%, 3%, 4%, 6%	bid to kid
	Pilocarpine hydrochloride	Piloptic	0.5%, 1%, 2%, 3%, 4%, 6%	bid to kid
	Pilocarpine hydrochloride	Pilostat	0.5%, 1%, 2%, 3%, 4%, 6%	bid to kid
	Pilocarpine nitrate		2%, 4%	
Cholinesterase inhibitors				
	Ecothiophate iodide	Phospholine iodine	0.125%	qd, bid
	Physostigmine	Eserine ointment	0.25%	
Carbonic anhydrase inhibitors				
	Acetazolamide	Diamox	125- and 250-mg tablet; 500-mg capsule	bid to qid
	Acetazolamide sodium	Diamox Parenteral	500 mg	
	Brinzolamide	Azopt	1%	bid, tid
	Dichlorphenamide	Daranide	50-mg tablet	bid, tid
	Dorzolamide hydrochloride	Trusopt	2%	bid, tid
	Methazolamide	Neptazane	25-, 50-mg tablets	bid, tid
Prostaglandins				
	Bimatoprost	Lumigan	0.03%	qd
	Latanoprost	Xalatan	0.005%	qd
	Travoprost	Travatan	0.004%	qd
	Unoprostone	Rescula	0.15%	qd
Hyperosmotics				
	Glycerin	Osmoglyn	50% solution	1-1.5 g/kg
	Mannitol parenteral	Osmitrol	5-25% solution	0.5-2 g/kg
Combination glaucoma agent				
	Dorzolamide/timolol maleate	Cosopt	2%/0.5%	bid

all are available in generic form, have a lower cost than newer glaucoma medications. Except for dry eye symptoms, local side effects from, and allergies to, the β-adrenergic antagonists are uncommon.

Each of the β-adrenergic antagonists can have beneficial effects in patients with systemic hypertension, migraine, angina, and mild to moderate congestive heart failure, as well as after myocardial infarction. Nonselective agents should be avoided in patients with asthma, and even betaxolol should not be used in patients with moderate to severe asthma or chronic obstructive pulmonary disease. All the β-adrenergic antagonists should be avoided in patients with heart block, bradyarrhythmias, severe myocardial dysfunction, or pulmonary edema. Depression, fatigue, confusion, and impotence may occur, and athletes may notice decreased exercise tolerance from reduced physiologic exercise-induced tachycardia during β-adrenergic antagonist therapy.

Nonselective Adrenergic Agonists

Epinephrine and dipivefrin (Propine), an epinephrine prodrug, reduce intraocular pressure less effectively than the nonselective β-adrenergic antagonist timolol. Frequent local and occasional systemic side effects have limited the usefulness of these drugs. Pupillary dilation, blurred vision, chronic red eye, ocular allergy, and conjunctival adrenochrome deposits are common. Side effects of epinephrine include headache, nervousness, tremor, increased blood pressure, palpitations, and tachycardia; these occur much less frequently with dipivefrin. Eyelid contact dermatitis is common with dipivefrin.

Selective α_2-Adrenergic Agonists

Apraclonidine (Iopidine) or brimonidine (Alphagan), used twice daily, reduces intraocular pressure about as effectively as timolol. Systemic side effects are infrequent but can include headache, dry mouth, and fatigue. Both agents cause red eye, and both have a fairly high incidence (12% to 18%) of ocular allergy and contact dermatitis. Patients taking apraclonidine frequently exhibit tachyphylaxis, an effect that limits its long-term use.

Carbonic Anhydrase Inhibitors

Oral and topical carbonic anhydrase inhibitors reduce aqueous production. Full-dose oral agents are more effective than two topical formulations, brinzolamide (Azopt) and dorzolamide (Trusopt), but oral formulations have a high incidence of systemic side effects including anorexia, fatigue, lassitude, paresthesias, confusion, depression, and urolithiasis. Oral carbonic anhydrase inhibitors may cause a mild metabolic acidosis, which can be problematic in patients with acid-base abnormalities or renal insufficiency, and concurrent use with high-dose salicylate therapy may potentiate metabolic acidosis. Potassium-depleting effects of acetazolamide (Diamox) are usually minor, but they can be substantial in patients receiving concurrent non–potassium sparing diuretic therapy. Acetazolamide is metabolized in the kidney, and methazolamide (Neptazane) is metabolized in the liver. The latter should be avoided in patients with liver disease.

The topical formulations cause few if any systemic side effects, but allergies do occur. Topical brinzolamide, with a more physiologic pH than dorzolamide, tends to sting less on instillation. The lower effectiveness of the topical carbonic anhydrase inhibitors and the need to administer these drugs twice daily have relegated their use to second- or third-line glaucoma medical therapy.

Cholinergic (Miotic) Agents

Cholinergic agents are effective and inexpensive, rarely cause systemic side effects, and have been available for many decades. However, frequent local ocular side effects and the need to be used three or four times daily have greatly reduced their use. These drugs induce miosis (pupillary constriction), which may cause dim night vision and, in patients with cataract, decreased visual acuity, and they also contract the ciliary muscle, which may cause eye ache, brow ache, and increased myopia.

Prostaglandin Analogues

Four prostaglandin analogues have become available. Three of these agents, bimatoprost (Lumigan), latanoprost (Xalatan), and travoprost (Travatan), are all highly effective, about 2 mm Hg more effective than timolol, and each is used once daily. Once-daily use and high effectiveness have led many ophthalmologists to use prostaglandin analogues as first-line agents in many patients with glaucoma. Unoprostone (Rescula) is used twice daily and is less effective than the other prostaglandin analogues. There is about a 30% nonresponse rate to latanoprost. Other patients demonstrate remarkable intraocular pressure lowering with latanoprost. Despite initial recommendations, latanoprost does not need to be refrigerated, but it should be kept from prolonged exposure to heat and light. Bimatoprost and travoprost cause more red eye than latanoprost, but they may have a lower nonresponder rate. Systemic side effects from any of the prostaglandin analogues are uncommon. A flulike illness has been reported. Local ocular side effects include eyelash lengthening and permanent darkening of the iris, more likely in a green or hazel-colored iris, and cystoid macular edema (fluid in the macula causing decreased visual acuity).

Hyperosmotic Agents

The use of osmotic agents has been largely relegated to ocular emergencies. Intravenous mannitol provides a dramatic and almost immediate reduction of intraocular pressure by ocular osmotic fluid reduction in acute glaucoma, and it can be useful in the nauseated patient. Mannitol (Osmitrol) is sometimes used preoperatively or intraoperatively during glaucoma and other eye surgery. Oral glycerin (Osmoglyn) has a similar but slower onset of effect. All osmotics can cause dramatic systemic fluid shifting and can be dangerous in patients with fluid retention and heart failure.

Other side effects include severe headache, dizziness, dehydration, and subdural hematoma. Mannitol and isosorbide are excreted unmetabolized by the kidney, but glycerin is metabolized to glucose and can cause severe hyperglycemia in patients with diabetes.

Other Medications

Cosopt (timolol and dorzolamide) is a fixed-combination glaucoma medication, which may improve compliance over the two agents used separately. Topical corticosteroids may cause significant intraocular pressure elevation in patients with glaucoma or ocular hypertension. However, topical corticosteroids and cholinergic antagonists (cycloplegic agents: atropine,* homatropine,* scopolamine*) play an important role in the management of glaucoma whenever there is active intraocular inflammation from uveitis or after recent ocular trauma or intraocular surgery. Successful reduction and elimination of inflammation may contribute to better intraocular pressure control in these patients.

Laser Therapy

Laser Trabeculoplasty

Argon or diode laser trabeculoplasty is an outpatient procedure performed with topical anesthesia, and it is a quick, safe, and convenient method for intraocular pressure reduction in patients with primary open-angle, pigmentary, and pseudoexfoliation glaucoma. Laser trabeculoplasty lowers intraocular pressure about as much as one glaucoma medication, but it is less effective in young patients and in traumatic glaucoma, and it is contraindicated in patients with active intraocular inflammation, angle neovascularization, or significant permanent angle closure. The effect of laser trabeculoplasty tends to wear off over time; re-treatments are less effective, and some patients have little, if any, response to the initial procedure. Selective laser trabeculoplasty allegedly can successfully be repeated, but there is a lack of evidence for this claim at this time.

Laser Peripheral Iridotomy

Early laser peripheral iridotomy is indicated in the management of angle-closure glaucoma with pupillary block or relative pupillary block. If treatment is substantially delayed, permanent angle closure will ensue, and intraocular pressure could be controllable only with glaucoma surgery.

Laser Cyclophotocoagulation

One method to reduce intraocular pressure is to destroy the aqueous-producing ciliary body. This has been performed using freezing (cyclocryotherapy) and with a noncontact (Nd:YAG), contact (Nd:YAG, diode), or intraocular laser probe. Ciliary body destruction is quicker than traditional glaucoma surgery, but it can cause pain, macular edema, and complete failure of aqueous production, leading to total loss of vision and collapse of the globe (phthisis bulbi).

*Not FDA-approved for this indication.

Surgical Therapy

Trabeculectomy

Glaucoma filtering surgery creates a fistula to divert aqueous from the interior to the exterior of the eye. Early glaucoma procedures were performed to create a full-thickness fistula, which, although successful, frequently caused short- or long-term problems from intraocular pressure that was too low postoperatively. Trabeculectomy is the most common glaucoma surgical procedure performed today. In this procedure, a partially covered fistula is produced to filter aqueous humor to the subconjunctival space. The partially covered fistula limits aqueous flow to prevent hypotony (too low eye pressure) postoperatively. This reduces the incidence of postoperative complications, but it also increases the long-term failure rate of the operation. Trabeculectomy is highly successful in eyes that have had no previous history of ocular surgery or trauma. For eyes with a higher risk of treatment failure after trabeculectomy, antifibrosing agents (adjunctive mitomycin C* or 5-fluorouracil*) can increase the chance of successful filtration by reducing postoperative scarring, the most common reason for filtering surgery failure. Nonpenetrating glaucoma surgery has the advantage of a lower incidence of hypotony than trabeculectomy, but it is associated with higher long-term postoperative intraocular pressure, a disadvantage for some patients.

Glaucoma Implants

For some patients whose eyes are a higher surgical risk, a glaucoma implant is the best option. This could include eyes with failed mitomycin C trabeculectomy or those with too much conjunctival scarring to allow the performance of a trabeculectomy. Current glaucoma implants combine a tube, with or without a pressure-sensitive valve, connected to a plate, to allow restricted scarring and to create a space around the plate for aqueous fluid collection and dispersion.

*Not FDA-approved for this indication.

OTITIS EXTERNA

method of
PETER S. ROLAND, M.D.
University of Texas Southwestern Medical Center
Dallas, Texas

Otitis externa can be divided into acute and chronic forms. Acute external otitis (AOE) is almost always of infectious etiology. Chronic forms of external otitis often include an infectious process, but are frequently complicated by underlying dermatopathology.

The normal external auditory canal (EAC) is a skin-lined cul-de-sac separating the pinna from the tympanic membrane. The lateral, cartilaginous third of the EAC contains sebaceous glands and modified apocrine sweat glands. Products of these glands, when mixed with desquamated epithelial cells, form cerumen. Cerumen has an acidic pH, and its presence produces acidification of the EAC. The pH of the normal EAC is around 6.1. Cerumen also contains lysozyme, immunoglobulins, and polyunsaturated acids, which together with its low pH, suppress bacterial growth. The waxy properties of cerumen produce a waterproofing effect, which prevents maceration of the skin of the EAC.

The EAC is colonized by skin organisms, notably diphtheroids, α-hemolytic streptococci, micrococci, and nonpathogenic staphylococci. Gram-negative organisms, notably *Pseudomonas*, are *not* recovered from the normal external auditory canal. A variety of fungal organisms are also found as normal flora of the external auditory canal including Curvularia and Alternaria.

ACUTE OTITIS EXTERNA

Anything that alters the integrity of the integumental barrier promotes the development of acute diffuse otitis externa. High temperature, high humidity, and exposure to water are uniformly recognized as important predisposing conditions, consequently its popular name, "swimmer's ear." Preexisting chronic dermatologic conditions (such as seborrheic dermatitis) and microtrauma also contribute to the development of acute otitis externa.

An important protective barrier is the "acid mantle," which creates a hostile environment for many causative organisms. Most of the organisms that cause external otitis grow best at a pH of 7.2 to 7.6, significantly higher than the normal pH of the EAC. The most common causative organisms in almost all studies have been *Pseudomonas aeruginosa* and *Staphylococcus aureus*. Together, *P. aeruginosa* and *S. aureus* account for 40% to 80% of recovered organisms in most large clinical series, but the relative incidence of these two organisms varies substantially. The remainder of infections are caused by a large variety of other organisms, generally gram-negative, none of which constitute a significant portion of cases. *Proteus* and *Klebsiella* spp. are fairly common and are usually responsible for as many as 3% to 4% of reported infections. Fungal external otitis is uncommon as a primary infection. It is reported as a causative agent in less than 2% of cases of acute otitis external in almost all large series.

Although historical features suggest the diagnosis and may explain the etiology of the disorder, the diagnosis rests almost entirely on the physical examination. Almost all patients will have edema of the EAC. Edema can be sufficiently severe so as to swell the canal entirely shut. Most will have some erythema. The tympanic membrane (TM), if it can be visualized at all, will be relatively normal. Otorrhea is frequently present but tends to be thin and milky rather than tenacious and purulent. Tenderness is almost always present and usually severe. Manipulation of the auricle or tragus can be exquisitely painful.

Treatment of AOE consists of aural toilet, reacidification of the external auditory canal, and the application of appropriate ototopical antimicrobial agents. Aural toilet can be achieved in several ways. The least desirable and least effective is "dry mopping." A cotton swab is used to gently remove as much debris from the EAC as possible. More effective are gentle irrigations of the EAC, which are often able to remove the majority of pus and debris. If the TM is intact, a solution of half rubbing alcohol and half white vinegar is useful. Otic Domeboro solution or H_2O_2 can also be used. The most reliable way to ensure good aural toilet is careful suctioning of the ear canal using the office microscope.

A variety of ototopical medicines are commercially available for the treatment of external otitis. Ototopic agents, which do not contain antibiotics, generally rely on low pH for their bacteriostatic and bacteriocidal properties. Based on the microbiology of the disorder, an appropriate antibiotic needs to be effective against both gram-positive and gram-negative organisms. Consequently, most ototopic antibiotic drops contain either an aminoglycoside or a quinoline.

Ototopic medications are effective only if they can be delivered to infected tissues. Even with aggressive canal cleansing, edema may be sufficiently severe as to compromise the canal lumen to such an extent that medications cannot effectively enter it. In such cases, a wick must be placed in the EAC to stent it open and ensure delivery of medication. Preformed and expandable Oto-Wicks are available commercially.

It is important to remember that sensitivity results from clinical laboratories should not be used as treatment guides when topical therapy is being utilized. Determinations of "sensitivity" and "resistance" are made on the basis of antibiotic tissue levels that can reasonably be expected after *systemic* administration of the antibiotic in question. This information is not relevant when topicals are being used. A 0.3% solution of topical antibiotic contains 3000 μg/mL. This is almost 1000 times higher than the level that can be achieved with systemic administration. Even organisms that are labeled "highly resistant" by clinical laboratories will succumb readily to these very high concentrations of antibiotic.

Systemic antibiotics should be used in individuals who are diabetic or otherwise immunocompromised, if there is spreading cellulitis onto the skin of the face or head, if there are systemic signs and symptoms, or if there is marked adenopathy. Oral quinolones (ofloxacin [Floxin Otic] ciprofloxacin [Cipro HC Otic]) provide the most appropriate antimicrobial spectrum for external otitis. Pain can be severe and must be treated. Oral narcotic agents are often required.

Treatment failures can arise for several reasons:

1. Poor compliance. Either failure to use the prescribed medication or constant re-exposure to water during the treatment period can result in persistant infection.

2. Topical sensitization. Topical sensitivity can arise to the antibiotic components of an ototopical medication or to excipients used in the vehicle. Topical sensitization to neomycin is especially common. Topical sensitivity may not result in a florid maculopapular and vesicular rash, but rather may manifest simply as failure of the condition to improve.

3. Acute external otitis may not respond to conventional therapy if necrotizing otitis media or "malignant otitis externa" has developed (see the following section).

4. Failure of effective delivery of a topical antibiotic medication. Aggressive aural toilet or placement of a wick will solve the problem.

5. The causative organisms are fungal and not bacterial. This is improbable (less than 2% of cases) unless the patient has been treated aggressively with topical antimicrobial agents in the recent past.

6. Infection is caused by a resistant bacteria organism. This is highly unlikely given the very high concentrations of antibiotic therapy in topical preparations. It is much more likely that the antimicrobial agent is not being effectively delivered to the infected tissue.

OTOMYCOSIS (FUNGAL EXTERNAL OTITIS)

AEO is only very rarely the result of fungal organisms. However, fungal organisms are recovered more commonly as a secondary pathogen after the use of broad-spectrum topical antibiotic drops, and fungi may play some role as copathogens along with *Pseudomonas* spp. or *S. aureus*. When interpreting positive fungal cultures obtained from patients with external otitis, it is critical to remember that fungi are normal saprophytes within the EAC. Only *Aspergillus* and *Candida* have been recovered more frequently from infected than from noninfected ears.

If fungi are suspected as the primary pathogen or as a significant copathogen, the same principles of aural toilet and reacidification that are used to treat bacterial external otitis should be applied and are frequently effective in eliminating the infection. If these measures are not adequate, a large number of antifungal antibiotics have been used to treat fungal external otitis, although none are Food and Drug Administration approved for this use. Nystatin (Mycostatin),* clotrimazole (Lotrimin),* ketoconazole (Nizoral),* tolnaftate (Tinactin),* and amphotericin (Fungizone)* have all been used and shown to be nonototoxic.

NECROTIZING EXTERNAL OTITIS

In immunocompromised patients, external otitis can spread to involve the underlying temporal bone and skull base. Skull-base osteomyelitis is most commonly seen in elderly diabetics and Pseudomonas is almost always the causative organism. When the disease occurs in nondiabetic, immunocompromised individuals, organisms other than *Pseudomonas* are sometimes encountered and fungal organisms constitute a meaningful subset of these cases.

Pseudomonas osteomyelitis of the temporal bone is often referred to as either "necrotizing" or "malignant" external otitis. There are a variety of reasons that diabetic patients appear to be prone to the disorder. The cerumen of diabetics is not as acidic as is that of normal individuals. It tends to have a pH of 7.4 rather than the usual pH of 6.1. As noted earlier, a pH of 7.4 is conducive to maximal growth of most of the causative organisms of external otitis. Moreover, it is well recognized that hyperglycemia produces impaired polymorphonuclear leukocyte function with impaired chemotaxis and phagocytosis. The microangiopathy associated with diabetes may also impair the delivery of inflammatory mediators and antimicrobials into the infected area. Decreased blood flow impairs healing and the immune response.

The diagnosis is clinical. Diabetics, especially elderly diabetics, who develop external otitis that fails to respond to the usual treatment measures should be considered to have early necrotizing external otitis. Unremitting pain is the common clinical feature. The erythrocyte sedimentation rate (ESR) is usually very high (80 mm/hour or greater). An elevated ESR supports the diagnosis and can be followed serially to document the effectiveness of treatment. The diagnosis should be confirmed using technetium-99m bone scans. When first described, the disease had a high mortality rate, but is now effectively treated with anti-*Pseudomonas* antibiotics. In the 1970s and 1980s, standard treatment for this disease consisted of a 6-week course of double-coverage therapy (usually an aminoglycoside and a semisynthetic penicillin). Double coverage was regarded as imperative to prevent the emergence of resistant strains. Over the last several years, it has been shown that the disease can be treated successfully with oral fluoroquinolones alone in 80% to 90% of cases. Outpatient fluoroquinolone therapy should generally be continued for 6 weeks. It should certainly continue until the patient has been pain free, the ESR has fallen to a near normal level, and there has been decrease activity in gallium-67 bone scanning. Ten to twenty percent of pHs will fail outpatient oral fluoroquinolone therapy and require long-term intravenous antibiotic therapy based on culture and sensitivity reports.

*Not FDA approved for this indication.

OTITIS MEDIA

method of
JAY A. WERKHAVEN, M.D.
Vanderbilt University
Nashville, Tennessee

The term *otitis media* is the name given to a spectrum of inflammatory diseases of the middle ear. This spectrum extends from acute otitis media (AOM) to otitis media with effusion (OME). AOM is defined as the rapid onset of signs and symptoms of acute infection within the middle ear. In OME, the signs and symptoms of AOM are absent, and the middle ear contains a collection of fluid that may vary in viscidity from serous to mucous.

SIGNIFICANCE

Otitis media is one of the most common infectious disorders of childhood. In the early part of the 20th century, otitis was the admitting diagnosis for almost 25% of pediatric admissions to the hospital. It is now second only to well child checkups in the number of office visits to the physician, an estimated 24.5 million visits in 1990. Otitis media generated the delivery of 18.7 million prescriptions for antibiotics in 1986. The average cost for treating otitis media has been estimated to be between $116 and $131 per episode. The direct and indirect (e.g., lost time from work, cost of babysitter) costs were estimated to have a $5 billion impact in 1996.

DIAGNOSIS

The diagnosis of otitis media is made by appropriate history and directed physical examination. Because many cases occur in younger children, direct history is unavailable. Otalgia is common, but the condition may also manifest as irritability or malaise, sleep disturbance, decreased appetite, or pulling or rubbing at the ear. Fever is not always present. Parents and older children may note a hearing loss. Older children may complain of a fullness or tinnitus in the ear. Associated signs and symptoms of upper respiratory tract infection may frequently be observed.

Examination of the patient begins with proper positioning. The infant may be laid on an examination table, whereas older children may sit on the parent's lap facing outward. Pulling upward and outward gently on the pinna straightens the external canal to allow direct visualization of the tympanic membrane. The external canal may need to be cleansed of obstructing cerumen, and I prefer a right-angle mastoid probe to accomplish this task. The probe is placed beyond the cerumen, rotated 90 degrees to engage the mass, and removed without contact with the external canal wall. The medial wall of the external canal is periosteum, and it is exquisitely sensitive to pressure. An ear loop or curet works to remove cerumen by compressing it against the canal wall and dragging it out of the canal, and thus this procedure may be very painful. The right-angle probe is also more effective in the removal of ear canal foreign bodies using a similar maneuver. Soft cerumen may be irrigated from the ear canal if the integrity of the tympanic membrane is known to be intact. Hydrogen peroxide* (3%) may be used to soften hard cerumen. A pneumatic otoscope employing the largest speculum that will comfortably fit the external canal is required. The examiner should brace the hand holding the otoscope against the patient's head, so that any motion of the patient does not cause the speculum to be driven into the sensitive periosteum of the external canal. A bright light is vital. The color of the tympanic membrane alone is not a reliable sign of otitis media, but frequently erythema is present in AOM. Assessment of the tympanic membrane for translucency may allow the observer to note the quality of the middle ear effusion. The status of the tympanic membrane light reflex is insignificant. Pneumatoscopy is vital in the diagnosis of otitis. Pneumotoscopy allows evaluation of the position of the tympanic membrane and its mobility. The tympanic membrane is frequently full in AOM and retracted in OME. Mobility is reduced in both conditions. In the infant, hypermobility of the external canal may confuse assessment of the tympanic membrane status.

EPIDEMIOLOGY AND RISK FACTORS

The average child has about three office visits per year for otitis-related illness in the first 2 years of life. An immature immune system and incompletely functioning eustachian tube are considered the most common factors associated with otitis in children. As circulating antibodies approach 85% of adult levels near 4 years of age, and eustachian tube function improves with increasing skull and midface growth around 6 years of age, most children outgrow otitis.

Some children, however, appear prone to increased episodes of otitis. Risk factors identified in these children include younger age, male sex, race (Native American and Inuit), lower socioeconomic status, daycare attendance, pacifier use, prone sleep position, winter season, passive smoke exposure, and lack of breast-feeding. In addition, various genetic and anatomic abnormalities such as Down's syndrome or cleft palate may also predispose a child to otitis.

PATHOGENESIS

Most episodes of otitis are bacterial in origin, although various viruses may be an inciting trigger or coexistent. The most common bacteria causing otitis are *Streptococcus pneumoniae*, *Haemophilus influenzae*, *Moraxella catarrhalis*, *Streptococcus* group A, and *Staphylococcus aureus*. Coexistent viruses include respiratory syncytial virus, rhinovirus, influenza virus, and adenovirus. Children with OME, although not appearing acutely ill, may still have identifiable bacteria in the middle ear effusion up to 42% of the time, in a pattern similar to that of AOM.

TREATMENT

Initial treatment of otitis media is directed at controlling both the symptoms and the pathogenesis. Fever, pain, and malaise are relieved with the use of acetaminophen (10 to 15 mg/kg every 4 hours), ibuprofen (Motrin) (10 mg/kg every 6 to 8 hours), or acetaminophen with codeine (1.0 mg/kg of the codeine component every 4 hours) in the case of severe otalgia.

*Not FDA-approved for this indication.

Topical warmth may be beneficial. The use of warmed oil instilled into the ear is discouraged because the presence or development of a tympanic membrane perforation would allow this oil to enter the middle ear and may provoke a granulomatous response. Topical anesthetic drops such as benzocaine only have effect on the tympanic membrane component of the otalgia and do not aid in relief of the pain from middle ear mucosal inflammation or pressure. Although decongestants and antihistamines may not have direct effects on the otitis, they may aid in symptomatic relief of the associated upper respiratory tract infection.

The antibiotic used in the initial treatment of AOM must be effective against the three major bacteria responsible for AOM. Amoxicillin (Amoxil) remains the first drug of choice. This drug is generally effective, safe, and inexpensive. Although 40% of *H. influenzae* organisms and more than 90% of *M. catarrhalis* organisms are resistant to amoxicillin, these bacterial infections have a high degree of spontaneous clearance. High-risk patients should be treated at a dose of 70 to 90 mg/kg/day, whereas low-risk patients may still be treated at a dose of 40 to 50 mg/kg/day. For those patients allergic to amoxacillin, an expanded macrolide such as azithromycin (Zithromax)* (10 mg/kg single dose on day 1, 5 mg/kg single dose on days 2 to 5) may be effective.

AOM not responding to initial therapy may result from drug-resistant *S. pneumoniae*. This bacterium is demonstrating resistance to high-level amoxicillin, and it may also be resistant to the macrolides and rarely to clindamycin (Cleocin).* There is wide geographic variability in resistance patterns, with a range of 15% to 45% of *S. pneumoniae* organisms showing resistance to amoxacillin at a dose of 50 mg/kg/day. Second-line antibiotic therapy includes the following:

1. Amoxacillin/clavulanate (Augmentin): 600 mg amoxacillin/5 mL concentration, dose calculated based on the amoxacillin component.
2. Cefuroxime axetil (Ceftin): 30 mg/kg/day given twice daily.
3. Clindamycin: 10 to 20 mg/kg/day given two or three times daily.
4. Cefdinir (Omnicef)*: 14 mg/kg/day given twice daily.
5. Intramuscular ceftriaxone (Rocephin): 50 mg/kg/day with a maximum volume of 1 mL per site.

Patients should demonstrate clinical improvement within 48 to 72 hours. If symptoms persist or worsen, reevaluation is necessary. Selection of a second-line antibiotic may be indicated. In severe cases, tympanocentesis may be needed. Indications for tympanocentesis include young age (children younger than 3 months have an increased risk of gram-negative otitis), immunodeficient status, impending complications (facial nerve paralysis or mastoiditis), unresponsive prolonged AOM, or the need for relief of pain. An otitis-prone child should be seen after the completion of therapy, and asymptomatic children should be seen at 10 to 12 weeks, to ensure clearance of effusion.

Prophylactic antibiotic use is generally discouraged because it may promote the further development of resistant bacteria, but it may be beneficial in the high-risk, medically complex patient. Amoxicillin at half the daily treatment dose is the preferred regimen. The administration of steroids in the treatment of AOM and OME is controversial and is incompletely supported in the literature. The consensus report from the National Institutes of Health does not support steroid use in OME.

*Not FDA approved for this indication.

Associated Management

Tympanic Membrane Perforation

Tympanic membrane perforation may occur in AOM. Topical antibiotic fluoroquinolone drops may then be used. The perforation most often spontaneously heals within 72 to 96 hours, so the window of efficacy for topical antibiotics is short.

Vaccines

The widespread use of *Haemophilus* vaccine has seen a decrease in otitis resulting from *H. influenzae* A and B, but nontypable *H influenzae* is still a significant cause of AOM. The large number of serotypes of *S. pneumoniae* (more than 90) has complicated development of an appropriate vaccine, but the heptavalent *S. pneumoniae* vaccine has been shown to be effective in reducing otitis caused by this organism in clinical trials.

Bilateral Myringotomy and Tube Insertion

Bilateral myringotomy and tube insertion may be beneficial in patients with recurrent AOM or persistent OME. Patients with AOM that occurs more frequently than three to four episodes in 6 months, especially with associated risk factors, achieve significant clinical improvement after tube placement. The average child in whom tubes are placed for recurrent AOM experiences 1.1 episodes of otitis per year while the tubes are functioning. The most prevalent styles of tubes remain in place for 1 year on average before spontaneous extrusion. Otitis occurring while tubes are functioning presents with otorrhea, and it may be treated with fluoroquinolone drops topically. Oral antibiotics are generally not used for isolated otitis after tube insertion, and topical antibiotics alone achieve a 95% cure rate.

OME after AOM has a spontaneous effusion clearance rate that may leave fewer than 10% of these children with effusion after 12 to 16 weeks. The effusion interferes with a child's hearing, both pure tone sensation and subtle language cues. Prolonged OME of greater than 16 weeks' duration may be associated with decrease speech and language acquisition and decreased cognitive skills. Some effusions cause otalgia because of the negative middle ear pressure; thus some children are symptomatic for several months. Referral to an otolaryngologist is indicated after bilateral OME has been observed for more than 12 to 16 weeks. Unilateral effusion may be observed for up to 6 months if it is asymptomatic. Publicity about office-based laser myringotomy for otitis has not been supported by published data. Adenoidectomy alone for the treatment of AOM or OME is also not supported.

EPISODIC VERTIGO

method of
JOSEPH M. FURMAN, M.D., PH.D.
University of Pittsburgh School of Medicine
Pittsburgh, Pennsylvania

Treatment of episodic vertigo and dizziness depends on the diagnosis. In many patients with episodic vertigo, a specific diagnosis can be reached; however, in others, although no specific diagnosis can be reached, a vestibulopathy that is a disorder of the peripheral vestibular system may be considered highly likely based on a thorough evaluation of the patient. Reaching an accurate diagnosis, if possible, is essential. A history, physical examination, and when appropriate, laboratory testing are the principal diagnostic tools. Obtaining the history of a patient with episodic vertigo is essential. By definition, vertigo is an illusory sensation of motion of self or surroundings and is much more likely to be the result of a vestibular system disorder and nonspecific dizziness. However, it may be very difficult for some patients to describe their abnormal sensations, in which case they may simply use the terms dizziness, lightheadedness, giddiness, or dysequilibrium. Physical examination of a patient with episodic vertigo should include a neurologic and otologic examination and, in addition, a neurotologic examination consisting of several specialized bedside evaluation methods. Laboratory testing of a patient with episodic vertigo may include vestibular laboratory testing, audiometry, and brain imaging.

TABLE 1. **Causes of Episodic Vertigo and Dizziness**

Diagnosis	Localization
Common	
Benign paroxysmal positional vertigo	Peripheral vestibular
Meniere's disease	Peripheral vestibular
Migraine-associated dizziness	Mixed
Anxiety-related dizziness	Mixed
Impaired vestibular compensation	Mixed
Nonspecific vestibulopathy	Unknown
Unusual	
Bilateral vestibular loss	Peripheral vestibular
Acoustic neuroma	Mixed
Vertebro-basilar insufficiency	Central vestibular
Recurrent vestibulopathy	Unknown
Multiple sclerosis	Central vestibular
Mal de debarquement syndrome	Central vestibular
Autoimmune inner ear disease	Peripheral vestibular
Horizontal semicircular canal benign paroxysmal positional vertigo	Peripheral vestibular
Epileptic vertigo	Central vestibular
Controversial Disorders	
Superior semicircular canal dehiscence syndrome	Peripheral vestibular
Cervicogenic dizziness	Other
Vascular cross-compression syndrome of the eighth cranial nerve	Peripheral vestibular

Some causes of episodic vertigo are relatively common, whereas others are unusual, and a few vestibular disorders that cause episodic vertigo are controversial. Some patients may suffer from more than one disorder simultaneously. Table 1 groups disorders that cause episodic vertigo as common, uncommon, and controversial and provides areas of localization for each disorder.

BENIGN PAROXYSMAL POSITIONAL VERTIGO

Now a well-defined disorder characterized by episodic vertigo induced by rolling in bed and looking up, benign paroxysmal positional vertigo is caused by free-floating debris in the posterior semicircular canal. The preferred treatment is a particle-repositioning maneuver (Figure 1). It is highly successful and provides complete relief in nearly all patients. Vestibular suppressant medications can be used early in the disorder, but after several days they should be used sparingly if at all. Approximately 15% of individuals with one episode of benign paroxysmal positional vertigo will have a recurrence within 1 year. Rarely, surgical procedures are required for patients refractory to nonsurgical treatment.

MÉNIÈRE'S DISEASE

Typical findings in patients with Ménière's disease include fluctuating aural fullness, tinnitus, hearing loss, and recurrent bouts of vertigo. Endolymphatic hydrops (swelling of the endolymphatic space) is the underlying pathophysiologic process of Ménière's disease. Medical treatment of endolymphatic hydrops includes administration of a diuretic and dietary sodium restriction. A combination of hydrochlorothiazide and triamterene (Dyazide)* is the diuretic of choice. Dietary sodium should be held below 2 g/d. About 20% of individuals with Ménière's disease will eventually fail medical therapy. Surgical treatment of Ménière's disease, discussed elsewhere in this volume, includes chemical labyrinthectomy, endolymphatic sac surgery, labyrinthectomy, and vestibular nerve section.

MIGRAINE-ASSOCIATED DIZZINESS

Migraine-associated dizziness is a diagnosis of exclusion and should be suspected in patients with nonspecific dizziness or vertigo associated with headache. A past history of migraine headaches or a positive family history of migraine increases the likelihood of this disorder. Patients with migraine-associated dizziness almost invariably report that their symptoms are exacerbated by viewing certain moving visual environments or that they are very sensitive to motion sickness. Treatment options for patients with

*Not FDA-approved for this indication.

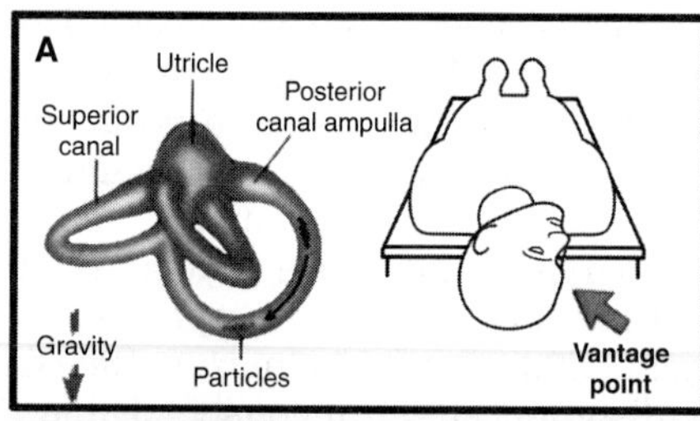

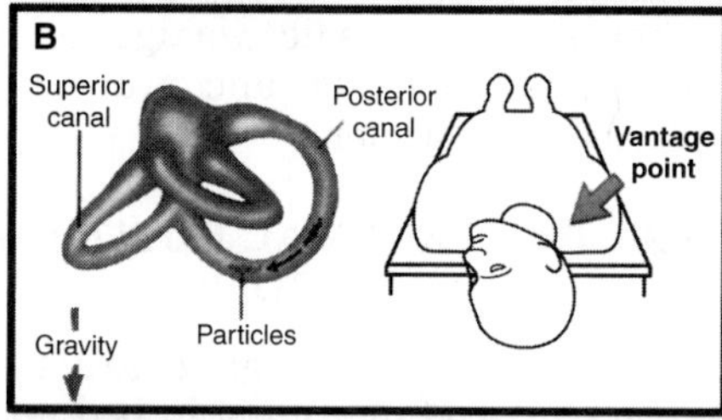

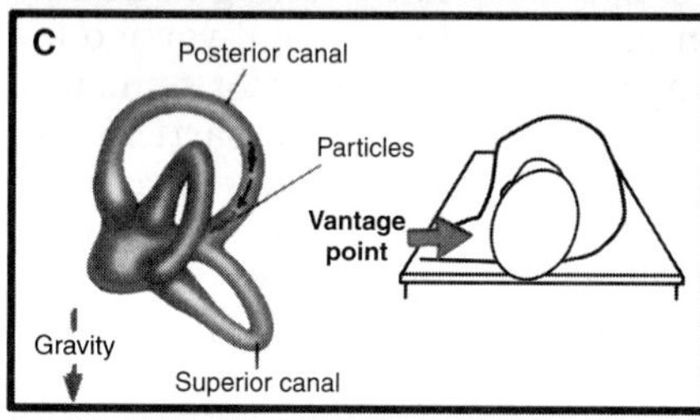

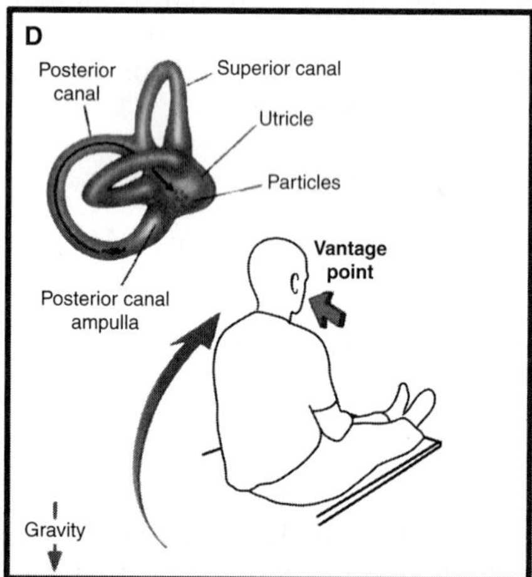

Figure 1. Bedside maneuver for the treatment of a patient with benign paroxysmal positional vertigo affecting the right ear. The presumed position of the debris within the labyrinth during the maneuver is shown in each panel. The maneuver is a three-step procedure. First, a Dix-Hallpike test is performed with the patient's head rotated 45 degrees toward the right ear and the neck slightly extended with the chin pointed slightly upward. This position results in the patient's head hanging to the right *(A)*. Once the vertigo and nystagmus provoked by the Dix-Hallpike test cease, the patient's head is rotated about the rostral-caudal body axis until the left ear is down *(B)*. Then the head and body are further rotated until the head is face-down *(C)*. The vertex of the head is kept titled downward throughout the rotation. The maneuver usually provokes brief vertigo. The patient should be kept in the final, face-down position for about 10 to 15 seconds. With the head kept turned toward the left shoulder, the patient is brought into the seated position *(D)*. Once the patient is upright, the head is titled so that the chin is pointed slightly downward. (Adapted from Furman JM, Cass SP: Benign paroxysmal positional vertigo. N Engl J Med 1999; 341(21):1590–1596.)

TABLE 2. **Treatment Options for Migraine-Related Vestibulopathy**

Avoid dietary triggers
Treat the underlying migraine phenomenon
Tricyclic antidepressants (e.g., imipramine (Tofranil),* 10–100 mg/d)
β-Blockers (e.g., propranolol (Inderal), 80–320 mg/d)
Calcium channel blockers (e.g., verapamil (Calan), 80–120 mg/d)
Treat movement-associated disequilibrium
Vestibular rehabilitation therapy
Treat space and motion discomfort
Clonazepam (Klonopin),* (0.25–0.5 mg bid)
Treat associated anxiety or panic disorder
Behavioral therapy
Pharmacotherapy
Tricyclic antidepressants

*Not FDA-approved for this indication.

migraine-associated dizziness are summarized in Table 2. First, the patient should be informed about the association between dizziness and an underlying migrainous condition and the importance of avoiding dietary triggers such as tyramine-containing food, alcohol, and caffeine. Second, the underlying migrainous condition should be treated with prophylactic antimigrainous medications even if headaches are not currently prominent. Third, if the most prominent vestibular symptom is movement-associated disequilibrium or unsteadiness, vestibular rehabilitation therapy is recommended. Fourth, if the patient reports severe space and motion discomfort, low-dose clonazepam (Klonopin),* 0.25 mg twice daily, should be prescribed. Finally, for patients with panic attacks or agoraphobia, psychiatric consultation should be obtained, and both behavioral therapy and specific medical therapy with antidepressant medications should be considered.

ANXIETY-RELATED DIZZINESS

Anxiety often accompanies dizziness. The cause-and-effect relationship between anxiety and dizziness is uncertain but may be related to a somatopsychic, a psychosomatic, or a common neurologic mechanism. The term "psychogenic dizziness" should be avoided in favor of the term "psychiatric dizziness." Psychiatric dizziness should be used to describe patients in whom dizziness occurs exclusively in combination with other symptoms as part of a recognized psychiatric symptom cluster. Hyperventilation is a maneuver that is commonly used to determine whether the dizziness is "psychogenic," but the test is actually quite nonspecific, and the results of such testing should be interpreted with great caution. Treatment of patients with a combined anxiety and vestibular disorder should include measures aimed at both conditions simultaneously. The vestibular disorder should be treated in whatever manner is appropriate. Treatment of anxiety disorders includes pharmacotherapy and behavioral therapy. Psychiatric referral is warranted for patients suffering from frequent panic attacks or from panic disorder with agoraphobia.

*Not FDA-approved for this indication.

IMPAIRED VESTIBULAR COMPENSATION

Vertigo, nausea, vomiting, blurred vision, and disequilibrium characterize an acute unilateral vestibular syndrome. Vestibular compensation rebalances the neural activity in central vestibular structures. This process causes a reduction in the symptoms and signs of acute vestibular syndrome. Through compensation, the vestibulo-ocular, vestibulospinal, perceptual, and autonomic symptoms and signs of acute vestibular syndrome largely resolve. Vestibular compensation occurs automatically in individuals with a normal central nervous system, normal vision, normal proprioception, and adequate physical activity. The process of vestibular compensation is thought to involve brainstem and cerebellar structures. Persistent dizziness that continues after an acute peripheral vestibular ailment may be the result of impaired vestibular compensation. Typical symptoms of impaired compensation include instability during standing and walking and blurred vision associated with quick head movements. Patients with impaired vestibular compensation often avoid vestibular stimulation by severely limiting head movement. Gait is often slow with a short stride length, and the head is held rigid during walking. Although limiting head movement reduces vestibular stimulation and thus sensations of dizziness, this strategy is maladaptive because vestibular stimulation is necessary to stimulate the process of vestibular compensation. Failure to compensate for a peripheral vestibular lesion can be the result of one or more factors, including fluctuating or aberrant peripheral vestibular activity; central nervous system abnormality; clinical or subclinical involvement of the contralateral ear; the presence of other sensory deficits, especially those involving vision and somatosensation; and a sedentary lifestyle. Central nervous system abnormalities that impair vestibular compensation include both structural abnormalities and dysfunction caused by certain drugs such as benzodiazepines. Treatment of patients with impaired vestibular compensation includes tapering vestibular suppressant medications and a course of rehabilitation therapy.

NONSPECIFIC VESTIBULOPATHY

Vestibulopathy of unknown origin and *nonspecific vestibulopathy* are terms used to describe a complex of nonspecific symptoms that are suggestive of some impairment in the balance system but do not fit any recognized vestibular syndrome. Nonspecific vestibulopathy is a diagnosis of exclusion. Conditions that should be considered and ruled out include Ménière's disease (endolymphatic hydrops), benign paroxysmal positional vertigo, migraine-related dizziness, anxiety and panic disorders, and potential central nervous system abnormalities such as multiple sclerosis, Chiari's malformation, and neoplasm. Follow-up care is important because a specific diagnosis may become evident

TABLE 3. **Medications Commonly Used to Reduce Dizziness, Vertigo, and Associated Nausea**

Generic Name	Trade Name	Class	Dosage	Primary Symptom Being Treated	Side Effects
Cyclizine	Marezine	Piperazine (H_1-blocking agent)	50 mg orally every 4 to 6 h	Dizziness	Drowsiness
Diazepam*	Valium	Benzodiazepine	1–10 mg orally, IM, or IV every 12 h	Dizziness	Lethargy
Dimenhydrinate	Dramamine	Ethanolamine (H_1-blocking agent)	50 mg orally, every 4 to 6 h	Dizziness	Drowsiness
Diphenhydramine	Benadryl	Ethanolamine (H_1-blocking agent)	25–50 mg orally, IM,* or IV* every 6 h	Nausea	Drowsiness
Droperidol*	Inapsine	Butyrophenone	2.5 or 5 mg IM	Nausea	Extrapyramidal reaction, drowsiness, respiratory depression
Hydroxyzine	Vistaril, Atarax	Piperazine derivative	25–100 mg orally every 8 h	Nausea	Drowsiness
Meclizine	Antivert, Bonine	Piperazine (H_1-blocking agent)	25 mg orally every 4 to 6 h	Dizziness	Drowsiness
Prochlorperazine	Compazine	Phenothiazine	10 mg orally or IM every 6 h or 25 mg rectally every 12 h	Nausea	Extrapyramidal reactions, drowsiness, anticholinergic effects
Promethazine	Phenergan	Phenothiazine	25 mg orally or rectally every 6 h	Nausea	Extrapyramidal reaction, drowsiness
			60 mg orally every 6 h (pseudoephedrine)		Restlessness
Scopolamine	Transderm Scōp	Amine antimuscarinic	1.5-mg adhesive skin patches every 3 d	Dizziness	Dry mouth, blurred vision, drowsiness, disorientation
Trimethobenzamide	Tigan	Substituted ethanolamine	250 mg orally every 6 to 8 h or 200 mg rectally or IM	Nausea	Extrapyramidal reaction (unusual)

*Not FDA-approved for this indication.

over time. Treatment options for nonspecific vestibulopathy include medications and a course of vestibular rehabilitation therapy. The choice of treatment depends on the physician's judgment regarding the importance and predominance of the symptoms of nausea, dizziness, anxiety, depression, or functional impairment in balance. Medications commonly used to decrease dizziness, vertigo, and nausea are listed in Table 3.

BILATERAL VESTIBULAR LOSS

Bilateral vestibular loss most commonly occurs as a result of aminoglycoside-induced ototoxicity, but other pharmaceutical agents such as cisplatin can also cause bilateral vestibular loss. In addition, the condition may be caused by bilateral Ménière's disease, autoimmune inner ear disease, otosyphilis, or bilateral acoustic neuromas, or it may be idiopathic. The combination of oscillopsia and ataxia (Dandy's syndrome) is pathognomonic for bilateral vestibular loss. Prevention is the best management for ototoxicity. Treatment of bilateral vestibular loss should include discontinuation of all vestibular suppressant medications and referral for a course of balance rehabilitation therapy. Patients should be taught how to use sensory input other than that from the vestibular system, such as from vision and proprioception. A properly fitted cane can provide increased proprioceptive input. The patient should also be cautioned to remove all loose rugs from the home, use night lights, and install handrails on stairways and in the bathroom. If at all possible, the patient should not receive further ototoxic medications.

ACOUSTIC NEUROMA

A lesion in the cerebellopontine angle should be suspected in the setting of dizziness associated with unilateral or asymmetric hearing loss or tinnitus. Diagnostic considerations should include a large acoustic neuroma or meningioma involving the posterior fossa. Large cerebellopontine angle tumors may produce a combination of peripheral and central vestibular abnormalities. Both vestibular nerve and cerebellar function may be impaired. The most common treatment of patients with acoustic neuroma is microsurgical excision of the tumor. Other treatment options include observation, planned subtotal removal, and stereotactic radiation. Selection of the appropriate treatment option depends on many factors and should be individualized. Patients should be counseled regarding the possible occurrence of vestibular symptoms after stereotactic radiation. Dizziness after stereotactic radiation may be related to reduced or aberrant vestibular nerve activity.

VERTEBROBASILAR INSUFFICIENCY

The blood supply of the vestibular system is derived from the basilar artery. The internal auditory artery arises from the anterior inferior cerebellar artery and gives rise to the anterior vestibular artery, which supplies the vestibular apparatus. Thus, ischemia in the vertebrobasilar artery system can cause vestibular symptoms on the basis of either peripheral vestibular dysfunction, central vestibular dysfunction, or both.

The diagnosis of vertebrobasilar insufficiency should be reserved for patients who have clearly defined episodes of transient neurologic symptoms and signs that can be localized to the posterior circulation. Isolated vertigo, especially if chronic, is rarely a symptom of vertebrobasilar insufficiency. Management of vertebrobasilar insufficiency includes a thorough cerebrovascular assessment and, often, administration of an antiplatelet agent.

RECURRENT VESTIBULOPATHY

Recurrent vestibulopathy is a clinical syndrome that consists of multiple episodes of vertigo lasting minutes to hours without auditory or neurologic signs or symptoms. Recurrent vestibulopathy is a diagnosis of exclusion. Several other disorders that can cause recurrent vertigo such as Ménière's disease (endolymphatic hydrops), recurrent vestibular neuritis, benign paroxysmal positional vertigo, perilymphatic fistula, migraine-related vestibulopathy, vertebrobasilar insufficiency, panic disorder, and seizure disorder should be excluded before diagnosing recurrent vestibulopathy. Recurrent vestibulopathy may be a provisional diagnosis. In approximately 30% of patients in whom recurrent vestibulopathy is diagnosed, a condition develops that warrants a more specific diagnosis, most commonly endolymphatic hydrops, benign paroxysmal positional vertigo, or migraine-related vestibulopathy. The cause of recurrent vestibulopathy is not known, and treatment is nonspecific. Antinauseant and antiemetic agents (see Table 3) should be prescribed for patients to have on hand in the event of an episode of acute vertigo.

MULTIPLE SCLEROSIS

Vertigo and imbalance in patients with multiple sclerosis may indicate a lesion in the central vestibular structures. A peripheral vestibular abnormality independent of multiple sclerosis should also be considered. Both peripheral and central vestibular symptoms and signs can be seen in patients with multiple sclerosis if they have a lesion that includes the root entry zone in addition to other brainstem structures. Prolonged recovery can be seen in those with root entry zone lesions caused by multiple sclerosis. Treatment of multiple sclerosis is discussed elsewhere in this volume.

MAL DE DEBARQUEMENT SYNDROME

Mal de debarquement syndrome is an unusual disorder defined as a sensation of motion experienced on return to stable land after sea or air travel. Normally, such sensations of motion last for hours to days. The pathophysiology of mal de debarquement syndrome is probably related to the capability of the vestibular system to adapt to various motion environments that include combinations of vestibular and visual stimuli. Treatment of mal de debarquement syndrome includes vestibular suppressants, anxiolytics, antidepressants, and acetazolamide (Diamox).* Most cases resolve spontaneously within weeks to months.

AUTOIMMUNE INNER EAR DISEASE

Autoimmune inner ear disease is a disorder characterized by auditory and vestibular dysfunction and is most often bilateral; it is thought to be produced by damage mediated by both cellular and humoral immune mechanisms. Autoimmune inner ear disease is usually bilateral but may begin unilaterally and rapidly progress to involve both sides. A diagnosis of autoimmune inner ear disease is difficult to confirm. A positive rheumatologic battery or elevated sedimentation rate may be suggestive. Autoimmune inner ear disease is often a diagnosis of exclusion and frequently depends on clinical criteria and response to a trial of corticosteroid therapy. Treatment usually includes corticosteroids, such as prednisolone, 1 mg/kg/d for 1 to 2 weeks, followed by a tapering dose and maintenance dose if a positive response has occurred. Cytotoxic agents such as azathioprine (Imuran)* and cyclophosphamide (Cytoxan)* have also been advocated as an adjunct if the disease stops responding to steroid therapy. Plasmapheresis may be effective.

HORIZONTAL SEMICIRCULAR BENIGN CANAL PAROXYSMAL POSITIONAL VERTIGO

Horizontal semicircular canal benign paroxysmal positional vertigo is a variant of typical benign paroxysmal positional vertigo. This entity is thought to result from debris in the endolymph of the horizontal semicircular canal rather than in the posterior semicircular canal as occurs in typical benign paroxysmal positional vertigo. The diagnosis of horizontal semicircular canal benign paroxysmal positional vertigo can be made by turning a patient's head to the right and to the left while the patient is supine. The patient will become vertiginous for 10 to 30 seconds, and a paroxysmal horizontal nystagmus will be observed for as long as the vertigo persists. Treatment of the condition consists of a special particle-repositioning maneuver. The patient is rolled 360 degrees from the supine position toward the unaffected ear, then to the prone position, then to the side-down position with the affected ear down, and then back to the supine position.

EPILEPTIC VERTIGO

Vestibular epilepsy, also known as tornado epilepsy, refers to a disorder in which vertigo occurs during seizures, presumably as a result of activation of cortical areas associated with the perception of motion. A diagnosis of vestibular epilepsy should be considered in any patient with a history of a seizure disorder who has vertigo of uncertain etiology. Careful inquiry regarding changes in level of consciousness during or after vertiginous episodes is essential. Prolonged video-electroencephalographic monitoring may be required to capture an ictal episode. Nystagmus may or may not be associated with vestibular epilepsy. Treatment of epilepsy is discussed elsewhere in this volume.

SUPERIOR SEMICIRCULAR CANAL DEHISCENCE SYNDROME

Superior semicircular canal dehiscence syndrome is a recently described disorder characterized by episodic vertigo induced by loud noises or pressure changes in the external auditory canal. This syndrome can be diagnosed by identifying a thinning (dehiscence) of the superior semicircular canal with careful imaging. Once the syndrome is identified, referral to a neurotologic surgeon familiar with the disorder is appropriate.

CERVICOGENIC DIZZINESS

Cervical vertigo is a poorly defined condition that refers to dizziness and disequilibrium thought to be caused by abnormal afferent activity from the neck. Cervical vertigo is a diagnosis of exclusion. Close temporal association of the symptoms of dizziness and neck pain after a neck injury should suggest a diagnosis of cervical vertigo. Cervical vertigo can be seen in association with flexion-extension (whiplash) injuries, severe cervical arthritis, herniated cervical disks, and head trauma, especially blunt trauma to the top of the head. Neck muscle spasm and pain are often associated with symptoms of dizziness. Some patients with cervical vertigo experience a "vicious cycle" of excessive neck muscle activity exacerbating their dizziness, which subsequently exacerbates their neck discomfort. Treatment of cervical vertigo includes muscle relaxants and physical therapy to improve range of motion of the neck and reduce neck muscle spasm and discomfort. Use of a cervical collar should be limited to no more than 1 to 2 hours per day.

VASCULAR CROSS-COMPRESSION SYNDROME OF THE EIGHTH CRANIAL NERVE

Vascular cross-compression syndrome of the eighth cranial nerve, which has been called disabling positional vertigo and vestibular paroxysmia, refers to a cochleovestibular syndrome caused by compression of the eighth cranial nerve by blood vessels within the cerebellopontine angle. The clinical description of vascular compression syndrome of the eighth cranial nerve is controversial, with no agreed-on set of diagnostic criteria. Treatment of vascular cross-compression syndrome of the eighth cranial nerve includes pharmacotherapy with carbamazepine (Tegretol),* baclofen (Lioresal),* or gabapentin (Neurontin).* Surgical treatment consists of microvascular decompression. A trial of

*Not FDA-approved for this indication.

*Not FDA-approved for this indication.

medical therapy is appropriate before referring a patient for a surgical opinion.

MÉNIÈRE'S DISEASE

method of
MICHAEL E. HOFFER, M.D., CDR, MC, U.S.N.,
RICHARD D. KOPKE, M.D., COL, MC, U.S.A.,
and
KIM R. GOTTSHALL, PH.D., COL, MC, U.S.A.
Naval Medical Center San Diego
San Diego, California

Ménière's disease is potentially disabling inner ear disorder that affects both hearing and balance. The disease was originally described by the French physician Prosper Meniere in 1861 in a series of reports to the Paris Academy of Medicine. Despite intensive early work on the disorder, it was not until 1938 that Hallpike and Cairns provided histopathologic evidence that the pathology of the disorder appeared to be endolymphatic hydrops, which is now the accepted pathologic change associated with Ménière's disease. Classic Ménière's disease is characterized by four symptoms as follows: (1) fluctuating hearing loss, (2) episodes of vertigo (usually lasting 20 minutes to 3 hours), (3) fluctuating tinnitus, and (4) fluctuating pressure. In the initial stages of the disease individuals have these symptoms together during an "attack." However, as the disease progresses, hearing loss and tinnitus can become constant, with intensifications before or during vertigo episodes. In addition, as the disease progresses, the individual's baseline balance function may not be completely normal between attacks. It is estimated that classic Ménière's disease occurs in anywhere from 3 to 14 per 1000 individuals, with some evidence for a genetic cause because the frequency has regional variation. In addition to classic Ménière's disease there are a number of variants of the disorder including both cochlear Ménière's disease (the auditory symptoms without the vertigo) and vestibular Ménière's disease (the vertigo without the auditory symptoms). The existence of these two variants is difficult to prove because Ménière's disease is primarily a diagnosis made by history and, without the classic four symptoms, it may be difficult to distinguish these variants from other disorders. Ménière's disease can be bilateral but the percentage of bilateral cases is a controversial. Reports vary from 5% to 70%, with most individuals assigning a 15% to 20% incidence of bilateral disease.

The mechanism whereby endolymphatic hydrops causes Ménière's disease is not completely understood. The most common explanation is that an increase in endolymphatic volume causes a break or a leak in one of the inner ear membranes, which causes mixing of endolymph and perilymph. Because the two fluids vary in electrolyte and protein compositions, the membrane break/leak causes a mixing of these components, which upsets the local milieu of the hair cells, causing an attack. The presumed etiology for the hydrops includes autoimmune, posttraumatic, or infectious causes, or anatomic abnormalities, but in most cases a direct cause cannot be determined.

DIAGNOSIS

The diagnosis of Ménière's disease is based on history. Many investigators treat Ménière's disease as a diagnosis of exclusion, but we feel that in classic cases a thorough history can provide the diagnosis by itself. In classic cases patients report vertigo episodes (true room spinning) lasting 20 minutes to 3 hours associated with pressure and tinnitus in one ear. In early states of the disease patients may or may not report hearing loss during the attack and should be instructed to attempt to notice a hearing loss during any future attacks (often putting a phone up to each ear and hearing the dial tone may allow patients to determine a unilateral loss). In the early states of the disorder patients may or may not notice hearing loss and tinnitus between attacks. In addition, individuals usually report having normal balance function between attacks. The frequency of the attacks varies and can be as frequent as once daily to as rare as one single attack. Attacks may or may not be triggered by food, stress, or other external factors and may vary in frequency and intensity over time. As the disorder progresses patients continue to have vertigo attacks associated with tinnitus, pressure, and hearing loss. However, they more commonly report hearing loss and tinnitus between attacks and begin to demonstrate balance disorders between attacks as well (usually expressed as unsteadiness). As the disorder progresses many patients experience a gradual reduction in hearing in the effected ear. In many cases over time (usually several years) the disease will "burn out." In this phase the patient no longer has spells of vertigo and has much less pressure, but is left with a baseline hearing loss (usually moderate to severe in nature) and some tinnitus. It is estimated that this "burn out" will occur in up to 70% of patients but may take 6 or more years to occur.

The physical exam of individuals with Ménière's disease is remarkable for what it does not show. Individuals should have a relatively normal otolaryngologic physical. In particular, individuals should have no obvious middle ear disease and no significant cerebellar or gross balance abnormalities. The one physical exam finding that some individuals have reported helpful in Ménière's disease is the presence of diplacusis. To test for diplacusis the examiner holds a tuning fork up to the patient's ears and the patient reports the tone (not loudness but frequency) of the tuning fork on each side. Diplacusis is said to be present if the patient reports the tone is higher or lower in one ear than the other. Unfortunately, this finding is not specific and the effected ear may hear the tone as higher or lower.

Many diagnostic tests have been for the evaluation of individuals with Ménière's disease. One of the most helpful tests is an audiogram. In classic cases the audiogram will show a flat low frequency hearing loss rising to less of a loss in the high frequencies. Initially this finding will only be present during or slightly after an attack, but as time progresses this finding may be seen on audiograms taken in between attacks. Over time the hearing loss may progress to involve more frequencies. A less specific audiometric finding is a compression of the dynamic range, meaning the amount of decibels between the patient's ability to hear at each frequency and the point at which the patient has discomfort (noise seems too loud) at each frequency is diminished. A variety of balance tests have been utilized in patients with Ménière's disease. Tests of the vestibule-ocular reflex including rotational chair sinusoidal testing and high speed head rotation testing demonstrate abnormalities in gain or symmetry, but these findings can be relatively nonspecific results. Tests of semicircular canal function including caloric testing, step-velocity testing, and head impulse testing usually indicate a peripheral vestibular weakness on the involved side. There has been a great deal of interest in electrodiagnostic testing for Ménière's disease. There is a growing body of literature to support the value of electrocochleography in the diagnosis of Ménière's disease. Although it is true that an increased summating to action potential ratio can indicate the presence of hydrops, it is not yet known what percentages of individuals with Ménière's disease do not have this finding and whether the finding will be present in individuals with early disease between their attacks.

The differential diagnosis for Ménière's disease is substantial. It can be especially difficult to distinguish nonclassic Ménière's disease (cochlear Ménière's disease or vestibular Ménière's disease) from a number of the diseases in the differential diagnosis. A full list of the differential diagnosis is beyond the scope of this discussion, but a number of disorders must be ruled out, particularly acoustic neuroma, multiple sclerosis, and transient ischemic attacks. Although none of these disorders truly mimic classic Ménière's disease, they can present with similar symptoms and can be relatively safely ruled out with a magnetic resonant imaging (MRI) scan that we obtain on all of our Ménière's disease patients. A number of peripheral disorders, most particularly vestibular migraines, atypical benign positional vertigo, and perilymphatic fistula, must be ruled out, and this is often possible with a combination of history, physical exam, and diagnostic testing but can be confusing in patients with nonclassical disease. To date there is no gold standard test to confirm the diagnosis of Ménière's disease. A good history and physical (journal entries from the patient are very helpful) and judicious use of diagnostic tests is still the most reliable way to make the diagnosis.

TREATMENT

The treatment of Ménière's disease has been very controversial. Although outcome-based studies are lacking, most physicians counsel patients to reduce their caffeine and salt intake. The degree of recommended reduction of both of these products varies from extremely low salt diets and no caffeine ingestion to simply no-added salt diets and one caffeinated beverage a day. Although extreme reductions may yield better results, they are rarely tolerated by patients, who may feel that the cure is worse than the disease. In addition to dietary restrictions, most physicians feel that medical therapy is an appropriate initial treatment step. We feel that a subset of individuals with unilateral disease (and most individuals with bilateral disease) has an autoimmune-mediated etiology for their Ménière's disease. Consequently we start all newly diagnosed patients on a 2-week regimen of corticosteroids. We treat the patients with 60 mg of prednisone* daily at approximately 9 AM (to minimize the steroid-axis suppression) for 14 days. Individuals who respond to this treatment are candidates for additional autoimmune therapy regimens. Those who do not respond are tried on more classic medicines for Ménière's disease. Although there are many medicines advocated, the mainstay of medical treatment for Ménière's disease is a combination thiazide and triamterene diuretic such as Dyazide.* This regimen may take several weeks to become effective. We do not advocate the long-term use of vestibular suppressants (such as meclizine [Antivert]* or diazepam [Valium]*) and feel that the role of these medicines as well as antiemetics is reserved for use during an acute attack. For those who fail medical therapy surgical or minimally invasive treatment options are available. In individuals with significant hearing loss a labyrinthectomy is relatively safe and highly effective. For those with usable hearing there are three basic surgical/procedural treatment options including transtympanic gentamicin (Garamycin) therapy, endolymphatic sac procedures, and vestibular neurectomy procedures. Each of these therapies has advantages and disadvantages. Endolymphatic sac procedures are nondestructive to hearing and balance function but are less successful than other surgical approaches. Vestibular neurectomy procedures are highly effective but do sacrifice vestibular function in the treated ear. Transtympanic gentamicin treatment is a minimally invasive way of treating Ménière's disease and is highly successful, but can have unpredictable results on hearing and balance function. Most recently, interest has been revived in devices and procedures that effect middle and inner ear pressure, and such devices will likely find a place in the treatment algorithm for Ménière's disease in the near future.

Regardless of the method chosen for invasive treatment of Ménière's disease, vestibular rehabilitation is an important part of the therapeutic regimens. Surgical and minimally invasive procedures, although very effective at controlling the vertigo associated with Ménière's disease, often produce a disequilibrium, which, while transient, can trouble patients for several months. Vestibular rehabilitation therapy dramatically reduces the length of posttreatment disequilibrium and can produce a better long-term functional outcome.

*Not FDA-approved for this indication.

SINUSITIS

method of
BRENT A. SENIOR, M.D.
University of North Carolina
Chapel Hill, North Carolina

Sinusitis is a disease with a long and sordid history. The ancient physician Hippocrates was well aware of this disease and was the first to coin the term "polyp" nearly 3000 years ago. This word meant "many footed" and was used by Hippocrates to refer to its intricate "roots" and propensity to recur if not completely removed during surgical management. Indeed, he described a surgical technique for managing nasal polyps and sinusitis that involved tying a ligature to a piece of cloth and dragging it through the nasal cavity, thereby amputating the polyps. It is no wonder that the great composer Joseph Haydn, after the performance of a similar procedure on him in 1783, suggested that his surgeon "putrify under the earth"!

Although the history of this disease is long, sinusitis remains extremely prevalent and has a significant economic impact. Community-acquired bacterial rhinosinusitis is estimated to occur 30 to 40 million times in the United States every year and result in nearly 18 million antibiotic prescriptions. Indeed, sinusitis is the second most common diagnosis resulting in the prescription of an antibiotic by physicians in the United States, behind only bronchitis.

Even though many people suffer at great cost to the health care system, it is important to realize just how badly people suffer. The Scottish anatomist John Bell, in his textbook of surgery in 1801–1808, described sinusitis as one of the most "loathsome and fatal diseases" and "one of the most horrible and incurable diseases." He wrote that patients become "waxen and pale"; they realize that they "will die and become resigned to [their] fate." Although many look at such descriptions as hyperbole, the afflicted will disagree. Data from the SF-36 has shown that individuals with chronic sinusitis have worse body pain, general health, vitality, and social functioning than the general population does. Indeed, they also exhibit worse body pain and social functioning than do individuals with congestive heart failure, angina, chronic obstructive pulmonary disease, and chronic back pain.

DIAGNOSIS OF SINUSITIS

Sinusitis, or better, rhinosinusitis, is actually a term referring to five separate entities as defined by the Rhinosinusitis Task Force established by the American Academy of Otolaryngology/Head and Neck Surgery in 1995. Acute rhinosinusitis is an inflammatory condition wherein nasal and sinus symptoms are present for less than 4 weeks. Chronic rhinosinusitis has symptoms persisting longer than 12 weeks, whereas the designation subacute rhinosinusitis requires symptoms lasting between 4 and 12 weeks. Patients with chronic rhinosinusitis may have a flare in their smoldering, ongoing, low-grade symptoms, a condition termed "acute flare of chronic rhinosinusitis." An additional entity has been defined, recurrent acute rhinosinusitis, that involves four discrete episodes of sinonasal inflammation interspersed with periods of relative normalcy.

The most common symptoms that people describe regarding their rhinosinusitis include nasal congestion, anterior nasal drainage (often discolored), postnasal drainage (often thick and bitter tasting), facial discomfort, and a decreased sense of smell. However, many of these symptoms are similar to those experienced in the presence of a viral upper respiratory tract infection or even allergy. To determine the presence of true bacterial rhinosinusitis, two features are helpful. Ideally, symptoms should be present for longer than 10 days or worsen after 7 days. Often, the symptoms will be more severe than those experienced with a typical "cold."

Regarding specific symptoms, the Rhinosinusitis Task Force has established a collection of "major factors" and "minor factors" to aid in diagnosis of the disease (Table 1). Major factors to be assessed are similar to those noted earlier: nasal obstruction or blockage, decreased sense of smell, pus in the nose on nasal examination, and facial discomfort. Minor factors include historical features that are a "soft call," including headache, fever, halitosis, fatigue, dental pain, cough, and ear pain or fullness. The diagnosis of rhinosinusitis is aided by the presence of two or more major symptoms or one major symptom combined with two or more minor symptoms.

Physical examination of a patient with rhinosinusitis will identify swelling and moisture over the inferior turbinates with occasional frank pus seen in the nasal cavity. The face may be tender to palpation. Transillumination is an old technique involving placement of a light source against the palate and assessing for decreased glow over the face in a darkened room. Unfortunately, this technique is plagued by low specificity and low sensitivity and often adds little to the diagnosis.

The value of obtaining plain radiographs is likewise probably minimal. Several authors have examined this issue, and the Agency for Healthcare Research and Quality published a meta-analysis on the topic in 1999. In that review of six studies, plain radiographs were found to have an overall sensitivity of 76% and a specificity of 79% for identifying rhinosinusitis when compared with maxillary sinus puncture and aspiration, considered by many to be the gold standard for the diagnosis of rhinosinusitis.

TABLE 1. **Diagnostic Criteria for Rhinosinusitis**

Major Signs/Symptoms	Minor Signs/Symptoms
Facial pain/pressure	Headache
Nasal obstruction	Fever
Purulent nasal discharge	Halitosis
Hyposmia/anosmia	Dental pain
Cough (children)	Cough (adults)
	Ear fullness/discomfort
	Fatigue

Computed tomographic (CT) examination of the sinuses can, however, provide valuable information. Mucosal thickening seen most commonly in the ethmoid sinuses, or in the "dependent" maxillary, frontal, or sphenoid sinuses, may indicate the presence of infection. This value is limited, however, to examination of an individual with chronic and not acute rhinosinusitis because the appearance of viral and bacterial inflammation will, in many cases, appear radiographically similar. Additionally, it has been clearly shown that viral "colds" may result in mucosal thickening on CT scans of the sinuses that persists, in some cases, for up to 6 weeks after the infection. Timing in obtaining the CT scan is therefore essential and best delayed until after at least 4 weeks of medical intervention.

Endoscopic examination, when performed by a skilled practitioner, can be very helpful in defining the presence of rhinosinusitis. Edema of the middle meatus can be readily identified, and purulence is often seen. Endoscopic evaluation has an added advantage that allows cultures to be obtained from purulence emanating from the middle meatus in a minimally invasive fashion. Studies of this technique have shown a very high correlation with the invasive maxillary sinus puncture procedure.

ETIOLOGY OF SINUSITIS

Acute rhinosinusitis in adults is a mucosal infectious disease that usually occurs in the setting of preceding viral infection or, occasionally, severe nasal allergy. Causative organisms, in order of prevalence, include *Streptococcus pneumoniae* (20% to 43%), *Haemophilus influenzae* (22% to 35%), and *Moraxella catarrhalis* (2% to 10%), with other streptococcal species, *Staphylococcus aureus,* and anaerobes being far less common. Mucosal infection results in edema and sinus ostial obstruction. These sequelae lead to mucus stasis, thereby potentiating greater infection. This chain of events corresponds to the "sinusitis cycle."

Chronic rhinosinusitis, however, has a decidedly different associated microbiology. The most common isolates include coagulase-negative staphylococci (36%), *S. aureus* (25%), *Streptococcus viridans* (8%), and *Corynebacterium* (5%). Some have also found high rates of anaerobic infection in chronic rhinosinusitis, whereas isolates in patients who have undergone previous sinus surgery often include gram-negative rods, most notably *Pseudomonas aeruginosa.*

Along with this decidedly different microbiology, mounting evidence is suggesting that chronic rhinosinusitis is not simply a mucosal infectious disease. Recent evidence has pointed to bone as a possible source of ongoing, overlying mucosal inflammation, although frank osteomyelitis has not been identified. Other research has suggested that the root cause of rhinosinusitis may exist in an eosinophilic-mediated immune response to mucosal fungus, which is found in nearly every human nose when carefully cultured. Research in both these areas continues.

TREATMENT OF SINUSITIS

Treatment of acute rhinosinusitis involves breaking the "sinusitis cycle." Chief in such treatment is killing of the causative bacteria via appropriate antibiotic therapy. Table 2 provides the recommendations of the American Academy of Otolaryngology/Head and Neck Surgery, the American Rhinologic Society, the American Academy of Otolaryngic Allergy, and the Centers for Disease Control and Prevention for antibiotic treatment of acute rhinosinusitis as determined by microbiology and emerging resistance patterns. For patients who have not received treatment within the previous 6 weeks and who are not penicillin allergic, amoxicillin is estimated to be effective in 89% of cases. Alternatives in order of estimated effectiveness include amoxicillin-clavulanate (Augmentin), cefpodoxime (Vantin), and cefuroxime (Ceftin). For those with penicillin allergy who have not been treated, trimethoprim-sulfamethoxazole (Bactrim) offers 81% effectiveness, with doxycycline and macrolides slightly less effective. For individuals who have recently been treated, fluoroquinolones, including gatifloxacin (Tequin), moxifloxacin (Avelox), and levofloxacin (Levaquin), are 95% effective. Similarly, amoxicillin-clavulanate is highly efficacious.

The typical treatment duration is suggested to be 10 days, although research to support this time frame is lacking.

Additional therapies that may be of benefit to patients include topical oxymetazoline (Afrin), phenylephrine (Neo-Synephrine), systemic decongestants (pseudoephedrine [Sudafed]), mucolytics (guaifenesin [Humibid]), and irrigation (saline). Providers are cautioned regarding the recommendation for topical decongestants because of the high risk of rhinitis medicamentosa with rebound nasal congestion if used for more than 72 hours. Although all these medications tend to provide symptomatic relief for patients, little experimental data exist to suggest more rapid resolution of the sinusitis.

Chronic rhinosinusitis, with its different microbiology and different clinical course, is best managed with a prolonged course of antibiotics (>21 days). Selection of an antibiotic should take into consideration its

TABLE 2. **Antibiotic Guidelines for the Treatment of Acute Bacterial Rhinosinusitis (Estimated Cure Rate)**

No Recent Treatment	Recent Treatment
Amoxicillin-clavulanate (Augmentin) (93%) Amoxicillin (89%) Cefpodoxime (Vantin) (87%) Cefuroxime (Ceftin) (84%)	Gatifloxacin (Tequim), moxifloxacin (Avelox), levofloxacin (Levaquin) (95%) Amoxicillin-clavulanate (93%)
Pencillin Allergic With No Recent Treatment	**Pencillin Allergic With Recent Treatment**
Trimethoprim/sulfamethoxazole (Bactrim) (81%) Doxycycline (Vibramycin) (80%) Macrolides (79%)	Gatifloxacin, moxifloxacin, levofloxacin (95%)

unique microbiology, particularly the possibility of *Pseudomonas* and anaerobic infection. Because these patients have commonly received extensive previous treatment with antibiotics, significant consideration should be given to otolaryngologic referral for endoscopically guided, culture-directed antibiotics.

All patients with chronic rhinosinusitis should also be managed with steroids, either intranasally, orally, or both. The steroids serve to reduce tissue edema and blunt the inflammatory response, which tends to be excessive in these individuals. Unless medically contraindicated, a short taper (2 weeks) starting at about 0.5 mg/kg/d prednisone is all that is needed to provide significant benefit. Steroids can be particularly helpful in an individual who has associated nasal polyps.

Nasal allergy is a common condition coexisting with rhinosinusitis, although causality is not clear. Thorough allergy evaluation with a skin–end point titration technique or radioallergosorbent testing is recommended as a component of successful medical therapy for an individual with rhinosinusitis.

Referral to an otolaryngologist/head and neck surgeon is necessary for any individual with complications of acute rhinosinusitis, including orbital (periorbital cellulitis, subperiosteal abscess, orbital abscess), intracranial (epidural abscess, meningitis), or facial (osteomyelitis) complications requiring urgent surgical management. Referral should also be considered for consideration of surgical intervention in any individual with chronic rhinosinusitis that is not responding to appropriate medical therapy. Only after thorough medical management as outlined earlier is surgery considered. With the modern techniques of functional endoscopic sinus surgery developed in the last 15 years, the chance of significant improvement in the patient's quality of life has been found to be over 90% in both the short and long term.

NONALLERGIC RHINITIS

method of
JOSE R. ARIAS, Jr. M.D., and
DENNIS K. LEDFORD, M.D.
University of South Florida College of Medicine and the James A. Haley V.A. Hospital
Tampa, Florida

Nonallergic rhinitis is an idiopathic syndrome of nasal symptoms without allergen specific IgE. Nonallergic rhinitis is a diagnosis of exclusion because of the lack of confirmatory tests. The symptoms are either sporadic or persistent and include nasal congestion, rhinorrhea, sneezing, and postnasal drip. Sneezing paroxysms and ocular and nasal itching, characteristic of allergic rhinoconjunctivitis, are not typical. Nonallergic rhinitis often is aggravated by environmental changes such as temperature, air movement, or odors. Subsets of nonallergic rhinitis have distinct features such as nasal eosinophilia or blood eosinophilia, but these reflect heterogeneity within the syndrome rather than a unifying pathophysiology.

DEMOGRAPHICS AND EPIDEMIOLOGY

The lack of definitive diagnostic criteria limits epidemiologic studies of nonallergic rhinitis. Prevalence estimates vary from 17% to 60% of subjects evaluated for rhinitis symptoms in specialty practices. Overlap between allergic and nonallergic rhinitis occurs commonly and has been designated mixed rhinitis by some authors. The prevalence of mixed rhinitis ranges from 16% to 34% in specialty practices. The majority of affected subjects are females. Age is also a factor in the prevalence and incidence of nonallergic rhinitis. One group reported that 70% of patients with a diagnosis of nonallergic rhinitis developed their symptoms as an adult (age >20 years) whereas allergic rhinitis usually occurred before the age of 20 years.

PATHOPHYSIOLOGY AND CLASSIFICATION

The pathophysiology of nonallergic rhinitis is poorly understood.

Nonallergic rhinitis is likely a syndrome with variable causes and a final common pathway of symptoms, including nasal congestion and increased secretions. A characteristic of the various forms of nonallergic rhinitis is nasal hypersecretion. Potential causes of this hypersecretion include sensory nerve receptor hypersensitivity, mast cell degranulation, neurogenic reflexes, and autonomic nervous system dysregulation. Characteristic nonimmunologic stimuli include strong odors (e.g., perfume, cologne, solvents), hair spray, beer or wine ingestion, temperature changes, cold air, increased humidity, cleaning products (e.g., detergents, window cleaners, disinfectants, soaps), spicy foods, and inhaled irritants (e.g., tobacco smoke, paint fumes, chlorine, gasoline fumes, automotive exhaust). Nasal challenges have demonstrated hyperreactivity with capsaicin, methacholine, and histamine. At least one group of investigators has described an increased number of nasal mast cells in subjects with perennial nonallergic rhinitis, without a difference between allergic and nonallergic patients. Other investigators have reported mast cell mediators following nasal challenges with nonspecific stimuli. Thus a variety of mechanisms is likely responsible for the various syndromes called nonallergic rhinitis.

The absence of a unifying pathophysiology has resulted in a descriptive classification scheme for nonallergic rhinitis. The stimuli clinically responsible or associated with symptoms are most often used to separate the various subtypes. Diseases or conditions associated with nonallergic rhinitis are listed in Table 1. Some of the more common will be reviewed.

Vasomotor Rhinitis

This term describes the most frequent form of nonallergic rhinitis. Vasomotor rhinitis is also designated

TABLE 1. **Classification of Nonallergic Rhinitis Related to Diseases or Conditions**

Atrophic rhinitis
Turbinectomy
Ozena (*Klebsiella ozaenae*)
Chronic sinusitis
Immunodeficiencies (IgA deficiency, CVID, HIV disease)
Osteomeatal obstructions
Cerebral spinal fluid rhinorrhea
Metabolic conditions
Acromegaly
Hypothyroid
Rhinitis with nasal polyps
Aspirin intolerance
Chronic sinusitis
Cystic fibrosis
Kartagener syndrome (bronchiectasis, chronic sinusitis, and nasal polyps)
Young syndrome (sinopulmonary disease, azoospermia, and nasal polyps)
Structurally related rhinitis
Choanal atresia
Nasal valve dysfunction
Obstructive adenoid hyperplasia
Septal deviation
Turbinate deformation
Vasculitis/autoimmune and granulomatous disease
Amyloidosis
Churg-Strauss syndrome
Midline granuloma
Relapsing polychondritis
Rhinoscleromatis (*Klebsiella rhinoscleromatis*)
Sarcoidosis
Sjögren syndrome
Systemic lupus erythematosus
Wegener granulomatosis

Adapted from Settipane RA and Lieberman P: Ann Allergy Asthma Immunol 86:494-508, 2001.

idiopathic perennial nonallergic rhinitis, a more descriptive term. This rhinitis is unrelated to allergy, infection, structural lesions, systemic diseases or drug abuse. The term vasomotor is misleading since it implies an unproven autonomic effect in the pathophysiology.

Patients with idiopathic perennial nonallergic rhinitis may be divided into two groups based upon nasal symptoms. One group is "runners" with "wet" rhinorrhea. The other is "dry" with nasal congestion and blockage to airflow as a predominant symptom and minimal rhinorrhea. Either type of patient experiences symptoms provoked by nonspecific triggers.

Nonallergic Rhinitis with Eosinophilia Syndrome

Nonallergic rhinitis with eosinophilia syndrome (NARES) is characterized by nasal eosinophils and perennial rhinitis symptoms. These symptoms include sneezing paroxysms, watery rhinorrhea, and nasal pruritus. Patients occasionally have hyposmia or anosmia. The prevalence of this syndrome is not known but estimates are that 15% to 20% of patients of nonallergic rhinitis have NARES. Despite nasal eosinophilia and occasional blood eosinophilia, allergic diseases, as determined by skin testing or serum IgE to specific allergens, are not typical. The etiology of NARES is unknown. NARES may be a precursor to the aspirin triad (asthma, aspirin sensitivity, and sinusitis).

Rhinitis Of Pregnancy (Hormonal Rhinitis)

Hormonal rhinitis occurs with pregnancy, puberty, the use of oral contraceptives, hypothyroidism, or female hormone replacement therapy. Of these, pregnancy is probably the most common association.

Rhinitis medicamentosa, allergic rhinitis, and sinusitis also cause nasal symptoms during pregnancy. Gastroesophageal reflux disease (GERD) may also be an aggravating factor, particularly during the latter stages of the pregnancy. GERD therapy may improve rhinitis but this treatment has not been studied in rhinitis of pregnancy.

Rhinitis symptoms in pregnancy usually intensify during the second month and persist to term, normally resolving shortly after delivery or termination of breast feeding. These symptoms may be due to progesterone and estrogen inducing glandular secretion, vasodilation and increased blood volume.

Rhinitis In The Elderly

Nonallergic rhinitis is progressively less common with advancing age.

Nasal complaints are frequently the result of cholinergic hyperactivity (gustatory rhinitis), antihypertensive medications, some of which are listed in Table 2, or nasal dryness resulting from Sjögren disease or idiopathic dryness. A change in antihypertensive therapy may be useful, particularly if α- or β-adrenergic antagonists are used.

Rhinitis Associated with Food

Gustatory rhinitis is a nonallergic syndrome with copious watery rhinorrhea associated with the ingestion or the odor of food or alcoholic beverages. Spicy foods typically trigger symptoms but any type of food may provoke rhinorrhea. Food allergy is a rare cause of rhinitis without other systemic symptoms, such

TABLE 2. **Antihypertensive Drugs Causing Nasal Congestion or Rhinitis**

Class	Trade Name Examples	Generic Name Examples
Angiotensin-converting enzyme inhibitors	Prinivil Zestril	Lisinopril
α-Blockers	Aldomet	Methyldopa
	Cardura	Doxazosin
β-Blockers	Corgard	Nadolol
	Normodyne	Labetalol
Calcium channel blockers	Adalat/Procardia	Nifedipine
	Cardizem/Tiazac	Diltiazem
Vasodilator	Apresoline	Hydralazine

as urticaria, lower airway complaints, angioedema, abdominal cramps, or diarrhea.

Rhinitis Medicamentosa

Rhinitis medicamentosa follows repetitive use of topical decongestants such as α-adrenergic agent phenylephrine (e.g., Afrin) or cocaine. Typically, regular use for more than 7 days is required before rebound symptoms develop. Rhinitis medicamentosa is also associated with systemic therapies, particularly antihypertensives (see Table 2), and in aspirin-sensitive subjects. Nasal congestion is the primary symptom and is often resistant to therapy. The nasal mucosa appears erythematous and congested, with bleeding resulting from tissue friability.

Gastroesophageal Reflux Disease And Rhinitis

Case reports and studies of patients with chronic upper airway symptoms describe a potential relationship between GERD and upper airway conditions. Theodoropoulos and colleagues statistically showed an association between GERD and an increased prevalence of upper airway complaints, including nasal congestion, postnasal drip, rhinorrhea, sneezing, nasal itching, sinus headaches, ear fullness, hoarseness, cough, or throat clearing. These symptoms overlap with those of nonallergic rhinitis. Neurogenic inflammation, which is implicated in lower respiratory complications of GERD, may be involved in the pathogenesis. Because GERD limited to the distal esophagus was associated with symptoms. This observation suggests that direct irritation of acid into the upper airway is not necessary.

Physical Rhinitis

Physical rhinitis describes nasal symptoms that occur in response to cold air (skier's/jogger's nose) or sunlight (reflex rhinitis). Neurogenic reflexes are probably responsible for symptoms, particularly the sneezing after exposure to sunlight. Cold air effects are partially the result of condensation forming during nasal exhalation.

MANAGEMENT

The mainstays of nonallergic rhinitis treatment are avoidance and pharmacologic management based upon symptomatology. The most common treatable symptoms are congestion or rhinorrhea. Sneezing and itching are less often a major problem in nonallergic rhinitis. Postnasal drip is usually poorly responsive to therapy.

AVOIDANCE

A variety of environmental factors may incite or worsen nonallergic rhinitis. The effects of these irritants are not mediated by specific IgE, but the patient's perception is usually an allergy to irritants. Reassurance to these patients that they are not allergic is helpful. Ventilation of the area in which exposures occurs, use of filters with absorbent, such as activated charcoal, or nasal saline irrigation are considerations when exposure is inevitable. Masking odors with menthol or eucalyptus products is also a consideration.

PHARMACOLOGIC

Anticholinergic Agents

Intranasal anticholinergic therapy, ipratropium bromide 0.03% (Atrovent) being the only approved agent, reduces rhinorrhea but has no effect on other nasal symptoms. Anticholinergics inhibit vagally mediated reflexes by antagonizing the action of acetylcholine at the cholinergic receptors of serous and seromucous glands. In contrast to tertiary amines like atropine, topical ipratropium, a quaternary amine, has a negligible systemic effect due to limited absorption. Topical side effects include nasal dryness and bleeding. Excessive dryness can usually be managed by reducing the dosage or dosing frequency. Combination treatment with antihistamine nasal spray azelastine (Astelin), nasal corticosteroids, or oral decongestant is an unstudied consideration. First-generation oral antihistamines, (e.g., chlorpheniramine [Chlor-Trimeton],* diphenhydramine [Benadryl],* clemastine [Tavist]*), and oral methscopolamine may relieve rhinorrhea or postnasal drip but are associated with limited systemic side effects of dry mouth, vaginal dryness, urinary hesitancy, tachycardia, and increased intraocular pressure.

Antihistamine Nasal Spray (Azelastine)

Azelastine (Astelin) is an antihistamine with probable anti-inflammatory properties that is available in the United States as a nasal spray formulation for the treatment of both seasonal allergic and perennial nonallergic rhinitis (Table 3). Two double-blind, placebo-controlled trials demonstrated efficacy in treating nonallergic rhinitis symptoms (rhinorrhea, sneezing, postnasal drip and nasal congestion). Azelastine has an onset of action less than 30 minutes in allergic rhinitis but onset of action in nonallergic rhinitis is not known. As-needed use is an option, but the published trial on nonallergic rhinitis is with regular therapy.

Dysgeusia and mild sedation, incidence of 5%–15%, the lower number in nonallergic subjects, are the most common side effect. Inhalation techniques to minimize aspiration of the spray into the throat, and foods with distracting taste, such as hard candy or chocolate, help alleviate the dysgeusia.

Corticosteroid Nasal Spray

Nasally inhaled corticosteroids are effective in controlling symptoms of nonallergic rhinitis. Beclomethasone (Beconase AQ, Vancenase AQ), budesonide

*Not FDA-approved for this indication.

TABLE 3. **FDA-Approved Nasal Sprays for the Treatment of Nonallergic Rhinitis**

Trade Name	Generic	Dose	Age
Astelin	Azelastine	2 sprays bid	>12 y
Atrovent	Ipratropium bromide	0.03% 2 sprays bid-tid	>6 y
Beconase AQ	Beclomethasone	1-2 sprays bid	>6 y
Flonase	Fluticasone	2 sprays qd or 1 spray bid	>4 y
Rhinocort Nasal Inhaler*	Budesonide	2 spray bid or 4 sprays qd	>6 y
Vancenase AQ	Beclomethasone	1-2 sprays qd	>6 y

*Contains chlorofluorocarbons and will be removed from the market when current supply is exhausted.

(Rhinocort Nasal Inhaler), and fluticasone (Flonase) have Food and Drug Administration (FDA) approval for nonallergic rhinitis but probably all topical corticosteroids are effective. The mechanism of action of nasal corticosteroids probably varies among different syndromes. For example, reduction of eosinophils may be important in NARES, whereas reduction in nasal blood or glandular secretion may be relevant in vasomotor rhinitis. Topical nasal corticosteroid side effects are usually limited to local irritation, with mucosal bleeding and very rarely nasal septal perforation. There is no evidence that prolonged use results in nasal mucosal atrophy, although the long-term studies are in allergic rhinitis. Patients should be instructed to direct the spray away from the nasal septum to minimize irritant side effects.

Cromolyn Sodium

Cromolyn* has not been studied in the treatment of nonallergic rhinitis. Mast cell mediators have been detected in nonallergic rhinitis, suggesting that topical cromolyn sodium may be effective.

Oral Decongestants

Oral decongestants, such as pseudoephedrine* (120 mg–240 mg/d) and phenylephrine* (4 mg every 4 hours), nonspecifically reduce congestion in nonallergic rhinitis. Decongestants have no effect on rhinorrhea or sneezing. Potential side effects include insomnia, loss of appetite, excessive nervousness, elevated blood pressure, urinary hesitancy, and palpitations. These side effects often limit effectiveness. If blood pressure is controlled and monitored, a continuous trial of oral decongestant may be reasonable in hypertensive subjects.

Saline

Topical, isotonic sodium chloride nasal sprays (e.g., Ocean Nasal Mist, Natru-Vent†) provide short-term moisturizing of nasal mucosa and irrigation of irritants. Homemade saline is equally effective but is not as convenient. Saline may reduce or remove dry crusted discharge. The irrigation effect may minimize the effect of odors, vapors, or aerosols. The necessity for frequent use with ongoing symptoms limits the acceptability of this therapy. Hypertonic saline solutions (e.g., Ocean Hypertonic Nasal Spray, ENTSol [available on the internet at www.ENTSolwash.com]) may decongest the nose without the problem of rebound congestion associated with topical α-agonists.

*Not FDA-approved for this indication.
†Not available in the United States.

Topical Decongestants

Topical α-adrenergic agonists, such as phenylephrine* (Neo-Synephrine), or imidazole agents, such as oxymetazoline (e.g., Afrin), vasoconstrict mucosal blood vessels and reduce nasal edema without affecting itching, sneezing, or rhinorrhea. They are usually not associated with systemic sympathomimetic effects. Topical decongestants should be used with caution or rebound nasal congestion occurs after more than 5–10 days of regular treatment (see rhinitis medicamentosa). Short term or intermittent use of these agents is safe and effective.

SPECIAL CONSIDERATIONS

Oral antihistamine therapy, including second and third generation agents, is unlikely to benefit patients with nonallergic rhinitis. The minimal itching and sneezing in these patients and the cost of sedating and nonsedating antihistamine therapy make therapeutic trials less appealing.

Oral leukotriene modifiers (e.g., zafirlukast [Accolate],* montelukast [Singulair],* zileuton [Zyflo]*) have not been studied in nonallergic rhinitis, but a treatment trial may be warranted in subjects with congestion. This suggestion is based upon the detection of leukotrienes in nasal lavage of some subjects with rhinitis. The cost of this therapy should limit use until data is available.

Specific subcategories of nonallergic rhinitis warrant consideration for individualized treatment strategies. Our recommended treatment of rhinitis in pregnancy is intranasal saline, steam inhalation, avoidance of irritants, intranasal cromolyn (NasalCrom),*

*Not FDA-approved for this indication.

and intranasal ipratropium (Atrovent) (both are FDA class B for pregnancy). Intranasal corticosteroids, topical azelastine, or oral pseudoephedrine* (all are FDA class C for pregnancy) may be useful for persistent rhinitis during the second or third trimester. Treatment for the primary complaint of congestion, with pseudoephedrine, should be avoided in the first trimester because of an association with gastroschisis. Other considerations are unapproved over-the-counter therapies such as oral garlic,‡ inhaled eucalyptus,‡ inhaled menthol,‡ or topical Shea butter *(Butyrospermum parkii).*‡

The symptoms of mucosal dryness and congestion seen in the elderly may be partially relieved with intranasal saline and topical ointments, such as petrolatum with eucalyptus,‡ menthol,‡ or Shea butter‡ applied to the septum. Continuous use of oral decongestants in elderly patients may not be tolerated because of urinary hesitancy, increased blood pressure, insomnia, or agitation. Nasal topical corticosteroids may be of value but are often associated with bleeding. Topical azelastine (Astelin) is also a consideration, but there is a 5% to 15% incidence of somnolence, which may be difficult to recognize in the elderly receiving multiple medications.

In patients affected by rhinitis medicamentosa, affected subjects should discontinue regular use of topical decongestants either acutely or over 7–10 days. High-dose (two times or more the dose used for allergic rhinitis) nasal corticosteroid may reduce the congestion, facilitating discontinuation of the topical decongestant. Oral corticosteroid, such as prednisone 40 mg/d with a tapering schedule over 7–10 days, may be helpful in refractory cases.

The rhinorrhea in skier's/jogger's nose usually responds to topical ipratropium bromide 0.03% (Atrovent). Optimum benefit is obtained when the nasal spray is used before participating in the physical activity.

SURGICAL MANAGEMENT

There is no surgical treatment for nonallergic rhinitis. Turbinectomy may be a last resort when all other medical management of nasal congestion has failed. The benefit of turbinectomy tends to be transient, lasting months to a year. Complications include dry nasal mucosa with recurrent bleeding. Other surgical approaches to reduce nasal secretion include vidian nerve section or electrocoagulation of the anterior ethmoidal nerve. These procedures are rarely recommended for nonallergic rhinitis.

---

*Not FDA-approved for this indication.
‡Not yet approved for use in the United States.

HOARSENESS AND LARYNGITIS

method of
ROBERT THAYER SATALOFF, M.D., D.M.A.
Jefferson Medical College, Thomas Jefferson University Graduate Hospital
Philadelphia, Pennsylvania
University of Pennsylvania
Philadelphia, Pennsylvania

Until the 1980s, most physicians who cared for patients with voice disorders asked only a few basic questions, such as: How long have you been hoarse? Do you smoke? The physician's ear was the sole instrument used routinely to assess voice quality and function. Visualization of the vocal folds was limited to indirect examination using regular light and looking through a mirror placed inside the patient's mouth, or by direct laryngoscopy with anesthesia in the operating room. Treatment of patients generally was limited to administration of medicines for infection or inflammation, surgery for masses, and no treatment if the vocal folds looked normal. Occasionally, voice therapy was recommended, but the specific nature of the therapy was not well defined or controlled, and results were often disappointing. Since the early 1980s, the standard of care for the diagnosis and treatment of voice disorders has changed dramatically.

WHAT KINDS OF QUESTIONS SHOULD BE ASKED?

Good medical diagnosis in all fields often hinges on asking the right questions, and listening carefully to the answers. This process is known as taking a history. Recently, medical care for voice problems has made use of a markedly expanded, comprehensive history that reflects new knowledge supporting the premise that there is more to the voice than simply the vocal folds. Virtually any body system may be responsible for voice complaints. In fact, problems outside the larynx often cause voice dysfunction in persons whose vocal folds appear fairly normal but function abnormally. These patients would have received no effective medical care for their voice problems just a few years ago.

What Is Hoarseness?

Most people with voice problems complain of hoarseness or laryngitis. A more detailed description of the problem (or the patient's chief complaints) is often helpful in identifying the cause. *Hoarseness* is a coarse, scratchy sound caused most commonly by abnormalities on the vibratory margin of the vocal fold. These may include swelling, roughness from inflammation, growths, scarring, or anything that interferes with symmetrical, periodic vocal fold vibration. Such abnormalities produce turbulence, which we perceive as hoarseness.

Breathiness is caused by abnormalities that keep the vocal folds from closing completely, including vocal fold paralysis, muscle weakness, cricoarytenoid joint injury or arthritis, vocal fold masses, or atrophy of the vocal fold tissues. These abnormalities permit air to escape when the vocal folds are supposed to be closed tightly. The air escape is perceived as breathiness.

Fatigue of the voice is the inability to continue to phonate for extended periods of time, with change in vocal quality. Often it is caused by misuse of abdominal and neck musculature, or overuse (singing or speaking too loudly or too long). Vocal fatigue may be a sign of general tiredness or serious illnesses such as myasthenia gravis.

Volume disturbance may appear as inability to speak or sing loudly or inability to phonate softly. Most volume problems are secondary to intrinsic limitations of the voice or technical errors in voice production, although hormonal changes, aging, superior laryngeal nerve paresis, and neurologic disease are other causes.

Even nonsingers normally require only about 10 to 30 minutes to warm up the voice. *Prolonged warm-up time*, especially in the morning, is caused most often by reflux laryngitis. *Tickling or choking* during speech or singing is associated with laryngitis or voice abuse. Often a symptom of pathology of the vocal fold's leading edge, this symptom requires that voice use be avoided until vocal fold examination has been accomplished. *Pain* while vocalizing can indicate vocal fold lesions, laryngeal joint arthritis, infection, or gastric (stomach) acid irritation of the posterior portion of the larynx; however, it is much more commonly caused by voice abuse with excessive muscular activity in the neck, rather than acute pathology on the leading edge of a vocal fold, and it does not usually require immediate cessation of phonation pending medical examination.

What Is Involved in a Physical Examination of a Person with Voice Problems?

Physical examination of a person with voice complaints involves a complete ear, nose, and throat assessment by an otolaryngologist and examination of other body systems. Subjective examination is supplemented by technologic aids that improve our ability to "see" the vocal mechanism, and allow quantification of aspects of its function. With phonation at middle C, the vocal folds come together and separate approximately 250 times per second. Strobovideolaryngoscopy uses a laryngeal microphone to trigger a strobe light that illuminates the vocal folds, allowing the examiner to assess them in slow motion. This technology allows visualization of small masses, vibratory asymmetries, adynamic segments caused by scar or early cancer, and other abnormalities that were simply missed under continuous light. The instruments typically found in a well-equipped clinical voice laboratory assess six categories of vocal function: vibratory, aerodynamic, phonatory, acoustic, electromyographic, and psychoacoustic. State-of-the-art analysis of vocal function is extremely helpful in diagnosis, therapy, and evaluation of progress during treatment of voice disorders (outcomes assessment).

COMMON DIAGNOSES AND TREATMENTS

After a thorough history has been obtained, and after physical examination and clinical voice laboratory analysis have been performed, it is usually possible for the physician to arrive at an accurate explanation for voice dysfunction. Treatment, of course, depends on the etiology. Fortunately, because technology has improved voice medicine, the need for laryngeal surgery has diminished. In a great many cases, voice disorders result from respiratory, neurologic, gastrointestinal, psychologic, or endocrine causes, or from some other treatable medical etiology.

Does Age Affect the Voice?

Age affects the voice substantially, especially during childhood and older age. Children's voices are particularly fragile. Voice abuse during childhood may lead to problems that persist throughout a lifetime. Any child with unexplained or prolonged hoarseness should undergo prompt, expert medical evaluation performed by a laryngologist who specializes in voice care.

In geriatric patients, vocal unsteadiness, loss of range, and voice fatigue may be associated with typical physiologic aging changes such as vocal fold atrophy. In routine speech, such vocal changes are the reason a person can be identified as old even over the telephone. With appropriate muscular conditioning of the body and voice, many of the characteristics associated with vocal aging can be eliminated, and a more youthful sound can be restored. Occasionally, surgery may be useful, as well.

Do Allergy and Postnasal Drip Bother the Voice?

Allergies and postnasal drip alter the viscosity of secretions and the patency of nasal airways, and have other effects that impair voice function. Many of the medicines used commonly to treat allergies (such as antihistamines) also have undesirable effects on the voice. If allergies are severe enough to cause persistent throat clearing, hoarseness, and other voice complaints, a comprehensive allergy evaluation and treatment by an allergy specialist is advisable. Postnasal drip, the sensation of having excessive secretions, may or may not be caused by allergy. Contrary to popular opinion, the condition usually involves secretions that are too thick rather than too abundant. If postnasal drip is not caused by allergy, it is usually managed best through hydration and by mucolytic agents such as guaifenesin (Humibid).* Reflux laryngitis can cause symptoms very similar to those of postnasal drip, and this diagnosis should always be considered in persons who have the sensation of throat secretions, and in those who feel a lump in the throat or who clear their throat excessively.

---

*Not FDA-approved for this indication.

What is the Effect of an Upper Respiratory Tract Infection without Laryngitis?

Although mucosal irritation usually is diffuse, patients sometimes have marked nasal obstruction with little or no soreness of the throat and a normal voice. If the laryngeal examination shows no abnormality, a person with a head cold should be permitted to speak or sing but advised not to try to duplicate his or her usual sound.

How about Laryngitis with Serious Vocal Fold Injury?

Serious vocal fold injuries, such as hemorrhage in the vocal folds and mucosal disruption (a tear), are contraindications to voice use. When these are observed, the therapeutic course of treatment includes strict voice rest (silence) in addition to correction of any underlying disease. Vocal fold hemorrhage is most common in premenstrual women who are using aspirin products or nonsteroidal medicines for cramps. Severe hemorrhage or mucosal scarring may result in permanent alterations in vocal fold vibratory function. In rare instances, surgical intervention may be necessary.

What about Laryngitis without Serious Vocal Fold Injury?

Mild to moderate edema and erythema of the vocal folds may result from infection or from noninfectious causes. In the absence of mucosal disruption or hemorrhage, these disorders are not absolute contraindications to voice use. If no pressing professional need for voice use exists, inflammatory conditions of the larynx are treated best with relative voice rest in addition to other modalities. However, in some instances speaking or singing may be permitted. The more good voice training a person has had, the safer it is to use the voice under adverse circumstances.

Does Voice Rest Help Laryngitis?

Voice rest (absolute or relative) is an important therapeutic consideration in any case of laryngitis. When no professional commitments are pressing, a short course (up to a few days) of absolute voice rest (silence) may be considered because as it is the safest and most conservative therapeutic intervention. Absolute voice rest is *necessary* only for serious vocal fold injury such as hemorrhage or mucosal disruption. Even then, it is virtually never indicated for more than 7 to 10 days. Other patients with vocal problems should also be instructed to speak softly and as infrequently as possible, often at a slightly higher pitch than usual, and with a slightly breathy voice; to avoid excessive telephone use; and to speak with abdominal support as they would in singing. This is relative voice rest, and it is helpful in most cases. It should be noted that voice rest is used based on anecdotal evidence, and evidence-based studies to confirm or refute its efficacy have not been performed.

What Are the Hazards of Laryngeal Trauma?

The larynx can be injured easily during altercations and motor vehicle accidents. Blunt anterior neck trauma may result in laryngeal fracture, dislocation of the arytenoid cartilages, hemorrhage, and airway obstruction. Late consequences, such as narrowing of the airway, also may occur. Hoarseness or other changes in voice quality after neck trauma should call laryngeal trauma to mind, with the first priority being the safety of the airway. Prompt evaluation by visualization and radiologic imaging should be performed. In many cases, surgery is needed.

Do Lung Problems Cause Voice Disorders?

Respiratory problems are especially problematic to singers and other voice professionals, but they may cause voice problems in anyone. Respiratory support is essential to healthy voice production. Obstructive pulmonary disease is the most common culprit in voice dysfunction. Even mild obstructive lung disease can impair support enough to cause compensatory increased neck and tongue muscle tension and abusive voice use, capable of producing vocal nodules and other structural lesions. Treatment of the underlying pulmonary disease to restore effective support is essential to resolving the vocal problem. Treating asthma is rendered more difficult in professional voice users because of the need in some patients to avoid not only oral steroid inhalers but also any bronchodilator medications that produce even a mild tremor.

How about Smoke and Pollution?

Exposure to *environmental irritants* is a well-recognized cause of voice dysfunction. Smoke, dehydration, pollution, and allergens may produce hoarseness, frequent throat clearing, and voice fatigue. These problems can generally be eliminated by environmental modification, medication, or simply breathing through the nose rather than the mouth since the nose warms, humidifies, and filters incoming air.

The deleterious effects of tobacco smoke upon the vocal folds have been known for many years. Smoking not only causes chronic irritation but cancer as well.

In addition to pollution-related voice disorders that may affect factory workers and the general population, singers, actors, and other performers may be exposed to a great many environmental irritants and pollutants and are at special risk for developing environmentally induced dysphonias. Some of these irritants and pollutants are encountered by almost all performers at some time during their careers. For example, theatrical halls are commonly not cleaned adequately. Hence, actors, singers, dancers, and others are exposed to dust and mold in high concentrations during rehearsals and performances. These conditions are aggravated if set construction is carried out coincident with rehearsals. Saw dust (often from wood treated with chemicals), fumes from oil-based paints, and other noxious substances are generated frequently only a few feet from performers. These exposures may result in mucosal and respiratory changes that affect voice performance adversely, and even may aggravate or cause health problems such as acute allergic episodes, asthma, cough and others.

Performers may be exposed to even greater hazards if they work around artificial fogs and smokes, or around pyrotechnic effects. Artificial fogs and smokes may be created using a variety of substances such as glycol-based products, oil-based products, organic chemicals, and inorganic chemicals. Often, the situation is aggravated by the addition of dyes or fragrances included for theatrical effect. Guidelines regarding use of artificially created smokes and fogs are controversial. Unfortunately, some of the substances still in common use contain materials that are toxic and can create substantial health problems. Pyrotechnic effects may be similarly troublesome. The explosives and colorants used to create pyrotechnic effects are potentially hazardous and include substances such as toxic metals (mercury and lead) and known carcinogens.

Can Foods or Drugs Affect the Voice?

The use of various *foods and drugs* also may affect the voice. Some medications may even permanently ruin a voice, especially androgenic hormones such as those given to women with endometriosis. Similar problems occur with use of anabolic steroids (also male hormones) that are used for postmenopausal loss of libido; these drugs are also used illicitly by body builders. More common drugs also have deleterious vocal effects. These include antihistamines; oral steroid inhalers; many neurologic, psychologic, and respiratory medications; and others. Some foods may also be responsible for voice complaints in people with normal vocal folds. Milk products are particularly troublesome to some people because the casein they contain increases and thickens mucosal secretions.

What about Hormones?

Endocrine problems have marked vocal effects, many by causing accumulation of fluid in the superficial layer of the lamina propria, altering the vibratory characteristics. Mild hypothyroidism typically causes a muffled sound, slight loss of range, and vocal sluggishness. Similar findings may be seen in pregnancy, during use of oral contraceptives (in about 5% of women), for a few days before menses, and at the time of ovulation. However, male hormones may actually cause laryngeal growth in women (as they do in boys at the time of puberty), permanently altering laryngeal structure and sound.

Do Stomach Problems or Hiatal Hernia Affect the Voice?

Gastrointestinal disorders commonly cause voice complaints. In *gastroesophageal reflux laryngitis*, stomach acid refluxes into the throat, allowing droplets of the irritating gastric juices to come in contact with the vocal folds, and even to be aspirated into the lungs. Reflux may occur with or without a hiatal hernia. Common symptoms are hoarseness, especially in the morning, prolonged vocal warm-up time, bad breath, sensation of a lump in the throat, chronic sore throat, cough, and a dry or "coated" mouth. Typical heartburn is frequently absent. Over time, uncontrolled reflux may cause cancer of the esophagus and larynx. Thus this condition should be treated conscientiously.

Does Anxiety Have Anything to Do with the Voice?

When the principal cause of vocal dysfunction is anxiety, the physician often can accomplish much by assuring the patient that no organic difficulty is present and by stating the diagnosis of anxiety reaction. Tranquilizers and sedatives are rarely necessary and are undesirable because they may interfere with fine motor control, affecting voice adversely. Recently, β-adrenergic blocking agents such as propranolol hydrochloride* (e.g., Inderal) have achieved some popularity in the treatment of preperformance anxiety in singers and instrumentalists. β-blockers should not be used routinely for voice disorders and preperformance anxiety. If anxiety or other psychologic factors are the cause of a voice disorder, their treatment by a psychologist or psychiatrist with special interest and training in arts medicine is extremely helpful. This therapy should occur in conjunction with voice therapy.

Can Abusing the Voice Create Problems?

Voice abuse through technical dysfunction is an extremely common source of hoarseness, vocal weakness, pain, and other complaints. It is seen routinely in vocally untrained singers, teachers, clergy, politicians, salespeople, secretaries, and others. In some cases, voice abuse can even create structural problems such as vocal nodules, cysts, and polyps. Now that the components of voice function are better understood, techniques have been developed to rehabilitate and train the voice for speech and singing. Voice therapy with a certified, licensed speech-language pathologist who specializes in voice is invaluable.

What Are Vocal Nodules?

Small, callous-like bumps on the vocal folds called nodules are caused by voice abuse. Occasionally, laryngoscopy reveals asymptomatic vocal nodules that do not appear to interfere with voice production; in such cases, the nodules need not be treated. However, in most cases, nodules are associated with hoarseness, breathiness, loss of range, and vocal fatigue. Voice therapy always should be tried as the initial therapeutic modality and often cures the majority of patients,

*Not FDA-approved for this indication.

even if the nodules look firm and have been present for many months or years. Even in those who eventually need surgical excision of the nodules, preoperative voice therapy is essential to prevent recurrence.

What Are Cysts?

Submucosal cysts of the vocal folds are usually also traumatic lesions that result from blockage of a mucous gland duct, although they may also occur for other reasons and may even be present at birth. They often cause contact swelling on the opposite vocal fold and are usually misdiagnosed initially as nodules. Often, they can be differentiated from nodules by strobovideolaryngoscopy revealing a mass that is obviously fluid-filled. They require voice therapy and usually surgery.

What Are Polyps?

These lesions are generally the result of trauma. In some cases, even sizable polyps resolve with relative voice rest and a few weeks of low-dose corticosteroid therapy. However, many require surgical removal. If unilateral polyps are not treated, they may produce contact injury on the contralateral vocal fold. Voice therapy should be used.

What about Vocal Fold Paralysis?

Paralysis or paresis may involve one or both vocal folds, and one or both nerves to each vocal fold. When paralysis/paresis is limited to the superior laryngeal nerve, the patient loses his or her ability to control longitudinal tension (stretch) in the vocal fold. Although superior laryngeal nerve paresis involves only one muscle (cricothyroid), the problem is difficult to overcome. The vocal fold sags at a lower level than normal, and the patient notices difficulty controlling pitch, controlling sustained tones, and projecting the voice. The recurrent laryngeal nerve controls all the other intrinsic laryngeal muscles. When it is injured, the vocal fold cannot move toward or away from the midline, although longitudinal tension is preserved and the vocal fold remains at its appropriate vertical level if the superior laryngeal nerve is not paretic. Compensation often occurs spontaneously during the first 6 to 12 months after paralysis, with the paralyzed vocal fold moving closer to the midline. At least 6 months (and preferably 12 months) of observation are needed prior to surgical intervention, unless it is absolutely certain that the nerve has been cut and destroyed, because spontaneous recovery of neuromuscular function is common. Laryngeal electromyography (EMG) is helpful in establishing the diagnosis and prognosis. Vocal fold paralysis should be treated initially with voice therapy. If voice therapy fails, vocal fold motion remains impaired, and voice quality or ability to cough or swallow normally is unsatisfactory to the patient, surgical treatments are generally quite satisfactory.

What Is Spasmodic Dysphonia?

Spasmodic (or "spastic") dysphonia is a diagnosis given to patients with specific kinds of voice interruptions. These patients may have a variety of diseases that produce the same vocal result, which is termed a laryngeal *dystonia*. There are also many interruptions in vocal fluency that are incorrectly diagnosed as spasmodic dysphonia. This error should be avoided because different types of dysphonia require different evaluations and treatments, and carry different prognostic implications. Spasmodic dysphonia is subclassified into adductor and abductor types.

Are There Other Neurologic Voice Disorders?

Many other neurologic problems commonly cause voice abnormalities. These include myasthenia gravis, Parkinson's disease, essential tremor, and numerous other disorders. In some cases, voice abnormalities are the first symptoms of a systemic problem.

What about Cancer of the Larynx?

Cancers of the larynx are common and are usually associated with smoking, although cancers also occur occasionally in nonsmokers, especially in persons with laryngopharyngeal reflux. Persistent hoarseness is one of the most common symptoms. Laryngeal cancers may also present with throat pain or referred ear pain. If diagnosed early, these cancers respond to therapy particularly well and often are curable. Treatment usually requires radiation, surgery, or a combination of the two modalities. It is usually possible to preserve or restore voice, especially if the cancer is detected early.

What Should Be Considered when Voice Surgery Is Contemplated?

Principles

Scar tissue occurs in response to trauma, including surgery. If scar tissue replaces the normal anatomic layers, the vocal fold becomes stiff and adynamic (nonvibrating). This results in asymmetrical, irregular vibration with air turbulence that we hear as hoarseness, or it results in microscopically incomplete vocal fold closure, allowing air escape which makes the voice sound breathy. Such vocal folds may look normal on traditional examination, but can be seen as abnormal under stroboscopic light. Conveniently, most benign pathology (e.g., nodules, polyps, or cysts) is superficial. Consequently, surgical techniques have been developed to permit removal of lesions from the epithelium or superficial layer of the lamina propria without disruption of the intermediate or deeper layers in most cases, thus reducing the risk of scar formation. All of these delicate microsurgical techniques are commonly referred to as *phonomicrosurgery*. Vocal fold "stripping" has not been an acceptable technique for more than a decade. Otolaryngologists with training in the new subspecialty of laryngology should be sought to provide patients with optimal results.

Precautions

A detailed discussion of laryngeal surgery is beyond the scope of this publication. However, a few points are worthy of special emphasis. Surgery for vocal nodules should be avoided whenever possible and should almost never be performed without an adequate trial of expert voice therapy, including patient compliance with therapeutic suggestions. In most cases, a minimum of 6 to 12 weeks of observation should be allowed while the patient is using therapeutically modified voice techniques under the supervision of a certified speech-language pathologist and possibly a singing or acting voice teacher. Proper voice use rather than voice rest (silence) is correct therapy.

What Can Be Done about a Voice that Is Worse after Surgery?

Too often, the physician is confronted with a desperate patient whose voice has been "ruined" by vocal fold surgery, recurrent or superior laryngeal nerve paralysis, trauma, or some other tragedy. Occasionally, the cause is as simple as a recently dislocated arytenoid cartilage that can be reduced. However, if the problem is an adynamic segment, decreased bulk and pliability of one vocal fold after "stripping," bowing caused by superior laryngeal nerve paralysis, or some other serious complication in a mobile vocal fold, great expertise is needed. Voice therapy is nearly always helpful in optimizing compensatory strategies and minimizing fatigue, but it usually will not restore the patient's normal voice. None of the available surgical procedures for these conditions is consistently effective in restoring normal voice, although improvements are obtained routinely. Tertiary subspecialty consultation should be obtained for such patients.

Are There Other New Developments in Surgical Technique?

New techniques of external laryngeal surgery to modify the laryngeal skeleton have become extremely useful in treatment of vocal fold paralysis, a common consequence of viral infection, surgery and cancer. Until the late 1980s, vocal fold paralysis was managed most often by endoscopic injection of Polytef (Teflon) into the tissues adjacent to the paralyzed vocal fold. This pushed the paralyzed side toward the midline, allowing the normal vocal fold to meet it, thus permitting glottic closure and improving voice. Although Polytef is relatively inert, granulomatous reactions to the foreign body are not uncommon, and stiffness of the vocal fold edge frequently impairs voice quality. Polytef infiltrated into tissues is hard to remove if the results are unsatisfactory, and injection of it has been largely replaced by autologous fat or facia injection or thyroplasty, which are better techniques. Thyroplasty is a technique in which a window is cut in the laryngeal skeleton, and tissues are depressed inward and held in place with a silicone block or Gore-Tex strip. This pushes the vocal fold toward the midline fairly reversibly, without injecting a foreign body into the tissues.

What about Singers, Actors, and Other Voice Professionals?

Professional singers, actors, announcers, politicians, and others put "Olympic" demands on their voices. These patients are often best managed by subspecialists familiar with the latest concepts in professional voice care.

How Can the Voice Be Kept Healthy?

Preventive medicine is always the best medicine. The more people understand about their voices, the more they will appreciate their importance and delicacy. Education helps us understand how to protect the voice, train and develop it to handle our individual vocal demands, and keep it healthy. Even a little bit of expert voice training can make a big difference. Avoidance of abuses, especially smoking, is paramount. If voice problems occur, expert medical care should be sought promptly. Interdisciplinary collaboration among family physicians, internists, laryngologists, speech-language pathologists, singing teachers, acting teachers, many other professionals, and especially voice users themselves, has revolutionized voice care since the early 1980s. Technologic advances, scientific revelations, and new medical techniques inspired originally by interest in treating professional opera singers have brought a new level of expertise and concern to the medical profession and improved dramatically the level of care available for all patients with voice dysfunction.

STREPTOCOCCAL PHARYNGITIS

method of
GRAHAM P. KRASAN, M.D.
University of Michigan
Ann Arbor, Michigan

Acute pharyngitis is an exceedingly common complaint in patients seeking medical attention at physician's offices, the emergency room, or other urgent care facilities. Viral pathogens are responsible for the overwhelming number of cases caused by infection. The most common bacterial cause of acute pharyngitis and tonsillitis is group A β-hemolytic streptococci (GABHS), or *Streptococcus pyogenes*, and children and young adults are at greatest risk for infection. In fact, GABHS account for 15% to 30% of the disease burden in all children with acute pharyngitis.

A major challenge for the clinician is distinguishing GABHS from viral causes of pharyngitis because findings on clinical examination are largely nonspecific, often reported between 68% and 86%. Diagnostic inaccuracy in this regard leads either to the indiscriminate use of antibiotics or, conversely, to an increased risk of suppurative and nonsuppurative complications as a consequence of untreated GABHS disease. Strict criteria that encompass both physical signs consistent with GABHS pharyngitis and confirmatory microbiologic laboratory data are required to arrive at definitive therapeutic decisions. To aid the clinician, the microbiology and epidemiology of GABHS disease, as well as current diagnostic and therapeutic strategies, will be reviewed herein.

MICROBIOLOGY

By microscopy, GABHS appear as gram-positive cocci, typically in pairs and chains, and they form gray-white colonies on 5% sheep blood agar plates with a circumferential rim of clear agar termed β hemolysis. In contrast, normal oral flora may be either α-hemolytic (greenish cast around colonies as a result of partial hemolysis) or γ-hemolytic (no hemolysis). β Hemolysis is largely due to the elaboration of streptolysin O, an oxygen-labile hemolysin expressed by almost all GABHS that lyses erythrocytes and has the capability of damaging the plasma membrane of a variety of mammalian cells. Group C and G streptococci are also β-hemolytic, and presumptive identification of GABHS is based on growth inhibition around a bacitracin susceptibility disk (0.04 U) placed on a freshly streaked plate.

Classification of streptococci into Lancefield serogroups is based on the reaction of extracted streptococcal cell wall carbohydrates against a panel of standard group-specific antisera. Individual GABHS strains are further subdivided by their M protein serotype (>100 serotypes described), a cell wall–associated virulence factor that inhibits phagocytosis. GABHS that express particular M protein serotypes can be epidemiologically segregated into those that predominantly cause throat infections and those that predominantly cause skin infections. The development of opsonic anti-M protein antibodies confers durable resistance to future infections with GABHS of the same M serotype. These anti-M protein antibodies also have a central role in the development of acute rheumatic fever (ARF) and acute poststreptococcal glomerulonephritis (APSGN) as a result of cross-reactivity with human structural proteins within a variety of target organs.

EPIDEMIOLOGY

GABHS are strictly human pathogens, and the mucous membranes and skin are the primary reservoirs. Although these organisms are not members of the normal nasopharyngeal flora, prolonged pharyngeal carriage without clinical manifestations is common. GABHS pharyngitis is a disease primarily of school-aged children (5 to 12 years of age) that occurs sporadically throughout the year with incidence peaks during the winter and early spring months in temperate climates. GABHS pharyngitis in children younger than 3 years is exceedingly uncommon, although a nasal streptococcosis syndrome manifested as purulent nasal discharge and excoriation of the nares has been described. The downward trend of GABHS pharyngitis cases as children age is probably due to immunologic protection after multiple infections during childhood.

Crowding is an important variable for person-to-person spread of GABHS in all age groups, and it is a risk factor for outbreaks in communities where close contact is common, such as daycare facilities, group homes, and military barracks. Transmission is usually via inhalation or other contact with infected droplets, although food-borne outbreaks have been well documented. Individuals are particularly contagious early in infection, and organisms can be present in the nares and throat weeks after symptoms resolve in those who are untreated. Patients who have received at least 24 hours of antibiotic therapy are considered noninfectious. During peak seasons, up to half of children may be asymptomatically colonized, and transmission rates upward of 30% may occur within the school setting or family household. Because spread among family members is extremely common, GABHS recolonization of a previously treated individual may account for a percentage of the presumed bacteriologic failures seen after therapy.

CLINICAL SYNDROMES

GABHS pharyngitis is typified by the abrupt onset of pharyngeal and tonsillar inflammation, which may be accompanied by palatal petechiae and yellowish nonadherent exudates. In addition to these local findings, tender anterior cervical lymph nodes are notable, as is fever, dysphagia, headache, and abdominal pain, with an absence of conjunctivitis, rhinorrhea, cough, hoarseness, and diarrhea. GABHS pharyngitis is a self-limited illness that develops after a 2- to 5-day incubation period and lasts 3 to 5 days; antibiotics will shorten the disease course if given within 24 to 48 hours after onset. Patients with symptoms persisting longer than a week or who do not improve with therapy are less likely to have true GABHS pharyngitis.

Unfortunately, a sizable number of individuals with GABHS pharyngitis have less classic manifestations, and differentiation from other etiologies cannot be accomplished on clinical grounds alone. Respiratory viral agents (coronavirus, influenza, parainfluenza, respiratory syncytial virus, rhinovirus) are among the most common causes of mild to moderate pharyngeal inflammation secondary to infection, and the inflammation is usually accompanied by coryza symptoms or an influenzal syndrome. In contrast, adenovirus may cause a frank exudative pharyngitis similar to GABHS in children, as can Epstein-Barr virus (EBV, the agent of infectious mononucleosis) in adolescents and adults. Clues to EBV infection on physical examination include the presence of relatively nontender enlarged posterior cervical lymph nodes and splenomegaly; EBV may be confirmed by either positive heterophil antibodies (Monospot) or elevated virus-specific antibody titers. Acute retroviral syndrome secondary to primary HIV infection must always be considered as an alternative diagnosis in this context. Herpes simplex virus and enteroviral (coxsackievirus, echovirus) infections predominantly cause vesicular or ulcerative lesions distributed over the posterior of the pharynx and soft palate, with accompanying high fever and dysphagia.

A variety of bacterial etiologies also cause pharyngitis, although they are relatively uncommon in clinical practice. An exudative pharyngitis indistinguishable from GABHS may occur as a consequence of infection with other β-hemolytic streptococci (groups C and G) or *Arcanobacterium haemolyticum*. A small fraction of patients may have *Neisseria gonorrhoeae* pharyngitis from oral-genital contact. *Mycoplasma pneumoniae* and *Chlamydia pneumoniae* are less common causes in the absence of lower respiratory tract symptoms. Impressive pharyngitis can be seen in the occasional case of *Corynebacterium diphtheriae*, *Francisella tularensis*, *Yersinia enterocolitica*, and synergistic anaerobic and spirochetal infections (Vincent's angina). Throat pain and erythema may also accompany chronic nasal drainage in those with sinusitis caused by nontypable *Haemophilus influenzae*, *Moraxella catarrhalis*, or *Streptococcus pneumoniae;* infectious or allergic rhinitis will also be manifested as a similar spectrum of symptoms. Finally, inflammatory disorders such as Behçet's disease, erythema multiforme, Kawasaki disease, and systemic lupus erythematosus should be considered in the differential diagnosis of pharyngitis.

Scarlet fever is due to an infection by GABHS strains that elaborate one or more erythrogenic exotoxins. Scarlet fever can accompany a number of superficial and deep-seated GABHS infections, including pharyngitis, impetigo, wound infections, and puerperal sepsis. Patients with scarlet fever typically have a blanching, diffuse fine red rash with a texture similar to sandpaper that erupts on the upper part of the chest 24 hours after symptoms begin. Other cardinal signs include circumoral pallor and, on the tongue, the development of prominent reddened papillae on a white-coated base ("strawberry tongue"). Areas of intense redness or petechiae (Pastia's lines) at flexural creases in the antecubital fossa, groin, and other regions may also be noticeable. After treatment is initiated, the rash typically fades within a few days, and subsequent exfoliation of the involved skin is common. The differential diagnosis for scarlet fever is broad and includes *A. haemolyticum*, viral exanthems, drug reactions, Kawasaki disease, and toxic shock syndrome.

Suppurative complications of GABHS pharyngitis include peritonsillar or retropharyngeal abscesses and cervical adenitis. Other localized infections caused by the contiguous spread of GABHS within the nasopharynx include sinusitis, otitis media, and pneumonia, although associated bacteremia, endocarditis, and sepsis are rare in immunocompetent patients. Nonsuppurative sequelae are the consequence of a vigorous immunologic response to GABHS and include ARF (arthritis, carditis, subcutaneous nodules, erythema marginatum, and Sydenham's chorea), reactive arthritis as a sole condition, APSGN, and neuropsychiatric disorders (pediatric autoimmune neuropsychiatric disorder associated with streptococcal infection—PANDAS syndrome). Although a marked resurgence of ARF occurred during the late 1980s and early 1990s, the incidence of this disease has again declined, and it is currently rare in the United States.

LABORATORY TESTING

Throat culture remains the gold standard for diagnosis and has a sensitivity of 90% to 97% when optimally performed. Poor recovery of GABHS from throat swabs is commonly due to inadequate sampling techniques, and a standardized culture method includes rubbing both tonsillar pillars and the posterior of the pharynx with a cotton- or synthetic fiber–tipped swab. Specimens should then be either immediately placed in transport media or inoculated onto 5% sheep blood agar plates and incubated in an aerobic chamber at 35°C to 37°C that contains a 5% to 10% CO_2 atmosphere for at least 24 hours. If no growth is apparent, plates should be reincubated for another day. Detection of β-hemolytic colonies may be improved either by stab inoculating the agar after streaking out the sample to cultivate subsurface growth or by incubating plates in an anaerobic environment.

For most routine GABHS culture, 5% blood agar will suffice, although recovery of low numbers of GABHS may be enhanced by preincubating swabs in Todd-Hewitt broth before plating on solid media (broth enrichment) or by using agar that contains inhibitors to suppress other flora (e.g., crystal violet, trimethoprim-sulfamethoxazole [Bactrim]); GABHS may, however, take longer to grow (48 to 72 hours) in the presence of inhibitors.

GABHS present in the pharynx are often rendered nonviable after only a few doses of an appropriate antibiotic, and false-negative throat cultures may also be due to surreptitious antibiotic use. False-positive results can occur as a result of misidentification of other β-hemolytic organisms such as group C, F, or G serotypes, *Staphylococcus aureus,* or *A. haemolyticum.*

Although throat culture is extremely sensitive, it is labor intensive, takes 24 to 48 hours to achieve a final result, and if done on site, requires trained personnel and maintenance of a diagnostic laboratory. Rapid detection systems have been developed as alternatives to culture methods and include genetic probe assays that detect streptococcal nucleic acids such as the Group A Streptococcus Direct Test (Gen-probe) and direct antigen tests (DATs). The sensitivity of genetic probe tests rivals that of conventional culture, although their use is largely limited by the need to invest in costly specialized equipment (luminometer). DATs are more practical solutions for the office setting because of their ease of use and rapid turnaround time; their introduction into clinical practice has revolutionized the outpatient diagnosis and management of GABHS pharyngitis.

DATs are generally two-step methods whereby group A carbohydrates are extracted from a clinical sample, antigens are bound by antibodies immobilized on a substrate, and antigen-antibody complexes are then visually detected. DATs are of no use in the diagnosis of group C or G streptococcal pharyngitis. Rapid antigen tests include the older latex agglutination method, enzyme-linked immunosorbent assay (ELISA), modified ELISA (single-step ELISA), and optical immunoassay (OIA). The specificity of all these tests is extremely high (90% to 98%), and a presumptive diagnosis of GABHS can be made with a positive DAT; a confirmatory throat culture is not recommended. In contrast, sensitivity estimates of specific DATs, when compared with routine throat culture, can vary widely in published studies (50% to >95%). Their performance characteristics may be greatly influenced by a number of factors, including capture of a sufficient quantity of organisms with the swab, experience of the technical personnel processing the sample or interpreting the DAT results, and the use of either routine culture or enrichment methods as a comparator.

In recent studies, the sensitivity of the OIA in particular has been reported to exceed the sensitivity of even routine culture. However, low GABHS colony counts can be directly correlated with false-negative OIA results, which also underscores the importance of collection techniques for ensuring accurate DAT-based therapeutic decisions. It is currently recommended that all patients with a negative DAT result have a confirmatory culture, although whether scant growth of GABHS (<10 colonies) represents true "strep throat" or streptococcal carriage in those with an intercurrent viral illness continues to be subject to some debate. This dilemma may be avoided to some degree by ensuring that patients with a viral syndrome (e.g., cough, rhinorrhea) do not undergo further workup because a positive culture would more likely identify streptococcal carriers, who are not at an increased risk for ARF. Some experts have advocated the use of high-sensitivity DAT methods without culture backup for most adults. One caveat to this strategy is that clinicians should reconfirm the advertised performance of a chosen test in their practice by using routine culture as the gold standard before relying on the stand-alone DAT approach and then institute quality control assessments in an ongoing manner. A confirmatory throat culture should, however, always follow a negative DAT result in those who have a personal or family history of ARF or if an outbreak of ARF is occurring in the community. Another exception would be pediatric patients because obtaining adequate throat swab specimens can be a significant challenge under the best of circumstances and the risk of ARF, though still remote, is considerably higher than in adults. As new antigen detection systems and improvements in current DAT technologies are introduced into the marketplace, the promise of a stand-alone rapid antigen test for GABHS diagnosis will soon come to fruition, although the current assays are insufficiently sensitive for this approach to be universally adopted.

Serologic testing has little role in the acute management of GABHS pharyngitis because antistreptococcal antibodies begin to rise significantly well after the onset of symptoms and peak 4 to 8 weeks after infection. Specific antibodies are typically raised against a number of extracellular streptococcal virulence factors, including streptolysin O (ASO), deoxyribonuclease B (DNase B), hyaluronidase, nicotinamide adenine dinucleotidase (NADase), and streptokinase. Most adolescents and adults have antibodies as a result of repeated episodes of GABHS disease throughout childhood, and infants may also have measurable titers as a consequence of maternal antibody transfer. Serologic diagnosis has its greatest utility in documenting past GABHS infection in those with poststreptococcal disease (e.g., ARF) because bacteria are rarely recoverable at that point. Serology may also be helpful in differentiating patients suffering true recurrent GABHS pharyngitis from carriers because predictable elevations in antistreptococcal antibodies would not typically occur as an immunologic response to intercurrent viral illnesses or to carriage. The ASO titer in particular is a commonly used, well-standardized assay, and a significant increase above age-related norms or between acute and convalescent titers is suggestive of recent GABHS infection. It should be underscored that young children may not have appreciable ASO titers during infection, and if clinical suspicion remains high, measuring other antibodies that may be more consistently elevated, such as anti-DNase B and anti-hyaluronidase, is often helpful. In addition, ASO titers may be spuriously low in individuals with GABHS skin infections, those who have had antibiotic treatment early in their course, and patients concurrently receiving immunosuppressive agents (e.g., steroids).

THERAPY

Antibiotic treatment shortens the duration of symptoms if given early, interrupts transmission of GABHS, and reduces the incidence of suppurative and nonsuppurative complications. Amazingly, in this era of emerging drug resistance, GABHS remains exquisitely sensitive to penicillin despite almost a half century of use, and it continues to be recommended by national advisory panels as first-line therapy for GABHS pharyngitis. Although all antibiotics that eradicate GABHS from the pharynx are assumed to interrupt the development of ARF, only penicillin has been rigorously studied in this regard. Prevention of ARF is most effective if therapy is initiated within 9 days of the onset of symptoms.

A single injection of benzathine penicillin G is recommended to ensure compliance, and it provides bactericidal levels for up to 28 days (Table 1). In children, benzathine penicillin G can be mixed with procaine penicillin G to lessen injection discomfort, although the efficacy of this regimen has not been

TABLE 1. **Treatment Regimens for GABHS Pharyngitis**

Drug	Adult Dosage	Pediatric Dosage	Duration
First-Line Therapy			
Benzathine penicillin G (Bicillin)	1.2 million U	1.2 million U (>27 kg) 600,000 U (<27 kg) *or* 900,000 U benzathine penicillin G + 300,000 U procaine penicillin	Single dose
Penicillin V (Pen-Vee K)	500 mg bid	250 mg bid or tid	10 d
Amoxicillin (Amoxil)	500 mg bid	50 mg/kg divided bid	10 d
Erythromycin estolate (Ilosone)	500 mg bid	40 mg/kg divided bid–qid	10 d
Alternatives			
Cefuroxime (Ceftin)	500 mg bid	20 mg/kg divided bid	10 d
Cephalexin (Keflez)	500 mg bid	25–50 mg/kg divided bid	10 d
Azithromycin (Zithromax)	500 mg qd day 1 250 mg qd days 2–5	12 mg/kg qd	5 d
Clarithromycin (Biaxin)	250–500 mg bid	15 mg/kg divided bid	10 d
Clindamycin (Cleocin)*	600 mg/d in tid/qid	20 mg/kg divided tid	10 d
For Eradication of GABHS Carriage, or Symptomatic Persons with Recurrent Episodes of Pharyngitis Proven by Culture			
Clindamycin	See above doses	See above doses	10 d
Amoxicillin-clavulanate	500 mg bid	45 mg/kg qd divided bid–tid	10 d
Benzathine penicillin G	See above doses	See above doses	
Benzathine penicillin G IM and rifampin PO	See above doses 300 mg bid (for 4 d)	See above doses 20 mg/kg qd divided bid (for 4 d)	

*May also be effective for eradication of streptococcal carriage.
Abbreviation: GABHS = group A β-hemolytic streptococci.

established in older adolescents and adults. Penicillin V is preferable as an oral alternative, and 10 days of therapy is essential for eradication of GABHS. Because the total duration of therapy cannot be shortened, alternative regimens of twice-daily and once-daily dosing have been studied in an attempt to improve compliance. Decreasing the frequency to once daily is inadequate, although twice-daily regimens of 500 mg in adults achieve similar cure rates for GABHS pharyngitis as thrice-daily schedules.

In the vast majority of those treated with penicillin, clearance of GABHS is achieved, although a 15% to 20% bacteriologic failure rate, defined as an inability to eradicate a particular strain from the pharynx after completion of an antibiotic regimen, has been observed. Because GABHS pharyngitis is a self-limited disease in the absence of suppurative complications, the greatest importance of bacteriologic failure is its potential impact on the risk of ARF. In fact, determining true penicillin failure is difficult and can be confounded by a number of clinical scenarios in which posttreatment recovery of GABHS occurs, such as noncompliance, inclusion of streptococcal carriers, and reinfection of an index patient with another GABHS strain via a family member or close contact. With these caveats in mind, a variety of mechanisms for penicillin failure have been proposed. Previous antibiotic therapy may select for β-lactamase–producing organisms, termed copathogens (*S. aureus*, nontypable *H. influenzae*, *M. catarrhalis*, anaerobes), within the pharyngeal compartment, which then locally inactivate the penicillin before it encounters GABHS. Eradication of copathogens with β-lactam/β-lactamase inhibitor combinations (amoxicillin-clavulanate [Augmentin]), cephalosporins, or macrolides is one rationale for the success of these antibiotics in patients with penicillin failure, although this mechanism has not been well substantiated. Suppression of commensal streptococci during penicillin therapy may lead to enhanced attachment of GABHS to epithelial cells previously shielded by the oropharyngeal flora and a decrease in the concentration of species-specific streptococcal antimicrobial compounds that have anti-GABHS activity. Finally, GABHS eradication may be incomplete as a result of poor penetration of penicillin into deep regions of the exudative tonsillar tissue.

Amoxicillin (Amoxil) is an attractive alternative to penicillin for GABHS pharyngitis because it is more palatable to children, its absorption is not inhibited by food, and it has a longer serum half-life. In addition, amoxicillin has a narrower spectrum of antibacterial activity than amoxicillin-clavulanate, oral cephalosporins, or macrolides do and would presumably contribute less to inadvertent selection for resistance in the resident microbial flora, such as *Streptococcus pneumoniae*. Recently, amoxicillin given as a single daily dose for 10 days has been found to be comparable in efficacy to 10 days of penicillin. Although further studies are necessary, these favorable results suggest that amoxicillin may replace penicillin as the first-line drug for GABHS pharyngitis.

One notable disadvantage of amoxicillin is the potential for morbilliform rash in patients with an exudative pharyngitis caused by EBV infection rather than GABHS.

A number of oral cephalosporins (e.g., cephalexin [Keflex], cefuroxime axetil [Ceftin], cefaclor [Ceclor], cefixime [Suprax], cefdinir [Omnicef], and cefpodoxime [Vantin]) are at least equivalent to penicillin in the treatment of GABHS pharyngitis and may be considered as alternative agents after bacteriologic failure. It is currently unclear why they may have this apparent superior activity, but it is potentially due to resistance to β-lactamase–producing copathogens or greater bacterial clearance in streptococcal carriers, an effect documented with this antibiotic class. A first-generation cephalosporin such as cephalexin (Keflex) is an acceptable alternative for patients with penicillin hypersensitivity that is not type I (IgE mediated). It has a relatively narrow spectrum of activity and is reasonably priced. Other generations of oral cephalosporins have been advocated as first-line options for GABHS pharyngitis, although it should be underscored that these drugs have unnecessarily broad antimicrobial activities and can be prohibitively expensive. Treatment with amoxicillin-clavulanate also leads to satisfactory GABHS clearance rates, but the same aforementioned considerations apply.

GABHS is susceptible to a variety of macrolides and to lincosamides (e.g., clindamycin), but they should be reserved for patients with severe type I (IgE-mediated) hypersensitivity to penicillin. Selection of a macrolide antibiotic versus clindamycin should be based on local susceptibility data if available. Erythromycin and clarithromycin should be given for 10 days, whereas azithromycin is approved by the Food and Drug Administration for a shorter 5-day course. Erythromycin is not tolerated as well as azithromycin (Zithromax) and clarithromycin (Biaxin) because of significantly greater associated gastrointestinal side effects. Clindamycin (Cleocin) is also effective in eradicating GABHS from the pharynx, although patients may have a greater risk for the development of pseudomembranous colitis as an adverse event.

Another caveat is that overuse of macrolide antibiotics for the treatment of respiratory infections is associated with the selection of drug-resistant isolates. High rates of resistance are common in many parts of the world, and cross-resistance among macrolides does occur. Certain European and Asian regions have reported erythromycin resistance rates exceeding 50%. Finland reported an incidence of erythromycin resistance as high as 17%, which then diminished to 8.6% after prescription rates of macrolide antibiotics for respiratory infections decreased by 42%. In the United States, rates of erythromycin resistance have been reported between 2.6% and 5.1%. In one recent longitudinal surveillance study of school-aged children in Pittsburgh, an erythromycin resistance rate of 48% was reported during the 2000–2001 season.

Resistance to macrolides is mediated either by constitutively expressed or inducible ribosomal methylases, or by antibiotic efflux pumps (M phenotype). These methylases, usually ermA, ermB in GABHS, mediate macrolide, lincosamide (clindamycin), and streptogramin B resistance (MLS_B phenotype) by altering the common 23S ribosomal binding site for these antibiotic classes. The efflux pumps, usually mefA, mediate resistance to macrolide antibiotics, while remaining sensitive to clindamycin. Regional differences exist in the prevalence of GABHS resistance mechanisms conferring different local resistance patterns. For example, in some European countries, a greater proportion of erythromycin-resistant strains of GABHS have the MLS_B phenotype, while surveillance studies in other countries have found a more equal distribution of the MLS_B phenotype and the M phenotype. The mechanism of resistance that predominates in the Pittsburgh area is the efflux pump (M phenotype), which is more common in the United States than the rRNA methylases.

Tetracyclines should not be used for GABHS pharyngitis because of widespread resistance. Although sulfonamides are recommended for GABHS chemoprophylaxis, they are inadequate alone, and in combination with trimethoprim, for therapy because of high relapse rates.

Individuals who are asymptomatic after completing one of the aforementioned antibiotic regimens should not be routinely reassessed with a throat culture to determine whether bacteriologic failure has occurred. Notable exceptions are in patients with a personal or family history of ARF, during community outbreaks of ARF, and in families in which a recurrent cycle of pharyngitis is attributable to GABHS. If an individual has a resumption of symptoms after therapy and remains positive for GABHS on culture, a repeat antibiotic course should be administered with an alternative drug such as a first-generation cephalosporin (e.g., cephalexin) or a macrolide. If compliance is a central issue, one can consider a single dose of benzathine penicillin G or use azithromycin, which can be given in an abbreviated course. Household members and other contacts of the index case who are ill should also be treated only if either DAT or culture is positive. Routine assessment of asymptomatic contacts is not recommended unless the risk of significant complications in these individuals is high, but if either ARF or APSGN has developed in the index patient, all contacts who are positive by throat culture should be treated to eradicate streptococcal colonization.

Carriers asymptomatically harbor GABHS and typically do not mount an associated rise in antistreptococcal antibodies, although early antibiotic treatment in patients with true acute disease may also abrogate normal elevations in antibody titer. In addition, many streptococcal carriers may already have measurable titers from previous GABHS infections, thereby adding to the inaccuracy of serologic criteria. Carriers are not at greater risk for either suppurative or nonsuppurative sequelae associated with GABHS, nor are they likely to transmit this organism to others. The mechanisms for pharyngeal carriage are not well understood, and some evidence suggests that organisms may attain an immunologically privileged niche by invading the surface epithelium. For example, in vitro experiments reveal that certain GABHS strains associated with oropharyngeal carriage can avidly invade human epithelial cells and that tonsils excised from patients with recurrent GABHS disease may contain viable intracellular organisms. Presumably, escape from the nasopharyngeal microenvironment provides a haven against both antibiotics and the mucosal immune response.

Eradication of chronic streptococcal carriage is difficult to achieve, although it may be a priority in a variety of clinical scenarios, including GABHS or ARF outbreaks in a closed community (e.g., military barracks), individuals who have had ARF, patients with a diagnostic dilemma because of recurrent pharyngitis, or those in whom tonsillectomy is being considered. In these situations, a number of therapeutic options are available, such as benzathine penicillin G or penicillin V combined with rifampin (Rifadin),* or clindamycin or azithromycin as single agents. The success of these regimens is predicated on ensuring that no one else in the household is also a GABHS carrier. Although clearance can be achieved, it is not usually a fruitful endeavor because established carriers often acquire another GABHS strain at a later date.

*Not FDA approved for this indication.

Section 4

The Respiratory System

ACUTE RESPIRATORY FAILURE

method of
ROBERT L. BURNAUGH, M.D., and
JOHN W. BRICE, M.D.
Augusta VA Medical Center and the Medical College of Georgia
Augusta, Georgia

The fact that the first two components of the emergency resuscitation algorithm, "A-B-C," have to do with restoration of normal respiratory function (Airway, Breathing, Circulation) confirms the importance of pulmonary function in maintaining homeostasis. Acute respiratory failure can occur by two mechanisms—from either a derangement in the uptake of oxygen from the atmosphere into the arterial blood or from the elimination of carbon dioxide from venous blood back into the atmosphere. Although the presence of acute respiratory failure can be suspected from the clinical appearance of the patient, analysis of arterial blood gases (ABGs) is necessary to confirm the diagnosis and to sort out the primary cause of dysfunction as either oxygenation failure or ventilation failure. An arterial oxygen tension ($Pa{O_2}$) of less than 55 torr or an oxygen saturation ($Sa{O_2}$) of less than 90% suggests hypoxemic respiratory failure, and an arterial carbon dioxide tension ($Pa{CO_2}$) of greater than 50 torr (with an associated drop in pH) indicates hypercapnic respiratory failure. Like many pieces of data, ABGs are best interpreted by comparison with the patient's baseline. A $Pa{CO_2}$ of 60 torr might be normal for a patient with established chronic obstructive pulmonary disease (COPD). In such a case, the pH should be near normal and the plasma bicarbonate elevated, signifying renal compensation for a longstanding respiratory acidosis.

PHYSIOLOGY OF RESPIRATORY FAILURE

Gas Exchange

As ambient air is inhaled, it is saturated with water vapor. Water vapor takes up space and thus decreases the space available for inspired gases. Upon entering the alveolar spaces of the lung, inspired air is further diluted by CO_2 diffusing in from the pulmonary capillaries. When these two factors are subtracted the alveolar oxygen tension ($P_A{O_2}$) can be estimated using the alveolar gas equation:

$$P_A{O_2} = F_I{O_2}\,(P_B - P_W) - (Pa{CO_2}/R)$$

where $F_I{O_2}$ is the fraction of inspired oxygen, P_B is barometric pressure, P_W is the vapor pressure of water (47 torr at sea level), and R is the respiratory quotient (the ratio of CO_2 production to oxygen consumption).

Several assumptions are made in this equation. One is that $Pa{CO_2}$ equals alveolar carbon dioxide tension ($P_A{CO_2}$), which is probably very close to the truth, as CO_2 is a very soluble gas. We also assume that R is 0.8 and, although this is an acceptable generalization, it is almost never exactly the case. Therefore, if we were breathing ambient air at sea level (P_B = 760 torr), then

$$P_A{O_2} = 0.21\,(760 - 47) - (40/0.8) = 100 \text{ torr}$$

Unlike the case with CO_2, there is normally a gradient between $P_A{O_2}$ and $Pa{O_2}$. This is due to the relative insolubility of oxygen. This gradient, the $P(A\text{-}a)O_2$, is normally less than 10 torr in healthy young adults but rises to around 30 torr in old age. Therefore, the normal patient breathing ambient air at sea level has a $Pa{O_2}$ of around 90 torr. The $P(A\text{-}a)O_2$, often called the A-a gradient, is calculated by subtracting the $Pa{O_2}$ obtained by ABG measurement from the $P_A{O_2}$ calculated by the alveolar gas equation (discussed previously).

Because alveolar hypoventilation will cause $Pa{O_2}$ to rise, there will be an increase in $P_A{CO_2}$. This extra CO_2 in the alveolus will occupy additional space; therefore, there will be a proportional decrease in $P_A{O_2}$ and thus a decrease in $Pa{O_2}$. The calculation of the A-a gradient can help determine whether hypoxemia is due to hypoventilation and increasing CO_2 (normal A-a gradient) or due to an impairment of oxygenation (elevated A-a gradient).

Acute respiratory failure can occur from failure of the lung as ventilatory pump, causing hypercapnia, or from inadequate oxygenation of arterial blood. There are multiple etiologies of both mechanisms, and the clinical scenario of concomitant hypercapnia and hypoxemia is not uncommon. It is imperative to seek out and treat the root causes of both problems.

Hypoxemic Respiratory Failure

Any process that impairs the transfer of oxygen from the atmosphere into the capillary blood in the lungs can cause hypoxemia. Hypoxemia is generally defined as a PaO_2 of less than 55 torr and/or a hemoglobin oxygen saturation (SaO_2) of less than 90%. Hypoxemic respiratory failure is a condition that develops when an acceptable PaO_2 or SaO_2 cannot be maintained despite the provision of supplemental oxygen.

Factors that are external to the patient, such as low partial pressures of inspired oxygen (PIO_2), can be the cause of hypoxemic respiratory failure. Low PIO_2 can occur at high altitudes and can be clinically important in management of some patients. A person with underlying lung disease and a low, but acceptable, PaO_2 while living on the coastal plain may have problems with hypoxemia if he or she travels to mountainous areas. Air travel can also induce problems in the patient with marginal baseline oxygenation. Although newer aircraft are more efficient at maintaining cabin pressure, they also fly at higher altitudes, causing an even lower PIO_2.

In typical clinical settings, abnormalities in the ventilation-perfusion ($\dot{V}/\dot{Q}$) equilibrium of the lung are the most common reasons for hypoxemia. If the perfusion and ventilation of lung tissue are not matched, the effectiveness of the lung as a gas transfer device becomes impaired. The causes for abnormal $\dot{V}/\dot{Q}$ relationships are protean. Common causes are COPD, pneumonia, pulmonary embolism, cardiogenic pulmonary edema (e.g., congestive heart failure) and noncardiogenic pulmonary edema (e.g., the acute respiratory distress syndrome).

If an area of lung has no ventilation (a $\dot{V}/\dot{Q}$ ratio of zero), then a shunt is said to exist. When extensive enough, this can cause hypoxemia resistant to treatment by supplemental oxygen alone. Hypoxemia in a patient with shunt is caused by the admixture of deoxygenated venous blood from unventilated lung with oxygenated blood from normally functioning areas of lung parenchyma. This causes a substantial drop in the final O_2 content of the arterial blood. To understand this, we need to look at the formula for the oxygen content of blood:

$$\text{Oxygen content} = (1.36 \times \text{Hgb} \times SaO_2) + (PaO_2 \times 0.003)$$

where Hgb is hemoglobin concentration (in grams per dL). The factor of 1.36 is the amount of O_2 (in mL) that 1 gram of hemoglobin can carry when fully saturated. Multiplying this factor by the hemoglobin concentration and then by the measured oxygen saturation will yield the amount of O_2 bound to hemoglobin (in mL of oxygen per dL of blood). Only a small quantity of O_2 is carried dissolved in plasma, due to the relative insolubility of oxygen (0.0031 mL per torr of oxygen tension). Shunted blood does not come into contact with any ventilated lung tissue, therefore an increase in FIO_2 will not affect its oxygen content. The blood leaving normal lung is already fully saturated, and an increase in FIO_2, while raising the PaO_2, will not significantly change the oxygen content.

Intrapulmonary shunt is common in patients with the acute respiratory distress syndrome (ARDS) and may rarely be due to pulmonary arteriovenous malformations. Extrapulmonary shunts do occur, as in atrial or ventricular septal defects, but these do not cause hypoxemia until right-sided pressures become so high that the shunt becomes right to left instead of left to right.

The inability of blood to reach equilibrium with the alveolar gases during its trek through the pulmonary vasculature can also cause hypoxemia. Normally the lung is quite efficient in this regard. Equilibration generally occurs in the pulmonary capillary bed with time to spare. Processes that cause thickening of the alveolar capillary membrane can reduce the efficiency of gas exchange. These processes can be inflammatory in nature, such as the interstitial pneumonias, or fibrotic processes, such as asbestosis. Interstitial edema from any cause will also impair diffusion. A reduction in the red cell transit time through the lung may also prevent full equilibration. This reduction must be relatively profound to have a noticeable effect and is generally not clinically important except in patients with widespread destruction of lung tissue and therefore a markedly reduced capillary bed or in cases of dramatically increased cardiac output. Some experts have postulated that a profound reduction in mixed venous oxygen content can be responsible for inadequate diffusion equilibrium.

As discussed earlier, alveolar hypoventilation can cause hypoxemia in the absence of other lung pathology by reducing the PAO_2, a pattern easily discerned by obtaining ABGs and calculating the A-a gradient, which will be normal if alveolar hypoventilation is the sole cause of hypoxemia. In addition to the aforementioned causes, hypoxemia can also be induced by excessive intrapulmonary oxygen consumption by leukocytes present in lung tissue in cases of severe pulmonary inflammation.

Hypercapnic Respiratory Failure

The level of CO_2 in arterial blood is very strictly maintained at 40 torr in healthy subjects. The hallmark of hypercapnic respiratory failure is an increasing PaO_2 and a decreasing pH. It is important to remember that patients with a chronic respiratory acidosis (e.g., patients with severe but stable COPD) will have a chronic elevation of PaO_2 but the pH will be normal by virtue of renal compensation. If a patient has had an ABG in the past (while stable), it is invaluable in determining what is normal for that patient. Overcorrection of PaO_2 is a common mistake in the treatment of COPD patients and can be avoided by working towards a normal pH instead of a PaO_2 of 40 torr in these cases.

Any factor that causes acute CO_2 retention can lead to hypercapnic respiratory failure. Reduced ventilatory drive is one cause of CO_2 retention. Causes of a reduced drive include drug overdoses (particularly narcotics or sedatives), trauma to or infarction of the mid or lower medulla, profound hypothyroidism, chronic malnutrition, and severe metabolic acidosis. Neuromuscular diseases (such as the muscular dystrophies, Guillain-Barré syndrome, myasthenia gravis, and amyotrophic lateral sclerosis) impair the function of the respiratory musculature even though respiratory drive is normal. Aminoglycosides and calcium channel blockers are weak neuromuscular blockers. This is rarely of clinical importance, but occasionally the failure of a patient to wean from mechanical ventilation is secondary to these drugs. Spinal cord injury in or above the thoracic levels can also lead to ventilatory pump failure.

Electrolyte imbalances, particularly hypophosphatemia, can cause dysfunction of respiratory muscles. Actual muscle atrophy can result from malnutrition and from disuse (as might occur with prolonged ventilatory support). Corticosteroid administration has also been associated with muscle weakness and atrophy.

Increased workloads from mechanical factors, however, are the most common cause of hypercapnic respiratory failure. These loads can be divided into four categories: inertial loads, threshold loads, resistive loads, and elastic loads. *Inertial loads* are imposed by the inertia of the respired gases themselves. The amount of work required to initiate or stop airflow is not generally of clinical importance. *Threshold loads* result from the prevention of air movement until a given pressure is obtained. These types of loads are sometimes intentionally applied to patients undergoing pulmonary rehabilitation. Threshold loads are often inadvertently imposed on patients being mechanically ventilated for respiratory failure if modes are used that require the patient to activate demand valves. This is frequently seen in older mechanical ventilators. Outside of such areas, threshold loads are not often significant.

Resistive loads, on the other hand, are quite clinically important and easy to understand. Fatigue from the increased resistive loads associated with obstructed airways, such as in COPD and asthma, is a common clinical scenario. *Elastic loads* are as important clinically as resistive loads. These are the result of abnormal pressure-volume relationships. Increased elastic loads are easy to see in patients with disease processes that cause stiff lungs, such as interstitial fibrosis and pulmonary edema. The work required to expand such stiff lungs is significantly higher than normal. In cases of kyphoscoliosis, the chest wall compliance is reduced, causing similar workload increases. What is less intuitively obvious is that elastic loads can be a problem in the patient with COPD. We are familiar with the idea that, from a pathologic sense, the lungs of a COPD patient are more compliant than normal. That is, a given amount of pressure will distend emphysematous lungs to a greater degree than it will normal lungs. This leads one to believe that elastic loads should be less in this setting. This would be true at low lung volumes; however, because of the loss of elastic recoil in the lung, these patients have hyperinflated lungs and their tidal breathing may be at volumes very near total lung capacity (TLC). Compliance is related to lung volume and at high volumes the compliance of the lung is actually quite low, and thus, the imposed elastic loads may contribute as much to the development of fatigue and respiratory failure as do resistive loads.

The $\dot{V}/\dot{Q}$ abnormalities discussed earlier can cause impairment to CO_2 excretion as well as O_2 uptake. Despite this, hypercapnia does not often result from $\dot{V}/\dot{Q}$ mismatch alone. This is due to the tight central control of Pa_{O_2}. Chemoreceptors respond to an increase in Pa_{O_2} by increasing minute ventilation, which stabilizes Pa_{O_2} but increases ventilation of nonperfused lung, often referred to as "wasted ventilation." If such compensatory mechanisms are pushed to their limits, fatigue and hypercapnia can occur.

Increased CO_2 production can be another cause of hypercapnia. High loads of carbohydrates will cause elevation of R values. While usually clinically unimportant, this can cause problems in the patient teetering on the verge of respiratory failure.

MANAGEMENT OF ACUTE RESPIRATORY FAILURE

Hypoxemic Respiratory Failure

Correction of the underlying cause is the treatment of choice in dealing with hypoxemia; however, the results of such treatment may take days or even weeks. In this interval, it is imperative that the oxygen content of arterial blood and the delivery of that oxygen to tissues be maintained at adequate levels. Supplemental oxygen can be provided by a variety of methods. Most simply, a nasal cannula can be utilized to deliver oxygen flows of 0.5 to 5 L per minute; however, F_{IO_2} is not precisely controlled. The minute ventilation of the patient will determine the actual F_{IO_2}. Minute ventilation is defined as the tidal volume multiplied by the respiratory rate. As minute ventilation rises, the supplemental O_2 provided will account for a lesser percentage of the total volume of ventilation, and, therefore, the F_{IO_2} will be less than expected.

Venturi masks produce a more reliable F_{IO_2} (ranging from 0.24 to 0.50); however, the higher one pushes the F_{IO_2} using a Venturi system, the lower the total produced gas flow will become. This will allow tachypneic patients to entrain a significant amount of room air around the mask, diluting the mixture and decreasing the F_{IO_2}. Aerosol units that connect directly to wall oxygen supply can generate a F_{IO_2} of up to 1.0, but such systems also produce lower flows as F_{IO_2} is increased. If a concentration of 50% or higher of oxygen is required, it is best to use two aerosol units and connect them both to the patient with a Y connector in order to produce flow rates that will match the patient's inspiratory flow rate.

Tight-fitting masks with reservoir bags and nonrebreathing valves can be used to approximate a F_{IO_2} of 1.0, but are generally not well tolerated by the patient. In addition, most commercially available nonrebreather masks have one of the exhalation ports open. This is done to prevent suffocation should the oxygen source become disconnected, but it allows significant entrainment of room air. A patient with hypoxemia that cannot be improved by a FIO_2 of less than 0.6 should be considered for intubation and mechanical ventilation, unless she or he has a process that can be easily reversed (e.g., congestive heart failure responsive to diuretics).

Noninvasive ventilation, employing cushioned masks held in place by specially designed straps, is a modality using bilevel positive airway pressure (BiPAP) to improve oxygenation without resorting to intubation. Patient tolerance and highly motivated nurses and respiratory therapists are essential to the success of this maneuver. Pulmonary medicine consultation is advised when considering noninvasive ventilation.

Hypercapnic Respiratory Failure

Hypercapnic respiratory failure from overdoses of narcotics and benzodiazepines is easily reversed by naloxone (Narcan) and flumazenil (Romazicon), respectively. Other overdoses may be problematic due to the lack of specific reversal agents. Mechanical ventilatory support may be required until respiratory depression resolves.

Respiratory failure caused by obstructive lung diseases (e.g., asthma and COPD) is a very common problem. In the COPD patient, mechanical ventilation is not required as long as the patient is reasonably oriented, hemodynamically stable, and able to protect his airway. Initial ABGs may look fairly horrendous, but a significant number of these patients can be managed without mechanical ventilation. Aggressive therapy should include:

1. Aerosolized β-agonists such as metaproterenol (Alupent) or albuterol (Proventil, Ventolin)
2. Aerosolized anticholinergics such as ipratropium (Atrovent)
3. Oxygen therapy as indicated
4. Intravenous methylprednisolone (Solu-Medrol) 125 mg intravenously, followed by 40 mg four times a day
5. Appropriate antibiotics for any respiratory infection
6. Vigorous pulmonary toilet, including chest physiotherapy if the patient cannot clear sputum.

Oxygen therapy must be applied thoughtfully in these patients but it is mandatory if the patient is hypoxemic. Supplemental O_2 can increase alveolar oxygen tensions in poorly ventilated areas of the lung, reducing autoregulation of blood flow away from these areas. The worsening $\dot{V}/\dot{Q}$ mismatch that results is the most important mechanism of worsening hypercapnia caused by O_2 therapy. The worry over increasing PaO_2 should *never* prevent the utilization of oxygen in a hypoxemic patient. If the hypercapnia and acidosis that result from reasonable O_2 therapy is too severe, then intubation and mechanical ventilation are required.

Intravenous aminophylline* has fallen out of favor with many physicians; however, it may still be a useful drug in some COPD patients with hypercapnic respiratory failure. Loading doses of aminophylline are no longer recommended. A continuous drip of 0.3–0.5 mg/kg/h is a reasonable starting point. Serum drug levels must be monitored closely. The therapeutic range should be 8–12 μg/mL. The mechanism of action of aminophylline is not known, and its bronchodilator action is minimal; however, it may act as a significant diaphragmatic inotrope. There is even some evidence that it may have an immune modulating effect.

Recent studies suggest that corticosteroid use reduces recovery time and hospital length of stay in COPD exacerbations. "Steroids are good unless they are bad," is an aphorism that should be in everyone's handbook of critical care medicine and one must be alert to the complications and contraindications of these agents whenever they are administered.

The management of refractory asthma leading to respiratory failure (status asthmaticus) is similar to that of COPD with several exceptions. The role of corticosteroids in this area is much clearer. Intravenous methylprednisolone (Solu-Medrol), in a dose of 125 mg (or equivalent) should be given as soon as possible and followed by 40 mg every 6 hours. Aminophylline is less likely to be of benefit, and β-agonists should be dosed as frequently as possible without inducing cardiac or other side effects.

In the usual asthma attack, hypocapnia is the rule. If an asthmatic in distress becomes hypercapnic, it may be a sign of impending respiratory failure. Although not all such patients will require intubation, the equipment and personnel should be standing by so intubation can be accomplished without delay if it becomes necessary. After being intubated, patients in status asthmaticus can be very difficult to manage because of very high peak inspiratory pressures. Heavy sedation and neuromuscular blockade are sometimes necessary. Recently, a new way of ventilating status asthmaticus patients has been investigated. Permissive hypercapnia uses lower pressures and accepts the hypercapnia and acidosis (which can be quite severe) that result. With vigorous therapy, these patients improve quickly and apparently tolerate the acidosis with fewer side effects than seen with the high peak pressures imposed by more standard therapy. Indeed a recent National Institutes of Health–sponsored study investigating permissive hypercapnia was halted early because of the lower mortality of critically ill mechanically ventilated patients who were exposed to lower positive pressure and lower volumes while on the ventilator. Tidal volume in the range of 5–10 mL/kg was used even if significant respiratory acidosis occurred in an effort to reduce barotrauma and volume trauma. Respiratory acidosis was permitted without correction as long pH remained above 7.20 with no apparent ill effect.

Respiratory failure from neuromuscular disease can create an ethical quagmire. Patients with the potential for developing irreversible respiratory failure should be queried about their desires for long-term life support measures before such measures

*Not FDA approved for this indication.

become necessary. If the episode of respiratory failure is due to an exacerbation of some other reversible process, then the use of BiPAP in a timed or synchronized mode can obviate the need for mechanical ventilation in some cases. BiPAP applies a higher pressure to the airway during inspiration and a lower pressure during expiration, creating a gradient and thus, airflow. It can be applied using a nasal mask identical to ones used for nasal continuous positive airway pressure (CPAP).

Mechanical Ventilation

Patients who have hypoxemia or hypercapnia (or both) who fail noninvasive therapy or who become unstable are candidates for mechanical ventilatory support. The ideal candidate for mechanical ventilation is someone with severe but reversible disease. Patients who develop respiratory failure as the terminal event in the natural history of their disease process should not be automatically intubated and supported. Time spent educating patients and their families on what to expect from any given disease process can prevent a great deal of unnecessary suffering as death approaches.

The goal of mechanical ventilation in acute respiratory failure is to return the patient to a stable condition with the minimum amount of nonphysiologic intervention. Remember, positive pressure ventilation is, by its very nature, nonphysiologic. The $Pa{O_2}$ should be kept above 60 torr and the $Sa{O_2}$ above 90%. There is no advantage to raising the $Pa{O_2}$ to abnormally high levels. The pH may be permitted to slowly decline (as discussed previously) in an effort to avoid parenchymal damage to the lung, though a value in the range of 7.35 to 7.45 is preferable.

Ventilator Modes and Settings

When treating acute respiratory failure, it is best to use a mode of ventilation in which all of a patient's attempts to breathe are fully supported. This goal can be accomplished in the majority of cases with assist/control mode ventilation (A/C), a mode that is relatively easy to understand and set. In the emergency situation, the $F{IO_2}$ should always be set at 1.0 and then adjusted down as quickly as clinically prudent. The short-term goal should be to get the patient to 60% or lower while maintaining adequate oxygenation. The tidal volume should be initially set between 5 and 10 mL/kg of ideal body weight and then adjusted based on the results of ABG analysis and peak airway pressure. If the patient is at risk of developing ARDS, then a lower tidal volume should be selected. If a patient has an alveolar filling process (e.g., pneumonia or pulmonary edema), a "normal" tidal volume might result in overdistention of otherwise normal alveoli. Such volume trauma has been identified as a major cause of ARDS. Use of lower tidal volumes can improve outcomes in critically ill patients on mechanical ventilation.

In A/C, the respiratory rate set will act as a backup if the patient's spontaneous rate falls. The rate should be set at a level that will assure that the patient receives an adequate minute ventilation. Remember, some acutely ill patients will require a dramatically increased minute ventilation. If a patient becomes suddenly more tachypneic, A/C, if set properly, will be able to keep up with patient demands.

The peak inspiratory flow rate is generally set between 60 and 80 L/min, but patients who are very tachypneic may require flow rates as high as 120 L/min. If high flow rates are used, they must be reduced as the patient improves and respiratory demands decrease. Dangerously high peak airway pressures can occur from inappropriately high flow rates. Some ventilators are time-cycled rather than volume-cycled and, because of this, have no independently controllable flow rate. To obtain an increased flow rate on such a machine, the inspiratory time can be decreased (less time for inspiration equals higher inspiratory flow rates) and the back-up rate can be adjusted closer to the actual respiratory rate.

The addition of a small amount (2 to 4 cm H_2O) of positive end-expiratory pressure (PEEP) has been shown to reduce the work of breathing. It is felt that this prevents microatelectasis and therefore reduces the shear forces caused by reopening collapsed alveoli. It will also keep COPD patients at a more favorable place on the Starling curve for their respiratory musculature by keeping them at a better functional residual capacity.

Higher levels of PEEP may be needed in patients with diffuse lung disease and refractory hypoxemia (e.g., ARDS). In such instances, PEEP can be increased slowly (in 2 to 3 cm H_2O increments) up to a maximum of 15 to 20 cm H_2O. If a PEEP of above 5 cm H_2O is required, a pulmonary artery catheter is useful to monitor cardiac output and mixed venous blood gases. As PEEP is increased, the intrathoracic pressure increases, and this may impede venous return to the heart. The result may be an improved $Pa{O_2}$ but decreased O_2 delivery to tissue due to impairment of cardiac output.

PEEP should not be used to treat focal processes because of the risk of hyperinflation of normal lung tissue and iatrogenic lung injury.

If peak inspiratory pressures exceed 40 to 45 cm H_2O or if a PEEP of above 15 to 20 cm H_2O is needed to oxygenate the patient, the risk of barotrauma and iatrogenic lung injury increases. Pressure-controlled ventilation (PC) can be used in this circumstance. PC functions very similarly to A/C, except an inspiratory pressure is set instead of a volume, and the machine cycles off when the set inspiratory time elapses rather than when a given volume is achieved. Damage from excessive pressures is less likely in this mode of ventilation, but delivered tidal volume becomes a variable. Close attention must be given to any patient on pressure-cycled ventilation. Analysis of pressure-volume waveforms can also help reduce the risk of air trapping and auto-PEEP, a potentially fatal complication. To obtain adequate ventilation in severe ARDS patients, PC can be used with the inspiratory to expiratory (I:E) ratio inverted; however, this is very nonphysiologic and requires sedation and usually use of nondepolarizing neuromuscular blockers to paralyze skeletal muscles. Consultation with an experienced intensivist is needed for such circumstances.

There continues to be a trend to use intermittent mandatory ventilation (IMV) with pressure support (PS) in patients presenting with acute respiratory failure. IMV gives a set number of ventilator-supported breaths per minute and allows all additional breaths to be spontaneous (with no ventilator support). When pressure support is used with IMV, all the spontaneous breaths are then supported by an applied pressure. While this method can certainly be used to ventilate a patient in respiratory failure, the variables that exist are much more complex, and it requires unfailing attention to detail. There are no data to show superiority of this to more standard modes of ventilation. Many other modes of ventilation exist and have very legitimate uses but are beyond the scope of this text.

Weaning from Mechanical Ventilation

The first question to be answered here is "Does the patient really need to be weaned?" Many patients intubated for respiratory failure can be simply extubated after the underlying pathology has been corrected. If the patient truly needs to be weaned from mechanical ventilation, then the question is more difficult. There is no consensus on how to wean. The medical literature has not been helpful—in fact, it is contradictory. There is no firm evidence that any method is superior to any other. Randomized, controlled trials have show intermittent T-tube trials and pressure support trials to be efficacious. These studies have consistently shown IMV to be less useful as a weaning tool.

Our approach is to place patients on a PS that will deliver a tidal volume of about 7 to 10 mL per kg of ideal body weight. The required PS level must be determined by close bedside observation of the patient. We do not use an IMV backup. If the patient is not breathing spontaneously, he or she is not a candidate to be weaned from support. We rest the patient regularly on A/C and slowly extend the time he or she is on PS and also slowly decrease the level of PS. Always rest the patient at night. Stressing a patient at night tends to cause undue agitation. After the patient can tolerate a PS of 8 to 10 cm H_2O, we attempt extubation.

Best results from weaning can probably be obtained by a consistent, thoughtful approach. If respiratory therapists and ICU nurses know what to expect and what to look for, the success rate will be higher, no matter what method is used. Appropriate psychologic support of the patient is often neglected. Weaning is very stressful. Frequent physician-patient and staff-patient interactions will assist the process.

ATELECTASIS

method of
MICHAEL B. GOTWAY, M.D.
University of California, San Francisco
San Francisco General Hospital
San Francisco, California

Atelectasis is diminished gas within the lung associated with reduced lung volume. Atelectasis is common in hospitalized patients, and may result in significant hypoxemia from ventilation-perfusion mismatching. Many conditions result in atelectasis, including bronchial obstruction, impaired diaphragmatic excursion (often the result of diaphragmatic paralysis or ascites), airway diseases, and pulmonary embolism, among others. Mechanisms that produce atelectasis may be classified into four different types: relaxation, resorption, adhesive, and cicatrization atelectasis (Table 1).

Relaxation atelectasis results from the presence of space-occupying conditions within the thorax, such as pleural effusion or pneumothorax. Normally, elastic recoil causes the lung to have a natural tendency to collapse, which is counteracted by the chest wall's natural tendency to expand. When a space-occupying process is present within the thorax, the lung retracts and relaxation atelectasis results. A mild form of relaxation atelectasis is commonly seen in the dependent lung regions in patients undergoing thoracic computed tomography.

Resorption atelectasis results from the resorption of gas from alveoli in the presence of bronchial obstruction. Collateral ventilation may limit the development of resorption atelectasis by allowing gas to move from ventilated to obstructed alveoli.

Adhesive atelectasis results from surfactant deficiency. Pulmonary surfactant diminishes surface tension within alveoli, allowing alveoli to remain patent at lower volumes. Conditions depleting pulmonary surfactant, including infantile respiratory distress syndrome, acute radiation pneumonitis, pneumonia, and pulmonary embolism, among other causes, promote development of adhesive atelectasis. Prolonged ventilation at low lung volumes, as in postsurgical patients, also promotes adhesive atelectasis. In this situation, adhesive atelectasis may cause significant hypoxemia through arteriovenous shunting, even in the presence of normal-appearing chest radiography.

Cicatrization atelectasis represents pulmonary parenchymal contraction resulting from localized or diffuse lung fibrosis. Localized lung fibrosis, as occurs after granulomatous infections, produces increased pulmonary elastic recoil, resulting in diminished pulmonary volume in the area of scarring. Diffuse cicatrization atelectasis is most frequently seen in patients with idiopathic pulmonary fibrosis, and manifests as diaphragmatic elevation with an overall diminished lung size.

Clinically, atelectasis may be asymptomatic, or the patient may be dyspneic and hypoxemic due to

TABLE 1. **Atelectasis: Etiologies by Mechanisms**

Relaxation	Resorption	Adhesive	Cicatrization
Pleural effusion	Mucous plug	Infantile respiratory distress syndrome	Old granulomatous infection
Pneumothorax	Endobronchial neoplasm	Adult respiratory distress syndrome	Chronic radiation fibrosis
Pulmonary mass	Aspirated foreign body	Pneumonia	Idiopathic pulmonary fibrosis
Mediastinal mass	Bronchial compression (lymphadenopathy, mass)	Pulmonary embolism	Stage IV sarcoidosis
Round atelectasis	Endotracheal tube malposition	Prolonged shallow breathing	
Dependent atelectasis	Blood clot	Toxic inhalation	
	Bronchial stricture	Acute radiation pneumonitis	

arteriovenous shunting. Patients may also experience cough because of activation of vagal stretch receptors in the lung. Low-grade fever is common, particularly in postsurgical patients. Tachypnea and tachycardia may occur if the atelectasis occurs abruptly. Physical examination may reveal dullness to percussion, egophony, decreased breath sounds, and elevation of the diaphragm. Arterial blood gas measurements may show hypoxemia and hypocapnia.

Radiographic patterns of atelectasis may be divided into complete lung collapse, lobar or segmental collapse, subsegmental ("plate-like") atelectasis, round atelectasis, or generalized atelectasis.

Round atelectasis is a distinctive form of atelectasis appearing as a rounded, subpleural opacity associated with pleural thickening, commonly within the lower lobes. Characteristically, bronchovascular bundles may be identified curving into the area of atelectasis, representing the so-called "comet tail" sign; this finding is most easily appreciated with computed tomography. Round atelectasis usually occurs in the setting of asbestos-related pleural disease, but may also be seen following tuberculous effusions, other infections, congestive heart failure, and pulmonary infarction. Round atelectasis is a form of relaxation atelectasis.

Radiographic signs of atelectasis may be divided into direct and indirect signs. Direct signs include displacement of interlobar fissures and crowding of bronchovascular bundles. Indirect atelectasis findings include locally increased opacity and compensatory mechanisms, such as mediastinal shift and tracheal deviation towards the side of atelectasis, elevation of the diaphragm, displacement of the hila, and compensatory hyperinflation of adjacent alveoli.

Prevention of atelectasis centers on achieving proper inspiratory effort and clearing pulmonary secretions. Postsurgical patients require adequate pain control, induced coughing, incentive spirometry every 2 to 4 hours as tolerated, periodic deep breathing, and mobilization. Occasionally bronchodilators such as albuterol (Proventil), 1.25 to 2.5 mg nebulized every 4 to 8 hours, may be useful. Chest physiotherapy may be used to stimulate secretion drainage and coughing. Intermittent positive-pressure breathing may be used to treat atelectasis, although this technique may produce gastric distention. Sterile catheter nasotracheal aspiration has been used to treat atelectasis, but may cause nasopharyngeal floral contamination of the lower airway, and is therefore not routinely recommended.

When routine measures fail to clear atelectasis, or secretions are too copious or thick to clear with conservative methods, fiberoptic bronchoscopy may be performed. Bronchoscopy may be performed earlier in critically ill patients who have little respiratory reserve, or when total lung atelectasis is present.

Atelectasis may cause significant hypoxemia, and should prompt a search for underlying causes. Risk factor identification is key to prevention, and initial treatment is conservative, but bronchoscopy may be required in refractory cases.

MANAGEMENT OF CHRONIC OBSTRUCTIVE PULMONARY DISEASE

method of
MITCHELL FRIEDMAN, M.D.
Tulane University Health Sciences Center
New Orleans, Louisiana

Chronic obstructive pulmonary disease (COPD) is a chronic disorder characterized by progressive ventilatory impairment, airway hyperreactivity, and partial reversibility to inhaled bronchodilators. Chronic bronchitis is clinically defined by the presence of cough and sputum production for at least 3 months in each of 2 consecutive years. Emphysema is a pathologic term that describes destruction of the gas-exchanging (i.e., alveolar surfaces) of the lung. Previous definitions of COPD have emphasized the terms "emphysema" and "chronic bronchitis," which are no longer included in the definition of COPD. The latest working definition of COPD was developed by the Global Initiative for Chronic Obstructive Lung Disease (GOLD, www.goldcopd.com) and defined as a disease state characterized by airflow limitation that is not fully reversible. The airflow limitation in COPD is progressive and associated with an abnormal inflammatory response throughout the airways, parenchyma, and pulmonary vasculature of the lungs to noxious particles or gases. The inflammation in COPD is characterized by an increase in neutrophils, macrophages, and T lymphocytes (especially $CD8^+$) in various parts of the lung. The predominant cytokine and chemokine mediators associated with COPD include TNF-α, IL-8, LTB4, and IL-1β and interferon γ. The chronic airflow limitation in COPD is due to a combination of small airway disease (obstructive bronchiolitis) and parenchymal destruction (emphysema). Chronic inflammation causes remodeling and narrowing of the small airways. The inflammatory response in COPD is markedly different from that in asthma. However, some patients with COPD also have asthma, and the inflammation in their lungs may show characteristics of both diseases. In addition to inflammation, an imbalance between proteinases and antiproteinases leads to destruction of the lung parenchyma, resulting in the loss of alveolar attachments to the small airways and decreases lung elastic recoil. These changes diminish the ability of the airways to remain open during expiration. Symptoms, functional abnormalities, and complications of COPD can all be explained on the basis on the underlying inflammation and the resulting pathology.

In the United States, COPD affects more than 16 million individuals and is the fourth leading cause of death behind cardiovascular disease, cancer, and cerebral vascular disease. More importantly, of these four disease groups, COPD is the one that continues to increase in prevalence. COPD has traditionally been thought of as a disease of the elderly, but data from the National Ambulatory Medical Care Survey demonstrated that approximately 70% of COPD patients were under the age of 65 and they consumed 67% of total COPD office visits and 43% of all hospitalizations. Thus COPD significantly affects the working age population. The high morbidity of this disease is demonstrated by the estimated 14 million office visits and 500,000 hospitalizations each year. The total economic impact of COPD in the United States in 1993 estimated to be more than $15.5 billion with office visits, hospitalization visits, and emergency department visits accounting for 17.3% of these direct costs.

The major environmental factors are tobacco smoke, occupational dusts and chemicals (vapors, irritants, fumes), and indoor and outdoor air pollution. Cigarette smoking is by far the most important risk factor for COPD, accounting for 80% to 90% of COPD. Cigarette smokers have a higher prevalence of respiratory symptoms and lung function abnormalities, a greater annual rate of decline in forced expiratory volume in 1 second (FEV_1), and a greater COPD mortality rate than nonsmokers. These differences between cigarette smokers and nonsmokers increase in direct proportion to the quantity of smoking. Age of starting to smoke, total pack-years smoked, and current smoking status are predictive of COPD mortality. The role of gender as a risk factor for COPD remains unclear. Recent studies show that the prevalence of the disease is almost equal in men and women, which probably reflects changing patterns of tobacco smoking. Some studies have in fact suggested that women are more susceptible to the effects of tobacco smoke than men. The death rate from COPD in women recently exceeded that in men in the United States. Pipe and cigar smokers have greater COPD morbidity and mortality rates than nonsmokers, although their rates are lower than those for cigarette smokers.

However, not all smokers develop clinically significant COPD. Although it is unclear what percentage of smokers develop the disease, the commonly cited figure is that 15% to 20% of cigarette smokers develop COPD. This percentage may be an underestimate because COPD is both underdiagnosed and underappreciated. Several family studies and case-control studies in twins have supported the hypothesis that there are genetic factors associated with the development of COPD. Recently it has been shown that the risk of development of COPD is increased in first-degree relatives of patients with COPD. Several potential candidate genes have been suggested that might predispose a cigarette smoker to the development of COPD. These include anti-elastase polymorphisms, gene polymorphisms of proinflammatory cytokines such as TNF-α and IL-1β, and antioxidant gene polymorphisms. A number of studies are now being undertaken to understand this more fully and it is likely that these studies will identify the genetic polymorphisms responsible for COPD and lead to identification of at-risk individuals and targets therapeutic interventions. Severe alpha antitrypsin deficiency is the only proven genetic risk factor in COPD.

The characteristic symptoms of COPD are cough, sputum production, and dyspnea on exertion. COPD has a variable natural history and not all individuals follow the same course. Chronic cough and sputum production often precede the development of airflow limitation, although not all individuals with cough and sputum production go on to develop COPD. Though an important part of patient care, a physical examination is rarely diagnostic in COPD and physical signs are usually not present until significant impairment of lung function has occurred. On auscultation of the lungs, patients with COPD often have reduced breath sounds, but this finding is not sufficiently characteristic to make the diagnosis. Wheezing during quiet breathing can be used to identify airflow limitation but wheezing heard only after forced expiration is of no diagnostic value. Common chest wall abnormalities, indicative of lung hyperinflation, include relatively horizontal ribs, "barrel-shaped" chest, and protruding abdomen. Detection of the heart apex beat and auscultation of heart sounds may be difficult due to pulmonary hyperinflation. Hyperinflation also leads to downward displacement of the liver and an increase in the ability to palpate the liver. In severe COPD, patients may demonstrate pursed-lip breathing and ankle or lower leg edema (a sign of right-sided heart failure).

The diagnosis of COPD is confirmed by spirometry. The presence of a postbronchodilator FEV_1 <80% of the predicted value or an FEV_1/forced vital capacity

(FVC) <70% confirms the presence of airflow limitation. A low peak flow is consistent with COPD but, in general, peak flow improvements are relatively small, compared with other diseases such as asthma. The progression of COPD is best tracked by periodic spirometry measurements (e.g., once a year or if there is a substantial increase in symptoms or complications). However, the management of COPD is largely symptom driven, and there is only an imperfect relationship between the degree of airflow limitation and the presence of symptoms. Other pulmonary function tests, such as flow-volume loops, diffusing capacity measurements, and lung volume measurements are not routinely necessary but can provide information in understanding of symptoms such as exercise intolerance as well as allowing for assessment of patients for surgery. Chest radiographs are seldom diagnostic early in COPD unless obvious bullous disease is present. Radiologic changes include flattened hemidiaphragms, increased retrosternal air space volume, hyperlucency of the lungs, and rapid tapering of the vascular markings. High resolution CT scanning might help in the differential diagnosis. In severe COPD, measurement of arterial blood gases is important.

There is a new classification of severity system proposed for COPD by the GOLD committee. The disease severity was divided into four stages. The staging is based on airflow limitation as measured by spirometry, which is essential for diagnosis and provides a useful description of the severity of pathological changes in COPD, as well as symptoms. The use of symptoms to help define COPD allows for the identification of those at risk for COPD and intervention at an early stage of the disease when the disease is not yet a health problem. The stages are:

Stage 0: At Risk—Characterized by chronic cough and sputum production. Lung function, as measured by spirometry, is still normal.

Stage I: Mild COPD—Characterized by mild airflow limitation (FEV_1/FVC <70% but FEV_1 >80% predicted) and usually, but not always, by chronic cough and sputum production.

Stage II: Moderate COPD—Characterized by worsening airflow limitation (30% <FEV_1 <80% predicted), and usually the progression of symptoms with shortness of breath typically developing on exertion. This is the stage at which patients typically seek medical attention because of dyspnea or an exacerbation of their disease. The division into stages IIA (<80% FEV_1 >50%) and IIB (<50% FEV_1 >30%) is based on the fact that exacerbations are especially seen in patients with an FEV_1 below 50% predicted.

Stage III: Severe COPD—Characterized by severe airflow limitation (FEV_1 <30% predicted) or the presence of respiratory failure or clinical signs of right-sided heart failure. Respiratory failure is defined as an arterial partial pressure of oxygen ($Pa{O_2}$) <60 mm Hg with or without arterial partial pressure of CO_2 ($Pa{CO_2}$) >50 mm Hg while breathing air at sea level. Respiratory failure may also lead to effects on the heart such as cor pulmonale (right-sided heart failure) Patients may have severe (Stage III) COPD even if the FEV_1 is >30% predicted, whenever these complications are present.

The main symptoms among patients in Stage 0 and Stage I are chronic cough and sputum production. These symptoms can be present for many years before the development of airflow limitation and are often ignored or discounted by patients. As airflow limitation develops in Stage II, patients often experience dyspnea, which may interfere with their daily activities. This is the stage at which they seek medical attention. However, some patients do not see a physician, unless the disease is being screened, until the airflow limitation worsens and the patient enters Stage III.

The general guidelines to management of COPD include the avoidance of risk factors to prevent disease progression and pharmacotherapy as needed to control symptoms. In addition, patient education including counseling about smoking cessation, instruction in physical exercise, nutritional advice are necessary components of a comprehensive COPD management plan. The goals of management are to relieve symptoms, increase exercise tolerance, improve quality of life, prevent and treat complications, and decrease disease progression.

Smoking cessation is the only intervention that has been shown to reduce the risk of developing COPD as well as stopping the progression of COPD. Smoking cessation measures include dependence counseling, nicotine replacement therapy, and antidepressants. Exclusive of smoking cessation, none of the existing pharmacologic therapy for COPD has been shown to modify the long-term decline in lung function. Pharmacologic management of COPD centers on improvements in lung function and symptoms such as dyspnea. Bronchodilator medications are central to the symptomatic management of COPD. The principal bronchodilator treatments are β_2-agonists, anticholinergics, theophylline (Slo-Phyllin), and a combination of these drugs. The inhaled bronchodilators (anticholinergics and β_2-agonists) form the cornerstone of therapy because they have the more rapid onset of action and least side effects compared with oral medications. Reduction of therapy once symptom control has been achieved is not normally possible in COPD. In fact, worsening of COPD usually requires the progressive introduction of more treatments, both pharmacologic and nonpharmacologic.

The anticholinergic bronchodilator, ipratropium bromide (Atrovent), which is the only anticholinergic bronchodilator approved for use in the metered-dose inhaler form, is available in a metered-dose inhaler or nebulized solution form. Ipratropium bromide is a quaternary amine compound that is not well absorbed, greatly minimizing adverse effects. The most important effect of anticholinergic bronchodilators appears to be their ability to block the effect of acetylcholine on muscarinic receptors, especially the M3 receptor. Ipratropium also blocks M1 and M2 receptors to modify transmission at the preganglionic junction, although these effects are probably less important in COPD. Ipratropium is administered four times daily. The bronchodilating effects of ipratropium last longer than short-acting β_2-agonists, such as albuterol (Proventil), with the effects remaining apparent for up to 8 hours after administration with increased dosing. Ipratropium has also been shown to decrease the frequency of exacerbations in COPD. Extensive use of ipratropium in COPD patients in a number of clinical trials over a wide range of doses has shown this agent to be very safe. Adverse effects that have been reported include dry mouth and a metallic taste that has been reported by some patients. Mucociliary defense is not affected by ipratropium. In patients using the nebulized solution, the direct effects of the drug may precipitate glaucoma, but this can be easily avoided by having the patients close their eyes during inhalation.

Short-acting β_2-agonists (e.g., albuterol [Proventil]) can be delivered by metered-dose inhaler, dry powder inhaler, orally, or in a nebulized solution. The inhaled route is preferable to the oral route, as it provides direct delivery to the airway mucus, offering a rapid onset of action (5 to 15 minutes), with fewer side effects than the oral form. The β_2-agonists induce bronchodilation by causing prolonged relaxation of airway smooth muscle due to β_2-adrenergic-mediated activation of adenylate cyclase in airway smooth muscle. The major drawback to albuterol is its short duration of action (4 to 6 hours) and the fact that the duration of action shortens within a few weeks. This is due to the development of tachyphylaxis, which occurs secondary to down-regulation of β-adrenergic receptors in the airways. There are also two long-acting β_2-agonists now approved for use in COPD: salmeterol (Serevent) and formoterol (Foradil). Both are delivered via dry-powder inhaler. Salmeterol, because of its lipophilic properties, partitions into the phospholipid membrane of the airway β_2-adrenergic receptor exosite. Binding to the exosite prevents the molecule from dissociating from the receptor, leading to a longer duration of action (approximately 12 hours), although the onset of action is longer than albuterol. Formoterol is an amphiphilic molecule that interacts with the β_2-adrenergic receptor lipid bilayer, but is also able to reach the receptor from the aqueous phase. Thus it exhibits both a rapid onset of action (similar to albuterol) and a prolonged duration of action (similar to salmeterol). There have been decreases in exacerbations with the use of long-acting β_2-agonists. The adverse effects of stimulation of β_2-adrenergic receptors can produce resting sinus tachycardia. In addition, ventricular rhythm disturbances can occur in very susceptible patients. However, these effects have been seen only rarely with inhaled therapy. When combined with diuretic therapy, hypokalemia can occur. Increases in O_2 consumption and mild decreases in $Pa{O_2}$ can also occur with the use of β_2-agonists, but the clinical significance of these changes are in doubt. Finally, musculoskeletal tremor is a reported adverse effect. The adverse effects of β_2-agonists are dose dependent.

Combining these two classes of bronchodilators with different mechanisms and duration of actions may increase the effects of these agents. Several studies have shown superior efficacy for either short- or long-acting β_2-agonists in combination with the anticholinergic ipratropium bromide. The combination of a short-acting β_2-agonists and anticholinergics (i.e., albuterol plus ipratropium [Combivent]) in stable COPD has been shown to produce greater and more sustained dilation than each of the individual components of therapy, without additional adverse effects or increased costs. With regard to combining long-acting β_2-agonists with anticholinergics, the concomitant use of salmeterol and ipratropium has been shown to significantly increase bronchodilation and decrease exacerbations compared with salmeterol alone. The combination of formoterol and ipratropium has also been shown to be more effective than albuterol and ipratropium in COPD.

Theophylline (Slo-Phyllin), the most commonly used methylxanthine, is metabolized by cytochrome P450 mixed function oxidases. Theophylline was a popular agent in the recent past, but its use has been declining due to potential toxic effects and the introduction of β_2-agonists and anticholinergics, which have, in comparison, minimal adverse effects. There is continuing controversy over the precise effects of this class of agents. They do cause bronchodilation secondary to nonselective inhibition of phosphodiesterase. In addition, a variety of nonbronchodilator activities (including changes in inspiratory muscle function) have been reported, but the clinical significance of these effects is not clear. Theophylline has the potential for serious adverse events because of its complex pharmacokinetics and narrow therapeutic index. Toxicity is dose-related. The potential problems associated with its use include atrial and ventricular arrhythmias, as well as seizures. More common but less serious adverse effects include headaches, insomnia, nausea, and heartburn, which can occur even in therapeutic dose ranges. Further, theophylline clearance declines with age, and there are a number of interactions with other commonly used drugs, which can alter drug levels of theophylline. Beneficial effects have also been shown with the combination of salmeterol, ipratropium, and theophylline, although combining all three classes of bronchodilators can be expected to increase the costs of therapy and the potential for adverse effects.

The efficacy of corticosteroid therapy in the chronic management of COPD is controversial. This is in contrast to asthma, in which the effects of corticosteroids in reducing inflammation are well accepted. The disparity is most likely due to the fact that the inflammation in COPD is relatively resistant to corticosteroid treatment, compared to asthma. In a meta-analysis of the effects of oral corticosteroids, only 10% of patients with COPD showed a clinically significant improvement in pulmonary function more often than patients receiving placebo. Furthermore, there are important risks associated with long-term oral corticosteroid treatment, including myopathy, glucose intolerance, decreased bone density, systemic hypertension, and cataract formation. Therefore, because of its relative lack of efficacy and evidence of adverse events, long-term treatment with oral glucocorticoids is not recommended in the treatment of stable COPD. Several large studies have recently assessed the long-term (up to 3 years) effects of inhaled corticosteroids in COPD. In these studies, no significant slowing of COPD disease progression was shown. Inhaled corticosteroid use has been shown to result in reductions in exacerbations of COPD leading to a recommendation in the GOLD management guidelines that treatment with inhaled corticosteroids be reserved for patients with FEV_1 <50% of predicted values and acute COPD exacerbations or for those with advanced disease who demonstrate improvement after steroid use. The long-term safety of inhaled corticosteroids remains unknown, particularly as it relates to decreases in bone density or cataract formation.

In regard to other pharmacologic interventions, influenza vaccines can reduce hospitalizations and serious illness and death in COPD and therefore are recommended. Young patients with severe hereditary α_1-antitrypsin deficiency and established emphysema may be candidates for α_1-antitrypsin augmentation therapy. However, this therapy is not recommended for patients with COPD that is unrelated to α_1-antitrypsin deficiency. The regular use of mucolytics in COPD has been evaluated in a number of long-term studies with the majority showing no effects on lung function or symptoms, although some have reported a reduction in the frequency of acute exacerbations.

In regards to nonpharmacologic management, COPD patients benefit from exercise training with improvements in exercise tolerance and symptoms. Nutritional state is another important determinant of symptoms, disability, and prognosis in COPD. A reduction in body mass index is an independent factor for increased morbidity and mortality in COPD patients. Approximately 25% of patients with Stage II to Stage III COPD show a reduction in both their body mass index and fat-free mass. Improving the nutritional state of weight-losing COPD patients can lead to improved respiratory muscle strength. The long-term administration of oxygen (>15 hours per day) to patients with chronic respiratory failure has been shown to increase survival. Oxygen therapy can be administered in three ways: long-term continuous therapy, during exercise, and to relieve acute dyspnea. The primary goal of oxygen therapy is to increase the baseline $Pa{O_2}$ to at least 60 mm Hg at sea level and rest or produce an $Sa{O_2}$ at least 90%, which will preserve vital organ function by ensuring adequate delivery of oxygen.

Noninvasive mechanical ventilation, using either negative pressure ventilation (nPV) or noninvasive intermittent positive pressure ventilation (NIPPV), has been used in COPD.

NIPPV can be delivered by different types of ventilators: volume-controlled, pressure-controlled, bilevel positive airway pressure, or continuous positive airway pressure. The use of NIPPV together with long-term oxygen therapy has been shown to result in a significant improvement in daytime arterial blood gases, total sleep time, sleep efficiency, quality of life, and overnight $Pa{CO_2}$ compared with oxygen therapy alone, indicating that NIPPV may be a useful addition to long-term oxygen therapy. However, NIPPV plus long-term oxygen therapy does not improve long-term survival. The combination of NIPPV with long-term oxygen therapy may be of some use in patients with pronounced daytime hypercapnia. Negative pressure ventilation via tank respirators, cuirass, or other devices has been shown not to improve shortness of breath, exercise tolerance, arterial blood gases, respiratory muscle strength, or quality of life, compared with standard therapy. There is no definitive guidelines as to the appropriateness of using invasive (conventional) ventilation in end-stage COPD.

Surgical treatments include bullectomy, lung volume reduction surgery, and lung transplantation. In carefully selected patients, bullectomy can be effective in reducing dyspnea and improving lung function. This procedure can also be used in COPD patients who have repeated episodes of hemoptysis, infection, or chest pain secondary to bullous disease. Lung volume reduction surgery (LVRS) is a surgical procedure in which parts of the lung are resected to reduce hyperinflation and increase the elastic recoil pressure of the lung. In some centers with adequate experience, perioperative mortality of LVRS has been reported to be less than 5% in those less severe patients (e.g., <Stage III). LVRS can be done by resection using median sternotomy or video-assisted thoracoscopy. LVRS is still an experimental palliative surgical procedure and several large randomized multicenter studies are presently being performed to investigate the effectiveness and cost of LVRS. Until the results of these controlled studies are known, LVRS cannot be recommended for widespread use. In appropriately selected patients with very advanced COPD, lung transplantation has been shown to improve quality of life and functional capacity. The 5-year survival rates are approximately 50%.

COPD is often associated with acute exacerbations of symptoms. Several studies have demonstrated that most patients with COPD have two or three exacerbations per year lasting on an average of 12 days each. The frequency of these exacerbations increases with the severity of the COPD. The most common causes of an exacerbation are infections of the tracheobronchial tree and air pollution. The cause of about one third of severe exacerbations cannot be identified. In regards to infection, in normal individuals the lower respiratory tract is sterile. Studies of lower airway secretions from patients with COPD have demonstrated that more than half have an identifiable tracheobronchial micro-flora. Transtracheal aspiration of patients with COPD has shown chronic colonization with bacteria including nonencapsulated strains of *Haemophilus influenzae, Moraxella catarrhalis,* and *Streptococcus pneumoniae*. Antibiotics administered as prophylaxis has been shown to have no effect on the frequency of acute exacerbations in COPD. Some exacerbations may be viral or mycoplasmal in origin. Both parenteral and inhaled corticosteroids have been shown to improve the inflammatory process and decrease exacerbations in COPD. It has been shown that parenteral corticosteroids need only to be given for relatively short periods of time (i.e., 2 weeks to be effective). More recent data have also suggested that high doses of inhaled corticosteroids may reduce the incidence of exacerbations.

Hospital assessment/admission should be considered for all patients with marked increase in symptoms, changes in physical findings, failure to respond to treatment, confusion, lethargy and coma, and worsening oxygenation or development of respiratory acidosis. Hospital mortality of patients admitted for an acute exacerbation of COPD is approximately 10%, and the long-term outcome is poor. Oxygen therapy is a useful adjunct and adequate levels of oxygenation are easy to achieve but may lead to CO_2 retention in patients with significant alveolar hypoventilation. Inhaled β_2-agonists are the preferred bronchodilators for treatment of acute exacerbations of COPD. The addition of Atrovent may be useful. Theophylline does not add any efficacy in the hospitalized patient with COPD. Parenteral glucocorticosteroids are recommended because short courses of less than 2 weeks improve function and symptoms. More prolonged treatment has not been shown to result in improved function and may increase side effects. Noninvasive intermittent positive pressure ventilation (NIPPV) can be used in selected patients with impending acute respiratory failure and those with life-threatening acid-base status abnormalities or altered mental status despite aggressive pharmacologic therapy. This modality has been shown to reduce morbidity and mortality. The use of invasive ventilation in end-stage COPD patients is influenced by the likely reversibility of the precipitation event, the patient's wishes, and the availability of intensive care facilities. Major hazards include the risk of ventilator-acquired pneumonia, barotrauma, and failure to wean back to spontaneous ventilation. Mortality among COPD patients with respiratory failure is no greater than mortality among patients ventilated for non-COPD causes. Weaning or discontinuation from mechanical ventilation can be a very difficult and prolonged process. NIPPV can be used during weaning to reduce weaning time, length of stay in the intensive care unit, and decrease the incidence of nosocomial pneumonia.

CYSTIC FIBROSIS

method of
LAURIE VARLOTTA, M.D.
St. Christopher's Hospital for Children
Drexel University College of Medicine
Philadelphia, Pennsylvania

Cystic fibrosis (CF) is the most common life-threatening, autosomal recessive disease in whites. Its incidence is 1 in 3200 newborns in the United States. CF is found in most ethnic groups, though less commonly in African Americans (1 in 15,000) and Asian Americans (1 in 31,000). This disease affects approximately 30,000 people in the United States. During the past 20 years, advances in the diagnosis and treatment of CF have improved the quality of life and survival, with a focus on early diagnosis, prevention of lung disease, and improved nutrition. The median survival is currently 33.4 years, up from 28.4 years in 1991 and 14 years in 1969. Approximately 40% of individuals with CF are adults.

PATHOPHYSIOLOGY

In 1989, investigators identified and cloned the CF gene, which is located on the long arm of chromosome 7. CF is caused by mutations in the gene encoding a protein product called the CF transmembrane conductance regulator (CFTR). This protein is located on the apical surface of all epithelial cell membranes. It acts primarily as a chloride channel regulator and secondarily regulates sodium channels. Epithelial cells are found in the sinorespiratory, hepatobiliary, and reproductive tracts, as well as the pancreas and sweat glands, thus involving these systems.

Over 1000 mutations are currently known to cause CF. Five different classes of mutations result in different degrees of chloride channel defects with differing severity of disease and clinical manifestations. Modifier genes and environmental factors play a role in clinical expression. Even within families with the same genetic mutations, clinical expression can vary significantly.

Lung Disease

The major cause of morbidity and mortality in individuals with CF is chronic, progressive lung disease. Chronic endobronchial infection and inflammation result in 2% to 4% loss of lung function per year. The abnormality in the gene leads to CFTR dysfunction, which causes abnormal airway secretions and inflammation and sets up a cycle of impaired mucociliary clearance, infection, inflammation, and increased mucus viscosity. This cycle causes airway obstruction with subsequent bronchiectasis, fibrosis, and ultimately, respiratory failure. *Staphylococcus aureus* and *Pseudomonas aeruginosa* (especially the mucoid type) are the most common bacteria involved in chronic infection (Fig. 1).

Gastrointestinal/Nutritional

Pancreatic exocrine dysfunction (pancreatic insufficiency) is present in approximately 93% of individuals with CF and can be correlated with specific mutations in CFTR. Occlusion of the pancreatic ducts causes insufficient or no secretion of pancreatic enzymes into the duodenum. Consequently, digestion of all types of food groups, particularly fat and protein, is abnormal, and malabsorption of fat mainly leads to steatorrhea with bulky, malodorous, greasy stools. Also associated

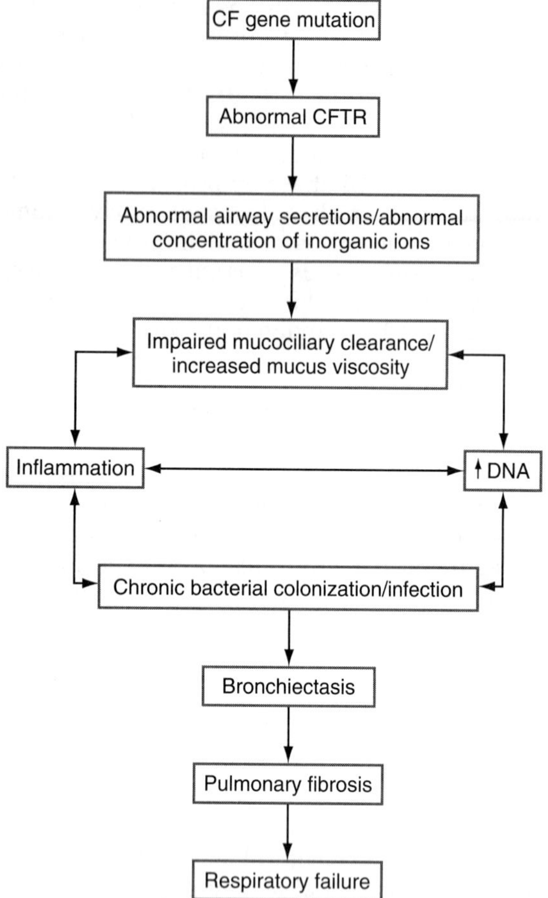

Figure 1. CFTR dysfunction causes an abnormality in airway secretions. This abnormality results in a cycle of impaired mucociliary clearance, infection, and inflammation, which gives rise to bronchiectasis, fibrosis, and ultimately, respiratory failure.

with the symptoms are abdominal distention and flatulence. Unchecked, this abnormal digestion can cause severe malnutrition and deficiency of fat-soluble vitamins (A, D, E, and K). It is known that malnutrition or even poor growth can be linked to loss of lung function.

DIAGNOSIS

The diagnosis is made in approximately 71% of individuals with CF by 1 year of age. However, CF has a number of different clinical manifestations, and the diagnosis should be considered despite physical appearances. CF is being diagnosed more often in adults.

In most cases, the diagnosis of CF is considered in a patient who has typical clinical features, such as chronic sinopulmonary disease and/or gastrointestinal and nutritional abnormalities, or a family history of CF. Confirmation of the diagnosis is by demonstration of an elevated sweat chloride concentration (>60 mmol/L) by pilocarpine iontophoresis (sweat test) twice on separate days. The diagnosis can also be confirmed by the presence of two known CF mutations or an abnormal nasal transepithelial potential difference, but an inability to find two mutations does not rule out the diagnosis. Currently, the mean age at diagnosis is 3.2 years. However, approximately 2% of patients have an "atypical" phenotype consisting of chronic sinopulmonary disease with chronic bacterial colonization by the typical bacteria found in CF, pancreatic sufficiency, and either borderline (40 to 60 mmol/L) or normal (<40 mmol/L) sweat chloride concentrations. Another clinical finding associated with CF is obstructive azoospermia or congenital absence of the vas deferens. In such individuals, the diagnosis is often made later in life (Table 1).

In recent years, newborns are frequently being tested through neonatal screening programs. In such cases the diagnosis is suggested by an elevated level of immunoreactive trypsinogen in blood and confirmed by mutation analysis. However, mutation analysis is limited, and results may be negative or inconclusive. These infants should have a sweat test to confirm the diagnosis.

MANAGEMENT

Individuals with CF should be cared for at a nationally accredited CF care center. A CF care center consists of a multidisciplinary team specially trained in the comprehensive care of patients with CF and their families. The team consists of physicians, nurses, nutritionists or dietitians, respiratory care therapists

TABLE 1. **Clinical Findings in Patients With Cystic Fibrosis***

TYPICAL FINDINGS
Sweat test >60 mmol/L
Usually diagnosed in younger individuals
Respiratory
Chronic sinopulmonary disease
Chronic cough/wheezing
Persistent chest radiograph changes
Bronchiectasis
Nasal polyposis/sinusitis
Gastrointestinal/Nutritional
Meconium ileus
Failure to thrive or malnutrition
Steatorrhea
Rectal prolapse
Electrolyte abnormalities
Genetics
Family history
Genotype
Prenatal diagnosis
Neonatal screening
ATYPICAL FINDINGS*
Sweat chloride test <60 mmol/L
Usually diagnosed in older individuals
Respiratory
Chronic bacterial colonization
Bronchiectasis
Sinusitis
Digital clubbing
Urogenital
Obstructive azoospermia
Congenital bilateral absence of the vas deferens

*Can have more than one clinical feature.

or physical therapists, social workers, and genetic counselors. The goal of the center is to provide quality medical care, educate the patient and family about CF, and help families emotionally with the diagnosis. On average, individuals older than 2 years with CF are seen every 3 months and more often if warranted. Patients younger than 1 year are seen monthly and those between 1 and 2 years, bimonthly. General pediatric or adult care should also be obtained, and the CF care center works closely with the general practitioner. Only the management of lung disease and nutritional issues will be discussed.

Management of Pulmonary Disease

The goals of therapy for lung disease are to prevent tissue damage, prevent the occurrence of pulmonary exacerbations, and restore lung function and clinical well-being by treating exacerbations. Pulmonary function testing is one of the most important parameters in evaluating lung function in individuals older than 5 years with CF. Spirometry measures airflow and is useful in determining the severity of lung disease. Often, large changes in lung function can occur without an increase in symptoms. Small airway obstruction occurs early, and for this reason, spirometry is performed at each visit. Infant pulmonary function testing may be performed in infants and toddlers.

Current therapies for the maintenance and treatment of CF lung disease include medications to reverse airway obstruction, antibiotics, mucolytics, airway clearance techniques, and drugs that control inflammation and modify the immune response. β-agonists and airway clearance are considered maintenance therapy and are performed one to two times per day, even in individuals without pulmonary symptoms. Airway clearance is increased, and antibiotics and other therapies are added during exacerbations.

Antibiotics

Antibiotic therapy is used to control the lung disease in individuals with CF. These drugs can be used intermittently or chronically, and the choice of antibiotic is based on oropharyngeal or sputum culture results. These cultures are specific for organisms found in the lower airways. If no organism is cultured, therapy is based on age-specific infection rates. Commonly, *S. aureus* is cultured in younger patients, whereas with increasing age, the incidence of infection with gram-negative organisms, especially *P. aeruginosa*, is increased.

In patients with milder lung disease, periodic use of oral antibiotics can curb symptoms and preserve lung function, but with increasing symptoms, chronic suppressive therapy is used. Aerosolized antibiotics may also be prescribed for exacerbations of symptoms or for chronic suppressive therapy. A study using a new formulation of tobramycin for inhalation, TOBI, 28 days on and 28 days off, showed improvement in lung function, even in individuals with mild disease. Other antibiotics are aerosolized, including semisynthetic penicillins, polypeptide antibiotics, and aminoglycosides. Even with the aggressive use of oral and aerosolized antibiotics, parenteral antibiotics may be necessary to improve lung function and symptoms. Generally, an aminoglycoside is used with an antipseudomonal penicillin or cephalosporin, depending on the bacteria found on sputum or oropharyngeal culture. Monotherapy is never used to avoid the development of bacterial resistance (Table 2).

β_2-Agonists

Symptoms of reversible airway obstruction are common in individuals with CF. The use of β_2-agonists has been debated, but patients often benefit from bronchodilator therapy in doses similar to those used for asthma.

Airway Clearance Techniques

A number of techniques can be used to enhance mucus clearance. Manual percussion and postural drainage have been the gold standard in the past for airway clearance. This procedure requires a trained caregiver and is effective, especially in infants and young children. With older children, adolescents, and adults, certain devices can be used to allow the individual to be more independent. Positive expiratory pressure devices (Therapep and Flutter), vibratory positive expiratory pressure devices (Acapella), and high-frequency chest wall oscillation ("vest") are some of the different devices available.

Mucolytics

The increased amount of neutrophil-derived DNA in CF mucus contributes to its viscosity. Dornase alfa (Pulmozyme) is a highly purified solution of recombinant human DNase I, an enzyme that cleaves extracellular DNA, thins the mucus, and allows it to be expectorated more easily. Studies have shown that Pulmozyme, given by inhalation once daily, improves sputum viscosity and airway flow and decreases the frequency of pulmonary exacerbations requiring intravenous antibiotic therapy in individuals with moderate lung disease. A recent study has demonstrated that the use of Pulmozyme once daily in individuals with mild pulmonary disease preserves lung function, including that of the small airways, and decreases the frequency of pulmonary exacerbations.

Anti-Inflammatory/Immune Modulators

Endobronchial inflammation is one of the hallmarks of chronic lung disease in CF. It contributes significantly to the lung disease and begins at an early age. Anti-inflammatory agents such as cromolyn (Intal), nedocromil (Tilade), and inhaled and oral corticosteroids are being used routinely, especially in patients with a large reactive airway component. A study using ibuprofen* for mild lung disease showed slowing of the progression of lung disease. However, because of side effects and issues with monitoring of levels, it is not used routinely. A multicenter trial using azithromycin*

*Not FDA-approved for this indication.

TABLE 2. **Antibiotics Commonly Used for Cystic Fibrosis**

Drug	Dosage
ORAL*	
Amoxicillin/clavulanate (Augmentin)	45 mg/kg/d of amoxicillin ÷ q12h (maximum, 875 mg q12h)
Azithromycin (Zithromax)	10 mg/kg/d on day 1 (maximum, 500 mg) 5 mg/kg/d on days 2-5 (maximum, 250 mg)
Cephalexin (Keflex)	25–100 mg/kg/d ÷ q6h (maximum, 4 g/d)
Cefuroxime (Ceftin)	30–40 mg/kg/d ÷ q12h (maximum, 1 g/d)
Ciprofloxacin (Cipro)[†]	40 mg/kg/d (maximum, 1 g q12h)
Clarithromycin (Biaxin)	15 mg/kg/d ÷ q12h (maximum, 500 mg q12h)
Clindamycin (Cleocin)	20–40 mg/kg/d ÷ q6–8h (maximum, 1.8 g/d)
Dicloxacillin (Dynapen)	25–50 mg/kg/d ÷ q6–12h (maximum, 4 g/d)
Doxycycline (Vibramycin)	2–5 mg/kg/d ÷ qd–q12h (used in patients older than 8 y) (maximum, 200 mg/d)
Levofloxacin (Levaquin)[†]	500 mg/d (dosage not established in children)
Minocycline (Minocin)	2 mg/kg/dose q12h (used in patients older than 8 y) (maximum, 200 mg/d)
Tetracycline (Sumycin)	25–50 mg/kg/d ÷ q6h (used in patients older than 8 y) (maximum, 2 g/d)
Trimethoprim/sulfamethoxazole (Bactrim)	8–10 mg/kg/d of trimethoprim ÷ q12h (maximum, 160 mg q12h) (used in patients over 2 months of age)
AEROSOLIZED[‡]	
TOBI	300 mg (1 vial) bid (specific compressor and nebulizer cup recommended by the manufacturer)
Amikacin (Amikin)[§]	300 mg bid
Ceftazidime (Fortaz)[§]	1 g bid
Colistin (colistimethate sodium) (Coly-Mycin)[§]	150 mg bid
Gentamycin (Garamycin)[§]	80 mg bid
PARENTERAL[‖]	
β-Lactam Penicillins	
Nafcillin (Nafcil)	50–100 mg/kg/d ÷ q6h (maximum, 12 g/d)
Ticarcillin (Ticar)	200–400 mg/kg/d ÷ q6–8h (maximum, 24 g/d)
Ticarcillin-clavulanate (Timentin)	200–400 mg/kg/d ÷ q6–8h (maximum, 24 g/d)
Piperacillin (Pipracil)	400–500 mg/kg/d ÷ q6h (maximum, 24 g/d)
Piperacillin/tazobactam (Zosyn)	400–500 mg/kg/d (piperacillin component) ÷ q6h (maximum, 24 g/d)
Other β-Lactams	
Ceftazidime (Fortaz)	150–200 mg/kg/d ÷ q6–8h (maximum, 6 g/d)
Meropenem (Merrem)	120 mg/kg/d ÷ q8h (maximum, 6 g/d)
Aztreonam (Azactam)	150–200 mg/kg/d ÷ q6–8h (maximum, 8 g/d)
Aminoglycosides[¶]	
Tobramycin (Nebcin)	7.5–10 mg/kg/d ÷ q8–12h or 10 mg/kg/d**
Amikacin (Amikin)	15 mg/kg/d ÷ q8–12h
Gentamicin (Garamycin)	7.5–15 mg/kg/d ÷ q8–12h
Other Antibiotics	
Ciprofloxacin (Cipro)[†]	30 mg/kg/d ÷ q8–12h. (maximum, 1.2 g/d)
Minocycline (Minocin)	2 mg/kg/dose q12h (used in patients older than 8 y) (maximum, 100 mg q12h)
Vancomycin (Vancocin)	40 mg/kg/d ÷ q6–8h (maximum, 4 g/d)
Trimethoprim/sulfamethoxazole (Bactrim)	10–20 mg/kg/d of trimethoprim ÷ q6–8h
Clindamycin (Cleocin)	25–40 mg/kg/d ÷ q6-8h (maximum, 4.8 g/d)

*Antibiotics can be used either for acute exacerbations for 2 to 3 weeks duration or as chronic suppressive therapy, depending on the clinical course.
†Not FDA approved for this indication in children.
‡Aerosolized antibiotics can be used in 2- to 3-week courses for acute exacerbations or for intervals of 28 days on, 28 days off, depending on the clinical course.
§Intravenous solution used.
‖Always give a combination of two or more antibiotics when treating exacerbations (see text). Treatment requires at least 10 to 14 days of intravenous therapy. Prolonged courses (3 to 4 weeks) may be needed to treat exacerbations, especially when treating resistant organisms.
¶Monitor for renal and ototoxicity. Monitor serum peak and trough levels closely.
**Monitor trough level only.

TABLE 3. **Complications in Patients with Cystic Fibrosis**

RESPIRATORY
Hemoptysis—massive
Allergic bronchopulmonary aspergillosis
Pneumothorax
Respiratory insufficiency
Respiratory failure
GASTROINTESTINAL
Distal intestinal obstructive syndrome
Malnutrition
Pancreatitis
Liver disease
Cirrhosis
Fibrosing colonopathy/colonic stricture
ENDOCRINE
Cystic fibrosis–related diabetes
Osteopenia
Osteoporosis
RHEUMATOLOGIC
Arthropathy
Arthritis
UROGENITAL
Obstructive azoospermia
Congenital bilateral absence of the vas deferens

given three times per week as an immune modulator is currently under way.

Nutritional Management

Nutrition is extremely important with regard to lung function and well-being. Pancreatic insufficiency occurs in 93% of individuals with CF, and these individuals require pancreatic replacement therapy to ensure adequate absorption of food.

Individuals with CF have increased caloric needs because of an increase in metabolism as a result of chronic infection and increased work of breathing, as well as loss of nutrients and calories from malabsorption. A diet high in calories and fat, vitamin and mineral supplementation, and increased salt intake are required to ensure good nutrition. Individuals often receive high-calorie oral supplements, but additional nutritional supplements, usually given at night via nasogastric or gastrostomy tube, may be needed to maintain good nutritional status.

Complications

A number of complications can occur in individuals with CF. They involve mainly the respiratory and gastrointestinal tracts, but a number of other organ systems may be affected as well, especially as the individual gets older. Table 3 lists some of the more common complications.

RESEARCH

A significant amount of research on CF is currently under way worldwide, including studies to correct the basic defect (i.e., gene therapy) or regulate ion transport. Other areas of research include better effort to understand the gene itself, as well as evaluation of other therapeutic modalities to improve quality of life and survival.

OBSTRUCTIVE SLEEP APNEA

method of
CHARLES A. POLNITSKY, M.D.
The Regional Sleep Lab
Waterbury, Connecticut
Quinnipiac University
Hamden, Connecticut

The partial or complete interruption of normal pharyngeal airflow during sleep, often associated with snoring, has only recently come to be recognized as more than a social annoyance. Sleep disordered breathing (SDB) is now understood to comprise a continuum of upper airway dysfunctional states that have a wide range of effects upon daytime psychologic and physiologic homeostasis. The vocabulary used in the evolving discipline of sleep medicine continues to be modified as the knowledge base expands.

TERMINOLOGY

Definitions in the sleep vocabulary vary from lab to lab. They should be noted when reading the literature as well as polysomnography (PSG) reports. Here is a general overview of common terms (Table 1). Obstructive sleep apnea (OSA) describes the objectively measured occurrence of a higher-than-normal number of SDB events per hour of sleep. These events include obstructive apneas, obstructive hypopneas, and respiratory effort-related arousals (RERAs), the hourly sum of which constitutes the respiratory disturbance index (RDI). Individuals who demonstrate an RDI or 5 or greater and who manifest excessive daytime somnolence (EDS), affective, or cognitive disorders (Table 2), are considered to have the obstructive sleep apnea-hypopnea syndrome (OSAHS or OSAS). Those who have few apneas and hypopneas, but who have a high number of RERAs are diagnosed with the upper airways resistance syndrome (UARS), which has similar medical implications.

Two other conditions are frequently encountered in the literature. Nonapneic snoring may be very loud and persistent, but not associated with airflow limitation or sleep fragmentation on PSG. Nonetheless, it may result in similar daytime complaints. At the other end of the severity spectrum, morbidly obese individuals whose respiratory excursion is limited by massive abdominal and chest inertia may exhibit OSAS plus the obesity-hypoventilation syndrome. They may have fixed nocturnal oxygen desaturation from pulmonary compressive atelectasis, chronic carbon dioxide retention with compensatory metabolic alkalosis, and cor pulmonale. These persons were originally thought to epitomize sleep apnea and historically were labeled "Pickwickian," after the now-famous Joe the Fat Boy in Dickens' "Pickwick Papers."

TABLE 1. **Sleep Apnea Terminology**

Obstructive sleep apnea (OSA)	General descriptive term for respiratory limitation caused by pharyngeal narrowing
Obstructive sleep apnea syndrome (OSAHS or OSAS)	Respiratory disturbance index of 5 or more in context of cognitive or affective complaints
Excessive daytime somnolence (EDS)	Increased sleep diurnal sleep pressure despite adequate nocturnal sleep based on history, Epworth sleepiness scale, and objective testing (multiple sleep latency or maintenance of wakefulness tests)
Upper airways resistance syndrome (UARS)	EDS in context of normal apnea-hypopnea index but frequent respiratory arousals and increased effort on polysomnography
Obstructive apnea (OA)	Pharyngeal airflow cessation for 10 seconds or more caused by airway narrowing; respiratory muscular efforts persist
Central apnea (CA)	Airflow cessation caused by loss of central drive; no muscular effort
Respiratory effort-related arousal (RERA)	Electroencephalogram arousal triggered by increased inspiratory effort detected by esophageal manometer or airflow sensor but not meeting apnea or hypopnea criteria
Apnea-hypopnea index (AHI)	Hourly average of apneas and hypopneas. Five or more considered abnormal
Respiratory disturbance index (RDI)	Hourly average of apneas, hypopneas, and RERAs

A brief mention of central apnea is necessary for completeness. Apnea can result from inadequate respiratory drive without pharyngeal obstruction. Among the various causes are brainstem lesions, metabolic alkalosis, anesthetic and narcotic administration, or overdose. Central apnea may also occur secondary to pharyngeal stimulation by continuous positive airway pressure (CPAP). It is extremely common in association with congestive heart failure, where it appears in the classic cyclic pattern known clinically as Cheyne-Stokes respiration. Some persons display both obstructive and central apnea.

PATHOPHYSIOLOGY

Most individuals with OSA have the condition because of a combination of several anatomic and physiologic aberrations (see Table 2). The final common pathway is the compromise of the pharyngeal airway cross sectional area and an increase in the critical pressure at which airway collapse occurs. In nonapneic persons, this critical pressure is subatmospheric; in OSA it frequently has a positive value. During wakefulness, a compensatory increase in pharyngeal constrictor tone maintains airway patency; in states of unconsciousness or sleep, this defense is attenuated and inspiratory collapse occurs. As seconds pass, hypercapnia, hypoxia, and the interruption of the normal inspiration/expiration rhythm result in increased respiratory effort, eventual electroencephalogram arousal, and reestablishment of the pharyngeal lumen. Airflow resumes, frequently with a gasp and resumption of snoring. The struggle to resume respiration may trigger bradycardia, tachycardia, or ectopy. On a humoral level, increased sympathetic discharge increases blood pressure and platelet aggregability and causes the release of inflammatory mediators implicated in atherogenesis.

Recurrent cycles such as this, sometimes occurring 100 times or more per hour, have effects that carry over into the next day. Sleep fragmentation results in EDS, which, in turn, affects driving and occupational safety as well as general job performance. Hypertension may become diurnal. Cognitive and affective abnormalities occur. There may be increased risk of cardiovascular events and stroke.

The condition also becomes self-propagating. As endless cycles of gasping and snoring progress, pharyngeal soft tissues become increasingly engorged. Vibratory neural damage also occurs. The result is further structural narrowing as well as increasing compromise of dilator neuromuscular control. Interestingly, most OSA sufferers are unaware of the snoring and terrifying pauses that keep their bedfellows awake. In contrast,

TABLE 2. **Clinical Features of OSA**

Signs and Markers	Symptoms and Complaints
Obesity (body mass index >28; neck >size 17, "metabolic syndrome")	Excessive daytime somnolence
Hypertension	Chronic fatigue
Male gender	Male impotence
Female postmenopausal state	Morning headache or fatigue
Craniofacial abnormalities (macroglossia, micro- or retrognathia, acromegaly)	Loud snoring
Nasopharyngeal narrowing	Gasping arousals
Adenotonsillar hyperplasia	Witnessed apnea
Engorged pharyngeal tissues	Sleep-associated motor vehicle accident or near-miss
High-arched hard palate	Somnolence on the job
History of chronic heart failure or cerebrovascular accident	Insomnia
Chronic renal failure	Restless sleep
Unexplained pulmonary hypertension	Poor memory or concentration ability
Smoking	Irritability
Alcohol or sedative use	Depression
Hypothyroidism	

others may complain of insomnia, restless sleep, gasping arousals, or nocturnal panic arousals with dyspnea or tachycardia.

DECISION TO TEST

Polysomnography remains the diagnostic gold standard. Because it is labor-intensive, expensive, and sometimes associated with long wait times, it would benefit all concerned if testing were ordered only on individuals most likely to have a positive result. Unfortunately, no screening criteria or algorithms have been validated. The likelihood that an individual has OSA increases in proportion to the number of complaints, signs, and symptoms that are listed in Table 2. EDS is the most common complaint to trigger a suspicion of OSA, especially in context of obesity, but specificity is low. Men commonly report snoring, apnea, and EDS; women are more likely to have morning headache, depression, and fatigue. The Epworth Sleepiness Scale (ESS) is a subjective but generally reliable indicator of EDS, but is an ineffective screening tool for OSA because the differential diagnostic list is long (Table 3). Overnight recording oximetry lacks both sensitivity and specificity. In-home, unattended multichannel screening devices are available, but remain unproven for a variety of technical reasons. In one study, 33% of data sets were uninterpretable; of the remainder, only 75% yielded decision-to-treat data matching results of the PSG controls.

Furthermore, because in-laboratory CPAP titration remains the gold standard, screening studies indicating an OSA diagnosis must be followed by a night in the lab, where a split-night study can usually provide both definitive diagnosis and CPAP titration data. The sleep lab stay also provides important additional information about the need for supplemental oxygen or bilevel positive airway pressure (BiPAP), quality and quantity of sleep, position dependency of apnea, cardiac dysrhythmias, abnormal limb movements, parasomnias, and seizure activity.

TABLE 3. **Differential Diagnosis—Excessive Daytime Somnolence**

Obstructive sleep apnea
Obesity-hypoventilation syndrome
Hypercapnic respiratory failure
Narcolepsy
Idiopathic or post-traumatic hypersomnia
Restless leg syndrome/periodic limb movement disorder
Circadian rhythm disturbances
- Frequent time zone crossing
- Rotating or night shift work
- Delayed sleep phase syndrome
- "24/7" global communications

Poor sleep hygiene
Secondary insufficient sleep syndrome
- Chronic pain
- Medical conditions, especially congestive heart failure, chronic obstructive pulmonary disease, nocturia
- Anxiety or depression
- Nocturnal gastroesophageal reflux disease
- Poor sleep environment

Chronic systemic disease
Prescription drug use, especially sedatives, hypnotics, narcotics, β-blockers, dopamine agonists
Illicit drug use
Alcoholism
Obesity or persistent snoring (even without obstructive sleep apnea)

POLYSOMNOGRAPHY

The full polysomnogram provides a 6 hour recording of multiple parameters (Table 4). After a minimum of 2 hours of diagnostic recording, if criteria establishing an OSA diagnosis are met, most labs proceed with CPAP titration-a split night study. Ideally, all sleep disordered breathing, nonspontaneous arousals, and oxygen desaturation events are eliminated by the end of the study night. The titration may be done manually employing a remote control, or by observation of an autotitrating CPAP (APAP) device. An attempt is made to have the patient achieve supine REM sleep, which usually results in the most severe OSA of the night.

TREATMENT

Current Medicare criteria for instituting treatment require an apnea-hypopnea index (AHI) of 5 or more plus one or more of the following: EDS, cognitive or affective complaints, hypertension, or cardiovascular disease. An AHI of 15 or more without complaints is also accepted. Many clinicians believe that these standards are too restrictive. They add RERAs into the calculation of events and report the sum as the RDI.

Continuous Positive Airway Pressure

Continuous positive airway pressure (CPAP), provided by a bedside blower connected to a variety of nasal and oronasal interfaces, provides definitive treatment for the majority of OSA patients. It is thought to work mainly by maintaining inspiratory airway pressure higher than the critical closing pressure discussed above. If applied with comfortable and leak-proof equipment, CPAP has been shown to be successfully employed on a nightly basis for at least 5 hours by more than 70% of individuals for whom it is prescribed. They experience nearly immediate

TABLE 4. **Standard Polysomnography Channels**

Lead	Parameter
Electroencephalogram—3 lead	Sleep stage/seizure
Electro-oculogram	Rapid eye movement (REM) identification
Electrocardiogram	Cardiac rate and rhythm
Chin electromyogram	Rapid eye movement (REM) identification
Leg electromyogram	Limb movement disorders
Oronasal airflow sensor	Breathing rate and depth
Thoracic and abdominal movement sensors	Respiratory effort
Oximeter	Oxygen saturation
Body position indicator	Position dependency
Microphone	Snoring

remission of EDS, snoring, cognitive, and affective complaints. Additional improvement may be seen over the first 2–4 weeks of use, as the pharyngeal engorgement caused by OSA remits.

Studies have shown that long-term success with CPAP is most likely when regular nightly use occurs within several weeks of institution. Achievement of this goal is enhanced by alleviation of several common sources of discomfort, including uncomfortable mask fit, air leaks (especially those leading to dry eyes), mucosal dryness or rhinorrhea, and nasal congestion. *Heated* humidification has been shown to improve most of the mucosal complaints; room temperature passive humidifiers are ineffective. Where necessary, topical nasal steroids and topical or systemic antihistamines control congestion from seasonal and perennial rhinitis. Unless otherwise contraindicated, oral sympathomimetic decongestant and antihistamine combinations given several hours before bedtime can be used in more refractory cases. For the specific complaint of morning rhinorrhea, topical ipratropium (Atrovent) nasal spray is effective.

Because the severity of apnea may vary even over the course of one night of sleep, a fixed CPAP setting may not suffice under all circumstances. Autotitrating CPAP devices (APAP) have been developed to follow changes in pharyngeal critical pressure. Caution must be exercised in the use of APAP devices for several reasons. First, at least four different sensor technologies are in use; some may not detect apnea unless it is accompanied by snoring; others do not adjust properly to mask leaks or central apneas. Studies comparing effectiveness of CPAP and APAP have yielded varying results. In general, the mean airway pressure applied by APAP during a given night may be slightly lower—and mean hours of use slightly greater—than with a fixed level of CPAP, but daytime clinical response is not necessarily improved. APAP is more expensive than CPAP and has greater potential for error in pressure delivery; more work is needed before the ideal population for its use has been identified. Current American Academy of Sleep Medicine guidelines exclude persons with chronic lung disease, congestive heart failure, and silent apnea. They also stress that, although APAP may be employed in the lab to facilitate CPAP titration, it must not be used in CPAP-naive individuals at home as a substitution for titration under PSG.

Bilevel Positive Airway Pressure

Bilevel positive airway pressure (BiPAP) couples a higher inspiratory pressure with a lower pressure on expiration. It is commonly employed in hospital as a form of noninvasive ventilatory support. BiPAP has also been used as a substitute for CPAP when patients complain of discomfort from high pressures and where maximum CPAP fails to control OSA fully. Controlled studies have failed to confirm increased comfort or compliance, however. BiPAP may be useful for patients who have both OSA and morbid obesity-associated hypoventilation.

Mandibular Advancement Devices

Mandibular advancement devices (MAD) have received considerable attention as alternative treatment for OSAS. They work by maintaining the mandible in a forward position, thereby increasing the pharyngeal cross-sectional area and inhibiting the tendency toward inspiratory collapse. Approximately 30 MADs of varying design and sophistication are available. Most must be fitted by a dentist with special interest in these devices. Although many clinical studies have established that patients prefer MADs over CPAP—and thus are more compliant—RDI reduction is much more variable, reducing the net positive advantage. In fact, some MAD users experience suboptimal control of OSA. Follow-up confirmatory PSG is therefore necessary.

Prescription of an MAD should be reserved for those individuals who have failed to comply with CPAP after appropriate efforts have been made by the patient, the equipment supplier, and the physician. Most studies have employed the MAD in context of mild or moderate OSA; one group of investigators has found similar results in persons with severe obstruction.

MADs may cause unacceptable side effects. Discomfort during use, increased salivation, temporomandibular joint pain, and dental malocclusion have been reported. There are few studies that have looked specifically at compliance over many years of use.

One additional potential for MAD use is in *combination* with CPAP when the latter is only partially effective in controlling apnea, or when the pressure is not tolerated well. Although rarely needed, this approach can potentially obviate the need for surgical treatment.

Surgical Procedures

Except for two specific subgroups of OSA, all operative procedures for OSA remain second line and are reserved for patients who fail both CPAP and MAD attempts. Juveniles with massive adenotonsillar hyperplasia may be cured by standard tonsillectomy and adenoidectomy. At the other end of the spectrum, morbidly obese persons in respiratory failure may require tracheostomy, which provides immediate relief of all levels of obstruction, and can be coupled with nocturnal ventilation when indicated.

Minimally invasive procedures such as laser-assisted uvulopalatoplasty (LAUP), palatal somnoplasty, and injection of sclerosing agents into the soft palate have no role in treatment of OSA, although they may provide temporary relief from snoring for 1–2 years. Of significant concern, they may convert noisy, snoring apnea into silent apnea without affecting the underlying physiologic consequences. PSG to rule out OSA is therefore necessary before snoring-specific treatments are offered. Radiofrequency lingual volume reduction is also under investigation, but remains unproven.

More invasive staged surgical procedures have been evaluated extensively and have been shown to be effective for about 50% of recipients—but success in many series has been defined by as little as a 50% reduction in the RDI. In order of complexity, conventional approaches include uvulopalatopharyngoplasty (UPPP), genioglossus advancement with hyoid fixation, and mandibulomaxillary advancement (MMA). The highest degree of success, approximately 90%, occurs with MMA. Because of the variable response, surgical procedures must be validated by PSG 3–6 months postoperatively.

All surgical procedures are associated with morbidity including bleeding, infection, and functional disabilities such as secondary nasal phonation and reflux on swallowing from palatal incompetence. CPAP application after LAUP may become impossible because of persistent air leak between tongue and the abbreviated soft palate.

Pharmacologic Therapy

No effective pharmacotherapy exists. Protriptyline (Vivactil),* progesterone,* aminophylline,* and acetazolamide (Diamox) have all been employed as respiratory stimulants for persons with reduced respiratory drive, but are of no use in the specific treatment of obstructive apnea.

Mention must be made of modafinil (Provigil).* This maintenance of wakefulness drug was initially indicated to treat the EDS component of narcolepsy. It is now being employed to counter daytime somnolence and fatigue in a variety of conditions including idiopathic hypersomnia, multiple sclerosis, muscular dystrophy, sleep deprivation in military combatants, and *residual* EDS in appropriately treated OSA. In this situation, patients have been placed on CPAP and have confirmed normalization of the RDI, yet continue to complain of significant sleepiness. The etiology of the condition remains unclear.

Extreme caution must be exercised in this circumstance. In the major study reporting this use of modafinil, the mean RDI on CPAP was still 5, which, under decision-to-treat criteria, is within the range that could cause EDS. It is clearly contraindicated to prescribe a CNS stimulant to a person still experiencing EDS secondary to inadequately treated OSA. Careful scrutiny of downloaded CPAP compliance data is essential on initiation and continuation of modafinil in this context. Furthermore, the temptation to prescribe this medication to untested individuals "clinically unlikely" to have OSA must be resisted; modafinil has no therapeutic action on OSA itself and may even have a negative impact.

Hypothyroidism is associated with OSAS. Although reestablishment of the euthyroid state may reduce SDB, it rarely is curative.

Weight Loss

Weight reduction is also helpful. Correction of morbid obesity can reverse the obesity-hypoventilation syndrome. A modest (10%–20%) weight loss has also been shown to reduce the RDI by as much as 50% in some individuals, although CPAP usually remains necessary. Although diet and exercise are frequently effective, surgical weight control procedures have been needed in selected cases. After the target weight has been achieved, repeat polysomnography should be done. Continued follow-up at 2–5 year intervals is essential; OSA may recur even if weight remains stable.

Diurnal hemodialysis usually does not correct apnea that has been described in up to 76% of persons with chronic renal failure. There is a report that switching to nocturnal dialysis provides effective control.

Sleep disordered breathing describes a continuum of circumstances under which partial or complete upper airway obstruction occurring repetitively during sleep may cause profound psychologic and physiologic daytime dysfunction. Some agreement on diagnosis and treatment has emerged within the past several years. Medical caregivers must continue to suspect and objectively confirm the problem in patients who present with a diversity of complaints. CPAP remains the initial treatment of choice for the majority of cases.

*Not FDA approved for this indication.

PRIMARY LUNG CANCER

method of
JACOB D. BITRAN, M.D.
Lutheran General Hospital
Park Ridge, Illinois

EPIDEMIOLOGY

Lung cancer is a health care problem of global proportions. Trillions of dollars are spent globally in providing care to victims of lung cancer and in lost wages that would be better spent on preventive medicine, prenatal care, and nourishing the world's youth.

Lung cancer is lethal. Within the United States, we are witnessing an epidemic of lung cancer. In 2002, it was estimated that lung cancer will be diagnosed in 169,400 individuals (90,200 men and 79,200 women) and 154,900 will die of it. Among U.S. women, lung cancer is the leading cause of cancer-related deaths and was projected to account for an estimated 65,700 deaths in 2002. Although the incidence of lung cancer has decreased in U.S. men, it is increasing at an alarming rate among U.S. women, with 79,200 cases in 2002 versus 73,000 in 1995. The increased incidence in women is clearly related to the fact that more women are smoking. In addition, given the popularity of smoking among teenage girls, it is likely that the epidemic of lung cancer will continue into the 21st century. Lung cancer is preventable in the majority of instances, and preventive efforts need to be redoubled to curb the rising tide of smoking among women and teenage girls.

Cigarette smoking accounts for 85% of all lung cancer; the remaining 15% is thought to be linked to either environmental exposure or genetic factors. Environmental exposure to arsenic, asbestos, *bis*(chloromethyl)ether, chromium, nickel, radon, and vinyl chloride and passive exposure to smoke (secondhand smoke) have been implicated in the increased risk for lung cancer. Most recently, an increased risk for primary lung cancer has been described in patients treated with external beam radiation therapy for Hodgkin's disease and breast cancer. Genetic factors that may contribute to an increased risk of lung cancer include genotypes inducing the synthesis of high levels of 4-debrisoquin hydroxylase and relative deficiency of the MU phenotype of glutathione transferase. Adults who survive childhood retinoblastoma have a 15-fold increased incidence of small cell lung cancer (SCLC) when compared with the general population. It is believed that the polycyclic aromatic hydrocarbons and *N*-nitrosamines in cigarette smoke lead to DNA damage by methylation. In turn, the DNA methylation leads to altered gene expression and contributes to the neoplastic process.

TABLE 1. **World Health Organization Histologic Classification of Epithelial Bronchogenic Carcinoma**

- I. Malignant
  - A. Squamous cell (epidermal) and spindle cell carcinoma
  - B. Small cell
    1. Oat cell carcinoma (lymphocytic-like)
    2. Intermediate cell type
    3. Combined oat cell carcinoma (mixed histologic types, small with squamous cell carcinoma or adenocarcinoma)
  - C. Adenocarcinoma
    1. Acinar
    2. Papillary
    3. Bronchoalveolar
    4. Mucinous secreting
  - D. Large cell
    1. Giant cell
    2. Clear cell
  - E. Adenosquamous carcinoma
    1. Carcinoid
    2. Bronchial gland carcinoma
    3. Adenoid cystic
    4. Mucoepidermoid
  - F. Others

Adapted from World Health Organization: Histological Typing of Lung Tumors, 2nd ed. Geneva, WHO, 1981.

SYMPTOMS AND SIGNS

The symptoms and signs of lung cancer can vary from complete absence of any symptoms or signs (an incidental lesion found on a chest radiograph that has been obtained for another reason) to the presence of a new or changed cough, dyspnea, hemoptysis, chest pain, shoulder pain, superior vena cava syndrome, Horner's syndrome, Pancoast's syndrome, supraclavicular or cervical lymphadenopathy, unresolving pneumonia or pneumonitis, bone pain, headache, paresis or paralysis, confusion, ataxia, or abdominal pain. Systemic symptoms can include fatigue, weight loss, or cachexia. Paraneoplastic syndromes that are often associated with primary lung cancer include ectopic adrenocorticotropic hormone (ACTH) syndrome, Eaton-Lambert syndrome, dermatomyositis, and acanthosis nigricans.

HISTOLOGIC CLASSIFICATION

It is likely that all lung cancers arise from a common pluripotent cell. Furthermore, it is likely that the phenotypic (histologic) appearance is a function of the altered gene expression associated with a variety of genetic mutations. The pathologic appearance of a primary lung cancer is of particular importance both for diagnostic purposes and in developing the therapeutic approach. Lung cancer is basically composed of four different subtypes: SCLC and squamous cell carcinoma, adenocarcinoma, and large cell lung cancer, all of which are referred to as non–small cell lung cancer (NSCLC). Most pathologists use the World Health Organization classification of lung cancer (Table 1). Many lung cancers, if examined closely, have mixed histologic features.

SCLC accounts for 25% of the lung cancer diagnosed in the United States. The presence of neurosecretory granules on electron microscopy and overexpression of the neural cell adhesion molecule (NCAM) is characteristic of SCLC. Most often, SCLC is manifested as a central (hilar) lesion. Adenocarcinoma accounts for 40% of all the lung cancer diagnosed in the United States, and it is the most frequent lung cancer in women. It is associated with cigarette smoking and pulmonary injury and can arise in a central or peripheral location. Squamous cell lung cancer accounts for 25% of all lung cancers and has been declining in the past 2 decades. It stains positively for keratin and is most often manifested as a central lesion. Large cell lung cancer accounts for about 3% of all lung cancers and has an anaplastic appearance. It is thought to represent a continuum of neuroendocrine tumors that include carcinoid and SCLC. Yet despite this view, large cell cancers are treated clinically as NSCLC. The use of immunohistochemical stains (carcinoembryonic antigen, cytokeratin-7, and TTF-1) permits accurate differentiation of poorly differentiated adenocarcinoma or anaplastic squamous cell lung cancer from large cell lung cancer. Bronchoalveolar carcinoma of the lung is classified as a subtype of adenocarcinoma. The neoplastic cells in bronchoalveolar carcinoma are type II pneumocytes. Patients with bronchoalveolar carcinoma usually have alveolar infiltrates or lobar consolidation that is often initially diagnosed as pneumonia. Unresolved pneumonia infiltrates in an adult may be a manifestation of bronchoalveolar carcinoma.

BIOLOGY OF PRIMARY LUNG CANCER

Lung cancers arise from mutations in the bronchial epithelium over the course of a person's life. Lung cancer represents the culmination of 10 to 20 such mutational events. In the past decade, scientists have begun to define these events and construct a hypothesis of how lung cancer develops. It appears that one of the earliest events that leads to bronchial epithelial hyperplasia is allelic loss on the short arm of chromosome 3 (3p), where at least three tumor suppressor genes are present. Allelic loss of 3p, coupled with allelic loss on the short arm of chromosome 9 (9p), leads to dysplasia. Mutational events that convert epithelial dysplasia into carcinoma in situ include mutation of the gene for p53 (chromosome 17) and mutational activation of the K-*ras* oncogene (chromosome 12). At this point, further mutational events and the loss of antecedent cytogenetic events will determine the progression of carcinoma in situ and the ultimate phenotypic appearance (histologic type) of the lung cancer. Deletion of 3p, coupled with *myc* oncogene (N-, c-, and L-*myc,* chromosome 8q24) activation, mutation of the gene encoding retinoblastoma (chromosome 13), and loss of K-*ras* activation, will lead to the SCLC phenotype. In contrast, persistence of K-*ras* activation, allelic loss of chromosome 1, and overexpression of c-*erb*-2 and/or *bcl*-2 will lead to the NSCLC phenotype.

Growth factors that serve as paracrine (autocrine) promoters of cellular growth include gastrin-releasing peptide (SCLC), epidermal growth factor (SCLC and NSCLC), insulin-like growth factor type I (SCLC and NSCLC), transforming growth factor-β1 (NSCLC), bombesin, and cholecystokinin (SCLC).

SCREENING FOR LUNG CANCER

Screening for lung cancer has been an area of investigation for almost 2 decades. Based on the findings of the Mayo Lung Project, screening of smokers by chest radiography and sputum cytology is not recommended. More recently, the Early Lung Cancer Action Project has published the results of low-dose computed tomography (CT) in patients at high risk for lung cancer. These results show that low-dose CT of the chest is superior to chest radiography at baseline. The results of this study have led to controlled clinical trials to evaluate whether low-dose spiral CT can decrease mortality from lung cancer in high-risk populations.

DIAGNOSTIC METHODS AND STAGING OF LUNG CANCER

Patients with lung cancer usually have an abnormal chest radiograph. Stage 0 lung cancer (carcinoma in situ) is exceedingly rare and represents an incidental finding in a patient undergoing bronchoscopy for another indication. If a suspicious lesion is found on chest radiography, obtaining old chest radiographs for comparative purposes is essential. If a lesion has been stable on the chest radiograph for 2 years, further workup is not necessary. New lesions need to be investigated, however. A thorough history and physical examination are key to the investigation of a pulmonary nodule or hilar mass. Particular attention should be paid to the lymph node examination (cervical and supraclavicular), the lung examination (localized rales or rhonchi, absent breath sounds), the abdomen (organomegaly), and the neurologic examination. The presence of lymphadenopathy or organomegaly will provide staging information and locate a potential area for biopsy to determine the histologic diagnosis. In the event that the findings on physical examination are entirely normal, CT of the chest to the level of the adrenals should be performed while the physician attempts to arrive at a histologic diagnosis. CT confirms the presence and extent of the pulmonary mass, evaluates the mediastinum for the presence or absence of any lymphadenopathy, and confirms or excludes the presence of other pulmonary nodules. Positron emission tomography (PET) with 2-fluorodeoxyglucose (2-FDG) is necessary for evaluating solitary pulmonary nodules and for staging of the lung cancer. PET scanning of the hilum and mediastinum is more sensitive than CT. The sensitivity and specificity of PET scans of the hilum and mediastinum are 85% and 89%, respectively. The absence of any uptake of 2-FDG on a PET scan excludes a malignant neoplastic process with a 99% level of confidence.

After a histologic diagnosis of lung cancer has been established, further workup is based on the symptoms and signs. Complaints of back pain should prompt a technetium Tc 99m bone scan. A complaint of headache should prompt CT or magnetic resonance imaging (MRI) of the brain. At the completion of clinical staging, patients are placed into a clinical stage as described in Table 2. Patients with clinical stage I and II NSCLC require further pathologic staging; patients with clinical stage IIIA, IIIB, and IV NSCLC will not require further pathologic staging, and treatment decisions can be based on the clinical stage. Patients with SCLC of any stage (with the exception of stage I) are treated with chemotherapy.

Pathologic Staging

Fiberoptic bronchoscopy is a very accurate and safe technique for rendering a diagnosis of lung cancer in patients with central (hilar) lesions. The bronchoscope can directly visualize the tracheobronchial tree, and hilar masses can be sampled by directed biopsy and/or brush biopsy. Location of the mass relative to the carina is noted, and the carina can be inspected and sampled. Clinical staging of the mediastinum is provided by CT of the chest. The presence of enlarged mediastinal lymph nodes (2 cm or larger) is considered pathologic, and histologic confirmation is not always necessary. Mediastinal lymph nodes that are 1 cm or smaller are considered normal, and mediastinoscopy is a low-yield procedure. Mediastinal nodes that are 1.1 to 1.9 cm are considered intermediate in size and represent a "gray area." Such nodes may be reactive or harbor metastases. PET scanning of the mediastinum in patients with nodes of normal or intermediate size can determine the presence or absence of metastases.

At present, patients with clinical stage I or II lung cancer and mediastinal nodes of indeterminate size and/or equivocal PET scans of the mediastinum

TABLE 2. **International Staging System for Lung Cancer**

PRIMARY TUMOR (T)	
T0	No evidence of primary tumor
TX	Cancer cell in bronchopulmonary secretions; no tumor seen on chest radiography or bronchoscopy
Tis	Carcinoma in situ
T1	Tumor ≤3 cm in greatest dimension, surrounded by lung tissue; no bronchoscopic evidence of tumor proximal to the lobar bronchus
T2	Tumor >3 cm in greatest diameter or tumor of any size that involves the visceral pleura or is associated with atelectasis extending to the hilum (but not involving the entire lung); must be ≥2 cm from the carina
T3	Tumor involves the chest wall, diaphragm, mediastinal pleura, or pericardium or is <2 cm from the carina (but does not involve it)
T4	Tumor involves the carina or trachea or invades the mediastinum, heart, great vessels, esophagus, or vertebrae; or malignant pleural effusion is present
NODAL INVOLVEMENT (N)	
N0	No demonstrable lymph node involvement
N1	Ipsilateral peribronchial or hilar nodes involved
N2	Metastases to the ipsilateral mediastinal nodes or subcarinal nodes
N3	Metastases to the contralateral hilar, mediastinal, or scalene or supraclavicular nodes
DISTANT METASTASIS (M)	
M0	No (known) distant metastasis
M1	Distant metastasis present—specify site(s)
Stage 0	Tis
Stage IA	T1, N0, M0
Stage IB	T2, N0, M0
Stage IIA	T1, N1, M0
Stage IIB	T2, N1, M0
Stage IIIA	T3, N0 or N1, M0; or T1-3, N2, M0
Stage IIIB	Any T, N3, M0; or T4, any N, M0
Stage IV	Any T, any N, M1

Adapted from Mountain CF: Revisions in the international staging system for lung cancer. Chest 111:1710-1717, 1997.

require mediastinoscopy (for right-sided lesions) or mediastinotomy (for the left hilar regions) for pathologic confirmation. Mediastinoscopy is a surgical procedure performed under general anesthesia in which a hollow, rigid instrument is introduced through a small incision in the suprasternal notch and advanced along the pretracheal plane to the level of the carina. Enlarged lymph nodes can be visualized and sampled for biopsy. On the right side, the upper margin of the hilum may be reached, whereas the aortic arch precludes access to the left hilum. Contraindications to mediastinoscopy include superior vena caval obstruction, mediastinal surgery, and previous radiotherapy. A limited parasternal mediastinoscopy can be performed for pathologic or diagnostic staging of left hilar or aortopulmonary window lesions. Figure 1 summarizes the clinical and pathologic staging of lung cancer.

Once pathologic staging has been completed and patients have been segregated into clinical/pathologic stages I to IV, the physician is ready to make treatment decisions regarding which patients are surgical candidates and which are better suited for alternative therapies.

PREOPERATIVE ASSESSMENT

It is obvious that in planning treatment, one needs to consider the overall health of the patient, the patient's age, and other co-morbid conditions that preclude lung resection. In patients who are identified as potential surgical candidates, preoperative assessment of pulmonary function and estimation of postoperative pulmonary function are necessary. All surgical candidates should have initial pulmonary function tests. Patients who have a preoperative forced expiratory volume in 1 second (FEV_1) of greater than 1.2 L and a diffusing capacity for carbon monoxide (DLCO) of greater than 80% and do not have hypercapnia or cor pulmonale are clearly surgical candidates, independent of the extent of lung resection (lobectomy versus pneumonectomy). Patients who have an FEV_1 of 0.5 L or less are inoperable, and no further assessment is required. Those with an FEV_1 of 0.8 to 1.2 L or a DLCO of less than 60% are considered borderline operative candidates in whom thoracotomy is deemed high risk. Such patients should undergo quantitative ventilation/perfusion lung scans to estimate postoperative pulmonary function. In general, patients who are estimated to have a postoperative FEV_1 of less than 0.5 L are not operative candidates.

NON–SMALL CELL LUNG CANCER

Treatment of Stages IA, IB, IIA, and IIB

Patients with stage I or II NSCLC account for only 20% to 25% of all patients with newly diagnosed NSCLC. The preferred treatment of such patients who are medically fit is surgical resection. The preferred surgical resection is lobectomy and a sampling of the mediastinal lymph nodes. Segmental pulmonary resection is an appropriate alternative if patients do not have the pulmonary reserve to undergo lobectomy; however, several series have reported a higher local recurrence rate after segmental resection. Pneumonectomy does not confer any advantage over lobectomy and is indicated only if lobectomy results in incomplete resection. The operative mortality (which includes the 30-day postoperative period) associated with pneumonectomy, lobectomy, and segmental resection is 6.2%, 2.9%, and 1%, respectively. Causes of death include pneumonia, respiratory failure, myocardial infarction, pulmonary embolism, bronchopleural fistula, and empyema. Video-assisted thoracoscopic lobectomy is undergoing evaluation, but at present, its role in the treatment of stages IA, IB, IIA, and IIB NSCLC is unclear.

Surgical resection in patients with stages IA, IB, IIA, and IIB NSCLC leads to an excellent disease-free survival rate of 60% to 80% for stage I NSCLC and 35% to 50% for stage II. Patients with stage I or II squamous cell carcinoma have better disease-free survival than do those with stage I or II adenocarcinoma. Additional prognostic factors that may predict recurrence and survival are the presence of K-*ras* mutations at codon 12 (adenocarcinoma, a factor indicating a poor prognosis) and overexpression of *bcl*-2 (positive prognostic factor).

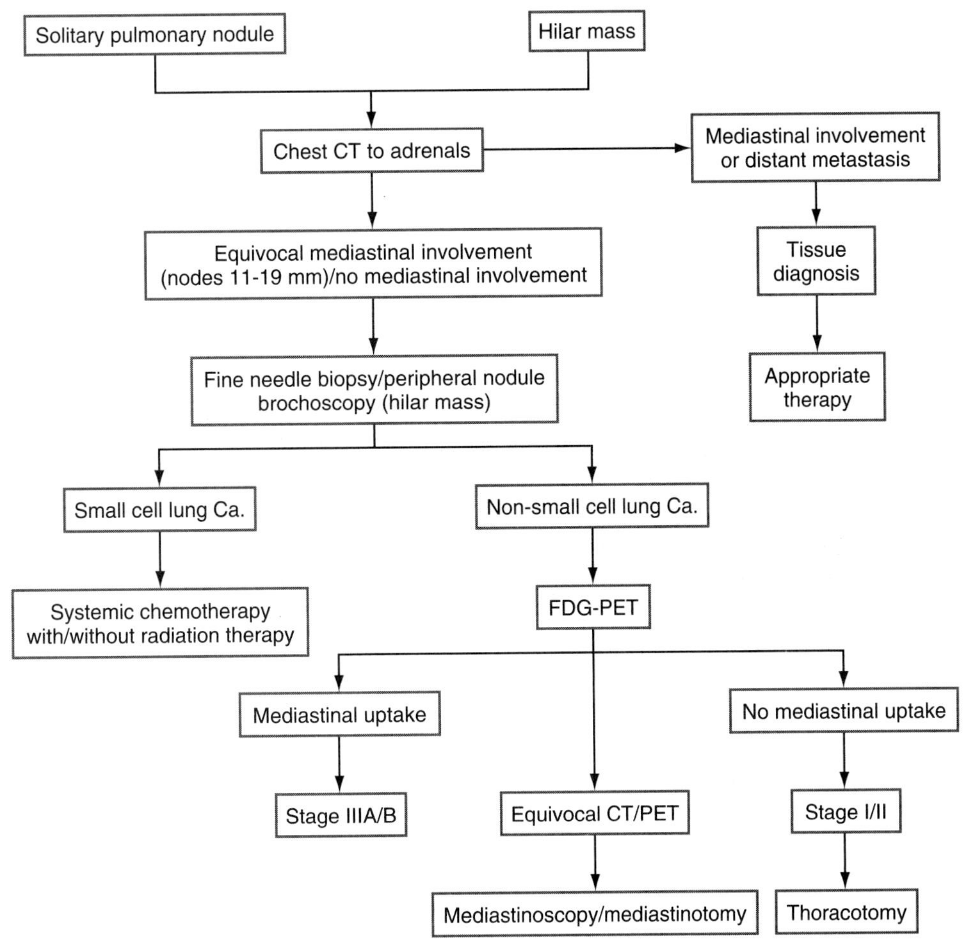

Figure 1. Clinical/pathologic staging of lung cancer. CT, computed tomography; FDG, fluorodeoxyglucose; PET, positron emission tomography.

Patients with stage I or II NSCLC who either are medically unfit or, for whatever reason, are not surgical candidates should be treated with radiotherapy, at least 60 Gy in 30 fractions (2-Gy fractions). The disease-free survival rate for patients with stage I or II NSCLC treated with radiotherapy is 17% to 32% at 5 years.

To date, adjuvant chemotherapy or postoperative radiotherapy has no role in patients with stage I or II NSCLC. Patients who have been successfully treated for stage I or II NSCLC have a 2% to 3% risk per year of a second primary lung cancer developing. In 10 years, the risk is 20% to 30%. Currently, ongoing studies are investigating neoadjuvant (preoperative) chemotherapy in stage I and II NSCLC. Because such patients represent a high-risk group, they should be monitored at a minimum of every 3 to 4 months for the first 24 months and then every 6 months thereafter.

Treatment of Stages IIIA and IIIB

Stage III:T3, N0-1, M0

Patients with stage IIIA NSCLC represent a subset of differing cohorts: T3, N0, M0; T3, N1, M0; T1-3, N2, M0; and T1-3, N3, M0. Accordingly, a uniform treatment approach to all patients with stage IIIA cannot be recommended. Rather, the treatment approach will vary with the subset of patients. For patients with NSCLC who have tumor directly extending into the chest wall (T3, N0-1, M0), it is generally agreed that surgical resection of the primary lung cancer and the involved chest wall is indicated. The 5-year survival rate of such patients is approximately 50%. To date, adjuvant postoperative radiotherapy to the chest wall or the resected tumor bed has had no role in management. For patients with Pancoast's tumor (superior sulcus tumors) (T3, N0-1, M0), treatment consists of preoperative radiotherapy of 30 to 45 Gy, followed if possible by lung resection along with resection of usually the first two ribs. The 5-year survival rate of patients with Pancoast's tumor is 35% to 45%. Whereas some reports advocate the use of radiotherapy and chemotherapy in the treatment of Pancoast's tumor, no randomized trials have compared the potential additive effect of chemotherapy, and its use cannot be recommended at this time.

Stage IIIA (T1-3, N2, M0) and Stage IIIB

Patients with mediastinal nodal (N2) involvement are detected in two ways. The most common is detection of mediastinal nodal involvement by chest radiography, chest CT, or mediastinoscopy. Such patients *are not candidates for surgery;* they have inoperable lung cancer and should be treated as described in the following paragraphs. The other smaller group of N2 patients are those who have clinical-pathologic stage I or II NSCLC and at the time of lung resection and are found on mediastinal nodal sampling to have involved mediastinal lymph nodes. The 5-year survival rate of this subset of patients is poor, 9% to 12%. No compelling data indicate that this subset of patients have had their natural history altered with the use of postoperative adjuvant chemotherapy, radiotherapy, or both. The recommendation for such patients is close follow-up, and treatment decisions can be made at the time of relapse.

As already stated, the vast majority of stage IIIA patients, T1-3, N2, M0, and stage IIIB patients are detected at the time of clinical staging. Patients with stage IIIA and IIIB NSCLC are best treated with either initial cisplatin-based chemotherapy followed by radiation therapy or concurrent chemotherapy and radiotherapy. Numerous prospective randomized trails and meta-analyses have demonstrated improved median survival when chemotherapy is added to radiation therapy. A recent prospective randomized study from Japan addressed the issue of whether chemotherapy should be used sequentially or concurrently with radiation therapy. The study showed that concurrent chemotherapy plus radiotherapy leads to improved median survival and 5-year relapse-free survival.

Patients with unresectable stage IIIA or IIIB NSCLC who have good overall physical status should be encouraged to participate in the current generation of clinical trials, which are designed to determine the optimal initial chemotherapy and optimal radiotherapy regimens. For patients who choose not to enroll in such studies, initial chemotherapy with a cisplatin- or carboplatin-based regimen followed by radiotherapy represents standard care. Patients who are debilitated from stage IIIA/IIIB NSCLC are best treated with palliative radiotherapy alone.

The concept of neoadjuvant chemotherapy (preoperative) is not new, and a number of feasibility studies have addressed this concept in stage IIIA patients with NSCLC. In most of these feasibility studies, surgical resection has been attempted after neoadjuvant chemotherapy. In 1994, two small prospective randomized studies showed a survival benefit with the use of neoadjuvant chemotherapy followed by surgical resection in a selected group of patients with stage IIIA NSCLC. Subsequently, two larger multi-institutional trials have confirmed the benefit of neoadjuvant chemotherapy followed by surgical resection versus surgery alone. Patients who received neoadjuvant chemotherapy had a median survival in the range of 26 to 64 months, and the 3- to 5-year survival rate was 25% to 30%. These results were better than those of the surgery control arm. Patients treated with surgery alone had a median survival of 8 to 12 months and a 3-year survival rate of 0% to 5%. However, this approach carries with it significant morbidity and a treatment-related mortality of 10% to 15%. Furthermore, it is unknown whether this treatment approach is better or worse than the sequence of chemotherapy followed by radiotherapy in patients with stage IIIA NSCLC. A large multi-institutional phase III trial is currently addressing this question. At present, the standard approach in patients with stage IIIA/IIIB NSCLC is initial chemotherapy followed by radiotherapy.

Treatment of Stage IV

After sequential staging, about 40%–50% of patients with NSCLC will be found to have stage IV disease. For such patients, no curative therapy is available, and the goal should be palliation and improved quality of life. Seven randomized clinical trials have attempted to answer the question of whether multiagent chemotherapy is better than best supportive care in NSCLC. These seven trials used a variety of chemotherapy regimens. During the past 8 years, three meta-analyses of these randomized trials have been performed, and the following conclusions have been reached:

1. Patients without debility from NSCLC (good performance status) have a 35% and 27% reduction in mortality from NSCLC at 3 and 6 months, respectively, which is statistically significant; however, the reduction in risk diminishes with time.
2. Median survival increases from 3.9 to 6.7 months, a net gain of 12 weeks.

Because none of the studies performed a quality-of-life analysis, conclusions cannot be drawn. However, a trial carried out by the National Cancer Institute of Canada and reported by Rapp and colleagues analyzed the cost of care and concluded that best supportive care was *more* expensive than one of the chemotherapy arms (CAP: cyclophosphamide [Cytoxan],* doxorubicin [Adriamycin],* and cisplatin [Platinol-AQ])*. Patients in the supportive care group required more radiotherapy and days in the hospital than did patients receiving CAP. The net savings with CAP chemotherapy was $6172 per year of life gained when compared with best supportive care. These data suggest that patients receiving chemotherapy experience palliation of symptoms and spend less time in the hospital. Thus, in patients who have a good performance status, the current recommendation is that they receive chemotherapy, preferably on an ambulatory basis. Such patients should be encouraged to enroll in clinical trials so that we can advance the state of the art. If patients decide to not enroll in such studies, medical oncologists can choose a variety of drugs in an attempt to provide palliation. During the past few years, many new chemotherapeutic agents have been developed and released. Many of these new drugs are active in NSCLC (>15% response rate) and include paclitaxel (Taxol), docetaxel (Taxotere), gemcitabine (Gemzar), irinotecan (CPT-11 [Camptosar]),* and topotecan (Hycamtin).* The current generation of clinical trials is exploring the use of small molecules that interfere with epidermal growth factor receptor (EGFR)

*Not FDA approved for this indication.

signal/transduction. IRESSA, an EGFR antagonist, interferes with the tyrosine kinase activated by EGFR. In phase II studies, it has provided clinical benefit, and Food and Drug Administration approved it recently. It is expected that better treatments will be forthcoming for stage IV NSCLC.

SMALL CELL LUNG CANCER

SCLC represents 20% to 25% of all lung cancers in the United States; the incidence of SCLC in 2002 was estimated to be between 33,000 and 42,000 men and women. SCLC is a distinct clinical-pathologic entity and is almost always associated with cigarette smoking. It has a characteristic histologic appearance consisting of the presence of neuroendocrine granules (electron dense) on electron microscopy and a distinctive cytogenetic alteration, deletion of the short arm of chromosome 3 (3p14-21), which in turn leads to overexpression of the c-*myc* oncogene. SCLC is associated with peptide secretion, such as gastrin-releasing peptide (bombesin), and it stains positively for neuron-specific enolase and chromogranin A. SCLS is characterized clinically by rapid tumor growth and progression. It is responsive to both chemotherapy and radiotherapy, and a large percentage of patients attain a complete response, which represents complete disappearance of all clinical disease. Other clinical features include ectopic production of hormones, such as antidiuretic hormone and corticotropin (ACTH). As stated previously, patients with SCLC may be characterized as having limited disease (encompassed within a single radiation therapy stage I, II, IIIA, IIIB) or extensive disease (stage IV).

Staging in SCLC consists of a thorough history and physical examination, chest radiography, CT of the chest to the level of the adrenals, bone marrow aspiration and biopsy (to detect occult bone marrow involvement), MRI or CT of the brain, and bone scanning. PET scans are sensitive in detecting occult metastases in patients with SCLC and thus complement the aforementioned staging procedures.

Treatment

Treatment of patients with SCLC is determined by whether they have limited or extensive disease. Patients with extensive disease represent about 67% of all those with SCLC, and treatment of such patients is chemotherapy with the intent of providing palliation. The chemotherapy regimens in clinical use include cisplatin (Platinol-AQ)* plus etoposide (VePesid)(PE), carboplatin* plus etoposide, and more recently, cisplatin* plus irinotecan.* A recent multicenter Japanese trial compared cisplatin plus weekly irinotecan with PE.

The cisplatin plus irinotecan combination led to superior median survival when compared when PE, 12.8 versus 9.4 months. Moreover, the 2-year survival rate for the cisplatin plus irinotecan combination was 19.5%, as opposed to 5.2% for the PE group. Clearly, patients with extensive SCLC and a good performance status should receive cisplatin plus irinotecan. For elderly patients or those debilitated by SCLC (poor performance status), a British trial conducted by the Medical Research Council Lung Cancer Working Party showed that oral etoposide resulted in greater toxic effects and an inferior survival than cyclophosphamide, Adriamycin (doxorubicin), and vincristine (CAV) did. Thus, even in the elderly or patients with poor performance status, multidrug chemotherapy remains the treatment of choice. The dismal survival of patients with SCLC underscores the importance of finding new and active agents. In the past 5 years, investigators have initiated phase II studies in previously untreated patients with extensive SCLC with the aim of identifying new agents. The design of these studies has been to use the single agent for three or four courses and obviously to continue its use if patients have a complete or partial response; however, if patients have either stable or progressive disease during the time that the phase II agent is administered, they rapidly cross over to a conventional chemotherapy program such as PE or CAV. It is clear from analyses of such trials that the use of a phase II agent in previously untreated patients with extensive SCLC does not jeopardize their ability to respond to a more conventional program, nor does it decrease their median survival. As a result of such studies, newer active chemotherapeutic agents for SCLC include paclitaxel (Taxol),* docetaxel (Taxotere),* topotecan (Hycamtin), JM-216† (an oral carboplatin analogue), and gemcitabine (Gemzar).*

Patients with SCLC who are found to have limited disease (approximately a third of patients with SCLC) are treated with concurrent chemotherapy and radiotherapy. In the past 9 years, a number of important trials have established the beneficial role of administering concurrent radiotherapy and chemotherapy in patients with limited SCLC. On the basis of a meta-analysis of 13 randomized trials that included over 2100 patients, the use of radiotherapy decreased mortality from SCLC by 14% and increased survival at 3 years by 5.4%. A randomized trial conducted in Canada addressed the issue of the timing of thoracic irradiation in limited SCLC and concluded that patients who received chemotherapy and radiotherapy beginning on the first day of treatment had better survival than when the thoracic radiotherapy was delayed. On the basis of the aforementioned meta-analysis and the Canadian trial, the current recommendation is to begin cisplatin (Platinol-AQ)* and etoposide (PE) (VePesid) with concurrent thoracic irradiation (through a portal that includes the chest primary, the mediastinum, and both supraclavicular fossae up to a total dose of 55 Gy). The PE regimen is given every 3 to 4 weeks for a total of six courses. Continuation of PE beyond six courses does not lead to a survival benefit as demonstrated by several

*Not FDA approved for this indication.

*Not FDA approved for this indication.
†Investigational drug in the United States.

randomized trials. Prophylactic cranial irradiation (PCI), 25 Gy in 10 fractions, is administered to these patients because the brain represents a pharmacologic sanctuary and numerous randomized studies have shown that PCI decreases the frequency and morbidity of central nervous system relapse. Concurrent radiotherapy and PE lead to a 70% to 90% complete response rate (complete clinical disappearance of all disease). The median survival for all patients with limited SCLC who are undergoing such treatment is 17 to 20 months; 2- and 4-year disease-free survival rates are 40% and 15% to 30%, respectively. This approach is not without toxic effects, including myelosuppression, esophagitis, and pulmonary fibrosis, which is usually radiographically apparent but generally asymptomatic. The use of PCI can lead to cognitive defects and a slight decrease in IQ. The 5-year disease-free survival rate for patients with limited SCLC is 12% ± 2%. A stepwise decrease in the disease-free survival rate is observed between years 2 and 5 as a result of the development of a second non–small cell primary lung cancer. Late relapse (>3 years) of SCLC is distinctly unusual. Patients with limited SCLC who do relapse usually do so within the first 24 to 36 months. Such patients may be candidates for phase II clinical trials or CAV if they have previously received PE. Survival after relapse is generally limited, 4 to 6 months.

The Role of Surgery

Ever since publication of the British Medical Research Council randomized trial in which surgical resection was compared with radiotherapy for SCLC, surgery has been abandoned as a mode of treatment for most patients with SCLC. To date, no study has demonstrated that the use of surgery in addition to chemoradiotherapy in patients with limited SCLC has conferred a survival advantage. The only subset of patients with SCLC who should be approached surgically are patients with small peripheral lesions (solitary pulmonary nodule). Such patients should undergo pulmonary resection even if preoperative biopsy shows SCLC. After resection, patients should receive postoperative adjuvant chemotherapy with either cisplatin (Platinol-AQ)* and etoposide (PE) (VePesid) or cyclophosphamide (Cytoxan),* doxorubicin (Adriamycin), and vincristine (Oncovin)* (CAV). The 5-year survival rate in this small subset of patients with SCLC is 50% to 60%.

CONCLUSION

The advances made in the past decade in the treatment of lung cancer have been small but incremental. The most fundamental advances have been in understanding the molecular events that lead to the malignant lung cancer phenotype. With a better understanding of the stepwise intracellular molecular events that result in a malignant phenotype, there is no doubt that novel compounds and treatments will be developed to delay and reverse the progression to malignant transformation. Clinical trials have brought about small, but significant incremental survival in stage IIIA and IIIB NSCLC. Clinical trials require the support of the entire medical community, including physicians, nurses, patients, insurers, and managed health care organizations. The sad comment is that only 1.4% of Americans in whom lung cancer is diagnosed participate in a clinical trial. Finally, identification of new drugs and novel antineoplastic compounds can only happen by supporting and enrolling patients in phase I and phase II studies. Progress in the treatment of lung cancer cannot occur without clinical research.

*Not FDA approved for this indication.

COCCIDIOIDOMYCOSIS

method of
ROYCE H. JOHNSON, M.D.
University of California Los Angeles
Los Angeles, California

Coccidioidomycosis was originally described in its disseminated form in the mid-1890's. In the early twentieth century the fungus was identified as *Coccidioides immitis* and is currently considered as one of the geographically defined endemic mycoses. More recently, a second species has been separated based on genomic differences of isolates from non-California sites. The fungus coccidioides is found only in the Western Hemisphere with small foci in South and Central America. The largest endemic focus is in northwest Mexico and the southwestern United States.

Coccidioides of both species are found in the native soils of the lower Sonoran life zone as mycelia. These mycelia produce specialized aerial structures, arthroconidia, that easily fracture and may travel as far as 75 or more miles from their point of origin. These arthroconidia may engender a new soil site or, if inhaled by susceptible human or animal host, produce a primary pulmonary infection.

In tissue, arthroconidia transform into spherular structures that reproduce by endosporulation. *Coccidioides* may be recovered on one of a number of media. It should be noted that this fungus is extraordinarily dangerous in the laboratory and special precautions should be taken or a serious laboratory accident with arthroconidial release could occur.

The host pathologic response is granulomatous inflammation similar to that seen with other endemic fungi, tuberculosis, or sarcoidosis. Spherules with endosporulation are specific; however, these structures are not always easily identified.

Sixty percent of healthy individuals with primary infection have no or trivial symptoms. The remainder develop pulmonary and/or systemic symptoms within one to four weeks of exposure. Cough and chest pain are the dominant pulmonary features. Some individuals will have relatively modest pulmonary symptomatology; fever, night sweats, and headache may be the symptomatic presentation. Erythema nodosum and less commonly erythema multiforme and other rashes

in association with significant arthralgia may occur with or without concomitant respiratory symptoms. The chest radiograph in mild cases may show no or very minimal changes. In more severe cases, especially those with respiratory symptoms, focal infiltrates predominate. A significant fraction of individuals will have perihilar and/or peritracheal lymphadenopathy. The disease may also present as an exudative pleural effusion with or without concomitant infiltrate, not unlike that seen in tuberculosis.

Chronic pulmonary involvement is not unusual. Residual fibrosis may occur. Pulmonary nodules may also represent a resolution of an acute infection; they are important only in that they may be confused with carcinoma in individuals who either live in or have visited the endemic area. Pulmonary cavities are frequently seen; these may be asymptomatic or cause persistent inflammatory symptoms. Complications of cavity include superinfection, hemorrhage, and rupture with the production of empyema.

Approximately 5% of all diagnosed symptomatic cases of coccidioidomycosis will disseminate. Approximately 50% of disseminated cases will not have a history of a diagnosed primary antecedent. Extrapulmonary foci include virtually every structure in the body. Infections of skin, subcutaneous tissue, lymph node, bone, joint, and meninges are most common.

Meningitis is the most serious manifestation of coccidioidomycosis. Without treatment, death usually occurs within one year. Presentation is often subtle with headache being the predominant manifestation. Cerebrospinal fluid analysis is compatible with chronic meningitis. MRI is more sensitive for defining meningeal inflammation than is CT scan. Alteration of consciousness, psychological disturbance, fever, stiff neck, and focal neurologic deficits are frequent, but not invariable. Cerebrospinal fluid analysis usually reveals a dominant lymphocytic pleocytosis, although

TABLE 1. **Chemotherapy for Coccidioidomycosis**

Drug	Route	Daily Dosage	Duration
Fluconazole (Diflucan)†	PO/IV	400-1200 mg‡	3 mo to years
Itraconazole (Sporanox)†	PO/IV	400-800 mg‡	3 mo to years
Ketoconazole (Nizoral)	PO	400 mg	3 mo to years
Amphotericin B Deoxycholate (Fungizone)	IV	0.7-1 mg/kg	7-17 wk*
Amphotericin B Lipid Complex (Abelcet)	IV	5 mg/kg	7-17 wk*
Amphotericin B Liposomal (Ambisome)	IV	3-5 mg/kg	7-17 wk*

*Based on 2 weeks of daily therapy and an additional 5-15 weeks of three times per week therapy. Particular clinical circumstance of an individual patient may dictate more intense or protracted therapy and/or repeat courses.

†Not FDA approved for this indication.

‡Exceeds dosage recommended by the manufacturer.

IV, intravenously; PO, by mouth.

TABLE 2. **Factors That Increase Risk for Dissemination of Coccidioidomycosis**

Age	Very young and very old
Sex	Male > Female
Race	African American, whites, Filipinos, and Latinos
Skin Test Response	Negative > Positive*
Serum Complement Fixation Titer	≥ 1:32†
Pregnancy	Mid-pregnancy until several months postpartum

*Skin test reagent currently not available.

†Titer may vary depending on laboratory.

in early infection, a moderate neutrophil predominance may occur. Cerebrospinal fluid eosinophilia may also be encountered and in the appropriate setting this finding is essentially diagnostic. Hypoglycorrhachia and increased cerebrospinal protein complete the typical analysis. Cerebrospinal fluid coccidioidal antibodies are usually, but not invariably, found at diagnosis.

Serum IgG, as detected by complement fixation or immunodiffusion antibodies is almost always present in disseminated coccidioidomycosis except in severely immunocompromised patients, especially those with human immunodeficiency virus. Diagnosis can also be made by culture of appropriate specimens. Histopathologic diagnosis can be made by identification of endosporulating spherules.

TREATMENT

The treatment of coccidioidomycosis in its myriad disease manifestations is currently clearly less than optimal. The majority of the therapy available is fungistatic and, therefore, unable to sterilize the patient with significant coccidioidomycosis. Currently available therapy includes amphotericin B (Fungizone), amphotericin B lipid complex (Abelcet), amphotericin B lipid complex (AmBisome), ketoconazole (Nizoral), fluconazole (Diflucan)*, and itraconazole (Sporanox)* (Table 1). There is some possibility that voriconazole (VFEND)* will have utility. At this point there is even more interest in the possibility that posaconazole, which is still an investigational agent, will have substantial anti-coccidioidal activity.

Primary Disease

It is well known that many cases of primary pulmonary coccidioidomycosis recover without chemotherapeutic intervention. Many authors, including the current guideline published by the Mycoses Study Group and the Infectious Disease Society of America, imply that treatment is not necessary in primary disease for low-risk individuals. In reality, however, most but perhaps not all individuals with primary disease receive therapy. It has long been agreed that pneumonia of substantial severity or

*Not FDA approved for this indication.

extent of duration of several weeks is an indication for therapy. The second indication is to diminish the risk for extrapulmonary dissemination (Table 2). No controlled trails for primary pulmonary disease have been undertaken. For disease of moderate extent, ketoconazole (Nizoral) 400 mg orally per day has been used and is the only FDA-approved azole for this indication. More commonly, fluconazole (Diflucan)* at doses of 400 mg orally per day or itraconazole (Sporanox)* 200 mg by mouth twice daily is initiated. Amphotericin products have been reserved for individuals with more severe clinical presentation with compromised gas exchange or in whom an azole has failed.

Pulmonary Nodule—Asymptomatic

If a solitary pulmonary nodule is found to be caused by *Coccidioides* by fine needle aspiration or surgical excision, therapy is not routinely advised. For an individual with underlying compromise with evidence of satellite disease that was not extirpated, a relatively short preventive therapy of an azole could be considered.

Pulmonary Cavity—Asymptomatic

Coccidioidal pulmonary cavities that are asymptomatic commonly can be diagnosed via sputum culture. Persistence of the cavity, especially if greater than 3 to 4 centimeters, the development of hemoptysis, or secondary infection may indicate the need for surgical intervention, usually with perioperative antifungal therapy. On occasion, such cavities can be followed for years with no therapy at all.

Symptomatic cavities such as those with concomitant pericavitary inflammation often benefit from antifungal therapy. In recent years azole therapy, particularly fluconazole, has been used in this circumstance. Alternatively, itraconazole or, less commonly, ketoconazole could also be used.

Rupture of a coccidioidal cavity into the pleural space that results in an empyema is a relatively uncommon, but serious, complication of cavitary lung disease. Intervention by a thoracic surgeon with experience with this disease is desirable. Some cases may be managed with chest tube drainage; others may require lobectomy and decortication. Antifungal therapy is usually given for an extended period perioperatively.

Chronic Fibrocavitary Pneumonia

Chronic fibrocavitary pneumonia often was a progressive and difficult to treat problem. While still representing a therapeutic challenge, the advent of azole therapy with protracted treatment courses has clearly changed the natural history of this disease, which previously often eventuated in death. Protracted courses of azoles should be undertaken.

*Not FDA approved for this indication.

Disseminated Infection—Nonmeningeal

Nonmeningeal extrapulmonary disease that is of limited extent and severity is usually managed with oral azoles: Fluconazole most commonly, alternatively itraconazole, or occasionally ketoconazole, all at doses of 400 mg by mouth daily. Some experts recommend initiating higher doses of fluconazole primarily. Amphotericin B and its congeners are alternative therapy, especially if the lesions appear to worsen rapidly, are in particularly critical locations such as the spine, or the disease is multifocal.

Surgical débridement, especially of osseous lesions, is occasionally important and sometimes is a critical adjunctive measure.

Meningitis

There are two main approaches to the treatment of coccidioidal meningitis. The classic therapy was with amphotericin B deoxycholate administered intrathecally, most commonly by direct cisternal puncture. At this time, therapy is usually initiated with fluconazole. Most experts use doses of 800 to 1200 mg** of fluconazole orally per day. Itraconazole may be an alternative, but in this circumstance may not produce the same salutary effects as fluconazole. Intrathecal amphotericin is usually reserved at this time for individuals who fail to respond to fluconazole therapy.

The most common complication of coccidioidal meningitis is hydrocephalus, which requires ventricular shunting, regardless of which medical therapy is being used. Vasculitic infarction is also a complication of coccidioidal meningitis. Steroid therapy with Decadron initiated at 20 mg per day and tapered over a period of 2 weeks may produce some improvement in this complication, as well as those with other focal neurologic deficits or profound encephalopathy.

REFERENCES

1. Galgiani JN, Ampel NM, Catanzaro A, et al: Practice guidelines for the treatment of coccidioidomycosis. Clin Infect Dis 30: 658-61, 2000.

**Exceeds dosage recommended by the manufacturer.

HISTOPLASMOSIS

method of
L. JOSEPH WHEAT, M.D.
MiraVista Diagnostics
Indianapolis, Indiana

The course of histoplasmosis is usually benign, clearing without therapy in the majority of cases. Severe or progressive illnesses have occurred primarily in persons who experienced a high-inoculum exposure or who had other diseases or conditions that may have affected their recovery from histoplasmosis. A few less common syndromes may result from the inflammatory response to the acute infection rather than from the infection per se: pericarditis and granulomatous mediastinitis are localized reactions to intrathoracic lymphadenitis, and rheumatologic syndromes are systemic immune responses to the primary infection. Other manifestations result from pulmonary damage caused by calcified rock-like pulmonary granulomas or lymph nodes (broncholithiasis) or from an exuberant fibrotic reaction (fibrosing mediastinitis). These findings have been reviewed elsewhere and are briefly summarized here as background for treatment recommendations.

The clearest indications for treatment, and ones for which clinical trials have demonstrated efficacy, are progressive disseminated and chronic pulmonary histoplasmosis. The role of therapy in the other forms of histoplasmosis is less certain and the benefit of therapy unclear. The recommendations that follow largely represent those of the author and differ somewhat from those of the expert panel of the Infectious Diseases Society of America. Reasons for the differences include the availability of new information and the author's prerogative to suggest personal recommendations rather than the expert consensus.

CLINICAL MANIFESTATIONS

Acute Pulmonary Histoplasmosis. Low-level exposure in a normal host may cause asymptomatic infection or a flu-like illness with enlarged hilar or mediastinal lymph nodes and localized pulmonary involvement (Table 1). Following heavier, point source exposure, patients are more often symptomatic and manifest diffuse pulmonary involvement, with diffuse infiltrates seen radiographically.

TABLE 1. **Indications for Antifungal Treatment in Histoplasmosis**

TREATMENT NOT INDICATED
Acute pulmonary, localized—resolves within 1 mo without therapy
Pericarditis—responds to anti-inflammatory therapy
Rheumatologic syndrome—responds to anti-inflammatory therapy
Fibrosing mediastinitis—not active infection or inflammatory reaction and does not respond to either form of therapy
Presumed ocular histoplasmosis—not clearly caused by *H. capsulatum*, and no evidence for active infection or responsiveness to therapy
TREATMENT INDICATED AND EFFECTIVE
Acute pulmonary, diffuse—evidence based upon case reports and author's experience
Progressive disseminated—evidence based upon clinical trials
Chronic pulmonary—evidence based upon clinical trials
TREATMENT SHOULD BE CONSIDERED, BUT EFFICACY UNCERTAIN
Acute pulmonary, localized without improvement after 1 mo
Granulomatous mediastinitis, without improvement after 1 mo
Immunosuppression in the presence of recent histoplasmosis infection
Pericarditis or rheumatologic syndromes treated with corticosteroids
Acute histoplasmosis within up to a year before immunosuppression for malignancy or organ transplantation

Pericarditis. Pericarditis occurs in 5% to 10% of symptomatic cases of acute histoplasmosis and represents a local inflammatory reaction to adjacent mediastinal histoplasmosis. Clinical findings resemble those of other types of pericarditis. Hemodynamic compromise complicates up to 40% of cases, but progressive disease resulting in constrictive pericarditis is rare. The presence of hilar or mediastinal adenopathy may offer a clue to the diagnosis of histoplasmosis.

Rheumatologic. Arthritis or arthralgia, often with erythema nodosum, occurs in 5% to 10% of patients with acute histoplasmosis and appears to represent a systemic inflammatory response to the acute infection. Symptoms may be moderately severe, limiting the patient's performance, and may persist for several months. The pulmonary component of the illness may not have been apparent.

Granulomatous Mediastinitis. Enlarged hilar or mediastinal lymph nodes are present in most cases of primary histoplasmosis and may be the cause of chest pain, a common complaint in acute cases. Enlarged nodes occasionally impinge upon the airways, pulmonary vessels, or vena cava or the esophagus, causing obstructive symptoms, often months after the acute infection. In such cases, a smoldering inflammatory process may cause the ongoing symptoms rather than persistent infection per se.

Fibrosing Mediastinitis. Fibrosing mediastinitis is thought to represent an exuberant fibrotic response to *Histoplasma capsulatum* antigens and is usually first recognized years after the initial infection. The superior vena cava, airways, pulmonary arteries or veins, or esophagus may be encased by the fibrotic mass. Active infection is absent, on the basis of the rarity of isolation of *H. capsulatum* from the tissues and the lack of response to therapy.

Chronic Pulmonary Histoplasmosis. Clinical and radiographic findings are similar to those seen in tuberculosis. Underlying emphysema appears to play an important role in the pathogenesis, perhaps by impairing pulmonary defenses or healing mechanisms. Fibrotic apical infiltrates with cavitation are seen on chest radiographs, and the illness is progressive, caused by ongoing infection.

Progressive Disseminated Histoplasmosis. Progressive disseminated histoplasmosis occurs mostly in patients with impaired cellular immunity, noted to include those treated for rheumatoid arthritis with tumor necrosis factor inhibitors. Patients exhibit febrile illnesses with weight loss, often accompanied by hepatosplenomegaly and laboratory evidence of bone marrow and liver involvement. Gastrointestinal, cutaneous, central nervous system, and adrenal lesions occur in 5% to 20% of cases.

TREATMENT RECOMMENDATIONS

Acute Pulmonary Histoplasmosis, Localized. Symptoms usually improve in a few weeks without therapy. Whether antifungal therapy hastens recovery or prevents complications is unknown, as clinical

TABLE 2. **Selection of Antifungal Agents in Histoplasmosis**

Severe disease	Amphotericin B 0.7-1 mg/kg/d or liposomal amphotericin B 3 mg/kg/d*
Mild disease	Itraconazole 200 mg once or twice daily†

*Preferred in disseminated histoplasmosis because of survival advantage.
†Dosage adjusted based upon results of blood level determination.

experience has not been reported and prospective trials have not been conducted. Treatment is not recommended unless the patient reports minimal improvement after several weeks of observation, in which case itraconazole (Sporanox) should be considered (Table 2). Guidelines for use of itraconazole are presented subsequently. The optimal duration of therapy is unknown, but a short course should suffice because of the favorable outcome of this type of histoplasmosis, reducing the cost of therapy and risk for toxicities.

Acute Pulmonary Histoplasmosis, Diffuse. Patients with diffuse radiographic involvement often experience protracted and even severe disease and should be treated. Case reports and unpublished experience of the author suggest that such patients benefit from therapy, but there have been no clinical trials or reports of observational cohorts. Amphotericin B (Fungizone) should be used initially in those with severe symptoms or pulmonary function impairment (Table 3). The inflammatory response may contribute to the pathogenesis of the respiratory compromise, supporting adjunctive corticosteroids for 1 to 2 weeks. Itraconazole should be used to complete a 6- to 12-week course after clinical response to amphotericin B.

Pericarditis. Pericarditis usually responds to anti-inflammatory medications without antifungal therapy. Corticosteroids can be used in more severe cases, perhaps combined with itraconazole to reduce the risks for progressive dissemination resulting from steroid-induced immune dysfunction. Drainage of pericardial fluid may be required if there is no response to corticosteroids or in patients with severe hemodynamic compromise. Outcome is excellent, only rarely resulting in constrictive pericarditis.

Rheumatologic Syndromes. The joint symptoms typically resolve over several weeks in response to anti-inflammatory therapy but may recur when treatment is stopped. In such cases anti-inflammatory treatment may be needed for 3 to 6 months. Antifungal therapy is not required unless corticosteroids are used for more than 2 weeks, in which case itraconazole may be given concurrently to prevent progressive disseminated histoplasmosis.

TABLE 3. **Duration of Therapy for Histoplasmosis**

Progressive disseminated	12 mo*
Chronic pulmonary	12–24 mo
Acute pulmonary	1.5–3 mo

*Lifelong maintenance therapy may be needed in patients with nonreversible immunosuppression, such as AIDS with persistent CD4 counts < 150 cells/mm^3.

Granulomatous Mediastinitis. Whether therapy improves the course in symptomatic patients is unclear, but there are reports suggesting benefit in some patients. Thus, a trial of itraconazole is reasonable, perhaps accompanied by a nonsteroidal anti-inflammatory agent. Resection of obstructive masses has been described but has never been required in the author's experience.

Antifungal or surgical therapy to prevent fibrosing mediastinitis is not recommended. Because hilar or mediastinal adenopathy is present in most cases of histoplasmosis and fibrosing mediastinitis is rare (<1 in 10,000 cases), unknown factors must play a role in the predisposition to this complication. The risk for serious adverse reactions to antifungal therapy or operative complications of surgery outweighs the potential for benefit. Until the pathogenesis of fibrosing mediastinitis is understood or at least the risk factors associated with it identified, preventive strategies cannot be proposed.

Fibrosing Mediastinitis. Fortunately, the functional impairment is often mild and nonprogressive and the long-term prognosis relatively good. Because the pathogenesis is fibrosis rather than ongoing infection or inflammation, there is no basis for anti-inflammatory or antifungal therapy or evidence that such therapy is helpful. Thus, therapy is not recommended for fibrosing mediastinitis. However, itraconazole may be tried if fibrosing mediastinitis cannot be distinguished from granulomatous mediastinitis. Placement of intravascular stents has been helpful in some patients. Surgery is hazardous and should be reserved for those who are expected to succumb without intervention. Only surgeons experienced with the surgical management of fibrosing mediastinitis should perform the operation and then only after fully informing the patient of the high operative mortality (up to 25%) and uncertain outcome of surgery.

Chronic Pulmonary Histoplasmosis. This infectious complication of histoplasmosis responds well to antifungal therapy. Treatment is indicated in all patients with chronic pulmonary histoplasmosis. Both amphotericin B and itraconazole are effective, and itraconazole is recommended. Itraconazole should be given for 12 to 24 months and until the radiograms show no evidence for continued improvement, to reduce the risk for relapse (~15%). Do not expect the radiogram to show complete clearing as residual scarring is very common.

Progressive Disseminated Histoplasmosis. Amphotericin B and itraconazole are both effective in disseminated disease, inducing remission in two thirds or more of cases. However, of patients with severe disease (hypotension or respiratory failure), nearly half died despite treatment with amphotericin B. Liposomal amphotericin B (AmBisome) was more effective than standard amphotericin B in a study in patients with AIDS with moderately severe or severe manifestations and was better tolerated. Thus, liposomal amphotericin B is preferred over the standard deoxycholate formulation. The other lipid formulations have not been studied and cannot be assumed to be as effective as liposomal amphotericin B, and they are not recommended. Following response to amphotericin B, treatment can be changed to itraconazole to complete 1 year of therapy. Treatment should be continued until antigen concentrations revert to negative or at least fall to below 2 units. Antigen concentrations in serum and urine should be monitored every 3 to 6 months during therapy, and rising levels should prompt evaluation for relapse.

Itraconazole is the drug of choice for treatment of disseminated histoplasmosis in patients with mild illnesses and induces clinical improvement within 2 weeks. Lifelong maintenance therapy may be needed in patients with irreversible immunosuppression or in whom relapse occurs after appropriate therapy—see the section on secondary prophylaxis later.

Central Nervous System Histoplasmosis. The response to therapy is inferior to that in other types of histoplasmosis: 20% to 40% of patients with meningitis die and up to half of responders relapse after therapy is stopped. The optimal treatment for *Histoplasma* meningitis is unknown, but an aggressive approach is recommended because of the poor outcome. Liposomal amphotericin B achieves higher concentrations in brain tissue than do other formulations, but none penetrate the cerebrospinal fluid (CSF). Itraconazole also fails to penetrate the CSF but was effective in a murine model of *Histoplasma* meningitis, as was amphotericin B. In that model, fluconazole antagonized the effect of amphotericin B.

Although the best therapy is unknown, the poor prognosis supports a recommendation for liposomal amphotericin B for 2 to 3 months and until CSF cultures are negative and CSF antigen levels are below 2 units. This should be followed by itraconazole for at least another year. Lifelong maintenance therapy may be needed in patients who relapse or in those whose CSF findings fail to normalize. Patients who do not respond to chronic itraconazole therapy have these options: high-dose fluconazole* (Diflucan) (800 mg daily†), voriconazole* (Vfend) (200 mg twice daily), and posaconazole‡.

Cerebritis or histoplasmomas in the brain or spinal cord, without meningitis, are perhaps more responsive to antifungal therapy. Liposomal amphotericin B for 2 to 3 months followed by itraconazole for at least a year is recommended, although a shorter duration of amphotericin B may suffice. Magnetic resonance imaging scans should be followed to affirm resolution before stopping therapy. Parenchymal lesions usually do not require surgical excision and resolve with antifungal therapy in most cases.

Guidelines for Use of Itraconazole in Histoplasmosis. Physicians must be familiar with the use of itraconazole to achieve the highest success rate and minimize toxicity. Given orally, the dose should be 200 mg three times daily for 3 days, then once or twice daily, depending on the blood levels. The capsule formulation should be given with food or an acidic beverage, and the suspension formulation should be given while fasting. The intravenous formulation can be used to reach steady state more rapidly and the dosage is 200 mg twice daily for 3 days followed by 200 mg once daily.

Itraconazole blood concentrations are highly variable, supporting a recommendation to measure them during the second week of therapy. The minimum effective concentration is unknown, but a trough level of 0.5 μg/mL is probably adequate because the concentration required to inhibit *H. capsulatum* is less than 0.02 μg/mL. The dosage may be reduced to 200 mg once daily if trough levels are at least 3 μg/mL. Levels should be rechecked after a dosage change. Blood concentration determination should be repeated if adherence is uncertain, interacting medications have been added or changed, or relapse is suspected.

As itraconazole is a potent P-450 3A4 inhibitor, it may elevate the concentration of other medications. The potential for drug interactions for all co-administered medications must be assessed. Concurrent treatment with the following drugs should be strictly avoided: astemizole* (Hismanal), cisapride (Propulsid), pimozide (Orap), quinine, and HMG coenzyme A reductase inhibitors. Drug levels of several other medications that are cleared by hepatic metabolism may be altered by itraconazole, making it essential to review the potential drug interactions before starting itraconazole or before adding other medications in patients who are already taking itraconazole. Drugs that induce P-450 3A4, such as rifampin (Rifadin), rifabutin (Mycobutin), and anticonvulsants, lower drug levels of itraconazole, potentially reducing its effectiveness, and they should be avoided in patients taking itraconazole. Symptoms or laboratory evidence for hepatitis should be monitored. Finally, itraconazole can cause congestive heart failure and should be used with caution in patients with impaired cardiac function.

Newer Agents in Histoplasmosis. *H. capsulatum* is highly susceptible to posaconazole† and has shown an excellent response to that agent in experimental infection. Conversely, *H. capsulatum* was not susceptible to caspofungin‡ (Cancidas), and caspofungin was ineffective in that model. Variable susceptibility and activity in the mouse model were observed to nikkomycin.† Others have shown voriconazole‡ (Vfend) to be active against *H. capsulatum*, but animal studies have not been conducted and experience in compassionate use studies in humans is too limited to assess its activity.

PREVENTION

Prevention of Reactivation. The questions are often asked: Are immunosuppressed persons with past histoplasmosis at risk for reactivation? Should they receive antifungal prophylaxis? Although there are reports of presumed reactivation in persons with AIDS

*Not FDA approved for this indication.
†Exceeds dosage recommended by the manufacturer.
‡Investigational drug in the United States.

*Not available in the United States.
†Investigational drug in the United States.
‡Not FDA approved for this indication.

who previously lived in endemic areas, reactivation appears rare. Histoplasmosis was not observed in over 500 patients who underwent immunosuppression for solid organ or bone marrow transplantation in a "hyper-endemic" area, emphasizing the rarity of reactivation. Prophylaxis is not recommended in persons with radiographic (calcified lung or spleen lesions) or serologic (complement fixation titers of <1:16 or M band by immunodiffusion) evidence of old histoplasmosis but should be considered if there is evidence for more recent infection (within the past year, for example).

Prevention of Exogenous Infection. The immunosuppressed patient is at greater risk for exogenous primary infection or reinfection upon exogenous exposure to *H. capsulatum*. Itraconazole, 200 mg daily, was more than 70% effective in persons with AIDS who had CD4 counts less than 150 cells/mm^3. Itraconazole prophylaxis is recommended if the case rate of systemic mycoses (histoplasmosis and other endemic mycoses or cryptococcosis) exceeds 10 cases per 100 patient-years.

Procedures to reduce exposure are appropriate for all individuals engaged in activities bringing them into contact with a contaminated site, for example, a cave or building proved or highly suspected as the source for exposure in a outbreak of histoplasmosis. Such individuals should be advised to wear protective clothing and approved breathing equipment, as reviewed elsewhere. Whether antifungal prophylaxis should be administered as well is unknown, but "preemptive" itraconazole therapy should be given at the first evidence of histoplasmosis. A 2-week course may be adequate for prophylaxis and a 6-week course for preemptive therapy.

Chronic Maintenance Therapy (Secondary Prophylaxis) to Prevent Relapse. Secondary prophylaxis to prevent relapse in persons with AIDS is also highly effective and was routinely recommended. More recently, maintenance therapy was shown to be unnecessary in patients who achieved CD4 counts above 150 cells/mm^3 in response to antiretroviral therapy if they had received at least 1 year of itraconazole and if *Histoplasma* antigen levels were below 4 units in the blood and urine. Secondary prophylaxis may also be appropriate in patients in whom immunosuppression is not reversible or patients who relapse after appropriate therapy.

BLASTOMYCOSIS

method of
CAROL A. KAUFFMAN, M.D.
Ann Arbor Veterans Affairs Healthcare System and University of Michigan Medical School
Ann Arbor, Michigan

Blastomycosis is an endemic fungal infection that is caused by the thermally dimorphic fungus *Blastomyces dermatitidis*. In the environment, *B. dermatitidis* exists as a mold that produces conidia (spores), which are aerosolized and subsequently inhaled to cause infection. At 37°C, the organism exists as a yeast that measures 5 to 20 μm in diameter, has a thick refractile cell wall, and produces single broad-based buds.

EPIDEMIOLOGY

Blastomycosis occurs mostly in the southeastern, south central, and north central United States and the Canadian midwestern provinces. It is highly endemic in Arkansas, Tennessee, Mississippi, and Wisconsin. However, *B. dermatitidis* can be found in many diverse geographic areas around the world, including the Middle East and Africa.

Soil is the presumed natural niche for *B. dermatitidis*, but the yield of soil cultures is quite low. In the largest outbreak, the source of the organism was traced to decaying wood and a beaver lodge on a pond in Wisconsin. The typical patient in whom blastomycosis develops is a middle-aged man who has an outdoor occupation or hobby. For most sporadic cases, a discrete point source of infection is not discovered.

PATHOGENESIS

Following inhalation, *B. dermatitidis* transforms into the yeast phase and causes pulmonary infection. It is likely that most patients have asymptomatic hematogenous dissemination after the initial pulmonary infection. Many patients manifest only pulmonary symptoms, others present with cutaneous lesions without other organ involvement, and a few have widespread disseminated infection. Cutaneous lesions should be viewed as a manifestation of hematogenous spread of the organism. Except in rare instances, cutaneous blastomycosis is not acquired by inoculation.

Cellular immunity involving T lymphocytes and macrophages is an important component of the host response to infection with *B. dermatitidis*. It is also likely that neutrophils play a role in host defense against this organism. Patients who are immunosuppressed are more likely to manifest severe pulmonary disease and disseminated infection. Infection in the immunosuppressed host has been documented either after a new exposure to *B. dermatitidis* or as a result of reactivation of a dormant focus of infection acquired years earlier.

CLINICAL MANIFESTATIONS

Most patients with acute pulmonary blastomycosis remain asymptomatic or are thought to have an "acute viral syndrome." It is likely that many are never diagnosed as having blastomycosis. Patients with acute pneumonia related to blastomycosis have fever, malaise, cough, and lobar or multilobar patchy or nodular infiltrates on a chest radiograph. Development of skin lesions in this setting should make one think of blastomycosis. The differential diagnosis includes bacterial causes of community-acquired pneumonia, mycoplasma pneumonia, and histoplasmosis.

Chronic pulmonary blastomycosis causes fever, night sweats, weight loss, fatigue, cough, sputum production, hemoptysis, and dyspnea. Chest radiography reveals cavitary, nodular, fibrotic or masslike lesions. Hilar and mediastinal lymphadenopathy and pleural effusions are uncommonly seen. Chronic blastomycosis must be differentiated from tuberculosis, other fungal infections, and lung cancer. Rarely, overwhelming pulmonary disease with acute respiratory distress syndrome occurs; this appears to be more common in older adults and immunosuppressed patients.

Cutaneous lesions are the most common manifestation of disseminated blastomycosis in both immunocompetent and immunosuppressed individuals. The typical lesions of blastomycosis are well-circumscribed painless papules, nodules, or plaques that become verrucous and develop multiple punctate draining areas. Cutaneous lesions may be solitary or multiple; rarely, many (even hundreds) of pustular or nodular lesions may develop in patients with disseminated infection. The skin lesions of blastomycosis can be mistaken for those caused by nontuberculous mycobacteria, other fungal infections, skin cancers, and bromide use.

Osteoarticular involvement is not uncommon with blastomycosis. Osteomyelitis can be found under contiguous skin lesions or at sites distant from cutaneous lesions. A bone scan should be obtained for all patients with disseminated blastomycosis; evidence of osteomyelitis necessitates prolonged therapy. Genitourinary involvement may be asymptomatic or associated with signs of prostatism; a prostatic nodule may be felt on digital rectal examination. Laryngeal and oropharyngeal blastomycosis almost always arises as a nodule or mass and is almost always thought to be cancer until the biopsy report shows granulomatous inflammation. Ocular lesions, meningitis, intracerebral mass lesions, and dissemination to liver, spleen, and lymph nodes occur infrequently but are more commonly noted in those who are immunosuppressed.

DIAGNOSIS

The definitive diagnostic test for blastomycosis is growth of the organism in culture. Aspirated purulent material, tissue biopsy material, sputum, or body fluid can be sent for culture. Urine obtained after prostatic massage may yield *B. dermatitidis* in those with disseminated blastomycosis. The mold phase takes several weeks for growth to occur at room temperature. Once growth occurs, highly specific and sensitive DNA probes are used for rapid identification of the mold as *B. dermatitidis*.

Cytologic examination of sputum or bronchoalveolar lavage fluid often shows the distinctive large thick-walled, broad-based, budding yeasts typical of *B. dermatitidis*. KOH smears of sputum or purulent material aspirated from pustular lesions are also helpful for visualizing the organism. Histopathologic examination usually reveals a mixed granulomatous-pyogenic inflammatory response. Cutaneous lesions characteristically show pseudoepitheliomatous hyperplasia; although suggestive, this finding is not specific for blastomycosis. Tissue should be stained with either periodic acid–Schiff (PAS) stain or methenamine silver stain to visualize the organisms. Identification of characteristic organisms allows a tentative diagnosis of blastomycosis and initiation of antifungal therapy while awaiting the results of cultures.

Standard serologic assays (complement fixation and immunodiffusion) have not proved helpful for the diagnosis of blastomycosis. Several different enzyme immunoassays have been reported to enhance specificity and sensitivity, but none of these assays have been made commercially available.

TREATMENT

Guidelines for the treatment of blastomycosis have been published by the Mycoses Study Group in conjunction with the Infectious Diseases Society of America. Many patients with acute pulmonary blastomycosis have resolution of all symptoms and signs before the diagnosis is established and do not need antifungal therapy. Except for this particular group, all other patients with blastomycosis should be treated with systemic antifungal therapy (Table 1).

The treatment of choice for patients who have mild to moderate pulmonary or disseminated blastomycosis is itraconazole (Sporanox), 200 to 400 mg daily. The 400-mg total daily dose should always be given as 200 mg twice a day to ensure maximum absorption. Children with blastomycosis should be treated with 5 to 7 mg/kg/day.* Cure rates of approximately 90% have been noted with itraconazole. The length of treatment is 6 to 12 months; this duration is necessary to achieve a cure and prevent relapse. Osteoarticular involvement requires therapy for at least a year. Absorption of the capsular formulation of itraconazole is problematic; patients should take the capsule with food and should avoid all acid-reducing agents, including proton pump inhibitors, H_2 blockers, and antacids. Alternatively, the oral suspension of itraconazole* allows improved absorption; this formulation should be given on an empty stomach and gastric acidity is much less important. An intravenous solution is also available for use for initial therapy for patients unable to take either oral formulation.

Fluconazole (Diflucan)* is not as effective as itraconazole and should be used only if the patient is unable to tolerate itraconazole; the dosage of fluconazole should be 400 to 800 mg daily for 6 to 12 months. Ketoconazole (Nizoral) is also effective for blastomycosis and is considerably cheaper than fluconazole or itraconazole. The dosage of ketoconazole should be 400 to 800 mg daily for 6 to 12 months; at the higher dosage, side effects, including gynecomastia and decreased libido, are common. Only a few patients have been reported who were treated with voriconazole* (Vfend) for blastomycosis; the role of this drug in treating endemic mycoses is unclear at this time.

---

*Not FDA approved for this indications.

TABLE 1. **Treatment of Blastomycosis**

Type of Disease	First-Line Therapy (Daily Dosage)	Second-Line Therapy (Daily Dosage)
Pulmonary		
Mild, moderate	Itraconazole (Sporanox), 200–400 mg*	Fluconazole† (Diflucan), 400–800 mg Ketoconazole, 400–800 mg
Severe	Amphotericin B (Fungizone), 0.7–1 mg/kg‡ Switch to itraconazole, 400 mg, when patient is stable§	Amphotericin B given as sole agent, total dose of 1.5–2.5 g‡
Disseminated		
Mild, moderate	Itraconazole, 200–400 mg*	Fluconazole,† 400–800 mg Ketoconazole, 400–800 mg
Severe	Amphotericin B, 0.7–1 mg/kg‡ Switch to itraconazole, 400 mg when patient is stable§	Amphotericin B given as sole agent, total dose of 1.5–2.5 g‡
Central nervous system	Amphotericin B, 0.7–1 mg/kg, 2 g total‡	After amphotericin B therapy suppress with fluconazole,† 800 mg or itraconazole, 400 mg if needed¶
Immunosuppressed Host	Amphotericin B, 0.7–1 mg/kg, 2 g total‡	After amphotericin B therapy itraconazole, 200–400 mg

*When a total daily dosage of itraconazole of 400 mg is required, dosing should always be 200 mg twice daily to ensure adequate absorption.
†Not FDA approved for this indication.
‡Lipid formulations of amphotericin B can be used if the patient cannot tolerate standard amphotericin B, but there is little clinical experience with any lipid formulation for this infection. The total dosage will be much greater because the daily dosage for lipid formulations varies from 3 to 5 mg/kg.
§Most patients can be switched from amphotericin B to itraconazole after their condition has stabilized.
¶Some patients with central nervous system blastomycosis may need lifelong suppressive azole therapy; others may require no therapy beyond initial therapy with amphotericin B.

For all patients treated with azoles, careful attention must be paid to drug-drug interactions. For example, concomitant administration of rifampin (Rifadin), carbamazepine (Tegretol), phenytoin (Dilantin), and long-acting barbiturates can lead to decreased serum levels of the azoles and failure of therapy. On the other hand, the azoles as a class lead to increased serum levels of warfarin (Coumadin), cyclosporine (Neoral), tacrolimus (Prograf), phenytoin, midazolam (Versed), triazolam (Halcion), oral hypoglycemic agents, and statin agents. Before use of any azole, careful perusal of the package insert is essential to avoid these sometimes life-threatening drug-drug interactions.

Patients who have severe pulmonary or disseminated blastomycosis, all patients who have central nervous system (CNS) infection, and immunosuppressed patients should be treated initially with amphotericin B (Fungizone) at a daily dosage of 0.7 to 1 mg/kg. If amphotericin B is used for the entire course of therapy, a total of 1.5 to 2.5 g should be given. It is now unusual for a patient to be treated solely with amphotericin B; almost all patients can be switched to itraconazole, 200 mg twice daily, after initial clinical improvement has occurred. Pregnant women must be treated with amphotericin B because azoles are teratogenic. Patients with CNS blastomycosis should be treated with at least 2 g of amphotericin B; some may then require suppressive azole therapy for an undefined period of time. It is not clear whether suppressive therapy should be with itraconazole, which enters the CNS poorly but is the most active azole, or fluconazole, which achieves excellent CNS levels but is a less active drug. With either regimen, the patient should be watched carefully for signs of relapse. AIDS patients and patients receiving immunosuppressive therapy have high relapse rates and should continue suppressive itraconazole therapy for life or until the immunosuppression is reversed.

PLEURAL EFFUSION AND EMPYEMA THORACIS

method of
MARK S. ALLEN, M.D.
Mayo Clinic and Mayo Foundation
Rochester, Minnesota

PLEURAL EFFUSION

Normally, only a few milliliters of fluid are present in the pleural space. An estimated 0.01 mL/kg/h enter the pleural space and lymphatics can absorb 0.20 mL/kg/h. When the rate of secretion from the pleural capillaries, pulmonary interstitial space, or peritoneal cavity exceeds the rate of reabsorption, an effusion occurs. Pleural effusions are classified as either a transudate or an exudate. If the fluid is protein poor, it is a transudate. Causes of a transudate, pleural effusion low in protein, include congestive heart failure, cirrhosis, nephrotic syndrome, peritoneal dialysis, hypoalbuminemia, constrictive pericarditis, malignancy, atelectasis, and urinothorax. If the effusion is protein rich, it is an exudate. Exudates occur from changes in capillary permeability caused by inflammation or infiltration of the pleura. Causes of an exudative effusion are more numerous and include infection, malignancy, and immunologic, inflammatory, iatrogenic, and subdiaphragmatic causes.

Symptoms of pleural effusion include dyspnea on exertion, pleuritic chest pain, fatigue, cough, weight loss, and fevers and chills. Physical examination usually reveals decreased breath sounds, dullness to percussion, and egophony over the affected area. A chest radiograph establishes the diagnosis; however, decubitus views, ultrasonography, or computed tomography (CT) may be necessary to localize and quantitate the effusion. Pleurocentesis should be the initial diagnostic test unless obvious congestive heart failure is present. The goal is to classify the effusion as a transudate or an exudate. Enough fluid should be removed for adequate analysis; however, if the patient is symptomatic, almost all of the fluid can be removed. The risk of re-expansion pulmonary edema is low as long as the pleural space is not connected to a high negative pressure and the volume removed is limited. The fluid need not be sent for every conceivable test; only those that will help determine the cause of the effusion are needed. It is helpful to save some of the fluid in a heparinized container, in the refrigerator, for future use as needed. Thoracentesis fluid should be sent for protein, lactate dehydrogenase, cell count, culture, pH, and cytology. The glucose level in pleural fluid is low in effusions caused by tuberculosis, rheumatoid arthritis, empyemas, or malignancies. The amylase is elevated in effusions secondary to pancreatitis, pancreatic pseudocyst, esophageal perforation, or malignancy. In addition to chemical analysis, the color of the fluid can help establish a diagnosis. Grossly bloody effusions are associated with trauma, pulmonary infarctions, malignancy, traumatic pleurocentesis, and, rarely, thoracic endometriosis. Brown fluid may represent a ruptured amebic abscess, black fluid an *Aspergillus* infection, tube-feed colored fluid a misplaced feeding tube, and white fluid a chylothorax. The smell of the fluid is also helpful; putrid-smelling fluid implies an anaerobic infection, and an ammonia smell is indicative of urinothorax.

Treatment of the effusion is usually directed toward the underlying cause. For symptomatic malignant effusions, talc pleurodesis through video-assisted thoracic surgery (VATS) or by talc slurry through tube thoracostomy is the preferred management. Repeated thoracentesis or other types of pleurodesis are usually less effective. If the lung parenchyma is trapped from a malignant peel, placement of a pleuroperitoneal shunt may help relieve symptoms.

EMPYEMA THORACIS

Pleural empyema is an accumulation of pus in the pleural space. Empyemas can be classified into three phases on the basis of the natural history of the disease. The first or acute phase is characterized by an expandable underlying lung surrounded by thin, purulent fluid. The second or transitional phase is characterized by turbid fluid with an increased cellular content and deposition of fibrin on the pleural surfaces. This forms a limiting peel, preventing extension of the empyema but also entrapping the underlying lung. The third or chronic phase is characterized by organization of the pleural peel and ingrowth of fibrous tissue, which entraps the lung.

Most empyemas are secondary to pneumonia. Other causes of empyema include lung abscess, chest trauma, subphrenic abscess, esophageal perforation, septic emboli, and postoperative infections. Empyemas occurring after a pulmonary resection can also be classified as pleural infections with or without a bronchopleural fistula.

The management of empyemas is related to etiology; however, adequate drainage of the empyema is important in all pleural space infections. As with any other collections of pus in the body, empyemas are seldom cured by antibiotic administration alone. Delay in treating empyemas, by administering prolonged antibiotic courses with inadequate drainage, significantly complicates subsequent treatment of an infected pleural space.

Early empyemas, without bronchopleural fistula, may be drained by thoracentesis. However, if there is a white blood cell count of more than $10{,}000/mm^3$, positive Gram stain or culture results, a glucose level less than 40, or a pH less than 7.2, the effusion should be defined as an empyema and probably needs to be drained by tube thoracostomy. In addition, if the pleural fluid is thick or incompletely drained after thoracentesis, a chest tube should be placed. Computed tomography (CT) is used to confirm adequate drainage of the pleural space. Appropriate antibiotics should be chosen to treat the acute phase of the pleural infection and any underlying pulmonary parenchymal infection.

With adequate drainage established, the patient's clinical course should improve, and after the underlying pneumonitis resolves, the antibiotics can be stopped. Patients who have inadequate evacuation of the empyema with tube thoracostomy or loculated collections may require further drainage to resolve the infection. This may include additional chest tubes, VATS, or thoracotomy and decortication. VATS can débride an empyema space, but when the empyema is large and well organized, it is tedious to perform a decortication with VATS. After the pleural space has been adequately evacuated and the acute inflammation resolved, a CT scan should be performed to detect any residual space in the pleural cavity. If no residual space exists, the chest tube can be removed. If there is a small or moderate residual space, a chest tube can be left in place to provide adequate drainage and slowly advanced out over a period of weeks. Occasionally, it is necessary to resect a rib and place a larger tube, an empyema tube, into the dependent portion of the cavity. Another option for long-term open drainage is an Eloesser flap. However, for most patients with an entrapped lung, thoracotomy with decortication provides quicker resolution and an Eloesser flap is rarely necessary. If a large residual space is present, closure is accomplished by mobilizing a chest wall muscle or the omentum into the cavity. Alternatively, a Clagett procedure, whereby the space is filled with antibiotic solution and closed, can be performed. As a last resort, a thoracoplasty is used to eliminate the space.

Patients who have bronchopleural fistulas associated with empyema require special management. Drainage and early antibiotics are the key points of treatment. Immediate drainage removes the collection of pus and prevents the purulent material from infecting the contralateral lung through the bronchopleural fistulas. The acute infection should be well controlled before undertaking repair of the bronchopleural fistulas. After drainage and resolution of the acute infection, plans for repair of the bronchopleural fistulas can be made; they rarely close spontaneously. The fistula can be repaired by direct suture closure and reinforced with a muscle or omental flap. A transsternal, transpericardial approach has been used for postpneumonectomy bronchopleural fistulas with long bronchial stumps. After the bronchopleural fistula is healed, the residual space can be closed with a Clagett procedure.

PRIMARY LUNG ABSCESS

method of
KENNETH V. I. ROLSTON, M.D.
University of Texas M.D. Anderson Cancer Center
Houston, Texas

A suppurative pulmonary infection with a cavity of 2 cm or more in diameter constitutes a *lung abscess*. Aspiration or necrotizing pneumonia with a high microbial load and failure to clear organisms secondary to bronchial obstruction are the most common predisposing factors. The infection is generally polymicrobial (mixed aerobic and anaerobic flora), and it can be associated with considerable morbidity and mortality despite aggressive treatment.

ETIOLOGY AND PATHOGENESIS

Conditions that alter mental status and lead to a reduced level of consciousness predispose to aspiration and lung abscess formation. These include alcoholism, cerebrovascular accidents, drug addiction, endotracheal intubation, esophageal disease, general anesthesia, nasogastric tube feeding, and seizure disorders. Organisms isolated most frequently are listed in Table 1. The principal anaerobes include *Prevotella, Fusobacterium, Bacteroides, Peptostreptococcus*, and *Clostridium* species. The principal aerobes include *Staphylococcus* and *Streptococcus* species and gram-negative bacilli such as *Klebsiella pneumoniae, Pseudomonas aeruginosa, Escherichia coli*, and

TABLE 1. **Organisms Most Commonly Isolated From Lung Abscesses***

ANAEROBES
Prevotella spp.
Fusobacterium spp.
Peptostreptococcus spp.
Bacteroides spp.
Clostridium spp.
AEROBES
Staphylococcus aureus
Coagulase-negative staphylococci
Streptococcus spp.
Klebsiella pneumoniae
Pseudomonas aeruginosa
Escherichia coli
Proteus spp.
OTHER ORGANIGMS†
Actinomyces spp.
Nocardia spp.
Rhodococcus spp.
Stenotrophomonas maltophilia
Candida spp.

*Most infections have mixed microbial flora.
†These organisms are uncommon and may be encountered in immunosuppressed hosts.

Proteus species. Less common organisms include *Actinomyces* species, *Nocardia* species, *Rhodococcus* species, *Stenotrophomonas maltophilia*, and *Candida* species. These are more frequent in immunosuppressed patients. Anaerobic organisms are present in more than 90% of cases, and aerobic organisms are found in more than half. Lung abscesses are primarily of endogenous origin. Some infections (*Staphylococcus aureus*, gram-negative bacilli) may be nosocomial.

The most common sites of lung abscesses are posterior segments of the upper lobes (right more common than left) and the apical segments of the lower lobes. These segments are dependent when the patient is horizontal. Ineffective clearing of aspirated material related to the risk factors listed earlier results in aspiration and subsequent necrosis and abscess formation. Infection also arises behind obstructions caused by enlarged lymph nodes or neoplastic lesions, initially giving rise to postobstructive pneumonia, followed by necrosis, cavitation, and abscess formation.

CLINICAL FEATURES AND DIAGNOSIS

The most common manifestations include low-grade fever, malaise, and a productive cough. Sputum production can be copious, it often smells foul, and hemoptysis may occasionally occur. The diagnosis is confirmed radiographically; the classic finding is a cavity with an air-fluid level. Associated findings may include mediastinal adenopathy and/or empyema. A microbiologic diagnosis is more difficult to make. Expectorated sputum is unreliable and often represents indigenous flora. Empyema fluid, if available, is a much more reliable source. Bronchoalveolar lavage using a protected specimen brush with quantitation of results may be useful in some patients.

TREATMENT

Prolonged antimicrobial therapy (1 to 3 months, based on response) and drainage constitute the primary modes of therapy for lung abscesses. Initial therapy is empirical and is generally based on Gram stain findings. Therapy can be tailored once microbiologic data become available. Penicillin has been the traditional agent of choice for infections that are predominantly anaerobic, but approximately 40% of gram-negative anaerobes are now resistant to penicillin because of β-lactamase production. Clindamycin (Cleocin) is preferable, although clostridia and some *Bacteroides fragilis* strains may be resistant. Most experts advocate sequential therapy (parenteral followed by oral antibiotics). Metronidazole (Flagyl) is less effective than clindamycin because anaerobic streptococci and *Actinomyces* species are resistant to it. For mixed infections requiring broader coverage, several agents have been shown to be effective. These include cefoxitin (Mefoxin), ticarcillin-clavulanate (Timentin), piperacillin-tazobactam (Zosyn), ampicillin-sulbactam (Unasyn), imipenem (Primaxin), and meropenem (Merrem). Newer-generation quinolones such as moxifloxacin (Avelox) have good activity against most anaerobes and aerobic gram-positive and gram-negative organisms of importance in lung abscess, but clinical data with these agents is lacking. Such agents may be particularly useful in patients who are allergic to β-lactam antibiotics or those who do not tolerate clindamycin. Trimethoprim-sulfamethoxazole (Bactrim, Septra) is the agent of choice for infections caused by *S. maltophilia* and *Nocardia* species.

Postural drainage is important and may hasten response to treatment. Bronchoscopy may be helpful in effecting drainage, particularly in the presence of partial obstruction or a foreign body.

Persistence of fever for more than 5 to 7 days and a lack of clinical or radiographic response should raise suspicions of undetected obstruction, empyema, or the presence of resistant organisms. Percutaneous drainage of the abscess or even surgical resection may be useful when response to antimicrobial therapy is deemed inadequate.

OUTCOME AND PROGNOSIS

Most patients with primary lung abscess respond to therapy, and the mortality rate ranges from 5% to 10%. Factors associated with poor responses include old age, chronic debilitation, immunosuppression, presence of obstruction, progressive pulmonary necrosis, large abscesses (larger than 6 cm), and resistant organisms causing infection.

ACUTE BRONCHITIS

method of
NELSON M. GANTZ, M.D.
Penn State College of Medicine
Hershey, Pennsylvania

Bronchitis refers to an inflammatory process involving the lower respiratory tract in which cough with or without sputum production occurs. In the United States, adults made more than 10 million office visits yearly for bronchitis, accounting for about 30% of all antibiotic prescriptions written for infections diseases. Bronchitis can be classified as either acute or chronic.

ACUTE BRONCHITIS

Acute bronchitis has been defined as an acute respiratory illness listing less than 3 weeks. Clinical features include cough with or without sputum production and substantial chest discomfort; wheezing may be present, and body temperature is usually normal. High fever (temperature >101°F) should prompt a search for other causes such as pneumonia. Patients with bronchitis lack the physical or radiologic findings of pneumonia. Acute bronchitis occurs more commonly during the winter months, and 90% of cases are viral in origin (Table 1). Treatable bacterial causes such as *Mycoplasma pneumoniae*, *Chlamydia pneumoniae*, or *Bordetella pertussis* account for only 10% of cases.

Pathophysiology of Acute Bronchitis

During acute bronchitis, the mucous membranes of the bronchial tree become hyperemic and edematous, resulting in bronchoconstriction. Increased mucus production occurs. Influenza virus can cause destruction of the respiratory tract epithelium, resulting in cough and substernal chest pain. Increased airway reactivity that mimics the pulmonary function changes with asthma may persist for 6 to 8 weeks.

Diagnosis

In evaluating an adult with an acute cough illness, the clinician should focus on excluding pneumonia. Clues to the presence of pneumonia include a heart rate greater than 100 beats/min, respiratory rate greater than 24 breaths/min, oral temperature above 38° C, and focal findings on chest examination. A chest radiograph should be obtained if these findings are present.

The diagnosis of acute bronchitis is one of exclusion. Other causes of acute cough include rhinosinusitis, nasopharyngeal infection, asthma, allergic rhinitis, aspiration of a foreign body, drugs, and inhalation of irritating substances.

The presence of sputum purulence based on color or consistency is not helpful concerning the cause of the infecting organism. Both bacteria and viruses can

TABLE 1. **Etiology of Acute Bronchitis**

Rhinovirus
Coronavirus
Influenza virus
Adenovirus
Respiratory syncytial virus
Parainfluenza virus
Herpes simplex virus
Mycoplasma pneumoniae
Chlamydia pneumoniae
Bordetella pertussis
Legionella pneumophila
SECONDARY BACTERIAL (?)
Haemophilus influenzae
Streptococcus pneumoniae

cause purulent sputum. A sputum Gram stain and culture are not recommended.

Blood streaks within the sputum can occur, but the presence of large amounts of blood should prompt the clinician to search for other causes.

Treatment

Antibiotic treatment is not recommended for patients with acute bronchitis because most cases are caused by viruses. Therapy should be directed toward symptom relief using analgesics, antipyretic agents, antitussives, β-agonist inhalers, hydration, vaporizers, and rest. Cessation of smoking and avoidance of other inhaled toxins are important. If bronchospastic symptoms are present, there is a role for bronchodilators. Patients with severe or persistent disease with a cough lasting more than 14 days may benefit from use of antibiotic therapy for mycoplasma or chlamydia infections as well as pertussis. Elderly persons or patients with co-morbid conditions with severe symptoms may benefit from antibiotics. For patients with suspected influenza, antiviral therapy is effective if initiated within 48 hours of symptom onset (Table 2).

Acute bronchitis resolves with or without antibiotics. The disease does not progress to pneumonia. Half the patients have a cough for about 2 weeks.

ACUTE EXACERBATION OF CHRONIC BRONCHITIS

Chronic bronchitis is defined as a productive cough on most days during 3 consecutive months for more than 2 consecutive years in the absence of other respiratory diseases. Chronic bronchitis is a major risk factor leading to the development of chronic obstructive pulmonary disease. The major risk factor for chronic bronchitis is smoking. Patients with chronic bronchitis often suffer an acute exacerbation of their illness related to bacterial infection.

TABLE 2. **Treatment of Influenza**

Amantadine* (Symmetrel) 100 mg PO qd or bid × 5 d
Rimantadine* (Flumadine) 100 mg PO qd or bid × 5 d
Oseltamivir† (Tamiflu) 75 mg PO bid with food × 5 d
Zanamivir† (Relenza) 10 mg bid by inhalation × 5 d

*Influenza A.
†Influenza A and B.

Pathophysiology

Smoking impairs mucociliary clearance. Bacterial and viral infection of the bronchial tree results in an increase in mucus volume and an inflammatory response that results in progressive airway damage. This damage predisposes the patient to more frequent infections and further airway damage. Although the role of bacterial infection in acute exacerbation of chronic bronchitis is controversial, meta-analysis has shown a benefit for patients treated with antibiotics. Patients with an acute exacerbation of chronic bronchitis benefit most if all three symptoms are present including increased dyspnea, increased sputum purulence, and increased sputum volume.

Diagnosis

Patients with chronic bronchitis who have an increase in dyspnea and increase in their sputum volume and purulence need to be evaluated. A chest radiograph is essential to exclude pneumonia. A sputum Gram stain and culture are not usually obtained for patients treated in the ambulatory setting. These studies may be obtained for hospitalized patients. Bacteria isolated in culture may reflect colonization of the true infecting pathogen. *Haemophilus influenzae* and *Streptococcus pneumoniae* are identified most frequently. As lung function deteriorates, gram-negative bacilli may be isolated.

Treatment

Patients with an acute exacerbation of chronic bronchitis should be treated with a course of antibiotics (Table 3). Although some patients improve without antibiotic treatment, other patients with reduced lung function are at increased risk for mortality.

Which antibiotic to administer is problematic. Factors to consider include bacterial resistance rates in the community for the likely infecting pathogens, drug allergies, drug adverse effects, and cost. Older agents still work, but the duration of therapy is longer. If failure occurs, consider the presence of drug-resistant pneumococci or *H. influenzae*. Although the newer agents may cost more, failure of an older drug could result in an expensive hospital stay.

Ancillary measures are important while treating patients with chronic bronchitis. Smoking cessation must be emphasized. Inhaled bronchodilators such as ipratropium and β_2-adrenergic agonists are indicated. Systemic and inhaled corticosteroids are often useful. Oxygen therapy and mechanical ventilation may be required for severe respiratory failure. It is important to review the status of both influenza and pneumococcal vaccines and administer these agents as needed.

TABLE 3. **Selected Oral Antimicrobials for Acute Exacerbation of Chronic Bronchitis**

Drug	Dosage	Duration (days)
Amoxicillin	500 mg tid	10
Amoxicillin	875 mg bid	10
Amoxicillin/clavulanic acid (Augmentin)	875/125 mg bid	7–10
Moxifloxacin (Avelox)	400 mg qd	5
Gatifloxacin (Tequin)	400 mg qd	7–10*
Levofloxacin (Levaquin)	500 mg qd	7
Doxycycline (Vibramycin)	100 mg bid	10
Clarithromycin (Biaxin XL)	1000 mg qd	7
Azithromycin (Zithromax)	500 mg qd*	3†
Azithromycin	500 mg day 1, 250 mg days 2 to 5	2–5
Cefprozil (Cefzil)	500 mg bid	10
Cefuroxime (Ceftin)	250–500 mg bid	10
Trimethoprim-sulfamethoxazole (Bactrim)	800/160 mg bid	10–14

*Exceeds dosage recommended by the manufacturer.
†FDA has given 3 d indication for otitis media but not bronchitis.

BACTERIAL PNEUMONIA

method of
PAUL G. AUWAERTER, M.D., M.B.A.
Johns Hopkins University School of Medicine
Baltimore, Maryland

The most common life-threatening infectious disease in the United States, bacterial pneumonia is listed as the fifth leading cause of death, especially among the elderly. Demographic projections predict that as an increasing proportion of U.S. society ages, the number of cases of pneumonia will likely rise from the 5.6 million cases annually, of which approximately 30% require hospitalization. Although health care costs related to pneumonia top $23 billion, perhaps because it is not a chronic disease, there has been little advancement over the past hundred years in the clinician's tools, which remain the chest radiograph and Gram stain sputum analysis to manage this infection. Because literally scores of pathogens may be responsible for causing pneumonia, clinicians are usually faced with scant specific information on which they must base therapeutic decisions.

Bacterial pneumonia may be defined as an acute infection of parenchymal lung tissue by microorganisms that also cause the host to respond with symptoms of illness. Within this broad definition, several categories exist that help clinicians to determine which bacterial pathogens may be most likely. *Community-acquired pneumonia* is the most common; however, local geography may dictate consideration of some organisms that fall outside the usual list of suspects. For example, residents of some urban locations with high prevalence of HIV infection may need to consider *Pneumocystis carinii* (actually a fungus) on their list of common pathogens, whereas patients presenting with pneumonia in Nova Scotia may well have acute *Coxiella burnetii* infection (Q fever). Residents of chronic care facilities have more gram-negative and staphylococcal infections than those with traditional community-acquired disease, and this illness deserves the separate category of *nursing home–acquired pneumonia*. Patients who develop pneumonia more than 48 to 96 hours after initial hospitalization have *nosocomial pneumonia,* with Enterobacteriaceae, *Pseudomonas aeruginosa,* and *Staphylococcus aureus* among the leading causative agents. *Aspiration pneumonia* denotes a clinical situation wherein recent seizure, altered mental status, or loss of consciousness may have predisposed the patient to inhalation of significant oral or gastric contents, thereby furnishing an environment likely to foster an anaerobic pulmonary infection.

DIAGNOSIS

A surprising number of patients labeled with pneumonia may actually have a more benign respiratory tract infection. Many practitioners prescribe antibiotics for routine viral infections such as acute bronchitis or rhinosinusitis, with the mistaken belief that either the patient requires these drugs or pneumonia will be prevented, although no study exists proving that point.

Pneumonia complicates fewer than 0.2% of acute bronchitic infections. Therefore, the presence of cough, which is among the most common complaints in patients presenting to either an emergency room or a primary care practice, must be distinguished between the potentially severe problem of bacterial pneumonia from a routine viral upper respiratory tract infection such as acute bronchitis. Although cough is the most common symptom of pneumonia and afflicts 90% of patients, sputum production may be lacking in up to half. In those who do produce sputum with their cough, even green or yellow phlegm is unhelpful because that can accompany either viral bronchitis or bacterial pneumonia.

Other respiratory symptoms may help to raise the concern of pneumonia. Fever higher than 102°F rarely accompanies viral respiratory infections (with the exception of influenza), and rigors should raise the suspicion of bacterial infection. Pleuritic chest pain and dyspnea often suggest a more concerning process. Other nonspecific symptoms may accompany pneumonia including headache, sweats, malaise, nausea, vomiting, and diarrhea. Occasional patients present confusingly with abdominal pain because of lower lobe pneumonia with overlooked or minimal respiratory complaints. Elderly and immunocompromised patients may have less prominent traditional signs of pneumonia such as fever or cough and instead may present with lethargy or altered mental status.

Pneumonia appears to be much more common in the elderly (more than 65 years old) than in younger age groups. Chronic health problems such as alcoholism, diabetes, HIV infection, congestive heart failure, malignant disease, and chronic obstructive pulmonary disease also appear to increase the frequency of pneumonia. Cigarette smokers are more prone to pneumonia because the habit disrupts normal mucociliary pulmonary defenses and macrophage function.

Unfortunately, physical examination findings do not lead to any firm conclusions regarding pneumonia even when they are combined with the medical history. Some patients may have minimal chest findings, although up to 80% of patients have some localized rales. Occasionally, findings on lung examination are detected before an abnormality is identified on the chest radiograph. Fewer than 25% have traditional signs of consolidation such as tactile fremitus, egophony, or tubular breath sounds. In the rare patient with splinting, a patient may favor bending the thorax on the side of a bacterial pneumonia to cause an inspiratory lag. Several prospective studies have failed to confirm that physical findings have much more than a 50% chance of supporting or excluding a diagnosis of pneumonia. Elevated respiratory rates are typically common in the elderly population. This population may have evidence of delirium or dehydration on examination secondary to pneumonia.

The chest radiograph remains the favorite arbiter of pneumonia, and because of the limitations of history and examination findings, it is critical to prevent overdiagnosis and overtreatment of nonpneumonia illness with antibiotics. The chest radiograph can also help the clinician to sort through some of the common items on the differential diagnosis list of pneumonia ranging from anodynic problems such as acute bronchitis (infiltrate negative chest radiograph) to more serious concerns such as congestive heart failure and septic or bland pulmonary emboli. Infiltrates on chest radiographs are often described in terms such as interstitial, reticulonodular, or patchy, although these terms are really not helpful for determining an etiologic diagnosis. A finding of lobar pneumonia, cavitation, or accompanying large pleural effusion generally is evidence of a traditional bacterial origin.

In the patient with cough and fever, a common problem facing the clinician is in whom do you order a chest radiograph? Studies examining this issue, usually in emergency department settings, have found that an absence of any vital sign abnormality (defined as temperature lower than 38.0°C, respiratory rate less than 30 breaths/minute, pulse slower than 100 beats/minute) means that there is a less than a 1% chance of finding pneumonia in a patient with no other concerning findings.

The chest computed tomography (CT) scan is clearly more sensitive than the chest radiograph in defining lung disease or in detecting subtle early infiltrates. This may be especially helpful in the immunosuppressed patient or in the patient with an equivocal chest radiograph. In smokers, CT scans may help to determine whether a tumor is causing obstructive pneumonia. However, although CT is more sensitive, clinicians ought not worry about ambulatory patients who may have CT findings but unremarkable chest radiographs because most of these patients appear to have minor infections that usually do not even require antibiotics. Moreover, because of both the extra radiation (approximately that of six to seven plain chest radiographs) and the extra expense, it is unlikely that CT scans will displace routine chest radiographs in the evaluation of most cases of pneumonia.

MANAGEMENT

In the patient with cough, fever, and infiltrate on chest radiograph, the next steps usually center on three important clinical decisions: whether additional diagnostic tests are pursued to define the cause, whether hospitalization is required, and which antibiotic to prescribe. For most patients with pneumonia, the decision regarding hospitalization tends to color further diagnostic evaluations and kinds of antibiotics prescribed. For the patient with pneumonia who remains ambulatory, most clinicians do not order additional tests but rather treat with an antibiotic for the expected pathogens (Table 1). Often referred as having *walking pneumonia*, these patients are usually less than 50 years old and frequently suspected of having viral or atypical bacterial pathogens such as *Chlamydia pneumoniae* or *Mycoplasma pneumoniae,* although antibiotic treatment should also cover the typical pathogens such as *Streptococcus pneumoniae, Haemophilus influenzae,* and *Morexella catarrhalis.* Good and relatively inexpensive choices for antibiotic treatment include macrolides or tetracyclines (Table 2). Fluoroquinolone drugs have exceptional activity against most routine bacterial pneumonic pathogens, but they are often reserved for older, sicker patients or for those with co-morbidities.

Approximately 18% to 30% of patients will require hospitalization for pneumonia. A large study performed in the 1990s examining clinical predictors of morbidity and mortality with pneumonia found an extremely low 30-day mortality rate (less than 0.1%) for patients less than 50 years of age who had no significant co-morbidities such as cancer, congestive heart failure, and renal or liver disease and who had normal vital signs. On a practical basis, normal respiratory status, normal mentation, and nontoxic appearance along with sufficient home support mean that the patient is a candidate for treatment as an outpatient. Compared with hospitalization for pneumonia

TABLE 1. **Microbial of Pneumonia Etiologies**

	Community-Acquired Pneumonia	Nursing Home–Related Pneumonia	Nosocomial Pneumonia/Ventilator-Associated Pneumonia
Streptococcus pneumoniae	15–35%	0–39%	<3%
Haemophilus influenzae	2–10%	0–22%	5–8%
Morexella catarrhalis	0–5%	0–5%	—
Legionella species	0–15%	0–6%	0–10%
Chlamydia species	5–15%	<6%	—
Mycoplasma species	1–10%	<1%	—
Gram-negative bacilli	5–10%	0–51%	30–60%
Staphylococcus aureus	1–5%	0–33%	20–40%
Viruses	2–10%	0–9%	<1%
Pneumocystis carinii	0–10%	—	—
Mycobacterium tuberculosis	0–5%	—	—
Aspiration	2–10%	6–20%	0–35%
Unknown	30–60%	0–74%	10–30%

of equivalent severity, studies suggest that ambulatory patients have shorter recovery periods, avoid nosocomial complications, and return to usual activities sooner.

Although algorithms exist to help decide which patients may benefit from hospitalization, in general, older patients and those with abnormal vital signs or laboratory abnormalities have higher associated mortalities. Most patients who are more than 65 years of age require hospitalization, because the average mortality rate in this group is 15% to 25%. Severe community-acquired pneumonia may represent about 10% of patients ill enough to require immediate intensive unit care or mechanical ventilation. These patients may be identified by respiratory rates greater than 30 breaths/minute, arterial oxygen tension less than 50 to 60 mm Hg on room air, multilobar pneumonia on chest radiograph, hypotension (less than 90 mm Hg systolic), requirement of vasopressors, oliguria, or abnormal mental status.

For patients admitted to the hospital, standard tests ordered include complete blood counts, comprehensive metabolic profiles, and blood cultures. Young adults or any patients with risk factors should have an HIV

TABLE 2. **Empirical Selection of Antibiotics for Bacterial Pneumonia**

COMMUNITY-ACQUIRED PNEUMONIA	
Outpatient	Doxycycline or macrolide
Older outpatient or with co-morbidities	Fluoroquinolone
Hospitalized (general medical ward)	Extended-spectrum cephalosporins with macrolide or β-lactam/β-lactamase inhibitor with macrolide or fluoroquinolone (alone)
Hospitalized (intensive care unit)	Extended-spectrum cephalosporins OR β-lactam/β-lactamase inhibitor with either macrolide or fluoroquinolone; consider antipseudomonal agents if structural lung disease exists
Aspiration	Fluoroquinolone with or without clindamycin, β-lactam/β-lactamase inhibitor
NURSING HOME–ACQUIRED PNEUMONIA	
Oral therapy	Amoxicillin/clavulanate or fluoroquinolone
Parenteral therapy	β-lactam/β-lactamase inhibitor or extended-spectrum cephalosporin with macrolide or fluoroquinolone (alone)
Aspiration	Fluoroquinolone with or without clindamycin or β-lactam/β-lactamase inhibitor
HOSPITAL-ACQUIRED PNEUMONIA (> 4 DAYS AFTER ADMISSION)*	
Intensive care unit	Cefepime or imipenem with or without aminoglycoside, with or without vancomycin
Other than intensive care unit	Extended spectrum cephalosporin with or without aminoglycoside, with or without vancomycin; may consider antipseudomonal agents with or without aminoglycoside, with or without vancomycin

Amoxicillin/clavulanate (Augmentin) 500 mg PO tid.
Clindamycin (Cleocin) 600–900 mg IV q 8h.
Doxycyline (Vibramycin) 100 mg PO bid.
Vancomycin (Vancocin) 1 g IV q12h.
Macrolide = clarithromycin (Biaxin) 500 mg bid; azithromycin (Zithromax) 500 mg day PO or IV qd.
Fluoroquinolone = moxifloxacin (Avelox) 400mg IV or PO qd; levofloxacin (Levaquin) 500 or 750 mg IV or PO qd; gatifloxacin (Tequin) 400 mg IV or PO qd.
Extended-spectrum cephalosporins = ceftriaxone (Rocephin) 1–2 g IV qd or cefotaxime (Claforan) 1–2 g IV q8h.
β-lactam/β-lactamase inhibitor = ampicillin/sulbactam (Unasyn) 1.5–3.0 mg IV q6h; ticarcillin/clavulanate (Timentin) 3.1–6.2 g IV q4–6h.
Antipseudomonal agents = piperacillin/tazobactam (Zosyn) 3.375 g IV q4–6h; imipenem/cilastatin (Primaxin) 0.25–1.0 g IV q6h; meropenem (Merrem) 1–2 g IV q8h; cefepime (Maxipime) 1–2 g IV q12h; ciprofloxacin (Cipro) 400 mg IV q12h.
Aminogylcosides = gentamicin or tobramycin 5mg/kg IV qd; amikacin 15 mg/kg/IV qd.
*Standard doses based on normal renal function.

serologic examination ordered as part of the evaluation of pneumonia. Although blood cultures offer the possibility of offering a definite diagnosis regarding cause of the pneumonia, the 24- to 72-hour incubation period means that any discrete information will not be available at the time of initial antibiotic selection.

The roles of the sputum Gram stain and culture remain controversial because the sensitivity and specificity of the tests are reduced by the potential for these samples merely to represent bacterial colonization of the oropharynx, rather than a true representation of the pneumonia. Sputum examined under low power (×100) microscopy showing more than 25 neutrophils and fewer than 10 epithelial cells per field is thought to minimize identification of pathogens representing the oropharyneal contamination. Purulent sputum without identification of a predominant organism should raise suspicion of an atypical bacterial infection with organisms such as *Legionella* or *Mycoplasma*. Sputum analysis may be helpful to offer guidance, but treatment decisions based solely on sputum results should not be entertained. Likewise, sputum culture results should not be offered as definitive proof, but they are helpful for suggesting types of infections as well as for information regarding local antimicrobial resistance.

Definitive microbiologic identification of the cause of pneumonia does offer the possibility for targeted antibiotic therapy. Most commonly, this is based on blood culture results, but any representative pathogen from a normally sterile body site qualifies, such as from pleural fluid. In many studies, up to 60% of patients have no identifiable cause of pneumonia. Although sputum results for traditional pathogens such as *S. pneumoniae* or *H. influenzae* can be considered only probable causes, certain organisms are not thought to colonize, and therefore their identification always qualifies as an implicated pathogen; examples include *Legionella* species, *Mycobacterium tuberculosis, P. carinii,* influenza virus, or endemic fungi such as *Histoplasma, Blastomyces,* or *Coccidioides*.

Besides standard bacterial, fungal, and viral stains and cultures, other tests may be used to help secure an etiologic diagnosis. *Legionella* urine antigen kits detect only the most common serotype 1 of *Legionella pneumophila*. The role of a new pneumococcal urine antigen is unclear, but it is positive in 80% of patients bacteremic with *S. pneumoniae*. Serologic studies for atypical pathogens such as *Chlamydia, Mycoplasma,* and *Legionella* are not especially specific even with a fourfold rise in titer using paired acute and convalescent sera, and of course they are only of help retrospectively. Cold-agglutinin or *Mycoplasma* IgM antibodies may support a suspicion of *M. pneumoniae* infection, but again they are prone to false-positive results.

Occasional patients may require invasive diagnostic procedures such as fiberoptic bronchoscopy with lavage or biopsy, although these techniques are usually reserved for patients with immunosuppressive conditions or those who do not respond to initial therapy. Most patients presenting with pneumonia and significant pleural effusions should undergo thoracentesis to determine whether empyema exists that may demand more definitive surgical drainage.

The clinician is therefore unlikely to know exactly what pathogen is the cause of pneumonia. Therefore, empirical decisions are often geared toward agents most commonly anticipated. For community-acquired pneumonia, these are typically *S. pneumoniae, H. influenzae, M. catarrhalis, C. pneumoniae, M. pneumoniae,* and *L. pneumophila*. For patients suffering from severe community-acquired pneumonia, *S. pneumoniae* and *L. pneumophila* are most commonly involved, although gram-negative bacilli are a significant cause, especially in patients with co-morbidities. Although commonly thought of causing a mild respiratory condition, *M. pneumoniae* has been described as causing up to 11% of community-acquired pneumonias requiring intensive unit care.

For the hospitalized patient with community-acquired pneumonia, empirical therapy is directed against the typical pathogens. Because *S. pneumoniae* remains a leading pathogen and the cause of most mortality, much has been written regarding the rise of penicillin resistance since the early 1990s. Although rates of resistance to both β-lactam and macrolide antibiotics have been rising, the clinical significance of the resistance has been difficult to define, even in patients who have received antibiotics for pathogens supposedly resistant in vitro. Although rates of resistance to penicillin and β-lactam drugs are up to 20% in many parts of the United States, resistance of *S. pneumoniae* to fluoroquinolones is generally less than 1% to 2%.

Despite the superiority of the fluoroquinolone class against respiratory pathogens, few data exist to show that patients receiving drugs for which the bacterium is resistant suffer any increased mortality or even added complications or longer lengths of stay. Therefore, although may organizations have written guidelines for the treatment of community-acquired pneumonia, no convincing data suggest that any one drug or drug regimen is superior. Table 2 reflects a set of recommendations balancing many of the considerations for the empirical treatment of pneumonia to cover both traditional bacterial pathogens and as well as atypical agents such as *Legionella, Mycoplasma,* and *Chlamydia*. The clearest impact on mortality demonstrated to date is not which antibiotic is given, but rather the timeliness of administration. For patients hospitalized, initiation of the antibiotic infusion within 8 hours of presentation to medical attention correlates with significantly reduced morbidity and mortality.

Certain subsets of bacterial pneumonia deserve special mention. Aspiration pneumonia may engender an infection rich in anaerobes and gram-negative bacilli, especially if the patient is from a nursing home environment (see Table 1). Patients from nursing homes who have pneumonia should have robust gram-negative antibiotic coverage in consideration of a likely aspiration event (see Table 2). Patients with severe community-acquired pneumonia should have therapy well directed against *Legionella* and gram-negative bacilli. Because these patients are critically ill, many clinicians use agents such as fluoroquinolones that are near certain to have antipneumococcal activity. If patients in the intensive care unit have severe chronic obstructive or other structural lung disease, antipseudomonal agents are used to broaden antimicrobial coverage.

Hospital-acquired pneumonia developing within 4 days of admission is usually due *S. pneumoniae,* methicillin-susceptible *S. aureus*, *H. influenzae*, or anaerobes much as in community-acquired pneumonia. Development of pneumonia after 4 days of admission or during prolonged hospitalization increases the risk of antibiotic-resistant organisms such as methicillin-resistant *S. aureus* and gram-negative bacilli such as *P. aeruginosa, K. pneumoniae,* and *Acinetobacter baumannii* (see Table 2). Development of pneumonia while the patient is on a ventilator (so-called ventilator-associated pneumonia) is tricky to diagnose conclusively and normally requires evidence of new infiltrate, worsening respiratory status, fever, and/or leukocytosis. The pathogens are much the same as those in nosocomially acquired pneumonia; however, endotracheal suction may represent only colonization. Few institutions practice quantitative bacterial cultures using a protected brush bronchoscope to define the offending pathogen specifically.

Most patients improve within 1 to 3 days of initial treatment. The average duration of fever is 2.5 days for pneumococcal pneumonia, although bacteremic pneumococcal pneumonia averages 6 to 7 days. *Mycoplasma*-based fevers absolve within 48 hours, whereas legionellosis tends to take 5 days or longer.

The duration of treatment is not well defined for pneumonia. Recommendations vary ranging from 7 to 10 days for most pneumonias to 14 days for illness caused by atypical agents such as *Mycoplasma* or *Legionella*. Pneumococcal pneumonia should be treated for 72 hours beyond the break of fever. For hospitalized patients, initial therapy is often parenteral, although there is little reason not to use agents with excellent bioavailability (e.g., fluoroquinolones) by the oral route in those without critical illness. Changing from parenteral to oral therapy is associated with numerous economic, health, and social benefits. Many randomized trials support the practice of switching to appropriate oral drugs when the patient has improved clinically and can take oral medicines, with the anticipation of a normally functioning gastrointestinal tract.

COMPLICATIONS AND EXPECTATIONS

Significant complications usually fall within the purview of those requiring intensive care unit support for respiratory failure or hypotension. Although hypoxemic respiratory failure is the most common reason for admission to the intensive care unit, adult respiratory distress syndrome may complicate up to 25% of cases. The development of adult respiratory distress syndrome prolongs hospital and intensive care unit stays considerably even when evidence indicates that the infection was sterilized within the first few days. Sepsis with multiorgan dysfunction is a frequent accompaniment of severe cases of pneumonia, especially those resulting from *S. pneumoniae*, *L. pneumophila*, and gram-negative bacilli. Occasionally, the pathogens causing pneumonia may have infected other organs, with resulting meningitis, endocarditis, septic arthritis, or purulent pericarditis.

Pleural effusions develop in up to 50% of patients with pneumonia. Most of these are sterile parapneumonic effusions, although perhaps 5% of patient will have empyema or complicated pleural effusion that will require drainage. The sicker a patient is, the greater the suspicion should be that the effusion should be aspirated diagnostically, although fluid levels of less than 1 cm on lateral chest decubitus radiographs have low chances of representing empyema. Thoracentesis that yields frank pus, bacteria identified on Gram staining, or a pH lower than 7.1 indicates a need for drainage.

Some patients do not respond to expected therapy. In these situations, careful thought should be given to whether pneumonia is an incorrect diagnosis. In these situations, congestive heart failure, embolus, neoplasm, sarcoidosis, drug-induced pneumonitis, or pulmonary hemorrhage should be entertained. If infectious pneumonia is indeed correct, then three possible arenas should be explored. Pathogen-based issues include drug-resistant organisms, unanticipated organisms such as *Nocardia* or *M. tuberculosis,* or nonbacterial infections that are fungal or viral. Drug-based issues include incorrect drug selection or dosing, problems with drug compliance especially in the ambulatory patient, and adverse reactions such as drug fever. Finally, host issues include local factors such as obstruction or foreign body mechanisms, development of superinfection or empyema, or suppressed immune status. Clinicians should note that mortality, especially in the elderly, for hospitalized patients with community-acquired pneumonia can easily range beyond 10% to 15% despite perfectly appropriate antibiotic administration and supportive care.

Workup of patients with poorly responsive pneumonia should cover both infectious and noninfectious issues. For example, chest CT scan, ventilation-perfusion scan, antineutrophil cytoplasmic antibody test, bronchoscopy, or open lung biopsy can especially help the clinician to sort through alternative diagnoses such as fungal pneumonias, tuberculosis, *Nocardia* infection, pulmonary emboli, alveolar cell carcinoma, Wegener's granulomatosis, and sarcoidosis.

Follow-up chest radiographs are not required when patients are improving as expected. Most patients clear their radiographs within 4 weeks if they are less than 50 years old; however, in older patients and in those with *L. pneumophila*, this may take substantially longer because only 55% of radiographic findings are resolved by week 12. Consideration of follow-up chest radiographs by week 7 to 12 should be entertained if there is any suspicion of neoplasia and probably in all smokers.

PREVENTION

Annual influenza immunization likely has the largest impact on community-acquired pneumonia by the prevention of both primary influenzal as well as secondary bacterial pneumonias. Although the vaccine offers only imperfect protection, at a minimum it lessens the severity of influenzal illness. Current recommendations suggest that all patients at risk of complications of influenza, health care workers, and all household members of patients at risk as well as all persons more than 50 years of age undergo annual vaccination.

The 23-valent pneumococcal capsular polysaccharide vaccine (Pneumovax) is approximately 60% effective in preventing bacteremic pneumococcal infection in immunocompetant adults. Although the protective effect wanes with advancing age and immunocompromising conditions, the vaccine is recommended for adults older than 65 years or an adult of any age with significant co-morbidities such as diabetes or pulmonary or cardiac disease. Both the influenza and pneumococcal vaccines can be given before hospital discharge, without risk of serious adverse reaction. Current guidelines suggest boosting the pneumococcal vaccine every 5 to 6 years. The conjugated pneumococcal vaccine (Prevenar) has been FDA-approved only for the prevention of pneumococcal bacteremia in children; its effect in adults is under study, and currently there are no recommendations for its use beyond childhood.

VIRAL UPPER RESPIRATORY TRACT INFECTIONS

method of
DIANE E. PAPPAS, M.D., J.D., and
J. OWEN HENDLEY, M.D.
University of Virginia Health Sciences Center
Charlottesville, Virginia

Viral respiratory infections are acute, self-limited infections of the respiratory tract that produce the familiar rhinorrhea, congestion, and cough of the common cold. Colds are the most common human illness and are a significant cause of absenteeism from both school and work. All ages are susceptible, but children are more frequently affected and experience more prolonged symptoms than adults.

Rhinovirus, with over 100 serotypes, is the most common pathogen, accounting for at least 50% of colds in both children and adults. But many other viruses may also cause the symptoms of the common cold, including respiratory syncytial virus (RSV), influenza viruses, parainfluenza virus, adenovirus, enteroviruses (echo- and coxsackieviruses), and coronaviruses. Colds may occur at any time, but there is an increased prevalence each fall and winter that occurs in a predictable fashion. It begins with an increased frequency of rhinovirus infections in September, followed by parainfluenza in October and November. Adenovirus infections are present at a low rate throughout the fall and winter months. RSV, influenza viruses, and coronavirus dominate the winter months. The cold season finally ends in March or April with a small increase in rhinovirus infections.

Viral transmission may occur through small-particle aerosol inhalation, large-particle droplet deposition on nasal or conjunctival mucosa, or direct transfer by hand-to-hand contact. Nasal secretions of infected individuals contain significant rhinovirus titers. Rhinovirus is commonly found on the hands of infected individuals, where it can live for up to 2 hours. Studies have shown that virus is efficiently transferred from hand to hand after contact as brief as 10 seconds; transmission is completed through subsequent contact with nasal or conjunctival mucosa and infection by self-inoculation results. In addition, contact with inanimate surfaces may spread infection, as rhinovirus may survive for several days on inanimate surfaces. Transmission through small-particle aerosol has not been demonstrated for rhinovirus or RSV, but both influenza virus and coronavirus can be transmitted by small-particle aerosol.

Cold symptoms usually appear within 24 to 48 hours after inoculation. This coincides with an influx of polymorphonuclear cells (PMNs) into the nasal submucosa and epithelium. The presence of colored nasal discharge also correlates with the presence of PMNs and may signify either the presence of PMNs or the presence of PMN enzymatic activity. At the same time, there is an increased concentration of albumin, kinins (bradykinin), and inflammatory mediators, including a potent chemoattractant for PMNs identified as interleukin-8, in the nasal secretions of infected individuals. Histologic studies have shown that the nasal epithelium remains intact during the course of the common cold and that rhinovirus replication occurs in only a small number of nasal epithelial cells.

The typical presentation of the common cold in children differs significantly from the illness seen in adults. Adults have an average of two to four colds per year, with nasal congestion as the prominent symptom. Fever is absent, and symptoms resolve within 5 to 7 days. Children younger than 6 years average eight colds per year, with colored nasal discharge as the prominent symptom. Children often have fever during the first 3 days of illness, and their symptoms are prolonged, lasting 10 to 14 days.

Abnormalities of the paranasal sinuses are common during the course of the common cold. In one study, 87% of healthy young adults with recent onset of cold symptoms had paranasal sinus abnormalities visible on computed tomography (CT) scan, with marked improvement or resolution in 79% of subjects evaluated at follow-up 2 weeks later (without antibiotic treatment). Similarly, in children, paranasal sinus abnormalities are commonly demonstrated in children undergoing head CT or magnetic resonance imaging for nonsinus diagnoses, especially in children who experienced cold symptoms in the preceding 2 weeks.

Abnormalities of the middle ear are also common. Two thirds of children aged 2 to 12 years had abnormal middle ear pressures at some time during the 2 weeks following onset of a cold, most often during the first week. The abnormal ear pressures were intermittent and shifted from ear to ear. In adults, 74% of subjects with rhinovirus infection had abnormal middle ear pressures, usually on days 2 to 5 of illness, with resolution in 2 to 3 weeks.

Complications of the common cold may include otitis media, asthma exacerbation, sinusitis, and pneumonia. Epistaxis, pharyngitis, and conjunctivitis may also occur.

TREATMENT

Antihistamines, decongestants, antitussives, and zinc lozenges are all marketed for symptomatic relief of cold symptoms in children and adults, but there are few studies that demonstrate any benefit of these products. Supportive therapy remains the mainstay of treatment.

In infants and children with fever during the first few days of illness, treatment with acetaminophen (or ibuprofen, in children older than 6 months) may be useful. Bulb suction with saline nose drops may be used for the temporary relief of nasal congestion in infants; the older child may use a saline nose spray. Children with asthma should use β-agonist medications to relieve bronchospasm, which may be triggered by viral upper respiratory tract infection.

The anticholinergic effects of first-generation antihistamines such as chlorpheniramine (Chlor-Trimeton Allergy) may help reduce the secretions of the common cold. In adults, several studies have found that treatment with chlorpheniramine may reduce cold symptoms, whereas treatment with diphenhydramine (Benadryl) or triprolidine hydrochloride (Zymine) did not. A study comparing an antihistamine-decongestant combination and placebo in children found that treatment provided no significant improvement in cold symptoms but that 46.6% of the subjects in the treatment group were asleep within 2 hours after treatment, compared with only 26.5% asleep in the placebo group. Side effects of first-generation antihistamines may include sedation, paradoxical excitability, respiratory depression, and hallucinations. Because of the lack of proven efficacy and the potential for serious side effects, antihistamines should not be used in children younger than 12 months.

Cough suppressants are commonly used in adults for symptomatic relief of the cough associated with the common cold. Narcotic cough syrups (such as codeine) and dextromethorphan (Benylin) (a narcotic analogue) are centrally acting cough suppressants. Both may cause respiratory depression. In children and adults with bronchospasm, effective cough suppression could result in mucus plugging and worsening respiratory symptoms. In children 18 months to 12 years old, codeine and dextromethorphan were shown to be no more effective than placebo in suppressing cough associated with the common cold; cough in all subjects was improved within 3 days. Because of the potential toxicity and the lack of proven efficacy, cough suppressants are not recommended for pediatric use.

Decongestants, either topical or systemic, are sympathomimetic medications that cause vasoconstriction of the nasal mucosa. In adults, oral pseudoephedrine (Sudafed) has been shown to reduce nasal congestion and sneezing, and phenylpropanolamine* has been shown to improve nasal patency temporarily. As many as 30% of adults reported side effects of these medications, including tachycardia, elevated diastolic blood pressure, and palpitations. There is an increased risk of hemorrhagic stroke with the use of phenylpropanolamine; the Food and Drug Administration has issued a public health advisory to consumers to avoid phenylpropanolamine. There are no studies demonstrating efficacy of these medications in children, and they are not recommended for pediatric use.

It remains unclear whether treatment with zinc gluconate† may shorten the duration of cold symptoms. Studies in adults are contradictory. In children, a randomized, double-blind, placebo-controlled trial in schoolchildren showed no benefit from treatment with zinc gluconate lozenges† (Halls Zinc Defense) but showed significant side effects including bad taste, nausea, throat irritation, and diarrhea.

Antibiotics are of no benefit in the treatment of viral respiratory infections or in the prevention of secondary bacterial complications. The unnecessary use of antibiotics may cause significant side effects and contribute to increasing antimicrobial resistance.

Patients should be encouraged to practice frequent hand washing and to avoid touching the nose and eyes in order to avoid transmission of viral respiratory infections from person to person. Annual influenza vaccination can prevent influenza infection and its complications. Treatment of high-risk infants with monthly injections of palivizumab (Synagis), a monoclonal antibody preparation, is available to prevent RSV infection.

---

*Not available in the United States.
†Not FDA approved for this indication.

VIRAL AND MYCOPLASMAL PNEUMONIAS

method of
RANDY A. TAPLITZ, M.D.
Oregon Health & Science University
Portland, Oregon

Viruses and *Mycoplasma* give rise to pneumonias historically described as "atypical" because their clinical, epidemiologic, and radiographic characteristics were believed to differ from those of "typical" bacterial pneumonias. Numerous studies have shown no convincing differentiating clinical or radiographic criteria between pneumococcal and atypical pneumonias; however, they are often considered separately to highlight differences in diagnostic tests and therapy.

MYCOPLASMA PNEUMONIA

Mycoplasma pneumoniae causes respiratory tract illness in children and in up to one third of adults with community-acquired pneumonia. It has been associated with outbreaks of respiratory disease in institutionalized settings, but it is responsible for only a small percentage of cases of community-acquired pneumonia requiring hospitalization. Clinical presentation, after a 2- to 4-week incubation period, is frequently with a prodromal illness with fever, chills, headache, and sore throat, followed by dry cough and radiographic evidence of pneumonia. Extrapulmonary manifestations may include nausea and vomiting and, rarely, rash, neurologic syndromes, or myocarditis. Cold hemagluttination and hemolytic anemia are sometimes observed. The chest radiograph may reveal interstitial or lobar disease. Laboratory tests to confirm *Mycoplasma* infection include serologic examination, culture, and DNA amplification. The most practical diagnostic test is immunoassay for the detection of *M. pneumoniae* IgM, which is rapid (less than 1 hour) and has a reported sensitivity and specificity of 90% and 93%, respectively. Cold agglutinin titers greater than 1:64 support the diagnosis, but they are neither sensitive nor specific. Because current commonly available tests are not very reliable or rapid in the detection of *Mycoplasma* pneumonia, therapy is usually empirical.

Treatment of *Mycoplasma* pneumonia involves supportive care and antimicrobial therapy, which is thought to shorten the duration of respiratory symptoms. *Mycoplasma* infections have traditionally been treated with erythromycin (E-Mycin) and tetracycline (Sumycin)/doxycycline (Vibramycin). Newer agents including azithromycin (Zithromax), clarithromycin (Biaxin), levofloxacin (Levaquin), sparfloxacin (Zagam), moxifloxacin (Avelox), and gatifloxacin (Tequin) also have good in vitro activity against this organism and are reasonable alternatives (Table 1). These antimicrobials also have activity against other community-acquired pneumonia pathogens including *Streptococcus pneumoniae, Chlamydia pneumoniae,* and *Legionella,* infection with which may be difficult to distinguish from *Mycoplasma* pneumonia on clinical grounds. When choosing an empirical regimen, one must consider the increasing resistance of the pneumococcus to macrolides and tetracycline/doxycycline; resistance to the fluoroquinolones, particularly levofloxacin, has also been reported. When the presentation is consistent with *M. pneumoniae* infection, empirical antibiotic treatment with a macrolide, doxycycline/tetracycline, or a fluoroquinolone is appropriate. For patients moderately to severely ill with pneumonia and in whom an etiologic agent cannot be confirmed, or in those who have comorbid conditions that put them at higher risk of complications, hospitalization should be considered. Such patients should receive either gatifloxacin or moxifloxacin *or* a macrolide or doxycycline *plus* a parenteral third-generation cepahalosporin to limit antibiotic failures related to pneumococcal resistance.

VIRAL PNEUMONIAS

Influenza

Influenza is the most common serious viral respiratory tract infection, and it is the one associated with the greatest morbidity and mortality. The risks for hospitalizations and deaths from influenza are higher among persons older than 65 years, in young children, and in those with chronic medical conditions such as cardiopulmonary disease. Influenza is characterized by the abrupt onset of fever, myalgia, headache, malaise, nonproductive cough, sore throat, and rhinitis. For most persons, this illness slowly resolves after several days; however, in some patients, influenza can exacerbate underlying medical conditions and can lead to secondary bacterial pneumonia, or it may be associated with primary influenza pneumonia. Primary influenza pneumonia begins as typical influenza, but it progresses rapidly to severe cough, dyspnea, and cyanosis. The chest radiograph reveals bilateral interstitial pneumonia or adult respiratory disease syndrome. Primary influenza pneumonia is rare between pandemics, but mortality is high.

Rapid tests for identification of influenza are available; these assays can detect influenza A and B in respiratory secretions in less than 1 hour, with a sensitivity of 70% to 90%. During epidemics, a diagnosis of influenza can often be made on clinical grounds in an unvaccinated patient with comparable sensitivity.

Patients with influenza pneumonia require supportive care to alleviate fever and cough and to maintain adequate hydration. Aspirin should be avoided, especially in children, because of the link with Reye's syndrome. Hospitalization is recommended for older or immunocompromised patients with influenza pneumonia.

Two classes of antivirals are approved for the treatment of uncomplicated influenza virus infection (see Table 1). The M2 ion channel inhibitors amantadine (Symmetrel) and rimantadine (Flumadine) are active

TABLE 1. **Diagnostic Tests and Recommended Drug Therapy for Mycoplasmal and Viral Pneumonias**

Pathogens	Rapid Diagnostic	Diagnostic Tests Serology, Culture, Other	*Recommended Antimicrobials (Adults)
MYCOPLASMAL			
Mycoplasma pneumoniae	PCR[a,b]	IgM, complement fixation, cold agglutinins	A macrolide or doxycycline or a fluoroquinolone[d]
VIRAL (COMMON)			
Influenza virus A and B	EIA, IFA[b], rapid culture method (shell vial assay)[c]	PCR[b], virus isolation from nasopharyngeal aspirate or swab or sputum	Oseltamavir or zanamavir, rimantadine or amantadine[e]
Respiratory syncytial virus	EIA, IFA, shell vial assay	PCR, virus isolation from nasopharyngeal washing, aspirate, or swab	Ribavirin[f]
Parainfluenza virus	IFA, shell vial assay	PCR, ELISA, shell vial culture, virus isolation from nasopharyngeal swab	—
Adenovirus	PCR, IFA, shell vial assay	ELISA, virus isolation from pharyngeal swab	—
VIRAL (RARE)			
Varicella-zoster virus	DFA from skin lesions, shell vial assay	Virus isolation, histopathology	— Acyclovir[g]
Herpes simplex virus	DFA from skin lesions, cytopathology	Virus isolation, histopathology	Acyclovir[h]
Cytomegalovirus	DFA, shell vial assay	Virus isolation, histopathology	Ganciclovir[i]
Hantavirus	PCR	EIA for IgM or IgG, histopathology	—
Measles (rubeola) virus	DFA	Virus isolation	—

[a]PCR assay available at selected references laboratories; reagents may not be FDA-approved for clinical use.
[b]IFA and PCR tests are available at some reference laboratories that use pooled reagents to detect multiple viruses in a single specimen.
[c]Rapid culture methods, such as shell vial assays, rely on detecting viral antigens expressed early in viral growth; results, often available in 24 to 48 hours, may not be available in all laboratories.
[d]Erythromycin 500 mg PO q6h; azithromycin (Zithromax) 500 mg PO day 1, then 250 mg/d PO; clarithromycin (Biaxin) 500 mg PO bid; doxycycline (Vibramycin) 100 mg PO bid; levofloxacin (Levaquin) 500 mg/d PO; gatifloxacin (Tequin) 400 mg PO qd; sparfloxacin (Zagam) 400 mg PO day 1, then 200 mg/d PO; moxifloxacin (Avelox) 400 mg qd; duration: 14 d for all except 5-7 d for azithromycin.
[e]Influenza A and B: oseltamivir (Tamiflu) 75 mg PO bid for 5 d; zanamivir (Relenza) 10 mg by inhalation q12h for 5 d; influenza A only: rimantadine (Flumadine) or amantadine (Symmetrel) 100 mg PO bid (qd in the elderly) for 7 d or until 1-2 d after cessation of symptoms.
[f]Ribavirin (Virazole) 20 mg/mL of diluent continuosly for 12-18 h with small particle aerosol generator.
[g]Acyclovir (Zovirax) 10-12 mg/kg IV q8h for at least 7 d.
[h]Acyclovir (Zovirax) 5-10 mg/kg IV q8h for at least 7 d.
[i]Ganciclovir (Cytovene) 5 mg/kg IV q12h for at least 14 d; consider addition of IVIG (intravenous immunoglobulin).
DFA, direct fluorescent antibody; EIA, enzyme immunoassay; ELISA, enzyme-linked immunosorbent assay; IFA, immunofluorescence assay; PCR, polymerase chain reaction.

only against influenza A and have been used to reduce the duration and severity of symptoms. The neuroaminidase inhibitors zanamivir (Relenza) and oseltamivir (Tamiflu) are active against influenza A and B, and they reduce the duration of illness and accelerate return to normal activity. Both classes of drugs must be given within 48 hours of illness onset to be most effective. Data do not exist to show that any of the drugs can prevent or treat influenza pneumonia. The most effective method of influenza prevention is yearly administration of the influenza vaccine.

Other Viral Causes of Pneumonia

Community-acquired pneumonia due to respiratory syncytial virus, parainfluenza, adenovirus and other viruses are infrequent in adults, and these viruses rarely cause severe pneumonia unless patients have significant immunosuppression or underlying medical problems. Other viral causes of pneumonia may be encountered in patients with particular epidemiologic risks (e.g., hantavirus pulmonary syndrome in patients with rodent exposure in endemic regions).

Respiratory syncytial virus is the leading cause of lower respiratory tract disease in infants and young children, and it can cause severe disease in immunocompromised adults. Clinical manifestations may range from mild upper respiratory infections to pneumonia, although bronchiolitis accounts for the majority of hospitalizations. Mortality is low among healthy children; children with underlying disease such as chronic lung disease or immunosuppression are at higher risk of severe disease. Ribavirin (Virazole) inhalation treatment is now rarely used in the United States because studies have not shown a decrease in mortality. Inhaled ribavirin has been used to treat immunocompromised patients with respiratory syncytial virus pneumonia, although controlled clinical trials are lacking. Adenovirus, picornavirus, coronavirus, and parainfluenza viruses have also been associated with lower tract respiratory diseases; no specific drugs have been shown to be effective for treatment of these viruses. Because of immunization and herd immunity, measles virus is now a rare cause of pneumonia. Members of the herpesvirus family including cytomegalovirus, herpesvirus, and varicella-zoster virus may cause pneumonia, particularly in transplant recipients or other immunocompromised patients (see Table 1).

LEGIONELLOSIS

method of
M.L. PEDRO-BOTET, M.D., PH.D.
Hospital Universitario Germans Trias i Pujol
Barcelona, Spain

and

VICTOR L. YU, M.D.
VA Medical Center
University of Pittsburgh
Pittsburgh, Pennsylvania

Legionnaires' disease is the designation for pneumonia caused by any of the *Legionella* species. *Legionella pneumophila* is the most common pathogenic species (accounting for 90% of human infections); 42 other species have been implicated in human disease. The other species most commonly implicated in pneumonias include *Legionella longbeachae*, *Legionella micdadei*, and *Legionella dumoffii*. Pontiac fever is an acute self-limited febrile illness without pneumonia.

CLINICAL PRESENTATION

The incubation period is 2 to 10 days. Fever is virtually always present. Symptoms of pneumonia are the predominant clinical manifestations, including nonproductive cough, dyspnea, and chest pain. Presence of upper respiratory symptoms, such as coryza are distinctly unusual. Gastrointestinal symptoms are often present. Diarrhea in a patient with pneumonia is a prominent symptom that should call attention to the possibility of legionnaires' disease.

Laboratory abnormalities are common, but hyponatremia, abnormal liver function tests, and elevated creatinine phosphokinase (CPK) occur more often in cases of legionnaires' disease than in pneumonias of other etiologies.

DIAGNOSIS

Radiograph almost always shows a pulmonary infiltrate at the time of clinical presentation. There is no distinct pattern, but nodular densities are often seen in immunosuppressed patients receiving corticosteroids.

Specialized microbiology tests are the definitive method for diagnosing legionnaires' disease. The Gram stain shows numerous polymorphonuclear leukocytes but organisms are few. The more specific laboratory tests include *Legionella* urinary antigen (which is sensitive for *L. pneumophila* serogroup 1 only), direct fluorescent antibody stain, and culture using multiple selective media. Seroconversion of antibodies to *L. pneumophila* are useful primarily in epidemiologic situations because of the necessity for convalescent sera after the patient has recovered.

Pontiac fever is diagnosed by seroconversion in a patient with the typical clinical manifestations of headache, fever, and myalgias.

THERAPY

As *Legionella* is an intracellular pathogen, the optimal antibiotic therapy for legionnaires' disease are those antibiotics that penetrate white blood cells and alveolar macrophages (Table 1). Beta-lactam antibiotics such as penicillins and cephalosporins are not effective because of their poor intracellular penetration. Macrolides, fluoroquinolones, rifampin (Rifadin),* trimethoprim-sulfamethoxazole (Bactrim) and tetracyclines have excellent intracellular penetration.

The newer macrolides (azithromycin [Zithromax], and clarithromycin [Biaxin]*) and quinolones (levofloxacin [Levaquin], moxifloxacin [Avelox],* or gemifloxacin)** are now the antibiotics of choice for legionnaires' disease. Azithromycin is more potent than erythromycin in vitro against *Legionella*, can be given once daily, and has few gastrointestinal side effects.

Quinolones are the most active drugs against *Legionella* in intracellular and animal models. Unlike the macrolides, they do not interact with cyclosporine (Sandimmune) or tacrolimus (Prograf), which are administered to transplant recipients. Compared with macrolides, there are no notable differences with respect to efficacy, but in one retrospective study comparing quinolones versus macrolides, times to apyrexia and hospital discharge were both shorter in patients receiving quinolones.

Other antibiotics that may be effective include tetracycline,* doxycycline,* and trimethoprim-sulfamethoxazole.* Rifampin* can be combined with another antibiotic to be used in patients with severe legionnaires' disease who are not responding to monotherapy.

The initial administration should be intravenous because the oral route may be unreliable in patients with gastrointestinal symptoms. Once an objective response has occurred (e.g., defervescence), oral therapy can be given. Duration of therapy can be 7 to 10 days and longer if the patient is immunosuppressed.

It should be noted that the newer macrolides and respiratory tract quinolones are also ideal antibiotics for empirical therapy of community-acquired pneumonia in the immunocompetent patient; they cover both the typical microorganisms, such as *Streptococcus pneumoniae* and *Haemophilus influenzae,* as well as the atypical microorganisms, such as *L. pneumophila*, *Chlamydia pneumoniae*, and *Mycoplasma pneumoniae*. Antibiotic therapy is not necessary for Pontiac fever.

*Not FDA approved for this indication.
**Investigational drug in the United States.

TABLE 1. **Antibiotic Selection for Legionella Infection**

Antimicrobial Agent	Dosage*
Macrolides	
Azithromycin (Zithromax)‡	500 mg orally or intravenously every 24 hours
Clarithromycin (Biaxin)	500 mg orally or intravenously† every 12 hours
Quinolones	
Levofloxacin (Levaquin)	750 mg intravenously every 24 hours 500 mg‡ orally every 24 hours
Ciprofloxacin (Cipro)¶	400 mg intravenously every 8 hours 750 mg orally every 12 hours
Ofloxacin (Floxin)¶	400 mg orally or intravenously every 12 hours
Moxifloxacin (Avelox)	400‡ orally every 24 hours
Tetracycline	
Doxycycline (Vibramycin)‡¶	100 mg orally or intravenously every 12 hours
Minocycline (Minocin)¶	100 mg orally or intravenously every 12 hours
Tetracycline (Sumycin)¶	500 mg orally or intravenously† every 6 hours
Others	
Trimethoprim-sulfamethoxazole (Bactrim)¶	160 and 800 mg intravenously every 8 hours 160 and 800 mg orally every 12 hours
Rifampin (Rifadin)‖¶	300–600 mg orally or intravenously every 12 hours

*The dosages are based on clinical experience and not on controlled trials.
†Intravenous form not available in some countries.
‡We recommend doubling the first dose.
‖Rifampin should only be used as part of combination therapy with a quinolone or a macrolide.
¶Not FDA approved for this indication.

PULMONARY EMBOLISM

method of
THOMAS M. HYERS, M.D.
St. Louis University School of Medicine
St. Louis, Missouri

Conventional therapy of pulmonary embolism (PE) is aimed at arresting growth of a thromboembolus to allow the body's adaptive mechanisms to organize and resorb the clot. In life-threatening PE, thrombolytic therapy is employed to lessen the clot burden and its attendant hemodynamic abnormalities. Under certain circumstances, surgical intervention is used to remove thromboembolus. Vena caval filters are used to reduce the risk of acute fatal PE. Long-term oral anticoagulation reduces the risk of recurrent venous thromboembolism. Duration of oral anticoagulation should be tailored to both the risk of recurrence and bleeding risk in individual patients. The rare syndrome of chronic thromboembolic pulmonary hypertension is a consequence of untreated or unresolved PE. It is insidious in onset and often occurs without a history of antecedent venous thromboembolism. When disease is present in proximal pulmonary arteries, it is amenable to treatment with pulmonary thromboendarterectomy.

INITIAL THERAPY

Unfractionated heparin (UH) and low-molecular-weight heparin (LMWH) are rapidly acting anticoagulants that provide effective treatment of acute PE and deep venous thrombosis (DVT). These drugs enhance the effect of a circulating coagulation inhibitor, antithrombin (formerly known as antithrombin III), so that the inhibitor combines with and inactivates thrombin, factor X, and factor IX. Both UH and LMWH must be given parenterally. When PE is suspected, anticoagulation with heparin or LMWH should be administered until the diagnostic evaluation is complete. If PE is confirmed, one or the other drug should be given in a therapeutic dose for at least 5 to 7 days or until an oral anticoagulant such as warfarin is fully effective on the basis of an international normalized ratio (INR) of 2.0 to 3.0 for 2 consecutive days.

UH is usually administered by intravenous infusion and its effect monitored by the activated partial thromboplastin time (APTT). The goal is to maintain the heparin infusion at a rate that keeps the APTT in the therapeutic range. This range is commonly cited as an APTT in seconds that corresponds to a plasma heparin level of about 0.3 to 0.6 U/mL (Table 1). Unfortunately, even the most experienced clinicians have great difficulty achieving this goal because UH is cleared rapidly and unpredictably from the circulation. Several nomograms and dosing schemes have been devised for administration of UH, but because of the unfavorable pharmacokinetic characteristics of the drug, achieving and maintaining a therapeutic effect continue to be a problem in many patients. Furthermore, because UH is usually given by intravenous infusion and requires monitoring and dose adjustment, most patients with PE must be hospitalized for at least 5 days if they are treated initially with UH.

LMWHs are fractionated from the parent heparin molecule to have mean molecular masses around 4 to 5 kDa. The smaller molecular size confers more favorable pharmacokinetic properties so that LMWHs can be administered subcutaneously on a body weight basis without subsequent monitoring or dose adjustment (Table 2). The only clinical caveat in this regard is that all LMWHs are cleared by the kidneys, and the dose of an LMWH should be monitored or reduced in patients with creatinine clearances below 30 mL/min.

TABLE 1. **Initiating Therapy with Unfractionated Heparin**

PULMONARY EMBOLISM SUSPECTED
Obtain baseline APTT, PT, CBC count
Check for contraindication to UH therapy
Order imaging study, give UH 5000 U IV

PULMONARY EMBOLISM CONFIRMED
Rebolus with UH 80 U/kg IV and begin infusion at 18 U/kg/h
Check APPT at 6 h (keep APTT in therapeutic range)
Check platelet count every 2-3 days
Start warfarin on day 1 at 5 mg and adjust dose by INR
Stop UH after at least 4-5 days of combined therapy when INR > 2.0
Give warfarin for appropriate duration at INR 2.0-3.0

APTT, activated partial thromboplastin time; CBC, complete blood count; INR, international normalized ratio; PT, prothrombin time; UH, unfractionated heparin.

Modified from Hyers TM, Agnelli G, Hull RD, et al: Antithrombotic therapy for venous thromboembolic disease. Chest 119(1 Suppl):180S, 2001.

TABLE 2. **Initiating Therapy with Low-Molecular-Weight Heparin**

PULMONARY EMBOLISM SUSPECTED
Obtain baseline APTT, PT, CBC count
Check for contraindication to therapy
Order imaging study, give LMWH in treatment dose

PULMONARY EMBOLISM CONFIRMED
Give LMWH in a treatment dose (enoxaparin or tinzaparin*)
Start warfarin on day 1 at 5 mg and adjust dose according to INR
Check platelet count every 2-3 days
Stop LMWH after 4-5 days of combined therapy when INR > 2.0
Give warfarin for appropriate duration at INR 2.0-3.0

*Enoxaparin at 1.0 mg/kg twice daily or 1.5 mg/kg once daily; tinzaparin at 175 IU/kg once daily.

APTT, activated partial thromboplastin time; CBC, complete blood count; INR, international normalized ratio; PT, prothrombin time; LMWH, low-molecular-weight heparin.

Modified from Hyers TM, Agnelli G, Hull RD, et al: Antithrombotic therapy for venous thromboembolic disease. Chest 119(1 Suppl):183S, 2001.

The convenience and portability of LMWH have allowed some patients with DVT to receive treatment at home or at least to be discharged from hospital earlier with a component of home therapy while waiting for the warfarin to achieve a therapeutic INR. Two LMWHs have been approved for treatment of DVT with or without PE. These are enoxaparin (Lovenox) and tinzaparin (Innohep).

The major complication associated with both UH and LMWH is bleeding. Patients can bleed from any location, but gastrointestinal and retroperitoneal bleeding seems to be most common. When localized bleeding occurs, the drug should be stopped and the cause investigated. Administration of packed red blood cells and other blood products may be necessary. UH can be neutralized with protamine sulfate administration, but this antidote is rarely necessary because the anticoagulant effect of heparin is rapidly cleared from the plasma. In this regard, protamine sulfate does not neutralize LMWH as effectively as it does UH.

Both heparin and LMWH can cause thrombocytopenia through an immune-mediated mechanism. Heparin-induced thrombocytopenia (HIT) can lead to paradoxical venous or arterial thrombosis because of intravascular consumption of platelets. UH appears to cause HIT in 2% to 3% of patients who receive the drug for more than 5 days. LMWH is less likely to cause this complication but should not be substituted for UH if HIT develops because LMWH cross-reacts with the HIT antibody in the majority of cases. A precipitous fall in platelet count, occurring usually between days 5 and 10 of therapy, signals the clinical onset of HIT. Although HIT usually occurs between day 5 and 10 of therapy with UH or LMWH, it can occur in the first day or two of therapy if the patient has been sensitized to heparin with prior treatment in the preceding 6 weeks. Two direct thrombin inhibitors, lepirudin (Refludan) and argatroban, have been approved for anticoagulation in patients with HIT and acute thrombosis (HITTS). When HITTS is suspected, UH or LMWH should be stopped immediately and one of the direct thrombin inhibitors should be started. If warfarin is also being given, it should be withheld until the platelet count has risen above 100,000/μL. At that point the warfarin can be restarted. The direct thrombin inhibitor should be continued until warfarin has prolonged the INR to greater than 2.0 on 2 consecutive days.

Long-term administration of UH in high dose can cause severe osteoporosis. This complication is particularly pertinent in pregnant women with venous thromboembolism (VTE) who cannot receive warfarin. LMWH appears to cause less osteoporosis than UH and should be considered in pregnant patients with VTE who require anticoagulation throughout pregnancy.

Thrombolytic agents dissolve fibrin thrombi by activating the plasma proenzyme plasminogen to the active enzyme plasmin. Plasmin then degrades fibrin, fibrinogen, and several other coagulation proteins. Currently, several thrombolytic agents are available for treatment of PE. These include streptokinase (Streptase), a bacterial product, and the human-derived products urokinase (Abbokinase) and tissue plasminogen activator (Activase). Each of these agents causes more thrombolysis than heparin or LMWH, although there is no clear evidence than one thrombolytic agent is preferred over another for treatment of PE. There is also no clear evidence that treatment of PE patients with thrombolytic agents improves survival. Furthermore, thrombolytic agents are more likely to cause bleeding than are the heparin products. Consequently, thrombolytic agents are usually reserved for patients with life-threatening PE or for those with massive iliofemoral thrombosis in whom compromise of the adjacent arterial circulation seems imminent. When a thrombolytic agent is infused, heparin or LMWH is held until the fibrinolytic effect has cleared. The heparin product is then restarted and given with warfarin as described previously.

SURGICAL METHODS

Various methods to remove pulmonary emboli have been utilized over the last 50 years. Direct surgical removal with cardiopulmonary bypass (pulmonary embolectomy) is rarely used because most patients who suffer PE either die or become stable before the operation can be undertaken. Several catheter-directed suction or fragmentation devices have also received sporadic usage. There are no controlled trials to make definitive statements about the value of any of these devices or procedures.

LONG-TERM ANTICOAGULATION

Warfarin (Coumadin) is an oral agent that interferes with effective synthesis of vitamin K–dependent coagulation factors II, VII, IX, and X. Warfarin also inhibits synthesis of the anticoagulant proteins C and S. The drug is given daily and monitored by the prothrombin time as standardized by the INR. Daily platelet counts should be monitored during administration of UH. Heparin or LMWH should be continued for at least 5 to 7 days until warfarin is fully effective as evidenced by an INR of 2.0 to 3.0 on 2 consecutive days. Warfarin is then given for at least 3 to 6 months and the INR maintained in the range 2.0 to 3.0. Because the therapeutic efficacy of warfarin declines rapidly when the INR falls below 2.0, clinicians are encouraged to target the INR to 2.5 when administering anticoagulation to patients.

As with the heparin products, bleeding is the most common complication of warfarin therapy. Bleeding risk is related to age, co-morbidity (particularly renal or hepatic disease and peptic ulcer), and to an inordinately prolonged INR. Because the anticoagulant effect of warfarin can be affected by numerous drug interactions and diet, therapy with this agent must be closely monitored with the prothrombin time and INR. Warfarin rarely causes a syndrome known as warfarin purpura. The syndrome is manifested by paradoxical subcutaneous thrombosis and is associated with congenital or acquired deficiency of protein C. This syndrome has become quite uncommon since physicians have stopped using large loading doses of warfarin.

Warfarin has fetopathic and teratogenic effects and should not be given during pregnancy or to women who might become pregnant. Pregnant women with VTE should receive either heparin or LMWH for the full term of pregnancy. At term, the drug is held for 24 hours and labor is induced. Heparin or LMWH should be restarted postpartum along with warfarin and the latter continued for at least 6 weeks after delivery. Warfarin has also been seen to fail to prevent recurrent PE in patients with VTE and cancer. In this circumstance, long-term therapy is usually given with UH or LMWH given subcutaneously in an anticoagulating dose.

Duration of warfarin therapy should be tailored to risk for recurrence of VTE (Table 3). Patients who experience a first episode of VTE after a time-limited risk factor such as surgery or transient immobilization probably need no more than 3 months of therapy. Patients who develop a first episode of VTE without a risk factor (idiopathic disease) should be treated for at least 6 months. Patients with a first episode of VTE and ongoing risk factors such as cancer, lupus anticoagulant, or one of the genetic predispositions (thrombophilia) listed in Table 3 should be treated for a longer period of time because the risk of recurrence is high. Patients with recurrent VTE, no matter what the putative risk factor, should receive long-term therapy. Well-designed randomized trials have established the duration of therapy in patients with transient risk factors and in those with idiopathic disease. The duration of therapy in patients with uncommon acquired or inherited predispositions is less clear as outlined in Table 3. In all situations, decision making about duration of therapy should include a careful assessment of bleeding and recurrence risks and of the individual patient's preference. On some occasions a prescription for anticoagulation of indefinite duration commits the patient to a lifetime of therapy. Therefore, the diagnosis of recurrent VTE should be firmly established before the recommendation is made.

TABLE 3. **Duration of Anticoagulant Therapy After Pulmonary Embolism***

3 to 6 months	• First event with reversible[†] or time-limited risk factor (patient may have underlying factor V Leiden or prothrombin 20210)
6 months or longer	• Idiopathic venous thromboembolism, first event
12 months to lifetime	• First event[‡] with Cancer, until resolved Anticardiolipin antibody Antithrombin deficiency • Recurrent event, idiopathic or with thrombophilia

*All recommendations are subject to modification by individual characteristics including patient's preference, age, co-morbidity, and likelihood of recurrence.

†Reversible or time-limited risk factors include surgery, trauma, immobilization, and estrogen use.

‡Proper duration of therapy is unclear in first event with homozygous factor V Leiden, homocystinemia, deficiency of protein C or S, or multiple thrombophilias and in recurrent events with reversible risk factors.

Modified from Hyers TM, Agnelli G, Hull RD, et al: Antithrombotic therapy for venous thromboembolic disease. Chest 119(1 Suppl):184S, 2001.

INFERIOR VENA CAVAL FILTERS

The major rationale for these devices is the presence of a contraindication to or a complication of anticoagulation in a patient with or at high risk for PE. These devices are also sometimes used in patients with massive, hemodynamically unstable PE and in chronic thromboembolic pulmonary hypertension (CTPH) after pulmonary endarterectomy, although the value of a filter is unclear in these circumstances. Whenever a filter is used, the sole benefit is reduction in risk of fatal PE in the ensuing 2 to 3 weeks. Filters do not prevent DVT and in fact seem to predispose to DVT over 1 to 2 years after insertion. When a filter is inserted in a high-risk patient, concomitant pharmacologic or mechanical prophylaxis should also be employed.

CHRONIC THROMBOEMBOLIC PULMONARY HYPERTENSION

Some patients do not resolve their PE even with proper treatment, and others seem to have episodes of PE that never come to medical attention. These individuals are at risk for development of CTPH, a syndrome that arises clinically as progressive dyspnea with a normal chest radiograph and pulmonary function tests. CTPH develops in less than 1% of patients who suffer PE. Half of patients with CTPH have never received medical care for PE, but, when questioned, some of these individuals remember a prior event that is compatible with the diagnosis. The presence of a lupus anticoagulant (anticardiolipin syndrome) appears to confer the highest risk, but this abnormality is present in only 10% to 15% of patients with CTPH. The hallmark of the syndrome is dyspnea, which progresses from dyspnea with exertion to continuous dyspnea that is present even at rest. The diagnosis is strongly suggested by an abnormal ventilation-perfusion lung scan that shows large perfusion defects with relatively normal ventilation. Medical therapy is ineffective, but pulmonary endarterectomy can be lifesaving when performed by an experienced surgeon with a skilled support team. A vena caval filter is usually placed during this surgery, and subsequent lifetime anticoagulation is prescribed.

NEW DIRECTIONS

Although LMWH offers greater convenience than UH, LMWH must still be given by parenteral injection. A small synthetic heparin-like molecule known as fondaparinux (1726 daltons) has been approved for prophylaxis of venous thromboembolism and will probably soon receive approval for treatment of DVT and PE. Fondaparinux (Arixtra) is given subcutaneously once daily without monitoring. Because of its small size, fondaparinux (with the antithrombin cofactor) inhibits factor Xa but not thrombin. An oral direct thrombin inhibitor known as ximelagatran (Exanta)* is in the final stages of evaluation for prophylaxis and treatment of venous thromboembolism. When approved, the drug will be given twice daily without monitoring or dose adjustment.

*Investigational drug in the United States.

SARCOIDOSIS

method of
ATHOL WELLS, M.D.
Royal Brompton Hospital
London, United Kingdom

Sarcoidosis is a multisystem disorder of unknown cause, most often occurring in young and middle-aged adults. The diagnosis is made when compatible clinicoradiologic features are associated with noncaseating granulomata on biopsy. Patients with sarcoidosis most frequently present with lung (hilar nodes and/or lung parenchyma), eye, and skin disease, but any organ may be affected, generally involving more than one site. The natural history is broadly bimodal. An acute onset (fever, erythema nodosum, arthralgia, and hilar lymphadenopathy) is usually indicative of a good outcome. However, an insidious onset may be followed, in a minority of patients, by inexorably progressive fibrosis of the lungs or other organs.

EPIDEMIOLOGY

The peak prevalence occurs in the third decade with, in Japan and Scandinavia, a second peak in women older than 50 years of age. Overall, there are marginally higher disease rates in women. There is a strikingly higher prevalence in African Americans (lifetime risk of sarcoidosis 2.4% compared with 0.8% for whites in the United States), and this is mirrored by a higher prevalence of more severe disease and a lower likelihood of presentation with asymptomatic disease.

Spatial clusters of sarcoidosis have raised the possibility of transmission of an infectious agent or a common environmental exposure, but data are inconclusive, due mostly to methodologic limitations (in disease classification and study design). Familial clustering of sarcoidosis has been documented in a number of studies, and early genetic data suggest a predisposition to an exaggerated cellular immune response with granuloma formation (a "sarcoid reaction"), probably triggered by a wide variety of environmental exposures.

CLINICAL FEATURES AND PROGNOSIS

The most frequent symptoms, present in up to 50% of patients, are cough, dyspnea, and poorly defined chest discomfort. The lungs are involved more frequently than other organs (in up to 90% of patients); however, in most cases, breath sounds are normal to auscultation. Chest radiographic appearances are staged as shown in Table 1. Pulmonary function tests may show lung restriction, airflow obstruction, a mixed ventilatory defect, or an isolated reduction in gas transfer.

Extrathoracic involvement is most commonly clinically significant in the eyes (25%), skin (25%), and lymph nodes (30%). *Ocular involvement* most frequently consists of acute anterior uveitis, which may clear spontaneously or require prolonged topical therapy, but lacrimal gland involvement, keratoconjunctivitis sicca, and, rarely, retinal vasculitis and optic atrophy, may all occur. All sarcoidosis patients should be evaluated by an ophthalmologist. *Cutaneous involvement* most frequently consists of erythema nodosum (which does not contain granulomas) and lupus pernio, consisting of chronic indurated plaques of the nose, cheeks, lips, and ears. Maculopapular eruptions, subcutaneous nodules, and hypo- or hyperpigmented areas also occur. *Lymph node involvement,* usually of cervical, axillary, or inguinal nodes, seldom requires treatment, but alternative diagnoses (tuberculosis and lymphoma) should be kept in mind.

Cardiac and central nervous system involvement are infrequent but clinically important when present. *Cardiac involvement* is clinically overt in 5%, ranging from benign rhythm disturbances to cardiomyopathy, or sudden death due to malignant arrhythmias. All sarcoid patients should have an electrocardiogram (ECG) at presentation. *Neurosarcoidosis* (5% to 10%) most commonly affects the base of the brain, causing facial palsy or diabetes insipidus with hypothalamic involvement. These early lesions tend to have a good outcome with treatment, whereas peripheral nervous involvement or space-occupying central nervous system lesions are more indicative of a chronic course.

Table 1. **Chest Radiographic Stages**

Stage 0	Normal appearances
Stage I	Isolated bilateral hilar lymphadenopathy (BHL)
Stage II	Pulmonary infiltration with BHL
Stage III	Pulmonary infiltration without BHL
Stage IV	Pulmonary fibrosis*

*Overt advanced fibrosis, as shown by honeycombing, hilar retraction, bullae, or cysts.

Clinically important extrathoracic disease may occur in any other organ, but the most frequent clinical problems are liver disease, musculoskeletal disease, and hypercalcemia. *Liver involvement* is evident in well over 50 % of biopsy specimens and liver function test abnormalities are common, but hepatomegaly is infrequent, and portal hypertension and liver failure are exceedingly rare. *Musculoskeletal involvement* consists of arthralgia (30% to 40%), usually affecting the knees, ankles, wrists, and small joints of the hands; this may be transitory or chronic. Deforming arthritis and bone cysts are rare but denote a worse prognosis. *Hypercalcemia* (up to 10%) or hypercalciuria (up to 20%) results from overproduction of active vitamin D by granulomas. Hypercalcemia requires treatment in its own right; undetected hypercalcemia or hypercalciuria may cause renal stones or, rarely, renal failure.

Nonspecific *systemic symptoms*, including fatigue, fever, drenching night sweats, weight loss, and generalized malaise may be sufficiently debilitating to require treatment and are thought to occur in one third of patients. The impact of fatigue tends to be underestimated by physicians; many patients do not mention fatigue unless prompted, but will often rate fatigue as their most disabling symptom on further discussion.

The natural history of sarcoidosis is highly variable. Prognostic evaluation is made more difficult by the tendency of the disease to wax and wane, and the need for early treatment in many cases also confounds definition of the natural history. Spontaneous remission occurs in two thirds of patients and the majority of the remaining patients stabilize, with or without treatment. However, inexorably progressive disease is fatal in 1% to 5% of cases (most commonly due to respiratory failure or cardiac disease).

Löfgren's syndrome (acute onset of fever, erythema nodosum, and arthralgia, with bilateral hilar lymphadenopathy) usually denotes a good long-term outcome. Chest radiographic appearances (see Table 1) provide additional prognostic information; the likelihood of spontaneous remission is 50% to 90% with stage I disease, 10% to 20% with stage III disease, and 0% with stage IV disease. An early distinction between progressive disease and chronic stable disease cannot be made with confidence and requires careful surveillance. Adverse prognostic indicators include chronic uveitis, lupus pernio, nasal mucosal involvement, cystic bone lesions, chronic hypercalcemia and ongoing disease progression in major organs (lungs, heart, central nervous system).

PATHOGENESIS

The key histologic lesion is the noncaseating granuloma (giant cells and macrophages and surrounding T lymphocytes, bearing the CD4 helper phenotype).

Cytokines produced in the lung suggest an antigen-triggered TH_1 immune response, and there is evidence of T-cell antigen-receptor stimulation. These findings, in conjunction with spatial clustering of illness and racial and familial predilection for disease, support the hypothesis that sarcoidosis results from the exposure of genetically susceptible hosts to unknown environmental agents.

DIAGNOSIS AND STAGING

In general, although the diagnosis is often highly likely on clinical grounds, the histologic confirmation of noncaseating granulomata is required. An important exception is the presentation of Löfgren's syndrome (fever, erythema nodosum, arthralgia, and bilateral hilar lymphadenopathy), in which rapid spontaneous remission may justify observation versus immediate biopsy. Overt skin disease should always be biopsied first, because a positive result may obviate more invasive procedures, such as transbronchial lung biopsy or liver biopsy. Even when granulomata are identified, the many causes of granulomatous responses must be kept constantly in mind. Tuberculosis and lymphoma (in which granulomatous reactions may occur in organs not directly infiltrated by lymphoma) are particularly important differential diagnoses in suspected pulmonary sarcoidosis.

A number of ancillary investigations may be helpful in individual cases, in helping to shift the balance of diagnostic probability, without providing a definitive answer in isolation. Tuberculin reactivity (Heaf or Mantoux testing) is typically negative in sarcoidosis: a positive tuberculin test should stimulate a vigorous search for tuberculosis. Kveim-Siltzbach skin testing is no longer performed because of concerns about transmissions of infectious agents. Increases in serum angiotensin-converting enzyme (ACE) levels, elevated 24-hour urinary calcium levels, a lymphocytosis on bronchoalveolar lavage (BAL) and positive signal on gallium scanning (especially increased uptake in the parotids, conjunctiva, and hilar nodes) may all provide useful ancillary diagnostic support. All of these tests have important sensitivity and/or specificity limitations, and their use is best reserved for patients in whom the diagnosis is uncertain. These tests (with the exception of BAL) may be useful when the diagnosis is secure, but the grounds for treatment for systemic symptoms, such as intractable fatigue, are marginal; in this scenario, the demonstration of objective evidence of ongoing disease activity may be invaluable.

In isolated pulmonary parenchymal sarcoidosis, the major differential diagnoses are other interstitial lung diseases, especially hypersensitivity pneumonitis and idiopathic pulmonary fibrosis. In chronic disease, appearances on chest radiography may be nonspecific, but high resolution computed tomography (CT) scan is often highly useful, either because appearances typical of sarcoidosis are disclosed, or because the picture is pathognomonic of an alternative diagnosis. The diagnostic value of CT in other contexts (and especially the vexing question of whether a typical CT scan appearance is an adequate substitute for biopsy confirmation) remains contentious. The presence of a BAL lymphocytosis may be an important ancillary diagnostic feature when patients present with advanced interstitial lung disease.

Diagnosis apart, the major purposes of investigation are to detect and quantify important complications (ECG, liver function tests, serum calcium levels, lung function tests, and so on) and to identify markers of active disease that might be used to monitor the disease.

TREATMENT

In many patients with self-limited disease, treatment is not required. The indications for treatment can be subdivided broadly into treatment of potentially dangerous disease (i.e., major end-organ damage or hypercalcemia) and treatment to relieve disabling symptoms.

Potentially dangerous disease, always requiring treatment, includes neurosarcoidosis, cardiac sarcoidosis, renal sarcoidosis, and hypercalcemia. Treatment of moderate to severe pulmonary, hepatic, and ocular involvement is also warranted, but in mild disease, therapeutic decisions may be a close call, especially in pulmonary disease. Evidence of ongoing progression of pulmonary disease (increasing dyspnea, declining pulmonary function indices, worsening disease on chest radiography) usually justifies intervention. Some physicians argue that stable pulmonary disease persisting for 1 year after presentation merits a period of treatment, in the hope of "switching off" disease activity and modifying the long-term outcome, but this approach is unproven.

The indications for treatment on "quality of life" grounds remain contentious and must be adapted to the individual patient. Symptoms (such as severe night sweats, disabling fatigue, and intractable arthralgia) may be unrelenting, despite the absence of a dangerous complication, and mild cutaneous sarcoidosis may have devastating psychological consequences. Often, no single laboratory parameter captures the overall life-impact of the disease, and thus, the decision to treat is necessarily subjective. This, in turn, requires the patient and physician, in partnership, to weigh the morbidity of sarcoidosis against the likely morbidity of treatment, with frank appraisal of the anticipated side effects of corticosteroid and immunosuppressive agents. In this scenario, early scrutiny of the treated outcome (degree of symptomatic improvement against severity of early corticosteroid side effects such as weight gain) is pivotal in justifying longer-term therapy. In patients presenting acutely with Löfgren's syndrome, with a good outcome identified by the presence of erythema nodosum, isolated hilar lymphadenopathy on chest radiography, and anterior uveitis, it is advisable to defer treatment if possible, to allow spontaneous remission.

Initial treatment always consists of corticosteroid therapy. The starting dose varies with the severity of disease and physician preference, but high starting doses (e.g., prednisone 60 mg daily or higher), once usual in sarcoidosis, should be reserved for potentially life-threatening disease (cardiac or central nervous system involvement). However, it is also important to achieve control of disease, before attempting to determine the minimum dose required to prevent relapse, and thus, an initial daily dose of prednisolone of 30 to 40 mg is usually warranted, often for four weeks. The dose is subsequently tapered, but the rapidity of this depends on the nature of the complication. In general, a slower reduction is advisable when there is major end-organ involvement, with careful re-evaluation before each reduction is effected (often every three months). In neurosarcoidosis and cardiac sarcoidosis, long-term maintenance treatment is usually needed. For treatment of symptoms, subsequent reductions should be tailored to the rapidity of the initial response. A striking symptomatic response within days or weeks of starting treatment usually justifies rapid reduction to a dose of prednisolone of 7.5 to 10 mg daily over 2 to 3 months, and attempted withdrawal of treatment within 12 to 18 months.

In severe disease that is resistant to high-dose oral corticosteroid therapy, it is occasionally necessary to introduce pulsed intravenous methylprednisolone (Solu-Medrol), usually at weekly intervals (500 mg to 750 mg, given over 1 hour), with prednisone 20 mg daily on intervening days. Any response is usually evident within 6 weeks, and is generally best maintained with the use of combination therapy (oral prednisone and an immunosuppressive agent). This approach is most often warranted in severe cardiac and neurologic disease.

Immunosuppressive drugs (especially azathioprine [Imuran],* methotrexate [Rheumatrex],* and hydroxychloroquine [Plaquenil],*) are the only widely used alternatives to corticosteroid therapy, but are more commonly used in combination with low-dose prednisone, as "steroid-sparing" agents. All of these agents are used in connective tissue diseases (rheumatoid arthritis, polymyositis, and so on); drug dosages and monitoring protocols for these diseases and for sarcoidosis are identical. However, anecdotal reports suggest that cyclophosphamide (Cytoxan),* which is also used in connective tissue diseases, is less effective than other immunosuppressive agents in sarcoidosis, except in chronic central nervous system involvement. Methotrexate and hydroxychloroquine are viewed as first-line therapies for skin disease. This context aside, the introduction of immunosuppressive therapy is usually reserved for patients requiring unacceptably high corticosteroid dosages in order to prevent relapse. A maintenance dose of 7.5 to 10 mg of prednisone daily seldom justifies the addition of an immunosuppressive agent, in the absence of important corticosteroid side effects (weight gain, hypertension, diabetes mellitus, depression, and osteoporosis).

A small minority of patients with pulmonary sarcoidosis progress to end-stage disease despite therapy. Vigorous continued treatment in the hope of preventing further decline is warranted, even in the absence of an initial response, because the only therapeutic alternative, single or double lung transplantation, carries a risk of recurrence of sarcoidosis in transplanted tissue, and requires aggressive immunosuppression in its own right. Stabilization of severe disease is always preferable to transplantation, which should be viewed as a treatment of last resort.

*Not FDA approved for this indication.

SILICOSIS

method of
H. ERHAN DINCER, M.D., and
RALPH M. SCHAPIRA, M.D.
Medical College of Wisconsin and
Milwaukee Veterans Affairs Medical Center
Milwaukee, Wisconsin

Exposure to inhaled silica or asbestos can result in numerous pleuropulmonary abnormalities. Silicosis and asbestosis refer specifically to the interstitial lung diseases resulting from the inhalation of the inorganic dusts silica and asbestos, respectively. Silicosis and asbestos represent two of the pneumoconioses that are defined as interstitial lung disease from the inhalation of inorganic dusts.

SILICOSIS

Silicosis refers to the potentially fatal interstitial pulmonary fibrosis resulting from the inhalation of crystalline silica (silicon dioxide [SiO_2]). Silica is a naturally occurring mineral oxide particle that is the cause of the most prevalent worldwide occupational lung disease, silicosis. The adverse health effects of silica exposure have been recognized for centuries, and legal limits on the exposure of industrial workers to airborne silica in the United States have been established. Nonetheless, nearly 15,000 silicosis-associated deaths were recorded in the United States during 1968 to 1994. Between the years 1987 and 1995, 577 people in the state of Michigan were reported to have met the clinical criteria of silicosis. Thus silicosis should always be considered in the differential diagnosis of an interstitial lung disease in a person who has had silica exposure, even if such exposure was in the distant past.

Several types of silica exist in both crystalline and noncrystalline structural forms. The noncrystalline forms of silica are not relevant to respiratory disease. Of the crystalline forms, quartz is the most common and is also the most important form of silica in terms of association with human pulmonary interstitial fibrosis. Numerous occupations are associated with the development of silicosis, including metal industries (foundries), surface and underground mining, construction (drilling and blasting), and sandblasting. Silica is related to asbestos in that asbestos is a naturally occurring fibrous mineral oxide. The parent structures of both silica and asbestos contain a silicon-oxide chemical group; both minerals also have associated transitional metals and similar chemical reactivity. However, silica and asbestos have important structural differences in size, shape, and chemical constituents.

After inhalation by humans, silica particles that are not trapped or cleared by the body's upper airway defense mechanisms accumulate in the lower respiratory tract, where the crystals mediate lung toxicity. Animal models of lung injury after exposure have been used to identify mechanisms by which silica causes lung injury and interstitial fibrosis. These studies demonstrate that silica exposure causes an accumulation of lung inflammatory cells composed of both neutrophils and macrophages. The inflammatory response can result in the generation of cytotoxic reactive oxygen products, including oxygen-based free radicals, such as the hydroxyl radical, which may injure the lung epithelium, potentially resulting in interstitial pulmonary fibrosis. Other inflammatory mediators from lung inflammatory cells have also been implicated in lung injury after silica exposure, including arachidonic acid metabolites and various cytokines and growth factors. Most recent evidence from these animal models shows that lung inflammatory cells that were isolated from silica-exposed lungs increase the production of nitric oxide, the latest mediator identified that may play a proinflammatory role in the pathogenesis of silicosis.

CLINICAL DISEASE

Silicosis is clinically divided into three categories: simple (or nodular) silicosis, complicated silicosis, and acute silicoproteinosis. The diagnosis is usually made by the history and clinical characteristics. Lung biopsy (usually requiring thoracotomy or video-assisted thoracoscopy) is needed only to evaluate for the presence of another interstitial lung disease when the diagnosis is in doubt.

Simple silicosis manifests in persons who have a significant occupational history of exposure to silica. Although most patients with silicosis have been exposed to silica for more than 20 years, silicosis can occur after far shorter exposures (termed *accelerated silicosis*). A study of silicosis in workers in Michigan (1985 to 1995) showed that 40 of the 567 reported cases of silicosis occurred in workers exposed to silica for less than 10 years. The intensity of exposure is believed to be related to the time course of disease expression (latency period) and progression. Patients with simple silicosis may be asymptomatic or have an occasional cough. Pulmonary function testing may be normal or demonstrate a mild restrictive abnormality (decrease in forced vital capacity [FVC] and total lung capacity [TLC]), usually in the absence of airway obstruction. The chest radiograph in patients with simple silicosis shows diffuse nodular opacities, usually most prominent in the upper lung zones. The opacities are small (<1 cm), in contrast to those in patients with complicated silicosis. Calcified hilar lymph nodes may be present. Computed tomographic scans confirm the presence of the nodular opacities, but these scans are not necessary to establish the clinical diagnosis. Histologic examination of the characteristic lesion in silicosis (the silicotic nodule) reveals concentric, acellular areas of collagen fibers, without necrosis, that may contain silica particles.

Complicated silicosis (also termed *progressive massive fibrosis*) is characterized by symptoms that can include progressive dyspnea and cough and by physical examination findings such as clubbing, cyanosis, and evidence of right-sided heart failure (cor pulmonale). Chest radiographs demonstrate opacities larger than 1 cm in diameter. Pulmonary function testing shows a restrictive abnormality that may be severe and can be accompanied by airway obstruction (decrease in 1-second forced expiratory volume [FEV_1]/FVC ratio). The diffusion capacity for carbon monoxide is usually decreased. In addition, significant hypoxemia that is aggravated by exercise may be present. The large opacities may obscure the radiographic evidence of tuberculosis, and many authorities believe that the incidence of *Mycobacterium tuberculosis* and nontuberculous mycobacterium is increased in patients with silicosis, particularly complicated silicosis. An increase in the incidence of bronchogenic carcinoma in patients with complicated silicosis has been suggested and the International Agency for Research in Cancer (IARC) has designated silica as a human carcinogen. Radiographic opacities in complicated silicosis can obscure the development of lung cancer or pulmonary tuberculosis, and these diseases must be considered when a change in the chest radiograph is noted. Weight loss, malaise, a decrease in appetite, or hemoptysis may be additional clues to the development of tuberculosis or lung carcinoma in patients with silicosis. Fiberoptic bronchoscopy with biopsies may be needed as part of the evaluation of potential lung cancer or tuberculosis. Caplan's syndrome is the development of pulmonary nodules, which may cavitate, in patients with rheumatoid arthritis, pneumonoconiosis, and silicosis.

Acute silicosis (also termed *silicoproteinosis*) clinically resembles pulmonary alveolar proteinosis and usually occurs within a few months after major, intense exposure to silica or years afterward. As such, acute silicosis is not truly a classic interstitial lung disease. Many reported cases have occurred in sandblasters. Acute silicosis represents an unusual pathologic reaction to the massive deposition of silica particles in the lungs and is characterized histologically by the presence of abundant granular eosinophilic material that accumulates in the alveoli. It is hypothesized that the silica disrupts normal surfactant metabolism, resulting in the abnormal accumulation of the proteinaceous material that disrupts the normal surface tension of the alveolar space and causes ventilation-perfusion mismatching and severe respiratory disease.

As is the case with most interstitial lung diseases, no specific treatment for the various forms of silicosis has proven efficacy. Thus silicosis is treated in much the same way as other interstitial lung diseases. The interstitial fibrosis characteristic of silicosis may progress even in the absence of continued exposure. Education and primary prevention is essential. Adherence to established occupational hygiene regulations, including legally enforceable limits of worker exposure, are mandatory in order to avoid concentrations of silica particles that can cause silicosis. The National Institute for Occupational Safety and Health (NIOSH) has set such exposure limits, and silicosis is reportable to the state health departments in many states. Patients at risk for silicosis as a result of type of employment should have a chest radiograph and pulmonary function testing at the start of employment and have these tests repeated every few years or sooner if clinically indicated. These tests are also important as tools for monitoring patients with an established diagnosis of silicosis in order to identify progression of the interstitial lung disease.

TREATMENT

Treatment of patients with silicosis is targeted at ameliorating symptoms; the physician must be vigilant for the development of tuberculosis, bronchogenic carcinoma (which may not be a direct effect of silica exposure), pulmonary arterial hypertension, and right-sided heart failure. Thus the treatment plan is not specific to patients with silicosis. Acute bacterial infections (pneumonia or bronchitis) should be treated with antibiotic choices targeted according to local bacteriologic patterns and severity of illness. A pneumococcal vaccination and annual influenza vaccination are highly recommended. Many authorities recommend that patients with silicosis receive an annual purified protein derivative (PPD) skin test and treatment of latent tuberculous infection (LTI) (formerly termed "chemoprophylaxis"), if indicated. Because silicosis is a risk factor for the development of pulmonary tuberculosis, the Centers for Disease Control and Prevention (CDC) recommends that treatment of LTI be considered in patients with silicosis (regardless of age) and a PPD skin reaction of greater than 10 mm (or >5 mm if a recent contact with a person with tuberculosis is infected with the human immunodeficiency virus [HIV], or has radiographic evidence of healed tuberculosis). Because a positive skin reaction may also indicate active pulmonary tuberculosis (and not simply LTI), patients with silicosis and a positive PPD must be carefully evaluated for active disease. If active tuberculosis is established, treatment with appropriate agents is indicated and prolonged therapy may be indicated, depending on the clinical response. Nontuberculous mycobacterial disease (such as with *Mycobacterium avium complex*) also warrants multidrug therapy. Patients with significant abnormalities in pulmonary function testing or evidence of cor pulmonale should be assessed both at rest and during exercise for the need for long-term oxygen therapy.

Pharmacologic therapy to interrupt the mechanisms of pulmonary inflammation with silicosis is not well established. Glucocorticoids are widely used in interstitial lung diseases, such as idiopathic pulmonary fibrosis, with mixed results. The role of glucocorticoids in silicosis is not well studied, and its use is reserved for patients with progressive pulmonary impairment. The use of other pharmacologic agents cannot be recommended. Another proposed approach is bronchoscopic lung lavage, which can be performed safely and is successful in removing silica from the lungs. However, the long-term benefits of lavage in influencing the course of silicosis is unclear.

ASBESTOSIS

Asbestos, an ancient mineral, is a generic term for several different forms of fibrous (in contrast to the crystalline structure of silica), hydrated magnesium silicates, including chrysolite, amosite, anthophyllite and crocidolite. Chrysolite asbestos accounts for more than 90% of the asbestos that had been in commercial use in the United States. The commercial use of asbestos rapidly expanded in the first half of the 20th century in the industrialized world because of its durability and heat resistance. With the recognition of the adverse health effects of asbestos exposure, the use of asbestos in the United States has been banned and asbestos has been replaced by synthetic silicates such as fiberglass. However, asbestos continues to pose a significant health threat in parts of the world where its use remains unregulated and to construction workers in the United States who can potentially come in contact with asbestos in demolition projects, given the ubiquitous presence of asbestos in building structures. Asbestos can also contaminate other currently used insulating products such as vermiculite, potentially leading to harmful exposure to inhaled asbestos.

Workers with potentially significant occupational exposure to asbestos include miners, millers and transporters of asbestos, or workers in fields such as the building trades and shipyards where asbestos was an essential material. During the time in which asbestos was in widespread use in the industrialized world, occupational hygiene regulations were lacking and many people were exposed to large numbers of inhaled fibers. The fate of inhaled asbestos fibers is determined mainly by fiber diameter and fiber length. Thinner fibers are more likely to be deposited in either the peripheral airways or distal airspaces. Fibers attract and activate lung macrophages, which release a host of chemotactic and proinflammatory factors, resulting in injury and fibrosis in the lung interstitium. It is also believed that reactive oxygen species such as the hydroxyl radical and nitric oxide may be involved in the pathogenesis of lung injury from asbestos.

CLINICAL DISEASE

Asbestosis tends to be prominent in the lower lobes and subpleural areas (in contrast to silicosis, which tends to involve the upper lobes). In advanced cases, it is difficult to distinguish asbestosis from fibrosis due to any other cause. Intensity and duration of exposure to asbestos are factors that determine the severity of the disease. Latency period, the duration between the initial exposure and the onset of asbestosis, depends on the level of exposure. However, the duration usually ranges from at least 10 to 30 years. Once the disease is established, asbestosis can be stable or progressive, but it rarely regresses. There has been no genetic predisposition identified so far.

The clinical presentation is nonspecific and similar to that of other forms of interstitial pulmonary fibrosis. The most common symptom is slowly progressive dyspnea, usually over a period of years. The physical examination findings are also nonspecific and include bibasilar fine end-inspiratory crackles (32% to 64%), finger or toe clubbing (32% to 42%) and the signs of cor pulmonale. Laboratory studies are generally nonspecific. Significant hypoxemia at rest or with exercise can be present, especially in advanced cases of asbestosis.

The diagnosis of asbestosis usually is based on an appropriate history of significant asbestos exposure, the physical examination, pulmonary function tests, and imaging studies. A lung biopsy (using an open thoracotomy or video-assisted thoracoscopic surgery) is rarely necessary and only utilized to help differentiate asbestosis from other causes of interstitial lung disease, such as idiopathic pulmonary fibrosis. Bronchoscopy has a highly limited role in the diagnosis of asbestosis. Biopsies obtained by bronchoscopy are too small to differentiate between the major types of interstitial fibrosis. The presence of asbestos bodies in lavage fluid obtained during bronchoscopy confirms exposure to inhaled asbestos but does not make the diagnosis of asbestosis.

The American Thoracic Society criteria for diagnosis of asbestosis includes: (1) a reliable history of nontrivial exposure to asbestos with an appropriate lag time from exposure to disease expression; (2) restrictive lung impairment on pulmonary function tests as well as a reduced diffusion capacity for carbon monoxide; (3) presence of bilateral fixed inspiratory crackles, not cleared with cough; and (4) imaging findings (chest radiograph or CT scan) revealing lung fibrosis. Exposure history and the findings on imaging studies are considered essential for the diagnosis. The most common chest radiograph abnormalities in people exposed to asbestos are calcified and noncalcified pleural plaques. However, pleural plaques represent a pleural abnormality, which is completely distinct from asbestosis. Unfortunately, there is some controversy in the value of radiographic interpretation in defining a population with asbestosis. Since 10% to 20% of patients with interstitial fibrosis of any cause may have a normal chest radiograph, the use of high resolution CT (HRCT) should be considered if the diagnosis is in doubt. HRCT both supine and prone position may be helpful to distinguish mild cases. Presence of parenchymal fibrosis can be diagnosed with HRCT. The earliest findings on HRCT include small subpleural nodules and with progression of disease, architectural distortion, traction atelectasis, and eventually, honeycombing. HRCT may also show curvilinear lines 5 to 10 cm in length parallel to the pleural surface, which is specific to asbestosis. Hilar and mediastinal lymphadenopathy are not seen with asbestosis and suggest another process. Asbestos exposure is associated with numerous other pleuropulmonary abnormalities distinct from asbestosis. The presence of such abnormalities, such as calcified and noncalcified pleural plaques, pleural fibrosis, pleural effusion, rounded atelectasis, lung cancer, and malignant pleural mesothelioma can also be suggested by HRCT. In addition, each of these abnormalities can coexist with asbestosis. Some authorities believe that asbestosis is an independent risk factor for lung cancer, even in the absence of smoking. However, there is a multiplicative risk of lung cancer in those who have had significant asbestos exposure and smoke, regardless of the presence of asbestosis. Thus, asbestosis is not a prerequisite for the development of lung cancer in asbestos-exposed individuals. The 10-year risk of death from asbestosis rises in proportion to the severity of interstitial fibrosis on chest radiograph (as assessed by the International Labor Office categories) to 35.4% for the most severe category.

TREATMENT

Similar to silicosis, there is no specific therapy for asbestosis and the care is the same as for those with other forms of interstitial lung disease. Avoidance of continued exposure to asbestos, in parts of the world where asbestos is still utilized, and smoking cessation are crucial. Glucocorticoids are widely used in the treatment of interstitial lung diseases, such as idiopathic pulmonary fibrosis, with mixed results, and they are occasionally prescribed in patients with progressive asbestosis. The appropriate treatment of respiratory tract infections, cardiopulmonary exercise program, long-term oxygen therapy in those with significant hypoxemia, and pneumococcal and influenza vaccinations are essential. Annual chest radiographs and spirometry are recommended for follow-up, although no survival benefit has been shown. The risk of tuberculosis does not appear to be increased in patients with asbestosis, unlike the situation in silicosis. Changes in the chest radiograph, such as the appearance of a new opacity, may suggest the development of lung cancer and an appropriate evaluation should be promptly undertaken.

HYPERSENSITIVITY PNEUMONITIS

method of
LESLIE C. GRAMMER, M.D., and
RACHEL E. STORY, M.D., M.P.H.
Northwestern University Medical School
Chicago, Illinois

Hypersensitivity pneumonitis (HP), also known as extrinsic allergic alveolitis, is the result of non–IgE-mediated inflammation of the lung parenchyma, alveoli, and terminal airways from inhaled antigens.

TABLE 1. **Selected Antigens Causing Hypersensitivity Pneumonitis**

Antigen Class	Antigen	Source of Antigen	Disease Name
Organic High-Molecular-Weight Compounds			
Bacteria	Thermophilic *Actinomyces*	Moldy hay, compost, mushroom compost	Farmer's lung, mushroom picker's lung
	Bacillus, Klebsiella	Air conditioner, humidifier	Ventilation pneumonitis
Fungi	*Aspergillus* species	Moldy malt in brewing	Malt worker's lung
	Penicillium casei, Penicillium roqueforti	Moldy cheese	Cheese worker's lung
	Trichosporon cutaneum	Japanese house dust	Summer-type hypersensitivity pneumonitis
Amebae	*Naegleria gruberi, Acanthamoeba castellani*	Contaminated humidifier or ventilation system	Ventilation pneumonitis
Animal protein	Avian protein	Dropping, feather bloom of pigeon, duck turkey, parakeet	Bird or pigeon breeder's lung, bird fancier's disease
	Rodent urine protein	Rat or gerbil urine	Laboratory worker's lung, gerbil keepers' disease
	Animal fur dust (cat)	Animal pelts, furs	Furrier's lung
Inorganic Low-Molecular-Weight Haptens			
Chemicals	Isocyanates	Paints, plastics	Paint-refinisher's lung
	Acid anhydrides	Plastics	Chemical worker's lung, plastic workers lung
Drugs	Amiodarone (Cordarone), gold, minocycline (Minocin), nitrofurantoin (Macrodantin)	Medications	Drug-induced hypersensitivity pneumonitis

Although exposure is historically associated with occupational activities such as farming and hobbies such as pigeon breeding, residential exposures of HP are becoming more common because of indoor molds. The mechanism of inflammation is not fully elucidated, but it is non–IgE mediated and is probably driven by activated macrophages and $CD8^+$ T cells.

EPIDEMIOLOGY AND CAUSATIVE AGENTS

The epidemiology of HP is antigen, population, and environment dependent. In the United States, the most common causes of HP include thermophilic *Actinomyces* and avian proteins. Thermophilic *Actinomyces* causes farmer's lung in 2% to 8% of the exposed population. The prevalence varies by region and change in season, with a higher incidence of disease in more humid areas and seasons. Avian proteins are the etiologic agents in pigeon breeder's lung, with disease developing in 6% to 21% of exposed individuals. The epidemiology in Japan is quite different; there, the most common cause of HP is summer mold contamination of homes with *Trichosporon cutaneum*.

Although a comprehensive list of etiologic agents is beyond the scope of this chapter, it is important to understand that causative antigens are either organic high-molecular-weight compounds or inorganic low-molecular-weight haptens. Examples of organic high-molecular-weight compounds include bacteria, fungi, amebae, and animal proteins. Inorganic haptens include chemicals such as isocyanates and acid anhydrides. Table 1 contains specific examples. Novel antigens responsible for HP are frequently reported in the literature, and therefore it is important to recall that any foreign protein or inorganic molecule capable of haptenization can potentially cause HP.

CLINICAL PRESENTATION AND DIAGNOSIS

HP occurs in acute, subacute, and chronic forms depending on the amount of antigen inhaled, the degree of host reactivity, and the duration of exposure. Patients with the acute form present with fever, dyspnea, and nonproductive cough within 6 to 12 hours after intense exposure to the inciting antigen. Symptoms resolve within several days if the patient is no longer exposed to the antigen. The chronic form is usually secondary to continuous low-level exposure to the antigen. Symptoms include insidious onset of shortness of breath, dyspnea on exertion, and productive cough and weight loss. The subacute form has features of both acute and chronic forms. Additional information distinguishing the three forms of HP is listed in Table 2.

The diagnosis of HP requires a high index of suspicion. History must focus on possible exposures and

TABLE 2. **Clinical Presentations of Hypersensitivity Pneumonitis**

Feature	Acute	Subacute	Chronic
Fever, chills	+	–	–
Dyspnea	+	+	+
Cough	Nonproductive	Productive	Productive
Malaise, myalgia	+	+	+
Weight loss	–	+	+
Rales	Dibasilar	Diffuse	Diffuse
Chest film	Nodular infiltrates	Nodular infiltrates	Fibrosis
PFTs	Restrictive	Mixed	Mixed
DLCO	Decreased	Decreased	Decreased

DLCO, diffusing capacity of lung for carbon monoxide; PFT, pulmonary function test.
From Grammer LC: Occupational allergic alveolitis. Ann Allergy Asthma Immunol 83:602-606, 1999.

temporal relation to symptoms. No single diagnostic test is definitive. Diagnosis requires exposure to an antigen capable of causing HP with an appropriate temporal relation to symptoms. Physical examination, chest radiography, and pulmonary function test results vary depending on the clinical presentation (see Table 2). High titers of serum precipitating IgG antibodies to the offending agent usually accompany HP. However, the presence of precipitins is not diagnostic and absence of serum precipitins does not rule out HP. For example, in pigeon breeders up to 50% of individuals with exposure have detectable precipitins but no symptoms of disease. If serum precipitins are negative in a patient with a suggestive history, the patient may need to be tested with antigens prepared from the suspected environment. Skin testing is not useful as HP is not an IgE-mediated disease. Bronchoalveolar lavage demonstrates a lymphocytosis with a CD8/CD4 ratio greater than 1. Lung biopsy is not diagnostic, but findings include small, poorly formed granulomas, patchy infiltration of alveolar walls with lymphocytes and plasma cells, and large histiocytes with foamy cytoplasm in the alveoli and interstitium. Inhalation challenges can be performed by reexposing a patient to the environment with the suspected antigen or inhaling the antigen in a hospital setting to demonstrate a relationship between exposure and symptoms. Inhalation challenge in a hospital environment is rarely done as there are no standard antigen preparations and severe respiratory reactions may occur.

TREATMENT, PREVENTION, AND PROGNOSIS

Early diagnosis and avoidance of the offending antigen are the cornerstones of management in HP. In occupational exposures such as farming, avoidance is difficult because it requires a significant change in lifestyle and occupation. Prednisone at a dose of 0.5 mg/kg/day for 2 to 4 weeks can decrease the symptoms of the acute and subacute stages of HP, but it does not seem to have any beneficial long-term effect on arresting disease progression. Industrial hygiene measures such as wetting compost to decrease dispersion of actinomycete spores and maintaining humidity in buildings at less than 60% have been reported to decrease the incidence of HP.

TUBERCULOSIS AND OTHER MYCOBACTERIAL INFECTIONS

method of
K. P. RAVIKRISHNAN, M.D.
William Beaumont Hospital
Royal Oak, Michigan

Tuberculosis (TB) is the deadliest infectious disease known to humans, with a very high mortality rate. The prevalence of TB is directly related to poor socioeconomic conditions, with high rates of infection in the overcrowded inner city population. In developing countries where the overall health of the population is extremely poor and health care resources are scarce, TB infection further impoverishes the society, causing a severe strain on the economy, welfare, and the health care control programs. The 2001 report of the Centers for Disease Control and Prevention (CDC) showed an all-time low incidence of TB in the United States. While enjoying the lowest incidence of TB, health agencies in the United States recognize the constant threat to our control program because of the uncontrolled state of global TB and the potential for a resurgence of TB. Stricter control and implementation of programs targeted toward high-risk groups will be necessary to achieve the U.S. Department of Health and Human Services goal of eradicating TB by the year 2010.

Of the 15,859 cases in the year 2001, about half were among foreign-born individuals, with a high incidence of multidrug-resistant tuberculosis (MDR TB). High-risk groups who are susceptible to the development of new infections and are likely to have high rates of reactivation have been identified (Table 1). Globally, over 8 million new cases occur every year, with over 3 million deaths from TB. The World Health Organization (WHO) has accepted control of TB as a global challenge and its main mission. Despite the resurgence of TB in the 1980s, there has been a steady

TABLE 1. **High-Risk Groups for Screening and Treatment with INH in case of positive PPD**

Household contacts to TB
Homeless
Low-income groups
Alcoholics and intravenous drug addicts
Institutionalized (nursing homes, prisons)
Recent travelers to endemic areas
Immigrants from endemic areas
Highly exposed (health care workers)
Medical conditions with high rates of infection and reactivation
- HIV infection
- Chest radiograph showing stigma tuberculosis
- Diabetes mellitus
- End-stage renal disease
- Prolonged steroid treatment and other immunosuppressive therapy
- Hematological and reticulo-endothelial malignancies
- Carcinoma of lungs, oro-pharynx and upper gastrointestinal tract
- Silicosis
- Postgastrectomy
- Intestinal bypass surgery
- Chronic malabsorption
- Being 10% or more below the ideal body weight

TABLE 2. **Causes of Resurgence of TB in the 1980s**

1. HIV/AIDS associated TB
2. Disparity in resource allocation
3. Poorly compliant patients
4. Drug resistant tuberculosis
5. Complex clinical presentations
6. Increase in the overall infection rate

further decline of TB in the new millennium. Renewed attention and public health awareness of this global problem will go a long way toward achieving the WHO goal of controlling TB in the coming decades. There is no safety provided by boundaries, and resurgence of TB from immigrant populations is a constant and costly threat to our population and public health resources. We should take every opportunity to support global programs because reduction of global TB will go a long way toward fulfilling our efforts to control and eradicate TB in the United States. This article is aimed at providing a comprehensive clinical perspective on TB with emphasis on awareness in the diagnosis, prevention, and management of TB.

There has been a steady decline in TB since the beginning of the last century, with sporadic uprisings during the great wars and during influenza epidemics. Since the 1950s, better public health care practices, advances in chemotherapy, and the use of isoniazid (INH) (Nydrazid) in management have led to a further dramatic decline of TB. Resurgence of TB in the 1980s is attributed to the HIV/AIDS epidemic and other factors including deficiencies and neglect in the health care system (Table 2). An additional 70,000 cases have been attributed to the HIV/AIDS epidemic in the 1980s. These cases brought about the overall increase in TB and the problems associated with an outbreak within the endemic problem. However, the renewed vigilant attack on TB was remarkable and has resulted in a dramatic decrease in case rates. Lessons learned from the outbreak and renewed enthusiasm are the silver lining in the cloud, which has helped to bring down the overall incidence of TB in the last decade.

The case rate of TB in the United States for the year 2001 was 5.6 cases per 100,000 population, a 40% reduction of case rate since its peak in 1992. Reactivated TB in the older population accounts for the majority of cases, but the distribution of new cases is among identifiable inner city populations and is due to overcrowding and a high density of high-risk groups including recent immigrants from highly endemic areas (i.e., Mexico, Philippines, Vietnam, China, and India). Latent TB infection is still a major problem in the general population, and the expertise of general practitioners in the treatment of TB is of great importance in the control of the disease. About 15 million people in the United States are infected with TB, and they serve as a reservoir capable of contributing to the annual reactivation cases of the disease in the elderly population.

TRANSMISSION, PATHOGENESIS, AND CLINICAL CHARACTERISTICS OF TUBERCULOSIS

Symptoms of TB are shared by many infectious and noninfectious inflammatory disorders. TB has earned its status as the "great mimic" as many clinicians have been misled by the lack of the classic presentation of TB as described and repeated in the medical literature. TB is a multiphasic disease with varying severity and extent of disease. Clinical manifestations of TB are closely tied to the pathogenesis of the disease, varying with the phase, intensity, and extent of disease. There is dramatic predictability and similarity in the pattern of presentation, but atypical presentations are seen in disseminated cases, especially in HIV/AIDS TB.

INFECTION

TB is transmitted by small particles, 1 to 2 μm in size, containing viable tubercle bacteria. Viable tubercle bacilli are highly infectious and, once deposited in the alveoli, cause an acute inflammatory process with local pneumonia and regional lymphadenopathy. In a normal host the infection is contained locally. The organisms are carried to vascular structures such as apices of the lungs, bone, kidney, adrenals, pericardium, meninges, peritoneum, and the systemic lymphatics. Host immunity develops within 3 weeks, keeping the organisms in check. The organisms remain dormant in the lung and the extrapulmonary sites with a potential to be reactivated when host immunity declines. In the majority of patients (>90%), with initial infection TB leaves behind the stigma of infection in the form of a positive tuberculin skin test or a granuloma in the chest radiograph (GOHN complex) without any clinical illness. For standardization, the American Thoracic Society defines a positive tuberculin skin test as follows:

15 mm	Non–immune-compromised U.S. population
10 mm	Patients from high-risk areas and patients who belong to high-risk categories
5 mm	Immunocompromised HIV/AIDS population

PRIMARY TUBERCULOSIS

Primary TB is a clinically manifest disease occurring in a small group of patients following the initial infection because of a high bacillary load or host factors. A patchy pulmonary parenchymal inflammation leads to pneumonic illness associated with regional lymphadenopathy and, at times, a pleural effusion. Cough, pleuritic chest pain, fever, anorexia, malaise, and weight loss are the predominant clinical findings. Chest radiographs may show a pulmonary parenchymal abnormality, lymphadenopathy, pleural effusion, and at times pericardial effusion. This often self-limited form of the disease is a common manifestation of childhood TB. In cases of a high bacillary load and in immunodeficiency states, disseminated infection is responsible for high infant and childhood mortality in developing countries. In places where drug-resistant TB is common, primary infection can be due to resistant strains of TB. In another group of cases, the latency is shorter and primary TB progresses to the reactivated form of TB. Progressive primary TB is indistinguishable from the reactivated form of TB, and the clinical features are as described subsequently for the reactivated form of TB. In children and in immunocompromised patients, primary TB can manifest as miliary TB, a hematogenously disseminated form of TB with a characteristic miliary nodular radiographic pattern and severe systemic illness. Fever, respiratory difficulty, pleuritis, pericarditis, myalgia, arthralgia, arthritis, and meningitis are due to granulomatous inflammation. Clinical manifestations of miliary TB are indistinguishable from those of other systemic illnesses such as bacterial endocarditis, systemic lupus erythematosus, vasculitis, and sarcoidosis.

REACTIVATION TUBERCULOSIS

This is the most common form of TB and accounts for the majority of cases. In about 5% of cases that have an acquired initial infection with TB, a symptomatic disease develops. The chance of clinical illness is highest in the first 2 years after initial infection. The majority of TB cases are due to reactivation of an acquired TB infection due to a decrease in cellular immunity, poor nutritional status, chronic debilitating disorders and other host factors (see Table 1). Pulmonary manifestations are due to ongoing inflammation and a parenchymal consolidative process in the lung. In its classic form, TB is unmistakable because of the chronic systemic symptoms of fever, malaise, weight loss, respiratory symptoms of cough, sputum production, and at times hemoptysis and chest radiograph with upper lobe cavitary lung disease. However, because of the similarity in clinical presentations and symptoms with many other chronic diseases, TB has earned special status as the great mimic among clinicians. The dictum in clinical medicine is, "Consider TB in the differential diagnosis in all cases of inflammatory disorders in the lung." Patients with diabetes, chronic renal failure, malignancies, and other immunocompromising diseases present with low-grade fever, malaise, loss of appetite, and weight loss. These symptoms are often distinguishable from their underlying disease process.

LATENT INFECTION

About 90% of patients who are infected with TB remain infected throughout life without ever manifesting clinical illness. In the United States there are about 15 million cases with latent infection. There is a threat of reactivation in this group, which serves as a reservoir capable of becoming active cases when host immunity wanes with old age, malnutrition, alcoholism, chronic debilitating illnesses such as diabetes, renal failure, immunosuppressive illnesses, medications, and HIV/AIDS. Identifying patients in this high-risk group with a positive tuberculin skin test and beginning chemoprophylaxis help to contain the infection and are the major components in the control of TB in the United States. Chemoprophylaxis with INH for 9 months is highly effective in preventing reactivation of TB in high-risk groups. INH is safe and effective with less than 1% chance of severe hepatotoxicity. Close clinical monitoring is necessary in older patients and those with chronic alcoholism. In patients who cannot tolerate INH, treatment with rifampin (RMP) (Rifadin) for 4 to 5 months is acceptable. Shorter duration of treatment with the combination of pyrazinamide (PZA) and RMP has been shown to be effective, but hepatotoxicity associated with this combination is unacceptable for prophylaxis. With the decrease in overall case rates of TB, today's clinicians will rarely see active cases of TB in their office practice. However, primary physicians will play a major role in the identification of high-risk groups with latent infection and treatment with INH in the coming years (see Table 1).

DIAGNOSIS AND LABORATORY METHODS

Early diagnosis of TB is an art, and an astute clinician with a keen clinical instinct looks for TB in high-risk groups and in patients with systemic, pulmonary, and extrapulmonary TB symptoms and signs. The tuberculin skin test (Mantoux test) is the initial diagnostic procedure and is the "gold standard" in detecting infection with TB, current or remote. Clinical examination, chest radiographs, and other imaging studies are helpful in the diagnosis of active infection. A standardized laboratory capable of microbiological studies, histopathology, and newer genetic probe techniques is extremely important in confirming the diagnosis promptly. In cases of MDR TB, sensitivity studies should be available promptly. All patients should be tested for HIV infection and other systemic diseases. Advances in liquid culture media and rapid diagnosis with amplification of RNA and DNA have become a standard in the early diagnosis and confirmation of the infection. This is extremely important in planning isolation and containing the infection, which helps in the control of TB by prompt drug treatment and avoiding unnecessary prolonged costly hospitalization.

TREATMENT

Management of TB has been simplified by TB control programs and by well-established guidelines and standards. Clinicians have to be familiar with the TB control programs in their region and currently accepted standards. Despite education in the community, there is a stigma associated with the disease and patients are often delinquent about follow-up after the initial diagnosis of TB. Local and regional health departments can be of great help, and these resources are often underutilized. Clinicians have to be familiar with the updated recommendations for prophylaxis of TB, chemotherapy for active disease, currently used medications, and their dose and side effect profiles, especially of the newer medications (Table 3). Treatment of TB is aimed at eradicating the illness with rapid clearance of the viable bacilli from the sputum and treating potential contacts in order to contain and control the infection and protect the society from the spread of the disease. The drug treatment has to be highly effective and the delivery of treatment should be efficient, cost effective, and acceptable, resulting in very high compliance by patients. Because the active disease is associated with many complex and confounding factors, the treatment program has to take into consideration the many factors that affect the success of the treatment programs. Complicating and confounding factors result in compliance.

TABLE 3. **The Common Antituberculous Drug, With Recommended Dosage and Common Side Effects**

Drugs	Dosage	Side Effects
Isoniazid	5–10 mg/kg up to 300 mg	Peripheral neuritis, hepatitis, elevated liver enzymes Serum sickness Skin rash
Rifampin (Rifadin)	10–20 mg/kg up to 600 mg	Hepatitis, febrile reaction thrombocytopenia
Ethambutol (myambutol)	15–25 mg/kg up to 1200 mg	Decrease visual acuity Color vision abnormality
Pyrazinamide	1.5–2.5 g	Hyperuricemia, hepatotoxicity GI disturbance
Streptomycin	15–20 mg/kg up to 1 g	Nephrotoxicity, auditory and vestibular toxicity

Innovative measures have been used to increase compliance and to achieve maximum cure rate by reducing the duration of therapy. Intermittent therapy and directly observed therapy have been extremely successful with good results in achieving good compliance and good outcome.

Initial Treatment

INH and RMP for 9 months have been an extremely effective combination in the initial management of TB. This effective combination renders the patient noninfectious in 10 days and sterilizes the sputum in 2 months with a cure rate of over 95% in cases of infection by drug-susceptible strains. There is no restriction of work and isolation of patients is unnecessary if the patients can resume activity in their own environment because the chance of new transmission is extremely rare in the presence of effective drug treatment. Clinical follow-up and close monitoring of liver enzymes are necessary to recognize the side effects and efficacy of treatment. Alternative to the conventional 9-month treatment regimen are designed to suit a variety of special groups to overcome the reasons for failure usually encountered in the treatment programs and to improve compliance.

Alternatives to Conventional Treatment Programs

- Initial treatment containing INH, RMP, ethambutol (EMB) (Myambutol), and pyrazinamide (PZA) given for 2 months followed by INH and RMP for 4 months is equally successful and has been helpful in reducing the duration with better compliance rates. The combination of RMP and PZA is capable of causing severe hepatotoxicity, and close monitoring and discontinuing the drugs promptly when the symptoms of side effects appear are necessary.
- INH, RMP, and PZA for 3 months followed by INH and RMP for 3 months daily, three times a week or twice a week, has improved compliance.
- INH, RMP, EMB, and streptomycin (SM) three times a week for 6 months has also been an effective regimen in poorly compliant groups.

Role of Corticosteroids in the Treatment of Tuberculosis

In acute overwhelming TB there is significant host response associated with tissue inflammation and fibrous proliferation. The heightened host response can lead to a poor clinical outcome in cases with acute respiratory failure; acute respiratory distress syndrome; involvement of extrapulmonary sites such as meninges, pericardium, peritoneum, and the adrenal glands. Corticosteroids with their anti-inflammatory properties can be used effectively in conjunction with anti-TB drugs especially in cases with pericarditis and meningitis. Methylprednisolone (Solu-Medrol) in doses of 1 mg/kg has been used with a tapering regimen after initial response to treatment. The clinician should recognize the potential for TB dissemination in the presence of corticosteroids.

EXTRAPULMONARY TUBERCULOSIS

In 10% to 15% of cases, reactivation occurs at extrapulmonary sites with or without the involvement of lungs. Because of the atypical manifestations and the lack of classical chest radiographic findings in over 50% of cases, extrapulmonary tuberculosis (EPTB) can be a challenge to clinicians in all specialties. In HIV/AIDS patients, other immunocompromised patients, intravenous drug addicts, and foreign-born patients, hematogenous spread is associated with a high incidence of EPTB. EPTB can be missed because of the atypical presentation and lack of expertise because TB is a rare disease in many areas of the United States. Despite the overall decrease in TB, the incidence of EPTB still remains high, especially in the case of HIV/AIDS TB, intravenous drug addicts, and foreign-born cases. Early diagnosis and careful handling of all specimens for microbiologic studies to assess drug sensitivity are important ingredients in the treatment of EPTB. INH and RMP have good tissue penetration, but the duration of treatment should be extended to 12 to 18 months depending on the clinical response. Because of lack of expertise among primary care physicians in this area, appropriate consultations should be obtained to avoid unnecessary diagnostic procedures, especially surgical interventions. Special imaging studies and adjustments in drug treatment including the use of corticosteroids as mentioned previously are necessary in special situations. Surgical interventions may be necessary in cases of constrictive pericarditis and in some cases of spinal TB with spinal cord compression.

MULTIDRUG-RESISTANT TUBERCULOSIS (MDR TB)

Drug-resistant TB is due to infection by organisms with primary drug resistance, ineffective initial drug treatment, poor compliance, and an overwhelming bacillary load as seen in cases of HIV/AIDS TB. MDR TB is a major problem in places where the incidence of TB is extremely high, such as New York City, Los Angeles, and Miami, and in the developing countries. Primary and acquired resistance places a strain on TB control programs. Early intervention with alternative treatment plans, tactful adjustment of drug regimens on the basis of microbial culture and sensitivity studies, and the use of available expertise from experienced centers are strongly recommended. Primary infection with MDR TB should be suspected in HIV/AIDS patients, drug addicts, institutionalized people, and patients from areas of heavy endemicity. Treatment of MDR TB should be designed carefully with at least three new anti-TB drugs the patients have not been exposed to previously; at times, six or more drugs have to be used in nonresponding patients. Clinicians and centers with experience in handling MDR TB can be a very useful resource in helping with difficult and complex cases. In a case of nonresponding MDR TB with poor tolerance to second- and third-line drugs, surgery should be considered if the disease is localized and if the patient is a candidate for resectional surgery.

HIV/AIDS TUBERCULOSIS

In the 1980s, resurgence of TB was mainly due to HIV infection. Immunosuppression associated with HIV infection changed the controlled formula in the pathogenesis of TB. There was an explosion of new cases, and the rapidity with which reactivation occurred was dramatic and added up to 60,000 new cases during this epidemic. HIV/AIDS and TB coexist in up to 40% of cases in developing countries, resulting in high morbidity and mortality. Many of the features of HIV/AIDS TB are likely to result in complexities, and special attention is necessary (Table 4). Early dissemination at the time of presentation, atypical clinical manifestations, higher incidence of drug intolerance, and higher mortality and morbidity rates are some of the features of HIV/AIDS TB. In most patients, initial treatment with INH, RMP, PZA, and EMB for 2 months followed by INH and RMP for 4 months is well accepted with good success. Patients who are receiving highly active antiretroviral therapy (HAART) should receive rifabutin* (Mycobutin) in place of RMP because RMP renders the HAART ineffective by causing rapid metabolism of protease inhibitors. There is a high chance of primary and acquired drug resistance in cases of HIV/AIDS TB, and early diagnosis and modification of treatment regimens are necessary to achieve optimal results.

TUBERCULOSIS—HOW TO AVOID PITFALLS

- A TB skin test should be mandatory in high-risk populations, institutionalized persons, and health care workers.

*Not FDA approved for this indication.

TABLE 4. **Common Differences TB vs AIDS/TB**

AIDS	Tuberculosis	AIDS/TB
PPD skin test	Positive in 80% cases	Variable
Location of infection	Upper lobes of lung	Any segment of lung, diffuse lung involvement, or extrapulmonary TB
Treatment	Predicted good responses to treatment in over 90%	Good response in early cases Unpredictable in overwhelming infections
Drug reactions	3-5%	Higher incidence
Other mycobacterial	Rare	Combined infections are common; i.e., *M. avium* infection

- Tuberculin skin tests should be a standard practice in all patients hospitalized for pulmonary and systemic infections to identify an infected high-risk patient.
- A neck mass in a foreign-born person could be due to a tuberculous lymphadenitis and should be evaluated for TB before invasive procedures—scrofula.
- Chronic back pain with minimal systemic manifestations could be due to spinal TB in patients coming from highly endemic areas—Pott's disease.
- Recurrent symptoms of urinary infections could be due to genitourinary TB—sterile acid pyuria of renal TB.
- In patients thought to have sarcoidosis, a caseating or noncaseating inflammatory process should raise suspicion for TB. TB should be excluded with appropriate special stains and tissue cultures. Patients should be treated with anti-TB drugs until the cultures are negative.
- In all high-risk patients with a positive tuberculin skin test, active TB should be excluded and TB treatment should be continued until culture results are known, especially in patients undergoing immunosuppressive treatment because the systematic manifestations can be indistinguishable from those of the primary illness.

PHYSICIANS' AND ALLIED HEALTH CARE PROFESSIONALS' RESPONSIBILITIES IN CONTROL OF TUBERCULOSIS

The Secretary of Health and Human Services endorsed a program to eradicate TB in the United States by the year 2010. A decrease from a current rate of 5.6 cases per 100,000 population (CDC data, 2001) to less than 1 case per 100,000 population is achievable by intensifying current treatment programs and control programs. Every primary physician should be knowledgeable about the diagnosis, management, and prevention of TB and the current standards recommended by the American Thoracic Society (ATS), the CDC, and the Infectious Disease Society of America (IDSA). Physicians should be aware of the regional programs and should use locally available resources such as health departments to enhance the knowledge and to provide optimal care for individual patients. The CDC (www.cdc.org), ATS (www.thoracic.org), and IDSA (www.idsociety.org) web sites are excellent resources for mycobacterial infections and management.

NONTUBERCULOUS MYCOBACTERIAL INFECTION

Infections with nontuberculous mycobacteria (NTMs) have been known for a long time as atypical mycobacterial infections and as mycobacteria other than tuberculosis (MOTT) in AIDS patients. Atypical mycobacteria share many common properties such as acid fastness in staining and the ability to cause pulmonary and extrapulmonary granulomatous disorders. As a group, they comprise diverse organisms with dissimilarities in their cultural characteristics and pathogenicity to humans compared with *Mycobacterium tuberculosis* (MTB). There are many organisms in this group capable of causing human infections (Table 5). *Mycobacterium avium-intracellulare* infections became common in patients with severe HIV/AIDS, and it is clear that immune defenses against these bacteria prevent us from developing infections with these ubiquitous acid-fast organisms. *M. avium* infection is quite predictable in HIV/AIDS patients with dropping CD4 counts and is an AIDS-defining disease. NTM causes significant clinical illness in patients with structural abnormalities and in patients with immunodeficiency syndrome. Patients with bronchiectasis and chronic obstructive pulmonary disease (COPD) with *Mycobacterium kansasii* infections are an example of the former, and HIV/AIDS patients with *M. avium* infection are an example of the latter. Mycobacteria are ubiquitous

TABLE 5. **Non-Tuberculous Mycobacterial Infections and Treatment**

Organism	Clinical Illness	Drug Treatment
M. avium	Pulmonary infection	Clarithromycin (Biaxin) 500 mg or azithromycin (Zithromax) 250 mg twice a day and rifampin* (Rifadin) 600 mg for 1 year
	Disseminated without HIV, *M. avium* in HIV/AIDS	Clarithromycin or azithromycin Ethambutol* (Myambutol) and rifampin* Prolonged course (lifetime)
M. kansasii	Cavitary lung disease Diffuse parenchymal disease	INH* 300 mg RMP* 600 mg and EMB* 800–1200 mg for 18 months
	Localized disease	Surgical resection
M. xenopi *M. chelonae* *M. abscesses* *M. scrofulaceum* *M. malmoense* *M. fortuitum*	Pneumonic illness Lymphadenitis Skin infections Abscesses and ulcerations Disseminated	Multi-drug treatment including macrolides, quinolones, amikacin* (Amikin) based on culture characteristics

EMB, Ethambutol; INH, Isoniazid; RMP, Rifampin.
*Not FDA approved for this indication.

organisms. Yet the prevalence and epidemiology of infections with NTMs in the environment are not clear. There are many examples of opportunistic pathologic processes resulting from exposure to environmental mycobacteria. These organisms are capable of causing granulomatous inflammation or an inflammatory hypersensitivity pneumonitis. Hypersensitivity pneumonitis caused by *M. avium* and *M. intracellulare* has been associated with disinfection of indoor swimming pools and public baths.

Pulmonary Nontuberculous Mycobacterial Infections

Colonization of the respiratory tract by NTMs, especially in patients with cystic fibrosis or COPD and immunocompromised patients, makes it difficult to determine the exact epidemiologic impact of pulmonary infections with NTMs. NTMs are estimated to occur in from 1 to 15 per 100,000 population in the United Stated with wide variability in geographic distribution. This variability is attributed to many factors such as differences in diagnostic capability and also the fact that these diseases, unlike TB, are not reportable. An increase in NTM infections, especially by *M. avium* and *M. kansasii*, has been reported when the incidence of TB decreases in a community. The risk factors are HIV/AIDS, bronchiectasis, COPD, advancing age, male sex, cystic fibrosis, previous TB, and silicosis. A disorder occurring in middle-aged women with poor cough and associated chronic bronchial inflammation with nodular bronchiectasis results from *M. avium* infection. This has been termed *Lady Windemere syndrome* and is characterized by chronic cough, bronchiolitis, and bronchiectasis caused by chronic *M. avium* infection and probably a hypersensitivity phenomenon. Use of macrolides, azithromycin (Zithromax), clarithromycin (Biaxin), and rifabutin (Mycobutin), a derivative of rifamycin S, has become the cornerstone of treatment of *M. avium* infection.

Despite advances in many areas of medicine, TB, a controllable infectious disease, still remains a major problem. Renewed enthusiasm among clinicians and allied health care professionals with a goal is key to eradicating TB by the year 2010. The challenge has to be accepted by clinicians with prompt diagnosis and management of TB. Health departments should be vigilant in case finding, reporting, and contact follow-up. Scientists should continue their diligent work with rapid diagnostic technology and development of newer therapeutic measures and vaccines. Genetic probing of the mycobacteria, genetic identification of the susceptible population, and development of new vaccines will enhance achieving control of TB in the United States and around the world.

Section 5

The Cardiovascular System

ACQUIRED DISEASES OF THE AORTA

method of
JEFFREY DATILLO, M.D., and
DAVID C. BREWSTER, M.D.
Massachusetts General Hospital
Boston, Massachusetts

Acquired diseases of the aorta include aortoiliac occlusive disease, aneurysmal disease, and aortic dissection. Although the origin of these entities is not entirely understood, the vast majority of information concludes that an arteriosclerotic degenerative process is the likely cause. Atherosclerosis is associated with well-known risk factors that include hypertension, hyperlipidemia, cigarette smoking, and genetic predisposition. Certain arteries are at a higher risk for the development of atherosclerosis, including the lower abdominal aorta, the carotid bifurcation, and the arteries of the lower extremities.

Ultimately, progression of disease leads to consideration of surgical therapy. The evolution of treatment modalities has become refined over the last 20 years. The modern vascular surgeon has not only open surgical options for treatment but also the newly acquired armamentarium of minimally invasive techniques including angioplasty and stenting at his or her disposal. Additionally, perioperative monitoring and anesthetic advances have contributed significantly to the success of aortic surgery. Intra-arterial blood pressure monitoring, central and pulmonary capillary wedge pressure, oxygen perfusion devices, and rapid transfusion equipment all have added valuable data and tools to the care of these patients.

ANEURYSMS OF THE AORTA

Abdominal Aortic Aneurysms

Aneurysms of the abdominal aorta (AAA) are increasing in incidence disproportionate to that of the aging population. Approximately 15,000 deaths per year in the United States are attributed to rupture of AAAs. In addition, it should be recognized that these numbers are probably an underestimate of the problem, mainly because most aneurysms are asymptomatic until they ultimately rupture and are misdiagnosed at the time of death as cardiac in origin.

Pathogenesis

Historically, aneurysmal disease was thought to be due to an atherosclerotic degeneration of the aorta. Recently, however, many researchers have documented several alternative hypotheses that may contribute to the underlying pathogenesis of aneurysmal formation. These include

- Genetic
- Proteolytic enzyme activity
- Hemodynamic influences
- Cystic medial necrosis
- Ehlers-Danlos syndrome
- Syphilis
- Dissection

Histologically, there are fewer medial elastic lamellae present in the infrarenal aorta, with a resultant decrease in elastic compliance of the aorta at that level. Additionally, there are profound alterations in hemodynamics at the flow divider (the bifurcation), which confer another potential mechanism for aneurysmal growth. As the aorta grows in diameter, the physical principle most commonly applied to the continued growth of aneurysms is the law of LaPlace. Simply stated, the radius is directly proportional to the tension applied to the vessel wall. Therefore, as the radius increases the tension on the vessel wall increases.

Diagnosis

An infrarenal abdominal aortic aneurysm larger than 5 cm in diameter can usually be diagnosed on physical examination, except in obese patients. The point at which to palpate an aneurysm is between the xiphoid process and the umbilicus. The clinical triad associated with rupture is pulsatile abdominal mass, back or abdominal pain, and hypotension. Plain film radiography is a simple modality of detecting aneurysms. In 60% to 70% of aneurysms, there is enough calcium present to detect the aneurysm on plain film. However, negative findings of plain film radiography cannot rule out the presence of an aneurysm.

The most commonly used imaging modalities to detect and document the size of AAAs are ultrasonography and spiral computed tomography (CT). Ultrasonography has been the diagnostic method of choice for initial diagnosis of pulsatile abdominal mass. Additionally ultrasonography is an effective tool used to periodically follow the size of the aneurysm. Ultrasonography offers a variety of advantages, including wide availability, relatively low cost, no need for contrast agents, and rapid performance. The accuracy of ultrasonography can be reproducible within 3 to 4 mm of actual size of the aneurysm. Limitations of ultrasonography include the respective location and measurements of branch vessels.

Spiral CT is the gold standard in accuracy for determining the size and location of aneurysms. It is a highly valuable tool in determining the relationship of the aneurysm to visceral vessels, venous anomalies, and topographic and vessel wall characteristics. Further, it is accurate in detecting leak, retroperitoneal hematoma, and rupture. Three-dimensional reconstruction is now possible in many modern centers to practically visualize any angle conceivable to plan reconstruction options.

Aortography can also be useful in selected patients with abdominal aortic aneurysms. In patients with normal renal function, aortography can delineate with accuracy the anatomy of angulations of the aorta, branch vessel relationships, and critical stenosis of these branch vessels. However, aortography is a poor diagnostic modality to delineate the size of the aneurysm because the size of the aneurysm is based on the largest outside diameter of the aneurysm.

Treatment

The goal of treatment is to prevent the rupture. The most important factor predicting rupture is aneurysm size. Aneurysms smaller than 4.5 cm in diameter have an annual risk of rupture of less than 2%, whereas the rupture rate for an aneurysm 5 to 7 cm in size is approximately 5% to 7% per year. This is a cumulative risk of 25% to 35% at 5 years. Furthermore, aneurysm rupture rates for aneurysms greater than 7 cm in size have been predicted to be around 20% per year. A clear indication for repair is when the risk of rupture exceeds the risk of the operation. Current perioperative mortality rates for open aneurysm repair average 2% to 5%. These risks rise when a patient has significant co-morbidities, including severe restrictive lung disease, renal failure, or untreated coronary artery disease.

Standard open repair of AAA has been well documented as a very effective and durable treatment that can be performed with highly acceptable morbidity and mortality rates in many experienced centers. The infrarenal aorta can be exposed via transperitoneal or retroperitoneal approaches. The aneurysmal section is then replaced with either Dacron or polytetrafluoroethylene. The transperitoneal approach offers greater access to the iliac arteries and the right renal artery. Conversely, the retroperitoneal approach offers distinct advantages such as access to the suprarenal aorta, avoidance of a scarred, previously operated upon abdomen, and access to the left renal artery. Relative contraindications to the retroperitoneal approach are large right iliac artery aneurysms, left-sided vena cava, and the distal right renal artery stenosis requiring bypass.

Another approach to repair of AAA has been the emergence of endoluminal techniques. Since the introduction of endoluminal repair in 1991, this technique has been eagerly accepted and used with rapidly increasing frequency in a growing number of centers in recent years. Complication rates of open repair increase substantially in elderly patients, or those patients with pulmonary, cardiac, or renal co-morbidities. The potential advantages of reduced risk, quicker recovery, and possibly diminished costs of care have generated intense interest on the part of patients, physicians, and industry. In September of 1999, two devices were granted U.S. Food and Drug Administration approval, and several devices currently in clinical trials will likely become commercially available within the next several years. The current wave of literature clearly documents the early feasibility and efficacy of endovascular repair of AAA. However, some reports of midterm experience have described a somewhat disturbing incidence of complications related to device failures, endoleaks, or other examples of treatment shortcoming, including continued AAA growth or even rupture despite endoluminal therapy.

Careful patient selection is paramount in the success of endovascular repair. One of the most important determinations lies in obtaining good quality imaging studies. The use of digital CT scanning with three-dimensional imaging capability is crucial. One must carefully evaluate three major criteria for consideration of stent grafting: (1) relationship of the aneurysm to the renal arteries for proximal attachment (length of neck, diameter of neck, and angulation of neck); (2) the distal attachment sites for diameter and involvement with other vessels; and (3) the diameter and quality of the vessels in which the device will be passed.

Our series review from our initial 7-year experience with 362 patients with AAAs treated by endoluminal stent-graft repair of the Massachusetts General Hospital indicates, like other reports, that endovascular AAA repair is safe and can be successfully performed in patients with suitable anatomy. The implant success in most centers is now approaching 98% to 99%, and this and other outcome parameters are likely to further improve with second- and third-generation devices. In addition to a low mortality rate of less than 1% and only a 1% early conversion rate, our results document quite effective treatment of the AAA relative to its anticipated natural history. The AAA has remained stable in size or actually diminished in maximal diameter in 94% of cases, and serious late problems such as conversion to open repair (2.2%) and AAA rupture (<1%) remain infrequent. The major disadvantage to our and other reports is the relatively short follow-up time when compared with conventional open repair.

Thoracic Aortic Aneurysms

Thoracic aneurysms can be divided into ascending or descending aneurysms. Aortic dissection, hypertension, smoking, hyperlipidemia, and familial trends are major risk factors in the development of thoracic aneurysms. Although most thoracic aneurysms are caused by atherosclerotic disease, aortic valvular disease may also be a contributing factor, especially with ascending aneurysms. The diameter at which a surgeon should consider repair is not well established. However, aneurysms larger than 6 cm in greatest diameter should be considered for repair. Diagnostic studies that are useful in delineating the extent of the aneurysm include spiral CT scanning, transesophageal echocardiography, and magnetic resonance angiography.

Treatment

Aneurysms of the ascending aorta and the arch vessels usually require cardiopulmonary bypass combined with hypothermic circulatory arrest. The aneurysm is resected and replaced, usually with a Dacron graft. The aortic valve is often replaced with an ascending aneurysm and the brachiocephalic vessels reimplanted with arch aneurysms. Descending aneurysms are repaired with standard aortic replacement techniques in which the aortic segment is replaced with a Dacron graft. The major risk is paraplegia caused by spinal cord ischemia. This occurs in up to 5% of patients. This risk can be reduced with reimplantation of unpaired intercostal muscles at the time of repair.

Thoracoabdominal Aortic Aneurysms

Thoracoabdominal aortic aneurysms (TAAs) extend from the chest and include the visceral vessels. The causes of TAAs include atherosclerosis, cystic medial degeneration, myxomatous degeneration, and dissection. The incidence of these aneurysms increases with age. Frequently, cystic medial necrosis is seen histologically and may accompany degenerative changes seen with atherosclerosis. As the process of atherosclerosis progresses, it causes occlusion of the vasa vasorum, which in turn causes medial necrosis and subsequent aneurysm formation. Aneurysms of the descending thoracic aorta compress and erode into adjacent structures, including the spine, airway, and esophagus. Patients may present with hoarseness, chest pain, cough, or hemoptysis as well as dysphagia.

The Crawford classification divides TAAs into types I through IV. Type I involves most of the descending thoracic and upper abdominal aorta. Type II involves most of the descending thoracic aorta and most, if not all, of the abdominal aorta. Type III involves the distal thoracic aorta and most of the abdominal aorta. Type IV involves all of the visceral abdominal aorta.

Diagnosis

Thoracoabdominal aneurysms can be diagnosed incidentally on plain chest radiographs in conjunction with workup of other clinical problems. Spiral CT scans and magnetic resonance imaging can be helpful in making specific anatomic diagnoses and further assist in details of sizing. The use of aortography can be helpful in determining the specific location of the aneurysm in relationship to branch vessels and detailing potential disease in those vessels that could require bypass. In general, for planning surgical resection, spiral CT in combination with aortography of the entire thoracic and abdominal aorta is essential for a well-planned resection. The combination of these two modalities will reveal critical anatomic considerations in planning the procedure and consideration of revascularization of the visceral vessels.

Treatment

The treatment is resection and grafting of the aneurysmal segment. A multidisciplinary approach is mandatory to maintain the morbidity and mortality rates as low as in the major centers. The mortality rate at our institution is approximately 8%. This rate is lower, 5%, if one considers the elective, nonurgent cases. Major complications of open repair of TAAs include respiratory failure, hemorrhage, renal insufficiency, paraplegia, and cardiac complications. Respiratory failure is the single most common complication following TAA repair. Preoperative predictive variables that can influence respiratory outcome include active cigarette smoking, chronic obstructive pulmonary disease, and significant reductions of forced expiratory volume in 1 second (FEV_1). Paraplegia is the most devastating nonfatal risk of TAA repair. A variety of strategies have been employed to reduce the risk of spinal cord ischemia and the resultant paraplegia. The tactics can be divided into surgical approaches to attempt to maintain the perfusion pressure to the cord, such as atrial-femoral bypass, or neuroprotective adjuncts to increase the tolerance of spinal cord ischemia during cross-clamping, such as spinal cooling. Despite these improvements, however, the paraplegia rate remains 5% to 10% in large-volume centers.

The operation is carried out generally through a standard posterolateral thoracotomy (fifth or sixth interspace) for type I and type II aneurysms. An eighth interspace incision is adequate for type III or IV aneurysms. Proximal control of the aorta in the chest is usually accomplished above the aneurysm without technical issues. Afterload reduction prior to clamping is critical and must be coordinated with the anesthesiologist. This can be done pharmacologically or with the use of an atrial-femoral bypass circuit. When the aneurysm is open, particular attention should be given to the critical zone of T9–L1 in which the vast majority of anterior spinal arteries arise from the aorta. Vessels in this area should be considered in reimplantation strategies and protected with balloon occlusion devices prior to re-establishment of arterial flow. The clamp is then moved down to prepare for the visceral and right renal segment, which is often included in an inclusion button. The left renal artery is addressed with a previously attached side arm anastomosis. Finally, the distal anastomosis is completed.

AORTIC DISSECTION

Acute aortic dissection is the most common catastrophic event involving the aorta. There are approximately 9000 patients who have dissecting aneurysms in the United States annually. Aortic dissections are three times more frequent in males; however, 50% of the dissections seen in females younger than 40 years of age occur in pregnancy. Acute dissection most frequently occurs in the sixth or seventh decade of life. A history of hypertension is present in 80% to 90% of patients.

When an aortic dissection occurs, the intimal layer of the artery suddenly tears away. The arterial blood then enters the space between the intimal and medial layers, creating a false lumen. The further shearing forces of the dissecting aorta can cause the dissection to progress into major branching vessels of the aorta. This, in turn, can lead to compromise in the arterial blood flow to the end organ, kidneys or visceral vessels.

Dissections are classified according to the location of the initial tear in the aorta. The two classifications used in clinical practice are the DeBakey and Stanford classifications. The Stanford classification is divided into two major groupings: A, which involves the ascending aorta, and B, which involves the descending aorta. The DeBakey classification includes type I, which involves the entire aorta originating in the ascending aorta; type II, which is limited to the ascending aorta; and type III, which is distal to the left subclavian artery extending distally, potentially to the abdominal aorta.

Diagnosis

The characteristic symptom of acute aortic dissection is a sudden onset of severe tearing pain in the back, chest, or abdomen. Diagnosis is particularly difficult at times because the symptom can arise from ischemia to end organs, leading the clinician into working up the symptom and not the original cause. Diagnostic imaging modalities include CT, magnetic resonance imaging, angiography, and transesophageal echocardiography. The important questions to be answered initially by diagnostic imaging are where the dissection is located proximally, where it extends to distally, and which lumen supplies which visceral vessels. Considerations for which study is to be performed should be determined by the particular clinical scenario; for example, elevated creatinine would obviate the use of contrast agents. The use of transesophageal echocardiography is particularly helpful in determining whether the dissection is proximal to the left subclavian artery.

Treatment

Initial treatment of any dissection is aggressive and vigilant medical control of hypertension. Type A or DeBakey I or II dissections are considered a surgical emergency, with rare exception. The mortality rate exceeds 50% if the dissection is not surgically corrected. Often the dissection will retrograde dissect and cause pericardial tamponade and coronary occlusion. Surgical repair of the proximal aorta will often redirect blood into the correct lumen distally. Careful monitoring, however, must be accomplished to ensure that conversion to a type B dissection does not occur. Furthermore, patients with a type B dissection with evidence of either rupture or end organ ischemia should be considered for urgent surgical correction.

Type III or type B dissections should initially be treated medically in an intensive care unit with central venous and arterial pressure monitors, an indwelling Foley catheter, or a cardiac rhythm monitor. Pharmacologic control of hypertension involves the use of β-blockade and nitrates. Currently, there are no data to support the idea that urgent surgical intervention in these patients is superior to medical therapy. When signs of organ or limb ischemia are detected, consideration for urgent surgical reconstruction, aortic fenestration, or endovascular therapy should undertaken.

AORTOILIAC OCCLUSIVE DISEASE

The infrarenal abdominal aorta and iliac arteries are common sites of atherosclerosis and lesion formation. Obliterative disease of the aortoiliac segment is accompanied usually with some form of infrainguinal peripheral vascular disease. The distribution of aortoiliac disease is often segmental and therefore quite amenable to treatment.

Diagnosis

In most cases, a detailed history and physical examination can establish the diagnosis of aortoiliac occlusive disease. Claudication of one or both legs with diminished or absent femoral pulses is often diagnostic. The distribution of the claudication is often important. Proximal symptoms such as buttock, thigh, or hip claudication certainly indicate inflow disease. More often, however, patients will have calf claudication, which indicates multilevel disease. In addition to a diminished pulse, the clinician can sometimes hear a bruit over the pelvis or the groin pulse.

The use of noninvasive hemodynamic studies can aid in the diagnosis of aortoiliac occlusive disease. These studies are frequently helpful in establishing the diagnosis and assessing the level of disease. Imaging studies such as magnetic resonance arteriography or conventional arteriography are extremely important in planning effective treatment. In addition to standard anteroposterior views, lateral and oblique films are often helpful in assessing possible visceral artery disease, pelvic circulation, and profunda femoral origin disease. Full lower extremity runoff studies are also advisable. Further, assessment of resting blood pressure gradients at the time of angiography is also useful. A lesion with a pressure gradient of 5 mm Hg or greater or with a 15% drop with pharmacologic vasodilatation is often diagnostic of a significant flow reducing lesion.

Treatment

Choices of proximal graft anastomotic configuration and distal configurations are the most important decisions to be made in regard to aortobifemoral bypass grafting. For most patients, an end-to-end aortic anastomosis is preferred for several reasons. First, there is less chance of competitive flow with the native aortoiliac system, which may lead to higher incidence of graft thrombosis. Second, an end-to-end anastomosis is superior from a hemodynamic and turbulence perspective. Further, the end-to-end configuration is less likely to cause distal atheromatous embolization and is easier to cover with retroperitoneal tissues after implantation. Although an end-to-end graft to aorta anastomosis is preferred in the majority of patients, certain anatomic patterns of disease are encountered that make an end-to-side configuration advantageous. These include patients with a sizable accessory renal artery arising from the infrarenal aorta. More commonly, however, is the patient with external iliac disease. These patients often have the common and internal iliac arteries preserved. In such a patient, an end-to-end proximal anastomosis with femoral bypass could lead to considerable devascularization of the pelvic area. Further, the incidence of male impotence and colonic ischemia is higher in this group of patients.

The long-term patency of aortobifemoral bypass grafting is greatly dependent on the completion of a technically perfect femoral anastomosis. Maintaining flow into the profunda femoris artery is critical to this end. Therefore, preoperative evaluation of the profunda femoris with assistance of an arteriogram or magnetic resonance angiography is imperative. Furthermore, an intraoperative examination of the profunda femoris is advised, with the passage of dilators to ensure the quality of the vessel. If the origin of the profunda is stenotic, the clinician should then be advised to consider bringing the anastomosis onto the profunda and performing a profundaplasty with the beveled tip of the anastomosis, thus allowing unimpeded flow into the profunda femoris.

The long-term patency rates are excellent. It is reasonable to expect 85% to 90% graft patency at 5 years, and 70% to 75% at 10 years. Perioperative mortality rates are 2% to 3% in most centers.

The role of catheter-based interventions may be a valuable treatment modality in some patients with aortoiliac occlusive disease. Careful evaluation of the lesions to be considered for treatment is critical in determining early and late success. For instance, usually lesions less than 5 cm in length in the common iliac artery are best suited for percutaneous transluminal angioplasty. Yet the long-term success rates of these procedures still appear to be less than those of conventional open repair. Controversy remains as to whether to use catheter-based therapies in the patient with milder symptoms who would not generally be considered for open surgical repair. Furthermore, patients with longer disease segments, multiple lesions, or total occlusions perhaps can benefit from the use of stents, although this hypothesis remains unproven at this time.

MANAGEMENT OF ANGINA PECTORIS

method of
ADAM BRODSKY, M.D., and
DAN FINTEL, M.D.
Northwestern University Feinberg School of Medicine
Chicago, Illinois

Angina pectoris is the cardinal symptom of myocardial ischemia. It is typically described as a pressure-like sensation in the chest that may radiate into the jaw, shoulder, or back or down the ulnar sides of the left arm and, less commonly, the right arm. Occasionally, angina pectoris may radiate to the throat, teeth, or ears. Angina is caused by an imbalance between oxygen demand and oxygen supply in the myocardium. The most common cause of this imbalance is obstructive epicardial coronary artery disease (CAD); however, other causes include microvascular disease, valvular disease, left ventricular hypertrophy, uncontrolled hypertension, and severe anemia.

Angina pectoris resulting from epicardial CAD may be classified as stable angina or unstable angina. Angina that occurs predictably with exertion and resolves predictably with rest is considered stable. *Stable angina* occurs with predictable frequency and intensity, depending on the frequency and intensity of the physical activity performed by the patient. The syndrome of stable angina is most often caused by fixed, flow-limiting atherosclerotic plaque in the epicardial coronary arteries. Coronary spasm may also disrupt blood flow either in addition to or independent of coronary atherosclerosis. When a patient's anginal pattern changes, becoming more frequent or more intense, occurring at a lower exercise threshold, or occurring at rest, it is referred to as *unstable angina*. Unstable angina occurs when a previously quiescent atherosclerotic plaque ruptures, exposing the lipid-rich core of the plaque to the bloodstream and causing platelet aggregation and clot formation. In addition to causing distal microembolization, the ruptured plaque may produce varying degrees of coronary obstruction resulting from the competing forces of intrinsic fibrinolysis and continued fibrin and platelet deposition. These factors are responsible for the varying and unpredictable nature of unstable angina. The clinical presentations of unstable angina and acute myocardial infarction are collectively referred to as the *acute coronary syndrome*.

Certain patients may not experience typical angina manifested by chest pain, but instead they may experience other symptoms such as nausea or shortness of breath. In the appropriate clinical setting, these symptoms may be considered anginal equivalents and thus carry the same prognostic value as typical angina. The Canadian Cardiovascular Society classified patients with angina into four groups. Class I patients have angina only with strenuous activity but not with ordinary activity. Class II patients have angina with ordinary activity such as climbing stairs or walking uphill. Class III patients have angina with minimal activity, such as walking one or two blocks on level ground. Class IV patients have angina with any physical activity at all and may also have angina when they are at rest.

STABLE ANGINA

Diagnosis

The patient's history, physical examination, laboratory tests, electrocardiogram (ECG), and other cardiac testing all contribute to the diagnosis of CAD and stable angina. The goal of each of these steps is to answer two questions: does the patient have CAD, and if so, what is the risk of having an adverse event in the future?

The initial patient history must focus on the nature of the patient's symptoms, including the quality, duration, and frequency, as well as factors that provoke or relieve the patient's symptoms. Historical symptoms considered to indicate higher risk include rest angina, nocturnal angina, or prolonged angina lasting longer than 20 minutes. Equally important as the patient's symptoms are the patient's risk factors for CAD. Recognized risk factors include age (greater than 45 years in men and less than 55 years in women), hypertension, hyperlipidemia, and family history of early CAD in a first-degree relative. Certain historical features such as a history of diabetes, cerebrovascular disease, or peripheral vascular disease are considered to be stronger than simple risk factors in that the risk of future adverse cardiac events in patients with these conditions is equivalent to the risk in patients with an established history of CAD (without these conditions). These conditions are therefore referred to as *CAD equivalents* and define a group of patients who should be treated as if they already have established CAD.

Physical examination features that increase the likelihood of having CAD include: hypertension, murmurs of aortic stenosis, abnormal apical impulse, other signs of heart failure (e.g., rales, S_3 gallop, elevated jugular venous pulse, edema), and other signs of vascular disease (vascular bruits, distal digital ulcerations, abnormal fundi, decreased peripheral pulses).

The resting ECG is very useful as well and can identify higher-risk patients (e.g., those with ST elevation or depression, dynamic T wave changes, left ventricular hypertrophy, pathologic Q waves, or new left bundle branch block) The ECG treadmill stress test is useful both for diagnosing angina resulting from flow-limiting coronary stenoses and for prognosis regarding the risk of future adverse cardiac events. Horizontal or downsloping ST depression or elevation greater than or equal to 1 mm extending at least 80 ms after the J point is considered a positive test, suggesting the presence of flow-limiting CAD. The duration of exercise and the maximum workload attained (measured in metabolic equivalents or as the rate-pressure product), as well as the hemodynamic response and symptomatic response, also yield important prognostic information. As a diagnostic test, the ECG treadmill test has a sensitivity of approximately 68% and a specificity of approximately 77%. ECG treadmill stress testing may be less accurate in women.

A stress test with myocardial imaging is indicated if the ECG is uninterpretable because of left bundle branch block, electronically paced ventricular rhythm, preexcitation (Wolf-Parkinson-White syndrome), or baseline ST segment deviation. An imaging modality is also indicated if the patient has had prior revascularization, in which case the additional information about ischemic territory and ischemic burden afforded by stress imaging is required. Because stress imaging testing may be performed using pharmacologic stressors instead of exercise, it is indicated for those patients who are physically unable to exercise to an adequate degree. Currently available imaging modalities include echocardiography and radionuclide imaging. The sensitivity and specificity of stress echocardiography are 82% to 85% and 85% to 86%, respectively. Radionuclide imaging has a slightly higher sensitivity (83% to 89%) and a slightly lower specificity (70% to 80%.) The various types of stress tests and their relative advantages and disadvantages are listed in Table 1.

The current gold standard for diagnosing epicardial CAD, the most common cause of stable angina, is the coronary angiogram. The angiogram visualizes only the lumen of the coronary arteries and therefore may underestimate diffuse disease or arterial segments in which atherosclerosis has led to positive remodeling while preserving the luminal area. By visualizing the entire coronary anatomy, angiography allows for risk stratification of patients based on their total burden of CAD.

Angiography is typically performed when the probability of CAD is high enough that specific therapy such as angioplasty or coronary artery bypass graft surgery is being contemplated. Most often, noninvasive stress testing is required to elevate the post-test probability of CAD to such a level; however, in certain cases, angiography may be performed as the initial test. Angiography is indicated as the initial test of choice for patients who have survived an episode of sudden cardiac arrest, in patients with severely reduced left ventricular function (ejection fraction less than 35%), for patients in whom a definitive diagnosis is necessary because of occupational requirements (e.g., airline pilots, firefighters), and for patients who are physically unable to undergo stress testing or in whom the accuracy of stress testing would be severely reduced (e.g. morbid obesity). Angiography is indicated after stress testing in patients with indeterminate stress test results or in whom left main or three-vessel disease is suspected.

Electron-beam computed tomography assesses the risk of epicardial CAD by measuring the amount of calcification in the coronary arteries. Several small studies have been performed showing sensitivities ranging from 85% to 100% and specificities ranging from 41% to 76%. Although this may be a useful test to exclude CAD in low-risk patients, the lack of large-scale trials and outcomes data makes it difficult to recommend widespread screening with this technique.

TABLE 1. **Characteristics of Various Types of Stress Tests**

			Imaging Modality →		
			Plain Electrocardiography	**Echocardiography**	**Radionuclide Imaging**
Stress Modality ↓	**Exercise**		Adequate initial test to rule out low-risk patients	Able to assess left ventricular structure and function; false-positive septal abnormalities in left bundle branch block and paced rhythms; able to assess functional capacity	Able to assess ejection fraction; false-positive septal abnormalities in left bundle branch block and paced rhythms; able to assess functional capacity
	Pharmacology	**Dobutamine**	X	Able to assess left ventricular structure and function; false-positive septal abnormalities in left bundle branch block and paced rhythms; may be performed in patients unable to exercise or tolerate vasodilators; no assessment of functional capacity	Able to assess ejection fraction; false-positive septal abnormalities in left bundle branch block and paced rhythms; may be performed in patients unable to exercise or tolerate vasodilators; no assessment of functional capacity
		Vasodilator	X	X	Able to assess ejection fraction; may be performed in patients unable to exercise or tolerate dobutamine; may be performed in patients with left bundle branch block and paced rhythms; no assessment of functional capacity

Once the diagnostic testing has taken place, the physician may appropriately stratify the patient's risk. Accurate risk stratification is important not only for future treatment decisions, but also for adequately addressing patients' expectations about prognosis. Certain historical features signify an increased risk of future events, such as the duration and frequency of anginal symptoms, as well as the presence of co-morbidities such as hypertension, diabetes, peripheral vascular disease, cerebrovascular disease, renal disease, or other cardiac disease. The patient's functional status also plays a role in determining the risk of future events. This may be assessed simply by history or more accurately by a treadmill stress test. The Duke treadmill score is a popular method of risk stratification. Using the Duke treadmill score, which is calculated on current stress test computer systems, the physician can predict the patient's future mortality risk from an annual mortality rate of 0.25% for the lowest scores to an annual mortality rate of 5% for the highest scores. Echocardiographic high-risk features include the presence of wall-motion abnormalities, low ejection fraction, concurrent severe valvular disease, and the presence of thrombus within the left ventricle. Radionuclide imaging also provides prognostic information, with the number and severity of myocardial perfusion defects resulting in a higher risk of future adverse cardiac events. Transient ischemic dilatation and lung uptake of radioisotope are also poor prognostic indicators. As described earlier, the angiographic severity of disease, including the number and severity of coronary lesions, the number of diseased vessels, and the location (proximal versus distal) of the lesions, also provides a basis for risk stratification. Table 2 lists several factors that may be used to stratify risk in patients.

Treatment

The treatment of chronic stable angina serves two purposes: to prolong life and to alleviate symptoms. It is therefore important to recognize that although certain therapies may have both mortality benefit and antianginal benefit, others may have only one or the other. The first line of treatment is risk factor modification. This primarily includes aggressive treatment of hypertension and diabetes, cessation of smoking, and treatment of dyslipidemia. Although these therapies have been clearly shown to reduce mortality, they are generally not directly antianginal and thus may not result in the patient's "feeling better." Nevertheless, physicians must strongly convey the lifesaving importance of these therapies to their patients. Several vitamins have also been studied in relation to heart disease. Despite earlier hopes that large doses of vitamins and antioxidants could have beneficial effects in CAD, more recent trials failed to find any such benefit.

TABLE 2. **Factors Used in Risk Stratification**

Historical	Functional	Echocardiographic	Nuclear	Angiographic
Age	Baseline activity level	Ejection fraction	Number/size of defects	Number of diseased vessels
Gender	Exercise capacity	Wall motion abnormalities	Severity of defects	Left main involvement
Frequency, duration, character of symptoms	Duke treadmill score	Left ventricular thrombus	Transient ischemic dilatation	Proximal location of lesions
Co-morbidities	Chest pain during stress test	Valvular disease	Lung uptake	Diffuseness of disease
Prior cardiac events	—	—	Ejection fraction	Ejection fraction

Lipid-Lowering Therapy

Lipid-lowering therapy is central to the treatment of atherosclerotic heart disease and stable angina. Several large-scale, randomized trials showed the benefits of low-density lipoprotein reduction for both primary and secondary prevention of cardiac events. The Heart Protection Study randomized more than 20,000 adults with CAD, other arterial occlusive disease, or diabetes to receive either 40 mg of simvastatin (Zocor) daily or placebo. The results showed a reduction in all-cause mortality for the simvastatin group, mainly resulting from a reduction in coronary deaths. This benefit was observed independent of initial low-density lipoprotein levels. All patients should follow the Adult Treatment Panel III guidelines regarding lipid-lowering therapy, which state that the goal low-density lipoprotein level for patients with CAD or CAD equivalents (diabetes, cerebrovascular disease, or peripheral vascular disease) is less than 100 mg/dL. Many patients with CAD have the metabolic syndrome, which is characterized by low high-density lipoprotein levels, hypertension, abdominal obesity, and insulin resistance. These patients must be treated aggressively using a multimodality approach including pharmacologic therapy, weight reduction, diet counseling, and exercise.

Antiplatelet Agents

Because of the central role of platelet activation in acute coronary syndromes, aspirin is clearly indicated for all patients with CAD at recommended doses of 75 to 325 mg/d. The use of aspirin has been shown in several trials to reduce by one third the incidence of adverse cardiac events. The Clopidogrel versus Aspirin in Patients at Risk of Ischemic Events trial showed an 8.7% relative risk reduction in ischemic stroke, myocardial infarction, or vascular death for clopidogrel (Plavix), a thienopyridine derivative, over aspirin. Clopidogrel may therefore be used in patients who are allergic to aspirin or in place of aspirin. There is also some evidence that low-intensity anticoagulation with warfarin (Coumadin) can reduce cardiac events; however, this is not common practice.

β-Blockers

β-Blockers are an important part of the pharmacotherapy of CAD. They act to decrease myocardial oxygen demand by lowering heart rate, contractility, and blood pressure. The lower heart rate also allows for a longer diastolic time interval, during which coronary perfusion occurs. Additionally, β-blockers have been shown to suppress ventricular arrhythmias. Typically, the dose of the β-blocker is titrated such that a resting heart rate of approximately 55 to 60 beats/minute is achieved. β-Blockers should be used cautiously in patients who have severe bradycardia at rest, and they are contraindicated in the presence of high-grade heart block. In rare instances, pacemaker implantation may be considered to allow the use of a β-blocker in a patient who would otherwise be intolerant because of severe bradycardia or heart block.

Angiotensin-Converting Enzyme Inhibitors

It has been known from the Survival and Ventricular Enlargement and Studies of Left Ventricular Dysfunction trials in the early 1990s that angiotensin-converting enzyme (ACE) inhibitors were beneficial in patients with decreased ejection fraction. In 2000, the Heart Outcomes Prevention Evaluation trial proved that the ACE inhibitor ramipril (Altace) had mortality benefit in patients either with or at high risk of vascular disease and with preserved ejection fraction. The blood pressure in this study was lowered by only 2 to 3 mm Hg, a finding suggesting that the ACE inhibitors have benefit beyond simple blood pressure lowering. Some ACE inhibitors are more lipophilic and therefore are theoretically better able to penetrate coronary atheroma. These have been referred to as tissue ACE inhibitors. Whether the full benefit of ACE inhibitors is restricted to the tissue ACE inhibitors or is a broader class effect remains controversial. Regardless, an ACE inhibitor should be standard therapy for all patients with CAD. For those patients experiencing cough, a common side effect of ACE inhibitors, an angiotensin-receptor blocker may be substituted. ACE inhibitors are particularly beneficial in patients with diabetes, because these drugs have been shown to delay the onset of overt proteinuria and renal failure. Angiotensin-receptor blockers may be used in patients who cannot tolerate ACE inhibitors owing to cough. Although angiotensin-receptor blockers have been shown to be beneficial in diabetic patients with microalbuminuria and in hypertensive patients with left ventricular hypertrophy, these drugs have not been specifically studied in patients with stable angina pectoris.

Calcium Channel Antagonists

Calcium antagonists may be divided into the dihydropyridines and the nondihydropyridines. All calcium antagonists lower blood pressure by decreasing peripheral vascular resistance and dilate the epicardial coronary arteries. The nondihydropyridine and older dihydropyridine calcium channel antagonists, such as verapamil (e.g., Calan, Isoptin), diltiazem (e.g., Cardizem, Tiazac), and nifedipine (e.g., Adalat, Procardia) are negatively inotropic, whereas the newer dihydropyridine calcium antagonists such as amlodipine (Norvasc) and felodipine (Plendil) are less negatively inotropic. This negative inotropy acts to reduce myocardial oxygen demand. Diltiazem and verapamil also slow the sinus rate and can slow conduction through the atrioventricular node, resulting in slower heart rates. By lowering peripheral vascular resistance, calcium antagonists may cause reflex activation of the sympathetic nervous system, resulting in higher levels of circulating catecholamines and reflex tachycardia. The concurrent use of β-blockers attenuates this effect. However, one must be cautious about combining β-blockers and calcium antagonists; generally, it is safer to use β-blockers with the newer dihydropyridine calcium antagonists, which have less nodal blocking and negative inotropic effects. Calcium antagonists are as effective as β-blockers in the symptomatic relief of angina; however, they have not been shown to decrease mortality and thus should only be used in conjunction with β-blockers for refractory anginal symptoms, for further blood pressure lowering in hypertensive patients, or as primary antianginal therapy in patients intolerant of β-blockers. Calcium blockers are also useful in patients with vasospastic angina. Moreover, short-acting dihydropyridine calcium antagonists have been shown to increase mortality in patients with unstable angina and should therefore be avoided.

Nitrates

Nitrates relieve ischemia through a dual mechanism. Vasodilation of the epicardial coronary arteries directly improves myocardial perfusion, whereas myocardial oxygen demand is reduced as a result of venodilation and subsequent preload and myocardial wall stress reduction. Nitrates are excellent antianginal agents; however, they have not been demonstrated to confer a mortality benefit. Short-acting sublingual tablets or sprays are commonly used as needed for periodic anginal episodes. Longer-acting preparations may be used on a regular basis for those patients who experience frequent angina despite the appropriate use of β-blockers. Nitrate tolerance will develop if a daily nitrate-free interval is not provided. Oral preparations are therefore given to provide such an interval, whereas transdermal preparations must be physically removed for an 8- to 12-hour period each day. Nitrates may cause headache when they are used acutely. These drugs may cause hypotension when they are used in higher doses. Nitrates should not be used with sildenafil (Viagra), because the combination of the two venodilatory agents may cause severe, potentially life-threatening hypotension.

Revascularization

Revascularization, either percutaneous or surgical, has the potential to improve symptoms as well as mortality. In general, higher-risk patients derive more benefit from revascularization than do lower-risk patients. The highest-risk patients include those with left main coronary artery stenoses, three-vessel disease with decreased left ventricular function, proximal left anterior descending stenoses, and high-risk stress test results with large areas of ischemic myocardium. Coronary artery bypass grafting has been shown to reduce mortality in such high-risk patients. The Asymptomatic Cardiac Ischemia Pilot Study included lower-risk patients and compared medical therapy with revascularization with either coronary artery bypass grafting or percutaneous coronary revascularization. At 2 years of follow-up, there was a significant mortality reduction in the revascularization group as compared with the medical therapy group. This trial suggests that even for lower-risk patients, a strategy of initial revascularization may be beneficial. For high-risk patients including those with three-vessel disease and left main CAD, and particularly in diabetic patients with multivessel disease, coronary artery bypass grafting has been shown to be superior to percutaneous coronary revscularization. However, in lower-risk patients, several trials failed to show a mortality difference between the two revascularization strategies. In general, patients who undergo percutaneous revascularization are more likely to need repeat revascularization than are those who undergo surgical revasculariztion. This may change in the near future with the introduction of drug-eluting coronary stents that reduce the incidence of in-stent restenosis, a major cause of repeat revascularization among percutaneously revascularized patients.

UNSTABLE ANGINA AND ACUTE CORONARY SYNDROME

Diagnosis

Unstable angina must be recognized separately from chronic stable angina because it defines a group of patients who are at increased risk of short-term adverse events and who therefore may benefit from more immediate and aggressive therapy. As discussed earlier, unstable angina and acute myocardial infarction, which comprise the acute coronary syndrome, represent a spectrum of disease etiologically defined by unstable atherosclerotic plaque. Historical features suggestive of acute coronary syndrome include recent worsening of anginal symptoms, changes in anginal patterns (e.g., frequency, duration, response to rest or sublingual nitroglycerin), or new angina at rest.

The physical examination is less helpful for diagnosing the acute coronary syndrome, but it is very useful for risk stratification. High-risk markers include hypotension, rales, presence of a third heart sound, new or worsening mitral regurgitation, and elevated jugular venous pulsations, ECG evidence of acute coronary syndrome includes new ST deviation or T wave inversion, as well as new left bundle branch block. Nonspecific T wave changes are less helpful in the diagnosis. Laboratory markers of myocardial injury such as troponin I, troponin T, and the MB fraction of creatine kinase (CK-MB) are useful in defining acute myocardial infarction. Typically, all these markers will be elevated in an acute myocardial infarction. Often, however, the troponins will be mildly elevated in patients with a normal CK-MB value. This may result from distal microembolization of plaque, thrombus, and/or platelet aggregates from the unstable or ruptured plaque.

Treatment

The treatment of the acute coronary syndrome is directed primarily at preventing thrombus formation on the unstable plaque, and in the case of acute myocardial infarction, restoring blood flow through the occluded coronary artery. Aspirin is an oral antiplatelet agent that should be given to all patients presenting with unstable angina, except those with documented aspirin allergy. For those patients with aspirin allergies, clopidogrel (Plavix), an adenosine diphosphate antagonist, should be used instead. Clopidogrel was shown in the Clopidogrel in Unstable Angina to Prevent Recurrent Ischemic Events (CURE) trial to be beneficial in patients presenting with an acute coronary syndrome who were treated with an initial conservative strategy and therefore may be used in addition to aspirin in patients who do not undergo early angiography. Anticoagulation with heparin or low-molecular-weight heparin should be used in combination with aspirin or clopidogrel. Low-molecular-weight heparins such as enoxaparin (Lovenox) and dalteparin (Fragmin) have become increasingly popular because of their easier dosing and more predictable effects, and they have been shown in large trials to be at least equivalent to (dalteparin) and probably superior to (enoxaparin) unfractionated heparin in the treatment of unstable angina. However, some interventional cardiologists prefer that low-molecular-weight heparin be discontinued 12 hours before angiography because of the difficulty both in monitoring and in acutely reversing its effects should a hemorrhagic complication arise.

The cardiovascular event rate associated with acute coronary syndromes has been reduced further through the use of intravenous platelet glycoprotein IIb/IIIa inhibitors. These agents bind to the glycoprotein IIb/IIIa receptor on the platelet surface and block platelet aggregation, thereby providing near total platelet inhibition. Glycoprotein IIb/IIIa inhibitors are used in high-risk patients who have signs of ongoing ischemia or injury. Because they are potent antiplatelet agents, they should not be used in patients with a history of recent stroke, surgery, or trauma. Special care must be taken in diabetic patients with proliferative retinopathy, to avoid retinal hemorrhage. Tirofiban (Aggrastat) and eptifibitide (Integrilin) are indicated for use in acute coronary syndromes, and abciximab (ReoPro) is indicated for use in conjunction with percutaneous coronary revascularization.

There have traditionally been two strategies regarding revascularization in the patient with unstable angina. The more conservative strategy suggests initial anti-ischemic, antithrombotic, and antiplatelet pharmacologic therapy, followed by noninvasive stress testing to stratify risk further in patients and to identify a subset of high-risk patients who would benefit from angiography and possible revascularization. The more aggressive strategy suggests similar pharmacologic therapy but with early angiography both to stratify risk in patients and to provide treatment with possible revascularization. Some more recent trials, such as the Treat Angina with Aggrastat (tirofiban) and Determine Cost of Therapy with Invasion or Conservative Strategy-18 trial, suggest that a strategy of early angiography may offer more benefit at less cost because patients with normal or low-risk angiograms may be safely discharged home earlier and higher-risk patients may be offered definitive treatment earlier. This approach may be more difficult in hospitals where angiography and/or percutaneous coronary intervention may not be available. In this case, high-risk patients should be transferred to another facility where early angiography may be performed. For lower-risk patients, the treating physician may decide, based on the patient's risk status and personal preferences, whether to treat the patient conservatively or to transfer the patient to another facility for more aggressive treatment. After an acute coronary syndrome, every patient should be treated with anti-ischemic therapy (β-blockers), lipid-lowering therapy (statins), an ACE inhibitor, and antiplatelet therapy (aspirin and/or clopidogrel). After percutaneous coronary intervention, clopidogrel has proven benefit for up to 9 months. The American Medical Association's Get With the Guidelines program aims to help physicians and hospitals to ensure that all patients are successfully treated with these proven, lifesaving therapies.

CARDIAC ARREST: SUDDEN CARDIAC DEATH

method of
BENZY J. PADANILAM, M.D.
The Care Group, LLC
Indianapolis, Indiana

and

ERIC N. PRYSTOWSKY, M.D.
St. Vincent Hospital and Health Care
Indianapolis, Indiana

The most recent estimates suggest that approximately 460,000 sudden cardiac deaths (SCDs) occur in the United States annually. The devastating nature of SCD to family and society has led to major public health initiatives for prevention and treatment of the events leading to SCD. Because coronary artery disease (CAD) is the most common etiology of SCD, a marked reduction in SCD will require efforts to curtail atherosclerotic heart disease. The immediate goal is to identify patients at high risk for sustained ventricular tachycardia (VT) or ventricular fibrillation (VF) and provide therapy to prevent SCD.

Definition. SCD is generally defined as "sudden and unexpected natural death from cardiac causes." Qualification of the terminology in the definition is important. "Sudden" is usually defined as occurring within 1 hour of the onset of symptoms. Whether SCD occurs in a person without previous symptoms of heart disease or in someone who has pre-existing cardiac disease, the key is that the event occurred unexpectedly at a point in time. Unfortunately, the terms cardiac arrest (CA) and SCD are frequently used interchangeably. The term SCD should be reserved only for people who die. This distinction would also make the commonly used term "resuscitated sudden cardiac death" rather inappropriate. CA may be defined as sudden cessation of cardiac function that is irreversible if not treated. VF, VT, asystole, and pulseless electrical activity (PEA) are the four cardiac rhythms that can result in CA. We suggest that one use CA for the event if the patient survives it.

Survival After Cardiac Arrest. Survival statistics are quite variable and depend importantly on the cause of CA and the time that it takes for cardiopulmonary resuscitation to begin. In a series of 352 out-of-hospital CA cases, the initial rhythm identified by paramedics was VF in 220 (62%), VT in 24 (7%), and bradycardia or PEA in 108 (31%). Although bradyarrhythmias can be the primary cause of CA, it can also be the end result of a sustained VT or VF episode. When the initial rhythm is VF or VT, resuscitation success and subsequent hospital discharge rates are much higher than for patients with PEA or bradycardia. In general, no more than 10% to 15% of patients are successfully resuscitated from out-of-hospital CA. These dismal statistics have prompted research into primary prevention of SCD.

MECHANISMS OF CARDIAC ARREST

Sustained VT and VF are the most common causes of CA. Analysis of intracardiac electrical activity from implantable cardioverter-defibrillators (ICDs) shows that many episodes of VF actually begin as rapid VT, often quite organized, that degenerates into VF. Reentry is considered the probable mechanism for most VT and VF episodes and typically occurs in the setting of *structurally abnormal* hearts. Structural abnormalities can be macroscopic, such as scar from previous myocardial infarction (MI), or be at a molecular level, such as the long QT syndrome (LQTS). When such hearts are subjected to transient *triggering factors* such as ischemia or electrolyte abnormalities, VF can ensue. Triggers for lethal arrhythmias are protean and temporally unpredictable, which is one major reason that therapy has centered on the ICD, a generic treatment that is immune to the whims of triggering events. Asystole and PEA are generally the end result of a mechanical cause of heart failure, such as massive MI or pulmonary embolism. It can also be the end-stage rhythm of a prolonged episode of sustained VT or VF.

Structural Cardiac Abnormalities Serving as Substrates

Atherosclerotic CAD, with its clinical consequences of myocardial ischemia, MI, and ventricular dilatation, is the structural basis for approximately 80% of cases of SCD in the United States. Cardiomyopathies account for 10% to 15% of cases, and the remaining small percentage is made up of a variety of other causes and includes patients without structural heart disease.

Coronary Artery Disease. CAD can cause acute ischemia that may result in life-threatening VT or VF. A healed MI may form the substrate for the development of reentry and sustained VT or VF, even years after the acute infarction. Although CAD is well accepted as the major heart disease associated with SCD, the exact cause-and-effect relationship of CAD to SCD has been difficult to establish. The incidence of acute coronary thrombosis in CA victims varies considerably, depending on the series quoted and how quickly the patient undergoes cardiac catheterization. The relationship of transient ischemia to SCD is even more difficult to ascertain. Because VF rarely occurs during stress tests, it is doubtful whether minor ischemia plays a significant role in SCD. Patients with a previous MI and a left ventricular ejection fraction (LVEF) of 0.40 or less are at particularly high risk for SCD, and primary prevention efforts are targeted to these individuals (see later).

Dilated Cardiomyopathy. Dilated cardiomyopathies account for approximately 10% of SCD cases. Both idiopathic dilated cardiomyopathy and dilated cardiomyopathy of defined cause have been associated with an increased risk for SCD. The different pathologic findings described in dilated cardiomyopathies such as interstitial fibrosis, perivascular fibrosis, myocardial hypertrophy, and degeneration may form the substrate for malignant ventricular arrhythmias.

Hypertrophic Cardiomyopathy. Hypertrophic cardiomyopathy is described in detail elsewhere in this book. The disease is caused by mutations in the contractile protein genes. Most patients have obvious hypertrophy of the left ventricle detected by echocardiography. In patients with cardiac troponin-T gene mutations, the hypertrophy may be subtle. The annual risk of death is 2% to 4% in adults and 4% to 6% in children and adolescents, but it varies according to the specific genetic mutation. Most SCD victims younger than 35 years have hypertrophic cardiomyopathy or another form of myopathy as the underlying cause.

Valvular Heart Disease. Aortic stenosis is well known to cause SCD. In severe aortic stenosis, the incidence of SCD is low in asymptomatic patients and relatively high in symptomatic patients. Mitral valve prolapse has also been reported to result in a low incidence of SCD. Typically, these patients have marked prolapse and significant mitral regurgitation. A 2% to 4% incidence of SCD has been reported over a 7-year period after prosthetic valve replacement. SCD is rare in patients with other valvular heart diseases.

Congenital Heart Disease. SCD is reported predominantly in patients with four congenital heart diseases: tetralogy of Fallot, transposition of the great arteries, aortic stenosis, and pulmonary vascular obstruction. A QRS duration of more than 170 msec has a positive predictive value for VT in patients after repair of tetralogy of Fallot. Congenital coronary artery abnormalities such as anomalous origin of the left main coronary artery from the right sinus of Valsalva can also result in SCD.

Wolff-Parkinson-White Syndrome. The estimated risk of SCD in patients with Wolff-Parkinson-White (WPW) syndrome is 1 in 1000 patient-years of follow-up. The mechanism of SCD in most patients is atrial fibrillation with a very rapid ventricular rate as a result of conduction over the accessory pathway, which degenerates into VF. Patients with a potential risk for SCD can be identified at electrophysiologic study. They typically have both inducible atrioventricular reentry and preexcited (conduction over the accessory pathway) ventricular rates higher than 230/min during atrial fibrillation.

Arrhythmogenic Right Ventricular Dysplasia. This disease is genetically heterogeneous, with defects recently localized to several chromosomes. One third of cases occur as a familial disorder with autosomal dominant inheritance. Fatty and fibrofatty infiltration develops in the right ventricle (apex, inflow, and outflow). The left ventricle can be involved in 50% to 67% of cases. The electrocardiogram (ECG) may reveal T wave inversion from V_1 to V_3, incomplete or complete right bundle branch block, and a terminal notch in leads V_1 and V_2 called an epsilon wave. The annual risk of sudden death is approximately 2%.

Long QT Syndrome. LQTS is a genetic abnormality of cardiac ion channels characterized by abnormally prolonged cardiac repolarization. QT intervals are prolonged on the surface ECG. Patients are at high risk for life-threatening VT (torsades de pointes), frequently in the setting of high adrenergic states such as physical or emotional stress. Two major forms of LQTS have been described: (1) the autosomal recessive form described by Jervell and Lange-Nielsen is characterized by congenital deafness and prolonged QT intervals, and (2) the autosomal dominant form described independently by Romano and Ward is characterized by prolonged QT intervals without associated deafness. In the autosomal dominant form, the majority of genetic defects are potassium channel mutations. Sodium channel mutations constitute approximately 10% of cases. LQT1 is due to mutations in the *KvLQT1* gene encoding I_{KS} current, LQT2 is due to mutations in the *HERG* gene encoding I_{KR} current, LQT3 is due to mutations in the *SCN5A* gene encoding Na^+ current, LQT4 is due to mutation of the ankyrin gene, LQT5 is due to mutation of the *minK* gene, and LQT6 is due to mutations in the *MiRP1* gene.

Brugada Syndrome. Described by Brugada and Brugada in 1992 as a syndrome of right bundle branch block, ST segment elevation in ECG leads V_1 to V_3, and SCD, the disease in some cases has been linked to mutations in the cardiac sodium channel gene *(SCN5A)*. The ECG changes can be transient in some patients, and sodium channel–blocking drugs can exacerbate or unmask the ECG changes. The disease is thought to account for a particularly pernicious sudden unexplained death syndrome (SUDS) that tends to occur during sleep in young men in Thailand. Polymorphic VT causes syncopal episodes and SCD.

Iatrogenic Causes. Electrolyte imbalances such as marked hypokalemia during aggressive diuresis can result in VF. CA can be induced by the use of antiarrhythmic drugs, usually torsades de pointes VT caused by marked QT prolongation. Female gender, older age, and ventricular hypertrophy are predisposing conditions for this problem. Non-antiarrhythmic drugs can, on occasion, produce marked QT prolongation and CA. Unfortunately, such drugs include a wide variety of agents from antibiotics to antipsychotics.

Other Diseases. Neuromuscular disorders, myocarditis, infiltrative myocardial disease, cardiac tumors, short-coupled torsades de pointes, catecholaminergic VT, coronary vasospasm, and idiopathic VF are some of the other disease states associated with SCD.

Triggering Factors

The concept of triggering factors is used to explain why a person with seemingly no change in cardiac function suddenly experiences CA or SCD. These physiologic or pathologic triggers can perturb the fine orchestration of the normal cardiac rhythm and initiate VT or VF. On rare occasion, these factors may lead to CA in a person with a normal heart, but we are continually learning that such individuals often have a previously unrecognized ion channel abnormality or other molecular defects. Commonly described triggers include myocardial ischemia, electrolyte abnormalities, hypoxia, autonomic nervous system dysfunction or imbalance, toxins such as cocaine, and ion channel–blocking drugs. Psychosocial factors and emotional stress may also play a role in triggering SCD.

PATIENT EVALUATION

All CA victims should be evaluated with a complete history, physical examination, and certain laboratory tests. The history should include the details of the event, including possible drug abuse, symptoms suggestive of cardiac disease or iatrogenic conditions known to cause sudden death, a family history of sudden death, and symptoms such as chest pain, shortness of breath, or palpitations. Most patients resuscitated from CA have at least some retrograde amnesia. Thus, whenever possible, additional history should be obtained from any witness to the CA.

Physical examination should be performed with particular emphasis on the cardiovascular and central nervous system. All patients should be evaluated with laboratory tests to rule out MI, a drug screen, and serum electrolyte assay. A 12-lead ECG should be performed and may provide evidence of acute MI or uncover rare conditions such as LQTS, Brugada syndrome, or WPW syndrome. We perform two-dimensional echocardiography and coronary angiography in all patients to determine the presence of structural heart disease and CAD. Electrophysiologic study occasionally provides additional useful information.

THERAPEUTIC OPTIONS

Implantable Cardioverter-Defibrillator. These devices can recognize and expeditiously treat life-threatening ventricular arrhythmias. Several studies have confirmed the efficacy of ICDs in preventing sudden death. The ICD lead systems are now transvenous, and the small size of the ICD generators allow pectoral implantation. Dual-chamber and biventricular pacing can be performed through currently available ICDs.

Pharmacologic Agents. None of the antiarrhythmic drugs have consistent efficacy in reducing mortality in CA survivors when compared with the ICD. Antiarrhythmic therapy with agents such as sotalol or amiodarone may still have a role in patients with recurrent sustained VT to reduce the incidence of frequent ICD shocks, but such drugs are not primary therapy for CA survivors. Drug therapy with β-blockers, angiotensin-converting enzyme (ACE) inhibitors, and aspirin should be used in appropriate patients as adjunctive therapy.

MANAGEMENT

Management of SCD may be considered under *secondary prevention* (management of CA victims) and *primary prevention* (strategies to predict and prevent SCD).

Secondary Prevention

Management of Out-of-Hospital Cardiac Arrest. Cardiopulmonary resuscitation by basic life support and advanced cardiac life support has been used to improve the survival of out-of-hospital CA victims. Early defibrillation of CA victims is key to a good outcome. Among antiarrhythmic medications, intravenous amiodarone has been shown to increase survival to hospital admission when administered during VF. Success in resuscitating a CA victim in the community depends on the layperson's understanding of basic life support. Early activation of the emergency medical system (EMS) followed by prompt initiation of cardiopulmonary resuscitation can improve the probability of survival. The steps in managing a CA victim have been likened to links in a chain. The following sequence of events should occur in quick fashion: (1) recognition of the early warning signs of CA, (2) activation of the EMS, (3) basic cardiopulmonary resuscitation (mouth-to-mouth breathing and chest compressions), (4) early defibrillation, (5) management of the airway and ventilation, and (6) intravenous administration of medications. If any of these links in the chain of management are missing, the victim's probability of survival diminishes.

Cobb and coworkers were pioneers in establishing community-based intervention for CA victims. They developed a rapid response system for emergency services in Seattle through the Seattle Fire Department. Approximately 60% of Seattle residents 12 years and older have had some training in cardiopulmonary resuscitation. Even in such an emergency care system, only about 30% of CA victims are discharged from the hospital alive. Most communities, especially in more rural areas of the United States, have far fewer successful resuscitations. In Memphis, only 10% to 13% of out-of-hospital CA victims given emergency care are discharged from the hospital alive. Such poor outcomes have prompted further refinement of resuscitation attempts, such as the availability of automatic external defibrillators (AEDs) in public places and homes of high-risk patients. AEDs allow people with minimal training to perform defibrillation because rhythm detection is automated.

In-Hospital Management. Our management approach is summarized in Figure 1. Patients with a clearly reversible etiology of CA are given specific therapy for that condition. An example is a patient in whom VF develops during or within the first 48 hours of acute MI. Successful radiofrequency ablation of an accessory pathway would be the therapy for a CA survivor with WPW syndrome, normal ventricular function, and documented rapid preexcited ventricular rates during atrial fibrillation at electrophysiologic study. The assumption is that VF was a consequence of the atrial fibrillation. One should be very careful in concluding that the VF has a reversible etiology in any given patient. Conditions such as significant hyperkalemia, hypokalemia, or hypoxia may be found during initial assessment of a resuscitated patient and may not be causative of the event. Data from follow-up of the Antiarrhythmics Versus Implantable Defibrillator (AVID) study registry population is interesting. All subgroups, including patients who had VF or sustained VT with apparent transient and correctable causes, had high mortality rates similar to the study group's. Most patients do not have an obvious reversible

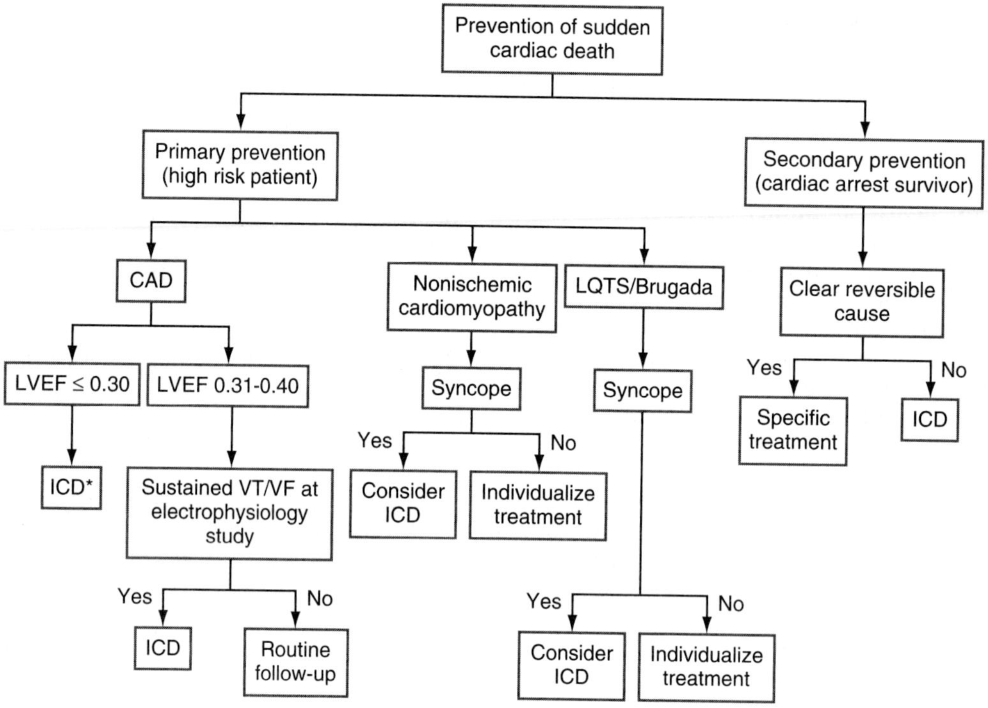

Figure 1. Algorithm for prevention of sudden cardiac death. CAD, coronary artery disease; EPS, electrophysiologic study; ICD, implantable cardioverter-defibrillator; LQTS, long QT syndrome; LVEF, left ventricular ejection fraction; VF, ventricular fibrillation; VT, ventricular tachycardia.

cause for the CA, and treatment depends in part on the type of heart disease present. Most patients will receive an ICD. An exception may be a patient with a structurally normal heart who has severe CAD and normal left ventricular function. Such individuals may do well with coronary artery bypass surgery and no ICD. Three major clinical trials (AVID, Canadian Implantable Defibrillator Study [CIDS], and Cardiac Arrest Study of Hamburg [CASH]) have established the superiority of ICD therapy over antiarrhythmic medications in improving long-term survival of CA survivors. Amiodarone treatment is inferior to ICD treatment in patients with an LVEF less than 35%, but it may be useful in selected patients with heart disease and better left ventricular function.

Primary Prevention

Risk Stratification. The relatively poor survival of CA victims has prompted the search for preventive approaches. The major task is to identify risk factors that select patients who are at higher risk for SCD. Some of the tests used in risk stratification are LVEF, signal-averaged ECG, T wave alternans, heart rate variability, baroreflex sensitivity, Holter monitoring, and programmed electrical stimulation. The LVEF is probably the most significant predictive test. In particular, an LVEF less than 0.40 in patients with CAD increases the risk for SCD. Data from the Multicenter Automatic Defibrillator Implantation Trial (MADIT) and the Multicenter Unsustained Tachycardia Trial (MUSTT) show that patients with CAD, an LVEF of 0.40 or less, nonsustained VT, and inducible sustained VT at electrophysiologic study are at high risk for SCD. Such patients require ICD implantation. Recent data from MADIT-2 demonstrate a survival advantage of the ICD in patients with previous MI and an LVEF of 0.30 or less. These patients do not require the presence of nonsustained VT or VT induced at electrophysiologic study to warrant ICD implantation. Although the aforementioned studies have established clinical guidelines for risk stratification in patients with CAD, no major risk stratification studies have been performed in patients with nonischemic cardiomyopathy.

Efficacy of Implantable Cardioverter-Defibrillators. In MADIT, the ICD decreased mortality by 54% when compared with "best medical therapy." In MUSTT, the primary endpoints of sudden death or resuscitated CA were statistically lower in patients who had electrophysiologically guided therapy. However, further analysis showed that the reduction in overall mortality and SCD was limited to patients who received an ICD and that neither amiodarone nor any other drug had a substantial impact on survival. Finally, the recently published MADIT-2 study involved 1232 patients randomized to receive an ICD or conventional therapy. The primary endpoint of overall mortality demonstrated a clear benefit for patients receiving an ICD. For the average follow-up of 20 months, mortality rates were 14.2% in the ICD group versus 19.8% in the conventional-therapy group. Overall, an approximately 31% reduction in the risk of death was noted. These results suggest that patients with similar clinical characteristics as those enrolled in MADIT-2 should be seriously considered for ICD therapy. It is quite possible that future studies may show that results from electrophysiologic testing may enable more precise risk stratification in these patients and that other factors such as QRS duration might also prove useful. Too few data are available to define which high-risk patients without symptoms who have nonischemic cardiomyopathy may benefit from ICD therapy. However, such patients who have unexplained syncope should be considered for electrophysiologic testing and possible ICD therapy.

Role of Pharmacotherapy. Administration of β-blockers after MI has been associated with a reduction in mortality and, in some studies, has reduced the incidence of sudden death. Primary prevention trials of β-blocker therapy for heart failure also have shown results similar to post-MI trials. Although ACE inhibitors have produced a decrease in total mortality in heart failure clinical trials, the reduction in sudden death has not been consistent. Regardless, ACE inhibitors are often beneficial in patients with heart disease. Amiodarone heart failure trials have produced mixed results. Whereas the Gruppo de Estudio de la Sobreviada en al Insuficiencia Cardiaca en Argentina (GESICA) trial showed beneficial effects with amiodarone therapy—a reduction in total mortality by 28%—the Amiodarone in Patients with Congestive Heart Failure and Asymptomatic Ventricular Arrhythmia Trial (CHF-STAT) demonstrated no significant benefit with amiodarone. Moreover, no survival benefit was seen with amiodarone in two large prospective post-MI trials.

CONCLUSIONS

CA and SCD continue to be a major public health problem in America. Several syndromes causing SCD have been described in the last few decades. CAD underlies the overwhelming majority of episodes. Risk stratification strategies are still being evolved for each syndrome known to result in SCD. Future research and clinical observations will undoubtedly result in the identification of new diseases that can cause SCD and, it is hoped, will also lead to novel therapeutic approaches. The advent of ICDs has facilitated both primary and secondary prevention of SCD and has thus improved the survival of patients.

ATRIAL FIBRILLATION

method of
MINA K. CHUNG, M.D.
The Cleveland Clinic Foundation
Cleveland, Ohio

Atrial fibrillation, the most common sustained arrhythmia seen in clinical practice, affects over 2 million patients in the United States. Its prevalence increases with advancing age such that 0.2% of the population 25 to 34 years old, 2% to 5% of those older than 60 years, and 6% to 10% of persons older than 80 years are affected.

Terminology. *Lone atrial fibrillation* is atrial fibrillation that occurs in the absence of cardiac or other conditions predisposing to atrial fibrillation. *Acute atrial fibrillation* generally refers to a duration of less than 48 hours. *Paroxysmal atrial fibrillation* is usually characterized by recurrent, transient episodes that revert to sinus rhythm spontaneously or with treatment. *Persistent atrial fibrillation* does not convert without intervention or cardioversion, and *permanent atrial fibrillation* is persistent despite cardioversion.

FACTORS PREDISPOSING TO ATRIAL FIBRILLATION

The most common cardiovascular diseases associated with atrial fibrillation are hypertension and ischemic heart disease. Other predisposing conditions include advanced age, rheumatic heart disease (especially mitral valve disease), nonrheumatic valvular disease, cardiomyopathies, congestive heart failure, congenital heart disease, sick sinus syndrome/degenerative conduction system disease, Wolff-Parkinson-White syndrome, pericarditis, pulmonary embolism, thyrotoxicosis, chronic lung disease, neoplastic disease, postoperative states, diabetes, and normal hearts affected by high adrenergic states, alcohol, stress, drugs (especially sympathomimetics), excessive caffeine, hypoxia, hypokalemia, hypoglycemia, or systemic infection.

MORBIDITY AND MORTALITY

Survival. Though not usually considered a life-threatening arrhythmia, atrial fibrillation has been associated with a 1.5- to 2-fold increase in total and cardiovascular mortality. Factors that may increase mortality in atrial fibrillation include age, mitral stenosis, aortic valve disease, coronary artery disease (CAD), hypertension, and congestive heart failure. Acute myocardial infarction or congestive heart failure is associated with higher mortality if atrial fibrillation is present.

Stroke/Thromboembolism. One of the most clinically important consequences of atrial fibrillation is its association with thromboembolic events and stroke. Atrial fibrillation is one of the most potent risk factors for stroke in the elderly and the most common cause of cardiogenic stroke. It carries a significant risk for silent cerebral infarction. Patients with nonvalvular atrial fibrillation have an approximately twofold to sixfold increased risk of stroke; the risk is increased 17-fold with rheumatic heart disease. The risk of stroke in nonvalvular atrial fibrillation increases with advancing age, the presence of concomitant cardiovascular disease, and other risk factors for stroke. In patients younger than 60 years without hypertension or cardiovascular disease, the risk of stroke is low. The estimated risk of stroke in patients younger than

65 years without the risk factors of hypertension, diabetes, or previous stroke or transient ischemic attack is approximately 1% per year. Patients who are older and have risk factors for stroke or concomitant cardiovascular disease have a rate of stroke of approximately 3% to 5% per year. Older patients (>75 years) with risk factors for stroke appear to be at particularly high risk (8% per year). Episodes of stroke are generally clustered at the onset of the arrhythmia.

Tachycardia-Induced Cardiomyopathy. Persistent rapid rates can lead to tachycardia-mediated cardiomyopathy with left ventricular dysfunction and congestive heart failure. The cardiomyopathy may be reversible with ventricular rate control and/or regularization of the rhythm, which may be achievable with medical rate control, atrioventricular (AV) node ablation, or attainment of sinus rhythm. Atrial cardiomyopathy can also occur with the structural remodeling during atrial fibrillation and lead to an increase in atrial size.

Symptoms and Hemodynamics. Atrial fibrillation may cause symptoms as a result of rapid ventricular rates, irregularity of ventricular rhythm, or loss of AV synchrony. Symptoms may include a limitation in functional capacity, palpitations, fatigue, dyspnea, angina, or congestive heart failure.

PATHOGENESIS

During atrial fibrillation, electrical activation of the atria occurs in rapid, multiple waves of depolarization, with continuously changing, wandering pathways determined by the local refractoriness, excitability, and conduction properties of the atrial tissue. Perpetuation of atrial fibrillation may be promoted by increasing atrial size and decreasing reentrant circuit wavelength (the product of conduction velocity and atrial refractory period), conditions that would support more reentrant wavelets. Therefore, structural enlargement of the atria can predispose to persistence of atrial fibrillation by allowing more reentrant circuits to be sustained in the atria. In addition, small reentrant circuits from shortened tissue refractoriness may enhance vulnerability to atrial tachyarrhythmias. During atrial fibrillation, electrical remodeling leading to shortening of atrial effective refractory periods and structural remodeling resulting in atrial enlargement can promote more wavelets and increased sustainability of atrial fibrillation.

More recently, *focal sources* that initiate and perhaps sustain atrial fibrillation have been identified, particularly in patients with lone atrial fibrillation in the absence of structural heart disease. These foci, which have been targets for curative ablation, most commonly arise from the ostia of the pulmonary veins, with some demonstrated to arise from the vein or ligament of Marshall, the right atrium, or the superior vena cava.

A dual substrate of sources initiating atrial fibrillation and electrical and structural substrates that promote maintenance of atrial fibrillation appears to underlie the spectrum of disease expression (Figure 1). Early manifestations may include frequent atrial ectopy, often initiated from a single focal source, which may then progress to repetitive bursts of atrial tachycardia and subsequent paroxysms of atrial fibrillation. These paroxysms may become more frequent and/or longer or even persistent as structural and electrical remodeling ensues. Factors that may promote remodeling include atrial stretch, calcium overload, left ventricular hypertrophy, ventricular dysfunction, valve disease, autonomic tone, inflammation, oxidative stress, fibrosis, and/or toxins.

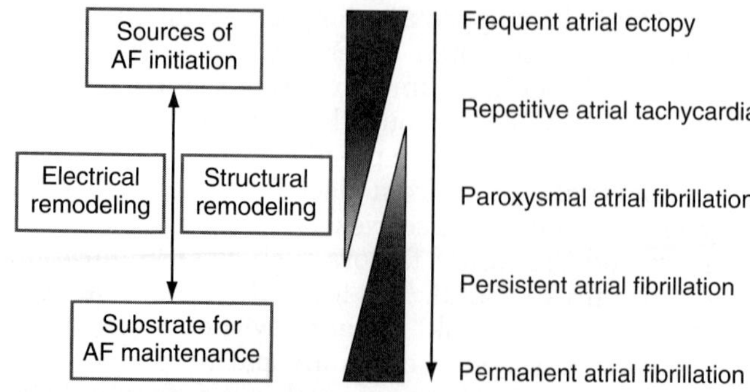

Figure 1. Dual-substrate model. The relative contribution of sources initiating atrial fibrillation (AF) and electrical and structural substrates that promote maintenance of AF underlies the spectrum of expression of atrial arrhythmia. Early manifestations may include frequent atrial ectopy or paroxysms of atrial tachycardia arising from focal sources. As structural and electrical remodeling ensues, paroxysms may evolve to persistent or permanent AF.

MANAGEMENT OF ATRIAL FIBRILLATION

History and Diagnostic Evaluation. Documentation of the actual occurrence of atrial fibrillation may be accomplished by electrocardiograms, rhythm strips, ambulatory monitors, or transtelephonic monitoring (Figure 2). Other potential underlying or precipitating conditions or factors should be sought, such as alcohol, caffeine, sympathomimetics, herbal supplements, or other drug use, as well as potential precipitating bradycardia or other primary arrhythmias.

Diagnostic testing for patients with atrial fibrillation usually includes thyroid function tests, exclusion of electrolyte imbalances, and an echocardiogram to evaluate ventricular function, atrial size, and the presence or absence of valvular disease. Functional stress testing or cardiac catheterization is often indicated, particularly to evaluate for CAD in patients with risk factors, determine candidacy for antiarrhythmic class 1C agents, or assess heart rate responsiveness.

Rate Versus Rhythm Control Strategies. The decision to pursue achievement and maintenance of sinus rhythm or to treat with ventricular rate control measures alone in an individual patient often involves a complex analysis of the risks and benefits of maintaining sinus rhythm. The benefits of maintenance of sinus rhythm versus control of heart rate alone include a potential for more complete relief of symptoms and hemodynamic improvement and avoidance

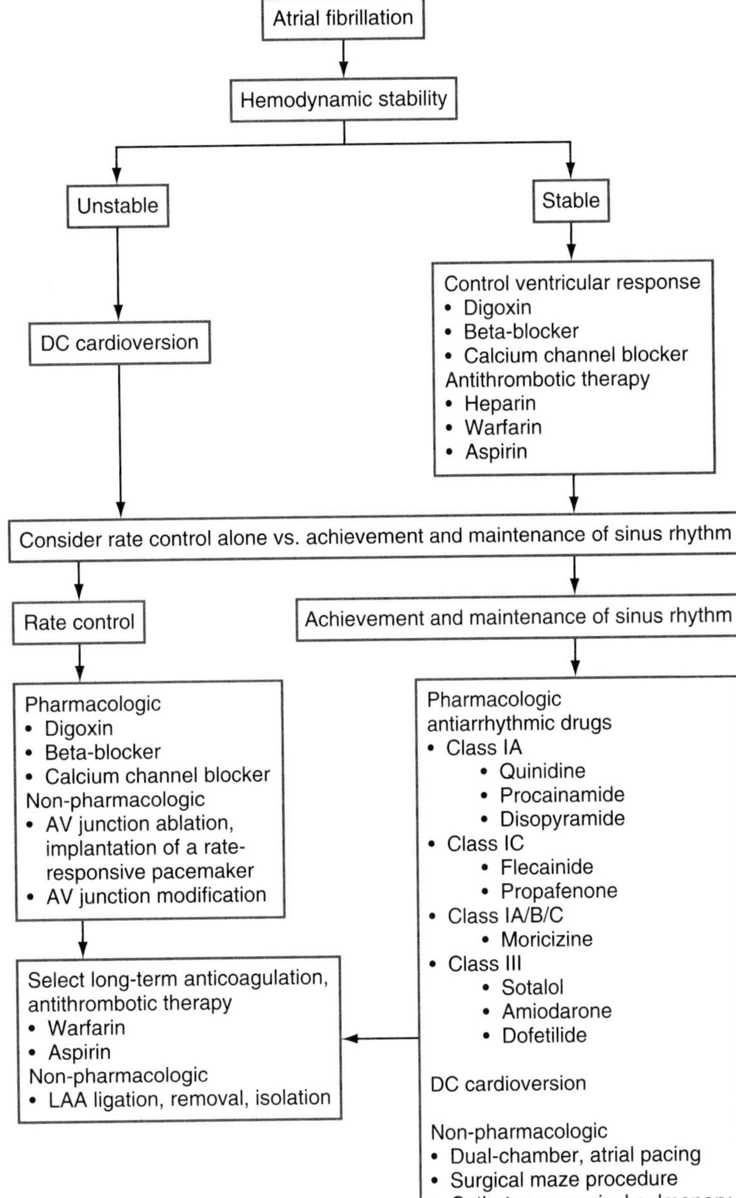

Figure 2. Strategies for management of atrial fibrillation. AV = atrioventricular; LAA = left atrial appendage.

of electrical and structural remodeling. However, even with antiarrhythmic therapy, recurrent atrial fibrillation will develop in approximately half the patients after cardioversion to sinus rhythm, and recent studies raise concern over the potential for increased mortality and proarrhythmia when antiarrhythmic agents are used. Potential benefits of a rate control strategy alone include a lower risk of adverse effects (including death and proarrhythmia) from therapy and possibly lower cost. However, symptom relief may be less complete.

In the largest trial to date of rate versus rhythm control strategies, the Atrial Fibrillation Follow-up Investigation of Rhythm Management (AFFIRM) randomized 4060 patients older than 65 years or with a risk factor for stroke to rate versus rhythm control strategies, with the primary endpoint being total mortality. No significant difference in total mortality was noted between strategies, although a trend toward better survival in the rate control arm was reported. Because the incidence of stroke was not lower in the rhythm control arm, another major finding was that continued anticoagulation remains important even with maintenance of sinus rhythm in the rhythm control arm.

Control of Ventricular Rate

Rapid ventricular rates can cause symptoms and/or ventricular dysfunction. Ventricular rate control therapy is achieved with AV node–blocking drugs or AV node modification or ablation with permanent pacing.

Pharmacologic Rate Control. Rate control (Table 1) is generally achieved with the use of agents that slow AV nodal conduction. Typical targets include a heart rate of 80 beats per minute (bpm) or lower at rest, 90 bpm average or lower on Holter monitoring, or 110 bpm or less on 6-minute walk testing and a peak heart rate 20% less than the maximal predicted heart rate on stress testing. Commonly used agents include digoxin, β-blockers, and calcium channel blockers.

Digoxin (Lanoxin) can be used safely in patients with heart failure and can be effective in controlling resting ventricular rates in patients with chronic, persistent atrial fibrillation. However, it has a delayed (1 to 4 hours) peak onset of its heart rate–lowering effect, has a narrow therapeutic window, and is less effective in rate control of paroxysmal atrial fibrillation or rapid rates during hyperadrenergic states, when vagal tone is low, such as during exercise or in acute and intensive care unit settings because of increased sympathetic tone. It must be used with caution in elderly patients and those with decreased renal function. Although digoxin has been tried in the past for conversion of atrial fibrillation, a randomized controlled study showed no significant effect of digoxin on conversion rate.

β-Adrenergic blockers are very effective in heart rate control, even with exercise, are available in intravenous form, and have a rapid onset of action. Potential side effects include bronchospasm, exacerbation of congestive heart failure as a result of negative inotropy, and a reduction in exercise tolerance as a result of negative inotropy and chronotropy. Nevertheless, β-blockers appear to produce long-term benefits in patients with left ventricular dysfunction.

Calcium channel blockers (e.g., *verapamil* [Calan, Covera, Verelan] and *diltiazem* [Cardizem, Tiazac]) can also slow ventricular rates during atrial fibrillation. Verapamil and diltiazem are available in intravenous formulations, have a rapid onset of action, and can be used safely in patients with chronic obstructive pulmonary disease and diabetes mellitus. Calcium channel blockers can have negative inotropic effects and can cause hypotension. In addition, the long-term safety of calcium channel blockers in patients has been questioned. Nonetheless, studies suggest positive benefits in reducing the electrical remodeling in the atrium that occurs with atrial fibrillation. Verapamil may attenuate the shortening of the atrial refractory period seen with even short-duration atrial

TABLE 1. **Pharmacologic Rate Control for Atrial Arrhythmias**

Agent	Loading Dose	Maintenance Dose	Side Effects/Toxicity	Comments
Digoxin (Lanoxin)	0.25-0.5 mg IV or PO, then 0.25 mg q4-6h to 1 mg in 1st 24 h	0.125-0.25 mg PO or IV qd	Anorexia, nausea; AV block; bradycardia; ventricular arrhythmias; accumulates in renal failure	Used in CHF; vagotonic effects on the AVN; delayed onset of action; narrow therapeutic window; less effective in postoperative, paroxysmal AF with high adrenergic states
β-Blockers			Bronchospasm, CHF, ↓BP, AV block, bradycardia	Effective in heart rate control, rapid onset of action
Propranolol *(Inderal)*	1 mg IV q2-5 min to 0.1-0.2 mg/kg	10-80 mg PO tid-qid		
Metoprolol *(Lopressor)*	2.5-5 mg IV over 2 min q5 min to 15 mg	25-100 mg PO bid-tid		
Esmolol *(Brevibloc)*	500 μg/kg IV over 1 min	50 μg/kg IV for 4 min; repeat load prn and ↑ maintenance to 20-50 μg/kg/min q5-10 min		Esmolol is a short-acting agent
Calcium channel blockers			↓BP, CHF, AV block	Rapid onset, can be used safely in COPD and DM
Verapamil *(Calan)*	2.5-10 mg IV over 2 min	5-10 mg IV q30-60 min, 40-160 mg PO tid, or 120-480 mg/d sustained release	↑ Digoxin level	
Diltiazem *(Cardizem)*	0.25 mg/kg over 2 min, repeat prn q15 min at 0.35 mg/kg	5-15 mg/hr IV, 30-90 mg PO qid, or 120-360 mg/d sustained release		Often well tolerated in patients with low LVEF

AF, atrial fibrillation; AV, atrioventricular; AVN, AV node; BP, blood pressure; CHF, congestive heart failure; COPD, chronic obstructive pulmonary disease; DM, diabetes mellitus; LVEF, left ventricular ejection fraction.

Table 2. **Pharmacologic Conversion Regimens**

Drug	Route	Dose	Success Rate (%)
Quinidine (Quinaglute)	PO	200-324 mg tid to 1.5 g/d	48-86
Procainamide (Procan)*	IV	1 g over 20-30 min	48-65
Propafenone (Rythmol)	PO	600 mg	55-87
	IV†	2 mg/kg over 10 min	40-90
Flecainide (Tambocor)	PO	300 mg	90
	IV†	2 mg/kg over 10 min	65-90
Amiodarone (Cordarone)	IV	1.2 g over 24 h	45-85
Sotalol (Betapace)	PO	80-160 mg, then 160-320 mg/d	52
Dofetilide (Tikosyn)	PO	125-500 μg bid based on creatinine clearance	30
Ibutilide (Corvert)	IV	1 mg over 10 min, repeat in 10 min × 1 prn	31

*Not FDA-approved for this indication.
†Not available in the United States.

fibrillation and has been associated with a lower incidence of early recurrence after cardioversion in some studies.

Nonpharmacologic Rate Control. For patients in whom adequate rate control cannot be achieved and for whom pharmacologic maintenance of sinus rhythm has been unsuccessful because of continued symptoms from the rapid rates, *AV node catheter ablation or modification* can be performed. Ablation of the AV node is one of the most effective methods of controlling ventricular rates during atrial tachyarrhythmias. Patients who have had complete AV junction ablation require a permanent rate-responsive pacemaker. AV junction ablation and pacing can provide superior symptom relief, a better quality of life, and improvement in left ventricular dysfunction caused by tachycardia-mediated cardiomyopathy in patients mainly disabled by rapid or irregular ventricular rates. The disadvantage is that patients become pacemaker dependent and require a permanent rate-responsive pacemaker. In addition, recent attention has highlighted the potential for right ventricular pacing to cause left ventricular dyssynchronous contraction that may lead to congestive heart failure. Early reports of an increased risk of late sudden death, primarily after early procedures using direct current (DC) ablation, have not been confirmed in recent studies with radiofrequency ablation. AV node modification without production of complete AV block may avoid the requirement for or dependence on a pacemaker. However, a significant rate of production of complete AV block during the procedure, a higher rate of recurrent rapid AV conduction, and less improvement in symptoms because of continued irregularity of ventricular rates can occur.

Rhythm Control—Achieving and Maintaining Sinus Rhythm

The mainstays of rhythm control therapy are antiarrhythmic drugs and electrical or pharmacologic cardioversion. Nonpharmacologic therapies include catheter or surgical ablation directed toward isolating pulmonary vein ostial or superior vena cava sources, catheter or surgical maze procedures, and permanent pacing or an atrial/ventricular defibrillator.

Restoration of Sinus Rhythm

In patients with a first occurrence of atrial fibrillation, spontaneous conversion to sinus rhythm may occur without any need for further therapy. If the atrial arrhythmia persists or remains symptomatic despite adequate rate control, the most effective method of restoring sinus rhythm is electrical cardioversion. Pharmacologic conversion can be attempted first with intravenous or oral regimens. Clinical instability manifested by hypotension, ischemia, or congestive heart failure, however, may prompt urgent electrical cardioversion.

Pharmacologic Conversion. Quinidine (Quinaglute, Quinidex), procainamide (Procan),* flecainide (Tambocor), propafenone (Rythmol), sotalol (Betapace), amiodarone (Cordarone, Pacerone), dofetilide (Tikosyn), and ibutilide (Corvert) have achieved success rates of 31% to 90% (Table 2).

Procainamide, amiodarone, and ibutilide have been studied in intravenous form for pharmacologic conversion. The drugs are more effective in patients with atrial fibrillation of shorter duration. *Procainamide* is a typical first-line intravenous antiarrhythmic drug chosen after rate control has been achieved because of the availability of an intravenous form and the ease of conversion to the oral form. Hypotension may necessitate a decrease in the infusion rate. Other potential side effects are QRS widening and proarrhythmia, including QT prolongation and torsades de pointes. Dosing should be modified and caution exercised in patients with renal insufficiency because an active metabolite, *N*-acetylprocainamide (NAPA), may accumulate to toxic levels in the presence of renal failure. Dosing should be adjusted according to serum levels, which should be checked daily during administration of intravenous procainamide. The use of procainamide may be acutely limited by hemodynamic effects in some patients with severe left ventricular dysfunction, by gastrointestinal side effects, or by fever. *Ibutilide* is an intravenous antiarrhythmic drug that has class III potassium channel–blocking activity. In one study, it has been shown to be more efficacious than

*Not FDA-approved for this indication.

procainamide in converting short-term atrial fibrillation/flutter to sinus rhythm. Patients should be monitored for QT prolongation and torsades de pointes. *Amiodarone* can also be used intravenously and may be helpful in patients with hemodynamic instability, recurrent atrial fibrillation despite cardioversion or other antiarrhythmic drugs, rate control refractory to conventional AV nodal–blocking drugs, or intolerance to standard antiarrhythmic or rate-controlling drugs as a result of negative inotropy. However, conversion rates may not be different from those of placebo-treated patients until after several hours of treatment.

Conversion may be achievable with oral loading regimens as well (see Table 2). *Flecainide*, 300 mg, and *propafenone*, 600 mg, have been used orally with comparable efficacy ("pill in the pocket" method). Flecainide and propafenone have usually been reserved for patients with no CAD and normal ventricular function. Rapid oral loading of *amiodarone* can generally be achieved in patients with intact gastrointestinal function. Oral *sotalol* can be used in patients who can tolerate β-blockade, but close attention to QT intervals and electrolyte balance is important because of the risk of proarrhythmia. *Dofetilide*, a new class III oral antiarrhythmic agent, has been studied for termination of atrial fibrillation/flutter. Dofetilide therapy should be initiated in the hospital so that patients can be monitored for QT prolongation and torsades de pointes. The dosage of dofetilide should be reduced if renal dysfunction is present. The use of quinidine is limited by proarrhythmia concerns, particularly in patients taking diuretics, at risk of electrolyte depletion.

Electrical Cardioversion. Electrical cardioversion is the most effective method of conversion to sinus rhythm and is the method of choice for hemodynamically compromising atrial fibrillation. Evaluation of the need for anticoagulation before cardioversion is essential (see later). Electrical cardioversion requires conscious sedation with a short-acting anesthetic such as etomidate or methohexital. An R wave–synchronized shock is delivered to defibrillation patches. Anterior-posterior patch positions (e.g., right parasternal–left paraspinal) are more optimal for atrial defibrillation than the anterior-anterior positions (e.g., right parasternal–left apical) that are often used for ventricular defibrillation. The standard initial monophasic shock energies used are 200 J for conversion of atrial fibrillation and 50 to 100 J for conversion of atrial flutter. If cardioversion is unsuccessful at the initial energies, an increase in energy is attempted. Newer *external biphasic defibrillators* have been successful at much lower energies in converting atrial fibrillation (e.g., median successful energy of 50 J) and flutter (median successful energy of 25 J) and may be used with success initially or after failed cardioversion. Sinus rhythm can be successfully achieved with biphasic defibrillation in over 99% of patients at our institution. For atrial fibrillation refractory to standard external cardioversion, high-energy, 720-J external shocks have been delivered successfully by synchronizing two monophasic defibrillators to the same QRS. Lower energies (2 to 10 J) with catheters placed in the right atrium and coronary sinus have been successful in achieving sinus rhythm.

Maintenance of Sinus Rhythm

Long-term maintenance of sinus rhythm (Table 3) often requires an oral antiarrhythmic agent, particularly in patients with frequent or resistant atrial fibrillation, underlying cardiovascular disease, enlarged atria, or other continuing disease factors that predispose to atrial fibrillation. The available antiarrhythmic agents that can be effective in maintaining sinus rhythm include class IA (quinidine, procainamide, disopyramide), IC (flecainide, propafenone), IA/B/C (moricizine), and III (sotalol, amiodarone, dofetilide) antiarrhythmic drugs.

Class IA Antiarrhythmic Drugs. Class IA drugs delay fast sodium channel–mediated conduction with depression of phase 0 and prolongation of repolarization. These agents can enhance AV nodal conduction and potentially increase the ventricular response during atrial fibrillation, but the concomitant use of AV nodal–blocking agents is usually required. The effects on repolarization with QT interval prolongation are associated with an increased incidence of torsades de pointes. *Quinidine* is one of the best-studied drugs used for atrial fibrillation. A meta-analysis showed that the proportion of patients remaining in sinus rhythm at 1 year was 50% with quinidine. However, total mortality was 2.9% in patients treated with quinidine versus 0.8% in the control group. The Stroke Prevention in Atrial Fibrillation (SPAF) trial also reported increased mortality with antiarrhythmic therapy, which usually consisted of quinidine; increased risk was seen in patients with a history of congestive heart failure. The use of quinidine has been limited by its potential for proarrhythmia, including torsades de pointes. If used, quinidine should be initiated in the hospital with continuous electrocardiographic monitoring and assessment of the QT interval. The risk is higher in patients taking diuretics and those with electrolyte depletion. Because quinidine increases serum digoxin levels, the concomitant digoxin dosage should usually be decreased. Other adverse effects include gastrointestinal symptoms, particularly diarrhea. *Procainamide,** which is available for intravenous use, is often a first-line antiarrhythmic agent for atrial fibrillation after cardiac surgery. However, its long-term use is often limited by a high incidence of drug-induced lupus, and long-term controlled trials are not available. *Disopyramide* (Norpace) has also been shown to be effective, with maintenance of sinus rhythm in approximately 50% of patients over a follow-up of 6 to 12 months. Its use is limited in older men because of anticholinergic side effects and urinary retention. The drug can also produce negative inotropic effects.

Class IC Antiarrhythmic Drugs. These agents markedly slow sodium channel–mediated conduction with a marked depression of phase 0 and only a slight effect on repolarization. *Flecainide* and *propafenone*

*Not FDA-approved for this indication.

TABLE 3. **Drugs for Maintenance of Sinus Rhythm**

Antiarrhythmic Drug	Dose	Maintenance of Sinus Rhythm (6-12 mo) (%)	Side Effects/Comments
Class IA			↑QT, proarrhythmia/TdP, potential ↑AVN conduction
Quinidine	200-400 mg PO tid-qid	30-79	Diarrhea, nausea, ↑ digoxin levels, thrombocytopenia
Procainamide	10-15 mg/kg IV at ≤50-mg/min load, then 1-4 mg/min IV; or 2-6 g/d PO bid or qid, sustained release	N/A	↓BP, CHF, drug-induced lupus, agranulocytosis; active metabolite NAPA with class III activity accumulates in renal failure
Disopyramide	100-300 mg PO tid	44-67	Anticholinergic effects (e.g., urinary retention, dry eyes/mouth, glaucoma), CHF
Class IC			Proarrhythmia, VT, conversion to atrial flutter
Flecainide	50-200 mg PO bid	34-81	Visual disturbance, dizziness, CHF; avoid in CAD or LV dysfunction
Propafenone	150-300 mg tid	30-76	CHF; avoid in CAD/LV dysfunction
Class IA/B/C			
Moricizine	200-300 mg tid	N/A	Proarrhythmia, dizziness, GI upset/nausea, headache; caution in CAD/LV dysfunction
Class III			
Sotalol	80-240 mg bid	37-70	CHF, bronchospasm, bradycardia, ↑QT, proarrhythmia/TdP
Amiodarone	600-1600 mg/d loading in divided doses, 100-400 mg/d maintenance	40-79	Pulmonary toxicity; bradycardia; hyperthyroidism or hypothyroidism; hepatic toxicity; GI (nausea, constipation), neurologic, dermatologic, and ophthalmologic side effects; drug interactions
Dofetilide	CrCl (mL/min) >60: 500 μg bid 40-60: 250 μg bid 20-40: 125 μg bid	58-71	↑QT, proarrhythmia/TdP, headache, muscle cramps. Exclude for use if CrCl <20 mL/min

AVN, atrioventricular nodal; BP, blood pressure; CAD, coronary heart disease; CHF, congestive heart failure; CrCl, creatinine clearance; GI, gastrointestinal; LV, left ventricular; NAPA, *N*-acetylprocainamide; TdP, torsades de pointes.

have been shown to be effective in the treatment of atrial fibrillation. Flecainide and propafenone have been equivalent in efficacy in comparative studies. Proarrhythmia in the form of ventricular tachycardia or wide complex tachycardia as a result of slow atrial flutter with 1:1 AV conduction can occur with flecainide or propafenone. Patients with underlying heart disease may be at higher risk for proarrhythmia with class IC agents. Flecainide and propafenone are usually avoided in patients with CAD or impaired ventricular function as a result of findings from the Cardiac Arrhythmia Suppression Trial (CAST), which showed increased mortality in patients treated with flecainide, encainide, and moricizine for ventricular arrhythmias after myocardial infarction. Flecainide is usually well tolerated, but noncardiac effects include visual disturbances, dizziness, and paresthesias. Propafenone contains weak β-blocking activity. *Moricizine* (Ethmozine)* is an antiarrhythmic agent with class I/IC properties, although controlled data on its efficacy in atrial fibrillation are sparse.

Class III Antiarrhythmic Drugs. Class III agents are potassium channel blockers that prolong repolarization. *Amiodarone* has effects on multiple ion channels. Its effects on sodium and potassium channels increase refractoriness in the atria, AV node, and ventricles. It also has noncompetitive β-adrenergic blocking and calcium channel–blocking activity, inhibits phospholipase, and antagonizes thyroid hormone. It is effective against atrial fibrillation and has a long half-life, with weeks to months required to achieve a steady state. Amiodarone has potential for toxicity when used long-term and has been associated with high discontinuation rates. However, the risk for pulmonary toxicity appears to be dose related, and maintenance doses when used for atrial arrhythmias are usually under 400 mg daily and often can be minimized to 200 mg or less. Other potential side effects include hypothyroidism or hyperthyroidism, elevated liver function test results or hepatic toxicity, bluish skin changes and photosensitivity, peripheral neuropathy, and very rarely, optic neuritis. Proarrhythmia is uncommon, but patients with congestive heart failure and previous proarrhythmia/torsades de pointes are at higher risk. Amiodarone can cause significant bradycardia. It has been reported to be superior to sotalol, propafenone, and flecainide for atrial fibrillation. *Sotalol* is a nonselective β-blocker with class III activity that has been effective in atrial fibrillation. It has been reported to be as efficacious as quinidine and propafenone. Monitoring for prolongation of the QT interval and torsades de pointes is recommended. The drug has significant β-blocking activity with a potential for bradycardia and negative inotropic effects as well. *Dofetilide* is a potent inhibitor of I_{Kr}, the rapid component of the delayed rectifier. Dofetilide did not increase mortality in the Danish Investigators of Arrhythmia and Mortality on Dofetilide (DIAMOND)

*Not FDA-approved for this indication.

trials in patients after myocardial infarction or in those with congestive heart failure. It was found to also be beneficial in maintaining sinus rhythm during these studies. The dosage should be adjusted in patients with renal insufficiency. In-hospital initiation is mandated.

Approach to Antiarrhythmic Drug Selection for Atrial Fibrillation

The antiarrhythmic drug chosen should provide adequate rate control and minimize the risk of thromboembolism. The decision to use an antiarrhythmic drug should include consideration of the frequency and duration of the atrial fibrillation, symptoms, reversibility of the arrhythmia, and the presence of structural heart disease. In addition, the risk of side effects, including organ toxicity and proarrhythmia, should be weighed against the benefit and efficacy rates of the drugs. In treating atrial fibrillation medically, it is often worthwhile to advise the patient that recurrences are expected (50% at 6 to 36 months), but not generally life-threatening. Total suppression of episodes may risk drug toxicity, and a reduction in symptoms and/or recurrences for improvement in quality of life is a reasonable goal. Above all, safety is emphasized.

Frequency, Duration, and Symptoms. With a *first episode* of atrial fibrillation, the future pattern of recurrence may not be well predicted. Although the conversion success rate and rate of recurrence are more favorable with an antiarrhythmic drug, it may be reasonable to avoid antiarrhythmic drug therapy for a first occurrence unless factors such as structural heart disease, large atria, or advanced age suggest a high risk of recurrence. Conversion may be attempted pharmacologically or electrically. Early recurrences of atrial fibrillation after cardioversion would prompt the use of an antiarrhythmic drug or verapamil in an attempt to attenuate the shortening of atrial refractory periods caused by electrical remodeling. However, after a first occurrence, it might be reasonable to stop the antiarrhythmic drug therapy after a period of a few weeks to months.

In patients with *recurring paroxysmal atrial fibrillation*, those with no symptoms might be adequately treated with rate control or antiarrhythmic therapy along with warfarin (Coumadin), if indicated. Patients with symptomatic occurrences might need further rate control or antiarrhythmic drug therapy. Infrequent episodes in a patient with a normal heart might be treatable with intermittent drug therapy (e.g., flecainide, 150 to 300 mg orally, or propafenone, 300 to 600 mg orally). Patients with frequent symptomatic episodes might require an antiarrhythmic drug.

Chronic, persistent atrial fibrillation should prompt consideration of cardioversion. Factors to be considered include duration of the atrial fibrillation, atrial size, and symptoms, as well as anticoagulation status, at least short-term, if not chronically. Antiarrhythmic therapy might be required for successful conversion and maintenance of sinus rhythm.

Structural Heart Disease. The presence of CAD and/or ventricular dysfunction limits consideration of some antiarrhythmic drugs because of a higher risk of proarrhythmia. Class IC drugs should be avoided in these patients (based on CAST). Dofetilide might be considered because no harmful outcomes have been reported from the DIAMOND myocardial infarction and congestive heart failure trials. Sotalol could be considered for patients with preserved left ventricular function who can tolerate the β-blocking activity of this drug, and it is often a first choice in patients with CAD. Amiodarone carries a low proarrhythmic profile and could be used as first- or second-line therapy, with safety based on the results of large randomized trials performed in patients after myocardial infarction (e.g., European Myocardial Infarction Amiodarone Trial [EMIAT], Canadian Amiodarone Myocardial Infarction Trial [CAMIT]) or in patients with heart failure (e.g., Congestive Heart Failure Survival Trial of Antiarrhythmic Therapy [CHF-STAT], Grupo de Estudio de la Sobrevida en al Insuficiencia Cardiaca en Argentina [GESICA]). Patients with left ventricular hypertrophy may have a higher risk of torsades de pointes, and class IC drugs or amiodarone may be the preferred first-line agents.

Efficacy, Organ Toxicity, and Proarrhythmia. As shown in Table 3, class IA and class IC drugs have an *efficacy* rate of approximately 50% in maintaining sinus rhythm at 6 months. Class IC agents have been more efficacious than class IA agents in some studies. Class III drugs may have a slightly higher efficacy rate at 50% to 70%. The Canadian Trial of Atrial Fibrillation (CTAF) showed that amiodarone was more effective than propafenone or sotalol in preventing recurrent atrial fibrillation. Comparative studies have not been sufficiently performed to conclude that specific agents within a class are more or less effective.

Side effects are common with antiarrhythmic agents, and the side effect profile often limits continuation, though not necessarily initiation of a drug. However, the risk for major *organ toxicity* does inhibit consideration of initiating certain drugs. Amiodarone has significant potential for organ toxicity, although this risk is dose and duration related. These side effects often limit use, particularly in younger patients. The high frequency of drug-induced lupus seriously precludes the long-term use of procainamide. A small risk of agranulocytosis has been noted with procainamide and a low risk of thrombocytopenia and lupus with quinidine. The negative inotropic, chronotropic, and bronchospastic side effects of drugs can also limit their use.

Proarrhythmia risk may be the most important factor to be considered. Despite being at low risk for proarrhythmia, patients with normal hearts and non–life-threatening atrial fibrillation should be treated with drugs that have the lowest risk of proarrhythmia or organ toxicity (Figure 3). Class IC drugs are often used as first-line agents for these reasons, with class IA drugs and sotalol being lower tier choices. Patients with CAD or ventricular dysfunction are at higher risk for proarrhythmia from class IC drugs and may be better treated with amiodarone or sotalol. Risk factors for proarrhythmia include structural heart disease (left ventricular dysfunction,

No structural heart disease
IC, amiodarone < sotalol, IA

Structural heart disease
Amiodarone < sotalol, 1A < 1C (except LVH)

Figure 3. Proarrhythmia risk by structural heart disease and antiarrhythmic drug. LVH = left ventricular hypertrophy.

congestive heart failure, CAD, previous myocardial infarction, left ventricular hypertrophy), female gender, older age, and for amiodarone, previous torsades de pointes and congestive heart failure.

The requirement for hospitalization for cardiac monitoring during initiation of therapy is controversial in some patients. Hospitalization is often recommended for initiation of antiarrhythmic drug therapy (Figure 4) in patients with structural heart disease, persistent atrial fibrillation, or therapy with certain antiarrhythmic agents, such as dofetilide (mandated in-hospital initiation), sotalol, quinidine, procainamide, and disopyramide. Inpatient initiation is also often suggested for heart failure patients with a history of torsades de pointes who are starting amiodarone therapy, patients with a previous history of proarrhythmia, prolonged QT at baseline in patients initiating class IA and class III drug therapy, patients with a propensity for bradycardia, or a history of ventricular arrhythmias in patients with significant left ventricular dysfunction and no implantable cardioverter-defibrillator.

Antiarrhythmic Drug Selection—Summary. Patients with ventricular dysfunction may be at higher risk for proarrhythmia. Patients who do not have any structural heart disease may respond well to class IC agents, which are well tolerated with few noncardiac side effects, have a low proarrhythmic risk, and are reasonably effective. For these patients, class IA and class III drugs carry a slightly higher risk of proarrhythmia and may have more side effects, and thus are used as second-line agents. In younger patients, amiodarone is usually a third-line drug because of the risk of organ toxicity. Patients with CAD but preserved left ventricular function may be treated first with sotalol and avoidance of class IC drugs. Amiodarone or dofetilide could be first- or second-line therapy. For patients with significant ventricular systolic dysfunction and severe congestive heart failure, amiodarone is often first-line therapy. Dofetilide could be tried as second- or first-line therapy.

Nonpharmacologic Therapies for Control of Atrial Fibrillation

Pacemaker Therapy

Permanent pacing may become necessary for sick sinus syndrome, for tachycardia-bradycardia syndromes, for bradyarrhythmias occurring as a result of drug therapy, or after AV junction ablation. Newer pacemakers may have sophisticated programming

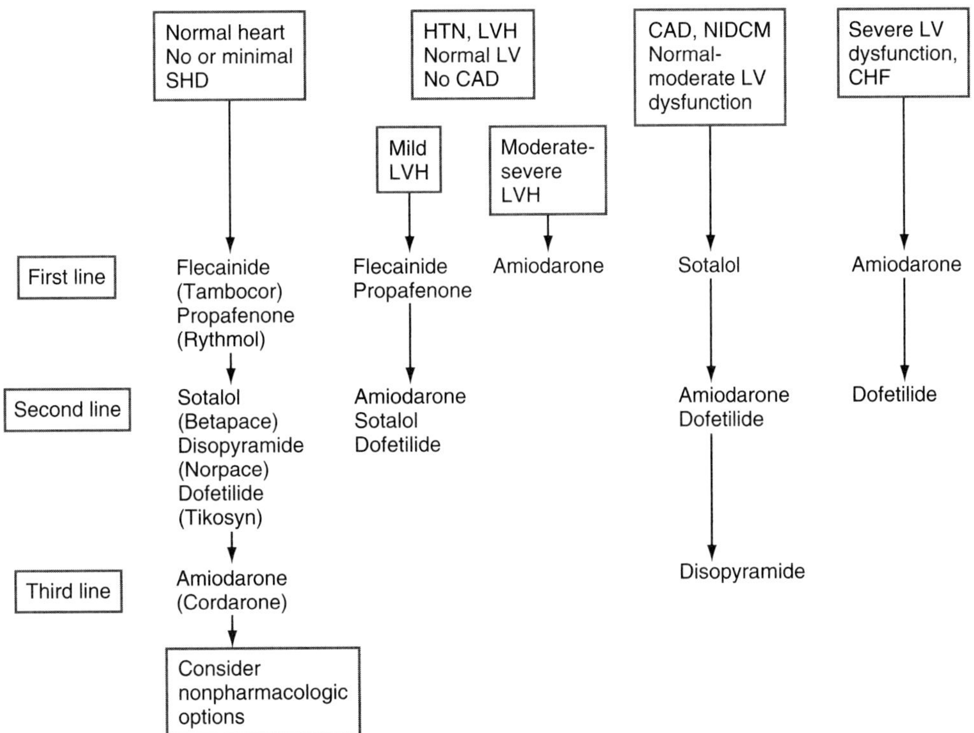

Figure 4. Antiarrhythmic drug selection—summary. CAD = coronary artery disease; CHF = congestive heart failure; HTN = hypertension; LV = left ventricular; LVH = left ventricular hypertrophy; NIDCM = non-ischemic dilated cardiomyopathy; SHD = structural heart disease. (Adapted from ACC/AHA Guidelines for the Perioperative Cardiovascular Evaluation for Noncardiac Surgery. *J AM Coll Cardiol* 1996;27:910-948. Copyright 1996 by the American College of Cardiology and American Heart Association, Inc.)

options that can restrict upper tracking limits during atrial arrhythmias, yet allow higher rate-responsive limits. In addition, pacemakers with "mode-switching" algorithms can change from dual-chamber pacing to single-chamber (VVI or VVIR) or DDIR pacing at the onset of atrial arrhythmias.

Several nonrandomized and randomized studies have suggested that the incidence of atrial fibrillation is lower with dual-chamber or atrial pacing that maintains AV synchrony than with single-chamber ventricular pacing. These benefits may be less in patients without sinus node dysfunction or bradycardia. Newer pacing approaches showing some promise in suppression of atrial fibrillation include the use of atrial overdrive pacing algorithms (variable results), site-specific pacing (e.g., at Bachmann's bundle, coronary sinus/right atrial septum), and dual–atrial site or bi-atrial pacing modalities.

Implantable Atrial Defibrillator

Implantable atrial defibrillator devices provid automatic or patient-activated, low-energy, ventricular-synchronous atrial defibrillation. Current devices provide ventricular and atrial defibrillation, as well as higher output shocks, which might be required, particularly if coronary sinus defibrillation leads are not implanted.

Catheter Ablation of Atrial Arrhythmias

Radiofrequency catheter ablation has been used not only for AV nodal ablation and modification but also for the *ablation of supraventricular tachycardias* that may degenerate to atrial fibrillation, such as AV nodal reentrant tachycardia or accessory pathway–mediated atrioventricular reentry. In addition, primary *radiofrequency ablation of typical atrial flutter circuits* can be successfully achieved in approximately 90% of patients by targeting an area of conduction that is present in the low right atrial isthmus between the tricuspid annulus, coronary sinus, and inferior vena cava. This approach has been used successfully, particularly in patients with concomitant atrial fibrillation that can be controlled with antiarrhythmic medication but whose recurrences while taking medication may be in the form of atrial flutter, which often occurs at a slow atrial rate that may facilitate 1:1 AV conduction. Atypical atrial flutter or tachycardias arising from the right or left atria have also been successfully ablated, especially those associated with atrial scars or incisions and those that can be mapped with newer mapping systems.

Catheter Ablation of Atrial Fibrillation

Catheter ablation of atrial fibrillation has targeted both the substrate for maintenance and the focal substrates initiating atrial fibrillation.

Catheter Maze—Right and Left Atrial Linear Ablation. Initially mimicking the surgical maze procedure, radiofrequency energy was delivered in linear applications to the right and left atria. Although moderate acute and long-term success rates were reported, the procedures were long, recurrence rates were high, and excessively high serious complication rates were reported. Right atrial linear ablation was studied as a potentially safer procedure but is associated with much lower success rates. Because of these factors and the higher success rates of ablation directed toward pulmonary vein foci, ablation for atrial fibrillation has generally progressed toward pulmonary vein isolation rather than linear ablation procedures.

Focal Atrial Fibrillation Ablation, Pulmonary Vein Isolation. Catheter ablation for atrial fibrillation has recently been primarily focused on the 89% to 95% of atrial fibrillation trigger foci that arise from pulmonary vein ostial foci. Radiofrequency ablation is delivered segmentally or circumferentially around the ostia to electrically isolate arrhythmogenic pulmonary vein foci. Reported acute success rates range from 87% to 95%, with long-term success ranging from 49% to 86%. Limitations of the current methods include a higher rate of recurrence and the risk of symptomatic pulmonary vein stenosis from ablation within the pulmonary vein (approximate risk, 4% to 5%), the latter leading to the use of intracardiac ultrasound and ring-type electrode catheters to isolate pulmonary vein ostia by the application of ablation energy to the left atrial side rather than inside the pulmonary vein ostia. These approaches have resulted in improved complication rates. Circumferential ablation methods using alternative delivery techniques and/or energy sources (e.g., ultrasound, microwave, or laser energy and cryoablation), as well as novel imaging and navigation methods, are under investigation. The success of applying this procedure to the spectrum of atrial fibrillation patients remains to be defined, although the procedure has been used with success, even in patients with chronic, persistent atrial fibrillation.

Surgical Approaches

Current surgical approaches to atrial fibrillation primarily use the *maze* procedure or variants of it. The Cox *maze procedure* was designed to cure atrial fibrillation by dividing the atria into "maze-like" corridors and blind alleys that control the development of reentry by limiting the available path length. Part of its success might be due to isolation of the pulmonary veins, which is part of the operation. The maze procedure has been used with a high degree of success (>90%), but it has seen limited use. However, it has been performed successfully in patients with symptomatic refractory atrial fibrillation or performed in conjunction with mitral valve surgery. Atrial transport function may be preserved but reduced. Newer methods of delivering radiofrequency energy, microwave energy, or cryoablation to isolate pulmonary vein ostia are also being performed. Surgical approaches may be combined with removal or ligation of the left atrial appendage.

CHRONIC ANTICOAGULATION AND ANTITHROMBOTIC THERAPY

One of the most clinically important consequences of atrial fibrillation is its association with thromboembolic events and stroke (see earlier). *Risk factors for stroke* or other thromboembolic complications associated with atrial fibrillation include previous transient ischemic attack or stroke, diabetes, hypertension, and age. In addition, other risk factors include left ventricular dysfunction, increased left atrial size, rheumatic mitral valve disease, prosthetic valves, women older than 75 years, mitral annular calcification, increased wall thickness, spontaneous echocardiographic contrast in the atrium, aortic atheroma, and thyrotoxicosis. Patients with lone atrial fibrillation (no risk factors, structural heart disease) who are younger than 65 years have a low stroke event rate of 1% per year.

Patients with *paroxysmal atrial fibrillation* also have an increased stroke rate of 3.7% per year. Clustering of events takes place at the onset of the arrhythmia, with a 6.8% incidence of embolism in the first month that decreases to 2% per year over the subsequent 5 years. Thus, patients with paroxysmal atrial fibrillation appear to have a risk similar to that of patients with chronic, persistent atrial fibrillation and are generally treated similarly with regard to anticoagulation.

Several *randomized, controlled trials*, summarized in Table 4A to C, have established the efficacy of *adjusted-dose warfarin* anticoagulation in the prevention of thromboembolic complications in patients with atrial fibrillation. The Atrial Fibrillation Investigators (AFI) pooled the results of five primary prevention trials and reported a 68% reduction in the risk of stroke with warfarin. The results with *aspirin* versus controls have been less solid. The AFI pooled analysis reported a borderline significant reduction in risk with aspirin. Overall, the results of studies comparing oral warfarin anticoagulation with aspirin show a larger reduction in relative risk with warfarin than with aspirin. A meta-analysis of these studies reported a 46% reduction in the relative risk for ischemic stroke and a 36% reduction in the relative risk for all strokes with warfarin versus aspirin. In addition, SPAF-3, in which atrial fibrillation patients with at least one risk factor for thromboembolism were randomized to low-intensity, fixed-dose warfarin (international normalized ratio [INR] of 1.2 to 1.5 for initial dose adjustment) and aspirin (325 mg/d) or adjusted-dose warfarin (INR of 2.0 to 3.0), reported significant superiority of adjusted-dose warfarin. Adjusted-dose warfarin has been compared with low-dose warfarin in several studies (Table 4C), with a meta-analysis of these studies showing a 38% reduction in relative risk

TABLE 4A. **Reduction of Stroke/Thromboembolism in AF: Warfarin Versus Control**

	Warfarin	Control	RRR (%)	*P* Value
AFASAK1	2.7	6.2	56	<.05
SPAF1	2.3	7.4	67	.01
BAATAF	0.4	3.0	86	.002
CAFA	3.4	4.6	26	.25
SPINAF	0.9	4.3	79	.001
AFI	**1.4**	**4.5**	**68**	**<.001**
EAFT	8.5	16.5	47	.001

TABLE 4B. **Reduction of Stroke/Thromboembolism in AF: Aspirin Versus Control**

	Aspirin	Control	RRR (%)	*P* Value
AFASAK1	5.2	6.2	16	NS
SPAF1	3.6	6.3	42	.02
EAFT	19.0	15.5	17	.12
AFI	**6.3**	**8.1**	**21**	**.05**
ESPS2	13.8	20.7	33	.16
LASAF Pilot				
125 mg qd	2.6	2.2	−18	NS
125 mg qod	0.7	2.2	68	.05

TABLE 4C. **Reduction of Stroke/Thromboembolism in AF: Warfarin Versus Aspirin and/or Low-Dose Warfarin**

	Warfarin	Aspirin	RRR (%)	*P* Value
AFASAK1	2.7	5.2	48	<.05
SPAF2				
<75 y old	1.3	1.9	33	.24
>75 y old	3.6	4.8	27	.39
EAFT	NA	NA	40	.008
AFASAK2	3.4	2.7	−21	NS
Hellemons et al.	2.5	3.1	19	NS
	Warfarin	**Low-Dose Warfarin + Aspirin**	**RRR (%)**	***P* Value**
SPAF3	1.9	7.9	74	<.0001
AFASAK2	3.4	3.2	−6	NS
	Warfarin	**Low-Dose Warfarin**	**RRR (%)**	***P* Value**
AFASAK2	3.4	3.9	13	NS
Hellemons et al.	2.5	2.2	−14	NS
Pengo et al.	3.6	6.2	42	.29

AF, atrial fibrillation; NS, not significant; RRR, relative risk reduction.
AFASAK, Atrial Fibrillation, Aspirin, Anticoagulation Study. Petersen P, Boysen G, Godtfredsen J, et al: Lancet 1:175-178, 1989.
SPAF, Stroke Prevention in Atrial Fibrillation Trial. Stroke Prevention in Atrial Fibrillation Investigators: Circulation 84:527-539, 1991.
BAATAF, Boston Area Anticoagulation Trial. Boston Area Anticoagulation Trial for Atrial Fibrillation Investigators: N Engl J Med 323:1505-1511, 1990.
CAFA, Canadian Atrial Fibrillation Anticoagulation Trial. Connolly SJ, Laupacis A, Gent M, et al: J Am Coll Cardiol 18:349-355, 1991.
SPINAF, Stroke Prevention in Non-rheumatic Atrial Fibrillation Study. Ezekowitz MD, et al: N Engl J Med 327:1406-1412, 1992.
AFI, Atrial Fibrillation Investigators (pooled analysis of first five studies in Table A, first three studies in Table B). Atrial Fibrillation Investigators: Arch Intern Med 154:1449-1457, 1994.
EAFT, European Atrial Fibrillation Trial. EAFT (European Atrial Fibrillation Trial) Study Group: Lancet 342:1255-1262, 1993.
ESPS, European Stroke Prevention Study. Diener H, Cunha L, Forbes C, et al: J Neurol Sci 143:1-13, 1996.
LASAF, Posada IS, Barriales V: Am Heart J 138:137-143, 1999.
SPAF2, Stroke Prevention in Atrial Fibrillation II. Stroke Prevention in Atrial Fibrillation Investigators: Lancet 343:687-691, 1994.
AFASAK2, Second Copenhagen Atrial Fibrillation, Aspirin, and Anticoagulation Study. Gullov AL, Koefoed BG, Petersen P, et al: Arch Intern Med 158:1513-1521, 1998.
Hellemons et al, Hellemons BSP, et al: BMJ 319:958-964, 1999.
SPAF3, Stroke Prevention in Atrial Fibrillation III. Stroke Prevention in Atrial Fibrillation Investigators: Lancet 348:633-638, 1996. SPAF III Writing Committee for the Stroke Prevention in Atrial Fibrillation Investigators: JAMA 279:1273-1277, 1998.
Modified from Albers et al: Chest 119(suppl):194-206, 2001; and Atrial Fibrillation Investigators: Arch Intern Med 154:1449-1457, 1994.

TABLE 5. **Risk Stratification Schemes for Nonrheumatic Atrial Fibrillation**

Atrial Fibrillation Investigators*		**SPAF3†**	
Risk Strata	*Annual Stroke Rate (%)*	*Risk Strata*	*Annual Stroke Rate (%)*
<65 y, no other RF	1.0	No RF, no history of HTN‡	1.1
<65 y, ≥1 other RF	4.9		
65-75 y, ≥1 other RF	4.3	No RF, history of HTN‡	3.6
>75 y, no other RF	3.5		
>75 y, ≥1 other RF	8.1	>1 RF§	7.9

*Atrial Fibrillation Investigators risk factors: previous transient ischemic attack/stroke, history of hypertension, diabetes mellitus, increasing age.

†SPAF3 risk factors: previous transient ischemic attack/stroke, systolic blood pressure over 160 mm Hg, impaired left ventricular function, women older than 75 years.

‡Patients taking aspirin.

§Patients taking aspirin plus low-dose warfarin.

HTN = hypertension; RF = risk factor.

From Laupacis A, Albers G, Dalen J, et al: Chest 114(suppl):579-589, 1998.

in favor of adjusted-dose warfarin, although this reduction did not reach statistical significance.

Recommendations for Antithrombotic Therapy. *Risk stratification schemes* and a *summary of recommendations* for antithrombotic therapy are shown in Tables 5 and 6. Anticoagulation is recommended if atrial fibrillation persists longer than 48 hours, especially if cardioversion is anticipated after this time, if atrial fibrillation continues to recur, or if the following risk factors are present. Anticoagulation with warfarin (target prothrombin time/INR, 2.5; range, 2.0 to 3.0 for atrial fibrillation) should be recommended for all anticoagulation-eligible patients with any of the following high-risk factors: age older than 75 years; previous transient ischemic attack, systemic embolus, or stroke; hypertension; poor left ventricular function; rheumatic mitral valve disease; or prosthetic heart valves. Patients with two or more moderate risk factors (age between 65 and 75 years, diabetes mellitus, CAD with preserved left ventricular function) should also be treated with warfarin. Those with one moderate-risk factor can be treated with aspirin or warfarin. Aspirin, 325 mg/d, can be recommended for patients younger than 65 years with no risk factors. These recommendations apply to paroxysmal as well as chronic, persistent atrial fibrillation.

Anticoagulation Before Cardioversion. The risk of emboli after cardioversion has been reported to be 0.6% to 5.6% without and 0.8% to 1% with anticoagulation. Anticoagulation recommendations for electrical cardioversion are as follows. For atrial fibrillation that has lasted over 48 hours, anticoagulation with warfarin (target INR, 2.5; range, 2.0 to 3.0) for 3 weeks should be provided before elective cardioversion. This regimen should be continued at least until sinus rhythm has been maintained for 4 weeks to allow time for mechanical atrial transport to resume and to assess for possible recurrence of atrial fibrillation. In some circumstances, a transesophageal echocardiography (TEE) protocol may be substituted for conventional therapy, but adjusted-dose warfarin should be continued until sinus rhythm has been maintained for at least 4 weeks. The role of TEE has been studied in the Assessment of Cardioversion Using Transesophageal Echocardiography (ACUTE) trial, which randomized 1222 patients undergoing cardioversion to conventional anticoagulation with therapeutic warfarin for 3 weeks before cardioversion or to a TEE-guided approach. The results showed no significant difference in thromboembolic complications occurring after cardioversion in the two arms. Consideration should be given to managing anticoagulation for atrial flutter similar to that for atrial fibrillation. Long-term anticoagulation beyond the 4 weeks after cardioversion should also be considered if the patient has cardiomyopathy, a history of previous embolism, mitral valve disease, or other indications for long-term anticoagulation as listed previously. The AFFIRM trial results highlight the importance of continuing long-term anticoagulation in patients with risk factors for stroke (as listed earlier), even in a rhythm control strategy with maintenance of sinus rhythm. Heparin anticoagulation followed by oral anticoagulation may be indicated for patients requiring emergency cardioversion for hemodynamic instability. For atrial fibrillation of less than 48 hours' duration, the risk of embolism after cardioversion appears to be low, but pericardioversion anticoagulation is recommended.

TABLE 6. **Guidelines for Antithrombotic Therapy for Atrial Fibrillation**

Risk Factors	**No.**	**Recommendation***
High†	1	Warfarin
Moderate‡	>1	Warfarin
	1	Warfarin or aspirin
None	0	Aspirin

*Warfarin target international normalized ratio: 2.5 (range, 2.0 to 3.0); aspirin, 325 mg/d.

†High risk factors: previous transient ischemic attack, systemic embolus, or stroke; hypertension; poor left ventricular function; rheumatic mitral valve disease; prosthetic heart valve; age older than 75 years.

‡Moderate risk factors: age 65 to 75 years, diabetes mellitus, coronary artery disease with preserved left ventricular systolic function.

Recommendations from Albers GW, Dalen JE, Laupacis A, et al: Antithrombotic therapy in atrial fibrillation. Chest 119(suppl):194-206, 2001.

SUMMARY

Atrial fibrillation remains a common clinical arrhythmia with a potential for the production of significant symptoms and morbidity, particularly from thromboembolic complications. Antithrombotic therapy is a cornerstone of management because anticoagulation has been demonstrated to be effective in reducing the frequency of stroke in patients at risk for thromboembolism. Rate and rhythm control strategies have been studied. Although a rhythm control strategy does not appear to confer any mortality advantage, individualized therapeutic approaches remain important, particularly in patients who remain symptomatic in atrial fibrillation. Recently, ablative therapies have produced cure in some patients with refractory atrial fibrillation, and advances in techniques for mapping and ablation are expected to continue to improve the safety and success of this procedure.

PREMATURE BEATS

method of
EZRA A. AMSTERDAM, M.D.
University of California School of Medicine
Davis, California
University of California Medical Center
Sacramento, California

Premature cardiac beats are the most frequent disturbances of cardiac rhythm and one of the most frequent causes of an irregular pulse. They originate from all areas of the heart; in descending order of frequency, they occur in the ventricles, atria, and atrioventricular (AV) junctional tissue. Although premature beats are a frequent manifestation of cardiac disease, they also occur in the absence of structural abnormalities of the heart and can be provoked by numerous cardiac and extracardiac factors. However, the prevalence and complexity of premature beats increase in the presence of heart disease, particularly in association with acute cardiac and noncardiac provoking factors. Although premature beats are frequently an incidental finding in both patients with cardiac disease and healthy persons, they commonly produce symptoms and can occasionally impair hemodynamic function. Moreover, they may also be harbingers of sustained tachyarrhythmias. Their prognostic importance varies from nil to ominous and depends on the setting—the presence or absence of cardiac disease—in which they occur. Symptomatic premature beats may be distressing to the patient, whereas asymptomatic premature beats may indicate increased prognostic risk to the physician if they are associated with structural heart disease. The essence of management of these rhythm disturbances is recognition that the patient, rather than the arrhythmia, is the primary consideration. Thus, depending on the circumstances of the individual patient, premature beats may require: (1) no specific treatment, (2) correction or elimination of cardiac or extracardiac provoking factors, or (3) pharmacologic or other therapy.

A *premature beat* is defined by its occurrence earlier in the cardiac cycle than the anticipated normal sinus beat, and it is further described by its origin from the atrium (atrial premature beat [APB]), AV junction (junctional premature beat [JPB]), or ventricle (ventricular premature beat or contraction [PVC]). Various terms, in addition to premature beats, have been applied to these ectopic forms, the most common of which are premature ventricular beat, premature ventricular depolarization, extrasystole, and ventricular ectopic depolarization. These alternative terms have also been applied to APBs and JPBs. Because an ectopic depolarization may be early (premature) or late (in which case it is an escape beat), and the prefix *extra* provides no information on timing, it is more precise to use the term *premature* to indicate an abnormally early beat.

Documentation of premature beats requires electrocardiographic (ECG) demonstration to determine their timing and morphology accurately. Morphology reflects their site of origin (atrium, junction, ventricle). By common consensus, three or more consecutive premature beats define *tachycardia*. For example, three consecutive PVCs comprise *ventricular tachycardia*. Two consecutive premature beats are referred to as *coupled premature beats* or *a couplet* (coupled PVCs). Single premature beats that occur after every other normal sinus beat are described as occurring in *bigeminy; trigeminy* and *quadrigeminy* indicate occurrence after every third and fourth normal beat, respectively. The focus in this chapter is on nonrepetitive premature beats.

MECHANISMS

Premature beats are caused by the same mechanisms that are primarily responsible for most cardiac arrhythmias: (1) disorders of impulse conduction, represented by reentry; and (2) disorders of impulse generation, comprising abnormal automaticity and triggered activity.

Reentry

This mechanism is generally considered to account for the majority of cardiac arrhythmias. It is considered an abnormality of impulse conduction and involves reexcitation of an area of myocardium by an impulse that returns to the latter focus after traversing a circuitous route. It requires unidirectional block and may include a region of inexcitable tissue, such as a myocardial scar. Reentry accounts for what has been classically termed the *circus movement* that underlies many arrhythmias. If the circus movement results in *endless loop impulse conduction*, a sustained arrhythmia will result. Isolated premature beats occur when the impulse following the reentry pathway dissipates after a single cycle. Reentry is associated with structural, functional, or metabolic abnormalities of the myocardium (e.g., ischemia, fibrosis, drug toxicity).

Abnormal Automaticity

This mechanism refers to: (1) the occurrence of spontaneous depolarization in cardiac tissue, such as atrial and ventricular muscle that normally lacks intrinsic automaticity; and (2) increased automaticity in the His-Purkinje system, which is automatic under physiologic conditions. Conditions that can cause an abnormal increase in automaticity include ischemia, metabolic abnormalities, and drug toxicity (e.g., digitalis, catecholamine, methylxanthines).

Triggered Activity

This mechanism is defined as the generation of action potentials resulting from *afterdepolarizations*. Triggered activity differs from automaticity in that it is dependent on the previous action potential rather than representing a spontaneous depolarization. Afterdepolarizations may occur during repolarization (early afterdepolarizations) or after repolarization (delayed afterdepolarizations). Afterdepolarizations may be subthreshold and not result in a premature beat. When individual triggered action potentials reach the threshold for depolarization of the cell, premature beats appear, whereas repetitive triggered activity results in a sustained arrhythmia. Triggered activity can be caused by ischemia, digitalis, and catecholamines.

GENERAL CONCEPTS

PVCs are detected during evaluation prompted by symptoms or as incidental findings on physical examination or ECG. Appropriate management is predicated on a thorough evaluation that includes a complete history, physical examination, and relevant laboratory studies, including a standard 12-lead ECG, and, in selected patients, special techniques such as ambulatory ECG monitoring and cardiac stress testing. These methods will provide evidence not only of the presence or absence of premature beats, but also of cardiac and noncardiac conditions that may be causative factors for ectopic beats.

History

Symptoms

Symptoms are frequently suggested by complaints of palpitations, variably described by patients as an irregularity, skipped beats, or pounding. Occasionally, symptoms of dizziness, presyncope, or syncope may be related to PVCs, although they are more likely to indicate sustained tachycardia or bradyarrhythmia.

Palpitation is defined as an unpleasant perception of the heartbeat as rapid or forceful. A "skipped beat" suggests an awareness of the compensatory pause frequently associated with premature beats, and a forceful sensation is commonly related to the increased contractility and augmented ejection of the post-extrasystolic beat.

There is a frequent discrepancy between palpitations and documented arrhythmia. Thus, in many patients with and without cardiac disease, palpitations do not correlate with premature beats, but rather, they represent an unpleasant awareness of the heartbeat unassociated with any abnormality of cardiac rhythm. In these cases, the symptom is commonly attributable to anxiety. Moreover, most patients with premature beats, even in relatively high frequency, are not aware of the irregular cardiac activity. By contrast, many more patients with sustained arrhythmias are aware of the abnormality. In this regard, one study that evaluated patients with palpitations reported that the symptom had a cardiac origin in less than one half of the group. The next largest category was psychiatric conditions, most of which were related to panic disorder.

Arrhythmogenic Factors

Important potential causes of premature beats revealed by the clinical evaluation include structural heart disease (ischemic, valvular, hypertensive, primary myocardial, right ventricular dysplasia, mitral valve prolapse), noncardiac disease (pulmonary disease, hyperthyroidism, electrolyte abnormalities), drugs (digitalis, diuretics, psychotropics, sympathomimetics), and habits (caffeine, nicotine, alcohol, cocaine, ampthetamines). Optimizing therapy and/or eliminating provoking factors may be sufficient to alleviate premature beats.

Physical Examination

The physical examination provides direct evidence of premature beats by detection of an irregular pulse, and therefore in selected patients it is important in indicating the need for further, objective evaluation by ECG and other methods. However, its utility resides in positive findings, because the brevity of the examination renders it insensitive to recognition of even relatively frequent premature beats. Isolated premature beats are distinguished by interruption of a regular rhythm by intermittent, singly occurring premature beats. However, the physical examination is limited beyond this point. It cannot provide the site of origin of the abnormal beat, because all types, by definition, occur early, and each may or may not be associated with a compensatory pause. The latter characteristic is worth emphasizing; it is a common misconception that a compensatory pause is diagnostic of PVCs. Moreover, frequent premature beats of any site of origin may result in an irregularly irregular rhythm indistinguishable from atrial fibrillation, atrial flutter with variable conduction, and multifocal atrial tachycardia. PVCs may be useful in the clinical diagnosis of hypertrophic obstructive cardiomyopathy. In this disease, the pulse of the post-PVC sinus beat, assessed by physical examination, is smaller than the pulse associated with sinus rhythm, whereas in physiologically normal persons and those with systolic murmurs not related to hypertrophic obstructive cardiomyopathy, the post PVC pulse is greater than that in sinus rhythm. This phenomenon is the result of the increased obstruction to left ventricular outflow caused by the augmented contractility of the post-PVC beat (a result of the force-frequency relation of cardiac muscle). The physical examination can reveal the characteristic click murmur of mitral valve prolapse, a condition commonly associated with premature beats.

Electrocardiogram and Ambulatory Monitoring

The definitive diagnosis of premature beats requires ECG documentation. The 12-lead ECG is a simple, relatively inexpensive office method by which abnormal beats may be detected. If the rhythm is regular and symptoms are intermittent, ambulatory monitoring is the most accurate means of detecting and quantifying abnormal cardiac rhythm and its relation to symptoms and daily activity. However, this is an expensive method and should be reserved for selected patients with significant symptoms or evidence of cardiac disease. In this regard, it has been found that the diagnostic yield and cost-effectiveness of transtelephonic event monitors are superior to those of 48-hour continuous ambulatory monitoring in the assessment of patients with palpitations. An event recorder provides direct correlation of symptoms and cardiac rhythm in that, rather than yielding a continuous record, it is an ambulatory monitor that is activated by the patient when symptoms occur. The resting ECG can also provide important evidence of cardiac abnormalities that are potential causes of premature beats. Thus, pathologic Q waves indicate prior myocardial infarction or cardiomyopathy. Enlargement of ventricles or atria can be detected, and ST-T abnormalities may indicate ischemia or fibrosis. Conduction abnormalities such as left bundle branch block are also suggestive of structural heart disease. It is essential to search for ECG patterns associated with arrhythmias (e.g., long QT syndrome, Brugada's syndrome, right ventricular dysplasia, Wolf-Parkinson-White syndrome).

Exercise Testing

This type of testing is useful in selected patients. It is indicated in those with symptoms related to exertion, in whom it provides objective evidence of exercise capacity; occurrence of symptoms; response of heart rate, rhythm, and blood pressure; and evidence of myocardial ischemia. It thereby can confirm or exclude, in a controlled setting, the presence or absence of cardiac rhythm abnormalities during exertional stress and their potential causes. Exercise testing is also useful in patients whose symptoms do not occur during exertion, to evaluate their threshold for arrhythmias and to detect evidence of cardiac disease. Premature beats in most patients, with or without cardiac disease, decrease during exercise and reappear as the heart rate declines after exercise. Exercise-induced reduction in premature beats, therefore, is not evidence of the absence of cardiac disease. However, an increase in the frequency of premature beats during exercise is associated with an increased probability of underlying cardiac disease.

Echocardiography

This method provides noninvasive evaluation of cardiac systolic and diastolic function, chamber dimensions, wall thickness, and valve structure and function. Intracardiac thrombi and percardial disease are also detectable by echocardiography. Abnormalities of all these aspects of cardiac structure and function may be relevant to the origin of premature beats. In addition, the single most important factor relative to the prognostic significance of PVCs is left ventricular systolic function. Therefore, this single test provides extensive information on cardiac status in a patient with premature beats. In selected patients, stress echocardiography provides a noninvasive approach to the detection of inducible myocardial ischemia and thereby evidence of coronary artery disease.

Summary of General Approach to the Patient

Evaluation should be thorough, to confirm or exclude the presence of premature beats in patients with compatible symptoms. The correlation between symptoms and objective evidence of premature beats is frequently weak. Patients with persistent symptoms and no evidence of premature beats on screening studies require further testing by methods such as an event recorder or ambulatory ECG monitoring. Exercise testing and echocardiography provide important information of value in selected patients. The former method is useful in patients with exercise-related symptoms suggestive of premature beats, and the latter provides noninvasive cardiac evaluation for detection of the cause of premature beats and the prognostic significance of PVCs. Elimination of provoking factors is essential and may obviate the need for further therapy in many patients.

ATRIAL PREMATURE BEATS

Clinical Features

APBs can be detected by prolonged ECG monitoring in approximately 10% of persons without evidence of cardiac disease. However, the prevalence of APBs rises to 80% or more in patients with disease involving the atria, such as dilation or fibrosis. The mechanism is usually automatic foci or reentry foci in the atrium, which are promoted by structural disease, but automatic foci may result from excessive adrenergic activity. Provoking factors include most of the causes enumerated earlier and, in addition, noncardiac conditions such as infection, fever, and emotional stress, which involve sympathetic stimulation. APBs may cause symptoms, but the patient is usually not aware of them unless they are of high frequency.

Electrocardiogram

APBs are recognized on the ECG by the premature appearance and altered morphology of the P wave compared with the sinus P wave. Depending on the site of origin in the atrium and the ECG lead, alterations may include increased or decreased amplitude, widening, notching, or superimposition on the preceding T wave. APBs may be associated with: (1) a compensatory pause before the next sinus P wave, (2) a pause that is greater than compensatory, or (3) no pause. These outcomes depend on the timing of the APB and on whether it penetrates and resets the sinus node. Very early APBs may be nonconducted (blocked) and hidden in the T wave. This can result in significant bradycardia if the APBs are bigeminal. Failure to recognize this abnormality may result in inappropriate therapy, such as a pacemaker, when the proper approach is an antiarrhythmic agent to abolish the APBs and to restore sinus rhythm. APBs may also result in aberrant conduction in the His-Purkinje system, owing to impulse conduction before these fibers are fully recovered from the preceding impulse. This yields a widened QRS complex that suggests a ventricular premature beat if the premature P wave is not identified.

Management

The clinical approach to most patients with APBs consists primarily of identifying and eliminating provoking factors and optimizing treatment of underlying cardiac disease, if present. Specific antiarrhythmic therapy is usually not required unless the APBs precipitate tachycardias, in which case digitalis, a β-blocker, or a calcium channel blocker that inhibits AV node conduction can be used.

JUNCTIONAL PREMATURE BEATS

Clinical Features

JPBs are less frequent than the other two forms of premature beats. They result from abnormal automaticity or reentry mechanisms and are induced by the previously noted provoking factors, most prominent among which are digitalis toxicity, myocardial infarction, and myocarditis. They may also occur in the absence of cardiac disease.

Electrocardiogram

Because the AV junction is located between the atria and ventricles, a JPB depolarizes in both anterograde (to the ventricles) and retrograde (to the atria) directions and can therefore produce both a P wave and a QRS complex. Their sequence on the ECG depends on both the site of origin of JPB in the junctional tissue and the conductivity of the pathways. If the retrograde impulse reaches the atria before the anterograde impulse reaches the ventricles, the result will be a premature, inverted P wave followed by a premature QRS complex; if the atria and ventricles are simultaneously depolarized, the P waves will be lost in the premature QRS complex; and if the ventricles are depolarized initially, a premature QRS complex will precede the premature, inverted P wave. Aberrant conduction within the ventricles may produce a wide QRS that is indistinguishable from a ventricular premature beat.

Management

Isolated JPBs are managed by correction of the underlying process. Specific antiarrhythmic therapy is usually not warranted unless sustained tachycardia occurs.

VENTRICULAR PREMATURE BEATS

Clinical Features

PVCs are the most frequent form of premature beat. They are associated with increased prognostic risk in patients with left ventricular dysfunction and are therefore a continuing therapeutic challenge. Drug therapy to suppress PVCs to prevent serious ventricular arrhythmias has been unsuccessful and is associated with increased mortality related to proarrhythmia. PVCs encompass the entire spectrum of provoking factors, but significant impairment of left ventricular function is the most important and most difficult to treat. PVCs originate at any site in the His-Purkinje (ventricular) conducting system and depolarize the right and left ventricles consecutively (rather than nearly simultaneously as occurs normally) by abnormal routes, thus accounting for the altered QRS complex in the ECG.

Electrocardiogram

A PVC is characterized on the ECG by a premature, bizarre, wide (0.12 seconds or longer) QRS complex. The ST segment and T wave are usually directed opposite to the dominant deflection of the QRS, representing a secondary repolarization abnormality. (In the simplest terms, abnormal depolarization results in abnormal repolarization.) A retrograde P wave may be seen but is commonly obscured in the wide QRS complex. Retrograde activation of the atria may also be precluded by their prior depolarization by the normal sinus beat before the arrival of the retrograde impulse. A PVC usually results in a compensatory pause before the next sinus beat, but depending on the timing of the PVC and conduction velocity of the impulses, there may be no pause.

A wide QRS complex may represent a beat of supraventricular origin when *aberrant conduction* is present. This phenomenon occurs when a premature beat arises from a supraventricular focus before the nodal and infranodal conducting pathways (AV node, junctional tissues, and bundle branches) are completely repolarized. This abnormal conduction is reflected by aberration—distortion and widening—of the QRS complex, which can be difficult to distinguish from PVCs. This is an important distinction because of the different clinical implications of supraventricular premature beats and PVCs. Morphologic criteria have been developed to aid in discrimination of aberrantly conducted beats and PVCs. Although these criteria are helpful, they are not definitive.

Descriptors favoring aberration include antecedent P wave, right bundle branch block pattern, triphasic QRS configuration in V_1 (rsRN), and initial QRS identical to the normally conducted beats. *Descriptors favoring ventricular origin* include fusion beats, capture beats, QRS complex 140 milliseconds or longer, left axis deviation, AV dissociation, and certain configurational characteristics of the QRS (V_1: monophasic or biphasic or R>R′; V_6: QS or rS; concordance: similar QRS polarity in V_1 to V_6).

Management

In patients with and without cardiac disease, symptoms from isolated PVCs are unusual, even when the abnormal beats are frequent. The therapeutic dilemma posed by PVCs is primarily related to their importance as a risk factor for sudden death in patients with left ventricular dysfunction, a finding indicating they may be triggers for initiating lethal ventricular tachyarrhythmias. Alternatively, PVCs may be markers of electrical instability and high risk without having an initiating role. In studies of survivors of myocardial infarction, it has been established that the presence of high-grade PVCs (more than 10 per hour) increases the risk of death. Thus, the long-term mortality rate in patients with the combination of left ventricular ejection fraction of less than 40% and greater than 10 PVCs per hour was 1.5 to 2.1 times higher than the mortality rate in patients with the same ejection fraction and fewer than 10 PVCs per hour. However, as previously indicated, drug therapy to reduce mortality by eliminating or decreasing the frequency of high-grade PVCs in patients with left ventricular dysfunction, with the goal of preventing lethal arrhythmias, not only has failed to achieve this end but also has been associated with an increase in mortality.

The deleterious outcomes of drug therapy were obtained in the Cardiac Arrhythmia Suppression Trial, and they resulted in a general policy of refraining from the use of antiarrhythmic therapy in patients with asymptomatic PVCs. Amiodarone (Cordarone) has the best record of efficacy and safety for drug therapy of high-grade PVCs but it is recommended only in high-risk patients. Noninvasive techniques such as the signal-averaged ECG have been useful in identifying those patients within this population who are at the highest risk. The approach to high-grade PVCs in patients with left ventricular dysfunction comprises vigorous management of the underlying disease with the appropriate cardioprotective agents (aspirin, β-adrenergic blockade, and lipid-lowering therapy for coronary artery disease; angiotensin-converting enzyme inhibitors, a diuretic, and digitalis for left ventricular dysfunction), optimization of anti-ischemic therapy, and correction of metabolic abnormalities.

In patients with acute coronary events (myocardial infarction, unstable angina), asymptomatic PVCs may presage the development of sustained ventricular arrhythmias. Therefore, in selected patients in this setting, it is reasonable to use antiarrhythmic drug therapy (e.g., β-blockade, amiodarone). However, the first approach is elimination of provoking factors (ischemia, pain, cardiac failure, metabolic abnormalities). Patients with PVCs that impair hemodynamic function require therapy.

In patients without evidence of structural heart disease, it is clear the PVCs impose no increase in prognostic risk. Distressing palpitation should be managed by correction of provoking factors and reassurance to the patient. This approach should result in the need for drug therapy in a very small minority of this group who have intolerable palpitations associated with anxiety. The most appropriate drug is a β-blocker because of its efficacy and safety. This approach is particularly useful in patients in whom PVCs are related to adrenergic stimulation associated with exercise or emotional stress.

In summary, specific drug therapy for asymptomatic, isolated PVCs is not currently indicated in patients with or without cardiac disease. In the former, drug therapy has not been beneficial and has been associated with increased mortality. In patients without cardiac disease, PVCs are not a risk factor for more serious arrhythmias, and drug therapy should be avoided in all but exceptional cases.

HEART BLOCK

method of
KELLEY P. ANDERSON, M.D.
Marshfield Clinic
Marshfield, Wisconsin

The clinical significance of heart block lies in the risk of sudden death from asystole- and bradycardia-related ventricular tachyarrhythmias, as well as a wide variety of other signs and symptoms. Although underdiagnosis or underassessment of risk can have serious consequences, overassessment of risk can also have adverse consequences as a result of the complications associated with unnecessary diagnostic procedures and treatments. A systematic evaluation is essential to accurately estimate the risk for future events, which is the basis for selecting the most appropriate therapy.

ELECTROCARDIOGRAPHIC PATTERNS

Heart block refers to an abnormality in conduction between the atria and ventricles. First-degree atrioventricular (AV) block is defined as a prolonged PR interval (>210 ms). Third-degree or complete AV block can be permanent or transient. The latter refers to failure of AV conduction of several (arbitrarily defined, usually ≥ 4) consecutive normal atrial impulses or asystole for 3 seconds or longer. Some authorities distinguish between "third-degree" and "complete" AV block. Second-degree AV block refers to failure of conduction of some (arbitrarily defined, usually ≤ 3) consecutive atrial impulses. Failure of conduction of two or more consecutive atrial impulses is called advanced second-degree AV block. Type I AV block refers to both the classic Wenckebach pattern (progressive PR prolongation, progressive shortening of the R-R interval, and an interval in which the blocked atrial complex is less than twice the preceding R-R interval) and atypical forms, which are as common as the classic form. The general definition of type I second-degree AV block is a single blocked P wave preceded by at least two consecutive conducted P waves, with variation in the PR interval of the conducted P waves before or after the blocked P wave. The criteria for type II second-degree AV block are (1) a single blocked P wave preceded by at least two consecutive conducted P waves and followed by at least one conducted P wave, (2) constant PR intervals of the conducted P waves before and after the blocked impulse, and (3) a constant interval between the P waves. Type I and type II AV blocks are electrocardiogram (ECG) patterns that represent only a fraction of the infinite number of sequences possible in second-degree AV block. Many sequences, such as two-to-one (2:1) AV block, do not fit either definition and therefore cannot be designated type I or type II. The critical distinction between type I and type II AV block is the variation in the PR interval. The reason for the criteria of constant P-P intervals is to avoid misdiagnosis when a pattern that resembles a type II AV block occurs in the context of a sudden increase in vagal activity and is accompanied by slowing of the sinus rate. The reason for specifying conducted P waves after the blocked impulse is to exclude misinterpretation of a PR segment interrupted by a junctional escape complex. Heart block is not said to be present when block of an atrial premature beat or pseudoblock is observed. Pseudoblock is a condition whereby an ectopic beat (which may be concealed, i.e., not manifested on the ECG) results in electrical activation of the AV conduction system and causes conduction failure of a subsequent beat.

The clinical significance of the ECG pattern of a block is its association with the site of the block, which is related to the prognosis. Type II second-degree AV block is almost always caused by a block in the His-Purkinje system. Other second-degree AV block ECG patterns (type I, 2:1, and other nondiagnostic sequences) have poor sensitivity and specificity for the site of block. If the QRS duration is prolonged (=120 ms), the site of block is more likely to be within the His-Purkinje system, and if the QRS complex is shorter than 120 ms, the site of block is more likely to be within the AV node. However, the specificity is insufficient to be the sole basis for management decisions. If the escape QRS complexes in third-degree AV block are narrow, they are likely to arise from the proximal portion of the AV conduction system and suggest that the level of block is within the AV node. If the escape QRS complexes are broader than the native complexes, the site of block is more likely to be in the His-Purkinje system. However, QRS widening may result from myocardial fibrosis despite a normal conduction system. Furthermore, bundle branch and fascicular block patterns can arise from delay in the conduction tissue and do not necessarily indicate an inability to conduct.

Unsustained polymorphic ventricular tachycardia in the context of heart block should be considered a sign of impending sustained ventricular arrhythmia. QT prolongation and postpause U wave accentuation may also indicate an increased risk of bradycardia-related sustained arrhythmias.

Definitions of ECG patterns in the literature are inconsistent and subject to debate. Therefore, diagnoses should be based on analysis of multiple ECG recordings. Documentation should include descriptions of the specific rhythms, including relevant measurements, copies of ECG tracings, and definitions used to arrive at the interpretations.

MECHANISMS

Conduction in the heart is unlike conduction in common electrical circuits, and heart block is unlike an open circuit. Electrical activity in the heart normally originates in pacemaker cells and passes from cell to cell via gap junctions. Movement of electrical activation within the cell involves active and passive components that depend on ion gradients, properties of ionic channels, and ion pumps, and such movement is modulated by sympathetic and parasympathetic activity. Conduction block occurs when one or more cells fail to activate normally. It can result from a variety of mechanisms, normal and abnormal, that alter cell function, cause cell death, or disrupt gap junctions (Table 1). Myocardial and conduction tissues consist of bundles of cells arranged in roughly parallel columns with many cross-links. Conduction block in a single cell has little impact because conduction occurring in adjacent parallel cells activates all downstream cells with almost no additional delay. Failure of activation of all cells at a particular level is necessary for complete block, which may explain the resilience of the AV node to permanent block because it is composed of a relatively large amount of tissue with multiple potential pathways. In contrast, the His bundle, bundle branches, and fascicles are comparatively narrow structures with little capacity for alternative conduction pathways

TABLE 1. **Mechanisms of Conduction Disturbances**

Prolonged refractory period (vagal activity, drugs, ischemia)
Sarcolemmal ion gradient disturbances (hyperkalemia, hypokalemia)
Sodium channel blockade (lidocaine, procainamide, flecainide, amiodarone, imipramine, etc.)
Calcium channel blockade (verapamil, diltiazem)
Energy depletion (ischemia, cyanide)
Cell dysfunction (inflammation, barotrauma, thermal injury)
Cell death (apoptosis, ischemic necrosis, inflammatory necrosis, surgical trauma, ablation)
Congenital structural defects (endocardial cushion defects)
Gap junction disturbances (fibrosis, edema, inflammation, genetic defects)

within each structure. If many but not all adjacent cells fail, a delay in activation of downstream tissue may occur because the conduction sequence follows a more circuitous route. Thus, a partial conduction block may appear as a delay in conduction. Conduction delay can also occur if the conduction velocity within the cell or across the gap junction is reduced. Slowing of conduction may be indistinguishable from conduction block if conduction through an alternate route is faster than through the damaged normal path. This mechanism explains why conduction may occur in a bundle or fascicle despite the appearance of a bundle branch block or fascicle block on the ECG.

The functional status of subsidiary pacemakers determines whether a complete AV block results in mild bradycardia or life-threatening asystole. Involvement in the pathologic process is suggested by frequent failure and slow rates of subsidiary pacemakers in patients with AV block, but the mechanisms are unknown. A number of drugs, including most antiarrhythmic agents, suppress subsidiary rhythms.

The mechanism of bradycardia-induced ventricular tachyarrhythmias is unknown. It is known that bradyarrhythmias precipitate torsades de pointes in the presence of electrolyte disturbances, genetic abnormalities in ion channel function, heart failure, and myocardial hypertrophy. Drug-induced torsades de pointes is more likely to occur during bradycardia. A comprehensive list of drugs that may account for bradyarrhythmia-related ventricular arrhythmias is available at *www.torsades.org*.

TABLE 2. **Etiologies of Heart Block**

Etiologies
Frequently Permanent or Progressive (Examples)
Alcohol septal ablation (acute, delayed)
Cardiomyopathies (hypertrophic, idiopathic, mitochondrial)
Catheter ablation (AV nodal reentry, accessory AV connections)
Congenital heart block (lupus)
Congenital heart disease (endocardial cushion defects)
Genetic disorders (sodium channel mutations)
Idiopathic fibrosis and calcification (Lev's disease, Lenègre's disease)
Infectious disorders—destructive (endocarditis)
Infiltrative disorders (amyloidosis)
Neuromyopathic disorders (myotonic dystrophy, Erb's dystrophy, peroneal muscular atrophy)
Noninfectious inflammatory disorders (HLA-B27–associated disorder, sarcoidosis)
Tumors (mesothelioma)
Frequently Transient or Reversible (Examples)
Blunt trauma (baseball)
Cardiac surgery (valve replacement)
Cardiac transplant rejection
Central nervous system
Drugs (antiarrhythmics, digoxin, edrophonium)
Electrolyte disturbances (hyperkalemia)
Metabolic disturbances (hypothermia, hypothyroidism)
Increased vagal activity
Infectious disorders—nondestructive (Lyme disease)
Myocardial ischemia
Myocarditis (Chagas' disease, giant cell myocarditis)
Rheumatic fever

ETIOLOGY

The list of disorders associated with heart block continues to expand. Several disorders result in progressive conduction system disturbances for which no cure has been identified. In clinical practice, however, the etiology is usually based on circumstantial evidence only. It is therefore difficult to exclude the presence of an occult disorder or two superimposed disorders. In individual circumstances, any of the etiologic classes listed in Table 2 could be permanent or transient, thus emphasizing the need to bring together all pertinent information when selecting treatment.

SIGNS AND SYMPTOMS

The duration of asystole or the heart rate during complete heart block depends on the rate of subsidiary pacemakers beyond the level of block. In second-degree AV block, the sinus rate, the conduction ratio, and the rate of subsidiary pacemakers all affect the resulting heart rate. Many patients with heart block have a reduction in the rate and reliability of subsidiary pacemakers. Asystole or severe bradycardia may cause sudden death by inadequate cerebral perfusion. The effects of bradycardia resulting from heart block depend on many factors, including body orientation, vasomotor tone, underlying cardiac function, the presence of valvular abnormalities, and the presence of cerebral vascular disease. Most signs and symptoms that occur shortly after the onset of heart block are due to reduced cerebral perfusion. However, inadequate cardiac output may affect other organs and cause metabolic changes that eventually produce symptoms. In some patients, symptoms attributable to conduction abnormalities have no obvious effect on cardiac output but probably cause changes in cardiac performance, to which some patients are unusually sensitive. Such abnormalities include PR prolongation, irregularities in rhythm, and atrial contraction against closed AV valves. Loss of the normal chronotropic response to exercise may also cause symptoms in some patients but not cause symptoms at rest. Conduction block may be rate dependent and occur in the presence of either bradycardia or tachycardia. Stress- or exercise-induced heart block may result from ischemia. Bradycardia-induced ventricular tachyarrhythmias are another frequent cause of sudden death, cardiac arrest, and syncope in patients with heart block. Patients at risk for heart block often have significant cardiovascular disease and may have symptoms for many other reasons.

METHODS USED IN THE ASSESSMENT OF HEART BLOCK

No laboratory or imaging tests are able to provide direct information about the pathologic state of the AV conduction system or reliably predict whether heart block will occur or, if present, whether it will be transient or permanent. Instead, these outcomes must be inferred from indirect evidence or past experience.

A comprehensive evaluation to exclude all causes of heart block includes invasive tests such as coronary angiography and myocardial biopsy, as well as a large number of specific laboratory tests. The objective of the initial evaluation is to obtain sufficient information to focus additional testing on a few specific disorders.

ECG recordings are used in patients with cardiac arrest, syncope, or transient symptoms to verify heart block and to exclude other mechanisms. Hospital monitoring is needed if immediate intervention is necessary, but subtle arrhythmias with prognostic significance, such as nonconducted P waves, may not be detected even by event detection algorithms or by human observers, who usually monitor many patients simultaneously. In contrast, Holter recordings are analyzed in detail to detect all arrhythmias on multiple channels by computer and a technician, and they are over-read by a cardiologist. Holter recordings are therefore indicated even in monitored hospitalized patients, as well as outpatients, when evidence of heart block is elusive. Holter monitoring may also provide important evidence that ambient arrhythmias are not causing significant symptoms. ECG documentation of the association (or lack of association) between heart block and symptoms provides the most reliable evidence for selection of therapy. The method used to obtain ECG documentation depends on the frequency of symptoms. Holter monitors provide high-fidelity recordings from multiple-lead sets but are inconvenient for recording periods longer than 48 hours. Most external loop recorders provide only a single ECG channel but can be used for periods of weeks to months. Implantable loop recorders provide continuous loop recording for 14 months or more.

Electrophysiologic studies allow precise measurement of AV node and His-Purkinje system function and can provide definitive information regarding the site of block if the conduction disturbance occurs during the study. Additional tests have been developed that "stress" the AV conduction system, including rapid atrial and ventricular pacing, administration of antiarrhythmic drugs such as procainamide and disopyramide, and combinations of drugs and pacing maneuvers. Provocation of conduction failures is assumed to indicate a propensity for spontaneous AV block. Unfortunately, the sensitivity is low, and a negative test does not imply a low risk of future episodes. Electrophysiologic studies have the additional advantage of providing immediate test results, as well as the results of programmed stimulation for provocation of supraventricular and ventricular tachyarrhythmias. Nevertheless, electrophysiologic studies do not provide the certainty and reliability of documented spontaneous arrhythmias.

THERAPY

Selection of the correct therapeutic approach should balance the risks and benefits of therapy against the risks of heart block for both immediate and long-term management. Pharmacologic agents are useful for emergency, temporary, and standby heart support in selected circumstances. The standby mode is accomplished by a prepared infusion at the bedside. To avoid excessive doses at the time of asystole or severe bradycardia, the optimal dose can be established in advance by test doses starting at low infusion rates. Atropine (0.5 to 3.0 mg or 0.04 mg/kg intravenously [IV]) is useful for the treatment or pretreatment of patients in whom heart block develops at the level of the AV node in the context of elevated vagal tone, such as in association with nausea or endotracheal tube suction. Atropine should be avoided in patients with an infranodal AV block because prolonged asystole may sometimes occur as a result of more frequent His-Purkinje system depolarization from an increased sinus rate. Vagal activity inhibits sympathetic activity, so a reduction in vagal tone by atropine disinhibits sympathetic activity and may account for the unpredictable effects of atropine on heart rate. Elevations in heart rate after atropine can persist for hours and cannot be readily reversed. Aminophylline* (2.5 to 6.3 mg/kg IV) is reported to reverse heart block resistant to atropine and epinephrine by antagonizing adenosine. Stimulation of β-adrenergic receptors increases sinus and subsidiary pacemaker rates, AV node and His-Purkinje system conduction velocities, and myocardial contractility. The effective refractory period is shortened in most tissue, but this effect varies with dose and the specific tissue type. Dobutamine (Dobutrex), 2.5 to 40 μg/kg/min, is a useful β-adrenergic receptor agonist because it increases cardiac output and lowers filling pressure without an excessive rise or fall in blood pressure. Isoproterenol (Isuprel), 0.02 to 0.06 mg as an IV bolus and then 0.5 to 10.0 μg/min by IV infusion, stimulates β_1- and β_2-adrenergic receptors and enhances vasodilation more than the other catecholamines do. This effect can result in unwanted hypotension in some circumstances, but isoproterenol is also less likely than other drugs to cause a reflex increase in vagal tone. Epinephrine (1-mg IV boluses for cardiac arrest, 0.2 to 1 mg subcutaneously, 0.5 to 5 μg/min IV) stimulates both α- and β-adrenergic receptors. It is recommended for asystolic cardiac arrest, in part because it increases myocardial and cerebral flow. However, the increase in systemic vascular resistance may be detrimental by augmenting metabolic acidosis and decreasing cardiac performance in patients with poor left ventricular function. The suggested dose ranges are broad because the response to β-adrenergic stimulants, such as improved AV conduction, varies widely and may be affected by β-adrenergic receptor down-regulation in patients with chronic elevations in sympathetic activity, such as those with long-standing heart failure. Any of the aforementioned agents may precipitate tachyarrhythmias by direct electrophysiologic effects mediated by adrenergic receptors and by indirect effects such as myocardial ischemia, and they may worsen hemodynamic status. The adverse effects of catecholamines are time dependent and cumulative.

*Not FDA approved for this use

Ischemia and receptor-mediated electrophysiologic effects occur immediately after administration, changes in gene expression of ion channels begin as early as several hours, and long-term alterations such as myocardial hypertrophy, apoptosis, and fibrosis usually begin to occur within 24 hours but may require much longer periods. The clinical significance of these effects is uncertain but suggests that the duration and dose of catecholamine infusions should be limited.

Temporary pacing can be achieved by transcutaneous, transvenous, transthoracic, transesophageal, and transgastric approaches. Transcutaneous pacing can be used in various standby modes, and the same cutaneous pads provide ECG monitoring and quick access to countershock. Although it avoids the risks of drugs and invasive methods, transcutaneous ventricular pacing cannot be accomplished in some patients despite the highest energies and multiple electrode positions. Furthermore, transcutaneous pacing is often painful, so most conscious patients require sedation. For these reasons, its principal uses are for short-term pacing during cardiopulmonary resuscitation and standby pacing in patients at risk for bradyarrhythmias. If the risk of bradycardia is high, ventricular capture should be verified in advance. Capture is often difficult to ascertain because transcutaneous stimuli cause large deflections on the ECG and pectoral muscle stimulation can be confused with a pulse. Capture should be verified by careful ECG analysis at subthreshold and suprathreshold stimulus amplitudes and confirmed by appropriately timed femoral artery pulses, Korotkoff sounds, or arterial pressure waveforms.

Transvenous insertion of an electrode catheter is the method of choice for most patients who require temporary pacing. This approach is reliable and safe when performed by competent staff with strict aseptic technique, fluoroscopic guidance, and appropriate catheters. Complications include inadequate pacing or sensing thresholds, vascular complications, pneumothorax, myocardial perforation, infection, and dislodgment. Small studies suggest that long-term (>5 days) temporary pacing can be safely and reliably accomplished with active-fixation permanent pacemaker leads attached to an external standard pulse generator. Tunneling the lead may enhance stability and reduce the risk of infection.

Permanent pacemakers are highly effective, safe, and cost-effective, with few contraindications. Although the complications are rarely life threatening, they should be carefully considered and acknowledged. Septicemia or endocarditis has been reported in 0.5% of patients. In patients with pacemaker-related endocarditis, in-hospital mortality is reported to be over 7% with a 20-month mortality of more than 25%. The rate of significant complications has been reported to be 3.5%. About 10% of pacemakers will become infected or have some other type of failure that may require extraction. In a recent series, the rate of major complications associated with extraction was 1.4%. Permanent pacemakers are associated with a long-term, continuous risk of infection, thrombosis, and erosion. In young persons, generators and leads need to be periodically replaced, which limits venous access sites while unused leads accumulate or must be extracted. Perhaps of greater consequence is the constant inconvenience of lifelong follow-up, electromagnetic interference, and false alarms from electronic surveillance devices, as well as exclusion from important procedures such as magnetic resonance imaging of the thorax. Moreover, pacing from the right ventricular apex, which is currently the most common ventricular pacing site, may have long-term detrimental effects.

APPROACH TO THE PATIENT

The objective of evaluation and management for heart block is to prevent adverse effects by (1) heart rate support in patients with poorly tolerated bradycardia; (2) monitoring and standby heart rate support in stable patients at high risk for asystole or severe bradycardia; (3) identification and treatment of reversible causes of heart block; (4) identification of patients at high risk for sudden death, syncope, or recurrent symptoms; and (5) selection and implantation of the appropriate rate support device as soon as safety permits.

Advanced cardiac life support guidelines apply to patients who are unresponsive or severely compromised by heart block. However, heart block is rarely the primary problem, so evaluation and treatment of other disorders should continue while efforts to increase the heart rate are under way.

The initial evaluation should include a thorough history and physical examination, review of current and previous ECGs and rhythm strips, and laboratory tests to determine whether heart block is present or whether the patient has a significant risk of heart block occurring in the future and, if so, a differential diagnosis of possible etiologies. The patient should then be stratified for the appropriate level of care: (1) an unstable patient who requires ongoing evaluation and treatment in an intensive care setting, (2) a stable patient at very high risk for asystole or complications who needs temporary transvenous pacing or other invasive procedures, (3) a patient at moderate risk who requires continuous monitoring and standby noninvasive heart rate support measures, (4) a patient at low risk who requires rapid but not immediate access to heart rate support measures that hospital monitoring provides, and (5) a patient at low risk who can be evaluated and managed as an outpatient.

Patients initially evaluated after resuscitated cardiac arrest, after syncope, or with ECG abnormalities that indicate conduction system abnormalities usually belong in one of the first four categories. The fifth category generally includes patients with mild symptoms and no suggestive ECG abnormalities and patients whose risk is estimated to be low after inpatient monitoring or previous evaluation. The most common scenario is a patient who has symptoms that could be due to heart block as well as other arrhythmic or nonarrhythmic causes. In such patients, ECG confirmation of the relationship between heart block and symptoms should be obtained.

Determination of the need for long-term heart rate support, as well as other issues that may affect the selection of implantable device (e.g., risk for ventricular tachyarrhythmias), should be accomplished as soon as possible because the risk of complications and the anxiety associated with temporary heart rate support measures increase over time. Major societies have developed guidelines for implantable rhythm management devices (*http://www.acc.org/clinical/statements.htm*). The reasons for the selected therapy, including the rationale for any deviation from established guidelines, should be documented and provided to the patient. This practice will reduce future confusion or misunderstanding about the original rationale for implantation, which can affect the management of patients with device complications and those with a compelling need for device upgrade or explantation.

Patients with acute coronary syndromes require special consideration. The incidence of heart block in patients with myocardial infarction (when creatine phosphokinase is used as the marker of necrosis) is approximately 10%. Although the incidence is probably lower when more sensitive markers such as troponin are used, heart block is still likely to be associated with increased in-hospital mortality because of larger infarct size. Bradycardia reduces myocardial oxygen consumption. Therefore, overcorrection of the heart rate must be avoided and ischemia should be relieved by increasing perfusion as soon as possible. Studies in the prethrombolytic era did not demonstrate a benefit in mortality with prophylactic temporary transvenous pacing, and complications were frequent. The risk of transvenous insertion may be higher in patients who require the administration of thrombolytics and other anticoagulants. Catheter-based revascularization methods should be given strong consideration because of their established effectiveness and the possible avoidance of thrombolytic drugs and because transvenous temporary pacing, if needed, is readily and safely accomplished during the procedure. Suggestions for standby temporary pacing (Table 3) should take into consideration the risk of transvenous pacing based on local circumstances (experience, fluoroscopic guidance, insertion site, use of anticoagulants, etc.). Most conduction disturbances associated with myocardial ischemia or infarction resolve quickly, but they can persist for days or weeks. The need for implantation of a permanent pacemaker as a consequence of myocardial infarction is rare, and prophylactic pacemaker implantation in high-risk subsets has not been shown to reduce mortality. Guidelines for temporary and permanent pacing in patients with acute myocardial infarction have been published (*http://www.acc.org/clinical/statements.htm*; *http://www.escardio.org*).

TABLE 3. **Suggestions for Temporary Pacing in Acute Myocardial Infarction**

Transvenous Pacing

Asystole or poorly tolerated bradycardia unresponsive to atropine or aminophylline
Persistent third-degree AV block
Alternating RBBB and LBBB, or RBBB and alternating LAFB and LPFB
Bifascicular block, new
Second-degree AV block (any type) and QRS ≥110 ms
Any indication listed below at the time of cardiac catheterization if performed

Standby Transcutaneous Pacing

Any indication listed above until a transvenous pacing system is inserted
Transient asystole or poorly tolerated bradycardia
Bifascicular block, uncertain time of onset or old
Second-degree AV block (any type) and QRS <110 ms
New first-degree AV block

Abbreviations: AV = atrioventricular; RBBB, LBBB = right, left bundle branch block; LAFB, LPFB = left anterior, left posterior fascicle block.

CONCLUSIONS

Heart block remains a challenge because prediction of symptomatic heart block (who and when) is still very limited and therapy guidelines are based on expert opinion or small studies. Although safe and effective treatments are widely available, they are associated with sufficient adverse effects that their use should be avoided in patients with minimal risk of asystole or clinically significant bradycardia. Fortunately, advances in molecular biology suggest that we are on the threshold of major advances in understanding the pathophysiology of cardiac conduction disturbances; this improved understanding should produce diagnostic tests and treatments that will relegate pacemakers to museum pieces.

TACHYCARDIAS

method of
KIMBERLY ANNE SELZMAN, M.D., and
MICHAEL J. REITER, M.D., PH.D.
University of Colorado Health Sciences Center
Denver, Colorado

Tachycardia, defined in adults as a heart rate exceeding 100 beats per minute (bpm), can be either a normal (i.e., physiologic) response or a nonphysiologic arrhythmia. Sinus tachycardia in the setting of physical exertion, emotional stress, or underlying fever, hypotension, or volume contraction is a normal response. In certain situations, however, sinus tachycardia is nonphysiologic (see later). Other supraventricular tachycardias (SVTs) and ventricular tachycardias (VTs), though sometimes precipitated by physiologic stress or sympathetic stimulation, are not considered normal, even in the absence of underlying heart disease.

SVTs are arrhythmias that originate proximal to the bifurcation of the bundle of His and typically involve the atria and/or atrioventricular (AV) node. VT is an arrhythmia that originates either in conduction tissue distal to the bifurcation of the His bundle or from one of the ventricles. VT most commonly occurs in the presence of underlying heart disease; SVT often occurs in its absence.

The first step in managing any tachycardia is to diagnose the arrhythmia. Distinction between SVT and VT can usually be made on the basis of the 12-lead echocardiographic (ECG) characteristics (Figure 1). It is critical to distinguish SVT from VT because management as well as prognosis are very different. Importantly, SVT and VT cannot be differentiated by symptoms, heart rate, or blood pressure during tachycardia. VT is invariably associated with a wide QRS complex (i.e., greater than 120 msec), whereas SVT usually has a narrow QRS complex. However, SVT may be associated with a wide QRS complex in the presence of a fixed or rate-related bundle branch block. A wide QRS complex tachycardia in a patient who has had a previous infarction or has significant left ventricular dysfunction is usually VT.

It is also important to examine the relationship between the P waves and QRS complexes during tachycardia. VT can be characterized by 1:1 ventriculoatrial (VA) conduction, some degree of VA block with more QRS complexes than P waves, or VA dissociation. Some types of SVT, such as atrial flutter and atrial tachycardia, have 2:1 AV conduction (or higher degrees of AV block) but not more QRS complexes than P waves. Adenosine typically has no effect on VT, but many SVTs are terminated with intravenous adenosine. With other SVTs, adenosine may cause AV block without terminating the tachycardia (Table 1).

Clinical tachycardias typically result from one of three electrophysiologic mechanisms: (1) *enhanced automaticity*—an acceleration or development of spontaneously firing cells that normally fire slowly or not at all; (2) *triggered activity*—a spontaneous firing of cells in response to a previous depolarization; or (3) *reentry*—a continuous, repetitive loop of myocardial activation. Although this classification may have some clinical utility (e.g., reentry tachycardias usually start and terminate abruptly and can be cardioverted), it is often not possible to distinguish a specific mechanism clinically.

In patients with episodic symptoms that may be secondary to a tachycardia, it is important to correlate their symptoms with an arrhythmia. A 24-hour Holter monitor or an event-recording monitor may be useful. Additional studies such as an echocardiogram to clarify the presence of underlying heart disease or an ischemia evaluation may also be beneficial.

Specific goals of therapy might include acute termination of tachycardia, prevention of recurrences, or amelioration of a chronic or recurring arrhythmia. Treatment options for acute termination include intravenous medical therapy or cardioversion if the patient is hemodynamically unstable. The approach to long-term treatment is influenced by many factors, including the patient's tolerance of the arrhythmia, the frequency of recurrence, and the expected course and prognosis of the particular arrhythmia, as well as the general medical condition of the patient. Most cases of VT are treated with antiarrhythmic therapy and automatic cardioverter-defibrillator implantation. For chronic treatment of SVTs, multiple options may be used, including oral AV node–blocking medications, antiarrhythmic agents, radiofrequency ablation, or rarely, surgery. Minimally symptomatic or infrequent tachycardias may not require any chronic therapy.

Radiofrequency ablation is an invasive procedure that uses radiofrequency energy to create a thermal lesion. The energy is delivered through a catheter tip placed in close proximity to the origin of the tachycardia under fluoroscopic and electrophysiologic guidance. Ablation is usually an outpatient or an overnight-stay procedure performed with conscious sedation. Success and complication rates depend on the specific tachycardia being ablated.

A general guide to the diagnosis and management of tachycardias is presented, but this area of cardiology is rapidly evolving. The use of antiarrhythmic agents has been supplanted, in many cases, by radiofrequency

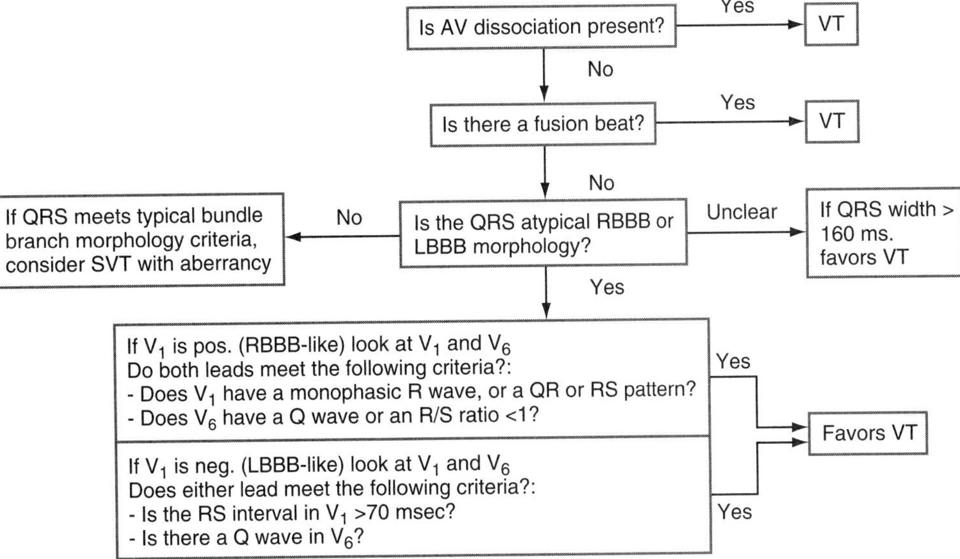

Figure 1. Algorithm to distinguish supraventricular tachycardia (SVT) from ventricular tachycardia (VT). AV, atrioventricular; LBBB, left bundle branch block; RBBB, right bundle branch block.

TABLE 1. **Electrocardiographic Features of Supraventricular Tachycardias**

Tachycardia	P Morphology	AV Relationship	RP Relationship*	AV Node Dependent†	Response To Adenosine (Adenocard)‡
Sinus Tach	Same as sinus	1:1	Long RP	No	Transient suppression of sinus and/or AV block
AVNRT	Retrograde,§ buried in QRS	Usually 1:1, may be 2:1 AV or VA block	Very short RP	Yes	Usually terminates with block in the AV node
AVRT	Retrograde	1:1	Short RP	Yes	Usually terminates with block in the AV node
ART	Retrograde	1:1	Short RP	Yes	Usually terminates with block in the AV node
Atrial Tach	Different from sinus	Usually 1:1 or 2:1 AV block	Usually long RP, can be short	No	Transient suppression, termination, or AV block
MAT	At least 3 different P waves	Usually 1:1	Long RP, variable	No	Transient AV block, will not terminate tachycardia
Atrial fibrillation	No discrete P waves	Variable	Not applicable	No	Increased AV block, will not terminate
Atrial flutter	Flutter, saw tooth	Usually 2:1, variable	Not applicable	No	Flutter waves with high-grade AV block

*The RP interval is termed *long RP* if the RP distance is greater than half the distance between the two QRS complexes. *Short RP* refers to an RP distance less than half the QRS-to-QRS interval.

†*AV node dependent* indicates that the AV node is an obligate component of the tachycardia mechanism.

‡Adenosine is not FDA-approved for diagnosing SVT.

§A retrograde P wave is a P wave, or atrial depolarization, caused by retrograde conduction from either the AV node or an accessory pathway and is negative in leads II, III, and aVF.

ART, antidromic reciprocating tachycardia; AV, atrioventricular; AVNRT, AV nodal reentry tachycardia; AVRT, AV reciprocating tachycardia; MAT, multifocal atrial tachycardia; Tach, tachycardia; VA, ventriculoatrial.

ablation or defibrillator implantation, for which referral to an electrophysiologist is appropriate.

SUPRAVENTRICULAR TACHYCARDIAS

Sinus Tachycardias

Sinus tachycardia originates from the sinus node and has a characteristic P wave morphology. As mentioned, it is most often an appropriate physiologic response, and treatment is directed toward the underlying condition. *Sinus node reentry tachycardia* is an unusual, nonphysiologic sinus tachycardia that is paroxysmal (abrupt in onset and termination) and without any correlation to physiologic conditions. This tachycardia terminates with intravenous adenosine (Adenocard) or esmolol (Brevibloc). Chronically, patients tend to respond to AV node–blocking agents (β-blockers or calcium channel blockers). *Inappropriate sinus tachycardia* is a nonparoxysmal sinus tachycardia in which the heart rate is dramatically exaggerated with exercise but the normal circadian rhythm is maintained with a decreased (and usually normal) heart rate during sleep. Treatment options include AV node–blocking medications (high-dose β-blocker therapy approaching or exceeding the recommended dosage may be required) or radiofrequency ablation in very symptomatic patients to modify the sinus node.

Paroxysmal Supraventricular Tachycardia

Paroxysmal SVT (PSVT) is a term used to describe a clinical syndrome encompassing recurrent episodes of SVT with an abrupt onset and termination, often in otherwise healthy patients without structural heart disease and with normal ECG findings during sinus rhythm. It is most frequently due to either AV node reentry tachycardia or AV reciprocating tachycardia, but it may be due to other tachycardia mechanisms as well. Although stress or excess caffeine intake can precipitate episodes, most often no particular activity is associated with the initiation of tachycardia in these patients. The frequency and severity of symptoms are variable and can range from mild palpitations to syncope.

Both AV node reentry tachycardia and AV reciprocating tachycardia are narrow complex, regular tachycardias (Figure 2). They are reentrant arrhythmias that use the AV node as part of the reentrant circuit. Therefore, maneuvers or medications that depress conduction through the AV node often terminate the episode. Vagal maneuvers such as carotid massage, the Valsalva maneuver, and the diving reflex (induced by putting the patient's face in cold water) are often successful. These maneuvers are an effective chronic strategy in certain patients. Intravenous adenosine or esmolol, by blocking conduction through the AV node, also terminate these tachycardias.

AV Nodal Reentry Tachycardia

AV nodal reentry tachycardia is due to a reentrant circuit within or around the AV node that conducts to the atria and ventricles almost simultaneously. Often, the P wave is not apparent (because it is simultaneous with the QRS complex), or it is seen at the tail end of the QRS. The P wave can deform the QRS and cause a pseudo R′ morphology in lead V_1 that is not present on the sinus rhythm electrocardiogram.

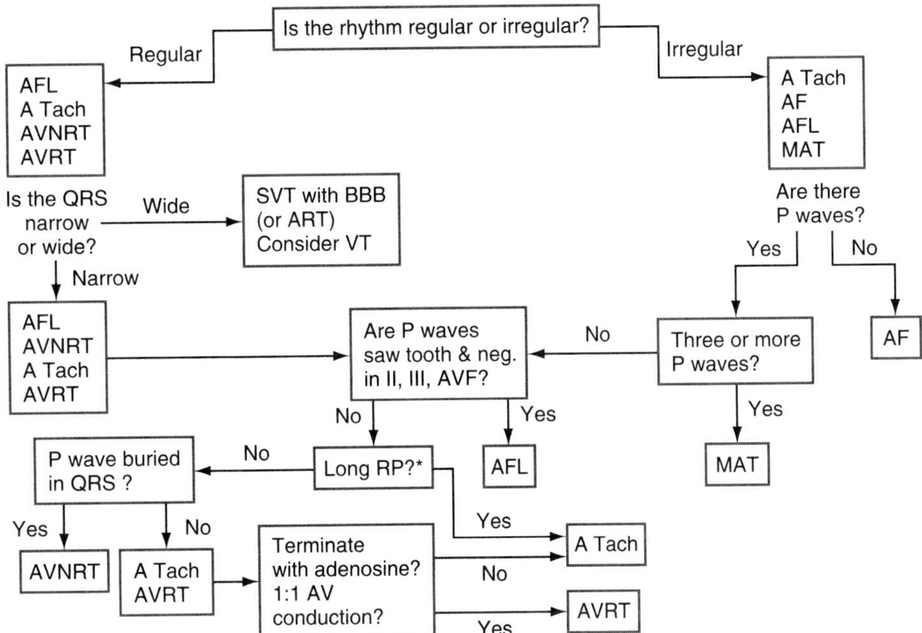

Figure 2. Algorithm for diagnosing supraventricular arrhythmias by electrocardiographic criteria.
*Long RP occurs when the distance from QRS to the next P wave is greater than half the distance between the two QRS complexes. AF, atrial fibrillation; AFL, atrial flutter; ART, antidromic reciprocating tachycardia; A Tach, atrial tachycardia; AV, atrioventricular; AVNRT, AV nodal reentry tachycardia; AVRT, AV reciprocating tachycardia; BBB, bundle branch block; MAT, multifocal atrial tachycardia; SVT, supraventricular tachycardia.

The ventricular rate is typically in the range of 150 to 250 bpm.

AV nodal reentry tachycardia is the most common type of PSVT. Although it can occur at any age, it usually becomes apparent in young to middle-aged adults. Initially, it is often infrequent and readily terminable with vagal maneuvers, but over time it may become more frequent, longer lasting, and more difficult to terminate. Adenosine is effective in terminating acute episodes. The long-term prognosis is excellent. In patients with infrequent episodes and known precipitants of episodes (e.g., nicotine or caffeine), avoidance of these offenders may be sufficient. For long-term treatment in more symptomatic patients, daily β-blockers or calcium channel blockers can be used to help prevent episodes. Class IC or IA agents may be used in patients without structural heart disease (Table 2), the former with usually fewer side effects. Class III agents may also be effective. Antiarrhythmics are rarely used now that radiofrequency ablation is so widely available and successful. Radiofrequency ablation is the treatment of choice in patients whose tachycardia has become drug resistant or in patients intolerant of drug therapy. In most centers, "cure rates" approach 95% to 98% and complication rates are approximately 1%.

AV Reciprocating Tachycardia

An accessory pathway is an AV connection that bypasses the AV node. It is due to abnormal embryologic development in which atrial tissue extends across the AV groove and allows electrical continuity. It is not usually associated with other congenital cardiac defects. If an accessory pathway conducts anterogradely (i.e., from atrium to ventricle), it is manifested by ECG changes referred to as "preexcitation," and the patient is said to have Wolff-Parkinson-White (WPW) syndrome (discussed later). If the accessory pathway only conducts retrogradely (i.e., from ventricle to atrium), it is referred to as a "concealed accessory pathway." Typically, patients with an accessory pathway can experience AV reciprocating tachycardia (also known as orthodromic reciprocating tachycardia), which is a reentrant rhythm with anterograde conduction over the AV node–His–Purkinje system and retrograde conduction over the accessory pathway.

Similar to AV nodal reentry tachycardia, AV reciprocating tachycardia is a narrow complex, regular tachycardia with ventricular rates ranging from 150 to 250 bpm. It is the second most common type of PSVT referred for electrophysiologic evaluation. Because the accessory pathway can conduct relatively quickly, the P wave is not usually too far from the preceding QRS complex, but it is often distinct and follows the QRS complex by approximately 60 to 90 msec. AV reciprocating tachycardia always has 1:1 AV conduction (Figure 3). Because the AV node is an obligate part of the circuit, initial long-term medical therapy in symptomatic patients is often with a β-blocker or calcium channel blocker. Approximately half the patients may respond to these safe and well-tolerated therapies. For more refractory patients, pharmacologic therapy may include class IC or IA agents (in patients without structural heart disease), sotalol (Betapace),* or amiodarone (Cordarone).* For patients unable or unwilling to undergo long-term medical therapy, radiofrequency ablation is appropriate. Ablation is 85% to 95%

*Not FDA-approved for this indication.

TABLE 2. **General Guide to Antiarrhythmic Therapy**

Vaughn Williams Class	Specific Agent	Preparation/Dosage	Typical Use	Comments
Class IA effect: Na channel blockade; used currently prolongs RP, QT interval			Prevention of SVT in patients without SHD	Rarely used currently to prevent VT Increased mortality has been found when used in patients with SHD
	Procainamide (Pronestyl)	IV: load = 1 g; infusion = 1-4 mg/min PO: 250-500 mg q6h	Termination of VT or AFib Prevention of SVT	Especially appropriate in patients with WPW and well-tolerated AFib
	Quinidine (Quinaglute)	PO: 324-648 mg q8-12h	Prevention of SVT	
	Disopyramide (Norpace)	PO: 200-400 mg bid	Prevention of SVT	
Class IB effect: Na channel blockade	Lidocaine (Xylocaine)	IV: load = 1 mg/kg; infusion = 1-4 mg/min	Termination or prevention of VT	Probably less effective than amiodarone or procainamide except during active ischemia
	Mexiletine (Mexitil)	PO: 200-300 mg q8h	Prevention of VT	Contraindicated if heart block is present
Class IC effect: Na channel blockade			Prevention of SVT in patients without SHD	Increased mortality has been found when used in patients with SHD or ischemia
	Flecainide (Tambocor)	PO: 50-150 mg q12h	Prevention of SVT	Contraindicated if heart block is present
	Propafenone (Rythmol)	PO: 150-300 mg q8h	Prevention of SVT	May be used orally on a prn basis to terminate AFib or flutter
Class II effect: β-blockade			Prevention of SVT Decrease VR in SVT	
	Metoprolol (Lopressor)	PO: 25-100 mg bid	Prevention of SVT	Multiple oral β-blockers are available. Metoprolol is shown as an example
	Esmolol (Brevibloc)	IV: load = 500 μg/kg; infusion = 50-200 μg/kg/min	Decrease VR in SVT Decrease VR in SVT	Esmolol is the preferred IV preparation due to its short half-life
Class III effect: prolongs RP, QT interval			Prevention of SVT or VT	These drugs can prolong the QT interval and be proarrhythmic; are often initiated in the hospital
	Sotalol (Betapace)	PO: 80-160 mg bid	Prevention of SVT or VT	Dosage interval decreased with renal failure
	Dofetilide (Tikosyn)	PO: 125-500 mg bid	Prevention of SVT	Dosage decreased with renal failure
	Amiodarone (Cordarone)	IV: load = 150 mg, then 1 mg/min × 6 h, then 0.5 mg/min × 18 h PO: 200-400 mg qd	Termination of VT Prevention of SVT or VT	Often started with an oral load (800-1200 mg qd)
	Ibutilide (Corvert)	IV: 0.01 mg/kg up to 1 mg over 10 min	Cardiovert AFib, atrial flutter	Best given through a central line
Class IV effect: Ca channel blockade			Prevention of SVT Decrease VR in SVT	Dihydropyridines have no significant AV nodal–blocking effect
	Verapamil (Calan)	PO: 120-240 mg bid		
	Diltiazem (Cardizem)	IV: 5- to 15-mg/h infusion PO: 120-360 mg qd		Should avoid if tachycardia is possibly VT
Miscellaneous	Digoxin (Lanoxin)	IV: load, 0.5 mg, then 0.25 mg q6h × 2 doses PO: 0.25-0.625 mg qd	Decrease VR in SVT	Should be avoided in patients with WPW
	Adenosine (Adenocard)	IV: 6- to 12-mg bolus	Termination of SVT	Diagnostically useful

AFib, atrial fibrillation; RP, refractory period; SVT, supraventricular arrhythmias; SHD, structural heart disease; VR, ventricular rate; VT, ventricular tachycardia; WPW, Wolff-Parkinson-White syndrome.

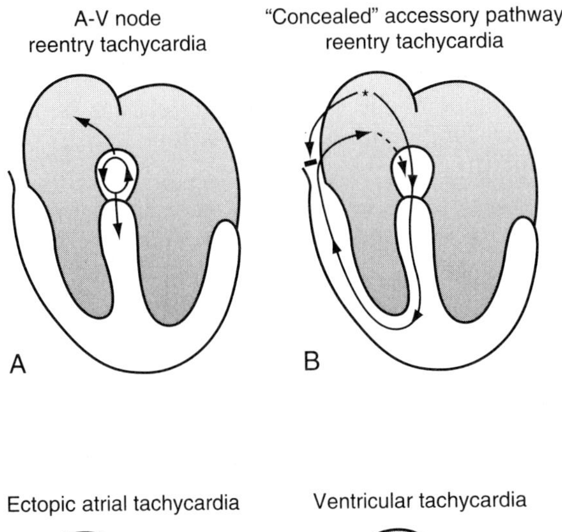

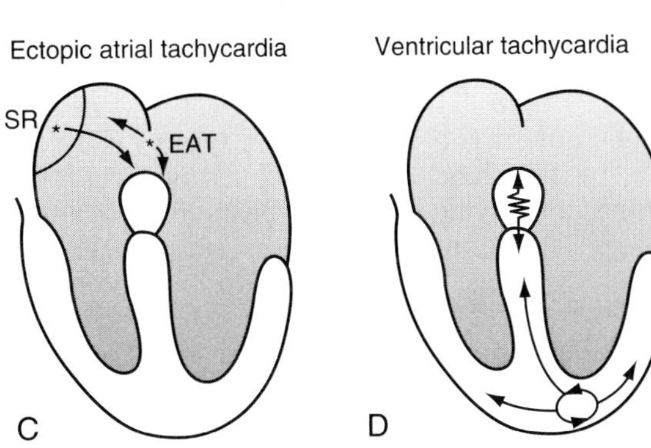

Figure 3. Mechanisms of selected tachycardias. See text for additional details. *A,* AV node reentry tachycardia; *B,* AV reciprocating tachycardia using a concealed accessory pathway; *C,* ectopic atrial tachycardia; *D,* ventricular tachycardia. EAT, ectopic atrial tachycardia; SR, sinus rhythm; *, the sinus node or area of impulse origination.

successful, depending on the location of the accessory pathway.

Wolff-Parkinson-White Syndrome

Patients with WPW syndrome have an accessory pathway that is capable of conducting anterogradely. This pathway results in an electrocardiogram with a short PR interval and a slurred initial QRS upstroke termed a *delta wave*. The delta wave is caused by fusion of normal AV node–His–Purkinje conduction and accessory pathway conduction. The accessory pathway can be located almost anywhere but is most commonly along the left lateral free wall.

The most frequent arrhythmia in these patients is AV reciprocating tachycardia, identical to the arrhythmia experienced by patients with a concealed accessory pathway. Because the accessory pathway is capable of conducting from the atria to the ventricles, these patients can rarely experience the reverse tachycardia (so-called antidromic reciprocating tachycardia) in which the reentry circuit travels anterogradely down the accessory pathway and retrogradely up the AV node. Such conduction results in a regular wide complex tachycardia in which each QRS is maximally preexcited. During the chaotic atrial activity of atrial fibrillation, patients with WPW syndrome can conduct to the ventricles via the AV node (typically with a narrow QRS complex), via the accessory pathway (with a wide QRS complex), or over both with varying degrees of fusion. In some patients, the accessory pathway can permit very rapid ventricular rates, which rarely can degenerate to ventricular fibrillation. A narrow QRS tachycardia in a patient with WPW syndrome may be treated acutely with intravenous adenosine or a β-blocker. A wide QRS tachycardia is more problematic given the possibility of atrial fibrillation or flutter with conduction over the accessory pathway. If urgent, the treatment of choice is cardioversion or, when intervention is less urgent, intravenous procainamide or amiodarone.

Chronic medical therapy in patients with WPW syndrome may include β-blocker therapy or a class IA, IC, or III antiarrhythmic drug to hinder accessory pathway conduction. Digoxin and possibly calcium channel blockers should be avoided because they may facilitate accessory pathway conduction. Radiofrequency ablation is often curative and is the treatment of choice, especially if the heart rate during atrial fibrillation exceeds 240 bpm. Success and complication rates depend on the location of the pathway; for left-sided pathways they are 90% to 95% and 1% to 2%, respectively.

Atrial Tachycardia

Atrial tachycardia results when the initial activation occurs somewhere in the atria other than the sinus node. The tachycardia requires only the involved portion of the atria and is therefore independent of the AV node. Suppressing AV nodal conduction with vagal maneuvers or adenosine will cause AV block and a slowed ventricular response, but not usually termination of the tachycardia. ECG features include a P wave morphology that differs from sinus rhythm and usually a narrow QRS complex. AV conduction can be 1:1, or some degree of AV block can be present. The rate is typically between 75 and 200 bpm.

Atrial tachycardia is more often associated with underlying structural heart disease (e.g., atrial dilatation or previous cardiac surgery) than are AV nodal reentry tachycardia or AV reciprocating tachycardia, but it can be seen in structurally normal hearts. Digoxin toxicity is a potential etiology and should be ruled out in appropriate circumstances.

Acutely, cardioversion can be performed, although the tachycardia frequently recurs. Prevention of recurrences is initially attempted with class IC agents. Class IA agents are not usually effective at the doses tolerated. Class III agents, especially amiodarone, may be the most effective, but complete suppression is generally difficult. Decreasing the ventricular rate (with oral or intravenous AV node–blocking agents) during tachycardia improves hemodynamics as well as symptoms. Chronic therapy can therefore consist of rate control with AV nodal blockers alone, maintenance of sinus rhythm with antiarrhythmic medication, or (most frequently) a combination of the two. Radiofrequency ablation is associated with success rates of approximately 75% to 85%.

Multifocal Atrial Tachycardia

This entity can be considered a variation of atrial tachycardia in which at least three different atrial foci appear to be involved. The electrocardiogram shows an irregularly irregular narrow complex tachycardia with three or more different P wave morphologies. It can be mistaken for atrial fibrillation. Multifocal atrial tachycardia is often first suspected when presumptive atrial fibrillation fails to respond to cardioversion. It is usually seen in patients with severe chronic obstructive pulmonary disease or cardiac failure. Acute therapy involves optimizing treatment of the underlying disease and slowing the ventricular rate with calcium channel blockers, digoxin, or β-blockers if the pulmonary process permits. Unfortunately, it is often refractory to pharmacologic therapy and difficult to treat. Long-term therapy should be directed toward improving the underlying medical condition.

Atrial Fibrillation

This tachycardia is covered elsewhere in this book and will not be reviewed here. In this arrhythmia, no organized atrial activity occurs, and it is distinguished from other SVTs by the absence of discrete P waves, the presence of an irregularly irregular rhythm, and a variable rate.

Atrial Flutter

Typical atrial flutter is a reentrant circuit in the right atrium with a regular atrial rate of about 300 bpm (can range between 250 and 305 bpm). The P waves are described as "saw tooth" and are usually best seen in leads II, III, and aVF. Flutter activity is often conducted to the ventricle with a 2:1 or higher AV block, and the heart rate is often 75 or 150 bpm. This tachycardia has a more organized atrial rhythm than atrial fibrillation does, and it is therefore often more difficult to control the ventricular rate. Atrial flutter can coexist with atrial fibrillation. If the diagnosis of flutter is uncertain, intravenous adenosine* can be administered. This agent will not terminate the arrhythmia but will prevent conduction to the ventricles and allow better visualization of the flutter waves. Chemical cardioversion under the auspices of continuous telemetry surveillance can be tried with intravenous ibutilide (Corvert) in patients without severely impaired ventricular function. Chronic treatment options include ventricular rate control with AV nodal blockers, maintenance of sinus rhythm with antiarrhythmic therapy, or radiofrequency ablation. Because many patients with atrial flutter have structural heart disease, the most commonly used antiarrhythmic medication is often a class III drug. The success of ablation is approximately 70% to 85%. Patients with atrial flutter who are at high risk for thromboembolic complications should be considered for long-term anticoagulation with warfarin (Coumadin).

*Not FDA-approved for this indication.

VENTRICULAR TACHYCARDIA

VT is defined as three or more consecutive beats of ventricular origin. It is considered sustained when it lasts longer than 30 seconds or is associated with hemodynamic instability. Most commonly, VT occurs in patients with a previous myocardial infarction or cardiomyopathy, but it is infrequently observed in patients with normal cardiac function.

The electrocardiogram during VT shows a regular, wide complex tachycardia with a rate anywhere from 120 to 220 bpm. The QRS is at least 120 msec wide and does not fit the criteria for a typical right or left bundle branch block. A QRS duration greater than 140 msec or atypical bundle branch morphology is very suggestive of a ventricular origin, whereas a QRS morphology more typical of bundle branch block should raise suspicion for SVT with aberrancy. VA dissociation (no consistent relationship between the P waves and the QRS complexes) is diagnostic of VT.

In the acute setting, cardioversion is the treatment of choice, especially in patients who are hemodynamically compromised. Even if the patient is stable, VT can degenerate to ventricular fibrillation and needs to be terminated. If the tachycardia is well tolerated, intravenous amiodarone, procainamide (Procanbid), or lidocaine may be effective in restoring sinus rhythm.

In a post–myocardial infarction patient, VT is associated with an increased risk of sudden death. In general, the worse the left ventricular function, the greater the risk of sudden death. Multiple studies have shown that an automatic implantable cardioverter-defibrillator (ICD) can reduce sudden death and mortality in selected patients. The currently accepted indications for ICD placement can be found in the most recent American Heart Association/American College of Cardiology guidelines. These guidelines encompass both primary prevention in patients who are thought to be at high risk for ventricular arrhythmia (postinfarction patients with ejection fractions <30% or postinfarction patients with ejection fractions <40%, nonsustained VT, and an inducible sustained VT) and secondary prevention in patients with a history of spontaneous VT or aborted sudden death. The utility of prophylactic defibrillator implantation in patients with nonischemic cardiomyopathy is under investigation.

Antiarrhythmic medications and radiofrequency ablation are sometimes used to reduce the frequency of VT episodes. Though inferior to the implanted defibrillator in terms of mortality and sudden death, ablation and antiarrhythmic agents have a role in patients with frequent VT episodes and subsequent shocks and in those who are unable to undergo ICD placement. The most widely used antiarrhythmic medications in this setting are amiodarone and sotalol.*

Idiopathic Ventricular Tachycardia

When VT occurs in patients with a structurally normal heart and normal electrocardiogram, it is termed *idiopathic ventricular tachycardia*. This uncommon entity typically originates from the right ventricular outflow tract but can originate elsewhere. Idiopathic VT has a better prognosis than VT does in patients with structural heart disease, and sudden death is infrequent. Workup of a patient with suspected idiopathic VT should include at least an echocardiogram and an evaluation for ischemic heart disease. Cardiac magnetic resonance imaging can rule out an isolated right ventricular cardiomyopathy known as arrhythmogenic right ventricular dysplasia. Symptomatic patients with idiopathic VT may respond to calcium channel*– or β-blocking* agents. For patients not wanting indefinite medical therapy, radiofrequency ablation is often curative.

Long QT and Torsades de Pointes

A prolonged QT interval during sinus rhythm can be inherited or acquired and predisposes the individual to a rapid polymorphic VT characterized by QRS complexes oscillating in amplitude and axis, a condition known as *torsades de pointes*. Because the QT interval is normally longer at slow heart rates, QT prolongation and torsades de pointes may be apparent only when the patient is bradycardic. Acquired long QT can be due to medications, an electrolyte imbalance, or an underlying medical condition. The list of QT-prolonging medications is extensive and includes many antiarrhythmic drugs (especially class IA and class III agents), tricyclic antidepressants, and some antibiotics.

Acute management of torsades de pointes consists of cardioversion for sustained tachycardia and intravenous magnesium. Pacing to increase the heart rate and decrease the effective QT interval may be helpful. Chronic treatment of acquired long QT syndrome requires the discontinuance and subsequent avoidance of any offending agents.

Congenital long QT syndrome is often manifested in childhood as syncope, episodes of polymorphic VT, or even sudden death. In young children, these spells can be misdiagnosed as seizures. It is frequently familial but may occur sporadically in some individuals. Family members of an affected individual should be evaluated with an electrocardiogram. Congenital long QT syndrome can be treated with β-blockade,* implantation of a pacemaker, and sometimes implantation of a defibrillator.

*Not FDA-approved for this indication.

Ventricular Fibrillation

This chaotic ventricular activity is always associated with hemodynamic compromise and is a medical emergency. It can be a primary arrhythmic event in the setting of cardiac ischemia or end-stage cardiomyopathy. It can also be due to degeneration of VT. Treatment is immediate defibrillation. Sometimes, repeated shocks are required, as well as intravenous amiodarone or lidocaine therapy.

CONGENITAL HEART DISEASE

method of
SCOTT E. FLETCHER, M.D.
Creighton University and University of Nebraska Children's Hospital
Omaha, Nebraska

Congenital heart disease is relatively uncommon with an incidence of approximately 8 cases per 1000 live births. Over the past several decades with improvement in surgical or catheter intervention, most children with congenital heart disease lead healthy lives long after their intervention. Despite this success, many require ongoing surveillance for long-term effects. The most common initial presentations are (1) an infant or child with a murmur, (2) a cyanotic newborn, and (3) an infant or child with congestive heart failure.

MURMUR EVALUATION

Most murmurs in pediatric patients are innocent and unrelated to any cardiac abnormality. Innocent murmurs can be made louder by conditions that increase cardiac output such as fever, exercise, or anemia. The most common innocent or functional systolic murmurs are (1) the branch pulmonary artery flow murmur in the newborn, (2) pulmonary outflow murmur, (3) Still's murmur, (4) supraclavicular bruit, and (5) cardiorespiratory murmur. A venous hum is a continuous murmur that can be made to disappear by supine positioning or jugular compression. Pathologic murmurs are often but not always present with congenital heart disease.

CYANOSIS

Cyanosis occurs when more than 5 g/dL of deoxygenated hemoglobin is present in blood. Cyanosis is usually respiratory in origin, with intrapulmonary right-to-left shunting because of ventilation-perfusion mismatch, but intracardiac right-to-left shunting related to heart disease must be considered. Cyanosis may be more apparent in the polycythemic child or the patient with poor cardiac output and increased oxygen extraction at the tissue level.

CONGESTIVE FAILURE

Major manifestations of congestive heart failure include tachypnea, tachycardia, excessive sweatiness, poor feeding, and failure to thrive. Rales and peripheral edema typically appreciated in adult patients with congestive heart failure are rare in infants. Hepatomegaly from passive congestion of a distensible liver capsule is a common but late finding in congestive heart failure. Cardiomegaly by chest radiography is the rule.

The following is a discussion of the more common congenital heart defects, their typical presentation, and current management strategies.

PULMONARY OVERCIRCULATION (LEFT-TO-RIGHT SHUNT)

Flow from the systemic circulation to the pulmonary circulation is described as a left-to-right shunt. This may be an intracardiac or extracardiac shunt. The four most common left-to-right shunts are VSD, ASD, AVSD, and PDA. Less common left-to-right shunts are AP window, coronary fistula, and partial anomalous pulmonary venous return.

Ventricular Septal Defect (VSD)

By far, the most common congenital heart defect is VSD. The typical presentation of a VSD is a murmur with or without signs of congestive heart failure. The manifestations, as well as management decisions, of a VSD are dictated by the relative pulmonary and systemic vascular resistances and the size and the location of the septal defect. The systolic murmur of VSD is usually harsh and can be best heard at the middle to lower left sternal border. When significant left-to-right shunting occurs, a diastolic flow rumble can also be heard across the mitral valve.

Four general types of VSD are encountered. Perimembranous VSDs account for nearly 80% of all significant communications within the ventricular septum. Infants with a large perimembranous VSD usually present between 2 weeks and 2 months of age with evidence of pulmonary overcirculation as pulmonary vascular resistance drops. In a subgroup of patients with large VSD, pulmonary vascular resistance remains high and the patient does not manifest signs of overt congestive heart failure. With advances in neonatal cardiac surgery, most infants with large perimembranous VSDs are operated on within the first 6 months of life for closure of their defect. Some perimembranous VSDs may close spontaneously or decrease in size over the first several years of life to a point of being hemodynamically insignificant. Spontaneous closure or decrease in size of the defect tends to occur by incorporation of tissue of the septal leaflet of the tricuspid valve into the defect. Small perimembranous VSDs can close spontaneously in the first several years of life.

All perimembranous VSDs place patients at risk of bacterial endocarditis, and bacterial endocarditis prophylaxis should be administered at times of risk. Perimembranous VSDs are occasionally associated with the development of progressive aortic insufficiency (AI) because of prolapse of the aortic valve into the septal defect. Reports of left ventricular–to–right atrial shunts have been described with spontaneous closure by septal tricuspid leaflet tissue ingrowth. Perimembranous defects are also associated with development of subaortic membranes.

The second most common location for VSD is the trabecular muscular septum. In early infancy, they are as common as perimembranous VSD. Muscular VSDs tend to close spontaneously in the first months of life with growth and thickening of the ventricular septum. Muscular VSDs may be associated with other forms of congenital heart disease. Rarely, an isolated muscular VSD is large enough to require intervention. Surgical closure can be difficult because of the heavy trabeculations within the right ventricle. Transcatheter closure techniques are used at some institutions.

A third location of VSD is in the inlet septum. Inlet VSDs also known as atrioventricular (AV) canal (AV septal) VSDs, tend to be large and do not close spontaneously. This subtype of VSD is commonly associated with Down syndrome. Usually, a cleft in the anterior mitral valve leaflet is associated. Inlet VSDs commonly occur in combination with primum ASDs. Surgical closure with or without repair of the mitral valve is generally required.

The fourth location of VSD is in the juxta-arterial position. These defects are also termed supracristal. Supracristal VSDs are most frequently seen in Asian populations. Supracristal VSDs are often complicated by significant aortic valve insufficiency. The mechanism of aortic valve insufficiency is prolapse of a valve cusp into the septal defect. Surgical therapy is usually warranted upon discovery of this rare VSD.

Atrial Septal Defect (ASD)

ASD is the second most common congenital heart lesion. It is the most common defect to be diagnosed after infancy. A systolic murmur may be heard over the pulmonary listening area secondary to increased flow. A fixed split second heart sound is classic. When significant left-to-right shunting occurs, a diastolic flow rumble across the tricuspid valve can be heard.

Except for mild growth deficiency, symptoms are unusual in the first decade of life. By the fifth decade of life, significant ASDs usually result in some exercise intolerance. Pulmonary vascular congestion, arrhythmias, and right ventricular failure are typical late symptoms.

The outcome of atrial septal communications discovered during the neonatal period is dependent on the size of the defect. Defects less than 3 mm universally undergo spontaneous closure or result in a probe patent foramen ovale. Defects between 3 and 8 mm in size have a 75% chance of decrease in size to a hemodynamically insignificant level. Generally, defects larger than 8 mm need surgical or transcatheter intervention.

Secundum ASDs account for more than 80% of ASDs, are located in the central region of the atrial septum, and usually arise with an asymptomatic heart murmur or cardiomegaly on screening radiograph. Atrial arrhythmias occur with increased frequency in patients with unrepaired ASD or those undergoing late closure. Surgical closure of secundum ASDs is accomplished with extremely low morbidity and mortality. Transcatheter therapy with several types of ASD devices has been successfully used in small to medium-sized atrial communications. In 2001, the Amplatz ASO device was approved by the Food and Drug Administration and is now used for many ASDs.

The second most common location of ASD is the ostium primum region. Often associated with VSD of the AV septal type, ostium primum ASDs do not close spontaneously. Primum ASDs are associated with clefts in the mitral valve, so mitral insufficiency may result. Because of associated mitral insufficiency, all primum ASDs require bacterial endocarditis prophylaxis when patients are placed at risk. Transcatheter closure techniques are not considered appropriate to close primum ASDs because of the proximity of the defect to the AV valves. Surgical repair before the age of 4 is usually recommended.

Less common, sinus venosus ASDs occur near the junction of the superior vena cava and the right atrium. This type of defect is almost always associated with anomalous connection of right-sided pulmonary veins. Physical findings and natural history are similar to those for secundum ASD. Sinus node disease following surgical closure and baffling of the pulmonary veins to the left atrium can rarely occur with closure of sinus venosus ASD.

The rarest atrial septal communication is in the coronary sinus. Coronary sinus ASDs occur in the region of the coronary sinus ostia through unroofing the sinus such that left atrial blood has easy access to the coronary sinus. Closure of the atrial septum (sinus os) leaving the coronary sinus unroofed results in a small residual right-to-left shunt but eliminates the right-sided volume load.

Patent Ductus Arteriosus (PDA)

PDA is a normal vascular structure in fetal life. The ductus arteriosus generally closes within the first 24 to 72 hours of extrauterine life. Persistent patency of the ductus is more common in premature infants and may impose a significant volume load on a relatively noncompliant left ventricle in these small neonates. Because of significant respiratory distress, some premature infants require pharmacologic ductus closure with prostaglandin inhibitors or surgical ligation.

In older children, a PDA is diagnosed by the presence of an asymptomatic continuous heart murmur, heard best in the left infraclavicular area. In large PDA, left ventricular enlargement and left atrial enlargement may be present. Untreated, the natural history of PDA includes congestive heart failure, endocarditis, and rarely pulmonary vascular disease. PDA closure is recommended at any age. In the asymptomatic patient, closure should be delayed until 1 year of age as spontaneous resolution of the left-to-right shunt has been reported. In the past, surgical ligation and division was the treatment of choice. During the 1990s, transcatheter occlusion of small to medium-sized ductus with Gianturco embolization coils became a suitable alternative. An Amplatz PDA device is promising for larger PDAs.

Atrioventricular Septal Defect (AVSD)

AVSD, also known as endocardial cushion defect or AV canal defect, is common among children with Down syndrome. In a complete AVSD, there is a large inlet muscular ventricular septal defect as well as an ostium primum ASD and a cleft in the anterior leaflet of the mitral valve. Symptoms are similar to those of a large ventricular septal defect. If the defect is unrepaired, these patients may have accelerated development of pulmonary vascular obstructive disease. In patients with persistent elevation of pulmonary vascular resistance, growth may be near normal; however, more commonly failure to thrive is seen. Repair of AV septal defect should be performed in infancy. In a minority of patients with AVSD, right or left ventricular hypoplasia is present and may preclude a biventricular repair. Surgery for AVSD is more difficult than for isolated ASD or VSD and success is often determined by postoperative mitral valve function.

OBSTRUCTIVE LESIONS

Obstructive lesions can occur to either the right or left ventricular outflow. Pulmonary valve stenosis, aortic valve stenosis, and coarctation of the aorta are most common. Less common is pulmonary artery stenosis that may occur with arteriohepatic dysplasia, with Williams' syndrome, or in association with complex congenital heart disease. Subvalve and supravalve AS are other examples of obstructive left heart lesions.

Pulmonary Valve Stenosis (PS)

PS may occur as an isolated defect and is a common component in complex congenital heart defects. A systolic murmur of variable intensity is heard at the upper left sternal border. A systolic ejection click is common. Isolated PS usually occurs at the level of the pulmonary valve. Typical stenotic pulmonary valves are thin and dome in systole. A subgroup of stenotic pulmonary valves are dysplastic, with characteristic supravalve narrowing and thickened "cauliflower-like" leaflets. Transcatheter therapy in the form of balloon valvuloplasty has become the treatment of choice for PS. Dysplastic pulmonary valves are less amenable to standard valvuloplasty techniques.

Severity of PS is graded into four categories. PS with a right ventricular–to–pulmonary artery gradient of less than 30 mm Hg and a right ventricular/aorta pressure rate less than 50% is considered mild. Mild PS rarely progresses and may actually improve with time. Most patients are asymptomatic, and the course is benign. PS is termed moderate when the right ventricular–to–left ventricular pressure ratio is between 50% and 80% and right ventricular–to–pulmonary artery pressure gradient is less than 80 mm Hg. Most patients have electrocardiographic evidence of right ventricular hypertrophy, which can lead to endocardial fibrosis and right ventricular dysfunction. Cardiac catheterization is warranted, and pulmonary balloon valvuloplasty is performed. PS is severe when right ventricular pressure is nearly equal to left ventricular pressure or the right ventricle–to–pulmonary artery gradient is greater than 80 mm Hg. The majority of children with severe PS have symptoms of exercise intolerance. Pulmonary balloon valvuloplasty is usually successful. If balloon valvuloplasty or surgical therapy is successful in achieving mild PS or better, the long-term course of PS is favorable.

Critical PS occurs in a small subgroup of pulmonary valves that arise in infancy with duct-dependent pulmonary blood flow. Transcatheter balloon valvuloplasty is often successful; however, the child may remain blue for a period of time secondary to right-to-left shunting at the atrial level. Some infants require palliative systemic–to–pulmonary artery shunts whereas other patients may be treated with balloon valvuloplasty alone. A combination of a palliative shunt and an outflow procedure is used in some patients. The size and function of the heavily hypertrophied right ventricle ultimately determine whether a complete two-ventricular repair is feasible. Similarly, a small group of patients with pulmonary atresia and intact septum can be initially treated with transcatheter therapy. The atretic valve membrane can be opened with a radio frequency catheter, laser, or stiff wire and then ballooned.

Aortic Stenosis (AS)

Aortic valve stenosis is the most common left heart obstructive lesion. From 1% to 2% of the general population has a bicuspid aortic valve, which may become dysfunctional and require surgical attention in middle to late adulthood. A smaller number of functionally bicuspid aortic valves cause significant obstruction to left ventricular outflow and require intervention during childhood years. Intervention in the form of balloon valvuloplasty or surgical valvuloplasty is usually performed in an effort to relieve left ventricular hypertrophy. The natural history of severe aortic valve stenosis suggests that sudden death in untreated AS is relatively common, as is endocarditis. With current management and antibiotic prophylaxis, these risks have significantly decreased. The typical presentation of AS is a systolic murmur, usually with a click, and heard best at the upper right sternal border.

In addition to auscultatory findings, the chest radiograph may show cardiomegaly. In the infant with poor left ventricular function, one may see pulmonary venous congestion. In the older child, the electrocardiogram may demonstrate left ventricular hypertrophy; however, the neonate with critical AS demonstrates right ventricular hypertrophy. Echocardiography is a reliable noninvasive method of assessing the severity of AS in children. Doppler-derived mean transvalvular gradients appear to correlate best with peak-to-peak left ventricular–to–aortic gradients measured in the cardiac catheterization laboratory. Significant ST-T wave changes during performance of a maximal exercise test may indicate a need for intervention in the patient with AS.

We define mild AS as a peak-to-peak pressure gradient of 40 mm Hg or less with minimal left ventricular hypertrophy in an asymptomatic patient. In general, no therapy is required except for the use of subacute bacterial endocarditis prophylaxis when placed at times of risk; however, these patients require diligent follow-up for worsening ventricular hypertrophy, ischemic symptoms, progressive stenosis, or severe ascending aortic dilation by noninvasive means.

Moderate AS, defined as a gradient less than 40 mm Hg with symptoms or between 40 and 70 mm Hg peak-to-peak gradient without symptoms, is generally treated. These catheter-measured gradients usually correlate with a mean transvalvar gradient of 25 mm Hg or more by Doppler echocardiography. Palliative therapy consists of balloon valvuloplasty in the catheterization laboratory or surgical valvotomy. Either can be associated with recurrence of stenosis as well as development of new AI.

In severe AS, there may be T wave changes in the lateral precordial leads suggesting ventricular strain or ischemia. Balloon valvuloplasty is our procedure of choice with a target result of 60% reduction in gradient. Greater relief of gradient may be associated with more severe AI.

Critical AS is seen exclusively in the neonatal period. Systemic cardiac output is dependent on right ventricular output through the PDA. Critical AS is associated with unicommissural aortic valves. Critical AS can be treated with balloon dilation through umbilical, femoral, or carotid artery approaches. Careful attention to balloon size (i.e., 90% annular diameter or less) should be observed because AI is poorly tolerated in this age group. Repeated valvuloplasty may be required at a later date.

Valve replacement is sometimes necessary in children with moderate to severe AS or AI. The Ross procedure with placement of a pulmonary autograft in the aortic position and a cadaveric homograft in the pulmonary position has been used with gratifying results. This procedure alleviates the need for long-term anticoagulation.

Coarctation of the Aorta (COA)

COA is due to medial thickening of the proximal descending aorta. The clinical presentation of COA depends on the severity of obstruction and the age of the patient. Neonates may present with congestive heart failure or even shock. Associated cardiac defects such as VSD are frequent. Neonatal coarctation is associated with hypoplasia of the transverse aortic arch and aortic isthmus. Although balloon angioplasty may be successful in relieving symptoms of congestive heart failure, recurrence of obstruction is common. We prefer an aggressive surgical approach with augmentation of the transverse aortic arch.

Children with COA outside the neonatal period generally present with upper extremity hypertension, decreased lower extremity pulsation, and possibly continuous murmurs from collateral blood flow around the COA. A systolic ejection click as a manifestation of frequently associated bicuspid aortic valve can be appreciated. Without intervention, greater than 90% of patients with COA die by age 50 years. Causes of death are aortic rupture, dissection, endocarditis, congestive heart failure, and intracranial hemorrhage. Successful repair reduces the risk of morbidity and mortality from all these causes. Intervention for COA should be undertaken when there is an upper–to–lower extremity resting blood pressure gradient of 15 to 20 mm Hg or greater in the presence of normal cardiac output. This degree of obstruction is generally associated with left ventricular hypertrophy by echocardiography and electrocardiography.

Surgical repair of COA using either an end-to-end anastomosis, subclavian flap, patch repair, or extended end-to-end anastomosis has been used for COA. Rarely, aneurysm formation at the site of repair has been described for all techniques but is more frequent when the patch repair is performed. Residual transverse arch hypoplasia may predispose to aneurysm formation. Balloon arterioplasty of discrete native coarctation has been well described and sometimes used with primary placement of endovascular stents. This may be the procedure of choice in patients of adult size. To avoid rare aortic aneurysm, balloon size should not exceed the diameter of the aorta at the level of the diaphragm.

Balloon arterioplasty is regarded as the treatment of choice for recurrence of COA after initial surgical repair. COA is a lifelong problem and requires intermittent imaging.

CYANOTIC DEFECTS

Cyanotic defects occur when deoxygenated blood is allowed to enter the systemic circulation. This may occur when there is some restriction to pulmonary blood flow, intracardiac shunting, or discordance between atrium, ventricle, and great vessels. The most common cyanotic defects with two functional ventricles are TOF, D transposition of the great vessels, and truncus arteriosus.

Transposition of the Great Arteries (TGA)

TGA arises in the first several weeks of life with moderate to severe cyanosis. The pulmonary artery arises from the left ventricle and the aorta from the right ventricle, giving rise to parallel circulations. In order to sustain life, a significant mixing lesion must be present at the atrial level, ventricular level, or PDA. Auscultation alone may be unimpressive except for a single second heart sound from the anteriorly malpositioned aorta. Electrocardiography may show right axis deviation and right ventricular hypertrophy. In newborns with an inadequate site of mixing, prostaglandin E1 (alprostadil [Prostin VR Pediatric]) infusion may be used to open the ductus arteriosus in order to stabilize the patient. A balloon atrial septostomy may also be used.

In simple TGA, most infants are currently managed with an arterial switch procedure. This surgical procedure involves transection above the level of the semilunar valves and moving the great vessels to their appropriate ventricle with transfer of the coronary arteries. The arterial switch is generally performed in the first several weeks of life. Intermediate-term follow-up of patients repaired by the arterial switch procedure is encouraging and supports continued use of this approach. In some patients with TGA, associated cardiac anomalies such as valvar or subvalvar pulmonary stenosis may necessitate an alternative surgical approach.

In the past, patients with TGA were managed with an atrial repair known as the Mustard or Senning procedure. Both consist of redirecting systemic venous return to the mitral valve so that deoxygenated blood may be pumped to the pulmonary arteries by a morphologic left ventricle and oxygenated blood pumped to the systemic circulation by a morphologic right ventricle. Although many patients having undergone the atrial baffle procedure continue to do extremely well, problems with the right ventricle serving as a systemic ventricular pump are increasingly encountered. Other postoperative problems include baffle obstruction, atrial and ventricular arrhythmias, and, rarely, sudden death.

Tetralogy of Fallot (TOF)

Malalignment ventricular septal defect, pulmonary stenosis, overriding aorta, and right ventricular hypertrophy make up TOF. In the extreme case, deviation of the outlet ventricular septum may be so significant as to result in pulmonary atresia. The degree of cyanosis is dependent on the amount of obstruction to pulmonary blood flow. Cyanosis is very severe in TOF with pulmonary atresia and absent in so-called pink tetralogy with mild pulmonary stenosis. Typically, the patient is suspected of having heart disease because of the systolic murmur of blood flow across the right ventricular outflow obstruction. The murmur is harsh and loudest at the left upper sternal border, with radiation into both lung fields. The electrocardiogram shows right ventricular hypertrophy, and the classic chest radiograph demonstrates a boot-shaped heart caused by right ventricular enlargement and hypoplasia of the main pulmonary artery segment.

The approach to TOF has undergone significant evolution since 1945, when Drs. Blalock and Taussig treated a TOF patient with a subclavian artery–to–pulmonary artery anastomosis. At present, palliative shunts to augment pulmonary blood flow are used only when associated anomalies preclude complete repair. Generally, closure of the ventricular septal defect and relief of the right ventricular obstruction can be performed with minimal morbidity and mortality in patients more than several months of age. In younger patients with marked cyanosis, patients with anomalous coronary arteries requiring cadaveric homograft placement, or patients with severe pulmonary artery hypoplasia, palliative shunts such as the modified Blalock-Taussig shunt to the central pulmonary arteries or palliative balloon valvuloplasty is used. In this selected group of patients, definitive repair is performed at a later date. The postoperative course in patients with TOF is frequently benign but may be complicated by residual pulmonary stenosis, pulmonary regurgitation, residual ventricular septal defect, right ventricular dysfunction, arrhythmias, and, on rare occasion, sudden death.

Truncus Arteriosus

Persistence of the common arterial trunk is a rare congenital malformation. Truncus is generally associated with a large VSD. Truncus is frequently associated with DiGeorge syndrome (22q$^-$). The single truncal valve is variably deformed and, when severely insufficient, can complicate management. Patients present with mild cyanosis at birth; however, as pulmonary vascular resistance falls, pulmonary overcirculation and congestive heart failure occur. Most centers now perform complete surgical repair in early infancy. Repair includes closure of the VSD to direct left ventricular output to the truncal valve and placement of a right ventricle–to–pulmonary artery connection. The right ventricle–to–pulmonary artery connection will need revision in childhood, secondary to the patient's growth.

FUNCTIONAL UNIVENTRICULAR HEARTS

A host of congenital cardiac lesions associated with hypoplasia of either the right or left ventricular chamber are now palliated with a univentricular repair. The Fontan procedure, initially described for tricuspid atresia, is used for double-inlet left ventricle, hypoplastic left heart, hypoplastic right heart, unbalanced AV canal, and other congenital cardiac defects in which two functional ventricles are not present. The Fontan procedure routes systemic venous return from the inferior and superior caval systems to the pulmonary arteries without a ventricular pump in this circulation. This procedure is usually staged such that pulmonary blood flow is initially delivered through a systemic artery–to–pulmonary artery shunt or through native circulation with pulmonary stenosis. Next, superior caval flow is directed to the pulmonary arteries at 4 to 6 months of age (hemi-Fontan or bidirectional Glenn). Following a period of adaptation, inferior caval flow is directed to the pulmonary arteries. The Fontan completion is performed at 18 to 24 months of age in our institution. Success of the Fontan procedure is dependent on adequate systolic function of the systemic ventricle, undistorted pulmonary artery anatomy, low pulmonary vascular resistance, normal diastolic relaxation of the systemic ventricle, and absence of significant AV valve regurgitation.

Hypoplastic Left Heart Syndrome (HLHS)

HLHS is a severe congenital heart defect that is characterized by hypoplasia of left-sided cardiac structures. The mitral valve and the aortic valve are critically stenotic or atretic. The left ventricle is of inadequate size to perform systemic work. With spontaneous constriction and ultimate closure of the PDA in the first several days of life, the left ventricle is asked to provide systemic cardiac output that was previously provided by the morphologic right ventricle. The left ventricle is inadequate for this purpose, and severe metabolic acidosis and shock occur. In patients diagnosed prenatally by fetal echocardiography or early postnatally, this insult of acidosis may be avoided by the use of prostaglandin E1 (Prostin VR Pediatric) to maintain ductal patency.

Without intervention, more than 95% of infants die in the first several months of life with only rare survivors beyond 1 year. If the family pursues medical treatment, two palliations are possible. One is heart transplantation, which requires lifelong immunosuppression and is limited by donor organ availability. A second option is a staged reconstructive palliation. The first-stage "Norwood procedure" is a high-risk operation, which prepares the morphologic right ventricle to perform as the systemic ventricular pump. This operation requires a great deal of expertise, but recent advances suggest greater than 80% survival for stage I Norwood. The second- and third-stage operations are the hemi-Fontan and Fontan.

CONCLUSION

Many other congenital heart defects are known but are beyond the scope of this brief discussion. Most defects warrant the use of bacterial endocarditis prophylaxis. In general, great strides have been made in the treatment of congenital heart disease. For most patients, the future is bright.

HYPERTROPHIC CARDIOMYOPATHY

method of
RAJESH THAMAN, M.D.
M. TERESA TOME, M.D., and
WILLIAM J. McKENNA, M.D.
Department of Cardiological Sciences
St. George's Hospital Medical School
London, United Kingdom

Hypertrophic cardiomyopathy (HCM) is the most common inherited cardiovascular disease, with an estimated prevalence of 1:500. Morphologically, hypertrophic cardiomyopathy is characterized by myocardial hypertrophy in the absence of a coexisting cardiac or systemic disease capable of producing ventricular hypertrophy, e.g., systemic hypertension or primary valvular heart disease. Familial disease with autosomal dominant transmission is recognized in about 50% of cases, and sporadic disease or milder forms of familial disease probably account for the rest. To date, over 100 mutations in 10 genes encoding cardiac sarcomeric proteins, which make up the basic contractile apparatus of the cardiac myocyte, have been linked to hypertrophic cardiomyopathy. The most common mutations identified are in the β-myosin heavy chain, cardiac troponin T, and the myosin-binding protein C. The other genes, namely cardiac troponin I, regulatory and essential myosin light chains, titin, α-tropomyosin, α-actin, and α-myosin heavy chain account for a minority of cases of HCM only. How these mutations give rise to the morphologic and phenotypic manifestations of hypertrophic cardiomyopathy is unclear; suggested mechanisms include alterations in the contraction-relaxation cycle and/or energy homeostasis of the heart.

PATHOPHYSIOLOGY

Microscopically, HCM is characterized by abnormal myocyte hypertrophy and disarray; other characteristic features include interstitial fibrosis and intramural coronary arteries with narrowed lumen. Macroscopically, hypertrophy usually develops during adolescence and normally affects the interventricular septum more than the free or posterior walls (asymmetric septal hypertrophy). Concentric and apical hypertrophy is also well recognized and right-sided involvement occurs in up to one third of patients, although never in isolation. Left ventricle systolic function is usually normal or hyperdynamic. With time, however, 5% to 10% of patients progress to an advanced stage characterized by progressive cavity enlargement, wall thinning, impaired systolic performance, and features of congestive cardiac failure. One third of patients have dynamic left ventricular outflow tract obstruction (LVOTO) secondary to the affect of systolic anterior motion of the mitral valve (SAM) on a narrowed left ventricular outflow tract. This is usually accompanied by mitral regurgitation. Diastolic dysfunction, caused by abnormal left ventricular relaxation and reduced left ventricular compliance, occurs frequently and a minority of patients have features resembling restrictive cardiomyopathy. Microvascular ischemia is common and thought to relate to abnormal intramural vessels, increased myocardial mass, elevated left ventricular filling pressures, and diastolic dysfunction.

CLINICAL PRESENTATION

Even within families with the same genetic defect, the clinical manifestations of hypertrophic cardiomyopathy are diverse, ranging from a benign asymptomatic course to severe heart failure, embolic stroke, and sudden cardiac death. The majority of patients however, do not experience disease-related symptoms or complications and may go unrecognized. When symptoms do occur the principal complaints are of chest pain, breathlessness, palpitations, and presyncopal or syncopal episodes. Sudden cardiac death is a well-recognized manifestation and hypertrophic cardiomyopathy is the most common cause of unexplained sudden cardiac death among young people and athletes.

DIAGNOSIS

HCM may be initially suspected because of a heart murmur, positive family history, new symptoms, or abnormal ECG pattern. Abnormal physical findings, which include forceful left ventricular impulse, rapid upstroke to the arterial pulse, a palpable left atrial beat, a fourth heart sound, and a mid-late systolic murmur tend to occur only in patients with outflow tract obstruction. The ECG is abnormal in 75% to 95% of patients with HCM. Left axis deviation, criteria for left ventricular hypertrophy with or without repolarization changes, left and or right atrial enlargement, and abnormal Q-waves are the most common features. The diagnosis of hypertrophic cardiomyopathy currently depends on the echocardiographic demonstration of a left ventricular wall thickness more than two standard deviations from the mean corrected for age, sex, and height (typically > 1.5 cm). For proper diagnosis of HCM, other conditions resulting in ventricular hypertrophy need to be ruled out (Table 1). DNA analysis is a more definitive method for establishing the diagnosis of HCM; however, this tends to be expensive and time consuming and is not yet routinely available.

TREATMENT

The clinical course in hypertrophic cardiomyopathy varies markedly; the vast majority of patients remain asymptomatic and, therefore, do not require treatment.

TABLE 1. **Differential Diagnosis of "Unexplained" Left Ventricular Hypertrophy**

Exaggerated "Physiologic" Response	Primary Genetic Disorders	Metabolic Disorders
Renal and Afro-Caribbean hypertension	Noonan's syndrome	Infants of diabetic mothers
"Athlete's" heart	Friedrich's ataxia	Amyloid
	Lentiginosis	Glycogen storage disease
		Mitochondrial myopathy
		Pheochromocytoma
		Inborn errors of fatty acid metabolism
		Fabry's disease

In patients with symptoms or significant exercise limitation, however, decisions regarding symptomatic treatment are generally guided by the presence or absence of left ventricular outflow tract obstruction.

Treatment of Obstruction

Beta-blockers are usually tried as first line therapy; the majority of patients show improvements on treatment, although high doses may be required. The beneficial effects of β-blockers appear largely to result from their negative inotropic actions, as well as prolongation of diastole, reduction in myocardial oxygen demand and outflow tract gradient, and increased passive ventricular filling. If β-blockers are ineffective disopyramide (Norpace),* can be tried. Disopyramide may reduce the gradient and relieve symptoms by virtue of its negative inotropic properties; however, the initial hemodynamic benefits often decrease with time. Patients are often unable to tolerate the high doses generally required for symptomatic improvement (up to 600 mg/d) due to the anticholinergic side effects. Because disopyramide may shorten the atrioventricular nodal conduction time and thus increase the ventricular rate during paroxysmal atrial tachycardia, which occurs commonly in hypertrophic cardiomyopathy, supplementary therapy with β-blockers in low doses is advisable. Verapamil (Calan),* is particularly effective in patients with chest pain and may also have beneficial effects on outflow tract gradient reduction by virtue of its negatively inotropic action; however, in some patients the vasodilatory effects may lead to serious hemodynamic compromise. Verapamil should, therefore, be used cautiously in patients with outflow tract obstruction.

For patients in whom medication proves unsuccessful or side effects become intolerable, ventricular septal myotomy–myectomy (Morrow's operation), alcohol septal ablation, or pacing may be considered. Myotomy–myectomy aims to widen the outflow tract, and therefore, reduce LVOTO and systolic mitral leaflet septal contact. Success rates of over 80%, perioperative mortality rates of 2% or less, and long-term symptom relief in up to 70% of patients have been reported. Similar success rates have been reported after alcohol septal ablation. This technique involves injection of alcohol into the septal perforators of the left anterior descending coronary artery to cause a limited myocardial infarction. Complication rates vary considerably, being closely related to the level of expertise at the center performing the procedure. The most common complication is that of high-grade atrioventricular block requiring permanent pacemaker. Use of dual chamber atrioventricular universal pacemaker (DDD) using a short-programmed atrioventricular delay leading to delayed activation and less vigorous contraction of the interventricular septum has a lower success rate, with gradient reduction reported in 30% to 50% of patients. Despite this, pacing may be useful in a subset of patients that are unsuitable for either surgery or alcohol septal ablation.

*Not FDA-approved for this indication.

Treatment of Nonobstructive Hypertrophic Cardiomyopathy

Patients without outflow tract obstruction constitute the majority of patients with HCM. In these patients β-blockers or calcium antagonists (verapamil* or diltiazem* [Cardizem]) can be used to optimize heart rate, leading to improvements in myocyte relaxation and cardiac filling and, possibly, a reduction in myocardial ischemia.

Heart Failure

In a small minority of patients, heart failure symptoms may accompany hypertrophic cardiomyopathy associated with ventricular enlargement and wall thinning or restrictive physiology. In these patients conventional heart failure treatment should be instigated, e.g., diuretics and angiotensin-converting enzyme inhibitors. Because many of these patients have diastolic dysfunction and require relatively high filling pressures to achieve adequate ventricular filling, it is advisable to administer diuretics with caution. Ultimately, heart transplantation may be the only option.

Supraventricular Arrhythmia/Rhythm Disturbance

Supraventricular arrhythmias, in particular atrial fibrillation and flutter, are common (20% to 30%) in patients with HCM and often develop in association with progressive atrial enlargement, secondary to obstruction, diastolic dysfunction, and/or mitral valve dysfunction. These arrhythmias can result in profound hemodynamic compromise, although they are usually well tolerated if the ventricular rate is adequately controlled. New-onset atrial fibrillation should be cardioverted, although if it is unsuccessful, β-blockers and verapamil are usually efficacious in controlling the heart rate. Ablation of the atrioventricular node and implantation of a pacemaker is occasionally necessary. Amiodarone (Cordarone) is the most effective antiarrthymic agent for the prevention of recurrent episodes of supraventricular tachyarrhythmia. Because recurrences or even brief episodes of atrial fibrillation/flutter in hypertrophic cardiomyopathy are associated with a significant risk of systemic thromboembolization, the threshold for the initiation of anticoagulation therapy should be low.

SUDDEN DEATH AND RISK STRATIFICATION

Sudden death is the most devastating consequence of hypertrophic cardiomyopathy and it often occurs in otherwise healthy individuals. Reported annual

*Not FDA-approved for this indication.

mortality rates from sudden death are 1% to 2% and are highest in adolescents and young adults. Sudden death occurs most commonly during mild exertion or at rest, but is not infrequently related to physical exertion. Ventricular tachyarrhythmia appears to be the final common pathway for sudden death in most patients. The exact trigger for this arrhythmia is unknown, but possible underlying etiologic factors include myocardial ischemia, diastolic dysfunction, outflow tract obstruction, inappropriate systemic arterial vasodilation, or supraventricular tachyarrhythmias. Bradyarrhythmias due to sinus node dysfunction or atrioventricular block may also be responsible in a minority of cases.

Patients who have survived a cardiac arrest are at highest risk and should be offered prophylactic therapy. Most other patients at risk can be identified by noninvasive assessment, which should include history, echocardiography, 48-hour Holter monitoring, and cardiopulmonary exercise testing. Established risk markers for sudden death include nonsustained ventricular tachycardia, left ventricular wall thickness equal to or greater than 30 mm, abnormal blood pressure response in those younger than 40 years of age, family history of sudden cardiac death, and unexplained syncope. Patients with none of the above risk factors have less than 1% estimated annual risk of sudden cardiac death and can generally be reassured. Patients who have two or more risk markers are at greatest risk, with a 4% to 6% annual risk of sudden death and prophylactic therapy should be considered. Although amiodarone* has been used extensively in the past to treat risk, evidence increasingly shows that the implantable cardioverter defibrillator (ICD) is more effective. Risk stratification is problematic in those patients with a single risk factor and at present, treatment is determined by the strength of the individual risk factor.

Although not yet routinely used in risk stratification, specific mutations may be associated with an adverse prognosis. For example, some β-myosin heavy chain mutations (e.g., Arg403Gln and Arg719Gln) and some troponin T mutations may be associated with a higher frequency of premature death.

SCREENING

Currently all first-degree relatives of affected patients should be offered screening; any identified affected family members should then undergo risk stratification. Currently, evaluation of family members relies on history, examination, and echocardiographic and electrocardiographic evidence of left ventricular hypertrophy. In the future, gene testing will enable a more reliable and conclusive diagnosis to be made and may identify patients at risk for sudden death prior the onset of hypertrophy.

*Not FDA-approved for this indication.

HEART FAILURE

method of
MARC A. SILVER, M.D.
Advocate Christ Medical
Oak Lawn, Illinois

Heart failure is epidemic in the United States. Every day, clinicians face the task of caring for more patients with heart failure in all its forms. Heart failure is the primary reason for hospitalization of Americans older than 65 years, and although 6 million Americans are estimated to have symptomatic heart failure, that number is expected to double over the next 7 years. Many millions more have asymptomatic left ventricular dysfunction or existing medical conditions that make it quite likely that heart failure will develop and they will die.

It is truly in the hands of primary care physicians, who care for most heart failure patients, as well as those with common precursors of heart failure, to better understand heart failure and its natural history and thereby make an impact on this challenging epidemic. Therefore, with this concept in mind, I will discuss heart failure from the perspective of understanding its natural history or stages, as well as a chronic disease process amenable to strategic planning.

DEFINITIONS

All clinicians define heart failure differently. Some choose to think about heart failure only when the patient has advanced disease characterized by significant volume overload and exercise limitation. Others consider heart failure to be present only when the left ventricle is dilated. Though broad by intent, heart failure is usually defined as a complex clinical syndrome that affects cardiac function (its ability to fill and/or eject blood) and is often preceded by and certainly accompanied by systemic neurohormonal abnormalities that participate in and perpetuate the dysfunction of the heart, as well as other target organs, including the vasculature and muscles.

Although a wide range of signs and symptoms may accompany the heart failure syndrome of whatever cause, once symptomatic, patients usually have evidence of dyspnea, fatigue, and sodium and water retention manifested as congestion in the lungs, legs, and gut.

It is useful, however, to think about heart failure not only as a symptomatic disease but also as a disease whose development begins decades before the patient crosses the threshold of clinical symptoms.

CLASSIFICATION AND STAGES OF HEART FAILURE

Although many clinicians bristle at the concept of prescribed sets of recommendations or guidelines to be applied to a diverse disease process such as heart failure, these guidelines are frequently a place where available evidence is evaluated in a critical way and balanced with consensus to provide the readers with a distillation of what might work for them when they are caring for a patient with a disease process.

Recently, one of the well-accepted standard guidelines for heart failure has been revised. Within the 2001 Revision of the American College of Cardiology/American Heart Association Guidelines for the Evaluation and Management of Chronic Heart Failure for the Adult (executive summary and full text available at http://www.acc.org/clinical/guidelines/failure/hf_index.htm), aside from detailed information on the testing and therapies currently supported by evidence, appears a new classification for heart failure (Table 1). The classification most clinicians are familiar with is that of the New York Heart Association (NYHA) (Table 2). The NYHA classification is generally applied to patients who at some point become symptomatic. Although they may revert to a symptom-free status (NYHA functional class I), it is still implied that the patient has overt heart failure. Even though the NYHA classification is of great value and carries prognostic value, it also tends to allow us to think of a patient with mild or moderate symptoms (i.e., NYHA functional class II to III) as having a mild or moderate disease, but indeed, patients in this category have a markedly shortened life span and by definition have less than optimal functional status.

The new classification, on the other hand (see Table 1), identifies four *stages* of heart failure based on the spectrum of common clinical syndromes from which they have evolved. By so doing, it is hoped that the clinician will recognize the patient's increased risk for the clinical syndrome and then act aggressively to reduce the risk and/or intervene earlier just as one would with a patient at risk for cancer.

TABLE 1. **Stages of Heart Failure**

Stage A

Patients who are at increased risk for heart failure because of associated medical conditions (e.g., hypertension, coronary artery disease, or diabetes mellitus)

Heart structure and function: Not yet affected

Potential therapies: Treatment of hypertension, smoking cessation, and weight loss; ACE inhibitors in appropriate patients

Stage B

Patients who have abnormal heart structure and/or function but who have not manifested signs or symptoms

Heart structure and function: Abnormal

Potential therapies: Same, plus ACE inhibitors and β-blockers in all appropriate patients

Stage C

Patients with symptomatic heart failure. These patients indeed have advanced heart failure. Note that signs and symptoms develop as late phenomena after significant perturbation of many homeostatic mechanisms and the consumption of large cardiac reserves

Heart structure and function: Abnormal

Potential therapies: Same, plus ACE inhibitors, β-blockers, and digoxin and diuretics in most patients; also, coronary revascularization and repair of mitral regurgitation in selected patients

Stage D

Patients with extremely advanced heart failure

Heart structure and function: Extremely abnormal

Potential therapies: Same, consideration of advanced therapies including investigational therapies, as well as end-of-life counseling and hospice

Abbreviation: ACE=angiotensin-converting enzyme.

TABLE 2. **New York Heart Associated Functional Classification of Heart Failure**

I. Symptoms occur only at a level that would cause normal individuals to become symptomatic
II. Symptoms occur with ordinary exertion or moderate levels of activity
III. Symptoms occur with less than ordinary degrees of activity
IV. Symptoms occur even at rest

This classification scheme is generally applied to patients once they are or have been symptomatic with heart failure (stages C and D). Note that in general, the classification implies the patient's worst level of functioning related to a heart failure symptom (e.g., fatigue, dyspnea, exercise intolerance).

The classification addresses four stages. Unlike the NYHA classification, in which a patient may easily pass back and forth through several functional classes over a period of days to weeks, as the patient passes through each stage of the new classification, there is no longer any hope of reverting to an earlier stage, which should act as an impetus to capture the patient at the earliest stage and prevent progression to the next stage by the use of proper diagnostics and therapeutics.

Stage A refers to patients who by virtue of having other common clinical conditions are at increased risk of heart failure ultimately developing. These conditions include hypertension, diabetes mellitus, and coronary artery disease. Similarly, patients with a family history of heart failure would have an increased risk. Clearly, the heart failure syndrome will not develop in all these patients, but acknowledging their "at-risk" status gives the clinician and the patient fair warning of the potential risk of development of heart failure and may serve as an early warning detection system for the insidious progression to more advanced heart failure. Progression to the next stage is preventable, and disease progression is usually measured in years or decades.

Stage B refers to patients in whom structural and even functional abnormalities in heart function have already developed, but because of enormous cardiac reserve, the signs or symptoms that usually bring these patients to medical attention have not developed. This stage has also been referred to as "asymptomatic left ventricular dysfunction." Progression to the next stage may be slowed and again may be measured in years.

Stage C represents most of what we call heart failure today, specifically, a patient who has structural and functional disease but who has now progressed and used up enough cardiac reserve to actually have signs and symptoms of the disease. By looking at heart failure in this perspective, it becomes clear that any symptomatic heart failure indeed represents a serious condition that the clinician must diagnose and treat accordingly. In this stage of the disease, clinicians can intervene to improve symptoms and quality of life, as well as improve, but not completely abolish the increased mortality. Progression to the next stage is quite variable but is usually measured in months to years.

Stage D represents very advanced disease in which even standard measures cannot overcome the severity of the disease and advanced measures need to be undertaken. During this stage, despite best efforts, patients usually have increased use of resources, decreased quality of life, and progressive limitation. Although many advanced resources are being applied during this stage, including heart transplantation and ventricular restraint and assist devices, generally, these patients ultimately die of either progressive heart failure or sudden cardiac death.

STEPS FOR APPROPRIATE HEART FAILURE MANAGEMENT

Physicians often take a reflex approach to initiating drug therapy in a patient with symptomatic heart failure. For example, a patient who is volume overloaded might be treated with diuretics as monotherapy while overlooking the need to not only treat the current symptoms but also plan a strategy to limit progression of disease. Therefore, a useful approach in planning patient care involves two broad steps. The first is assessment of the information needed to create a management plan, and the second is an understanding of the therapeutic targets in heart failure treatment.

An assessment of what is known or yet needed to be known to best make the diagnosis and treat a patient with heart failure is a very useful step. This assessment generally involves an understanding of the etiology of the heart failure, the current stage or functional class, and so forth. However, even after a detailed history and physical examination and collection of some diagnostic data, a gap can remain in the information needed to complete the therapeutic plan. Generally, the clinician can group the areas that need to be completed into three main categories: diagnostics, therapeutics, and prognostics. In fact, it is useful to consider these three areas each time a patient is seen in the office or hospital. Even though one often initiates treatment without complete information in each of these areas, not asking what other information is needed often leads to an incomplete understanding of the disease syndrome, as well as suboptimal therapy.

Diagnostics refers to any additional information that allows a better understanding of the etiology, status, degree of limitation, and signs and symptoms of a patient. For example, an echocardiogram allows assessment of the nature and degree of left ventricular function and may lead to consideration of myocardial ischemia (wall motion abnormalities) or valvular disease (valvular regurgitation or stenosis) as a therapeutic target. Often, in this category are tests that might reveal an easily addressable cause of the heart failure and even a form of heart failure that is potentially reversible (such as hyperthyroidism).

Therapeutics refers to the design of the treatment strategy based on what is currently known about the patient and that patient's disease. It is also useful to write down a therapeutic plan, including the one or two next steps one might take for the patient should the signs or symptoms not abate with the current regimen. For example, one might begin with using angiotensin-converting enzyme (ACE) inhibitors but indicate that if the patient is found to have underlying coronary artery disease, the addition of long-acting nitrates will be considered.

Prognostics refers to focusing in on what is known about the patient's heart failure in terms of predicting what might be the path of progression in the near future. Though imperfect, many pieces of information are closely linked to survival and disease progression, including functional status, exercise tolerance, and left ventricular ejection fraction. In considering any additional prognostics, the clinician should always ask what might be done differently given the result. Over the years we have become more willing to intervene earlier with therapeutics, which can alter progression of the disease, and we are therefore less dependent on a bad set of prognostic markers to make these decisions. Nevertheless, awareness of a low peak oxygen consumption, a low right ventricular ejection fraction, or a markedly elevated neurohormonal marker often serves to alert the physician and the patient and family to review the current therapeutic plan and broaden considerations to include the next level of care and treatment, which might consist of investigational therapies and evaluation for heart transplantation. The role of measurement of B-type natriuretic peptide in this regard is of some interest and may prove to be a prognostic marker against which we target our therapies.

Treatment Targets

In designing the drug treatment plan, we take into consideration the following treatment targets for patients with heart failure: improved survival, improved symptoms, slowing and/or reversal of disease progression, improved functional status and quality of life, avoidance of troublesome adverse events, and decreased use of resources, including hospitalization. With the recognition that not all these targets are concordant or attainable, the drug regimen reflects these targets and our understanding of the ability of drugs to address them.

In general, patients with symptomatic heart failure are managed with a core group of four drug classes, including diuretics, an ACE inhibitor, a β-blocker, and usually digoxin. The former and the latter are generally applied to relieve symptoms or to improve functional status or exercise tolerance, whereas the middle two are also administered with the specific intention of altering disease progression, reversing the structural and/or functional abnormalities of the heart and other target organs, and improving medium- and long-term survival.

Increasing evidence supports the initiation of ACE inhibitors and β-blockers jointly when caring for a symptomatic patient. Diuretics often need to be adjusted up or down, depending on a patient's level of

TABLE 3. **Common Heart Failure Drugs and Their Therapeutic Targets**

Drug	Dose	Comment
Loop diuretics (expressed as furosemide [Lasix] equivalent units)	40-100 mg once or twice daily	Many factors affect the doses required, such as patient compliance with dietary restrictions, fluid intake, and associated titration of other medication, including ACE inhibitors and β-blockers
ACE inhibitors (expressed as enalapril [Vasotec] equivalent units)	10-20 mg twice daily	Higher doses seem to be have an impact on hospitalization rates. Be aware of adverse events that will limit use, including hyperkalemia. To allow adequate titration of β-blockers, reduced doses may be used
β-Blockers (expressed as carvedilol [Coreg] equivalent units)	25-50 mg twice daily	Dependent on body size. Although data suggest clinical improvement and decreased mortality with smaller doses, the target remains full dose
Digoxin	0.125-0.25 mg daily	Adjustment needed for renal function. Routine measurement of serum levels is not required unless done to confirm toxicity

compensation, as well as where they are in terms of other (β-blocker) titration. Target doses for most of the commonly used drugs come from clinical trials suggesting their benefit (ACE inhibitors) or from tradition, as well as from attempts to balance drug efficacy with drug safety (digoxin and diuretics). Target doses are listed in Table 3. Excellent details and practical considerations of implementing and titrating heart failure drugs can be found in recent guidelines (http://www.acc.org/clinical/guidelines/failure/hf_index.htm).

Nonpharmacologic Measures

An enormous armamentarium outside routine drug therapy is available to clinicians caring for patients with heart failure. In general, most nonpharmacologic measures should be used in a simultaneous fashion with the initiation and titration of drug therapy. Although most of these therapies either have not or will not undergo rigorous clinical investigation, they nonetheless remain therapeutic cornerstones of complete heart failure care. Often, dramatic functional improvement can be observed with more careful attention to nonpharmacologic therapies. Of particular interest is an understanding that sleep-disordered breathing (including obstructive and central forms of sleep apnea) may be present in nearly 40% of heart failure patients. Increasing evidence suggests that therapy that includes continuous positive airway pressure may alter symptoms, disease progression, and even survival (Table 4). As far as dietary advice, generally admonitions for avoidance of excessive sodium intake and fluid are given along with specific information on lowering dietary saturated fat. However, emerging information is that the patient with heart failure suffers a significant energy imbalance and may well benefit from nutritional assessment, including measurement of nitrogen balance.

TABLE 4. **Nonpharmacologic Therapies for Patients With Heart Failure**

Definitely Helps Reduce Symptoms or Improve Functional Status
Salt restriction (target, 2.3 g of salt/d)
Exercise
Stress reduction
Screening for depression
Smoking cessation
Weight loss
Treatment of documented sleep-disordered breathing
May Be of Use in Selected Patients
Fluid restriction
Avoidance of alcohol

USE OF DISEASE MANAGEMENT AND OTHER RESOURCES

Perhaps one of the greatest tools at hand for clinicians caring for patients with heart failure, as well as for their families, is provision of a thorough understanding of the heart failure syndrome and how self-empowered actions might have a significant impact on how they feel, what they can do, and how long they might live. Studies have repeatedly demonstrated the benefits of a structured disease management program in reducing symptoms, improving functional status, and in particular, reducing heart failure hospitalizations. Frequently, the clinician can best serve the patient by fostering and supporting a heart failure disease management program. Though not present in all communities yet, the resources required (a physician and/or a nurse champion) are often available everywhere. Abundant educational, patient-oriented books and material are available to support these programs.

Disease management programs are often part of a larger specialized heart failure center. Within these structures abide advanced strategies, including investigational therapies. It is incumbent on the clinician to be aware of these local and regional resources and refer patients when appropriate. Even with advanced disease, these centers can often offer improved outcomes and strategies not available to all clinicians.

Another area within the disease management spectrum that can be used is the home care programs that exist in most communities. These services frequently provide a link between intensive hospital-based care and infrequent, less intensive office-based care. In addition, for many patients with advanced disease, home care meets the constraints of patients and families.

For patients with advanced disease, physicians often begin discussions surrounding end-of-life issues too late. Generally, patients who have advanced disease requiring frequent hospitalization and treatment are aware of their likelihood of death and, in fact, value regaining some of the mastery and control of their lives through discussion of end-of-life planning and preferences. For some, hospice care will be the choice made, whereas for others, referral to specialized centers and participation in emerging therapies through clinical trials might be the correct choice. Understanding comes only with an open and frank discussion with each patient and family.

EMERGING AND EMERGED NEW THERAPEUTIC AREAS

Because of the intense interest in heart failure, a variety of additional therapies have recently undergone or are currently undergoing clinical investigation that the clinician should be aware of. These therapies include new application of biventricular pacemakers, aggressive mitral valve repair for patients with ongoing mitral valve regurgitation, and the use of left ventricular assist devices as bridges to heart recovery, as well as destination or permanent therapies. Moreover, several new cardiac restraint devices are being applied with some success. Within years, genomic therapies will broaden, as will areas of vascular and myogenic regeneration. Again, although most clinicians will not be aware of all these newly emerging therapies, what they can offer their patients is interest and referral to a specialized center where suitable therapies can be sought.

MITRAL VALVE PROLAPSE

method of
TSUNG O. CHENG, M.D.
The George Washington University
Washington, DC

Mitral valve prolapse (MVP) is one of the commonest diagnoses made in everyday clinical practice. However, despite voluminous literature on the subject (as of June 9, 2003 this author found 4098 citations in a Medline PubMed search using MVP as the key word), clinicians remain interested in it because of its increasing prevalence, various etiologies, divergent clinical manifestations, new echocardiographic techniques for diagnosis, and improved surgical results. Therefore, I find it necessary and important to update my original article published here in 2001.

PREVALENCE

MVP has become the most common valve anomaly in the United States and is also frequently found throughout the world. Its prevalence varies from less than 1% to 38%, differing not only between countries but also within the same country. The prevalence depends on whether the study is clinical or echocardiographic, based on autopsy or surgical material, or in a hospital or non–care-seeking population. Other explanations for the varying prevalence are the age, sex, and weight differences of the study population, imprecise terminology, the care with which auscultation or echocardiography or both are carried out and interpreted, and some selection biases.

ETIOLOGY

Patients with MVP have an anatomically "floppy" mitral valve. The mitral valve shows redundant leaflets with domes protruding toward the left atrial cavity. When the domes show a distinct overshoot, the condition produces an anatomic substrate for mitral regurgitation. However, not all floppy mitral valves diagnosed either by the pathologist in the autopsy room or by the surgeon in the operating room have necessarily been regurgitant during life.

The essential pathologic process in MVP is collagen dissolution with myxomatous degeneration in the principal support structures of the valve—a continuous complex of chordae tendineae and pars fibrosa—the so-called dyscollagenosis. Characteristically, the affected leaflets are voluminous, redundant, and thickened. Not only is the surface area of anterior and posterior cusps of myxomatous mitral valves from patients with MVP, especially those with significant mitral regurgitation, much larger than in normal controls, but also the mitral anulus is greatly dilated. The gross morphology of increased surface area, decreased density, and dilated anulus of the mitral valve explains the characteristic appearance of large, voluminous, and ballooning cusps seen on echocardiograms and angiocardiograms and in the operating or autopsy room.

PATHOPHYSIOLOGY

MVP is more frequent in women than men. There is also an inverse relation between the incidence of MVP and the body weight of the subject; in general, females tend to be thinner than males. That it is the female leanness rather than the female gender that determines the high prevalence of MVP is shown by the high prevalence among both male and female ballet dancers, who must stay lean throughout their professional career. Additional support for the strong association of body weight with the prevalence of MVP is furnished by studies of patients with anorexia nervosa. Several studies reported a high incidence of MVP among patients with anorexia nervosa. Of particular interest was the observation that, in patients with anorexia nervosa and MVP, after the patients received treatment and regained weight, their MVP disappeared only to recur during the follow-up period in the patients who lost weight again. Finally, the disappearance of MVP with weight gain could also account for the striking decline in the prevalence of MVP in women with increasing age, in the Framingham study, from 17% in women 20 to 29 years of age to 1.4% in women older than 80, because an increase in age is generally accompanied by an increase in weight.

All of these observations render strong support to the concept that MVP results from a valvular-ventricular disproportion. The mitral valve apparatus and left ventricular cavity have to be proportionate in size in order to maintain a delicate balance. If there is too much of the mitral valve apparatus or too little of the cavity size, then during systole the mitral valve by necessity prolapses from the left ventricle to the left atrium because of the simple law of geometry. Conditions in which there is too much valve tissue include the floppy mitral valve, Marfan syndrome, rheumatic valvulitis with collagen deposition, papillary muscle dysfunction in coronary artery disease, and lupus erythematosus with Libman-Sacks verrucous endocarditis. If the size of the left ventricular cavity is too small in relation to the mitral valve apparatus, such as in hypertrophic cardiomyopathy, atrial septal defect, anorexia nervosa, straight back syndrome, pectus excavatum, or pulmonary hypertension with right ventricular enlargement ("reverse Bernheim syndrome"), MVP also occurs. On the other hand, with increasing age, scarring of chordae or fibrosis of leaflets or both may occur and the left ventricular cavity tends to enlarge with or without associated systolic hypertension; both tend to reduce the extent of MVP, thus accounting for the decline in prevalence of MVP with age in women.

CLINICAL MANIFESTATIONS

The high prevalence of symptoms in patients with MVP in most reported series contrasts sharply with the low prevalence of symptoms in subjects with MVP in population-based studies and other studies of healthy volunteers. This discrepancy may partly be explained by selection and ascertainment bias. The clinical presentations may range from such nonspecific symptoms as chest pain, palpitation, dizziness, and dyspnea to more pronounced manifestations of significant mitral regurgitation, cerebral ischemic events, infective endocarditis, and, rarely, sudden death.

The mechanisms of chest pain in patients with MVP are multifactorial: chest wall syndrome, mechanical stress on papillary muscle, coronary artery spasm, left ventricular dysfunction, myocardial supply-demand imbalance, coexisting coronary artery disease, panic attacks, and esophageal dysfunction. One or more of these mechanisms may be responsible for chest pain in patients with MVP. Of particular interest are the last two: panic attacks and esophageal dysfunction.

The link between MVP and panic disorders was somewhat controversial. Although MVP may be associated with panic attacks and although β-adrenergic hyperactivity plays an important role in the pathogenesis of symptoms in patients with MVP, there is an apparent contrast in patterns of autonomic dysfunction between patients with MVP and patients with panic attacks. Nevertheless, panic attacks should be considered in evaluating patients with MVP and chest pain.

It has also been shown that in patients with MVP the chest pain may be esophageal in origin. One study showed that out of 18 patients with MVP and normal coronary arteriograms 14 had esophageal motility disorders. Response to sublingual nitroglycerin is not helpful because esophageal spasm responds to such a treatment too. Therefore, not all chest pains in patients with MVP are cardiac in origin.

DIAGNOSIS

The characteristic cardiac findings on physical examination in patients with MVP are the midsystolic click or clicks and a late systolic murmur. Auscultation remains the most sensitive and specific method of detecting MVP. Repeated and systematic auscultation of the patient in the supine, left lateral, sitting, standing, and squatting positions and following a Valsalva maneuver may be necessary to detect or bring out both the midsystolic click and the late systolic murmur. The intensity with which clinical auscultation is pursued is probably the main reason for the reported differences in prevalence of MVP in the various population-based studies. The late systolic murmur may vary markedly in intensity from being barely audible to a loud whoop; the variation may be either spontaneous or induced by a Valsalva maneuver or held expiration. Of historical interest was the report by Osler in 1880 of a 12-year-old girl whose "remarkable whistling sound ... was distinctly audible at a distance of 3 feet 2 inches by measurement." Osler further stated that there were times when the murmur completely disappeared. This elusive behavior of the auscultatory findings of MVP intrigued another physician, Sir Arthur Conan Doyle, enough to include it in one of his stories about Sherlock Holmes and Dr. Watson:

> *"Have you your stethoscope? Might I ask you—would you have the kindness? I have grave doubts as to my mitral valve, if you would be so good. The aortic I may rely upon, but I should value your opinion upon the mitral." I listened to his heart, as requested, but was unable to find anything amiss, save, indeed that he was in an ecstasy of fear...*
>
> *Sir Arthur Conan Doyle*
> *The Sign of Four*

Yet, puzzling as the condition can be, it is also true that a constellation of telltale symptoms and signs can be so typical of MVP that a computer can make an accurate diagnosis.

The impetus to the escalating diagnosis of MVP really began with the introduction of echocardiography, first the M-mode and then two-dimensional. The sensitivity and specificity of both methods varied among different studies. Some of the reported differences in prevalence of MVP between various studies may reflect variable criteria for selection of the study population, differences in diagnostic criteria, availability of optimal resources for performance of high-quality echocardiograms, and interobserver variability in echocardiographic interpretations. Another explanation for the unusually high prevalence of MVP—35% in one study of apparently normal children—is the nonplanar, hyperbolic-paraboloid or saddle shape of the mitral anulus, which allows mitral leaflets that are on the left ventricular side of the mitral anulus in the long-axis view to appear to be on the left atrial side of the anulus in the apical four-chamber view. Thus, it is now customary to rely only on the long-axis view to diagnose MVP.

More recently, by using the techniques of three-dimensional and four-dimensional (or dynamic three-dimensional) echocardiography, I and my colleagues from Wuhan, China studied patients with MVP by transthoracic and transesophageal approaches. We were able to observe the stereoscopic structure and the motion of a normal mitral valve (Figure 1) and the prolapsing leaflets of the mitral valve (Figures 2 and 3) with its regurgitant jet in patients with MVP. These techniques are of great value in evaluating patients with MVP, increasing the diagnostic sensitivity and specificity, and giving assistance to surgeons in making preoperative therapeutic decisions and assessing the intraoperative and postoperative results.

MANAGEMENT

General Measures

The most important principle in management of patients with MVP is to avoid overdiagnosis. Dynamic auscultation and strict echocardiographic criteria are essential. Not all midsystolic clicks or late systolic murmurs are due to MVP. When the echocardiographic findings are equivocal, clinical follow-up in a few years, perhaps with a repeated echocardiogram by a well-trained technician, is appropriate.

Anxiolytic drugs may suppress many of the nonspecific symptoms of MVP, but they do not alter the underlying pathophysiology of the mismatch in size between the mitral valve apparatus and the left ventricular cavity. β-Blockade not only abates the anxiety and other manifestations of excessive catecholamine effect but also controls most of the supraventricular and ventricular arrhythmias.

MVP, in general, is a benign condition unless complications occur. Although rare, they may cause concern. Of all the complications of MVP, the three most important ones are infective endocarditis, sudden death, and progressive mitral regurgitation.

Infective Endocarditis

Patients with MVP are at increased risk for infective endocarditis and therefore should receive antibiotic prophylaxis before any bacteremia-producing procedures. The American Heart Association in its latest recommendation published in 1997 devoted a considerable amount of discussion to this matter.

The old teaching of "no murmur, no prophylaxis" has been challenged because murmurs of mitral regurgitation in patients with MVP can come and go. Furthermore, unless the clinician performs dynamic auscultation, many patients with MVP may not reveal a late systolic murmur at a given time.

Infective endocarditis complicating MVP causes considerable cumulative morbidity and incremental health care costs, but antibiotic prophylaxis against infective endocarditis is highly cost-effective. Therefore, all patients with MVP should receive antibiotic prophylaxis whether or not mitral regurgitation is evident on routine physical examination.

Sudden Death

Although occasional cases of sudden death have been reported in patients with MVP, current available data indicate that the incidence is extremely rare.

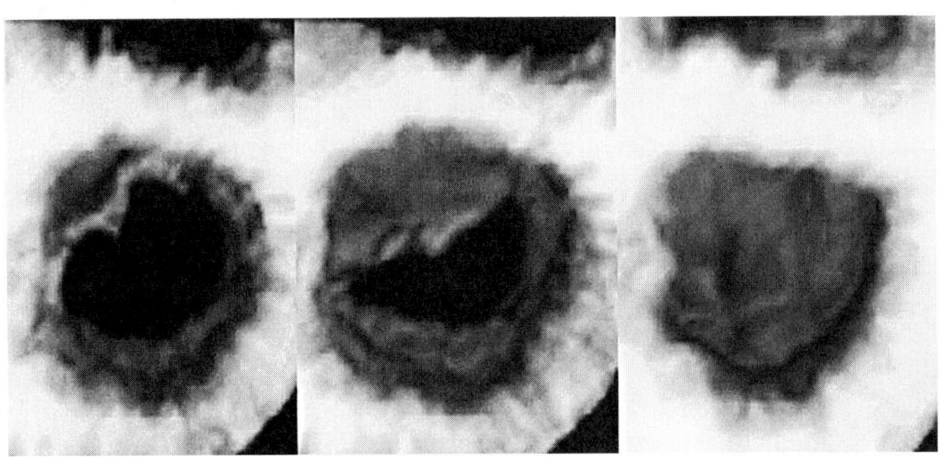

Figure 1. Three-dimensional echocardiograms of a normal mitral valve viewed from left ventricle: when fully opened during diastole (left), partially closed during early to mid systole (middle), and fully closed during late systole (right). (Courtesy of Professor X. F. Wang, Wuhan, China.)

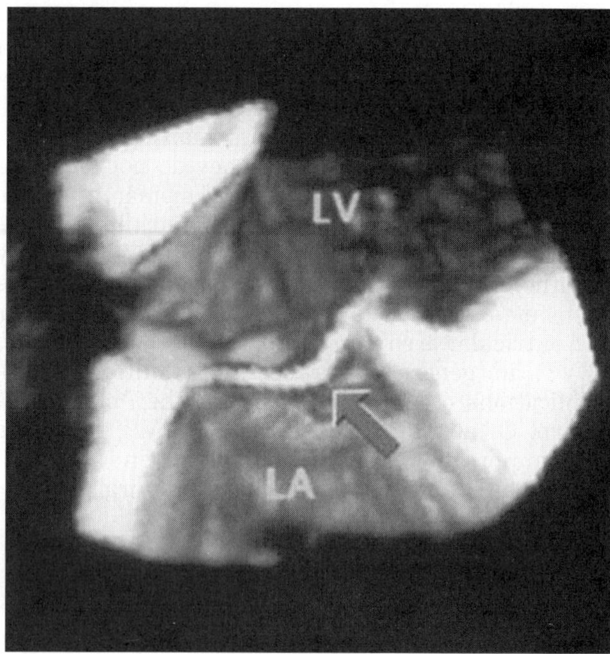

Figure 2. Three-dimensional echocardiogram of a prolapsing mitral valve (arrow). LA, left atrium; LV, left ventricle. (Courtesy of Professor X. F. Wang, Wuhan, China.)

Despite the presumption that the basis for sudden death in MVP is arrhythmic, it is clear that the number of patients with MVP with complex arrhythmias greatly exceeds the number who die suddenly. Furthermore, it is unclear whether the presence and severity of mitral regurgitation add any risk of sudden death to patients with MVP. In both the autopsy study reported in 1995 by Dollar and Roberts and the clinical prospective study reported in 1995 from the New York Hospital–Cornell Medical Center, mitral regurgitation was not an evident risk factor for sudden cardiac death in patients with MVP. On the other hand, prolongation of QT interval and increased QT dispersion might be useful markers of arrhythmogenic mortality. The most important prognostic markers for sudden cardiac death in patients with MVP are previous cardiac arrest, a family history of sudden death at a young age, and mitral valve redundancy on echocardiograms. Patients with a history of cardiac arrest should be considered for implantable cardioverter-defibrillator therapy. Because cases of sudden death are so rare, a cooperative study with a centralized registry seems indicated to collect these otherwise isolated instances and also pool prospective observations in patients, especially athletes, with MVP with potential markers of risk for sudden death.

Surgical Intervention

MVP is the leading cause of mitral valve surgery for isolated mitral regurgitation. Whereas MVP with or without mitral regurgitation is more common in young women, MVP with significant mitral regurgitation is more common in elderly men. A small percentage of patients, male or female, with MVP develop progressive mitral regurgitation that eventually needs surgical intervention. From both the Framingham study and the community study of Olmsted County, Minnesota, residents reported by the Mayo Clinic, at least 10% (probably more when the lifetime risk is considered) of patients ultimately require valve surgery for correction of mitral regurgitation in addition to being at risk for all of the other complications of MVP.

Mitral valve repair is preferred to replacement. Advantages of repair over replacement are as follows:

1. Better preservation of postoperative left ventricular function through preservation of the chordae tendineae.
2. Operative mortality with repair is about half that with valve replacement.
3. Long-term survival with repair is superior to that after valve replacement.
4. Thromboembolism is about four times less frequent after repair than after replacement, with the most striking differences reported when mechanical valves were compared with repair; thus, repair

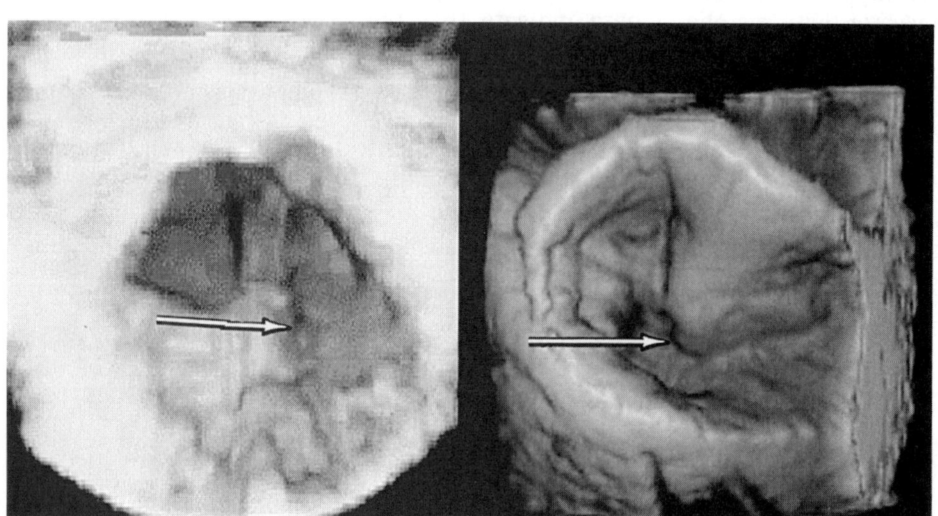

Figure 3. Three-dimensional echocardiograms of a prolapsing mitral valve as viewed from left ventricle (left) and left atrium (right), showing the prolapse (arrow in both). (Courtesy of Professor X. F. Wang, Wuhan, China.)

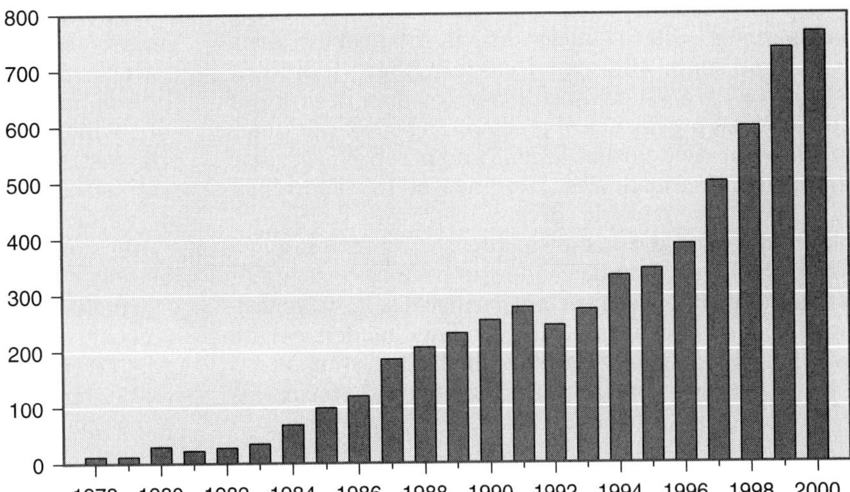

Figure 4. Progressive increase in the number of mitral valve repairs for mitral regurgitation from 1978 to 2000 at the Cleveland Clinic, Cleveland, Ohio. (Courtesy of Dr. Delos M. Cosgrove, Cleveland Clinic.)

obviates the need for long-term anticoagulation in patients with sinus rhythm.

5. Postoperative infective endocarditis is less frequent after repair than after replacement.

Therefore, there has been a progressive increase in the number of mitral valve repairs performed in major medical centers for MVP patients with mitral regurgitation (Figure 4). It is essential that, when referring patients with MVP for surgical treatment, the referring physician choose the surgeon with the most experience in mitral valve repair rather than the surgeon who has replaced the most mitral valves.

Because the most important predictors of postoperative outcome are left ventricular ejection fraction and end-systolic diameter, all patients with signs of left ventricular dysfunction (ejection fraction less than 60% or left ventricular end-systolic dimension greater than 45 mm, or both) should be considered for surgery. Surgery is of debatable value in asymptomatic patients with no signs of left ventricular dysfunction. In patients with MVP and preserved left ventricular function with recurrent ventricular tachyarrhythmias despite medical therapy, early surgery is also controversial because solid data on the value of "prophylactic" surgery are currently lacking.

Asymptomatic patients with MVP and moderate mitral regurgitation and preserved left ventricular function can be observed medically on a yearly basis. Echocardiography should be performed every 2 years to monitor the size and function of the left ventricle, the severity of mitral regurgitation, the size of the left atrium with and without atrial fibrillation, and the degree of pulmonary hypertension. Asymptomatic patients with severe mitral regurgitation and preserved left ventricular function should be seen every 6 months and echocardiography repeated every 12 months. The follow-up should be closer in patients with borderline values such as left ventricular ejection fraction of 60% to 65% and left ventricular end-systolic diameter of 40 to 45 mm. These patients should be instructed to report promptly any deterioration of functional status. Today, the results of mitral valve repair are so good that there is no reason to hesitate recommending surgery to patients with MVP and significant mitral regurgitation when the previously enumerated indications exist.

INFECTIVE ENDOCARDITIS

method of
MATTHEW E. LEVISON, M.D.
Medical College of Pennsylvania/Hahnemann University
Philadelphia, Pennsylvania

DEFINITION

A vegetation, or a lesion resulting from the deposition of platelets and fibrin on the endothelial surface of the heart, is the hallmark of endocarditis. Infection is the most common cause, and the usual pathogen is one of a variety of bacterial species, in which case microscopic bacterial colonies are buried beneath the surface of fibrin, in the absence of an inflammatory reaction. Other types of microorganisms such as rickettsiae, chlamydiae, and fungi may also be involved, so the more general term *infective* rather than bacterial endocarditis is preferred. Usually, the heart valve is the site of the vegetation, but in certain instances, vegetations may occur on other parts of the endocardium. Involvement of extracardiac sites, which can produce an illness clinically similar to endocarditis, is properly termed *endarteritis*.

HOST

In population-based studies, the age- and sex-adjusted incidence of endocarditis is about 5 per 100,000 person-years. The incidence rate in the Philadelphia region is approximately 12 per 100,000 person-years, with the excess incidence attributed almost entirely to the increased frequency of intravenous drug use in this region, where endocarditis in intravenous drug users represents 46% of all cases. Other significant risk factors are (1) advancing age (in part because of the increased prevalence of predisposing cardiac lesions, e.g., degenerative cardiac lesions and prosthetic cardiac valves, and circumstances that may lead to bacteremia, e.g., invasive urologic procedures, anorectal and colonic disease, and use of intravascular catheters in the elderly) and (2) male gender (in part because of the increased prevalence of certain cardiac lesions in males, such as bicuspid aortic valves). The incidence rate ratio for those 65 years or older is almost 9 times that of those younger than 65 years, and the rate for males is 2.5 times that for females.

PATHOGENESIS OF BACTERIAL ENDOCARDITIS

The following sequence of events is thought to result in endocarditis: the normal endothelium is nonthrombogenic, but when damaged, the endothelium is a potent inducer of blood coagulation. The turbulent blood flow produced by certain types of congenital or acquired heart disease, especially flow from a high- to a low-pressure chamber or across a narrowed orifice, traumatizes the downstream endothelium. Such blood flow creates a predisposition for the deposition of platelets and fibrin on the surface of the endothelium, the so-called nonbacterial thrombotic endocarditis lesion (NBTE). Episodes of bacteremia with microbial species capable of survival in the bloodstream, adherence to the NBTE, and proliferation at this site can then result in infective endocarditis.

Risk Factors for Bacteremia. Trauma to mucosal surfaces populated with a dense endogenous flora (including the gingival crevice, oropharynx, terminal ileum, colon, distal part of the urethra, and vagina) releases many different microbial species into the bloodstream. The intensity of the resulting bacteremia is directly related to the magnitude of the trauma, the density of the microbial flora, and the presence of inflammation or infection at the site of skin or mucosal injury. For example, spontaneous and procedure-induced bacteremia occurs more frequently in the presence of periodontal and periapical infection and is a likely consequence of the hyperemia and more abundant microflora in infected tissues surrounding the teeth. Optimal oral hygiene fostered by regular personal and professional care is therefore important in patients who are at risk for endocarditis.

The specific microbial species entering the circulation depend on the unique endogenous microflora colonizing the particular traumatized site. However, only a few bacterial species that gain access to the bloodstream in this manner—specifically, viridans streptococci, staphylococci, and enterococci—are commonly capable of causing endocarditis. Viridans streptococci and enterococci account for about 65% of cases of bacterial endocarditis.

Bacteremia caused by viridans and other oral streptococci occurs in 18% to 85% of dental extractions and periodontal procedures sufficiently extensive to cause gingival bleeding. Bacteremia caused by oral streptococci also follows esophageal dilation and sclerotherapy for esophageal varices. Enterococcal bacteremia occurs somewhat less frequently and follows genitourinary and gastrointestinal invasive procedures such as prostatic surgery, endoscopic retrograde cholangiopancreatography for biliary obstruction, biliary tract surgery, surgery on the lower intestinal mucosa, and urethral dilation.

A history of such procedures within the preceding 2 months has been found in 25% of patients with viridans streptococcal endocarditis and in 40% of those with enterococcal endocarditis. However, these procedures (particularly dental procedures) are common in the general population, which makes assessment of the risk of the procedure for the development of endocarditis difficult; the mere temporal association of a particularly common procedure, such as a dental procedure, with a rare disease such as endocarditis does not necessarily infer causation. Minor mucosal trauma as routine as bowel movements, brushing teeth, chewing hard candy, or other everyday experiences causes an asymptomatic bacteremia characterized by small numbers (usually <10 colony-forming units [CFU]/mL of blood) and very short duration (15 to 30 minutes). Although transient bacteremia is a common, everyday event and each event may be associated with only a very small risk for endocarditis, the cumulative risk of these transient episodes of low-grade bacteremia may be sufficient to account in large part for the 75% of patients with viridans streptococcal endocarditis or the 60% of patients with enterococcal endocarditis who fail to recall a medical or dental procedure that preceded the onset of their endocarditis. Indeed, transient bacteremia from everyday events may additionally be responsible for some cases of endocarditis in patients who give a history of a preceding procedure. One recent study of patients with endocarditis that used age- and sex-matched, population-based controls and sought to quantify the risk attributable to various procedures failed to demonstrate a relationship between recent dental procedures and endocarditis from oral organisms.

Cardiac Risk Factors. Predisposing cardiac lesions are found in about three fourths of patients with infective endocarditis. Patients without a predisposing cardiac risk factor more likely have nosocomial endocarditis, have endocarditis caused by more virulent organisms such as *Staphylococcus aureus*, or are intravenous drug users.

The degree of risk for endocarditis in these cardiac lesions has commonly been inferred from the relative frequencies at which particular cardiac lesions occur in patients with endocarditis. However, inferring risk from these distributions can be problematic. Mitral valve prolapse (MVP) is now among the more frequent cardiac lesions found in patients with endocarditis. Various degenerative valvular lesions, cyanotic congenital heart disease, bicuspid aortic valves, rheumatic valvular heart disease, prosthetic cardiac valves, and previous endocarditis are other conditions that have been identified as cardiac risk factors for

TABLE 1. **Cardiac Conditions Associated With Endocarditis**

High Risk	Moderate Risk	Low Risk
Prosthetic Valve	Valvular RHD	Nonvalvular RHD
Previous endocarditis	Other CHD	Secundum ASD
Cyanotic CHD	Marfan's syndrome	Surgery>6 mo ago, no residua of ASD, VSD, PDA
Surgical conduits or systemic/ pulmonary shunts	Hypertrophic cardiomyopathy	
	MVP with regurgitation	Kawasaki disease
		Pacemakers, CABG
	MVP/thick leaflets	MVP/no regurgitation

Abbreviations: ASD = atrial septal defect; CABG = coronary artery bypass graft; CHD = congenital heart disease; MVP = mitral valve prolapse; PDA = patent ductus arteriosus; RHD = rheumatic heart disease; VSD = ventricular septal defect.

endocarditis (Table 1). However, because the relative frequency of various lesions in case series of endocarditis also reflects the prevalence of the particular cardiac abnormality in the general population, the lesions found more frequently in the population at large are also most likely to be common in case series of patients with endocarditis. The high prevalence of MVP in the general population, estimated to be between 2% and 21%, will lead to a greater representation in series of patients with endocarditis than will a rarer, but more risky cardiac abnormality such as valvular rheumatic heart disease.

The true degree of the risk for endocarditis of a cardiac lesion can be determined only by measuring the incidence rate of endocarditis in those who have a particular cardiac abnormality. The highest incidence rates (300 to 740/100,000 patient-years) occur in persons with previous native valve endocarditis and prosthetic cardiac valves. For prosthetic valve endocarditis (PVE), the risk is greatest during the first few postoperative months as a result of intraoperative and perioperative contamination, and it probably does not vary by site of placement or type of prosthetic valve material. The incidence rate is approximately 400/100,000 patient-years for those with valvular rheumatic heart disease; 100 to 200/100,000 patient-years for individuals with uncorrected congenital lesions, especially those associated with cyanosis, including single-ventricle states, transposition of the great arteries, patent ductus arteriosus, ventricular septal defects, tetralogy of Fallot, and tricuspid or pulmonary stenosis or atresia; and 50/100,000 patient-years (only about 10-fold higher than that of the general population) for patients who have MVP *with* murmur. Other lesions associated with endocarditis include Marfan's syndrome and hypertrophic cardiomyopathy.

Cardiac lesions that pose no greater risk than that of the general population include secundum atrial septal defects, atherosclerosis, previous coronary artery bypass graft surgery, MVP *without* murmur, previous rheumatic heart disease without valvular dysfunction, cardiac pacemakers and implanted defibrillators, and syphilitic aortitis.

CLINICAL FEATURES

Symptoms usually begin within 2 weeks of the inciting bacteremia. In the preantibiotic era, when endocarditis was uniformly fatal, a short duration of illness of less than 6 weeks before death was typical for acute endocarditis; in contrast, subacute and chronic endocarditis had a more indolent course, with death occurring in 6 weeks to 2 years. Such a distinction based on chronicity has continued to prove useful in the antibiotic era. Chronicity is now used in reference to the duration of illness before diagnosis. Acute endocarditis is usually caused by *S. aureus,* especially when accompanied by marked signs of general infection and suppurative embolic phenomena, and it has a rapidly fatal course if treatment is delayed. Infection may develop on a previously normal valve. Therefore, a diagnosis of acute endocarditis can serve as an effective guide to empirical antibiotic therapy, even before the results of blood culture are available. In contrast, subacute endocarditis, commonly caused by streptococci and enterococci, often develops on previously damaged endocardium, has less dramatic clinical manifestations of general infection, and is characterized by nonsuppurative peripheral vascular phenomena.

Clinical manifestations result from (1) the valvular infection itself, (2) embolization of fragments of the vegetation, (3) suppurative complications that result from hematogenous spread of infection, or (4) an immunologic response to the infection in the form of immune complex vasculitis. Systemic manifestations of endocarditis most commonly include fever and other symptoms that may accompany fever, such as drenching night sweats, arthralgia, myalgia, pain in the low back region and thighs, and weight loss. Fever is usually low grade, with temperature peaks rarely exceeding 39.4° C, but may be high and spiking in acute endocarditis. Fever may be absent in a few patients, such as those who are very elderly or severely debilitated, have significant renal or heart failure, or are taking antipyretics or antibiotics.

Cardiac manifestations include murmurs, valve ring abscess, myocardial infarction, myocardial abscess, and diffuse myocarditis. Murmurs of valvular insufficiency can be due to destruction or distortion of the valve and its supporting structures or, more rarely, valvular stenosis as a result of large vegetations. Murmurs are likely to be absent in tricuspid endocarditis or may be absent when a patient is first seen with acute endocarditis. PVE may result in regurgitant systolic or diastolic murmurs as a result of dehiscence of the valve at the annulus, the usual site in PVE, or muffling of the usual crisp prosthetic valve clicks. Valve ring abscesses may result from local extension of the infection from the valve ring of the noncoronary cusp of the aortic valve. A valve ring abscess can lead to (1) persistent fever despite appropriate antimicrobial therapy, (2) heart block as a result of the destruction of conduction pathways in the area of the atrioventricular node and bundle of His in the upper interventricular septum, (3) pericarditis or hemopericardium as a result of burrowing abscesses into the pericardium, or (4) shunts between cardiac chambers or between the heart and aorta as a consequence of burrowing abscesses into other cardiac chambers or the aorta. Myocardial infarction can result from coronary artery embolization, and myocardial abscess can occur as a consequence of bacteremia. Diffuse myocarditis is possibly due to immune complex vasculitis.

Congestive heart failure, the most common complication of endocarditis, develops in about 60% of patients as a consequence of valvular or myocardial involvement, or it may precede the onset of endocarditis and be caused by the underlying cardiac lesion. Congestive heart failure may develop dramatically in patients with acute *S. aureus* endocarditis with the sudden onset of an aortic diastolic murmur or rupture of the mitral valve chordae. It occurs more frequently with left-sided than right-sided endocarditis and more often with aortic involvement than mitral involvement.

Extracardiac manifestations include (1) embolic events that result in infarction of numerous organs, such as the lung in right-sided endocarditis or the brain, spleen, or kidneys in left-sided endocarditis; (2) suppurative complications, such as abscesses, septic infarcts, and mycotic aneurysms; and (3) immunologic reactions to the valvular infection, including glomerulonephritis, sterile meningitis or polyarthritis, and a variety of vascular phenomena such as mucocutaneous petechiae, splinter hemorrhages, Roth's spots, and Osler's nodes. The development of clinically apparent splenomegaly and many of the various nonsuppurative peripheral vascular phenomena is related to the duration of illness before diagnosis. The frequency of these clinical manifestations (<50%) is currently less than in the past because of an earlier diagnosis and a consequent shorter duration of illness before initiation of antimicrobial therapy.

Systemic embolization, often a devastating complication when the cerebral circulation is involved, occurs in about 20% to 40% of patients with left-sided endocarditis. Embolization is more frequent with *S. aureus* and fungal endocarditis, vegetations of the anterior leaflet of the mitral valve, and vegetations larger than 1 cm in diameter. Frank cerebral abscess is rare but occurs in 1% to 5% of patients with *S. aureus* endocarditis. Septic pulmonary emboli that appear as multiple round infiltrates commonly occur in patients with tricuspid valve *S. aureus* endocarditis and may cavitate or be complicated by empyema. The frequency of embolization decreases dramatically during the first 2 weeks of antimicrobial therapy as the vegetation heals.

Mycotic aneurysms are an unusual but important complication of endocarditis. Mycotic aneurysms are commonly asymptomatic but can become clinically evident in 3% to 5% of patients, even months or years after completion of successful therapy. These aneurysms characteristically develop at arterial bifurcations, such as in the middle cerebral, splenic, superior mesenteric, pulmonary, coronary, and extremity arteries, the abdominal aorta, and the sinus of Valsalva. In a patient with endocarditis, unremitting headache, visual disturbance, cranial nerve palsy, meningeal signs, or a focal neurologic deficit is suggestive of impending rupture of a cerebral mycotic aneurysm. Signs of blood loss at any site in a patient with endocarditis should suggest rupture of a mycotic aneurysm.

Nosocomial Endocarditis. Nosocomial endocarditis, defined as endocarditis following a hospital-based procedure performed within 4 weeks before the onset of symptoms, accounts for 10% to 30% of cases of endocarditis. The clinical features of nosocomial endocarditis are similar to those of community-acquired endocarditis. The source of the bacteremia can be identified in more than 90% of cases of nosocomial endocarditis. The most important bacteremia-inducing event during hospitalization that results in endocarditis is the use of an intravascular device, which is present in up to 50% of cases. *S. aureus* bacteremia is much more frequently complicated by endocarditis (10% to 30% of the time) than nosocomial enterococcal bacteremia is (<1%). A major predisposing cardiac lesion for nosocomial endocarditis is a prosthetic cardiac valve. Although blood cultures are usually positive, the diagnosis of endocarditis is frequently delayed because of failure to recognize the presence of endocardial infection, which frequently is evident only on transesophageal echocardiography (TEE).

ECHOCARDIOGRAPHY

Echocardiography has become second only to culture of blood in the investigation of patients who are clinically suspected of having endocarditis. Echocardiography can visualize valvular vegetations, satellite vegetations, flail valves, ruptured chordae, perivalvular abscesses, fistulas, valvular perforations, and mycotic aneurysms. Echocardiography is also relied on to identify predisposing cardiac lesions and the causes and severity of congestive heart failure by assessment of ventricular size, wall motion, and dynamic function. Two-dimensional transthoracic echocardiography (TTE) and TEE, the two types of echocardiography currently in use, are safe and may be performed at the bedside. TTE is rapid, noninvasive, and relatively inexpensive. TEE is invasive, requires sedation, and is slightly more expensive. TTE can give more general information regarding cardiac structure and function that cannot be obtained with TEE; however, TEE is frequently helpful in situations where TTE is not, such as in the presence of obesity, emphysema, and prosthetic cardiac valves, which may obscure the TTE image. Hemodynamic complications such as central or perivalvular regurgitant flow in the presence of a prosthetic valve can easily be detected and semiquantitated by the addition of color-flow Doppler. The sensitivity of TEE is greater (90% to 100%) than that of TTE (<80%), and vegetations as small as 1 mm can be detected. TEE also has a specificity (i.e., true-negative rate), positive predictive accuracy (the probability of endocarditis when the

TABLE 2. **Modified (Duke) Criteria for the Diagnosis of Infective Endocarditis**

1. *Definite diagnosis of infective endocarditis*
   A. Pathologic criteria
      a. Microorganisms demonstrated by culture or histologic examination of vegetations, vegetations that have embolized, or an intracardiac abscess specimen
      b. Pathologic lesions: vegetations, vegetations that have embolized, or intracardiac abscess confirmed by histologic examination showing active endocarditis
   B. Clinical criteria
      a. 2 major criteria *or*
      b. 1 major/3 minor *or*
      c. 5 minor
2. *Possible diagnosis*
   a. 1 major and 1 minor criterion *or*
   b. 3 minor
3. *No endocarditis*
   a. Firm alternative diagnosis
   b. Clinical resolution after ≤4 d of antimicrobial therapy
   c. No pathologic evidence of infective endocarditis at surgery or autopsy with ≤4 d of antimicrobial therapy *or*
   d. Does not meet criteria for possible infective endocarditis, as above

Major Criteria

1. Blood Culture
   a. 2 separate blood cultures positive for
      i. Viridans streptococci, *Streptococcus bovis,* HACEK, *Staphylococcus aureus*
      ii. Community-acquired enterococci in the absence of a primary focus
   b. Microorganisms consistent with endocarditis isolated from at least 2 blood cultures drawn >12 h apart
   c. Positive blood cultures: 3 of 3, most of >4 with 1st and last ≥1 h apart
   d. Single positive blood culture for *Coxiella burnetti* or antiphase 1 IgG antibody titer>1:800
2. Endocardial involvement
   a. Echocardiography: oscillating intracardiac mass on a valve or supporting structure, in the path of a regurgitant jet stream, or on implanted material in the absence of an alternative anatomic explanation, valve ring abscess, or new partial dehiscence of a prosthetic valve
   b. New regurgitant murmur (increasing or changing pre-existing murmur not sufficient)

Minor Criteria

1. Predisposing heart condition or intravenous drug use
2. Fever, temperature >38° C
3. Major arterial emboli, septic pulmonary infarcts, mycotic aneurysm, intracranial hemorrhage, conjuctival hemorrhage, and Janeway's lesions
4. Immunologic phenomena: glomerulonephritis, Roth's spot, Osler's node, and rheumatoid factor
5. Positive blood culture, but does not meet major criterion, or serologic evidence of active infection by organism consistent with infective endocarditis

Modified from Li JS, Sexton DJ, Mick N, et al: Proposed modification to the Duke criteria for the diagnosis of infective endocarditis. Clin Infect Dis 30:633–638, 2000.

echocardiogram is positive), and a negative predicative accuracy (the probability of no endocarditis when the echocardiogram is negative) of 95% to 100%. However, the frequency of a falsely positive finding of vegetations, such as nonspecific valvular thickening or rupture of a valve leaflet or the mitral valve chordae, which can simulate a vegetation in patients likely to be studied by echocardiography, though very low, may be greater than the frequency of endocarditis in low-risk populations. Therefore, echocardiography should be performed only for the diagnosis of endocarditis in patients in whom such a diagnosis is likely on clinical grounds. The use of TEE as the initial diagnostic test is recommended in patients with at least "possible endocarditis" according to clinical criteria (see Duke criteria, Table 2), in patients with suspected complicated infective endocarditis (i.e., paravalvular abscess), and in those with suspected PVE.

Sequential echocardiography during the course of antimicrobial therapy is used to assess healing of vegetations, detect the development or progression of complications, and guide decisions regarding the necessity and timing of surgery. The finding of early closure of the mitral valve as a consequence of elevated left ventricular end-diastolic pressure in association with acute aortic valve endocarditis has been used to predict the need for surgery, and detection of a vegetation, especially a large one (i.e., >10 mm in largest dimension), has been found to signify a poorer outcome, such as a greater likelihood of embolization, congestive heart failure, the need for surgery, and death. However, for assessment of the need for surgical intervention, echocardiographic results must be viewed in light of the specific clinical situation, especially the patient's hemodynamic status, previous embolic events, and the type of pathogen involved, such as antibiotic-resistant gram-negative bacilli or fungi.

Other Investigative Procedures. Cardiac catheterization can provide important information and should not be avoided when indicated in selected patients with endocarditis for fear of dislodging emboli. Coronary angiography is used to assess the presence of significant coronary artery disease before elective placement of prosthetic cardiac valves in patients who are older than 40 years and have additional atherogenic risk factors. Contrast-enhanced computed tomography (CT) or magnetic resonance imaging (MRI) can best evaluate abscesses or infarcts of the intra-abdominal organs (spleen or liver). Contrast-enhanced CT or MRI of the head may provide evidence of a bleeding mycotic aneurysm. Magnetic resonance angiography for the detection of intracranial aneurysms is promising, but four-vessel cerebral angiography is the standard for detection of aneurysms smaller than 5 mm.

ELECTROCARDIOGRAPHIC MANIFESTATIONS

A baseline electrocardiogram (ECG) should be obtained to assess the presence of conduction abnormalities, which develop in about 10% to 20% of patients with endocarditis as a consequence of burrowing valve ring abscesses. Prolongation of the PR interval may be the initial indication of the sudden development of more severe conduction abnormalities, such as complete heart block. Other abnormalities that can be detected by ECG include myocardial infarction and pericarditis.

HEMATOLOGIC MANIFESTATIONS

Progressive anemia of chronic disease with normochromic, normocytic indices routinely develops in patients with subacute endocarditis, and normal platelet, white blood cell, and differential counts. In acute endocarditis caused by *S. aureus*, anemia may be initially absent, although the white blood cell count is usually elevated with a shift to the left and the platelet count is often low. PVE with an unstable prosthesis may cause acute hemolysis. The erythrocyte sedimentation rate is routinely elevated in endocarditis, except in those with hypofibrinogenemia secondary to disseminated intravascular coagulation or congestive heart failure.

RENAL MANIFESTATIONS

Proteinuria and microscopic hematuria are common findings that occur in up to 50% of patients. Renal emboli or focal glomerulonephritis can cause microscopic hematuria, but gross hematuria usually indicates renal infarction. Renal failure that develops in a patient with endocarditis is usually due to diffuse immune complex glomerulonephritis.

OTHER LABORATORY MANIFESTATIONS

Serologic evidence of circulating immune complexes, as detected by Raji cell radioimmunoassay, may be found in patients with endocarditis, the frequency of which is related to the duration of illness. Occasional false-positive nontreponemal serologic tests for syphilis occur. Cerebrospinal fluid may show polymorphonuclear leukocytes and a moderately elevated protein concentration in up to 15% of patients, but a normal glucose value. Frank bacterial meningitis, though unusual, occurs in *S. aureus* endocarditis.

DIAGNOSIS

Definitive diagnosis of infective endocarditis depends on microbiologic or pathologic proof of infection by histology or culture of vegetations obtained at the time of surgery or autopsy or by histology or culture of vegetations obtained at the time of surgical removal of an arterial embolus. In lieu of surgery or autopsy, a definitive diagnosis can be established by demonstration of (1) a characteristic vegetation, valve ring abscess, or new prosthetic valve dehiscence with echocardiography and (2) intravascular infection with multiple blood cultures obtained over an extended period that are positive for a microorganism consistent with endocarditis. However, blood culture or echocardiography is usually performed only after the diagnosis is suspected on the basis of the history and physical findings. Because the clinical manifestations are numerous and no single clinical finding is pathognomonic of endocarditis, a constellation of signs and symptoms, in addition to the presence of certain risk factors, has been suggested as a set of diagnostic criteria for general clinical use. Risk factors include the presence of a prosthetic cardiac valve or other predisposing cardiac conditions and intravenous drug use. The diagnosis can be ranked in order of the probability that endocarditis is present by distinguishing between major and minor criteria, which allows for weighting of clinical, microbiologic, and echocardiographic findings, as has been done by the Duke endocarditis group (see Table 2).

Microbiologic Investigation

Isolation of a pathogen from several blood cultures obtained over an extended period is important both to confirm the diagnosis of endocarditis and to enable determination of the optimal antibiotic regimen. Bacteremia in endocarditis is characterized by a constant number of organisms per milliliter of blood (usually 20 to 200CFU/mL), unrelated to the height of the patient's temperature or the site of blood sampling (e.g., arterial versus venous blood), except for a slight fall in numbers across the hepatic or splenic circulation. Less than 5% of patients with endocarditis have sterile blood cultures if adequate culture methods are used. The proper method of obtaining blood for culture includes (1) disinfection of the skin with 70% isopropyl alcohol and then 2% iodine or iodophor solution, with the disinfectant allowed to remain on the skin for at least 1 minute, and (2) withdrawal of 10mL to 20mL of blood per blood culture in an adult through the least contaminated site, preferably an antecubital vein rather than, for example, the femoral vein. Three blood cultures should be obtained in this manner at least 1 hour apart to demonstrate that the bacteremia is continuous. The clinical microbiology laboratory should be advised of the suspected diagnosis of endocarditis because some organisms require special media or more prolonged incubation (up to 3 weeks) for detection. In the absence of previous antibiotic therapy, the first three blood cultures are expected to be positive in over 95% of patients. Previous antibiotic therapy and infection with fastidious bacteria (such as *Abiotrophia* species, the HACEK group of organisms, *Neisseria, Brucella*, and *Legionella*), fungi, *Bartonella, Tropheryma, Chlamydia, Coxiella*, and *Rickettsia* can result in negative cultures. Gram stain of the blood cultures may identify some pathogens that may not otherwise be apparent. *Abiotrophia* species require subculture on pyridoxal- or L-cysteine–enriched agar or on plates streaked with *S. aureus*. Serology will be required for *Bartonella, Brucella, Chlamydia, Mycoplasma, Legionella,* and *Coxiella* (although antibodies for *Bartonella* and *Chlamydia* are often cross-reactive); polymerase chain reaction on cardiac valvular tissue for *Bartonella, Tropheryma,* and *Coxiella*; special stains or fluorescent antibody staining on tissue for *Bartonella, Tropheryma, Legionella, Coxiella, Chlamydia*, and fungi; and special media or the lysis centrifugation system for *Bartonella, Legionella, Brucella,* and fungi. Fungal endocarditis, which is likely to have negative blood cultures, tends to be complicated by large vegetations and embolization, in which case the organisms can be identified by Gram stain and culture of the surgically removed emboli.

In acute endocarditis, for which empirical antibiotic therapy should be initiated as soon as possible, two to three blood samples should be drawn 1 hour apart for culture before initiation of empirical therapy. In the face of a preceding course of antibiotic therapy, further antibiotic treatment should be withheld and blood cultures repeated until positive if clinical conditions permit. The longer the duration since the last dose of antibiotic or the shorter the preceding course of the antibiotic, the more likely that the blood culture will be positive. Bacteriuria with either enterococci or *S. aureus* occurs in endocarditis caused by the respective organism.

A variety of in vitro tests must be performed on the pathogen isolated from blood to assess its susceptibility to potential bactericidal drugs (Table 3). Enterococci are routinely tested for β-lactamase production (which predicts resistance to penicillin and ampicillin) and for high-level gentamicin and streptomycin resistance (which predicts lack of synergy with a combination of

TABLE 3. **In Vitro Assays**

Organism	Test	Result
Viridans streptococci	Broth dilution test	Penicillin MIC
Enterococci	Broth dilution test	Penicillin MIC Vancomycin (Vancocin) MIC
	Growth in 500 μg/mL of gentamicin 1000 μg/mL of streptomycin	High-level resistance* Gentamicin (Garamycin) Streptomycin
	Nitrocefin degradation	β-Lactamase production
Staphylococcus aureus, coagulase-negative staphylococci	Nitrocefin degradation	β-Lactamase production
	Oxacillin/methicillin sensitivity	MRSA/MRSE
	Broth dilution test	Vancomycin MIC Rifampin (Rimactane) MIC TMP/SMX (Bactrim) MIC
Other pathogens	Broth dilution tests	Antibiotic MIC/MBC† Time-kill studies†
All pathogens	Serum antibiotic concentrations	Peak and trough vancomycin‡ and aminoglycoside§ concentrations

*The choice of an aminoglycoside should be based on in vitro high-level aminoglycoside susceptibility testing. If the strain is susceptible to high levels of gentamicin, gentamicin is preferred because determination of gentamicin serum levels is more generally available.

†May be useful for nonstandard antimicrobial regimens or unusual pathogens.

‡Vancomycin peak serum levels obtained 1 hour after completion of a 1- to 2-hour infusion should be in the range of 30 to 45 μg/mL. Vancomycin trough levels obtained just before the next dose should be 10 to 15 μg/mL.

§Gentamicin peak serum levels obtained 1 hour after the start of a 20-to 30-minute IV infusion or IM injection should be about 3 μg/mL, and the trough level should be less than 1 μg/mL. The streptomycin peak serum level 1 hour after IM administration is about 15 to 20 μg/mL, and the trough should be about 5 μg/mL.

Abbreviations: MBC = minimal bactericidal concentration; MIC = minimal inhibitory concentration; MRSA = methicillin-resistant *S. aureus*; MRSE = methicillin-resistant coagulase-negative staphylococci; TMP/SMX = trimethoprim-sulfamethoxazole.

From Levison ME: In vitro assays. In Kaye D (ed): Infective Endocarditis, 2nd ed. New York, Raven, 1992, pp 151–167.

the respective aminoglycoside and a cell wall–active drug such as vancomycin, penicillin, or ampicillin), in addition to susceptibility to penicillin and vancomycin. Synergism between cell wall–active antibiotics and aminoglycosides has been demonstrated for other microorganisms, including viridans streptococci, staphylococci, *Pseudomonas aeruginosa,* and aerobic enteric gram-negative bacilli, and its presence can be assessed by a special in vitro test, the so-called time-kill assay.

For nonstandard regimens or unusual pathogens, peak serum bactericidal activity may be assayed against the patient's pathogen early in the course of therapy, and if inadequate, the dose of antibiotic is increased (though not at the cost of toxicity) and the serum retested. Measurement of vancomycin or aminoglycoside serum levels is helpful to ensure adequate but nontoxic antibiotic levels.

Organisms should be retained in the laboratory for susceptibility testing of additional antibiotics if the need arises, and organisms obtained at surgery or relapse should be retested for antimicrobial susceptibility.

Diagnostic Strategies in Special Situations

Intravenous Drug Users. Because outpatient follow-up in this population is rarely possible, admission of febrile intravenous drug users without a clinically apparent source for their fever is indicated for at least a week until the results of blood culture are available. Blood cultures will usually become positive within 1 week if fungi, fastidious gram-negative bacilli or streptococci, or anaerobes are involved or the patient has recently taken antibiotics. After obtaining blood for culture, empirical antimicrobial therapy should be initiated. Once the blood cultures are found to be positive, evidence of endocarditis should be sought initially by TTE and, if negative, by TEE. Even if the patient has another potential source for the bacteremia and no echocardiographic or clinical evidence of endocarditis, but the organism isolated is likely to be a cause of endocarditis, such as *S. aureus,* the diagnosis of endocarditis should nevertheless be suspected. If no apparent source for the bacteremia can be found, the patient should still be considered to possibly have endocarditis even if echocardiographic and clinical evidence is lacking. In patients with negative echocardiographic results, if the clinical course dictates and another diagnosis is still not apparent, TEE should be repeated in about 1 week. If blood cultures remain negative after 1 week of incubation, the patient may be discharged from the hospital without echocardiography, unless clinical evidence of left-sided or right-sided endocarditis is detected, in which case the diagnosis of endocarditis should nevertheless be suspected.

Nosocomial Native Valve Endocarditis. In patients with bacteremia related to intravascular devices, such as an arteriovenous graft for hemodialysis, indwelling central intravenous catheter, cardiac assist balloon pump, or pacemaker wire, removal of the intravascular device is usually required, especially with *S. aureus* or fungi or if a tunnel or exit site infection is present. In patients with *S. aureus* bacteremia, echocardiography should be performed to detect vegetations and to assess for complications of valve infection because of the high frequency of endocarditis in these patients. Catheter-associated, coagulase-negative staphylococcal nosocomial bacteremia, which rarely eventuates in native valve endocarditis, should not be investigated with echocardiography after the initiation of antibiotic therapy unless the patient has a prosthetic cardiac valve. Indeed, catheter removal may not be necessary to cure coagulase-negative, staphylococcal catheter-associated bacteremia. The necessity of echocardiography to detect occult native valve endocarditis after catheter removal and initiation of antibiotic therapy for nosocomial fungemia or enterococcal bacteremia is unresolved.

Prosthetic Valve Endocarditis. The diagnosis of PVE is usually suspected because of fever and confirmed by the presence of multiple blood cultures positive for the same microorganism. In a recent study, 43% of patients with a prosthetic valve in whom fever and bacteremia developed had PVE, or it developed later. Any organism in blood cultures in these patients must be taken seriously as a potential cause of endocarditis, including streptococci, enterococci, staphylococci, enteric gram-negative bacilli, atypical mycobacteria, and fungi, regardless of whether a portal of entry can be identified (such as an intravascular device, undrained abscess, wound infection, or genitourologic or gastrointestinal disease or procedure). In those with clinical evidence suggestive of PVE, empirical antibiotic therapy can be initiated after three to four sets of blood cultures are obtained. After antimicrobial therapy is started, blood cultures should be repeated to assess for clearance of bacteremia. The source of the bacteremia should be sought and eliminated (e.g., drainage of abscesses or removal of intravascular devices). Echocardiographic evidence of endocarditis, such as valvular vegetations, new prosthetic valve dysfunction, and perivalvular infection, should be sought by TEE. New conduction abnormalities, which can occur as a result of perivalvular extension of infection, should be sought by ECG. Serial ECG and echocardiograms should be obtained if initially unrevealing. An annular location and perivalvular extension of the infection are likely when the aortic valve is involved and when infection develops within the first 12 months after surgery.

ANTIBIOTIC THERAPY

Principles. Effective antimicrobial therapy for endocarditis optimally requires identification of the specific pathogen and assessment of its susceptibility to various antimicrobial agents. Therefore, every effort must be made to isolate the pathogen before initiation of antimicrobial therapy, if clinically feasible. In patients who are in immediate danger of death, empirical antibiotic therapy should be started as soon as possible after obtaining blood cultures. Empirical therapy should be targeted at the most likely pathogens in that particular clinical setting. Specific antimicrobial therapy that is anticipated to be the most effective and least toxic, inconvenient, and costly is instituted once the results of antimicrobial susceptibility testing of the isolated pathogen become available. Minimal requirements for an effective antimicrobial regimen include the following:

Bactericidal Activity. Bacteriostatic agents are not able to clear pathogens from infected tissues unaided by host defenses, such as polymorphonuclear leukocytes, antibody, and complement. Because host defenses are not thought to operate within vegetations (except in tricuspid valve vegetations, where polymorphonuclear leukocytes may aid the effect of an antimicrobial agent), clearance of bacteria from these vegetations requires a bactericidal antibiotic. In fact, complete eradication of pathogens from the vegetation is thought to be essential to cure endocarditis. If any bacteria remain after completion of antibiotic therapy, the residual organisms will multiply and cause a relapse. If the pathogen cannot be eliminated completely by antimicrobial therapy, the infected vegetation may need to be excised surgically to effect a cure. For microorganisms without predictable susceptibility, the bactericidal activity of an antimicrobial agent for the particular patient's pathogen must be assessed by determination of the minimal inhibitory (MIC) and minimal bactericidal (MBC) concentrations of the antimicrobial agents in vitro (see Table 3).

High Concentrations of the Antimicrobial Agent in the Vegetation. Optimally, the antimicrobial agent should have a minimal "inoculum effect"; specifically, it should exhibit the least reduction in potency when tested against microbial inocula, such as the microbial densities of 10^8 to 10^{10} CFU/g that exist in vegetations, which are higher than the standard inocula of 10^5 to 10^6 CFU/mL used to perform the MIC and MBC tests. If the inoculum effect is considerable, such as a rise in MIC and MBC at high inocula, as is usually seen with β-lactam antibiotics, the doses of the antimicrobial agent must be adjusted to compensate for the reduction in potency that would be anticipated in vivo in the vegetation. Doses of the antimicrobial agent must also be large enough to achieve concentrations of the antimicrobial agent in blood to facilitate passive diffusion of the agent into the depths of the vegetation where the microcolonies of the pathogen are located. Dosing that is sufficiently large to attain bactericidal activity against the patient's pathogen in a greater than 1:8 dilution of the patient's serum at the peak time after administration of the antimicrobial agent has traditionally guided therapy (although more recent data suggest that dilutions >1:64 have more predictive accuracy for bacteriologic cure). Serum bactericidal activity can be quantitated by the in vitro serum bactericidal test. However, the methodology of the test in general has not been well standardized, and scant clinical data are available to validate this recommendation. Despite high concentrations in blood, some antimicrobial agents fail to penetrate vegetations deeply enough (e.g., amphotericin B), or they penetrate vegetations unevenly (e.g., teicoplanin). Because amphotericin B is the only fungicidal agent, cure of fungal endocarditis usually requires surgery.

Prolonged Duration of Antimicrobial Therapy. Over 90% of the microbial population in the vegetation are nongrowing and metabolically inactive once the infection has become well established. Nongrowing organisms are more likely to be found in the central portions of the microcolonies in the deeper regions of the vegetation. Because bactericidal drugs such as the β-lactam are active only against growing microorganisms, each dose is able to effect a reduction in microbial count in only that minor portion (less than 10%) of the population that happens to be growing at the time of drug administration. The duration of drug therapy must therefore be prolonged to result in complete clearance of the pathogen from the vegetation.

The duration of therapy varies with the specific pathogen, the site of the infection, and the type of antibiotic. For example, bacterial clearance is more rapid for viridans streptococci than for staphylococci, in tricuspid than in aortic vegetations, with antistaphylococcal β-lactams than with vancomycin, and with combinations of a cell wall–active agent plus an aminoglycoside than with a single drug. More rapid clearance in these special circumstances may permit a shorter course of therapy to achieve cure.

The duration of antimicrobial therapy after valve replacement depends to some extent on evidence of active infection at the time of surgery. In patients with positive intraoperative cultures or Gram stain, a full course of postoperative therapy is reasonable; otherwise, an additional 2 weeks plus the time remaining on the regimen is routinely recommended for that type of endocarditis.

Dosing Should Be Frequent Enough to Prevent Regrowth of Microorganisms Between Doses. The organisms that remain after brief in vitro exposure to an aminoglycoside or a β-lactam antibiotic frequently exhibit a postexposure delay in further growth in vitro, the so-called postantibiotic effect. Unfortunately, no such effect occurs with enterococci or *P. aeruginosa* in the rat model of endocarditis despite a postantibiotic effect in vitro. Thus, even though a bactericidal effect can be achieved in the vegetation in the early portions of a dosing interval when levels of the drug are high, if antibiotic levels are not maintained in the vegetation at least above the MIC during the rest of the dosing interval, regrowth of residual organisms may occur and efficacy may be compromised.

Standardized regimens have been recommended for the most common pathogens on native and prosthetic valves—viridans streptococci, enterococci, staphylococci, and HACEK organisms (Table 4). Staphylococci that are sensitive to methicillin or oxacillin can be treated with an antistaphylococcal β-lactam such as nafcillin or cefazolin, or vancomycin; a β-lactam is always preferable over vancomycin because of the relatively slow bactericidal action of vancomycin. Ceftriaxone has relatively poor antistaphylococcal activity and should not be used for this indication despite the ease of its once-daily regimen. Methicillin (or oxacillin)-resistant *S. aureus* (MRSA) is cross-resistant

TABLE 4. **Standard Antibiotic Therapy for Infective Endocarditis Caused by Common Pathogens (Doses Are for Adults With Normal Renal Function)**

A. *Penicillin-susceptible streptococci, i.e., viridans streptococci,* Streptococcus bovis, Streptococcus pneumoniae, *group A and B streptococci (MIC ≤0.1 μg/mL)*

1. Aqueous penicillin G, 12–18 million U daily IV continuously or every 4 h, cefazolin (Kefzol), 1 g IV q8h, ceftriaxone (Rocephin), 2 g IV q24h, or vancomycin (Vancocin), 15 mg/kg IV q12h for 4 wk (Vancomycin: for patients with immediate-type allergic reactions to penicillin, i.e., urticaria, angioedema, or anaphylaxis. These regimens are preferred in patients ≥65 y old and those with 8th nerve or renal impairment)
2. Aqueous penicillin, 12–18 million U daily IV continuously or q4h, or ceftriaxone, 2 g IV q24h, plus gentamicin, 3 mg/kg IV* or IM q24h for 2 wk (This last regimen is appropriate for uncomplicated cases of endocarditis in patients at low risk for adverse events from aminoglycosides. For prosthetic valve endocarditis: a 6-wk course of penicillin plus gentamicin [Garamycin] for at least the first 2 wk)

B. *Relatively penicillin-resistant streptococci, i.e., viridans streptococci,* S. bovis, S. pneumoniae, *group A and B Streptococci (MIC >0.1–0.5 μg/mL)*

1. Aqueous penicillin, 18 million U daily IV, or cefazolin, 1 g IV q8h for 4–6 wk, plus gentamicin, 1 mg/kg IV or IM q8h for the first 2 wk (For prosthetic valve endocarditis: a 6-wk course of penicillin plus gentamicin for at least the first 4 wk[§])
2. Vancomycin, 15 mg/kg IV q12h (For patients with immediate-type allergic reactions to penicillin, i.e., urticaria, angioedema, or anaphylaxis. Vancomycin use may enhance the nephrotoxicity of gentamicin. When vancomycin is chosen, the addition of gentamicin is not recommended)

C. *Penicillin-resistant streptococci (MIC >0.5 μg/mL), non-VRE, non–β-lactamase–producing enterococci, Abiotrophia[†] (nutritionally variant streptococci)*

1. Aqueous penicillin, 18–30 million U daily IV plus streptomycin, 7.5 mg/kg (max, 500 mg/dose) q12h, or gentamicin, 1 mg/kg IV or IM q8h for 4–6 wk (For prosthetic valve endocarditis, a minimum of 6 wk of combined penicillin [or vancomycin] and aminoglycoside is recommended[§])
2. Vancomycin, 15 mg/kg IV q12h, plus streptomycin, 7.5 mg/kg (max, 500 mg/dose) q12h, or gentamicin, 1 mg/kg IV or IM q8h for 4–6 wk (For patients with immediate-type allergic reactions to penicillin, i.e., urticaria, angiodema, or anaphylaxis. For prosthetic valve endocarditis, a minimum of 6 wk of combined penicillin [or vancomycin] and aminoglycoside is recommended[§]).

D. *Methicillin/gentamicin-susceptible staphylococci—uncomplicated right-sided disease, native valve only*

Nafcillin (Unipen) or oxacillin, 2 g q4h IV, *with* gentamicin, 1 mg/kg q8h IV/IM for 2 wk (Vancomycin is less rapidly bactericidal than antistaphylococcal β-lactam antibiotics, as reflected by slower clearance of staphylococci from vegetations and blood. Consequently, vancomycin is not effective in the short-course [2-wk] regimen and, similarly, should not be used in other antistaphylococcal regimens unless the organism is methicillin resistant or the patient has an immediate-type penicillin allergy that precludes use of β-lactam antibiotic)

E. *Methicillin-susceptible staphylococci—native valve*

Nafcillin or oxacillin, 2 g q4h, cefazolin (Ancef), 2 g q8h IV, or vancomycin, 15 mg/kg q12h IV for 4–6 wk, *with or without* gentamicin, 1 mg/kg q8h IV/IM for the first 3–5 d only. (The additional benefit of an aminoglycoside has not been clearly established. Use gentamicin only if the isolate is gentamicin susceptible. Cefazolin [Kefzol] or vancomycin should be used in penicillin-allergic patients. Cefazolin should be avoided in those with immediate-type penicillin hypersensitivity)

F. *Methicillin-resistant staphylococci—native valve*

Vancomycin, 15 mg/kg q12h for 4–6 wk

G. *Methicillin-resistant staphylococci—prosthetic device*

Vancomycin, 15 mg/kg q12h, *plus* rifampin (Rifadin)[‡] 300 mg q8h for 6 wk or longer, *plus* gentamicin, 1 mg/kg q8h IV/IM for the first 2 wk (Rifampin should be added in cases of rifampin-susceptible, staphylococcal PVE; combination therapy is essential to prevent the emergence of rifampin resistance. If the isolate is gentamicin resistant, use another aminoglycoside to which the isolate is sensitive. If resistant to all aminoglycosides, substitute a fluoroquinolone to which the isolate is sensitive)

H. *Methicillin-susceptible staphylococci—prosthetic device*

Nafcillin or oxacillin, 2 g q4h IV for 6 wk or longer, *plus* rifampin,[‡] 300 mg for q8h for 6 wk or longer, *plus* gentamicin, 1 mg/kg q8h IV/IM for the first 2 wk (Rifampin should be added in cases of rifampin-susceptible, staphylococcal PVE; combination therapy is essential to prevent the emergence of rifampin resistance. If gentamicin resistant, an alternative third agent should be added after in vitro susceptibility testing results are known. Cefazolin or vancomycin should be used in penicillin-allergic patients. Cefazolin should be avoided in those with immediate-type penicillin hypersensitivity)

I. *HACEK organisms*

Ceftriaxone,[‡] 2 g IV q24h for 4 wk

*Exceeds dosage recommended by the manufacturer.

[†]Because of technical difficulties in susceptibility testing of *Abiotrophia* species, many experts recommend treating infection by these strains with the standard regimen recommended for enterococci. Six weeks of therapy is recommended for patients with enterococcal endocarditis who have had more than 3 months of symptoms before therapy. Six to 8 weeks of therapy is recommended for prosthetic valve endocarditis. Cephalosporins are not acceptable alternatives for treatment of enterococcal endocarditis.

[‡]Not FDA-approved for this indication.

[§]If gentamicin is administered in three equally divided doses per day, adjust dose to achieve peak and trough serum levels of ~3μg/mL and <1 μg/mL, respectively. The dose of streptomycin administered q12h is adjusted to achieve peak and trough serum levels of ~20 μg/mL and <5 μg/mL, respectively.

Abbreviations: PVE = prosthetic valve endocarditis; VRE = vancomycin-resistant enterococci.

Adapted from Wilson WR, Karchmer AW, Dajani AS, et al: Antibiotic treatment of adults with infective endocarditis due to streptococci, enterococci, staphylococci and HACEK microorganisms. JAMA 274: 1706, 1995.

to all β-lactams; in addition, these strains are frequently resistant to other classes of antibiotics, except vancomycin. In the event that vancomycin is not tolerated, many MRSA are sensitive to trimethoprim-sulfamethoxazole, which has been shown to be effective in one series of cases. Strains should be tested for susceptibility to rifampin or gentamicin if the use of these drugs is planned. Linezolid and quinupristin-dalfopristin (Synercid) may be active against MRSA, but linezolid has limited bactericidal activity and Synercid is not bactericidal against strains that have MLSb-type resistance, a frequent finding in MRSA. MSLb resistance is due to methylation of the ribosomal target that results in decreased affinity of this target that is common to antibiotics of these classes.

Ticarcillin, aztreonam, antistaphylococcal penicillins such as nafcillin and methicillin, the cephalosporins, and the carbapenems have no or limited activity against enterococci. Linezolid and Synercid have only inhibitory activity against enterococci, and the activity of Synercid is limited to *Enterococcus faecium*. Enterococci should be routinely tested for high-level resistance to gentamicin and streptomycin because they frequently exhibit this type of resistance to one or both aminoglycosides. Only the aminoglycoside to which the enterococcal strain is sensitive should be chosen for combination with a cell wall–active antimicrobial agent (penicillin, ampicillin, or vancomycin). β-Lactam–gentamicin combinations are preferable to vancomycin-gentamicin because of the increased risk of nephrotoxicity with the vancomycin-gentamicin combination. No reliable bactericidal regimen is available to treat infective endocarditis caused by enterococcal strains that are resistant to high levels of both aminoglycosides in vitro and thus lack penicillin-aminoglycoside synergy. Endocarditis from these strains can be treated with penicillin or vancomycin alone for 8 to 12 weeks, but the relapse rate is high. If the enterococcus is β-lactamase positive (detected by a nitrocefin strip because MIC testing of β-lactamase–positive strains may fail to disclose this type of penicillin resistance), ampicillin-sulbactam or vancomycin can be used alone for 8 to 12 weeks because most of these strains are also highly aminoglycoside resistant. If the enterococcus has a penicillin MIC greater than 16 μg/mL, vancomycin can be used in combination with an aminoglycoside if the strain is highly aminoglycoside susceptible. If the enterococcus is vancomycin resistant (MIC >4 μg/mL), infectious disease consultation should be sought because these strains are usually multidrug resistant.

In vitro susceptibility testing should be performed on gram-negative bacilli, anaerobes, and diphtheroids and the patient treated with the regimen that demonstrates the best bactericidal activity. Therapy for endocarditis attributable to these organisms should be developed in consultation with an infectious disease specialist. Bactericidal activity against anaerobic gram-negative bacilli can frequently be achieved with metronidazole, aerobic enteric gram-negative bacilli or *P. aeruginosa* is often cleared with a cell wall–active agent–aminoglycoside combination or ciprofloxacin, and bactericidal activity against diphtheroids can frequently be attained with a vancomycin-aminoglycoside combination. *Bartonella* endocarditis has been treated with doxycycline and aminoglycoside plus valve replacement, and doxycycline* plus hydroxychloroquine and valve replacement have been successful in treating *Coxiella* endocarditis (although reinfection of the prosthetic valve is common). Blood culture–negative endocarditis is generally treated empirically with vancomycin, ceftriaxone, and gentamicin.

SURGICAL THERAPY

Replacement of an infected valve with a prosthesis is indicated in the following situations:

1. Increasing or refractory congestive heart failure secondary to valvular dysfunction. The prognosis of patients with congestive heart failure and infective endocarditis is grave. In patients who are hemodynamically unstable, emergency cardiac valve replacement should not be delayed to allow further antibiotic therapy. Delayed surgery in conjunction with worsening of congestive heart failure increases operative mortality from 6% to 8% in patients with mild or no congestive heart failure to 17% to 33% in those with severe congestive heart failure. The incidence of reinfection of a newly placed cardiac valvular prosthesis is estimated to be 2% to 3%, far less than the mortality associated with uncontrolled congestive heart failure. Although the frequency of operative mortality and PVE is higher when a prosthetic valve is implanted in the presence of active infection, the overall outcome is better if the valve replacement is prompt, before the development of severe congestive heart failure or spread of the infection into perivalvular tissue. If the patient is hemodynamically stable, valve replacement is best delayed until a course of antimicrobial therapy is completed, or at least until after 7 days of antibiotic therapy has been given.
2. Multiple clinically significant emboli despite antibiotic therapy for 2 weeks. However, the first or second embolic episode may so impair the patient that prosthetic valve replacement at that point may be futile. The use of a variety of factors, such as the large size or continued enlargement of vegetations with medical therapy, location on the anterior leaflet of the mitral valve, and fungi or *S. aureus* as the pathogen, to predict significant embolization as an indication for valve replacement remains unresolved.
3. Endocarditis caused by certain pathogens that rarely respond to medical therapy alone, such as fungi, enterococci for which no synergistic bactericidal combination is available (e.g., high-level ampicillin/aminoglycoside/vancomycin–resistant enterococci or β-lactamase–producing/high-level aminoglycoside–resistant *Enterococcus faecalis*), and β-lactam– or fluoroquinolone-resistant gram-negative bacilli.
4. Uncontrolled bacteremia despite optimal antibiotic therapy. However, it should be remembered that the

*Not FDA approved for this indication.

average duration of *S. aureus* bacteremia in patients receiving vancomycin therapy is 8 days, with bacteremia persisting for several weeks in some patients before its ultimate resolution.

5. Indications for surgical treatment of a valve ring abscess, which may heal with antimicrobial therapy alone, include further extension of infection into the myocardium, the development of prosthetic valve dehiscence, heart block, congestive heart failure, or persistence of bacteremia despite medical therapy. Patients with valve ring abscess should be monitored for the development of conduction abnormalities, which may require placement of a transvenous pacemaker because of the risk of a high-grade heart block.

6. The surgical indications for PVE are the same as those outlined for native valve endocarditis. Some patients without evidence of infection at the annulus may be treated medically. To avoid the complications of prosthetic valve replacement (e.g., PVE, bleeding, thromboembolic events, and valve deterioration), new surgical options that have been proposed as an alternative to a prosthetic valve include valve débridement, valvuloplasty, and repair or replacement of the paravalvular structure with a pulmonary root autograft. Prosthetic valve replacement in an intravenous drug user is problematic because the prosthetic valve places the patient at continued risk for PVE. Alternatively, tricuspid valve resection without prosthetic replacement can be tolerated hemodynamically for extended periods in many of these patients.

Intrathoracic, intra-abdominal, or peripheral mycotic aneurysms usually require surgical excision, whereas cerebral aneurysms may heal with medical therapy alone. Cerebral aneurysms should be monitored closely with serial angiograms and generally require surgery if accessible and enlarging or bleeding. Myocardial revascularization should be performed at the time of elective valve surgery if significant coronary artery disease is present. However, patients who require emergency placement of a prosthetic valve for hemodynamic decompensation secondary to acute endocarditis cannot usually tolerate the dye load necessary for coronary angiography and the additional bypass surgery.

ANTICOAGULANT THERAPY

Although anticoagulant therapy may impede further enlargement of a vegetation, it is relatively contraindicated in endocarditis because of the increased risk of intracranial hemorrhage from either occult mycotic aneurysms, cerebral emboli, or cerebral immune vasculitis. Anticoagulation may be used for an over-riding indication that is separate from endocarditis, but for deep vein thrombophlebitis of the lower extremities, an inferior vena cava filter would be preferable to anticoagulation. Anticoagulation may be continued with caution during treatment of PVE; however, anticoagulation is particularly problematic when *S. aureus* is the pathogen because of the increased risk of cerebral embolism with this organism, in addition to being problematic in patients with endocarditis who undergo prosthetic valve replacement within 1 month after a neurologic event. In these latter patients, use of a bioprosthesis that will not require anticoagulation is preferable to a mechanical prosthesis.

SHORTER INPATIENT THERAPY

The use of shorter courses of antibiotic therapy and oral regimens and the administration of parenteral antibiotic therapy at home have been investigated in selected patients as a means of shortening the duration of hospitalization. The usual candidate for outpatient therapy is a patient with endocarditis due to a highly penicillin-sensitive viridans streptococcus, when the duration of illness is less than 3 months, and when there is low risk for serious complication, such as CHF or emboli. Such patients can be treated with 4 weeks of a β-lactam alone or 2 weeks of a β-lactam plus an aminoglycoside (see Table 4). Close monitoring on a regular basis is required to assess response to therapy and possible development of adverse drug effects. Easy access to medical care in the event of complication and a support system at home are essential. Having a focal infection that would require more than 2 weeks of antimicrobial therapy, PVE, or significant renal or eighth nerve impairment would preclude the use of short-course β-lactam–aminoglycoside combination therapy. Absorption of orally administered agents may be unreliable, so the oral route is not generally recommended. Before considering outpatient therapy, most patients should first be evaluated and stabilized in the hospital; only rarely can some patients be managed entirely as outpatients. The standard regimens used to treat penicillin-sensitive streptococci require either continuous infusion of penicillin or frequent intravenous administration. A single daily dose of ceftriaxone is an attractive alternative to penicillin. Because of its long half-life and good potency against these streptococci, serum levels of ceftriaxone remain well above the MIC and MBC for over 24 hours.

RESPONSE TO THERAPY

Once receiving appropriate antimicrobial therapy, most patients will note a sense of well-being, lessened fatigue, and improved appetite, and their temperature will usually fall to normal levels within 2 to 5 days. The erythrocyte sedimentation rate, anemia, and renal function may take weeks to months to improve. Circulating immune complexes and related serologic findings, including hypocomplementemia, mixed cryoglobulinemia, and rheumatoid factor, also tend to resolve gradually with effective antibiotic therapy. A variety of tests are performed to monitor both the antimicrobial effects (see Table 3) and the potential toxicities of the drugs used to treat the infection. Blood cultures for streptococci and enterococci should become sterile after 1 to 2 days of appropriate therapy and cultures for *S. aureus*, after 3 to 5 days; however, with vancomycin therapy, blood cultures for *S. aureus*

TABLE 5. **Reasons for Inadequate Clinical Response**

Inadequate therapy: wrong drug, wrong dose
Infarcts secondary to emboli
Metastatic abscesses of the spleen, kidney, brain etc., which may require surgical drainage
Suppurative thrombophlebitis at the site of an IV catheter, with or without superinfecting endocarditis
Other superinfections, e.g., *Clostridium difficile* colitis, urinary tract infection
Febrile reaction to the antimicrobial agent or another drug
Another unrelated febrile illness

may take 10 to 14 days to become sterile. Blood cultures are performed daily until sterile. If no organism is isolated from blood but the patient has a good clinical response to an empirical antimicrobial regimen, the empirical therapy should be continued. If no organism is isolated and no clinical response to empirical therapy is seen after 1 to 2 weeks, endocarditis from a fastidious pathogen, or a diagnosis other than infective endocarditis should be considered, such as antiphospholipid antibody syndrome, which requires anticoagulants rather than antibiotic therapy.

If the pathogen is initially isolated from blood and appropriate antimicrobial therapy is started but fever persists or recurs, blood cultures should be repeated to assess for persistent or relapsing infection, among other possibilities (Table 5), most commonly pulmonary or systemic embolization. Blood cultures are repeated 2 and 4 weeks after therapy has been completed because relapse is most common within 1 month. The relapse rate is less than 1% to 2% for native valve endocarditis caused by viridans streptococci, 8% to 12% for enterococci, and higher for *S. aureus* and other pathogens or PVE.

OUTCOMES

Factors that affect mortality include the infecting organism (the mortality of endocarditis from fungi, *P. aeruginosa,* and aerobic enteric gram-negative bacilli > staphylococci > enterococci > streptococci), the site of infection (aortic > mitral and left-sided > tricuspid infection), PVE versus native valve endocarditis (early-onset PVE > late-onset PVE > native valve endocarditis), age (higher in the elderly and very young), gender (men > women), and the presence of certain complications such as heart or renal failure, rupture of a mycotic aneurysm, cardiac arrhythmias and conduction abnormalities, perivalvular extension, cerebral emboli, and perhaps, severe immunosuppression from HIV infection. Heart failure remains the leading cause of death. However, with increasing use of prosthetic valve replacement for heart failure, the leading cause of death may shift to neurologic complications from embolic episodes or mycotic aneurysms or to uncontrolled infection with antibiotic-resistant microorganisms. After cure of one episode of endocarditis, patients still have a greatly increased risk of reinfection.

PREVENTION

The effect of endocarditis prophylaxis with antimicrobial agents has been estimated to be modest, with less than 10% of all cases being preventable by prophylaxis. For example, only about half of cases have recognizable predisposing cardiac lesions, most cases do not follow an invasive procedure, and only about two thirds of cases are due to microorganisms (viridans streptococci and enterococci) against which prophylactic regimens are directed. However, in patients who are

TABLE 6. **Chemoprophylaxis of Endocarditis**

Chemoprophylaxis Recommended for High- and Medium-Risk Patients

Dental procedures
- Dental and periodontal procedures known to induce mucosal bleeding
- Dental implant placement and reimplantation of avulsed teeth
- Endodontic instrumentation or surgery only beyond the apex
- Subgingival placement of antibiotic fibers or strips
- Initial placement of orthodontic bands but not brackets
- Intraligamentary local anesthetic injections

Respiratory tract
- Tonsillectomy and adenoidectomy
- Bronchoscopy with a rigid bronchoscope
- Surgery on the respiratory mucosa

Genitourinary tract
- Prostate surgery
- Cystoscopy or urethral dilation

Chemoprophylaxis Recommended for High-Risk, Optional for Medium-Risk Patients

- Esophageal dilation or sclerotherapy for esophageal varices
- Biliary tract surgery
- Endoscopic retrograde cholangiography with biliary obstruction

Surgery on the intestinal mucosa

Chemoprophylaxis Optional for High-Risk Patients

- Bronchoscopy with a flexible bronchscope, with or without biopsy
- Transesophageal echocardiography
- Endoscopy with or without gastrointestinal biopsy
- Vaginal hysterectomy
- Vaginal delivery

Continued

TABLE 6. **Chemoprophylaxis of Endocarditis—Cont'd**

Prophylactic Regimens	
*Dental, Oral, Respiratory Tract, and Esophageal Procedures in Patients at High and Moderate Risk**	
STANDARD REGIMEN	
Amoxicillin (Amoxil)†	2.0 orally 1 h before the procedure
AMOXICILLIN/PENICILLIN-ALLERGIC PATIENTS	
Clindamycin (Cleocin)†	600 mg orally 1 h before the procedure
or	
Cephalexin (Keflex)† or cefadroxil (Duricef)†‡	2.0 g orally 1 h before the procedure
or	
Azithromycin (Zithromax)† or clarithromycin (Biaxin)†	500 mg orally 1 h before the procedure
PATIENTS UNABLE TO TAKE ORAL MEDICATIONS	
Ampicillin†	IV or IM administration of ampicillin, 2 g within 30 min before the procedure
AMPICILLIN/PENICILLIN-ALLERGIC PATIENTS UNABLE TO TAKE ORAL MEDICATIONS	
Clindamycin†	IV administration of clindamycin, 600 mg within 30 min before the procedure
or	
Cefazolin (Kefzol)‡	IV administration of cefazolin, 1.0 g within 30 min before the procedure
Genitourinary/Gastrointestinal (Excluding Esophageal) Procedures in Patients at High Risk§	
STANDARD REGIMEN	
Ampicillin,† amoxicillin,† plus gentamicin (Garamycin)	IV or IM administration of ampicillin, 2 g, plus gentamicin, 1.5 mg/kg (not to exceed 120 mg) within 30 min of starting the procedure; 6 h later, ampicillin, 1.0 g IV/IM, or amoxicillin, 1 g orally
AMPICILLIN†/AMOXICILLIN/PENICILLIN-ALLERGIC PATIENTS	
Vancomycin (Vancocin) plus gentamicin	IV administration of vancomycin, 1.0 g over 1–2 h, plus gentamicin, 1.5 mg/kg IV/IM (not to exceed 120 mg); complete infusion or injection within 30 min of starting the procedure
Genitourinary/Gastrointestinal (Excluding Esophageal) Procedures in Patients at Moderate Risk	
STANDARD REGIMEN	
Ampicillin† or amoxicillin†	IV or IM administration of ampicillin, 2 g within 30 min of starting the procedure, or amoxicillin, 2 g orally 1 hr before the procedure
AMPICILLIN/AMOXICILLIN/PENICILLIN-ALLERGIC PATIENTS	
Vancomycin	IV administration of vancomycin, 1.0 g over 1–2 h; complete infusion within 30 min of starting the procedure

*Doses in the table are for adults.
†Not FDA-approved for this indication.
‡Cephalosporins should not be used in individuals with immediate-type hypersensitivity reactions to penicillin (urticaria, angioedema, or anaphylaxis).
§No second dose of vancomycin or gentamicin is recommended.
Adapted from Dajani AS, Taubert KA, Wilson W, et al: Prevention of bacterial endocarditis. Recommendations of the American Heart Association. JAMA 277: 1794, 1997.

known to have a risky cardiac lesion and are about to undergo a procedure that is likely to induce bacteremia with organisms having predictable susceptibility to antibiotics with minimal inconvenience, toxicity, and cost, the American Heart Association has made the recommendations shown in Table 6. Additional preventive measures are to minimize invasive procedures; avoid unnecessary use of intravascular catheters, a major predisposing event for nosocomial endocarditis; aggressively treat focal infections; and maintain good dental hygiene in patients at increased risk for endocarditis.

HYPERTENSION

method of
WILLIAM J. ELLIOTT, M.D., PH.D.
Department of Preventive Medicine
RUSH Medical College of RUSH University at RUSH-Presbyterian-St. Luke's Medical Center
Chicago, Illinois

High blood pressure (BP), or hypertension, is a major contributor to premature morbidity and mortality in many countries, and is expected to increase in importance worldwide by 2010. Compared with other known risk factors for acute myocardial infarction, heart failure, stroke, and end-stage renal disease, hypertension is perhaps the simplest to diagnose, easiest to treat, and one of the most cost-effective preventive strategies. Because of its high prevalence (e.g., 24% of adults aged 18–74 years) in the United States, hypertension generates more office visits than any other chronic condition. Successful treatment of hypertension has been a major contributor to the impressive reduction in age-adjusted stroke mortality (≈62%) and coronary heart disease mortality (≈45%) in the United States since 1972, when the National High Blood Pressure Education Program began. Because so much information about hypertension has been derived from clinical trials, many evidence-based recommendations can now be made about its diagnosis and management.

DEFINITION AND CLASSIFICATION OF HYPERTENSION

Hypertension is currently diagnosed if the systolic BP is 140 mm Hg or higher, the diastolic BP is 90 mm Hg or higher, or the person is taking antihypertensive medications. The current classification system (Table 1) for BP uses only two "stages" for hypertension. Stage 1 encompasses about 70% of the people diagnosed with hypertension, and accounts for well more than half the deaths and disability ultimately attributed to hypertension. The "cut-points" for the stages of hypertension (see Table 1) reflect roughly equal future cardiovascular risk: a diastolic reading of 100 mm Hg carries about the same prognostic importance as a systolic reading of 160 mm Hg. When the systolic and diastolic readings for a given patient fall into different stages, the BP is classified into the higher stage. For instance, both 182/94 mm Hg and 142/112 mm Hg are properly placed in stage 2, the former because of the systolic reading, and the latter because of the diastolic elevation. The correct classification of a patient's hypertension is likely to become more important if current proposals are implemented that make the amount of payment to health care providers directly proportional to the absolute risk (and BP stage) of the individual being treated.

TABLE 1. **Classification of High Blood Pressure**

Category	Systolic (mm Hg)	Diastolic (mm Hg)
Normal	<120	and <80
Pre-hypertensive	120–139	or 80–89
Stage 1 hypertension	140–159	or 90–99
Stage 2 hypertension	≥160	or ≥100

The Seventh Report of the Joint National Committee on Prevention, Detection, Evaluation, and Treatment of High Blood Pressure (JNC 7) has now combined the categories of what was formerly called "normal" and "high-normal" blood pressures. Individuals with systolic blood pressures between 120 and 139 mm Hg or diastolic blood pressures between 80 and 89 mm Hg (see Table 1) are now said to have "pre- hypertension," and should adopt lifestyle modifications to prevent crossing the 140/90 mm Hg border into hypertension. This category change was warranted because about 90% of 55 to 65-year-old people in the Framingham Heart Study with "pre-hypertension" became hypertensive after 25 years of follow-up.

Although hypertension is most common in older women, neither age nor gender alters this classification scheme for hypertension. As people ascend in age past the sixth decade, systolic BP typically increases, but diastolic BP decreases. In some studies, pulse pressure (systolic minus diastolic BP), when widened (typically >70 mm Hg), is a marker for noncompliant and often atherosclerotic blood vessels. Pulse pressure in older people is a better predictor of heart failure, mortality, heart attack, stroke and all cardiovascular events than either mean arterial or systolic BP alone.

MEASUREMENT OF BLOOD PRESSURE

Although BP is traditionally measured in the medical office using a stethoscope and sphygmomanometer, home (self) BP monitoring and ambulatory BP monitoring are now quite easily and frequently performed. Both home and ambulatory measurements can be useful, primarily to supplement office BP readings; no clinical trials involving morbidity or mortality endpoints have relied only on BP measurements outside the medical office.

Office BP Measurements

Proper BP measurement technique should be routinely followed. The most common mistakes include: using an undersized BP cuff (<80% of the arm circumference), deflating the mercury column faster than 2–3 mm Hg/sec, having the patient rest for <5 minutes before cuff application, not inflating the cuff high enough, and readings influenced by caffeine, tobacco, alcohol, or pain.

Home and Ambulatory BP Measurements

Many convenient, inexpensive, and accurate machines are available to estimate home BP. Even persons with visual or auditory impairment or problems with hand-eye coordination can use semiautomatic devices with digital readouts and printers. Home BP monitoring allows the patient (and physician) to be more informed about BP readings, improves medication and office visit adherence in our clinic, and can reduce health care expenditures for frequent office visits. Ambulatory BP monitoring (ABPM), formerly used mostly in research, allows frequent, automated measurements of BP over a 24-hour period, during a person's usual daily activities, including sleep. The utilization of ABPM devices is expected to increase, because the Center for Medicare and Medicaid Services authorized (in 2002) a small payment for it when performed for its most common indication outside research settings, to diagnose "white-coat hypertension."

Both home and ambulatory BP readings are typically lower than office readings. Home readings correlate better with the extent of target-organ damage than do traditional readings taken in a health care provider's office; ABPM is even better. Both home and ABPM readings can be helpful in evaluating symptoms suggestive of intermittent hypotension. People who routinely measure BP at home probably have a better prognosis than those who do not, both because of greater interest in their BP and from increased social support, when a friend or spouse becomes involved in BP measurement and overseeing pill-taking and appointment-keeping behaviors. In several studies, ABPM measurements have been better predictors of death, myocardial infarction, or stroke than office or home BP readings.

Home BP readings should be interpreted cautiously, carefully, and conservatively. Many factors that contribute to BP variability are more difficult to control in the home, including circadian variation, food and alcohol ingestion, exercise, and stress. Before home readings are accepted, the instrument should be calibrated against a standard sphygmomanometer using a Y-tube, and the technique of the measurer checked. Although there are no data from long-term clinical studies basing all treatment decisions solely on home readings, supplementing office BP measurements with home readings is beneficial, especially when the two are widely disparate. People who have much lower home BP readings (compared with the office) suffer fewer major cardiovascular events than people who have elevated readings in both places do.

ABPM has reawakened interest in the circadian variation of pulse and BP. Most normotensive people and perhaps 80% of hypertensives have at least a 10% drop in BP during sleep, compared with the daytime average. Individuals who lack this BP pattern are at increased risk of cardiovascular events; blacks and elderly people may have smaller nocturnal BP drops. Elderly persons with *more* than a 20% difference between nighttime and daytime average BPs have more unrecognized ischemia in "watershed areas" (of the brain and other organs) during sleep, if the BP declines below the autoregulatory threshold.

White-Coat Hypertension

About 20% of American hypertensives have substantially lower BPs outside than in the health care provider's office (so-called "white-coat hypertension"). The white coat itself is unlikely to be the only factor that increases BP. Definitions of "white coat hypertension" vary; differences of more than 10% (comparing several office BPs obtained during installation of the ABPM device with the daytime average) are certainly suggestive.

The clinical consequences and prognostic significance of white-coat hypertension are controversial. One school of thought suggests that if a person has an acute rise in BP because of an approaching physician, similar elevations in BP are likely whenever any stressful stimulus is encountered. In several studies, people with white-coat hypertension had a greater prevalence of subclinical risk factors for cardiovascular disease, including left ventricular hypertrophy, family history of hypertension and heart disease, dyslipidemia, and elevated fasting insulin levels. These considerations argue for drug therapy in "white-coat hypertensives," because many with the diagnosis would be expected to develop sustained hypertension in the future.

A minority view, based on more conservative definitions of "white-coat hypertension," proposes that some individuals consistently show a persistent, marked elevation in BP in response to the health care environment. These people have a very reduced risk of either target-organ damage or major cardiovascular sequelae, compared with people with sustained hypertension. Whether such individuals have a similar (or even identical) risk for cardiovascular events, compared with completely normotensive people, is unlikely, but is still open to question.

The best treatment for white-coat hypertension is still unresolved. Clearly these individuals should benefit from therapeutic lifestyle changes, which could reduce the probability of progression to sustained hypertension. Completely abstaining from antihypertensive medication in white-coat hypertensives appears unwise. Whether intensive treatment with continuous antihypertensive medication is warranted for only temporary increases in BP is debatable. Antihypertensive drug treatment *and* repeated ABPM sessions required to assess the adequacy of therapy in white-coat hypertensives would certainly not be very cost-effective.

INITIAL EVALUATION OF THE HYPERTENSIVE PATIENT

There are four key issues to address during the initial office evaluation of a person with elevated BP readings:

- Documenting an accurate diagnosis of hypertension.
- Stratifying the person's risk for cardiovascular events, which involves: (1) defining the presence or absence of existing cardiovascular or renal disease, or "target-organ damage" related to hypertension and (2) screening for other cardiovascular risk factors that often accompany hypertension.
- Assessing whether the person is likely to have an identifiable cause for the elevated BP (i.e., secondary hypertension), and should have further diagnostic testing for it.

- Obtaining information that may be helpful in choosing effective therapy.

Documenting the Diagnosis

To diagnose hypertension, elevated BP measurements should generally be documented at least twice, at visits separated by a week or more. Patients who exhibit wide fluctuations in BP, or who are hypertensive at some evaluations, but normotensive at others, may need additional measurements, either in the office, at home, or by ABPM. Treatment should generally *not* be instituted until the diagnosis is clearly proved. In rare circumstances, such as when target-organ damage is noted, treatment may begin after a single set of measurements.

Stratifying Risk for Cardiovascular Disease

Before beginning treatment for hypertension, an assessment of the person's risk for cardiovascular and renal events is warranted. Although several evidence-based algorithms for estimating absolute risk for a given patient exist, most were thought to be too complicated to use in everyday medical practice. In the very simple scheme recommended by the Sixth Report of the Joint National Committee on Prevention, Detection, Evaluation, and Treatment of High Blood Pressure (JNC VI) for risk assessment, people with elevated BPs were divided into three general categories, designated A, B, or C. In the 1971-74 iteration of the National Health and Nutrition Examination Survey (NHANES I), 19.2% of the people with either high-normal BP or hypertension fell into risk group C, with either diabetes mellitus, target-organ damage (TOD), or existing cardiovascular disease. The lowest risk group, making up 9% of the at-risk population in NHANES I, was risk group A; these women have neither cardiovascular disease nor risk factors. More than 70% of hypertensives have one or more risk factors (but not diabetes) and no TOD or cardiovascular disease; they are at intermediate risk, and were in risk group B. This scheme emphasizes the importance of TOD and existing disease as indicators of a patient's absolute risk, which affects the decision about initial drug therapy. This simple three-category system for estimating cardiovascular risk has been largely superseded by more quantitative methods, most of which are based on the Framingham risk equations; one of these was included in the 2001 guidelines from the National Cholesterol Education Program, and is widely available on the internet and in other easy-to-use formats.

The people with the highest short-term risk of a stroke, heart attack, or renal disease are those who already have evidence of disease; for instance, history of a recent transient ischemic attack, previous myocardial infarction, or renal impairment. Hypertensive people with TOD are at the next highest level of absolute risk. Subclinical TOD is detected by physical examination or laboratory tests that indicate a derangement of structure or function in the eyes, heart, kidneys, or blood vessels related to prolonged periods of uncontrolled hypertension. Nearly equal to these two categories in absolute risk are diabetics, who have about twice the risk of cardiovascular events as nondiabetic hypertensive people. Both JNC VI and the National Cholesterol Education Program placed diabetics in the highest category of risk. JNC VI and 7 recommend that a diabetic with a BP higher than 129/84 mm Hg should receive antihypertensive drug therapy, even though the diagnosis of hypertension is *not* confirmed. This is perhaps the most striking example of how we should treat individual patients according to their absolute risk for cardiovascular and renal events, and *not* by BP levels alone.

Unlike its predecessor, JNC 7 avoided a discussion of cardiovascular risk as a basis for beginning therapy. Instead, lifestyle modifications are now recommended for both pre-hypertensive and hypertensive people. Drug therapy is reserved for those with hypertension and high-risk people (e.g., diabetics and those with chronic kidney disease) whose blood pressure is above goal (see below).

Considering Secondary Hypertension

More than 95% of Americans with hypertension have no specific cause for their elevated BPs (i.e., primary hypertension). It is important, however, to consider the possibility that newly diagnosed hypertension has a specific cause, for three reasons. First, BP control is often difficult to achieve in those with secondary causes of hypertension; diagnosing it early is likely to get BP to goal more quickly. Second, and particularly important in younger people, diagnosing and treating secondary hypertension will reduce the future burden of treatment (both expenditures for pills and follow-up, adverse effects of therapy, and quality of life). For some secondary causes, specific and potentially curative therapy is available. Last, routine consideration of secondary causes when the diagnosis of hypertension is made will assure that at least once during the person's lifetime, a potential diagnosis will be entertained and the risks and benefits of further testing are critically evaluated.

Guiding Therapy

Many of the nearly 90 antihypertensive agents currently available in the United States differ in efficacy in various conditions. It is often helpful to discuss these potential confounders of treatment with the patient, in an effort to "individualize" treatment according to the patient's specific dietary, medical, and personal considerations. For example, diuretics and calcium antagonists are more effective than angiotensin-converting enzyme (ACE) inhibitors and angiotensin II receptor blockers (ARBs) when dietary sodium is excessive. Some drugs have "compelling conditions" for which the drug improves cardiovascular morbidity and mortality (Table 2). Also, some patients are fearful of specific adverse effects of certain drugs (e.g., male

TABLE 2. **Compelling Conditions for which Specific Antihypertensive Drug Therapy Has Reduced Morbidity and Mortality in Clinical Trials**

Compelling Condition	Indicated Therapy	Clinical Trial(s)
Postmyocardial infarction with left ventricular dysfunction or heart failure	β-blocker ACE inhibitor	Norwegian Timolol (Blocadren) Survival Study; Beta-Blocker Heart Attack Trial (BHAT), others Survival And Ventricular Enlargement (SAVE) trial, others
Heart failure	ACE inhibitor, then β-blocker	CONSENSUS (COoperative New Scandinavian ENalapril SUrvival Study), many others; MERIT-HF (MEtoprolol (Lopressor, Toprol XL) Randomized Intervention Trial in Heart Failure), many others
Left ventricular dysfunction	ACE inhibitor	SOLVD (Study on Left Ventricular Dysfunction), others
Type 1 diabetes with renal dysfunction	ACE inhibitor	Captopril (Capoten) Cooperative Study Group
Renal impairment with proteinuria	ACE inhibitor	REIN (Ramipril [Altace] Evaluation in Nephropathy), others
Established vascular disease	ACE inhibitor	HOPE (Heart Outcomes Prevention Evaluation)
Type 2 diabetes with 1 additional risk factor	ACE inhibitor	HOPE (Heart Outcomes Prevention Evaluation)
Type 2 diabetic with renal impairment	ARB	IDNT (Irbesartan [Avapro] Diabetic Nephropathy Trial), RENAAL (Reduction of Endpoints in Non-insulin dependent diabetes mellitus with the Angiotensin II Antagonist Losartan [Cozaar])
Type 2 diabetic with microalbuminuria	ARB, or ACE inhibitor	IRMA-2 (IRbesartan [Avapro] MicroAlbuminuria trial #2); Diabetes Substudy of HOPE (Heart Outcomes Prevention Evaluation)
Poststroke/TIA	ACE inhibitor ± diuretic	PROGRESS (Perindopril [Aceon]) pROtection aGainst REcurrent Stroke Study
Isolated systolic hypertension	Diuretic or dihydropyridine calcium antagonist	SHEP (Systolic Hypertension in the Elderly Program), Syst-EUR (Systolic Hypertension in Europe), Syst-China (Systolic Hypertension in China)
Left ventricular hypertrophy (using strict criteria)	ARB	LIFE (Losartan [Cozaar] Intervention For Endpoint reduction)

ACE, angiotensin-converting enzyme; ARB, angiotensin receptor blocker.

sexual dysfunction). Sharing this information with the physician can help avoid medications with a higher incidence of the problem.

Medical and Social History

In addition to assessing the absolute risk of cardiovascular and renal disease, a careful drug, environmental, and nutritional history should be obtained during the initial evaluation of a hypertensive patient, and intermittently during subsequent management. It is particularly important to ascertain whether the patient is taking any drug (by prescription or over-the-counter) or other substance that might elevate BP. Of particular concern are the nonsteroidal anti-inflammatory drugs and sympathomimetic amines (once commonly found in weight loss, cold, and allergy preparations). Other drugs can either elevate BP or interfere with some antihypertensive agents, including cyclosporine (Sandimmune, Neoral, Gengraf), erythropoietin (Epogen, Procrit), corticosteroids, cocaine, theophylline (Uniphyl, Uni-Dur), and monoamine oxidase inhibitors.

A focused dietary history is very important, because the most effective therapeutic lifestyle changes involve limiting either calories or sodium. A sensible target is 100 mEq (2.4 gm or 2400 mg) of sodium per day. The caloric intake, eating pattern, and changes in weight should be noted, because weight loss remains the most successful of all therapeutic lifestyle changes, and should be part of the therapeutic plan for *all* overweight hypertensive people.

The patient's alcohol consumption, tobacco habit, and exercise pattern should be determined. Restricting alcohol, eliminating tobacco, and physical activity are all recommended, although beneficial long-term effects on cardiovascular morbidity and mortality mediated through BP lowering are unlikely to ever be proven in clinical trials.

In addition, the medical history should carefully ascertain the patient's prior experience with, and attitudes toward, antihypertensive drugs, and be sensitive to cultural factors or health beliefs that could hinder diagnostic or therapeutic plans.

Physical Examination

The "directed" physical examination of the hypertensive patient should pay special attention to weight, TOD, and features suggestive of secondary hypertension.

- The optic fundi (graded on the Keith-Wagener-Barker scale of hypertensive retinopathy) provide clues to the duration and severity of hypertension.
- The neck may disclose an enlarged thyroid gland, abnormalities of the venous circulation, or carotid bruits.

- Auscultation of the chest can provide evidence of heart failure or bronchospasm; the latter would make β-blocker therapy relatively contraindicated.
- Cardiomegaly, cardiac murmurs, and extra sounds should be sought.
- Abdominal bruits are probably the most cost-effective evidence for renovascular hypertension. An abdominal mass may indicate pheochromocytoma or polycystic kidney disease.
- Bruits, absent or decreased pulses, and abnormal hair growth patterns in the lower extremities should be noted. Edema can be a sign of heart failure or renal disease.
- The brief neurologic examination should be more complete if there is a history of stroke or transient ischemic attack.

Laboratory Testing

In most hypertensive patients, only a few inexpensive and simple laboratory tests are needed initially: serum glucose (preferably fasting), creatinine, total cholesterol, high-density lipoprotein cholesterol, triglycerides, a 12-lead electrocardiogram, and a complete urinalysis. When the probability of secondary hypertension is high, based on the history and physical examination, additional tests may support or reject a specific cause. Echocardiography, 24-hour urine collections, or quantitation of urinary protein excretion may be useful in occasional patients.

SECONDARY HYPERTENSION

Patients with an identifiable secondary cause of hypertension usually present with a relatively abrupt onset of hypertension, typically presenting at a higher stage and with considerable target-organ damage. They typically do not respond as well to antihypertensive drug therapy as patients with primary hypertension. The response to specific antihypertensive drugs may also offer important clues to the presence and type of secondary hypertension. The most common forms of secondary hypertension and useful tests for each are shown in Table 3. The choice of tests, and the order in which they are obtained, depends not only on the pretest probability of the disease, but also on safety, availability, local expertise with the test, and its cost.

MANAGEMENT

Successful management of hypertension requires a major commitment from the patient, the provider and the health care system. The patient must continue to take a potentially costly medication with known side effects and see a physician frequently for an asymptomatic condition, hoping to reduce the risk of a major complication. The provider must help the patient achieve and maintain goal BP (and control other cardiovascular risk factors), without being sure that such treatment will prevent an event that would have occurred without it. The health care system must fund both pharmacy and physician benefits, with the realization that many people require treatment, some for many years, before a single catastrophe will be prevented.

Therapeutic Lifestyle Changes

Nearly all hypertension guidelines recommend nutritional-hygienic measures to control BP, despite the absence of clinical trial evidence demonstrating they reduce cardiovascular morbidity or mortality. There is, however, good public health rationale for advocating weight loss, dietary salt restriction, and other nonpharmacologic methods as preventive, adjunctive, and occasionally definitive treatment for hypertension. Weight loss is the most effective single nondrug modality to reduce BP in overweight people, followed by dietary salt restriction. Although long-term adherence to therapeutic lifestyle change is uncommon, most individuals should restrict alcohol to one to two drinks/day, avoid tobacco, exercise (30 minutes most days of the week), reduce caffeine (if excessive), and supplement potassium, calcium, or magnesium (if a deficiency state is present).

In the Treatment of Mild Hypertension Study (TOMHS), a vigorous program of therapeutic lifestyle changes, executed by experts with very motivated participants, was *inferior* to antihypertensive drug therapy *plus* therapeutic lifestyle changes in both

TABLE 3. **Screening and Other Tests for Common Forms of Secondary Hypertension**

Diagnosis	Preferred Screening Test(s)	Other Tests
Renovascular hypertension	Captopril (Capoten) scintigraphy	Doppler ultrasound of renal arteries, magnetic resonance angiography, renal angiogram
Mineralocorticoid excess states	24-hour urinary aldosterone during salt loading, plasma aldosterone/renin ratio	Computed tomographic scan of adrenals
Pheochromocytoma	24-hour urine for vanillylmandelic acid, and metanephrines	Plasma metanephrines, plasma catecholamines, T_2 weighted magnetic resonance imaging
Sleep apnea	Formal sleep study	
Cushing's syndrome	8 AM plasma cortisol	Dexamethasone suppression test(s)
Hypothyroidism	Thyroid-stimulating hormone	Serum thyroxine, triiodothyronine levels

reducing BP and preventing overall cardiovascular events. Because of difficulties in sustaining initial therapeutic lifestyle changes alone, many patients and most clinicians prefer a strategy that adds antihypertensive drug therapy earlier than older national guidelines recommend, particularly when initial efforts at weight loss and sodium restriction are unsuccessful or troublesome.

Choice of Initial Drug Therapy

Initial Antihypertensive Drug Therapy for "Complicated Patients"

Both JNC VI and 7 recognized that many hypertensive people begin treatment after they have already developed cardiovascular disease or other medical conditions that may be positively affected by specific antihypertensive drug therapies. JNC VI divided these situations into "compelling indications" or "clinical conditions." In the former, an agent from a specific class of antihypertensive drugs should be prescribed for a given patient if there is clinical trial evidence for that kind of antihypertensive drug to reduce morbidity or mortality for a condition that is also present in the patient. Thus, for a hypertensive person with systolic heart failure, an ACE inhibitor should not only lower BP, but also reduce mortality and hospitalizations. Table 2 provides examples of antihypertensive drugs that have demonstrated benefits in improving prognosis in conditions commonly found in hypertensive people. There are also some contraindications for specific antihypertensive drugs that limit their use (Table 4). A guide to the choice of an antihypertensive drug is provided in Table 5.

JNC VI and 7 also recognized clinical situations in which specific antihypertensive drug therapy may be beneficial in improving *symptoms* of, or surrogate markers for, another condition, but might not have a major effect on reducing morbidity or mortality. Two examples are a diuretic or a β-blocker for a hypertensive person with either osteoporosis or an essential tremor (respectively). Although it is likely that the person's cardiovascular risk will improve if the hypertension is successfully treated, the symptomatic benefit of the drug on osteoporosis or essential tremor itself will not necessarily reduce the associated morbidity and mortality. Most patients, however, are pleased to see symptomatic improvement in their tremor, or a stabilization in bone density, when taking these drugs; this may enhance medication adherence. Similarly, some medical conditions can be caused or exacerbated by certain antihypertensive drugs, or can be remedied by others. If the physician can identify these situations in a given patient, such considerations may be sufficient reason to favor or avoid specific medications, even if they would be routinely preferred for other patients with similar problems.

TABLE 4. **Contraindications for Specific Antihypertensive Drug Classes (see JNC VI)**

Antihypertensive Drug Class	Contraindication(s)
Thiazide diuretic	Allergy
β-Blocker	Asthma; diabetes with frequent hypoglycemia
Angiotensin-converting enzyme inhibitor	Angioedema resulting from angiotensin-converting enzyme inhibitor; pregnancy; renal artery stenosis
Calcium antagonist	Allergy
Angiotensin II receptor blocker	Pregnancy; renal artery stenosis
α-Blocker	Orthostatic hypotension with frequent falls
Alpha$_2$ agonist (centrally acting drug)	Allergy

Initial Antihypertensive Drug Therapy for "Uncomplicated Hypertensives"

At the time JNC VI was written, only diuretics or β-blockers had been used in clinical trials in otherwise *uncomplicated hypertensives*, and had demonstrated a reduction in cardiovascular morbidity or mortality compared with placebo. For ethical reasons, we will *never* have direct evidence, in a broad range of hypertensive patients, to prove that newer classes of drugs are superior to placebo. A meta-analysis that included 27 trials and 136,124 patients concluded that all observed differences in cardiovascular outcomes could be explained by the achieved differences in systolic blood pressure. More recently completed large clinical trials indicate that most differences across various classes of antihypertensive agents in the prevention of all cardiovascular events are small (Table 6).

The only major exception is initial treatment with an α-blocker, which was associated with an *increased* risk of cardiovascular events (mostly heart failure) in ALLHAT (Antihypertensive and Lipid-Lowering [Treatments to Prevent] Heart Attack Trial). Although systolic BP was higher (by 3 mm Hg) in the patients randomized to doxazosin (Cardura) than in those given chlorthalidone (Thalitone), the investigators implicated the initial drug, rather than the differential BP lowering resulting from it, as the reason for the observed differences in prognosis. Most authorities, therefore, have removed α-blockers from the list of recommended initial therapies for uncomplicated hypertension.

Whether a β-blocker can be recommended as routine initial antihypertensive therapy is debatable, especially for older hypertensive patients. A meta-analysis that included only two trials of an initial β-blocker against placebo concluded that these drugs significantly reduced only stroke, whereas an initial diuretic provided impressive protection against all cardiovascular events. Many recent clinical trials that included a physician's choice of either a diuretic or a β-blocker as the initial treatment option (see Table 6) have not reported results according to these subgroups, possibly because of an inherent "indication bias" that may well confound the results.

The controversy about calcium antagonists as possible initial treatment for hypertension has been largely resolved by the final results of ALLHAT. Since

TABLE 5. **Advantages and Disadvantages of Specific Classes of Antihypertensive Medications with Medical Conditions Commonly Found in Hypertensive Patients**

Condition	Diuretic	β-Blocker	Calcium Antagonist	ACE Inhibitor	Angiotensin Receptor Blocker
COPD/asthma	-	----	±	± or - (?)	±
Heart failure (systolic type)	+++	-- (or +?)	+ or -	+++	++
Heart failure (diastolic type)	++	++	+ or ++	±	±
Type 2 diabetes mellitus	-	--	±	++	+
(prone to hypoglycemia)	±	----	±	++	+
(with renal impairment)	++	±	±	+++	+++
(with microalbuminuria or proteinuria)	±	±	±	+++	+++
Dysrhythmias	- (?)	+++	+++ or ±	± or +	±
Angina pectoris	±	+++	+++	±	±
Postmyocardial infarction	± (?)	+++	+ or - (?)	+++	±
"Silent ischemia"	± or - (?)	++	++	±	±
Degenerative joint disease (NSAID usage)	--	--	±	---	---
Renal impairment	+++	+	±	++	+
Renovascular hypertension	±	±	+	----	----
Pregnancy	-	±	±	----	----
Benign prostatic hypertrophy	--	-	±	±	±

ACE, angiotensin-converting enzyme; COPD, chronic obstructive pulmonary disease; NSAID, nonsteroidal anti-inflammatory drug; ----, severely contraindicated; ---, moderately contraindicated; --, mildly contraindicated; -, possibly contraindicated; ±, no major effect; +, possibly beneficial; ++, mildly beneficial; +++, FDA-approved for this use; (?), uncertainty exists.

1995, many reports have suggested that calcium antagonists are associated with increased all-cause mortality, myocardial infarctions, bleeding and cancer. In ALLHAT, the 9,048 hypertensive patients randomized to the calcium antagonist, amlodipine (Norvasc) had *no* significantly increased risk of fatal or nonfatal myocardial infarction compared to the 15,255 people given the diuretic, chlorthalidone (Thalitone, Hygroton). There were similarly no significant differences across these randomized groups in death, bleeding, or cancer. As in previous studies, however, amlodipine was associated with a significantly *higher* risk of heart failure than chlorthalidone. Previous claims of a significantly lower risk of stroke with an initial calcium antagonist were not corroborated by a recent meta-analysis that included results from both ALLHAT and CONVINCE (Controlled ONset Verapamil INvestigation of Cardiovascular Endpoints). After completion of several more ongoing clinical trials (Table 7), there will be even more data, but it is very unlikely that calcium antagonists will be significantly better than an initial diuretic in preventing cardiovascular events.

Recent nationwide pharmacy dispensing data indicate that hypertensive American patients are now receiving more ACE inhibitors than calcium antagonists. Many patients and physicians have been favorably impressed with recent hypertension trials that included an ACE inhibitor. Both the Heart Outcomes Prevention Evaluation (HOPE) Study and the Second Australian National BP Trial showed that the ACE inhibitor was better than a regimen without an ACE inhibitor (placebo in the former, a diuretic in the latter). In ALLHAT, perhaps because blood pressure was significantly higher in the group randomized to lisinopril (Prinivil, Zestril) than those given chlorthalidone, and because a second-step diuretic was prohibited, cardiovascular events, stroke and heart failure were all slightly, but significantly, worse with the ACE-inhibitor than with the diuretic.

Most health care providers working in cost-sensitive clinical environments are encouraged to use the cheapest initial drug that will lower BP and prevent cardiovascular events. In most circumstances this will be a low-dose thiazide or thiazide-like diuretic. This strategy was verified by the final ALLHAT data, which showed no significant overall benefit to the newer and more expensive agents, leading to the conclusion that thiazide-type diuretics "should be preferred for first-step antihypertensive therapy." Figure 1 shows one approach to assembling an antihypertensive drug regimen. JNC 7 recommended a thiazide-type diuretic as first-line therapy for most individuals with Stage 1 hypertension, followed (if needed) by an ACE-inhibitor, angiotensin II receptor blocker (ARB), β-blocker, or calcium antagonist. For those with Stage 2 hypertension, or if the blood pressure is more than 20/10 mm Hg over goal, JNC 7 recommended initial two-drug therapy (one of which should usually be a diuretic).

Target BPs Based on Absolute Risk of Cardiovascular and Renal Disease

Probably the most prescient recommendation made by JNC VI was the suggestion that the BP target during treatment should *not* be the same for all hypertensive patients. Although a BP goal of <140/90 mm Hg had been advanced by several previous reports, this goal is now recommended for uncomplicated patients. Even before the Hypertension Optimal Treatment (HOT) study showed (in 18,790 hypertensive patients) the benefit of reducing the diastolic BP to 83.6 mm Hg to "optimally reduce cardiovascular risk," the JNC VI report had suggested such a target. The HOT study

TABLE 6. **Recent Clinical Trials That Showed Small and Nonsignificant Differences in Major Adverse Cardiovascular Events (MACE: Stroke, Myocardial Infarction, or Cardiovascular Death) between Drug Classes**

Name (acronym)	Test Agent(s)	Comparator(s)	Patients	Results
Swedish Trial in Old Patients with Hypertension #2 (STOP-Hypertenstion 2)	Calcium antagonist or ACE-inhibitor	Physician's choice of diuretic or β-blocker	6614 hypertensive Swedes, 70-84 years old	No significant differences in MACE ($P = 0.89$ for ACE-I vs. Comparator, 0.97 for CA)
NORdic DILtiazem Trial (NORDIL)	Diltiazem (Cardizem, Tiazac, Dilacor)	Physician's choice of diuretic or β-blocker	10,881 hypertensives, aged 50-74 years in Sweden or Norway	No Significant difference in MACE ($P = 0.97$)
International Nifedipine GITS Study: Intervention as a Goal in Hypertension Treatment (INSIGHT)	Nifedipine GITS (Procardia XL)	HCTZ + Amiloride (Moduretic)	6321 hypertensive patients in Europe or Israel	No significant difference in MACE or HF ($P = 0.35$)
National Intervention Cooperative Study in Elderly Hypertensives (NICS-EH)	Nicardipine (Cardene)	Trichlormethiazide (Naqua, Metahydrin)	414 Japanese>60 years old with BP 160-220/<115 mm Hg	No significant difference in MACE ($P = 0.92$)
United Kingdom Prospective Diabetes Study #39 (UKPDS 38)	Captopril (Capoten)	Atenolol (Tenormin)	1148 hypertensive type 2 diabetics	No significant differences in diabetes-related endpoints ($P = 0.43$)
CAPtopril Primary Prevention project (CAPPP)	Captopril (Capoten)	Diuretic or β-blocker	10,985 hypertensive Swedes or Finns, aged 25-66 years	No significant difference in MACE ($P = 0.52$)
Verapamil in Hypertension and Atherosclerosis Study (VHAS)	Verapamil SR (Calan SR, Isoptin SR)	Chlorthalidone (Thalitone)	1414 hypertensive Italians	No significant difference in MACE (42 vs. 43, NS, P not given)
European Lacidipine Study of Atherosclerosis (ELSA)	Lacidipine (Lacipil, not yet available in USA)	Atenolol (Tenormin)	2,259 European patients with known carotid stenosis	No significant difference in MACE (31 vs. 27, NS, P not given)
Antihypertensive and Lipid Lowering [prevention of] Heart Attack Trial (ALLHAT)	Amlodipine (Norvasc) Lisinopril(Prinivil, Zestril)	Chlorthalidone (Thalitone, Hygroton)	33,357 in 623 centers in USA and Canada	No significant differences in composite MACE for amlodipine or lisinopril vs. chlorthalidone
Controlled ONset Verapamil INvestigation of Cardiovascular Endpoints (CONVINCE)	COER-Verapamil (Covera-HS)	HCTZ (Hydrodiuril, Esidrex) or Atenolol (Tenormin)	16,602 hypertensives older than 55 years, with ≥1 additional risk factor	No significant difference in MACE ($P = 0.77$)
Study on COgnition and prognosis in the Elderly (SCOPE)	HCTZ + Candesartan (Atacand/HCT)	HCTZ[Hydrodiuril, Esidrex]+ any other non-ARB, non-ACE-Inhibitor	4937 European patients aged 70-89 with uncontrolled BP on HCTZ 12.5 mg/d	No significant difference in MACE ($P = 0.19$)
INternational VErpamil SR/Trandolapril study (INVEST)	Verapamil SR (Calan SR, Isoptin SR) (± trandolapril [Mavik]	Atenolol [Tenormin] (± HCTZ [Hydrodiuril, Esidrex]	22,576 hypertensive patients with coronary heart disease	No significant difference in MACE ($P = 0.62$)

TABLE 7. **Important Ongoing Clinical Trials in Hypertension**

Acronym (Name)	Test Agent(s)	Comparator(s)	Patients	Primary Endpoint	Duration; Completion Year
ASCOT (Anglo-Scandinavian Cardiac Outcomes Trial)	Amolodipine [Norvasc] (± Perindopril [Aceon])	Atenolol [Tenormin] (± diuretic)	19,342 residents of Scandinavia or the U.K.	Fatal coronary heart disease or non-fatal myocardial infarction	5-year follow-up planned, expected completion in 2005
HYVET (HYpertension in Very Elderly Trial)	Indapamide (Lozol) ±Perindopril (Aceon)	Placebo	~2,100 patients>80 years old	Fatal or non-fatal stroke	5-year follow-up planned; excepted completion in 2006
ON-TARGET (ONgoing Telmisartan Alone and in combination with Ramipril Global Endpoint Trial)	Telmisartan (Micardis)	Ramipril (Altace)	~28,400 hypersensitive patients at high risk for cardiovascular events (like HOPE)	Stroke myocardial infarction, cardiovascular death	5-year follow-up planned; expected completion in 2006
SHELL (Systolic Hypertension in the Elderly Long-term Lacidipine) Trial	Lacidipine (Lacidipil, not yet available in U.S.)	Chlorthalidone (Thalitone, Hygroton)	4,800 Italians with isolated systolic hypertension	Stroke, myocardial infarction, cardiovascular death	5-year follow-up planned, expected completion in 2003
TROPHY (TRial Of Prevention of HYpertension	Candesartan (Atacand)	Placebo	803 people with high-normal BP	Incidence of hypertension	2-year treatment, then 2 years of observation, excepted completion in 2005
VALUE (Valsartan Amolodipine Long-term Utilization Evaluation)	Amlodipine (Norvasc) (±HCTZ [Hydrodiuril, Esidrex])	Valsartan (Diovan) (±HDTZ [Hydrodiuril, Esidrex])	15,314 patients in 31 countries	Actual or aborted myocardial infarction, hospitalization for heart failure, or CHD death	6-year follow-up planned, expected completion in 2004

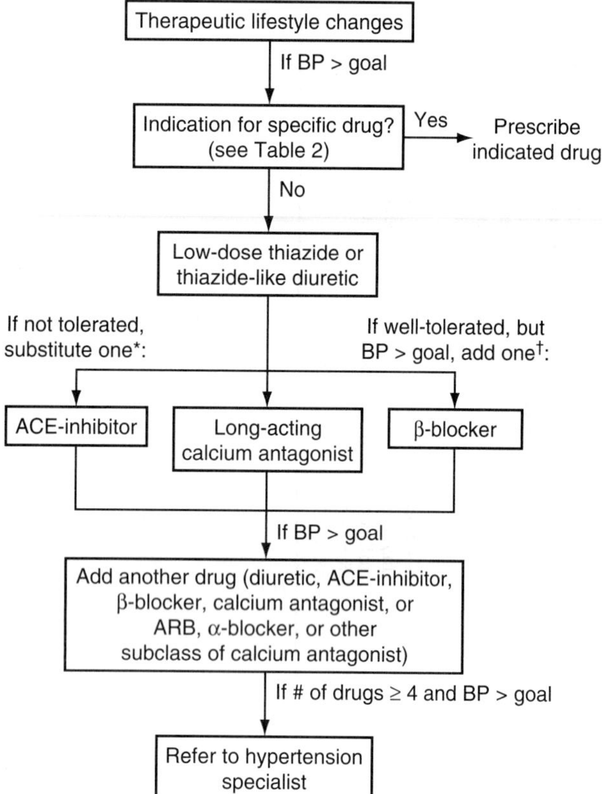

Figure 1. One algorithm for constructing an effective antihypertensive drug regimen.
*A β-blocker is usually not recommended as initial therapy for hypertensive patients older than age 60, but is an acceptable add-on to a diuretic in this age group.
†The combination of a β-blocker and an angiotensin-converting enzyme inhibitor typically lowers blood pressure less effectively than other two-drug combinations, and is usually not recommended. The combination of a diuretic and a calcium antagonist may lower blood pressure, but has not yet been shown in clinical trials to reduce morbidity and mortality in hypertensives.

results suggest that there is no significant *increase* in risk by lowering BP to a diastolic target of ≤80 mm Hg, but there appears to be little further benefit, either. Because the probability of drug-related side effects often increases as the doses are increased, it is likely that the target BP of <140/90 mm Hg will be defensible for uncomplicated hypertensive patients for some time.

Both JNC VI and 7 recommended that diabetic patients, and those with renal impairment, should have a lower BP treatment target than individuals with lower absolute risk. JNC VI suggested a BP of <130/85 mm Hg, without *any* clinical trial data on which to base this recommendation. At least two important studies have since corroborated this recommendation. The first clinical trial to demonstrate the benefit of a lower BP target for diabetics was the United Kingdom Prospective Diabetes Study (UKPDS) #38. Over 8.4 years of follow-up, 1,148 type 2 diabetics randomized to two different BP goals (<150/85 mm Hg or <180/105 mm Hg) did much better if treated to the lower goal. Interestingly, the achieved BP difference between groups was 10/5 mm Hg (154/87 versus 144/82 mm Hg), which when subtracted from the usual current BP goal for nondiabetic patients (140/90 mm Hg) gives a target for diabetics that is *identical* to the 130/85 mm Hg recommended in JNC VI! The HOT study's 1,501 diabetics showed the lowest risk of stroke, heart attack, or cardiovascular death, even in intent-to-treat analyses, if randomized to a diastolic BP ≤80 mm Hg. These data have led to more recent recommendations from several expert panels, including JNC 7, to lower diabetics' goal BP to <130/80 mm Hg.

Those responsible for health care financing were initially concerned that the lower BP goal recommended for diabetics would require more antihypertensive pills and more visits to health care providers, and therefore would lead to a large increase in medical costs. Cost analyses taken directly from the UKPDS clinical trial, however, show an overall cost-saving with the lower BP goal. Despite higher drug and provider costs in the first few months, the strategy of the lower BP goal *saved* lives, strokes, limbs, *and money* over the long term. The cost-effectiveness ratio for the lower BP goal was –£720 per year of life saved, and an even more impressive –£1049 year of life without diabetic complications. We reached a similar conclusion from an economic analysis of US epidemiologic and clinical trial data for older (≥60 years) diabetics treated to a goal of <130/85 mm Hg, compared with leaving the target BP at <140/90 mm Hg. Because the lower BP goal impressively reduces the risk of expensive cardiovascular events, including stroke, heart attack, heart failure, and renal replacement therapy, the incremental cost-effectiveness ratio for the lower BP goal is negative (meaning more intensive treatment *saves* money!), just as in UKPDS.

Most authorities recommend that one of the drugs (if not the initial drug) used to lower BP in diabetics should be an antagonist of the renin-angiotensin-aldosterone system. In HOPE, an impressive reduction in nearly all types of *cardiovascular* morbidity or mortality was seen among diabetic patients randomized to ramipril (Altace), which the authors attributed more to the ACE-inhibitor than to the ≈3/1 mm Hg difference in BP between the randomized groups; that conclusion remains to be proved. HOPE did show a 30% reduction in dialysis in diabetics, but the difference was not significant, as the totals were only 8 (given ramipril [Altace]) and 10 (on placebo). Very recently, two clinical trials using an ARB have successfully reduced the long-term risk of a composite *renal* endpoint (death, dialysis, transplantation, or doubling of serum creatinine) in type 2 diabetics. In IDNT (Irbesartan [Avapro] Diabetic Nephropathy Trial), the ARB was about 20% or 23% more effective than either placebo or amlodipine (Norvasc) (respectively) in preventing renal events. In RENAAL (Reduction of Endpoints in Non-insulin dependent diabetes mellitus with the Angiotensin II Antagonist Losartan [Cozaar]), the ARB was about 16% more effective than placebo in preventing the primary endpoint when added to any antihypertensive drug therapy except an ACE inhibitor or an ARB. Although neither of the ARB studies was powered to show a difference in cardiovascular events between the ARB and other arms, the American Diabetes Association has recommended that either an ACE-inhibitor or an ARB be part of the treatment regimen for all hypertensive type 2 diabetics.

Recent clinical trial data from the African American Study of Kidney Diseases (AASK) and REIN (Ramipril [Altace] Evaluation In Nephropathy) trials suggest that an ACE inhibitor is a good initial choice for most nondiabetic patients with renal impairment. In the AASK study, patients receiving ramipril (Altace) did better than with either amlodipine (Norvasc) or metoprolol (Lopressor, Toprol XL), particularly in patients with greater degrees of proteinuria, even though BP reductions were very similar. Some have suggested that the results of this study reinforce another recommendation made by JNC VI: to consider protein excretion as a valuable surrogate endpoint for future renal and cardiovascular risk. Because BP reduction itself typically reduces proteinuria, there has been controversy about whether ACE inhibitors or ARBs should be recommended specifically for this "benefit." In AASK, ramipril (Altace) significantly reduced both protein excretion and clinical outcomes, compared to amlodipine (Norvasc). On the other hand, few individuals with hypertension and renal impairment will achieve a BP goal of <130/80 mm Hg using only an ACE inhibitor (with or without a diuretic). The strategy of adding a calcium antagonist to this regimen has been successfully studied, and is currently recommended by the National Kidney Foundation. The IRMA-2 (IRbesartan [Avapro] MicroAlbuminuria) study recently reported that, in a dose-dependent fashion, an ARB can protect type 2 diabetic patients with microalbuminuria (urinary albumin excretion between 30 and 300 mg/d) from progressing to frank proteinuria (>300 mg/d of proteinuria).

JNC VI recommended the lowest BP target (<125/75 mm Hg) for hypertensive individuals with renal impairment and proteinuria be 1 gm/24 hours. Although partially successful in the Modification of Diet in Renal Disease study, the more recent AASK study showed *no* benefit with such a low target. As a compromise, JNC 7 suggested the same blood pressure target (<130/80 mm Hg) for patients with chronic kidney disease as with diabetes.

Constructing A Regimen

Because most hypertensive patients will require more than a single drug to achieve the more intensive treatment goals recommended recently, one probably needs to worry less about the initial choice of therapy (e.g., top of Figure 1) than choosing appropriate combinations of drugs to achieve the goal BP. The choice should be based on the clinician's assessment of which potential complication of hypertension poses the greatest risk to the individual patient. For example, a type 2 diabetic at high risk for renal failure should receive an ARB (with or after the diuretic), whereas a similar type 2 diabetic without microalbuminuria, who is otherwise at high risk for cardiovascular events, should have an ACE inhibitor with or after the diuretic. A hypertensive patient with a previous myocardial infarction should begin with a β-blocker; a person who survived a stroke probably should start with an ACE inhibitor with or without a diuretic.

One of the attractive features of Figure 1 is that, if the combination of a diuretic and another drug does not lower BP to goal, an appropriate choice for the third-line agent is found adjacent to the agent chosen as the second drug. Similarly, if the initial diuretic is not tolerated, it might be recommended as the second-line choice; otherwise, the second choice is again found adjacent to the initial agent chosen. This avoids the combination of an ACE inhibitor and a β-blocker, which lowers blood pressure less effectively than other two-drug combinations, including a diuretic and a calcium antagonist.

The ideal drug regimen would have many characteristics. In addition to lowering the BP to goal, the regimen should be administered once daily, without regard to meals, be relatively inexpensive, cause few adverse effects (and perhaps even result in fewer side-effects than a single-drug therapy), and be widely available in all pharmacies and benefits plans. Several of the newer fixed-dose combination products have several of these attributes (Table 8). Combinations including a dihydropyridine calcium antagonist and an ACE inhibitor, for instance, cause less pedal edema than the calcium channel blocker alone, even at the same doses. It is unfortunate that, since the late 1960s, only a single triple-drug combination has existed in the United States, containing hydrochlorothiazide, reserpine, and low-dose hydralazine (Ser-Ap-Es).

Follow-Up and Drug Withdrawal

Semi-annual office visits are recommended for even well-controlled hypertensive patients to confirm the adequacy of BP control, maintain surveillance of weight and other modifiable risk factors, review and renew prescriptions, and sustain motivation for therapeutic lifestyle changes and medication compliance. Every 3 months might even be more appropriate.

When BP is not at goal, the patient should return at much shorter intervals; 1 month is probably sufficient for most patients. Weekly visits for dose titration are too frequent, because most popular antihypertensive agents have long serum elimination half-lives. Once-daily antihypertensive agents require at least 5 days of administration before achieving a reasonable steady-state plasma level, and achieving a stable pharmacodynamic effect typically takes twice as long. After the BP target is achieved, visits may be spaced less frequently.

Although JNC VI recommended "step-down therapy" for hypertensive patients whose BPs have been controlled effectively for more than 1 year, more recent data question the wisdom of that advice. Some currently used antihypertensive drugs have been available for decades, and after patients are on a well-tolerated, stable regimen, it might not be useful to step down treatment if retitration to goal is frequently required. In the Trials of Nutrition in the Elderly (TONE) Study, the majority of the volunteers resumed

TABLE 8. **Combination Products Currently Approved for Hypertension in the USA (Listed, Within Subtype, in Chronological Order of FDA Approval)**

Diuretic/Diuretic Combinations[†]	Trade Name(s)
Triamterene/hydrochlorothiazide (37.5/25, 50/25, 75/50)	Dyazide**, Maxzide**
Spironolactone/hydrochlorothiazide (25/25, 50/50)	Aldactone**
Amiloride/hydrochlorothiazide (5/50)	Moduretic**
β-blocker/Diuretic Combinations	
Propranolol/hydrochlorothiazide (40/25, 80/25)	Inderide
Metoprolol/hydrochlorothiazide (50/25, 100/25)	Lopressor/HCT
Atenolol/chlorthalidone (50/25, 100/25)	Tenoretic
Nadolol/bendroflumethiazide (40/5, 80/5)	Corzide
Timolol/hydrochlorothiazide (10/25)	Timolide
Propranolol LA (long-acting)/hydrochlorothiazide (40/25, 80/25)	Inderide LA
Bisoprolol/hydrochlorothiazide (2.5/6.25, 5/6.25, 10/6.25)	Ziac*
Centrally Acting Drug/Diuretic Combinations	
Guanethidine/hydrochlorothiazide (10/25)	Esimil
Methyldopa/hydrochlorothiazide (250/15, 250/25, 500/30, 500/50)	Aldoril
Methyldopa/chlorothiazide (250/150, 250/250)	Aldoclor
Reserpine/chlorothiazide (0.125/250, 0.25/500)	Diupres
Reserpine/chlorthalidone (0.125/25, 0.25/50)	Demi-Regroton
Reserpine/hydrochlorothiazide (0.125/25, 0.125/50)	Hydropres
Clonidine/chlorthalidone (0.1/15, 0.2/15, 0.3/15)	Combipres
ACE Inhibitor/Diuretic Combinations	
Captopril/hydrochlorothiazide (25/15, 25/25, 50/15, 50/25)	Capozide*
Enalapril/hydrochlorothiazide (5/12.5, 10/25)	Vaseretic
Lisinopril/hydrochlorothiazide (10/12.5, 20/12.5, 20/25)	Prinzide, Zestoretic
Fosinopril/hydrochlorothiazide (10/12.5, 20/12.5)	Monopril/HCT
Quinapril/hydrochlorothiazide (10/12.5, 20/12.5, 20/25)	Accuretic
Benazepril/hydrochlorothiazide (5/6.25, 10/12.5, 20/12.5, 20/25)	Lotensin/HCT
Moexipril/hydrochlorothiazide (7.5/12.5, 15/25)	Uniretic
Angiotensin II Receptor Antagonist/Diuretic Combinations	
Losartan/hydrochlorothiazide (50/12.5, 100/25)	Hyzaar
Valsartan/hydrochlorothiazide (80/12.5, 160/12.5, 160/25)	Diovan/HCT
Irbesartan/hydrochlorothiazide (75/12.5, 150/12.5, 300/12.5)	Avalide
Candesartan/hydrochlorothiazide (16/12.5, 32/12.5)	Atacand/HCT
Telmisartan/hydrochlorothiazide (40/12.5, 80/12.5)	Micardis/HCT
Eprosartan/hydrochlorothiazide (600/12.5, 600/25)	Teveten HCT
Calcium Antagonist/ACE-Inhibitor Combinations	
Amlodipine/benazepril (2.5/10, 5/10, 5/20, 10/20)	Lotrel
Verapamil (extended release)/trandolapril (180/2, 240/1, 240/2, 240/4)	Tarka
Felodipine (extended release)/enalapril (5/5)	Lexxel
Diltiazem/enalapril (180/5)	Teczem
Vasodilator/Diuretic Combinations	
Hydralazine/hydrochlorothiazide (25/25, 50/25, 100/25)	Apresazide
Prazosin/polythiazide (1/0.5, 2/0.5, 5/0.5)	Minizide
Triple Combination	
Reserpine/hydralazine/hydrochlorothiazide (0.10/25/15)	Ser-Ap-Es

*Approved for initial therapy.
**Indicated for initial therapy only for individuals in whom the development of hypokalemia cannot be risked.
[†]Numbers in parentheses indicate the strength (in mg) of each drug in a particular combination product.

drug therapy or had a clinical event during 30 months of follow-up. For most patients, continuing antihypertensive drug therapy would have been more cost-effective than the TONE program of intensive and extensive nutritional and behavioral counseling and frequent physician visits, and probably safer because BP control was maintained without interruption.

Management in Special Circumstances

More medical attention and closer follow-up should be provided to hypertensive patients with increased cardiovascular risk, including those of an older age, with diabetes, hypertensive crisis, renal impairment, refractory hypertension, pregnancy, or expecting impending surgery.

Older Patients with Hypertension

For many years, there was controversy as to whether (not how!) older hypertensive people should be treated with antihypertensive drug therapy. This question has now been answered with a resounding affirmative, both because clinical trials in older patients demonstrate the overwhelming benefits of treatment for essentially all important endpoints, including all-cause mortality (Figure 2). Although many recent trials in

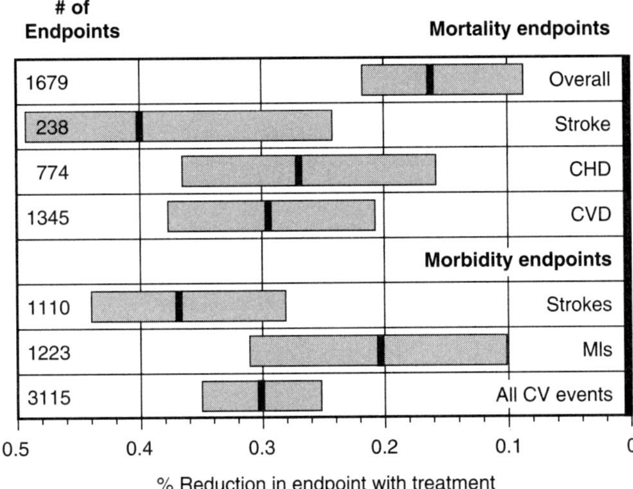

Figure 2. Results of a meta-analysis of 14 controlled treatment trials of antihypertensive drug therapy compared to placebo or no treatment in ≈23,996 older adults. The number of each type of endpoint is given in the left column. The dark vertical bars indicate the point estimate of the risk reduction with antihypertensive drug therapy; horizontal bars indicate the limits of 95% confidence intervals. In this meta-analysis, because the odds ratios for all cardiovascular events are significantly lower than 1.00, antihypertensive drug therapy was associated with a statistically significant reduction in all endpoints, including all-cause mortality.
CHD, coronary heart disease; CVD, cardiovascular disease (includes cerebrovascular and heart disease); MIs, myocardial infarctions.

older hypertensive patients show that successfully lowering BP is probably more important than which drug is used initially to lower it, an initial diuretic is preferred. At least in meta-analyses, thiazide or thiazide-like diuretics are unsurpassed in preventing cardiovascular events; they also have the lowest acquisition cost, and a relatively low frequency of predictable adverse effects in older people.

Because, by design, many of the early clinical trials in hypertension excluded patients older than 74 years of age, there had been little evidence to show that people age 75 and older benefit from antihypertensive drug therapy. Some have argued that the lack of such evidence should preclude antihypertensive drug therapy in older hypertensive people. A recent meta-analysis that included all 1,870 patients older than age 80 enrolled in eight clinical trials showed that, among those randomized to antihypertensive medications, substantial and significant reductions occurred in stroke (–34%), cardiovascular events (–22%), coronary heart disease events (–22%), and heart failure (–39%).

Diabetic Patients with Hypertension

Because diabetes doubles cardiovascular risk, all diabetic patients should be treated to a lower BP goal than usual. The challenge to attaining this goal (<130/80 mm Hg, as recommended by JNC 7, the National Kidney Foundation, the American Diabetes Association, the British Hypertension Society, and the Canadian Consensus Conference on Hypertension) is substantial. Many surveys of BP control in large groups of patients have shown much worse control of BP in diabetic subjects, as compared to non-diabetics, even when equivalent target BPs (<140/90 mm Hg) are used.

For patients who begin treatment at more than 15/10 mm Hg over their goal BP, the National Kidney Foundation's Consensus Statement recommends an ACE inhibitor and a diuretic (thiazide or thiazide-like, if the serum creatinine is ≤1.5 mg/dL, or a loop diuretic if higher). If the BP goal is not achieved, sequential addition of a long-acting calcium antagonist (with a non-dihydropyridine type preferred over a dihydropyridine type), a β-blocker (or α-β-blocker) if the pulse is ≥84 beats/minute, or the other type of long-acting calcium antagonist (if the pulse is <85 beats/minute), and finally an α-blocker. If this five-drug strategy does not achieve the goal BP, referral to a hypertension specialist is often helpful.

These recommendations were made before publication of the results of three important clinical trials, IDNT, IRMA 2, and RENAAL. The use of an ARB to prevent renal complications of type 2 diabetes in patients with microalbuminuria, or those with renal impairment, can now be endorsed without reservation.

Patients with Hypertensive Crises

The term *hypertensive crisis* blurs the distinction between what was formerly called "hypertensive emergency" (typically defined as "very high BP with evidence of acute target-organ damage") and "hypertensive urgency." The major important difference between the two conditions is the rapidity and setting of their treatment. Hypertensive emergencies are best treated in hospital (typically in the intensive care unit) with a short-acting, rapidly reversible, intravenously administered antihypertensive drug. Hypertensive urgencies may be routinely treated in the outpatient setting with any one of a number of oral antihypertensive agents, including captopril (Capoten), labetalol (Normodyne, Trandate), or clonidine (Catapres). Nifedipine capsules (Procardia), which had been widely used in this setting for nearly 20 years, are now to be used "with great caution, if at all," according to a Food and Drug Administration advisory, because of their propensity to cause quick and excessive hypotension. Perhaps the most important aspect of the treatment of hypertensive urgency is to arrange quick follow-up for the patient where better long-term management of BP can be assured.

When a patient presents with a very high BP and the physician is concerned about hypertensive emergency, there are four types of "acute target-organ damage" that should be sought. Various neurological emergencies should be considered (Table 9), and appropriate steps taken to distinguish among them, since the treatment is different. Hypertensive encephalopathy (typically a diagnosis of exclusion) improves dramatically and quickly after BP is reduced acutely. During a stroke-in-evolution, hypertension is typically *not* treated with BP-lowering drug therapy

TABLE 9. **Types of Hypertensive Crises, with Suggested Drug Therapy and BP Targets**

Type of Crisis	Drug of Choice	BP Target
Neurological		
Hypertensive encephalopathy	Nitroprusside* [Nipride]	25% reduction in mean arterial pressure over 2-3 hours.
Intracranial hemorrhage or acute stroke in evolution	Nitroprusside* [Nipride] (controversial)	0-15% reduction in mean arterial pressure over 6-12 hours, if BP persists at >180/110 mm Hg (controversial)
Acute head injury/trauma	Nitroprusside* [Nipride]	0-25% reduction in mean arterial pressure over 2-3 hours (controversial)
Subarachnoid Hemorrhage	Nimodipine [Nimotop]	Up to 25% reduction in mean arterial pressure in previously hypertensive patients, 130-160 systolic in normotensive patients
Cardiac		
Ischemia/infarction	Nitroglycerin [Nitrobid IV, others] or Nicardipine [Cardene]	Reduction in signs of ischemia (e.g., chest discomfort, EKG changes)
Heart failure	Nitroprusside* [Nipride]or nitroglycerin [Nitrobid IV, others]	Improvement in signs of heart failure (typically only 5-10% decrease in BP)
Aortic dissection	β-Blocker + nitroprusside* [Nipride]	**<120 mm Hg systolic in 20 minutes** (if possible)
Renal		
Hematuria or acute renal impairment	Fenoldopam [Corlopam]	0-25% reduction in mean arterial pressure over 1-12 hours
Catecholamine Excess States		
Pheochromocytoma	Phentolamine [Regitine]	To control paroxysms
Drug withdrawal	Drug withdrawn	Typically only one dose necessary
Pregnancy-Related		
Eclampsia	Magnesium sulfate, methyldopa [Aldomet], hydralazine [Apresoline]	Typically <90 mm Hg diastolic, but often lower

*Some physicians prefer an intravenous infusion of either fenoldopam [Corlopam] or nicardipine [Cardene], neither of which has potentially toxic metabolites, over nitroprusside [Nipride]. Recent studies have also shown improvements in renal function during therapy with the former, as compared to nitroprusside [Nipride].

unless it exceeds 180/110 mm Hg. Cardiac and vascular emergencies include acute myocardial infarction (and myocardial ischemia), pulmonary edema (and acute heart failure), and acute aortic dissection. The latter is the condition that has the lowest target BP (<120/80 mm Hg), and the least time to achieve it (typical recommendation: 20 minutes). Renal target-organ damage is manifested as either acute hematuria or acute elevation in serum creatinine; access to medical records to ascertain prior creatinine levels is very helpful. Catecholamine-related hypertensive emergencies include either pheochromocytoma, drug withdrawal (usually clonidine [Catapres]), or a crisis resulting from monoamine oxidase inhibitors. Although eclampsia includes many other criteria besides elevated BP, one of the most important early treatments for this disorder is an appropriate antihypertensive drug regimen, which makes delivery of the infant much less dangerous. The recommended drug for each type of emergency, and the BP target most frequently cited are found in Table 9. For most hypertensive emergencies, reduction of mean arterial pressure by 10% in the first hour, and another 10% to 15% during the next few hours is appropriate; the exceptions are stroke-in-evolution, aortic dissection, and eclampsia. Nitroprusside (Nipride) is the drug most commonly used for treatment of hypertensive emergencies, although fenoldopam (Corlopam) has both theoretic and practical advantages for renally impaired patients, and shares (with nicardipine [Cardene]) a lack of potentially toxic metabolites (cyanide, thiocyanate) associated with high doses or long infusions of nitroprusside (Nipride).

Hypertensive Patients with Renal Impairment

Chronic renal impairment may be either a cause of hypertension, or a consequence of undertreated hypertension. People with hypertension and chronic renal impairment differ in two important ways from those with normal renal function: their renally excreted antihypertensive drugs should be reduced in dose (or less commonly, in frequency of administration), compared with people with normal renal function. Those with renal impairment should also have a lower BP target, especially because reduction in BP may be the most important intervention to prevent or delay the onset of dialysis or renal transplantation.

ACE inhibitors play a special role in the management of hypertensive patients with nondiabetic renal impairment. Although serum creatinine often rises during the first few weeks after starting an ACE inhibitor, this should generally not be of concern unless the increase is more than 25% higher than the baseline (i.e., pre-ACE inhibitor) measurement. Although African Americans have a greater incidence of cough or angioedema with ACE inhibitors than whites, the recent AASK trial showed that the ACE inhibitor was *more* effective in preventing death, dialysis, or renal transplantation than either the calcium antagonist or the β-blocker. These data suggest that an ACE inhibitor (or perhaps an ARB, if there is cough) should be part of the antihypertensive drug regimen for African Americans and perhaps other hypertensive patients with renal impairment.

Evidence to answer the question of which BP target should be achieved in hypertensive patients with nondiabetic renal impairment is still being gathered in prospective clinical trials. JNC VI recommended <130/85 mm Hg for the goal BP of patients with renal impairment, but the lower target of <125/75 mm Hg was not beneficial in AASK, even for those with more than a gram of proteinuria/day. Until further studies prove otherwise, JNC 7 now recommends achieving a BP target of <130/80 mm Hg for both diabetics and nondiabetics with renal impairment, regardless of the degree of proteinuria.

Patients with Refractory Hypertension

Although definitions of what constitutes "refractory hypertension" vary (usually BP >140/90 mm Hg despite two or three appropriately chosen antihypertensive drugs in proper doses), there is general agreement about the treatment and evaluation of these patients. The more common causes of refractory hypertension are listed in Table 10. Identification of people with white-coat hypertension may be important, because this condition responds less well to antihypertensive drug therapy than the much more common primary hypertension. Medicare recently began reimbursement for ABPM, and this may make the procedure more widely available; home BP monitoring may be a viable substitute.

Many physicians believe the primary reason for refractory hypertension is the failure of the patient to take medications as prescribed. Probably the simplest method of assessing adherence to pill-taking is to ask routinely about it. The physician may discover evidence for nonadherence by one of several methods. Inspecting pill bottles for dates of dispensation and performing pill counts, a telephone call to the pharmacist to ascertain the number of refills during the previous year, and using simple clinical measurements (e.g., heart rate and orthostatic BP readings in patients prescribed a β-blocker or an α-blocker, respectively), can be very useful.

BP control is often compromised by other drugs the patient may be taking. Nonsteroidal anti-inflammatory drugs, including the new COX-2 (cyclooxygenase-2) inhibitors, are likely the most common offenders, but steroids, cyclosporine (Sandimmune, Neoral, Gengraf), nicotine, caffeine, and erythropoietin (Epogen, Procrit) can also raise BP. Efforts to reduce the exposure to these medications can be attempted, but many times the therapeutic effects of these other medications are more important than their BP-raising effects, and additional antihypertensive drug therapy must be given.

Secondary hypertension is much more common in individuals with refractory hypertension. In our clinic, renovascular disease is approximately three times more common in referred patients who have refractory hypertension than in the self-referred population, even after controlling for differences in initial BPs. Pheochromocytoma and mineralocorticoid-excess states are less common causes of refractory hypertension. The most common successful intervention for patients with resistant hypertension in our clinic is modification of the drug regimen. Adding or switching to an appropriate diuretic (a thiazide if the glomerular filtration rate is higher than 49 mL/min, or loop diuretic if lower than 50 mL/min), and adding an α-blocker are the most frequently successful changes.

Pregnant Patients with Hypertension

Over the last few decades, hypertension has been seen more commonly in pregnant women, perhaps because obstetricians are more aware of the short- and long-term risks of elevated BP. There are few other situations in medicine when only an elevated BP (in the absence of target-organ damage) routinely precipitates hospitalization, bedrest, and the institution of drug therapy. Although chronic hypertension (before pregnancy) increases both maternal and fetal risk, it seldom increases the risk of pre-eclampsia or eclampsia.

The management of hypertension during pregnancy is challenging because many of the drugs usually used in therapy are either contraindicated or a potential threat to the mother or fetus. Diuretics, which are the preferred first-line therapy for nonpregnant hypertensive patients, are generally avoided during pregnancy (unless the woman had been taking them before conception) because of the risk of oligohydramnios. ACE inhibitors and ARBs are contraindicated in pregnancy because of the risk of renal and other fetal malformations. Nitroprusside (Nipride) is contraindicated because of its metabolic transformation to cyanide, which is very toxic to the fetus.

Most physicians caring for hypertensive pregnant women fall back on time-tested and traditional antihypertensive drugs, including, in order, methyldopa (Aldomet), hydralazine (Apresoline), a β-blocker (typically labetalol [Trandate, Normodyne] in the United States), and then perhaps a calcium antagonist. These agents have the advantage of many years of use, and in the case of methyldopa (Aldomet), outcome studies showing no increased risk of either fetal or maternal morbidity or mortality.

Hypertensive Patients with Impending Surgery

The American Society of Anesthesiologists recognizes uncontrolled hypertension as a risk factor for peri- and postoperative morbidity and mortality. Accordingly,

TABLE 10. **Common Causes of "Resistant Hypertension"**

Pseudo-resistant Hypertension

"White-coat hypertension" (clinic responder)

Non-adherence to Antihypertensive Therapy

Dietary indiscretion to salt, ethanol, or other dietary stimulus
Poor adherence to drug treatment, due to:
- Side-effects of antihypertensive agents
- Excessive cost of medication(s)
- Inconvenient or inappropriate dosing schedules
- Organic brain syndrome (e.g., impairment of memory, forgetfulness)

Poor understanding of the importance of taking pills as directed
- Inadequate patient education
- Instructions not understood
- Lack of continuing, consistent primary source of medical care

Drug-Related Causes

Inadequate doses of antihypertensive drugs
Inappropriate combinations of antihypertensive drugs (e.g., clonidine [Catapres], methyldopa [Aldomet])
Rapid metabolism (e.g., rapid acetylators of hydralazine [Apresoline])
Drug-drug interactions
- Nonsteroidal anti-inflammatory drugs
- Sympathomimetic agents (e.g., nasal decongestants, appetite suppressants, cocaine, caffeine)
- Oral contraceptive pills (more of a problem with older, high-dose agents)
- Corticosteroids
- Licorice (and similarly-flavored chewing tobacco)
- Cyclosporine [Sandimmune, Neoral, Gengraf]/tacrolimus [Prograf]
- Erythropoietin [Epogen, Procrit]
- Cholestyramine [Questran, LoCholest, Prevalite] (or other resin-binding agents, taken simultaneously with antihypertensive drugs)
- Antidepressants (monoamine oxidase inhibitors, some tricyclics {e.g., venlafaxine [Effexor]})
- Rebound hypertension after abrupt discontinuation of centrally acting drugs, β-blockers, or occasionally, calcium antagonists

Associated Medical Conditions

Tobacco use (especially cigarette smoking during the 15 minutes before BP measurement)
Increasing weight (and obesity)
Chronic pain
Intense, acute vasoconstriction (e.g., Raynaud's phenomenon)
Insulin resistance/hyperinsulinemia
Anxiety-induced hypertension, hyperventilation, and/or panic attacks

Secondary Hypertension

Renovascular hypertension
Chronic renal impairment
Sleep apnea
Pheochromocytoma
Mineralocorticoid excess states

Volume Overload

Excessive sodium intake
Progressive renal damage and impairment (e.g., hypertensive nephrosclerosis)
Fluid retention due to direct (or indirect) vasodilators (e.g., minoxidil [Loniten])
Inadequate or inappropriate diuretic therapy

most hypertensive patients receive closer scrutiny when elective surgery is planned; occasionally the procedure must be postponed to achieve better BP control. Because of the large armamentarium of intravenously available antihypertensive drugs, however, even emergency operations can usually be performed without incident, since most anesthesiologists are very well-acquainted with intraoperative antihypertensive therapy.

Because major surgery (especially vascular surgery) carries a high risk of postoperative complications in hypertensive patients with unrecognized heart disease, preoperative cardiac testing of hypertensive patients well before the planned operation is often recommended. Much has been written about the proper sequence of such tests; in our center and in some of the recent literature, dobutamine echocardiography has become the favored test. For individuals who show no wall-motion abnormalities and whose tests are not otherwise suggestive of major coronary disease, short-term treatment with a β-blocker is often given. The impressive efficacy of this therapy, administered during hospitalization or for 30 days after the operation has been seen in two randomized trials. Such short-term β-blocker use is an excellent example of how cardiovascular risk can be reduced by treatment that is given only for a few days, rather than for a lifetime (as is more typical in treated hypertensive patients).

Organizing for Successful Management

The goal of hypertension management is to prevent the morbidity and mortality associated with it, and to do so in the "least intrusive" manner (both physiologically and fiscally). Because hypertension is not a disease, but a condition that increases cardiovascular and renal risk, its long-term control is a continuing challenge. For many years, most patients with hypertension were thought to have no noticeable symptoms. Recently, however, a significant decrease in headache has been seen when antihypertensive drugs without appreciable side effects are compared with placebo. Similarly, quality of life was best among those who achieved the lowest BPs in both HOT and TOMHS, suggesting that subtle symptoms *may* be attributable to elevated BP that improve when BP is lowered. It is nonetheless often difficult to convince a person with hypertension that taking a pill or changing one's lifestyle will result in tangible short-term benefits. Unfortunately, treating hypertension (even successfully) does not reduce cardiovascular risk to the level of a normotensive person. This provides strong impetus for initiating therapeutic lifestyle changes early, even before the levels of BP we call hypertension are present.

It is difficult to continuously motivate patients to sustain their therapeutic lifestyle changes and adhere to prescribed medications. National survey data indicate that about 34% of America's hypertensive people had their home BPs lower than 140/90 mm Hg in 1999–2000; other countries have even worse results. Economically, medication nonadherence is a very important issue, because about 10% of the money spent on hypertension is wasted by people not taking a physician's advice, and not taking pills. This nonadherence results in unnecessary hospitalizations, preventable strokes and myocardial infarctions, and admissions to nursing homes (where drug-taking can be more carefully and efficiently supervised). Individuals who are nonadherent have an infinite cost-effectiveness ratio, because they incur all of the cost, but none of the benefit of treatment.

Education of the patient (and family) is the cornerstone of improving adherence; patients with educational or cognitive deficits about hypertension and its treatment are unlikely to follow instructions for very long. Some clinics have improved their hypertension control rates after a health educator or a pharmacist was added to the hypertension treatment team. Behavioral suggestions are often useful: integrating pill-taking into the activities of daily living (e.g., taking pills when caring for teeth) or using a pillbox to organize pills according to days of the week they are to be consumed. Increasing social support appears to be a beneficial strategy, especially for older individuals. The family member or caretaker can remind the patient of the need to take pills and keep office visits, as well as actually measure BP with a home device. Several studies now show a higher rate of BP control among patients who have (and use) home BP monitors. Pills that are taken once per day, without regard to food intake, and that are well-tolerated, lead to better long-term adherence. Avoiding large, bad-tasting, or hard-to-swallow pills is important for many patients. Sensitivity of the physician to the patient's out-of-pocket expenses for medication is also important: many patients prefer fixed-dose combination pills because this strategy reduces the pharmacy copayment.

Missing one's appointments for follow-up care and monitoring of hypertension treatment has been associated with poorer outcomes. Several routine procedures can help to minimize this. Appointment reminders (either by telephone or by mail) increase return visit rates. Scheduling a specific time and date with a known health care provider, at the end of the office visit, is more successful than "calling in for a future appointment." Decreasing waiting times, having convenient office hours, and having a solicitous, caring office staff are also helpful.

Several characteristics of physicians impact on patients' adherence to medications and willingness to keep appointments. Physicians who are willing to involve the patient (when appropriate) in medical decision-making are more successful in controlling BP. A common example is asking whether the patient would prefer to take a less expensive pill more often or a more expensive pill just once a day. Physicians who are perceived as having effective communication skills, who encourage questions from the patient and appropriate family members, and who provide feedback about the patient's progress also achieve better results.

Most health care systems have accepted the treatment of hypertension as a worthwhile endeavor, which is actually cost-saving in high-risk patients and relatively cost-effective in others (when compared with many other common medical interventions). Recent efforts by some health care systems to reduce health care costs by restricting pharmacy benefits, limiting the range and doses of drugs on an accepted formulary, and reducing accessibility of health care services have generally been ineffective in the long-term. Systemwide efforts (often called "disease management programs") to encourage acceptance of generic drugs, increase the threshold for beginning antihypertensive drug therapy in low-risk patients, use one drug to treat both hypertension and a concomitant medical condition, and to encourage adherence to medication-taking have been more successful. The workload of the health care provider involved in these efforts can be increased by some of these procedures, but is sometimes offset by case managers and other allied health professionals who perform some of these important tasks.

Hypertension control is an important public health goal that requires a long-term commitment from the patient, the physician, and the health care system. When all work together toward a common goal, recent progress in demonstrating the benefits of hypertension therapy in clinical trials can be easily and effectively translated to the daily practice of medicine. This will eventually reduce the burden of disease from adverse cardiovascular and renal outcomes formerly associated with untreated elevated BP.

ACUTE MYOCARDIAL INFARCTION

method of
LAURA MAURI, M.D., M.Sc. and
PATRICK T. O'GARA, M.D.
Brigham and Women's Hospital
Boston, Massachusetts

Approximately 800,000 myocardial infarctions (MIs) occur yearly in the United States, and of these more than 25% are fatal. The majority of these deaths are due to arrhythmias prior to hospital arrival. Mortality rates are disproportionately higher among elderly persons and patients with diabetes. Early recognition, risk stratification, and timely treatment are critical elements of any clinical care pathway. Management decisions made within the first 1 to 2 hours after symptom onset are the most important in determining patients' survival.

PATHOPHYSIOLOGY

The underlying pathophysiologic mechanism of acute myocardial infarction (AMI) is rupture of the fibrous cap of an atherosclerotic plaque. Plaque rupture activates platelets, endothelium, and clotting factors, leading to rapid formation of thrombus that occludes the coronary artery lumen and results in myocardial necrosis. The clinical spectrum of acute coronary syndromes, from ST elevation myocardial infarction (STEMI) to non–ST elevation myocardial infarction (NSTEMI) and unstable angina, is based on this common pathophysiologic substrate. The majority of culprit plaques are not obstructive before rupture; thus, MI is not always preceded by a history of angina.

Some MIs may occur by a mechanism other than plaque rupture. One common mechanism is increased myocardial oxygen demand, which may be caused by fever, anemia, hyperthyroidism, tachycardia, or significant hypotension or hypertension. Patients with left ventricular hypertrophy or fixed coronary stenoses may be especially susceptible to AMI in this setting. Treatment of demand-related myocardial ischemia should be focused on reversing the underlying stimulus.

Other rarer causes of myocardial necrosis include primary coronary vasospasm (associated with ST elevation), coronary embolism (from intracardiac or valvular sources), spontaneous coronary dissection, myocardial bridging (causing external systolic compression of the coronary lumen), congenital coronary anomalies, blunt chest wall trauma, and myocarditis.

DEFINITION

The World Health Organization definition of MI requires the presence of at least two of the following criteria: (1) chest discomfort consistent with myocardial ischemia, (2) changes on serial ECGs, and (3) rise and fall of serum markers of myocardial necrosis. Because only 50% of patients who subsequently have elevation in cardiac enzymes manifest diagnostic electrocardiographic changes at presentation, the diagnosis cannot always be made immediately, and often requires 12 to 24 hours of observation. With widespread use of serum markers more sensitive than creatine kinase (CK), the definition of MI has been extended to include infarctions detectable by troponin elevation only (European Society of Cardiology–American College of Cardiology consensus document 2000).

CLINICAL PRESENTATION

History

Patients presenting with typical chest discomfort at rest lasting for 30 minutes or more should be suspected to have MI. Other classical symptoms include jaw or arm pain, throat tightness, nausea, and diaphoresis. Many patients with MI, however, do not have these classical symptoms, particularly elderly persons, women, and patients with diabetes. Patients with a history of prior angina often present with symptoms of infarction that are similar in nature but more severe than those of their prior angina and less likely to be relieved with nitroglycerin.

Physical Examination

Just as the extent of MI may range from minute to extensive, the physical examination on presentation may range from well compensated to one of cardiogenic shock. Key signs of extensive infarction include sinus tachycardia, hypotension, rales, and an S_3 gallop. An S_4 gallop may be a sign of ongoing ischemia but may also be associated with isolated hypertension. Peripheral edema may be a clue to subacute or chronic right ventricular dysfunction. In the patient with inferior MI, the presence of elevated venous pressure with Kussmaul's sign (a paradoxical increase in jugular venous pressure with inspiration), clear lungs, and hypotension should suggest right ventricular involvement. Low-grade fever is not unusual following STEMI and does not necessarily signify infection. The physical examination is also especially useful in distinguishing other causes of chest pain and assessing for mechanical complications of MI.

LABORATORY EVALUATION

Electrocardiogram

An electrocardiogram (ECG) should be obtained within 10 minutes of presentation and serves as the main triage point in the acute care of the patient with suspected MI. The ECG serves to diagnose, risk-stratify, and aid in definition of the coronary anatomy of the patient with AMI. The standard ECG criterion for STEMI is the presence of ST elevation of 0.1 mV or more in two or more contiguous leads. ST depression and T wave inversion are less specific findings. ST elevation in non–Q wave leads suggests ongoing injury and requires triage to a strategy of acute reperfusion; in contrast, ST depression usually suggests myocardial ischemia or "subendocardial" infarction. The classical ST elevation pattern in AMI is concave down ("tombstone") and may be associated with loss of R wave voltage and terminal T wave inversion or with eventual Q wave formation in the same leads. The number of leads with ST elevation correlates with the extent of infarction and the associated mortality risk. The absence of ST elevation, however, does not always signify a lack of coronary occlusion. Classically, infarctions in the territory of the distal left circumflex artery may be electrocardiographically "silent." The differential diagnosis of ST elevation on ECG includes coronary vasospasm, pericarditis, myocardial aneurysm, and early repolarization.

The location of the culprit artery can be inferred from the ECG leads showing ST elevation. ST elevation in leads V_1 to V_3 suggests injury to the anterior wall of the left ventricle, supplied by the left anterior descending (LAD) artery. ST elevation in leads V_4 to V_6, I, and aVL suggests lateral wall injury caused by left circumflex artery (LCX) occlusion. ST elevation in leads II, III, and aVF suggests inferior wall injury, most commonly caused by right coronary artery (RCA) infarction. In the case of a left dominant circulation, inferior MI may be caused by LCX artery infarction. Recognition of inferior infarction should prompt examination of the ECG for ST depression in V_1 and V_2 that may reflect posterior involvement and ST elevation in right-sided lead V_4, reflecting right ventricular infarction. ST changes in multiple anatomic territories connote left main, multivessel disease or an extensive distribution of a single coronary artery, such as when the LAD also supplies the inferior septum.

Other critical ECG features are the presence of Q waves signifying prior MI and abnormalities of cardiac rhythm and conduction. In some patients, the presenting ECG may demonstrate a life-threatening arrhythmia such as ventricular fibrillation or tachycardia or complete heart block. In these patients, once sinus rhythm is established by standard advanced cardiac life support protocols, the immediate next step should be to repeat the 12-lead ECG to determine whether infarction is the underlying cause of arrest. Intraventricular conduction delays deserve special mention. The presence of a new left bundle branch block in the setting of recent ischemic chest pain is consistent with LAD artery occlusion and carries a mortality rate of 25%. The presence of a new right bundle branch block in the setting of anterior ST elevation carries a 20% increased risk of mortality and connotes extensive proximal LAD artery infarction. New atrial fibrillation may also signify cardiac decompensation secondary to a large territory of infarction with heart failure.

Serum Cardiac Markers

Myocyte necrosis results in the release of markers of cardiac injury from the cytoplasm into the bloodstream. These markers are used to (1) detect MI in the absence of diagnostic ECG changes, (2) estimate the extent of myocardial injury, and (3) assess for reinfarction. Commonly used markers include myocardial specific creatine kinase (CK-MB), cardiac troponin I, cardiac troponin T, and myoglobin. Because of the different patterns of release, a selective combination of markers may be most useful in clinical practice. CK-MB is released from cardiac myocytes within 3 to 4 hours of infarction, peaks in 10 to 24 hours, and is cleared within 2 to 4 days. Cardiac troponins are detectable at 2 to 4 hours, peak at 10 to 24 hours, but remain elevated for 5 days to 2 weeks. In contrast, myoglobin peaks earliest (4 to 8 hours) and is the most quickly cleared (within 1 day). Troponins may detect infarction that has occurred prior to presentation and in addition are more sensitive for the detection of smaller amounts of myocardial injury. Because they are released only from cardiac myocytes, troponins are also the most specific markers of myocardial necrosis. For the detection of recurrent ischemia, however, CK-MB or myoglobin is preferable.

CK-MB has been correlated with patient outcomes in AMI, and cardiac troponin, in acute coronary syndromes. It must be stressed, however, that because there is a time delay between the onset of myocardial necrosis and serum detection, lack of elevated serum markers at presentation in patients with characteristic symptoms or ECG changes, or both, should not dissuade the clinician from diagnosing and treating AMI. Several other biomarkers, such as B-type natriuretic peptide and C-reactive protein, do not measure myocardial injury but do correlate with risk in acute coronary syndromes.

Differential Diagnosis

The differential diagnosis of acute chest discomfort is broad and includes both benign and dangerous conditions that may be distinguished by the history and physical examination. Chest pain related to infarction is not usually fleeting, discretely localized, pleuritic, or positional. Pleuritic chest pain should prompt evaluation for pulmonary embolism, pneumonia, spontaneous pneumothorax, or pleurisy. Positional chest pain with PR depression or diffuse ST elevation and a rub should suggest pericarditis, either viral or after MI. Sudden onset of severe chest pain with hypertension but no ECG changes may indicate aortic dissection. Chest radiography should be performed in all patients with suspected MI. Chest pain that is reproducible with upper extremity movement or palpation by the examiner is unlikely to be ischemic in origin. A difficult diagnosis to make is early herpes zoster, in which patients may present with unilateral chest discomfort before the characteristic skin lesions erupt. Other causes of chest discomfort that may appear similar to MI include anxiety attack and gastroesophageal reflux or spasm. In summary, it is essential to consider quickly the differential diagnosis in all patients presenting with chest pain, prior to initiating reperfusion therapies that could seriously complicate nonischemic chest pain syndromes, such as aortic dissection or pericarditis.

TREATMENT—IMMEDIATE

The cornerstones of AMI treatment are rapid restoration of normal blood flow, reduction of myocardial supply-demand mismatch, and prevention of acute complications.

The patient should have an ECG within the first 10 minutes of arrival at the emergency room in order to differentiate ST elevation from NSTEMI. Establishment of intravenous access, application of low-flow oxygen, and initiation of cardiac monitoring occur concurrently. If ST elevation is present, reperfusion therapy (thrombolysis versus primary angioplasty) should be initiated without delay.

Aspirin

Aspirin has been shown in large trials to reduce mortality from AMI by 22% (International Study of Infarct Survival 2) and should be given at a dose of 160 to 325 mg immediately on presentation. If aspirin cannot be given orally, it can be given as a suppository with similar efficacy.

Nitroglycerin

Nitroglycerin may be used to relieve chest pain associated with MI, to alleviate hypertension, and to decrease preload in patients with concomitant congestive heart failure. It may started at sublingual doses of 1/150 grain (0.4 mg) given every 5 minutes for 3 doses to relieve chest pain, followed by an intravenous nitroglycerin infusion if necessary. It should be avoided in the patient who is hypotensive and be used with caution in inferior MI, where it may unmask right ventricular dysfunction.

β-Blockade

β-Blockade has been shown to decrease the likelihood of ventricular arrhythmias and recurrent ischemia in AMI. In the absence of contraindications, such as bradycardia or congestive failure, β-blockers should be initiated. We use a dosage of metoprolol (Lopressor) 5 mg IV every 5 minutes for 3 doses, followed by oral dosing as needed for a target heart rate of 50 to 60 beats per minute and systolic blood pressure of 100 to 120 mm Hg.

Morphine

In the patient who continues to have chest discomfort, morphine may be required for analgesia. It has the additional benefit of pulmonary vasodilation, useful in patients presenting with congestive heart failure.

Reperfusion Therapies in ST Elevation Myocardial Infarction

The presence of ST elevation should prompt immediate institution of a strategy aimed at opening the infarct-related artery and restoring normal coronary blood flow at the epicardial and microvascular levels. The choice between thrombolysis and percutaneous coronary intervention depends on characteristics of the patient and hospital resources. Primary angioplasty has been shown to be superior to thrombolysis, with decreased mortality, recurrent ischemia, and stroke, when performed quickly by experienced operators. For logistic reasons, however, in hospitals far from a qualified catheterization laboratory, thrombolysis may achieve more rapid reperfusion. Successful efforts to decrease the time to reperfusion include emergency medical service–initiated triage and establishment of hospital-specific clinical practice guidelines. Prehospital thrombolysis is not recommended as a routine strategy, but in settings where prehospital transport time is greater than 90 minutes and a physician is present in the ambulance, this therapy may offer benefit.

Thrombolysis

Thrombolytic agents activate endogenous plasminogen, thereby increasing the rate of fibrinolysis of formed thrombus. When given within 6 hours of symptom onset, these agents have been shown to reduce mortality in AMI by 20% to 30%. The most feared complication of thrombolysis is hemorrhagic stroke, occurring in 0.5% to 1% of cases. This complication is fatal in at least 50% of patients and results in substantial long-term morbidity among survivors.

Currently, the three relatively fibrin-specific thrombolytic agents used most often are front-loaded alteplase (Activase) (tissue plasminogen activator), 15 mg IV bolus, followed by up to 50 mg over 30 min, then up to 35 mg over the next 60 min; single-bolus tenecteplase (TNKase), 30 to 50 mg based on weight; and double-bolus reteplase (Retavase), 2 doses of 10 U each separated by 30 minutes. These therapies are combined with aspirin 325 mg and heparin* (60 U/kg intravenous bolus followed by 12 U/kg/h infusion, to a target activated partial thromboplastin time of 50 to 70 seconds) or, in the case of tenecteplase, the low-molecular-weight heparin enoxaparin (Lovenox) (30 mg IV bolus followed by 1 mg/kg every 12 hours, Assessment of the Safety and Efficacy of a New Thrombolytic Regimen [ASSENT]-3). The adjunctive use of glycoprotein IIb/IIIa inhibitors has been associated with improved rates of angiographic reperfusion (Thrombolysis in Myocardial Infarction [TIMI] 14) and decreased rates of recurrent ischemia; however, their addition to half-dose thrombolysis does not decrease mortality and may increase bleeding complications (Global Use of Strategies to Open Occluded Coronary Arteries [GUSTO]-V).

Before initiating thrombolysis, the contraindications should be reviewed. These include: previous hemorrhagic stroke, known intracranial neoplasm, active internal bleeding, suspected aortic dissection, severe hypertension in excess of 180/110 mm Hg, current use

*Not FDA-approved for this indication.

of anticoagulants, recent trauma, surgery, prolonged cardiopulmonary resuscitation, and pregnancy. Elderly patients (older than 75 years) have represented less than 10% of patients in trials of thrombolysis but form a larger proportion of the patients presenting with AMI. Although advanced age is associated with higher rates of intracranial hemorrhage, older patients may derive a greater absolute survival benefit from thrombolysis.

When thrombolysis is chosen, the goal should be a "door-to-needle" time of 30 minutes or less. Clinical signs of reperfusion include resolution of chest pain and a fall of 70% or greater from peak ST elevation. The median time to reperfusion following successful thrombolysis is approximately 45 minutes. Signs of ongoing infarction after that interval should prompt an alternative plan for reperfusion, such as rescue angioplasty.

Primary Angioplasty

Primary angioplasty is the use of angioplasty or stenting as first-line treatment of STEMI. Its advantages when compared with thrombolysis are a higher rate of reperfusion (90% versus 60% to 80%), a significantly lower rate of stroke (0.1%), and a significant reduction in mortality. When a strategy of primary angioplasty is undertaken, the goal is a "door-to-balloon" time of less than 60 to 90 minutes.

Trials of angioplasty versus thrombolysis have generally involved a selected group of eligible patients cared for in high-volume centers with specialized expertise. Several areas of debate remain. There is evidence suggesting that patients who present with STEMI to community hospitals may benefit from rapid transfer to tertiary hospitals for primary angioplasty, compared with a strategy of thrombolysis in the community, despite the increased time to therapy (Air Primary Angioplasty in Myocardial Infarction [Air-PAMI], Danish Multicentre Randomized Trial on Thrombolytic Therapy versus Acute Coronary Angioplasty in Acute Myocardial Infarction [DANAMI-2]). Other trials have shown that some qualified community hospitals can achieve acceptably low mortality rates with primary angioplasty even in the absence of on-site cardiac surgical backup (Cardiovascular Patient Outcomes Research Team [C-PORT]). There is consensus, however, that primary angioplasty requires access to a dedicated 24-hour on-call team with experienced high-volume operators and a minimum door-to-balloon time.

Patients targeted for angioplasty should be treated with intravenous heparin, dose adjusted during the procedure to an ACT of 300 to 350 seconds in the absence of IIb/IIIa inhibition and 250 to 300 in the presence of IIb/IIIa inhibition. The use of low-molecular-weight heparin during angioplasty has been shown to be safe (National Investigators Collaborating on Enoxaparin [NICE 1]), but many operators still have concerns about its efficacy given the lack of randomized trials during coronary intervention. The addition of thrombolysis prior to transfer for angioplasty has thus far not been shown to reduce mortality and is associated with higher bleeding complications. Glycoprotein IIb/IIIa inhibitors may be associated with higher rates of early reperfusion when given before arrival in the catheterization laboratory. They are also frequently started during AMI angioplasty, and although they reduce early rates of subacute stent thrombosis, glycoprotein IIb/IIIa inhibitors do not decrease total major adverse cardiac events Controlled Abciximab and Device Investigation to Lower Late Angioplasty Complications (CADILLAC).

Non–ST Elevation Myocardial Infarction: Early Invasive versus Conservative Strategies

NSTEMI must be distinguished from STEMI. First, thrombolysis in NSTEMI is associated with *increased* mortality and is not recommended except in the specific circumstance of true posterior MI manifested as precordial ST segment depression. Second, if infarction is not ongoing, the decision to pursue an invasive strategy can be made over the first 24 to 48 hours rather than in the first hour. It should also be noted that on initial presentation, NSTEMI cannot be distinguished from unstable angina unless serum markers are already elevated.

Formerly, many cardiologists favored an initial conservative strategy for the treatment of NSTEMI and unstable angina that involved medical stabilization, with cardiac catheterization performed for recurrent spontaneous ischemia or a positive predischarge exercise test. This strategy was supported in the prestent era by the results of the TIMI 3B trial. However, two large trials in the stent era have demonstrated benefit of an early invasive strategy in intermediate- to high-risk patients (Fast Revascularisation during InStability in Coronary artery disease [FRISC II] and Treat angina with Aggrastat and determine Cost of Therapy with an Invasive or Conservative Strategy [TACTICS]-TIMI 18). This strategy consisted of routine angiography during the first days after presentation followed by revascularization as indicated. An early invasive strategy is favored in patients with recurrent ischemia, elevated troponin, new ST depression (≥0.5 mV), evidence of congestive heart failure or hemodynamic instability, depressed systolic function, ventricular tachycardia, or prior revascularization. In such patients, the invasive approach is associated with a further relative reduction in the composite endpoint of death, recurrent MI, and rehospitalization for refractory angina, when compared with a conservative strategy.

The choice of pharmacologic therapy for NSTEMI depends on the management strategy chosen. In all cases, aspirin is essential and should be started early and continued indefinitely following MI. In the patient with a true aspirin allergy, the thienopyridine clopidogrel (Plavix) may be substituted. The combination of clopidogrel and aspirin has been shown to decrease the rate of death, MI, and stroke in patients with unstable angina for whom invasive procedures are not planned

(Clopidogrel in Unstable Angina to Prevent Recurrent Events [CURE]). However, because it increases rates of perioperative bleeding, clopidogrel should be withheld from patients for whom coronary artery bypass graft surgery is likely, for up to 5 to 7 days prior to operation. The use of glycoprotein IIb/IIIa inhibitors should be reserved for patients with continuing ischemia, elevated troponin, ST segment depression, or other high-risk features that would prompt intervention. Intravenous unfractionated heparin is recommended for patients managed with an invasive strategy, but enoxaparin, the low-molecular-weight heparin, may be preferred for patients managed conservatively unless renal failure or obesity is present.

COMPLICATIONS

Mechanical Complications

Mechanical complications of AMI include mitral regurgitation secondary to papillary muscle rupture, ventricular septal rupture, and left ventricular free wall rupture or pseudoaneurysm formation. These complications should be suspected in the patient with sudden hemodynamic deterioration following AMI. In the thrombolytic era, these events have become less frequent and appear to occur earlier—as early as 24 hours rather than the classical 5 to 7 days after infarction. For acute mitral regurgitation or ventricular septal rupture, intra-aortic balloon counterpulsation may provide beneficial afterload reduction. Myocardial free wall rupture is usually fatal even if emergent pericardiocentesis is performed. Emergent cardiac surgical consultation is recommended for these complications as mortality rates with medical therapy approach 90%.

Severe Ventricular Dysfunction

The presence of pump failure leading to cardiogenic shock should prompt early coronary angiography, with invasive hemodynamic monitoring and consideration of early revascularization. Severe left ventricular dysfunction may require inotropic support, intra-aortic balloon counterpulsation, and, in some cases, consideration for cardiac transplantation. Severe right ventricular dysfunction accompanying inferior MI may also lead to cardiogenic shock and is associated with increased mortality. Such patients are markedly preload dependent and benefit from volume loading but may also require inotropic support.

Left Ventricular Thrombus

Formation of left ventricular thrombus occurs in the setting of large anterior infarction and may be detected on echocardiography. The risk of stroke from left ventricular thrombus is highest in the first 21 days, and a period of warfarin (Coumadin) anticoagulation (3 months) should be considered if new anterior akinesis is present.

SECONDARY PREVENTION

β-Blockers

β-Blocker therapy decreases mortality after AMI and should be continued indefinitely in most patients. Patients with severe left ventricular dysfunction may not be able to begin this therapy until after medical stabilization has been achieved.

Angiotensin-Converting Enzyme Inhibition

Angiotensin-converting enzyme inhibitors are recommended for all MI survivors. The magnitude of their benefit is highest among patients with depressed left ventricular function or anterior MI. After initiating an ACE inhibitor, it is necessary to monitor serum creatinine and potassium.

Aspirin

Long-term use of aspirin after AMI reduces mortality, reinfarction, and stroke. It is recommended at a dose of 81 to 325 mg daily.

Lipid-Lowering Therapy

Lipid-lowering therapies, specifically HMG coenzyme A (CoA) reductase inhibitors, have been shown to decrease mortality following MI (Scandinavian Simvastatin Survival Study [4S], Cholesterol and Recurrent Events [CARE]). The fasting lipid profile should be checked within 24 hours of presentation. We recommend that all patients be started on HMG CoA reductase inhibitors after MI with a low-density lipoprotein goal of less than 100 mg/dL. It is necessary to monitor subsequent liver enzyme tests and CK.

Smoking Cessation

Smoking cessation is of proven benefit after MI and should be emphasized by all clinicians. Referral to smoking cessation programs may increase compliance. After recovery from MI and in the absence of recurrent ischemia, pharmacologic intervention may also be useful.

Cardiac Rehabilitation

If revascularization has not been performed, the patient should undergo a submaximal exercise test to assess the short-term risk of recurrent ischemia prior to hospital discharge. After 4 to 6 weeks, a symptom-limited exercise test should be performed, and a program of cardiac rehabilitation that includes education regarding risk factor modification and exercise should be initiated.

Mortality from MI has decreased substantially over the past five decades because of early recognition, aggressive reperfusion, rhythm management, and application of appropriate secondary prevention strategies.

PERICARDITIS

method of
IGNACIO INGLESSIS, M.D.
Harvard Medical School
Massachusetts General Hospital
Boston, Massachusetts

Pericarditis, or inflammation of the pericardium, results in three distinctive syndromes:

- Acute noneffusive pericarditis
- Pericardial effusion with or without pericardial tamponade
- Constrictive pericarditis

ACUTE NONEFFUSIVE PERICARDITIS

This condition is classically defined as acute pericardial inflammation without pericardial effusion. However, the widespread use of echocardiography has shown that most patients have small pericardial effusions.

Etiology

The etiology of acute pericarditis is summarized in Table 1. Most patients with acute pericarditis have viral or idiopathic pericarditis. Tuberculous pericarditis remains a significant problem in developing countries and should be in the differential diagnosis of patients with HIV infection.

Clinical Features

Chest Pain

It is of sudden onset, pleuritic, located in the anterior chest, and increases with deep inspiration or cough or by lying flat. Pain radiation to the left trapezius ridge is characteristic. Occasionally, respiratory or gastrointestinal symptoms precede the development of pain.

Pericardial Friction Rub

Usually, this is heard as a high-frequency scratchy or rough sound, best noticed at the left sternal border. Pericardial rubs may vary in intensity and may even disappear, depending on the respiratory phase or body position, which is a useful way of distinguishing rubs from heart murmurs. Although pericardial rubs tend to decrease in intensity as fluid accumulates in the pericardial sac, they may persist despite the presence of large pericardial effusions.

Electrocardiography

There are four consecutive phases:

- Phase 1: ST-segment elevation with upper concavity, upright T waves, and PR-segment depression in most leads
- Phase 2: Resolution of ST- and PR-segment changes
- Phase 3: Diffuse T-wave inversions
- Phase 4: Normalization of the electrocardiogram

Additional Findings

Half of these patients have elevation of troponin levels and transient wall motion abnormalities on echocardiography, findings reflecting variable degrees of coexistent myocarditis. Echocardiography may also show pericardial effusion, most of them small. Leukocytosis and elevation of acute phase reactants (C-reactive protein and erythrocyte sedimentation rate) are also seen.

Evaluation

The initial evaluation includes electrocardiogram, chest radiograph, tuberculin skin test, antinuclear antibody test, and rheumatoid factor test. Echocardiography should be done routinely. Blood

TABLE 1. **Etiology of Acute Pericarditis**

Common Causes	Uncommon Causes	Rare Causes
IDIOPATHIC CAUSES	MYOCARDIAL INFARCTION	INFECTIONS
VIRAL INFECTIONS	Hemopericardium	Pyogenic
Coxsackievirus	Dressler's syndrome	Tuberculoous
Echovirus	DRUGS	Fungal
COLLAGEN VASCULAR DISEASE	Procainamide	Parasitic
Rheumatoid arthritis	Hydralazine	PRIMARY NEOPLASIA
Systemic lupus erythematosus	CHEST TRAUMA	Mesothelioma
Scleroderma	Pentrating	Sarcoma
METASTATIC NEOPLASIA	Blunt	RADIATION
Lung	PLEUROPULMONARY DISEASE	INTRAPERICARDIAL ELECTRODES
Breast	Pneumonia	Automatic implanted cardioverter defibrillator
Lymphoma	Pulmonary emboli	Pacemakers
UREMIA	Acute pleuritis	PANCREATITIS
	AORTIC DISSECTION	MYXEDEMA
	CARDIAC SURGERY	

cultures should be obtained if there is a suspicion of bacterial pericarditis.

Most patients with acute pericarditis have idiopathic or viral pericarditis with a benign course and therefore do not warrant further evaluation. Pericardiocentesis should be performed in those patients who present with pericardial tamponade, in those suspected to have bacterial pericarditis, and in those who have persistent symptoms and significant pericardial effusion after 1 week of therapy. Finally, pericardial biopsy should be considered in those patients who remain clinically active for more than 3 weeks without an established diagnosis.

Treatment

Nonsteroidal anti-inflammatory drugs (NSAIDs) are the mainstay of treatment. Ibuprofen (Motrin)* is the first choice, 300 to 800 mg every 6 to 8 hours, depending on severity. Indomethacin (Indocin),* 25 to 50 mg every 8 hours, or aspirin,* 325 to 650 mg every 4 to 6 hours, are valid alternatives. Corticosteroids are used in cases refractory to NSAIDs and in pericarditis resulting from collagen vascular disease. Prednisone* is started at 60 mg daily and is tapered promptly to the minimally effective dose. Finally, colchicine, 0.6 mg every 12 hours, has been used alone or in combination with NSAIDs for the treatment and prevention of recurrent pericarditis.

PERICARDIAL EFFUSION

Pathologic *pericardial effusion* is defined as the accumulation of greater than 35 mL of fluid in the pericardial sac.

Etiology

All causes of acute pericarditis can result in significant pericardial effusion. However, large pericardial effusion are usually caused by malignant disease, tuberculosis, connective tissue disease, uremia, cardiac perforation, aortic dissection, cholesterol pericarditis, and myxedema.

Pathophysiology of Pericardial Tamponade

Pericardial tamponade is defined as a hemodynamic abnormality produced by the accumulation of pericardial fluid that impairs diastolic filling of the ventricles. Initially, there is shifting of the interventricular septum toward the left ventricle as the right ventricular filling increases during inspiration, leading to reduction in left ventricular filling, decreased stroke volume, and decreased systolic arterial pressure. As fluid accumulates, left ventricular filling is impaired in both respiratory phases, and severe hypotension ensues.

*Not FDA-approved for this indication.

Clinical Presentation

The clinical presentation of patients with pericardial effusion varies from patients who are completely asymptomatic to those presenting with pericardial tamponade and cardiovascular collapse. Presentation is not necessarily related to the size of the effusion but rather to the rate of fluid accumulation, because the pericardium grows to accommodate its content when it is subjected to chronic stretching. Hence, whereas the rapid accumulation of 150 to 200 mL may result in cardiac tamponade, the slow accumulation of larger effusions may be well tolerated.

Classic cardiac tamponade presents as dyspnea, elevated systemic venous pressure, tachycardia, distant heart sounds, systemic hypotension, and arterial *pulsus paradoxus* (defined as an inspiratory drop in systolic arterial pressure of more than 10 mm Hg). Some patients may have a more subacute presentation characterized by dyspnea and peripheral edema without circulatory collapse.

Chest Radiography

An unexplained increase in heart size suggests pericardial effusion. However, the sensitivity and specificity of radiography are low. The lung fields are typically without significant pulmonary edema.

Electrocardiography

The electrocardiogram can be entirely normal but most frequently shows nonspecific ST-segment and T-wave changes. Sinus tachycardia, low voltage, and electrical alternation of the QRS complexes are also seen.

Echocardiography

This is the procedure of choice for the diagnosis and follow-up of pericardial effusion. This technique provides excellent sensitivity and specificity. The signs of cardiac tamponade are right atrial and right ventricular diastolic collapse and dilation of the inferior vena cava with lack of inspiratory collapse. Doppler studies show marked increase in right-sided valve flow velocities and a marked decrease in left-sided valve velocities during inspiration.

Additional Imaging Studies

Computed tomography and magnetic resonance imaging are useful is in detecting pericardial effusion, as well as for assessing pericardial thickness, masses, and cysts.

Cardiac Catheterization

This technique is used to confirm the diagnosis of cardiac tamponade if doubts persist after echocardiography, and it also allows the evaluation of hemodynamic changes after pericardiocentesis. The hallmark findings are elevation and diastolic equalization of all cardiac chambers and intrapericardial pressures. Cardiac tamponade also produces characteristic changes in the waveform of the cardiac chambers: the right atrial "Y descent" and the early diastolic dip in the ventricular pressure tracings are gradually obliterated and are finally abolished.

Treatment

Once the diagnosis of pericardial effusion has been made, it is important to determine whether the effusion is creating significant hemodynamic compromise. Asymptomatic patients without hemodynamic compromise, even with large pericardial effusions, do not need to undergo drainage procedures unless there is a need for fluid analysis for diagnostic purposes. Conversely, when the diagnosis of cardiac tamponade is made, there is a need for emergency pericardiocentesis to relieve hemodynamic compromise. Patients with pericardial tamponade awaiting fluid drainage should undergo aggressive intravascular fluid expansion, and one should avoid drugs that may impair cardiac output such as diuretics, β-blockers, or calcium channel blockers. Pressors may be needed to maintain adequate tissue perfusion.

Pericardiocentesis can be done percutaneously or surgically. Most patients are initially treated with catheter pericardiocentesis, because it has the advantages of being a faster procedure performed using local anesthesia and allowing precise hemodynamic evaluation. However, surgical drainage should be performed when biopsy sampling is required for the diagnosis, when there is suspected brisk pericardial bleeding suggestive of myocardial rupture or aortic dissection, in patients with significant coagulopathy or thrombocytopenia, and when fluid reaccumulates after a percutaneous attempt.

Fluid Analysis

Basic fluid analysis includes hematocrit and cell count, Gram and Ziehl-Neelsen stains, cultures, glucose, protein, pH, lactate dehydrogenase testing, and immunocytochemistry. Depending on clinical suspicion, additional tests may be required, such as rheumatoid factor, antinuclear antibody, complement levels, amylase, adenosine deaminase, and cholesterol levels. Pericardial fluid may consist of transudates, exudates, hemopericardium, or a combination of these. Table 2 summarizes the differences between transudative and exudative fluids.

Management After Pericardiocentesis

Based on the cause of the effusion and the patient's clinical and hemodynamic condition, the pericardial catheter may be removed or left in the pericardial space for 48 to 72 hours. Recurrences after catheter drainage have been reported in up to 50% of patients, most commonly in those with malignant pericardial effusions. Patients who continue to drain more than 100 mL per 24 hours 3 days after the procedure should be considered for more aggressive therapy, including intrapericardial instillation of sclerosing agents (e.g., tetracycline), systemic chemotherapy, radiotherapy, percutaneous balloon pericardial window procedures, and surgical intervention.

CONSTRICTIVE PERICARDITIS

Constrictive pericarditis is an unusual cause of congestive heart failure characterized by a thickened and fibrotic pericardium that limits diastolic filling of the heart.

Etiology

Constrictive pericarditis is common sequela of most of the acute and chronic inflammatory processes that affect the pericardium; however, its cause is unknown in the majority of cases. Unrecognized viral pericarditis probably does play a major role. Other frequent causes include mediastinal radiation therapy, cardiac surgery, infection, chest trauma, neoplasia, uremia, and collagen vascular disease.

Pathophysiology

An initial inflammatory insult results in fibrin deposition with subsequent adherent fibrosis, obliteration of the pericardial space, and sometimes late calcification as the entire heart becomes encased in a noncompliant pericardium. Characteristically, in early diastole, the heart volume is less than pericardial volume, so ventricular filling is unimpeded and occurs rapidly; however, it is halted in mid-diastole once the rigid pericardium limits further expansion. Consequently, diastolic pressures are elevated in all four chambers of the heart, and the stroke volume is both reduced and fixed. Biventricular systolic function

TABLE 2. **Distinction Between Exudative and Transudative Pericardial Fluid**

Parameter	Exudate	Transudate
Appearance	Turbid, purulent, or bloody	Clear, straw, or amber
Total protein	>30 g/L	<30 g/L
Lactate dehydrogenase	>200 IU/L	<200 IU/L
Glucose	Lower than blood glucose	Equal to blood glucose
Cholesterol	>45 mg/dL	<45 mg/dL
Cells	Many (leukocytes, lymphocytes, neoplasic)	Few (usually mesothelial)
Microorganisms	Present in cases of infectious origin	Absent

is normal or nearly normal in most cases. Tachycardia becomes the major mechanism for maintaining cardiac output.

Clinical Presentation

The patient has predominant systemic venous congestion (peripheral edema and fluid retention) and low cardiac output symptoms (fatigue and weakness). Symptoms of pulmonary congestion are seen less frequently. Elevation of jugular venous pressure with rapid Y descent, Kussmaul's sign (lack of normal jugular venous pressure collapse during normal inspiration), and a pericardial knock are frequently appreciated.

Chest Radiology

The cardiac silhouette is usually normal in size. Pericardial calcification is now seen less frequently than in the past. The lung fields show mild pulmonary venous hypertension; however, frank pulmonary edema is rare.

Electrocardiogram

There is mild low voltage with nonspecific T-wave abnormalities. Biatrial enlargement is sometimes seen. Atrial arrhythmias, particularly atrial fibrillation, frequently develop in the late stages.

Echocardiography

Biatrial enlargement, preserved ventricular dimensions, normal systolic function, and often some degree of pericardial thickening are noted. Doppler studies demonstrate significantly increased respiratory variations in flow measured at the mitral and tricuspid valves and at the hepatic and pulmonary veins, findings reflecting the lack of normal transmission of intrathoracic pressures to the heart.

Cardiac Catheterization

One sees elevation and equalization of all diastolic pressures with early rapid and late impeded diastolic filling shown by the prominent Y descent in the right atrial pressure tracing and the "dip and plateau" diastolic waveform in both ventricular pressure tracings.

Additional Studies

First-pass radionuclide angiography typically shows early rapid diastolic filling and decreased atrial systole contribution to late filling. Magnetic resonance imaging or computed tomography studies are additional means of detecting pericardial thickening.

Prevention of Pericardial Constriction

Corticosteroids have been shown to improve the condition in patients with subacute constrictive pericarditis early after heart surgery or with tuberculous pericarditis. Intrapericardial urokinase* has also been reported to be successful in the treatment of several cases of exudative fibrinous pericarditis, and it may have a role in preventing constriction. In patients with tuberculous pericarditis, the effectiveness of specific pharmacologic therapy in preventing constriction is controversial.

*Not FDA-approved for this indication.

Treatment

Treatment of established constriction is based on control of congestive symptoms and definitive surgical resection of the diseased pericardium. Judicious use of salt restriction and diuretics may offer relief of congestive symptoms; however, most patients have a progressive and irreversible course and eventually require pericardial resection. Careful titration of diuretics is mandatory to avoid further reduction in stroke volume and hypoperfusion to vital organs, particularly the liver and kidneys. Thiazides (chlorothiazide [Diuril], 500 to 1000 mg/d) are usually effective in patients with mild (New York Heart Association class II) symptoms. In more advanced cases (NYHA class III or IV), the use of loop diuretics (furosemide [Lasix]), 20 to 400 mg/d alone or in combination with thiazides, is often necessary.

Many patients with mild disease are asymptomatic or have minimal symptoms and may remain stable for months to years on diuretic therapy alone; in such patients, pericardiectomy can be safely deferred. Conversely, the surgical mortality rate is increased in patients with advanced symptoms. Consequently, the procedure is safest and most beneficial for patients with progressive class II symptoms that persist despite optimized diuretic therapy, provided the pericardium is widely resected. The surgical mortality rate is low; most patients show prompt hemodynamic improvement postoperatively that is maintained in the long term.

PERIPHERAL ARTERIAL DISEASE

method of
GLENN FUSONIE, M.D., and
JOHN D. EDWARDS, M.D.
University of Cincinnati
Cincinnati, Ohio

Peripheral arterial disease (PAD) traditionally refers to diseases of blood vessels outside the heart and brain. PAD is further classified into either a functional disorder such as Raynaud's or vasospastic disease, or an organic disorder caused by structural changes to the blood vessel from inflammation or fatty deposits that ultimately affect blood circulation. The diagnosis and management of PAD has undergone tremendous change since the 1980s. Increasingly prevalent are less invasive screening examinations and procedures for management such as angioplasty and stenting.

The following discussion will cover the most common peripheral arterial conditions likely to be encountered.

LOWER EXTREMITY ARTERIAL OCCLUSIVE DISEASE

Atherosclerosis

There are multiple reasons for lower limb occlusive disease. The most common is atherosclerosis, which is a disease of the intima of the vessel wall that causes luminal narrowing and progresses to thrombosis and occlusion. The exact reason for this fatty build-up that eventually forms the dense, occlusive plaque is not fully elucidated. The most important risk factors its development and progression include smoking, hypertension, diabetes, and hyperlipidemia. Elevated homocysteine, hypercoagulable states, or even infectious agents may participate.

In the outpatient setting, early recognition of these risk factors with behavioral modification or medical management can help prevent the progression of atherosclerosis. Three critical behavioral modifications include: cessation of smoking, altering diet, and starting an exercise program. Aside from these behavioral changes, metabolic factors, such as hypertension and hyperlipidemia, should be closely monitored and managed.

The most common symptomatic manifestation of mild to moderate peripheral atherosclerosis is intermittent claudication. This condition occurs with an annual incidence of 2% in persons over 65. Approximately 12% of the adult population is affected. It is pain that develops during or after exercise when oxygen supply does not meet the tissue demands. It is relieved by rest and is highly reproducible. It most commonly affects the calves, but patients can also present with buttock or hip pain depending on the level of the arterial disease. The physics of resistances helps to explain how the tissue oxygen demands are not met. Normal arteries dilate with exercise to increase the delivery of blood and therefore oxygen to the periphery where it is needed. If there is a tight stenosis, the resistance of that artery is fixed. Therefore, with exercise, the vessel cannot dilate. The supply of oxygen filled blood cannot be increased. There is effectively a decrease in the delivery of oxygen. This physiology helps explain the pain that develops as well as the finding of a reduction in a patient's Ankle Brachial Index (ABI) with exercise.

The pain of claudication is usually described as muscle cramps or fatigue. With a careful history, it can be distinguished from neurogenic causes, which are often variable in presentation and affected by positional changes on examination. The examination is also a key component toward determining the presence of significant peripheral arterial disease. Many patients with claudication will have an abnormal pulse. When a pulse is absent or diminished, the disease is usually one level proximal.

When a pulse cannot be appreciated, a hand-held Doppler can be used to quickly and easily assess blood flow transcutaneously. Here, an ultrasonic beam at a frequency of 2 to 10 MHz is reflected by red blood cells proportional to their velocity, producing an audible frequency. Normal arterial flow is triphasic, or has three reflections. Mild to moderate disease leads to a biphasic signal. With more severe disease, only monophasic signals can be obtained. With the Doppler, an ABI can be obtained at the bedside by comparing the pressure at the ankle with the pressure of the arm. Normally, this index is greater than 1. A normal ABI performed at rest does not consistently rule out arterial disease because some fixed stenoses may only produce a reduction in the ABI with exercise. Furthermore, many calcified arteries produce falsely elevated ABIs, which is commonly seen in diabetics and renal failure patients.

The vascular laboratory can be a helpful adjunct to the examination. Segmental pressures can be obtained as well as an ABI. The symptomatic patient whose ABI is nondiagnostic can be placed on the treadmill with repeating the ABI following exercise. If the patient has significant claudication, pain onset and cessation of exercise will be associated with a decrease in their ABI. Patients who have had prior vascular interventions, such as leg bypasses should be periodically assessed in the noninvasive laboratory. Early detection of a graft stenosis may lead to an intervention that prevents graft failure.

Patients with more severe PAD may present with rest pain, ulceration, or tissue necrosis. Rest pain is pain in the toes or dorsum of the foot when in a recumbent position that is relieved by dependency. It usually occurs at night, preventing the patient from falling asleep. The patient will often report getting up during the night to walk around, or dangle the symptomatic leg over the side of the bed. Any patient with rest pain or a foot ulcer with evidence of arterial insufficiency should be referred to a vascular surgeon. Many of these patients may require only angioplasty and/or stenting of a severe, short-segment stenosis in the common iliac artery to alleviate their rest pain. Surgery may be necessary for some.

Diabetics deserve special mention. Because many have peripheral neuropathy, they are at much higher risk of foot complications. They should be warned of this potential and taught to closely monitor their feet. Any complaint about swelling, redness, blistering, purulent drainage, fever, worsening glucose control, or malodorous change warrants a physical evaluation. Diabetic foot infections need to be identified early and managed aggressively to avoid limb amputation. Aside from neuropathy, diabetics have a two- to fourfold increase in the rate of PAD. Diabetics more commonly have infrapopliteal occlusive disease and vascular calcification. The duration and severity of their diabetes correlates with the incidence and extent of PAD. Because of the incidence of foot infections and the nature of the disease affecting infrapopliteal arteries, there are higher rates of limb amputations in diabetics. Still, distal bypasses in these individuals can be quite effective.

Nonatherosclerotic Disease

Although atherosclerosis is responsible for most arterial abnormalities, there are various other nonatherosclerotic causes. These disorders will be briefly mentioned here.

Fibromuscular dysplasia is characterized by multiple areas of eccentric arterial stenosis alternating with segments of arterial dilation, leading to an angiographic appearance of a string of beads. It most commonly involves the renal artery. The carotids and iliac arteries are the next most common. Ninety percent occur in females. Surgery for this disorder is primarily indicated for symptomatic lesions.

Buerger's disease or thromboangiitis obliterans is a syndrome characterized by segmental thrombotic occlusions of small and medium arteries. Affected patients are predominantly young male smokers.

Raynaud's syndrome characterizes all patients with vasospastic disease of the hands. If no underlying condition is found that might be causing the syndrome, then it is called Raynaud's disease. It is a diagnosis of exclusion in which symptoms are usually triggered by cold or emotions.

The term *immune arteritis* applies to necrotizing transmural inflammation of the arterial wall. These conditions include radiation-induced arteritis, polyarteritis nodosa, Kawasaki disease, Cogan's syndrome, Behçet's disease, hypersensitivity angiitis, and giant cell arteritis.

ANEURYSMS

An aneurysm is defined as a localized enlargement of an artery such that its diameter is more than 1.5 times the caliber of the surrounding normal artery. This dilation occurs following arterial wall tensile strength weakening and decreased wall resilience. The exact mechanism is not fully elucidated. However, a change in the extracellular matrix proteins, elastin and collagen, is certainly part of the process. The importance of elastin in the maintenance of arterial wall structure is emphasized by the high frequency of aneurysms in patients with Marfan's syndrome, an inherited disorder with mutations in fibrillin-1 and associated elastins. The importance of fibrillar collagens is illustrated by the arterial fragility found in patients with Ehlers-Danlos syndrome, an inherited disorder with mutations in type III procollagen.

Abdominal Aortic Aneurysms

Abdominal aortic aneurysms (AAA) currently affect about 6% to 9% of men older than age 65. A family history of AAA may be found in as many as 20%, suggesting a genetic component. AAA is the most common true aneurysm and has a high propensity to rupture. Death from rupture currently ranks 15th of leading causes in the United States. Only 50% of individuals whose aneurysm ruptures make it to a hospital, and only 50% will survive the emergent operation. These statistics are obviously dreadful. However, mortality for elective surgical repair is less than 5% in most cases. This illustrates the importance of detection before rupture.

Aside from family history (twofold), increasing age, and male gender (four- or fivefold), the various other risk factors that have been identified include cigarette smoking (five- to sixfold), hypertension, and white race (twofold). Because most AAAs are asymptomatic, early detection can be difficult. A thorough physical examination is crucial. However, the sensitivity of detecting aneurysms on routine physical examination is only 50%. A strong case can be made for routine noninvasive screening ultrasound.

The majority of patients are aymptomatic at the time their AAA is identified. These patients are managed according to the natural history of AAAs. The major risk factor for rupture is the size or diameter of the aneurysm. Annual rupture risk is estimated to be 20% per year for a 6.5 cm AAA and 30% per year for a 7.5 cm AAA. Generally, it is felt that risk transitions between 5 and 6 cm from low to high risk. Because of this belief, many vascular surgeons offer repair to their patients with AAAs greater than 5 cm in diameter. Other surgeons look at the relative size or the rate of expansion. Patients with AAAs that increase in size more than 0.5 cm in 6 months are offered repair. This expansion rate is greater than the expected 0.2 to 0.4 cm per year. A patient whose aneurysm is less than 5 cm is followed every 6 months to 1 year with ultrasound or CT scan surveillance.

Endovascular repair is now a potential option. The durability of these repairs is still under investigation. However, it is a less invasive tool that may be of particular benefit to patients previously considered inoperable because of their medical history. Not all patients are endograft candidates. If by history a patient is a candidate, then a CT scan with 3 mm cuts and an aortogram are used to evaluate whether or not an endograft repair is feasible. These studies are used to estimate the size and length of the neck of the aneurysm, the degree of tortuosity of the neck and iliac vessels, and the degree of calcification, and to determine if the iliac arteries are aneurysmal or not.

Symptoms are often present only because of rupture or acute expansion. Patients with a ruptured AAA experience abrupt onset of abdominal pain, which often radiates into the flank or groin. The majority of symptomatic aneurysms are palpable. An aneurysm that has ruptured leads to at least transient hypotension. If the patient is hypotensive and has a palpable abdominal mass, the management is straightforward. That patient needs emergent exploration. There are some institutions now that manage ruptured aneurysms endovascularly. If the patient is not hypotensive and does not have an obvious pulsatile mass, there may be time to obtain a CT scan. If acute expansion is determined to be the cause of the patient's symptoms, the patient should be admitted and have their AAA repair expeditiously during that admission.

Peripheral Aneurysms

Popliteal artery aneurysms are the most common peripheral arterial aneurysm. They occur almost exclusively in men. Atherosclerosis is thought to be the cause in the majority. Most are fusiform. Popliteal aneurysms are bilateral in more than 50% of cases and up to 80% of patients with bilateral popliteal aneurysms have other aneurysms. Unlike AAAs, up to 80% of patients with popliteal aneurysms are symptomatic at the time of presentation. The most common presentation is lower extremity ischemia from thrombosis of the aneurysm. Rupture rarely occurs. Other symptoms may be caused by local compression of adjacent nerves and veins. Up to 55% of these aneurysms thrombose. Distal embolization is common.

Diagnosis is made by careful examination and is confirmed by duplex ultrasound. Surgical repair is undertaken for all patients with symptomatic aneurysms, asymptomatic aneurysms greater than 2 cm in diameter, or aneurysms of any size that contain intramural thrombus. Limb salvage is excellent for elective repair but outcome worsens significantly when revascularization is undertaken in the setting of severe ischemia. In the setting of thrombosis and limb ischemia, thrombolytics with slow revascularization followed by traditional surgery may improve the limb salvage rate.

Isolated iliac artery aneurysms are rare. When they do occur, they are bilateral in 50% of the cases. They are usually asymptomatic until rupture. Occasionally they produce unique signs due to local compression of adjacent pelvic structures, such as the ureter. Although the natural history is not well known, most surgeons offer surgical repair at 3 cm or greater. Endovascular repair is an evolving option.

CAROTID ARTERY DISEASE

Stroke remains the third leading cause of death trailing only heart disease and cancer. According to the American Heart Association (AHA), 158,448 American adults died from stroke in 1998. An incidence of about 195 per 100,000 population. There are approximately 4.5 million stroke survivors alive today. Eighty-three percent of strokes are ischemic: 32% are embolic, 20% are small-vessel thrombotic, and 31% are large-vessel thrombotic. The remaining 17% are hemorrhagic. One third of survivors require prolonged inpatient rehabilitation. The AHA estimated that in the year 2002, the direct and indirect costs of stroke could be 49.4 billion dollars.

The various risk factors for stroke include smoking, hypertension, obesity, physical inactivity, diabetes, age, sex, and race. Overall cardiovascular mortality rates are declining for men but increasing for women. Clearly diet modification, exercise, smoking cessation, and better control of blood pressure and diabetes can help prevent stroke and other cardiovascular-related morbidity.

Carotid artery disease is the cause of stroke in 30% to 40% of victims. This fact was better appreciated in the 1950s. The first thromboendarterectomy was performed in the early 1950s. In the 1980s, several articles questioned the appropriateness of the surgery and asked whether or not it works. These articles helped lead to three randomized trials in the early 1990s that looked at symptomatic patients and stratified the degree of carotid stenosis and compared medical management alone to aspirin and surgical intervention. These trials include: North American Symptomatic Carotid Endarterectomy Trial (NASCET), European Carotid Surgery Trial (ECST), and Veterans Administration Trial. NASCET and ECST found a relative risk reduction of nearly 50% in favor of surgical intervention for symptomatic patients with greater than 70% stenosis when looking at stroke and/or death as the outcome. The VA study was stopped shortly after the other two study results were published.

In 1995, the Asymptomatic Carotid Atherosclerosis Study (ACAS) documented a 57% relative reduction in perioperative stroke or death. It looked at asymptomatic patients with 60% or greater carotid stenosis. There are a few criticisms of this study. First, it did not stratify the degree of stenosis. Further, the relative risk reduction was obtained with an average perioperative stroke rate of 2% to 3% in centers of excellence. There are concerns that these outcomes would be difficult to duplicate. Still, if the surgical complication rate can be maintained around 2% to 3%, then operating on a 60% asymptomatic carotid stenosis is supported by this data.

An interesting fact from the ACAS results is the 1% stroke rate following angiography. This number is higher than expected and probably does not represent the true risk of stroke associated with cerebral angiograms. However, it does further emphasize the invasiveness of angiography. Today, the diagnosis is most often confirmed by carotid duplex ultrasound. Some centers evaluate patients with duplex ultrasound alone and others supplement magnetic resonance angiography and reserve conventional angiography for equivocal findings on the former two studies.

Carotid angioplasty and stenting may represent a less invasive way to prevent stroke from carotid disease. Similar to surgery in the 1990s, angioplasty and stenting must be scrutinized. These procedures are offered in certain centers, but the prospective, randomized comparisons to surgery are not complete. There are ongoing studies such as CAVATAS, CREST, and CASET. These ongoing trials and the newer trials investigating stenting with neuroprotective devices may someday obtain results that support their use. However, for now, angioplasty and stenting should be performed only in high-risk patients or at centers involved with these randomized, prospective trials.

VENOUS THROMBOSIS

method of
THOMAS G. DELOUGHERY, M.D.
Oregon Heath and Science University
Portland, Oregon

It is estimated that pulmonary emboli hospitalize at least 250,000 people in the United States per year and that at least 32,000 of those die from thrombosis. It is estimated that the mortality rate of untreated pulmonary embolism is 30% to 40%, and the risk of pulmonary embolism from untreated proximal deep venous thrombosis (DVT) is 50% to 80%.

DIAGNOSTIC TESTS FOR PULMONARY EMBOLISM AND DEEP VENOUS THROMBOSIS

Clinical Signs and Symptoms

Patients first notice dyspnea and cough following a pulmonary embolism. Chest pain occurs hours to days after the event with development of lung infarction. One third of patients have hemoptysis, and 10% to 20% have syncope. Most patients on examination have tachypnea (70% to 92%) but less than half have tachycardia. Chest radiographs are normal in only 30%. A nonspecific infiltrate is seen in 50% to 70% and an effusion in 35%. In the Prospective Investigation of Pulmonary Embolism Diagnosis (PIOPED) study, *15%* of patients had Po_2 greater than 90 mm Hg and *20%* had alveolar-arterial gradients less than 20 mm Hg. These results demonstrate that patients with pulmonary embolism need not be hypoxic or have an abnormal alveolar-arterial gradient.

Prediction Rules

There has been great interest in clinical prediction rules for DVT and pulmonary embolism. Using these rules, clinicians can better predict which patients are at higher risk of thrombosis. Several examples exist. The best validated for DVT are the Wells criteria (Table 1), and two prediction rules have also been validated for pulmonary embolism (Table 2). These prediction rules help in interpreting nondiagnostic studies and may be used as described in the following along with the D dimer to determine whether patients should be evaluated for thrombosis.

D Dimer

A major advance in evaluation of patients with DVT–pulmonary embolism is the wide availability of rapid D-dimer assays. Thrombi have areas that are growing and other areas that are undergoing fibrinolysis. It has been shown that all patients with clinically significant thrombosis have levels of D dimers above 500 ng/mL. Confusion arises because three different types of D-dimer assays are available, all with different abilities to help in diagnosing DVT–pulmonary embolism.

TABLE 1. **Clinical Probability Score for Deep Venous Thrombosis**

Variable	Points*
Active cancer	+1
Paralysis or recent plaster immobilization of lower extremity	+1
Recently bedridden for > 3 days or major surgery within 4 weeks	+1
Local tenderness	+1
Calf swelling greater than 3 cm compared with asymptomatic side (measured 10 cm below tibial tuberosity)	+1
Pitting edema in symptomatic leg	+1
Dilated superficial veins (nonvaricose) in symptomatic leg only	+1
Alternative diagnoses as likely as or more likely than deep venous thrombosis	–2

*Low probability <0, moderate probability 1-2, and high probability >3.
From Wells PS, Hirsh J, Anderson DR, et al: J Intern Med 243:15-23, 1998.

The D-dimer study used for diagnosis of disseminated intravascular coagulation is the *latex agglutination test*. It is designed for high levels of D dimers seen with disseminated intravascular coagulation and is not sensitive enough for DVT diagnosis.

TABLE 2. **Clinical Probability Score for Pulmonary Embolism**

Variable	Points
Rule 1*	
Clinical signs and symptoms of DVT	+3
PE as likely as or more likely than alternative diagnosis	+3
Immobilization or surgery in past 4 weeks	1.5
Previous PE or DVT	1.5
Heart rate more than 100/min	1.5
Hemoptysis	1
Active cancer	1
Rule 2†	
Previous DVT or PE	+2
Heart rate > 100	+1
Recent surgery	+3
Age:	
60-79	+1
>80	+2
$Paco_2$	
<36 mm Hg	+2
36-40 mm Hg	+1
Po_2	
<50 mm Hg	+4
50-59 mm Hg	+3
60-69 mm Hg	+2
70-79 mm Hg	+1
Atelectasis	+1
Elevated hemidiaphragm	+1

*Low probability <2, moderate probability 2-6, and high probability >6.
†Low probability 0-4, intermediate probability 5-8, high probability >9.
Abbreviations: DVT = deep venous thrombosis; PE = pulmonary embolism.
Rule 1 from Wells PS, Anderson DR, Rodger M, et al: Excluding pulmonary embolism at the bedside without diagnostic imaging: management of patients with suspected pulmonary embolism presenting to the emergency department by using a simple clinical model and D-dimer. Ann Intern Med 135:98-107, 2001.
Rule 2 from Wicki J, Perneger TV, Junod AF, et al: Assessing clinical probability of pulmonary embolism in the emergency ward: A simple score. Arch Intern Med 161:92-97, 2001.

This type of D-dimer assay should never be used in the diagnostic evaluation of DVT–pulmonary embolism.

"Rapid" point of care D-dimer assays such as the SimpleRed are slide assays devised to read positive if the D dimer is above 500 ng/mL. These types of assays are less sensitive (80% to 90%) than the rapid enzyme-linked immunosorbent assay (ELISA) but are simple to use and require no special equipment to run. The rapid D dimer is most effective when used with a clinical prediction rule. Thus, a patient with a negative D dimer and low probability of a thromboembolic event has a low chance of having thrombosis and need not be evaluated further. If a patient has either "not low" probability or a positive D dimer, the patient needs further workup for DVT–pulmonary embolism (Figure 1).

The *"rapid ELISA"* or *"high-sensitivity"* assay for D dimer offers nearly 100% sensitivity for DVT. Accordingly, a patient with a negative ELISA D dimer requires no further evaluation. The rapid ELISA assay requires special equipment to perform the test (Figure 2).

The other drawback of the D-dimer test is its lack of specificity coupled with its high sensitivity. Therefore, patients with positive D-dimer assays require further testing to establish the presence of thrombosis. Patients with recent trauma or recent surgery, pregnancy, or who are older than 70 have a higher baseline D-dimer level, which greatly limits the use of D dimers in these patients.

Computed Tomography Scan

The newer high-resolution computed tomography (CT) scanners such as helical CT have demonstrated the ability to image pulmonary emboli in the larger pulmonary vessels. In many institutions CT scans are rapidly replacing other methods for diagnosing pulmonary embolism. CT scans have high specificity for pulmonary embolism but are highly sensitive only

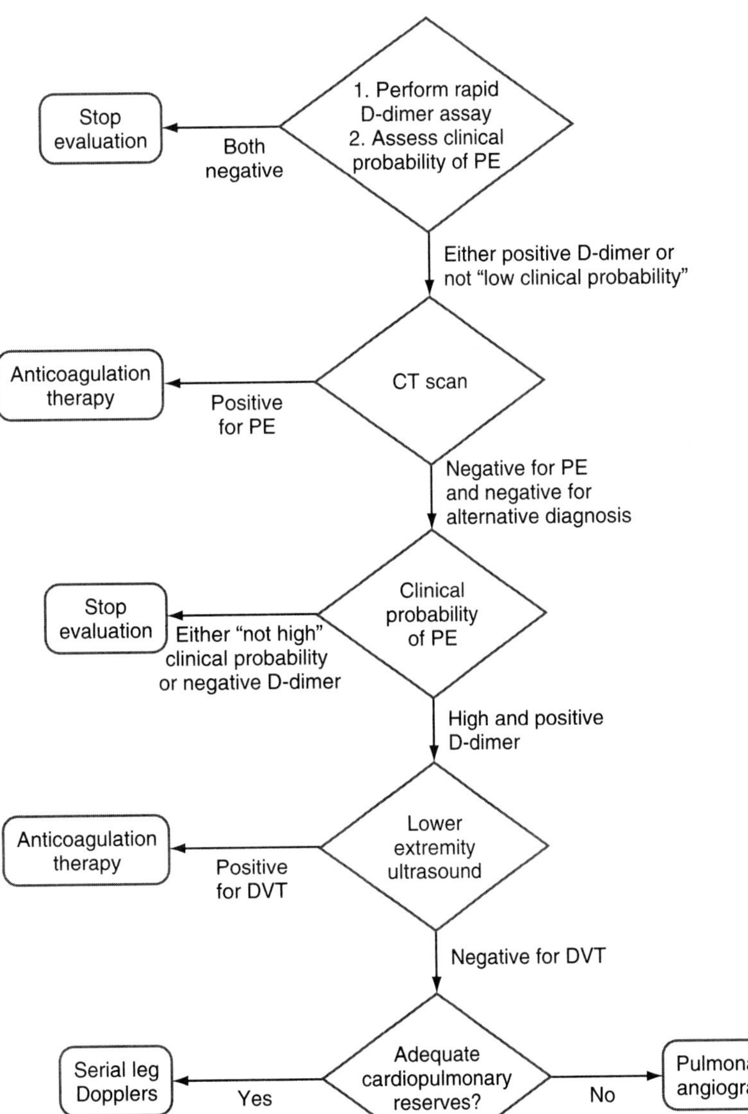

Figure 1. Diagnostic flow chart for pulmonary embolism using *point of care* D dimer. CT, computed tomography; DVT, deep venous thrombosis; PE, pulmonary embolism.

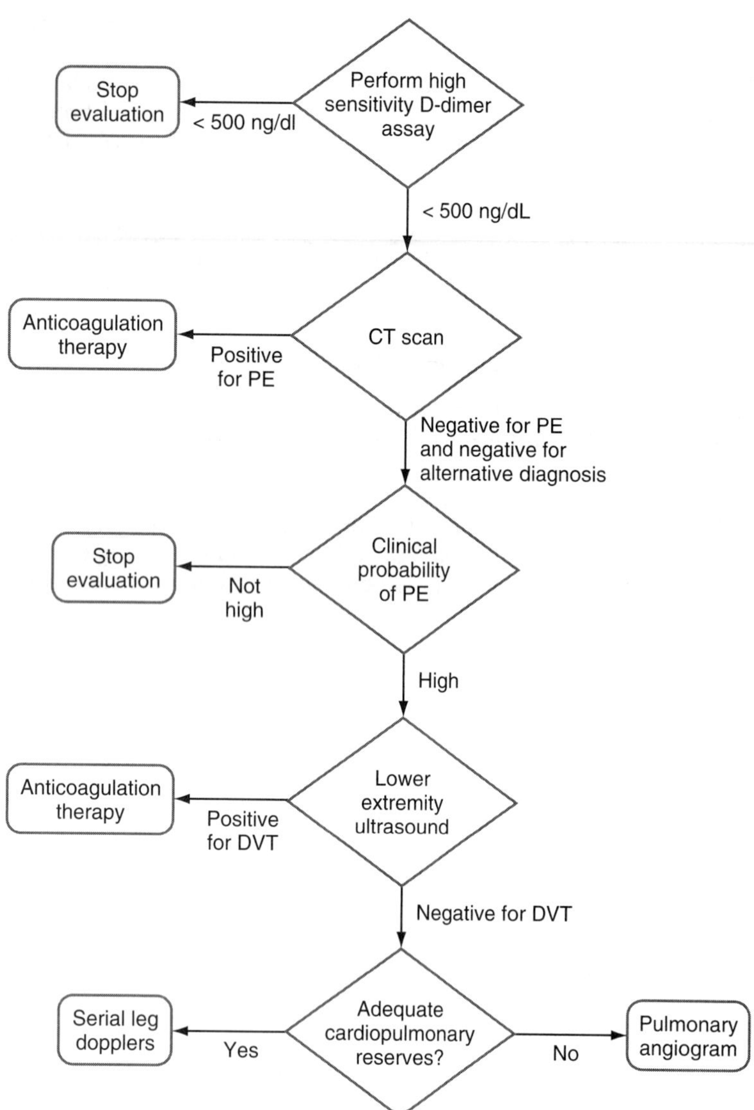

Figure 2. Diagnostic flow chart for pulmonary embolism using *high-sensitivity* D dimer. CT, computed tomography; DVT, deep venous thrombosis; PE, pulmonary embolism.

to central and segmental pulmonary arterial embolism. The overall sensitivity of CT for pulmonary embolism appears to be as low as 70%. Therefore, a negative CT scan *does not* rule out the diagnosis of pulmonary embolism. Also, the specificity of CT for pulmonary embolism is lower for clots in the subsegmental distribution. These caveats must be balanced by the fact that CT scans are often readily available and may also lead to diagnosis of nonthrombotic causes of pulmonary symptoms.

Ventilation-Perfusion Scans

Ventilation-perfusion ($\dot{V}/\dot{Q}$) scans are sensitive but not specific for pulmonary embolism. Interpretation is best viewed as "high probability," "negative," and "nondiagnostic." High-probability scans are specific if the patient has not had a previous pulmonary embolism (90%), but this falls to 73% in patients with previous pulmonary emboli. The specificity is 83% in patients with cardiac or pulmonary disease. Only 40% to 50% of patients with pulmonary emboli have high-probability scans. An abnormal chest radiograph is found in 70% of patients with pulmonary embolism. Unless the chest radiograph defect is small or not in a nonperfused area, this makes the scan an intermediate- or low-probability one. Low-probability scans *do not* rule out pulmonary embolism. As many as 20% to 36% of patients with pulmonary embolism have low-probability scans. In PIOPED, high clinical suspicion coupled with a low-probability scan yielded a 40% rate of pulmonary embolism. Generally, 15% to 25% of patients with low-probability scans have pulmonary emboli. In a prospective study, 7.8% of sick patients with low-probability scans died of autopsy-proven pulmonary embolism. An absolutely normal scan does confidently rule out pulmonary embolism. Unless a patient has a high-probability scan or a normal scan, one needs to do further studies to establish the diagnosis of pulmonary embolism. Furthermore, a high-probability scan is diagnostic for pulmonary embolism only in patients with a high pretest probability of pulmonary emboli.

Leg Studies

Leg studies are the definitive diagnostic test in patients with symptoms of DVT. Furthermore, leg studies aid in the diagnosis for the patient with a nondiagnostic $\dot{V}/\dot{Q}$ scan or negative CT scan. DVT is present in 50% to 70% of patients with proven pulmonary embolism. If DVT is present, this establishes the need for anticoagulant therapy and eliminates the need for angiography. In one study the use of leg studies reduced the need for angiography from 43% to 26% after indeterminate $\dot{V}/\dot{Q}$ scans.

Venogram

The venogram used to be the "gold standard." Venograms visualize both the calf and deep veins. Drawbacks of venography include dye load and a 5% risk of actually causing thrombosis. Given that few venograms are currently obtained, the accuracy and ability to perform technically adequate studies are greatly reduced.

Duplex Ultrasonography

Duplex ultrasonography has 93% sensitivity and 98% specificity for diagnosing proximal DVT in symptomatic patients. Duplex has lower sensitivity (6% to 70%) for detection of calf DVT. In cases of a negative study and suspicion of pulmonary embolism, one needs either to perform follow-up duplex ultrasonography to rule out clot extension or perform angiography if the suspicion of DVT or pulmonary embolism is high.

Pulmonary Angiography

Pulmonary angiography is the gold standard for diagnosis of pulmonary embolism. Angiography is invasive with a mortality rate of 0.5% and morbidity of 2% to 4%. These risks are lower than those of empirical anticoagulation or of ignoring a pulmonary embolism.

DIAGNOSTIC APPROACH

Deep Venous Thrombosis

If available, a negative rapid high-sensitivity D-dimer assay eliminates the need for further evaluation of patients suspected of having DVT. If the high-sensitivity assay is not available, the clinical probability of DVT should be assessed. If the clinical probability is not low, Doppler ultrasonography of the lower extremities is performed. If this is positive, the patient requires antithrombotic therapy. If it is negative and the patient had a low pretest probability of DVT, no further scans are done. Otherwise, the scan should be repeated in 1 week.

Pulmonary Embolism

Unfortunately, there are still many approaches to the diagnosis of pulmonary embolism. If a high-sensitivity D-dimer assay is available and it is negative or the patient has a low probability of pulmonary embolism *and* a rapid D-dimer assay is negative, no further studies are needed.

If further evaluation is required, one approach is to obtain a CT scan. If this is positive for embolism, treatment can be started. Because a negative CT scan does not rule out embolism, further testing is needed. In this case leg studies are useful. If they are positive for DVT, the need for therapy is established. If negative, the test can be repeated in 1 week or, if the patient is very ill, angiography can be done. The patient with a negative CT scan and low clinical probability of PE need not be studied further.

If a $\dot{V}/\dot{Q}$ scan is obtained and is normal, an embolus is ruled out. If the scan is read as high probability in a previously healthy patient with a high pretest probability, this is diagnostic. For indeterminate scans, the legs should be studied. A positive leg scan mandates therapy, and no further testing is required. If the leg scan is negative, the approach is tailored to the patient's state of health. For patients with good cardiopulmonary reserve who are also reliable, angiography can be avoided by repeating the leg scan 1 day and 1 week later. Studies have shown that patients with indeterminate $\dot{V}/\dot{Q}$ scans and persistently negative leg scans have a low risk of recurrent thrombosis. Patients who are ill should undergo pulmonary angiography.

IMMEDIATE THERAPY

Heparin

See the following section.

Thrombolytic Therapy

Given the natural history of pulmonary embolism, the role of thrombolytic therapy is uncertain. That thrombolytic therapy lyses clots faster than heparin was of no clinical significance in the large trials of the early 1980s or in more recent trials. For example, 24-hour lung perfusion improved by 2.7% in a group treated with heparin and 6.2% in a urokinase (Abbokinase) group, but both groups were equal in perfusion by day 5. Another trial showed that patients with right ventricular dysfunction related to pulmonary embolism failed to show an improvement in death rates with thrombolytic therapy. Many patients with pulmonary embolism are poor candidates for lytic therapy because of recent surgery or other reasons. Also of concern is the 1% to 2% risk of intracranial hemorrhage that accompanies thrombolytic therapy. The vast majority of patients with pulmonary embolism who live long enough to be diagnosed survive. Therefore, only a small number of patients would benefit from thrombolytic therapy. However, for the patient *in extremis* because of a pulmonary embolism who is *not* a candidate for embolectomy, fibrinolytic therapy is an option.

If thrombolytic therapy is required, the dosing for the agents is the same as for cardiac indications. Plasma fibrinogen and the activated partial thromboplastin time (aPTT) should be measured every 4 hours after treatment. When the aPTT is below two times normal and the fibrinogen is over 100 mg/dL, heparin should be started.

Thrombolytic therapy for DVT has little effect on long-term outcomes such as postphlebitic syndrome. It therefore has little role in management of these patients. One situation in which lytic therapy may be useful is in massive DVT involving the common femoral or iliac system. One approach is to use catheter-guided lytic therapy to recanalize the vessel. Typically, this is done when the vein does not recanalize spontaneously and the patient has severe and persistent symptoms.

Embolectomy

Embolectomy may be useful in the small subset of patients who are in unresponsive shock. Some series claim up to 70% survival. It has been suggested that if after an hour of medical management, a patient has persistent signs of massive pulmonary embolism such as a systolic blood pressure less than 90 mm Hg, urine output less than 20 mL per hour, and/or Po_2 less than 60 mm Hg, that patient is a candidate for embolectomy. This approach obviously requires the presence of a qualified cardiac surgeon.

Vena Cava Filter

The role of filters in treatment of thromboembolic disease is unclear because of lack of good trials. A strong indication for filter placement would be pulmonary embolism–DVT in a patient in whom anticoagulant therapy is contraindicated. A trial showed that patients at high risk for pulmonary embolism who were treated with heparin had fewer pulmonary emboli with filter placement. This trial did not demonstrate any improvement in survival with filter placement. Some people have used filters as prophylaxis in patients unable to undergo anticoagulation. The role of filters in long-term prevention is unknown. The risk of DVT is doubled with long-term filter placement. It is unclear whether patients with filters require lifelong anticoagulation. The disadvantages of filters are leg edema from filter thrombosis, no protection against thrombosis, and venous collateral formation years after filter placement. A trend toward widespread clinical use of removable inferior vena cava filters has been seen, and these may prove to be useful for patients who transiently cannot undergo anticoagulation or who are at high risk for thrombosis and need surgery.

Compression Stockings

Compression stockings are extremely useful in the prevention of postphlebitic syndrome. A randomized trial demonstrated halving of the rate of postphlebitic syndrome with compression stocking use. Patients should be advised that they should wear stockings most of the day, every day for best effect.

TREATMENT OF DEEP VENOUS THROMBOSIS

There is now abundant evidence that use of low-molecular-weight heparin (LMWH) for therapy in DVT–pulmonary embolism treatment is both safer and more effective than use of standard heparin. Evidence is also clear that stable patients with DVT–pulmonary embolism can be treated at home with LMWH. There are two LMWHs approved for therapy, enoxaparin (Lovenox) 1 mg/kg every 12 hours or tinzaparin (Innohep) 175 units/kg every day. For patients with a low thrombotic burden one may use enoxaparin 1.5 mg/kg every day. For short courses of therapy, most patients do not need to have LMWH levels determined. Patients who are very obese (more than two times ideal body weight), pregnant, those with severe liver or heart failure, and those receiving long-term heparin therapy should have levels measured. In patients with renal failure, dosing should be once per day. Levels are determined 4 hours after injection, and the therapeutic range for enoxaparin is 0.7 to 1.2 anti-Xa units.

These regimens may be used with either inpatients or outpatients. Although LMWH is more expensive than standard heparin, inpatient savings can be realized because multiple aPTTs or platelet counts are unnecessary. In addition, in inpatient populations the early trials demonstrated that LMWH was more effective and safe than standard heparin.

The ability to give LMWH subcutaneously has opened the door to outpatient therapy. Careful selection of patients is crucial. A patient should be considered for outpatient therapy if the only thing that would lead to the patient's admission was administration of intravenous heparin. The first dose of LMWH is given as soon as possible, and warfarin is started the first evening of diagnosis. The second dose of LMWH should be a "transition" to have the patient on an 8 AM and 8 PM schedule. This is derived by adjusting the second dose of LMWH for the difference between the first and second doses. It is done by multiplying the patient's usual dose of 1 mg/kg by the difference in time between the first two doses divided by 12. For example, if a 60-kg patient received the first dose at midnight, at 8 AM the patient would receive 40 mg and from then on 60 mg every 12 hours. Patients should be observed every day with a visit or telephone check. One still needs to overlap LMWH and warfarin by 24 hours when the International Normalized Ratio (INR) is in the therapeutic range.

Standard heparin is fading from use because of its unfavorable pharmacokinetics and the demonstration of better outcomes with LMWH. If it is used, the absolute key in standard heparin use is to give enough. The standard bolus should be 5000 units (10,000 for larger thrombi or pulmonary embolism). The initial drip should be 1400 units/hour. The aPTT should be checked 4 to 6 hours after the bolus and the drip adjusted accordingly. A supratherapeutic aPTT may just reflect the bolus. The drip should never be turned down until two consecutive aPTTs are supratherapeutic. Therapeutic range varies with different aPTT reagents and must be standardized at each laboratory with heparin levels. One must be aggressive in rapidly achieving the proper aPTT.

All patients should receive at least 5 days of heparin therapy. Some authorities recommend that 10 days of heparin should be given for large pulmonary embolisms because it has not been proved that 5 days is sufficient therapy.

Warfarin (Coumadin) is started the evening of diagnosis (or day 5 of therapy if heparin is being used for 10 days) with a loading dose of 2.5 to 10 mg orally. A dose of 5 mg is recommended in most patients. Young (younger than 60) healthy patients may need a 10-mg loading dose, whereas frail elderly persons (older than 85) should start with 2.5 mg. Warfarin is titrated to an INR of 2 to 3. Use of warfarin affects all the vitamin K–dependent proteins. Factor VII falls first, resulting in prolongation of the INR. However, the full antithrombotic effect of warfarin does not occur until factors X and II have fallen. This fall takes an additional 24 to 48 hours after factor VII levels fall. This is why heparin and warfarin therapy should overlap for at least 24 hours.

Special Situations

Patients with Cancer

The hypercoagulable state associated with malignancy (especially adenocarcinomas) can be refractory to warfarin therapy. Long-term LMWH is a useful alternative in these patients. Patients should have LMWH levels checked weekly until the dose is stable. Rarely, patients may have tumors that secrete heparinases. These patients may require higher doses of heparin. Clinical trials suggest that any patient with a diagnosis of cancer may benefit from being treated for the full 6-month course with just LMWH. Cancer patients treated with LMWH have significantly lower rates of recurrent thrombosis.

Calf Vein Thrombosis

Patients with calf vein thrombosis are at risk for extension to proximal vein thrombosis and subsequent pulmonary embolism. These patients should have anticoagulation with heparin and then with warfarin for 6 weeks. Patients with thrombosis in the muscular veins of the calf (soleal, gastrocnemial) can be treated just with 10 days of therapeutic LMWH or, if stable, simply observed with serial ultrasonography.

Superficial Venous Thrombosis

Most superficial venous thrombosis can be treated with heat and anti-inflammatory agents. However, 20% to 30% of patients with greater saphenous vein thrombosis go on to have thrombosis of the deep system. These patients may be treated with a short course of heparin or monitored with serial ultrasonography. Data have been presented in abstract form showing that a 10-day course of enoxaparin (Lovenox) 40 mg/d is effective at both reducing symptoms and preventing progression and should be considered for very proximal saphenous vein thrombosis or for very symptomatic superficial thrombosis.

Duration of Therapy

Most patients with a first proximal DVT and no underlying hypercoagulable state should receive anticoagulation for 6 months. The risk for recurrent thrombosis levels off in 6 months. Patients with idiopathic thrombosis continue to be at higher risk of thrombosis, with 10% to 30% of patients having recurrent thrombosis during the next 8 years. Patients should be informed about the risk of recurrent events, and a joint decision about therapy should be made. Patients with pulmonary embolism appear to be a higher risk of recurrence, and these patients should receive anticoagulation for 1 year.

Patients with a second thrombosis, even without a demonstrable hypercoagulable state, have a high risk of recurrence without anticoagulant. They should be maintained with lifelong anticoagulation.

Patients with first thrombosis and "strong" hypercoagulable states (antiphospholipid disease, antithrombin III, protein C or protein S deficiency) should receive lifelong anticoagulation. There is mounting evidence that patients with idiopathic pulmonary embolism should also receive lifelong therapy. Patients with a "weak" hypercoagulable state (e.g., actor V Leiden) and a removable risk factor can receive anticoagulation for just 6 months. However, patients with two or more weak states or a severe idiopathic thrombosis should be considered for indefinite anticoagulation.

Section 6

The Blood and Spleen

APLASTIC ANEMIA

method of
STEPHEN D. NIMER, M.D., and
DAVID J. ARATEN, M.D.
Memorial Sloan-Kettering Cancer Center
New York, New York

Aplastic anemia (AA) is characterized by low peripheral blood cell counts accompanied by a hypocellular bone marrow. Normal or increased bone marrow cellularity, an inaspirable (dry tap) or fibrotic marrow, an elevated reticulocyte count, abnormal lymphocyte populations, lymphadenopathy, or splenomegaly suggest alternative diagnoses. A diagnosis of severe AA requires a cellularity less than 25% and two of the following abnormalities: an absolute neutrophil count (ANC) less than 500/mm^2, a platelet count less than 20,000/mm^2, a reticulocyte count less than 20,000/mm^2. A patient meeting these criteria with an ANC less than 200/mm^2 would be classified as having very severe AA.

The presence of a normocellular or hypercellular marrow, cytogenetic abnormalities, excess blasts (greater than 5% of the nucleated marrow cells) or morphologic abnormalities in the bone marrow are features of the myelodysplastic syndromes—a group of diseases that should be differentiated from AA. There is a hypocellular variant of myelodysplasia, which commonly responds to treatments for AA, such as immunosuppression. Up to 25% of patients with typical MDS (e.g., those with the refractory anemia subtype) may also respond to such treatments. Other conditions that can (rarely) masquerade as AA (shown in Tables 1 and 2) should be excluded by a careful history, physical examination and review of the peripheral blood smear.

TABLE 1. **Aplastic Anemia—Differential Diagnosis**

Hairy cell leukemia
Hypersplenism
Myelofibrosis
Ionizing radiation
Systemic lupus erythematosus
Vitamin B_{12} deficiency
Alcoholism
Ehrlichiosis
Sarcoidosis
Tuberculosis
Hyperthyroidism

It is critical to differentiate acquired AA—an autoimmune disease responsive to immunosuppression—from hereditary forms of AA, such as Fanconi's anemia, dyskeratosis congenita, or Schwachman-Diamond syndrome. Presentation in youth, congenital abnormality of the limbs or kidneys, short stature, café au lait spots, pancreatic insufficiency, nail dystrophy, oral leukoplakia, or a family history of the disease would mandate a search for a congenital cause. The diagnosis of Fanconi's anemia is based on demonstrating increased spontaneous and diepoxybutane (DEB)-induced chromosomal breaks. It is crucial not to miss this diagnosis prior to allogeneic BMT, because a unique chemotherapy-radiation conditioning regimen must be used and the diagnosis must be excluded in potential sibling donors. The remainder of this chapter will focus on patients with the acquired form of AA.

PATHOGENESIS

There are two pathologic derangements in acquired AA: (1) an autoimmune assault mediated by T-cells (or NK-like T-cells) targeting the hematopoietic stem cell, and (2) a variable paucity of stem cells—which is a direct consequence of (1). It is important to determine whether medications or other possibly inciting or perpetrating factors are present in a patient with peripheral blood cytopenias (Table 3), because occasionally patients may recover on discontinuation of an inciting medication. Recovery of counts after discontinuation of medication more commonly occurs in patients with mild cytopenias, and is extremely rare in patients with pancytopenia or agranulocytosis. As described below, both immunosuppressive therapy (IST) and allogeneic bone marrow transplantation (BMT) are effective treatments for AA. IST treats derangement (1) and depends upon the recovery of endogenous stem cells to reverse derangement (2)—a process that can take months. In contrast, BMT addresses both (1) and (2) and provides normal stem cells immediately.

TREATMENT: BLOOD OR MARROW TRANSPLANTATION

Blood or marrow transplantation (BMT) from an HLA-identical sibling is a potentially curative treatment for severe AA, a previously uniformly fatal

TABLE 2. **Diagnostic Tests in the Workup of Aplastic Anemia**

DEB test
HIV test
Flow cytometry to rule out PNH cell population
B_{12} folate
Iron, TIBC, ferritin
Bone marrow examination with karyotype and trephine biopsy
Reticulocyte count
LDH
Review of peripheral smear to evaluate for large granular lymphocytes
HLA typing of patient and siblings

DEB, diepoxybutane; HLA, histocompatibility leukocyte antigen; LDH, lactate dehydrogenase; TIBC, total iron-binding capacity.

disorder. Prior to transplantation, candidates for BMT should minimize transfusions and especially avoid receiving blood products obtained from family members because this increases the risk of rejection. Only CMV-negative blood products should be given to transplant candidates who are CMV negative or whose CMV status is not yet known. HLA typing of all siblings should be performed urgently to expedite BMT. A well established conditioning regimen is: cyclophosphamide (Cytoxan),* 50 mg/kg intravenously daily, beginning on day −5 and continuing until day −2, for a total dose of 200 mg/kg, based on ideal body weight, with hyperhydration to prevent hemorrhagic cystitis, and antithymocyte globulin (ATGAM),* 30 mg/kg via central line intravenously, given daily beginning on day −4 and continuing until day −2. Due to the risk of anaphylaxis, ATG should be given under direct physician supervision, with a test dose and medications, including steroids, to prevent or treat allergic reactions, including anaphylaxis. Unmodified donor marrow from an HLA-matched sibling is infused on day 0. Graft versus host disease (GVHD) prophylaxis, such as cyclosporine (Sandimmune),* must be started prior to the infusion of donor stem cells. It is generally continued for at least 90 days to avoid acute GVHD. This conditioning regimen is generally used for unmodified grafts, which are the standard of care. T-cell depleted grafts, which are used to prevent life-threatening GVHD, may require a more intensive conditioning regimen, such as one that includes total body irradiation.

TABLE 3. **Etiologic Agents in Acquired Aplastic Anemia**

Pharmacologic agents*
Cancer chemotherapeutic agents
Alkylating agents (e.g., busulfan), anthracyclines (e.g., daunorubicin), antimetabolites (e.g., methotrexate), antimitotic agents (e.g., colchicine), levamisole†
Antibiotics
Chloramphenicol, penicillins, cephalosporins, sulfonamides†
Anti-inflammatory drugs
Phenylbutazone§, indomethacin, ibuprofen, sulindac, diclofenac, gold compounds, penicillamine
Antiepileptic agents
Felbamate, phenytoin, carbamazepine, ethosuximide, and others
Antithyroid agents
Methimazole, propylthiouracil
Hypoglycemic agents
Chlorpropamide, tolbutamide
Antimalarial agents
Quinacrine§, chloroquine
Neuroleptic agents
Chlorpromazine,† clozapine†
Cardiac medications
Captopril,† procainamide†
Chemicals and toxins
Pesticides, benzene, other aromatic hydrocarbons
Infections
Viral hepatitis, Epstein-Barr Virus (infectious mononucleosis), cytomegalovirus, brucellosis, miliary tuberculosis, parvovirus B19††
Rheumatologic and autoimmune diseases
Systemic lupus erythematosus (SLE), rheumatoid arthritis, cryoglobulinemia, graft versus host disease
Paroxysmal nocturnal hemoglobinuria
Ionizing radiation
Thymoma
Pregnancy
Idiopathic

*Listed are agents more commonly associated with aplastic anemia. The list is not intended to be exhaustive.
†More commonly associated with agranulocytosis than with aplastic anemia.
††More commonly associated with aplastic crises in patients with underlying hemolytic disorders.
§Not available in the United States.

Transplants using matched sibling donors are highly successful, with approximately 80% survival at 5 years. Relapse after engraftment is rare, but there may be an increased risk of developing a malignancy.

IMMUNOSUPPRESSIVE THERAPY

Except for those patients with the most severe form of the disease (very severe AA), there are generally sufficient residual stem cells to mediate a hematopoietic recovery without providing allogeneic stem cells. This requires that the autoimmune process be halted, and this is generally accomplished using immunosuppressive therapy (IST), which is now the mainstay of treatment for AA patients, especially for those without a donor or those of older age. Antithymocyte globulin (ATG),* is the most frequently used form of IST. ATG is derived from the serum of a horse (or rabbit) that has been immunized with human thymocytes. The serum is enriched in polyclonal antibodies that are reactive to a broad array of human lymphocyte antigens. The preparation is absorbed with human red cells to remove nonspecific antibodies and lyophilized. It can be given alone or with cyclosporine (CSA)*, and can be supported by the use of hematopoietic growth factors, such as G-CSF (Neupogen). Equine ATG (ATGAM) can be given in a number of different acceptable schedules, in the hospital under physician supervision, with a test dose and the premedications and precautions described above, including high-dose steroids. A typical schedule would be 40 mg/kg, intravenously per day, by slow infusion, for 4 days, with 1 mg/kg of methylprednisolone premedication and 1 mg/kg methylprednisolone infusion concurrently with the ATG. ATG acutely results in antibody-mediated

*Not FDA approved for this indication.

peripheral destruction of neutrophils, red cells, and platelets. Therefore, platelet transfusions may need to be given daily or even twice daily (after each ATG infusion is completed) to all thrombocytopenic patients (<50,000 per microliter). Patients often develop worsening neutropenia after treatment with ATG, thus fever should be treated with broad-spectrum antibiotics, even when febrile infusional reactions are suspected. Red blood cell transfusions are also commonly required. A course of corticosteroids is given to patients after ATG to prevent serum sickness, which is manifested by fever, rash, and joint pain, and can occur 10 to 30 days post-ATG infusion. Asymptomatic ALT (SGPT) elevations are common after ATG. Hematologic responses may take 3 months or longer, necessitating excellent supportive care. Of note, some patients will respond only after a second infusion of ATG, given months after the initial treatment. Paroxysmal nocturnal hemoglobinuria (PNH) or myelodysplastic syndrome (MDS) may also develop after ATG, especially in patients with partial responses. Relapse after IST is not uncommon, but it can respond to re-treatment. Relapses (responsive to re-treatment with ATG) have been reported in up to 19% of women who become pregnant after having been treated for AA. Rabbit-derived ATG (Thymoglobulin) is effective in AA, but it is not known how this preparation compares with the equine product (ATGAM), which is known to have an excellent (upwards of 80%) response rate. Therefore, the use of rabbit ATG is typically reserved for patients previously treated with equine ATG, or those with a history of allergies to equine products, or those with life-threatening reactions to the equine product.

CYCLOSPORINE

In clinical trials, the addition of cyclosporine (CSA) (Neoral, Sandimmune) shortly after completion of ATG decreases the median time required to respond to ATG, with particular advantages for those patients with very low neutrophil counts (very severe AA). CSA should be given in effective doses with monitoring for side effects, such as hypertension, renal and hepatic dysfunction, tremor, and hirsutism. Cyclosporine is not given concurrently with ATG because it antagonizes the killing of lymphocytes by ATG in vitro. It should be initiated after the ATG has been completed; magnesium oxide* 400 mg twice a day is often given to ameliorate renal toxicity. Patients receiving the combination of ATG, cyclosporine, and steroids are immunosuppressed and require aerosolized pentamidine or alternative strategies to prevent *Pneumocystis* pneumonia. All symptomatic complaints and fevers should be investigated to rule out opportunistic infections. Blood pressure, creatinine, and liver functions must be monitored closely as well as the trough cyclosporin level. The patient should be counseled regarding numerous food and drug interactions with CSA and the potential lack of bioequivalence among the generic and the two distinct brand formulations. For nonsevere AA, CSA can be used as a single agent with significant efficacy.

BONE MARROW TRANSPLANT VERSUS IMMUNOSUPPRESSIVE THERAPY

For those patients with an HLA-identical sibling, a crucial decision between BMT and IST must be made (Table 4). (Those without a matched sibling donor should be treated initially with IST.) Younger patients tolerate BMT better than do older patients, and patients with higher neutrophil counts are more likely to have sufficient hematopoietic recovery after IST. Based on the patient's age and neutrophil count, it may be possible to predict which is the better initial therapy. However, treatment decisions must be individualized based on access to an experienced transplantation center, CMV status, and other factors. The presence of a large population of PNH cells identified by flow cytometry may also influence this decision, because these patients are more likely to develop clinical PNH after IST (PNH does not occur after BMT). Conversely, small PNH cell populations may be an indicator of immunologic-mediated marrow failure and thus may predict a good response to IST.

HLA typing should be performed on all newly diagnosed patients, with unrelated donor searches initiated for those with very severe AA without a related donor, even when IST is planned as the initial therapy. HLA typing—even when BMT is not immediately planned—may provide some additional useful information. For instance, AA is associated with the HLA-DR2 (DR15) allele, which may predict a response to IST.

*Not FDA approved for this indication.

TABLE 4. **Transplantation versus Immunosuppression**

	Transplantation	Immunosuppression
PROS	Curative Prevents PNH and MDS Efficacious in all severities of AA	Less intensive, less short-term mortality Equally effective in all age groups Brief hospitalization
CONS	Graft rejection is rare Regimen-related mortality Infertility	Incomplete and delayed recovery Relapse Can develop PNH and MDS Serum sickness

AA, aplastic anemia; MDS, myelodysplastic syndrome; PNH, paroxysmal nocturnal hemoglobinuria.

CYTOKINE THERAPY

Granulocyte colony stimulating factor (G-CSF [Neupogen]),* may play a role in the supportive care of some patients with AA treated with IST, because it prolongs the circulating half-life and increases the function of mature neutrophils. G-CSF is typically given to patients with severe neutropenia or those who develop neutropenic infections. Cytokine therapy should not be used as a substitute for definitive therapy of AA. Most patients with AA with normal renal function have elevated levels of erythropoietin and do not benefit from pharmacologic doses. Stem cell factor (kit ligand) has been used experimentally to treat AA patients, and it has shown limited efficacy.

ANDROGENS

Although used extensively in the era prior to the advent of IST, androgens do not increase peripheral blood counts in those also receiving IST. They should not be used as a substitute for definitive therapy for acquired AA. Androgens are helpful in the supportive management of Fanconi's anemia, but side effects can be profound, including hepatotoxicity, hepatic adenomas, or androgenization in females.

PREGNANCY AND APLASTIC ANEMIA

The initial presentation of AA has long been thought to be associated with pregnancy and the peripartum period. Recurrences of AA during pregnancy occur at a rate much higher than expected, confirming this association. Nonetheless, most pregnant women with recurrent AA have a good outcome with IST administered during pregnancy. Both CSA and ATG are pregnancy category C medications. There is extensive experience with CSA during pregnancy in renal graft recipients with no evidence of fetal harm and ATG and cyclosporine should be used in pregnancy when clinically indicated. Women who have had AA should be monitored with regular complete blood cell counts (CBCs) during and after pregnancy. Women who have had AA and have a large PNH cell population (>10% of red cells) have a high likelihood of life-threatening thromboses as a result of increased estrogens and compression of a gravid uterus on intra-abdominal vessels. In such patients, pregnancy should be attempted only with great caution, with low-molecular-weight heparin administered starting very early in pregnancy and continuing for several months afterward, with regular monitoring of the peak anti-factor Xa activity targeting the upper end of the therapeutic range.

*Not FDA approved for this indication.

FOLLOW-UP OF SUCCESSFULLY TREATED PATIENTS

Patients treated with IST are at risk of developing PNH, myelodysplastic syndrome (MDS), and to a lesser extent, acute myelogenous leukemia (AML). An elevated LDH and reticulocyte count, anemia, darkened urine, and decreased haptoglobin would suggest PNH and should be investigated with flow cytometry of peripheral blood cells using antibodies specific for GPI-linked proteins. Patients with PNH are particularly prone to the development of venous thrombosis. If the diagnosis of PNH is made, a search for occult thromboses and additional thrombotic risk factors should be initiated and anticoagulation considered. Falling peripheral blood counts are suggestive of either recurrent AA or the development of MDS or AML. A bone marrow examination should be performed to assess these possibilities. Patients who develop MDS or AML after IST should be considered for allogeneic transplantation if the patient is a suitable candidate and a donor is available.

Patients with features indicative of recurrent AA, particularly a hypocellular marrow, should be treated again with IST. If the peripheral blood counts are trending downward but are not in a life-threatening range, cyclosporine (Neoral, Sandimmune),* can be considered as a single agent. Similarly some patients will relapse after tapering the CSA after initial treatment and rapidly recover after restarting the CSA; such patients may demonstrate dependence on CSA

*Not FDA approved for this indication.

TABLE 5. **Supportive Care for Bone Marrow Failure**

Cytopenia	Treatment
Neutropenia	GCSF,* "neutropenic diet", emergent management of any febrile episode with empirical broad-spectrum antibiotics chosen based on community resistance patterns, avoidance of rectal exams, suppositories, enemas. Avoidance of fungal spores (e.g., gardening and wood chopping). Granulocyte donations from GCSF-primed donors for refractory, established infections.
Thrombocytopenia	Platelet transfusions (irradiated, leukocyte depleted) if platelet count <10,000 or if <50,000 prior to surgery. Use CMV seronegative units for CMV seronegative recipients. Avoid antiplatelet or anticoagulant agents. Activity modification to prevent head trauma.
Anemia	Transfusion of irradiated, leukocyte-depleted, packed cells. For transplant candidates: avoidance of direct donations from family members. Use CMV-seronegative units for CMV-seronegative recipients. Exogenous erythropoietin* for those with renal insufficiency and low erythropoietin. Correction of concurrent iron and/or B_{12} deficiency. Folic acid to avoid megaloblastic crisis, especially in PNH.
Transfusional iron overload	Phlebotomy as tolerated after response to IST or after complete donor engraftment.

*Cytokines should not be used as a substitute for definitive therapy.
CMV, cytomegalovirus; GCSF, granulocyte colony stimulating factor; IST, immunosuppressive therapy; PNH, paroxysmal nocturnal hemoglobinuria.

for maintenance of their remission. Otherwise, ATG* should be given for recurrent and clinically significant cytopenias. Those who have had a life-threatening reaction to either the rabbit or equine product in their initial treatment should be given the other product on relapse. Otherwise, it is unclear whether it is preferable to use the same product that achieved the initial response.

SUMMARY

Once a nearly universally fatal disorder, severe AA is now successfully treated in perhaps 80% to 90% of patients with the disorder. Advances in supportive care and in transplantation may result in even higher rates of success in the future (Table 5).

*Not FDA approved for this indication.

IRON DEFICIENCY

method of
JAMES C. BARTON, M.D.
Southern Iron Disorders Center and University of Alabama at Birmingham
Birmingham, Alabama

Iron deficiency is common worldwide. In developed countries, iron requirements of reproduction in women (menstruation, pregnancy, lactation) and the increased iron requirements for growth in infants and children often exceed dietary iron availability and absorption. Pathologic blood loss in men and postmenopausal women, especially that from the gastrointestinal tract, is also a common cause of iron deficiency. In less well developed areas, diets poor in absorbable iron, vegetarianism, intestinal parasitism, chronic diarrhea, and multiparity are common causes of iron deficiency. Successful treatment of iron deficiency depends on identification and management of its cause or causes and administration of a regimen that takes into account the cause and severity of iron deficiency, co-morbid disorders, and concomitant medications.

NORMAL IRON METABOLISM

Body iron quantities are regulated by controlled absorption that responds directly to body demands and the rate of erythropoiesis. Quantities of total body iron in healthy adults are approximately 4.0 g in men and 3.5 g in women. Hemoglobin represents about 2.0 g in men and 1.5 g in women. Storage sites contain approximately 1.0 g in men and 0.3 g in women. The remaining iron, about 6% of total body quantities, is incorporated in myoglobin, heme enzymes, transferrin, and other compounds.

Dietary iron typically consists of heme iron derived from animal products, nonheme ionic iron in vegetable foods, and inorganic iron added to fortify certain foodstuffs. Iron compounds must be soluble for absorption to occur. Heme iron is readily soluble. Nonheme iron absorption is facilitated by gastric acid and other molecular species such as ascorbic acid (vitamin C) and certain amino acids that maintain iron solubility at acid values of pH. Other substances commonly present in food, such as tannate in tea and phytates in vegetables, inhibit iron absorption. Iron is absorbed only from the small intestine, especially the duodenum. Transport of nonheme iron across the microvilli of absorptive enterocytes requires its reduction to a soluble ferrous form and binding to DCT1 (divalent cation transporter), quantities of which are increased in iron deficiency. Subsequent transfer of iron to the blood is modulated by a complex of *HFE* protein, transferrin receptor, and β_2-microglobulin that regulates the affinity of transferrin receptor on the basolateral surfaces of enterocytes for transferrin. On average, 5% to 10% of ingested iron in food is absorbed.

Iron is highly conserved because of phagocytosis and digestion of senescent erythrocytes by macrophages in the spleen, marrow, and liver and iron storage in ferritin molecules (or degraded ferritin aggregates known as hemosiderin). Conserved iron is released into the circulation as needed and is delivered by transferrin to erythrocytes and other cells through their surface transferrin receptors. Unavoidable iron losses of approximately 1.0 mg daily occur because of exfoliation of skin and gastrointestinal tract cells, perspiration, and minor trauma. In menstruating women, there are additional average daily iron losses of 0.5 to 1.0 mg. Average net iron losses with normal term pregnancy are about 700 mg. If insufficient quantities of iron are presented to the gastrointestinal tract in a form acceptable for absorption or if iron absorptive mechanisms are not intact, iron depletion, iron-deficient erythropoiesis, and iron deficiency anemia develop sequentially in accordance with the rate of net iron loss.

CAUSES OF IRON DEFICIENCY

Infants and adolescents sometimes become iron deficient because dietary iron intake is insufficient to meet physiologic demands of rapid growth. Women of childbearing age frequently develop iron deficiency because of the high iron requirements of menstruation, pregnancy, and lactation. Iron deficiency in other circumstances is typically associated with pathologic blood loss from gastrointestinal tract lesions of diverse etiologies. These include erosion or ulceration of the esophagus, stomach, or duodenum; malignant neoplasms (particularly those of the colon, esophagus, or stomach); microangiopathy (inherited or acquired); inflammatory disorders (especially Crohn's disease); diverticula; and polyps. Chronic intestinal blood loss related to hookworms is a common cause of iron deficiency in certain parts of the world. Some patients who receive chronic warfarin or aspirin therapy develop iron deficiency as a result of gastrointestinal blood loss without demonstrable "anatomic" lesions.

Less frequently, iron deficiency is due to urinary tract blood loss from lesions within the kidneys, ureters, or bladder or to conditions that cause hemoglobinuria (e.g., defective heart valve prostheses, paroxysmal nocturnal hemoglobinuria). Chronic blood loss from the respiratory tract related to recurrent epistaxis or hemoptysis (e.g., idiopathic pulmonary hemosiderosis, lung fluke infestation) is unusual. Many regular blood donors and highly trained athletes develop iron deficiency. Most persons treated with chronic hemodialysis develop iron deficiency because of blood retained in dialysis apparatus, hemolysis, and laboratory testing. "Nonbleeding" gastrointestinal causes of refractory iron deficiency anemia in patients without gastrointestinal symptoms include atrophic gastritis, celiac disease, and *Helicobacter pylori* gastritis. Antitransferrin antibodies have been reported as rare causes of iron deficiency.

SIGNS AND SYMPTOMS OF IRON DEFICIENCY

Many persons with iron deficiency experience weakness, ease of fatigue, or dyspnea with exertion, often before the development of anemia. Pica, the compulsive ingestion of (often) non-nutritive substances, is a common and distinctive consequence of iron deficiency that occurs in approximately one half of persons with iron deficiency. Pica occurs more frequently in women than men. Ice eating (pagophagia), the most common form of pica, can cause significant damage to teeth. Some patients prefer dirt or clay, salt, sand, paper, cold fruit or lettuce, laundry starch, or other substances. Some patients report evidence of bleeding that explains the development of iron deficiency. In severe, chronic iron deficiency, sore mouth or tongue, nail and hair changes, dysphagia, paresthesias, and loss of memory and normal affect sometimes occur. However, many persons are incidentally discovered to have iron deficiency. The most common physical sign of iron deficiency is pallor, although some patients have angular stomatitis, glossitis, koilonychia, or cricoid or esophageal web.

LABORATORY ABNORMALITIES ASSOCIATED WITH IRON DEFICIENCY

Routine clinical laboratory abnormalities associated with iron deficiency and other forms of anemia that must often be considered in the differential diagnosis are displayed in Table 1. Because iron deficiency is more common in women, many laboratories report lower statistical reference limits for iron measures in women than men. Nonetheless, astute clinicians recognize that serum iron measures that probably indicate the presence of iron deficiency are equally applicable to men and women. Persons with serum ferritin less than 50 ng/mL often have iron depletion or deficiency by bone marrow examination criteria, regardless of the laboratory's lower reference limit for serum ferritin. Further, anemia or abnormal serum iron measures related to chronic inflammation, renal insufficiency, malignancy, or deficiency of other micronutrients sometimes occur coincidentally with iron deficiency. Thus, some patients require testing for other disorders before an appropriate treatment regimen for iron deficiency can be recommended.

GENERAL PRINCIPLES OF IRON REPLACEMENT THERAPY

Treatment should not be undertaken until the diagnosis is firmly established and potential adverse effects of therapy have been considered (Table 2). In all cases, therapy must be monitored regularly. There is no established indication for administering iron therapy other than the treatment of iron deficiency. Most patients can be treated safely and adequately with oral iron preparations. Hematinic combinations should be avoided. Intravenous iron therapy should be reserved for noncompliant patients, those unable to take oral iron, patients who absorb iron poorly, or

TABLE 1. **Laboratory Assessment of Iron Deficiency***

Stage of Iron Deficiency	Laboratory Measurement	Diagnostic Result
Depletion of iron stores	Serum ferritin concentration	<50 ng/mL
	Serum total iron-binding capacity	Increased
	Stainable marrow iron	Absent
Iron-deficient erythropoiesis	Serum transferrin saturation	<15%
	Mean corpuscular volume	<80 fL
	Red cell distribution width	Increased
	Free erythrocyte protoporphyrin concentration	Increased
	Serum transferrin receptor concentration	Increased
Iron deficiency anemia	Hemoglobin concentration	<13.0 g/dL (men) <12.0 g/dL (women)

*Laboratory-specific reference ranges for all measurements should be consulted. The differential diagnosis of iron deficiency often includes anemia of chronic inflammation, renal insufficiency, or malignancy. In the latter forms of anemia, total iron-binding capacity is usually decreased, serum ferritin concentration is normal or increased, and red cell distribution width is normal. These forms of anemia may also occur concomitantly with iron deficiency. In some patients, the differential diagnosis of iron deficiency may include forms of thalassemia minor, hemoglobinopathy E, Lepore hemoglobinopathy, forms of sideroblastic anemia, anemia of chronic liver disease, anemia of chronic hemolysis, hypoplastic and aplastic anemia, myeloproliferative and myelodysplastic disorders, congenital dyserythropoietic anemias, anemia of myxedema, and megaloblastic anemia.

TABLE 2. **Potential Adverse Effects of Iron Replacement Therapy***

Adverse Effect	Form of Iron Therapy	Relative Frequency	Susceptible Patients
Black discoloration of stools	Iron salts, carbonyl iron	Very common	Children, adults
Epigastric pain, nausea, constipation, abdominal cramps, metallic taste	Iron salts (more likely, especially with ascorbic acid), carbonyl iron (less likely), intravenous iron (unlikely)	Common	Children, adults
Acute iron poisoning	Iron salts	Common in children; rare in adults	Children (accidental, (ingestion), adults (accidental ingestion, suicide attempts)
Arthralgias, myalgias, bone aches, low-grade fever	Intravenous iron (likely with doses >500 mg Fe), oral iron (less likely)	Uncommon	Children, adults
Decreased absorption of other medications	Iron salts, carbonyl iron	Uncommon	Children, adults
Flushing, hypotension	Intravenous iron	Uncommon with proper administration	Children, adults
Skin discoloration related to extravasation	Intravenous iron	Very uncommon with proper administration	Children, adults
Tooth discoloration	Liquid oral iron	Very uncommon with proper administration	Children
Severe hypersensitivity, anaphylaxis	Intravenous iron	Very uncommon with proper administration	Children, adults
Increased susceptibility to infections with *Vibrio vulnificus*, other bacteria	Intravenous iron (dose related)	Probably uncommon	Adults receiving hemodialysis who consume raw shellfish
Iron overload	Intravenous iron (more likely), oral iron (less likely)	Rare	Adults

*We do not recommend single intravenous doses >500 mg Fe because of an increased likelihood of adverse effects. We do not recommend intramuscular iron therapy, the adverse effects of which include: increased frequency of severe allergy or anaphylaxis; pain, discoloration, and atrophy of subcutaneous tissues at injection sites; therapy failure related to limitations of iron doses; and occurrence of sarcomas at injection sites (rare). Intravenous iron therapy should not be administered to pregnant women unless the benefit outweighs the potential risk to the fetus. Intravenous iron therapy for children should be undertaken only by pediatricians experienced in such management. Iron replacement is usually contraindicated for persons with hemochromatosis, hemosiderosis, or inherited hemolytic anemia.

patients in whom recurrent bleeding causes iron loss in excess of that which can be replaced at an acceptable rate with oral therapy. However, intravenous iron therapy does not induce a more rapid erythropoietic response than is possible with oral iron replacement. Intravenous iron therapy should be given only by physicians experienced in such treatment who are prepared to treat severe hypotension or hypersensitivity sometimes caused by such treatment. Physicians sometimes delay the recovery of patients unnecessarily because they do not understand the indications, proper administration, and safety of intravenous iron replacement. For persons treated with chronic hemodialysis, intravenous administration is the only suitable route of replacement. Nonetheless, we do not recommend single intravenous doses greater than 125 mg of Fe because of an increased likelihood of adverse effects (see Table 2). We do not recommend intramuscular iron therapy (see Table 2).

Dietary change to increase the quantity of food iron ingested is usually ineffective as treatment for iron deficiency. Similarly, multivitamins that contain "daily" amounts of iron (usually 10 to 20 mg Fe as inorganic iron salts) are usually inadequate for replacement therapy in adults. There is no basis for advising patients to take "multivitamins with iron" routinely unless they are premenopausal women or are vegetarians with proven, uncomplicated iron depletion. However, infants and some children may benefit from iron supplements prescribed by an experienced pediatrician. Transfusion of erythrocytes is indicated to elevate the circulating red blood cell mass in persons with iron deficiency anemia who have vigorous bleeding or cardiac or respiratory compromise, but this is not an acceptable means by which to replace iron.

ORAL IRON THERAPY

Carbonyl Iron

We recommend this as the oral therapy of choice for most persons. Carbonyl iron consists of microspheres of pure iron precipitated from the gas iron pentacarbonyl and is widely used for food iron fortification. As replacement therapy, carbonyl iron causes less gastrointestinal toxicity than iron salts and is equally effective in correcting iron deficiency. The usual adult dosage is 50 mg three times daily (Feosol caplets), preferably taken on an empty stomach. Other doses (to be divided into three or four equal portions) include: adolescent boys 18 years of age or younger, 120 mg daily; menstruating adolescent girls 12 to 18 years of age, 60 to 120 mg daily; preadolescent school-age children, up to 6 mg/kg/d; and infants and young children, 3 mg/kg/d as oral suspension (Icar).

In persons with anemia, the hemoglobin concentration usually increases about 1 g/dL weekly. Treatment should be continued until anemia is corrected and serum ferritin concentration is greater than 50 ng/mL. In patients who have objectionable gastrointestinal symptoms, administration with meals or reduction of daily dosing frequency may be necessary, although this may delay correction of iron deficiency. Completion of therapy in patients without continuing iron loss typically requires 4 to 6 months.

Iron Salts

Iron salts, inexpensive and available without prescription, are suitable for many children and adults. The most frequently used preparation is ferrous sulfate (325-mg tablets; 65 mg Fe per tablet). In adults, the dose is one tablet three times daily, preferably on an empty stomach. In older children, the dose is 5 mg/kg of iron daily as tablets or elixir (administered by an adult). Rate of response of anemia, monitoring of hemoglobin and ferritin concentrations, and dose adjustments for adverse gastrointestinal symptoms associated with treatment are similar to those for carbonyl iron therapy. Ferrous gluconate, ferrous fumarate, polysaccharide-iron complex, and enteric-coated iron preparations can be used similarly. However, many contain less iron per tablet than ferrous sulfate or are less absorbable and thus induce therapeutic responses less rapidly; most are more expensive.

INTRAVENOUS IRON THERAPY

Iron Dextran

This preparation (InFeD; 50 mg Fe/mL) is indicated in the treatment of iron deficiency in persons with normal renal function who fail to respond to or do not tolerate oral iron supplementation. Although therapy has been associated with adverse effects (see Table 2), iron dextran is safe and effective when administered properly by skilled persons. Each infusion in adults should consist of 500 mg Fe in 500 mL of normal saline. We recommend premedication with intravenous diphenhydramine (Benadryl) (25 mg), cimetidine (Tagamet) (400 mg), or famotidine (Pepcid) (20 mg) and dexamethasone (10 mg) and a test dose of approximately 5 mL over 10 to 15 minutes in a freely flowing intravenous line. If no adverse effect occurs, the remaining dose should be infused over 2 to 3 hours. Infusions are repeated every 2 to 3 weeks until correction of anemia and reconstitution of iron stores occur as described for oral iron preparations. Many patients who require intravenous iron dextran for initial management have recurrent bleeding and iron deficiency and thus require periodic maintenance infusions.

Iron Sucrose

This product (Venofer; 20 mg Fe/mL) is indicated for treatment of iron deficiency in patients undergoing chronic hemodialysis who are receiving supplemental erythropoietin therapy. Doses of 100 mg Fe administered intravenously over 2 hours during hemodialysis appear to be safe and effective. Typically, goals of therapy include maintenance of serum transferrin saturation 30% or higher, serum ferritin concentration 300 ng/mL or higher, and hemoglobin greater than 11.0 g/dL. Most hemodialysis patients require ongoing or recurrent therapy.

Iron Gluconate

This product (Ferrlecit, Schein; 12.5 mg Fe/mL) is indicated for treatment of iron deficiency in patients undergoing chronic hemodialysis who are receiving supplemental erythropoietin therapy. Typical treatments consist of 125 mg of Fe administered intravenously at each of sequential hemodialysis treatments to achieve maintenance of serum transferrin saturation, serum ferritin concentration, and hemoglobin similar to those goals of iron sucrose therapy.

FAILURE OF IRON REPLACEMENT THERAPY

The most common cause of unsuccessful therapy is poor compliance, often related to adverse gastrointestinal effects of oral iron preparations. Another common cause is unrecognized or uncorrectable chronic or recurrent blood loss. Gastrectomy, duodenectomy, achlorhydria, and intestinal bypass are often associated with iron malabsorption. Some commonly used drugs decrease iron absorption, including antacids, histamine H_2 antagonists, proton pump antagonists, calcium supplements, and tetracycline. Other persons suspected to have suboptimal iron absorption benefit from evaluation of other micronutrients and from gastrointestinal tract endoscopy and associated testing. The occurrence of anemia other than that of iron deficiency should be considered. In persons with chronic disease or renal insufficiency or in those receiving anticancer chemotherapy, erythropoietin therapy is often necessary to induce a satisfactory erythropoietic response to otherwise adequate supplies of iron. Regardless of the cause of initial treatment failure, many patients require subsequent intravenous iron replacement.

AUTOIMMUNE HEMOLYTIC ANEMIA

method of
KAREN E. KING, M.D., and
PAUL M. NESS, M.D.
Johns Hopkins Medical Institutions
Baltimore, Maryland

The autoimmune hemolytic anemias (AIHAs) are characterized by two features: (1) shortened red blood cell survival and (2) evidence of autoantibodies directed against red blood cell antigens. The incidence of AIHA is approximately 1 to 2 cases per 100,000 per year. Approximately 30% to 50% of AIHAs are idiopathic or primary. The remaining cases are secondary to underlying diseases, such as lymphoproliferative diseases, immunodeficiency states, solid tumors, connective tissue disorders, or infectious diseases. AIHA is seen in all races. Although all ages can be affected, the incidence of AIHAs increases with age. Women are more often affected than men.

CLASSIFICATION AND SEROLOGIC DIFFERENTIAL DIAGNOSIS

Immune hemolytic anemia (IHA) can be classified into three major groups: (1) alloimmune IHA, including hemolytic transfusion reactions and hemolytic disease of the newborn; (2) drug-induced IHA; and (3) AIHA. On the basis of the in vivo and in vitro characteristics of the causative autoantibody, AIHA can be subdivided into those associated with warm antibodies, reacting optimally at 37°C, and those associated with cold antibodies, reacting optimally at 0°C to 5°C. The AIHAs associated with cold antibodies can be further subdivided into the more common cold agglutinin syndrome and the rare paroxysmal cold hemoglobinuria. Typically, warm AIHA results from IgG autoantibodies, whereas cold agglutinin syndrome is caused by IgM autoantibodies. Paroxysmal cold hemoglobinuria results from an IgG autoantibody known as a biphasic hemolysin or the *Donath-Landsteiner antibody*; this antibody binds to red blood cells at low temperatures, activates complement, and leads to hemolysis at 37°C. Both the warm and cold types of AIHA can be idiopathic, or they can be secondary to infection or diseases such as leukemia or systemic lupus erythematosus.

The diagnosis of AIHA is usually made by taking into account the clinical findings and the results of laboratory testing and serologic evaluations. The clinical severity varies based on the time course of the disease. Patients may present with fatigue, weakness, dizziness, fever, dyspnea on exertion, and even angina. On physical examination, patients may have jaundice, pallor, and/or hepatosplenomegaly. A peripheral blood smear classically reveals microspherocytosis, reticulocytosis, and nucleated red blood cells. Laboratory tests may reveal an elevated total bilirubin, increased serum lactate dehydrogenase, and decreased haptoglobin. Patients with a brisk hemolytic process may even have hemoglobinuria and hemoglobinemia.

The serologic evaluation of AIHA begins with routine pretransfusion testing including determination of ABO group, Rh type, and antibody screening tests. A direct antiglobulin test (DAT) using anti-IgG and anti-C3 (C3d) will identify IgG and/or complement coating of the red blood cells. Eluate studies can further elucidate the nature and specificity of the red blood cell–bound IgG. Serum studies including the indirect antiglobulin test using either untreated or enzyme-treated homologous red blood cells at 20°C and 37°C will demonstrate antibody present in the serum, and selected cell panel studies may reveal a specificity of the antibody.

For cold AIHA, a cold agglutinin titer and thermal amplitude studies are helpful in determining and confirming the clinical significance of the cold autoantibody. In general, the cold autoantibodies that clinically cause cold agglutinin syndrome have a high titer (greater than 1000), and serum studies using 30% bovine albumin show reactivity at 30°C. If paroxysmal cold hemoglobinuria is suspected, a Donath-Landsteiner test must be performed to identify the biphasic hemolysin or Donath-Landsteiner antibody. The results of such serologic tests allow classification into warm AIHA, cold agglutinin syndrome, or paroxysmal cold hemoglobinuria (Table 1).

Occasionally, unusual patients may not be classifiable into one of the three types of AIHA. Some patients appear to have a combination of warm and cold AIHA, or mixed-type AIHA. These patients may have the classic serologic features of both (e.g., IgG and complement on the red blood cells and serum revealing a high-titer IgM cold antibody together with an IgG warm autoantibody) or IgG and C3 on the red blood cells with low-titer IgM cold autoagglutinins of high thermal amplitude in the serum. Another group of unusual patients with hemolytic anemia and all the clinical and hematologic features of warm AIHA present with a negative DAT and no detectable serum antibodies—so-called Coombs'-negative or DAT-negative AIHA. In these patients, more sensitive testing, such as the enzyme-linked antiglobulin test or radiolabeled antiglobulin tests, may be necessary to identify red blood cell–bound IgG.

TABLE 1. **Autoimmune Hemolytic Anemias: Serologic Findings**

Parameter	Warm Autoimmune Hemolytic Anemia	Cold Agglutinin Syndrome	Paroxysmal Cold Hemoglobinuria
Direct antiglobulin test	IgG, IgG and C3; less commonly C3 only; negative (2%–4% of cases)	C3 only	C3 only
Immunoglobulin type	IgG (sometimes IgA, rarely IgM)	IgM	IgG
Eluate	IgG	Nonreactive	Nonreactive
Serum	IgG agglutinating red blood cells at the antihuman globulin phase (panagglutinin)	IgM agglutinating antibody, usually titers >1000, reacting at 30°C in albumin	IgG biphasic hemolysin (Donath-Landsteiner antibody)
Specificity	Rh specificity common	Anti-I, anti-i	Anti-P

TRANSFUSION THERAPY

Blood transfusion may be required for patients with AIHA who present with fulminant hemolysis or patients with chronic hemolysis who become symptomatic while they are awaiting response to primary modes of therapy. The presence of red blood cell autoantibody coating the patient's red blood cells or appearing as a panagglutinin in the serum contributes additional risks of blood transfusion to the general risks of infectious disease transmission and transfusion reaction. Like the patient's autologous red blood cells, donor red blood cells will be destroyed by the autoantibody and will not have normal survival. The autoantibody can make it difficult to detect coexisting or underlying clinically significant red blood cell alloantibodies that can cause severe hemolytic transfusion reactions. Despite these concerns, transfusion may be required in AIHA, and it may be lifesaving. Some patients with AIHA have reticulocytopenia despite intense erythroid hyperplasia in the bone marrow. In these patients, transfusions may be required as a life-sustaining measure for profound anemia. Reticulocytopenia may persist for long periods before the onset of adequate erythropoiesis or control of the hemolytic process with corticosteroids or splenectomy. These cases emphasize that transfusion should not be avoided in AIHA, despite old dogma to the contrary.

The transfusion management of patients with AIHA requires careful communication between the clinician and the transfusion service. It is important to know the capabilities of the transfusion service for performing specialized immunohematologic procedures or where these procedures may be available on a referral basis. It is also critical for the clinician to assess the patient's history of pregnancies and previous transfusions with great care; it is unlikely that a previously untransfused male patient will have masked alloantibodies.

At the Bench

Although patients with AIHA can present as an ABO discrepancy (the standard cell and serum typing procedures producing discrepant results), ABO typing can usually be performed after removal of IgG autoantibody in warm AIHA or warm washing red blood cells to remove IgM autoantibody in cold agglutinin syndrome. In an emergency or if ABO results are not clear, then group O donor blood can be used. Rh typing can also be difficult if the patient's cells are heavily coated with autoantibody. Low-protein, monoclonal reagents are available for Rh typing in the setting of immunoglobulin-coated red blood cells. Procedures to dissociate antibody may be helpful in these situations.

The most pressing problem in a patient with previous pregnancies or transfusions is detecting or identifying alloantibody that may be hidden or masked by the autoantibody. The exclusion of underlying clinically significant alloantibodies is time-consuming, and the clinical situation may not allow for completion of these studies before transfusion is needed. In the untransfused patient, autologous adsorption studies are required to investigate the presence of underlying alloantibody. If the patient has been transfused in the preceding 3 months, more complex differential allogeneic adsorption studies are required. In the untransfused patient, determination of the red blood cell phenotype is invaluable. Procedures are available to dissociate autoantibody so that phenotyping can be performed. Not only can the patient's phenotype guide the exclusion of alloantibodies by indicating which antigen specificities are at risk of eliciting an alloantibody, but also it has been shown that when available, phenotypically matched red blood cells are an efficient method of providing safe red blood cells for transfusion in this setting. Additionally, patients with AIHA are candidates for a long-term transfusion program, in which case a phenotype would be helpful. If time does not allow for phenotyping, a pretransfusion aliquot of red blood cells can be frozen so that phenotyping can be performed in the future if the need arises.

At the Bedside

When the decision has been reached to begin transfusions, several additional steps can enhance patient safety. In some cases, transfusions of small aliquots of blood may be sufficient to provide relief of symptoms while avoiding the complications of fluid overload. The use of leukocyte-reduced red blood cells is useful to avoid febrile, nonhemolytic transfusion reactions whose initial presentation can suggest a hemolytic reaction with more severe consequences. In cases of transfusion for patients with cold agglutinin syndrome, blood warmers are often suggested, but there are limited data to support or refute this recommendation.

THERAPY

The approach to the management of AIHA depends, in part, on whether the disease is primary or secondary to disorders such as B-cell malignant diseases and systemic lupus erythematosus. Other factors that determine the initial therapy include the temperature at which the antibody binds to the red blood cell (warm or cold reactive) and the isotype (IgG versus IgM) of the autoantibody. The endpoint of therapy is not the normalization of the DAT. Patients may have positive DATs without hemolysis or without anemia, or, alternatively, patients may have symptomatic AIHA with a negative DAT. Finally, the most common forms of therapy, detailed in the following sections, may raise the level of hemoglobin, whereas the DAT may remain positive.

Warm Autoimmune Hemolytic Anemia

Corticosteroids

For adult patients with either idiopathic or the secondary forms of warm AIHA, corticosteroids are the initial therapy of choice. The clinical response to corticosteroids results primarily from their effect on tissue macrophages, which become less efficient in clearing IgG or C3-coated cells. Only after several weeks of therapy is a significant fall in antibody production observed. Among adults, permanent remissions of AIHA are observed in fewer than 20% of cases. Therefore, subsequent therapy is based on the presumption that clinical relapse is likely.

Splenectomy

Approximately 50% to 60% of patients will have a good to excellent initial response to splenectomy and will require less than 15 mg/d of prednisone to maintain an adequate level of hemoglobin. Late relapses do occur, presumably caused by enhanced antibody synthesis and hepatic sequestration. The role of splenectomy in patients with mixed IgG/IgM, or coexisting IgM and warm-reactive IgG antibodies requires further definition.

The subsequent therapeutic decisions in warm AIHA are based on the need to maintain an adequate level of hemoglobin and the need to avoid the complications of long-term steroid administration or immunosuppression. After splenectomy, there is a low risk of developing the overwhelming postsplenectomy sepsis syndrome, a risk that may be reduced further by the use of pneumococcal and meningococcal vaccines and by the prompt use of antibiotics for each febrile illness.

Immunosuppressive Therapy

The use of immunosuppressive therapy should be considered only for the following symptomatic patients: (1) those who fail to respond to splenectomy or who have a relapse after splenectomy; (2) those for whom splenectomy represents an unacceptable medical risk; or (3) those who have serious side effects of corticosteroids. Cyclophosphamide (Cytoxan)* has gained favor in several other hematologic disorders caused by autoantibodies. Azathioprine (Imuran)* is also a commonly used immunosuppressive agent. These agents are cytotoxic, and white blood cell and reticulocyte counts should be closely followed. Therapy should be continued as tolerated for at least 3 months, to ensure maximal inhibition of antibody synthesis. These agents may lead to an increased risk of neoplasia; consequently therapy should not be extended for prolonged periods. Cyclosporine (Sandimmune)* has been used with success; however, the use of cyclosporine requires the monitoring of kidney function. High-dose cyclophosphamide followed by granulocyte colony-stimulating factor (filgrastim [Neupogen]) has been used with success in a few patients who were refractory to other therapies. Another newer treatment option is the use of anti-CD20 monoclonal antibody, rituximab (Rituxan),* which has been associated with successful treatment of both idiopathic AIHA and AIHA secondary to lymphoproliferative diseases.

Additional Forms of Therapy

Plasma Exchange. The efficacy of plasma exchange is limited in warm AIHA by the continuous antibody production and the large extravascular distribution of IgG. In general, plasma exchange of 1 to 1.5 plasma volumes is effective in lowering the serum level of antibody by a least 50%. On cessation of therapy, the return to preapheresis levels of antibody will depend on the rate of autoantibody production and the rate of equilibration between the extravascular and intravascular compartments. Occasional dramatic responses have been reported in patients who are being prepared for surgery or as a temporizing measure after the initiation of immunosuppressive therapy.

Vinca Alkaloids. Responses in a few patients with warm AIHA have been reported after infusion with vincristine*-laden, IgG-coated platelets as a vehicle for delivery of the drug to the macrophage.

Other Modalities. Danazol (Danocrine),* an attenuated synthetic androgen, has proved to be of benefit in some patients with refractory warm AIHA. In view of the relatively low risk of long-term side effects, danazol may be used in the future with increasing frequency in the management of steroid-dependent patients. Intravenous gamma globulin (Gamimune N)* at 400 mg/kg/d for 5 days or 1 g/kg for 2 days, has been shown effective for managing subacute emergencies in idiopathic thrombocytopenic purpura. It is possible that the drug may bind to Fc receptors on macrophages and thereby increase the life span of circulating cells coated with IgG antibody. Therefore, this drug may prove to have an adjunctive roll in the management of warm AIHA as well.

Cold Agglutinin Syndromes

The preferred therapy for the cold agglutinin syndromes depends on the severity of the patient's symptoms, the serologic characteristics of the autoantibody, and the nature of the underlying disease, if present. Patients with idiopathic cold AIHA often have moderately severe, partially compensated anemia, and medical therapy is generally unsatisfactory. Steroids have been successful in occasional patients with cold agglutinins when the antibody has a high thermal amplitude but is present only in low titer or when an IgG cold-reactive antibody is found. Consequently, steroids are not efficacious in most patients with cold AIHA. Similarly, splenectomy is not usually effective, presumably because the liver is the dominant site of sequestration of red blood cells heavily sensitized with C3. Long-term administration of oral alkylating agents helps many patients with the secondary forms of cold AIHA but is only occasionally successful in patients with the idiopathic form of the disease who have high titers of circulating IgM antibody. Plasma exchange may be effective in acute situations and can be considered as a temporizing measure. The use of in-line blood warmers is advisable, and more elaborate measures to perform the entire exchange process at 37°C are occasionally required. When the presence of cold agglutinins is part of an established B-cell malignant disease, the severity of hemolysis often waxes and wanes in parallel with the underlying process. Therapy for the malignant

*Not FDA approved for this indication.

*Not FDA approved for this indication.

disease with prednisone and an alkylating agent is often sufficient to control the rate of hemolysis as well.

Because most of these therapies have little practical impact on the management of cold AIHA, patients with mild, compensated anemia are often not treated for long periods or may require only episodic transfusions. If transfusion is required, the use of a blood warmer is generally recommended. Many patients do well by merely avoiding exposure to the cold.

NONIMMUNE HEMOLYTIC ANEMIA

method of
CARLO BRUGNARA, M.D.
Children's Hospital Boston and Harvard Medical School
Boston, Massachusetts

Several congenital and acquired diseases lead to premature destruction of the erythrocyte in the absence of antibody-mediated hemolysis. I address here congenital anemias characterized by abnormal red cell morphology or abnormal metabolism and acquired nonimmune hemolytic anemias.

CONGENITAL NONIMMUNE HEMOLYTIC ANEMIAS

Hemolytic Anemias Caused by Red Cell Membrane Abnormalities

The functional integrity and proper survival of the human erythrocyte are critically dependent on several integral membrane proteins and their interaction with the underlying cytoskeleton. Genetic alterations in these critical components result in chronic hemolytic anemia, reduced red cell survival, and characteristic morphologic abnormalities of the erythrocyte.

Hereditary Spherocytosis and Elliptocytosis

CLINICAL MANIFESTATIONS

Hereditary spherocytosis (HS) arises as a chronic hemolytic anemia, with jaundice and splenomegaly. Severity of this disease varies from mild to severe. Thirty percent of the cases are mild, with Hb levels higher than 11 g/dL, reticulocyte counts below 6%, and bilirubin levels around 1 to 2 mg/dL. In neonates with HS, early neonatal icterus is common; Hb values are usually normal at birth but decrease sharply in the first 3 weeks of life, frequently to levels that require blood transfusion. The erythropoietic response to hemolysis is delayed in neonatal HS; reticulocytosis appropriate for the level of anemia appears only several months after birth. Bilirubin gallstones are a frequent and sometimes early complication. Severe anemia caused by acute red cell aplasia (parvovirus B19 infection) is another potential complication.

Hereditary elliptocytosis (HE) is characterized by chronic hemolysis and elliptic erythrocytes. In some cases elliptocytes coexist with spherocytes or poikilocytes. A subtype of HE is hereditary pyropoikilocytosis, with extreme poikilocytosis and bizarre-shaped erythrocytes. Most cases of HE are clinically mild and asymptomatic.

MOLECULAR AND CELLULAR BASES OF THE DISEASE

Mutations affecting ankyrin, band 3 anion exchanger, β- or α-spectrin, and protein 4.1 or 4.2 have been shown to produce HS or HE. One person in every 5000 in Europe or North America is born with HS. However, a large number of mild cases are undiagnosed and the incidence could be as high as 1 in 2000. The incidence of HS is lower in blacks. Seventy-five percent of the HS-HE cases display an autosomal dominant pattern of transmission (one parent carries the abnormality). In the remaining cases of HS, both parents are clinically and hematologically normal. Most of these cases are autosomal recessive, although de novo mutations resulting in dominant HS have been demonstrated. Coinheritance of HS and Gilbert's syndrome results in higher levels of bilirubin and greater risk for developing gallstones.

LABORATORY DIAGNOSIS

HS and HE are chronic hemolytic anemias with abnormal erythrocyte morphology (presence of hyperchromic spherocytes, uniformly dark and round cells, and/or microspherocytes for HS; presence of elliptocytes in HE). High mean corpuscular hemoglobin concentration (MCHC) indicates the presence of spherocytes and low mean cell volume (MCV) in conjunction with high MCHC that of microspherocytes, the latter being a good indicator of disease severity. Osmotic fragility (un-incubated) is characteristically increased in HS; in borderline cases overnight incubation (incubated osmotic fragility) can demonstrate increased fragility. Marked reticulocytosis or the presence of a significant number of fetal erythrocytes, which are more osmotically resistant than adult erythrocytes, may mask the increased fragility of HS erythrocytes. Additional biochemical markers of hemolysis are decreased haptoglobin and increased serum lactate dehydrogenase (LDH) and bilirubin levels.

All cases of hereditary pyropoikilocytosis and many of HE exhibit abnormal erythrocyte thermal sensitivity, with increased fragmentation at temperatures of 44°C to 46°C.

TREATMENT

Because shortened red cell survival and anemia are due to the splenic sequestration of spherocytes, splenectomy is the preferred therapy for severe HS. To prevent postsplenectomy infections, vaccination against pneumococcus, *Haemophilus influenzae*, and meningococcus should be performed before surgery, with boosters every 5 years. Oral penicillin* should be administered for at least 1 year after surgery and in very young children continued up to 5 to 6 years of age. The surgical risk associated with splenectomy, the risk of postsplenectomy sepsis, and the higher incidence of

*Not FDA approved for this indication.

myocardial infarction in splenectomized patients after age 40 should be carefully considered in patients with mild to moderate anemia. For young patients and adults with gallstones and mild HS, the best therapeutic strategy involves combination of prophylactic splenectomy and satellite cholecystectomy. Isolated cholecystectomy should be performed laparoscopically.

Subtotal splenectomy has emerged as a treatment option for young children with HS. This procedure removes approximately 90% of the enlarged spleen, leaving a remnant that is approximately one quarter of a normal spleen. Subtotal splenectomy leads to a therapeutic decrease of hemolytic rate in most cases while at the same time maintaining adequate phagocytic function. Although there is some regrowth of the remaining spleen, this does not diminish the beneficial effects of subtotal splenectomy.

Hereditary Stomatocytosis and Xerocytosis

Hereditary stomatocytosis and xerocytosis are rare genetic disorders of still unidentified membrane proteins, mostly dominantly inherited. The severity of hemolysis can range from mild to severe. There have been reports of several cases of strikingly severe thrombotic complications following splenectomy in patients with hereditary stomatocytosis. Iron overload is a common complication of hereditary stomatocytosis.

Hemolytic Anemias Caused by Red Cell Metabolism Abnormalities

The two genetic defects in red cell metabolisms associated with significant hemolysis affect either glucose-6-phosphate dehydrogenase (G6PD) or pyruvate kinase (PK). The production of reduced nicotinamide adenine dinucleotide phosphate (NADPH) by the pentose phosphate pathway plays a central role in providing this essential coenzyme to reductive processes and to protect against oxidant damage. G6PD catalyzes the first step of this pathway. NADPH is the essential hydrogen donor that supports the regeneration of reduced glutathione (GSH) from oxidized glutathione and the activity of catalase, which degrades H_2O_2.

PK catalyzes an essential step in ATP synthesis. PK defects result in (1) ATP deficiency with early demise of reticulocyte and erythrocytes and (2) marked increases in glycolytic intermediates above the defect, resulting in a marked elevation in 2,3-diphosphoglycerate that favors the compensation of the anemia.

Glucose-6-Phosphate Dehydrogenase Deficiency

CLINICAL MANIFESTATIONS

At steady state, in the absence of offending agents, no hematologic or serum biochemical abnormalities are present. A typical presentation is that of a hemolytic crisis, with anemia, jaundice, and dark urines, precipitated by a variety of offending agents, including antimalarial drugs (primaquine, pamaquine*), sulfonamides and sulfones, nitrofurans, and antihelmintics. Hemolysis usually resolves in a few days, with return to baseline Hb levels in a few weeks. An acute hemolytic attack after ingestion of fava beans (favism) is typical in children, with severe symptomatic anemia, fever, abdominal pain, nausea, and more rarely vomiting.

Severe neonatal jaundice is a frequent neonatal complication of G6PD deficiency. A small fraction of patients present with chronic hemolytic anemia, with reticulocytosis and normal red cell indices.

*Not available in the United States.

MOLECULAR AND CELLULAR BASES OF THE DISEASE

The gene of G6PD resides toward the end of the long arm of chromosome X. Approximately 500 mutations have been described that result in qualitative or quantitative changes in G6PD. High-incidence areas for G6PD deficiency are Africa, the Mediterranean countries, the Middle East, and Southeast Asia. Although this X-linked disease mostly affects males, the incidence of G6PD deficiency is sufficiently high to produce cases of symptomatic females. G6PD deficiency cells are unable to regenerate large quantities of GSH and thus compensate the increased generation of oxidized glutathione by an oxidizing agent. When GSH is depleted, SH residues of Hb are oxidized and denatured Hb precipitates on the inner side of the membrane.

LABORATORY DIAGNOSIS

Moderate to severe anemia characterizes hemolytic attacks; staining with methyl violet reveals the presence of Heinz bodies (precipitates of denatured Hb, more prominent within the first 24 hours of an acute episode). Haptoglobin levels are extremely low, free Hb may be present in serum, unconjugated bilirubin is elevated, and urines are dark because of the presence of hemoglobinuria. The direct antiglobulin test is negative, ruling out autoimmune hemolysis.

Several semiquantitative screening tests are available for the initial identification of a deficiency in G6PD. Samples with less than 30% of the normal activity should be considered deficient. Specific quantitative determination of G6PD activity is available in several reference or specialized laboratories. However, false-negative results may be obtained in the presence of reticulocytes or leukocytes (increased G6PD activity) and immediately after acute hemolysis because the destruction of older cells leaves behind a relatively "young" population with higher G6PD activity. After a severe hemolytic episode, it may be necessary to wait 2 to 3 weeks before performing G6PD activity studies.

TREATMENT

Transfusion should be considered if the anemia is severe and the hemolysis is persistent (continuous hemoglobinuria). Acute renal failure may complicate a severe hemolytic episode. Drugs and/or food known to generate oxidative insults should be avoided.

Pyruvate Kinase Deficiency

PK deficiency affects mostly people of northern European and Mediterranean ancestry. Transmission is autosomal dominant. Anemia is seen only in the presence of homozygous defects. The clinical severity of the chronic hemolysis varies, with exacerbations of hemolysis during pregnancy or infections; aplastic crises related to parvovirus infections are a potential complication.

ACQUIRED NONIMMUNE HEMOLYTIC ANEMIAS

Paroxysmal Nocturnal Hemoglobinuria

CLINICAL MANIFESTATIONS

Paroxysmal nocturnal hemoglobinuria (PNH) is a rare acquired disease that usually arises as hemolytic anemia in a previously healthy subject, in many cases associated with the report of dark urine (sign of hemoglobinuria and intravascular hemolysis). Anemia is characterized by paroxysmal hemolytic crises and in less than half of the cases is accompanied by the classical nocturnal hemoglobinuria. Deep vein thrombosis can be the initial presentation and less frequently cytopenia and bone marrow failure, from mild degrees all the way to severe aplastic anemia. In "florid PNH," hemolysis and thrombotic complications are prominent; in "aplastic anemia with a PNH clone" the picture is that of severe aplastic anemia with the incidental finding of a PNH clone. PNH is a chronic disorder, with a median survival time of 8 to 10 years.

MOLECULAR AND CELLULAR BASES OF THE DISEASE

PNH erythrocytes lack membrane proteins, which use a glycosyl phosphatidylinositol (GPI) anchor embedded into the membrane to attach to the cell membrane. Acquired mutations in the *PIG-A* gene (phosphatidyl inositol glycan complementation group A), a critical component in the biosynthetic process of GPI anchors, have been demonstrated in most patients with PNH. The *PIG-A* gene is located on the short arm of the X chromosome, and a single (one-hit) mutation can induce the PNH phenotype. Thus, PNH is a clonal disorder. However, because PNH clones and *PIG-A* mutations can be seen in hematologically normal subjects, it is possible that additional factors determine the expansion of these clones in PNH. The absence of proteins that limit complement activation and insertion in red cells (CD55, CD59, C8-binding protein) explains the chronic intravascular hemolysis of PNH and its exacerbation with concomitant viral or bacterial infections. The pathophysiology of thrombotic complications of PNH is not clear: the hypercoagulable state of PNH seems to be due to platelet hyperactivity (platelets also arise from the PNH clone) rather than activation of the coagulation factors cascade because it is not prevented by warfarin (Coumadin) or heparin prophylaxis. The aplastic anemia associated with PNH is most likely due to autoimmunity because it responds to immunosuppressive therapy in the majority of cases.

LABORATORY DIAGNOSIS

The classical tests based on the hemolysis of PNH erythrocytes in the presence of acidified serum or low ionic strength (Ham test, sugar-water test, sucrose hemolysis) have been replaced by specific flow cytometric determination of CD59/55 on red cells. On the basis of the expansion of the PNH clone, the proportion of cells defective in CD59/55 and the extent of CD59/55 depletion vary among subjects and in the same subject over time. The severity of the disease is usually related to the proportion of CD59/55-deficient cells.

TREATMENT

Allogeneic bone marrow transplantation (BMT) should be considered in young patients, especially if an HLA-identical sibling is available. A less aggressive treatment course, which is the only option for patients who are not candidates for BMT, is based on immunosuppressive therapy with antilymphocyte globulin (ALG) or antithymocyte globulin (ATG)* and cyclosporine (Neoral).* Supportive treatment with chronic red blood cell transfusion is another therapeutic option for PNH patients. If PNH arises as "aplastic anemia with a PNH clone," the therapy should be similar to that of other aplastic anemias and is detailed elsewhere.

Traumatic (Angiopathic) Hemolytic Anemias

CLINICAL MANIFESTATIONS

Erythrocytes undergo mechanical damage when exposed to disturbances of the blood flow, which generate high shear stress. Traumatic hemolysis can be seen in 5% to 15% of heart valve surgical replacements, more commonly with mechanical (carbon alloy) valves. Rarely, traumatic hemolysis may be seen in congenital heart defects, such as patent ductus arteriosus or ventricular septal defects. These clinical situations are defined as macroangiopathic hemolytic anemias to distinguish them from traumatic anemias associated with disseminated intravascular coagulation and thrombotic thrombocytopenic purpura–hemolytic-uremic syndromes (microangiopathic anemias). In microangiopathic anemias, intravascular activation of the coagulation cascade in small vessels leads to formation of fibrin aggregates that disrupt blood flow and cause traumatic hemolysis. Acute, self-limited traumatic hemolysis can be seen after strenuous physical exercise or activities that impose local damage on circulating blood cells (long-distance running, drumming, karate).

*Not FDA approved for this indication.

LABORATORY DIAGNOSIS

The hallmark of traumatic hemolysis is the presence on the peripheral smear of schistocytes (fragmented red cells) and sometimes "helmet," "burr," or "triangle" cells. Haptoglobin is decreased and indirect bilirubin and serum LDH are increased. Additional laboratory abnormalities may be present depending on the underlying disease.

TREATMENT

Severe anemia may require transfusion. Anemia usually resolves with the resolution of the underlying disease.

PERNICIOUS ANEMIA AND OTHER MEGALOBLASTIC ANEMIAS

method of
LENEE A. LANE, PHARM.D.
Norman Regional Hospital
Norman, Oklahoma

Megaloblastic anemias most frequently result from a deficiency in either vitamin B_{12} (cobalamin) or folic acid (folate). Pernicious anemia is one form of cobalamin-deficient anemia in which patients lack intrinsic factor (IF) necessary for cobalamin utilization. Many other physiologic abnormalities may potentially lead to these vitamin deficiencies despite proper dietary intake. The highest risk population for these deficiencies is older adults. Diagnostic advances over the past 20 years have improved the ability to identify and treat more patients for these deficiencies, thereby avoiding permanent neurologic damage and improving quality of life.

EPIDEMIOLOGY

Tissue cobalamin deficiency is more commonly observed in older adults, with an estimated prevalence of nearly 40% in some studies. It is rare to see folate deficiency in this population without accompanying cobalamin deficiency. The 1994 Framingham study, an epidemiologic investigation of heart disease, broke down the original cohort of 5209 subjects aged 29 to 63 to 548 patients between 67 and 96 years of age. Almost 20% of these patients had laboratory findings suggestive of cobalamin deficiency. Folate deficiency alone was present in less than 1% of the older cohort.

Since the addition of folate to whole-grain products in 1998, the overall percentage of folate deficiency has declined from 13% in 1994 to less than 0.5% today. A growing concern is masked cobalamin-deficient anemia with folate food fortification. Folate supplementation at therapeutic dosages can partially correct the megaloblastic presentation, making diagnosis of cobalamin deficiency more challenging. The continued cobalamin deficiency may progress to irreversible neurologic symptoms. On the opposite side, folic acid deficiency in pregnancy leading to permanent neural tube defects in children can be minimized by the food fortification.

PATHOPHYSIOLOGY AND ETIOLOGY

Megaloblastic anemias most commonly result from impaired production of tetrahydrofolate necessary for proper DNA synthesis. Cobalamin and folate are necessary cofactors in the enzymatic cycle for tetrahydrofolate production. A deficiency of either of these cofactors impairs cell division in the bone marrow while RNA and protein synthesis continues, resulting in enlarged erythrocytes. Cobalamin deficiency also impairs the synthesis of *S*-adenosylmethionine (SAM) necessary for proper nervous system functioning. Folate is also involved in this pathway but does not seem to impair SAM production at times of deficiency (Figure 1).

Cobalamin is obtained mostly from meat, eggs, and milk. The recommended dietary allowance is 2.4 μg per day and the average liver reserve is 2 to 5 mg. It may take years to deplete this reserve and for cobalamin deficiency to become evident.

There are different causes for cobalamin-deficient anemia originating from different physiologic abnormalities in the cobalamin transport system. Ingested dietary cobalamin is first displaced from its protein binding sites through the activity of pepsin at an acidic pH and bound to haptocorrin in the stomach and small intestine. Pancreatic enzymes cleave this bond, allowing cobalamin binding to IF that is produced by parietal cells in the gastric mucosa. The IF allows absorption of cobalamin through the terminal ileum. Serum cobalamin binds to transcobalamin II (TCII), allowing cell absorption and utilization.

The most common cause for cobalamin deficiency is food cobalamin malabsorption resulting from the inability to displace the vitamin from protein food sources. These patients may take medications that alter gastric acid secretion (e.g., H_2 blockers, proton pump inhibitors, colchicine, neomycin, and aminosalicylic acid), have a history of gastric surgery, or have atrophic gastritis with hypochlorhydria or achlorhydria. *Helicobacter pylori* has been associated with producing food cobalamin malabsorption through less clear mechanisms. Patients with food cobalamin malabsorption have functional IF for the absorption of free cobalamin supplementation but have difficulty with dietary sources.

Pernicious anemia is a form of cobalamin malabsorption caused by a lack of IF. IF may be lost following injury to the parietal cells or by autoantibodies binding to the cobalamin binding site of IF. Other reasons for cobalamin-deficient anemia include ileal disease, pancreatic insufficiency, strict vegetarianism, TCII deficiency, and fish tapeworm infestation.

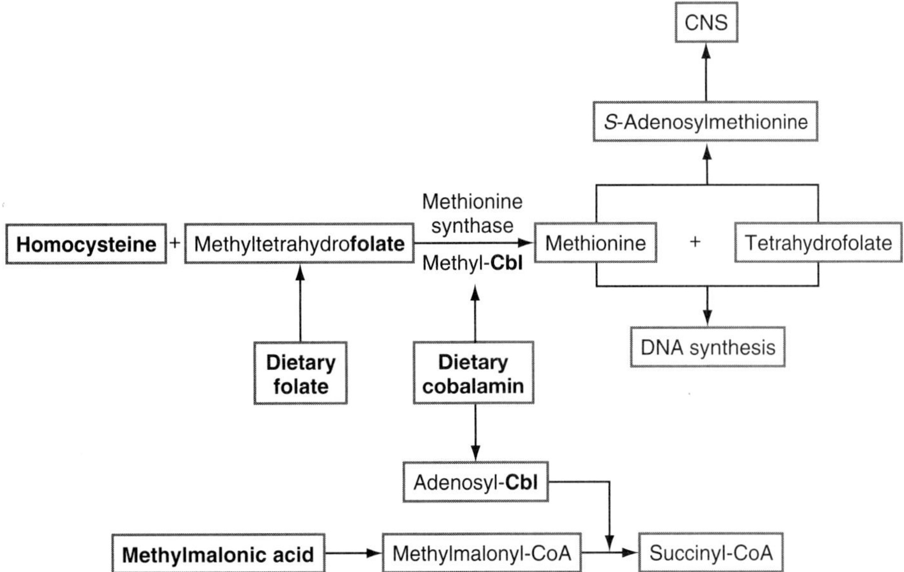

Figure 1. The role of cobalamin, folate, homocysteine, and methylmalonic acid in the synthesis of tetrahydrofolic acid, methionine, and succinyl-CoA. Cbl, cobalamin; CNS, central nervous system; CoA, coenzyme A.

Dietary folate is obtained primarily from vegetables, fruit, dairy products, and cereal. The recommended dietary allowance is 400 μg per day and the average body reserve is only 5 to 10 mg, which can be rapidly depleted in 2 to 4 months. Folate-deficient anemia most commonly develops with inadequate dietary intake. Other causes include increased demand in pregnancy and infancy, malabsorption in jejunal disease or short-bowel syndrome, impaired folate metabolism in alcoholic patients, and impaired folate absorption seen in tropical and nontropical sprue. Drugs that may induce a folate deficiency include anticonvulsants, oral contraceptives, triamterene, sulfasalazine, and methotrexate.

An acute and potentially fatal megaloblastic anemia may result from prolonged inhalation of nitrous oxide anesthesia, most commonly occurring with recreational abuse. Adenosylcobalamin, SAM, and total folate are depleted rapidly and methylcobalamin is quickly destroyed.

CLINICAL SIGNS AND SYMPTOMS

Cobalamin-deficient anemia becomes apparent after liver stores have been exhausted. It may take 5 to 15 years, depending on the etiology of the deficiency, for clinical symptoms to arise. Anemia may be moderate to severe by the time a patient seeks medical attention. Cobalamin deficiency affects all cells, but the cells that undergo rapid turnover are most likely to display abnormalities initially, for example, the gastrointestinal tract and bone marrow. A patient may present with a smooth and sore beefy red tongue from atrophic glossitis, loss of appetite, weakness, and diarrhea or constipation. Depending on which enzymatic cycle is more strongly disrupted, neurologic complications such as paresthesias, numbness, ataxia, and dementia can be evident first, especially in older adults.

Folic acid–deficient anemia can occur more rapidly because body folate stores remain adequate for only 2 to 4 months after the deficient state. The presentation may be similar to that of cobalamin deficiency, with diarrhea more common than constipation and usually without the neurologic symptoms. The weakness may progress slowly and is accompanied by headache, dyspnea, syncope, and palpitations. If neurologic symptoms are present, the patient may have an underlying cobalamin deficiency.

LABORATORY FINDINGS

Hematologic findings are identical in both cobalamin- and folate-deficient anemias. Declines in hemoglobin (Hb) and hematocrit (Hct) may be the initial laboratory finding in many patients after routine screening, but this usually follows an increase in mean corpuscular volume (MCV) of greater than 100 fL. A normal MCV may be present in coexisting iron deficiency, renal insufficiency, or an inflammatory process. Other findings include an elevated red cell distribution width (RDW), elevated mean corpuscular hemoglobin (MCH), and normal mean corpuscular hemoglobin concentration (MCHC).

Serum cobalamin is not a definitive diagnostic test because it may not be low in all patients with cobalamin deficiency. Clinically significant cobalamin deficiency has been found in 2.9% of patients with serum cobalamin levels greater than 200 pg/mL. Low serum cobalamin may be present in as many as 2.5% of normal healthy subjects who are not anemic.

Serum folate may be decreased for a variety of reasons including alcoholism, hemodialysis, or chronic disease. It is not an independent indicator of folate-deficient anemia but reflects only an imbalance between blood level and tissue deficiency. Red blood cell (RBC) folate decreases after body stores are depleted and reflects folate status at the time RBCs were produced.

Methylmalonic acid (MMA) and homocysteine (Hcy) serum levels have been markedly elevated in more than 90% of cobalamin-deficient patients before abnormalities in serum cobalamin. Elevated Hcy levels alone have been seen in approximately 80% of cases of strict folic acid deficiency and can accompany elevated MMA in 12% of these patients. They may be more sensitive markers than serum cobalamin or folate. L-Methylmalonyl-coenzyme A (CoA) mutase and methionine synthetase are cobalamin-dependent enzymes. Without cobalamin, methylmalonyl-CoA accumulates and eventually hydrolyzes to methylmalonic acid. Both folate and cobalamin play a role in homocysteine's conversion into methionine; therefore, homocysteine may be elevated in either folate or cobalamin deficiency (Table 1; see Figure 1).

Changes in the bone marrow occur because of maturation arrest of the immature cells. Megaloblastic changes in erythrocytes and white blood cells can be seen on peripheral blood and bone marrow smears. Besides being macrocytic, the neutrophils have hypersegmented nuclei. When greater than five lobes are present, a megaloblastic disorder is strongly suggested, and with greater than six lobes a diagnosis can be made. Mild pancytopenia is more commonly observed in cobalamin deficiency than folate deficiency.

The Schilling test can be used to differentiate between pernicious anemia and other causes of anemia. It is a less utilized tool because of the difficulty in performing the procedure and regulatory issues involving the use of a radioactive substance. The patient must initially ingest cobalt-labeled cyanocobalamin. Unlabeled cyanocobalamin is then injected intramuscularly (IM) at 1000 μg 1 hour later. A 24-hour urine collection begins at this time. The amount of oral cyanocobalamin absorbed in 1 hour can be measured by the total amount excreted in 24 hours because absorption ceased after the IM injection saturated all the tissue binding sites. A normal result is 8% to 40% elimination of the given oral dose.

When an abnormal result is obtained, a second test is performed to determine whether a lack of IF is responsible. The procedure is identical to the first test except that the IF is administered with the oral cyanocobalamin. If a normal result is obtained, a diagnosis of pernicious anemia is likely. If an abnormal result continues, the malabsorption may be attributed to other bowel disorders such as inflammatory bowel disease or following small-bowel resection.

A more frequently utilized test for pernicious anemia is the detection of parietal cell and/or IF antibodies. This test lacks specificity because these

TABLE 1. **Laboratory Findings for Cobalamin- and Folate-Deficient Anemias***

Hematologic Findings (Normal Range)	Cobalamin	Folate Deficiency Deficiency
Hemoglobin (14-18 g/dL males, 12-16 g/dL females)	⇓	⇓
Hematocrit (42-52% males, 37-47% females)	⇓	⇓
Mean corpuscular volume (80-90 fL males, 82-98 fL females)	⇑	⇑
Red cell distribution width (11.5-14.5%)	⇑	⇑
Mean corpuscular hemoglobin (27-33 pg/cell)	⇑	⇑
Mean corpuscular hemoglobin concentration (31-35 g/dL)	∅	∅
Serum cobalamin (190-900 ng/L)	⇓ or ∅	∅
Serum folate (≥3.5 μg/L)	∅	⇓
Red blood cell folate (5-15 ng/mL)	∅	⇓
Reticulocyte count (0.5-2.5%)	⇓ or ∅	⇓ or ∅
Methylmalonic acid (73-271 nmol/L)	⇑	∅
Homocysteine (5.4-16.2 μmol/L)	⇑	⇑

*⇑, increased; ⇓, decreased; ∅, within normal range.

autoantibodies are frequently detected in older adults and those with other autoimmune disorders.

TREATMENT

Cobalamin Deficiency

The goal of treatment is to replace liver stores and improve neurologic symptoms when present. Cyanocobalamin and hydroxocobalamin are the available derivatives of cobalamin for replacement therapy. Cyanocobalamin formulations include parenteral, administered IM or deep subcutaneously (SC), intranasal gel, and over-the-counter oral (PO) or sublingual tablets. Hydroxocobalamin is available only as an IM formulation. Cyanocobalamin has been the "gold standard" of treatment.

The patient with neurologic manifestations of cobalamin-deficient anemia may be treated with 1000 μg IM cyanocobalamin per day for 7 days, then weekly for 1 to 2 months until resolution of neurologic symptoms and normalization of Hb and Hct. Some experts recommend the continuation of 1000 μg IM injections every 2 weeks for 6 months.

It was well documented in the late 1950s that approximately 1% of an oral cyanocobalamin dose was absorbed by simple diffusion. Many small studies provide enough evidence to support the use of PO cyanocobalamin at 1000 to 2000 μg a day for initial treatment in patients without neurologic symptoms and as maintenance therapy in all patients with cobalamin-deficient anemia.

Patients should be counseled to avoid drinking ethanol with their cyanocobalamin replacement because ethanol decreases its absorption. Caution is also recommended with concurrent administration of aminosalicylic acid, chloramphenicol, cholestyramine, cimetidine, colchicine, neomycin, potassium, and ranitidine, which may also reduce absorption.

Optic atrophy has been reported to progress rapidly in some patients with early Leber's disease treated with cyanocobalamin. Hydroxocobalamin is the preferred supplement in these patients.

Folic Acid Deficiency

Before treating only folic acid deficiency, one must rule out the risk of underlying cobalamin deficiency. In an acutely ill patient, folic acid (folate, pteroylglutamic acid) may be administered IM at 1 to 5 mg and with cyanocobalamin if a combined deficiency exists. A dose of 1 to 2 mg PO daily is adequately absorbed in most patients, but 5 mg per day may be required for patients with a malabsorption syndrome.

Caution should be used when folate supplementation is necessary with phenytoin or fosphenytoin. Subtherapeutic serum phenytoin levels may result, placing patients at risk for seizure. Folate decreases the antiparasitic effect of pyrimethamine and should be avoided. Sulfasalazine has been shown to decrease the absorption of folate supplementation.

MONITORING

Reticulocyte counts normally begin to rise after a few days and peak in 1 week, whereas Hb continues to rise over 6 to 8 weeks. RBC, Hct, and MCV become normal in 1 to 3 months. MMA and Hcy tend to normalize in 7 to 14 days and are equated with evident deficiency. It has also been reported that Hcy may remain elevated in folic acid–deficient patients inappropriately treated with cyanocobalamin and MMA may remain elevated in cobalamin-deficient patients inappropriately treated with folic acid.

With initial cyanocobalamin replacement therapy for severe megaloblastic anemia, it is important to monitor serum potassium levels for the first 48 hours. Hypokalemia has resulted from increased potassium requirements by erythrocytes during conversion to normal erythropoiesis.

Other improvements include rapid resolution of classical symptoms of fatigue, glossitis, loss of appetite, and other gastrointestinal symptoms. Neurologic impairments should continue to improve over 1 to 2 months.

Monitoring continues to be lifelong. It is important that all patients understand the typical signs and symptoms of megaloblastic anemia and the importance of compliance with prescribed treatment. An initial 3- and 6-month laboratory evaluation assists in determining whether current supplementation is adequate.

THALASSEMIA

method of
SYLVIA TITI SINGER, M.D.
Children's Hospital Oakland
Oakland, California

The thalassemias, inherited disorders of hemoglobin synthesis, are the most common single gene diseases worldwide. Most forms are inherited in a mendelian recessive fashion from asymptomatic parents who are the gene carriers and have one chance in four of having an affected child. The disease results from a defective synthesis of one of the two globin chains, alpha (α) or beta (β), that constitute adult hemoglobin. More than 100,000 affected babies and several million heterozygotes are born annually. The highest incidence is in the "malaria belt," around the equator, as it reflects an advantage of the heterozygous form against *Plasmodium falciparum* malaria; however, as a result of population migration, it is found throughout the world. Clinically, there is a large variation, ranging from silent, asymptomatic carriers to those who depend on transfusions for survival. The latter, a severe form of the β-globin deficiency, is sometimes referred to as Cooley's anemia.

The last two decades have resulted in a broader understanding of the molecular mechanisms and pathophysiology of thalassemia, leading to successful prenatal diagnosis and improved supportive care as well as cure with bone marrow transplantation (BMT). These major advances have resulted in decreased morbidity and prolonged life expectancy, yet the issues of determining optimal care of the disease complications and choosing the best treatment option continue. In addition, prevention and treatment for patients in developing countries, where conventional treatment is often unavailable, are still a challenge.

PATHOPHYSIOLOGY

Formation of fully balanced normal hemoglobin requires tetramers consisting of two types of globin chains and a heme moiety. Different types of globin chains, classified as α-like or β-like, are synthesized and sequentially expressed in the embryo and fetus, declining after birth and replaced by the adult types α2β2 (hemoglobin A) and α2δ2 (hemoglobin A_2). The mechanisms that control the hemoglobin switch from fetal to adult hemoglobin, around 38 weeks of gestation, are not fully understood.

Thalassemia is caused by defective or absent synthesis of either of the two chains, α or β, of the adult hemoglobin tetramer as a result of a gene deletion or mutation. Classification is according to the particular globin chain that is ineffectively produced; α- and β-thalassemias are the more common and important types. Other, less common types include δβ-thalassemia and γδβ-thalassemia. Other hemoglobinopathies involve genes for structural hemoglobin variants, such as hemoglobins S, C, and E. Frequently, a gene for thalassemia from one parent is inherited along with one of these structural variants from another parent. The important diseases of this type are hemoglobin E-β thalassemia and sickle cell–thalassemia (S-β thalassemia), with the latter having clinical manifestations of sickle cell disease.

Decreased or absent globin chain synthesis results in a diminished amount of normal functional hemoglobin, increased hemolysis resulting in anemia, and an imbalance between the two globin types as the unaffected chain is continuously produced. The unpaired globin chain alters red cell cellular and membrane properties, leading to early destruction of cells in the bone marrow or ineffective erythropoiesis. Ineffective erythropoiesis is mainly a feature of β-thalassemia as the relative excess unstable α chains precipitate and disintegrate, causing oxidative damage to the red cell membrane. The excess of β chains in α-thalassemia is a more stable globin chain aggregate, resulting in less intramedullary cell death, accounting for the differences in disease symptoms and severity. The mutations causing β-thalassemia can be classified as resulting in either a complete absence of β-globin production—β zero thalassemia (β0)—or a reduction in synthesis—β plus thalassemia (β+). Over 200 different mutations have been described; the majority are nucleotide substitutions. In addition to the underlying β mutation, which affects the level of β-globin chain synthesis, other globin chain factors and gene modifiers are involved in altering the phenotype.

α-Thalassemia is caused by a different mechanism, as normal individuals inherit two α-globin genes from each parent, resulting in an α,α/α,α genotype. The majority of mutations are gene deletions, and phenotypic expression is dependent on the number of available α genes: Homozygous state, deletion of four α-globin genes (– –/– –), results in hydrops fetalis, a severe, usually fatal disease in utero or shortly after birth. The excess γ chains in the hydropic fetus form tetramers named hemoglobin Barts, which can be detected on hemoglobin electrophoresis in the newborn. It is a useless type of hemoglobin as it cannot deliver oxygen. The few cases that have survived the perinatal period are transfusion dependent and have a high prevalence of malformations. Hemoglobin H disease, characterized by three α-globin gene deletions, is a combination of a *cis* deletion and a single α-globin gene deletion (α–/– –), resulting in a moderately severe anemia. The remaining unpaired β-globin chains form tetramers named hemoglobin H. Hydrops fetalis and hemoglobin H disease are generally found in Southeast Asian individuals because both require *cis* α gene deletion, known as (– –SEA), which is endemic to that area. The α-thalassemia trait is expressed by two α gene deletions, a *trans* deletion (α–/α–) or a *cis* deletion (α,α/– –), causing mild microcytic hypochromic anemia. Silent carriers have one gene deletion and three intact α-globin genes (α,α/α–) and are clinically and hematologically undetectable. One important nondeletion α mutation, termed Constant Spring, results in an elongated α chain because of a mutation in the stop codon of the α gene and is inherited in conjunction with two other deleted α genes.

CLINICAL PRESENTATION

α-Thalassemia

Hemoglobin H disease, involving three α gene deletions, is common in people of Asian descent and causes a chronic moderately severe hemolytic anemia. Patients may have splenomegaly or cholelithiasis and may require transfusions during episodes of oxidative stress induced by infections, fever, or certain medications. Hemoglobin H–Constant Spring, the co-inheritance of a nondeletional α gene variant, arises with more severe hemolytic anemia and hypersplenism requiring more frequent transfusions. Patients are observed periodically, at 3- to 6-month intervals, for monitoring of spleen size, hemoglobin level, and growth pattern. Special attention is required during febrile episodes, when the hemoglobin can drop precipitously. The main treatment measures are supplementation with daily folic acid and family education on the potential hemolytic risks involved with high fevers and the use of certain medications. A partial list includes sulfa, antimalaria agents, aspirin, and naphthalene.

β-Thalassemia Major and Thalassemia Intermedia

The important forms of β-thalassemia are classified on the basis of their clinical severity into thalassemia major and thalassemia intermedia. However, even within these categories there is a remarkable variability from a mild anemia to complete transfusion dependence for survival. Patients with thalassemia major usually develop severe anemia (hemoglobin less than 5 g/dL) within the first 6 months of life because the decreasing levels of fetal hemoglobin cannot be replaced by normal adult hemoglobin. Transfusion therapy is usually initiated to "turn off" the marrow and halt continuous marrow expansion. If regular transfusion therapy is not initiated, a clinical picture of severe untreated β-thalassemia, typical Cooley's anemia, develops: profound anemia, splenomegaly, progressive bone changes, and masses of extramedullary hematopoiesis caused by marrow expansion. β-Thalassemia intermedia arises later, usually during the second year of life, not requiring early intervention with blood transfusions. These patients with a moderate but well-compensated anemia usually grow and develop well. However, not infrequently symptoms of progressive anemia, heart failure, pulmonary hypertension, hypersplenism, and bone expansion evolve during the second and third decades of life. These clinical developments essentially categorize the patient as having thalassemia major, frequently necessitating initiation of regular transfusion therapy. Identifying the β genotype molecular defect alone cannot fully predict the phenotype—major versus intermedia—as other genetic and environmental factors can modify the severity of the disease. β-Thalassemia trait, the heterozygote or carrier state, is generally asymptomatic and has mainly a screening and diagnostic significance for genetic counseling. In clinical practice it occasionally needs to be distinguished from iron deficiency.

Hemoglobin E/β-thalassemia is one of the most common types of β-thalassemia, prevalent primarily in Southeast Asia and in other countries because of population migration. Double heterozygotes for both β and E mutations have a clinically severe thalassemia. However, a large clinical variability ranging from severe transfusion-dependent thalassemia major phenotype to a mild anemia exists. The majority of patients have a thalassemia intermedia phenotype and do not always require early transfusion treatment. Confusion can occur in newborn hemoglobin electrophoresis between the mild form of EE and the severe form of E/β-thalassemia as both have no hemoglobin A present and similar hemoglobin E and F levels; therefore, parental testing is occasionally required.

DIAGNOSIS

Newborn screening, if implemented, detects new cases, which are then referred for laboratory and clinical follow-up. In older children and adults, especially women of reproductive age and belonging to ethnic groups at high risk for thalassemia, alertness concerning the carrier state with a microcytic, hypochromic anemia is important. Further screening with hemoglobin electrophoresis and quantitative hemoglobin A_2 should be performed, and other causes for microcytic anemia need to be ruled out first. If α-thalassemia is suspected, usually with a mildly elevated hemoglobin F level or presence of hemoglobin Barts, referral to centers that can identify the different forms by DNA testing is recommended. Table 1 presents general guidelines for clinical and laboratory screening for thalassemia. When a couple at risk for having a child with thalassemia has been identified, genetic counseling and education regarding prenatal testing should be offered. Prenatal testing is accomplished by fetal DNA polymerase chain reaction (PCR) methods or

TABLE 1. **Diagnostic Features for α and β Carrier State and Hemoglobin H Disease**

Diagnosis	Red Blood Cell Parameters	Hemoglobin Electrophoresis*	DNA Testing	Treatment
Silent carrier (–α/αα) or α-Thalassemia trait (– –/αα) or (–α/–α)	Normal Hb/slightly low Low MCV for age Normal RDW	HbF normal $HbA_2 < 3\%$	Diagnostic	No treatment. Screen partner, genetic counseling
HbH disease (–α/– –)	Low Hb (7–9 g/dL) Low MCV (50–65 fL) Hypochromia, fragmented cells	Hb Bart's 5% (higher in newborn) HbH (~10%) HbF mildly elevated 1%–3%	Diagnostic	Screen partner, genetic counseling Avoid oxidative stress–inducing medications Transfusions or splenectomy may be clinically indicated
HbH-(CS) (– –/$\alpha\alpha^{cs}$)	Low Hb (7–8 g/dL) Moderately low MCV Severe hypochromia	HbH (~10%) HbCS (2%–3%) occasionally found	Indicated For diagnosis	
β-Thalassemia trait	Normal-low Hb Low MCV Normal RDW Elevated RBC	HbF elevated (2%–7%) HbA_2 3.5%–7%	Gene mapping recommended	No treatment. Screen partner, genetic counseling

*Hemoglobin electrophoresis, the initial test for detection of the variant hemoglobin, can also detect β hemoglobin variants, such as HbE, S, or the Constant Spring α globin variant. Other techniques can further specify type and severity of disease.

Abbreviations: CS, Constant Spring; Hb, hemoglobin; MCV, mean cell volume; RDW, red cell distribution width.

later by direct fetal hemoglobin testing. The relation between genotype and phenotype enables prediction of the likely prognosis for a particular genotype a child may inherit, although it is difficult to predict with certainty.

TREATMENTS AND DECISION MAKING FOR TREATMENT OPTIONS

The standard of treatment for a child with newly diagnosed β-thalassemia major is still regular transfusion therapy along with an iron-chelating agent. The decision to start transfusions is a difficult one; it is usually a lifelong commitment and has its own risks and side effects beside the emotional impact. Although usually signs of worsening anemia, splenomegaly and poor growth, determine the need for the start of transfusions, other considerations must be addressed as well. Patients may be classified as having thalassemia intermedia on the basis of the level of anemia and DNA mutation, requiring close follow-up for timing and type of treatment intervention but not necessarily early initiation of chronic transfusions. Furthermore, occasional worsening anemia is a result of a superimposed nutritional deficiency such as folic acid or iron deficiency or an infectious complication, and unnecessary premature start of transfusion therapy can be avoided. Other treatment modalities such as BMT or drugs aimed at increasing the fetal and total hemoglobin should be considered if indicated. Table 2 lists laboratory tests and considerations prior to the start of transfusions.

Transfusions

Anemia and erythropoiesis, the main complications of thalassemia, are ameliorated by chronic transfusion therapy. Current goals of chronic transfusion also include lessening iron intake as opposed to the earlier approach, in which an attempt was made to suppress marrow erythropoiesis completely by maintaining a higher post-transfusion hemoglobin. Patients receive transfusions every 3 to 4 weeks and maintain baseline pretransfusion hemoglobin of 9.5 to 10.5 g/dL and post-transfusion hemoglobin of 13 to 13.5 g/dL. This adequately eradicates the consequences of anemia and erythropoiesis, yet minimizes iron accumulation. Baseline iron level and liver function, as well as blood safety, need to be considered for any patient starting transfusions (Table 3; see Table 2).

Considerations for Splenectomy

Without transfusion therapy, or occasionally even with chronic transfusions, extramedullary hematopoiesis leads to splenomegaly and hypersplenism. It was generally thought that splenectomy may decrease the transfusion requirements by increasing red cell survival and has been recommended when the total yearly red blood cell use exceeds 200 mL/kg. However, spleen removal does not always result in sustained reduced blood consumption and/or a substantial decrease of iron burden. In young children, a known risk of overwhelming sepsis exists. In addition, it is possible that pulmonary vascular disease and thrombosis may be long-term problems in splenectomized patients. If splenectomy is planned, vaccination with 23-valent (Pneumovax 23) and/or 7-valent pneumococcal vaccine (Prevnar) and *Haemophilus influenzae* (Comvax) and meningococcal vaccines (Menomune), ideally 3 to 6 weeks prior to splenectomy, is required along with family education concerning the risk of life-threatening infection. After splenectomy, lifelong penicillin prophylaxis* is recommended, and a low-dose antiplatelet agent should be considered, especially in older splenectomized patients.

Fetal Hemoglobin Augmentation

Induction or reactivation of γ-globin synthesis, which combines with α chains to produce hemoglobin F, can result in a higher fetal hemoglobin and may

*Not FDA approved for this indication.

TABLE 2. **Recommended Measurements prior to the Initiation of Transfusion Therapy**

Measurement	Test	Significance
Thalassemia mutation	DNA mapping (α and β)	1. Prediction of clinical phenotype (limited) 2. Future genetic counseling
RBC phenotype	ABO + RBC minor antigen determination	Provide phenotypically matched blood to avoid future alloimmunization.
HLA typing	Patient and full siblings	Identify potential BMT donor and inform the family about this therapeutic option
Screening for hepatitis, baseline liver status	Liver function tests, hepatitis A, B, and C serology. Obtain PCR if serology is positive for hepatitis B or C	Increased risk for liver disease Treatment intervention if PCR positive
Assessment of immunization records and vaccination as needed	Hepatitis A and B	Avoid blood-transmitted hepatitis
	Streptococcus pneumoniae	Obtain immunity prior to possible splenectomy 1. Valent conjugate pneumococcal vaccine (Prevnar) 2. Booster with 23-valent vaccine (Pneumovax 23) at age 5 to 10 years
	Influenza	Immunize annually—decrease infectious risk
	Haemophilus influenzae	Obtain immunity prior to splenectomy

TABLE 3. **Guidelines for Monitoring Patients Receiving Transfusion and Chelation Therapy**

Blood transfusion
Prestorage leukoreduced packed red blood cells every 2–4 wk
Target pretransfusion hemoglobin at 9–10 g%
Mean hemoglobin 12–12.5 g%
Total annual transfusion requirement ~200 mL/kg/y
Consider immune hemolysis with a Coombs test in case of unusually low pretransfusion hemoglobin
Iron load and chelation
Quarterly ferritin level
Initiate chelation: ~age 3 y. Ferritin level ~1000 μg/dL in two or three measurements or at approximately 3.2–7 mg iron per gram liver dry weight
Liver iron assessment every 1–2 y
Deferoxamine toxicity
Quarterly hearing and vision screen
Annual audiology and ophthalmology evaluation
Growth measurement: monthly height, biannual sitting height, annual growth velocity
Annual measurement of chelatable trace elements and antioxidant elements: zinc, copper, selenium, vitamins C and E

improve overall hemoglobin production and reduce ineffective erythropoiesis. This cost-effective investigational approach can in some cases decrease transfusion dependence or increase hemoglobin in nontransfused patients. The most frequently used compounds, hydroxyurea* and butyrate, have demonstrated remarkable effectiveness in subgroups of patients with specific mutations and resulted in milder or no responses in many others. Several studies have used high-dose erythropoietin (Epogen)* as a single agent or in combination with hydroxyurea.* Patients with thalassemia intermedia and those with E-β thalassemia mutation should be considered for a trial of drug treatment that in some cases can reduce or delay the need for transfusions and chelation therapy and improve quality of life. More research on other pharmacologic compounds, combination therapy, and best patients as candidates is required.

Bone Marrow Transplantation

Although somewhat debatable because of the procedure's usual toxic and infectious risks from the myeloablative pretransplantation conditioning regimens, transplantation from an HLA-matched sibling donor is the only available cure of thalassemia at this time. Obtaining HLA typing for patients and their siblings and discussing BMT if applicable are important in the early stages of the disease course. More than a thousand HLA-identical successful transplantations have been performed. However, only a small percentage (estimated at 30%) of patients who have a matched donor, as well as low risk factors, can undergo the procedure. Studies from the early 1990s showed that transplant outcome is based on the risk categories of adequacy of chelation, degree of hepatomegaly, and hepatic portal fibrosis. Overall, younger patients and those lacking complications of the disease or its treatment, in particular chronic hepatitis, have the best outcome. BMT from alternative donors such as HLA-matched unrelated donors and HLA-nonidentical relatives is not routinely used and has involved high rates of graft failure and graft-versus-host disease. More recent promising investigational approaches include nonmyeloablative, chimer-inducing regimens to reduce the transplant-related toxicity and the use of umbilical cord blood stem cells, which may yield improved results even in high-risk patients. After a successful BMT, patients need to continue iron chelation therapy for removal of the preexisting iron load.

ASSESSMENT OF BODY IRON BURDEN AND CHELATION THERAPY

Iron overload is a major complication of β-thalassemia and unless adequately removed is the cause of organ damage, morbidity, and mortality. A packed red blood cell unit of 250 mL delivers approximately 175 mg of iron. As iron accumulates in the parenchyma and non–transferrin-bound iron is present in plasma, progressive dysfunction of the heart, liver, and endocrine organs occurs. A single method for measuring body iron load does not exist. Periodic assessment of ferritin levels is most commonly used, but it is a poor indicator of iron load. Measuring hepatic iron concentration by liver biopsy is considered the most sensitive method, providing quantitation of iron concentration and extent of liver damage as well as predicting the threshold for risk of cardiac disease and early death (levels of 15 mg/g dry weight or more). It is recommended that biopsy be performed every 1 to 2 years or more frequently if liver pathology related to hepatitis needs to be assessed. Magnetic susceptometry using a superconducting quantum interference device (SQUID) is not generally available but provides an excellent noninvasive correlation with liver biopsy–determined iron concentration. When liver iron is unavailable, persistent ferritin levels over 2500 μg/L can assist in predicting development of cardiac disease.

Methods for removal of the tissue iron with chelation therapy are a major aspect of thalassemia management, as no physiologic mechanism for excreting excess iron exists. Optimal body iron corresponds to a hepatic iron range of approximately 3 to 7 mg iron per gram liver dry weight. Subcutaneous deferoxamine (Desferal) administration is the best means of iron chelation at this time, requiring continuous infusion given with a portable pump. It can also be given as an intravenous infusion but not orally because of its poor gastrointestinal absorption. A dose of 20 to 50 mg/kg/day (lower doses for young children and higher for patients with severe iron overload) given over 8 to 10 hours, usually 5 nights a week, is recommended. Higher doses are given to patients with life-threatening iron-induced organ damage. Oral vitamin C (250 mg) given with deferoxamine chelation optimizes the mobilization of iron. Periodic monitoring for potential side effects is recommended (see Table 3) as dose reduction or stopping treatment is sometimes needed. Although it is an effective chelator, compliance

*Not FDA approved for this indication.

remains poor in approximately 50% of patients because of its cumbersome, uncomfortable, and expensive mode of administration. Alternative approaches, aimed at decreasing the frequency and duration of administration, are under investigation, including a long-acting hydroxyethyl starch deferoxamine. Extensive research for developing an effective oral iron chelator is under way with several agents having reached clinical trials. The most extensively evaluated is deferiprone (Ferriprox, L1).* Data have shown its short-term efficacy at a dose of 75 mg/kg/d, although variation in response and relation of efficacy to the iron load have been reported. Controversy over its toxicity and effectiveness and lack of controlled studies have limited its widespread use. Studies have suggested an additive effect of using deferoxamine with deferiprone,*,† especially for cardiac iron chelation. More studies are under way for assessment of L1 with Desferal effectiveness and toxicity. Another oral chelator currently entering a clinical trial phase in North America is the tridentate synthetic chelator ICL670.‡

MONITORING AND TREATMENT OF DISEASE COMPLICATIONS IN CHRONICALLY TRANSFUSED PATIENTS

Many of the classical Cooley's anemia manifestations are not apparent in developed countries where patients typically receive transfusions from infancy; hence, the disease expression becomes the consequences of chronic blood transfusions, namely those of iron overload and blood-transmitted infections. Thus, although thalassemia major is a treatable condition with regular transfusions and lifelong iron chelation, it remains a complex, multiorgan disease requiring close monitoring and treatment interventions (Table 4).

The Heart

Mortality from cardiac disease (heart failure or fatal arrhythmia) remains the main cause of death in patients with transfusion-induced iron overload. However, as patients' life expectancies have improved, it has become evident that early and effective chelation can prevent death from cardiac disease. Quantitation of cardiac iron has been difficult, although a technique using T2-weighted magnetic resonance imaging showed good correlation with cardiac iron stores. Regular monitoring for cardiac function and arrhythmias with annual echocardiography, electrocardiography, and 24-hour Holter monitoring is important, although not sufficiently sensitive for early detection of disease. When cardiac dysfunction is diagnosed, aggressive chelation along with cardiac medications should be started as it can still be reversed and improved.

*Not available in the United States.
†Not FDA approved for this indication.
‡Investigational drug in the United States.

TABLE 4. **Guidelines for Screening and Monitoring Organ Dysfunction in Patients Receiving Regular Transfusions**

CARDIAC DISEASE
Annual echocardiography, electrocardiography, Holter monitoring for those older than 10 years
Antioxidants: Annual vitamin C and E levels
LIVER DISEASE
Quarterly liver function tests, bilirubin
Annual hepatitis serology, or sooner if liver function tests elevated
Hepatitis C or B polymerase chain reaction (if serology is positive)
ENDOCRINOPATHIES
Annual thyroid function: triiodothyronine, free thyroxine, thyroid-stimulating hormone*
Annual parathyroid function: parathyroid hormone, calcium, ionized calcium*
Annual fasting glucose, add oral glucose tolerance test if abnormal*
Assess for osteopenia and osteoporosis: Annual bone density (starting at age ~10 years)†
Annual testosterone—males*
Luteinizing hormone, follicle-stimulating hormone, estradiol as clinically indicated—females*
Referral to a fertility clinic and infertility workup when indicated
GROWTH DELAY
Bone age, Tanner stage
Assess for growth hormone deficiency: insulin-like growth factor (IGF) 1, IGF binding protein 3

*Hormone replacement as indicated.
†Calcium 1000–1400 mg/d, with vitamin D (400 U/d), consider biphosphonates to inhibit bone resorption.

Liver Damage and Hepatitis

Iron-induced hepatic disease is frequently worsened by coexistence of hepatitis C. Most hepatitis C–infected patients have chronic hepatitis; however, cirrhosis, liver failure, or hepatocellular carcinoma may develop and therefore regular monitoring of liver function tests and antibody for hepatitis C and hepatitis C PCR are essential if indicated. Treatment with interferon alfa-2b (Intron A), 3 million units by subcutaneous injection three times a week, or combination treatment using interferon alfa and ribavirin (Rebetron) 1000 to 1200 mg daily, resulted in clearance of hepatitis C virus RNA and improved liver histology. Studies under way are looking at the effect of pegylated alpha interferon (PEG-Intron, Pegasys), which has the advantage of once-a-week treatment and fewer side effects.

Endocrinopathies

Iron deposition in the anterior pituitary gland, thyroid, and parathyroid glands as well as pancreatic cells and adrenal cells can result in endocrine dysfunctions; delayed puberty, short stature, and hypogonadism. In addition to chelation therapy, close monitoring of growth pattern, pubertal stage, and laboratory tests can assist in early intervention with specific therapy (see Table 4). Specific treatments are available: Growth hormone shots, estrogen replacement for early menopause and loss of bone mass in women, and testosterone for men are often needed. Impaired glucose tolerance with progression to diabetes mellitus is another serious complication requiring routine testing and standard diabetes treatment when diagnosed.

Bone Disease

Bone complications, osteopenia and osteoporosis, affect a majority of adult patients, even those who have adequate transfusion or chelation status. Persistent backache, scoliosis, fractures, cord compression, and spinal deformities can occur. The patients with diabetes, pubertal delay, or male gender appear to be most frequently and severely affected by osteoporosis. Inadequate calcium and vitamin D levels, hypoparathyroidism, lack of physical activity, iron deposition in the bone matrix, and long-term deferoxamine (Desferal) chelation are all contributing factors. Early diagnoses of low bone mass and treatment intervention are extremely important. Yearly screening starting in the second decade with dual-energy x-ray absorptiometry (DEXA), a low-irradiation safe technique, is the preferred method for bone density assessment. Treatment measures include calcium supplementation (1000 mg/d, 1200 to 1400 mg/d for adolescents), maintenance of normal levels of vitamin D, and nutritional counseling as well as hormone replacement therapy for hypogonadism to achieve a normal peak bone mass. Biphosphonates such as sodium alendronate (Fosamax), 5 mg/d or 35 mg weekly inhibit osteoclastic bone resorption and have been reported to improve bone density.

FUTURE PERSPECTIVES AND CHALLENGES

Thalassemia is a widespread, highly prevalent disease. Thanks to improved medical and health care, life expectancy for both affected infants and young adults has improved. With current research advances, we can expect improvements in standards of treatment for the management of thalassemia: improved screening of involved organs such as the heart and endocrine organs, development of new iron chelators, and prevention and early treatment of transfusion-transmitted hepatitis C disease. In addition, advances in prenatal screening using DNA mutation analysis are likely. Further research investigating new methods for BMT and stem cell transplantation, gene therapy, and gene manipulations is also anticipated.

SICKLE CELL DISEASE

method of
KATHRYN L. HASSELL, M.D.
University of Colorado Health Sciences Center
Denver, Colorado

The term sickle cell disease refers to a group of inherited hemoglobinopathies in which one gene for the β-globin chain of hemoglobin has the sickle cell mutation (valine for glutamine at the sixth position) and the other gene is abnormal in some way. Sickle cell anemia (hemoglobin SS [HbSS]), occurs when both genes that produce β-globin chains have the sickle mutation. Other common variants include sickle cell hemoglobin C disease (HbSC disease), in which one β-globin gene has the sickle mutation and the other β-globin gene produces hemoglobin C. Sickle cell disease also occurs when one β-globin gene has the sickle mutation and the other underproduces normal β-globin chain; the defect is called β-thalassemia. If the thalassemic gene produces some normal β-globin, the disease sickle β^+-thalassemia is present. If the thalassemic gene produces no β-globin chains, the disease sickle β°-thalassemia is present. Less common variants of sickle cell disease include sickle hemoglobin D (HbSD), sickle hemoglobin E (HbSE), and sickle hemoglobin O_{Arab} ($HbSO_{Arab}$).

If a person inherits one β-globin gene that has the sickle cell mutation and a normal β-globin gene, the person has sickle cell trait. This genetic carrier state results in normal hematologic parameters and no significant health effects.

PATHOPHYSIOLOGY OF SICKLE CELL DISEASE

The underlying pathophysiology of sickle cell disease begins when a gene controlling hemoglobin production switches from producing fetal hemoglobin (which does not contain β-globin chain) to adult hemoglobin (which contains β-globin chains). In the case of sickle cell disease, β-globin chains have the sickle mutation. This switch usually occurs between 2 to 6 months of life.

CHRONIC HEMOLYSIS

It is important to recognize the different variants of sickle cell disease as the severity of the illness and age of onset of some complications are, to some extent, related to the underlying genetic abnormality. Sickle hemoglobin forms long, rodlike polymers within red blood cells (RBCs) when there are changes in intracellular factors, including oxygenation, hydration, and ion content. These polymers distort RBCs into different shapes, including the typical sickle cell. This polymerization is initially reversible, and cells "sickle" and "unsickle" for a number of cycles until the polymerization becomes irreversible. This irreversibly sickled cell is fragile and susceptible to hemolysis, leading to the chronic hemolytic anemia seen in sickle cell disease.

The propensity to and frequency of polymerization of sickle hemoglobin depend on the nature and concentration of the hemoglobin in the RBC. The prototypic example is sickle cell anemia, in which the RBC content predominantly sickles hemoglobin and the chronic hemolytic anemia is severe, resulting in low baseline hemoglobin values, increased indirect bilirubin, increased aspartate transaminase (AST), increased lactate dehydrogenase (LDH), and a compensatory elevation of baseline reticulocyte count. In sickle β°-thalassemia, in which the only functional gene is a sickle cell gene, the hemolytic anemia is similarly severe, but the RBCs are microcytic because

TABLE 1. **Hematologic Characteristics of Common Sickle Cell Diseases and Sickle Cell Trait**

Disease	Baseline Hemoglobin Concentration (g/dL)	Mean Corpuscular Volume	Baseline Reticulocyte (%)	Relative Clinical Severity
HbSS (sickle cell anemia)	6.0–9.0	Normal	5–30	++++
HbSβ°-thalassemia	6.0–9.0	Low	5–30	++++
HbSC (sickle hemoglobin C disease)	10–13	Normal	3–4	+++
HbSβ$^+$-thalassemia	10–14	Low	3–4	++
HbAS (sickle cell trait)	14–16	Normal	Normal	0

Hb, hemoglobin.

of the underproduction of hemoglobin with the thalassemia defect. In other variants of sickle cell disease, the relative degree of anemia and reticulocytosis depends on how readily sickle polymers form in the RBC. For example, hemoglobin C and hemoglobin A (normal adult hemoglobin) tend to interfere to some extent with polymerization, so the degree of hemolytic anemia is generally less in patients with hemoglobin SC disease and sickle-β$^+$-thalassemia. Table 1 depicts some of the common sickle cell variants and their usual hematologic parameters.

CHRONIC MICROVASCULAR INJURY

Even when not sickled, RBCs that contain sickle hemoglobin are abnormal. These RBCs have damaged membranes and adhesion molecules on their surface that lead to adhesion to vessel walls, especially in the postcapillary venules, even when they are not sickled. If they are retained in the vessel and accumulate, they are susceptible to deoxygenation, sickling, and hemolysis. If they detach from the vessel wall, chronic vessel wall injury occurs. Chronic microvascular injury contributes to splenic infarction, retinopathy, chronic renal disease, osteonecrosis of the humeral or femoral heads, chronic lung injury, and other chronic complications seen in sickle cell disease. This ongoing injury is often clinically silent until overt organ damage is apparent and occurs even in patients who have infrequent or rare pain events.

ACUTE VASO-OCCLUSIVE EVENTS

A sickle cell pain event probably occurs when RBCs (unsickled or sickled) attach and accumulate in an area of activated or damaged endothelium, leading to temporary vaso-occlusion. Transient endothelial injury may be induced by infection or inflammation associated with cytokine release, dehydration, hypoxia, chemical or severe metabolic abnormalities, or other stimuli, resulting in increased adherence of RBCs and compromise of flow with downstream ischemia and pain. Therapy is directed at reversal of endothelial injury and RBC adhesion, as well as minimizing sickle hemoglobin polymerization. It is not always possible to identify the acute changes that lead to a clinical pain event.

ACUTE COMPLICATIONS ASSOCIATED WITH ACUTE PAIN EVENTS

The acute complications that occur in patients with sickle cell disease and their treatments are summarized in Table 2.

Acute Vaso-Occlusive Pain Event

In the majority of patients with sickle cell disease, including those with sickle cell anemia, care for an acute pain event is sought from health care providers less than once per year. The majority of pain events are actually experienced by a minority of patients with sickle cell disease and not always by those with apparently more severe forms of the disease.

As described in the pathophysiology section, a pain event occurs when RBCs adhere to damaged or activated endothelium leading to transient vaso-occlusion. The pain tends to occur in a pattern characteristic for each patient, although severe pain events may result in diffuse pain or pain in atypical locations. Despite the acute nature of vaso-occlusive pain, hematologic parameters including hemoglobin, hematocrit, and reticulocyte count often do not significantly change. A significant change in these parameters may indicate additional complication of sickle cell disease, such as an aplastic crisis or the presence of acute end-organ damage. Underlying conditions, including infection, dehydration, hypoxia, or other stressors, should be carefully sought and reversed if present.

There are no data demonstrating the benefits of excessive intravenous hydration and excessive supplemental oxygen. The goal of these interventions is to maintain adequate hydration and adequate oxygenation. Excessive intravenous hydration may be associated with the development of acute syndrome.

Prompt aggressive therapy of pain is critical in minimizing the duration of an event. For mild pain events, adequate therapy may include rest, oral hydration, and oral non-narcotic pain medication including acetaminophen or ibuprofen. Moderately severe pain may require oral medications containing narcotics, such as acetaminophen with codeine, or even short-term intravenous fluids and doses of parenteral narcotic medications. For pain events that fail to resolve with conservation management or are quite severe from the outset, intravenous fluids to maintain

TABLE 2. **Acute Complications Associated with Sickle Cell Disease**

Complications	Affected Patients (Age, Disease Type)	Features	Treatment
Pain event	All	Pain	Standing dose or PCA narcotics Fluids if needed to maintain hydration Oxygen if needed to maintain normal O_2 Reversal of any triggering factors
Dactylitis	Young children	Painful swollen hands or feet	As above
Acute chest syndrome (ACS)	All	Hypoxia, chest pain, infiltrate, or chest radiograph	Standing dose or PCA narcotics Judicious use of fluids Oxygen to maintain normal O_2 Empirical antibiotic therapy Transfusion therapy
Acute multiorgan failure syndrome	All	ACS ± acute hepatic ± acute renal failure Rhabdomyolysis	As above
Splenic infarction	Sickle cell anemia: <age 2 Milder sickle cell diseases: into adulthood	Left upper quadrant (LUQ) pain, nausea, vomiting, left plural effusion	Standing dose or PCA narcotics Maintain hydration Oxygen if needed to maintain normal O_2 Careful monitoring for ↓hemoglobin/platelets
Priapism	All	Painful sustained erection	Standing dose or PCA narcotics Hydration Oxygen if needed to maintain normal O_2 Transfusion therapy (exchange) Irrigation with phenylephrine Drainage/shunt procedure
Splenic sequestration	Sickle cell anemia: <2-3 y of age Milder forms of sickle cell disease into adulthood	Signs/symptoms of anemia LUQ discomfort, enlarged spleen Shock	Volume resuscitation Simple transfusion if needed
Aplastic crisis	All	Signs/symptoms of anemia	Simple transfusion if necessary
Ischemic stroke	Children, most common ages 5-10 Less common in adults	Focal neurologic symptoms Headache Seizures	Exchange transfusion Supportive neurologic care
Hemorrhagic stroke	Adolescents and adults	Headaches Seizures Focal neurologic symptoms	Exchange transfusion Supportive neurologic care
Bacterial sepsis	Children <5 y old All	Signs/symptoms infection Fever	Antibiotic therapy
Cholecystitis	All	Right upper quadrant pain ↑ Bilirubin, alkaline phosphatase	Antibiotic therapy Supportive care Elective cholecystectomy after first episode

PCA, patient-controlled analgesia.

normal hydration and parenteral narcotics through a patient-controlled analgesia device or intravenous narcotics administered on a regular schedule are necessary. Pain medication should be offered around the clock, *not* per required need ("prn"). Use of prn scheduling allows the pain to rebuild again rather than maintaining adequate pain control. Anti-inflammatory medication may be a useful adjunct to narcotic therapy.

Pain events often last 5 to 10 days and resolve gradually. Between episodes, most patients are pain free and do not require chronic pain medication unless a chronic pain syndrome has developed

Dactylitis (Hand-Foot Syndrome)

This unique manifestation of sickle cell disease tends to occur in infants and children younger than 3 years and may be the first clinical manifestation. This generalized osteitis causes painful swelling of the hands and feet and is treated with pain medication.

ACUTE COMPLICATIONS ASSOCIATED WITH END-ORGAN INJURY

Acute Chest Syndrome

The development of hypoxia, chest pain, shortness of breath, and an infiltrate on chest radiography is characteristic of acute chest syndrome. Fifteen percent to 40% of sickle cell disease patients experience this acute complication. Sequestration of RBCs in the pulmonary circulation, with endothelial injury, results in vasoconstriction and interstitial edema and may be accompanied by fever, a fall in hemoglobin, and thrombocytopenia. This complication may be triggered by a number of events, including pulmonary infection and fat embolism from areas of infarcted bone marrow. Empirical antibiotic therapy should be given. Early recognition and therapy probably reduce the mortality and morbidity associated with this syndrome. Treatment includes adequate oxygen supplementation, adequate pain control to reduce splinting, avoidance of excessive intravenous fluids, incentive spirometry, and in many cases transfusion therapy (see "Transfusion Therapy"). Use of inhaled nitric oxide resulted in improvement in some anecdotal cases and is under investigation.

Acute Multiorgan Failure Syndrome

Patients who present with severe diffuse pain events, especially if they have a relatively high baseline hemoglobin (≥9 g/dL), may develop acute multiorgan failure syndrome. Acute chest syndrome, acute hepatic, and/or renal failure develops rapidly over 6 to 12 hours, often heralded by the development of fever, mental status changes, and a fall in hemoglobin and platelet count. As this syndrome clinically resembles sepsis, empirical antibiotic therapy should be given. Early recognition and aggressive supportive care, including transfusion, can reverse this potentially fatal complication of sickle cell disease.

Splenic Infarction

The process of autosplenectomy, which generally occurs before the age of 2 in children with sickle cell anemia and sickle β°-thalassemia, is generally clinically silent. In patients with less severe sickle cell diseases, however, the spleen is more variably affected and may survive chronic injury from sickle RBCs into adulthood. In these patients, focal acute occlusion may result in areas of infarction, which manifest with pain in the left upper quadrant, nausea, vomiting, and occasionally a sympathetic left pleural effusion. Treatment is supportive, with aggressive pain management, adequate intravenous hydration, and careful observation for fall in hemoglobin and/or platelet count that may herald splenic sequestration (see the section on splenic sequestration). Splenic infarction has occurred rarely in persons with sickle cell trait, usually those of non-African descent, when they are exposed to high altitude.

Priapism

Adherence and sickling of RBCs in the sinusoids of the corpora cavernosa of the penis, with secondary stasis, hypoxia, and sickling, can lead to a painful sustained erection. Recurrent priapism or even a single sustained event (>24 hours) may result in impotence. Immediate treatment includes intravenous pain medication and hydration. The goal is to obtain resolution of pain and detumescence. If conservative measures are ineffective after 6 to 12 hours, exchange transfusion therapy replacing sickle RBCs with normal RBCs that will not be trapped in the penile circulation is performed. If symptoms persist, direct corporeal irrigation with an α-adrenergic agonist such as phenylephrine or a glans-cavernosum shunt may be helpful. Case reports suggest that sildenafil (Viagra)* may be effective in promoting detumescence. A rare syndrome in which neurologic events, including stroke, occur within 1 to 2 weeks of exchange transfusion for priapism is seen in children with sickle cell disease.

*Not FDA approved for this indication.

ACUTE COMPLICATIONS ASSOCIATED WITH SIGNIFICANT ANEMIA

Mild worsening of anemia may be seen during a pain event, but transfusion therapy is not generally required unless there is evidence of associated acute end-organ injury. A significant fall in hemoglobin from baseline values may herald the development of a severe sickle cell complication, such as acute chest syndrome. However, other complications result in severe anemia by other mechanisms.

Acute Splenic Sequestration

The spleen is composed of sinusoids in which sickle RBCs are trapped. In patients with severe forms of sickle cell disease (sickle cell anemia and sickle β°-thalassemia), the spleen is generally infarcted and involutes by the age of 3 to 5 years. Prior to autosplenectomy, in young children, and in patients with milder forms of sickle cell disease in whom splenic function is retained into adulthood, acute sequestration of sickle RBCs can result in abrupt enlargement of the spleen with a sudden drop in hemoglobin. In small children, this sequestration can result in hypovolemia, shock, and death. Splenic sequestration may occur in the setting of a recent infection and is recognized by a newly palpable or increased spleen in the setting of lethargy, pallor, and reduction in hemoglobin. Prompt treatment should include volume support with intravenous fluids and transfusion therapy. Recurrent splenic sequestration may be treated with chronic transfusion therapy or splenectomy, although the latter is usually deferred if possible in children younger than 5 years.

Transient Aplastic Crisis

The development of viral or other infections that severely compromise bone marrow function may temporarily reduce RBC production, resulting in acute anemia caused by continued hemolysis without appropriate marrow compensation. Parvovirus B19 is the most common infectious agent associated with aplastic crisis and is also the etiology of erythema infectiosum ("fifth disease"). Aplastic crisis is recognized by a fall in hemoglobin associated with a markedly diminished reticulocyte count. Management of this complication is supportive, with the use of transfusion if the anemia is severe and/or the suppression is prolonged.

Older children and adults may also experience a relative aplasia if they become severely folic acid deficient or experience severe bone marrow suppression associated with infections, other medical conditions, or medications.

ACUTE NEUROLOGIC COMPLICATIONS

Cerebrovascular Accident (Stroke)

Macrovascular events are uncommon in sickle cell disease. The notable exception is ischemic stroke, which affects up to 10% of children with sickle cell anemia, occurring frequently between the ages of 5 and 10 years. This event probably occurs in the setting of chronic endothelial injury with gradual stenosis of large cerebral vessels. Evidence of this stenosis may be detectable by transcranial Doppler sonography, and a randomized study has demonstrated that chronic transfusion therapy may reduce the risk of stroke in children with abnormal findings.

Ischemic stroke is characterized by focal neurologic deficits, which may be subtle and transient. More overt events may be associated with headache or seizure activity. A computed tomographic scan and/or magnetic resonance imaging (MRI) identifies the intracerebral pathology, and magnetic resonance angiography (MRA) can be used to identify damaged vessels. Treatment for acute stroke is immediate exchange transfusion and careful observation for increased intracerebral pressure. Chronic transfusion therapy is offered to reduce significantly the risk of recurrent stroke, as thus far no other therapy has been demonstrated to be as effective in reducing recurrence. The long-term duration and intensity of transfusion therapy have not been conclusively determined.

Intracerebral Hemorrhage

In older children and adults, the more common acute neurologic event is intracerebral hemorrhage, occurring at sites of chronic vessel injury with or without aneurysm formation. MRA or traditional angiography should be performed to evaluate for sites of abnormal vasculature. Clinical management is similar to that of ischemic cerebral events, although the benefits of long-term transfusion therapy are less clear.

OTHER ACUTE COMPLICATIONS

Bacterial Sepsis

One of the leading causes of mortality in young children with sickle cell disease is pneumococcal sepsis. When functional asplenia occurs in patients with sickle cell anemia and sickle β°-thalassemia, usually within the first year of life, the child is susceptible to overwhelming infection. This risk is highest in children 5 years of age and younger. A randomized study has demonstrated marked reduction in this mortality with the daily use of prophylactic oral penicillin,* which is now offered to all children with sickle cell anemia and sickle β°-thalassemia until the age of 5 years.

The need to initiate prophylactic penicillin* in very young children has been a major impetus for newborn screening to identify the presence of sickle cell disease in infants. Recognition of these children and their families also presents an opportunity for family education about the need to seek immediate medical attention for fever and how to palpate an increase in spleen size in an effort to reduce morbidity and mortality associated with splenic sequestration.

The presence of fever in a patient with sickle cell disease should be assumed to represent potentially severe bacterial infection until proved otherwise. Immediate evaluations, including blood cultures, and prompt administration of a parenteral antibiotic, often a cephalosporin, are critical for fever in children with sickle cell disease. Empirical antibiotic coverage in adults should also be considered. Fever is not a characteristic of an uncomplicated pain event.

Acute Cholecystitis

Lifelong hemolysis in patients with sickle cell disease results in the formation of bilirubin gallstones and/or sludge that can cause acute cholecystitis. Right upper quadrant pain, nausea, vomiting, and increased bilirubin and alkaline phosphatase may indicate this complication. Generally, therapy is the same as for any patient with acute cholecystitis, with appropriate attention to empirical antibiotic coverage, adequate intravenous hydration, and pain control. Elective cholecystectomy may be necessary for patients with recurrent cholecystitis.

CHRONIC COMPLICATIONS

Even in the absence of acute pain events, chronic vascular injury results in a number of chronic manifestations of sickle cell disease.

Retinopathy

Chronic microvascular injury to the retinal vessels can occur in patients with any form of sickle cell disease. This injury results in neovascularization and sea fan formation and can lead to retinal detachment and blindness. Ophthalmologic evaluation, with a dilated retinal examination, should be performed at least once a year beginning at age 10.

Osteonecrosis of the Femoral and Humeral Heads

The microcirculation of the femoral and humeral heads is susceptible to chronic injury by circulating sickle RBCs, leading to osteonecrosis. The principal manifestation is initially intermittent, then eventually constant, pain in the true hip area with progressive limitation of range of motion and mobility. The most common intervention is total hip replacement, which is delayed as long as possible because the patients are generally young and active and tend to wear out the prosthetic joint. Chronic nonsteroidal anti-inflammatory medication use and joint rest by the temporary use of crutches may provide symptomatic relief. Study is under way to investigate the benefits of core decompression in this population.

Chronic Lung Injury

One of the leading causes of severe morbidity and mortality in adults with sickle cell disease is the development of chronic lung disease with associated cor pulmonale. Sickle lung disease begins in early stages

*Not FDA approved for this indication.

with a restrictive pattern on pulmonary function tests. Microvascular injury progresses until pulmonary hypertension develops, resulting in exercise intolerance, shortness of breath, hypoxia, palpitations, and atypical chest pain. Death may result from complications of end-stage right-sided heart failure or arrhythmias. Although chronic lung injury is believed to occur as a complication of recurrent acute chest syndrome, patients with sickle cell disease who have not had acute lung complications may develop chronic lung injury. Therapy has included chronic transfusion therapy, but there is currently no well-established treatment approach.

Chronic Renal Disease

Another significant cause of morbidity and mortality in patients with sickle cell disease is chronic renal disease. All persons with sickle cell disease, and even sickle cell trait, experience ischemia in the renal medulla, resulting in a limited ability to concentrate the urine. Sickle cell disease patients may develop a glomerulonephropathy characterized by hypercellularity and focal and segmental glomerulosclerosis. Microalbuminuria and proteinuria may be early indications of sickle nephropathy, along with the development of hypertension. Limited data suggest that treatment with an angiotension-converting enzyme inhibitor* may lessen the proteinuria and perhaps retard the progression of sickle nephropathy and should be considered in patients with proteinuria even in the absence of hypertension. Renal transplantation has been used successfully in patients with sickle cell disease, although there may be an increased rate of graft failure and pain events after transplantation.

Papillary Necrosis

Persons with both sickle cell disease and sickle cell trait may develop ischemia in the renal papillae, resulting in necrosis. The usual manifestations are flank pain and hematuria, with blunting or cavitation of the papillary tip on radiographic studies. Treatment is supportive, including adequate hydration and pain management. Painless hematuria of unclear etiology may also occur in the absence of papillary necrosis. A thorough evaluation for the etiology should be undertaken, including a search for common genitourinary malignancies and the rare renal medullary carcinoma, which appears to be more common in patients with sickle cell trait and hemoglobin SC disease.

*Not FDA approved for this indication.

Bone Infarct or Osteomyelitis

With prolonged ischemia, focal areas of bone may become infarcted, resulting in prolonged severe focal pain. Sympathetic joint effusions may form if the infarct is located near a joint space.

If fever and leukocytosis are associated with a focal area of bone pain, osteomyelitis should be considered. Infectious agents are most commonly gram-positive organisms, although *Salmonella* is another less common etiologic agent. Diagnosis may be made with bone scan, MRI, and/or biopsy, and treatment involves appropriate long-term antibiotic therapy.

Leg Ulcers

Leg ulcers may develop with occlusion of small skin vessels, although there is often a chronic inflammatory component. Treatment includes local wound care and antibiotic therapy for associated cellulitis. Refractory ulcers may respond to transfusion therapy.

TRANSFUSION THERAPY

As depicted in Table 3, the use of transfusion should be limited to treatment of severe acute complications of sickle cell disease or to preclude the recurrence of such events. There is no evidence that transfusion is necessary or helpful in uncomplicated pain events, even if the hemoglobin falls below baseline values.

TABLE 3. **Indications for Transfusion Therapy**

Acute Simple Transfusion	Acute Exchange Transfusion
1. Patient's hemoglobin is below baseline value AND patient has a. splenic sequestration b. aplastic crisis c. mild acute chest syndrome (mile hypoxia, chest pain, mild chest radiographic changes) d. early multiorgan failure syndrome e. acute high-output heart failure 2. Patient is in chronic transfusion program where goal is to sustain hemoglobin ≥ 10 g/dL. 3. Preoperatively for elective surgery (sickle cell anemia patients and S β°-thalassemia) Transfusion is NOT INDICATED if the patient has only typical pain, but no other acute complication of sickle cell crisis, EVEN IF the hemoglobin falls below baseline. AVOID transfusion to hemoglobin >10 g/dL and/or significantly above patient's baseline values as hyperviscosity may result.	Stroke Priapism Severe acute chest or multiorgan failure syndrome Stroke or central nervous system bleeding Sustained priapism after local drainage has failed Emergency surgery in patients with sickle cell anemia or history of acute chest syndrome

Acute Transfusion Therapy

Severe acute anemia, as seen in splenic sequestration or aplastic crisis, may necessitate transfusion support if the episode is prolonged and high-output heart failure develops.

Severe acute end-organ injury, including acute chest syndrome, acute multiorgan failure syndrome, strokes, and priapism, is an indication for transfusion therapy. If the patient's hemoglobin falls significantly below baseline values and/or is below 10 g/dL, simple transfusion of packed RBCs can be given until the hemoglobin is back to baseline values or to about 10 g/dL. Exceeding these values may result in increased blood viscosity and exacerbation of the acute injury.

If the patient's hemoglobin has not fallen significantly below baseline or the event is severe (as for stroke or priapism), an RBC exchange transfusion should be performed. Except for infants and small children, an RBC exchange transfusion can be performed using an apheresis instrument. For very small patients, a manual exchange may need to be performed. The goal is to reduce the percentage of cells containing sickle hemoglobin to less than 30%.

Chronic Transfusion Therapy

When the percentage of sickle hemoglobin has been reduced to less than 30%, the bone marrow's production of new sickle RBCs can be suppressed by maintaining the patient's hemoglobin above their baseline value, generally at a value of approximately 10 g/dL. Simple transfusion is given every 3 to 5 weeks to maintain bone marrow suppression.

In patients with a baseline hemoglobin above 10 g/dL or for those who have had recurrent events despite simple transfusion, chronic exchange transfusions can be performed every 4 to 5 weeks in an effort to suppress effectively bone marrow production of sickle RBCs.

Extended chronic transfusion therapy is recommended for patients who have had ischemic stroke and may also be used for patients with other recurrent acute events such as acute chest syndrome, priapism, or splenic sequestration. A limited course of chronic transfusion therapy (e.g., 3 to 6 months) may be used after a severe acute event to facilitate recovery from end-organ damage. The role of chronic transfusion therapy to prevent development or progression of chronic complications, including chronic lung disease, chronic renal disease, retinopathy, or avascular osteonecrosis, has not been well established.

Complications of Transfusion Therapy

Three main complications of transfusion therapy limit broader application.

The first complication is the risk of transmission of viral and other infectious agents. Although the risks are relatively small, they must be weighed when considering a chronic transfusion program.

The second complication is the development of multiple alloantibodies that preclude further transfusion. Sickle cell disease patients, often with ethnic origins in areas where malaria is prevalent, have relatively few antigens on their RBC surfaces. In contrast, blood donors, especially in the United States, tend to have European ancestry and have relatively more antigens on their RBC surface. When blood with these antigens is given to patients who do not have the same antigens in their RBCs, the recipient can develop multiple antibodies, making it difficult or impossible to find compatible blood in the future. This complication can be virtually eliminated by providing blood matched for these antigens (not just ABO and Rh blood type) so that antibodies never develop. Unfortunately, the availability of matched blood is limited in many areas, leading to either alloimmunization or hesitation in offering chronic transfusion therapy.

The third complication of transfusion therapy is the accumulation of iron, with secondary hemosiderosis and the potential for severe organ damage and premature death. With every milliliter of packed RBCs given, the patient receives 1 mg of iron. Thus, a typical unit of packed RBCs contains 250 mg of iron. The iron is retained in the body and eventually accumulates pathologically, inducing dysfunction of critical organs including the liver and heart. Therapy for iron overload in sickle cell disease is currently limited to parenteral chelation therapy using deferoxamine.* Deferoxamine (Desferal) is commonly delivered subcutaneously or intravenously as a 12-hour infusion taken 3 to 7 days a week. Compliance with such a regimen can be difficult, and for intravenous therapy an indwelling catheter is required. In the United States, there are currently no available oral chelation agents.

In order to avoid initial or additional iron accumulation, some providers elect to switch from simple transfusion to chronic exchange transfusion therapy. Because as much blood is removed as is given, there is little or no net gain of iron and iron accumulation is markedly reduced.

PREGNANCY AND SICKLE CELL DISEASE

Women with sickle cell disease of all types are able to have successful pregnancies. Most women with milder sickle cell diseases, such as hemoglobin SC disease and sickle β^{+}-thalassemia, have maternal and fetal outcomes similar to those of women without sickle cell disease. It is unclear whether miscarriages are more frequent in women with sickle cell disease. There is an increased risk of some maternal and fetal complications as pregnancy progresses, but cooperative management by both a high-risk obstetric provider and a sickle cell disease specialist can significantly reduce these complications.

Labor and delivery should be managed according to obstetric considerations, and there is no advantage to induction of labor or delivery by cesarean section. Awareness of possible increased tolerance of narcotic

*Not FDA approved for this indication.

therapy facilitates appropriate pain medication dosing during labor.

Maternal Complications

Pregnant women with sickle cell disease are more susceptible to the development of bacteriuria and urinary tract infections. Some data suggest that there is an increased risk for preeclampsia, placenta previa, placental abruption, and preterm labor. The use of chronic transfusion therapy does not affect these complications.

Fetal Complications

Intrauterine growth retardation and small-for-gestational-age births may occur more frequently in women with sickle cell anemia. Chronic transfusion therapy with correction of anemia does not affect these complications, and the occurrence of these complications does not correlate with the degree of anemia. Ultrasound surveillance can be conducted to monitor for these complications. Biophysical profile and measures of fetal activity must be interpreted with caution when the mother has received narcotic therapy.

Sickle Cell Complications during Pregnancy

Some women experience an increase in the frequency and severity of pain events during pregnancy. Vigilance should be maintained for the development of acute complications of pain events, such as acute chest syndrome. The use of chronic transfusion therapy does affect the frequency and severity of sickle cell complications during pregnancy and may be warranted in women with a marked increase in severity of their underlying sickle cell disease during pregnancy.

SICKLE CELL DISEASE AND SURGERY

Patients with sickle cell disease may experience acute sickle-related complications when undergoing major surgery. A preoperative transfusion study demonstrated that reduction of the percentage of sickle RBCs to less than 60% by giving simple blood transfusion for 2 to 3 weeks prior to surgery was as effective as reducing the percentage of sickle cell hemoglobin to less than 30% using an exchange transfusion in ameliorating the frequency and severity of postoperative pain events and acute chest syndrome in patients with sickle cell anemia and sickle β°-thalassemia. Maintenance of hydration, adequate pain control, and careful attention to adequate oxygenation are also critical.

In patients with other forms of sickle cell disease, there are fewer data to address the importance of preoperative transfusion. A patient who has a history of severe pain events or acute chest syndrome may benefit from preoperative transfusion therapy.

THERAPY FOR SICKLE CELL DISEASE

Hydroxyurea Therapy

Hydroxyurea (Droxia) is an oral chemotherapy agent that has been demonstrated to reduce the frequency and severity of sickle cell pain events and acute chest syndrome in adult patients with sickle cell anemia and sickle β°-thalassemia. Hydroxyurea induces the production of fetal hemoglobin, which partially inhibits the polymerization of sickle hemoglobin. Other changes with hydroxyurea therapy include an increased mean cell volume and reduction of the white blood cell count, which may also affect the pathophysiology of sickle cell disease. Hydroxyurea doses are titrated upward until hematologic toxicity (neutropenia) is approached; complete blood counts are monitored every 2 weeks. Response may take several months and is assessed by measurement of fetal hemoglobin and improvement in clinical course. It is unclear whether long-term hydroxyurea is leukemogenic, and pregnancy should be avoided while either a man or woman is receiving therapy; thus, the anticipated benefits of therapy need to be carefully weighed against the disadvantages and risks.

The use of hydroxyurea in older children* (≥5 years) does not appear to be associated with short-term adverse effects, but the efficacy and long-term effects are under investigation. The use of hydroxyurea in infants* is also under study.

There are no data available yet that demonstrate that hydroxyurea is effective in the primary or secondary prevention of severe acute complications (e.g., stroke) or chronic complications (e.g., chronic lung or renal disease).

Bone Marrow Transplantation

Allogenic bone marrow transplantation has been successfully performed in patients with sickle cell disease, and both cord blood and miniallogenic techniques are under investigation. One of the major limitations of transplantation is the determination of who is best served by transplantation because there are significant risks including mortality and morbidity from graft-versus-host disease and other transplant complications. Current programs focus on bone marrow transplantation for patients who have demonstrated sufficiently severe disease, as marked by stroke or recurrent acute complications, to warrant the risks but are not so severely compromised by these complications as to be poor transplant candidates. An additional limitation is the lack of matched siblings, unaffected by sickle cell disease, to serve as donors. To overcome this problem, some programs are investigating the use of cord blood and/or unrelated donors.

Gene Therapy

Because the origin of sickle cell disease is a single point mutation in the β-globin gene, it would seem

*Not FDA approved for this indication.

simple to overcome. However, techniques to either insert corrected genes or alter the simple mutation remain elusive. One limitation is the need to affect the majority of cells in the bone marrow so as to achieve sustained production of normal RBCs. However, encouraging animal models of cell transfection with antiretroviral vectors have been developed and application to humans may begin in the near future. A combination of gene therapy with autologous bone marrow transplantation, or other combination of approaches, may offer the best hope for cure of this complex disease.

NEUTROPENIA

method of
AYALEW TEFFERI, M.D., and
COSTAS L. CONSTANTINOU, M.D.
Mayo Clinic
Rochester, Minnesota

Circulating white blood cells, also called leukocytes, consist of granulocytes, monocytes, and lymphocytes. Granulocytes include neutrophils, eosinophils, and basophils. Accordingly, *neutropenia* refers to an absolute decrease in circulating neutrophils. Approximately 90% of peripheral blood neutrophils display segmented nuclei (polymorphs), whereas the nucleus in the remaining 5% to 10% (band neutrophils) is C-shaped. The absolute neutrophil count (ANC) is calculated by multiplying the total white blood cell count by the sum of the percentages of polymorphs and band neutrophils.

In white adults, the reference ranges for white blood cells and ANC are approximately 3.5 to 10.5 and 1.7 to 7.0×10^9/L, respectively. However, the corresponding values for persons of African ancestry are significantly lower, and this *ethnic neutropenia* has been attributed to diminished bone marrow granulocyte reserve. Nevertheless, neutropenia is currently defined as an ANC of less than 1.5×10^9/L. Furthermore, depending on the degree of neutropenia, the process is subclassified as mild (ANC, 1 to 1.5×10^9/L), moderate (ANC, 0.5 to 1.0×10^9/L), or severe (ANC lower than 0.5×10^9/L). *Agranulocytosis* is a term that refers to severe neutropenia that is associated with either a maturation arrest or a reduced pool affecting bone marrow granulocyte progenitors. The risk of neutropenic infection is highest in severe neutropenia and is negligible in mild neutropenia.

GRANULOPOIESIS

All blood cells, including neutrophils, are derived from hematopoietic stem cells that are both pluripotent and capable of self-renewal. During granulopoietic differentiation of hematopoietic stem cells, the granulocyte undergoes several stages of differentiation starting with the myeloblast and ending with the polymorph. The first stages of differentiation (myeloblast, promyelocyte, myelocyte) are accompanied by cell division (mitotic pool), but the latter stages (metamyelocyte, band neutrophil, polymorphs) are not (postmitotic pool). The average time the granulocyte takes to mature from the myeloblast stage into a polymorph and to egress from the marrow is 10 to 14 days. Once released into the circulation, the neutrophil remains in circulation for an average of 7 hours before migrating into other tissues (diapedesis).

Under normal conditions, there are 10- to 20-fold more neutrophils in the bone marrow (storage pool) than in the peripheral blood. Furthermore, approximately 50% of peripheral blood neutrophils are found embedded in the vascular wall (marginal pool). There is a dynamic equilibrium among the storage, marginal, and circulating pools of neutrophils that may be influenced by several factors including exercise (catecholamine release), infection, and treatment with corticosteroids.

CLASSIFICATION

A practical way of classifying the causes of neutropenia is based on the underlying mechanism: reduced production (hypoproliferative), peripheral destruction (hyperproliferative), and shifts from the circulating pool to other neutrophil compartments (Table 1). Hypoproliferative neutropenia may be further subclassified into congenital and acquired forms (see Table 1).

TABLE 1. **Classification of Causes of Neutropenia**

Hypoproliferative Causes
Congenital
Kostmann's syndrome (autosomal recessive)
Shwachman-Diamond syndrome (autosomal recessive)
Chédiak-Higashi syndrome (autosomal recessive)
Dyskeratosis congenita (X-linked)
Cartilage-hair hypoplasia (autosomal recessive)
Myelokathexis (autosomal dominant)
Congenital immunodeficiency syndromes (hyper-IgM syndrome, reticular dysgenesis)
Glycogen storage diseases (GSD1b)
Cyclic neutropenia (autosomal dominant)
Benign chronic idiopathic neutropenia including pseudoneutropenia
Ethnic neutropenia
Acquired
Drug-induced conditions
Toxic exposure (benzene, radiation)
Postinfectious disorders (HIV, Epstein-Barr virus, cytomegalovirus, parvovirus)
Myelophthisis
Clonal myeloid disorders
Large granular lymphocyte leukemia
Hyperproliferative Causes
Autoimmune neutropenia (drug-induced, associated with collagen vascular disease, idiopathic)
Isoimmune neutropenia
Circulating Pool Shifts
Hypersplenism
Sepsis

Hypoproliferative Neutropenia

Congenital Neutropenia

As illustrated in Table 1, certain congenital syndromes are associated with neutropenia. These include Kostmann's syndrome (a maturation defect at the promyelocyte stage), Shwachman-Diamond syndrome (pancreatic insufficiency), Chédiak-Higashi syndrome (large inclusion bodies in neutrophils, albinism, bleeding diathesis), dyskeratosis congenita (epiphora, short stature, dental caries), cartilage hair hypoplasia (short-limb dwarfism), myelokathexis (neutrophil hypersegmentation), congenital immunodeficiency syndromes (X-linked hyper-IgM syndrome), and glycogen storage diseases.

Cyclic neutropenia is a poorly understood congenital disorder that presents with recurrent episodes (every 2 to 6 weeks) of neutropenia associated with symptoms of fever and mouth lesions. Between episodes, patients are generally well. *Chronic idiopathic neutropenia* is a milder phenotype of congenital neutropenia and includes the ethnic neutropenia that is often seen in African and American blacks, West Indians, and Yemenite Jews. Some cases of chronic benign neutropenia may involve increased margination without affecting the total pool of peripheral neutrophils (*pseudoneutropenia*). The degree of neutropenia is mild to moderate, and there is no predisposition to infection.

Acquired Hypoproliferative Neutropenia

DRUG-INDUCED NEUTROPENIA

Drug-induced neutropenia is the most common cause of neutropenia encountered in routine clinical practice. Although neutropenia is an expected and predictable occurrence with the use of cancer chemotherapy, it is the unexpected occurrence with many other drugs that is diagnostically challenging. First, all drugs must be suspected of contributing to the cause of new-onset, otherwise unexplained, neutropenia regardless of whether the particular drug has neutropenia as a common side effect (Table 2).

TABLE 2. **Noncytotoxic Agents that May Be Associated With Neutropenia***

Antibiotics (penicillins, cephalosporins, sulfonamides, chloramphenicol)
Antiretroviral therapy (zidovudine)
Hypoglycemic agents
Antimalarials (quinine, pyrimethamine)
Antiarrhythmics (procainamide, tocainide, quinidine)
Anti-inflammatory agents (indomethacin, phenylbutazone, gold salts)
Antithyroid agents (carbimazole, propylthiouracil)
Anticonvulsants (phenytoin, carbamazepine)
Phenothiazines
α-Methyldopa
Diuretics (spironolactone, chlorothiazide, ethacrynic acid)
Clozapine
Cimetidine
Penicillamine

*This is not a complete list of drugs that may be associated with neutropenia. Consultation with the *Physicians' Desk Reference* is encouraged.

Second, treatment duration, although a very helpful piece of information, does not reliably exclude the possibility of drug-induced neutropenia. As a general principle, when faced with a list of medications, a drug that has recently been added is more likely to be the offender, especially if it is associated with a considerable risk of neutropenia.

POSTINFECTIOUS NEUTROPENIA

Postinfectious neutropenia is most common after viral infections (HIV, Epstein-Barr virus, cytomegalovirus, parvovirus, the hepatitis viruses, varicella, measles, rubella). Other offending infectious agents and diseases include *Rickettsia rickettsii*, the cause of Rocky Mountain spotted fever, tularemia, *Salmonella typhi*, ehrlichiosis, and *Staphylococcus aureus*.

MYELOPHTHISIS

Myelophthisis refers to a bone marrow infiltrative process including metastatic cancer, granulomatous infection, and collagen fibrosis. Neutropenia associated with myelophthisis is always associated with other cytopenias (pancytopenia) as well as a peripheral blood smear showing immature myeloid cells and nucleated red cells.

CLONAL MYELOID DISORDERS

The term *myeloid disorders* refers to hematologic malignant diseases characterized by the proliferation of nonlymphoid lineage cells. Myeloid disorders are clonal stem cell processes that may be associated with ineffective hematopoiesis that results not only in neutropenia but also in anemia and thrombocytopenia. In general, myelodysplastic syndrome, aplastic anemia, and paroxysmal nocturnal hemoglobinuria are also associated with other cytopenias. A rarer syndrome is pure white cell aplasia, which is associated with thymoma in most cases.

LARGE GRANULAR LYMPHOCYTE LEUKEMIA

Large granular lymphocyte leukemia is a clonal T or natural killer cell disorder that is often associated with moderate to severe neutropenia, with or without other clinical manifestations including anemia, constitutional symptoms, and splenomegaly. The disease-associated neutropenia is usually asymptomatic, but it may result in life-threatening infection. Large granular lymphocyte leukemia sometimes occurs in association with rheumatoid arthritis and Felty's syndrome.

Hyperproliferative Neutropenia

Autoimmune Neutropenia

Autoimmune neutropenia implies the involvement of antibodies that sensitize neutrophils for peripheral destruction by the reticuloendothelial system. The production of such antibodies may be triggered by drugs, viral infections, or unknown stimuli. Autoimmune neutropenia is also frequently seen in association with collagen vascular diseases. In drug-induced autoimmune neutropenia, antibodies are produced when a complex between the drug (hapten) and a leukocyte surface protein becomes antigenic. The onset of neutropenia after drug (usually antibiotic) exposure may be immediate, in the presence of previous exposure, or it may take a few days. Antineutrophilic antibodies can be detected in autoimmune diseases such as systemic lupus erythematosus, rheumatoid arthritis, and its variant, Felty's syndrome (rheumatoid arthritis, splenomegaly, pigmented spots in lower extremities, and neutropenia).

Isoimmune Neutropenia

The pathogenesis of this disease is similar to that of hemolytic disease of the newborn. During pregnancy, the mother may be exposed to foreign neutrophil antigens (from the fetus) either during pregnancy or at the time of delivery. This results in production of IgG antibodies, which then cross the placenta and cause severe immune-mediated neutropenia.

Neutropenia Associated With Circulating Pool Shifts

Hypersplenism

Neutropenia of usually mild to moderate severity may accompany *splenomegaly* from various causes including liver disease. The exact underlying mechanism is not known but may involve abnormal splenic sequestration of neutrophils and other blood components. Hypersplenic neutropenia is often associated with moderate thrombocytopenia.

Sepsis

Overwhelming *sepsis* can accentuate peripheral utilization as well as vascular margination of neutrophils, with resultant pseudoneutropenia.

DIAGNOSIS

A bone marrow examination is often performed early in the diagnostic workup of a patient with pancytopenia but not in the patient with isolated neutropenia. Regardless, the first step in the approach to the patient with neutropenia is to determine whether the patient is symptomatic (fever, physical or laboratory signs of infection). In case of symptomatic neutropenia, the patient must be managed with antibiotics and other appropriate measures concomitant with the evaluation of the underlying neutropenia. In this regard, examination of the oral cavity, perianal region, and skin is essential.

In isolated neutropenia, review of medication history is the most important first step of the diagnostic workup. Recently prescribed drugs are best discontinued. In the presence of a medication list that includes drugs that are used on a long-term basis and before the onset of neutropenia, drug modification can await other diagnostic evaluations. Alternatively, essential medications may be substituted, and use of nonessential medications can be deferred. In drug-induced neutropenia, recovery of the ANC after cessation of drug use is usually prompt (within a few days), whereas in the case of bone marrow suppression, the ANC may be slower to recover (usually weeks).

A thorough history and physical examination are also essential to rule out the possibilities of congenital neutropenia, history of toxin exposure, infection-associated neutropenia, autoimmune neutropenia, and hypersplenism. The incidental finding of isolated mild to moderate neutropenia in persons of certain ethnic background does not require any further evaluation other than a repeat complete blood cell count in a few weeks.

Laboratory tests that are usually ordered in the setting of isolated neutropenia include serum vitamin B_{12} and folate levels (nutritional deficiencies usually cause pancytopenia), antineutrophil antibodies (lack both sensitivity and specificity), antinuclear and antiphospholipid antibodies (to look for association with collagen vascular diseases), rheumatoid factor (to look for association with rheumatoid arthritis), and peripheral blood smear (to look for large granular lymphocytes or other clues to an associated hematologic disorder). We recommend consultation with a hematologist before a bone marrow examination is ordered.

TREATMENT

Specific treatment for neutropenia is not recommended in the presence of an ANC greater than 1×10^9/L. Management of chemotherapy-induced neutropenia is different from that of other types of neutropenia and is best directed by a hematologist or oncologist. In all other instances, the treatment of both moderate (ANC, 0.5 to 1×10^9/L) and severe (ANC lower than 0.5×10^9/L) neutropenia depends on whether the patient is symptomatic (fever, active infection, a history of recurrent infection).

General recommendations for the asymptomatic patient with moderate to severe neutropenia include attention to dental care and high-fiber diet and the possible use of a stool softener to prevent rectal mucosal tears. Selective decontamination of the skin and bowel flora and prophylactic antibiotic use are no longer advisable.

In symptomatic neutropenia, the myeloid growth factors granulocyte colony-stimulating factor (filgrastim [Neupogen]) and granulocyte-macrophage colony-stimulating factor (sargramostim [Leukine])* and antimicrobials may be used either in the setting of prophylaxis or during active infection. *Febrile neutropenia* and *neutropenic fever* are terms that are used interchangeably and refer to the presence of fever in a patient with moderate to severe neutropenia. In general, such patients are comprehensively evaluated for the source of infection (blood and urine cultures, chest radiograph) and are given empirical intravenous antibiotics with full gram-negative coverage. Additional gram-positive and fungal antibiotic coverage may be necessary, depending on the clinical situation.

---

*Not FDA approved for this indication.

Infections in neutropenic patients may not be characterized by inflammatory reactions (e.g., abscess, pulmonary infiltrates) because of the absence of an adequate inflammatory response mediated by neutrophils. The source of fever in febrile neutropenia is often elusive. Blood cultures are positive only in a few cases. The responsible organisms usually are derived from endogenous flora (gastrointestinal tract and skin).

Myeloid growth factors (granulocyte colony-stimulating factor, granulocyte-macrophage colony-stimulating factor) are increasingly used in patients with neutropenia. However, these drugs are very expensive, and an increase in neutrophil count does not always translate into clinical benefit. Rather, physicians should base their decisions on results of randomized clinical trials that are designed to examine important clinical endpoints such as morbidity and mortality. At this juncture, evidence supports the use of myeloid growth factors in symptomatic congenital neutropenia and in the setting of hematopoietic stem cell transplantation but not in febrile neutropenia or afebrile chemotherapy-induced neutropenia.

HEMOLYTIC DISEASE OF THE FETUS AND NEWBORN

method of
AHMET A. BASCHAT, M.D., and
CARL P. WEINER, M.D.
University of Maryland
Baltimore, Maryland

The combination of hydrops, jaundice, and anemia as a disease entity has been recognized for centuries. Yet hemolytic disease of the perinate has had a unique place in fetal medicine since it became the first treatable fetal disease. In 1961, Liley reported its natural history and the successful antenatal treatment with adult red blood cells. In 1964, Freda and colleagues prevented sensitization in Rh-negative persons by passive immunization with anti-D antibodies. In 1981, Rodeck reported high survival rates for hydropic fetuses after intravascular transfusion. Despite the introduction of these effective preventive and therapeutic strategies, fetal and neonatal hemolytic disease remains a condition with serious perinatal consequences.

PATHOPHYSIOLOGY OF HEMOLYTIC ANEMIA

Fetal hematopoiesis occurs at three principal sites during overlapping gestational epochs. Beginning by day 21 (mesoblastic period) in the yolk sac, erythropoiesis slowly shifts to the liver and spleen (hepatic period) and then to the bone marrow by 16 weeks. Erythropoiesis takes place predominantly in the bone marrow (myeloid period) by 28 weeks and is under the humoral control of erythropoietin. Fetal hemoglobin consists of two α and two γ chains (hemoglobin F), and constitutes 60% to 90% of neonatal hemoglobin at term. It is almost completely replaced by adult hemoglobin (two α and two β chains) by 4 months of age.

Hemolytic anemia can occur whenever the erythrocyte life span declines to less than 70 to 90 days and the hematopoietic system can no longer meet the demands. The loss of oxygen-carrying capacity triggers erythropoietin release. Erythropoietin stimulates red blood cell production initially in the bone marrow, and is eventually supplemented by the recruitment of long-inactive sites of red blood cell production (extramedullary hematopoiesis). From sites such as the liver, spleen, kidneys, and adrenal glands, immature red blood cells (erythroblasts) enter the fetal circulation, hence the name *erythroblastosis fetalis*. The severity of anemia reflects the rate, rapidity, and site of red blood cell destruction. Hemolysis may be confined to the bloodstream (red blood cell membrane defects), may occur in the reticuloendothelial system (isoimmunization), or may even affect the burst-forming units at the sites of red blood cell production (e.g., in Kell anemia).

Although hypoxemia is perhaps the principal risk of severe anemia, the impact is worsened because red blood cells are the principal buffers in the fetus. Hypoxia-mediated metabolic acidemia and cardiac dysfunction result in the clinical finding of hydrops, with its attendant high mortality if untreated.

Hyperbilirubinemia secondary to erythrocyte hemolysis is an important component of hemolytic disease, and bilirubin levels usually rise before the onset of anemia (except for Kell isoimmunization; see later). Because of reduced glucuronyl transferase and limited placental transport, most bilirubin in the fetus is albumin bound and lipid soluble. This "indirect" bilirubin penetrates the blood-brain barrier, enters neurons, preferentially in the basal ganglia and the auditory center, and causes cell death. Neonates with severe hyperbilirubinemia are at risk of encephalopathy (kernicterus), a risk more pronounced in preterm infants. The clinical picture includes lethargy progressing to hypotonia, poor sucking, and eventually the development of apneic episodes. Mortality approaches 90% with severe toxicity. Survivors typically have profound neurosensory deafness and choreoathetoid spastic cerebral palsy.

The heterogeneous disorders capable of causing hemolytic anemia may be grouped into four broad categories (Table 1). Of these, the inherited defects of red blood cell enzymes and shape are rare and are evident through the family history and inheritance pattern. Isoimmunization, conversely, is responsible for most cases of fetal and neonatal hemolytic disease.

RHESUS ISOIMMUNIZATION

Maternal red blood cell isoimmunization results from exposure and response to a foreign red blood cell antigen. Whereas more than 400 red blood cell antigens are described, only a few are clinically relevant causes of hemolytic anemia. The D antigen is most antigenic, and it remains the prototype for maternal

TABLE 1. **Differential Diagnosis of Hemolytic Anemia**

Immune-mediated anemia	Common Rhesus family (D,C,E,c,e) Kell Uncommon JK^a (Kidd) Fy^a (Duffy) $Kp^{a\ or\ b}$ k S Rare Do^a, $Di^{a\ \&\ b}$, Fy^b, Hutch, JK^b, Lu^a, M, N, s, U, YT
Hemoglobinopathies	Homozygous α-thalassemia: Bart's hemoglobin H disease Hemoglobin H disease
Erythrocyte enzyme deficiencies	Glucose-6-phosphate dehydrogenase deficiency Pyruvate kinase deficiency
Erythrocyte membrane defects	Hereditary spherocytosis, elliptocytosis, among others

red blood cell isoimmunization, although immune prophylaxis has enhanced the importance of other antigen groups (see Table 1). Antibodies to D remain the most common cause of fetal hemolytic anemia.

Although several nomenclatures are used for the Rhesus blood group system, the one by Fisher and Race is confirmed genetically and works best in clinical practice. The Rh system is composed of three antigen pairs (Cc, Dd, and Ee) that are encoded by two homologous genes on the short arm of chromosome 1—the Dd and CcEe genes. A person may be heterozygous or homozygous for each of the three alleles. The principal Rh phenotype is determined by the D/d genotype. The presence of the D antigen determines a person as Rh positive (Rh^+ phenotype). The d antigen has never been demonstrated, and its existence is questionable. Thus, the absence of the D antigen determines a person as Rh negative (Rh– phenotype). Because certain combinations of phenotypes are more common than others, the genotype may be predicted from the red blood cell phenotype obtained using antisera specific for C, c, D, E, and e (there is no antiserum to d). Because the genes for the Rh alleles are sequenced, polymerase chain reaction is often used, with the recognition that serologic and genotypic typing are not 100% concordant.

The Rh blood group contains more than 35 other antigens of lesser clinical importance. The most common is the D^u variant, of which there are two types. In the D^{u+} variant, D expression is weakened by the presence of a C allele. These patients are actually Rhesus positive. In the second variant (D^{u-}), part of the antigen is missing. These women are phenotypically Rh negative and therefore are at risk of isoimmunization.

PATHOPHYSIOLOGY

Fetal hemolytic disease has several prerequisites. The maternal blood type must be negative and the fetal blood type positive to the corresponding allele. The mother must have been sensitized by exposure to the antigen, and she must have the capacity to mount an adequate IgG response. Transplacental passage of IgG with subsequent attachment to fetal erythrocytes results in hemolysis.

Transplacental fetal-maternal hemorrhage is the most common cause of isoimmunization. Heterologous blood transfusion is second overall, but it is the most common cause of sensitization to uncommon antigens. Based on Kleihauer-Betke staining of maternal blood smears, fetal-maternal hemorrhage occurs in at least 75% of women. Microscopic hemorrhage is detectable in virtually all women when flow cytometry is used. Both the frequency and magnitude of bleeding are related to the fetal-placental blood volume, and they increase from 3% and 0.03 mL in the first trimester to 45% and 25 mL in the third trimester. Contrary to ABO antigens, which are weakly expressed on fetal red blood cells, Rh antigens are well developed by 30 days of gestation. Therefore, fetal-maternal hemorrhage can potentially cause maternal isoimmunization by 4 weeks after conception.

Primary sensitization after exposure is characterized by IgM production against the D antigen, and it is dose dependent to the quantity of Rhesus-positive red blood cells that enter the circulation of a susceptible individual. The primary sensitizing immune response occurs over 6 weeks to 12 months, and it remains predominantly IgM, which cannot traverse the placental barrier. Fifteen percent of Rhesus-negative volunteers will become sensitized after a 1-mL exposure of Rhesus-positive red blood cells. The proportion increases to 30% after 40 mL and to 65% after 250 mL. Three percent of women with uncomplicated pregnancies become sensitized after a small fetal-maternal hemorrhage (0.1 mL). A second antigenic challenge stimulates a rapid (amnestic), maternal IgG response. Thus, the first pregnancy is generally not at great risk. The magnitude of the IgG response and avidity of binding to the red blood cell increase with the time between antigen challenges. The small molecular weight of IgG allows appreciable transplacental passage from the early second trimester onward.

Transferred IgG binds to the D antigen on the surface of fetal erythrocytes. The avidity and degree of binding are determined by the quantity as well as the subclass of IgG (e.g., IgG_1 and IgG_3), and they may be further modified by maternal HLA type and fetal sex. Fetal red blood cell aggregates are formed by chemotactic adherence to macrophage rings. These large rosettes are trapped and destroyed in the reticuloendothelial system by extravascular hemolysis at a rate much faster than simple complement-mediated hemolysis. The anemia may develop slowly over months in association with a low reticulocyte count and normal bilirubin. Conversely, it may progress rapidly over a week, with reticulocytosis and hyperbilirubinemia. The clinical picture can thus range from mild anemia to fetal hydrops and stillbirth, depending on the antigenicity of the fetal red blood cell antigens, the magnitude of transplacental IgG transfer, the density of the antigens on the fetal red blood cell membrane, the avidity of antigen binding and the functional efficiency of the fetal reticuloendothelial system, and the protective effects of ABO incompatibility.

INCIDENCE

The natural incidence of Rhesus isoimmunization is determined in part by the incidence of a Rhesus-negative blood type and the predilection of carrying a fetus with Rhesus-positive blood type. The prevalence of Rhesus-negative status is lowest in Chinese and Japanese persons (approximately 1%), and is highest in Basques (up to 100%), where the mutation most likely originated. In North America, the incidence of the Rhesus-negative genotype is 15% in whites, 8% in African Americans, and 2% among Native Americans. The likelihood for a Rhesus-negative mother (d/d genotype) carrying a Rhesus-positive fetus is determined by the zygosity of the father. If the father is homozygous Rhesus positive (DD), all children will be Rhesus positive, whereas if he is heterozygous (D/d), only 50% of his children will be Rhesus positive.

The natural incidence of Rhesus isoimmunization at term in Rhesus-negative women with ABO compatibility is 16%. ABO incompatibility decreases the incidence almost tenfold (1.5% to 2%). This natural risk is further modified by precipitating factors. First trimester abortion, chorion villous sampling, amniocentesis, external cephalic version, blunt abdominal trauma, and ectopic pregnancy are all associated with significant transplacental hemorrhage and maternal exposure to the fetal D antigen. In the absence of immunoprophylaxis, the risk of Rhesus disease is 2% to 5%. Passive immunization is the primary means to decrease the incidence of hemolytic disease of the fetus and newborn.

PREVENTION

Successful passive immunization with anti-D immunoglobulin (RhoGam) to prevent Rhesus isoimmunization was first achieved in 1964. The U.S. Food and Drug Administration approved its use in 1968 after confirming efficacy in male prisoners. Anti-D immunoglobulin is extracted by cold alcohol fractionation from the sera of persons with high titers. This extraction process removes viral pathogens such as HIV and hepatitis B, and an infectious risk from anti-D immunoglobulin has not been substantiated.

Anti-D immunoglobulin binds D antigen sites on fetal red blood cells present in the maternal circulation. Presumably, blockade of these sites prevents their recognition by B lymphocytes and transformation of activated B lymphocytes to IgG producing plasma cells. Anti-D immunoglobulin has a half-life of 24 days, and a standard 300-μg dose provides 12 weeks of protection against exposure to up to 30 mL of blood, or 15 mL of erythrocytes. Before the introduction of anti-D immunoglobulin, 10% of susceptible pregnancies developed hemolytic disease of the fetus and newborn. Approximately 90% of these resulted from a fetal-maternal hemorrhage during a prior pregnancy at term. Administration of anti-D immunoglobulin within 72 hours of delivery reduces the incidence by 90%. The administration of an additional dose at 28 weeks produces a further decline in incidence from 2% to 0.1%. Although the 72-hour limit is based on the original study protocol evaluating the efficacy of anti-D immunoglobulin, beneficial effects may still be obtained after administration up to 28 days postpartum.

Current guidelines for management of Rhesus-negative women with uncomplicated pregnancy focus on the prevention of isoimmunization from physiologic fetal-maternal hemorrhage (Table 2). If a patient is Rhesus negative and the antibody screen is negative on the first prenatal visit, the screen is repeated at

TABLE 2. **Preventive Guidelines for Rhesus-Negative Women in Pregnancy**

Time	Test	Anti-D-Ig Dose
First prenatal visit	ABO and Rhesus blood typing Direct and indirect Coombs' test	None
28–29 wk	Direct and indirect Coombs' test for newly developed antibodies	300 μg
32 wk	Direct and indirect Coombs' test for newly developed antibodies	None
At birth	Neonatal cord blood for ABO and Rhesus type Direct Coombs' test for red cell bound antibodies	—
Within 72 h of delivery	Rosette test Kleihauer-Betke estimate of fetoplacental hemorrhage	300 μg (individualize for Kleihauer-Betke result)
First trimester spontaneous miscarriage	—	50–200 μg
First trimester therapeutic abortion	—	300 μg
After prenatal diagnosis by chorion villous sampling of amniocentesis	—	300 μg
Other high risk situations: abdominal trauma, placental abruption, antepartum hemorrhage	Rosette test, Kleihauer-Betke estimate of fetoplacental hemorrhage	300 μg (individualize for Kleihauer-Betke result)

28 weeks, and anti-D immunoglobulin administered if the test result is still negative. Another antibody screen is repeated when the woman is in labor. If the father is Rhesus negative and there is no question about paternity, the prophylactic doses of anti-D immunoglobulin can be omitted. Postpartum, mothers of Rhesus-positive newborns are treated with an additional 300 μg of immunoglobulin.

Approximately 1 in 1300 pregnancies has a fetal-maternal hemorrhage during delivery in excess of 30 mL. Risk factors such as placental abruption, abdominal trauma, intrauterine manipulation, placenta previa, fetal demise, multiple gestation, and manual removal of placenta identify only half these women. In such high-risk circumstances, estimating the amount of transplacental bleeding with the Kleihauer-Betke test may refine the recommended 300-μg dose of anti-D immunoglobulin. This test makes use of the relative resistance of fetal hemoglobin to acid denaturation. Acid citrate buffer is used to remove adult hemoglobin, leaving red cell ghosts. After fixation with 80% ethanol and hematoxylin-eosin staining, the maternal blood is examined on a counting chamber. The amount of fetal blood in the maternal circulation can be approximated from the number of fetal red blood cells per grid using the following formula:

Fetal cells/number of maternal cells = estimated blood loss/estimated maternal blood volume in mL (85/kg)

After delivery, anti-D immunoglobulin may be withheld, provided the last administration was less than 21 days earlier and passively acquired antibodies are still demonstrable on the antibody screen. One in 400 women has a transplacental hemorrhage greater than 30 mL, and the rosette test may be performed in maternal blood to assess the need for further administration of anti-D immunoglobulin. Rosette formation indicates the presence of fetal red blood cells, and the dose of anti-D immunoglobulin may have to be adjusted, guided by the Kleihauer-Betke test.

MANAGEMENT OF RHESUS ISOIMMUNIZATION IN PREGNANCY

The diagnosis of isoimmunization in a Rhesus-negative mother requires demonstration of an IgG antibody in her plasma that can bind to Rhesus-positive cells. The indirect Coombs' test verifies the presence of antigen-specific IgG, and it is expressed as a fractional titer based on the greatest dilution where this antibody is still demonstrated. The direct Coombs' test is positive when IgG-coated red blood cells are demonstrated using antihuman antiglobulin, and it is performed on either fetal or neonatal blood samples. If the indirect Coombs' test is positive at any prenatal visit not related to prophylactic immunoglobulin, the fetus is Rhesus positive and at risk of hemolytic disease. The goal of management is to identify the fetus or neonate at risk of significant anemia, to institute adequate therapy ending with vaginal delivery of a nonanemic baby. Elimination of the anemia and the suppression of fetal erythropoiesis remove the adverse effects of the disease. Such management requires maternal and fetal evaluations at referral centers that have considerable experience with the specialized investigation techniques and interpretation of test results.

Identification of the fetus at risk requires verification of the fetal blood type. If the father is Rhesus negative, there is no doubt about paternity, and isoimmunization followed the administration of blood products or occurred during a prior pregnancy with different paternity, then the fetus is probably not at risk. If such an approach is not practical clinically, the fetal blood type should be ascertained. One sequence is to begin with testing paternal zygosity using antisera against C, c, E, e, and D. After determination of parental zygosity is completed, the fetal genotype is estimated based on established distribution tables for genotypes in ethnic groups. If the father is homozygous Rhesus positive, then all the children will be affected, whereas heterozygosity halves that risk. If the father is also ABO incompatible with the mother, there is a 60% chance that the fetus will be ABO incompatible with the mother, thus reducing the risk of hemolytic disease from 16% to 2%. Other investigators proceed directly to fetal blood sampling when the maternal indirect Coombs' test result is greater than 1:16 and the obstetric history is compatible with isoimmunization.

Once a fetus is confirmed to be either at risk or affected, the stage of pregnancy when the disease last manifested guides the timing of invasive fetal testing in the current pregnancy. The patient's past history and antibody titer provide estimates of the anticipated disease severity and onset, whereas peak blood flow velocities in the middle cerebral artery, as measured by Doppler ultrasound, provide a reasonable noninvasive means of evaluation for anemia. Although fetal disease severity typically increases from one affected pregnancy to the next, the risk of hydrops may be as high as 10% even in the first pregnancy. Prior hydrops carries a 90% repeat risk. If the maternal indirect Coombs' antibody titers are performed in a laboratory with a reproducible, clinically validated technique, the results will be both reproducible and of relative value in predicting fetal disease during the first sensitized pregnancy only. Fetal hydrops generally does not occur with titers lower than 1:32, but familiarity with a laboratory's critical cutoff values for hemolytic disease is essential to avoid clinical error. The development of fetal anemia is associated with increased middle cerebral artery peak systolic velocities. Although a normal value does not exclude anemia, an elevated peak blood flow velocity above the gestational norm strongly suggests fetal anemia. Anticipation of the disease onset or ultrasound evidence of fetal anemia determines the timing of invasive fetal testing. The approach depends on the number of previously affected pregnancies.

The titer should be determined on a monthly basis during the first sensitized pregnancy, and invasive testing should be initiated once the critical titer is reached. If this is the second or higher affected pregnancy, the gestation of onset for the previously affected pregnancy guides the timing of invasive testing, and the titers are not helpful. In either situation, an elevated middle cerebral artery peak systolic velocity should prompt earlier fetal testing. Other ultrasound markers such as increased amniotic fluid volume, liver and spleen size, placental thickness, bowel echogenicity, increased cardiac diameter, and pericardial effusion are not reliable for the prediction of anemia. Sonography is but an adjunct and not a replacement for invasive studies. There are several approaches once the decision for invasive testing is made. Some clinicians continue to rely on amniotic fluid spectrophotometric testing (see later) despite its high error rate, whereas others use fetal blood sampling. Regardless of the approach, almost all groups now use the peak middle cerebral artery velocity to refine the testing intervals.

Fetal hemolysis and hyperbilirubinemia increase bilirubin content in amniotic fluid through tracheal and pulmonary secretions. The presence of bilirubin in the amniotic fluid alters spectrophotometric light absorption at 450 nm wavelength. The shift in optical density of amniotic fluid at 450 nm (delta O.D. 450) is proportional to the amount of bilirubin and can be plotted against a semilogarithmic reference range determined by Liley in 1961 for pregnancies between 27 and 41 weeks' gestation. The graph can be used to categorize amniotic fluid bilirubin levels into three ascending zones of severity. Zone 1 indicates mild or no fetal disease, zone 2 indicates intermediate disease, and zone 3 indicates severe disease with a risk of hydrops within 1 week. The normal delta O.D. 450 in the second trimester is in zone 2. Thus, in the absence of overtly abnormal results, the overall accuracy of the delta O.D. 450 in predicting anemia or hydrops is poor. Therefore, determination of serial values at 1- to 2-week intervals or direct sampling of fetal blood is necessary when results are equivocal, particularly if the middle cerebral artery peak systolic velocity is elevated.

Whereas amniotic fluid sampling allows the determination of fetal karyotype and blood type and provides an indirect measure of the degree of hemolysis, fetal blood sampling allows additional determination of the complete blood and reticulocyte counts, bilirubin level, electrolytes, and blood gas values. Fetal blood sampling is carried out by ultrasound-guided cordocentesis, using a 22-gauge needle, of the umbilical vein. The disease severity, anticipated progression, and degree of metabolic compromise can be accurately determined, and fetal transfusion therapy is planned accordingly.

Two techniques available for fetal transfusion are intraperitoneal and intravascular. The latter has essentially replaced the intraperitoneal technique, which relied on the absorption of red blood cells through subdiaphragmatic lymphatic vessels during fetal respiration. Additional disadvantages of the intraperitoneal technique include the possibility of local trauma, limitation of transfusion volume because of the risk of obstructing cardiac venous return, and slow absorption, particularly with hydrops.

Fetal intravascular transfusion is indicated when the fetal hematocrit is less than 30% and the fetus is less than 35 weeks' gestation or when there is evidence of hydrops. Blood group O, Rhesus-negative, irradiated, cytomegalovirus-negative blood with a hematocrit approximating 75% is used for this purpose. Blood with a lower hematocrit requires a higher transfusion volume, whereas blood with a hematocrit higher than 85% mixes poorly. At the end of the transfusion, a repeat fetal sample is obtained. The goal is a closing value of 50% to 55%. This supraphysiologic goal is selected to reduce the number of transfusions while suppressing fetal erythropoiesis. The transfusion volume is typically in the range 50 mL/kg of nonhydropic fetal body weight, but it can vary greatly for a given fetus, depending on the starting hematocrit, fetal condition, presence of hydrops, and sonographically estimated fetal weight. Hydrops is proof of fetal cardiac dysfunction, and these fetuses tolerate intravascular volume poorly. Yet even partial correction of the fetal oxygen-carrying capacity is rapidly accompanied by normalization of cardiac function, long before the hydrops resolves sonographically. These fetuses should begin treatment with a partial transfusion. Knowledge of the closing hematocrit and realization that the fetal hematocrit will decline approximately 1 hematocrit point per day permit one to predict when the fetal hematocrit will reach 30%. Allowing the fetus to decline further risks the resumption of fetal erythropoiesis. Survival rates in large, experienced centers approach 100% for nonhydropic fetuses, and they exceed 90% when hydrops is there at presentation. Risks of transfusion such as fluid overload, umbilical cord laceration or thrombosis, umbilical artery spasm with bradycardia, graft-versus-host disease, and fetal demise are minimized if the procedure is carried out at experienced referral centers.

The last transfusion is planned at 34 to 35 weeks' gestation, to allow a normal vaginal delivery between 37 and 38 weeks. There is no reason to confirm pulmonary maturity. The mode of delivery is governed by obstetric factors. Delivery should be conducted at a medical center experienced with caring for neonates with potentially severe hyperbilirubinemia.

TREATMENT OF THE NEONATE

In the absence of adequate prenatal therapy, some 50% of neonates have mild disease with a hematocrit higher than 36% and bilirubin values lower than 20 mg/dL. Twenty-five percent of these neonates have moderate disease or hydrops. Exchange transfusion is rarely necessary if the fetus has received at least two intrauterine transfusions and the targeted hematocrit values were achieved. Hyperbilirubinemia can usually be managed by phototherapy, which converts indirect bilirubin to a more water-soluble isomer.

ABO INCOMPATIBILITY AND MINOR BLOOD GROUP ANTIGENS

ABO incompatibility rarely causes fetal disease because the antibodies are IgM and because these antigens are not strongly expressed on the fetal erythrocyte. Isoimmunization to minor blood group antigens is usually the result of blood transfusion. Although Lewis antibodies are most common, they are almost always IgM. Further, the antigen is poorly expressed on the fetal erythrocyte. Therefore, the risk of hemolysis is low.

Kidd, Kell, and Duffy are the most common minor blood group antigens to which isoimmunization causes perinatal hemolytic disease. Kell isoimmunization is of particular interest because its pathophysiology differs from that of the others. The clinical course is particularly unpredictable by indirect fetal assessment because the anti-Kell IgG antibodies damage or inhibit erythrocyte progenitors. Severe anemia and hydrops may develop rapidly, with low antibody titers and delta O.D. 450 values. Management is similar to that of Rhesus isoimmunization, with monitoring and intervention tailored to the individual circumstances.

OTHER CAUSES OF HEMOLYTIC DISEASE

Rare causes of fetal and neonatal hemolytic disease include hemoglobinopathies, red blood cell membrane defects, and red blood cell enzyme deficiencies. Because thalassemia can affect the α and β hemoglobin chains, it may result in disease in utero. Bart's hemoglobin (deletion of all four α chain genes) is the most severe form and causes hydrops fetalis. Hemoglobin H disease (deletion of three α chain genes) is less severe, but it requires lifelong transfusion treatment. In contrast, sickle cell disease (defective β chain) does not manifest in utero, owing to the protective effect of fetal hemoglobin.

Inherited defects in cell membrane proteins cause abnormally shaped red blood cells vulnerable to hemolysis. Diseases such as hereditary spherocytosis, elliptocytosis, poikilocytosis, and stomatocytosis are named after the shape of the erythrocyte.

Defective enzymes in the two major metabolic red blood cell pathways, the hexose monophosphate shunt and the Embden-Meyerhof pathway, predispose to hemolysis under certain conditions. Glucose-6-dehydrogenase deficiency is the most common defect, inherited in an X-linked fashion and partially expressed in females and fully in males. The prevalence is highest among African American, Southeast Asian, Native American, and Mediterranean ethnic groups. Severe hemolysis may occur with oxidant stress, and it can occasionally affect newborns.

HEMOPHILIA AND RELATED DISORDERS: A PRACTICAL APPROACH

method of
CLODAGH RYAN, M.B., and
BARRY WHITE, M.D., M.Sc.
National Centre for Coagulation Disorders, St. James's Hospital
Dublin, Ireland

HEMOPHILIA A (FACTOR VIII DEFICIENCY) AND HEMOPHILIA B (FACTOR IX DEFICIENCY)

Hemophilia is an X-linked bleeding disorder caused by a deficiency of factor VIII (FVIII) or factor IX (FIX) coagulant activity, and it has a prevalence in all racial groups of approximately 1:10,000 and 1:50,000 respectively.

Clinical Presentation

The clinical manifestation of hemophilia varies depending on the concentration of the deficient clotting factor. Patients with severe hemophilia (FVIII:C or FIX:C levels lower than 1 U/mL) usually present in the first 2 years of life with spontaneous bleeding involving joints and muscles. More severe bleeding involving the central nervous system, the head and neck, and the gastrointestinal tract occurs less frequently. Patients with moderate hemophilia (FVIII:C or FIX:C levels of 1 to 5 U/mL) usually bleed after trauma, surgical procedures, or dental extractions, but they may occasionally have spontaneous bleeding. Patients with mild hemophilia (FVIII:C or FIX:C levels greater than 5 U/mL) usually present only after a hemostatic challenge, and the disorder is often not diagnosed until teenage years or adulthood.

Diagnosis

FVIII and FIX deficiency is associated with a prolongation of the activated partial thromboplastin time (aPTT), which corrects on mixing studies. The prothrombin time (PT) and the thrombin clotting time (TCT) are normal. The diagnosis is made on specific FVIII and FIX assays, which should be repeated on separate occasions to confirm the diagnosis.

There is a family history in two thirds of patients with hemophilia, and the inheritance pattern is similar to that of other X-linked disorders. If a patient with hemophilia has children, all the daughters will be carriers, and no son will be affected. If a hemophilia carrier has children, there will be a 50% chance that a male child will have hemophilia and a 50% chance that a female child will be a carrier. Female carriers of severe hemophilia mutations frequently have reduced FVIII or FIX levels, with a range of 30 to 70 U/mL (normal more than 50). Reduced FVIII levels are also seen in von Willebrand disease (vWD), and consequently this should be considered in the differential diagnosis of mild to moderate hemophilia.

The strategies for the identification of carrier status include family pedigree, measurement of coagulant factor levels, linkage analysis, and direct mutation analysis. A detailed family pedigree may identify obligate carriers. Daughters of men with hemophilia are obligate carriers, as are women with two children with hemophilia or one child with hemophilia and a family history of hemophilia. FVIII or FIX levels should be measured in potential carriers to identify those at risk of bleeding. However, the measurement of factor levels alone is an unreliable guide to carrier status. Direct mutation analysis has now replaced linkage analysis as the investigation of choice. This involves the identification of the mutation in the affected male or obligate carrier, followed by screening for this mutation in potential carriers. The identification process is simplified by the finding that an inversion within intron 22 of the FVIII gene is noted in more than 40% of patients with severe FVIII deficiency. Prenatal diagnosis using chorionic villous sampling after 10 weeks can be used to determine both the sex of the fetus and the presence of a specific hemophilia mutation.

Management

The key to the effective treatment of hemophilia is the prompt administration of the deficient clotting factor. This can be achieved by the administration of clotting factor concentrates, which are available as plasma-derived or recombinant products. Recombinant factor concentrates are the treatment of choice because they are associated with a reduced risk of blood-borne infection. Desmopressin (1-deamino [8-D-arginine] vasopressin [DDAVP]) is useful in responsive patients with mild FVIII deficiency.

Factor concentrates can be given as a bolus or by continuous infusion. The use of continuous infusion is preferable in major bleeding and surgical procedures because it provides sustained normalization of factor levels and reduces overall product requirement. Otherwise, convenience dictates that treatment be administered by bolus infusion. The desired factor rise depends on the severity of the bleeding. Acute hemarthrosis usually requires factor levels of 30 to 50 U/mL, whereas severe bleeding episodes require factor levels of 100 U/mL, followed by a continuous infusion.

The dose of the factor concentrate is calculated on the basis of the patient's weight, the estimated plasma volume, and the severity of the bleeding. Pharmacokinetic studies have demonstrated that the following simple formula can be used to calculate the appropriate treatment dose:

FVIII: Percentage of factor rise desired × patient's weight × 0.5
Repeated every 12 hours or followed by a continuous infusion of 4 IU/kg/hour

FIX: Percentage of factor rise desired × patient's weight × 1 (1.2 for recombinant FIX)
Repeated every 24 hours or followed by a continuous infusion of 6 IU/kg/hour

Pretreatment and posttreatment FVIII and FIX levels, along with daily levels during continuous infusion, should be monitored to ensure adequate treatment and to allow dose adjustment.

In addition to treatment at the times of surgical procedures or bleeding, there is clear evidence to support the use of prophylactic factor replacement in children. Primary prophylaxis with FVIII and FIX concentrate significantly reduces joint damage in children with severe hemophilia. The recommended treatment schedule is FVIII 20 to 40 IU/kg three times per week or FIX 20 to 40 IU/kg twice per week.

DDAVP, a synthetic analogue of vasopressin, is the drug of choice in responsive patients with FVIII deficiency because it avoids exposure to blood products. The doses and side effects are similar to those used in vWD and are outlined later in this chapter.

Adjunctive Therapy

Antifibrinolytic agents such as tranexamic acid (15 mg/kg every 6 to 8 hours) and ε-aminocaproic acid (60 mg/kg every 4 to 6 hours) can be administered orally, intravenously, and topically, and they are particularly effective in oral cavity and uterine bleeding. Analgesia may be required, especially for the pain associated with chronic arthropathy. In general, aspirin and other nonsteroidal anti-inflammatory drugs are contraindicated. However, the newer cyclooxygenase II inhibitors do not appear to affect platelet function and have been used in patients with severe hemophilia.

Inhibitors

One of the most serious complications of hemophilia treatment is the development of an inhibitor, which is usually an IgG antibody directed against FVIII or FIX. The incidence of inhibitor development is up to 33% in FVIII deficiency and 7% in FIX deficiency. The median number of factor exposure days before the development of an inhibitor is 9 to 12 days, and the median age is 2.5 years. A family history of inhibitors increases the likelihood of their development. The Bethesda assay is the standard method for measuring the inhibitor titer. Patients should be screened for inhibitors annually, preoperatively, and in the setting of a poor response to therapy.

Immune tolerance induction is effective in eradicating FVIII inhibitors in up to 80% of patients with severe hemophilia. The optimum approach to immune tolerance induction has not been determined, and differing regimens for the administration of FVIII concentrate vary from 50 IU/kg three times per week to 300 IU/kg/d. The most important predictor of success is the inhibitor titer before commencement of immune tolerance induction, with a titer of less than 10 Bethesda units (BU)/mL associated with a higher and quicker response rate.

The management of acute bleeding depends on the severity of the hemorrhage and whether patients are low or high responders. Low responders have inhibitor levels of less than 5 BU/mL, and they do not develop an amnestic response on further exposure to FVIII. In low responders, higher doses of human FVIII or porcine FVIII can be effective. For all other inhibitor patients, recombinant FVIIa (NovoSeven), at a dose of 90 μg/kg every 2 to 4 hours, or FEIBA (FVIII inhibitor bypassing activity), at a dose of 50 U/kg every 6 to 12 hours, can be effective in achieving hemostasis.

Acquired Hemophilia

Acquired hemophilia is rare, with an incidence of 1 to 4 cases/million per year, and it usually presents in the seventh or eighth decade. It can be associated with autoimmune disease, malignant disease, and pregnancy, but in 50% of patients, no cause is found. Mucocutaneous bleeding and soft tissue bleeding are more prominent features than in patients with inherited severe hemophilia. Immunosuppressive therapy including steroids, cyclophosphamide (Cytoxan), and intravenous immunoglobulin is successful in eradicating the inhibitor in 60% to 70% of cases. Recombinant FVIIa and FEIBA are effective in the management of acute bleeding episodes, at doses similar to those given in patients with severe hemophilia who develop inhibitors.

Gene Therapy

Gene therapy may hold the key to a cure for hemophilia. However, to date, this treatment is restricted to clinical trials.

VON WILLEBRAND DISEASE

Von Willebrand disease (vWD) is the most common bleeding diathesis, with an estimated prevalence of 0.1% of the general population. It results from either a quantitative deficiency (types 1 and 3) or a qualitative defect (type 2) of von Willebrand factor (vWF). This protein is synthesized by endothelial cells and megakaryocytes, and it mediates platelet adhesion to the subendothelium and platelet-platelet cohesion in vessels with high shear stress. It also acts as a protective carrier for FVIII. Type 1 vWD is the most common subtype and accounts for approximately 80% of cases. It is usually inherited in an autosomal dominant pattern with variable penetrance and expression. Type 2 vWD is further divided into four subgroups, as outlined in Table 1. Type 3 vWD is a recessive condition resulting from a complete absence of vWF in plasma and platelets and is extremely rare, with an incidence of 3 to 5 cases per million.

TABLE 1. **Current Classification of von Willebrand Disease**

Type	Description
1	Partial quantitative deficiency of von Willebrand factor
2	Qualitatative deficiency of von Willebrand factor
2A	Decreased platelet-dependent von Willebrand factor function, with lack of high-molecular-weight multimers
2B	Increased platelet dependent von Willebrand factor function, with lack of high-molecular-weight multimers
2M	Decreased platelet dependent von Willebrand factor function, with normal multimeric analysis
2N	Decreased von Willebrand factor affinity for factor VIII
3	Complete deficiency of von Willebrand factor

Clinical Presentation

The most common manifestations of vWD are easy bruising, epistaxis, menorrhagia, and bleeding after surgical procedures and dental extractions. The clinical presentation of type 3 vWD is similar to that of severe hemophilia.

Diagnosis

A detailed personal and family history is an essential component in the diagnosis of vWD and must always be considered in conjunction with the laboratory investigations. Investigations include a full blood count, blood group determination, FVIII:C, vWF antigen, vWF functional activity (ristocetin cofactor), and ristocetin-induced platelet aggregation. Multimeric analysis is required for the subclassification of type 2 vWD.

Environmental factors such as age, menstruation, estrogen therapy, and stress all increase vWF levels and should be considered in the interpretation of the results. The baseline variation in vWF necessitates repeated testing before a diagnosis can be made. The mean vWF levels in persons belonging to blood group O are 25% to 30% lower than in members of other blood groups.

Management

The treatment options for patients with vWD include DDAVP, vWF concentrates, and antifibrinolytic agents. DDAVP is a synthetic analogue of vasopressin, which increases FVIII and vWF levels transiently by releasing these proteins from their storage sites. It is inexpensive, relatively well tolerated, and carries no risk of viral transmission, and it is the drug of choice in responsive type 1 vWD. It is administered intravenously at a dose of 0.3 μg/kg diluted in 50 to 100 mL of saline over 30 minutes, and this results in a three- to fivefold increase in FVIII within 1 hour of completion of the infusion. Treatment can be repeated every 24 hours depending on the response and indication, although the response is reduced with repeated infusions. A test dose of DDAVP at the time of diagnosis establishes the individual response pattern. DDAVP is not useful in type 3 vWD, and many investigators believe that it is contraindicated in type 2B vWD. In other vWD subtypes the response is variable and requires individual assessment.

Common side effects include facial flushing and headaches that often resolve on slowing the infusion rate. Hyponatremia resulting from the antidiuretic effect is important, and patients must be advised to avoid excessive fluid intake. DDAVP is contraindicated in patients with a history of seizures, arterial disease, and hypersensitivity reactions to DDAVP, as well as in children less than 2 years of age. DDAVP can also be administered intranasally, and this method of administration has been used for the self-treatment of women with menorrhagia.

Replacement Therapy

Approximately 15% of patients with vWD will require replacement therapy with plasma derived concentrates. These patients include those who do not respond to DDAVP or who have a contraindication to its administration. Virally inactivated FVIII-vWF concentrates are the products of choice. Once-daily infusion is usually sufficient to control hemostasis. FVIII levels should be measured every 12 hours on the day of the surgical procedure and then every 24 hours. The FVIII:C response can be predicted on the basis that 1 IU/kg will increase the level by approximately 2 U/mL (1.5 U/mL in children). However, vWF and FVIII levels may be discrepant, and measurement of vWF antigen and activity should be considered in the event of continued bleeding during treatment with vWF concentrate.

Patients with type 3 vWD may require prophylactic treatment with vWF concentrate at a frequency of two to three times weekly. Purified vWF is currently under assessment in clinical trials.

Adjunctive Therapy

Tranexamic acid (Cyklokapron; 15 mg/kg every 6 to 8 hours) and ε-aminocaproic acid (Amicar; 60 mg/kg every 4 to 6 hours), as outlined previously, may be clinically effective. Tranexamic acid should not be used if there is a history of urinary tract bleeding or thrombosis. Estrogen therapy is useful in managing menorrhagia.

Pregnancy

During normal pregnancy, the FVIII and vWF levels rise from the tenth week of gestation, with the greatest rise in the last trimester. This results in the correction of vWF and FVIII levels in most patients with type 1 vWD, and consequently they usually do not require treatment at the time of delivery. vWF levels should be assessed at approximately 28 weeks' and 34 to 36 weeks' gestation to determine whether treatment is required at the time of parturition. vWF concentrate or DDAVP (in responsive patients) may be required for those patients with low vWF levels. Patients with type 3 vWD require replacement therapy.

Acquired von Willebrand's Disease

Acquired vWD has occurred in the setting of autoimmune disease, particularly hypothyroidism, in lymphoproliferative disorders, in patients with solid tumors, and in drug-related (valproic acid) conditions. Treatment of the underlying condition may correct the laboratory parameters. Treatment options to prevent or treat bleeding include vWF concentrate, DDAVP, intravenous immunoglobulin, recombinant FVIIa, and plasma exchange.

RARE FACTOR DEFICIENCIES

Other deficiencies of coagulation factors that cause a bleeding disorder, such as deficiencies of fibrinogen, FII, FV, FVII, FX, FXI, FXII, and FXIII, are inherited as autosomal recessive traits, with prevalences of between 1:500,000 and 1:2,000,000. Clinical symptoms are usually restricted to those patients who are homozygous or compound heterozygous for the factor deficiency.

Fibrinogen Deficiency

Deficiencies of fibrinogen can be divided into two groups phenotypically. In *afibrinogenemia,* fibrinogen activity and antigen level (type I) are decreased or absent. *Dysfibrinogenemia* is characterized by decreased fibrinogen activity and normal or moderately reduced antigen level (type II). Patients with afibrinogenemia usually have a significant bleeding tendency. Approximately 50% of patients with dysfibrinogenemia are symptomatic, with either bleeding problems or thrombotic events. In afibrinogenemia, the PT, aPTT, and TCT are all prolonged and correct on mixing studies. Clotting and immunologic assays are required to measure the fibrinogen. Replacement therapy with fibrinogen concentrate or cryoprecipitate is the treatment of choice in the management of bleeding episodes or surgical procedures.

Prothrombin Deficiency

The clinical manifestations of severe prothrombin deficiency range from mild to moderate mucosal bleeding to life-threatening bleeding complications. The PT and aPTT are prolonged, and the TCT is normal. Specific assays for prothrombin clotting activity are required to make the diagnosis. Replacement therapy with prothrombin complex concentrate is the treatment of choice, and it can be used both prophylactically and therapeutically.

Factor V Deficiency

Patients with severe FV deficiency frequently present with mucosal bleeding or postoperative or oral cavity bleeding. However, spontaneous life-threatening bleeding complications are rare. The PT and aPTT are prolonged. The TCT is normal, and a diagnosis of FV deficiency is confirmed by specific FV clotting assays. Bleeding episodes require treatment with 10 to 15 mL/kg plasma, and this approach may also be required at the time of surgery to increase the FV level to more than 10%.

Factor VII Deficiency

There is a relatively poor correlation between the FVII level and bleeding tendency because even levels lower than 10% are effective in controlling hemorrhage. There is a prolonged PT with normal aPTT and TCT. A specific assay for FVII clotting activity is used for the diagnosis. FVII has a short half-life of 4 to 6 hours and therefore must be administered regularly. Treatment options include FVII concentrate and recombinant FVIIa (NovoSeven).

Factor X Deficiency

The clinical manifestations of severe FX deficiency are similar to those of severe FVIII or FIX deficiency. The PT and aPTT are prolonged. The TCT is normal. Diagnosis is confirmed by a specific FX assay. The treatment of choice is prothrombin complex concentrate, and this can be used both for prophylaxis and the management of acute bleeding and surgery.

Factor XI Deficiency

The Ashkenazi Jews of Eastern European descent have a high frequency of heterozygosity for this condition, at 8%. There is a poor correlation between the FXI level and bleeding tendency, and most patients with severe FXI deficiency are only mildly affected and are usually only symptomatic after trauma or surgical procedures. There is a prolonged aPTT, with a normal PT. TCT is normal. A specific FXI clotting assay is used to make the diagnosis. The management of surgery or acute bleeding may require treatment with plasma or FXI concentrate.

Factor XII Deficiency

The exact role of FXII in the coagulation cascade has not been clearly elucidated, but it is recognized that a deficiency is not associated with bleeding problems. Laboratory investigations reveal a prolonged aPTT, with a normal PT. A specific FXII assay confirms the diagnosis. Because there are no bleeding complications, no specific therapy is required

Factor XIII Deficiency

Patients with severe FXIII deficiency frequently have a severe clinical phenotype. Umbilical stump bleeding occurs in 80% of neonates, and central nervous system bleeding is not uncommon. Investigations reveal normal PT, aPTT, and TCT. A specific FXIII assay is required to identify patients with FXIII deficiency. FXIII concentrate is the treatment of choice for the management of surgical procedures and bleeding episodes. The long half-life of FXIII allows monthly prophylactic infusions.

PLATELET-MEDIATED BLEEDING DISORDERS

method of
JOEL S. BENNETT, M.D.
University of Pennsylvania School of Medicine
Philadelphia, Pennsylvania

Platelets provide primary hemostasis by forming hemostatic plugs at sites of vascular injury. Accordingly, insufficient numbers of circulating platelets and inherited and acquired disorders of platelet function can result in bleeding. These situations are encountered frequently in clinical practice, engendering substantial and appropriate concern about the risk and prevention of bleeding.

ELEMENTS OF PLATELET FUNCTION

Circulating platelets are maintained in a nonreactive state by nitric oxide and prostacyclin secreted by endothelial cells until they are needed for hemostasis. In addition, the intact endothelium forms a barrier separating platelets from adhesive substrates in subendothelial connective tissue. Disruption of this barrier allows platelets to come in contact with, and adhere to, collagen, fibronectin, and laminin. However, at the higher shear rates of blood in arteries and the microcirculation, platelet adhesion requires that the platelet membrane glycoprotein (GP) Ib-IX complex bind to subendothelial von Willebrand factor (vWf). Collagen is also an important substrate for platelet adhesion, not only because it is the binding site for vWf in the subendothelium but also because it is an agonist for platelet aggregation and secretion.

Platelets form a hemostatic plug by aggregating on the layer of adherent platelets. Aggregation is an active metabolic process in which agonists such as thrombin, ADP, thromboxane A_2, and collagen initiate signaling pathways that enable the platelet membrane GPIIb-IIIa complex (also known as αIIbβ3) to bind soluble fibrinogen or vWf. Fibrinogen and vWf bound to GPIIb-IIIa cross-link platelets into a hemostatic plug.

Platelets are also secretory cells and contain four types of granules: dense (δ) granules containing ADP, ATP, calcium, serotonin, and pyrophosphate; α granules containing a variety of proteins including fibrinogen, vWf, factor V, platelet-derived growth factor (PDGF), and IgG; lysosomes containing acid hydrolases; and microperoxisomes containing peroxidase activity. The δ granule ADP is thought to propagate primary platelet responses, α granule PGDF participates in wound repair, and α granule factor V contributes to thrombin generation. However, the function of many of the other α and δ granule substances is unclear. Nonetheless, disorders of platelet secretion produce mild to moderate bleeding, indicating that platelet secretion plays a role in hemostasis.

The plasma membrane of activated platelets provides an essential procoagulant surface for the assembly of the tenase and prothrombinase complexes that activate coagulation factor X and prothrombin, respectively. This activity, formerly known as platelet factor 3, occurs when an agonist-stimulated rise in intraplatelet Ca^{2+} induces the exposure of anionic phospholipids on the platelet surface, a reaction mediated by a membrane-associated phospholipid scramblase.

QUANTITATIVE PLATELET DISORDERS

Adequate numbers of functional platelets are required to support primary hemostasis. A decreased number of platelets (thrombocytopenia) results from decreased platelet production by bone marrow megakaryocytes, accelerated platelet removal, or platelet sequestration in an enlarged spleen. Unfortunately, there is no readily available test to differentiate between these possibilities, so that the clinical context in which thrombocytopenia occurs can be important in deciding which mechanism pertains. However, in the absence of splenomegaly, the presence of megakaryocytes in an otherwise normal bone marrow suggests that thrombocytopenia is due to accelerated platelet removal.

The cutaneous bleeding time is a measure of platelet function in vivo and is sensitive to platelet number. Bleeding time prolongation occurs when the platelet count declines to less than 100,000/μL. However, hemorrhage following trauma or surgery generally does not occur if the platelet count is greater than 50,000/μL. Moreover, when a patient's only hemostatic abnormality is thrombocytopenia, significant spontaneous bleeding generally does not occur until the platelet count declines to less than 5000 to 10,000. Nonetheless, there is no absolute threshold for spontaneous bleeding related to thrombocytopenia and it can occur at higher platelet counts when fever, sepsis, severe anemia, and other hemostatic defects are present or when platelet function is impaired by medication.

Thrombocytopenia Related to Decreased Platelet Production

Platelet production decreases when the number of bone marrow megakaryocytes decreases in diseases such as acute leukemia and aplastic anemia; myelophthisic processes in which bone marrow is replaced by metastatic carcinoma, fibrosis, or multiple myeloma; following chemotherapy and/or radiation therapy; when the number of marrow megakaryocytes is decreased by ethanol toxicity; and during infections with viruses such as HIV, measles, cytomegalovirus, and varicella. Thrombocytopenia also occurs when megakaryocyte proliferation is impaired by diseases such as myelodysplasia and paroxysmal nocturnal hemoglobinuria. Overt bleeding in all of these disorders, when clearly related to thrombocytopenia, is treated by platelet transfusion. The use of prophylactic platelet transfusion to prevent bleeding, however, is an area of controversy. Platelet transfusion is complicated by the short life span of circulating platelets (10 days), by the 5-day shelf life of untransfused platelets, and by platelet immunogenicity. Thus, when the conditions responsible for decreased platelet production cannot be readily reversed, long-term prophylaxis would require frequent platelet transfusions and the risk of developing refractoriness to transfusion because of platelet alloantibodies. Studies performed primarily in patients undergoing treatment for acute leukemia have shown that in the absence of overt bleeding, outcome is unchanged when platelet counts of 5000 to 10,000/μL are used as the threshold for prophylactic transfusion. Because most chronic conditions rarely result in this level of thrombocytopenia, regular prophylactic platelet transfusions are not usually necessary. When prophylactic platelet transfusion is required, using single-donor apheresis platelets and/or platelet donors who are HLA identical to the recipient must be considered to prevent the development of refractoriness.

Thrombocytopenia Related to Increased Platelet Destruction

Both nonimmune and immune processes can lead to thrombocytopenia related to a shortened platelet life span. Nonimmune causes of accelerated platelet clearance include sepsis, disseminated intravascular coagulation, thrombotic thrombocytopenic purpura–hemolytic-uremic syndrome (TTP-HUS), preeclampsia or eclampsia, cardiopulmonary bypass, and the Kasabach-Merritt syndrome of giant cavernous hemangiomas. Thrombocytopenia in these disorders generally resolves as the disorders resolve and platelet transfusion is rarely necessary. It is noteworthy that in TTP-HUS, thrombocytopenia is associated with thrombosis rather than bleeding and there are reports of clinical deterioration, even death, following platelet transfusion. On the other hand, excessive bleeding following cardiopulmonary bypass may respond to platelet transfusion when all of the other hemostatic defects associated with bypass have been corrected.

Immune-mediated platelet destruction can be due to hypersensitivity to medication, alloimmune sensitization following transfusion or pregnancy, and autoimmunity. The list of medications reported to cause antibody-mediated platelet destruction is long, but in many cases the supporting evidence is scant. Drugs that definitely cause antibody-mediated thrombocytopenia include quinine and quinidine, sulfonamides, and gold salts. Nonetheless, medications must always be considered as a possible etiology for thrombocytopenia. Besides stopping the offending medication, emergent treatment for severe thrombocytopenia with bleeding in this situation includes platelet transfusion, as well as corticosteroids and intravenous immunoglobulin (IGIV), similar to emergent treatment for autoimmune thrombocytopenia (see later).

Heparin-induced thrombocytopenia (HIT) is a special case of drug-induced thrombocytopenia. HIT is the most common cause of drug-induced thrombocytopenia in hospitalized patients, occurring in up to 5% of patients given unfractionated heparin for 5 to 10 days by any route. HIT results from the formation of antibodies to a complex between heparin and the platelet α granule protein platelet factor 4. It is a unique form of thrombocytopenia because patients with HIT rarely bleed; rather the HIT immune complex activates platelets by binding to the platelet Fc receptor, thereby causing thrombosis in both the arterial and venous circulations. HIT must always be considered when thrombocytopenia is detected in a hospitalized patient. It is mandatory that all heparin administration be stopped when HIT is considered and alternative anticoagulation instituted, at least until the platelet count returns to normal and perhaps for as long as 30 days. Alternative anticoagulants currently approved for HIT include the direct thrombin inhibitors recombinant hirudin and argatroban. Warfarin (Coumadin) should not be used for acute HIT because several days of treatment are required for its anticoagulant effect and because its use has been associated with a syndrome of venous limb gangrene that has led to amputation.

Alloimmune thrombocytopenia is due to sensitization to platelet alloantigens such as Pl^{A1} (HPA-1a) and results from either transfusion (post-transfusion purpura, PTP) or maternal sensitization during pregnancy (neonatal alloimmune thrombocytopenia, NATP). PTP causes profound thrombocytopenia and bleeding 7 to 10 days following blood transfusion and can be treated with IGIV or plasma exchange. NATP can cause severe thrombocytopenia and bleeding in neonates and is treated with platelet transfusion, corticosteroids, and IGIV.

Autoimmune thrombocytopenia is related to circulating antiplatelet autoantibodies. Although platelet autoantibodies and thrombocytopenia can occur in autoimmune diseases such as systemic lupus erythematosus and in low-grade lymphoproliferative disorders such as chronic lymphocytic leukemia and well-differentiated lymphocytic lymphoma, they frequently occur in otherwise healthy individuals as a disease known as idiopathic thrombocytopenic purpura (ITP). Patients with ITP, often young women (although ITP can occur at any age in either sex), present with spontaneous mucocutaneous bleeding or with unexplained asymptomatic thrombocytopenia. Red cell and white cell counts are usually normal, splenomegaly is not present, and peripheral blood smears are remarkable only for a decreased number of platelets, many of which may be larger than normal. Megakaryocytes are present and often plentiful in ITP bone marrow, but because the differential diagnosis for typical ITP is usually limited to ITP and myelodysplasia, a bone marrow examination is rarely necessary in the absence of findings suggesting myelodysplasia. On the other hand, HIV infection can initially present with an ITP-like picture, and HIV infection must at least be considered when evaluating a patient for possible ITP. Although assays are available to detect antiplatelet antibodies, the assays lack sensitivity and specificity and are rarely helpful diagnostically.

Treatment of ITP is guided by symptoms and platelet count. Because bleeding symptoms are usually minimal to absent until platelet counts decline below 30,000/μL, asymptomatic patients with platelet counts greater than 30,000 can be carefully observed without treatment. When bleeding is present and/or the platelet count is less than 30,000/μL, treatment is initiated with prednisone at a dose of 1 mg/kg body weight. Most patients respond favorably to prednisone and platelet counts increase toward normal over the course of days to weeks. When the platelet count increases to greater than 100,000, a slow prednisone taper is initiated with three possible outcomes. First, the platelet count may remain normal after prednisone is discontinued. Second, the platelet count may decrease during the taper but it remains greater than 30,000 at prednisone doses of 10 mg or less. Third, the disease relapses and either fails to re-respond to prednisone or prednisone doses greater than 10 mg daily are required to maintain an acceptable platelet count. The latter group of patients, as well as patients who initially fail to respond to prednisone, are candidates for splenectomy because 60% to 75% enter remission following this procedure. The small number of patients continuing to experience symptomatic thrombocytopenia after splenectomy are candidates for trials of various immunosuppressive agents including azathioprine (Imuran),* cyclophosphamide (Cytoxan),* rituximab (Rituxan),* and cyclosporine (Neoral).*

Occasionally, patients with ITP present emergently with severe thrombocytopenia (<5000/μL) and/or internal bleeding. These patients should be treated with high doses of corticosteroids (methylprednisolone [30 mg/kg/d] and IGIV [1 g/kg daily times 2]). Platelet transfusion can be given concurrently with IGIV for critical bleeding. Anti-D immune globulin may be substituted for IGIV in Rh-positive patients who have not undergone splenectomy.

Thrombocytopenia Related to Platelet Sequestration in an Enlarged Spleen

Approximately 30% of the circulating platelet mass is normally present in the spleen. Additional platelets may be sequestered in the spleen when it enlarges because of portal hypertension or infiltrative diseases. Thrombocytopenia related to hypersplenism generally produces platelet counts in the range of 40,000 to 50,000/μL, bleeding related to thrombocytopenia alone

*Not FDA approved for this indication.

is unusual, and in most patients thrombocytopenia associated with hypersplenism requires no specific treatment.

QUALITATIVE PLATELET DISORDERS

A prolonged bleeding time in a patient with a normal platelet count suggests a diagnosis of von Willebrand disease or of an acquired or a hereditary qualitative platelet disorder.

Acquired Qualitative Platelet Disorders

Acquired disorders of platelet function frequently cause abnormal platelet function in vitro and prolong bleeding times in vivo but only occasionally induce a mild bleeding diathesis. However, they can become clinically important when thrombocytopenia or other hemostatic disorders are present. Acquired platelet function disorders can be classified into those in which platelet function is impaired by medication and those in which platelet function is impaired by nonhematologic and hematologic diseases. Although a wide variety of medications impair platelet function in vitro, only a small number actually produce clinically significant bleeding. These include aspirin, the thienopyridines ticlopidine (Ticlid) and clopidogrel (Plavix), and the GPIIb-IIIa antagonists abciximab (ReoPro), tirofiban (Aggrastat), and eptifibatide (Integrilin). Aspirin is an important cause of platelet dysfunction. It irreversibly inactivates the enzyme prostaglandin endoperoxide H synthase-1 (PGHS-1, cyclooxygenase-1), thereby preventing platelet synthesis of thromboxane A_2. In adults, platelet prostaglandin synthesis is nearly completely inhibited by a single 100-mg dose of aspirin. Aspirin has a minimal effect on hemostasis in normal individuals. However, it causes a substantial prolongation of the bleeding time and can precipitate hemorrhage in individuals with preexisting hemostatic defects such as von Willebrand disease, hemophilia A, warfarin ingestion, uremia, and other disorders of platelet function.

Nonhematologic disorders in which platelet dysfunction can be a prominent feature include uremia and cardiopulmonary bypass. Platelet dysfunction in uremia is usually corrected by dialysis. When it persists, the vasopressin analog desmopressin (DDAVP)* is the treatment of choice, but conjugated estrogens* and cryoprecipitate can also improve hemostasis in uremic patients. DDAVP causes the release of vWf from tissue stores and has been reported to shorten the bleeding time in 50% to 75% of patients with uremia. It is usually administered intravenously at a dose of 0.3 μg/kg over 15 to 30 minutes (maximum dose 20 μg). Improvement in the bleeding time occurs within 30 to 60 minutes and lasts for approximately 4 hours. Dosing can be repeated at 12- to 24-hour intervals, but tachyphylaxis may occur with repeated dosing. The prolonged bleeding time in uremia can also be shortened, and hemostasis may be improved, by the correction of anemia using red cell transfusion or erythropoietin. Platelet dysfunction following cardiopulmonary bypass can result from the interaction of platelets with the bypass circuit and from the hypothermia induced during bypass. Although platelet dysfunction generally resolves spontaneously 2 to 24 hours after bypass, persistent bleeding may require platelet transfusion. DDAVP and the protease inhibitor aprotinin (Trasylol)* have been used prophylactically to diminish mediastinal bleeding and transfusion requirements, but reported results have been inconsistent.

*Not FDA approved for this indication.

Platelet dysfunction can occur in chronic myeloproliferative disorders such as polycythemia vera and essential thrombocythemia, in dysproteinemias such as multiple myeloma and macroglobulinemia, in myelodysplasia and leukemia, and in acquired forms of von Willebrand disease. Platelet dysfunction in the myeloproliferative disorders is due to intrinsic platelet defects as well as to substantial increases in platelet count and can result in both bleeding and thrombosis. Reducing the platelet count with hydroxyurea (Droxia)* or anagrelide (Agrylin) reduces the risk of bleeding or thrombosis in patients older than 60 and in patients with symptomatic platelet dysfunction regardless of age. Aspirin can be helpful in patients with thrombosis, but its routine use in asymptomatic patients can increase the risk of bleeding. Platelet dysfunction in dysproteinemia can result from an inhibitory effect of a paraprotein on platelet function and improves when the concentration of protein is decreased by plasmapheresis or chemotherapy. Thrombocytopenia is clearly the most common cause of bleeding in patients with leukemia and myelodysplasia, but platelet dysfunction has also been described. Acquired von Willebrand disease is a rare complication of myeloproliferative disorders, autoimmune diseases, and dysproteinemias. DDAVP, infusions of vWf concentrates, and IGIV* (especially in patients with monoclonal paraproteins) have been reported to improve hemostasis in these patients, whereas treatment of the primary disease alone may not.

Hereditary Qualitative Platelet Disorders

The Bernard-Soulier syndrome (BSS) and Glanzmann's thrombasthenia (GT) are rare autosomal recessive disorders of the platelet membrane glycoproteins GPIb-IX and GPIIb-IIIa, respectively. These disorders arise in infancy or childhood with characteristic platelet-type bleeding: ecchymoses, epistaxis, and gingival bleeding. Patients with BSS are thrombocytopenic and have very large platelets that do not agglutinate when exposed to ristocetin because they are unable to bind vWf. Platelet counts and platelet morphology are normal in GT, but the platelets cannot aggregate in response to ADP and thrombin because they lack a sufficient number of functional fibrinogen receptors. Treatment of bleeding in both conditions requires platelet transfusion.

*Not FDA approved for this indication.

Hereditary disorders of platelet secretion are not uncommon causes of easy bruising, menorrhagia, and excessive postoperative and postpartum blood loss. The disorders can be due to a deficiency of platelet granules (gray platelet syndrome–α granule deficiency; δ storage pool disease (δSPD)–dense granule deficiency) or to aspirin-like defects resulting from abnormalities of the platelet secretory mechanism. δSPD is the most common platelet secretion disorder and can be further subclassified into δSPD associated with albinism (the Hermansky-Pudlack and Chédiak-Higashi syndromes) and δSPD in otherwise normal individuals. Patients with δSPD have normal platelet counts and often, but not always, have prolonged bleeding times and abnormal platelet aggregation studies. An increased ratio of platelet ATP to ADP, because of the absence of platelet dense granule ADP, however, is diagnostic. Although bleeding in patients with secretion disorders can be controlled by platelet transfusion, this is seldom necessary because DDAVP inexplicably shortens bleeding times and improves hemostasis in these patients.

DISSEMINATED INTRAVASCULAR COAGULATION

method of
CHENG HOCK TOH, M.D.
Royal Liverpool University Hospital
Liverpool, United Kingdom

Disseminated intravascular coagulation (DIC) represents the loss of a normally localized and exquisitely controlled hemostatic process that complicates well-recognized conditions such as sepsis and trauma. With widespread microvascular–reticuloendothelial system involvement in the inflammatory reaction to the initiating stimulus, in vivo thrombin generation becomes greatly enhanced and actively sustained. It is in this context that targeting of the coagulant-inflammatory interface has seen the emergence into clinical practice of successful modulatory therapy in sepsis per se and DIC in general. In addition, the shift of emphasis in better understanding the mechanisms that sustain thrombin generation (Table 1) rather than its initiation promises to deliver better tools that can monitor the progress and pace of DIC. A combination of diagnostic and therapeutic advances promises to improve on the prognosis for the patient with DIC into the future.

DIAGNOSIS

As subclinical coagulopathy is common in sepsis and this could be a basis for identifying at-risk patients, the International Society of Thrombosis and Haemostasis Standardisation Sub-Committee on DIC has put fresh emphasis on defining this nonovert stage of DIC. The working diagnosis for nonovert DIC scores for both abnormal coagulation results and the abnormal trends in these results. As the practical management of critically ill patients requires assays that are simple and rapid in performance, the current basis for testing in nonovert DIC emphasizes the use of simple global tests of coagulation, such as the prothrombin time and the platelet count (Table 2). An advantage is the greater worldwide applicability of these tests and the ability to standardize definitions for future multicenter therapeutic trials in this area. However, the recognition that these tests may be insufficiently robust on their own suggests the inclusion of more specific indicators of thrombin generation or ones that mark the link between coagulation and inflammation. Hence, the template for scoring nonovert DIC builds in the use of such tests provided they fulfill evidence-based criteria of usefulness in both being prognostic and diagnostic. Such a strategy would ensure systematic improvements in the diagnosis of DIC to best achieve progressive improvement in clinical outcome.

TABLE 1. **Mechanisms Sustaining Thrombin Generation**

Activation of intrinsic pathway of coagulation
Reduction in levels of endogenous anticoagulant factors (e.g., protein C, antithrombin)
Increased availability of negatively charged phospholipid surfaces:
Externalization of inner cellular membrane leaflet
Cellular microparticle formation
Circulating lipoproteins

TREATMENT

Although the mainstay of DIC management is to remove the primary inciting cause, this is often inadequate at the point of severe sepsis or trauma. Although blood product support with fresh frozen plasma, cryoprecipitate, and platelets has been used, this offers supportive treatment at best. The principle of thrombin suppression has been tried with heparin with little evidence of benefit, in part because of the complication of excessive bleeding.

Activated Protein C

Among the myriad of strategies tried in severe sepsis, a recombinant form of human activated protein C (rhAPC), called drotrecogin alfa activated

TABLE 2. **Practical Markers of Nonovert Disseminated Intravascular Coagulation**

Coagulation Test	Finding
PT	Increasing clot time
Platelets	Falling count
APTT	Increasing transmittance waveform abnormality
Fibrin-related marker	Rising levels

APTT, activated partial thromboplastin time; PT, prothrombin time.

(Xigris), has emerged as the first successful treatment. A large multicenter randomized controlled trial demonstrated that drotrecogin alfa activated (Xigris) (24 μg/kg/hour continuous infusion over 96 hours) significantly reduced mortality from 30.8% to 24.7% at 28 days. Protein C (PC) deficiency was not a criterion for enrollment and 13% of patients had normal PC levels on treatment entry, suggesting that intervention was frequently at a nonovert phase of DIC. Although APC is well known as an anticoagulant by inactivating factors VIIIa and Va and therefore limiting thrombin generation, there is also evidence of anti-inflammatory properties. APC can attenuate the inflammatory response by modulating nuclear factor κB. Certainly, suppression of APC activity in baboon models of sepsis led to increased microvascular thrombosis and neutrophilic infiltration within tissue sections of affected animals.

In practical terms, care should be exercised when drotrecogin alfa activated (Xigris) is used in the presence of thrombocytopenia. In the trial, there was a nonsignificant increasing trend toward intracranial hemorrhage with drotrecogin alfa activated (Xigris) treatment, particularly with coincident thrombocytopenia of less than 50×10^9/L. Platelet transfusion in this group during drotrecogin alfa activated (Xigris) treatment would therefore be particularly important.

Protein C

Use of zymogen blood-derived PC (Ceprotin) replacement therapy has been reported to reduce significantly morbidity and mortality in series of patients with meningococcal septicemia in one nonrandomized trial. PC levels are low in sepsis and correlate with mortality. PC binds to the endothelial protein C receptor (EPCR) and is then activated to APC by the thrombin-thrombomodulin (TM) complex. Hence, the efficacy of this therapeutic regimen depends very much on adequate levels of TM and EPCR at the cell surface. However, these are often diminished in severe sepsis. At present, PC (Ceprotin) treatment is used mainly for purpura fulminans in the pediatric setting.

Antithrombin

Antithrombin (AT), like APC, has been shown to have both anticoagulant and anti-inflammatory properties. Similarly, levels are markedly reduced in sepsis: swamped by rapid thrombin generation, increased degradation from a variety of serine proteases, and a reduction in hepatic synthesis. A large randomized controlled trial using high-dose AT failed to demonstrate a significant mortality reduction, although subgroup analysis suggested that this may be primarily due to the adverse outcome of the arm involving heparin coinfusion with AT. Certainly, at the cellular level there is experimental evidence that the microcirculatory benefits of AT during endotoxemia can be adversely effected by the presence of heparin in either unfractionated or low-molecular-weight forms. Thus, there is no present role for AT therapy on its own outside the confines of a clinical trial.

Tissue Factor Pathway Inhibitor

As the tissue factor (TF)–factor VIIa pathway is a potent driver of the coagulant process, strategies to nullify this pathway have also been applied in the treatment of sepsis and DIC. Tissue factor pathway inhibitor (TFPI) is the physiologic inhibitor of this pathway and binds TF-VIIa. The full results of its therapeutic use in a large randomized controlled trial of sepsis are awaited, but it has become apparent that no overall efficacy has been demonstrated. As the TF–factor VIIa pathway is integral in initiating rather than sustaining the coagulant process, this strategy may not be as successful if it is thrombin sustenance rather than thrombin initiation that has greater pathogenic consequence in sepsis and DIC. Indeed, TFPI levels are not depressed in DIC and conversely increase with sepsis severity. Another issue may be the uncertainty over the anti-inflammatory properties of TFPI. Certainly, studies in human endotoxemia models have not substantiated the case for this adjuvant property.

SUMMARY

There is now cautious optimism about an improved prognosis in DIC, hitherto associated with impending death. Although thrombin suppression appears key to this preliminary success, it seems likely that the intrinsic anti-inflammatory properties of APC itself are important too. However, there is still considerable progress to be made as mortality in the drotrecogin alfa activated (Xigris) therapeutic arm was still high at 25%. The future may see improvements through the use of combination therapies, but such trials are not yet currently under way. For the present, an important focus for improving prognosis is earlier detection of the DIC process at a nonovert phase to enable therapeutic intervention prior to irreversible decompensation.

THROMBOTIC THROMBOCYTOPENIC PURPURA

method of
LESLEY A. KRESIE, M.D.
Baylor University Medical Center
Dallas, Texas

Thrombotic thrombocytopenic purpura (TTP) is an occlusive disorder of the systemic microvasculature characterized by platelet aggregation, red blood cell fragmentation, and thrombocytopenia. TTP has classically been associated with a pentad of signs and symptoms: thrombocytopenia, microangiopathic hemolytic anemia, neurologic findings, decreased renal function, and fever. It is not uncommon for patients to lack one or more of these findings at initial presentation; therefore, it is now recommended that TTP be suspected in any patient who has acute, severe thrombocytopenia and microangiopathic hemolytic anemia without any other explanation. If untreated, TTP is fatal in 80% to 90% of patients. Initiation of timely plasma exchange can decrease the mortality rate to about 20%, but as many as 40% of patients may have relapses after initial, successful treatment.

ETIOLOGY AND PATHOPHYSIOLOGY

TTP was first described in the early 1920s, but its etiology had been a mystery until now. The discovery of a protease deficiency has given us new insight into the cause and potential avenues for treatment of this disorder. The presence of a plasma protein defect was first suspected after observations of successful treatment with plasma transfusions and plasma exchange. Unusually large von Willebrand factor (ULvWF) multimers were then discovered in the plasma of patients with chronic relapsing TTP.

Under normal conditions, vWF is released from the endothelial cells and binds platelets to exposed subendothelium at sites of vascular injury. The larger the vWF multimer, the higher is its capacity for promoting platelet aggregation. In order to maintain normal levels of platelet aggregation, any ULvWF multimers released into the circulation are quickly broken down into smaller units. In patients with TTP, this control process is defective. The ULvWF multimers remain in the circulation and promote systemic platelet clumping. Microvascular thrombi, containing platelets and vWF with little or no fibrin, are formed in most organs. Platelet counts drop and red cells are damaged as they attempt to pass through the thrombi. Occlusion of the microvasculature leads to ischemia and organ dysfunction, most notably in the central nervous system (CNS) and kidneys.

The enzyme involved in cleaving these ULvWF multimers has now been identified. This protease is designated ADAMTS13 and the corresponding gene has been localized to chromosome 9q34. The name stands for the family of proteases, "*a* *d*isintegrin-like *a*nd *m*etalloprotease with *t*hrombo*s*pondin type 1 repeats." A constitutional deficiency of the protease has been identified in patients with the rare, familial form of chronic relapsing TTP. Acute, acquired TTP, however, has been associated with the transient development of IgG autoantibodies that inhibit protease activity. Inhibitors of ADAMTS13 have also been observed in drug-induced TTP related to ticlopidine (Ticlid) and possibly clopidogrel (Plavix). Of interest, patients with hemolytic-uremic syndrome (HUS), a condition with presenting features similar to those of TTP, have levels of protease activity within the normal range.

Approximately 1000 new cases of acute idiopathic TTP occur each year in the United States, and the disease has been increasing in prevalence. This rise in prevalence is greater than can be accounted for simply by increased recognition of the disease. TTP can occur at any age but is most common in young adults (median age ~ 40 years) and occurs more frequently in women. The adult form of TTP has been associated with numerous clinical situations including bone marrow transplantation, pregnancy (75% occurring in the peripartum-postpartum period), and various autoimmune disorders. Drugs that have been associated with TTP include quinine, ticlopidine (Ticlid), clopidogrel (Plavix), mitomycin C (Mutamycin), cyclosporine (Sandimmune), and other chemotherapeutic and immunosuppressive agents.

DIAGNOSIS

There is no gold standard for the clinical diagnosis of TTP. Only a minority of patients present with the classical pentad of signs and symptoms. However, all patients with TTP show signs of thrombocytopenia and fragmentation anemia. As these are rather nonspecific findings, the diagnosis of TTP usually requires a high index of suspicion and the exclusion of other causes of microangiopathic hemolytic anemia (Table 1). Neurologic symptoms are noted in about 70% of patients and initially arise as confusion, delirium, or focal seizure activity. These abnormalities may wax and wane during the course of the illness. Renal failure may not be immediately evident in the patient; however, some patients have proteinuria and elevated blood urea nitrogen on initial presentation.

Laboratory findings in TTP include: anemia, thrombocytopenia (often below 20,000/mm^3), fragmented red blood cells (schistocytes) on peripheral blood smear, and elevated serum lactate dehydrogenase (LDH). Serum LDH elevation is a hallmark of red cell destruction and tissue injury related to ischemia. Tests of the coagulation system including prothrombin time, partial thromboplastin time, fibrinogen, and fibrin split products are usually normal or only mildly abnormal and exclude the presence of disseminated intravascular coagulation. Evans' syndrome (autoimmune hemolytic anemia with concurrent autoimmune thrombocytopenia) can be excluded from the differential by performing a direct antiglobulin test (direct Coombs' test), which should be negative in TTP. As some opportunistic infections associated with HIV

TABLE 1. **Differential Diagnosis of Thrombotic Thrombocytopenic Purpura**

Disseminated intravascular coagulation
Sepsis
Evans' syndrome
Hemolytic-uremic syndrome
Preeclampsia/eclampsia, HELLP
Vasculitis
Scleroderma, SLE
Disseminated malignancy
Malignant hypertension

HELLP, hemolysis, elevated liver enzymes, low platelet count; SLE, systemic lupus erythematous.

infection may mimic TTP, a test for HIV should also be considered upon initial presentation. At present, there are no confirmatory tests to establish the diagnosis of TTP. Current tests for ADAMTS13 deficiency or inhibitors of ADAMTS13 are not readily available and lack standardization.

MANAGEMENT

When the diagnosis is established (or strongly suspected), plasma exchange should be initiated as soon as possible. The patient should undergo daily plasmapheresis with fresh frozen plasma (FFP) replacement. The apheresis procedure removes the ULvWF multimers to prevent further platelet aggregation while infusion of fresh frozen plasma replaces the deficient vWF-cleaving protease. If immediate plasma exchange is not available, simple transfusion of FFP should be initiated until the patient can be transferred to another facility. Response to therapy should be monitored by disappearance of neurologic symptoms (if present); normalization of LDH, platelet count, and hemoglobin; and disappearance of schistocytes from the peripheral smear. Patients may require daily plasma exchange for days or even weeks. When the patient shows a sustained response, plasma exchange can be tapered down to three times a week and then once a week before complete discontinuation of therapy.

Corticosteroids are frequently used in addition to plasma exchange. The identification of autoantibodies to ADAMTS13 in patients with acute TTP supports the administration of corticosteroids. However, many patients respond fully to plasma exchange therapy alone. Corticosteroids are recommended for patients who appear to be refractory to treatment. These patients may also show improved response if the cryosupernatant fraction of plasma is used in place of FFP. Removal of the cryoprecipitate from the donor plasma results in removal of the largest vWF multimers. Case reports of refractory patients also document successful treatment by administration of chemotherapeutic and immunosuppressive agents such as rituximab (Rituxan),* vincristine (Oncovin, Vincasar),* and cyclophosphamide (Cytoxan).* Splenectomy has also been used with varying success.

Although extreme thrombocytopenia is the hallmark of this disorder, platelet transfusions should be avoided unless life-threatening bleeding (particularly CNS) is present. The infusion of platelets may only provide additional substrate for the formation of thrombi. Myocardial infarction and strokes have reportedly occurred after platelet transfusion.

After successful therapy, patients should be monitored on a regular basis. The frequency of follow-up visits can be steadily decreased as the patient remains stable. A complete blood count and LDH should be performed at each visit. If either the platelet count starts to drop or the LDH begins to rise, another course of plasma exchange should be initiated. Relapse has been reported in 10% to 40% of patients. Most relapses occur within the first year, but relapses have occurred as many as 10 years after remission. Mortality associated with relapse is minimal as the patients are usually responsive to retreatment.

The effects of the systemic ischemia may take months or years for full recovery, and persistent neurologic abnormalities have been noted that may be the result of actual stroke. However, continued observations suggest gradual improvement in most patients. The majority of patients suffer no long-term complications after successful treatment of acute TTP.

*Not FDA approved for this indication.

HEMOCHROMATOSIS

method of
BRUCE Y. TUNG, M.D., and
KRIS V. KOWDLEY, M.D.
University of Washington School of Medicine
Seattle, Washington

Hereditary hemochromatosis (HHC), the most common genetic disorder in persons of northern European descent, is inherited as an autosomal recessive trait. Discovery of the hemochromatosis gene, *HFE*, in 1996 has led to significant advances in the diagnosis and management of HHC patients.

A specific missense mutation of *HFE* that leads to a cysteine-to-tyrosine substitution at amino acid 282 (C282Y) has been found to be homozygous in 82% to 100% of HHC patients. A second missense mutation with a histidine-to-aspartate substitution at amino acid 63 (H63D) has also been described. Only C282Y homozygotes and some C282Y/H63D compound heterozygotes appear to be at risk for significant iron overload.

Population-based studies have demonstrated that the prevalence of the C282Y homozygous genotype is approximately 1 in 200 in patients of northern European descent. However, iron overload does not develop in all homozygotes. Great controversy has arisen regarding penetrance of the C282Y homozygous genotype, which has been reported to be as low as 1% and as high as 80%.

CLINICAL FEATURES

Hemochromatosis is a multisystem disease. Iron accumulation may lead to dysfunction of the liver, heart, joints, pancreas, pituitary, and other endocrine organs. The clinical features of HHC are not typically present until the fourth or fifth decades of life. Phenotypic expression of the disease is influenced by dietary intake of iron, alcohol intake, and pathologic or physiologic blood loss. Consequently, HHC develops in men at a younger age than in women because menstruation delays iron loading in women.

With the advent of screening programs and genetic testing, the clinical features of HHC are changing.

Increasingly, HHC patients are identified from abnormal serum iron studies or genetic testing before the development of signs or symptoms. When symptoms are present, weakness, arthralgia, and impotence are the most common. Hepatomegaly is present in over 50% of probands with newly diagnosed HHC; skin pigmentation and arthritis are also frequently observed. Diabetes mellitus typically does not arise until after the development of cirrhosis.

DIAGNOSIS OF HEMOCHROMATOSIS

Serum Iron Studies

Serum iron studies, including the serum iron concentration, total iron-binding capacity, and serum ferritin, are usually the first tests ordered when the diagnosis of HHC is considered. A threshold fasting transferrin saturation of 45% is sensitive and specific in identifying asymptomatic individuals with HHC (Figure 1). Serum ferritin is frequently elevated; however, elevated levels are not specific for the diagnosis of HHC because serum ferritin may be falsely elevated by many inflammatory conditions.

Genetic Testing

Genetic testing for both the C282Y and H63D mutations of *HFE* is available as a diagnostic test for HHC. The C282Y mutation is homozygous in 82% to 100% of patients in whom HHC is clinically diagnosed. However, the clinical penetrance of iron overload in C282Y homozygotes is highly variable and depends on the population studied and the definition of iron overload used. Nonetheless, the presence of the C282Y homozygous mutation in a patient with elevated serum transferrin saturation and ferritin levels establishes a diagnosis of hemochromatosis. In addition, clinical iron overload may develop in approximately 1% to 5% of patients who are compound heterozygotes (C282Y/H63D).

Liver Biopsy

With the advent of genetic testing, the role of liver biopsy in the management of HHC is evolving. Liver biopsy in patients with HHC has two primary indications: when the diagnosis of HHC is still in doubt despite biochemical and genetic testing and to evaluate for the presence of cirrhosis for prognostic information. Liver biopsy is indicated for HHC patients with serum ferritin levels greater than 1000 ng/mL because such patients are at higher risk for the development of cirrhosis. In HHC, the overall prognosis is directly related to the presence or absence of cirrhosis.

Quantitation of hepatic iron remains the gold standard for the diagnosis of phenotypic iron overload. In homozygotes for HHC who express the phenotype, the hepatic iron concentration is often greater than 4000 μg/g dry weight. The hepatic iron index is helpful in distinguishing patients with homozygous HHC from those with lesser degrees of iron loading, such as heterozygotes for HHC or patients with alcoholic or chronic viral liver disease. The hepatic iron index is calculated by dividing the hepatic iron concentration (in μmol/g dry weight) by patient age (in years). The hepatic iron index is usually higher than 1.9 in HHC homozygotes and less than 1.9 in patients with iron loading from other causes. It is important to remember that phenotypic criteria for HHC, such as the hepatic iron concentration and hepatic iron index, were established before the introduction of *HFE* gene testing. As noted earlier, it is now recognized that many C282Y homozygotes have milder phenotypic expression and thus lower hepatic iron levels.

Quantitative Phlebotomy

In situations in which the diagnosis of HHC remains equivocal and liver biopsy is contraindicated, quantitative phlebotomy can be useful to confirm the presence of significant iron overload. Freely expressing

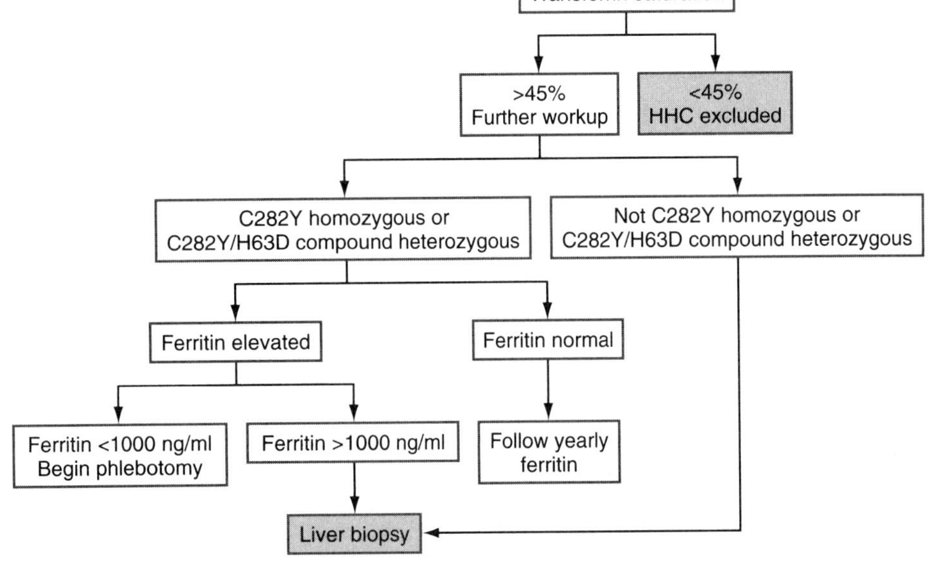

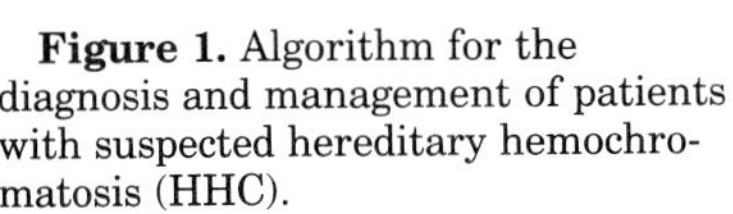
Figure 1. Algorithm for the diagnosis and management of patients with suspected hereditary hemochromatosis (HHC).

HHC homozygotes almost always have more than 4 g of excess body iron. Because each unit of blood contains approximately 250 mg of elemental iron, a minimum of 16 to 20 phlebotomies may be needed to achieve iron depletion. However, as noted before, homozygotes with incomplete expression may have lower mobilizable iron stores.

SCREENING

Family screening is an important part of the care of patients with HHC because discovery of the disease before the development of cirrhosis is associated with a normal life expectancy if patients are compliant with phlebotomy. The disorder is inherited as an autosomal recessive trait, so all first-degree relatives, especially siblings, should be screened. For a C282Y homozygous proband, first-degree relatives should be screened with *HFE* genotyping and serum iron studies. For a C282Y homozygous proband with children, *HFE* genotyping of the spouse is an alternative strategy to screening each child. For probands who lack the C282Y homozygous mutation, relatives should be screened with serum iron studies and liver biopsy performed if the iron studies are abnormal.

HHC appears to be an ideal disease for population-based screening because it is a common disorder, has a long asymptomatic period, is treatable if detected early, leads to significant morbidity and mortality if untreated, and has a readily available screening test. Several studies have demonstrated that population screening with transferrin saturation is both feasible and cost-effective. Population-based genetic screening cannot be recommended at the current time because of the variable clinical penetrance of the C282Y homozygous genotype, the lack of proof of cost-effectiveness, and the multiple societal ramifications of widespread genetic testing.

THERAPY FOR HEMOCHROMATOSIS

The goal of therapy for HHC is to prevent or reverse the organ damage associated with excess iron accumulation. Part of this goal must be achieved through establishment of a timely diagnosis because hepatic cirrhosis and diabetes mellitus are irreversible complications of HHC and do not improve with iron reduction therapy. Once cirrhosis is present, life expectancy is reduced, and the risk of hepatocellular carcinoma developing may be increased up to 200-fold. By contrast, patients who are iron depleted before the development of cirrhosis have a normal life expectancy.

Phlebotomy is the mainstay of iron reduction therapy and is divided into *induction* and *maintenance* phases. The goal of phlebotomy therapy is to achieve and maintain serum ferritin levels less than 50 ng/mL. Transferrin saturation will often remain elevated and does not need to be monitored during phlebotomy therapy. Induction phlebotomy is begun weekly, with 250 mg of iron in 500 mL of whole blood removed per session. For patients in whom significant anemia develops, the interval between phlebotomy sessions may require lengthening. Induction phlebotomy is continued until iron depletion is attained, as confirmed by a reduction in serum ferritin below 50 ng/mL. Depending on the initial body iron load, iron depletion may take 1 to 2 years to achieve in some HHC patients. After a state of iron depletion is reached, lifelong maintenance phlebotomy is necessary, but only three to four phlebotomies per year may be required, with a goal of maintaining serum ferritin at less than 50 ng/mL.

Iron chelation therapy with deferoxamine (Desferal) has a limited role in the treatment of patients with HHC. Chelation therapy with deferoxamine in HHC patients is reserved for those with severe cardiomyopathy or cardiac arrhythmias. In these selected patients, the combination of chelation therapy and phlebotomy promotes accelerated iron reduction.

A considerable proportion of patients with clinically evident HHC, perhaps as high as 20% to 30%, have a significant history of alcohol intake. Alcohol is not necessary for development of the clinical manifestations of HHC, but significant alcohol intake does accelerate the clinical expression of HHC. All HHC patients should be strongly encouraged to avoid or at least severely limit alcohol intake.

It is difficult to assess how large a role dietary iron plays in the iron accumulation of HHC. Once patients have started phlebotomy therapy, the effect of changes in dietary iron are likely to be negligible. Therefore, patients who have started phlebotomy therapy should be counseled to avoid supplemental iron, but significant dietary changes to reduce iron intake are unnecessary. Vitamin C supplements do increase iron absorption and should generally be avoided with HHC.

C282Y homozygous and C282Y/H63D compound heterozygous individuals who are nonexpressing (normal serum ferritin) should have serum ferritin levels monitored yearly to check for iron accumulation.

MANAGEMENT OF SPECIFIC COMPLICATIONS OF HEMOCHROMATOSIS

Liver Disease

HHC patients with cirrhosis are at high risk for the development of hepatocellular carcinoma, which may account for up to 30% to 45% of deaths in these patients. Serial measurements of α-fetoprotein coupled with abdominal ultrasonography or computed tomography are indicated for cirrhotic patients. For end-stage liver disease associated with HHC, orthotopic liver transplantation is the only effective therapy, although survival rates are poorer after liver transplantation for HHC than for most other indications.

Arthropathy

Joint involvement is very common in HHC and may be the major symptom affecting quality of life.

Typically, an osteoarthritis-like degeneration of the metacarpophalangeal joints is seen, although symmetric polyarthropathy involving the proximal and distal interphalangeal joints, wrists, knees, and hips may also occur. Management of the arthropathy associated with HHC does not differ significantly from the management of degenerative osteoarthritis. The joint disease does not typically improve with iron depletion therapy.

Cardiac Disease

Initially, iron accumulation results in clinically silent increases in left ventricular wall thickness, which may progress over time to dilated cardiomyopathy manifested echocardiographically by left ventricular enlargement and a reduced ejection fraction. Electrocardiographic abnormalities have been described in up to 30% of patients with HHC. The most common arrhythmias associated with cardiac iron overload are atrial tachyarrhythmias, ventricular premature beats, and rarely, ventricular tachycardia. Phlebotomy therapy has been shown to improve the structural and functional cardiac abnormalities, although improvements in cardiac disease are more pronounced if iron reduction is undertaken before the development of dilated cardiomyopathy.

Diabetes Mellitus

Diabetes is typically a late manifestation of HHC; it is present in 70% of cirrhotic patients but only in 10% of noncirrhotics. With earlier diagnosis and treatment of HHC through family and population screening, the prevalence of overt diabetes in patients with newly diagnosed HHC is declining. Medical therapy for the diabetes associated with HHC does not differ significantly from standard therapy for diabetes mellitus. Phlebotomy does not reverse insulin dependence, but approximately a third of patients are able to reduce their insulin requirements.

Other Endocrine Abnormalities

Impotence and amenorrhea are common symptoms of HHC and are usually caused by secondary hypogonadism. Unfortunately, phlebotomy does not lead to improvements in serum luteinizing hormone, follicle-stimulating hormone, testosterone, or impotence. Therapy with intramuscular testosterone injections may be beneficial. Clinical hypothyroidism or adrenal failure are uncommon and usually due to involvement of the pituitary gland.

Skin Pigmentation

Bronze pigmentation of the skin is caused by melanin deposition in the basal layers of the epidermis. The pigmentation is most prominent in sun-exposed areas, but it may also occur in mucous membranes and sun-protected regions. Skin pigmentation typically improves with phlebotomy therapy.

Infectious Complications

Patients with iron overload have an increased susceptibility to certain bacterial infections. Although *Yersinia enterocolitica* is a frequent cause of self-limited enterocolitis in normal hosts, in patients with iron overload it may cause septicemia and multiple hepatic abscesses. Septicemia with unusual organisms such as *Yersinia pseudotuberculosis, Vibrio vulnificus,* and *Listeria monocytogenes* has also been reported in patients with iron overload. Infections with these unusual pathogens should prompt a search for the diagnosis of HHC.

HODGKIN'S DISEASE: CHEMOTHERAPY

method of
KRISTIE A. BLUM, M.D., and
NANCY L. BARTLETT, M.D.
Washington University
Siteman Cancer Center
Division of Oncology
St. Louis, Missouri

In the early 1950s and 1960s, Hodgkin's lymphoma (HL) accounted for 30% of the total lymphoma deaths, compared with only 6% today. Advances in chemotherapy and radiation therapy are primarily responsible for this improvement; however, these advances have also led to increasing reports of serious delayed toxicities. Coronary artery disease and second malignancies have been observed in patients cured of their HL 15–20 years ago and have had a significant impact on long-term survival. Newer chemotherapy regimens, limited radiation doses and fields, and in some cases, elimination of radiation are now being explored in an effort to reduce late treatment mortality. Greater knowledge of prognostic features in HL helps identify patients suitable for these reduced intensity approaches. Patients with poor prognostic features or relapsed disease may benefit from treatment with novel therapeutic agents. Therefore, despite the remarkable improvement in the survival of patients with HL over the last 50 years, the optimal management of HL remains controversial.

Although HL was first described in the nineteenth century, it has proven difficult to characterize molecularly. Hodgkin's Reed-Sternberg (HRS) cells represent less than 1% of the cellular infiltrate, and are hard to isolate from the extensive background inflammatory cells (plasma cells, macrophages, T-cells, and granulocytes). Immunophenotyping has not elucidated the cellular origins of classical HL, because HRS cells express CD30, CD70, and CD15, and heterogeneously express both T-cell and B-cell markers such as CD3 and CD20. CD30 expression does not clarify the cellular (B or T cell) origin of HL, because it is normally present on both activated B and T cells.

CD15 positivity is also not helpful, because it is widely expressed on epithelial cells, macrophages, some B cells and neoplastic T cells. In addition, the clonality of HL has been difficult to ascertain. HRS can be positive for both λ- or κ-light chains, unusual in clonal lymphoid malignancies that usually express one of these light chains exclusively. In 1996, single-cell micromanipulation techniques permitted the use of polymerase chain reaction (PCR) assays to demonstrate the presence of IgH rearrangements in single CD30+ HRS isolated from immunostained paraffin blocks or frozen tissue. Although time-consuming, these single-cell isolation techniques assured that the DNA of HRS used in PCR assays was not contaminated by DNA from the surrounding inflammatory stromal cells. Analysis of these miromanipulated HRS cells indicates that most patients have a clonal rearrangement of IgH genes, consistent with a B-cell origin. This discovery influenced the World Health Organization's (WHO) decision to encourage use of the term Hodgkin's lymphoma in place of Hodgkin's disease, although both are listed and accepted in current classification systems. Hopefully, continued progress in understanding the origins and characteristics of HRS cells will eventually lead to new therapeutic approaches for this disease.

The division of HL into early stage (Ann Arbor stage I-II) or advanced stage (Ann Arbor stage III-IV) disease (Table 1) has prognostic and therapeutic implications. Although some authorities now advocate similar therapy for all stages of HL, staging remains an important prognostic factor with survival rates as high as 90% for patients with early stage HL, compared with 50% in the advanced setting. Yet stage alone is insufficient to predict outcomes. For example, patients with early stage HL and bulky disease, B-symptoms, or high tumor burden (more than three nodal sites of involvement) have 10-year relapse-free survivals (RFS) of only 50% to 70% after treatment with extended field radiotherapy. As in non-Hodgkin's lymphoma (NHL), the development of an international prognostic factors index for HL facilitated characterization of a patient's risk for relapse. In a review of 1618 patients with advanced-stage disease, seven adverse prognostic factors were identified (Table 2). Using these risk factors, a prognostic model was developed in which 5-year freedom from progression (FFP) was 84% for patients with no risk factors, compared with 42% for five or more risk factors (see Table 2). The situation is less clear in early-stage disease, in which no such model exists. Instead, a variety of publications have recognized several unfavorable features in early stage disease, which include B-symptoms, bulky adenopathy (a mediastinal mass ratio [MMR] ≥0.33 by chest x-ray or ≥0.35 by chest CT, or a nodal mass ≥10 cm), extranodal involvement, elevated erythrocyte sedimentation rate (ESR), or age greater than 60. In addition, biologic parameters may also affect prognosis. For example, overexpression of bcl-2 (an anti-apoptotic protein) or reduced p53 (a tumor suppressor) correlates with reduced survival. Efforts have been made to group patients with early stage HL into very favorable, favorable, and unfavorable risk groups. Unfortunately, such categories vary by treatment center. Refinement of such prognostic models will further guide efforts to minimize therapy in low-risk patients and intensify or develop new therapies for the highest risk groups.

TABLE 1. **Ann Arbor Staging System for Hodgkin's Lymphoma**

Stage I	Involvement of a single lymph node region or lymphoid structure, or involvement of a single extralymphatic site (I_E).
Stage II	Involvement of two or more lymph node regions on the same side of the diaphragm, which may be accompanied by localized contiguous involvement of an extralymphatic site or organ (II_E).
Stage III	Involvement of lymph node regions on both sides of the diaphragm, which may also be accompanied by involvement of the spleen (III_S) or by localized contiguous involvement of an extralymphatic site or organ (III_E).
Stage IV	Diffuse or disseminated involvement of one or more extralymphatic organs or tissues, with or without lymph node involvement.

*The absence or presence of fever (>38°C), unexplained weight loss (>10% body weight), or night sweats should be designated by the suffix letters A or B, respectively.

EARLY STAGE HL

As early as 1960, extended field radiotherapy (mantle irradiation or subtotal nodal irradiation) was the mainstay of therapy for early stage HL. Before the advent of MOPP (nitrogen mustard, vincristine, procarbazine, and prednisone; Table 3) chemotherapy in the late 1960s, radiotherapy (RT) was the only curative treatment for HL. The predilection for a pattern of contiguous spread favored this approach of irradiation to involved lymph nodes and prophylactic RT to uninvolved adjacent nodes. With extended field radiotherapy (EFRT), 77% to 85% 10-year overall survival (OS) rates have been reported. MOPP chemotherapy alone appears to be either equivalent or even inferior to EFRT in early stage HL. An NCI-supported trial found similar 7-year OS rates of 85% and 90%, respectively,

TABLE 2. **Prognostic Factors in Advanced Stage Hodgkin's Lymphoma**

Age ≥45 years
Stage IV
Male gender
Hemoglobin <10.5 g/dL
Serum albumin <4 g/dL
Leukocytosis (white blood cell count ≥15,000/mm³)
Lymphocytopenia (ALC <600/mm³ or lymphocyte count <8% of white blood cell count)

No. of risk factors	Freedom from progression at 5 years
0	84%
1	77%
2	67%
3	60%
4	51%
≥5	42%

TABLE 3. **Chemotherapy Regimens in Hodgkin's Lymphoma**

ABVD		
Doxorubicin (Adriamycin RDF)	25 mg/m^2 IV days 1 and 15	Repeat cycle every 28 days
Bleomycin (Blenoxane)	10 mg/m^2 IV days 1 and 15	
Vinblastine (Velban)	6 mg/m^2 IV days 1 and 15	
Dacarbazine	375 mg/m^2 IV days 1 and 15	
MOPP		
Nitrogen mustard	6 mg/m^2 IV days 1 and 8	Repeat cycle every 28 days
Vincristine (Vincasar PFS)	1.4 mg/m^2 IV days 1 and 8	
Procarbazine (Matulane)	100 mg/m^2 PO days 1–14	
Prednisone	40 mg/m^2 PO days 1–14	
MOPP/ABVD		
Nitrogen mustard	6 mg/m^2 IV days 1 and 8	
Vincristine	1.4 mg/m^2 IV days 1 and 8	
Procarbazine	100 mg/m^2 PO days 1–14	
Prednisone	40 mg/m^2 PO days 1–14	
	Alternate every 28 days with:	
Doxorubicin	25 mg/m^2 IV days 1 and 15	
Bleomycin	10 mg/m^2 IV days 1 and 15	
Vinblastine	6 mg/m^2 IV days 1 and 15	
Dacarbazine	375 mg/m^2 IV days 1 and 15	
MOPP/ABV Hybrid		
Nitrogen mustard	6 mg/m^2 IV day 1	Repeat cycle every 28 days
Vincristine	1.4 mg/m^2 IV day 1	
Procarbazine	100 mg/m^2 PO days 1–14	
Prednisone	40 mg/m^2 PO days 1–14	
Doxorubicin	35 mg/m^2 IV day 8	
Bleomycin	10 mg/m^2 IV day 8	
Vinblastine	6 mg/m^2 IV day 8	
Stanford V		
Doxorubicin	25 mg/m^2 IV days 1 and 15	Repeat cycle every 28 days for a total of 3 cycles
Vinblastine	6 mg/m^2 IV days 1 and 15	
Nitrogen mustard	6 mg/m^2 IV day 1	
Vincristine	1.4 mg/m^2 IV days 8 and 22	
Bleomycin	5 units/m^2 IV days 8 and 22	
Etoposide (VePesid)*	60 mg/m^2 IV days 15 and 16	
Prednisone	50 mg/m^2 PO every other day	
BEACOPP		
Bleomycin	10 mg/m^2 IV day 8	Repeat cycle every 21 days
Etoposide	100 mg/m^2 IV days 1–3	
Doxorubicin	25 mg/m^2 IV day 1	
Cyclophosphamide	650 mg/m^2 IV day 1	
Vincristine	1.4 mg/m^2 IV day 1	
Procarbazine	100 mg/m^2 PO days 1–7	
Prednisolone	40 mg/m^2 PO days 1–14	
Escalated BEACOPP		
Bleomycin	10 mg/m^2 IV day 8	Repeat cycle every 21 days
Etoposide*	200 mg/m^2 IV days 1–3	
Doxorubicin	35 mg/m^2 IV day 1	
Cyclophosphamide (Cytoxan)	1250 mg/m^2 IV day 1	
Vincristine	1.4 mg/m^2 IV day 1	
Procarbazine	100 mg/m^2 PO days 1–7	
Prednisolone	40 mg/m^2 PO days 1–14	
GCSF	SC days 8+	
ESHAP		
Etoposide*	40 mg/m^2 IV days 1–4	Repeat cycle every 21–28 days
Methylprednisolone	500 mg IV days 1–5	
Cytarabine (Cytosar-U)	2000 mg/m^2 IV day 5	
Cisplatin (Platinol-AQ)*	25 mg/m^2 CIVI days 1–4	
ICE		
Ifosfamide (Ifex)*	5000 mg/m^2 CIVI over 24 hours day 2	Repeat cycle every 14 days
Mesna (Mesnex)*	5000 mg/m^2 CIVI over 24 hours day 2	
Carboplatin (Paraplatin)*	AUC = 5 (maximum 800 mg), day 2	
Etoposide (VePesid)*	100 mg/m^2/day IV days 1–3	

*Not FDA approved for this indication.

ABVD, doxorubicin, bleomycin, vinblastine, and dacarbazine; IV, intravenous; MOPP, nitrogen mustard, vincristine, procarbazine, and prednisone; PO, by mouth; BEACOPP, bleomycin, etoposide, doxorubicin, cyclophosphamide, vincristine, procarbazine, and prednisone; CIVI, continuous intravenous infusion; ESHAP, etoposide, methylprednisolone, high-dose cytarabine, and cisplatin; ICE, ifosfamide, carboplatin, and etoposide.

for patients with stage I-IIIA HL randomized to EFRT or MOPP. Patients with bulky mediastinal masses, stage IIIA disease, elevated ESR, or more than four sites involved were noted to have superior outcomes with MOPP. An Italian study reported an 8-year OS of 56% using MOPP compared with 93% with EFRT ($P < .001$). Perhaps this discrepancy is due to the inclusion of patients with poor prognostic features in the NCI trial, whereas the Italian trial was limited to IA and IIA HL only. In addition, the Italian group's outcomes with MOPP are lower than those attained in other trials, even trials for patients with advanced-stage HL.

Combined Modality Therapy

With MOPP's proven efficacy, the addition of chemotherapy to EFRT (so-called combined modality therapy or CMT) was examined in an attempt to further improve outcomes in patients with early stage HL, particularly patients with poor prognostic features. Initial studies evaluated a full course of MOPP or MOPP-like chemotherapy either before or after EFRT. A meta-analysis of several randomized trials showed a 54% reduction in the odds of failure with the addition of chemotherapy, but no difference in OS. More recently, more effective, less toxic chemotherapy regimens have been successfully combined with EFRT. The European Organization for Research and Treatment of Cancer (EORTC) compared six cycles of MOPP plus mantle RT to six cycles of ABVD (doxorubicin, bleomycin, vinblastine, and dacarbazine) plus mantle RT, with the ABVD arm demonstrating a superior RFS. The German Hodgkin's Study Group (GHSG) recently reported 2-year FFP rates of 96% with two cycles of ABVD and EFRT, compared with 87% with EFRT alone. In a United States Intergroup study of 348 patients, 3-year failure free survival (FFS) rates were 94% with three cycles of AV (doxorubicin and vinblastine) combined with subtotal lymphoid irradiation (STLI), compared with 81% with STLI alone ($P < .001$).

In addition to the use of less toxic chemotherapy, efforts have been made to reduce the dose and field of radiation in CMT. Replacement of EFRT with involved field radiotherapy (IFRT) limits cardiopulmonary toxicities and may minimize the rate of breast and lung carcinoma, because less pulmonary parenchyma and ductal breast tissue are exposed to ionizing radiation. In a Stanford study, patients were randomized to receive either EFRT or IFRT after six cycles of VBM (vinblastine, bleomycin, methotrexate*). FFP was similar at 92% and 87% between the EFRT and limited field groups, respectively. A randomized trial of four cycles of ABVD followed by either IFRT or STLI demonstrated identical 7-year disease-free survival rates of 94% and 97%, respectively. In a Canadian study of non-bulky stage IA or IIA HL, no patients have relapsed at 2 years follow-up with two cycles of chemotherapy with COPP (cyclophosphamide, vincristine, procarbazine, and prednisone)/ ABV or ABVD followed by IFRT. Ongoing trials are evaluating lower doses of radiation (20 Gy) compared with standard doses of 35–40 Gy in the combined modality setting.

*Not FDA approved for this indication.

Chemotherapy Alone

Potential long-term toxicities of even IFRT have encouraged investigators to consider chemotherapy alone in patients with favorable early-stage disease, particularly women ages 15 to 30 years who are at greatest risk for secondary breast cancers after mediastinal and axillary irradiation. A small study of ABVD alone for patients with stage I-II HL resulted in 42-month progression-free survival (PFS) and OS rates of 84% and 95%, respectively. At Memorial Sloan Kettering, 152 patients with stage I-IIIA non-bulky HL were randomized to six cycles of ABVD alone or to six cycles of ABVD plus RT (mantle field used from 1990 to 1999 and IFRT from 1999 to 2000). No statistically significant differences in FFP or OS were noted in the two groups. The 5-year FFP and OS rates were 81% and 92% for ABVD, and 86% and 97% for ABVD + RT. Because of small patient numbers, as much as an 18% difference in FFP and OS could have been missed. Results of recently completed randomized trials by the EORTC and the NCI of Canada comparing chemotherapy alone to EFRT or CMT will be important in helping to answer the current controversy of chemotherapy alone versus CMT for patients with early stage HL.

Bulky or Unfavorable Early Stage Disease

For early stage patients with high-risk features, four to six cycles of ABVD with IFRT are appropriate. RT is necessary in patients with bulky disease because of the patients' high risk of relapse after chemotherapy alone. However, some concern exists that the combination of RT, bleomycin, and doxorubicin will increase the risk of cardiopulmonary disease in these patients, so newer regimens such as Stanford V (doxorubicin, vinblastine, nitrogen mustard, vincristine, bleomycin, etoposide,* and prednisone; see Table 3) are being developed that limit the cumulative doses of these drugs. Stanford V has demonstrated 5-year FFS rates of 96% in patients with bulky stage II HL. With the Stanford V regimen, chemotherapy is administered weekly over 12 weeks and is followed by consolidative IFRT. Stanford V has 50% and 75% less doxorubicin and bleomycin, respectively, than does six cycles of ABVD. A large US Intergroup group trial comparing Stanford V to six cycles of ABVD in patients with bulky stage I/II, stage III, and stage IV HL is under way. Until this trial is completed, either Stanford V or six cycles of ABVD with IFRT is appropriate for patients with early stage, bulky HL.

In summary, either chemotherapy alone with six cycles of ABVD or CMT with four cycles of ABVD and IFRT are considered acceptable standard approaches for early stage HL. Patients to bulky disease should receive CMT. Results with less than six cycles of ABVD alone or less than four cycles of ABVD with IFRT are not yet available.

*Not FDA approved for this indication.

ADVANCED STAGE HL

The mainstay of therapy for advanced HL is combination chemotherapy. Six to eight cycles of ABVD is currently the standard of care for patients with advanced stage HL. In a randomized trial comparing ABVD, MOPP/ABVD, and MOPP in stage III-IV HL, both 5-year OS and FFS rates were superior for ABVD (OS 73%, FFS 61%) and MOPP/ABVD (OS 75%, FFS 65%) compared with MOPP alone (OS 66%, FFS 50%). In a US Intergroup study, there was no difference in 5-year FFS or OS for ABVD versus MOPP/ABV hybrid; however, febrile neutropenia, anemia, thrombocytopenia, fatigue, and hypotension occurred more frequently with the hybrid regimen. Inexplicably, the MOPP/ABV group had more pulmonary toxicity than the ABVD arm (30% versus 24%, respectively, $P < .06$), which resulted in seven deaths, although patients on the ABVD arm received higher cumulative doses of bleomycin. In addition, there were 28 (6.8%) second malignancies and 11 cases (2.7%) of myelodysplasia or acute leukemia in the hybrid arm, compared with 18 (4.2%) second malignancies and 2 (0.5%) cases of myelodysplasia with ABVD. Therefore, ABVD appears to be the optimal therapy for advanced stage HL, similar in efficacy to, but less toxic than, MOPP/ABVD combinations.

Two new regimens, Stanford V and BEACOPP (see Table 3), are being compared with ABVD for advanced stage HL in randomized trials. The GHSG has piloted the BEACOPP regimen (bleomycin, etoposide,* doxorubicin, cyclophosphamide, vincristine, procarbazine, and prednisone), administered on a 21-day schedule, with the hypothesis that a shortened treatment interval may improve outcomes. In addition, an escalated BEACOPP regimen (30% dose escalation of BEACOPP with G-CSF support) has been explored. BEACOPP is the first regimen tested in a phase III trial that appears to be superior to an ABVD-containing regimen, with 5-year FFP rates of 87% for escalated BEACOPP, 76% for BEACOPP, and 69% for COPP/ABVD ($P < .05$). These benefits appeared to be limited to patients younger than age 65 and were tempered by the development of myelodysplasia or secondary acute leukemia in 4 of 469 patients treated with BEACOPP and 9 of 466 patients treated with escalated BEACOPP, compared with 1 of 260 patients treated with COPP/ABVD at a median follow-up of 56 months. Dose-escalated BEACOPP led to sterility in nearly all treated patients. BEACOPP did appear to be superior in patients with adverse prognostic features, particularly in those with four or more risk factors (see Table 2), suggesting that chemotherapy for advanced HL may be tailored by prognostic group in future trials.

A single institution phase II trial has found a 5-year OS rate of 96% and FFP rate of 89% using Stanford V in 142 patients with stage II-IV HL. However, these results are dependent on prognostic group. Using the international prognostic index for advanced stage HL, 5-year FFP reached 100% for patients with zero risk factors, 91% for one risk factor, 95% for two risk factors, 86% for three risk factors, and 65% for patients with four or more risk factors following Stanford V therapy. Toxicities consisted primarily of myelosuppression, constipation, fatigue, and sensory peripheral neuropathy. With greater than 5 years of follow-up, only one second malignancy has occurred (lung cancer in a patient with an extensive smoking history). In a recent Italian study of 275 patients with advanced stage HL, Stanford V appeared inferior to ABVD and MEC (mechlorethamine, CCNU, vindesine,† chlorambucil, prednisone, epirubicin,* vincristine, procarbazine, vinblastine, and bleomycin), with 3-year FFS rates of 53.4% for Stanford V, 81.4% for ABVD, and 86.6% for MEC. However, this study only provided RT to those patients with bulky disease or patients who failed to attain a complete remission with chemotherapy. Only 65% of patients on the Stanford V arm received RT, which may explain the lower FFS seen in this series of patients, compared with the results reported at Stanford University in which 85% of patients received consolidative RT. Hopefully, an ongoing US Intergroup trial randomizing patients with either bulky stage II HL, stage III HL, or stage IV HL to Stanford V (with IFRT) or ABVD will help delineate the role of Stanford V in the advanced setting.

The role of RT in advanced disease is less clear. Both Stanford V and the BEACOPP regimens incorporate IFRT. In a study by the Southwestern Oncology Group, the addition of consolidative RT to MOP/BAP (mechlorethamine, vincristine, prednisone, bleomycin, doxorubicin, and procarbazine) chemotherapy demonstrated no significant advantage over chemotherapy alone. A GHSG trial randomized patients with a complete response after six cycles of COPP/ABVD to either two additional cycles or consolidative RT—again, with no difference seen in disease-free survival between the two groups. Additional studies are planned through the EORTC to assess if 24 Gy of RT to all involved sites will benefit those patients with a partial remission only after 6 cycles of MOPP/ABVD. It is possible that RT may have a greater impact in patients with advanced stage HL who have bulky disease at diagnosis or who have less than a complete response after combination chemotherapy. In fact, the improvement in FFS seen with the Stanford V and BEACOPP regimens may be due in part to the addition of RT to these regimens, rather than the chemotherapeutic drugs or intensive schedules.

Because of the high risk of relapse in patients with advanced stage HL, particularly those patients with multiple risk factors, some consideration has been given to transplanting these patients in first remission. A randomized, multicenter European study found no differences in OS or RFS among 205 patients receiving four courses of standard ABVD chemotherapy followed either by autologous stem cell transplant or by four additional courses of an ABVD-containing regimen. All patients had to have at least two poor prognostic features including anemia, an elevated

*Not FDA approved for this indication.

*Not FDA approved for this indication.

†Investigational drug in the United States.

lactate dehydrogenase (LDH), bulky mediastinal disease, extranodal involvement, or inguinal disease. Five-year FFS reached 85% in the transplant arm and 83% in the conventional treatment arm. Likewise, a study from the French GOELAMS group found no difference in four-year FFP or OS rates in high risk patients with HL randomized either to four cycles of ABVD plus high-dose BEAM (BCNU, etoposide,* cytarabine, and melphalan*) chemotherapy with autologous transplant or to three cycles of VABEM (vindesine,† doxorubicin, BCNU, etoposide,* and methylprednisolone) plus IFRT without transplant. Therefore, preliminary data do not support the use of autologous transplant in first remission for high-risk HL.

RELAPSED OR REFRACTORY HL

For patients who fail to obtain a complete response with induction therapy or relapse after chemotherapy or combined modality therapy, two to four cycles of salvage chemotherapy followed by an autologous hematopoietic stem cell transplant should be considered. Non–cross-resistant salvage regimens are favored. ESHAP (etoposide,* methylprednisolone, high-dose cytarabine, and cisplatin*) and ICE (ifosfamide,* carboplatin,* and etoposide*) have response rates of 70% to 88% in the salvage setting. Fifty percent of patients with HL who respond to salvage chemotherapy will achieve a long-term remission after autologous transplantation. High-dose therapy with autologous transplantation improves OS and event-free survivals by 7% and 26%, respectively, at the time of first relapse. Patients with a first remission lasting longer than 12 months, no bone marrow or pulmonary involvement at relapse, no B-symptoms, and chemosensitive disease at the time of transplant have the most favorable outcome with high-dose therapy. In a study from Stanford, only 10% of patients achieving a partial remission with salvage chemotherapy and 0% of nonresponders were alive at 4 years, compared with 68% of patients achieving a complete response.

Those patients who are ineligible for high-dose therapy and autologous transplant due to age or comorbidities should be considered for clinical trials with novel investigational agents (see Table 3 and discussion of New Agents and Advances in the Treatment of HL later in this chapter). If novel agents are unavailable, several chemotherapeutic drugs including etoposide (VP-16),* gemcitabine,* chlorambucil, cyclophosphamide, vinorelbine,* and vinblastine all have single-agent activity in the relapsed setting and can often be used as palliative therapy for an extended period of time. Gemcitabine and vinorelbine both can lead to 40% to 50% response rates in heavily pretreated patients, with median remission durations of 6 to 7 months.

A special situation arises for those patients with favorable stage HL treated with RT only or chemotherapy only before relapse. It is possible that EFRT or six cycles of salvage therapy alone may be adequate to cure these patients at relapse, particularly when the recurrence is limited to only a few nodal sites and the recurrence occurs more than a year from initial therapy. At Stanford, 10-year disease-free survivals for patients treated with combination chemotherapy after failing RT were 88%, 58%, and 34%, respectively, for patients with stage IA, IIA, or IIIA-IVB disease at relapse. A review of primary chemotherapy failures at Stanford University suggests that half of patients (n = 13) can have prolonged remissions following salvage RT, usually in the setting of prolonged first remission durations and good response (i.e., CR) to front-line chemotherapy.

*Not FDA approved for this indication.
†Investigational drug in the United States.

NODULAR LYMPHOCYTE-PREDOMINANT HL

As early as 1960, a subtype of HL characterized by an extensive infiltrate of small lymphocytes with scattered larger cells ("popcorn cells"), without classic HRS cells, was described. Although some trials suggested that this subtype followed a more indolent course than classical HL and had a natural history similar to follicular NHL, these results could not be confirmed because of the differing classification schemes employed by each institution. With the development of the Revised European-American Lymphoma (REAL) classification scheme, lymphocyte-predominant HL (LPHL) was formally described. In the REAL and WHO classifications, LPHL has distinct phenotypic and immunohistochemical characteristics, namely the presence of "popcorn cells" with folded, lobulated nuclei and inconspicuous nucleoli that are CD20 positive, CD30 negative, and CD15 negative.

LPHL has some unusual features that are not commonly seen in classic HL; for example, it affects middle-age men (median age 35), it typically involves lymph nodes outside of the mediastinum, and it does not spread predictably from one adjacent lymph node group to the next. OS ranges from 80% to 90% at 10 years, and late relapses are common. In addition, there is an increased risk of developing secondary NHL, usually diffuse large B-cell NHL, after LPHL. Because of its CD20 expression, high OS rate, frequent late relapses, and association with diffuse large-cell lymphoma, some authors suggest that this form of HL is more similar to indolent NHL, rather than classic HL.

Historically, LPHL has been treated with EFRT or regional radiation, similar to early stage classic HL. However, retrospective studies have consistently shown that at least half of all deaths in LPHL are potentially treatment related, primarily resulting from cardiac disease or second malignancies. This finding, in conjunction with the lack of a contiguous spread pattern, makes this approach difficult to justify. Treatment is controversial, with some authors recommending therapy with IFRT, rituximab (Rituxan),* or even conventional combination chemotherapy regimens used for NHL such as CVP (cyclophosphamide, vincristine, and prednisone).

*Not FDA approved for this indication.

However, no clear data exist to suggest that these regimens improve outcomes over standard HL therapies. Some authors recommend IFRT for patients with early stage LPHL because of its propensity to induce prolonged remissions with minimal toxicity. Combination chemotherapy can be reserved for relapsed disease. Promising results have also been seen with single-agent rituximab, with response rates as high as 100% in the relapsed setting. However, because median remission durations are less than 1 year after a single course of rituximab,* maintenance rituximab* is now being evaluated. Monoclonal antibody therapy is appealing in this disease, because it may minimize the risks of myelodysplastic syndrome, cardiac disease, or secondary malignancies associated with classic HL therapy. Rituximab's* efficacy needs to be confirmed in larger trials and further explored in untreated LPHL. Therefore, although no standard therapy for LPHL exists, emphasis has been placed on using well-tolerated regimens with little long-term toxicity such as IFRT or single agent rituximab* resulting from the excellent outcomes and prolonged survivals of this histologic subgroup.

ACUTE TOXICITIES OF THERAPY FOR HL

Common toxicities associated with ABVD include nausea, vomiting, fever, alopecia, and myelosuppression. Less commonly, pulmonary compromise related to the bleomycin, cardiotoxicity resulting from the doxorubicin, and phlebitis related to the dacarbazine can be noted. Bleomycin should be discontinued from all subsequent cycles in the event that a patient develops shortness of breath or cough that is not disease related. A decline in diffusing lung capacity for carbon monoxide (DLCO) on pulmonary function tests or parenchymal abnormalities on chest radiograph also necessitates discontinuation of bleomycin. In addition, all patients should be counseled about smoking cessation and avoiding secondhand smoke, as this can exacerbate any pulmonary complications. Doxorubicin associated cardiomyopathy is rare, but can be seen in patients receiving a cumulative dose >400 mg/m^2 or who have underlying cardiac disease. Symptomatic declines in cardiac ejection fraction will also necessitate discontinuation of doxorubicin. Dacarbazine-related phlebitis can be minimized by administration via a central venous catheter.

Leukopenia and neutropenia are common findings with ABVD administration. However, life-threatening infections are rare, occurring in fewer than 2% of patients. Although hematologic growth factors should not be used routinely, they can be used to maintain dose intensity and schedule. To prevent frequent treatment delays, GCSF can be administered for 3 to 5 days between the day 1 and 15 treatments of ABVD.

Depending on the radiation field, RT can lead to esophagitis, dry mouth, fatigue, skin irritation, and nausea. Most of these toxicities resolve within 2 to 4 weeks of completing the RT. Radiation pneumonitis can occur within 2 to 6 months of therapy and occasionally requires steroid therapy for symptomatic relief.

DELAYED TOXICITIES OF THERAPY FOR HL

Several devastating complications have been associated with MOPP chemotherapy and EFRT. Beyond 15 years of follow-up, death from other causes surpasses that from HL. These toxicities include cardiopulmonary complications (myocardial infarctions, valvular disease, pericarditis, and pneumonitis), along with second malignancies that include acute myeloid leukemias, myelodysplasia, breast carcinoma, and lung carcinoma. Mediastinal RT increases the risk of cardiac death more than threefold. Nearly every solid tumor has been reported following HL. Relative risks for these malignancies after therapy for HL include lung (10.3), breast (4.1), melanoma (11.6), soft-tissue sarcoma (24.3), salivary gland (37.9), and thyroid (10.6). The risk of breast cancer can be correlated with the age of the patient at the time of HL treatment; with a 40-fold increase for those younger than age 20, compared with only a slight elevation for women older than 30. The risk of secondary malignancy continues to climb even after 30 years have elapsed from the time of initial therapy for HL. Because most patients are quite young at the time of diagnosis, this represents a serious complication of therapy, for which oncologists and primary care physicians must remain vigilant. The myelodysplasia and secondary leukemias have been attributed to the MOPP regimen and will hopefully be less common with the use of ABVD. Use of reduced radiation doses and fields will hopefully decrease cardiopulmonary complications and the risk of second solid tumors.

Mediastinal and neck RT also leads to hypothyroidism in more than half of patients treated with RT. Therefore, yearly thyroid function tests are recommended in those patients receiving IFRT or EFRT to the neck. Infertility was also commonly seen after therapy with intensive regimens including MOPP or pelvic irradiation. The widespread use of ABVD and limited radiation fields has minimized this complication. However, infertility may again become a problem if more intensive regimens such as BEACOPP are routinely used. Patients who have relapsed disease and are candidates for stem cell transplantation should be routinely counseled regarding fertility options, because all of these patients will become infertile after the transplant.

NEW AGENTS AND ADVANCES IN THE TREATMENT OF HL

Despite the advances in the care of HL since the advent of EFRT and MOPP chemotherapy in the 1960s, there are still many unresolved issues regarding the care of these patients. In particular, the number of chemotherapy cycles and minimal radiation dose required to maintain high FFS rates while

*Not FDA approved for this indication.

minimizing long-term toxicity must be further investigated. In addition, the role of alternative chemotherapy regimens (i.e., Stanford V and BEACOPP) for both early and advanced stage disease must be further explored. Several large randomized studies in progress in both Europe and the United States will hopefully address these issues.

Novel alternative therapies are needed for patients with relapsed or refractory HL, particularly those patients who are not candidates for high-dose therapy with stem cell transplant or for those who relapse after such therapy. Several newer "targeted therapies" may have a role in this setting. For example, monoclonal antibodies directed at the CD30 antigen are in clinical trials. In addition, proteasome inhibition with drugs such as PS-341† may have activity in this disease. Finally, conventional chemotherapeutic agents with single agent activity in HL (i.e., gemcitabine*) need to be incorporated into new combination regimens that could be used as salvage therapy.

SPECIAL SITUATIONS IN HL

HL in Pregnancy

The development of HL during pregnancy poses many therapeutic challenges. In the first trimester, the fetus is at an increased risk of developmental anomalies or early miscarriage when exposed to either therapeutic or diagnostic radiation or when exposed to chemotherapy. Therefore, management is based primarily on the women's symptoms at diagnosis and the age of the fetus. Occasionally, depending on the mother's symptoms at diagnosis and the length of the pregnancy, it is possible to delay therapy until delivery or at least the third trimester, when chemotherapy can be administered safely. Full combination chemotherapy with ABVD generally does not harm the fetus after the third trimester is reached. Partial or even full-dose RT can also be given safely to the neck, axilla, and upper mediastinum in the last 3 months of the pregnancy, if needed to palliate bulky adenopathy. Whenever possible therapy should be delayed until after delivery, but options are available, particularly in the third trimester. Therefore, in the setting of pregnancy, a full discussion with the patient and the obstetrician regarding the patient's options and the risks of therapy or delay of therapy must take place before initiating a treatment plan.

Clinical Emergencies: Superior Vena Cava Syndrome, Airway Obstruction, Spinal Cord Compression, or Biliary Obstruction

Although clinical emergencies related to the compression of the superior vena cava, trachea, spinal cord, or biliary tract are relatively rare in HL, they do occasionally occur. When these are the presenting symptoms of the disease, a quick and accurate diagnosis is always the first order of business. Although a core needle biopsy or excisional biopsy is always preferred, a fine-needle biopsy may be acceptable if warranted by the patient's clinical situation. It is almost never necessary to initiate therapy without an accurate diagnosis. After the diagnosis is obtained, treatment with chemotherapy or combined modality therapy is preferred. In general, HL is very chemosensitive, and most of the symptoms related to these presentations will improve after the first cycle of therapy. If a patient is very unstable or has additional comorbid conditions making chemotherapy more risky, RT alone may be considered.

HIV Infection and HL

When HL occurs in patients with HIV, it is generally more advanced and more difficult to cure because of the patient's underlying immune suppression and increased risk of infection. Most patients with HIV and HL present with B symptoms, advanced stage, and extranodal involvement (usually the bone marrow, liver, and spleen). In addition, contiguous spread of tumor to adjacent lymph node regions does not occur as in classic HL. Occasionally, HL has been found to involve unusual sites such as the central nervous system, skin, tongue, or esophagus in patients with HIV. HL, in contrast to NHL, frequently occurs relatively early in HIV disease; that is, with CD4 counts higher than $200/mm^3$.

For patients with no prior opportunistic infections who are relatively healthy, standard therapy with either combined modality therapy or six to eight cycles of ABVD is recommended, depending on the stage. However, dose reductions or administration of growth factors (i.e., GCSF) may be required in this setting because of the patient's immunocompromised state. For patients with evidence of immunocompromise (a history of opportunistic infection or a low CD4 count), ABVD at a 25% to 50% dose reduction is recommended. Even with full-dose chemotherapy, outcomes are poor in the HIV setting, with a median survival of 16 months and a 53% 3-year disease-free survival. The addition of antiretroviral therapy to chemotherapy may improve outcomes as has been seen in NHL; however, further studies must be done to confirm this.

*Not FDA approved for this indication.
†Investigational drug in the United States.

HODGKIN'S DISEASE: RADIATION THERAPY

method of
RICHARD W. TSANG, M.D., and
MARY K. GOSPODAROWICZ, M.D.
University of Toronto
Princess Margaret Hospital
Toronto, Canada

The term Hodgkin's lymphoma (HL) is now used synonymously with Hodgkin's disease. It has distinct clinical, biologic, and pathologic features that set it apart from the more heterogeneous non-Hodgkin's lymphomas. The treatment program and prognosis are also distinctively different. The successful treatment of HL has often been cited as an example of the success of modern cancer treatment. This is exemplified by the evolution in the use of curative radiation therapy (RT) and multiagent chemotherapy, by the concept of accurately defining the anatomic extent of the disease through clinical and surgical-pathologic staging, and by the use of combination therapy to achieve the best therapeutic ratio. With cure being a reality for most patients, observed late effects of treatment, such as second cancers, are the main challenges. Therefore, the more recent efforts in stage I and II disease have focused on lowering treatment intensity, to reduce the dose and extent of RT, and on the use of short-course chemotherapy. This article discusses the current use of RT for HL, with special attention to the management of stage I and II disease. Patients with HL presenting in childhood, during pregnancy, in old age, and in the setting of HIV infection may need various modifications to the treatment protocol and are beyond the scope of this discussion.

INCIDENCE AND EPIDEMIOLOGY

HL is less common than the non-Hodgkin's lymphomas (NHLs), and for every seven cases of NHL, there is only one case of HL. The American Cancer Society estimated that, in 2002, 7000 new cases of HL were diagnosed (3700 males, 3300 females), and 1400 deaths (800 males, 600 females) occurred. The incidence is bimodal, with the first peak in the third decade in life and a second smaller peak after the age of 50 years. Although the incidence has remained stable since the 1970s, the 5-year relative survival rates have improved significantly from 71% in 1974 to 1976 to 83% in 1992 to 1997. The origin of HL is unknown, but factors documented to be associated with a higher risk include a positive family history, higher socioeconomic status, and prior Epstein-Barr virus infection, such as infectious mononucleosis.

PATHOLOGY AND BIOLOGIC CHARACTERISTICS

The three cardinal morphologic features of HL are: effacement of the involved lymph node with destruction of its normal architecture; infiltration of inflammatory cells such as lymphocytes, histiocytes, plasma cells, and fibroblasts; and the presence of the malignant cell, the Reed-Sternberg (RS) cell. The Rye classification with its four subtypes of HL (lymphocytic predominance, nodular sclerosis, mixed cellularity, and lymphocytic depletion) has been replaced by the World Health Organization classification (Table 1). In the World Health Organization classification, classic HL is considered separately from nodular lymphocyte-predominant HL. The most common subtype is nodular sclerosis, accounting for 70% to 80% of cases in North America, with the lymphocyte-depleted type being the least common. Mixed-cellularity histology is more common in developing countries and in patients infected with HIV.

HL differs from other malignant diseases in that the malignant cells, the RS cells, are typically sparse within the tumor. In most cases, the RS cell is of B-cell origin. The various subtypes of HL (see Table 1) have distinct morphologic, immunophenotypic, and clinical characteristics.

Nodular lymphocyte-predominant HL comprises less than 5% of the cases, and it usually presents with localized involvement of peripheral lymph node areas such as cervical, axillary, and inguinal regions. Morphologically, it has a nodular pattern and is characterized by the presence of a RS cell variant known as an L&H cell or "popcorn cell." These cells have a typical immunophenotype of B cells (CD20+, CD79a+, CD45+, J chain positive, and immunoglobulin light and/or heavy chain positive), and are negative for CD15 and CD30. Epstein-Barr virus antigens are usually absent in L&H cells. Nodular lymphocyte-predominant HL carries a good prognosis when the disease is localized at presentation, although multiple relapses tend to occur. The disease commonly remains responsive to therapy, however.

In classic HL, the typical immunophenotype for the RS cells are positivity for CD30 and CD15, and negativity for CD45 and the J chain. B-cell markers such as CD20 and CD79a are usually absent. Epstein-Barr virus–related proteins are detected in approximately 40% of cases.

The lymphocyte-rich subtype represents approximately 5% of HL. Its clinical features are similar to those of nodular lymphocyte-predominant HL, with localized disease at presentation involving a peripheral lymph node region.

The nodular sclerosis subtype is characterized by a nodular growth pattern, the presence of collagen

TABLE 1. **World Health Organization Classification for Hodgkin's Lymphoma**

Nodular lymphocyte predominant Hodgkin's lymphoma	(NLPHL)
Classic Hodgkin's lymphoma	(CHL)
Nodular sclerosis classic Hodgkin's lymphoma	(NSHL)
Mixed-cellularity classic Hodgkin's lymphoma	(MCHL)
Lymphocyte-rich classic Hodgkin's lymphoma	(LRCHL)
Lymphocyte-depleted classic Hodgkin's lymphoma	(LDHL)

Adapted from Jaffe ES, Harris NL, Stein H, et al (eds): Pathology and Genetics of Tumours of Haematopoietic and Lymphoid Tissues. World Health Organization Classification of Tumours. IARC Press, Lyon, France, 2001.

bands, and an RS cell variant known as the lacunar cell. It is the most common subtype of HL, accounting for 65% to 70% of cases, and is the only subtype without a male predominance (male-female ratio approximately 1:1). Typically, the cervical and mediastinal areas are involved.

Mixed-cellularity subtype represents 10% to 15% of cases; 70% are male, and a bimodal distribution is not observed. Patients more commonly present with stage III or IV disease, with peripheral lymph node involvement and mediastinal disease being less common.

The lymphocyte-depleted subtype is very rarely seen, and many previous cases have now been recognized as being NHLs. Rare cases may still be seen in association with HIV infection. This subtype is less well characterized because of its rarity, but it usually affects male patients, it is present in advanced stages with systemic symptoms, and it involves abdominal lymph nodes and organs with relative sparing of peripheral lymph nodes. It has a worse prognosis than the other subtypes.

CLINICAL PRESENTATION, PATIENT EVALUATION, AND STAGING

Clinical Presentation

The most common presentation is with an asymptomatic lymph node enlargement in supradiaphragmatic areas, typically in the neck, that may wax and wane. Approximately 70% of patients present with stage I or II disease. Only 5% of patients with stage I or II disease present with involvement of infradiaphragmatic sites. Mediastinal lymph node involvement is common, occurring in 80% of cases, and when the disease is bulky it may cause symptoms (chest pain, cough, dyspnea). Systemic symptoms of night sweats, fever, and weight loss are reported in approximately 30% of patients. Generalized pruritus and alcohol-induced pain localized over the involved lymph node tissue are also characteristic but less frequent.

Patient Evaluation

The goals of staging investigations are to determine disease extent, to assess its anatomic distribution, and to ascertain normal organ function relevant to the choice of therapy. A complete history and physical examination with special attention to the lymphoid system are performed, including Waldeyer's ring structures. The location and size of lymph node masses should be documented. This is especially important for the subsequent determination of RT target volume because after chemotherapy, no gross disease may be present at the time of RT planning. Histologic confirmation of the diagnosis by an experienced hematopathologist is mandatory. Minimum laboratory tests include a complete blood count and lactate dehydrogenase, bilirubin, transaminase, and creatinine levels. An HIV serology test should be performed when risk factors of HIV infection are present. A unilateral bone marrow biopsy is necessary only if the complete blood count is abnormal, in stage III and IV disease, or if B symptoms are present. Imaging tests are the key to defining the anatomic extent of disease; computed tomography of the head and neck, thorax, abdomen, and pelvis is the standard staging procedure. Special attention is paid to document areas of bulky disease, such as mediastinal involvement and whether the disease has infiltrated extranodal tissues such as lung parenchyma, chest wall, and pericardium. A bulky mediastinal mass is defined as a transverse mediastinal diameter exceeding one third of the transthoracic diameter or a maximum mediastinal diameter measuring 10 cm or more. Total body gallium 67 scanning is useful in staging because of its high sensitivity and specificity for active HL, and it also serves as a follow-up test to document response to therapy or recurrence in patients with gallium-avid tumors. Positron emission tomography with fluorine 18–labeled deoxyglucose is a promising tool for staging

TABLE 2. **Ann Arbor Staging Classification for Hodgkin's Lymphoma**

Clinical Stage	Hodgkin's Lymphoma
Stage I	Involvement of a single lymph node region
Stage I_E	Localized involvement of a single extralymphatic organ or site
Stage II	Involvement of two or more lymph node regions on the same side of the diaphragm
Stage II_E	Localized involvement of a single extralymphatic organ or site and its regional lymph nodes with or without involvement of other lymph node regions on the same side of the diaphragm
Stage III	Involvement of lymph node regions on both sides of the diaphragm and a localized single extralymphatic organ or site
	If accompanied by:
Stage III_E	Same as stage III plus localized involvement of an associated extralymphatic organ or site
Stage III_S	Same as stage III plus involvement of the spleen
Stage III_{E+S}	Same as stage III plus involvement of both an extralymphatic organ or site and the spleen
Stage IV	Disseminated (multifocal) involvement of one or more extralymphatic organs, with or without associated lymph node involvement; or isolated extralymphatic organ involvement with distant (nonregional) nodal involvement
All stages divided	
A	Without weight loss, fever, or night sweats
B*	With one or more of: 1. Unexplained weight loss of more than 10% of the usual body weight in the 6 months before first attendance 2. Unexplained fever with temperature higher than 38°C 3. Night sweats

Pathologic Stages

The definitions of the four stages follow the same criteria as the clinical stages but with the additional information obtained after laparotomy. Splenectomy, liver biopsy, lymph node biopsy, and bone marrow biopsy are mandatory for the establishment of pathologic stages. The results of these biopsies are recorded as indicated above.

*Pruritus alone does not qualify for B classification, nor does a short, febrile illness associated with a known infection.

and assessment of response, and it can be used instead of gallium scans.

Staging Classification

The American Joint Committee on Cancer and the International Union Against Cancer TNM classifications both endorse the Ann Arbor staging classification (Table 2). Treatment decisions are based on the Ann Arbor classification supplemented by other prognostic factors and pathologic findings.

PROGNOSTIC FACTORS

Although the anatomic extent of disease reflected by Ann Arbor stage is an important prognostic factor, many other factors are known to influence the outcome in patients with HL. These include histologic type, tumor bulk, and the number of involved nodal regions and extranodal sites, as well as age, gender, erythrocyte sedimentation rate, and various hematologic and biochemical parameters. Given the increased use of combined-modality therapy (chemotherapy followed by RT), the importance of some of these variables has decreased in significance. However, even with routine use of combined-modality therapy, a large mediastinal mass, the presence of B symptoms, or unexplained anemia is associated with poor prognosis. A full study of prognostic factors in advanced stage HL was reported by Hasenclever and colleagues. Seven factors identified to have an independent adverse effect on the freedom from disease progression were: male sex, age 45 years or more, stage IV disease, hemoglobin less than 105 g/L, serum albumin less than 40 g/L, leukocyte count 15×10^9/L or greater, and lymphocyte count less than 0.6×10^9/L (or less than 8% of leukocyte count). Patients with none of these factors had a 5-year freedom from disease progression of 84%, compared with 67% for those with two factors and 42% for those with five or more factors.

PRINCIPLES OF MANAGEMENT

All patients with HL are treated with curative intent. Historically, the treatment of stage I and II disease was based on RT, and treatment of stage III and IV disease was based on chemotherapy. RT is an exceedingly effective treatment modality in HL. Moderate doses (35 to 40 Gy) result in local control of disease in more than 95% of patients. Lower doses (25 to 30 Gy) are adequate for microscopic disease or for disease sites showing response to chemotherapy. The current optimal treatment involves combined-modality therapy in stage I and II, except for nodular lymphocyte predominant HL, in which RT alone is used. The standard chemotherapy regimen is doxorubicin, bleomycin, vinblastine, and dacarbazine (ABVD). Substitution of different drugs may lead to inferior results (e.g., replacing doxorubicin with epirubicin) and is not recommended outside a clinical trial.

TABLE 3. **Principles of the Management of Hodgkin's Lymphoma**

Basis for Therapeutic Decisions
Histology
Stage
Tumor burden (e.g., bulk of tumor and location and number of involved nodal regions)
Other prognostic factors (see text)
Therapeutic Recommendations
Stage IA Nodular Lymphocyte-Predominant Hodgkin's Lymphoma
Recommend
Involved-field radiation therapy (35 Gy)
Stage I and II (Favorable)*
Recommend
Chemotherapy (ABVD for three cycles) followed by involved-field radiation therapy (35 Gy)
Stage I and II (Unfavorable)*
Recommend
Chemotherapy (ABVD for four to six cycles) followed by involved field radiation therapy (35 Gy)
Stage III and IV
Recommend
Chemotherapy (ABVD for six to eight cycles)
Involved-field radiation therapy (35 Gy) for initial sites of bulky disease (maximum tumor diameter ≥10 cm), if present

*For Stage I and II disease, the presence of one or more of the following adverse factors will place the patient in the "Unfavorable" group; all others will be considered "Favorable":
Systemic symptoms (Stage IB or IIB)
Bulky mediastinal disease or peripheral site with bulk ≥10 cm
Extranodal extension (stage I_E, or II_E)
Unexplained anemia (<105 g/L)
ABVD, doxorubicin, bleomycin, vinblastine, and dacarbazine.

The approach to the management of HL used in the Princess Margaret Hospital in Toronto is summarized in Table 3. Patients with stage III and IV disease are treated with ABVD chemotherapy alone. Those with large mediastinal mass or bulky disease receive adjuvant involved-field RT. When RT follows chemotherapy in combined-modality therapy protocols, RT is usually started 3 to 4 weeks after the last course of chemotherapy to minimize the drug-radiation interaction. The successful treatment of a patient with HL involves multidisciplinary care with involvement of the general practitioner, hematologist or medical oncologist, pathologist, and radiation oncologist. The support of allied health care disciplines including dental, nutritional, and physical therapy and social and psychology services is also essential to good patient care.

PRINCIPLES AND TECHNIQUES OF RADIATION THERAPY

The aim of RT is to deliver an adequate dose of radiation to the target volume to ensure a high rate of local control with acceptable acute and long-term toxicity. Custom-designed shaped fields are used to conform to the tumor to reduce the volume of irradiated normal tissues. The common terms used to describe the extent of RT are *involved-field, extended-field, and total lymphoid (or nodal) irradiation.* The use of these terms varies considerably in the literature. Generally, involved-field RT defines treatment limited to the clinically involved lymph node region. In contrast, extended-field RT includes RT given also to uninvolved adjacent lymph node regions. An example of extended-field RT for a patient with a stage I or II supradiaphragmatic presentation would be treatment with the mantle technique and prophylactic irradiation of the upper abdominal lymph nodes and the spleen. This is also termed *subtotal nodal irradiation.* The *mantle technique* covers all lymph node regions of the neck (submandibular, anterior cervical, supraclavicular), axillae, both lung hila, and the mediastinum. Shaped shielding blocks for the lung and heart are routinely used. The *inverted-Y fields* cover the para-aortic lymph nodes below the diaphragm and the bilateral pelvic and inguinal-femoral lymph nodes. *Total lymphoid RT* implies treatment to all the major lymphoid regions, with the mantle and the inverted-Y fields, with or without Waldeyer's ring fields. Its use at present is uncommon in HL. The RT planning process requires simulation in the desired treatment position with an appropriate immobilization device. Simulation with computed tomography allows accurate delineation of target volume coverage and normal tissue shielding with a three-dimensional perspective. Treatment is delivered with megavoltage linear accelerators with radiograph beam energy of 6 MV, and a fractionated course of treatment is typically of 4 weeks' duration, given 5 days a week (e.g., 35 Gy in 20 fractions over 4 weeks, at 1.75 Gy per fraction).

MANAGEMENT OF STAGE I AND II HODGKIN'S LYMPHOMA

Radiotherapy Alone

For many years, extended-field RT has been the standard treatment for patients with favorable clinical stage I and II HL. Extended-field RT for these patients with favorable disease features resulted in a relapse rate of 15% to 20%, with 5-year overall survival of 90% to 95%. Patients who had a disease recurrence after extended-field RT usually had a relapse outside the radiation field, and they were successfully salvaged with chemotherapy. The concerns about this policy included the knowledge that potentially serious late effects of therapy occurred with such treatment. This prompted a move to treatment with a short course of chemotherapy with reduced RT fields. In the past, the use of limited RT (e.g., mantle fields) alone led to an unacceptably high recurrence rates (30% to 50%). The modern treatment with ABVD chemotherapy and involved-field radiation leads to disease control in excess of 90% of patients. RT alone is still used in nodular lymphocyte-predominant HL, because the curative potential of ABVD chemotherapy is uncertain in this disease, and the indolent course of the disease and the tendency to multiple late relapses are present regardless of the initial treatment approach.

Combined-Modality Therapy

Our present recommendations for stage I and II HL are detailed in Table 3. In patients with favorable disease, treatment consists of planned combined-modality therapy, with ABVD for three cycles, followed by involved-field RT. Staging laparotomy is not performed. Several clinical trials have shown a lower recurrence rate with this approach compared with extended-field RT alone, and the use of involved-field RT in the setting of combined-modality therapy was validated in a prospective randomized trial. Combined-modality therapy results in superb disease control (more than 95% at 5 years) and allows for a reduction of the RT volume, thereby reducing the potential for late effects. The 5-year survival is expected to be 98% to 99%. The exact number of chemotherapy cycles in favorable stage I and II HL is still a matter of debate, ranging between two and four cycles. The recommended involved-field RT dose is 30 to 35 Gy, and whether a lower dose (20 Gy) is adequate is a question being addressed in clinical trials. It is not known to what extent involved-field RT is of benefit in patients with stage I or II favorable HL treated with six cycles of ABVD. In patients with unfavorable stage I and II HL, typically those with bulky mediastinal disease or B symptoms, a full course of ABVD (six to eight cycles) is followed by involved-field RT (35 Gy). This approach results in a very low recurrence rate (8% to 10%) and 5-year survival rates of 85% to 94%. An alternate combined-modality therapy program in common use is the Stanford V protocol, which involves weekly chemotherapy treatments for 12 weeks, followed by RT (36 Gy) to areas of initial tumor bulk of 5 cm or more.

ROLE OF RADIATION THERAPY IN STAGE III AND IV HODGKIN'S LYMPHOMA

The primary treatment for stage III and IV HL is chemotherapy. The standard regimen is ABVD for six to eight courses. The routine use of RT does not improve survival in stage III to IV HL and is not indicated. However, for patients with bulky sites of disease, typically a large mediastinal mass, the addition of RT improves local tumor control. For this reason, we recommend involved-field RT to the bulky site of disease (see Table 3). If the Stanford V protocol is used in stage III to IV HL, regional RT (36 Gy) is prescribed to initial lymph node sites with a tumor bulk of 5 cm or larger.

SIDE EFFECTS OF RADIATION THERAPY

Acute side effects are those occurring during or within a few weeks of completion of treatment, and they include general symptoms of anorexia, fatigue, and possibly nausea. Specific effects depend on the normal tissues irradiated. Skin erythema and alopecia of the local area are common; skin desquamation is rare. If the midline neck structures are treated, dysphagia and laryngitis will occur, but they will be transient, lasting 1 to 3 weeks. If the high cervical area is treated, change in taste and dryness of the mouth can occur because of exposure of the salivary glands. All these symptoms can be managed conservatively, with oral rinses, analgesics, and good dental hygiene. If a large volume of the bone marrow is irradiated, for example in the inverted-Y technique, transient myelosuppression will occur and can result in pancytopenia lasting a few weeks.

Subacute side effects occur 1 to 4 months after completion of RT. *Radiation pneumonitis* occurs in fewer than 5% of patients and generally only in those who had large volumes of lung tissue irradiated are at risk. It is characterized by cough, dyspnea, and low-grade fever. It is important to rule out and treat infection. Chest radiography or computed tomography typically shows pulmonary infiltrates in the distribution of the irradiation portals. Treatment consists of supportive care with the addition of glucocortocoids if symptoms are severe. Radiation pericarditis is rare, and patients are only at risk if a large volume of the heart is radiated to a higher dose. Lhermitte's sign is a transient shocklike sensation experienced in the spine and radiating to the extremities, triggered by flexion of the neck, occurring 2 to 4 months after completion of treatment. It is observed in 25% to 30% of patients receiving the mantle treatment fields, and it typically resolves in about 6 months. The toxicity of RT may be exacerbated in patients receiving chemotherapy.

ASSESSMENT OF RESPONSE AND FOLLOW-UP

Cure requires disease eradication, and therefore it is the first step to attain complete remission. In patients completing the treatment program for HL, response is usually assessed 6 to 8 weeks afterward. Because the RT dose fractionation schedule is determined before treatment and is based on the dose-response relationship and tolerance of tissues within the treatment volume, the presence of residual abnormality at the end of the treatment course is not an indication for additional RT. The assessment of response includes a physical examination and repeat imaging studies with computed tomography, gallium scanning, or positron emission tomography. In nodular sclerosis HL, persistent abnormalities may be present at the completion of treatment, with residual fibrosis noted. These features gradually resolve over a period of months. Residual mediastinal abnormalities are especially common, particularly if a bulky mass was present before treatment. Resolution of gallium avidity and a negative positron emission tomography scan are useful in distinguishing viable lymphoma from fibrosis. Although most recurrences in patients with HL occur within 2 to 3 years after the diagnosis, late relapse is infrequent (less than 5%). Accordingly, patients are assessed three to four times per year for the first 2 to 3 years, with a decreasing frequency, and usually yearly after 5 years. Follow-up assessment consist of a history, physical examination, blood count, and attention to possible late effects of treatment and its management (see later). Routine imaging for screening of HL recurrence is not useful beyond the first 2 to 3 years.

LATE EFFECTS OF TREATMENT

Late effects occur months to years after treatment. In contrast to acute effects, which are reversible, most late effects are permanent, although most are treatable. The mantle technique exposes a significant volume of lung tissue to RT, in the apices and lateral to the mediastinum. These areas usually become fibrotic over 6 to 18 months, and changes can be appreciated on chest radiographs. Patients are rarely symptomatic, but pulmonary function tests may show mild abnormalities. Toxicity of chemotherapy drugs such as bleomycin is additive. Late cardiac complications may include valvular disease, ischemic heart disease, and pericarditis. The relative risk of a fatal cardiac event after RT to the heart is approximately two to three times that of an age-adjusted healthy population. With modern RT technique, the risk is expected to be lower. The thyroid gland is often directly exposed to radiation, and thyroid nodules and hypothyroidism are present in up to 30% to 50% of patients. Hypothyroidism is easily managed with thyroid replacement therapy. Gonadal dysfunction is associated only with pelvic radiation such as the inverted-Y technique, and it can be minimized in men with scrotal shielding and in women with consideration of pretreatment oophoropexy. Infectious complications include a significant risk of developing herpes zoster, and for patients who had splenectomy, risk of severe sepsis with encapsulated organisms such as *Streptococcus pneumoniae*. Because of this risk, pneumococcal revaccination is recommended every 5 years. Long-term complications of the gastrointestinal, genitourinary, skeletal, and central nervous systems are rare with modern techniques. Psychosocial problems, including chronic fatigue, are also common in long-term follow-up of patients with HL, with many contributing factors including RT, chemotherapy, and the overall impact of the diagnosis and its treatment. Survivors of HL are known to have an increased risk of mortality compared with the general population, and this effect becomes dominant 10 to 15 years after treatment, when death resulting from HL becomes extremely unlikely. The cause is multifactorial, with second malignant disease the main contributing factor. Approximately 45 to 70 excess second malignant diseases per year are seen among 10,000 patients treated for HL (absolute excess risk), and about two thirds or more of these are solid cancers. This finding translates to an alarming statistic of a 25-year cumulative actuarial risk of 20% to 30% for the development of a second cancer in a survivor of HL. Although leukemia and myelodysplasia are chiefly related to alkylating agent–based chemotherapy (e.g., the MOPP regimen [nitrogen mustard, vincristine, procarbazine, and prednisone]), solid cancers result from the carcinogenic effects of radiation. Secondary breast cancers are more common in women who were treated when they were less than 30 years old, with the highest risk for patients treated as adolescents. The lung cancer risk is highest for smokers. These two cancers account for most second solid cancers. Other cancers seen at increased incidence include: thyroid, salivary gland, oral cavity, gastrointestinal, cutaneous, and connective tissue tumors and NHLs. The magnitude of the late effects observed has been the driving force behind the change in the treatment approach to the reduction of RT volumes and dose. Whether these approaches will have a significant impact on the incidence of late effects is too early to determine. However, given a large cohort of long-term survivors of HL at present, much can be achieved at the time of follow-up visits to detect, counsel, and treat the late effects of therapy, to reduce the risk of treatment-related morbidity and mortality. Screening for hypothyroidism should be performed at each visit. Patients who had splenectomy should undergo vaccination to protect against pneumococcal, meningococcal, and *Haemophilus influenzae* infections, and this is preferably done before treatment. Patients should receive counseling regarding health and psychological issues, including the impact of treatment on quality of life, reproduction, cardiovascular fitness, and risk of a second malignant disease. Smoking cessation is a must. Sun protection practices and avoidance of sunburn are encouraged. Risk factors for ischemic heart disease should be minimized, for example with a heart-healthy diet, control of body weight and blood pressure, and monitoring of cholesterol and lipid profile. For women who had RT to breast tissue, regular self-examination and screening mammography should start 7 to 8 years after treatment, or at age 40 years, whichever comes first.

SALVAGE THERAPY AND THE ROLE OF RADIATION

Patients in whom initial chemotherapy or combined-modality therapy fails will receive salvage chemotherapy and autologous stem cell transplantation (ASCT) in a second attempt to achieve cure. The disease-free survival rate is 30% to 55% at 5 years after ASCT. RT is commonly incorporated into the high-dose protocols. After chemotherapy, HL tends to recur in previously involved sites, particularly if the disease was bulky. Before the routine use of high-dose chemotherapy and ASCT in the late 1980s, selected patients in whom initial chemotherapy failed were given RT as salvage treatment. The techniques used varied from mantle fields to extensive fields up to total nodal irradiation. Patients were usually selected to receive RT because the disease at the time of relapse was predominantly localized, nodal, and amenable to coverage with radiation. The in-field control rate was approximately 90%, and one third of the patients survived 5 years with control of disease. Patients were more likely to have a durable response if the disease-free interval was longer than 12 months from completion of initial chemotherapy. Although these data cannot be directly compared with results of ASCT, they nevertheless show that RT alone could salvage a small proportion of patients who would now be routinely considered candidates for ASCT. These data also show that certain patient characteristics predict a favorable response to RT: predominantly nodal disease, no systemic symptoms, favorable histologic features, and a long disease-free interval. Thus, failure of chemotherapy does not necessarily imply radiation resistance, and applying RT judiciously in sequence with high-dose chemotherapy and ASCT may improve disease control and survival.

RT can be given before ASCT, either to the involved field or to extended fields up to total nodal irradiation. The conditioning regimen should not include total body irradiation. Another approach is to deliver involved-field radiation 2 to 3 months after ASCT. The indications for posttransplant RT include previous bulky disease (5 cm or larger), disease responding incompletely to salvage chemotherapy, residual abnormalities after ASCT, and limited-stage disease in which the original treatment plan had included RT. The extent of radiation fields and dose are individualized, depending on prior exposure to radiation, anatomic distribution of the disease, and normal tissue toxicity. Doses of 25 to 35 Gy are associated with a high rate of in-field control and with minimal short- and long-term toxicity. Several institutional series reported the benefits of involved-field radiation given after ASCT. For patients who have recurrent or progressive disease despite ASCT, RT can remain an extremely useful modality of treatment for locoregional control.

UNRESOLVED ISSUES IN THE RADIATION THERAPY MANAGEMENT OF HODGKIN'S LYMPHOMA

The efficacy of RT in achieving local disease control has been accepted for many years. With excellent local control rates, attention has been focused on reducing the long-term toxicities such as second malignant diseases and cardiac complications. In the setting of combined-modality therapy, current ongoing clinical trials are addressing optimal RT target volume and total dose. Some of the controversies in the RT management of HL are as follows:

1. The necessity of coverage of a whole nodal region versus just the initially involved node, after a complete response to chemotherapy, is debated.
2. Optimal RT dose in combined-modality protocols: Excellent results are obtained with doses ranging from 30 to 40 Gy. Trials are ongoing to examine whether a lower dose (e.g., 20 Gy) can be given without compromising efficacy. Finally, is RT required at all for patients treated with optimal chemotherapy?
3. Role of RT in stage III or IV HL: The routine use of RT after chemotherapy results in a slight increase in tumor control rates but not survival. Is there a subgroup of patients who will benefit from RT, other than those with bulky disease?

4. Optimal RT in the setting of high-dose chemotherapy and stem cell support: The role of radiation in the setting of ASCT requires further refinement. This relates to the indications, selection of patients for therapy, dose-fractionation parameters, and timing with chemotherapy and ASCT.

ADDITIONAL INFORMATION ACCESSIBLE THROUGH THE WORLD WIDE WEB

1. National Comprehensive Cancer Network Clinical Practice Guidelines in Oncology: http://www.nccn.org/physician_gls/index.html
2. National Cancer Institute's Physician Data Query (PDQ): http://www.cancer.gov/cancerinfo/pdq/treatment
3. Active clinical trials: http://www.clinicaltrials.gov/

ACUTE LEUKEMIA IN ADULTS

method of
ELIHU ESTEY, M.D.
University of Texas M. D. Anderson Cancer Center
Houston, Texas

Acute leukemia results from genetic alterations in normal hematopoietic stem cells. These alterations reduce the ability of stem cells to differentiate normally into red cells, platelets, and granulocytes, and they produce a survival and proliferative advantage relative to the residual normal stem cells. The consequent accumulation of abnormal cells, known as "leukemic cells" or "blasts," interferes with the ability of residual normal stem cells to differentiate. The result is bone marrow failure, the clinical manifestations of which, primarily anemia, lead patients to seek medical attention. A hemoglobin concentration of less than 12 g/dL is present at diagnosis in 95% of patients with acute myeloid leukemia (AML), which accounts for 80% of cases of acute leukemia in adults. Pancytopenia is typical in such patients. Less commonly, symptoms reflect tissue invasion as a result of the excess proliferation. The sites most commonly affected are the gum, skin, lymph nodes, spleen, kidney, and most ominously, the lung.

DIAGNOSIS AND CLASSIFICATION

The diagnosis of acute leukemia rests on demonstrating an accumulation of blasts in marrow or, less frequently, in peripheral blood. The presence of more than 30% blasts in a marrow aspirate was previously required to make the diagnosis. The minimal criterion has recently been changed to 20%, however, which suggests that any such criterion is essentially arbitrary. After establishing the diagnosis, the lineage of the blasts is assessed (myeloid = AML, lymphoid = acute lymphoid leukemia [ALL], and undifferentiated = acute undifferentiated leukemia). The distinction is important because many cases of AML are unlikely to respond as well to ALL-type therapy as to AML-type therapy and vice/versa. If Auer rods are present in the blasts, the diagnosis is AML. If not, lineage determination is based on whether the blasts express surface antigens associated with the myeloid (equivalently monocytic, erythroid, or megakaryocytic) or lymphoid immunophenotype. Myeloid antigens are CD13, CD33, c-kit, CD14, CD64 (the latter two are monocytic markers), glycophorin A (an erythroid marker), and CD41 (a megakaryocytic marker). Lymphoid markers are CD10, CD19, and CD20 (pre-B or B cells) and CD2, CD3, CD4, CD5, and CD8 (T cells). Alternatively, lineage determination can be accomplished with histochemical stains. If the blasts stain for myeloperoxidase, the diagnosis is AML. If the blasts are peroxidase negative but stain for butyrate or nonspecific esterase, acute monocytic leukemia (a variant of AML) is diagnosed. If the blasts are peroxidase and butyrate negative and express none of the myeloid or lymphoid antigens noted earlier, the diagnosis is acute undifferentiated leukemia, which is commonly treated like AML.

The initial marrow aspirate may be "dry," which is indicative of marrow fibrosis. In this case, biopsy is mandatory to exclude, in particular, acute megakaryocytic leukemia. If the marrow contains more than 50% normoblasts and pronormoblasts, the blast percentage is based only on the nonerythroid cells; in such cases, the diagnosis is typically acute erythroid leukemia, which can be confirmed if glycophorin A is expressed on the blasts' surface.

SUPPORTIVE CARE

Therapy for acute leukemia often results in rapid reduction of an elevated white blood cell count (WBC). This reduction is often associated with the development of a "tumor lysis syndrome" characterized by hyperuricemia, hyperphosphatemia, and renal failure. Prevention of tumor lysis syndrome rests on administration of intravenous fluid and allopurinol (Zyloprim) (or rasburicase) if the blast count is over 10,000. If the count is higher than 10,000 to 50,000, the patient, particularly if elderly or with monocytic leukemia, is at risk for chemotherapy-associated pulmonary failure. Bronchoalveolar lavage typically shows hemorrhagic fluid in these cases; treatment consists of fluid restriction, high-dose steroids, and continuous venovenous dialysis, which may remove the inciting cytokines. Dialysis is also used to treat severe cases of tumor lysis syndrome.

The myelosuppressive nature of typical antileukemic therapy puts a premium on prevention/treatment of infection and hemorrhage. Although antibiotic prophylaxis is controversial, the development of fever (>101°F), unrelated to the administration of chemotherapy, calls for the use of broad-spectrum antibiotics such as imipenem* or a third-generation cephalosporin.

*Not FDA approved for this indication.

If pneumonia is documented (by computed tomography in cases in which the chest radiograph is unrevealing), a lipid amphotericin* preparation and/or candicidin* is begun. Otherwise, these antifungals are administered if culture-negative fever persists for 3 days. If infection (pneumonia, sepsis) persists, granulocyte-macrophage (GM-CSF) or granulocyte colony-stimulating factor (G-CSF) should be started, and if possible, granulocyte transfusions should be administered, with G-CSF used to increase the donors' granulocyte counts.

Red cells are transfused to keep the hemoglobin concentration higher than 8 g/dL (lower in a young patient, higher in the presence of coronary artery disease). Platelets are administered if the platelet count is less than 10,000, unless it has been this low for weeks without improvement after previous transfusions, the patient is not bleeding, and disseminated intravascular coagulation (DIC) is not present. If the count does not increase significantly after transfusions of pooled platelet concentrates, family members are used as donors. Transfusions of cryoprecipitate are used to attain a fibrinogen level greater than 150 mg/dL, and fresh frozen plasma is administered to keep the prothrombin time less than 16 seconds. All blood products are filtered to reduce the risk of alloimmunization.

Patients are weighed daily. Fluid retention is common and can produce a radiographic pattern similar to that of pneumonia.

TREATMENT OF ACUTE MYELOID LEUKEMIA

Treatment of AML is intended to produce and maintain a complete remission (CR). Criteria for CR are a platelet count greater than 100,000/μL, a neutrophil count greater than 1000/μL, and a bone marrow that has less than 5% blasts. Patients who achieve a CR live longer than patients who do not. The difference is largely attributable to the time spent in CR, thus suggesting a correlation between achievement of CR and survival time. In general, once 3 years has elapsed from the CR date, the probability of recurrence sharply declines and becomes less than 10%. Accordingly, patients who have been in continuous CR for 3 years can, for operational purposes, be considered "potentially cured." Only patients who reach CR are potentially cured.

Once AML is diagnosed and the decision to treat is made, the need for emergency therapy must be assessed. Emergency treatment is required if the circulating blast count is rising rapidly or is over 100,000. Other indications for immediate therapy are DIC and organ dysfunction, especially pulmonary dysfunction, which is attributed to leukemic infiltration (most commonly seen in patients with greater than 10,000 circulating blasts). In the latter situation, it is more important to initiate chemotherapy than to perform leukapheresis, the value of which is controversial.

Standard Therapy

Remission induction therapy for newly diagnosed AML usually consists of a combination, commonly called 3 + 7—3 days of an anthracycline and 7 days of ara-C (cytarabine [Cytosar-U]) at 100 to 200 mg/m^2 daily, days 1 through 7. The results of randomized trials suggest that at the doses compared, idarubicin (Idamycin), 12 mg/m^2 daily on days 1 through 3, is the anthracycline of choice. However, differences between idarubicin and daunorubicin (Cerubidine), though statistically significant, are not necessarily medically significant; thus, survival differences are measured in months. In clinical practice, a bone marrow aspirate is usually obtained 2 to 3 weeks after beginning therapy. Biopsy is needed only if the quality of the aspirate does not permit determination of cellularity. If the marrow continues to show blasts and is cellular, a second course of the same therapy is often given, sometimes at reduced total dose (e.g., 2 + 5). If the day 14 or 21 marrow is hypoplastic, therapy is usually delayed until it is clear that leukemia has reappeared, at which time the second course begins. A second repeated course of therapy can certainly produce remissions, but they are usually shorter in duration than remissions produced after one course of therapy, thus illustrating the connection between the results of induction therapy and the results of postremission therapy. It is important to recognize that the initial marrow obtained after a period of hypoplasia may demonstrate up to 30% to 50% blasts as a reflection of the regeneration of normal, not "leukemic" marrow. In this circumstance, follow-up (e.g., at 1- to 2-week intervals) examination of marrow shows a reduction in the blast percentage concomitant with a rise in neutrophils and platelets.

Three types of postremission therapy can be distinguished. *Maintenance* therapy is usually defined as therapy less myelosuppressive than that used to produce remission. The doses used in *consolidation* therapy usually approach the doses used during induction, whereas those in *intensification* therapy may surpass them. Typically, once in remission after treatment with the 3 + 7 regimen, patients receive maintenance therapy with the same drugs given during induction but administered at approximately monthly intervals for 4 to 12 months. It is likely that the need for a prolonged duration of maintenance therapy depends on the intensity of induction and post-remission therapy. For example, whereas a randomized German AML Cooperative Group trial noted that the addition of 3 years of maintenance lengthened the median duration of remission from 8 to 13 months and the improved probability of 3-year relapse-free survival (RFS) to 30% from 7%, a similarly randomized trial by the same group found no difference in RFS or survival when patients in the no-maintenance arm received a more intensive induction treatment and one intense post-remission course. *Some* maintenance therapy is needed if intensive post-remission therapy is not contemplated. It seems clear, however, that any benefit from traditional maintenance after the administration

*Not FDA approved for this indication.

of 3 to 4 months of consolidation is relatively small and perhaps nonexistent with respect to survival.

Prognostic Factors With Standard Therapy

Standard therapy (i.e., 3 + 7, followed by varying lengths of consolidation or maintenance therapy) results in 60% to 70% CR rates and median remission durations of approximately 1 year, but with less than 20% of all patients achieving long-term RFS. It must be stressed that all these results are averages. Departures from these averages are common, so speaking of an average outcome is potentially misleading. It is incumbent on physicians treating AML to define the prognosis of the specific patient for whom they are caring. This prognosis dictates whether that patient might appropriately receive palliative care or standard therapy or (much more frequently) might be considered a candidate for a clinical trial involving investigational therapy.

Prognostic factors can be divided into those primarily associated with early death and those primarily associated with resistance to chemotherapy. Rates of therapy-induced mortality increase with increasing age, abnormal organ function, and in particular, poor performance status. An ambulatory (Zubrod performance status <3) adult would be expected to have an induction mortality rate of less than 5% to 10% if younger than 50 years, but it rises to 30% to 40% if 80 years or older. The profound effect of performance status is illustrated by noting that a bedridden (Zubrod performance status >2) adult younger than 50 years has a probable mortality rate of 40%, with mortality rates of 60% in bedridden patients 70 years or older. Except for infirm patients older than 50 years or so, the primary cause of treatment failure with 3 + 7 is resistant AML, either manifested as failure to enter initial CR despite having lived long enough to do so or, more often, manifested as a CR that is only transient. The principal predictor of resistant AML after 3 + 7 is the karyotype of the AML cells. Three groups can be distinguished. A *better-prognosis group* (Table 1) consists of patients with pericentric inversion of chromosome 16 (inv[16], associated with French-American-British [FAB] subtype M4EO) or a translocation between chromosomes 8 and 21 (t[8;21], associated with FAB subtype M2). Each of these abnormalities disrupts the function of a transcription factor (so-called core-binding factor [CBF]) that regulates the expression of genes important in hematopoietic differentiation. At most, 10% of unselected patients have CBF AML; typically, such patients are younger than 60 years. A *worse-prognosis group* (Table 1) comprises patients with monosomy of chromosomes 5 and/or 7 (−5, −7), deletions of the long arms of these chromosomes (5q−, 7q−), or abnormalities involving three or more chromosomes ("complex abnormalities"). These patients, who constitute about 30% to 40% of all patients, are on average older (>50 to 60) and disproportionately have either a history of abnormal blood counts before the diagnosis of AML (antecedent hematologic disorder [AHD]) or have "secondary AML," in which they have received alkylating agents for other conditions. The remaining 50% to 60% of patients, including the approximately 5% in whom no metaphases can be recovered for analysis, fall into an *intermediate-prognosis group* (Table 1), whose prognosis in most cases bears more resemblance to the worse than to the better group. Independent of cytogenetics, resistance is also more common in patients with AHD or in those whose blasts have an internal tandem duplication of the *flt3* gene or the multidrug resistant *(MDR1)* phenotype, which leads to more rapid egress of drugs such as anthracyclines (Table 1).

TABLE 1. **Predictors of Failure With Standard Therapy**

Factor	CR Rate (%)	Long-Term RFS Rate (%)
Cyto inv(16), t(8;21) (i.e., CBF AML)	>90	40–50
Cyto −5/−7, complex	30–50	<5
Cyto normal or other	50–75	10–30
History of abnormal counts (AHD)	40–70	<10
De novo AML	50–80	<10–50
MDR⁺ (age >55 y)	35	Depends on Cyto, AHD, flt3, ITD
MDR⁻ (age >55 y)	60	Depends on Cyto, flt3, ITD
flt3 ITD⁺ (age <60 y)	78	36
flt3 ITD⁻ (age <60 y)	84	56

AHD, antecedent hematologic disorder; AML, acute myeloid leukemia; CBF, core-binding factor; CR, complete remission; Cyto, cytogenetics; ITD, internal tandem duplication; MDR, multidrug resistance protein; RFS, relapse-free survival.

Effect of High-Dose Ara-C or Stem Cell Transplantation in Various Prognostic Groups

High-dose ara-C (HDAC) in general denotes daily doses of 2 to 12 g/m^2, in contrast to standard-dose ara-C (SDAC), which consists of daily doses of 100 or 200 mg/m^2. HDAC can produce CRs in patients who relapsed after maintenance with SDAC. Numerous randomized trials have compared HDAC and SDAC in untreated patients, either as induction therapy or as post-remission therapy, or both. These trials have concluded that (1) the toxicity of HDAC (e.g., cerebellar and cerebral) outweighs anti-AML effect in patients older than 65 years; (2) patients younger than 60 years benefit from HDAC given during induction, in CR, and perhaps both; and (3) *this benefit is proportional to the patient's probable sensitivity to SDAC, as determined by blast cell karyotype.* Specifically, HDAC at, for example, 3 g/m^2 every 12 hours on days 1, 3, and 5 repeated for four cycles, increases potential cure rates to 70% to 80% in patients with inv(16) or t(8;21) and to 30% to 40% in patients with a normal karyotype, but very little, if at all, in patients with prognostically worse karyotypes. Intermediate doses of ara-C at 0.4 to 1.0 g/m^2 daily (IDAC) for 4 days seem to be equivalent to HDAC in patients with a normal karyotype and, possibly, in those with inv(16) or t(8;21).

European and American trials have investigated allogeneic and autologous transplantation in first CR by assigning patients with HLA-matched sibling donors to allogeneic transplantation and randomizing patients without such donors between autologous transplantation and either continued chemotherapy or no further therapy. The proportion of patients assigned to chemotherapy who actually receive it is higher than the corresponding proportion of patients assigned to allogeneic or autologous transplantation. Because it has been demonstrated that patients with a donor who do not receive a transplant are prognostically worse than patients who do receive a transplant, comparisons between allogeneic transplantation and chemotherapy are performed by comparing patients assigned to allogeneic transplantation with patients assigned to chemotherapy rather than by comparing patients according to the treatment actually received. The same "intent-to-treat principle" governs analyses of autologous transplantation versus chemotherapy. Such comparisons invariably demonstrate decreased relapse rates with allogeneic transplantation and less strikingly with autologous transplantation. In addition, more deaths occur in CR (i.e., procedure-related deaths), particularly with allogeneic transplantation. Nonetheless, superior RFS is still seen with allogeneic transplantation and less frequently with autologous transplantation because the reduced frequency of relapse more than compensates for the increased frequency of death in CR. However, in no trials does the group assigned to either allogeneic or autologous transplantation have longer survival. Do any subgroups do better with allogeneic transplantation than with chemotherapy or vice versa? It has generally been accepted that patients older than 60 years have an excess mortality rate if given allogeneic transplantion. However so-called mini-transplants, in which patients receive reduced amounts of chemotherapy and/or radiation before allogeneic transplantation, thus relying on an immunologically mediated and readily demonstrable "graft-versus-leukemia" effect, can be performed in patients up to 75 years of age. However, the relative effectiveness of mini-transplants is uncertain. It has also been accepted that allogeneic transplantation should be performed in the first CR in patients younger than 20 years. However, the results with HDAC- or IDAC-containing chemotherapy are such that some doubt has been cast on the need for allogeneic transplantation. The largest study to examine the effect of cytogenetics found a trend for patients with inv(16) or t(8;21) to live longer if assigned to chemotherapy rather than allogeneic transplantation, whereas patients with prognostically intermediate karyotypes lived longer with allogeneic transplantation, but only if younger than 35 years. Most importantly, outcome was similarly poor in the adverse karyotype group regardless of whether patients were assigned to allogeneic transplantation or chemotherapy. Similarly, nothing has been found to suggest that autologous transplantation affects the prognosis in these patients.

Use of Prognostic Factors in Planning Treatment

Physicians seeing patients with AML should make management decisions based on analysis of the aforementioned prognostic factors. The three general options are standard therapy extended to include HDAC/IDAC or transplantation, investigational therapy, and palliative care:

Standard Therapy. Although standard therapy should naturally be considered first, the data just presented and in Table1 indicate that it is satisfactory for only a minority of patients (a third to two fifths). Candidates for standard therapy include patients with inv(16) or t(8;21), who if younger than 60 to 65 years, have a high probability of potential cure if therapy includes HDAC or IDAC, as described before. Given the increasing likelihood of complications as age increases, the dose of ara-C should be reduced (e.g., to 0.5 to 1.0 g/m^2) in patients older than 60 years. Another group in whom standard therapy could be considered appropriate are ambulatory patients younger than 60 to 70 years in the intermediate karyotype group, provided that they do not have AHD, *flt3* mutation, or MDR1 positivity (Figure 1). Here the probability of potential cure may approach 30%, again particularly if HDAC or IDAC is used during post-remission therapy. However because the probability of eventual treatment failure in these patients is 70% and because the median remission lasts at most 1 to 2 years, investigational approaches should also be offered.

Investigational Therapies. In the remaining patients, expectations with standard therapy are so low that its use can readily be questioned. Such patients have a substantial probability of either death during remission induction (if bedridden and older than 50 years or older than 80 years regardless of performance status, see Table 1) or resistance to therapy (if in the worse-prognosis cytogenetic group or in the intermediate-prognosis cytogenetic group but with AHD, *flt3* mutation, or MDR1 positivity).

Palliative Care. If investigational therapy is not feasible, palliative care should be strongly considered in patients older than 65 years with a performance status greater than Zubrod 2 or in patients older than 80 years regardless of performance status. Median survival in such patients after standard therapy is only about 2 months. In other patients for whom investigational therapy is not an option, the choice between standard therapy and palliative care should be made on a case-by-case basis.

Acute Promyelocytic Leukemia

Acute promyelocytic leukemia (APL) results from translocations between the retinoic acid α (RARα) locus on chromosome 17 and the "promyelocytic leukemia" (PML) protein locus located on chromosome 15. This PML-RARα fusion is responsible for the 15;17 translocation (t[15;17]) demonstrable in 95% to 100% of cases. APL represents less than 10% of unselected cases of AML; independent risk factors for a

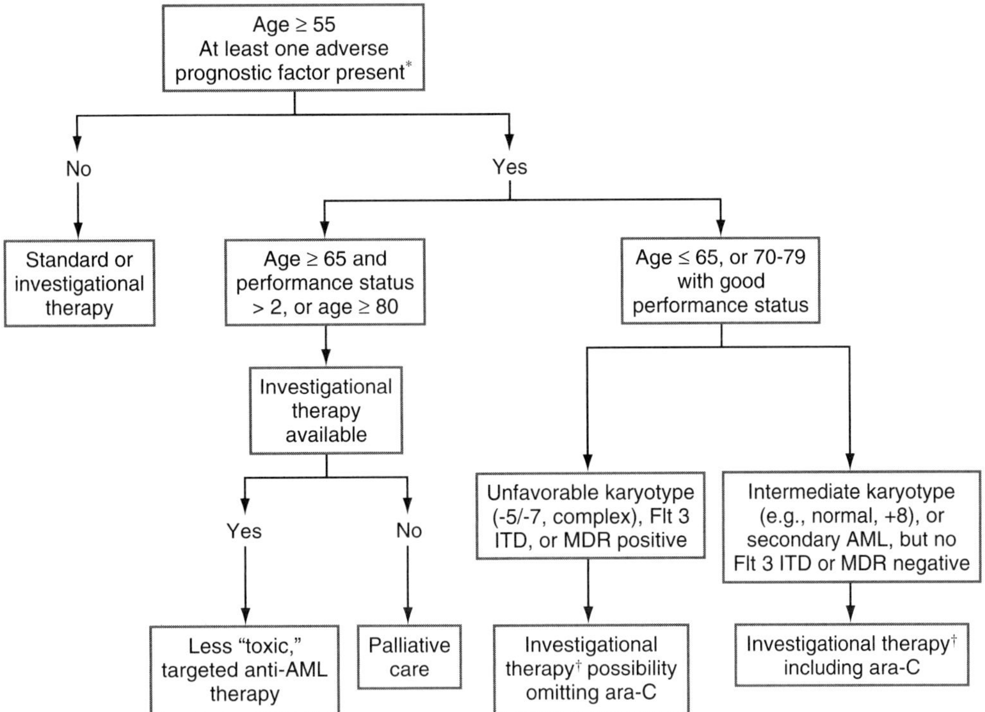

Figure 1. Approach to an older patient with untreated acute myeloid leukemia (AML). *Adverse prognostic features are age 65 years or older, performance status greater than Zubrod 2 or abnormal organ function (e.g., bilirubin >2, creatinine >2), abnormal cytogenetics (excluding inv[16], t[8;21], MDR1 expression, flt3 ITD, or mutation. †If investigational therapy is unavailable, decide on palliative versus standard therapy options on a case-by-case basis. ITD, internal tandem duplication; MDR, multidrug-resistant mutation.

diagnosis of APL in a patient with AML are younger age, Hispanic background, and obesity. The chief clinical feature is a bleeding diathesis resulting both from plasmin-dependent primary fibrinolysis and DIC. In any case of untreated AML, particularly when a patient is initially seen with such features, it is crucial to perform cytogenetic analysis to detect the distinctive t(15;17). In the rare case in which such analysis does not show the t(15;17) but the clinical or morphologic picture is suggestive, a molecular test, which can be performed in a few hours, can detect the characteristic disruption of PML in virtually all cases. Either demonstration of t(15;17) or a positive molecular test is requisite for the diagnosis. Recognition of APL is crucial because appropriate treatment is both different from that used for other types of AML and curative in most patients.

Several findings have contributed to these results. Anthracyclines are so effective that there is probably no reason to administer ara-C,* the use of which necessitates a reduction in the dose of idarubicin* or daunorubicin.* The addition of all-trans-retinoic acid (ATRA, 45 mg/m^2 daily) to chemotherapy (e.g., idarubicin, 12 mg/m^2 on days 2, 4, 6, and 8) increases the CR rate and more dramatically reduces the relapse rate (Figure 2). Current data suggest that ATRA should be used together with anthracyclines during induction and probably during post-remission therapy as well. The major toxicity of ATRA is a potentially fatal syndrome (APL differentiation syndrome [APLS]) characterized by fever and leakage of fluid into the extravascular space producing fluid retention, effusions, dyspnea, and hypotension; it is effectively treated with dexamethasone* (10 mg intravenously twice daily for 3 to 5 days, with a rapid taper). The use of frequent transfusions of platelets, cryoprecipitate, and fresh frozen plasma makes the use of heparin unnecessary. A molecular test (polymerase chain reaction [PCR]) that detects molecular evidence of t(15;17) provides a relatively sensitive and highly specific means of detecting impending hematologic relapse. After three cycles of anthracycline-containing post-remission therapy, over 90% of patients should be "PCR negative." If not or if molecular relapse occurs during follow-up, therapy should be changed. Arsenic trioxide (ATO) is the treatment of choice for relapsed APL (either molecular or hematologic). ATO can also cause the APLS. A stratification system has been developed that distinguishes patients with newly diagnosed disease who are at low, intermediate, or high risk. Low-risk patients have WBCs less than 10,000 and platelet counts higher than 40,000; a WBC over 10,000 identifies a patient at high risk, whereas others are at intermediate risk. Anticipated cure rates are close to 100%, 90%, and 70%. Low-risk patients may require only three to four courses of post-remission therapy (e.g., idarubicin* + ATRA), after which PCR tests can be performed every 3 months for 1 year, with ATO

*Not FDA approved for this indication.

*Not FDA approved for this indication.

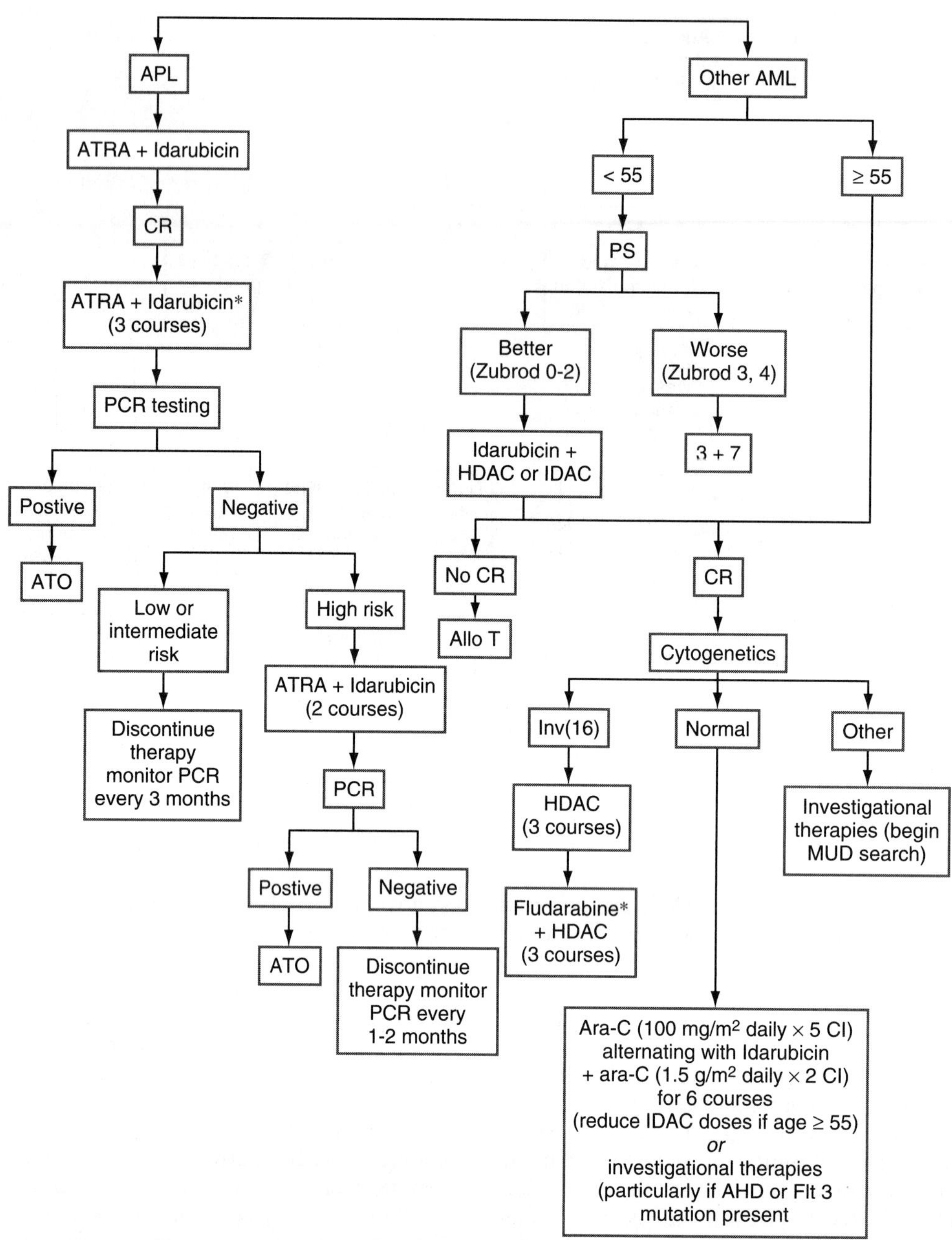

Figure 2. Suggested management of patients with untreated acute myeloid leukemia (AML). *Not FDA-approved for this indication. AHD = antecedent hematologic disorder; Allo T, allogeneic transplantation; APL, acute promyelocytic leukemia; ATO, arsenic trioxide; ATRA, all-trans-retinoic acid; CI, continuous infusion; CR, complete remission; HDAC, high-dose ara-C; IDAC, intermediate-dose ara-C; MUD, matched unrelated donor; PCR, polymerase chain reaction; PS, performance status.

given if the PCR reverts to positivity. Intermediate-risk patients may require a longer duration of post-remission treatment (e.g., 6 months). High-risk patients have both a higher early death rate from hemorrhage and a higher risk of relapse. These patients might benefit from more intense post-remission therapy or the use of ATO, gemtuzumab ozogamicin (Mylotarg),* or HuM195; the latter two agents, directed at the CD33 surface antigen, which is highly expressed on APL cells, have shown activity in APL. More frequent PCR testing (e.g., monthly in CR) may also be advisable.

*Not FDA approved for this indication.

Treatment of Relapsed/Refractory Acute Myeloid Leukemia

Recurrent AML will develop in most patients who achieve a CR. Ten percent to 50% of patients with newly diagnosed AML, depending on the prognostic factors noted earlier, will never enter CR ("primary refractory disease"). The most important factor predicting the outcome of therapy for relapsed/refractory AML (salvage therapy) is duration of the first CR (DurCR1), with primary refractory AML given a DurCR1 of zero (Figure 3). Table 2 illustrates the use of DurCR1 in planning salvage therapy; the data reflect M.D. Anderson results. Allogeneic transplantation

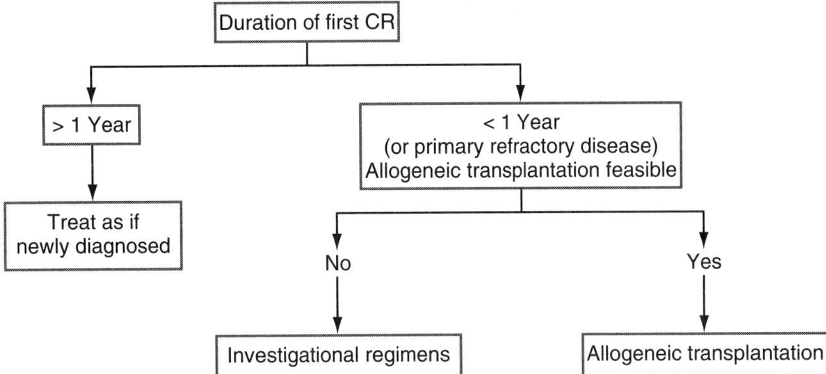

Figure 3. Suggested management of relapsed or refractory acute myeloid leukemia. CR, complete remission.

appears to be superior to HDAC- or IDAC-containing regimens in patients with a DurCR1 of less than 1 year; the great majority of these transplants were from an HLA-matched sibling donor. The same is true if attention is restricted to HDAC- or IDAC-treated patients who would have been candidates for an allogeneic transplant (less than 50 years old, etc.).

Newer or Investigational Agents

Combinations of topotecan* with ara-C or fludarabine* with ara-C (FLAG), with or without idarubicin, do not appear to be superior to more standard regimens. Gemtuzumab ozogamicin* may be marginally superior to HDAC regimens in patients with a DurCR1 of less than 6 months, but it seems inferior in patients with a DurCR1 longer than 12 months. It also seems to be inferior in untreated patients older than 65 years. Combinations with ara-C and idarubicin are under investigation. Other investigational agents include new nucleoside analogues or are intended to block the function of MDR1, cause re-expression of silenced tumor suppressor genes, inhibit the abnormal tyrosine kinase arising from *flt3* mutations, inhibit the farnesyl transferases that are needed for the functioning of RAS pathways, or block the function of proteins associated with resistance to chemotherapy-induced cell death.

*Not FDA approved for this indication.

TREATMENT OF ACUTE LYMPHOID LEUKEMIA

Vincristine (Oncovin), corticosteroids, L-asparaginase (Elspar), cyclophosphamide, methotrexate, and 6-mercaptopurine (6-MP) have considerably more activity in ALL than in AML; ara-C and anthracyclines are also effective in ALL. Given this number of drugs and the relatively younger age of adults with ALL than with AML, average CR rates are higher in ALL, typically 80% to 90%, with numerous induction regimens probably similarly effective. Two other differences from AML are the use of prolonged (e.g., 2 years) maintenance therapy, frequently using 6-MP, methotrexate, vincristine, and prednisone, and the need for central nervous system prophylaxis with intrathecal ara-C and/or methotrexate. However, as with AML, the prognosis has considerable variability, although most adults relapse. Perhaps the most commonly seen adverse prognostic feature is the presence of the Philadelphia chromosome (t[9;22], Ph′), which

TABLE 2. **Treatment of Relapsed or Refractory Acute Myeloid Leukemia**

Duration of 1st CR (wk)	HDAC- or IDAC-Containing Regimens, All Patients	HDAC- or IDAC-Containing Regimens, Patients <50 Years Old With Good Performance Status, Creatinine and Bilirubin Each <2	Allogeneic Transplant	Recommended Salvage Treatment
0 (primary refractory)	11/72 (15%)	6/19 (32%)	11/19 (58%)	Allogeneic transplant; investigational therapy if donor not available
1–26	10/44 (23%)	8/21 (38%)	7/12 (58%)	Allogeneic transplant; investigational therapy if donor not available
27–52	13/63 (21%)	6/24 (25%)	6/8 (75%)	Allogeneic transplant; investigational therapy if donor not available
>52	39/74 (53%)	22/32 (69%)	7/11 (64%)	HDAC/IDAC or allogeneic transplant

CR, complete remission; HDAC, high-dose ara-C; IDAC, intermediate-dose ara-C.

is found in 20% to 30% of cases of adult ALL; the presence of t(4;11) is similarly unfavorable. Whereas 3-year survival rates are 50% in patients with a normal karyotype, they are less than 20% in Ph′-positive ALL. It is generally accepted that allogeneic transplantation should be performed in the first CR in Ph′ patients. A longer time to CR, older age, higher initial WBC, and a non–T cell immunophenotype also affect the prognosis unfavorably, and allogeneic transplantation is also reasonable in these patients. However, as in AML, changes in the effectiveness of chemotherapy could influence these recommendations. For example, the addition of imatinib mesylate (STI571, "Gleevec")* to standard chemotherapy appears to delay relapse in Ph′ patients. Consolidation with ara-C, cyclophosphamide, and L-asparaginase has converted the prognosis of T cell ALL from unfavorable to favorable, with the need for maintenance therapy under investigation. Dose-intensive regimens featuring cyclophosphamide, methotrexate, and ara-C have eliminated the need for maintenance in B cell (Burkitt type) ALL. Dose intensification of anthracyclines, methotrexate, and L-asparaginase is also being studied, as are new agents such as anti-CD20 monoclonal antibodies, a liposomal preparation of vincristine, and "compound 506" for T cell ALL.

*Not FDA approved for this indication.

ACUTE LEUKEMIA IN CHILDREN

method of
JEFFREY E. RUBNITZ, M.D., PH.D.
St. Jude Children's Research Hospital
Memphis, Tennessee

Acute leukemia, the most common malignant disease in children, accounts for approximately one third of all childhood cancers. *Acute lymphoblastic leukemia* (ALL) predominates during childhood, with 2500 new cases diagnosed in the United States each year. In contrast, only 500 new cases of *acute myeloid leukemia* (AML) occur annually in the United States. Certain environmental factors, such as exposure to ionizing radiation, benzene, and specific chemotherapeutic agents, are associated with a higher risk of acute leukemia. Alkylating agents can induce secondary AML that is characterized by a prior myelodysplastic syndrome and abnormalities of chromosomes 5 and 7, whereas exposure to topoisomerase II inhibitors, especially the epipodophyllotoxins teniposide and etoposide, can lead to the rapid development of secondary AML with rearrangements of the *MLL* gene. Similarly, genetic diseases associated with chromosomal instability (Bloom's syndrome, Fanconi's anemia, and ataxia-telangiectasia) or with immunodeficiencies (Wiskott-Aldrich syndrome) are characterized by an increased risk of acute leukemia. However, most cases of childhood acute leukemia have no clearly identifiable cause, although many cases are believed to arise in utero.

PRESENTATION AND DIAGNOSTIC WORKUP

Children with acute leukemia often present with signs and symptoms of bone marrow failure, such as pallor, fatigue, bleeding, bruising, and fever. Bone pain, hepatosplenomegaly, and adenopathy are also common. Initial laboratory findings may include anemia, thrombocytopenia, neutropenia, and leukemic blasts on a peripheral blood smear. Complete morphologic, immunologic, and genetic examinations of the bone marrow are necessary to diagnose and to characterize fully each case of leukemia. Historically, acute leukemias were classified morphologically by the French-American-British system, which identified three types of ALL (L1 through L3) and eight types of AML (M0 through M7). Current classification systems rely more heavily on the immunophenotypic and genetic characteristics of each type of leukemia, rather than on morphology. For example, ALL is broadly classified as B-precursor, T-cell, or mature B-cell leukemia, based on the expression of surface antigens.

Leukemic blasts in most cases have specific genetic alterations, many of which have prognostic implications (Table 1). These alterations include changes in chromosome number (ploidy) and structure; about half of all cases of childhood ALL have recurrent translocations. Therefore, standard cytogenetic analysis

TABLE 1. **Frequency of Particular Genetic Abnormalities in Pediatric Patients With Acute Leukemia and Their Outcome**

Subgroup	Frequency (%)	5-Year Event-Free Survival Estimate (%)
Acute Lymphoblastic Leukemia		
B cell (rearranged *MYC* gene)	2–3	75–85
B precursor		
Hyperdiploid*	25	80–90
TEL-AML1	22	85–90
E2A-PBX1	5	75–85
BCR-ABL	3	20–40
MLL-AF4	2	20–35
Hypodiploid†	1	25–40
Rearranged *MLL*	5	30–50
T cell		
MLL-ENL	1	85–95
HOX11	3	80–90
TAL1	6–7	30–40
LYL1	1	30–40
Acute Myeloid Leukemia		
AML1-ETO	10–15	50–70
CBFβ-MYH11	8–10	50–70
MLL-AF9	5–10	40–60
PML-RARα	5–10	70–80

*More than 50 chromosomes
†Fewer than 45 chromosomes

and molecular methods, including reverse-transcriptase polymerase chain reaction, Southern blot analysis, and fluorescence in situ hybridization, are essential to the workup of all patients.

SUPPORTIVE CARE

At the time of diagnosis and during treatment, the most common complications in children with acute leukemia are fever, metabolic abnormalities, and hyperleukocytosis. In addition, the bone marrow failure that accompanies leukemia results in anemia and thrombocytopenia.

Fever

Infectious complications, both at diagnosis and during therapy, remain a major cause of morbidity and mortality in children with leukemia. Although leukemia itself can cause fever, all fevers in patients with leukemia should be presumed to be infectious. In the setting of neutropenia (defined as fewer than 500 neutrophils/mL), patients with fever should be started on broad-spectrum antibiotics after cultures are obtained. Although some studies suggest that certain patients with cancer who have fever and neutropenia may be treated with oral antibiotics, we currently admit all children with febrile neutropenia and begin intravenous antibiotics. We treat all such patients with at least a third- or fourth-generation cephalosporin (e.g., ceftazidime [Fortaz] or cefepime [Maxipime]). Because of the high incidence of α-hemolytic streptococci infection in patients with AML who have received high-dose cytarabine (Cytosar-U), we recommend the empiric use of vancomycin (Vancocin)* as well. For patients who have evidence of sepsis, are colonized with *Pseudomonas aeruginosa*, or who have recently received cephalosporins, we add an aminoglycoside, such as tobramycin (Tobrex). We treat children who have severe abdominal pain, radiologic evidence of typhlitis, or known infection with *Bacillus cereus* with a carbapenem (imipenem or meropenem) rather than a cephalosporin.

Patients who receive very intensive therapy, such as children with AML or high-risk ALL, are at increased risk of fungal infections, most commonly candidiasis and aspergillosis. Therefore, patients who remain febrile after 3 to 5 days of antibiotic therapy should receive empirical antifungal therapy. Currently available antifungals include traditional amphotericin B, lipid formulations of amphotericin B (AmBisome and Abelcet), azoles (fluconazole, itraconazole, and voriconazole), and echinocandins (caspofungin and FK463). Several studies suggest that voriconazole may be as effective as amphotericin for empirical antifungal treatment of neutropenic patients with persistent fever and for the treatment of invasive aspergillosis. Because of the high morbidity and mortality associated with invasive fungal infections, we are currently treating all patients with AML with prophylactic voriconazole in an attempt to reduce the incidence of these devastating events.

*Not FDA approved for this indication.

Metabolic Abnormalities

The lysis of leukemic blasts can cause hyperphosphatemia, hyperuricemia, hyperkalemia, and secondary hypocalcemia. In patients with high tumor burdens and rapid tumor growth, these abnormalities may be present at the time of diagnosis. More commonly, they occur soon after therapy is started. These abnormalities are referred to as tumor lysis syndrome and can lead to acute renal failure. To prevent tumor lysis syndrome, all patients should receive aggressive hydration at 3 L/M^2/d. Patients at high risk of tumor lysis syndrome and those with signs of the syndrome should receive recombinant urate oxidase to prevent obstructive uric acid nephropathy. To prevent or treat hyperphosphatemia and hypocalcemia, patients should also receive oral phosphate binders, such as aluminum hydroxide, or calcium carbonate.

Hyperleukocytosis

Patients with very high leukocyte counts are at risk of *leukostasis*, the sludging of leukemic blasts in small vessels. Stasis is more common in AML and may lead to infarction and hemorrhage in the lungs or central nervous system (CNS). In such cases, leukapheresis in older children or exchange transfusions in infants can be used to reduce the leukocyte count rapidly before chemotherapy is begun. However, the criteria for leukapheresis are controversial, and chemotherapy may sometimes be more efficacious at rapidly lowering the leukocyte count.

TREATMENT OF ACUTE LYMPHOBLASTIC LEUKEMIA

Mature B-cell ALL does not respond well to the chemotherapy used for other types of childhood ALL. However, outstanding results, with event-free survival estimates of nearly 90%, have been obtained with treatments that emphasize cyclophosphamide and the rapid rotation of antimetabolites in high doses. Thus, B-cell ALL was the first form of ALL to be recognized as a distinct clinical entity and the first to be treated by separate protocols designed specifically for the leukemia's unique features.

Modern trials for all other types of childhood ALL emphasize risk-based therapy to reduce toxicity in good-risk patients and to ensure appropriate therapy for patients at a high risk of relapse. In more recent clinical trials, risk classification strategies have been based on the presenting features and response to therapy. The use of such strategies has resulted in 5-year event-free survival rates greater than 70%. Although particular genetic features such as t(4;11) and t(9;22), confer a poor prognosis, others, including hyperdiploidy and the t(12;21), are associated with an excellent outcome (see Table 1). However, the best predictor of outcome is early response to therapy, which is influenced by the sensitivity of the leukemic cells to chemotherapy and by host characteristics. Simple morphologic examination of peripheral blood cells after 1 week of therapy is a relatively good indicator of ultimate outcome. However, morphologic examination tends to be subjective and imprecise, whereas minimal residual disease assays provide objective and sensitive measurements of low levels of leukemic cells. Current methods for assessing minimal residual disease are DNA-based polymerase chain reaction analysis of rearrangements of clonal antigen receptor genes, RNA-based polymerase chain reaction analysis of leukemia-specific gene fusions, and flow cytometric detection of aberrant immunophenotypes. In addition to the clinical importance of minimal residual disease measurement in the treatment of ALL, host factors such as pharmacodynamics and pharmacogenomics also have significant effects on treatment outcome.

With the exception of B-cell ALL, the treatment of childhood ALL includes four components: remission induction, consolidation, continuation, and treatment of subclinical CNS leukemia. Induction therapy generally consists of three or four drugs, which may include a glucocorticoid, vincristine, asparaginase, and an anthracycline. This type of therapy induces a complete remission in more than 95% of patients. Although glucocorticoids are an essential component of induction therapy, the optimal steroid has not yet been determined; dexamethasone* may provide better leukemic control than does prednisone,* but it may also be associated with greater toxicity when it is used in induction therapy. In some regimens, patients are given up to seven drugs during induction in an attempt to induce a faster and deeper reduction in leukemic cell burden and thereby to prevent the development of drug resistance. Intensive regimens of remission induction seem to have improved the outcome for some subsets of patients.

Consolidation, or intensification, therapy is given soon after remission has been achieved in an attempt to reduce the leukemic cell burden further before the emergence of drug resistance. In this phase of therapy, the drugs are used at higher doses than during induction, or different drugs are used, such as high-dose methotrexate (Rheumatrex) and 6-mercaptopurine (Purinethol), epipodophyllotoxins with cytarabine, or multiagent combination therapy. Consolidation therapy, first used successfully in the treatment of patients with high-risk disease, also appears to improve the long-term survival of patients with standard-risk disease. Similarly, the addition of intensive reinduction therapy is beneficial for patients in both risk groups. An alternative type of intensification therapy involves the prolonged, intensive use of L-asparaginase to deplete serum continuously of asparagine. The prolonged use of L-asparaginase and doxorubicin (Adriamycin) in some protocols has contributed to excellent overall outcome, especially for patients with *TEL-AML1*–positive B-lineage ALL and for patients with T-cell ALL.

*Not FDA approved for this indication.

The most intensive form of intensification is allogeneic stem cell transplantation (SCT). Patients with ALL blast cells positive for the Philadelphia chromosome are candidates for allogeneic SCT during first remission; an international collaborative study showed that patients who had this type of ALL and received stem cell transplants from an HLA-matched related donor had an outcome that was better than that for the same group who received only intensive chemotherapy. In contrast, allogeneic SCT has failed to improve the outcome for infants with ALL or for patients with t(4;11)-positive ALL.

Whereas B-cell ALL is treated with 2 to 8 months of intensive therapy, continuous postremission therapy is required to achieve an optimal outcome for pediatric patients with B-precursor or T-cell ALL. High-dose pulse therapy with intermittent rest periods is associated with an inferior outcome. Continuation therapy should be prolonged, because attempts to reduce the length of therapy to 12 or 18 months have resulted in overall outcomes that are less than optimal. Although a subset of patients may be cured with a shorter duration of therapy, patients in most clinical trials receive therapy for at least 2 to 2.5 years.

Most continuation regimens for ALL comprise weekly low-dose methotrexate and daily oral mercaptopurine. Outcome is improved by the addition of intermittent pulses of steroids and vincristine to the antimetabolite backbone; therefore, these components are included in most modern regimens of continuation therapy. Because the antileukemic effect of dexamethasone* is greater than that of prednisone,* dexamethasone is currently the steroid of choice; however, dexamethasone is associated with increased risks of avascular necrosis, osteoporosis, and fractures. Patients with high-risk ALL may also benefit from intensified continuation therapy that includes the rotational use of drug pairs. The improvements in relapse-free survival gained by intensification with anthracyclines or epipodophyllotoxins must be weighed against the late sequelae of these agents, which include cardiotoxicity and treatment-related acute myeloid leukemia.

The treatment of subclinical or overt CNS leukemia has tremendously affected the overall cure rates for childhood ALL. The risk of CNS relapse is higher for particular patients, including those with high leukocyte counts at diagnosis, T-cell disease, or leukemic blasts in the cerebrospinal fluid; therefore, such patients require more intensive CNS-directed therapy, which includes cranial irradiation, intrathecal chemotherapy, and systemic chemotherapy with dexamethasone* and high-dose methotrexate. Although the most effective modality is cranial irradiation, it is associated with significant morbidity such as neurotoxicity, endocrinopathy, and second malignant neoplasms. Therefore, intrathecal therapy has largely replaced cranial irradiation in the treatment of all patients except those at very high risk of CNS relapse. In fact, in three studies in

*Not FDA approved for this indication.

which cranial irradiation was not given to any patient, the CNS relapse rates were less than 10%.

TREATMENT OF ACUTE MYELOID LEUKEMIA

The treatment of AML consists of remission induction therapy and postremission consolidation, or intensification, therapy. Some trials have also included a maintenance phase; however, the effectiveness of maintenance therapy in AML has not been proved. Remission induction regimens typically include cytarabine (Cytosar-U) and an anthracycline, such as daunorubicin (Cerubidine). Some regimens also contain etoposide, thioguanine, or dexamethasone.* Approximately 90% of children with AML will achieve remission, but nearly half will suffer a relapse of their disease. More recent attempts to induce a deeper remission and better long-term outcome have included the use of newer agents, the use of alternative anthracyclines, and intensification of induction therapy. Evidence from several trials suggests that intensification of therapy by increasing drug doses, prolonging drug exposure, or decreasing the interval between courses of therapy may improve outcome.

Although extended maintenance therapy as the only postremission treatment is ineffective for AML, intensive postremission regimens decrease relapse rates. Today, most cooperative groups have abandoned the use of maintenance therapy for AML and rely on a short period (two to four courses) of intensive consolidation therapy that includes high-dose cytarabine. The only exception to this is the treatment of acute promyelocytic leukemia, which is treated with conventional chemotherapy plus all-trans-retinoic acid.* The use of all-trans-retinoic acid has dramatically improved the prognosis for this subtype of AML.

Studies performed in the 1980s demonstrated that allogeneic SCT is a feasible and effective alternative to chemotherapy as postremission treatment for AML. Many studies have demonstrated that relapse-free survival rates for patients receiving stem cell transplants from matched related donors are better than those for patients who receive only chemotherapy. Some studies have also shown an overall survival advantage associated with SCT; however, others have shown no such advantage, primarily because of transplant-related mortality. Therefore, considerable controversy exists regarding which patients should undergo SCT during first remission. Some investigators recommend allogeneic SCT during first remission for all patients who have a matched related donor, whereas others suggest that only intermediate-risk and high-risk patients should undergo SCT in first remission.

FUTURE DIRECTIONS

Gene expression profiling, the process in which the expression of thousands of genes in a particular cell type is analyzed, has the potential to predict relapse and the development of secondary cancers more accurately than do current methods. Therefore, gene expression profiling may allow the construction of more precise risk classification schemes and more specific tailoring of the intensity of therapy than is currently possible. More important, gene expression profiling may identify new targets against which novel and specific therapies may be developed.

Because cure rates for AML remain unacceptably low, novel therapies are urgently needed. Gemtuzumab ozogamicin (Mylotarg), an anti-CD33-calicheamicin conjugate designed to target AML blasts, has shown activity as a single agent and is now being tested in combination with conventional chemotherapeutic agents. Because abnormal methylation of tumor suppressor genes has been implicated in the pathogenesis of AML, demethylating agents are also being investigated for the treatment of AML. Similarly, histone deacetylase inhibitors have a profound impact on gene expression and may, alone or in combination with demethylating agents, retinoids, or conventional chemotherapy, play a role in the treatment of AML by relieving the differentiation block that characterizes the leukemic blast.

More promising, however, is the development therapies targeted to specific abnormalities in the leukemic cell. Imatinib mesylate (Gleevec), a selective inhibitor of the BCR-ABL tyrosine kinase, induces durable responses in patients with chronic-phase chronic myelogenous leukemia (CML). The inhibitor also has activity in accelerated-phase or blast-crisis CML, although the results are not as long-lived. Similarly, a phase II study demonstrated that imatinib induced complete bone marrow responses in about one third of patients with relapsed or refractory Philadelphia chromosome–positive ALL. Other kinase inhibitors under development include selective inhibitors of FLT3, which is mutated or overexpressed in subsets of ALL and AML. Like BCR-ABL in CML, FLT3 represents a specific and rational target for therapeutic intervention. In this regard, several FLT3 inhibitors have been developed. These agents selectively inhibit autophosphorylation of wild-type and mutant FLT3 in preclinical models, inhibit downstream targets of FLT3, induce apoptosis in cell lines and primary AML samples harboring FLT3 mutations, and have a therapeutic effect in mouse models of AML. In addition, these inhibitors may be able to overcome the differentiation block caused by FLT3 activation. It is our hope that these kinase inhibitors, which are now in phase I and II trials, will lead to less toxic and more effective cures.

ACKNOWLEDGMENTS

I thank Julia Cay Jones for expert editorial review. This work was supported by the Cancer Center Support Grant CA21765 from the National Cancer Institute and by the American Lebanese Syrian Associated Charities (ALSAC).

*Not FDA approved for this indication.

CHRONIC LEUKEMIAS

method of
TARIQ I. MUGHAL, M.D. and
JOHN M. GOLDMAN, D.M.
Department of Haematology
Hammersmith Hospital at Imperial College, London
London,
United Kingdom

CHRONIC MYELOID LEUKEMIA

Although chronic myeloid leukemia (CML) was the first human leukemia to be identified as a distinct entity almost 160 years ago, it was not until 1960 that the first important clue to its pathogenesis was recognized. It was discovered at that time that CML cells had a consistent cytogenetic abnormality—the Philadelphia (Ph) chromosome. Later the Ph chromosome was found to carry a *BCR-ABL* fusion gene, and the encoded oncoprotein is now considered to be the principal cause of the chronic phase (CP) of CML as a consequence of its enhanced tyrosine kinase activity. Until now, only allogeneic stem cell transplantation (SCT) using HLA-matched donors could induce long-lasting hematologic and cytogenetic remission for patients with CML. However, in the 1990s it was recognized that the kinase activity of the *Bcr-Abl* protein could be inhibited in a highly specific manner by a small molecule of the phenylaminopyrimidine family, now known as imatinib mesylate (Gleevec). This discovery proved to be a major landmark in the treatment of patients with CML in both the chronic and advanced phases, although patient follow-up is still short. Almost all chronic phase patients achieve hematologic remissions, and the incidence of complete cytogenetic remissions exceeds 50%. Other important therapeutic advances in the last 20 years were the introduction of interferon-alfa (IFN-α) in the early 1980s and the discovery that adoptive immunotherapy with donor-derived lymphocytes can restore complete remission for patients who relapse after allogeneic SCT.

CML accounts for about 15% of all adult leukemias, with an annual incidence of 1 to 1.5 per 100,000 of population and a median age of onset of 50 to 55 years. Currently the only definite predisposing factor is radiation as exemplified in survivors of Hiroshima and Nagasaki atomic bombs in 1945, though other agents, such as benzene, may possibly increase the risk of acquiring CML. The initial transforming event must occur at the level of a multipotential hematopoietic stem cell, which then proliferates to produce the clinical features of CML in CP (Figure 1). The leukemic clone has a tendency to undergo further "spontaneous" molecular changes that lead to so-called advanced phase disease. About half of the patients in the CP transform directly into "blastic transformation," whereas the remainder do so after an intermediate period of "accelerated" phase disease.

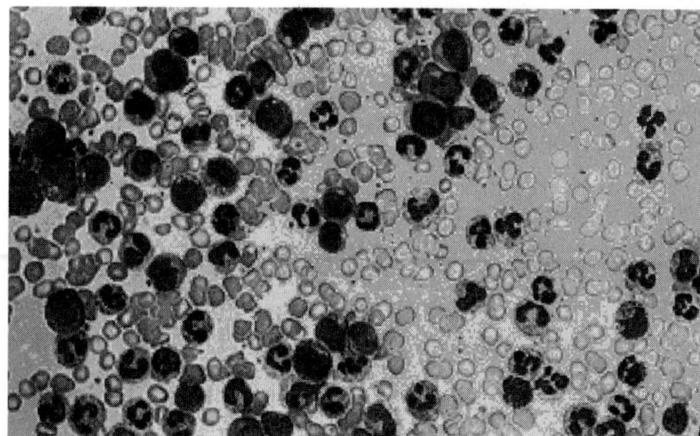

Figure 1. Peripheral blood film: CML in CP.

Molecular Pathogenesis

About 90% of CML patients have a Ph chromosome in all cells of the myeloid series and in some B lymphocytes. This acquired cytogenetic abnormality is the result of a reciprocal translocation of chromosomal material involving the long arm of one 9 chromosome and one 22 chromosome, referred to as t(9;22)(q34;q11) (Figure 2). The remaining 10% of patients with hematologically "acceptable" CML lack the Ph chromosome and are described as Ph negative CML. About half of such patients have a cytogenetically occult *BCR-ABL* gene and are referred to as Ph-negative, *BCR-ABL* positive cases; the remainder are *BCR-ABL* negative and some of these have mutations in the *RAS* gene.

The Bcr-Abl oncoprotein must play a central role in the pathogenesis of CML, though the precise mechanism is not known. It may act by constitutively activating mitogenic signaling, by reducing apoptosis, or by impairing adhesion of CML cells to the stroma and extracellular matrix. The deregulation of the ABL tyrosine kinase facilitates autophosphorylation, resulting in a marked increase of phosphotyrosine on Bcr-Abl itself, which creates binding sites for the SH2 domains of other proteins. A variety of such substrates, which can be tyrosine phosphorylated, have now been identified. Although much is known of the abnormal interactions between the Bcr-Abl oncoprotein and

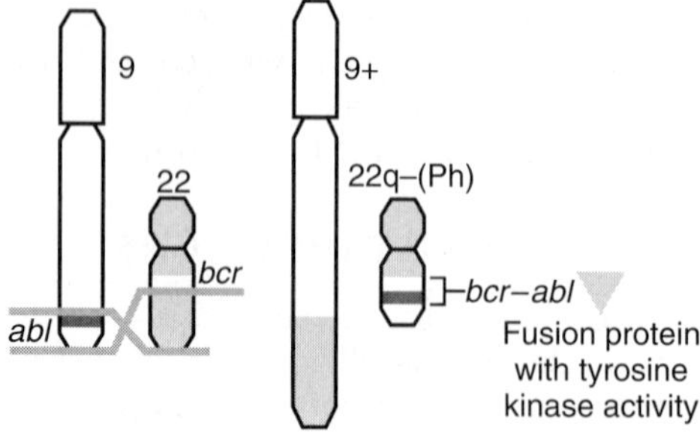

Figure 2. Ph chromosome.

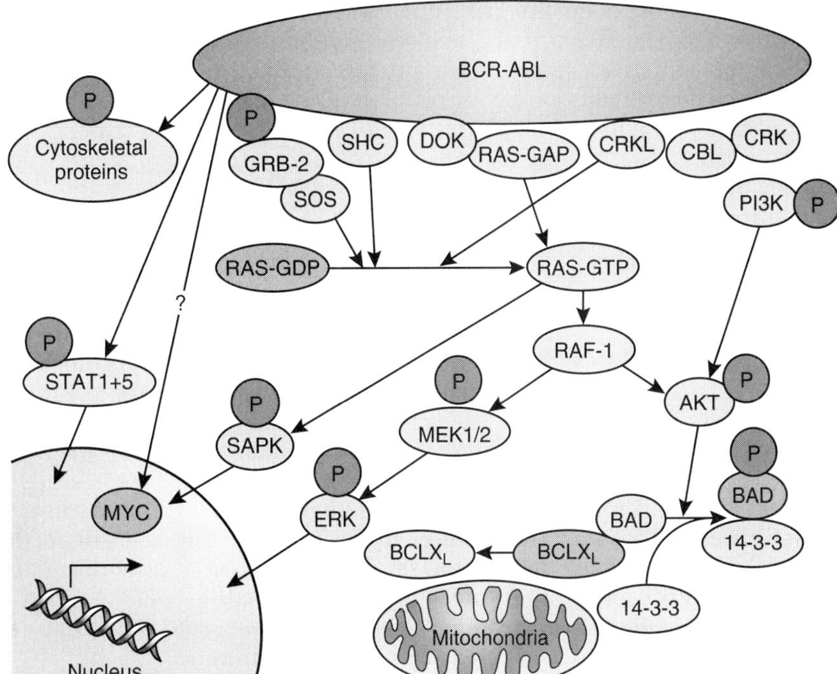

Figure 3. Molecular basis of *BCR-ABL*.

other cytoplasmic molecules, the precise details of the pathways through which the "rogue" proliferative signal is mediated, such as the RAS-MAP kinase, JAK-STAT, and PI3 kinase pathways, are incomplete and their respective contributions to the leukemic "phenotype" are still ill-defined. Much also remains to be learned about the role of the tyrosine phosphatases in the transformation process.

The genetic events resulting in the production of the Bcr-Abl oncoprotein can be summarized as follows. There are three separate DNA breakpoint locations in the *BCR* gene on chromosome 22 (Figure 3), but only the *major* breakpoint cluster region (M-BCR) is important in the genesis of CML. In CML the actual break in DNA occurs usually either in the intron between exon e13 and e14 or in the intron between exon e14 and e15 (toward the telomere). By contrast, the position of the breakpoint in the *ABL* gene on chromosome 9 is highly variable and may occur at almost any position upstream of exon a2. The Ph translocation results in the juxtaposition of 5′ sequences from the *BCR* gene with 3′ sequences from the *ABL* gene. This event results in the generation of the *BCR-ABL* fusion gene transcribed as an 8.5-kb mRNA, which encodes a protein of 210 kD ($p210^{BCR\text{-}ABL}$) that has much greater tyrosine kinase activity than its normal Abl counterpart. The different breakpoints in the M-BCR result in two slightly different chimeric *BCR-ABL* genes, which generate mRNA with e13a2 or e14a2 junctions. The type of *BCR-ABL* transcript has no prognostic significance.

At the cytokinetic level, the mechanism by which the Bcr-Abl oncoprotein results in the preferential proliferation and differentiation of myeloid progenitors is quite unclear. It is likely that normal myeloid progenitor cells are preferentially maintained in G_0 as a result of proliferation of leukemic cells, but conversely, there are also quiescent Ph-positive progenitor cells that can, under certain circumstances, be induced to proliferate.

Treatment Options for CML in Chronic Phase

A newly diagnosed patient whose disease is still in chronic phase may be faced with starkly contrasting approaches to initial therapy. It is now widely accepted that allogeneic SCT can, if successful, cure patients with CML, but only a minority of patients are eligible for this procedure and the risks of morbidity and mortality attributable to the transplant are still appreciable. Conversely conventional anti-CML drugs such as busulfan [Myleran], hydroxyurea [Hydrea], and IFN-α are palliative and do not entirely eradicate the CML even in patients with the most sensitive disease. Thus the patient who does have a possible SCT donor may have to decide soon after diagnosis whether or not to submit himself or herself to the risk of the transplant procedure. The patient may be helped to a certain degree by efforts made over the last 20 years to predict outcome with transplant and with nontransplant therapy.

Nontransplant Treatment Options

Criteria definable at diagnosis can help to predict prognosis for CML patients and thus assist in the clinical decision-making process. The index devised by Sokal and colleagues in 1984 on the basis of patient cohorts treated with busulfan divides patients into various risk categories based on a mathematical formula that takes into account the patient's age, spleen size, peripheral blood blast cell percentage, and platelet count at diagnosis. An updated version of this, known as the Hasford or Euro score, is based on survival of patients treated with interferon-alfa; it employs the factors considered by Sokal but adds assessment of basophil and eosinophil numbers. Future prognostic scoring systems may also take into account the presence or absence of small deletions on the derivative 9q+ chromosome, the rate of shortening of telomeres in the leukemia cell population, or the pattern of gene expression as assessed by micro-array technology.

IMATINIB MESYLATE

Imatinib mesylate (Gleevec), previously known as STI571, is a 2-phenylaminopyrimidine compound that occupies the kinase pocket of the Bcr-Abl oncoprotein and thus blocks access to ATP and prevents phosphorylation of any substrate. It entered clinical trials in 1998 for patients with CML refractory to or intolerant of IFN-α, and the preliminary results were impressive. It was then used as a single agent in a prospective multicenter study involving 1106 patients in which newly diagnosed chronic-phase patients were randomly allocated to receive imatinib or the combination of INF-α and cytarabine. Imatinib was given at a starting dose of 400 mg daily by mouth. A preliminary analysis at a median follow-up of 18 months showed that the incidence of hematologic responses was significantly higher with imatinib than with the two-drug combination (95% versus 56%). The incidence of complete cytogenetic responses was also significantly higher with imatinib than with the control combination (76% versus 15%). Progression-free survival was significantly better with the imatinib arm (97.7% versus 91.5%). In general the hematologic and cytogenetic responses occurred very much more rapidly than in comparable patients treated with the two-drug combination, but it is still too early to say whether imatinib confers an overall survival advantage in comparison with other agents, and if so, to what extent. The toxic effects so far were in most cases relatively minor and infrequent. Some patients developed significant cytopenias. Rashes, bone pains, and fluid retention were seen, but less than 2% of patients discontinued treatment because of imatinib-related side effects. Thus imatinib has effectively replaced other agents as initial treatment for patients who are not eligible for "up-front" allogeneic SCT.

BCR-ABL-positive cells can become resistant to imatinib as a result of various mechanisms, including (1) *BCR-ABL* overexpression that may be associated with *BCR-ABL* gene amplification, (2) P-glycoprotein overexpression resulting in reduced uptake or increased cellular elimination of imatinib, and/or (3) the selection in favor of cell populations containing Abl kinase domain point mutations that impair imatinib binding but allow ATP to continue to act as phosphate donor. There must also be other mechanisms by which a cell can overcome imatinib effects.

IFN-α

Until the recent introduction of imatinib, the standard treatment for patients with CML in CP was IFN-α either alone or in combination with cytarabine. IFN-α largely replaced hydroxyurea and busulfan in the 1980s. The agent is usually administered by subcutaneous injection at daily doses ranging from 3 to 5 MU/m^2. IFN-α offers a survival advantage that is maximal for those achieving a cytogenetic remission, compared with hydroxyurea. Toxicity is quite common, but in general quite mild and reversible. Most patients suffer from flulike symptoms, lethargy, and weight loss that lasts 1 to 3 weeks after starting treatment; these usually subside spontaneously. Less common but more troublesome side effects include anorexia, weight loss, depression, alopecia, and immune-mediated complications, such as thrombocytopenia and hypothyroidism. In one French study published in the late 1990s, the addition of cytarabine to IFN-α appeared to offer superior survival compared with IFN-α alone. A more recent study from Italy did not confirm this result. A long-acting form of IFN-α—pegylated IFN-α—has been introduced to reduce the toxicity of the unpegylated form and retain its efficacy.

HYDROXYUREA

Hydroxyurea (Hydrea), an inhibitor of RNA reductase, became gradually more popular for the management of CML in the chronic phase when the toxicity of busulfan came to be recognized in the 1980s. The drug is usually given by mouth at a daily dose 1.0 to 2.0 gm typically 1.5 gm. In newly diagnosed patients hydroxyurea usually restores spleen size and blood counts to normal within 4 to 8 weeks. Treatment may then be maintained for many years. Toxic effects are rare but include mouth ulcers, rashes, leg ulceration, and various nonspecific gastrointestinal disturbances. These are all reversible on reducing or stopping the drug. The drug remains valuable today for rapid cytoreduction in the newly diagnosed patient but should be replaced as soon as convenient by use of interferon-alfa or imatinib or by an allogeneic SCT if appropriate.

BUSULFAN

Busulfan (Myleran), a modified alkylating agent, was the mainstay of treatment for CML between 1960 and 1980. It was usually given as a single agent at a daily dose of 2–4 mg by mouth. Side effects included marrow aplasia, skin pigmentation, irreversible gonadal failure, and, rarely, a progressive pulmonary fibrosis referred to as busulfan lung. The drug is still used on occasion in older patients who cannot tolerate hydroxyurea or interferon-alfa.

Stem Cell Transplantation

Allogeneic SCT using blood- or marrow-derived hematopoietic stem cells performed in the CP can eradicate all evidence of leukemia (and thus presumably cure) selected patients with CML. This cure depends on the contribution of a "graft-versus-leukemia" (GvL) effect mediated by T-lymphocytes. Current experience suggests a probability of event-free survival (EFS) at 5 years of 60% to 70% for patients transplanted in CP using an HLA-identical sibling donor; the corresponding figure for patients transplanted with cells from matched unrelated donors is 45% to 55%. There is still an appreciable risk of morbidity and mortality principally because of graft-versus-host disease (GvHD) and opportunistic infection, in particular that resulting from cytomegalovirus (CMV). The major factors determining the outcome for a given transplant procedure are patient age, disease phase, disease duration, patient-donor histocompatibility, and patient-donor gender combination. Using these five factors a system has been devised to predict the probability of survival after allo-SCT in a given clinical situation. Thus, ascribing a score of 0, 1, or 2 to each of five principal factors one can derive at a total score that, to a large extent, correlates inversely with the probability of survival at 5 years posttransplant. For example, survival appears to be best for patients younger than 40 years of age who are still in chronic phase and are transplanted within 1 year of diagnosis with stem cells from a male sibling. For such a cohort, the 5-year EFS is probably 70% to 80% and the relapse rate 10% to 20%.

It is probable that the precise details of the transplant procedure including the choice of stem cell source (i.e., marrow vs. peripheral blood) also influence the outcome. After a peripheral blood SCT the patients achieve more rapid engraftment but there may be a slight excess of chronic GvHD, perhaps because of the increased T-cell numbers in the peripheral blood compared with bone marrow. It has been suggested that prior treatment with IFN-α might increase the risk of treatment related mortality (TRM) after allo-SCT, but recent data show that stopping the drug 3 months or longer before the transplant eliminates any possible added risk. It is not known if prior use of imatinib affects a subsequent transplant.

A number of groups have tried to minimize the toxicity of conditioning regimens to make SCT more available to higher risk and perhaps older patients. Such procedures are termed "reduced intensity conditioning," "nonmyeloablative" SCTs or "mini-SCTs." The conditioning includes very little or no radiotherapy and is based on the use of purine analogues, notably fludarabine, which are potent immunosuppressive agents. Myeloid engraftment is facilitated by use of relatively large numbers of blood derived CD34+ cells. The antileukemic effects of these reduced-intensity conditioning regimens depend on the GvL effect mediated by donor-derived lymphocytes. Some CML patients are able to achieve sustainable molecular remissions with this procedure. For those patients who fail to achieve remission or relapse posttransplant after initial benefit, cytogenetic or molecular remission can be induced by the transfusion of donor lymphocytes.

Autologous SCT has been tested in nonrandomized trials over the past two decades. Originally the procedure involved use of peripheral blood stem cells collected at diagnosis and stored until required; more recently, Ph-negative progenitor cells were "mobilized" into the peripheral blood by use of high dose chemotherapy and G-CSF, which were collected by use of the cell separator. The technique can induce long periods of Ph-negative hematopoiesis but does not cure. It may have a useful palliative role for selected patients with advanced phase CML.

Treatment Options for CML in Advanced Phase

It is difficult to make precise recommendations for management of advanced phase disease but some general principles can be suggested.

Accelerated Phase Disease

It may be possible to control or reverse the features of accelerated phase (AP) disease by altering the dosage of cytotoxic drugs employed or by adding a drug, such as hydroxyurea, to which the patient has not previously been exposed. Imatinib has shown impressive activity in AP and may be valuable as a single agent or combined with other drugs such as cytarabine, doxorubicin (Adriamycin), or homoharringtonine. Patients whose symptoms are due predominantly to splenomegaly resistant to standard anti-CML agents may benefit from splenectomy; this applies particularly if they are thrombocytopenic before surgery. Allogeneic SCT should be reconsidered for the younger patient, although it may have been ruled out while he or she was in the chronic phase. Autografting is a reasonable option as palliation but does not definitely prolong life.

Blastic Transformation

It has, recently, been usual to classify the blastic transformation as myeloid or lymphoid by immunophenotyping and then to start treatment with combination chemotherapy appropriate to acute myeloid or to adult acute lymphoblastic leukemia, respectively. Remission of the acute phase with restoration of CP hematopoiesis can be obtained in 10% to 30% of cases, but the majority of patients obtain little benefit from this approach. Patients who respond well to treatment for lymphoid transformation should, however, be offered neuroprophylaxis because neuroleukemia as the first sign of relapse is otherwise not uncommon. The approach to managing patients in blastic transformation has changed somewhat since the introduction of imatinib. This agent is able to control the disease for a finite period in the majority of cases and it is reasonable therefore to start treatment for blastic disease with imatinib at a dose of 600, or better 800 mg, daily. The overall treatment strategy should however incorporate use of standard cytotoxic drugs. Patients who respond well to the sequence of imatinib followed by other cytotoxic drugs should be considered for allogeneic SCT.

CHRONIC LYMPHOCYTIC LEUKEMIA

Chronic lymphocytic leukemia (CLL) consists of a monoclonal expansion of mature, long-lived, functionally deficient B-lymphocytes that express high levels of two anti-apoptotic proteins, BCL-2 and BCL-$_{XD}$, and low levels of the pro-apoptotic protein BAX and are therefore resistant to apoptosis. Rarely it can also affect

T-lymphocytes. CLL is the most common type of leukemia in the Western world, accounting for more than 30% of all leukemias and has a median age of occurrence of 60 years. It is more prevalent in males, with a male:female ratio of 2:1. There are no known risk factors for CLL, though one study has observed a slight increase in CLL among persons chronically exposed to electromagnetic fields. Recently there was also speculation that CLL might be causally linked to infection by HTLV-1, based upon a small Jamaican study, but this remains unconfirmed. A second related retrovirus, HTLV-2, has been identified in some cases of related disorders, the T-cell prolymphocytic leukemia (PLL) and T-cell hairy cell leukemia.

Clinically, about 40% to 50% of all patients with CLL have no symptoms when diagnosed. Most come to medical attention after a blood test for unrelated reasons. The remainder present with fever, weight loss, lymphadenopathy, hepatosplenomegaly, and infections—particularly opportunistic infections.

Molecular and Diagnostic Features

The characterization of CLL is based on cell morpholoy and immunologic markers as proposed by the French-American-British group. Immunophenotyping is useful in distinguishing B- from T-cell disorders and from a variety of the related lymphoproliferative disorders such as hairy cell leukemia, PLL, lymphoplasmacytoid lymphomas, and the leukemic phase of follicular non-Hodgkin's lymphoma. Current guidelines for the minimum diagnostic criteria for CLL are: a blood lymphocytosis (absolute lymphocyte count of at least $5000/mm^3$) with mature appearing lymphocytes and a characteristic immunophenotype of monoclonal B cells. This is described as: Surface immunoglobulin (most often IgM or IgM and IgD) of low intensity with either κ or λ light chain, expression of pan-B cell antigens (CD19, CD20, and CD23), and the co-expression of CD5 on the leukemic B cell. CLL cells are typically negative for surface CD22 and FMC7. Most cells are in the G_0 phase of the cell cycle and are unresponsive to standard mitogenic stimuli.

Cytogenetic abnormalities occur in about 50% of all patients, with trisomy 12 and 13q14 deletions being the most frequent. Molecular evidence of a minimal region of deletion (MRD) spanning <300 kb and common to all CLL cell lines with 13q14 deletions has been identified, suggesting that the abnormalities at 13q14 may represent a common event in the pathogenesis of CLL. Immunoglobulin genes appear to play an important prognostic roll in CLL. For example, it has been observed that patients with unmutated V genes (both V_H and V_L) display higher percentages of $CD34^+$ cells compared with those with mutated V genes and were more likely to have trisomy 12, advanced stage, and a significantly poorer survival. Moreover, the patients with unmutated V genes expressed a higher level of the surface protein ZAP-70, which is therefore an additional marker of poor prognosis. Very recently it was confirmed that $CD34^+$ expression and immunoglobulin variable-region mutations are independent prognostic variables in CLL, but $CD34^+$ expression may vary during the course of the disease.

Treatment

Some patients with CLL have an indolent disease and may not require any specific therapy because this would not prolong survival, though more than 50% of all early stage patients with CLL eventually progress and require treatment. Treatment should also be offered when patients become symptomatic, even though they may still have early stage disease. There are a number of well-recognized prognostic factors in CLL, principally the rate of doubling of the lymphocyte counts in less than 12 months, a diffuse pattern of involvement on the trephine biopsy, and an abnormal karyotype. To these have recently been added the poor prognosis associated with the presence in the leukemia cell of the unmutated V genes and overexpression of CD38. Currently there are two well-defined staging systems: the Rai staging system, which is based on Dameshek's proposed model of orderly disease progression in CLL and consists of five stages, and the Binet staging system (also known as the international staging system), which comprises three stages. Both systems are shown in Table 1. The Rai system has recently been revised to include three stages: low risk (Rai 0-1), intermediate risk (Rai 2), and high risk (3–4). In contrast to CML, both allogeneic and autologous SCT procedures remain under investigation at present.

Nontransplant Options

Chlorambucil (Leukeran), either alone or with a glucocorticoid steroid, usually prednisolone, has been the most frequently used first-line drug in the treatment of CLL for almost four decades and remains the first-line treatment in many countries today. Cyclophosphamide orally is an equivalent drug. For patients presenting with more advanced disease, combination chemotherapy is used. The most common regimens are cyclophosphamide (Cytoxan), vincristine (Oncovin), and prednisolone; sometimes an anthracycline is also added. Although these latter regimens have resulted in higher responses, there are no major durable responses or survival advantages compared with chlorambucil.

TABLE 1. **Rai and Binet Staging Systems for Chronic Lymphocytic Leukemia**

Stage	Description
Rai staging system	
0	Lymphocytosis
1	Lymphocytosis and lymphadenopathy
2	Lymphocytosis and splenomegaly or hepatomegaly
3	Lymphocytosis and anemia (hemoglobin <11 g/dL)
4	Lymphocytosis and thrombocytopenia (platelets <100,000/μL)
Binet staging system	
A	Two or fewer lymphoid-bearing areas
B	Three or more lymphoid-bearing areas
C	Presence of anemia (hemoglobin <10 g/dL) or thrombocytopenia (platelets <100,000/μL)

Fludarabine (Fludara), (9-β-D arabinofuranosyl 2-fluroadenine monophosphate) is a purine analogue, which is very effective treatment for CLL patients resistant to chorambucil. The drug is generally myelosuppressive and may be associated with an increased risk of viral infections. A randomized trial in the United States comparing fludarabine with chorambucil in newly diagnosed patients with CLL confirmed a higher incidence of CR (27% vs. 3%) overall responses (70% vs. 43%), and duration of these responses (2.75 years vs. 1.4 years) in the fludarabine-treated cohorts, but no evidence of prolongation of survival. A smaller French randomized study of fludarabine versus CAP (cyclophosphamide, adriamycin, and prednisolone) revealed similar findings. Currently most specialists use fludarabine for second-line therapy of CLL patients. Other new drugs that have now entered the clinics include cladribine (Leustatin) (2′-chlorodeoxyadenosine) and pentostatin (Nipent) (5′-deoxycoformycin).

Other investigational therapies include the use of monoclonal antibodies, in particular Campath-1H, an immune antibody against CD52 and the heavy and light chain constant regions of human IgG1 and kappa, respectively. Preliminary results from several small phase I/II studies have demonstrated its effectiveness as salvage therapy in about one third of patients who relapsed after an initial response with fludarabine. Some of the current studies are also assessing the role of Campath-1H as a first-line therapy compared with chorambucil. Combination therapy of fludarabine, Campath-1H, and rituximab (Rituxan) (mabthera) is also being considered as potential investigational second-line treatment based on small pilot studies. Campath-1H is also being investigated as an in vivo purging agent in patients being considered for autologous SCT. Gene transfer of CD40-ligand has been shown to induce autologous immune recognition of CLL cells and is being developed further for the treatment of CLL.

Transplant Options

Preliminary results with allogeneic and autologous SCT for the treatment of advanced stage CLL in young adults demonstrate high response rates with durable CR. Long-term follow-up using PCR amplification and sequencing of the rearranged IgH from the original malignant clone show that most of the patients remain disease-free and free of PCR-detected MRD, suggesting that this treatment may offer the chance of cure to selected patients with poor-risk CLL. Recent results collated by the European and international registries confirm the applicability of SCT, both allogeneic and autologous for the treatment of patients with Rai poor-risk CLL who are younger than age 50 years. The 5-year EFS for the patients who were allografted was 34% and for those who were autografted was 28%. The risk of relapse for the allografted group was 40%, and 70% for the autografted group. These preliminary experiences are encouraging and further studies are in progress. The recognition of GvL effect in allogeneic SCT in patients with CML has also led to the nonmyeloablative allogeneic SCT being explored in suitable patients with CLL. Some patients appear to have achieved hematologic remissions but the longer term results have not been assessed.

Disorders Related to CLL

T-Cell Chronic Lymphocytic Leukemia

Although T-CLL is a rare disease in the Western countries, its prevalence in Asian countries is quite high. Morphologic and immunophenotyping studies suggest this disease to be a subtype of the prolymphocytic leukemias. Patients often present with pancytopenia and prominent splenomegaly, and the lack of lymphadenopathy is noteworthy. The general prognosis is similar to poor-risk CLL and most patients tend to be refractory to fludarabine treatment.

Prolymphocytic Leukemia

PLL can be *de novo* or arise as a consequence of CLL transformation. PLL cells are larger and less homogeneous than CLL cells, and have a clear and more abundant cytoplasm, clumped nuclear chromatin, and a single prominent nucleolus. The immunophenotype of a PLL cell is FMC7+, CD22+ and surface IgM+. Cytogenetic analysis often reveals 14q+ and t(11;14)(q13;q32). Most patients have a clinical course similar to poor-risk CLL and respond to fludarabine. A minority of patients has an indolent course.

Large Granular Lymphocytic Leukemia

Large granular lymphocytes (LGL) are a heterogeneous group of large lymphocytes, which express CD8 and CD56 (previously known as natural killer or NK) surface antigens and are associated with antibody-dependent cell-mediated cytotoxicity. LGL leukemia, also described as Tγ lymphoproliferative disorder, has a varied natural history, ranging from an indolent condition to one reminiscent of ALL. Most patients present with recurrent infections, anemia, and splenomegaly; significant lymphadenopathy is unusual.

The majority of patients with LGL leukemia do not require any specific treatment at presentation, and various strategies have been offered on an ad hoc basis, including prednisolone,* cyclophosphamide (low dose), IFN-α, splenectomy, and intensive chemotherapy for the more aggressive forms. The factors associated with poor prognosis are fever, low CD56 expression, and LGL counts.

Hairy Cell Leukemia

Hairy cell leukemia (HCL) is a mature B-lymphoproliferative disorder characterized by distinct clinical, morphologic, and histologic features. It is characterized by splenomegaly and marrow failure in conjunction with infiltration of myeloid tissues by a lymphoid cell with villous processes that project from the cytoplasm of the cell. Immunophenotyping is useful to distinguish HCL from B-cell disorders with hairy or villous lymphocytes, such as the variant form

*Not FDA approved for this indication.

of HCL or splenic lymphoma with villous lymphocytes (SLVL). Typically HCL cells express the following markers: CD11c, CD25, HC2, and B-ly-7. A scoring system based on these four markers was introduced recently to facilitate a more accurate diagnosis of HCL.

The identification and precise diagnosis of these disorders is important because of the prognostic and therapeutic implications. Whereas patients with typical HCL (Catovsky Score 4) respond to IFN-α and 5′-deoxycoformycin (pentostatin), these drugs are less useful in the variant form of HCL and splenectomy is the treatment of choice for SLVL.

Adult T-Cell Leukemia/Lymphoma

Adult T-cell leukemia/lymphoma (ATL) is a distinct form of leukemia/lymphoma first described on the island of Kyushu in south Japan and subsequently found to occur in the Caribbean, United States, and other countries. Epidemiologic studies have described the causal association between ATL and HTLV-1. The disease appears in people at a median age of 40 years. ATL cells typically have the phenotype of mature helper T cells and express CD2, CD3, and CD4 antigen. They also express CD25 and clonal rearrangement of the T-cell receptor β chain is often present. Cytogenetic abnormalities are common and include trisomy 3q or 6q, 14q, and inv 14.

ATL is characterized by lymphadenopathy and hepatosplenomegaly. There is a high incidence of cutaneous involvement, which may take a variety of forms. Lytic bone lesions and hypercalcemia occur commonly. Standard therapy is similar to that employed in the management of poor-prognosis high-grade lymphoma, but the outcome is generally unsatisfactory. Allogeneic SCT could be contemplated if a suitable donor is available.

NON-HODGKIN'S LYMPHOMA

method of
AUAYPORN NADEMANEE, M.D.
City of Hope National Medical Center
Division of Hematology and
Bone Marrow Transplantation
Duarte, California

The incidence of non-Hodgkin's lymphoma (NHL) has been rising and currently NHL accounts for almost 5% of all cancers occurring in the United States, with 53,900 new cases expected in the year 2002, including 28,200 in men and 25,700 in women. NHL consists of a group of heterogeneous lymphoproliferative malignancies with varied clinical behaviors and underlying biology. The etiologies of most NHLs continue to be poorly understood. Unlike Hodgkin's disease, the age-incidence curve in NHL increases exponentially with NHL being relatively rare before the age of 10 years, and increases very gradually through age 25 years, then the rates begin to rise more steeply, with the sharpest increases occurring after age 55 years.

RISK FACTORS FOR NHL

Immune dysfunction, congenital or acquired, is a well-described condition associated with NHL, and the incidence of NHL is elevated among persons with severe immune deficiencies. Recipients of organ transplant have a 2- to 15-fold increased risk of NHL. The increased risk of NHL in human immunodeficiency virus 1 (HIV)-infected persons is well-documented and the risk increases in parallel with length of survival among persons with HIV. The incidence of NHL is also twofold increased among persons with autoimmune disorders, including rheumatoid arthritis and Sjögren's syndrome.

Several oncogenic viruses have been linked to the occurrence of NHL. Epstein-Barr virus was found in a variety of subtypes of NHL, but more commonly in T-cell subtypes and more frequently with higher grade NHL. Molecular and epidemiologic studies have confirmed that human T-cell lymphotropic virus type 1 (HTLV-1) is the infectious agent associated with adult T-cell lymphoma (ATL). Human herpesvirus 8 has been found consistently in pleural effusion lymphomas or body cavity–based lymphoma in HIV patients. A number of studies conducted in Italy and Japan have suggested an association of hepatitis C virus (HCV) and NHL. However, studies performed in Northern Europe and North America, where HCV is less prevalent than in Southern Europe and Asia, have not found excessive HCV infection among persons with NHL.

A number of chemical exposures have been weakly associated with an increased risk of NHL in epidemiology studies: solvents, pesticides, herbicides, fuels and oils, and dusts. Farming/agriculture is one of the few occupations that is consistently associated with a mildly increased risk for NHL. In one meta-analysis study, a 30% increase in risk of NHL was reported among farmers in the United States.

Classification of NHL

The classification of NHL has been modified several times over the last four decades and has been a source of confusion and frustration for clinicians. Rappaport's classification subdivided the NHL based on the morphology of lymphoma cell growth pattern and its clinical importance. In the 1970s, it became apparent that NHLs were tumors of the immune system and were derived from B or T lymphocytes. This led to the classification of Lukes and Collins and Lennert and colleagues (Kiel Classification). The Working Formulation was proposed in 1982 in an attempt to unify the complex and confusing lymphoma terminology and improve communication between pathologists and clinicians. With an increase in knowledge of the biology of immune system and the introduction of the new techniques for immunophenotyping and molecular genetic analysis, many new disease entities of NHL were described in the 1980s and 1990s that were not included in the previous classification. In 1994, the International Lymphomas Study Group recognized the existence of

TABLE 1. **WHO/REAL Classification of Non-Hodgkin's Lymphoma**

B-Cell Neoplasms

Precursor B-Cell Neoplasm

Precursor B-lymphoblastic leukemia/lymphoma (precursor B-acute lymphoblastic leukemia)

Mature (Peripheral) B-Neoplasms

B-cell chronic lymphocytic leukemia/small lymphocytic lymphoma
B-cell prolymphocytic leukemia
Lymphoplasmacytic lymphoma*
Splenic marginal zone B-cell lymphoma (± villous lymphocytes)†
Hairy cell leukemia
Plasma cell myeloma/plasmacytoma
Extranodal marginal zone B-cell lymphoma of MALT type
Nodal marginal zone B-cell lymphoma (± monocytoid B cells)†
Follicular lymphoma
Mantle cell lymphoma
Diffuse large B-cell lymphoma
  Mediastinal large B-cell lymphoma
  Primary effusion lymphoma‡
Burkitt's lymphoma/Burkitt cell leukemia§

T and NK-Cell Neoplasms

Precursor T-Cell Neoplasm

Precursor T-lymphoblastic leukemia/lymphoma (precursor T-acute lymphoblastic leukemia)

Mature (Peripheral) T Neoplasms

T-cell chronic lymphocytic leukemia/small lymphocytic lymphoma
T-cell prolymphocytic leukemia
T-cell granular lymphocytic leukemia¶
Aggressive NK leukemia¶
Adult T-cell lymphoma/leukemia (HTLV-1+)
Extranodal NK/T-cell lymphoma, nasal type¶
Enteropathy-like T-cell lymphoma**
Hepatosplenic γδ T-cell lymphoma†
Subcutaneous panniculitis-like T-cell lymphoma†
Mycosis fungoides/Sézary syndrome
Anaplastic large cell lymphoma, T/null cell, primary cutaneous type
Peripheral T-cell lymphoma, not otherwise characterized
Angioimmunoblastic T-cell lymphoma
Anaplastic large cell lymphoma, T/null cell, primary systemic type

*Formerly known as lymphoplasmacytoid lymphoma or immunocytoma.
†Provisional entities in the REAL classification.
‡Not described in REAL classification.
§Includes the so-called Burkitt-like lymphomas.
¶Entities formally grouped under the heading large granular lymphocyte leukemia of T- and NK-cell types.
¶Formerly known as angiocentric lymphoma.
**Formerly known as intestinal T-cell lymphoma.

these new entities and proposed a new classification called the "Revised European-American Classification of Lymphoid Neoplasms" (REAL). By combining morphologic, immunophenotypic, cytogenetic, molecular biologic features and clinical features, REAL classification proposed 34 biologically well-defined lymphoma entities (Table 1). Recently, this REAL classification has been modestly revised to take an even more global stature as the World Health Organization (WHO) classification (see Table 1).

Chromosome Abnormalities in NHL

With continued improvement in techniques of molecular diagnosis, it is becoming increasingly clear that most NHLs exhibit distinct nonrandom chromosomal abnormalities that are associated closely with morphologically and clinically distinct subtypes of NHL. Chromosomal aberrations in NHL include translocation and, less frequently, deletions and mutations. The major chromosomal abnormalities in NHL are shown in Table 2.

Staging of NHL

After diagnosis of NHL is made, a variety of tests are performed to identify all sites of known disease and determine prognosis based on known clinical risk factors. The staging of NHL has become more accurate and more complicated with the advent of noninvasive studies and availability of more sophisticated tools such as positron emission tomography. In addition, certain presentations of NHL require specific testing, such as lumbar puncture, to rule out central nervous system involvement in patients with lymphoblastic lymphoma or those who present with testicular involvement. The goal of staging is to define the extent of the disease, which will help clinicians in making decisions about treatment and in defining the prognosis. However, in certain NHLs, stage may be less important than the measures of tumor burden such as bulky mass or elevated serum lactate dehydrogenase (LDH). The true benefit of thorough staging is to permit a comparison of results from various treatment studies and to allow for uniform treatment plan and study groups. The diagnostic tests used for staging of NHL are listed in Table 3.

TABLE 2. **Chromosomal Abnormalities in Non-Hodgkin's Lymphoma**

Abnormality	Oncogene	Disease	Percentage of Cases Positive
t(11;14)(q13;q32)	*Bcl*-1	Mantle cell NHL	>95
t(14;18)	*Bcl*-2	Follicular NHL	80–90
		DLCL	35
3 q27	*Bcl*-6	DLCL	40
15 q11-13	*Bcl*-8	DLCL	4
1 q21	*Bcl*-9	Marginal zone NHL	40
t(1;14)(p22; q32)	*Bcl*-10	MALT	5–7
t(9;14)(p13;q32)	PAX5	Lymphoplasmacytoid NHL	50
t(8;14)(q24;q32)	C-*myc*	Burkitt NHL	100
t(2;5)(p23;q35)	ALK	Anaplastic large cell NHL	40–60

NHL, non-Hodgkin's lymphoma; DLCL, diffuse large cell lymphoma; MALT, mucosa-associated lymphoid tissue; ALK, anaplastic lymphoma kinase.

TABLE 3. **Ann Arbor Staging System**

Stage	Area of Involvement
I	Single lymph node group
II	Multiple lymph node groups on same side of diaphragm
III	Multiple lymph node groups on both sides of diaphragm
IV	Multiple extranodal sites or lymph nodes and extranodal disease
X	Bulk >10 cm
E	Extranodal extension or single isolated site of extranodal disease
A/B	B symptoms: weight loss >10%, fever, drenching night sweats

From Lister TA, Crowther D, Sutcliffe SB, et al: Report of a committee convened to discuss the evaluation and staging of patients with Hodgkin's disease: Cotswolds meeting. J Clin Oncol 7:1630-1636, 1989.

The Ann Arbor staging system (Table 4), originally designed to assess anatomic spread of Hodgkin's disease, remains the most widely used staging system for NHL despite its deficiencies. This system defined the distribution of lymphatic involvement and therefore may not be applicable in some NHLs in which dissemination may be noncontiguous and more hematogenous than lymphatic. In addition, the bulky disease and kinetics of disease are not addressed. Furthermore, Ann Arbor staging is of little use in lymphoblastic lymphoma or Burkitt's lymphoma. Nevertheless, advanced stage III/IV correlates with a worse outcome than is seen with more limited stages of disease.

Treatment

The treatment of NHL is evolving with the addition of new therapeutic agents, monoclonal antibodies, and innovative therapy such as radioimmunotherapy in the armamentarium. Only treatment of certain NHLs will be discussed here.

TREATMENT OF DIFFUSE LARGE CELL LYMPHOMA

Localized Stage Diffuse Large Cell Lymphoma

Localized disease is commonly used in reference to stage I or II (IE or IIE, when present with extralymphatic organ involvement). Radiation therapy alone provides initial disease control but with a very high risk of relapse resulting in a 5-year disease-free survival (DFS) of only 35%, therefore it is not recommended. Combined modality approach with anthracycline-based combination chemotherapy and involved-field radiation (IFRT) has emerged to be treatment of choice in most localized diffuse large cell lymphoma (DLCL). Two randomized studies have demonstrated the superiority of combination chemotherapy of CHOP (cyclophosphamide [Cytoxan], doxorubicin [Adriamycin RFG],* vincristine [Vincasar

*Not FDA approved for this indication.

TABLE 4. **Staging Workup for NHL**

Diagnosis

Essential:

Hematopathology review of all slides with at least one paraffin block representative of the tumor.
Rebiopsy if consult material is nondiagnostic
Adequate immunophenotyping to establish diagnosis*
- Paraffin panel: CD45 (LCA), CD20 (L26/Pan B), CD3, CD5, CD10, bcl-2; cyclin D1; (optional kappa/lambda)
- Cell surface marker analysis by flow cytometry: kappa/lambda, CD45, CD3, CD5, CD19, CD10, TdT, CD14, CD13, CD33, CD20, CD23, CD43

Useful Under Certain Circumstances:

Additional immunohistochemical studies to establish lymphoma subtype
- DLBCL:
- CD10, bcl-6, bcl-2, MIB1

Molecular genetic analysis to detect antigen receptor and oncogene rearrangements; bcl-2, bcl-1, c-myc rearrangements
Cytogenetics

Workup

Essential:

Physical exam: attention to node-bearing areas, including Waldeyer ring, and to size of liver and spleen
Performance status
B symptoms
CBC, differential, platelets
LDH
BUN/creatinine
Albumin, aspartate transaminase, bilirubin, alkaline phosphatase
Serum calcium, uric acid
Chest radiograph, PA and LAT
Chest/abdominopelvic CT scan
Unilateral or bilateral bone marrow biopsy ± aspiration
Calculation of International Prognostic Index (IPI)
MUGA scan
Beta-2-microglobulin

Useful in Selected Cases:

Gallium-67 scan (planar and SPECT) double dose with delayed images or PET scan
Neck CT
Head CT or MRI
Pregnancy test
Stool guaiac, if anemic
HIV
Lumbar puncture, if paranasal sinus, testicular, parameningeal, orbit, CNS, paravertebral, or HIV lymphoma, or high-grade NHL

CBC, complete blood count; LDH, lactate dehydrogenase; PA, posterior-anterior; LAT, lateral; CT, computed tomography; MUGA, multiple gated acquisition; SPECT, single photon emission computed tomography; PET, positron emission tomography; MRI, magnetic resonance imaging; HIV, human immunodeficiency virus; CNS, central nervous system; NHL, non-Hodgkin's lymphoma.

PFS], and prednisone*) plus IFRT over CHOP alone in the treatment of stage I and II DLCL. In the Southwestern Oncology Group (SWOG) trial, patients with non-bulky stage I or II DLCL were randomized to three cycles of CHOP followed by IFRT or to eight cycles of CHOP alone. In the Eastern Cooperative Oncology Group trial, patients were randomized to eight cycles of CHOP with or without IFRT. Based on these results, patients with non-bulky localized disease have an extremely good prognosis and may be treated with three to four cycles of CHOP combined

*Not FDA approved for this indication.

with IFRT. Patients who present with bulky disease or local extranodal disease may be more effectively treated with a full six to eight cycles of CHOP and IFRT.

Advanced Stage DLCL

Several combination chemotherapy regimens for treatment of DLCL have been developed. The first-generation chemotherapy regimen, CHOP, has been shown to produce complete remission (CR) rates of 45% to 53% with 30% to 37% long-term survivors. In an attempt to improve the response rate and survival, second- and third-generation combination chemotherapy regimens were developed based on the concept of dose intensity and alternate drug schedule to prevent drug resistance. These regimens were designed to deliver six to eight active anti-lymphoma drugs at the highest possible drug dose per unit time. All of the phase II trials had shown that these regimens were at least 20% to 30% better than CHOP. However, in a randomized setting, all of these therapies were equivalent. Fisher and others reported the results of SWOG intergroup study, which compared CHOP with the second- and third-generation chemotherapy regimens. After more than 6 years, there was no difference in PFS and overall survival (OS) between CHOP and the newer regimens but fewer patients died from toxicity in the CHOP arm. Thus CHOP has remained to be the current standard chemotherapy for advanced stage DLCL.

With the introduction of anti-CD20 monoclonal antibody, IDEC-C2B8 (rituximab, [Rituxan], IDEC Pharmaceuticals, CA), treatment of advanced stage B-Cell DLCL is evolving. When rituximab was given as single agent in DLCL patients, an overall response rate of 37% was reported by Coiffier and colleagues. Given the low toxicity associated with rituximab and the different mechanism of action, rituximab has been added to CHOP in phase II studies for B-cell DLCL. The combination was well-tolerated without increased toxicity, other than symptoms during rituximab infusion, and the response rates were high. This has led to phase III randomized trials comparing CHOP and CHOP plus rituximab in advanced stage DLCL. The first and important landmark study was reported recently by Coiffier and others for the Group d'Etude des Lymphomes de l'Adulte (GELA). In this study, 399 newly diagnosed, stage II-IV, DLCL patients aged 60–80 years who were randomized to receive eight cycles of CHOP every 3 weeks or eight cycles of R-CHOP (CHOP combined with rituximab 375 mg/m^2 the same day). The R-CHOP arm was clearly superior, with a CR rate of 76% compared with 62% for CHOP. Twenty-two percent of patients in the CHOP arm progressed during treatment compared with 10% in the R-CHOP arm, and the relapse rate was also significantly higher in CHOP arm (23% versus 13%). In addition, R-CHOP improves OS and event-free survival for patients with either low or high age-adjusted IPI (Table 5). Therefore, based on the GELA trial, R-CHOP has become the standard of care for elderly patients with advanced stage B-cell DLCL.

TABLE 5. **International Prognostic Index***

All Patients:	International Index, All Patients:
Age >60 years	Low 0 or 1
Serum LDH >1x normal	Low intermediate 2
Performance status 2–4	High intermediate 3
Stage III or IV	High 4 or 5
Extranodal involvement >1 site	
AGE-ADJUSTED INTERNATIONAL PROGNOSTIC INDEX*	
Patients ≤60 Years:	**International Index, Patients ≤60 Years:**
State III or IV	Low 0
Serum LDH >1x normal	Low intermediate 1
Performance status 2–4	High intermediate 2
	High 3

*Table adapted from data published in The International Non-Hodgkin's Lymphoma Prognostic Factors Project. A predictive model for aggressive non-Hodgkin's lymphoma. N Engl J Med. 329:987-994, 1993.

Because the GELA study only includes patient's age older than 60 years of age, a randomized study for younger patients may be required. Nevertheless, given the superior outcome of R-CHOP in older patients, R-CHOP combination has also become the standard of care even for younger patients.

Treatment options for patients with advanced-stage DLCL also vary depending on additional prognostic information provided by the age-adjusted International Prognostic Index (see Table 5). Patients who fall into a low or low-intermediate risk category have a very good prognosis, whereas patients who have advanced stage and elevated LDH level or poor performance status (high-intermediate or high-risk category) have less than a 50% chance of being cured with standard CHOP chemotherapy. Several phase II studies have shown that high-dose therapy (HDT) and autologous stem cell transplant (ASCT) during first CR/partial remission can improve prognosis and survival of these poor-risk patients. However, not all the randomized studies comparing standard chemotherapy to chemotherapy followed by HDT and ASCT, have confirmed the benefit of HDT and ASCT during first remission. Therefore, given the toxicity associated with high-dose therapy, this treatment should be recommended in the context of appropriate clinical trials.

Patients who relapse after initial complete response or who never achieve remission with induction chemotherapy have a very poor prognosis. HDT and ASCT are recommended because they are the only treatments that can induce long-term disease control. These patients should be treated with a non–cross-resistant combination chemotherapy regimen, such as ICE (ifosfamide,* carboplatin,* and etoposide*), or ESAP (etoposide,* methylprednisolone, cytarabine arabinoside,* and cisplatin*) in an attempt to achieve a second response then proceed to HDT and ASCT. Patients with recurrent disease after HDT and ASCT, or those failing multiple chemotherapy regimens, are not likely to benefit from currently available standard therapy.

*Not FDA approved for this indication.

TREATMENT OF FOLLICULAR LYMPHOMA

The treatment approach to follicular lymphoma depends on the extent of initial disease involvement. Patients with non-bulky, localized (stage I-II) follicular lymphoma are candidates for potentially curative infrared (IF)-RT with or without chemotherapy, or extended-field RT. The addition of chemotherapy or more extended-field RT can improve failure-free survival, but has not been shown to improve OS. In circumstances where toxicity of IF-RT outweighs the potential clinical benefit, observation is recommended. Patients who relapse after initial RT should be treated as advanced stage follicular lymphoma.

Standard approaches to advanced stage follicular lymphoma are evolving and may change in the next few years based on improvement in response seen with monoclonal antibodies. Because follicular lymphoma is currently incurable with standard therapy, the approach has been one of "watch and wait" until disease progression or symptoms occur. There are multiple options of therapy and the choice of therapy is highly individualized depending on age, performance status, goals of therapy, and physician's preference. Alkylating agents (chlorambucil, cyclophosphamide) with or without steroid, is the old standard. Overall response rates of 50% to 70% with CR rates of 15% to 20% were reported with CVP (cyclophosphamide,* vincristine, and prednisone*). Higher response rate and CR were reported with fludarabine (Fludara)*-containing combinations as outlined in Table 6, but no proven increased OS.

Rituximab (Rituxan) alone has been shown to be effective front-line and maintenance therapy in previously untreated follicular lymphoma. Based on the synergy between chemotherapy drugs and the antibody, several trials of chemotherapy plus rituximab have been studied in follicular lymphoma. The results of these trials are shown in Table 6. Thus far, concurrent use of rituximab with CHOP reported by Czuczman and others produced the highest response rate, which also translated into prolonged progression-free survival. Fludarabine combinations also have high response rate but are associated with greater degree of low blood count and increased risk of opportunistic infections.

At the time of disease recurrence, a repeat lymph node biopsy should be performed to rule out histologic transformation, which occurs in 10% to 70% of patients with low-grade NHL. If transformation into DLCL is documented, treatment should be directed toward DLCL and HDT followed by stem cell transplant should be considered.

*Not FDA approved for this indication.

TABLE 6. **Summary of Studies In Patients with Previously Untreated Follicular or Low-Grade Non-Hodgkin's Lymphoma**

Reference	No. of Patients	Study Design	Regimen	Objective Response (Complete), %	Duration
FLUDARABINE (FLUDARA)					
Hagenbeek et al., 1998	381	Randomized	Fludarabine* CVP	69 (39)† 53 (17)	TTP: 16.8 mo TTP: 13.2 mo
Klasa et al., 1999	91 (previously treated)	Phase III, randomized	Fludarabine* CVP	62 (5) 52 (7)	PFS: 11 mo† PFS: 9 mo
Velasquez et al., 1999	81	Phase II	Fludarabine* + mitoxantrone*	91 (43)	2-y PFS: 63% 2-y OS: 93%
Hochster et al., 2000	27	Phase I	Fludarabine* + Cyclophosphamide*	100 (89)	DFS: >60 mo OS: >60 mo
RITUXIMAB (RITUXAN)					
Czuczman et al., 2001	40	Phase II	Rituximab + CHOP	100 (63)	TTP: >65 mo
Hainsworth et al., 2002	62	Phase II	Rituximab (induction + maintenance)	73 (37)	PFS: 34 mo
Maloney et al., 2001	85	Phase II	CHOP × 6 followed by rituximab	72 (44)	2-y FFS: 76% 2-y OS: 95%
FLUDARABINE + RITUXIMAB					
Cabanillas et al., 2000	39 32	Randomized	FND + rituximab FND followed by rituximab	73 (73)‡ 67 (67)‡	2-y FFS: 88% for responders versus 34% for nonresponders
Czuczman et al., 2001	40	Phase II	Rituximab + fludarabine	90 (82.5)	Response: >15+ mo

†$P < .05$.
‡Molecular response in blood (in marrow) at 12 months, $P = .32$ ($P = 1.0$).
CHOP, cyclophosphamide, doxorubicin, vincristine, prednisone; CVP, cyclophosphamide, vincristine, prednisone; DFS, disease-free survival; FFS, failure-free survival; FND, fludarabine, mitoxantrone, dexamethasone; OS, overall survival; PFS, progression-free survival; TTP, time to progression.

For patients with relapsed follicular lymphoma, options of therapy have evolved over the last few years and include rituximab alone, salvage chemotherapy with or without rituximab, radioimmunotherapy, and HDT followed by autologous or allogeneic stem cell transplant. The result of radioimmunotherapy is encouraging. Zevalin (yttrium-90-labeled anti-CD20 monoclonal antibody, IDEC Pharmaceutical, CA), the first radioimmunotherapy for NHL approved by the Food and Drug Administration, produces overall response rate of 80%, and 34% CR in previously treated patients with relapsed or refractory CD20+ low-grade follicular and transformed NHL. Therefore, given the available options, the decision to proceed to treatment and the choice of therapy should also be individualized.

TREATMENT OF MANTLE CELL LYMPHOMA

Mantle cell lymphoma (MCL) is currently an area of intensive investigation. It may be distinguished from other B-cell NHL on the basis of its unique immunophenotypic profile (CD5+, CD20+, CD23–, CD10+, and CD43+) and cyclin D1 expression. Patients with MCL tend to be older, with an average age of 61 to 68 years. Most patients present with advanced stage IV disease with peripheral blood, bone marrow, and gastrointestinal involvement. The prognosis is very poor and it is incurable with standard conventional chemotherapy. Higher response was reported with CHOP in combination with rituximab; however, the median PFS was only 16.6 months. More aggressive regimens, higher dose Cytoxan, vincristine, Adriamycin, and Decadron (hyper-CVAD) and M-A (escalated cyclophosphamide,* vincristine,* doxorubicin,* and dexamethasone,* alternating with high-dose methotrexate [Rheumatrex]* and cytarabine [Cytosar-U]*) have been reported from the M. D. Anderson Cancer Center. The response rate was 94%, with 38% CR. However, the curability of this regimen could not be assessed because most patients underwent HDT and ASCT after hyper-CVAD induction. Recently, the addition of rituximab* to hyper-CVAD and M-A have produced a fairly high response rate of 72% and a 2-year failure-free survival of 90%. Despite the encouraging results, the data need to be confirmed.

The role of HDT and autologous or allogeneic SCT in patients with MCL is actively being investigated. Overall experiences of HDT and ASCT have indicated that relapse continues to occur after ASCT and there was no survival plateau, especially for those who were transplanted in relapse or subsequent remission. However, selected patients with MCL may benefit from HDT and ASCT during first CR. Therefore, patients with MCL should be enrolled in clinical trials of investigational therapies or high-dose and SCT in an attempt to improve DFS and cure for MCL.

*Not FDA approved for this indication.

LYMPHOMA OF MUCOSA-ASSOCIATED LYMPHOID TISSUE

Mucosa-associated lymphoid tissue (MALT) lymphoma, also known as extranodal marginal zone B-cell lymphoma, represents a distinct subset of B-cell NHL that differs from other low-grade B-cell lymphomas in its morphologic, immunophenotypic, and clinical characteristics. The most commonly involved site is the stomach. Other nongastric MALT lymphomas can arise from the skin, lung, salivary gland, conjunctiva, orbit, breast, prostate, ovary, small bowel, and colon. The disease tends to be localized at presentation, although it may involve draining lymph nodes.

Patients with gastric MALT lymphoma usually present with gastrointestinal bleeding, dyspepsia, and epigastric pain. Endoscopic findings include ulcers, gastritis, or diffuse gastric thickening, which are often associated with the presence of *Helicobacter pylori* bacterium. About two thirds of patients with localized gastric MALT lymphoma can achieve remission after eradication of *H. pylori* infection. Therefore, for clinical stage IE, treatment with antibiotics in combination with a proton pump inhibitor is recommended. For patients with stage IE *H. pylori* negative, or stage II disease, or those who fail to respond to antibiotics, excellent results have been reported with localized radiation. For patients with advanced stage III/IV, systemic chemotherapy used for low-grade lymphoma is recommended.

Radiation therapy is also recommended for localized nongastric MALT lymphomas. Advanced stage patients should be managed the same way as patients with follicular lymphoma. In situations where MALT lymphoma coexists with large cell lymphoma, patients should be managed as DLCL.

TREATMENT OF HIGH-GRADE NHL

Burkitt's lymphoma and lymphoblastic lymphoma have very aggressive clinical courses and typically involve extranodal sites such as bone marrow and meninges. The clinical characteristics are sometimes overlapping with acute lymphoblastic leukemia (ALL). Because Burkitt and Burkitt-like lymphomas are frequently associated with HIV infection, HIV serology should be part of the diagnostic workup. Because of high tumor turnover and rapid doubling time, tumor lysis syndrome occurs frequently at initiation of therapy. Several intensive short-course chemotherapy regimens have been proven effective in treatment of Burkitt's lymphoma, including CODOX-M/IVAC protocol (cyclophosphamide, vincristine, doxorubicin,* methotrexate, ifosfamide,* etoposide,* and cytarabine) from the National Cancer Institute, and the "Vanderbilt regimen" (a brief. high-intensity cyclophosphamide, etoposide,* vincristine, bleomycin, methotrexate, and prednisone*). Because of the high incidence of leptomeningeal involvement, intrathecal chemotherapy is also incorporated into the regimen.

*Not FDA approved for this indication.

Lymphoblastic lymphoma is a T-cell malignancy that occurs more often in young men and typically presents with mediastinal mass, pleural effusion, bone marrow, and leptomeningeal involvement. In general, treatment with ALL-like regimen including induction, consolidation, central nervous system prophylaxis, and maintenance therapy, is recommended. Excellent results have been reported from the M. D. Anderson Cancer Center using hyper-CVAD alternating with high-dose methotrexate and cytarabine (see MLC). High-dose therapy and SCT have been performed during first remission in selected patients. Patients with relapsed or refractory disease have extremely poor prognosis because they may not respond to salvage therapy and therefore are not candidates for HDT and stem cell transplant.

MULTIPLE MYELOMA

method of
FAITH E. DAVIES, M.B.B.Ch., M.D., and
PETER J. SELBY, M.D.
University of Leeds
Leeds, England

Multiple myeloma represents 10% to 15% of all hematologic malignancies and 1% of all cancers. The incidence increases with age, with approximately 40% of patients being younger than 60 years. The clinical picture involves a combination of bone destruction, immune deficiency, bone marrow failure, and renal failure. The diagnosis requires the presence of at least two of three characteristic features: a paraprotein or monoclonal immunoglobulin in the blood and/or the urine, bone marrow infiltration by malignant plasma cells, and the presence of osteolytic bone lesions. The outlook for patients is poor, with a median survival of approximately 3.5 years.

Myeloma must be distinguished from other disorders characterized by monoclonal gammopathies, including monoclonal gammopathy of undetermined significance (MGUS), Waldenström's macroglobulinemia, non-Hodgkin's lymphoma, light chain amyloid, idiopathic cold agglutinin disease, essential cryoglobulinemia, and heavy chain disease. MGUS describes a condition characterized by the presence of a low level of paraprotein in the absence of other clinical features of multiple myeloma. Demonstration of a paraprotein in the serum or urine is often an incidental finding, and patients are typically asymptomatic. Clonal plasma cells are present within the bone marrow but represent less than 5% to 10% of the total nucleated cells. Long-term surveillance is recommended because an overt plasma cell disorder will develop in approximately 25% of cases.

STAGING AND PROGNOSTIC FACTORS

Two traditional staging systems reliably separate multiple myeloma patients into prognostic groups by using simple laboratory measurements. Performance status, renal function, and the hemoglobin level form the basis of the Medical Research Council staging system. The extent of the bone lesions and the presence of hypercalcemia are also thought to reflect the aggressiveness of the disease, and these elements are incorporated in the Durie-Salmon staging system. These systems remain widely used in the clinic to determine which patients should receive therapy, although few physicians would use them to direct specific therapeutic decisions.

At present, β_2-microglobulin is the single most important prognostic variable in multiple myeloma, with serum levels correlating with tumor stage and response to therapy. The extent and type of bone marrow infiltration also have prognostic significance: patients with a plasmablastic morphology have a shorter survival. In addition, measures of tumor cell proliferation such as the plasma cell labeling index (PCLI) are useful: a high PCLI correlates with a shorter survival time independent of tumor cell mass. The percentage of circulating plasma cells at diagnosis has also been shown to be an independent prognostic variable. The presence of certain cytogenetic abnormalities likewise has prognostic significance: patients with partial or complete deletions of chromosome 13 or abnormalities of 11q have an adverse outcome.

TREATMENT

The clinical picture of myeloma both at diagnosis and during its clinical course is a complex of bone destruction leading to pain or fracture with hypercalcemia; infection as a result of immune deficiency; marrow failure leading to anemia and, less commonly, thrombocytopenia; and renal failure caused by hypercalcemia, direct damage from paraprotein, or precipitation of light chain in renal tubules. Other features include plasmacytoma, hyperviscosity, and biochemical disturbances.

Current therapy for multiple myeloma includes the use of conventional low-dose chemotherapy or high-dose chemotherapy with autologous or allogeneic stem cell transplantation. Although these regimens are able to reduce the tumor burden, complete molecular remission of disease is rare, and almost all patients eventually relapse. Novel treatment approaches are currently being evaluated and will be used either alone or in combination with conventional or high-dose chemotherapy to improve response and outcome.

General Principles

The first priorities in the management of a patient with multiple myeloma are alleviation of pain and treatment of infection, together with careful assessment for hypercalcemia and renal failure and correction of anemia. The most important aspect of the management of renal failure is preventive with maintenance of high fluid throughput. Acute renal failure must be managed by a careful search for precipitating factors such as hypercalcemia, dehydration, hyperuricemia, and infection. When these conditions are corrected, patients' renal function often improves. Chronic renal failure can be improved by vigorous hydration, dialysis, and reduction of the myeloma cell mass by intensive chemotherapy. Hypercalcemia should also be managed by rehydration, and if this measure is insufficient, the addition of corticosteroids or bisphosphonates is helpful. Symptoms of hyperviscosity improve with vigorous plasmapheresis to reduce both the paraprotein concentration and serum viscosity.

The choice of specific therapy to control the underlying disease depends on biologic factors, the presence of other serious medical conditions, and patient choice. Intensive approaches are often associated with procedure-related toxicity resulting in morbidity and mortality. To minimize morbidity and mortality, most physicians would set an upper age limit of 70 years for autologous transplantation and 45 years for allogeneic transplantation. Although it is suggested that these intensive approaches may result in improved quality of life and overall survival, some patients may prefer to adopt a lower dose regimen. The different approaches to therapy need to be discussed at diagnosis because the use of alkylating agents as induction therapy can affect the yield of peripheral blood stem cells.

Conventional Treatment

For patients not considering a high-dose procedure, many physicians will use oral melphalan (Alkeran) because it is well tolerated, especially in the elderly, and alopecia is rare. The standard regimen is 7 mg/m^2/d for 4 days every 3 weeks, but bioavailability is variable, and patients should be carefully monitored for myelosuppression. Response to treatment is gradual, and maximal response may take several months. Approximately 50% of patients will respond. However, only a minority attain a true complete response consisting of the disappearance of paraprotein and a normal marrow. Most patients reach a "plateau phase," during which the paraprotein level is stable and the patient has minimal symptoms and does not require a blood transfusion. Continuing therapy during this phase has no effect on survival. Some physicians add prednisolone (Delta-Cortef),* 20 mg twice daily, to the melphalan, although the results of a number of trials suggest that it has no survival benefit. Weekly oral cyclophosphamide (Cytoxan),* 400 or 300 mg/m^2 intravenously, is an alternative to melphalan because it produces similar results in terms of response rates and survival but is less myelotoxic and therefore useful for patients with cytopenia.

A recent overview of worldwide randomized trials (a total of 27 trials) suggests that no significant difference in mortality is seen in patients treated with melphalan/prednisolone therapy versus combination chemotherapy regimens including cyclophosphamide, melphalan, carmustine (BCNU), lomustine (CCNU),* doxorubicin (Adriamycin),* vincristine (Vincasar PFS),* and prednisolone. However, an improved response rate was observed in the combination chemotherapy group, which may translate to improved quality of life. We therefore recommend the use of a combination regimen such as ABCM (day 1: Adriamycin [doxorubicin], 30 mg/m^2 intravenously, and BCNU, 30 mg/m^2 intravenously; days 21 to 24: cyclophosphamide, 100 mg/m^2 orally, and melphalan, 6 mg/m^2 orally), until a plateau is achieved, in patients younger than 70 years who are not considering a high-dose procedure.

In the early eighties it was noted that high doses of glucocorticoid steroids were capable of producing remission in patients with refractory or relapsed disease. The addition of doxorubicin and vincristine given as a continuous infusion over a 4-day period to dexamethasone (Decadron)* (intravenous vincristine, 0.4 mg, and Adriamycin, 9 mg/m^2, given over a period of 24 hours for 4 days, along with 4 days of oral dexamethasone, 40 mg/d [VAD]) or to 4 days of methylprednisolone (Solu-Medrol),* 1 mg/m^2/d with a maximum of 1.5 g/d (VAMP), achieved high responses in these patients. Both these regimens (VAD and VAMP/c-VAMP) have now been used as primary therapy in myeloma patients and have achieved high overall (70% to 80%) and complete (8% to 28%) response rates. These regimens do not damage stem cells, thus making them the treatment of choice for patients proceeding to stem cell harvest and a high-dose procedure. VAD is also suitable for patients with severe renal impairment because no dosage modification is required and toxicity is not increased in these patients. The disadvantage of these regimens is the requirement for a central line, although current studies are evaluating an oral regimen with idarubicin (Idamycin)* rather than intravenous doxorubicin.*

High-Dose Therapy with Autologous Transplantation

For patients younger than 70 years with multiple myeloma, high-dose therapy with autologous bone marrow transplantation (ABMT) or peripheral blood stem cell transplantation (PBSCT) should be considered. Most centers use intravenous high-dose melphalan alone at a dose of 200 mg/m^2 and prefer peripheral blood cells rather than bone marrow cells as support. Some centers also give total body irradiation; however, the available data suggest that this conditioning regimen has greater toxicity and no survival benefit. A number of groups have shown an improvement in response rates and survival with high-dose melphalan in both relapsed/refractory patients and those with newly diagnosed multiple myeloma when compared with historical controls. The results of a number of ongoing prospective randomized trials comparing high-dose therapy with either PBSCT or ABMT support and conventional combination therapy in patients with newly diagnosed disease are just becoming available. Early reports suggest improved

*Not FDA approved for this indication.

*Not FDA approved for this indication.

response rates and a small, but significant survival advantage in patients undergoing high-dose treatment versus conventional treatment, as well as a procedure-related mortality less than 5%. A randomized study comparing transplantation in first remission with transplantation at relapse showed no significant difference in survival but an improvement in quality of life in the early-transplant cohort. Although the results from these studies of autografting in myeloma are encouraging, the survival curves show no obvious plateau and suggest that high-dose therapy with stem cell support is not a curative procedure.

A number of additional strategies have been evaluated to improve outcomes. Methods to either deplete tumor cells or select normal hematopoietic progenitor cells from autologous bone marrow or peripheral blood stem cells before transplantation result in up to a 5-log depletion of tumor cells without affecting engraftment. However, this strategy does not appear to have any clinical benefit because residual tumor cells are detectable within both the graft and the patient after transplantation. Another approach has been to use multiple high-dose therapies with stem cell transplantation. Although some evidence indicates an increase in response rates with this sequential approach, the effect on overall survival remains unclear.

High-Dose Therapy with Allogeneic Transplantation

Allogeneic bone marrow transplantation has not been widely used in the treatment of multiple myeloma because of its high associated morbidity and mortality (up to 40%), especially in older patients. It is because of this high transplant-related mortality that many physicians place an upper age limit of 45 years for allogeneic transplantation in myeloma. However, a number of reports show a high complete response rate, with some of the responses being durable. The stage at diagnosis, preconditioning remission status, extent of previous treatment, gender, and serum β_2-microglobulin level are important prognostic factors. Residual clonal myeloma cells are, however, still detectable by polymerase chain reaction after transplantation, consistent with the lack of a plateau in the survival curves and the continued late relapses.

The assumption that this mode of treatment is most likely to eradicate myeloma cells and the possibility of a significant graft-versus-myeloma effect have encouraged further consideration of this therapy. Data from a number of centers have shown that patients with relapsed multiple myeloma after allogeneic bone marrow transplantation can achieve marked clinical responses after infusions of lymphocytes collected from the marrow donor because of a graft-versus-myeloma effect. However, graft-versus-host disease may occur and contribute to the procedure-related mortality.

More recently, low-dose radiotherapy in combination with chemotherapy or chemotherapy alone is undergoing evaluation in the setting of nonmyeloablative transplantation or "mini-allografting." The goal of this strategy is to reduce toxicity related to the conditioning regimen while attempting to take advantage of the graft-versus-myeloma effect of allogeneic transplantation. This approach can be used in older individuals or patients who would otherwise not be eligible for conventional high-dose transplantation because of underlying morbidity. Initial reports in myeloma suggest a lower procedure-related mortality, although the incidence of graft-versus-host disease varies. At present, it is recommended that patients wishing to undergo such an approach be encouraged to enter a clinical trial so that toxicity and response data can be collected.

One of the major obstacles to curing myeloma is the persistence of minimal residual disease after high-dose therapy and stem cell transplantation, and a number of approaches are being developed for the generation and enhancement of allogeneic and autologous antimyeloma immunity after transplantation. These approaches include vaccination strategies with patient-specific idiotype, tumor RNA or DNA, or CD40-activated autologous myeloma cells. Immunization with dendritic cells pulsed with patient-specific idiotype or tumor cells and fusion of myeloma cells with autologous dendritic cells are also being investigated. A number of ongoing phase I/II clinical trials are offering such approaches, and patients should be encouraged to partake.

Radiation Therapy

Radiation therapy is an effective treatment modality in myeloma. Its role in established disease is for the palliation of disease-related skeletal complications, including impending cord compression, pathologic fractures, and pain related to bone lesions, and for the treatment of localized extramedullary plasmacytomas.

Bisphosphonate Therapy

Skeletal complications are a major source of morbidity in myeloma. A number of randomized clinical trials have demonstrated the efficacy of bisphosphonates in reducing the incidence of skeletal complications, including a decrease in bone pain, hypercalcemia, and vertebral and long bone fractures. Bisphosphonates are known to inhibit osteoclastic activity and reduce bone resorption. Recent in vitro reports suggest that these drugs also have a direct antimyeloma effect resulting in apoptosis of myeloma plasma cells and that they induce the inhibition of cytokines important for myeloma growth and survival and have an immunomodulatory effect. It is therefore recommended that all patients receive bisphosphonate therapy (oral or intravenous) during active treatment and, when appropriate, during the plateau phase.

Interferon Therapy

A recent meta-analysis of a number of clinical trials using interferon alfa-2a (Roferon-A)* in myeloma has demonstrated a small, but significant survival

*Not FDA approved for this indication.

advantage for patients when the drug is used as maintenance therapy or in combination with conventional chemotherapy for induction of remission. This treatment is recommended for all patients in a stable plateau phase, although a proportion of patients will find compliance difficult because of side effects.

Biologically Based Novel Therapies

Recent advances in understanding the biology of multiple myeloma have led to the development of a number of novel therapies that are currently in phase I/II clinical trials. These therapies not only target the myeloma plasma cell directly but also the bone marrow microenvironment, including cytokines, bone marrow stromal cells, and blood vessels. It is important to encourage patients to partake in such trials so that efficacy, dosage, and appropriate regimens can be determined.

Recent reports of increased bone marrow angiogenesis, coupled with the known antiangiogenic properties of thalidomide (Thalomid),* provided the rationale for the use of this drug in the treatment of relapsed or refractory myeloma, and a number of studies have reported impressive response rates around 30%. Thalidomide has also been used as front-line therapy in combination with other agents; however, although a good response rate has been reported, concern has been expressed regarding the high incidence of venous thrombotic events. The role of the cytokine vascular endothelial growth factor (VEGF) as a growth, survival, and migration factor has also recently been reported and has resulted in the use of VEGF and other tyrosine kinase inhibitors in the relapse setting. Another exciting drug undergoing trial is the proteasome inhibitor. Proteasomes are important in cell cycle regulation and the ubiquitinization of proteins. Inhibition of proteasomes stabilizes a number of proteins and confers growth arrest to the cell and, ultimately, apoptosis. In multiple myeloma, proteasome inhibition leads to deregulation of the nuclear factor NFκB, which is important in growth, survival, and drug resistance, as well as interleukin-6 (IL-6) transcription and secretion from bone marrow stromal cells.

The introduction of therapeutic monoclonal antibodies has permitted the development of effective tumor-targeted therapies with minimal host toxicity. In myeloma, a number of antibody-based therapies are being investigated that either target antigens on the myeloma cell surface (CD38, CD138, MUC1, HM1.24) or inhibit cytokine-mediated growth and survival signaling (antibodies directed against IL-6 and the IL-6 receptor complex).

Solitary Plasmacytoma

Some patients initially have a single solitary painful osteolytic lesion caused by a plasma cell infiltrate, and further investigations reveal no evidence of systemic disease, although some patients will have a low level of paraprotein. Local control is achieved in 90% of patients with radiotherapy, but overt myeloma will eventually develop in two thirds of these patients.

Extramedullary Plasmacytoma

Isolated extramedullary plasmacytoma may also occur and affects the nose, nasopharynx, and paranasal sinuses in particular. Radiotherapy is the treatment of choice, with less than a 5% chance of disease recurrence, provided that the adjacent lymph nodes are included in the irradiated field. It is, however, extremely important to distinguish patients with this condition from those with widespread myeloma because of the big difference in the clinical disease course.

POLYCYTHEMIA VERA

method of
STEVEN M. FRUCHTMAN, M.D., and
CELIA L. GROSSKREUTZ, M.D.
Mount Sinai Medical Center
New York, New York

Polycythemia vera (PV) is a hematologic malignancy involving an abnormal clone of the pluripotent marrow stem cell. It evolves as a chronic, slowly progressive disorder characterized by panhyperplasia of the bone marrow involving the erythroid, myeloid, and megakaryocyte series. The hyperplastic marrow leads to elevation of the red cell mass, considered essential for the diagnosis of the disease, and varying degrees of leukocytosis and thrombocytosis.

The stem cells from these patients are capable of forming in vitro erythroid colonies without the addition of erythropoietin to the culture system. These "endogenous" erythroid colonies arise from the abnormal clone and suggest autonomous cell growth.

Patients with PV left untreated do poorly; 50% are reported to die within 18 months of the first sign or symptom. Death is frequently related to thrombosis, especially of the cerebral, coronary, and pulmonary circulations. Unusual sites for thrombosis are also seen, such as the hepatic circulation. With appropriate therapy median survival is between 8 to 15 years, but PV is typically a disease of the elderly, with a mean age at diagnosis of 60 years. Thus, younger patients with appropriate therapy can have a much longer survival.

DIAGNOSIS

By using the proposed modified criteria for the diagnosis of PV shown in Table 1, the diagnosis of PV can be made with great confidence.

*Not FDA approved for this indication.

TABLE 1. **Proposed Modified Criteria for the Diagnosis of Polycythemia Vera**

A1 Raised red cell mass (>25% above mean normal predicted value, or PCV ≥ 0.60 in males or 0.56 in females)
A2 Absence of cause of secondary erythrocytosis
A3 Palpable splenomegaly
A4 Clonality marker, (i.e., acquired abnormal marrow karyotype)
B1 Thrombocytosis (platelet count >400 × 10^9/L)
B2 Neutrophil leucocytosis (neutrophil count >10 x 10^9/L; >12.5 × 10^9/L in smokers)
B3 Splenomegaly demonstrated on isotope or ultrasound scanning
B4 Characteristic BFU-E growth or reduced serum erythropoietin
A1 + A2 + A3 or A4 establishes PV
A1+ A2 + two of B establishes PV

BFU-E, burst-forming unit–erythroid; PV, polycythemia vera.

It is important to exclude secondary causes of erythrocytosis (Table 2) that are caused by increased erythropoietin, which may be physiologically appropriate (e.g., high altitude, smoking) or physiologically inappropriate (e.g., erythropoietin-secreting renal tumors). The measurement of serum erythropoietin level is very useful in the differential diagnosis. In PV, erythropoietin production is down-regulated by a negative feedback mechanism and serum levels are usually low or normal. In contrast, the secondary erythrocytosis has elevated erythropoietin levels.

TREATMENT

Therapy consists of controlling the elevated red cell mass with phlebotomy. Some patients require cytoreductive drugs to control the number of circulating blood elements. The only potentially curative therapy is allogeneic stem cell transplantation. This is a consideration only in patients who develop high risk postpolycythemic myeloid metaplasia with myelofibrosis.

Phlebotomy

Once the diagnosis of PV is established, it is important to reduce the increased blood volume by repeated phlebotomy to prevent thrombotic or hemorrhagic complications. This is best accomplished by phlebotomies of 250 to 500 mL every other day until a hematocrit of between 40% and 45% is obtained. In the elderly, or those with a compromised hemodynamic status, blood should be withdrawn only twice weekly, and only 250 to 300 mL should be removed at each session.

TABLE 2. **Common Causes of Secondary Erythrocytosis**

CONGENITAL
Mutant high oxygen affinity hemoglobin
Congenital low 2,3-diphosphoglycerate
Autonomous high erythropoietin production

ACQUIRED
Arterial hypoxemia (high altitude, cyanotic congenital heart disease, chronic lung disease)
Other causes of impaired tissue oxygen delivery (smoking)
Renal lesions (renal tumors, cysts diffuse parenchymal disease, hydronephrosis, renal artery stenosis, renal transplantation)
Endocrine lesions (adrenal tumors)
Miscellaneous tumors (cerebellar hemangioblastoma, uterine fibroids, bronchial carcinoma)
Drugs (androgens)
Hepatic lesions (hepatoma, cirrhosis, hepatitis)

Once a normal hematocrit is achieved, blood counts should be obtained every 4 to 8 weeks to determine the frequency of phlebotomies. A phlebotomy should be performed whenever the hematocrit is equal to or greater than 45%. When a state of sufficient iron deficiency has been reached, the frequency of phlebotomies will decrease. Iron supplementation should be avoided because this will stimulate erythropoiesis and, thus, red cell production. Iron deficiency is reported to produce symptoms unrelated to anemia, such as dysphagia, soreness of the tongue, koilonychia, and pica. These problems are rare and patients typically feel better after adjustment to their normal red cell mass.

Phlebotomy alone is the treatment of choice in young patients, to avoid the concern of an increased incidence of neoplastic transformation associated with the long-term use of myelosuppressive therapy.

Patients under the age of 50 and all women in the childbearing years should be managed with phlebotomy unless there are specific thrombosis-related risk factors. The most significant risk factor is a prior thrombotic event, including myocardial infarction, peripheral arterial occlusion, pulmonary infarction, and venous thrombosis. In such cases, myelosuppression is indicated. Intermittent phlebotomy is used as adjuvant therapy in patients requiring myelosuppression whenever the hematocrit is above 45% in order to minimize the amount of myelosuppression used.

Myelosuppression

Phlebotomy will not control the thrombocythemia, leukocytosis, hyperuricemia, hypermetabolism, pruritus, and complications of splenomegaly seen in PV patients. Patients treated with phlebotomy alone have a higher incidence of serious thrombotic complications during the first 3 years of therapy when compared to patients treated with myelosuppression. Thus, elderly patients who are more prone to thrombotic disease should be treated with myelosuppression in addition to phlebotomy.

Hydroxyurea (Hydrea)

This antimetabolite prevents DNA synthesis by inhibiting the enzyme ribonucleoside reductase. Hydroxyurea* (HU) is a frequently used drug for patients requiring myelosuppression. The initial dose is 15 mg/kg daily orally and subsequent adjustment of the dose is based on initial weekly blood counts for a month, to control the hematocrit without causing leukopenia or thrombocytopenia. If the white cell count falls below 3500 cells per mm^3 or the platelet count falls to less than 100,000 per mm^3, HU is

*Not FDA approved for this indication.

withheld until these elements normalize and then is reinstituted at 50% of the prior dose. When the peripheral blood count is maintained within an acceptable range on a stable dose of HU, the interval between blood counts is lengthened to 2 weeks and then to every 4 weeks.

For patients who require frequent phlebotomies or who have platelet counts greater than 600,000 per mm^3, the dose of HU can be increased by 5 mg/kg daily at monthly intervals, with frequent monitoring until control is achieved. The majority of patients will be controlled with doses between 500 and 1000 mg daily. Supplemental phlebotomy is preferable to increased myelosuppression to control the hematocrit.

In emergency situations, particularly those presenting with signs of decreased cerebral perfusion in the setting of an elevated hematocrit or marked thrombocytosis, more rapid control of disease may be crucial. Daily phlebotomy to a hematocrit of 45% should be accompanied by a loading dose of HU of 30 mg/kg/d for 7 days, followed by the maintenance dose of 15 mg/kg daily.

Besides the requirement for close observation to prevent excessive marrow suppression, acute toxicity is rare; occasionally rash, fever, nausea, and oral or lower extremity ulcerations may be seen.

Studies have reported variable results regarding the leukemogenic potential of hydroxyurea, and the issue remains unsettled. This has prompted trials with other agents considered safe for long-term use, such as interferon-α and anagrelide (Agrylin).

Interferon-α (IFN-α)

IFN-α* is a biologic response modifier that suppresses the proliferation of hematopoietic progenitors. In PV patients, IFN-α reduces the hematocrit to below 45% in 60% of the cases and reduces the spleen size and controls the pruritus in 75% of the patients. It is also highly effective in controlling the platelet counts. The initial dose of IFN-α is 3 million units subcutaneously three times a week but dose modifications may be required. Full response to IFN-α usually requires 6 months to a year of treatment.

The major problem with IFN-α therapy, apart from its cost and parenteral route of administration, is the incidence of acute side effects leading to cessation of treatment in about one third of patients. These include flulike symptoms, fever, and joint pain that sometimes can be controlled with prophylactic acetaminophen. Liver function abnormalities and depression are also seen.

The role of IFN-α in PV therapy is uncertain although promising for the management of young patients who require myelosuppression and those with intractable pruritus. It does not cross the placenta and thus may be used in pregnant women who may have an indication for myelosuppression.

The recent development of pegylated-IFN, because of its slower clearance, permits once-weekly dosing.

*Not FDA approved for this indication.

Anagrelide

Anagrelide* (Agrylin) is an oral quinazoline derivative that has a profound effect on the maturation of megakaryocytes resulting in a reduction of platelet production. It controls thrombocytosis in 66% of patients with PV. Time to response is between 17 and 25 days. It is also reported to cause a minimal decrease in hematocrit.

The dose is 0.5 to 1.0 mg orally four times daily. Typically steady state doses are 2.2 to 2.5 mg daily. The most significant side effects include palpitations, fluid retention, dizziness, and headaches; these are related to the drug's vasodilatory and inotropic properties. They can be minimized by initially starting with a low dose, such as 0.5 mg twice daily, and gradually increasing the dose until control of the platelet count is achieved. Patients with lactose intolerance may have diarrhea due to its packaging with lactose. This can be treated with lactase supplements.

Because of its primary effects on platelets, anagrelide (Agrylin) has been used primarily in essential thrombocytopenia; however it can be also used in PV in conjunction with phlebotomy to control thrombocytosis. Its use avoids the development of leukopenia typically seen with other myelosuppressive agents; this permits easier control of the platelet number without the risk of causing a low white cell count.

Antithrombotic Therapy

The use of aspirin or other antiplatelet agents in patients with PV and other myeloproliferative disorders remains controversial.

Low-dose aspirin 80 to 325 mg daily seems reasonable to recommend for patients who have a prior history of thrombosis or cardiovascular disease, such as myocardial infarction or ischemic stroke, for which antiaggregating therapy would be prescribed in any event, irrespective of the presence of PV. In addition, aspirin is effective for the treatment of erythromelalgia and other microvascular, neurologic, and ocular disturbances.

In patients with PV who continue to have thrombotic or vascular symptoms, despite aspirin and good control of the hematocrit and platelet count, clopidogrel (Plavix),* 75 mg daily or ticlopidine (Ticlid),* 250 mg orally twice daily should be considered.

*Not FDA approved for this indication.

THE PORPHYRIAS

method of
JEAN-CHARLES DEYBACH, M.D., and
HERVÉ PUY, M.D.
Hôpital Louis Mourier
Colombes, France

The *porphyrias* are a group of inherited metabolic disorders of heme biosynthesis in which specific patterns of overproduction of heme precursors are associated with characteristic clinical features: acute neurovisceral attacks, skin lesions, or both. Each type of porphyria is the result of a specific enzymatic defect in the heme pathway (Table 1). Acute intermittent porphyria and the rare 5-aminolevulinic acid (ALA) dehydratase deficiency porphyria are associated with acute attacks only. Variegate porphyria and hereditary coproporphyria are associated with both acute attacks and skin lesions. Congenital erythropoietic porphyria, porphyria cutanea tarda (PCT), and erythropoietic protoporphyria present with skin lesions only.

REGULATION OF HEME SYNTHESIS

Heme is synthetized from succinyl coenzyme A and glycine in all tissues, but mostly in liver and bone marrow, for the synthesis of hemoproteins such as hemoglobin, myoglobin, cytochromes, catalase, peroxidase, nitric oxide synthase, and tryptophan pyrrolase. Control of this heme biosynthesis differs between liver and bone marrow. The first-step enzyme 5-aminolevulinic acid (ALA) synthase is coded for by two genes: one erythroid-specific gene (ALA synthase-2 on chromosome X) and one ubiquitous (ALA synthase-1 on chromosome 3).

In the erythroid cell, erythropoietin and iron are involved in the control of the enzymes participating in heme formation. In the liver, the hemoproteins formed, including cytochrome P-450, are rapidly turned over in response to current metabolic needs. The free cellular heme pool retroinhibits ALA synthase-1 activity by negative-feedback regulation.

EXCRETION OF PORPHYRINS AND PORPHYRIN PRECURSORS

The intermediates (porphyrinogens) are unstable and rapidly oxidize to their corresponding porphyrins. Enzyme defects give rise to a characteristic biochemical profile of porphyrins and porphyrin precursors, ALA and porphobilinogen (PBG), and to accumulation in urine, feces, plasma, and/or erythrocytes that allow the type of porphyria to be accurately identified in patients (see Table 1). Enzyme or DNA analysis is used for family studies.

ACUTE HEPATIC PORPHYRIAS

Acute attacks are identical in four of the hepatic porphyrias: acute intermittent porphyria, hereditary coproporphyria, variegate porphyria, and ALA dehydratase deficiency porphyria. Except for ALA dehydratase deficiency porphyria, an autosomal recessive disorder, the acute hepatic porphyrias are autosomal dominant conditions in which a 50% reduction in enzyme activity is brought about by a mutation in one of the alleles of the corresponding gene (see Table 1). The penetrance is low, and about 90% of affected persons never experience an acute attack. Variegate porphyria and hereditary coproporphyria may also be associated with skin lesions, and such lesions are the only manifestation of the condition in 60% of patients with variegate porphyria (see Table 1). In most countries, acute intermittent porphyria is the most common of the acute porphyrias.

Clinical Features

Acute attacks are precipitated by events that increase the demand for heme synthesis. These include hormonal fluctuations, stress, fasting, infection, and exposure to porphyrinogenic drugs. Acute attacks are rare before puberty (except in ALA dehydratase deficiency porphyria) and after menopause, with a peak occurrence in the third and fourth decades; women are five times more likely to be affected than men. Most patients suffer one or possibly two acute attacks and are then symptom free for the rest of their lives. A few patients have recurrent acute attacks, which may require a special treatment regimen.

The acute porphyrias may present with a sudden, life-threatening crisis characterized by severe abdominal pain, neuropsychiatric symptoms, autonomic neuropathy, and electrolyte disturbances. All these clinical features of an acute attack can be explained by lesions of the nervous system. The mechanism of neural damage in these disorders is poorly understood. Various hypotheses that are not mutually exclusive have been proposed. The leading hypothesis is that ALA or PBG overproduced by the liver is neurotoxic. Conversely, formation of hemoproteins may be compromised by the inherited enzyme deficiency.

Acute attacks usually begin with generalized abdominal pain. Constipation, nausea, vomiting, and insomnia may precede and accompany the abdominal crisis. Examination does not show signs of peritoneal irritation; radiographic films of the abdomen usually disclose a normal pattern of bowel gas. Tachycardia, excess sweating, and hypertension are often associated with abdominal pain. Acute attacks are more commonly observed in women (18 to 40 years old), and recurrent exacerbations of the disease may occur periodically (mostly during the week preceding the menses). Occasionally, the presence of red or dark urine may help in the diagnosis.

In 20% to 30% of patients, signs of mental disturbance such as anxiety, depression, disorientation, hallucinations, paranoia, or confusional states are observed. Abdominal pain may disappear within a few days, generally when no harmful drug has been used. When acute attacks last several days, the gastrointestinal manifestations frequently lead to weight loss,

TABLE 1. **The Main Types of Porphyrias: Synopsis of Symptomatology and Biochemistry**

Porphyria Type (OMIM)	Affected Enzyme (EC)	Clinical Presentation	Inheritance	Biochemical Findings			
				Urine	***Stool***	***Erythrocytes***	***Plasma Peak*† *at***
ALA dehydratase porphyria (ADP) [125270]	ALA dehydratase (ALAD; EC 4.2.1.24)	Acute neurovisceral attack	AR	ALA, Copro III		Zn-Proto	
Acute intermittent porphyria (AIP) [176000]	PBG deaminase (PBGD; EC 4.3.1.8)	Acute neurovisceral attack	AD	ALA, PBG, Uro III			615–620
Congenital erythropoietic porphyria (CEP) [606938]	Uroporphyrinogen III synthase (UROS; EC 4.2.1.75)	Cutaneous photosensitivity Skin fragility, bullae with or without anemia	AR	Uro I, Copro I	Copro I	Uro I, Copro I	615–620
Porphyra cutanea tarda (PCT) [176100]	Uroporphyrinogen decarboxylase (UROD; EC 4.1.1.37)	Cutaneous photosensitivity Skin fragility, bullae	AD	Uro III, Hepta	Isocopro, Hepta‡		615–620
Hepatoerythropoietic porphyria (HEP) [176100]	Uroporphyrinogen decarboxylase (UROD; EC 4.1.1.37)	Cutaneous photosensitivity Skin fragility, bullae with or without anemia	AR	Uro III, Hepta	Isocopro, Hepta‡	Zn-Proto	615–620
Sporadic porphyria cutanea (sPC) [176090]	ND	Cutaneous photosensitivity Skin fragility, bullae	ND	Uro III, Hepta	Isocopro, Hepta‡		615–620
Hereditary coproporphyria (HC) [121300]	Coproporphyrinogen oxydase (CPO; EC 1.3.3.3)	Acute attack only (72%) Skin lesions only (7%) Both (21%)	AD	ALA, PBG, Copro III	Copro III		615–620
Variegate porphyria (VP) [176200]	Protoporphyrinogen oxydase (PPOX; EC 1.3.3.4)	Acute attack only (20%) Skin lesions only (59%) Both (21%)	AD	ALA, PBG, Copro III	Proto IX > Copro		624–627
Erythropoietic protoporphyria (EPP) [177000]	Ferrochelatase (FECH; EC 4.99.1.1)	Acute photosensitivity	AD*		Proto IX	Free-Proto IX	626–634

*Erythropoietic protoporphyria is mainly related to the co-inheritance of both a *FECH* gene mutation and a weak normal *FECH* allele — autosomal recessive inheritance has also been reported in a few families.

†Fluorescence emission peak in nm.

‡Heptacarboxyl-porphyrin.

AD, autosomal dominant; ALA, δ aminolevulinic acid; AR, autosomal recessive; Copro, coproporphyrin; EC, enzyme classification; I or III: type isomers; Isocopro, isocoproporphyrin; ND, not defined; OMIM, Online Mendelian Inheritance in Man; PBG, porphobilinogen; Proto, protoporphyrin; Uro, uroporphyrin.

whereas prolonged vomiting may cause oliguria and hyperazotemia.

Porphyric neuropathy often occurs when harmful drugs have not been avoided during an acute attack; however, neurologic manifestations are also a problem in the differential diagnosis and treatment when the type of porphyria is not known (e.g., an acute attack of porphyria may begin with seizures, and all antiseizure drugs can potentially adversely affect this disease).

Neuropathy is primarily motor: in the early stages pain in the extremities is very common ("muscle pain"); weakness often begins in the proximal muscles, more commonly in the arms than in the legs. Paresis in the extremities may occur and can also be strikingly local. Muscle weakness may progress and may lead to tetraplegia with respiratory and bulbar paralysis and death. After a severe attack, complete or partial muscle function can improve over a period of months. Recovery from paralysis may be incomplete, with sequelae mostly in the extremities. It is very difficult to foresee the long-term evolution of an acute crisis with neuropathy. The central nervous system is seldom involved; pyramidal signs, cerebellar syndrome, transitory blindness, or consciousness abnormalities can occur. The cerebrospinal fluid is usually normal. In general, neuropathy is now far less common than in the past.

During acute attacks, dehydration and electrolyte imbalance occur frequently and should be looked for and treated appropriately. Hyponatremia occurs in 40% of patients, and, when severe, it can lead to convulsions. Patients with acute hepatic porphyrias are at increased risk of developing chronic renal failure with progressive tubulointerstitial nephropathy and hepatocellular carcinoma.

Clinical manifestations are usually nonspecific, even in the presence of cutaneous lesions; only biologic data allow a precise diagnosis of the type of acute hepatic porphyria. Care should be taken not to ascribe all bouts of abdominal pain to acute porphyria because other acute abdominal conditions may be missed in these patients.

Laboratory Diagnosis

Attacks of acute porphyria are characterized by increased excretion of urinary ALA and/or PBG (20- to 200-fold higher). In ALA dehydratase deficiency porphyria and lead intoxication, the overexcretion is restricted to ALA. Treatment can be instituted immediately, while further laboratory investigations precise the porphyria type by analyzing porphyrin excretion patterns in urine, feces, and plasma (see Table 1).

Urinary uroporphyrin and coproporphyrin may be secondarily increased in acutely ill patients or in several other conditions such as hepatobiliary disease, alcohol abuse, and infections. Excess urinary porphyrin excretion alone lacks diagnostic specificity and is therefore insufficient evidence for symptoms to be ascribed to porphyria, even in a patient with known porphyria. High levels of precursors (ALA and mostly PBG), are the most important diagnostic indicators.

Treatment

Supportive Treatment

A careful search should be made for any precipitating factors, especially drugs (including oral contraceptives), underlying infection, and a hypocaloric diet. These precipitants should be withdrawn as soon as possible. Analgesia is a major component of supportive treatment. Opiates are usually required, often in high doses, together with an antiemetic and a phenothiazine such as chlorpromazine for anxiety and restlessness and to decrease the analgesic requirement. The danger of addiction in patients who experience frequent attacks must always be considered. Adequate fluid intake is essential, with regular monitoring of electrolyte status. Attention should also be paid to calorie intake. Both these requirements can be accommodated using 2 L of normal saline per day to which 5% glucose has been added. Other complications such as persistent hypertension and tachycardia, severe motor neuropathy, and seizures should be treated as they occur using drugs recommended as safe in these situations (Table 2).

Specific Treatment

Two specific therapies are mainly used: glucose and hematin. Before heme became available, carbohydrate loading was the only treatment for an acute attack. An adequate supplement (100 to 300 g/d) should be administered usually by slow intravenous perfusion. To minimize the danger of precipitating hyponatremia, glucose must be administered with careful management of intravenous fluids, including electrolyte measurement at least daily, and avoidance of hypotonic solutions.

Treatment of a porphyric attack was greatly improved by the introduction of hematin. Urinary ALA and PBG levels decrease dramatically in 2 to 3 days, a finding showing that feedback control of ALA synthase has become efficient. In the United States, lyophilized heme (Panhematin) is available, whereas a more stable preparation of human hemin (heme arginate [Normosang]) is widely available. Heme arginate is supplied as a concentrated solution that requires dilution in normal saline immediately before use. This solution should be infused at a dose of 3 to 4 mg/kg body weight per 24 hours over 20 minutes, and usually over 4 days. In practice, adults usually receive the entire contents of a single vial for each dose. An increased incidence of thrombophlebitis at the infusion site has been reported. Therefore, the following are recommended: the vein used for infusion should be changed every day, the infusion site should be flushed thoroughly with saline after heme arginate administration, and 5% human serum albumin may be included in the solution. Hematin has never been associated with serious hemorrhage; however, it should not be used in conjunction with

TABLE 2. **Management Summary for Acute Attacks and Cutaneous Porphyria**

	Treatment	Indication	Safe Drugs	Porphyria Information Resources
Acute Attacks (acute intermittent porphyria, variegate porphyria, hereditary coproporphyria)	Preventive	Prescribe drugs from safe drug list Avoid alcohol, Avoid smoking and cannabis Avoid dieting, fasting		United States: American Porphyria Foundation P.O. Box 22712 Houston, TX 77227 Web site: www.enterprise.net/apf/index.html
	Specific	Repress heme synthesis	Heme arginate, hematin	Europe: European Porphyria Initiative Web site: www.porphyria-europe.com
	Supportive	Stop porphyrinogenic drugs Maintain fluid, calorie intake	2 L normal saline containing 5% dextrose or glucose	Heath Park
		Treat symptoms		Cardiff CF 14 4XN (including a list of safe drugs) British Porphyria Association
		Pain	Aspirin, paracetamol, dihydrocodeine, pethidine, morphine, diamorphine	
		Vomiting/sedation	Promazine, chlorpromazine, cyclizine, ondansetron	14 Mollison Rise Gravesend, Kent DA 12 4QJ
		Constipation	Bulk laxatives, senna	
		Hypertension and tachycardia	Propranolol, atenolol, labetalol	France: Centre Français des Porphyries CHU Louis Mourier 92701 Colombes Cedex Web site: www.porphyries.com (including a list of safe drugs)
		Convulsions	Monitor and correct hyponatremia Diazepam (IV 10 mg once only), clonazepam, magnesium sulphate	
Cutaneous porphyria	Supportive	Sunlight avoidance Protective clothing Sunblocks (opaque sunscreens)		South Africa: Liver Research Centre University of Cape Town Cape Town Web site: www.uct.ac.za/depts/liver/porphpts.htm (including a list of safe drugs)
Porphyria cutanea tarda	Preventive	Prescribe drugs from safe drug list Avoid alcohol, Avoid smoking and cannabis Avoid dieting, fasting		
	Specific	Iron and porphyrin depletion	Venesection 500 mL twice weekly until remission Chloroquine 125 mg twice weekly until remission	
Congenital erythropoietic porphyria	Specific	Hemolytic anemia Restore erythroid heme synthesis	Blood transfusion Bone marrow transplantation	
Erythropoietic protoporphyria	Specific	Increase tolerance to sunlight Deplete hepatic protoporphyrin Hepatic failure	β-carotene 100–300 mg/d Activated charcoal 40-50 g/d Liver transplantation	

anticoagulant therapy. Other side effects are negligible, and heme arginate has been used successfully during pregnancy.

All the types of treatment described must be used early in the attack before any nervous or respiratory complication develops. Neither carbohydrate loading nor intravenous heme will reverse an established peripheral neuropathy.

Recurrent Acute Attacks

A few patients have repeated acute attacks. Women with cyclical premenstrual attacks may respond to suppression of ovulation with gonadotropin-releasing hormone analogues. If this treatment is successful, it can be continued for up to 2 years before attempting withdrawal. Otherwise, management of repeated attacks severe enough to require hospitalization is difficult. It may be possible to abort the development of an attack by prompt administration of heme arginate without the need of a full course: regular once-weekly administration of a single dose may help control the disease. Such patients are likely to require permanent indwelling venous catheters, with all their attendant complications. A few patients have now received very large cumulative doses of heme arginate without serious side effects, although hepatic iron overload has been observed.

Prevention

Symptomatic patients and those who are diagnosed after screening of the family should avoid predisposing factors such as drugs, alcohol, fasting, or hormones that are known to precipitate acute attacks. Benefit versus risk should always be considered in conjunction with the severity of the disorder requiring treatment and the disease activity of the porphyria. When difficult treatment decisions have to be made, consideration should be given to contacting a national center with expertise in managing porphyria for advice.

CUTANEOUS PORPHYRIAS

The cutaneous porphyrias present with photosensitivity, with symptoms restricted to sun-exposed skin. Two groups can be defined, based on their clinical features: those presenting with skin fragility and blisters (the bullous porphyrias) and those with acute photosensitivity (erythropoietic protoporphyria). Porphyrin-induced photosensitivity results from the absorption of light (wavelength 400 to 410 nm) at the surface of the skin and the subsequent production of reactive oxygen species that induce the inflammatory response and damage the skin.

General Supportive Treatment

Avoidance of sunlight and wearing of appropriate clothing to cover the skin decrease skin symptoms. Absorbent sunscreens are of little help because they are designed to block ultraviolet A and B radiation. Reflecting sunscreens containing zinc oxide or titanium dioxide are more effective, but their use is limited by their lack of cosmetic appeal.

Bullous Porphyrias

The skin lesions of PCT, hereditary coproporphyria, and variegate porphyria are quite similar; those of hepatoerythropoietic porphyria and congenital erythropoietic porphyria are more severe and present earlier. The lesions of photosensitivity affect areas exposed to light such as the backs of the hands, face, and neck and, in women, the legs and backs of the feet. Skin fragility is perhaps the most specific feature: minimal trauma is followed by a superficial erosion soon covered by a crust. Bullae or vesicles usually appear after exposure to the sun and take several weeks to heal, leaving hypopigmented or hyperpigmented atrophic scars. White papules (milia) may develop in areas of bullae, particularly on the backs of the hands. Hypertrichosis is often seen on the upper cheeks, ears, and arms. Increased pigmentation of sun-exposed areas is common.

Porphyria Cutanea Tarda

PCT results from decreased activity of urodecarboxylase (see Table 1). This most common form of porphyria is a heterogeneous group including three types:

1. The sporadic type (sPCT, type I; 80% of cases) is often observed in male patients without a family history of the disease. Its development appears to be related to an inducing compound such as alcohol, estrogens, iron overload, or hepatitis C virus (HCV). In this sporadic type, urodecarboxylase activity is deficient only in the liver.
2. The familial type (fPCT, type II, 20% of cases) has an earlier onset and is observed equally in both genders. In fPCT, there is a 50% reduction of urodecarboxylase activity in all tissues, and this defect is inherited in an autosomal dominant fashion.
3. Hepatoerythropoietic porphyria is the rare homozygous form of type II that presents in infancy or childhood and causes severe, blistering skin lesions.

Several risk factors are known to predispose patients to develop the enzyme deficiency associated with PCT. Variable degrees of liver dysfunction are common among patients with PCT, particularly in association with excessive alcoholic intake. The incidence of hepatic cancer among patients with PCT seems to be greater than in the general population. Among the precipitating factors, estrogens, iron overload, HCV, and, to a lesser extent, hepatitis B virus (HBV) and HIV, are most frequently incriminated. Many drugs classified as porphyrinogenic in acute porphyrias will also precipitate or exacerbate PCT; however, most patients receive these drugs (or alcohol) for several years before they develop PCT. Abnormal iron metabolism appears to be another precipitating factor in the clinical onset, probably related to oxidative radicals produced by reactive intracellular iron. Mutations of the *HFE* gene associated with hemochromatosis are found in fPCT and sPCT more commonly than in control populations, a finding indicating that genetic factors unrelated to the heme biosynthesis pathway can predispose to PCT. A strong association has been found between HCV and PCT in several countries. HBV and HIV are not as closely associated with PCT as HCV, but antibodies to HCV, HBV, and HIV should be evaluated in each patient with PCT at the time of diagnosis. These precipitating factors act either alone or in combination.

Urine contains increased concentrations of uroporphyrin and 7-carboxy-porphyrin; levels of coproporphyrin, 5-carboxylic-porphyrin, and 6-carboxylic-porphyrin are moderately increased. In the feces, the dominant porphyrin excreted is often isocoproporphyrin. During clinical remission, total porphyrin excretion decreases progressively, and measurement of urinary porphyrins and ferritin is one of the best methods for following the effects of treatment. After a few months, urinary porphyrin levels appear normal, but in the feces, coproporphyrin and isocoproporphyrin levels may remain increased for a long period.

All patients with PCT should first be advised to treat infectious disease (e.g., HCV, HIV) and to avoid precipitating factors (e.g., alcohol, pills, porphyrinogenic drugs) and exposure to sunlight until clinical and biologic remission has been obtained by treatment. Phlebotomy is at present the treatment of choice, even when serum iron or ferritin levels are not increased. A unit of blood (350 to 450 mL) is removed at 1-week intervals until transferrin saturation reaches 16% or less or the ferritin level is reduced to the lower limit of normal. Urine porphyrin levels are monitored every 3 months: clinical and biologic remissions are usually obtained within 6 months.

When phlebotomy is contraindicated (anemia, cardiac or pulmonary disorders, age) low-dose chloroquine therapy (200 mg weekly), which complexes with porphyrin and slowly mobilizes it from the liver, is the best alternative. The duration of treatment and relapse rate are only marginally greater than with venesection. High-dose treatment must be avoided because it causes a hepatitis-like syndrome in patients with PCT. In severe cases, combined phlebotomy and chloroquine therapy is often used with good results. Because of the high incidence of liver disease, liver function should be followed.

Skin blisters in patients receiving long-term dialysis may be caused either by PCT or pseudoporphyria. The differential diagnosis should be performed by porphyrin analysis in plasma or feces. In these cases, erythropoietin supplementation, in gradually increased doses, is given to increase erythropoiesis and thereby deplete excessive body iron stores.

The skin lesions of hereditary coproporphyria and variegate porphyria are quite similar. However, patients with variegate porphyria and hereditary coproporphyria may also suffer from neurovisceral symptoms. Treatment of skin manifestations in these two disorders is based purely on skin protection and removal of precipitating factors; phlebotomies and hydroxychloroquine are not helpful in these porphyrias.

Congenital Erythropoietic Porphyria

Congenital erythropoietic porphyria is a rare autosomal recessive disorder resulting from a marked deficiency of uroporphyrinogen III synthase activity (see Table 1). Skin blisters are observed in the neonatal period or in early infancy both in congenital erythropoietic porphyria and in hepatoerythropoietic porphyria, the rare homozygous form of type II PCT. Both are serious, chronic, progressive, and mutilating disorders associated with hemolytic anemia. Urine is reddish brown from the first day of life and exhibits a purple fluorescence under long ultraviolet light. The diagnosis is confirmed by a characteristic porphyrin pattern in urine, plasma, and feces. Treatment of hepatoerythropoietic porphyria and congenital erythropoietic porphyria involves skin protection and blood transfusions to maintain the hemoglobin concentration. Allogeneic bone marrow transplantation has been successful in several patients with moderate to severe disease.

Acute Photosensitivity Porphyria

Erythropoietic Protoporphyria

Erythropoietic protoporphyria results from decreased activity of the final enzyme in the heme synthetic pathway, ferrochelatase (see Table 1). It is an autosomal dominant disorder, with variable penetrance. The variable penetrance is the result of the co-inheritance of a low-expression allele, which, in addition to the abnormal allele, results in decreased ferrochelatase activity lower than the 50% threshold. Clinical manifestations of erythropoietic protoporphyria begin in childhood, with acute and severely painful photosensitivity and a history of burning in areas of skin exposed to sunlight. Pain is usually followed by edema, erythema, and swelling. Repeated exposures lead to chronic changes giving the skin a waxy, thickened appearance with faint linear scars.

Urine porphyrin levels are normal. The diagnosis is based on increased free protoporphyrin levels in erythrocytes and in plasma, which has a characteristic fluorescent emission peak (see Table 1). Patients often exhibit slight microcytic, hypochromic anemia. Liver dysfunction has been reported in up to 20% of patients with erythropoietic protoporphyria and hepatic failure in less than 5%. The liver dysfunction is caused by the accumulation of protoporphyrin in hepatocytes that results in cell damage, cholestasis, and further retention of protoporphyrin. Patients with erythropoietic protoporphyria may develop gallstones composed of protoporphyrin and are at increased risk of cholelithiasis.

Acute burning pain is ameliorated by the application of cold water. Avoidance of sunlight is the mainstay of management. Oral β-carotene (75 to 200 mg/d; optimal blood concentration of 11 to 15 μmol/L), which acts as a singlet oxygen trap, improves light tolerance in about one third of patients. It is impossible to predict which patients will develop severe liver disease, and management should include annual biochemical assessment of liver function. When liver dysfunction appears, treatment with cholestyramine, which depletes hepatic protoporphyrin, or activated charcoal, which binds protoporphyrin in the gut and interrupts the enterohepatic circulation, should be attempted, but the efficacy of these agents is not proved. Once liver failure is advanced, liver transplantation is usually the only treatment likely to ensure the patient's survival.

SUGGESTED READINGS

Anderson KE, Sassa S, Bishop DF, et al: The porphyrias. In Scriver CR, Beaudet AL, Sly WS, Valle D (eds): The Metabolic Basis of Inherited Disease, vol 1, 8th ed. New York, McGraw-Hill, 2001.

Deybach JC, H Puy: Acute intermittent porphyria from clinical to molecular aspects. In Kadish KM, Smith KM, Guilard R (eds): Porphyrin Handbook, vol 14. San Diego, Academic Press, 2003, pp 23–41.

Elder GH: The cutaneous porphyrias. In Hawk JLM (ed): Photodermatology. London, Chapman and Hall, 1998.

THERAPEUTIC USE OF BLOOD COMPONENTS

method of
EDWARD C. C. WONG, M.D., and
NAOMI L. C. LUBAN, M.D.
Children's National Medical Center
Washington, DC

Very rarely does transfusion of whole blood occur nowadays. It is necessary to have a well-grounded understanding of the biology and physiology of the individual cellular and liquid components of whole blood to prescribe the proper component for patients. Transfusion should be undertaken only if the anticipated benefit outweighs the potential risk. A sound decision by the physician whether to transfuse a particular product can come only through knowledge of the many blood components now available.

ADMINISTRATION OF BLOOD COMPONENTS

Responsibilities of the physician include explaining the benefits and risks of transfusion to the patient and obtaining informed consent in accordance with institutional guidelines. The transfusion process is initiated when a physician writes an order specifying the component and the volume to be given. In addition, pretransfusion medication, if indicated, rate and duration of administration, and use of a blood warmer or electromechanical device should be specified. The identity of the blood unit and the recipient must be verified at each step, starting from the collection of the sample for group, type, and crossmatch and continuing through release from the blood bank to the final infusion of the component. This verification may be done by using bar code or other identifier system. The patient's pretransfusion and post-transfusion vital signs must be recorded. All blood components must be administered through a macroaggregate particulate filter (170 to 260 μm), and the transfusion must be completed within 4 hours of the time of release from the blood bank.

Special infusion sets for high flow typically have large filter surface areas and large-bore tubing, and they include an in-line hand pump rapid infuser. For massive transfusion, as in cases of trauma, rapid infuser/blood warmers are available. Other special sets include mechanical infusers, gravity drip sets, and, for transfusion of small volumes of blood products, syringe-push sets. Microaggregate filters can be used for red blood cells to screen out microaggregates, which typically consist of degenerating platelets, leukocytes, and fibrin strands. Third-generation leukoreduction filters are used for white blood cell reduction of both red blood cell and platelet products. Presumed benefits include a reduced risk of cytomegalovirus (CMV) transmission, HLA alloimmunization, and febrile, nonhemolytic transfusion reactions. These filters may be used before storage of blood products, before transfusion, in the blood bank, or at the bedside.

Solutions that can be co-administered with red blood cells include normal saline (0.9% USP) and, under rare circumstances, 5% albumin, ABO-compatible plasma, or plasma protein fraction. Hypotonic or hypertonic saline, lactated Ringer's solution, 5% dextrose, and medications must not be administered with blood or blood components, to avoid hemolysis and loss of anticoagulation and to distinguish transfusion-mediated reactions from reactions mediated by other causes. Red blood cells and whole blood can be safely warmed to 37°C, but not more than 42°C using specifically designed devices. These devices are indicated for adults receiving rapid and multiple transfusions of red blood cells or whole blood at a rate of more than 50 mL/kg/hour, infants receiving rapid transfusions of more than 15 mL/kg/hour, adults or infants receiving exchange transfusions, and patients with cold agglutinin disease.

Blood or blood components can be modified in several ways to accommodate the patient's clinical situation. Red blood cell and platelet products can be issued in smaller amounts either to reduce donor exposure or to decrease the probability of volume overload. Washing of red blood cells or platelets may be necessary to reduce anaphylactoid reactions from foreign plasma protein exposure. For those patients who have a history of anaphylactic reaction to blood or blood components and who have demonstrable anti-IgA antibodies, IgA-deficient blood or blood components can be obtained. Similarly, those patients with antibodies to red blood cell antigens must receive red blood cell units negative for the antigens to which the patient has developed antibodies. Consultation with a transfusion medicine physician may be necessary in these cases.

RED BLOOD CELL PRODUCTS

Whole Blood

Allogeneic whole blood units are rarely used in the United States because they lack the advantages offered by component therapy. More frequently, whole blood units are collected for autologous transfusion. The standard single unit of whole blood contains 450 mL collected into 63 mL of anticoagulant-preservative solution. The hematocrit is usually between 36% and 44%, and the whole blood unit must be stored at 1°C to 6°C. Depending on the anticoagulant-preservative solution, the shelf life will range between 21 and 35 days. However, after 24 hours of storage, few functional platelets or granulocytes remain, and amounts of factors V and VIII are significantly decreased.

Whole blood units, when available, may be used in patients who are actively bleeding, with massive volume loss (more than 25%), and who need both oxygen-carrying capacity and blood volume expansion. However, these units should not be used for patients who are normovolemic because red blood cells are preferred in this setting. In an average-sized adult, 1 U of whole blood should increase the hemoglobin concentration by 1 g/dL and the hematocrit by 3% to 4%.

Other uses of whole blood units include blood prime for therapeutic procedures in patients with small blood volumes, neonatal exchange transfusions, and primes for devices such as selected cardiac bypass procedures and continuous hemoperfusion. However, whole blood units are often not available or are unsuitable because of decreased coagulation factor concentrations, especially of factors V and VIII. In these cases, reconstitution using red blood cell units and plasma-compatible fresh frozen plasma (FFP) or 5% albumin often suffices.

Red Blood Cells

Red blood cells are prepared by removal of 200 to 250 mL of plasma from 1 U of whole blood. Various anticoagulant-preservative solutions are used that influence the shelf life and hematocrit of the final product. Units prepared in citrate–monobasic sodium phosphate–dextrose (CPD) are approximately 250 mL in volume, with a hematocrit of 70% to 80% and a 21-day shelf life when they are stored at 1°C to 6°C. Units prepared in citrate–monobasic sodium phosphate–dextrose-adenine (CPDA-1) have a longer, 35-day shelf life with a similar volume and hematocrit as CPD-prepared units. More commonly in the United States and Canada, additive red blood cell units are available. Additive solutions such as AS-1 (Adsol: dextrose, adenine, mannitol, sodium chloride) and AS-3 (Nutricel: dextrose, adenine, monobasic sodium phosphate, sodium chloride) are available to extend the shelf life further, to 42 days at 1°C to 6°C. After hard packing of a whole blood unit, the additives are added using sterile technique. Units prepared with 100 mL of additive solution are approximately 350 mL in volume with a hematocrit of 50% to 60%. They have essentially no plasma, and they flow rapidly.

Red blood cells are indicated for patients with anemia who require an increase in oxygen-carrying capacity and red blood cell mass. As with whole blood, 1 U of red blood cells in an average-sized adult will usually raise the hemoglobin concentration by 1 g/dL and the hematocrit by 3% to 4%. In pediatric patients, a volume of 10 mL/kg (with an adjusted hematocrit of 80%) can be anticipated to raise the hemoglobin concentration by 3 g/dL. For additive units (which have an adjusted hematocrit of 65%), a volume of 10 mL/kg can be expected to result in a less than 3 g/dL increment.

LEUKOCYTE-REDUCED RED BLOOD CELLS

One unit of red blood cells contains approximately 10^8 white blood cells. This is approximately a log less than that contained in whole blood units. Current third-generation leukocyte reduction filters can provide a 3 log or 99.9% reduction of white blood cell content to less than 5×10^6 white blood cells and, with some filters, less than 1×10^6 per product. This leukocyte reduction step can be performed at the bedside or, preferably, shortly after collection at the blood center. However, many studies have found that more consistent transfusion of quality-controlled leukocyte-reduced products occurs when the red blood cells are leukocyte-reduced in the blood bank or blood center, where problem units and filter failure can be better identified.

Leukocyte-reduced red blood cells are indicated for patients with repeated febrile nonhemolytic transfusion reactions to cellular blood components or to minimize alloimmunization to foreign HLA antigens. Febrile nonhemolytic transfusion reactions are typically caused by reactions to donor white blood cells or to cytokines present in the product. Patients who have persistent febrile nonhemolytic transfusion reactions to bedside leukocyte-reduced products may benefit from the lower levels of cytokines present in prestorage leukocyte-reduced products. Alloimmunization to foreign HLA class I antigens is of significant concern for patients who may require repeated platelet transfusions. Because platelets also possess HLA class I antigens, patients sensitized to such antigens can become refractory to platelet transfusions. If the decision is made to use leukocyte-reduced red blood cells to prevent alloimmunization, it should be made before the first transfusion, and leukocyte-reduced platelets should also be used.

Controversial and unproven indications for leukocyte-reduced red blood cells include reduction of immunomodulation that may lead to an increased risk of cancer recurrence or bacterial infections, reduction in prion-transmitted disease, and reduction in *Yersinia entercolitica* contamination of red blood cells. Canada and many countries in Europe have already initiated universal leukocyte reduction. In the United States, the Food and Drug Administration (FDA) is in the process of creating a regulatory requirement or endorsing it as a product standard.

WASHED RED BLOOD CELLS

Red blood cell washing involves the use of sterile saline to rinse away the plasma remaining in a red blood cell unit. The procedure removes more than 98% of the plasma, including plasma proteins, microaggregates, and cytokines, as well as up to 20% of the red blood cells. The procedure takes approximately 1 to 2 hours with an automated cell washer, and the resultant product (about 180 mL) is suspended in sterile saline to a hematocrit of 70% to 80%. This product is indicated for severe, recurrent allergic reaction to blood components not prevented by premedication with an antihistamine. Typically, such reactions are caused by an allergy to plasma proteins. Patients known to be severely IgA-deficient with a circulatory anti-IgA antibody may have anaphylactic reactions to IgA present in blood components and should receive either red blood cells from IgA-deficient donors (ordered well in advance) or washed red blood cells. Because the washing process creates an open system, this component has a shelf life of only 24 hours at 1°C to 6°C. Washed red blood cells are not a substitute for leukocyte reduction because washing reduces the white blood cell content by only 1 log.

FROZEN-DEGLYCEROLIZED RED BLOOD CELLS

A freezing process involving a high glycerol concentration is used by most blood centers for long-term storage (up to 10 years at −65° or colder temperatures) of red blood cell units with rare phenotypes. Preparation requires thawing and deglycerolization using a series of saline-glucose solutions. The final hematocrit is between 55% and 70%, with a 94% to 99% reduction of white blood cell content and at least 80% of the original red blood cell mass remaining. If the units are thawed using a closed system, the shelf life is 2 weeks; however, in most blood centers, units are thawed using an open system mandating a shelf life of only 24 hours at 1°C to 6°C.

PHYSIOLOGIC BASIS FOR RED BLOOD CELL TRANSFUSIONS

Because of the risk of adverse reactions to blood transfusion, the American College of Physicians recommends that transfusion of allogeneic blood be avoided whenever possible. The primary indication for red blood cell transfusions is to restore or maintain oxygen-carrying capacity to meet tissue demands for oxygen. *Oxygen delivery* is the product of arterial oxygen content and cardiac output. *Critical oxygen delivery* is oxygen delivery below which organ function can no longer be maintained. The overall goal of intensive care support of the patient is to maintain an oxygen delivery reserve such that the critical oxygen delivery is never reached, and oxygen demand never exceeds supply in any critical tissue.

The ability of each individual patient to compensate for acute anemia and an alteration in oxygen demand by increased oxygen delivery to organs cannot be adequately determined in a practical manner aside from invasive monitoring. A National Institutes of Health panel in 1988 concluded that the traditional perioperative practice of transfusion of red blood cells at hemoglobin levels less than 10 g/dL should be replaced in the stable patient with no signs of end-organ hypoxia with a standard of 7 g/dL. Patients with hemoglobin levels between 7 and 10 g/dL may require red blood cell transfusions if signs of tissue hypoxia, such as tachycardia, chest pain, or shortness of breath, or electrocardiographic changes consistent with ischemia are present. A 1996 guideline by the American Society of Anesthesiologists states that a hemoglobin lower than 6 g/dL is "almost always" indicative of the need for transfusion, with clinical judgment reserved for patients with hemoglobin concentrations between 6 and 10 g/dL. A College of American Pathologists 1998 task force came up with similar recommendations and proposed using tachycardia, hypotension in the presence of normovolemia, mixed venous oxygen tension of less than 25 mm Hg and an oxygen extraction ratio greater than 50%, or a total oxygen consumption of more than 50% of baseline as indicators of transfusion. More recent studies of adult patients in intensive care units suggest that transfusion is associated with higher mortality rates, a finding that makes the judicious use of red blood cell transfusion all the more necessary.

PLATELET PRODUCTS

Whole Blood–Derived Platelets

Platelets prepared by centrifugation of individual (often termed *random donor*) units of whole blood must contain at least 5.5×10^{10} platelets in 50 to 70 mL of plasma. They must be stored at 20°C to 24°C under constant agitation because storage at cold temperatures has been shown to be detrimental to platelet function. As a result of these warmer storage temperatures, the shelf life of these products is only 5 days because the risk of bacterial contamination rises significantly during storage. Whole blood–derived platelet transfusions are indicated for: (1) bleeding caused by insufficient numbers of normal platelets or platelets with abnormal function, and (2) prophylactic use in patients with severe thrombocytopenia who are at risk of spontaneous hemorrhage or are undergoing an invasive procedure.

Thresholds for prophylactic transfusion vary depending on the circumstance and have come under increased scrutiny. In general, a platelet count greater than 50,000/μL is sufficient for primary hemostasis during most surgical and/or invasive procedures. A threshold of 100,000/μL may be indicated for procedures in which even minute bleeding can prove deleterious, such as complex neurosurgery and surgery of the retina or trachea. Historically, prophylactic transfusion of platelets was considered for patients with platelet counts lower than 20,000/μL associated with bone marrow hypoplasia as a result of primary disease or myeloablative chemotherapy. More recent studies have shown that hospitalized patients with platelet counts higher than 10,000/μL who are otherwise stable and who have no symptoms of clinical bleeding may not need prophylactic transfusion. This lower threshold of 10,000/μL for prophylactic platelet transfusions in stable patients is being adopted widely. Modification of this policy may be needed if a patient has other risk factors that may deleteriously affect platelet function such as fever, sepsis, or antibiotic therapy or if bleeding may result in severe clinical sequelae (i.e., central nervous system bleeding in a patient with a tumor of the central nervous system).

Platelet transfusions are often ineffective in certain conditions associated with accelerated platelet destruction or consumption, such as immune thrombocytopenic purpura, disseminated intravascular coagulation, sepsis, uremia, and hypersplenism. Platelet transfusions in these conditions may be tried in the setting of active bleeding. Platelet transfusions are contraindicated except in life-threatening hemorrhage for patients with thrombotic thrombocytopenic purpura/hemolytic uremic syndrome and heparin-induced thrombocytopenia. Platelet transfusions in these patients may promote platelet thrombus formation and serious thrombotic complications.

The conventional wisdom is that 1 U of random donor platelets raises the platelet count by 5000/μL in an average-sized adult in the absence of factors leading to increased platelet consumption or destruction. A standard adult dose of 1 U/10 kg and a pediatric dose of 5 to 10 mL/kg are commonly used. Traditionally, individual units of platelets have been pooled into a single bag for ease of administration. The pooling process decreases the shelf life to 4 hours. The standard number of units pooled at a given institution is often determined more by custom than by science. Standard pools of 6, 8, and, rarely, 10 U are used. Regimens decreasing the standard pool size to 5 or even 4 U and increasing the frequency of platelet transfusion are becoming more common based on studies in oncology patients.

Pheresis Platelets

Pheresis platelets are collected from a donor during a 2- to 3-hour cytapheresis procedure in which platelets are selectively removed in a volume of 200 to 400 mL plasma while the rest of the blood components are returned to the donor. This technique allows an increased yield of platelets from that single donor. Single pheresis platelet units contain approximately the same number of platelets as a pool of six to eight random donor platelets (minimum of more than 3×10^{11} platelets). Clinicians often prefer these products for the patient who requires long-term hemotherapy (i.e., those receiving high-dose chemotherapy) because these products expose the recipient to fewer donors, presumably decreasing the risk of acquiring transfusion-transmitted disease and reducing the risk of alloimmunization to foreign HLA antigens. More recent scientific studies, however, do not support these theoretical advantages of pheresis platelets. The indications for the use of pheresis platelets are essentially the same as for random donor platelets.

Leukocyte-Reduced Platelets

Current third-generation leukocyte reduction filters provide 3 log or 99.9% reduction of leukocytes present in either a pool of random donor platelets or pheresis platelet unit. After leukocyte reduction, these platelet products should contain fewer than 5×10^6 and often less than 1×10^6 white blood cells. Now available with current pheresis technology are prestorage leukocyte-reduced pheresis platelets in which the leukocyte reduction step is accomplished during the collection procedure. As with leukocyte-reduced red blood cells, leukocyte-reduced platelets presumably help to prevent or decrease febrile nonhemolytic transfusion reactions, alloimmunization to HLA antigens, and CMV transmission.

Platelet Refractoriness

Patients who fail to obtain an adequate increment in response to two sequential platelet transfusions are termed *refractory*. To assist in the diagnosis and treatment of such patients, it is useful to calculate the corrected count increment with the following formula:

$$\frac{(\text{Plt increment}/\mu\text{L}) \times \text{body surface area (m}^2)}{\text{Platelet dose (in multiples of } 10^{11})}$$

Two consecutive transfusions with a corrected count increment less than 7500/μL are presumptive evidence of the refractory state. This may be the result of either immune or nonimmune causes. Nonimmune causes (i.e., increased platelet sequestration, consumption, or destruction) include splenomegaly, fever, sepsis, disseminated intravascular coagulation, bleeding, antibiotic therapy, and use of immunosuppressive agents. No special platelet product can improve platelet increments in cases of nonimmune refractoriness. The underlying cause must be resolved, if possible, while the patient is supported with standard platelet products. Immune causes include autoantibodies, such as immune thrombocytopenic purpura or alloantibodies to HLA class I antigens (most common) or platelet-specific antigens (less common). Patients with immune thrombocytopenic purpura generally have broadly reactive autoantibodies that rapidly destroy transfused platelets as well. No special platelet products offer any improved benefit, and these patients should be supported with usual platelet products only in cases of active life-threatening bleeding. Patients shown to have alloimmune refractoriness can be supported with special platelet products (discussed later).

To distinguish immune from nonimmune causes, it is important to obtain post-transfusion platelet counts not later than 60 minutes after a platelet transfusion. Immune causes typically result in rapid destruction of transfused platelets, whereas nonimmune causes typically lead to lowered platelet counts over a period of hours. If an alloimmune refractory state is suspected, a specimen from the patient should be sent for evaluation of alloantibodies to HLA class I antigens. If the testing is negative, it is likely that the patient's refractory state has a nonimmune cause, and the patient should be supported with pooled random donor or pheresis platelet products. Rarely, the patient may have an antibody to a platelet-specific antigen. If this is suspected, a reference laboratory can identify those antibodies directed at specific platelet antigens.

If the screen for HLA alloantibodies is positive, the alloantibody specificity should be determined. If the number of specificities detected is limited, pheresis platelets that lack the antigens corresponding to the patient's alloantibodies (HLA antigen-negative pheresis platelets) may be tried. If the number of the specificities detected is great, then pheresis platelets that possess HLA antigens closely related or identical to the patient (HLA-matched pheresis platelets) should be tried. Not all HLA-matched pheresis platelets are equivalent, and their degree of identity with the patient is graded on a scale of A (most identical) to D (least identical). This must be considered when one judges responses to HLA-matched pheresis platelets. An alternative to HLA-matched platelets is the use of crossmatched platelets that produce negative reactions when the patient's specimen is crossmatched against specific HLA phenotyped donor platelets. The crossmatch technique requires screening for HLA or platelet-specific antibodies and a large number of phenotyped donors and hence is available only at major blood centers. Other measures that can be tried in refractory patients include using ABO-matched platelets and fresher platelets. Excellent communication between clinicians and transfusion medicine specialists is critical for success in managing refractory patients.

Pheresis Granulocytes

Granulocytes are the least used blood component, owing to the logistics of collection and the limited benefit with current collection methods. This component has limited storage viability and is prepared only when requested by the clinician through the recruitment and cytapheresis of a volunteer donor. Because granulocytes have a high specific gravity, white blood cell separation is enhanced during the collection process using a sedimenting agent such as hydroxyethyl starch. Corticosteroids are traditionally administered to the donor to mobilize white blood cells and to increase the yield. The component contains at least 1×10^{10} granulocytes with variable numbers of lymphocytes, platelets, and red blood cells in 200 to 300 mL plasma and is stored at 20°C to 24°C without agitation.

Granulocytes must be infused as soon as possible but no later than 24 hours after collection (stored at 20°C to 24°C). Depending on institutional protocols, this may require that the attending physician waive, in writing, viral serologic testing of the product and obtain separate consent from the recipient. Granulocytes are indicated for patients with severe neutropenia and overwhelming infection (bacterial or fungal) with a lack of response to prolonged antibiotic therapy and bone marrow demonstrating myeloid hypoplasia with a chance of future recovery. Although no general standard dose and duration of granulocyte transfusion therapy are recommended, a minimum of 1 to 2×10^{10} granulocytes/d is used as a guideline. Studies demonstrating the efficacy of the granulocytes for either treatment or prophylaxis of infections in neonates failed to show efficacy in a meta-analysis.

Several studies used recombinant granulocyte colony-stimulating factors in normal donors to increase collections to 6 to 8×10^{10} granulocytes per procedure. These granulocytes have the added benefit of improved function. The efficacy and potential toxicity of growth factor–stimulated products still await randomized clinical trials.

PREVENTION OF TRANSFUSION-ASSOCIATED GRAFT-VERSUS-HOST DISEASE

Foreign T lymphocytes are present in all cellular blood components and have the potential to cause transfusion-associated graft-versus-host disease in immunocompromised and non-immunocompromised recipients of HLA-haploidentical blood components. This disease has an up to 90% mortality and is characterized by fever, skin rash, diarrhea, hepatitis, and marrow aplasia. Transfusion-associated graft-versus-host disease can be prevented by gamma irradiation of cellular blood components with 2500 cGy. Donor units intended for blood relatives, intrauterine transfusion, neonatal exchange transfusions, premature infants, congenital acquired immunocompromised patients, and solid organ or stem cell transplant recipients should be irradiated. HIV-infected patients do not require irradiated blood. All HLA-matched products should be irradiated as well. Leukocyte-reduced products do not prevent transfusion-associated graft-versus-host disease because they still contain sufficient residual T lymphocytes to induce the graft-versus-host reaction.

PREVENTION OF CYTOMEGALOVIRUS DISEASE

Certain selected immunocompromised populations at risk of severe disease caused by primary infection with CMV should receive blood products that are less likely to transmit the virus. Cellular components from CMV-seronegative or, alternatively, leukocyte-reduced cellular blood components can be used. Patient populations at risk include CMV-seronegative stem cell or solid organ transplant recipients, CMV-seronegative pregnant women, low-birth-weight premature infants born to CMV-seronegative women, recipients of intrauterine transfusions, and those rare patients with acquired immunodeficiency syndromes who are CMV seronegative. HIV-infected patients do not benefit from CMV-negative blood components.

FRESH FROZEN PLASMA

FFP is plasma that is separated from a donated unit of whole blood and is frozen within 8 hours of collection. Plasma obtained by apheresis equipment can also be made into FFP. Each unit of FFP (220 to 250 mL volume) has a shelf life of 1 year when it is stored at −18°C or colder. These collection and storage conditions result in minimal loss of factors V and VIII.

FFP is indicated for patients with documented multiple coagulation factor deficiencies who are actively bleeding or at risk for bleeding before an invasive procedure. An unexplained prolonged prothrombin time or partial thromboplastin time should be confirmed to result from a factor deficiency before FFP infusion is considered. Prolonged prothrombin time and partial thromboplastin time resulting from heparin therapy or a circulating coagulation inhibitor are not indications for FFP therapy. FFP is, however, indicated on an emergency basis for reversal of bleeding associated with oral anticoagulant therapy if vitamin K replacement has failed or is untimely. FFP is also used during plasma exchange therapy for patients with thrombotic thrombocytopenic purpura/hemolytic uremic syndrome, congenital deficiencies of C1 esterase inhibitor, proteins C and S, antithrombin III, and isolated or combined factor deficiencies of factor II, V, VII, X, or XI. Recombinant or commercially available pooled plasma concentrates should be used whenever available in place of FFP. FFP should not be used for patients with minimal prolongation of coagulation testing (less than 1.5 × midpoint of normal range) before invasive procedures; there is little evidence that FFP prevents bleeding in this setting. FFP should not be used for volume expansion, as a nutritional source, or to enhance wound healing.

Because normal plasma contains a multiplicity of interrelated coagulation factors, the concentration of a single coagulation factor needed to maintain hemostasis ranges from 10% to 50% of normal levels. Factor levels of 50% are generally considered adequate for surgical hemostasis. For men, the volume FFP volume to infuse can be calculated using the following formula:

Estimated plasma volume (mL) = weight (kg) × 66 mL/kg × (1.0 − hematocrit)*

Factor level of hemostasis (%) = desired (%) − actual (%)

Volume FFP (mL) = % factor level for hemostasis × estimated plasma volume (mL)

*For neonates, children and adult females, this formula becomes slightly modified because the number of mL/kg is age and gender dependent. (For preterm infants, use 108 mL/kg; for term birth, use 100 mL/kg; for patients 2 to 10 years old, use 80 mL/kg; for adolescents, use 70 mL/kg; and for women, use 60 mL/kg.)

FFP is thawed at 30°C to 37°C. Thawed FFP has a shelf life of 24 hours when it is stored at 1°C to 6°C. Post-transfusion assessment of coagulation status is critical for determining efficacy.

Not all frozen plasma provided for component use is FFP. Some institutions stock only 24-hour frozen plasma, and others thaw plasma with a 5-day shelf life. Levels of factors V and VIII are lower in such products.

CRYOPRECIPITATE

When units of FFP are thawed at 1°C to 6°C, a precipitate of select plasma proteins forms. After expressing the cryo-poor supernatant plasma, the precipitate is refrozen at −18°C and has a shelf life of 1 year. This product, termed *cryoprecipitate*, contains 150 to 250 mg of fibrinogen and at least 80 IU of factor VIII, as well as high concentrations of von Willebrand factor, factor XIII, and fibronectin compared with the original FFP unit.

Cryoprecipitate is indicated for patients with bleeding who have severe congenital or acquired hypofibrinogenemia (less than 100 mg/dL), dysfibrinogenemia, or factor XIII deficiency. It may also be used as the basis for a topical fibrin sealant in certain surgical settings. It should be used for hemophilia A or von Willebrand's disease only if recombinant or virus-inactivated concentrates containing factor VIII or von Willebrand factor, respectively, are not available or for the rare variant form of von Willebrand's disease in which such concentrates are contraindicated. Cryoprecipitate is thawed at 30°C to 37°C. Thawed cryoprecipitate has a shelf life of 6 hours when it is stored at 1°C to 6°C. Typically, units of cryoprecipitate are pooled before transfusions, thus decreasing the shelf life to 4 hours. The dosage for treating hypofibrinogenemia (less than 100 mg/dL) can be estimated by the following formulas for men:

Estimated plasma volume (in dL) = weight (kg) × 0.66 dL/kg × (1.0 − hematocrit)*

Fibrinogen (mg) = [desired fibrinogen level (mg/dL) − initial fibrinogen level (mg/dL)] × estimated plasma volume in dL.

Units cryoprecipitate needed = fibrinogen (mg)/250 mg fibrinogen/U cryoprecipitate.

PLASMA DERIVATIVES

Plasma derivatives are concentrates of plasma proteins prepared from large donor pools (10,000 to 60,000) of plasma or cryoprecipitate. The specific protein of interest is purified, concentrated, and subjected to various procedures designed to inactivate or remove contaminating cell fragments, cytokine, and viruses. There are significant differences in the manufacture and viral inactivation or removal among different manufacturers of plasma derivatives.

*Again, this formula is slightly modified as for coagulation factor replacement (see earlier) for neonates, children, and women.

Methods of viral inactivation or removal include solvent-detergent (SD) treatment, 60°C to 80°C dry heat, 60°C heat in solution (pasteurization), immunoaffinity chromatography (monoclonal), and nanofiltration. There are rare reports of hepatitis B and hepatitis C transmission by 60°C heat-inactivated coagulation factor concentrates. There have been no reports of lipid-enveloped virus (HIV, hepatitis B and C viruses) transmission with products inactivated by SD treatments. Transmission of nonenveloped viruses such as hepatitis A and parvovirus, however, has been reported for SD-treated coagulation factor concentrates. Recombinant DNA technology has advanced the treatment of coagulation defects dramatically; albumin stabilization is used in some products, whereas newer products contain no albumin. To date, no transfusion-transmitted viral diseases have been identified in patients receiving these products. Nucleic acid testing of plasma pools for HIV, hepatitis C, and, with increasing frequency, parvovirus B19 and hepatitis A add a safety margin. SD plasma, called PLAS+SD, a pooled plasma product for more generic use, has become unavailable in the United States.

Human-derived and recombinant factor VIII preparations are available for short-term and prophylactic treatment of bleeding in hemophilia A and B patients. Certain selected human-derived factor VIII preparations (Humate-P, Alphanate, and Koate-HP) contain significant amounts of von Willebrand factor. They should be used for treatment of significant bleeding in von Willebrand's disease in place of cryoprecipitate.

Several different human-derived preparations of factor IX are available. Factor IX complex contains 1% to 5% of factor IX and some quantities of factors II, VII, and X. These additional factors, some of which become activated during preparation, increase the risk of thrombosis. Coagulation factor IX contains 20% to 30% of factor IX and only trace amounts of factors II, VII, and X, with less risk of thrombosis. These products have been used for factor IX–deficient patients and those with inhibitors to factor VIII during acute bleeding episodes. Recombinant formulations of factor IX (e.g., Benefix) are now available for acute and prophylactic use in congenital factor IX deficiency.

Recombinant factor VIIa (NovoSeven) is currently licensed for patients with inhibitors to factor VIII and IX. Off-label use for global coagulation deficiencies and platelet dysfunction syndrome has also been reported. Antithrombin III and protein C concentrates may be used for patients with congenital deficiency of these proteins who are at risk of thrombosis, but these concentrates are often in short supply or unavailable. Human albumin (5% and 25%) preparations are commonly used to provide colloid replacement. They contain 96% albumin with 4% globulin and other proteins and are heated in solution at 60°C for 10 hours to inactivate viruses. The 5% solution is osmotically and oncotically equivalent to human plasma. Albumin given to correct nutritional hypoalbuminemia or to treat ascites in patients with portal hypertension is of questionable benefit. Intravenous γ-globulin preparations contain 90% IgG and trace quantities of IgA and IgM; all manufacturers use one or more viral inactivation steps. These preparations are administered to provide IgG replacement for patients with immune deficiencies and are also used as immunomodulatory agents for autoimmune disorders such as immune thrombocytopenic purpura and Guillain-Barré syndrome. FDA advisories have warned of a thrombotic risk with IgG solutions.

ADVERSE REACTIONS TO BLOOD TRANSFUSIONS

method of
GERALD L. LOGUE, M.D.
Department of Medicine
State University of New York at Buffalo
Buffalo, New York

Transfusion medicine has developed as a clinical discipline with a strong scientific base over the past century. Advances in immunology and blood resource management have allowed transfusion therapy to become standard treatment for many medical conditions. Adverse reactions to blood transfusion therapy range from severe life threatening emergencies to those posing only minor inconvenience. These reactions may be immediate, occurring during or within hours of transfusion, or delayed, occurring days to months after transfusion.

IMMEDIATE TRANSFUSION REACTIONS

Immediate Hemolytic Transfusion Reactions

Transfusion of ABO-incompatible red blood cells, such as type A or B cells, into a type O recipient, results in the most dangerous and most preventable of immediate reactions. Naturally occurring complement-activating antibodies usually cause rapid intravascular hemolysis producing hemodynamic shock, disseminated intravascular coagulation, and acute renal failure. The prevention of acute hemolytic reactions requires special care to identify the blood drawn from the patient for analysis, as well as the blood products to be transfused. These identification procedures must be taken seriously, because clerical errors account for the majority of acute hemolytic transfusion reactions.

Effective therapy requires rapid diagnosis. All transfusions must be stopped immediately if there is a suspicion of such a reaction. Steps must be taken to identify the cause of this reaction.

Signs and symptoms of an acute hemolytic reaction in a conscious patient include fever, chills, pain at the site of infusion, back or chest pain, flushing, and generalized bleeding. In an unconscious patient, signs may include a falling blood pressure, increased bleeding or oozing, and hemoglobinuria. When an immediate hemolytic transfusion reaction is suspected, a sample of blood should be drawn from the patient and sent immediately to the blood bank with the donor blood. After infusion of ABO incompatible blood, the plasma is usually red. Fresh urine should be examined for hemoglobin.

If an acute hemolytic reaction is verified, therapy must begin immediately to maintain blood pressure, intravascular volume, blood pH, urine alkalinity, and urine output. Hypotension should be treated with volume replacement, and a screen for disseminated intravascular coagulation should be ordered. If the patient has overt disseminated intravascular coagulation, therapy with cryoprecipitate, 2 to 4 units, should be given if the fibrinogen level is less than 100 mg per dL; platelets, 4 to 6 individual units, should be given if the platelet count is less than 50,000 per mm^3 and fresh-frozen plasma, 1 to 3 units as tolerated by fluid volume status, given if the partial thromboplastin time is elevated. Mannitol or furosemide (Lasix) should be used as necessary to prevent acute tubular necrosis. Urine output and serum electrolyte and creatine levels should be monitored closely. Immediate hemodialysis may be required.

Acute Febrile Reactions

Febrile nonhemolytic reactions are characterized by fever and tachycardia. These reactions occur in previously transfused or multiparous patients and are caused by antileukocyte antibodies. When fever occurs during a blood transfusion, the transfusion should be stopped and the patient studied for a hemolytic reaction. If a hemolytic reaction has not occurred, antipyretics such as acetaminophen may be administered. If a patient has recurrent febrile reactions, it may be necessary to premedicate with antipyretics before the transfusion. White blood cell antibodies can rarely produce a transfusion-associated acute respiratory distress syndrome that is characterized by pulmonary edema with normal cardiac function. Microaggregate filters are useful to prevent febrile transfusion reactions as well as transfusion-associated acute respiratory distress syndrome.

Rarely, blood products become contaminated with bacteria. Some gram-negative organisms such as *Yersinia spp.* and *Pseudomonas spp.* can survive and multiply under refrigerated conditions. If this complication is suspected, the transfusion must be discontinued and the blood product must be cultured and Gram stained immediately. If a contaminated transfusion is suspected, therapy should include support of the patient's blood pressure, kidney function, and tissue oxygenation. Shock, if present, is caused by infusion of endotoxin, but broad-spectrum antibiotics should also be initiated pending the results of culture.

Acute Urticarial Reactions

Hives occur in approximately 3% of patients who receive blood transfusions and usually are caused by a reaction to plasma antigens present in the transfused blood. Such reactions are rarely serious. To treat this reaction, the transfusion is stopped and an antihistamine such as diphenhydramine administered. The patient is then watched carefully for 10 to 30 minutes. If further signs and symptoms of allergic reaction such as dyspnea, wheezing, chills, or fever ensue, epinephrine may be given.

Congestive Heart Failure

Hypervolemia may occur when blood is rapidly given to patients with compromised cardiovascular status. Such patients obviously should receive packed red blood cells rather than whole blood. For patients with severe chronic anemia who have evidence of congestive heart failure, packed red blood cells should be infused slowly with the patient in a semi-upright position. Packed red blood cell transfusions are usually well tolerated, and the increased oxygen-carrying capacity of the blood hastens the patient's overall improvement.

Anaphylactic Reactions

Anaphylactic reactions to blood are extremely rare. Patients who are IgA deficient may experience anaphylactic reactions after receiving blood products. These reactions are caused by antibiotics against IgA, usually in individuals previously exposed to blood products. The incidence of severe IgA deficiency in the general population is approximately 0.1%. If an anaphylactic reaction to blood products is suspected, the patient should have quantitation of serum IgA levels before further transfusion therapy is attempted.

Complications of Massive Blood Product Transfusion

Other immediate reactions include the potential for citrate toxicity. With massive infusions of large volumes of blood products containing citrate, it is potentially possible to decrease ionized calcium levels. When massive transfusions are being given, it is important to continue careful cardiac monitoring, and if arrhythmias related to calcium occur, it is important that intravenous calcium be administered. Also, hypothermia can be produced with massive blood transfusions of cold blood. Acute vascular hypothermia may affect platelet function and produce cardiac arrhythmias. In all situations of massive transfusion, temperature-controlled warming devices should be used to warm blood before infusion. With large-volume transfusion it is also theoretically possible to produce hyperkalemia by potassium leakage from stored red blood cells. Transfusion-associated hyperkalemia is rare, but in a large-volume transfusion situation, careful monitoring for cardiac arrhythmias related to hyperkalemia is also essential. Dilutional coagulopathy and thrombocytopenia are occasionally seen when massive transfusion requirements are met by transfusion of packed red blood cells alone. It is useful to transfuse fresh-frozen plasma and platelets along with red blood cells if the blood loss exceeds an entire blood volume.

DELAYED TRANSFUSION REACTIONS

A variety of complications may occur days to months after transfusion of blood products. Some of these reactions are immune, but the largest number of reactions occur as the result of the transfusion of infectious agents. The blood supply in the United States is safe because blood is collected from volunteer donors whose history is carefully evaluated and the blood is tested for markers of infectious disease including HIV and hepatitis.

Delayed Hemolytic Transfusion Reactions

Delayed hemolytic reactions occur in patients who have previously been sensitized to minor blood group antigens but whose antibody levels have fallen below detectability by routine screening procedures. After transfusion, an anamnestic antibody response occurs, usually within 2 weeks after transfusion of red blood cells containing the offending antigen. These reactions are characterized by a falling hemoglobin level and a rise in the bilirubin concentration. The direct antiglobulin test may or may not become positive transiently, but plasma antibody against the antigen usually becomes detectable in 1 to 2 weeks. Although the hemolysis remains limited to the transfused cells that possess the antigen, delayed transfusion reactions may rarely produce abrupt intravascular hemolysis with the risk of renal failure. It is important to identify delayed hemolytic transfusion reactions because on subsequent transfusion, the antibody may again have disappeared, and blood bank records are the only method of identifying the antibody and preventing recurrent, delayed hemolytic transfusion reactions.

Post-Transfusion Purpura

Post-transfusion purpura is a rare, delayed reaction of blood transfusion that occurs most commonly after packed red blood cell transfusions. Patients with post-transfusion purpura usually lack a common "public" platelet antigen such as PL^{A1} (HPA-1A). When these individuals are transfused with the antigen, an immune thrombocytopenic syndrome that destroys the patient's own platelets is triggered. The reaction is characterized by the abrupt onset of severe thrombocytopenia, usually with bleeding, 3 to 14 days after the transfusion of blood products. Treatment is empirical and includes the use of high-dose intravenous immune globulin (2 grams per kg) and plasmapheresis.

Transfusion-Associated Graft-Versus-Host Disease

Because blood products contain circulating stem cells, a transfusion recipient, especially if immunocompromised, may be inadvertently engrafted with the donor stem cells and develop graft-versus-host disease. The clinical complex of rash, mucositis, diarrhea, and abnormal liver functions from this disease may not be recognized in transfusion recipients. Although such complications usually occur in patients with recognized immunosuppression, they have been described in patients with no known predisposing conditions. Clinical symptoms usually occur 1 to 2 weeks after transfusion and are almost invariably fatal. Thus, it is extremely important that patients with known or suspected immunodeficiency syndromes receive irradiated blood products. It is also recommended that blood irradiation be used for directed donations from first-degree relatives.

Viral Agents

Hepatitis Viruses

Hepatitis B and C can be transmitted by transfusion of blood products. Screening of blood for hepatitis B virus is well characterized and effectively eliminates the transfusion of this agent by blood products. Hepatitis C testing eliminates the vast majority of hepatitis C transmissions. Thus, with the advent of rigorous testing for the various hepatitis viruses, the likelihood of transmitting viral hepatitis has been reduced to the range of 1% or less in most areas.

Retroviruses

Human immunodeficiency virus types 1 and 2 (HIV1 and HIV2) and human T cell lymphotropic virus types I and II (HTLV) may be transmitted by blood products. Prevention of transmission of HIV in blood products is accomplished by several mechanisms. The first includes rigorous questioning to exclude individuals likely to be infected with the virus and immunologic screening, including testing for HIV antibodies and, most recently, HIV antigen testing in transfusion products. These testing procedures make the transmission of HIV by transfusion extraordinarily rare. HTLV screening also occurs. As in other situations described previously, leukodepletion may markedly reduce the transmissibility of agents such as HTLV.

Herpesvirus

The herpesvirus cytomegalovirus and Epstein Barr virus are known to be transmitted by blood products. Most individuals receiving transfusion therapy are immune to Epstein-Barr virus, so the significance of transmission of this virus is questionable. Cytomegalovirus can also be transmitted by transfusions of blood products, and cytomegalovirus-negative blood is used in certain restricted situations such as for low-birth-weight infants and bone marrow transplant recipients. It is also clear that leuko-depletion of blood products markedly reduces the transmissibility of cytomegalovirus infection.

Parvovirus

Parvovirus, an agent that produces erythroid hypoplasia, may be transmitted by transfusion. Parvovirus-induced aplastic anemia is a risk in patients with underlying hematologic diseases with increased red blood cell production such as patients with sickle cell disease. There is no effective method to screen transfusion products for this virus.

Transmission of Other Infections

Rare diseases transmitted by transfusion therapy include malaria, trypanosomiasis, babesiosis, and syphilis. Transmission of falciparum, vivax, and ovale malaria has been controlled by deferring the donation of blood by potentially exposed individuals for 6 months. Persons who have been infected with *Plasmodium malariae* are excluded from blood donation because of the high incidence of asymptomatic carriers of this disease. *Trypanosoma cruzi* causes Chagas' disease in Latin America. Transmission in developed countries has occurred through blood donations from immigrants from areas endemic for this agent. Creutzfeldt-Jakob disease could theoretically be transmitted by transfusion, but no cases of such transmission have been clearly proved. Epidemiologic studies continue in this area. Finally, transmission of *Treponema pallidum*, the causative agent of syphilis, is possible through blood transfusion. Current serologic testing includes studies to detect circulating antibodies to these agents. Although some have suggested that syphilis screening is no longer necessary for blood products, it is likely that identifying individuals who have been exposed to syphilis is also a surrogate marker for other sexually transmitted infections and, therefore, a useful means of excluding blood donors who are potentially infectious with retroviruses.

Immune Modulation

Controversy exists regarding the role of transfusion of blood products in modulation of the recipient's immune system. This immune modulation probably occurs through exposure of the individual to donor leukocytes. Some retrospective clinical studies suggest that recurrence of tumors is increased after resection in individuals who have received blood products. Also, both retrospective and prospective human studies have found an increase in postoperative bacterial infections in individuals receiving transfusion therapy. This increased risk of bacterial infection appears to be reduced with leuko-depleted blood products. Clinical studies in this area are continuing. Leuko-reduced blood products are also useful for reducing primary HLA alloimmunization in transfusion recipients. Leuko-reduction is clearly most beneficial for prevention of recurrent febrile nonhemolytic transfusion reactions as described previously.

Iron Overload

Chronic transfusion therapy carries the long-term risk of iron overload. Transfusions in the range of 50 to 100 units of red blood cells carry the risk of tissue damage similar to that seen with idiopathic hemochromatosis, including endocrine, hepatic, and cardiac failure. Symptoms of iron overload may be insidious, and the clinical diagnosis may not be established early. The iron chelation agent deferoxamine (Desferal) is available but difficult to use. Clearly, the judicious use of chronic transfusions is indicated, including erythropoietin administration whenever possible.

Section 7

The Digestive System

CHOLELITHIASIS AND CHOLECYSTITIS

method of
ROBERT V. REGE, M.D.
The University of Texas Southwestern Medical Center
Dallas, Texas

Gallstones may be found in up to 10% of individuals younger than 50 years and are one of the most common disorders in human beings. Their incidence increases with advancing age, and they are even more common in obese patients, diabetic patients, and individuals with a family history of gallstones. A genetic influence on gallstone formation and growth is clearly operative because some ethnic groups (e.g., American Indians) have extremely high rates of gallstone formation. Gallstone formation has also been associated with parenteral nutrition, rapid weight loss, and ileal diseases. Most gallstones remain asymptomatic for long periods and never cause clinical disease, but some become symptomatic and induce severe attacks of abdominal pain or lead to serious complications such as acute cholecystitis, obstructive jaundice, pancreatitis, gallstone ileus, and ascending cholangitis. More than 600,000 operations are performed each year in the United States for symptomatic gallstone disease.

Cholecystectomy remains the treatment of choice for the great majority of patients. Currently, laparoscopic cholecystectomy is possible in 95% of patients with uncomplicated disease and 60% to 90% of patients with advanced disease, depending on the severity of inflammation or fibrosis. When successful, laparoscopic cholecystectomy decreases the length of hospital stay and time to complete recovery when compared with open surgery. However, other modalities, such as endoscopic retrograde management of bile duct stones, percutaneous approaches to the biliary tract, lithotripsy, and gallstone dissolution also play a key role in the treatment of select patients, and a comprehensive approach to biliary tract disease requires a team of well-trained surgeons, interventional gastroenterologists, and interventional radiologists.

TYPES OF GALLSTONES

Gallstones are classified as cholesterol, mixed, and pigment gallstones by gross and compositional analysis. Cholesterol and mixed gallstones are largely composed of cholesterol, but they usually contain calcified shells or pigmented centers that preclude dissolution therapy. Together, they account for 80% of gallstones in the West. Pigment gallstones are found in 10% to 27% of gallstone patients. Black pigment gallstones are composed mainly of an amorphous bilirubin polymer and calcium salts or calcium bilirubinate. Black pigment gallstones are more common in the elderly and in patients with hemolytic anemia or cirrhosis. Calcium bilirubinate stones usually form behind biliary strictures or in bile containing bacteria or parasites.

ASYMPTOMATIC GALLSTONES

In the past, it was thought that patients with asymptomatic gallstones were at great risk for the development of symptoms or complications, and prophylactic operations were uniformly offered to these patients. Longitudinal studies with ultrasound corrected this misconception by showing that symptoms or complications developed in only 1% to 2% of patients per year. The risk of observation of patients with asymptomatic gallstones is less than the risk of prophylactic surgery, which is therefore no longer recommended. Select groups of patients with gallstones may have a higher risk of problems developing and deserve prophylactic surgery. The cumulative risk of symptoms or complications developing over many years is thought to justify cholecystectomy in children. Symptomatic disease develops at a higher rate in patients with congenital hemolytic anemia, in individuals with large gallstones (greater than 2.5 cm), and in morbidly obese patients who undergo rapid weight loss after surgery than in the general population, and these individuals may benefit from prophylactic surgery. In the past, it was taught that gallstones, complications of gallstones, and complications after emergency/urgent surgery were more likely to develop in diabetic patients. Recent studies have demonstrated similar outcomes for diabetic and nondiabetic patients, and prophylactic surgery for diabetic patients is no longer recommended.

Removal of a gallbladder containing asymptomatic gallstones at an operation performed for another reason must weigh the risks and benefits of an added procedure. Incidental cholecystectomy seems to be justified in conjunction with colectomy because symptoms develop in as many as 20% of these patients within 5 years. Removal of the gallbladder adds no significant morbidity or mortality to the primary operation. Little data exist regarding incidental cholecystectomy during other abdominal operations. It may not be prudent in some situations (e.g., prosthetic material required), and the decision to perform incidental cholecystectomy in most circumstances must be left to the discretion of the surgeon.

SYMPTOMATIC GALLSTONES

Right upper quadrant and epigastric pain beginning 15 to 60 minutes after meals is quite specific for gallstone disease and is termed "biliary colic." Colic is, however, a misnomer because the pain is usually constant, not colicky. Ingesting fatty foods, onions, cabbage, spicy foods, or dairy products may trigger an episode of pain that lasts from 20 minutes to several hours. Pain lasting longer than 3 hours suggests complicated gallstone disease or pain from another abdominal disease process. Patients with symptomatic gallstones or chronic cholecystitis can expect episodes to increase in frequency and severity, and complications of gallstone disease are more likely to develop than in those with asymptomatic gallstones. By 2 to 5 years, at least 50% of symptomatic patients require operative treatment. The risk of observation of symptomatic gallstones is higher than the risk of surgery. Cholecystectomy is clearly indicated in these patients if co-morbidities do not make operative treatment prohibitive.

A group of patients with gallstones who have vague mild pain, indigestion, flatulence, and nausea without vomiting are now classified as being mildly symptomatic or having atypical symptoms. These symptoms are not specific for gallstone disease and may be caused by a multitude of other gastrointestinal disorders. Patients with mildly symptomatic gallstones act more like asymptomatic than symptomatic patients; only 1% to 2% per year require cholecystectomy. Surgery should be recommended only for persistent symptoms after other upper gastrointestinal disorders such as ulcer disease and gastroesophageal reflux disease are excluded. Cholecystectomy may be used to relieve symptoms in 50% to 70% of patients with persistent symptoms, especially if they significantly interfere with their lifestyle, but patients must understand that they have a considerable chance that surgery will not relieve their symptoms.

Chronic acalculous cholecystitis and cholesterolosis of the gallbladder may cause symptoms typical of gallstone disease, but specific tests do not exist for these disorders. Obviously, ultrasound will not reveal gallstones, but it may reveal a gallbladder polyp or "sludge." An oral cholecystogram may reveal no or only faint visualization of the gallbladder and can therefore demonstrate impaired gallbladder function. Impaired gallbladder emptying measured with ultrasound or gallbladder scintigraphy (hepatic 2,6-dimethyliminodiacetic acid [HIDA] scanning) after the administration of cholecystokinin may suggest gallbladder disease in some of these patients, but the specificity and sensitivity of this test is low. The diagnosis is thus most often made clinically, with the imaging studies supporting but not ensuring the diagnosis. Similar to patients with mildly symptomatic disease, relief of symptoms in patients undergoing operative therapy after this test ranges from 50% to 70%.

CHRONIC CHOLECYSTITIS

Patients with a clear history of biliary colic and the presence of gallstones on an imaging study meet the criteria for surgery. Cholecystectomy will relieve symptoms in 90% to 95% of patients with typical symptoms. Ultrasonography is the imaging study of choice because it is noninvasive and successfully demonstrates the gallstones in 90% to 95% of patients. Plain films of the abdomen and computed tomography (CT) are not very sensitive and demonstrate gallstones in only 20% of patients when they are present. However, if these studies detect gallstones, they are very accurate. On the other hand, when gallstone disease mimics another abdominal disease or when other gastrointestinal disorders mimic gallstone disease, extensive testing may be required before surgery is recommended. Upper and lower gastrointestinal endoscopy or radiologic barium studies, liver function tests, 24-hour pH monitoring, CT, oral cholecystography, ultrasonography, or gallbladder scintigraphy (HIDA scan) may be needed to exclude gastroesophageal reflux, peptic ulcer disease, hepatitis, pancreatitis, intestinal pathology, and malignant tumors of the stomach, bile duct, duodenum, or pancreas, or these studies may be necessary to document gallbladder abnormalities.

Operative Treatment of Chronic Cholecystitis

Cholecystectomy is the treatment of choice for patients with symptomatic cholelithiasis. This operation can be performed with a mortality rate less than 0.3%, and it relieves symptoms in 95% of patients either laparoscopically or by the open method. Overall, only about 5% to 10% of patients require open surgery, although conversion rates may reach 30% to 40% in patients with severe acute cholecystitis or gangrene of the gallbladder. Bile duct injury is reported to occur in 1 in 800 patients treated by open surgery and in 1 in 400 to 800 patients treated laparoscopically. Experienced laparoscopic surgeons report complication rates with laparoscopic cholecystectomy comparable to those of open cholecystectomy. The laparoscopic approach is not safe or prudent in 5% to 10% of patients, and the surgeon should convert to an open operation liberally. Safety is the primary concern of the surgeon, and conversion of the operation to open cholecystectomy should not be considered a failure.

ACUTE CHOLECYSTITIS

Acute cholecystitis is the most common complication of gallstones and occurs in about 10% of patients. It is caused by cystic duct obstruction by a gallstone, tumor, or swelling. Bacteria in bile infect the gallbladder wall and, if unchecked, lead to gallbladder perforation, pericholecystic abscess, or peritonitis. As the process progresses, inflammation, swelling, and fibrosis increase and make surgery more difficult. Patients may be successfully treated medically with bowel rest and antibiotics, but they will eventually require cholecystectomy. Operative treatment remains the treatment of choice, although the timing of surgery is still controversial.

Patients are initially seen with unremitting right upper quadrant pain. Most patients also have fever, an elevated white blood cell (WBC) count, and/or nausea and vomiting. Ultrasonography is the most common test for confirming the presence of gallstones, and the gallstones are often accompanied by a thickened gallbladder wall, a gallbladder "rim" sign, or an ultrasonographic Murphy sign (pain when the gallbladder is compressed with the ultrasound probe). Gallbladder scintigraphy (HIDA scan) is helpful in those in whom the signs and symptoms are less typical. HIDA scans are very sensitive and specific for acute cholecystitis in that the gallbladder will not be visualized in 98% of patients because of cystic duct obstruction. Gallbladder visualization occurs in a few patients with acute acalculous cholecystitis (false-negative result). HIDA scans are not reliable in critically ill patients and patients maintained by parenteral nutrition who have not emptied their gallbladders. Percutaneous aspiration of the gallbladder, along with Gram stain and culture of the aspirate, may be helpful in these latter patients and is therapeutic if a gallbladder drain is left in place.

Patients with acute cholecystitis should be admitted to the hospital, given nothing by mouth, and treated with broad-spectrum parenteral antibiotics. A second-generation cephalosporin or a combination of ampicillin-sulbactam and an aminoglycoside will suffice and should be continued postoperatively. A nasogastric tube is placed if the patient has persistent vomiting. In the past, patients were treated until resolution, and cholecystectomy was performed in 4 to 6 weeks. However, worsening symptoms or complications such as gallbladder perforation develop during treatment in up to a third of patients, and they require urgent cholecystectomy. Therefore, medical treatment with delayed cholecystectomy is not the treatment of choice, although it is still indicated for patients with significant co-morbidities precluding operative therapy. High-risk patients who fail medical therapy may be successfully treated with percutaneous cholecystostomy.

Surgery is now more often performed within 24 to 72 hours because the complication rate and chance of successfully performing the procedure are not improved by delaying cholecystectomy for 6 weeks. The likelihood of successfully performing a laparoscopic procedure is related to the duration of symptoms experienced by the patient. Success is highest if surgery is performed when the onset of symptoms is less than 72 hours earlier; conversion rates during this period approximate those for elective cases. Conversion rates may be as high as 30% to 40% if surgery is performed 7 to 14 days after the onset of symptoms, a period sufficient for the initiation of severe inflammation and fibrosis. Laparoscopic cholecystectomy for gangrenous cholecystitis results in similar conversion rates. It is important to understand that patients who are successfully treated with the laparoscope derive the benefits of this minimally invasive approach and that patients converted to an open operation fare no worse than those who are treated from the onset with open surgery. It is thus prudent to attempt laparoscopic cholecystectomy in these patients and convert to an open operation if the dissection does not progress satisfactorily or if the biliary tract anatomy cannot be clearly defined.

About 5% of patients with acute cholecystitis do not have gallstones, and these patients are often critically ill. The diagnosis is frequently delayed because the signs and symptoms of cholecystitis cannot be elicited because of the patient's medical condition, ultrasound findings may be unremarkable, and HIDA scanning is not reliable in those who have not eaten and emptied their gallbladder. Urgent cholecystectomy or percutaneous cholecystostomy is warranted in patients with acalculous cholecystitis because this disease may rapidly progress to gangrene and perforation.

COMMON BILE DUCT STONES

Common bile ducts stones are present in as many as 10% to 20% of patients undergoing cholecystectomy. Only about 4% without preoperative risk factors will have "silent" common bile duct stones. Intraoperative cholangiography can be performed either routinely or selectively with the laparoscope, but it should always be performed in patients at high risk for choledocholithiasis (Table 1) and whenever the biliary anatomy is not well defined by operative dissection. Choledocholithiasis also causes obstructive jaundice, usually associated with pain. Ultrasonography is used to document stones in the gallbladder and dilated intrahepatic and extrahepatic ducts. It will occasionally demonstrate a stone in the common bile duct. CT also demonstrates dilated intrahepatic and

TABLE 1. **Criteria for Intraoperative Cholangiography**

Clinical history	Jaundice Pancreatitis
Abnormal laboratory values	↑ Bilirubin ↑ Alkaline phosphatase ↑ γ-Glutamyltransferase
Preoperative imaging	
Ultrasound or CT	Dilated extrahepatic ducts (common bile duct >7 mm) Dilated intrahepatic ducts
ERCP	Choledocholithiasis
MRCP	Choledocholithiasis
Intraoperative indicators	Palpable stone Dilated common bile duct Large cystic duct/small stones

Abbreviations: CT = computed tomography; ERCP = endoscopic retrograde cholangiopancreatography; MRCP = magnetic retrograde cholangiopancreatography.

extrahepatic bile ducts, and it excludes mass lesions in the pancreas. The cause of jaundice may best be ascertained by directly imaging the biliary tract. Endoscopic retrograde cholangiopancreatography (ERCP) is the procedure of choice because it is successful in 90% to 95% of patients and has low complication rates. It may also be therapeutic. Percutaneous transhepatic cholangiography is reserved for patients in whom ERCP cannot visualize the proximal biliary tract. It is successful and safe in more than 90% of patients with dilated intrahepatic ducts, but it is more likely to result in complications such as bile leakage and hemorrhage.

Surgeons have several options for the treatment of patients with suspected common bile duct stones: routine preoperative ERCP with or without sphincterotomy plus stone removal when present, intraoperative cholangiography followed by common duct exploration (laparoscopic or open) or intraoperative ERCP, or postoperative ERCP with or without sphincterotomy plus stone removal. In addition, small stones (<5 mm) may be observed, with intervention reserved for patients with symptoms.

The routine use of preoperative ERCP in all patients at risk for common bile stones incurs the highest cost per residual stone avoided. It is cost-effective if the risk of a common bile duct stone is greater than 80%, which is the case if the patient has cholangitis, persistent jaundice, or unresolving pancreatitis or, of course, if a common bile duct stone is visualized by another test. Intraoperative cholangiography with laparoscopic common bile duct exploration either by the transcystic duct method or via choledochotomy is effective, safe, and cost-effective. Success rates between 90% and 97% and morbidity less than 5% are the norm. Although results are comparable, transcystic duct exploration is performed much more frequently than laparoscopic choledochotomy. Because open common bile duct exploration is associated with greater morbidity, length of hospital stay, and recovery time than postoperative ERCP is, it is now primarily reserved for very large common bile duct stones.

Intraoperative ERCP is technically difficult and advocated by a few. The logistics of performing this procedure in the operating room are complex. Observation of small (<5mm), asymptomatic common bile duct stones is reasonable and rarely associated with complications. Contrast should be seen to flow into the duodenum on cholangiography. Patients in whom symptoms develop require prompt ERCP with stone removal, which is almost always successful.

OTHER COMPLICATIONS OF GALLSTONES

Gangrenous cholecystitis, gallbladder empyema, emphysematous cholecystitis, and gallbladder perforation are advanced manifestations of acute cholecystitis. Patients with these complications frequently have higher than expected WBC counts, severe abdominal pain often associated with abdominal guarding or rebound, high fever, and failure to respond to medical therapy. Unfortunately, complicated gallbladder disease may have a minimum of findings and can be very difficult to diagnose. A high index of suspicion must be maintained, especially in patients who are initially seen late after the onset of symptoms. A typical patient with complicated disease is a man older than 60 years who has a history of cardiovascular disease. Although the patient may not have a significant fever, the WBC count is often greater than 16,000.

Imaging studies are helpful if they reveal significant findings, but such is often not the case. Abdominal radiographs or CT scans show air in the gallbladder wall or lumen with emphysematous cholecystitis. Ultrasonography or CT demonstrates pericholecystic fluid, subhepatic fluid, or an abscess with gallbladder perforation. Urgent abdominal exploration is indicated if advanced disease is suspected because these complications are associated with significant mortality and morbidity.

Acute gallstone pancreatitis results when a gallstone passes into and through the common bile duct. Patients have severe epigastric pain, left upper quadrant pain, elevated values of serum amylase or lipase, gallstones, and no other obvious cause for the pancreatitis. Attacks range from very mild and transient to life threatening. The gallstone usually passes into the duodenum when the attack is transient, but 20% to 30% of patients have a gallstone retained in their common bile duct. Cholecystectomy with intraoperative cholangiography in these patients is reasonable from a medical and cost perspective. Retained stones may be managed as described earlier (see Common Bile Duct Stones). ERCP is indicated in patients with persistent or severe attacks of pancreatitis.

Gallstone ileus refers to intestinal obstruction caused by a gallstone that has eroded from the gallbladder into the intestinal tract. The gallstone usually creates an obstruction at the ileocecal valve or in the sigmoid colon. By necessity, a fistula is present between the gallbladder and the stomach, duodenum, or colon. Besides dilated loops of bowel, abdominal films demonstrate air in the biliary tract. Occasionally, the gallstone will be seen if it is calcified. Treatment should relieve the bowel obstruction by removing the gallstone. The fistula is treated later, although such treatment is often not necessary when the patient does not have subsequent symptoms.

CIRRHOSIS

method of
PONSIANO OCAMA, M.D., and
WILLIAM M. LEE, M.D.
University of Texas, Southwestern Medical Center at Dallas
Dallas, Texas

Cirrhosis is defined histologically as fibrosis of the liver with formation of regenerative nodules. Pathophysiologically, cirrhosis follows chronic liver injury leading to activation of perisinusoidal stellate cells, which undergo transition from a quiescent state into proliferative, fibrogenic, and contractile myofibroblasts. Viable hepatocytes are replaced with connective tissue, and the degree of architectural distortion and the remaining amount of functional hepatic mass largely determines the liver's ability to function. Due to increased resistance to blood flow through the liver and increased hepatic inflow, portal hypertension develops. The loss of functional mass causes impairment in synthetic, metabolic, and excretory functions of the liver.

Cirrhosis represents the end stage of fibrogenesis and regeneration of the liver tissue. At the cirrhotic stage, the liver disease is considered irreversible.

Etiology

Various conditions may lead to cirrhosis. Common causes include infections with hepatitis B, C, and D viruses; alcohol; autoimmune liver disease and nonalcohol steato-hepatitis (NASH)—a condition that occurs primarily in patients with diabetes mellitus; obesity; and hyperlipidemia. Other causes of cirrhosis include primary biliary cirrhosis, primary sclerosing cholangitis, hemochromatosis, Wilson's disease, and α_1-antitrypsin deficiency.

Clinical Features

Most patients usually have no or few symptoms at first. Patients may present with fatigue, weakness, exhaustion, nausea, loss of appetite and loss of weight, jaundice, easy bruising, or generalized pruritus. As more complications begin to emerge, symptoms specific to the complications appear. Patients can therefore present with hematemesis and/or melena due to bleeding esophageal and, occasionally, gastric varices; alteration of sleep patterns and other neuropsychiatric manifestations due to hepatic encephalopathy; increase in abdominal girth: and abdominal pain constituting symptoms of ascites.

Diagnosis

The diagnosis of cirrhosis can be presumed from the symptoms and physical findings at presentation. The findings of silky hair, jaundice, parotid gland enlargement, gynecomastia, spider nevi, caput medusae, ascites, leg edema, and palmar erythema may suggest cirrhosis. Liver function tests may be deranged. Depending on the cause, aminotransferase or alkaline phosphatase levels are increased but do not connote the presence of cirrhosis, only damage to hepatocytes or bile ducts, respectively. Serum albumin levels and prothrombin time (INR: international normalized ratio) reflect the ability of the liver to synthesize important serum proteins. The albumin level is low and INR increased in the presence of cirrhosis. A diffuse (polyclonal) increase in immunoglobulin levels in serum is often seen. Serum bilirubin levels are not raised in most patients with cirrhosis, but may be in late stage or in particularly cholestatic diseases. A complete blood count in the cirrhotic patient will often reveal a decrease in neutrophil and platelet counts as evidence of splenic sequestration of these formed elements.

Imaging studies such as an abdominal computerized tomography, magnetic resonance imaging, or ultrasonogram of the liver may reveal abnormalities in its size, shape, and architecture. The presence of a nodular contour, increase in size, and number of intra-abdominal veins (varices), and the presence of ascites or splenomegaly all point to a likely cirrhotic physiology. The definitive diagnosis is made from liver biopsy showing nodules and an advanced-stage fibrosis. Biopsies are performed under local anesthesia by the percutaneous Menghini method unless coagulopathy or the presence of ascites or encephalopathy makes the risk excessive. In these instances, an open biopsy or transjugular approach may be used.

Classification of Severity of Cirrhosis

The Child-Pugh classification is used to grade severity of cirrhosis and it is shown in Table 1. In this system, 1 to 3 points are given for each of five criteria, with the total score used to determine the class or severity of the disease. This system, originally used to stratify risk in patients preparing for shunt surgery, has achieved a more general application in recent years. The higher the score, the more severe the condition of the patient. Life expectancy in Child class A may be 15 to 20 years, whereas those in class C may have a life expectancy of 1 to 3 years. The development of features reflecting Child class B is an indication to consider transplant evaluation.

Management

There is no specific treatment to prevent or resolve hepatic fibrosis. The management of cirrhosis,

TABLE 1. **Child-Pugh Classification**

Findings	1 Point	2 Points	3 Points
Serum albumin (g/dL)	>3.5	2.8-3.5	<2.8
Serum bilirubin (mg/dL)	<2.0 (for PBC, <4.0)	2.0-3.0 (for PBC, 4-10)	>3.0 (for PBC, >10)
Prolongation in prothrombin	1-4	4-6	>6
time(s) or INR	<1.7	1.7-2.3	>2.3
Ascites	None	Slight or controlled on diuretics	Moderate or severe
Encephalopathy	None	Mild or moderate	Severe

Class A, 5-7 points; Class B, 8-10 points; Class C, 11-15 points; INR, International Normalized Ratio; PBC, primary biliary cirrhosis.

therefore, lies in the treatment of the etiology (if known), preferably before late-stage disease is present. In many instances, the first presentation of a patient with cirrhosis is with a complication, evidence of hepatic decompensation. Treatment of the complications of cirrhosis can be lifesaving as well as palliative.

MANAGEMENT OF CAUSES OF CIRRHOSIS

Viral hepatitis

Viral hepatitis is now the most common cause of cirrhosis in the United States.

Two viruses, designated B and C, are responsible for most of the cirrhosis found worldwide. Hepatitis B is a DNA virus of the hepadnavirus family and is spread largely by sexual means and injection drug use. Hepatitis C is an RNA virus related to yellow fever virus. It affects more than 3 million people in the United States, roughly twice the number infected with hepatitis B. Both viruses replicate within hepatocytes, with liver injury related to the host immune attack on virus-infected cells. Cirrhosis evolves over many years, and the rate of evolution is quite variable. Factors known to be associated with more rapid progression of cirrhosis in hepatitis C include male gender, concomitant use of alcohol, and older age. Therapy is directed at disrupting viral replication and stimulating the immune system. For hepatitis B, interferons have been effective as have oral nucleoside analogues. For hepatitis C, interferon therapy may be given alone or combined with another antiviral, ribavirin, (Rebetron), which appears to improve the rates of sustained viral response, defined as the absence of detectable HCV RNA in serum at 24 weeks following treatment. A sustained viral response is associated with an approximate 98% likelihood of similar findings at 5 years following treatment.

For chronic HBV infection, IFN-α-2b (Intron A) may be given at a dose of 10 million units three times a week or 5 million units daily for a period of 16 weeks. The end point of treatment is loss of HBeAg and seroconversion to anti-HBe, loss of viral DNA, and a return of the liver enzymes to normal. The response rate in selected patients is about 40%, but due to the high dose of interferon, side effects are felt more frequently than with treatment for hepatitis C virus. Selection criteria for this treatment is also more strict and require that the patient should have high ALT levels of more than 100 to 200 IU, a low HBV viral count of less than 200 pg/mL, and no evidence of decompensated liver cirrhosis. For patients who do not meet these criteria, response rates are less than 5%. Other factors sometimes associated with a favorable response include absence of immunosuppression, female sex, history of acute icteric hepatitis, short known duration of hepatitis, wild-type (HBeAg-positive) virus, and horizontal (other than perinatal) acquisition of the virus. Lamivudine (Epivir-HBV), at a dose of 100 mg daily is a nucleoside analogue that is effective for treating HBV. It is taken orally and does not require the use of strict selection criteria as is the case with IFN-α-2b. It has minimal side effects and responses to lamivudine are quite uniform, resulting an approximate 3 to 4 log decrease in HBV DNA and improvement in aminotransferase levels. Resistance to lamivudine is a serious problem, developing at a rate of 25% at one year, 40% at 2 years, and greater than 50% in the third year of therapy. Resistance is due to the appearance of specific point (YMDD) mutations in the polymerase gene. Adefovir dipivoxil (Hepsera) 10 mg daily is effective both against lamivudine-resistant virus and the wild virus, and has been approved recently by the Food and Drug Administration for treatment of hepatitis B viral infection. No mutation has been demonstrated against adefovir up to this time.

Nucleoside analogues do not typically eradicate the virus although seroconversion to the HBeAg negative, anti-HBe positive state occur in 15% to 20% of patients over each year of treatment. In those who do not seroconvert, cessation of medication results in return of viral DNA to pretreatment levels. For hepatitis C viral infection, the genotype of the virus tends to influence response to treatment with IFN-α-2b and ribavirin. Only about 40% of patients with genotype 1, which is the most common in the United States, respond to a once a week treatment with 1.5 μg/kg of pegylated IFN alfa-2b (PEG-Intron) and daily 600 to 1200 mg of ribavirin (Virazole). Those with genotypes 2 and 3 show up to 80% response to the above treatment. Treatment is taken up to 24 weeks, at which time in all the genotypes the viral RNA should not be detected in blood by qualitative testing. Treatment is then stopped for patients with genotypes 2 and 3 and the patient is monitored at 1, 3, and 6 months for the viral RNA and liver enzymes. For genotype 1, absence of detectable RNA at 24 weeks means treatment may be effective but must continue for another 24 weeks. Thereafter monitoring can be done as for genotypes 2 and 3 above.

In all the genotypes, if virus is detected at 24 weeks of treatment, then the treatment is discontinued because the patient will probably not respond thereafter if no response has been obtained at this point.

Side effects of interferon include flu-like symptoms, headache, generalized body ache, depression, and loss of appetite and weight. It causes bone marrow suppression and the blood counts tend to fall. Other side effects include seizure disorders and thyroid dysfunction. Ribavirin causes hemolytic anemia, which is quite variable between patients. These effects are usually tolerated by most patients but in 10% to 15% of cases dose adjustments are required, and in 5% to 10% of patients treatment may need to be discontinued.

Alcohol-Induced Liver Disease

Excessive alcohol intake over time causes steatohepatitis and eventually cirrhosis at a variable rate depending on the quantities and other presumably genetic factors. Although it is stated that at least 80 g of alcohol daily for at least 20 years is required to induce these changes in the liver, the required dose tends to vary. Even in the most incorrigible alcoholics only about one third to one half develop cirrhosis. Women and people who are overweight appear to be more prone to severe alcoholic liver disease and may progress significantly at a smaller daily dose than other alcohol consumers.

Abstinence remains the most effective treatment for patients with alcohol-induced liver disease. This is true not only for patients with alcoholic fatty liver and alcoholic hepatitis but also for those with alcoholic cirrhosis. Patients with alcoholic cirrhosis who have not developed jaundice, ascites, or GI bleeding have a 5-year survival of almost 90% if they can stop drinking. These patients are frequently malnourished, with significant protein-calorie malnutrition found in 75% of the patients. Deficiencies of vitamins and minerals require replacement. Thiamine 50 to 100 mg daily may be required with pyridoxine, 100 mg daily. Folic acid is almost always needed at 1 to 5 mg daily.

Nonalcoholic Steato-Hepatitis (NASH)

The diagnosis of nonalcoholic steato-hepatitis is usually suspected in persons with asymptomatic elevation of aminotransferase levels, radiographic findings of fatty liver, or unexplained persistent hepatomegaly in persons who do not consume alcohol. This clinical suspicion of NASH and the severity of the condition can be confirmed with a liver biopsy. Patients typically are obese, diabetic, or on corticosteroid medication.

Management of NASH depends on the cause, although in some cases no specific etiology of NASH can be found. Other drugs associated with NASH include high-dose estrogen, tamoxifen, methotrexate, and amiodarone.

Proper management of diabetes mellitus together with weight reduction has been found to lead to improvement in the liver histology and liver enzymes. The rate of weight loss is important and may have a critical role in determining whether liver histologic findings will improve or worsen. In patients with a high degree of fatty infiltration, rapid weight loss may promote necro-inflammation, portal fibrosis, and bile stasis. A weight loss of about 500 g per week in children and 1600 g per week in adults is advocated.

Patients with hyperlipidemia may require treatment with lipid-lowering drugs. Gemfibrozil (Lopid),* 600 mg twice a day, has been reported to improve liver test results.

In patients with drug-induced NASH, modification of the drug dose or stopping the drug altogether may be required in order to have an improvement in the liver structure and function. Ursodiol (Actigall),* has been suggested as a possible treatment for NASH, but well-controlled long-term studies are not available to support its use. Recent evidence suggests that steato-hepatitis is a common antecedent to cryptogenic cirrhosis.

Autoimmune Liver Diseases

These include the autoimmune cholestatic liver diseases—primary biliary cirrhosis (PBC) and primary sclerosing cholangitis (PSC)—and autoimmune hepatitis, formerly called chronic active or lupoid hepatitis.

PBC and PSC are chronic, slowly progressive cholestatic liver diseases that occur primarily in adults. PBC primarily affects middle-aged women and is characterized by ongoing destruction of the interlobular and septal bile ducts. PSC principally affects young men and is characterized by diffuse inflammation and fibrosis of the entire biliary tree. Diagnosis is made for PBC by the constellation of cholestatic liver disease, exclusion of extrahepatic biliary disease, a positive anti-mitochondrial or antinuclear antibody test in serum, and a compatible liver biopsy showing bile duct injury or destruction. Diagnosis of PSC is most easily made using endoscopic cholangiopancreatography, which shows stricturing, beading, and dilation of the intra- and extrahepatic biliary tract. The exact etiology and/or pathogenesis of PBC and PSC are not understood. The natural history of these autoimmune-mediated conditions is one of slow progression with eventual development of cirrhosis, portal hypertension (with its attendant complications), and death unless liver transplantation intervenes. Patients present with pruritus and eventually jaundice, although this is rarely present in early stage disease. Ursodiol (Actigall),* 13-15 mg/kg/d has been found to slow the progression of PBC, but results with PSC have been more equivocal. Cholestyramine (Questran) 4 g three to four times a day with meals relieves itching and lowers serum bile acids. It also increases intestinal excretion of bile acids by preventing their reabsorption. If cholestyramine is not effective, then phenobarbital* 120 mg/d may be added. Rifampin (Rifadin),* has also been effective in treating pruritus. Lowered bile acid production coupled with the use of cholestyramine may result in diminished absorption of fat-soluble vitamins. Vitamin D, 50,000 U weekly, prevents osteopenia in these patients. Vitamin A deficiency causes night blindness and is corrected by 25,000 to 50,000 U twice weekly and 5 to 10 mg/d of oral vitamin K (Mephyton) may improve the prothrombin time. Vitamin E deficiency is replaced by 400 IU of the vitamin daily. If a patient has steatorrhea, fat intake can be restricted to less than 40 g/d; if this is not considered adequate for energy requirements, then medium chain fatty acids (MCT oil 1 tablespoon three to four times a day) is given. These do not require bile salts for absorption.

PSC is associated with ulcerative colitis in 90% of cases and cholangiocarcinoma occurs in 10% to 15%. The treatment of choice in patients with end-stage PSC and PBC is liver transplantation.

Autoimmune hepatitis is characterized by autoimmune clinical and serologic features including the presence of circulating autoantibodies, a high serum globulin level, and a strong therapeutic response to glucocorticosteroids. Antinuclear antibodies, anti-smooth muscle antibodies, antiactin antibodies, and antineutrophil cytoplasmic antibodies have been

*Not FDA approved for this indication.

*Not FDA approved for this indication.

found in this condition, which tends to affect mainly women. Antiliver kidney antibody (anti-LKM) has also been demonstrated (type II autoimmune hepatitis).

Most patients with autoimmune hepatitis are responsive to corticosteroids with a 10-year survival after diagnosis of 90% in treated patients. Most of the patients require long-term maintenance therapy, particularly if cirrhosis is present at diagnosis. Some patients however, remain in remission when drugs are withdrawn after initial suppression with anti-inflammatory therapy. All patients in whom the histologic appearance shows severe hepatitis with or without fibrosis or cirrhosis may be started on corticosteroid therapy. Azathioprine (Imuran),* is most frequently employed as a steroid-sparing agent. It can be used alone, after weighing the side-effects of the steroids against that of azathioprine. As a single drug therapy, prednisone 20 to 30 mg is given in the initial course of treatment, and treatment is maintained with a daily dose of prednisone 5 to 15 mg or azathioprine 100 to 200 mg. In the combination regimen, an initial course of prednisone 10 to 20 mg and azathioprine 50 to 100 mg is given, with a maintenance therapy using prednisone 5 to 10 mg and azathioprine 50 to 150 mg daily.

Hereditary Hemochromatosis

Hereditary hemochromatosis (HH) is a genetic disease most commonly associated with mutation in the *HFE* gene (C282Y gene homozygosity or C282Y/H63D compound heterozygosity). In HH, the liver is the recipient of an excess amount of absorbed iron. The excess iron affects other organs, including the heart, joints, skin, and endocrine glands (pancreas and pituitary glands) in addition to the liver. Diabetes mellitus develops in 30% to 60% of patients with advanced disease. Excessive skin pigmentation is also present in most symptomatic patients but is absent in the early stages of iron accumulation.

Males are affected most frequently, and they tend to present at 40 to 60 years of age with symptoms and signs due to the affected organs mentioned. Patients may present with fatigue, loss of libido, or symptoms related to diabetes or cardiac failure. Skin pigmentation, testicular atrophy, loss of body hair, and arthropathy may be observed in these patients.

The diagnosis is made by the finding of excess iron as high serum iron, high serum ferritin levels, or increased iron on liver biopsy. In addition, a gene test, which identifies the presence of the abnormal genotypes listed above, can be performed. At diagnosis, most patients have 15 to 20 g of storage iron, whereas normal total body iron stores are approximately 2 to 4 g in women and 6 to 8 g in men. Repeated phlebotomy is the desired treatment. Each unit of blood contains 200 to 250 mg of iron. Most patients can tolerate a weekly phlebotomy of one unit. Once iron stores have returned to normal, reflected by serum ferritin level of less than 50 ng/mL and a transferrin saturation of less than 50%, maintenance phlebotomy every 2 to 6 months is done. Iron chelators, such as desferrioxamine (Desferal),* are used in patients who cannot tolerate phlebotomy, but are much less effective than phlebotomy.

*Not FDA approved for this indication.

Wilson's Disease

Like HH, Wilson's disease (WD) is a hereditary condition with autosomal recessive inheritance. There are a variety of genes involved so that there is not one genetic test for the condition. In WD there is defective biliary excretion of copper, resulting in excess deposition in the liver. It is a disease of adolescents and young adults in which copper is deposited in the eyes and the brain in addition to the liver. Patients may have hepatosplenomegaly, features of chronic liver disease, hypersplenism, ascites and/or encephalopathy. In the eyes, Kayser-Fleischer rings or sunflower cataracts may be seen. Neurologically, WD can manifest as rigidity, tremors, or unsteady gait due to involvement of the basal ganglia. In some instances, a fulminant form of Wilson's disease can be seen with hemolysis and rapid downhill course requiring transplantation. Ceruloplasmin level is typically less than 20 mg/dL with high urine copper level, although occasionally normal values are seen. Copper is demonstrated on liver biopsy, generally in excess of 250 μg/g of dry weight (normal hepatic copper is 15 to 55 μg/g dry weight).

D-Penicillamine (Cuprimine), 250 to 500 mg three to four times/day increases excretion of copper. Improvement is slow. D-Penicillamine has bothersome side effects, such as skin rash, arthralgias, proteinuria, and an SLE-like reaction. Trientine (Syprine), is an alternative treatment.

MANAGEMENT OF COMPLICATIONS OF CIRRHOSIS

Portal Hypertension

Increased pressure in the portal venous circuit is the result of increased vascular resistance to blood flow in the disorganized liver architecture, as well as vasodilation in the splanchnic circulation. This leads to the formation of ascites, esophageal varices, hepatic encephalopathy, and hepato-renal syndrome. Evidence of any of these clinical organ failure syndromes constitutes hepatic decompensation. Although patients with established cirrhosis may live normal lives with a low (<20%) 10-year mortality, the presence of any of these signs of decompensation increases mortality to 50% at 5 years.

Ascites

In addition to the hypertensive, hyperdynamic portal circulation, the presence of hypoalbuminemia and increased renal sodium absorption play roles in ascites formation. Development of ascites is associated with a poor prognosis. In diuretic-sensitive ascites there is a 50% 2-year survival rate, and those with diuretic-resistant ascites have a 50% 6-month survival and a 25% 1-year survival.

*Not FDA approved for this indication.

The first evidence of ascites is an increase in abdominal girth and gain in weight. Peritoneal fluid of less than 2 liters is difficult to detect clinically, and ultrasonography may be a more accurate test to confirm the diagnosis.

Bed rest and salt restriction to 2 g/d of sodium alone may induce a modest diuresis and minimize the accumulation of ascitic fluid. The aim is to achieve a weight loss of 0.5 kg/d. Patients with peripheral edema can lose up to 1 kg/d. Fluid restriction to 1500 mL/d may be required but if there is dilutional hyponatremia (serum sodium <120 mmol/L), restriction to less than 1000 mL/d is advised. Spironolactone (Aldactone) 100 to 200 mg/d is added to the treatment. Side effects may include painful gynecomastia and hyperkalemia. Amiloride (Midamor),* 5 to 10 mg/d or triamterene (Dyrenium) 50 to100 mg/d may be used. Furosemide (Lasix) 40 to 80 mg/d can be added to the treatment if there is no adequate response to spironolactone alone. In diuretic-resistant ascites (not responding to 400 mg/d of spironolactone or 30 mg/d† of amiloride plus 160 mg/d of furosemide for 2 weeks), large-volume paracentesis is performed with 6 to 8 g of albumin given intravenously for every unit of ascitic fluid removed. Other modes of treatment include the peritoneovenous shunt, which requires surgery and is not commonly performed now, and the transjugular intrahepatic portosystemic shunt (TIPS), which is associated with an encephalopathy rate of at least 25%.

When ascites becomes resistant to diuretics, the patients should be considered for transplantation. The current use of the Mayo end-stage liver disease score (MELD score) gives precedence to evidence of renal insufficiency, such as that seen in patients refractory to diuretics.

Spontaneous Bacterial Peritonitis

Spontaneous bacterial peritonitis (SBP) is a puzzling condition that occurs in 10% to 30% of patients with cirrhosis and ascites. Patients may present with fever, abdominal pain, and worsening of encephalopathy, or they can remain silent. Aerobic gram-negative organisms account for about 70% of the cases, with *Escherichia coli* and *Klebsiella* predominating. Gram-positive cocci are found in about 30% of cases, with streptococci predominating. Anaerobes are rare; when they are found it is usually in patients with surgical peritonitis as is seen in perforated viscus. The usual source of the organism is the intestinal tract, but the urinary tract has also been implicated.

SBP is diagnosed when ascitic fluid polymorphonuclear (PMN) cell count is greater than 200 cells/mL, there is a pure growth of bacteria in culture, and there is no surgically treatable source of the infection. Empirical treatment should be started as soon as an elevated PMN count is detected in order to reduce mortality, which approaches 40%. Cefotaxime (Claforan) 2 g every 8 hours is started immediately before the diagnosis is made. Aminoglycosides should not be used in such cases because of increased nephrotoxicity. Secondary prophylaxis with norfloxacin 400 mg daily or ciprofloxacin 750 mg once weekly is started in these patients.

*Not FDA approved for this indication.

†Exceeds dosage recommended by the manufacturer.

Portasystemic Encephalopathy (PSE)

Portasystemic encephalopathy (PSE) is a neuropsychiatric syndrome that occurs in 28% of patients with liver cirrhosis and portal hypertension within 10 years after diagnosis of cirrhosis. It is thought to be caused by absorption of toxins from the gut and the shunting of these sedating toxins past the liver to the brain. It is precipitated by gastrointestinal bleeding, increased protein intake, infections, azotemia, and hypokalemia. Other precipitants are sedatives, hepatic failure from all causes, and constipation. The severity of PSE varies from barely detectable subclinical encephalopathy to flaccid coma as shown in Table 2.

In the treatment of PSE it is important to identify the precipitating factor, if possible, and correct it. Limit the protein intake to 0.8 to 1 g/kg. Lactulose (Cephulac) 30 mL every 8 hours is given and titrated to produce two to four loose stools per day. It is a laxative and creates an acidic environment to neutralize the ammonia in the gut, thus preventing resorption across the colonic mucosa. About 90% of patients respond to lactulose. In the remaining 10% who are refractory to lactulose, neomycin 500 to 1000 mg twice a day may be added to treatment. Neomycin is ototoxic and potentially (though rarely) nephrotoxic. Metronidazole (Flagyl),* 250 to 500 mg orally three times a day can also be used in place of neomycin.

Hepatorenal Syndrome

Hepatorenal syndrome (HRS) is an acute, progressive, oliguric renal failure occurring in patients with advanced liver damage who have no clinical, laboratory, or anatomic evidence of other causes of renal failure and who have been shown to have an adequate intravascular volume. The mechanism is not fully understood. There is decreased renal blood flow, decreased glomerular filtration rate, and decreased cortical perfusion. Urinary sodium secretion is less than 10 mmol/L and urinary volume less than 500 mL/d. The prognosis is very poor and patients require liver transplantation. Potentially nephrotoxic drugs, such as nonsteroidal anti-inflammatory drugs (NSAIDs) or aminoglycosides, should be avoided and a search for

*Not FDA approved for this indication.

TABLE 2. **Grades of Portasystemic Encephalopathy**

Grade	Level of Consciousness	Neurologic Findings
0	Normal	Normal
Subclinical	Normal	Prolonged trail test
1	Restless, mild confusion	Prolonged trail test Tremor (asterixis)
2	Lethargic	Prolonged trail test Asterixis
3	Somnolent but arousable	Unable to do trail test
4	Comatose	May be decerebrate

sepsis made. Ascites is tapped for white cell count, Gram stain, and culture. Blood, urine, and cannula tips are cultured. A broad-spectrum antibiotic may be started, irrespective of the proof of infection. Dialysis can give temporary relief as patients await transplantation. Full recovery of the kidneys should be expected once the liver disease is managed by transplantation.

Hepatocellular Carcinoma

Cirrhosis from any cause increases the risk of developing hepatocellular carcinoma (HCC). One to 5% of patients with cirrhosis develop HCC annually. Patients should be monitored by α-fetoprotein and ultrasonography every 6 months for early detection of the tumor, though careful studies to confirm the cost-effectiveness of this strategy have not been performed. Ultrasound or a CT-guided biopsy can be performed on suspicious lesions. Once diagnosis is confirmed, surgical resection provides the only hope of cure. Other modes of treatment include tumor chemoembolization via the hepatic artery, transplantation, and percutaneous ethanol injection. Outcome is generally poor if the tumor is multifocal, invades blood vessels, or is more than 5 cm.

OTHER CONSIDERATIONS IN LIVER CIRRHOSIS

Vaccination

Hepatitis A and B vaccines should be given to all patients with cirrhosis who are found to be non-immune to these viruses. All patients with cirrhosis should receive a single dose of polyvalent pneumococcal vaccine. This protects against infections such as pneumonia and peritonitis because *Streptococcus pneumoniae* is a very common cause of pneumonia and spontaneous bacterial peritonitis. An annual injection of influenza vaccine protects against influenza.

Avoidance of Medication Toxicity

Patients with cirrhosis may have their condition worsened by most drugs. Strict selection of drugs used for treating various conditions have to be made according to the knowledge of their effects on patients with cirrhosis. A number of drugs are metabolized by the liver and because of abnormal liver function, these drugs tend to accumulate in the body in unmetabolized forms which are either not active or toxic to the body. In patients with coagulopathy and portal hypertension, nonsteroidal anti-inflammatory drugs make bleeding more likely by inhibiting platelet function and causing gastrointestinal ulceration. In patients with portal hypertension, renal blood flow depends significantly on prostaglandins. NSAIDs inhibit prostaglandins causing decreased renal blood flow due to afferent arteriolar vasoconstriction. This can cause acute renal failure. NSAIDs should therefore be avoided in patients with cirrhosis.

The effect of acetaminophen on the liver is dose dependent. It can be used safely in doses not exceeding 3 g/d. Alcohol may lead to acetaminophen hepatotoxicity at lower doses.

Hepatic Osteodystrophy

Bone disease is a complication of chronic liver disease, especially chronic cholestasis as seen in PBC and PSC. Bone pain and bone fractures occur, possibly due to osteomalacia and osteoporosis. In osteoporosis, there is loss of bone (both matrix and its mineral) whereas in osteomalacia there is defective mineralization of osteoid laid down by osteoblasts. The majority of patients with hepatic osteodystrophy have osteoporosis as the cause of osteopenia. Patients with chronic liver disease are at an increased risk of developing osteodystrophy for a variety of reasons including the effect of alcohol on bone mass, malnutrition, vitamin malabsorption, sedentary lifestyle, and use of corticosteroids. Women with clinically evident cirrhosis may have early menopause, and this increases the risk of osteoporosis. Tobacco use also increases risk of osteoporosis.

Bone mineral density should be measured by dual energy x-ray absorptiometry (DEXA), and levels of serum calcium, phosphate, and vitamin D should be assessed in these patients, who may present with bone pain and deformity due to fractures. They may require 0.5 to 2.0 g/d of calcium carbonate or calcium citrate plus vitamin D 400 to 2000 IU/d. In some patients 100 IU/d of calcitonin (Miacalcin) may be added to the treatment. Perimenopausal women and postmenopausal women should receive hormone replacement if not contraindicated. Corticosteroids should be kept to the minimum and exercise should be encouraged. Bisphosphonates such as etidronate (Didronel),* 5 to 10 mg/kg/d or alendronate (Fosamax) 5 to 10 mg/d may be administered. Alendronate is contraindicated in patients with esophageal varices due to risk of esophageal ulceration. Alcohol and tobacco use should be eliminated.

Liver Transplantation

Liver transplantation is the definitive treatment for a variety of irreversible problems associated with chronic liver disease. Patients with cirrhosis who are in Child's class B, and those with refractory ascites, hepatorenal syndrome, and any other condition that is irreversible and progressive should be referred early for liver transplant evaluation. Orthotopic liver transplantation (OLT) offers overall 5-year survival rates of greater than 60% to 70%. Unfortunately, OLT is limited by the number of donor organs, leading to prolonged waiting periods for most patients. As a result, the MELD score has been developed to replace the Child-Turcotte-Pugh (CTP) score as a disease severity score. The change is designed to improve the organ allocation system, such that available organs are directed to patients based on the severity of their liver disease rather than the total time on the waiting list. The MELD score uses serum creatinine (mg/dL), total bilirubin (mg/dL) and international normalized ratio (INR). The minimum acceptable value for any of the variables is 1, the maximum acceptable value for

*Not FDA approved for this indication.

serum creatinine is 4, and the maximum value for MELD score is 40. It requires regular assessment of the variables and the higher the score, the higher the patient position on the waiting list. Using this scoring system, organs are allocated according to the medical urgency.

Palliative Care

Many patients with advanced cirrhosis may not be candidates for liver transplantation. This could be due to various reasons including multifocal, large hepatocellular carcinomas, other life threatening medical conditions, alcohol abuse, and chronic infections. Such patients develop worsening conditions with ascites, irreversible coagulopathy, encephalopathy, and spur-cell anemia. Survival is generally measured in weeks or months. They need supportive care and at appropriate time, hospice care.

BLEEDING ESOPHAGEAL VARICES

method of
MARIA MELA, M.D., and
ANDREW BURROUGHS, MB, CHB HONS
Royal Free Hospital NHS Trust
London, United Kingdom

At the time of diagnosis of cirrhosis, varices are present in about 60% of decompensated and 30% of compensated patients. In most patients, esophageal varices enlarge over time, although regression has also been observed particularly in alcoholic cirrhotic patients who abstain. Acute variceal bleeding in cirrhotics can be life threatening with a mortality 30% to 50%. Although overall survival is improving because of new therapeutic approaches, mortality is still closely related to failure to control hemorrhage or early rebleeding, which is a distinct characteristic of portal hypertensive bleeding and occurs in as many as 50% of patients in the first days to 6 weeks after admission. Recent interest has been directed at identifying hemodynamic factors that correlate with the absence of variceal bleeding (e.g., hepatic venous pressure gradient [HVPG] below 12 mmHg), and a hypothesis has been described with bacterial infection as a trigger for bleeding. Recent advances include the very early administration of drug therapy and antibiotic prophylaxis in acute variceal bleeding and the evidence for nonselective β-blockers,* as therapy of first choice for secondary and primary prophylaxis, with banding as an alternative for contraindications or intolerance to β -blockers. HVPG monitoring with a target reduction of equal to or greater than 20% of the baseline or an absolute reduction of HVPG to less than or equal to 12 mmHg has been shown to correlate with bleeding and early rebleeding, but the clinical applicability still needs evaluation.

*Not FDA approved for this indication.

ACUTE VARICEAL BLEEDING

Effective resuscitation, accurate diagnosis, and early treatment can reduce mortality due to variceal bleeding. The aims are not only to stop bleeding as soon as possible but also to prevent early rebleeding, which is associated with worsening mortality. The *initial resuscitation* of the patient is as important as the other specific measures to promote hemostasis. Overtransfusion must be avoided and blood should be replaced to a modest target hematocrit of 25% to 30%. The optimal use of clotting factors has been little studied; a practical approach is to give 2 units fresh frozen plasma (FFP) after 4 units of blood when the prothrombin time (PT) is more than 20 seconds and platelets if the count is less than $50{,}000 \times 10^6/mm^3$ in an actively bleeding patient. Endotracheal intubation must be considered for encephalopathic patients or those with massive hematemesis to avoid aspiration.

Bacterial infections occur in 35% to 66% of cirrhotics with variceal bleeding, and their presence has been identified as predictive of early rebleeding and death. *Antibiotic prophylaxis* significantly increases the mean survival rate and the mean percentage of patients free of infection. Therefore, prophylaxis with an oral or intravenous (IV) quinolone,* or IV cephalosporin* is mandatory in cirrhotics with gastrointestinal bleeding, irrespective of the suspected presence of sepsis.

The currently recommended treatment schedule for acute variceal bleeding also includes the administration of a vasoactive drug at the time of admission followed with endoscopic treatment at the time of diagnostic endoscopy. Pharmacologic treatment is aimed at arresting hemorrhage by decreasing pressure and blood flow within the esophageal varices, thus allowing hemostasis at the bleeding point. *Terlipressin (Glypressin),** a synthetic analogue of vasopressin, is one of the agents of first choice for the treatment of acute variceal bleeding and should be administered as soon as possible before endoscopic investigation and maintained for at least 2 days (2 mg every 4 hours for the initial 24 hours; 1 mg every 4 hours for the next 24 hours), preferably 5 days, to prevent early rebleeding. It produces decreases in portal pressure of 16% to 35% and significantly reduces the failure of initial hemostasis and the overall mortality. Compared with endoscopic therapy (the gold standard therapy for acute variceal hemorrhage) it is equally effective in the initial control of bleeding and the prevention of early rebleeding. When used as an adjuvant to emergency sclerotherapy, terlipressin improves hemostasis and reduces mortality at a level that approaches statistical significance. It has also been used in cirrhotics with hepatorenal syndrome type 1 and found to improve the renal function and survival; its renal protective role may also favor it as the drug of first choice. *Somatostatin*,*,† (SMS) can also be used for the control of bleeding and prevention of early rebleeding from

*Not FDA approved for this indication.
†Not available in the United States.

esophageal varices. SMS increases splanchnic vascular resistance mainly by inhibiting the release of vasodilatory peptides such as glucagon, vasoactive intestinal peptide, and substance P. Therefore it reduces splanchnic and azygos blood flow and portal pressure. Early administration of SMS (250 μg bolus injection followed by 500 μg/hour infusion) has proved safe and very effective on its own, and as adjuvant therapy to sclerotherapy during the critical 5-day period following variceal bleeding. The evidence currently demonstrating efficacy of octreotide (Sandostatin)* in acute variceal bleeding is less than that for SMS. The optimal dose, route, and duration of treatment are not adequately determined.

In terms of *endoscopic therapy*, sclerotherapy or band ligation represent the gold standard in the management of acute variceal bleeding because they stop bleeding in 80% to 100% of the patients, prevent early rebleeding, and significantly increase survival. Various sclerosants have been used with no difference in efficacy. Band ligation results in fewer complications but requires a second intubation after the diagnostic endoscopy. Therefore, many endoscopists prefer to perform emergency sclerotherapy and use ligation at subsequent treatment sessions.

Transjugular intrahepatic portosystemic stent shunt (TIPSS) is indicated in patients in whom bleeding cannot be controlled or recurs after two sessions of endoscopic treatment. It has largely replaced esophageal transection for cases of uncontrollable variceal bleeding and it is particularly useful for bleeding fundal varices.

Balloon tamponade can be applied in cases of uncontrollable bleeding. It is highly effective in arresting hemorrhage but it carries a very high risk of complications. It should always be used as a bridge until more definite endoscopic/TIPSS/surgical treatment is applied. Use of tubes that can be applied over an endoscope (Zimmon tube) may reduce the complication rate.

SECONDARY PREVENTION

Patients surviving the first episode of variceal bleeding are at a very high risk of recurrent bleeding (70% or more in the first year). Therefore, the consensus is that all patients who survive an episode of variceal bleeding must receive some effective long-term therapy to prevent further variceal bleeding. There is no role for observational policy; active therapy has proved superior to none.

Nonselective β-blockers (NSBBs), *propranolol* (Inderal),* and *nadolol* (Corgard),* constitute the first-line treatment for prevention of recurrent variceal bleeding. They decrease the splanchnic blood flow by reduction of cardiac output and reflux splanchnic arterial constriction and reduce HVPG by 12% to 16% in one third to one half of treated patients. β-Blockers decrease the risk of rebleeding and improve survival, especially in patients with more advanced liver disease. Adverse events are generally mild and occur in 17% of patients. Treatment with β-blockade should be continued indefinitely. Given the low cost of propranolol,* it should always be considered the initial treatment of choice for patients who survive the initial few days following variceal bleeding (starting dose 40 mg twice daily). Some studies suggest that hemodynamic response to pharmacotherapy (absolute reduction of HVPG to ≤12 mmHg or ≥20% of the baseline) is predictive of clinical response and that alternative therapies (i.e., banding or TIPSS) should be offered to nonresponders whose risk of rebleeding is considered high. However, the interval to repeat measurements may need to be very short to identify patients before they rebleed. Since HVPG measurement is invasive, costly, and involves hospital stay, other methods have been investigated, namely Doppler ultrasonography and direct variceal pressure measurement. Until their accuracy is further assessed the hemodynamic assessment of pharmacotherapy is not currently standard practice.

Variceal band ligation should be used for secondary prevention if there are contraindications or an intolerance to β-blockers. It has replaced sclerotherapy because it is better tolerated with fewer complications and it is more efficacious in the secondary prophylaxis. Recent trials of β-blockers versus banding show no difference of the two treatment modalities, and in one study the combination of *β-blockers* and *nitrates* was also as effective as band ligation in preventing re-bleeding and survival. The use of isosorbide mononitrate,* on its own, is contraindicated as it may worsen ascites and survival.

TIPSS reduces the risk of rebleeding but increases the risk of hepatic encephalopathy without effect on survival.

PRIMARY PREVENTION

In patients with cirrhosis, the risk of gastrointestinal bleeding is approximately 30% and the initial episode will prove fatal in 30% to 50%. Consequently, the primary prevention of variceal hemorrhage is an important therapeutic goal.

In cirrhotics with large varices, prophylactic nonselective β-blockers (NSBBs)* therapy should be given. NSBBs have greater potential in primary rather than secondary prophylaxis because the hemodynamic response after administration of β-blockers is better in compensated patients without previous episodes of variceal bleeding. They significantly reduce the bleeding risk and the mortality rate due to bleeding with a strong trend to reducing overall mortality. NSBBs are effective independent of cause and severity of cirrhosis, presence of ascites, and variceal size, and they also prevent bleeding from the gastric mucosa. However, 15% to 25% of patients have contraindications or develop side effects precluding their use.

ISMN as monotherapy is contraindicated, as it is ineffective in the setting of primary prevention and is associated with increased mortality. The available evidence does not support the routine use of combined β-blocker and ISMN.

*Not FDA approved for this indication.

*Not FDA approved for this indication.

As in secondary prevention, the hemodynamic response appears to be the main factor predicting bleeding. However, HVPG monitoring is less feasible when considering a universal use of β-blockade for all patients with varices. Currently, the maximum tolerated dose of β-blockers is titrated according to the resting heart rate (25% reduction) and the development of symptoms.

Primary prophylaxis with *variceal ligation* appears to be safe and may be a reasonable alternative for patients who have contraindications and are intolerant or noncompliant to β-blockers. It is unlikely that ligation will become a routine prophylactic treatment because it is much more expensive and less available than β-blockers and it does not prevent the bleeding from gastric mucosa.

PREVENTION OF THE DEVELOPMENT OF VARICES

One published study does not support the use of propranolol* for the prevention or development of large esophageal varices in cirrhotics with or without small varices. However, timolol (Blocadren)* appears to be more effective in reducing the portal pressure in cirrhotics without varices compared with those with varices, suggesting greater effect of pharmacotherapy when administered in the early stages of portal hypertension, before the formation of varices. Until further encouraging results become available, the usefulness of prevention of formation/growth of varices (pre-primary prophylaxis) in clinical practice is yet to be proved.

DRUGS FOR FUTURE TRIALS

Recent evidence indicates that in the context of liver injury, hepatic stellate cells (resident perisinusoidal mesenchymal cells with a microanatomic position in the sinusoids analogous to vasoregulatory pericytes), respond to endothelins (ET) and transform into myofibroblasts. In this form they may lead to a perisinusoidal constriction and increased intrahepatic resistance. A mixed ET_A/ET_B receptor antagonist, Bosentan* has been shown to reduce portal pressure by 15% to 20% when administered to isolated perfused cirrhotic livers. Similar compounds are currently undergoing phase I clinical trials, opening new perspectives for the treatment of portal hypertension.

Nitric oxide (NO), a vasodilatory molecule, has also been of intense interest. In the cirrhotic liver there is a deficit in the NO levels and experimental enhancement of the expression of NO synthase in liver cells reduces the portal pressure for short periods.

A number of vasoactive compounds (angiotensin II, endothelins, and NO) play a major role in the injured liver, not only by regulation of the intrahepatic blood flow but also by direct modulation of extracellular matrix production and fibrogenesis. Losartan (Cozaar),* (antagonist of angiotensin II), captopril (Capoten),* (ACE inhibitor) and ET-A receptor* blockade have all been suggested as putative *antifibrotic agents,* based on animal experiments. Interestingly, modification of the microcirculation may well have a secondary effect on the fibrogenesis and, therefore, the interaction of vasoactive drugs/receptor antagonists, stellate cells, and microcirculation fibrogenesis becomes much more complex.

Angiotensin-II (ANG-II) is considered a potential mediator of intrahepatic portal hypertension, because its plasma levels are elevated in cirrhosis and its administration induces a rise in portal pressure. Despite some initial encouraging results, more recent studies showed that ANG-II receptor antagonists only marginally reduce the portal pressure while they cause hypotension and renal impairment. Therefore they may prove to be useful in early, but not in late, cirrhosis for their antifibrotic potential. Because of effects on the kidneys they should not be used in cirrhosis.

Prazosin (Minipress), clonidine (Catapres),* carvedilol (Coreg),** and *5-HT receptor antagonists* have all been reported to reduce the portal pressure, but they also reduce the mean arterial pressure, which limits their clinical use.

Based on the hypothesis that bacterial infection, through the increased release/synthesis of endothelin due to endotoxemia and subsequent contraction of stellate cells may trigger variceal bleeding in cirrhotics, *antibiotics* have been suggested as therapeutic agents in the prevention of bleeding. However, this remains to be tested in clinical trials.

The therapeutic role of hemostatic agents in acute bleeding and particularly of *recombinant factor VIIa* has been studied in a randomized trial, but the results are not yet available.

CONCLUSION

In *acute variceal bleeding*, initial resuscitation of the patient is of major importance; administration of antibiotics should be routine, whether sepsis is suspected or not. Endoscopic therapy is the gold standard and should be associated with administration of terlipressin or somatostatin (to be started before endoscopy and continued for five days). TIPSS is effective for failed endoscopic treatment. The first line treatment for *secondary prevention* of variceal hemorrhage is nonselective β-blockers. The combination of β-blocker and nitrates* is another alternative. In patients who have contraindications to β-blocker therapy or who have bled while on β-blockers, band ligation is the preferred treatment. For *primary prevention* of variceal bleeding, the current treatment of choice is β-blockers. Again, variceal ligation is a reasonable alterative for patients who cannot tolerate or who have contraindications to β-blockers.

Currently there is no standardization of screening practices for the presence of varices. In the absence of compelling data suggesting otherwise, we suggest that every patient with cirrhosis (except those with short life expectancy) should be offered a one-time screening endoscopy to screen for varices, given the low risk of endoscopy, the high prevalence of varices, and the

*Not FDA approved for this indication.

*Not FDA approved for this indication.

proven efficacy of primary prophylaxis. Because most liver diseases are progressive and liver function is an independent predictor of the risk of first bleeding, the presence of varices, even if small ones, is sufficient indication in the authors' practice to prescribe β-blockers, provided the patient is tolerant of therapy. This avoids the use of repeated endoscopy, usually at 1 to 2 years to monitor varices.

DYSPHAGIA AND ESOPHAGEAL OBSTRUCTION

method of
ROBIN D. ROTHSTEIN, M.D.
Pennsylvania Hospital
University of Pennsylvania Health System
Philadelphia, Pennsylvania

Dysphagia is the sensation of difficulty swallowing and may include either motility problems or mechanical obstruction. Abnormalities can be classified by location as either oropharyngeal or esophageal. Although the differential diagnosis is broad, a thorough history often is predictive of the underlying disorder. It is essential that the clinician be familiar with both intrinsic and extrinsic disorders of the esophagus to assist in the evaluation of dysphagia.

MOTOR ABNORMALITIES

Disturbances in motor function of the esophagus range from reduced motor activity to hyperactivity or incoordination. Examples of these distinct motor disturbances include gastroesophageal reflux, achalasia, and diffuse esophageal spasm, respectively. In general, patients who suffer from motility disorders have greater sensitivity to balloon distention and a greater percentage of swallow-related symptoms.

Primary achalasia is the classic motor abnormality of the esophagus, often affecting young adults in their 20s and 30s. Symptoms often precede the diagnosis by many years. Despite dysphagia, afflicted patients usually maintain their weight. Pulmonary complications may be a prime factor leading to medical attention. Patients may have recurrent pneumonia, aspiration, or, infrequently, lung abscess. Halitosis, recurrent belching, and the presence of regurgitated material on the pillow in the morning may impel some to seek medical attention. Although dysphagia is the primary symptom, early in disease, chest pain may be present. The features of achalasia progress over time and result in more severe symptoms, greater dilation and tortuosity of the esophagus, and worsening morbidity.

Pseudoachalasia or *secondary achalasia* cannot be manometrically differentiated from primary achalasia. However, this syndrome is associated with an underlying malignant disease or other pathologic abnormality. A rare form of achalasia is *congenital cricopharyngeal achalasia,* which presents in the newborn with dysphagia, choking, and nasal reflux. Myotomy of the cricopharyngeus effectively resolves the problem.

Less specific motor abnormalities are the spastic disorders of the esophagus, including diffuse esophageal spasm, the nutcracker esophagus, and nonspecific esophageal motility disorder. Many clinicians have abandoned the term *nutcracker esophagus* and categorize it as another form of nonspecific motor abnormalities. These entities are benign and nonprogressive, and manometry often depicts nondiagnostic and nonspecific abnormalities.

Oropharyngeal dysphagia is common in the elderly and is associated with high morbidity, mortality, and cost. Difficulty with swallowing frequently occurs in patients who have had a stroke; it is a common malady in nursing home residents, and it often leads to feeding difficulties. Parkinson's disease and oculopharyngeal muscular dystrophy are other maladies that may lead to oropharyngeal dysphasia. Correct diagnosis of dysphagia in the elderly helps one to recognize those patients at risk of malnutrition and pulmonary complications.

Motor abnormalities may accompany structural damage to the esophagus after *caustic ingestion.* Low-amplitude contractions and absent peristalsis occur within a week of caustic ingestion. These abnormalities may persist for months.

OBSTRUCTION

Obstructive lesions of the esophagus include both benign and malignant abnormalities involving any portion of the esophagus. Extrinsic lesions may also cause obstruction. The severity of symptoms often correlates with the degree of narrowing. This has been well established with *esophageal rings.* Rings with a diameter less than 13 mm are associated with solid-food dysphagia, and patients with rings over 20 mm are generally asymptomatic.

Esophageal strictures may result from either benign or malignant conditions and require different therapeutic approaches. Although *reflux* is the most common cause of benign strictures, corrosive damage, rings, and radiation may also constrict the esophagus. In general, reflux-induced strictures are located at the squamocolumnar junction and consist of mucosa and submucosa. *Schatzki's ring* is a discrete distal esophageal narrowing that can cause intermittent dysphagia. Gastroesophageal reflux may be a precursor for its development. Classic reflux-induced strictures consist of fibrous tissue, and they are often slowly progressive, with solid-food dysphagia preceding difficulty with liquids. These strictures are often smoothly tapered and are found in the distal esophagus.

The *lower esophageal muscular ring* has been less well studied. Rings are identified as a circumferential distal narrowing, approximately 1.5 cm above the squamocolumnar junction. These rings are thicker than mucosal rings and are often associated with motor disorders. Esophageal motility testing has revealed peristaltic, high-amplitude, long-duration, and multiple peaked contractions and hypertensive lower esophageal sphincter pressures. Patients with muscular rings may respond less well to dilation than do patients with mucosal rings.

Webs of the esophagus are thin mucosal membranes generally located in the postcricoid region. They are more frequently found in the elderly. In the rare disorder *Plummer-Vinson syndrome,* there is an association of iron deficiency anemia with cervical webs. The risk of pharyngeal and esophageal cancers is increased in this condition.

Dysphagia may occur in the *postoperative setting.* Esophagogastric banding, a relatively new technique for treatment of obesity, may cause dysphagia because the band acts as a site of obstruction. Postoperative dysphagia occurs commonly after a Nissen fundoplication. Most patients improve over the first 6 weeks after the surgical procedure. Persistent and severe symptoms are more likely if patients had intraoperative difficulties or in patients with an increased body mass index. Preoperative manometry does not consistently identify those patients at risk.

Primary tumors of the esophagus that cause stricturing are adenocarcinomas and squamous cell carcinomas. Contiguous primary carcinomas, typically lung, or neighboring malignant lymph nodes can cause extrinsic compression. Metastastic lesions, including from lung and breast cancer, are extremely rare causes of esophageal narrowing and may cause occlusion by either compression or submucosal spread.

Benign extrinsic lesions may lead to dysphagia. Hypertrophic anterior cervical osteophytes or diffuse skeletal hyperostosis may be associated with dysphagia and esophageal obstruction. Dysphagia lusoria results from an anomaly of the aortic root and may consist of an aneurysm or occlusive disease that can cause esophageal compression. An aberrant subclavian artery courses behind the esophagus.

Foreign body ingestion occurs in both children and adults. Children are more likely to suffer from non–food-related dysphagia from various accidental ingestions. The type of foreign body swallowed varies with age. In younger children, coins are commonly encountered. Chicken and fish bones are more typical in older children and in adults. In elderly persons, dentures are the more commonly accidentally ingested items. Children usually have a normal esophagus. Adults frequently have an underlying abnormality. Up to one third of adults have an underlying stricture.

Irritants to the esophagus may lead to problems with mechanical obstruction. Accidental exposures typically occur with children and are often household items, including cleaners and adult medications. Suicidal gestures are more frequent in adults, generally with ingestion of alkali, sodium hydroxide, or sulfuric acid. Tissue destruction occurs by liquefaction or coagulation. Progression to stenosis is common after caustic-induced esophagitis, and the severity correlates with the amount of alkali ingested.

DIAGNOSIS

Although historical features are essential in evaluating the symptom of dysphagia, the site where patients sense dysphagia does not necessarily correlate with the location of the problem. Patients with distal obstruction may have symptoms referred proximally. Various modalities are available for diagnostic evaluation, and it is essential the clinician have a thorough understanding of their different utilities to assist in establishing a diagnosis. Multiple tests may be required to assess the patient's condition. Radiologic studies (videoesophagography or scintigraphy), endoscopy, and manometry are often complementary for the evaluation of dysphagia.

Videofluoroscopic swallowing or cine-esophagography is a well-established method for evaluating patients with oropharyngeal dysphagia. It is safe, it allows for visualization of pharyngoesophageal function and structure, and it enables one to assess risk of aspiration in both benign and malignant conditions of the esophagus. In large studies, findings on videofluoroscopy have included the following: mass lesions from the oral cavity, larynx, and pharynx; diverticula; strictures, webs, and rings; and extrinsic lesions. Various dilutions of barium can be used to assess the consistencies of foods that can be safely swallowed without aspiration. Videoesophagography is the most cost-effective and accurate for patients with achalasia, diffuse esophageal spasm, and scleroderma, in addition to being better tolerated than manometry.

Barium-contrast esophagography is especially useful in evaluating and localizing most anatomic causes of dysphagia and is superior for extrinsic or intramural lesions compared with endoscopy. However, for evaluation of esophageal dysphagia, especially in patients with a history of gastroesophageal reflux, upper endoscopy is the preferred modality. Pathologic diagnosis can be achieved for obstructive lesions. Additionally, endoscopy allows for therapeutic intervention, including dilation of a stricture, stent placement, or removal of foreign bodies.

Esophageal manometry should be considered when structural lesions have been eliminated and there is a concern about motility disorders. This technique has proven utility for diagnosis of motor abnormalities, especially achalasia. Specific patterns can be identified with scleroderma, hypertensive lower esophageal sphincter, and diffuse esophageal spasm. The usefulness of pharyngeal and upper esophageal manometry has been less well established. Technologic advances have improved these recordings. At present, oropharyngeal manometry is probably best suited for unusual clinical presentations and for clinical research.

Scintigraphic studies are occasionally used for evaluation of the esophagus. Technetium 99m–labeled sucralfate can be used to assess injury because it has an affinity for injured mucosa. Scintigraphic labeling is nonspecific and can be used for caustic injury and reflux-induced damage. Occasionally, scintigraphic studies using labeled water are used to assess esophageal transit.

TREATMENT

Therapy is aimed at the individual patient and is affected by patient and physician choice, cost consideration, concurrent disease, and underlying esophageal pathologic features. For malignant strictures, both surgical and endoscopic options exist. Nonresectable malignant esophageal strictures may be recanalized with photodynamics, endoluminal laser, or bipolar electrocoagulation. Various types of stents have been developed, including those with antireflux valves and forms capable of bridging and maintaining placement at the gastroesophageal junction. The decision regarding the type of stent employed varies and is dependent on local availability, familiarity, and expertise. Costs of self-expanding metal stents may initially be high, but these stents may reduce the need for multiple procedures and hospitalizations. Both short-term and long-term risks remain high and include bleeding, overgrowth by tumor, food impaction, perforation, and migration of stents, particularly those placed at the gastroesophageal junction. Self-expanding metal stents may be preferable to plastic types because of easier implantation and greater longevity. Symptom relief may be incomplete, and patients may need to maintain a semisoft diet.

Laser coagulation has been used for unresectable gastroesophageal junction tumors. Multiple endoscopic sessions may be needed, but hospitalization rates are similar to those in patients with self-expanding metallic stents. Some studies suggest a higher morbidity and hospital mortality rate with self-expanding stents, but similar rates of palliation using laser. Most patients are able to ingest at least soft or solid foods. Operator skill and experience are most likely significant factors for success and complication rates.

High-dose intraluminal brachytherapy can be used as palliative therapy for advanced or recurrent carcinoma. The risk of complications is high, but patients experience a long dysphagia-free period. Brachytherapy can be used alone or with a combination of external and intraluminal radiation therapy.

Esophageal dilation is frequently used to treat benign strictures of the esophagus. Most benign strictures are secondary to peptic disease and involve the distal esophagus. Schatski's rings often require one dilation with a large-bore dilator. For the rare patient with a persistent distal esophageal ring, endoscopic incision may be helpful. Empirical dilation has been used successfully in patients with solid-food dysphagia but an endoscopically normal appearance. Patients with solid and liquid dysphagia are less likely to benefit. Cervical webs are frequently treated with dilation with tapered dilators. For the occasional patient with Plummer-Vinson disease, dysphagia may improve with iron repletion. If not, dilation can be used.

Esophageal dilation can be performed using various techniques, often based on operator training and experience and the availability of specific equipment. Hydrostatic and pneumatic balloons and wire-guided polyvinyl bougies have nearly replaced mercury-filled rubber bougies, especially for dilation of more complex and tight stenotic strictures. The rate of perforation is greater in blind passage of mercury-weighted bougies compared with directed techniques. Complications of the procedure are low, with a less than 0.5% risk of perforation and bleeding and a 0.01% risk of death. Dilations of the esophagus using an over-the-wire technique may be safely performed without fluoroscopy.

Rigid dilators and balloons appear to be equally safe and effective for dilation of distal esophageal rings and peptic strictures. More severe strictures may require repeat sessions. Treatment of refractory benign strictures with esophageal stents remains controversial.

Removal of foreign objects in both children and adults can be achieved by endoscopic manipulation. Items lodged in the cervical esophagus may require examination while the patient is under anesthesia, and possible surgical intervention. If clinically appropriate, a plain neck and chest radiograph should be obtained to exclude perforation. Computed tomography may be necessary for more subtle tears and should be considered in every symptomatic patient with unremarkable plain films.

In children, typical foreign bodies removed include coins, toy parts, jewels, batteries, sharp materials such as needles and pins, and fish and chicken bones. Most children do well, without the need for future endoscopic intervention. Children who have had repair of atresia or tracheoesophageal fistulas are at higher risk of foreign body impactions. In contrast, adults are more likely to require subsequent esophageal dilation for strictures or, less likely, to need treatment for motor abnormalities. Unfortunately, the history is often unreliable in children, and the decision to remove a coin should not depend on the child's memory of its denomination. Coins ingested by older children and those located at the gastroesophageal junction are more likely to pass spontaneously. The use of intravenous glucagon has not demonstrated promise in promoting coin passage.

Choices of treatment of achalasia include pneumatic dilation, surgical myotomy, medications, botulinium toxin injection, and esophagectomy. Pneumatic dilation and surgical myotomy provide either good or excellent relief in up to 90% of patients. In the few patients with advanced disease and a severely dilated esophagus, esophagectomy may be indicated. A gastric pull-up is performed for continuity of the gastrointestinal tract or, less likely, a jejunal or colonic interposition. Cost analysis of the various treatments has been done, and pneumatic dilation is more cost-effective than surgery or botulinum toxin injection, depending on the number of repeat dilations required. Laparoscopic esophagomyotomy is the most effective treatment option, but it has the highest initial cost.

Physical therapy and dietary management have been used to improve pharyngeal dysphagia. Head-raising strengthening exercises have been shown to improve upper esophageal sphincter function and to reduce aspiration. Some patients are able to resume eating.

Treatment of dysphagia after fundoplication is frequently necessary in patients with persistent or severe symptoms. Tapered dilators have been safely used in this population of patients. Successful treatment correlates with lower esophageal sphincter pressure. Those with higher lower esophageal sphincter pressure are more likely to benefit from therapy.

DIVERTICULA OF THE ALIMENTARY TRACT

method of
CHARLES CHAPPUIS, M.D.
University Medical Center
Lafayette, Louisiana

Although most often found in the colon, *diverticula* can be found in virtually all segments of the gastrointestinal tract including esophagus, stomach, small intestine, and colon. True diverticula contain all layers of the bowel wall including mucosa, submucosa, and muscular wall. *False diverticula* or *pseudodiverticula* are herniations of mucosa and submucosa through the muscular wall of the bowel, often at the site of a penetrating blood vessel. Various theories regarding the pathogenesis of alimentary tract diverticula have been proposed and include pulsion, traction, abnormalities of the muscular coat, and congenital abnormalities. Complications associated with diverticula of the alimentary tract include bleeding, pain, and perforation.

ESOPHAGEAL DIVERTICULA

Esophageal diverticula are outpouchings containing one or more layers of the esophageal wall. They may occur in the upper, middle, or lower esophagus.

Zenker's Diverticulum

Pharyngoesophageal diverticulum, or *Zenker's diverticulum,* the most common diverticulum of the esophagus, usually occurs in patients older than 60 years of age. These pulsion diverticula usually arise between the inferior pharyngeal constrictor muscle and the cricopharyngeus muscle, the result of increased pressure secondary to motility disorder. The diverticulum typically dissects toward the left and inferiorly into the superior mediastinum.

Symptoms include intermittent cough, excessive salivation, halitosis, and intermittent dysphagia, especially with solids. Other problems include gurgling sounds when swallowing and regurgitation of previously ingested food. The most significant problem associated with Zenker's diverticulum is aspiration, often nocturnal, which may lead to pneumonia.

Plain films of the chest or neck may reveal an air-fluid level in the diverticulum. A barium esophagram is usually diagnostic, revealing the diverticulum, often located posteriorly and on the left. Fiberoptic endoscopy is indicated if the contrast study reveals a mass or ulceration, to rule out malignant disease.

Treatment

Surgical therapy is indicated in symptomatic patients and is directed primarily toward the underlying motility disorder. The most common approach in dealing with this problem is the combination of a cervical esophagomyotomy with resection of the diverticulum. The procedure is usually performed through an oblique left neck incision that parallels the sternocleidomastoid muscle. It is recommended that a No. 40 to No. 50 French bougie be inserted in the esophagus before resection of the diverticulum, to avoid narrowing the esophagus. The myotomy is performed from the base of the diverticulum and extending 7 to 10 cm proximally and distally. Small diverticula often blend into the exposed mucosa after the esophagomyotomy. Excision of larger pouches is best done with the surgical stapler.

Recurrence is rare, and most patients have an excellent result after the procedure. Success rates are lower if diverticulectomy is performed without myotomy.

Midesophageal Diverticula

Midesophageal diverticula are usually found within 4 to 5 cm of the carina. Although frequently asymptomatic, they can result in dysphagia, retrosternal pain, regurgitation, belching, and heartburn. Most of these diverticula are discovered as incidental findings on barium esophagram. In the past, these true diverticula were often caused by traction in patients with inflammatory disease in the mediastinum such as lymphadenopathy from tuberculosis or histoplasmosis. Neuromuscular dysfunction is now thought to play a role in the development of midesophageal diverticula, the result of pulsion forces.

Treatment

Treatment is directed at the underlying disease because simple excision of the diverticulum will not relieve patients' symptoms in most cases. Esophageal manometry should be performed before surgical treatment is undertaken, to rule out motility disorders.

Epiphrenic Diverticula

Epiphrenic diverticula are pulsion diverticula that develop in the distal third of the esophagus, often within 10 cm of the gastroesophageal junction. These diverticula are often found on the right side, the result of esophageal motility disorders. They are multiple in 19% of these patients. Symptoms are those common to motility disorders of the esophagus such as dysphagia, vomiting, epigastric or chest pain, anorexia, and weight loss. As is true for other diverticula of the esophagus, barium esophagram is best for detecting epiphrenic diverticula.

Treatment

Symptomatic patients often require surgical intervention. Along with resection of the diverticulum, esophagomyotomy is performed. If an antireflux procedure is indicated after myotomy, a partial fundoplication (Belsey type) should be performed, rather than a full 360-degree Nissen fundoplication. Most patients report good long-term relief after treatment.

GASTRIC DIVERTICULA

Both true and false diverticula can be found in the *stomach*. Most are discovered on upper gastrointestinal contrast studies, and almost all of them are asymptomatic. Although complications are rare, when they do occur, they are similar to those associated with diverticula in other parts of the gastrointestinal tract, such as bleeding, diverticulitis, and perforation. Gastric diverticula may occur at any age, but most appear between the ages of 20 and 60 years.

Treatment

In the absence of complications associated with gastric diverticula, treatment is not indicated. If complications do occur, resection of the diverticulum is usually sufficient. Occasionally, partial gastric resection may be necessary for lesions such as those located in the pyloric area.

DUODENAL DIVERTICULA

Duodenal diverticula are rarely found before the age of 40 years, and they are usually false diverticula located in the second portion of the duodenum, near the ampulla of Vater. The common bile duct and pancreatic duct may occasionally open into the diverticulum itself. Most of these diverticula are asymptomatic and are discovered on upper gastrointestinal contrast study or endoscopic examination of the duodenum for unrelated problems. Potential complications include obstruction of the biliary or pancreatic ducts with associated cholangitis or pancreatitis, perforation, or hemorrhage. Periampullary duodenal diverticula may be perforated during the course of endoscopic retrograde cholangiopancreatography, especially when the test is combined with endoscopic sphincterotomy.

Treatment

Surgical treatment of duodenal diverticula is indicated only when complications occur. Diverticula found on routine examination require no specific therapy. When operative intervention is undertaken, care should be taken to preserve the integrity of the biliary and pancreatic ducts.

JEJUNAL AND ILEAL DIVERTICULA

Diverticula of the jejunum and ileum are much less common than diverticula of the duodenum. Most occur in the jejunum, are false diverticula, and are found in older age groups. The cause of diverticulosis of the jejunum and ileum is thought to be motor dysfunction resulting in uncoordinated contractions of the small bowel. Acute complications include bleeding, obstruction, and perforation. More chronic complaints include abdominal pain, malabsorption, chronic gastrointestinal hemorrhage, and intestinal obstruction.

Treatment

No treatment is indicated for asymptomatic, incidentally identified diverticula. Treatment of complications such as bleeding, diverticulitis, or hemorrhage often requires resection and anastomosis. Patients who present with malabsorption secondary to bacterial overgrowth in a diverticulum can initially be treated with antibiotics, followed by resection of the diverticulum.

MECKEL'S DIVERTICULUM

Meckel's diverticulum is a remnant of the vitelline duct that connected the yolk sac to the midgut of the embryo. Failure of the vitelline duct to become obliterated accounts for the anomaly. Although the size and shape of the diverticulum may vary greatly, the diverticulum is usually 3 to 5 cm long. The incidence of this condition in various autopsy series is 2% to 3%. The diverticulum is usually situated 40 to 50 cm from the ileocecal valve. It is a true diverticulum containing all layers of the bowel wall and is found on the antimesenteric side of the ileum. Most of these diverticula are lined with ileal mucosa, and 15% to 30% of them are lined with heterotopic tissue including gastric, pancreatic, colonic, and/or jejunal tissue.

Diverticula lined with gastric mucosa may develop into a chronic peptic ulcer, either in the diverticulum itself or in the adjacent ileal mucosa. Ectopic gastric mucosa can often be identified by a technetium scan of the abdomen. Complications other than bleeding include diverticulitis, which often mimics appendicitis, intestinal obstruction, perforation, and carcinoma.

A standard upper gastrointestinal contrast study rarely demonstrates Meckel's diverticulum. Enteroclysis or the introduction of barium directly into the small bowel through a nasogastric tube positioned beyond the ligament of Treitz is often a useful diagnostic adjunct.

Treatment

Surgical resection is the treatment for symptomatic Meckel's diverticulum. Resection of the adjacent segment of ileum is often indicated when peptic ulceration is present. There is no clinical evidence to support resection of asymptomatic Meckel's diverticula discovered either at laparotomy or by contrast study.

COLONIC DIVERTICULA

Colonic diverticulosis is estimated to occur in approximately 5% of the population. Although it is uncommon before the age of 40 years, the incidence increases with advancing age, so by the ninth decade, it is present in two thirds of the population. There is no sex predilection because both men and women are affected equally. Most colonic diverticula are the acquired pulsion type, the result of herniation of mucosa and submucosa through the circular muscle layer of the colon. The diverticula are usually located between the mesenteric and antimesenteric taenia. Segmentation and muscular contraction in the colon result in high intraluminal pressures, the pulsion force that results in herniation of the mucosa. Right-sided or cecal diverticula are usually true diverticula containing all layers of the colonic wall. These right-sided diverticula are thought to be congenital. It is suggested that colonic diverticular disease is the result of a lack of dietary fiber. High-fiber diets are thought to decrease segmentation and intraluminal pressure and thereby decrease the impetus for herniation.

Bleeding and diverticulitis are the most common clinically significant sequelae of colonic diverticulosis. Hemorrhage associated with diverticular disease is thought to be related to the association of the diverticulum and the adjacent penetrating mural vessels. Diverticula were once thought to be the most common cause of lower gastrointestinal hemorrhage. Angiodysplasia, primarily in the right colon, is now thought to be as common a source of hemorrhage, if not more so.

Perforation of a single diverticulum is thought to be the initial event that results in peridiverticulitis. The perforation may be contained within the mesocolon, or it may freely perforate the peritoneal cavity, resulting in peritonitis. Abscess may develop that either extends into the mesentery or to adjacent organs such as the small bowel or urinary bladder. Fistulas may also form involving adjacent organs such as small bowel, bladder, and uterus. Occasionally, patients with delayed presentation may be found to have a colocutaneous fistula. The sigmoid colon is involved with diverticulits in more than 90% of cases, and it is the sole segment of bowel involved in 50%.

Diverticulitis typically presents with left lower quadrant abdominal pain, low-grade fever, leukocytosis, nausea with occasional vomiting, and mild to moderate abdominal distention. Occasionally, one may appreciate a palpable mass in the left lower quadrant on physical examination.

Treatment

Gastrointestinal hemorrhage should be managed first with fluid resuscitation to achieve hemodynamic stabilization and treat and/or prevent hypovolemia. The diagnostic approach depends on whether the bleeding ceases spontaneously or is persistent or recurrent. Attempts should be made to identify the source of hemorrhage, and this can be aided with the use of colonoscopy, nuclear medicine scanning, and angiography. In cases of persistent or recurrent bleeding in which the site of bleeding has been identified, a segmental colectomy can be performed. Persistent hemorrhage and inability to localize the site of bleeding may necessitate subtotal colectomy.

Mild attacks of diverticulitis can be treated with bowel rest, intravenous fluids, and parenteral antibiotics. Some cases may be amenable to management on an outpatient basis with a clear liquid diet and oral antibiotics with broad spectrum coverage to include *Bacteroides fragilis*. Most patients requiring hospitalization will show improvement in 3 to 5 days.

Patients with severe cases of diverticulitis or with associated complications may require more prolonged hospitalization. Computed tomography may often demonstrate the extent and complications of diverticulitis, and a scan should be obtained early in patients with suspected complications of diverticular disease. Patients with recurrent attacks of diverticulitis should undergo elective primary resection of the involved segment of colon.

Diverticulitis complicated by the development of an abscess may require drainage, either by computed tomography–guided percutaneous drainage or by operation. Operation is also indicated in patients with peritonitis secondary to perforated diverticulitis. The involved segment of perforated colon is resected, often with formation of a temporary colostomy.

Most fistulas form secondary to abscess rupture into a contiguous hollow viscus. Colovesical fistula is the most common type of spontaneous internal fistula, occurring in 2% to 4% of patients who develop diverticulitis. Often, the patient presents with symptoms of a urinary tract infection. Patients with more advanced cases may describe passage of feces or air through the urethra. Most patients with colovesical fistula are male. The uterus interposed between the bladder and sigmoid colon provides protection in women.

Colovesical fistula can usually be treated with primary resection of the involved segment of bowel and fistula tract with anastomosis. Obvious defects in the bladder wall are sutured with layered absorbable suture in conjunction with urethral catheter drainage. If neoplasm is suspected as a cause of the fistula, a segment of bladder including the fistula should be resected en bloc with the colon.

INFLAMMATORY BOWEL DISEASE

method of
CHRISTOPHER E. SHIH, M.D., and
MARY L. HARRIS, M.D.
Johns Hopkins Medical Institutions
Baltimore, Maryland

Inflammatory bowel disease (IBD) is a chronic gastrointestinal disorder that consists of two major entities: *ulcerative colitis* and *Crohn's disease*. Ulcerative colitis is characterized by inflammation limited to the mucosal layer of the colon. *Ulcerative proctitis* refers to disease confined to the rectum, *distal colitis* (or *proctosigmoiditis*) extends into the midsigmoid colon, *left-sided colitis* extends to the splenic flexure, and *pancolitis* encompasses any disease proximal to the splenic flexure. Crohn's disease, in contrast, is characterized by transmural inflammation, skip lesions, and granulomas, rather than continuous disease. It can involve the entire gastrointestinal tract from mouth to anus. Most patients have small bowel disease, approximately 20% have disease limited to the colon, about one third have perianal disease, and a few patients have oral, esophageal, gastric, or duodenal involvement.

Both ulcerative colitis and Crohn's disease can present with abdominal pain, diarrhea, fever, and weight loss. Because Crohn's disease is transmural, it can also present with strictures, fistulas, and abscesses. Although there is much individual variability in the natural history of IBD, most patients suffer from a chronic, intermittently relapsing course. The treatment of IBD has several goals: induction of disease remission; maintenance of disease remission; improvement in quality of life; and avoidance of long-term complications such as malnutrition, osteoporosis, and colon cancer. Advances in the understanding of the mechanisms and pathogenesis of IBD have expanded the list of drugs available to combat the disease. Therapeutic agents currently available focus on reducing inflammation, altering luminal bacteria, modifying the immune system, and targeting specific immune processes.

DRUG THERAPY

Aminosalicylates

Sulfasalazine (Azulfidine) and 5-aminosalicylic acid (5-ASA) are the mainstays of outpatient treatment for mild to moderately active IBD. Sulfasalazine is a composite molecule composed of 5-ASA linked by an azo bond to sulfapyridine. It possesses both anti-inflammatory and antibacterial properties. Because colonic bacteria are necessary to reduce the inactive parent drug to its active moieties, this drug is mainly effective in patients with colonic disease. Most of the side effects associated with aminosalicylate use are the result of sulfapyridine;* therefore, certain 5-ASA compounds have been developed with an efficacy equal to that of sulfasalazine but with fewer side effects. Mesalamine (Asacol, Pentasa, Salofalk*) is formulated for delivery into the distal small bowel and colon by either an acrylic resin or encapsulation in ethylcellulose granules; olsalazine (Dipentum) consists of two 5-ASA molecules joined together; and balsalazide (Colazal) contains one 5-ASA linked to a carrier molecule. The latter two are mainly active in the colon. The precise mechanisms of action of aminosalicylates are unknown, although in vitro studies suggest that inhibition of prostaglandin and cytokine synthesis, free radical scavenging, immunosuppressive activity, and impairment of white cell adhesion and function all play a role.

In ulcerative colitis, aminosalicylates are useful for the treatment of mild to moderate disease and for maintenance of remission. Dosages range from 2 to 4 g/d of sulfasalazine, 2 g/d of olsalazine, 2.4 to 4.8 g/d of Asacol, and 4 g/d of Pentasa. All aminosalicylates have similar efficacy, although one report suggested that balsalazide (6.75 g/d) may be more effective than mesalamine in the treatment of left-sided active disease. Higher doses are more effective in inducing and maintaining remission, but they also carry a greater side effect burden; therefore, therapy should begin at lower doses and titrated upward as needed. For active distal colitis, topical therapy with 5-ASA enemas (Rowasa) and suppositories (Canasa) may be beneficial. Several studies have confirmed the superiority of 5-ASA enemas over placebo and steroid enemas, with remission and maintenance rates of 90% and 75%, respectively.

*Not available in the United States.

In Crohn's disease, sulfasalazine† is effective in active colonic disease and benefits some patients with arthritis. 5-ASA† is effective for the treatment of small bowel or colonic disease and for maintenance of remission. Pentasa† at 4 g/d has been proved to decrease the Crohn's disease activity index dramatically and to induce remission more frequently than placebo. Several meta-analyses favor mesalamine† over sulfasalazine for maintenance therapy, especially in patients with ileitis. 5-ASA has also been proved to prevent postoperative recurrences in patients undergoing surgery for Crohn's disease.

Common side effects of sulfasalazine include nausea, headache, fever, rash, and male infertility. These effects are dose related, although most patients tolerate 2 to 4 g/d without problems. Agranulocytosis is a rare but serious side effect, usually occurring within the first 2 months of therapy (but may occur after several years) and typically resolving within 1 to 2 weeks of discontinuation. Sulfasalazine is a competitive inhibitor of folate absorption, so folic acid supplementation (1 mg/d) should be instituted. Common side effects of the 5-ASA preparations include fever, rash, and diarrhea, although they are generally much better tolerated than sulfasalazine. Rarely, acute interstitial nephritis, hypersensitivity pneumonitis, pancreatitis, or neutropenia can occur. Side effects of the topical drugs are few and consist mainly of anal irritation and pruritus. Current data demonstrate that all aminosalicylate preparations are safe in pregnancy and lactation.

Corticosteroids

Corticosteroids are highly effective in treating active IBD but have no proven benefit for maintenance of remission, and their prolonged use is associated with well-known toxicity. For ulcerative proctitis, topical steroids in the form of hydrocortisone enemas (Cortenema) or foams (Cortifoam) are effective, although one meta-analysis concluded that 5-ASA enemas are superior to steroid enemas. For more severe proctitis, left-sided ulcerative colitis, or pancolitis, oral or parenteral steroids are used. A typical regimen is oral prednisone, at 40 mg/d, and for more severe or fulminant disease, hydrocortisone (Solu-Cortef, 100 mg intravenously every 8 hours) or methylprednisolone (Solu-Medrol, 40 mg/d intravenously) can be used. Many physicians believe that a 24-hour continuous infusion may be more effective than bolus dosing, although this has not been proven. Side effects of high-dose intravenous steroids include hyperglycemia, hypertension, and acute psychosis. Gradual tapering should begin after the patient has been stable for 2 to 4 weeks. A common method is to decrease the dose by 5 mg every 1 to 2 weeks down to a dose of 20 mg/d, with further reduction based on the patient's ability to tolerate the regimen.

Active inflammatory Crohn's disease responds well to oral prednisone (40 mg/d). As in ulcerative colitis, the goal should be tapering and discontinuation of

†Not FDA-approved for this indication.

steroids, although many patients are unable to be weaned from the drugs definitively and are considered to be *steroid-dependent*. Steroids may be used in combination with other drugs; one study demonstrated that sulfasalazine* and prednisone together were better than either alone. Budesonide (Entocort EC),* administered at 9 mg/d orally, is a glucocorticoid with low systemic activity resulting from extensive hepatic first-pass metabolism that has demonstrated efficacy similar to that of conventional steroids, with less toxicity and impact on the hypothalamic-pituitary-adrenal axis. Studies suggest that this drug is effective for inducing remission in ileal or ileocecal disease, but it is probably ineffective for maintaining steroid-induced remission. Budesonide enemas† are available as well and are comparable to conventional steroid enemas with less endogenous cortisol suppression.

Antibiotics

Studies in animals suggest that *dysbiosis*, or altered balance of protective bacteria and aggressive commensal organisms, plays a role in the pathogenesis of IBD. In multiple animal models that lack luminal bacteria, there is a total absence of immune activation and colitis. Several antibiotics have proven to be beneficial in Crohn's disease. Ciprofloxacin (Cipro),* 500 mg orally twice daily, is similar in efficacy to mesalamine and is superior to placebo in the treatment of small bowel and colonic disease. Side effects include headache, rash, nausea, arthralgias, and tendinitis. Metronidazole (Flagyl),* 250 mg orally three or four times daily, is probably the best studied of the available antibiotics and is useful in treating patients with active small bowel and colonic Crohn's disease. It is also effective in treating perianal disease and may delay recurrence after ileocolonic resection. Side effects include nausea, metallic taste, and peripheral neuropathy. Other effective antibiotics are clarithryomycin (Biaxin),* tetracycline,* and cephalexin (Keflex).* Several studies have demonstrated that ciprofloxacin* may have short-term and long-term benefits in the treatment of ulcerative colitis.

Immunomodulators

Azathioprine and 6-Mercaptopurine

Azathioprine (Imuran)* is a purine analogue interfering with nucleic acid metabolism and cell proliferation; its principal metabolite is 6-mercaptopurine (6-MP [Purinethol*]). Both azathioprine and 6-MP can be used interchangeably, although the latter is often better tolerated. In Crohn's disease, these drugs are indicated for induction of remission in steroid-dependent or steroid-refractory disease, in fistulizing disease, as maintenance therapy, and possibly in preventing relapse after surgical treatment. Studies have suggested a role for monitoring enzyme and metabolite concentrations in guiding dose administration of azathioprine and 6-MP. Thiopurine methyltransferase is one of the enzymes involved in the metabolism of 6-MP to 6-thioguanine and 6-methylmercaptopurine. Low 6-thioguanine levels may guide dose adjustment in nonresponding patients, whereas low thiopurine methyltransferase activity may identify patients at risk of bone marrow toxicity. Dose ranges for azathioprine* and 6-MP* are 1.5 to 2.5 mg/kg/d, according to enzyme and metabolite concentrations. A full therapeutic response can vary from 6 to 8 weeks to 4 to 6 months. Approximately 30% of patients will have a relapse despite therapy. Risk factors for relapse include female gender, younger age, and time for achieving remission longer than 6 months. The optimal duration of maintenance therapy is unclear; one study suggested that continued therapy beyond 4 years may not be beneficial. Azathioprine and 6-MP are also effective in treating ulcerative colitis refractory to conventional therapy and should be considered before colectomy. These drugs are effective in 60% to 70% of patients with refractory disease, and they also maintain remission and may spare the patient steroid dosing.

Side effects include allergic reactions, leukopenia, pancreatitis, and elevation of aminotransferases. Therefore, careful monitoring of the patient, including monthly complete blood counts with differentials (weekly during the first month of treatment) and liver function tests, is warranted. Other side effects include opportunistic infections, particularly in patients concurrently taking corticosteroids, and a theoretical risk of neoplasia, although studies have not substantiated this risk at doses used to treat IBD. The safety of azathioprine and 6-MP in pregnancy is poorly understood. 6-MP has teratogenic properties in animal models, but several series and anecdotal evidence suggest that it and azathioprine are probably safe.

Methotrexate

Methotrexate* is a folic acid analogue that inhibits binding of dihydrofolic acid to dihydrofolate reductase. Its utility in induction of remission in Crohn's disease is well established, but studies for maintenance therapy have been mixed. Some physicians select methotrexate if a patient is intolerant to azathioprine or 6-MP or if therapy with these agents fails. The usual dosage is 25 mg/week intramuscularly. A response can be observed in 3 to 12 weeks, and the drug should be discontinued if no therapeutic gain is achieved by week 16. Side effects include hepatotoxicity, interstitial pneumonitis, opportunistic infections, and bone marrow suppression. In the past, some authors advocated liver biopsies after 500 to 1000 mg of total drug to monitor hepatotoxicity (fibrosis and/or cirrhosis), although increasing evidence suggests that this recommendation may not be justified. Folic acid (Folvite),* 1 mg/d, should be given routinely to reduce side effects, and patients must abstain from alcohol for further prevention of fibrosis or cirrhosis. In ulcerative colitis, methotrexate may be an alternative treatment in patients who are intolerant of or refractory to azathioprine or 6-MP.

*Not FDA-approved for this indication.
†Not available in the United States.

*Not FDA-approved for this indication.

Cyclosporine

Cyclosporine (Sandimmune)* is a cyclic polypeptide that inhibits T-cell function and proliferation. It is most commonly used in severe steroid-resistant ulcerative colitis but is not indicated for long-term therapy. One study demonstrated that its use enabled 60% of patients presenting with severe steroid-resistant ulcerative colitis to avoid colectomy for 1 year. The drug may be given as a continuous or 4-hour infusion (4 mg/kg/d). Blood levels must be carefully monitored, with a 12-hour trough monoclonal antibody level goal of 300 to 400 ng/mL during the acute phase. Serum cholesterol should be checked before initiating cyclosporine; a level lower than 120 mg/dL is a contraindication because of the risk of seizures. For responding patients, oral cyclosporine* (5 to 7 mg/kg/d) should be continued for 3 to 4 months, and trough levels should be maintained at 150 to 300 ng/mL. Cyclosporine is not usually prescribed for Crohn's disease, with the exception of fistulizing disease, in which intravenous cyclosporine may be effective in reducing fistula drainage. Side effects include hypertension, seizures, neuropathy, opportunistic infections, multiple drug interactions, and nephrotoxicity, which is usually reversible. An increase in the serum creatinine of more than 30% requires a decrease in dosage or temporary discontinuation. Trimethoprim-sulfamethoxazole (Bactrim, Septra)* is advocated for prophylaxis against *Pneumoncystis carinii* pneumonia.

Infliximab

Infliximab (Remicade) is a chimeric monoclonal antibody targeting tumor necrosis factor-α (TNF-α). Growing evidence suggests that TNF-α plays a pivotal role in the pathogenesis of Crohn's disease and possibly ulcerative colitis. Infliximab is indicated for induction and maintenance of remission in moderately to severely active Crohn's disease unresponsive to conventional treatment. For induction, the dose used is 5 mg/kg intravenously given as a single infusion at 0, 2, and 6 weeks. For maintenance, the dose is 5 mg/kg given every 8 weeks, although some patients may require a decrease in the administration interval or an increase in the dosage to 10 mg/kg. Data exist for use up to 54 weeks (the ACCENT trials), although longer use is reportedly safe and effective for maintenance therapy beyond 1 year. In active inflammatory disease, infliximab may be steroid-sparing. In fistulizing disease, ongoing trials have demonstrated efficacy in closing or decreasing drainage of fistulas. Nonsmokers and those receiving concurrent immunomodulator therapy are more likely to respond. Side effects include infusion reactions (pruritus, rash, headaches) that usually respond to acetaminophen (Tylenol) or diphenhydramine (Benadryl), development of anti-chimeric antibodies (which may increase the risk of infusion reactions), and infections such as pneumonia, abscesses, or tuberculosis. A PPD skin test and chest radiograph are recommended in all patients before infliximab therapy is initiated. Small bowel obstruction has been described with infliximab use, so caution is warranted in patients with stricturing or fibrostenotic disease. In pregnancy, preliminary reports suggest that infliximab is probably safe, although extensive data are lacking. Studies are currently under way for use of infliximab in ulcerative colitis.

*Not FDA-approved for this indication.

Other Agents

Nicotine

The observation that smokers are at decreased risk of ulcerative colitis led to two placebo-controlled trials of transdermal nicotine (Nicotrol)* in active mild distal and left-sided ulcerative colitis. Both trials demonstrated the efficacy of this agent, although its use may be limited by nausea and headache. It is not effective in maintaining remission and is contraindicated in Crohn's disease. Transdermal nicotine is probably most useful in patients with ulcerative colitis exacerbations and recent smoking cessation.

Heparin

Heparin* has anti-inflammatory and antithrombotic properties. Data are mixed regarding its efficacy in the treatment of ulcerative colitis. It may be indicated as short-term, adjunctive therapy in patients with refractory disease or as a bridge to immunomodulator treatment. Data suggest that low-molecular-weight heparin (enoxaparin [Lovenox]*) may be useful in steroid-refractory ulcerative colitis. Caution is warranted in patients with active gastrointestinal bleeding.

Investigational Drugs

Numerous agents are currently being evaluated, particularly in refractory IBD unresponsive to conventional treatment. Recombinant human interleukin-11 (oprelvekin [Neumega])* is a cytokine with multiple biologic effects including thrombocytopoietic properties and enhancement of intestinal mucosa barrier function. It is safe and effective in a subset of patients with Crohn's disease. Fish oil–derived eicosapentaenoic acid inhibits leukotriene activity and may be effective in both ulcerative colitis and Crohn's disease. Thalidomide (Thalomid)* may be of benefit in steroid-refractory and fistulizing Crohn's disease, but it has teratogenic side effects. Mycophenolate mofetil (CellCept)* is an immunosuppressant used more often in the setting of organ transplantation, and it may be an alternative agent in patients with Crohn's disease who are intolerant of or unresponsive to azathioprine (Imuran)* or 6-MP.* Probiotics are emerging as potentially useful in certain diseases, and preliminary observations in ulcerative colitis suggest that these agents may be as effective as mesalamine. Other drugs currently under investigation include adhesion molecules involved in lymphocyte-endothelial recognition, inhibitors of lymphocyte trafficking (e.g., natalizumab,†

*Not FDA-approved for this indication.
†Investigational drug in the United States.

LDP-2, Isis 2302), inhibitors of Th1 polarization (e.g., anti–IL-12,† interferon-γ,* anti–interferon-γ†), inhibitors of TNF (e.g., etanercept [Enbrel]* and CDP571,† both with negative studies in Crohn's disease), inhibitors of T-cell activation, anti-CD4 antibodies, and growth hormone (somatropin [Genotropin]*).

MEDICAL MANAGEMENT

Medical management of IBD is dictated by the site, extent, and severity of disease, as well as by the side effect profile of the medications used (Tables 1 and 2). Disease activity may be defined as mild to moderate (local symptoms with no overt systemic disturbances) or severe (fever, weight loss, anemia, hypoalbuminemia).

Ulcerative Colitis

Proctitis

Approximately 30% of patients with ulcerative colitis present with proctitis, although subsequent proximal spread of disease can occur. Typical presenting symptoms include rectal bleeding, tenesmus, diarrhea, mucus, and rectal pain. The mainstay of treatment is topical 5-ASA suppositories or steroid foams. Usually, 5-ASA suppositories (Canasa) 500 mg given twice a day will work within 3 weeks, and this dose is continued until the patient is in remission. In patients who cannot tolerate topical therapy, oral 5-ASA agents can be substituted with similar efficacy. Systemic steroids are rarely required in ulcerative proctitis, and they should be reserved for patients with severe or refractory disease.

*Not FDA-approved for this indication.
†Investigational drug in the United States.

Proctosigmoiditis

Patients with proctosigmoiditis, or distal colitis, also generally respond to topical therapy. Presenting symptoms include bloody diarrhea, abdominal pain, and possibly fever, weight loss, or anorexia. Therapy for mild to moderate disease should begin with 5-ASA or hydrocortisone enemas. As with suppository therapy, 5-ASA is preferred because of its proven benefit in maintaining remission. For patients not tolerating or responding to topical therapy, oral 5-ASA agents can be used. Evidence suggests that the combination of oral and topical 5-ASA may be more effective than either preparation alone in the treatment of distal colitis. Three to 6 weeks of treatment may be required before a response is seen. For patients with a more severe clinical presentation, oral prednisone* (40 to 60 mg/d) may be given for 10 to 14 days, followed by a taper of 5 mg per week. Trials have demonstrated that budesonide (Entocort)* enemas are effective in inducing remission in distal ulcerative colitis and produce less endogenous cortisol suppression than conventional corticosteroids.

Left-Sided Colitis and Pancolitis

Therapy in patients with left-sided colitis or pancolitis should be tailored based on the clinical picture. As with proctosigmoiditis, oral and topical 5-ASA, oral or systemic steroids in more severe disease, and maintenance 5-ASA are standard measures. Other considerations include supplemental iron for

*Not FDA-approved for this indication.

TABLE 1. **Treatment of Ulcerative Colitis**

	Proctitis	Left-sided Colitis	Pancolitis
Mild	Topical aminosalicylates[1] Topical steroids	Oral and topical aminosalicylates	Oral and topical aminosalicylates Oral steroids[2] Steroid-sparing agent[3]
Moderate	Oral and topical aminosalicylates Topical steroids	Oral and topical aminosalicylates Oral steroids Steroid-sparing agent[3]	Oral and topical aminosalicylates Oral steroids Steroid-sparing agent[3]
Severe	Oral and topical aminosalicylates Oral steroids Hospitalization[4] Immunosuppressive agent[3,5]	Hospitalization Oral aminosalicylates Intravenous steroids Immunosuppressive agent[5]	Hospitalization Oral aminosalicylates Intravenous steroids Immunosuppressive agent[5]
Fulminant		Hospitalization Oral aminosalicylates Antibiotics Intravenous steroids Immunosuppressive agent[5] Surgical intervention[6]	Hospitalization Oral aminosalicylates[7] Antibiotics Intravenous steroids[7] Immunosuppressive agent[5] Surgical intervention[6]
Maintenance	Oral aminosalicylates Topical steroids	Oral aminosalicylates Azathioprine/6-MP[7]	Oral aminosalicylates Azathioprine/6-MP[7]

[1]Aminosalicylate enemas and/or suppositories; not FDA-approved for this indication.
[2]Low threshold for oral steroid; not FDA-approved for this indication.
[3]Azathioprine/6-MP; not FDA-approved for this indication.
[4]Hospitalization is uncommon.
[5]Cyclosporine; not FDA-approved for this indication.
[6]If no clinical improvement in 24 to 72 hours, then surgical intervention is indicated. Surgical consultation should occur early in the evaluation of patients with severe or fulminant disease.
[7]Not FDA-approved for this indication.

TABLE 2. **Treatment of Crohn's Disease**

Mild CDAI[1] 150-220	Oral aminosalicylates[2] Antibiotics[2, 3]
Moderate CDAI 220-400	Oral aminosalicylates Antibiotics[3] Oral steroids Consider immunosuppressives[4]
Severe CDAI >400	Hospitalization Oral aminosalicylates[2] Intravenous antibiotics Intravenous steroids[2] Immunosuppressives[4]
Maintenance and prevention of postoperative recurrence	Oral aminosalicylates[2] Antibiotics[2, 3] Azathioprine/6-MP (Purethinol)[2] Infliximab[2]
Perianal disease and fistulas	Antibiotics[2, 5] Immunosuppressives[2, 4] Infliximab[2]

[1]The Crohn's Disease Activity Index (CDAI), as part of a 7-day diary, measures disease activity based on constitutional symptoms, extraintestinal manifestations, and severity of pain. Objective factors of body weight, frequency of bowel movements, hematocrit, and the use of antidiarrheal medications are also measured.

[2]Not FDA-approved for this indication.

[3]Metronidazole has demonstrated the best efficacy in clinical trials. Alternative antibiotics, especially ciprofloxacin (not FDA-approved for this indication), are appropriate.

[4]Azathioprine/6-MP (not FDA-approved for this indication), cyclosporine (not FDA-approved for this indication), methotrexate (not FDA-approved for this indication), infliximab (not FDA-approved for this indication).

[5]Metronidazole with or without ciprofloxacin.

patients with iron deficiency anemia resulting from long-term blood loss and antidiarrheal agents such as loperamide for patients with persistent diarrhea. Antidiarrheal agents and narcotics should not be used in the acute setting because of the risk of toxic megacolon.

Severe or Fulminant Colitis

Presenting symptoms of severe or fulminant ulcerative colitis include frequent bloody stools, dehydration, fever, anorexia, weight loss, and abdominal pain. Patients with fulminant disease are at risk of developing toxic megacolon and perforation and should be immediately hospitalized. Primary therapy involves bowel rest, intravenous steroids, and prompt surgical consultation. Broad-spectrum antibiotics should be given to all patients with high fever, leukocytosis, bandemia, megacolon, or peritoneal signs. Patients with intestinal dilation should undergo decompression with a nasogastric tube and possibly a rectal tube. It may be helpful to have patients roll from supine to prone every 2 hours, to redistribute gas. Narcotics are contraindicated in the setting of severe or fulminant colitis because they may predispose patients to toxic megacolon.

Patients who do not respond to intravenous corticosteroids are candidates for intravenous cyclosporine (Sandimmune IV).* Response is usually seen in 3 to 5 days. For those who respond, oral cyclosporine (Neoral)* should be continued for 3 to 4 months while steroids are being tapered, with careful monitoring of trough levels. Because cyclosporine is not effective for maintenance, azathioprine (Imuran)* or 6-MP (Asacol)* should be introduced (or continued in patients already taking them) at the beginning of oral cyclosporine treatment. Patients with toxic megacolon that fails to resolve within 72 hours, those in whom a 7- to 10-day regimen of cyclosporine* therapy fails, or those in whom cyclosporine* is contraindicated should be considered for colectomy.

*Not FDA-approved for this indication.

Refractory Colitis

Regardless of the extent of colonic involvement, some patients remain refractory despite conventional treatment. Infliximab's efficacy has been reported for some of these patients, but phase III multicenter studies are pending. Colectomy should be a consideration in chronic symptomatic disease when all medical avenues have been exhausted.

Crohn's Disease

Oral Lesions

Oral lesions can complicate the clinical picture by causing severe pain and potentially impairing nutrition. Aphthous ulcerations are the most common, followed by cheilitis, sialadenitis, and granulomatous masses. These lesions usually coexist with intestinal disease and may respond to appropriate intestinal therapy. Topical therapy with prednisolone slurries (10 mg swish and spit twice daily) reduces pain and enhances resolution of ulcers, while minimizing systemic adverse effects.

Gastroduodenal Involvement

Fewer than 5% of patients with Crohn's disease have gastroduodenal involvement. Presenting symptoms include epigastric pain, nausea, and vomiting and may be confused with peptic ulcer disease. Proton pump inhibition, histamine-2 receptor antagonists, or sucralfate (Carafate)* may be added to mesalamine (Pentasa),* formulated for proximal small bowel delivery. For more severe or refractory disease, prednisone,* azathioprine,* or 6-MP* may be required.

Ileitis

The ileum is the most common region of small bowel involvement and patients may present with abdominal pain, diarrhea, fever, anemia, and potentially weight loss. In mild to moderate disease, initial treatment should begin with oral mesalamine (Asacol or Pentasa),* along with antibiotics such as metronidazole (Flagyl)* or ciprofloxacin (Cipro).* For refractory disease, oral prednisone* may be initiated at 20 to 40 mg in single morning dosing. After resolution of symptoms, a taper schedule by 5 mg/week is used. The role of alternate-day steroid therapy after long-term use allows for pituitary-adrenal axis recovery. An alternative to prednisone is budesonide* controlled ileal release at 9 mg/d. Once remission is obtained, long-term maintenance therapy with mesalamine (Asacol),* 2.4 to 4.8 g/d, is recommended.

*Not FDA-approved for this indication.

Complications of ileal disease include partial or complete bowel obstruction, perforation with abscess formation, or frank peritonitis with fever, chills, abdominal pain, and leukocytosis. Management involves complete bowel rest, broad-spectrum antibiotics, and possible catheter or surgical drainage with resection.

Ileocolitis and Colitis

Patients with active ileocolitis or disease limited to the colon can present with abdominal pain, usually nonbloody diarrhea, fever, or weight loss. Therapy in mild to moderate disease is initiated with oral sulfasalazine (Azulfidine),* 2 to 4 g/d, or mesalamine,* 2.4 to 4.8 g/d. As with ileitis, antibiotics followed by oral prednisone should be considered in patients unresponsive to aminosalicylates. Once remission is achieved, maintenance therapy should be continued with an oral 5-ASA agent. Patients with active distal Crohn's colitis can benefit from topical therapy with mesalamine or hydrocortisone enemas. Patients with severe or fulminant Crohn's colitis should be treated in a manner similar to patients with ulcerative colitis, with bowel rest, parenteral corticosteroids, and immunomodulator therapy.

Refractory Disease

In addition to steroids, mesalamine, and antibiotics, azathioprine,* 6-MP,* methotrexate (Rheumatrex),* and infliximab are available for patients with refractory disease. Optimistically, steroids can be tapered as these immunomodulators exert their therapeutic effects. Monitoring of hepatic and renal function as well as bone density in long-term immunomodulator and steroid use is important. Prolonged bowel rest with total parenteral nutrition may improve surgical outcomes. Risks of total parenteral nutrition include potential line sepsis, thrombophlebitis, and, rarely, pulmonary embolism as a consequence of a hypercoagulable state.

Perineal or Fistulizing Disease

Perineal (rectovaginal and perianal) fistulas and abscesses may occur in one third of patients with Crohn's disease. Ideally, treatment consists of synergistic metronidazole (Flagyl),* 10 to 20 mg/kg/d, and ciprofloxacin (Cipro),* 500 mg twice daily. Because of a high relapse rate after cessation of antibiotic therapy, some patients will require long-term treatment with azathioprine, 6-MP, and/or surgical seton placement. In addition, enterocutaneous, enterovesicular, and rectovaginal fistulas are treated with azathioprine* or 6-MP* and infliximab (at weeks 0, 2, and 6, followed by every 8 weeks). A relatively new treatment option is injection of fibrin glue while the patient is under general anesthesia, although studies are lacking regarding long-term outcomes.

SURGERY

Indications for urgent surgical treatment in IBD include hemorrhage, perforation, and toxic megacolon.

*Not FDA-approved for this indication.

Elective indications include chronic disease refractory to medical therapy, moderate to high-grade dysplasia, frank malignancy, or dysplasia-associated lesions or masses found on surveillance endoscopy. Dysplasia-associated lesions or masses are nonadenomatous lesions seen in IBD that may have underlying malignancy not detectable by endoscopic biopsy. In ulcerative colitis, the preferred method for elective colectomy is the ileal pouch–anal canal anastomosis. This procedure improves the quality of life for patients and reduces the risk of colonic malignancy. An ileostomy may be unavoidable in patients who are not candidates for this operation or in whom a continence-preserving operation fails because of, for example, obesity or rectal malignant disease. Complications include urinary and sexual dysfunction and a potential reduction in female fertility. Other complications include bowel obstruction, anastomotic leak, irritable bowel syndrome, and pouchitis. Pouchitis, leading to increased urgency, bowel movements, and incontinence, may respond to antibiotics and topical mesalamine,* and on occasion it may require surgical diversion.

In Crohn's disease, the surgical approach is focal, targeting sites of bleeding, obstruction, perforation, abscesses, or fistula formation. In addition to resection, other therapeutic options include strictureplasty, balloon dilation, or stenting. Surgery for Crohn's disease is not curative; postoperative recurrence rates are very high and may lead to subsequent reoperations.

NUTRITIONAL SUPPORT

Malnutrition is a common feature in IBD. Mechanisms include decreased oral intake, malabsorption, increased energy expenditure, and enteral protein loss. Specific nutrients at risk for deficiency include vitamin B_{12}, calcium, fat-soluble vitamins, folic acid, iron, protein, and trace minerals. Consequences of malnutrition include growth retardation and pubertal delay in children and adolescents, osteoporosis and osteomalacia, anemia, and postoperative morbidity. Parenteral nutrition is indicated in preoperative management and on a long-term basis in the unfortunate patient with short bowel syndrome (loss of more than 70% of bowel). Closure of fistulas may be induced by total parenteral nutrition and bowel rest with aggressive medical therapy, although this beneficial response may be lost on resumption of oral feeding. Patients with IBD should be carefully monitored for nutrient deficiencies and should be supplemented as necessary.

Specific foods that trigger intestinal symptoms should be avoided. For example, lactose intolerance is common, and patients often benefit from dietary fat and dairy restriction. Those with small bowel strictures should follow a low-residue diet and should avoid nuts, seeds, and corn. Calcium oxalate nephrolithiasis is common in patients with Crohn's disease with an intact colon because of absorption of unbound oxalate. Medium-chain triglyceride supplements may be

*Not FDA-approved for this indication.

helpful in patients with short bowel syndrome and diarrhea.

Osteoporosis is particularly prevalent in the IBD population owing to corticosteroid use, calcium and vitamin D malabsorption, and proinflammatory mediators. Bone loss begins within the first 3 months of corticosteroid use. All patients taking steroids should undergo baseline bone densitometry and should be followed yearly while they are taking steroids. Vitamin D (400 IU/d) and calcium supplementation (1000 to 1500 mg/d) are requisite, and bisphosphonate therapy (alendronate [Fosamax] 70 mg/week orally, risedronate [Actonel] 35 mg/week orally, or pamidronate [Aredia] 30 mg intravenously every 3 to 4 months) is indicated for patients with abnormal bone density.

COLON CANCER SURVEILLANCE

The increased risk of colorectal cancer in IBD is related to the duration and extent of disease, with mortality occurring at younger ages than in the general population. Routine endoscopic cancer surveillance is recommended at 8 to 10 years after the onset of symptoms of pancolitis and left-sided colitis. Proctitis appears to carry a risk similar to that of the general population. Although less clear, Crohn's colitis should be treated similarly to ulcerative colitis, particularly if the colonic disease is extensive. Dysplasia may precede colorectal cancer. In ulcerative colitis, total colectomy is standard for moderate to high-grade dysplasia, dysplasia-associated lesions or masses, or frank malignancy, whereas segmental resection is recommended in Crohn's colitis. In surveillance colonoscopy, the mucosa is sampled every 10 cm in 8 regions, for a minimum of 32 biopsies. Folate* supplementation has been reported to decrease the incidence of dysplasia in chronic ulcerative colitis, and long-term control of disease with mesalamine may reduce the risk of colorectal cancer.

SUPPORTIVE THERAPY

Patients with IBD often have chronic, refractory diarrhea and may benefit from antidiarrheal agents such as loperamide (Imodium). However, antidiarrheals are contraindicated in acute disease because of the risk of ileus or toxic megacolon. In patients with ileal resections of less than 100 cm, diarrhea is caused by bile salt malabsorption. A bile acid–binding resin, cholestyramine (Questran),* 4 g/dose, is recommended. In addition, coexistent irritable bowel syndrome may occur in 20% of patients with IBD; antispasmodic agents such as hyoscyamine (Levsin) or dicyclomine (Bentyl) may be beneficial when symptoms persist in the absence of active inflammatory disease.

PSYCHOSOCIAL SUPPORT

A positive, supportive approach by the physician is important in reassuring and easing patients' anxieties regarding chronic pain, impaired quality of life, depression, fear of surgery, and risk of malignancy. A multidisciplinary approach may be necessary, with referrals to dietitians, social workers, or psychiatrists in appropriate cases. Information and resources available to patients and families include the Crohn's and Colitis Foundation of America (Web site: http://www.ccfa.org), which can provide education and information on local support groups.

*Not FDA-approved for this indication.

IRRITABLE BOWEL SYNDROME

method of
SANJAY NANDURKAR, M.B.B.S., and
PETER GIBSON, M.D.
Monash University
Box Hill Hospital
Box Hill, Victoria, Australia

Irritable bowel syndrome (IBS) is classified as a functional gastrointestinal disorder characterized by symptoms of abdominal pain and discomfort and disturbances in defecation. The diagnosis of IBS is not laboratory based but rests mainly on identifying patients with a particular symptom complex. IBS is a highly prevalent disorder and can have a significant impact on quality of life. The pathophysiology of this condition remains poorly understood. However, recent renewed interest has led to well-designed studies that are attempting to explain the basic mechanisms underlying this chronic disorder. The last 5 years have also seen the introduction of newer pharmacologic agents aimed at management of this condition.

DIAGNOSIS

IBS is a chronic disorder with a female preponderance. It is unclear whether the curiously high proportion of males with IBS noted in certain Asian countries (such as Pakistan and Bangladesh) is related to differences in health care–seeking attitudes within the population. IBS usually develops early in life with a history of unexplained abdominal discomfort associated with irregular bowel habits; ancillary symptoms such as bloating, lower back pain, or urogynecologic symptoms may also be present. The original definition of IBS put forth by Manning was based on a symptom cluster that included the following: abdominal pain with relief after defecation, more frequent stools occurring at the onset of pain, looser stools occurring at the onset of pain, visible abdominal distention, passage of rectal mucus, and a sensation of incomplete evacuation after defecation. Furthermore, based on the type of alteration in bowel habits observed, the disorder was classified into diarrhea- and constipation-predominant subtypes.

An international consensus meeting of experts in this field put forth the ROME classification system wherein the disorder is defined essentially according to its main attributes, that is, abdominal discomfort and altered bowel pattern. These criteria were recently modified (ROME II) and validated in prospective clinical studies. Adoption of the ROME II criteria (Table 1) has been helpful in standardizing the definition of IBS across clinical studies and therapeutic trials. However, it should be emphasized that no structural lesion is pathognomonic of this disorder.

EPIDEMIOLOGY

IBS is a common disorder. In the Western population, prevalence estimates vary widely (3% to 20%), depending on the criteria used; in North America, using cutoffs of two, three, and more than four of the six established Manning criteria yielded prevalence estimates of 17, 13, and 9 per 100, respectively. Lower estimates (3%) were obtained when the modified ROME definition was applied. Recent data report a prevalence of 4% to 7% in Asian populations; in most patients (80%) referred to specialists, IBS was not diagnosed by their referring general practitioners. The prevalence is clearly greater in women but appears to be equal in whites and blacks. Women tend to have more constipation-predominant IBS. The prevalence of IBS does not appear to change significantly with age. Longitudinal studies have shown that symptoms tend to fluctuate over the years. Indeed, a proportion of patients (up to a third) who earlier met the criteria for IBS may not do so the following year.

PATHOPHYSIOLOGY

Although the exact pathophysiologic mechanisms underlying this disorder still need to be clarified, several key observations made to date suggest that an interaction between psychologic factors and an alteration in gut sensitivity, gut reactivity, and regulation of the brain-gut axis may be responsible for the production of symptoms.

Altered Gut Sensitivity

IBS patients have enhanced perception of visceral activity. Moreover, this heightened perception is not restricted to the colon but also applies to the esophagus, stomach, and small bowel. However, they do not exhibit increased sensitivity to somatic pain stimuli; indeed, their peripheral somatic thresholds may be elevated.

TABLE 1. **ROME II Criteria for Diagnosing Irritable Bowel Syndrome**

Twelve weeks or more of abdominal discomfort or pain in the past 12 months that has 2 of 3 features:

Relief with defecation and/or
Association with a change in the frequency of stools and/or
Association with a change in the form (appearance) of stools

Symptoms that cumulatively support the diagnosis of irritable bowel syndrome:

Abnormal stool frequency (for research purposes, abnormal frequency may be defined as more than 3 bowel movements per day and fewer than 3 bowel movements per week)
Abnormal stool form (lumpy/hard or loose/watery)
Abnormal stool passage (straining, urgency, or feeling of incomplete evacuation)
Passage of mucus; bloating or a feeling of abdominal distention

Altered Gut Reactivity

Emerging data suggest that inflammatory models may explain some of the pathophysiology underlying this disorder. An increase in mast cells in the terminal ileum and colon has been demonstrated in patients with IBS by some investigators, but not by others. Recent research has shown that in patients with IBS, full-thickness biopsy specimens of the jejunum demonstrate low-grade infiltration of the myenteric plexus by $CD3^+$ T lymphocytes, along with neuronal degeneration. IBS-type symptoms may develop in up to a quarter of patients who have recovered from bacterial gastroenteritis (especially that caused by *Campylobacter*); female gender, longer duration of illness, and stress may be predictors for the acquisition of postinfectious IBS. An increased number of $CD3^+$ T cells, intraepithelial lymphocytes, and enterochromaffin cells have been observed in the colon of subjects with postinfectious IBS. However, no population-based studies have been conducted to prove that these inflammatory findings can be used as diagnostic markers for IBS.

Altered Regulation of the Brain-Gut Axis

Communication between the central nervous system and the gut is bidirectional. Visceral afferent signals are filtered and modulated by the brain. Perception thresholds vary according to the emotional state, and stress and anxiety can up-regulate perception. Conversely, relaxation can down-regulate visceral perception. Recent data derived from functional brain imaging techniques have shown that (1) viscera have a greater representation on the limbic cortex than somatic structures do (thereby explaining the greater autonomic responses evoked by visceral sensation than by somatic sensation) and (2) colonic stimulation of IBS patients causes greater activation of the limbic system than in healthy controls (thus suggesting altered processing in IBS patients as opposed to controls).

Altered Psychologic State

IBS patients report more psychologic or psychiatric disturbances (such as depression, anxiety, personality disorder) and major life stress events (such as abuse) than healthy controls do. Prevalence estimates for psychiatric disorders in IBS range from 40% to 90%; a higher prevalence is seen in those who seek health care, especially in tertiary institutions. Psychologic stress, in turn, has been shown to exacerbate gastrointestinal symptoms in IBS patients. Moreover, IBS patients may also have a maladaptive coping style that may adversely affect their clinical outcome.

APPROACH TO INVESTIGATION

After positively identifying patients fulfilling the requisite diagnostic criteria (see earlier), further tests are carried out mainly to exclude other disease processes that may mimic IBS symptoms. The extent of such investigation depends largely on the clinical scenario. Laboratory testing includes a complete blood count, routine serum chemistry panel, C-reactive protein, and thyroid function tests. Whether serologic screening for celiac disease should be carried out in all patients is controversial, but up to 5% of patients with IBS (diarrhea or constipation predominant) have celiac disease. Certainly, if upper gastrointestinal endoscopy is performed, harvesting of multiple duodenal biopsy samples is mandatory. Colonoscopy is generally indicated to rule out a neoplasm (especially in patients older than 50 years) in constipation-predominant IBS, but it is also helpful in patients with diarrhea to rule out inflammatory bowel disease and microscopic and collagenous colitis. In such a situation, biopsy of the terminal ileum, right and left colon, and rectum should be performed for histopathologic assessment. Routine use of ultrasound and computed tomography is not indicated. The absence of other diseases helps firmly establish the diagnosis. Finally, "alarm" features such as fever, weight loss, and blood in the stool suggest that alternative diagnoses should be sought.

TREATMENT

One of the main goals of therapy in IBS is to provide the patient with adequate information about this disorder and to direct treatment toward their most dominant symptoms. The steps in therapy (Figure 1) can be outlined as follows:

Explanation of the Disorder

Patients often seek health care to obtain reassurance that they are indeed suffering from a genuine medical condition and that it is not "all in their mind." To that end, it is imperative to spend adequate time during the consultation to address their concerns and assure them that IBS is in fact a highly prevalent condition and that their symptoms are quite typical of this disorder. Moreover, the absence of other medical conditions that were sought by blood tests and endoscopy helps strengthen the diagnosis. Furthermore, it needs to be stressed that this condition is not associated with any long-term sequelae such as bowel cancer. Finally, the fluctuating nature of this disorder needs to be explained along with the fact that most therapies are not aimed at a "cure" but essentially at symptom control. In addition, it needs to be stressed that in spite of adequate therapy, symptoms may flare up for reasons not entirely understood.

Lifestyle Modification

At the initial visit, the severity of the condition and its impact on quality of life need to be ascertained. Lifestyle modification is usually chosen as the first step in management, either on its own or combined with other pharmacologic and nonpharmacologic therapies (see later). Although replenishment of adequate fiber and water in the diet is usually emphasized as good clinical practice, data to support its efficacy in IBS are lacking. The addition of commercially manufactured fiber (20 to 30 g/d) can be useful in a subgroup of patients with constipation-predominant IBS. It is prudent to start with small amounts of supplemental fiber and then gradually increase the dose; patients should be warned of increasing flatulence and bloating, which are side effects of excess fiber intake, and be advised to increase fluid intake.

A food diary may help identify specific dietary items that provoke symptoms. Such food items may need to be avoided if they consistently precipitate symptoms. Stress plays a major role in precipitating symptoms in many patients with IBS. A careful history of potential stressors in the home and office environment needs to be explored and adequately addressed.

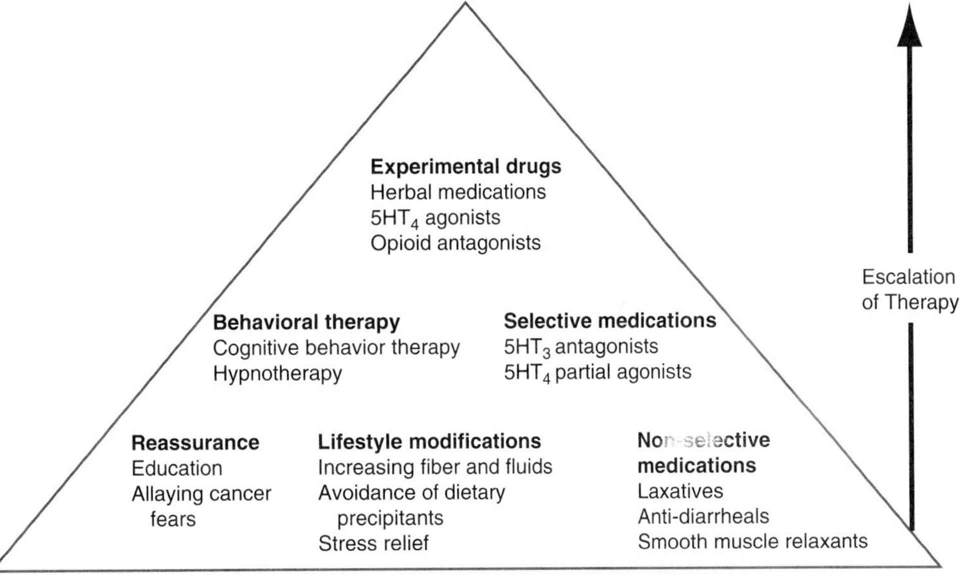

Figure 1. A therapeutic approach to irritable bowel syndrome.

Pharmacologic Therapies

Pharmacologic therapy should be directed at the patient's most dominant symptom. Drug therapy can be broadly divided into nonselective and selective agents.

Nonselective agents include antidiarrheals, laxatives, antispasmodics, and anticholinergics, the use of which is not restricted to IBS. For patients with diarrhea-predominant IBS, antidiarrheals such as loperamide (Imodium), 2 to 4 mg taken half an hour before meals, is quite effective in decreasing the frequency of bowel movements. Depending on the severity of the diarrhea, antidiarrheals can be used regularly or on demand. In patients with constipation-predominant IBS, apart from fiber supplementation, osmotic laxatives may be useful. Sorbitol or magnesium-containing laxatives (such as Epsom salts, 1 to 2 teaspoons in the morning) are generally considered safe for long-term use. Stimulant laxatives such as senna should be reserved for intermittent use only. In patients in whom the predominant symptom is crampy abdominal pain, smooth muscle relaxants such as dicyclomine (Bentyl) or mebeverine,*† anticholinergics, or even peppermint oil show modest benefit in selected cases, but the overall results from randomized trials have been disappointing. Antidepressant medications may be useful in patients with predominantly pain and bloating, and they ppear to work independently of their antidepressant effect. Tricyclic antidepressants such as amitriptyline (Elavil),* 30 to 150 mg/d, tend to constipate, whereas selective serotonin reuptake inhibitors (SSRIs) such as sertraline (Zoloft),* 50 to 150 mg/d, may be more useful in patients with a tendency for constipation.

Specific pharmacologic agents used in IBS have targeted serotonin receptors. Alosetron (Lotronex), a selective 5-HT_3 antagonist (1 mg twice daily), is effective in treating women (but not men) with diarrhea-predominant IBS. It reduces the sensation of urgency and abdominal discomfort and improves stool consistency. However, its use has been associated with severe constipation and the uncommon but potentially fatal development of ischemic colitis. The latter side effect prompted its earlier withdrawal from the market, but it has recently been reinstated. Extreme care needs to be exercised in patient selection and monitoring. Tegaserod (Zelnorm), a 5-HT_4 partial agonist, has proven benefit in constipation-predominant IBS. At a dose of 6 mg twice a day, it is significantly better than placebo in treating multiple symptoms of IBS (abdominal pain, bloating, irregular bowel movements) and promoting general well-being. Clinical experience indicates that about 50% to 60% of patients benefit from tegaserod and that the benefit is gratifyingly marked in some.

Behavioral Therapies

In a subset of patients with IBS, stress plays an important role in exacerbation of symptoms. In these patients, psychologic treatment should be sought, especially when an adequate response to standard medical therapy is lacking. Cognitive behavior therapy or relaxation therapy can be useful if patients are motivated and a proper explanation about the nature of the therapy is provided. Preliminary data suggest that hypnosis may be effective in treating IBS symptoms by decreasing psychologic stress, although it appears to have little effect on physiologic parameters.

*Not FDA-approved for this indication.

†Not available in the United States.

Experimental Drugs

Several new drugs such as cholecystokinin antagonists, antimuscarinic agents, and opioid agonists are currently undergoing trials. Alternative therapies such as herbal medicines are also being explored.

HEMORRHOIDS, ANAL FISSURE, PERIANAL ABSCESS, AND FISTULA IN ANO

method of
FABIO M. POTENTI, M.D., and
MATTHEW D. VREES, M.D.
Brown University
Providence, Rhode Island

HEMORRHOIDS

Although the prevalence of hemorrhoids is not known precisely, the literature has reported a range from 4.4% to 80%, depending on the population studied. Regardless of the exact incidence, it is one of the most common medical complaints.

Anatomy

Hemorrhoids are submucosal cushions of tissue that lie both above and below the dentate line of the anal canal. Although many variations exist, hemorrhoids most commonly receive their blood supply from: (1) the superior rectal artery (mesenteric), (2) the middle rectal arteries (systemic), and (3) the inferior rectal artery (systemic) allowing for natural portosystemic shunts. They are typically located in the right anterior, right posterior and left lateral positions of the anal canal. These cushions of tissue not only are made up of arterial and venous plexuses but also have a rich supply of nerves, connective tissue, and smooth muscle.

Classification

Understanding the classification system of hemorrhoids is essential to their proper diagnosis and treatment, as well as for differentiating hemorrhoids from other common anorectal disorders. Hemorrhoids are divided into two categories: internal and external.

Internal hemorrhoids arise above the dentate line, are covered by transitional or columnar epithelium, and are classified based on the degree of prolapse (Table 1). External hemorrhoids are distal to the dentate line and are covered with anoderm. They are separate from skin tags, which are covered by true squamous epithelium.

Etiology

We have observed that one of the biggest contributing factors to the development of hemorrhoids is a low-fiber diet. The unproved theory is that small-caliber stools fail to activate the rectoanal inhibitory reflex. In turn, the internal sphincter fails to relax and thus creates an environment of high intraluminal pressures that, combined with hard stools, is responsible for mucosal surface injury. Other investigators have demonstrated that patients with hemorrhoids have increased activity of the internal anal sphincter, although it has not been shown whether the changes to the sphincter are causative or a result of the hemorrhoids. Certainly, the development of hemorrhoids is multifactorial, and it is unlikely that any single change in lifestyle would eliminate the disease.

Evaluating the Patient With "Hemorrhoids"

When evaluating a patient who complains of hemorrhoids, one must keep in mind that patients brand all disorders in the perianal region as "my hemorrhoids," and clinicians must be careful not to misdiagnose the complaint by ignoring less common and potentially more dangerous conditions. As with most diseases, the diagnosis can be made in most cases by the history of symptoms, and a properly performed examination is all that is needed to verify the diagnosis.

Symptoms

Internal Hemorrhoids

Bleeding is the most common symptom associated with internal hemorrhoids. The bleeding is typically episodic and is described as bright red blood seen in the toilet bowl after an otherwise normal bowel movement. The blood may or may not be mixed with the stool, may be found just on the toilet paper, or it can be massive. If it is ignored long enough, patients can present with any degree of anemia. In the evaluation of rectal bleeding, we must always consider other causes of hematochezia and perform colonoscopy when indicated. Prolapse or protrusion of hemorrhoids may produce a feeling of pressure or a mass in the anal area. Patients may also complain of moistness or itchiness from the irritation caused by the normal mucus produced by the columnar or transitional epithelium of the hemorrhoidal mucosa. Fourth-degree internal hemorrhoids lead to thrombosis and potentially infarction, which are associated with severe pain. The pain is throbbing and constant. It is not relieved unless manual reduction or excision of the hemorrhoid is performed. If patients complain of pain and thrombosis is not found, a diagnosis other than hemorrhoids exists.

External Hemorrhoids

Complaints from external hemorrhoids range from acute to chronic symptoms. Unlike with internal hemorrhoids, bleeding is not a symptom associated with external hemorrhoids in the acute phase. Almost exclusively, patients complain of severe pain, again associated with thrombosis. These lesions may resolve on their own with time when the overlying anoderm sloughs, at which time some bleeding may be observed. With healing, redundant skin may develop, creating anal skin tags, which become the complaint of patients in the later phase. Except in rare cases of associated dermatitis, the significance of skin tags is limited to cosmesis and hygiene.

Examination

Examination of the perianal area, the anus, and the rectum is best performed and is most comfortable to the patient on a proctologic examination table with the patient in a prone or left lateral decubitus position. The first part of every examination of this area is a complete inspection of the perianal region. This part of the examination is often overlooked but is crucial to appropriate diagnosis. Part of the inspection includes spreading of the patient's buttocks, to allow good exposure to the distal anus, most fissures, external hemorrhoids, skin tags, and dermatitis. After this inspection, the patient should be made aware that the next portion of the examination is the digital rectal examination. Because many patients present with a

TABLE 1. **Classification of Internal Hemorrhoids**

Degree	Description	Symptoms	Treatment
First	Prolapse of hemorrhoid cushion into the lumen of the rectum and anal canal	Bleeding	Conservative rubber band ligation*
Second	Prolapse out of the anal canal with pressure and spontaneous reduction	Discomfort, swelling, and bleeding	Conservative rubber band ligation;* hemorrhoidectomy excision/stapled
Third	Prolapse out of the the anal canal with pressure and requiring manual reduction	Pain when prolapsed and with thrombosis, bleeding	Conservative treatment; hemorrhoidectomy excision/stapled
Fourth	Prolapsed out of the anal canal and unable to be reduced	Severe pain with thrombosis or infarction	Hemorrhoidectomy

*When conservative management fails.

complaint of pain in the area of the anus, reassurance is imperative. Internal hemorrhoids are not typically palpable. The digital examination allows for estimation of sphincter tone, detection of the presence of low rectal or anal cancer, diagnosis of an abscess, and assessment of the patient's pain. After the digital examination, anoscopy should be performed. Anoscopy is the best maneuver for visualization of internal hemorrhoids. Second- and third-degree hemorrhoids are easily observed, whereas first-degree hemorrhoids may require the patient to perform Valsalva's maneuver. Furthermore, carcinoma of the anus can be observed during anoscopy. Other tests such as rigid or flexible sigmoidoscopy, colonoscopy, barium enema, or defecography should be performed on a patient-to-patient basis.

Treatment: Conservative, Destructive, and Restorative

Conservative Treatment

The initial treatment for all patients with nonthrombosed hemorrhoids should be the addition of fiber to the diet. In addition, we insist that patients increase their water intake to at least eight glasses of water a day, and we also prescribe sitz baths, which help with pain and hygiene. Sitz baths consist of soaking the perianal region in warm water. No other topical remedy has ever been shown to reduce the pain or duration of symptoms produced by hemorrhoidal disease significantly. We do not recommend any of the innumerable over-the-counter products to our patients and discourage the prolonged use of products that contain steroids because they may contribute to the risk of fungal infections.

Destructive Treatment

RUBBER BAND LIGATION

Rubber band ligation is one of the most frequently used methods of hemorrhoidectomy in the United States. This procedure is best used in the office setting in patients with symptomatic first- and second-degree hemorrhoids. Care must be taken to place the band high above the dentate line to minimize any pain associated with the procedure. Over a 5- to 7-day period, the rubber band strangulates the tissue, at which time the banded hemorrhoid will slough. Complications associated with rubber band ligation are uncommon when the procedure is performed correctly but include pain, bleeding, and urinary retention. To minimize the risk of bleeding, patients should be advised not to take antiplatelet medication (e.g., aspirin, clopidogrel [Plavix]) for at least 1 week after the ligation, and the procedure is contraindicated in patients receiving heparin or warfarin (Coumadin). Pelvic sepsis has been reported and should be considered when pain and urinary retention are associated with fever.

INFRARED PHOTOCOAGULATION AND SCLEROTHERAPY

Infrared photocoagulation and sclerotherapy are two methods that obliterate the hemorrhoid and scar the tissue by using heat or a sclerosing agent, respectively. Infrared photocoagulation has never been shown to be superior, although the cost is greater. Sclerotherapy may be safe in patients who require anticoagulation, but it can cause oleomas and abscesses.

HEMORRHOIDECTOMY

Surgical hemorrhoidectomy should be reserved for patients with third- and fourth-degree hemorrhoids. Although the surgical therapy for acutely thrombosed hemorrhoids has not changed since the 1970s, there has been an evolution or perhaps a revolution in the treatment of nonthrombosed third- and fourth-degree hemorrhoids.

ACUTELY THROMBOSED HEMORRHOIDS

Conservative nonsurgical methods for the management of acutely thrombosed hemorrhoids have not been shown to be advantageous, when compared with surgical excision. Ice packs and analgesics may reduce the pain temporarily, but the time to complete symptom resolution is greatly prolonged. For acutely thrombosed external hemorrhoids, excision in the office with local anesthesia is the preferred treatment because it will alleviate the pain immediately and will eliminate recurrence. Some authors describe incision and drainage of the hemorrhoid. We do not recommend this treatment because it may lead to persistent pain, drainage and superinfection of retained clot, and almost certain development of an unsightly skin tag.

The treatment of acutely prolapsed and thrombosed internal hemorrhoids is best achieved by operative hemorrhoidectomy with some form of systemic anesthesia. Extreme care to maintain sufficient intact anoderm between hemorrhoid columns is paramount to avoid anal stricture.

CHRONIC SYMPTOMATIC HEMORRHOIDS

Hemorrhoidectomy is performed after all previously described conservative treatments have failed. Hemorrhoidectomy is best performed with the patient in the prone jack-knife position and using local, spinal, or general anesthesia. It is crucial to minimize the amount of intravenous fluids administered during the procedure, to reduce the incidence of urinary retention associated with this operation. We perform a closed hemorrhoidectomy as described by Ferguson. The Ferguson-Hill retractor allows continuous exposure to the hemorrhoid complex being excised while preserving internal sphincter fibers. We choose to close the mucosal defect with absorbable suture. None of the different tools for cutting, including laser, harmonic scalpel, or cautery instrument, have been proved to be superior to scissors.

MANAGEMENT OF THE PATIENT AFTER HEMORRHOIDECTOMY

Complications of hemorrhoidal surgery include severe pain, bleeding, urinary retention, constipation, infection, fecal incontinence, and anal stenosis. All patients should consume high-fiber diets and should take sitz baths. Patients should be immediately examined if fever or urinary retention is observed.

Restorative Treatment

STAPLED HEMORRHOIDECTOMY

Stapled hemorrhoidectomy is a revolutionary approach to treating third- and fourth-degree hemorrhoids. Longo first described the technique in 1998, and although it is referred to as a "hemorrhoidectomy," it is really an anopexy with division of the vessels supplying the hemorrhoids. The hemorrhoids are not excised but are restored to their normal physiologic position using a circular stapling device. Randomized trials have demonstrated that the stapled hemorrhoidectomy offers many advantages over the standard (Ferguson or Milligan-Morgan) hemorrhoidectomy, including a shorter hospital stay, less postoperative pain, and a quicker return to normal activity. Opponents to this technique refer to the added expense of the equipment and the lack of long-term follow-up.

ANAL FISSURE

Anal fissures are simply splits in the anoderm beginning at the level of the dentate line and thought to be caused by tearing as a result of the passage of a hard stool. They are most commonly located in the anterior or posterior midline position and are classified as either acute or chronic. In contrast, anal fissures associated with Crohn's disease and AIDS are found in atypical positions and are secondary to the disease and not to mucosal tearing.

Symptoms

Patients with fissure in ano classically report excruciating pain on defecation, with blood found on the toilet paper. After defecation, the patient describes a dull ache or spasm in the anal canal. This pain typically resolves within a few hours and is rarely associated with significant bleeding.

Diagnosis

The diagnosis of fissure in ano can be made by spreading the patient's buttocks and examining the distal anal canal. If the fissure is noticed, no further examination, including a digital rectal examination, should be attempted at this time because of the patient's severe pain.

Treatment

Most patients with anal fissures will respond to medical therapy. Medical management consists of sitz bath and stool-bulking agents; "stool softeners" are avoided. With these techniques, more than 90% of acute anal fissures will heal. To prevent recurrence, patients should continue taking stool-bulking agents indefinitely. Surgical management is reserved for patients with chronic anal fissures, which do not respond to medical management. Although sphincter stretching and fissure excision have been described, neither has been shown to be beneficial, and both techniques are clearly potentially dangerous. Lateral sphincterotomy is the standard surgical technique. Biopsies are reserved for atypical fissures, to rule out an underlying pathologic process. In women in whom a preexisting occult sphincter injury from childbirth is likely, we prefer to cover the fissure with a cutaneous advancement flap. Before sphincterotomy, the patient should be made aware of the high rate of incontinence observed in the early postoperative period and up to a 13% incidence of long-term incontinence. Surgical treatment of fissures is contraindicated in patients with Crohn's disease and AIDS. Physiologic sphincterotomy can be accomplished with botulinum toxin* injections or topical nitroglycerin.* Both modalities have been shown to reduce the pain associated with the fissure, but nitroglycerin does not appear to increase fissure healing significantly.

ABSCESS AND FISTULA IN ANO

Abscess

Etiology

Perirectal abscesses result from obstruction of the anal glands found in the anal canal. These glands pass into the submucosa, internal sphincter, and intersphincteric plane, and this anatomic arrangement explains why the abscess may occur in multiple locations. If the tract between the gland and the abscess is covered with epithelium, a fistula will develop.

Classification

Abscesses are classified based on their location. The most common location is the perianal region, followed by the ischiorectal and intersphincteric regions, and, least commonly, the supralevator region. The horseshoe abscess is rare but important. It is believed to begin as a posterior intersphincteric abscess, which spreads to the ischiorectal and supralevator spaces.

Diagnosis

The symptoms and findings of an abscess depend on its location. Inevitably, the patient complains of pain in the area of the abscess. Examination demonstrates erythema, swelling, and a tender mass with perianal and ischiorectal abscesses. Intersphincteric abscesses are associated with extreme tenderness on digital rectal examination, without any external signs of infection. Either endorectal ultrasound or computed tomography can be helpful in diagnosing these more complex abscesses, but a rectal examination while the patient is under general anesthesia is often the only sure diagnostic method.

---

*Not FDA-approved for this indication.

Treatment

The treatment of all abscesses consists of incision and drainage, no matter the location. This approach alone is adequate to treat most abscesses and should be performed as soon as the diagnosis is made, to eliminate the risk of necrotizing infections. Antibiotics are not normally required and should be reserved for patients with extensive cellulitis or those with prosthetic heart valves, prosthetic joints, diabetes, or immunosuppression. Perianal abscesses can usually be drained in the outpatient setting, whereas more complex abscesses should be managed in the operating room. The key to good drainage includes keeping the abscess cavity open, and it can be accomplished with a simple gauze wick; conversely, a mushroom-shaped catheter can be placed and secured with a simple suture.

Fistula in Ano

A *fistula in ano* is an abnormal tract between the anal canal and the perineum. A fistula, usually diagnosed after drainage of an abscess, is complicated by continued drainage or recurrence. Fistulas do not heal on their own, and management is determined by the type of fistula (Table 2).

Classification

Fistulas are classified in relation to the anal sphincter. Fistulas can run between the internal and external anal sphincter (intersphincteric fistulas), through the sphincters (transphincteric fistulas), or above the sphincter complex (suprasphincteric). Extrasphincteric fistulas are likely to originate from parts of the gastrointestinal tract other than the anus, and their diagnosis and treatment are beyond the scope of this discussion.

Treatment

Treatment of fistula in ano requires good understanding of the anatomy. The keys to treatment are to create good drainage, to obliterate the internal opening, and to accomplish both without injuring the external anal sphincter. Depending on the location of the fistula (classification), this may be accomplished with a simple fistulotomy and obliteration of the epithelial tract, or it may require seton drainage with a delayed anal mucosal flap. A newer technique that uses placement of a seton followed by injection of fibrin glue has been shown to be successful in approximately 50% of patients.

TABLE 2. **Fistula in Ano**

Type	Treatment
Superficial perianal	Fistulotomy
Intersphincteric	Seton
	Fibrin glue* versus mucosal flap
Transphincteric	Seton
	Fibrin glue versus mucosal flap
Suprasphincteric	Seton and mucosal flap

*Not FDA-approved for this indication.

GASTRITIS AND PEPTIC ULCER DISEASE

method of
SRIPATHI R. KETHU, M.D., and
STEVEN F. MOSS, M.D.
Division of Gastroenterology
Brown Medical School
Providence, Rhode Island

GASTRITIS AND PEPTIC ULCER DISEASE

Gastritis is a histopathologic diagnosis and peptic ulcer disease (PUD) is an endoscopic or radiologic diagnosis. Neither of these conditions has a specific symptom complex to help the clinician arrive at a diagnosis. Instead, physicians encounter patients with symptoms of dyspepsia that may or may not be secondary to gastritis or PUD. Thus for the primary care provider the discussion of gastritis and PUD must be prefaced by first considering the approach to the patient with dyspeptic symptoms.

DYSPEPSIA

Dyspepsia refers to pain or discomfort centered in the upper abdomen, which may be intermittent or continuous, and may or may not be related to eating meals. The symptoms may be described by several other terms, including: bloating, fullness, belching, and nausea or simply as indigestion. The prevalence of uninvestigated dyspepsia in the general population is not well documented. However, up to 25% of people in the community each year report chronic or recurrent pain or discomfort in the upper abdomen and approximately 2% to 5% of family practice consultations are for dyspepsia.

Etiology and Differential Diagnosis

Dyspepsia can result from an identifiable cause such as peptic ulcer disease, malignancy, gastroesophageal reflux, or the use of specific medications. Other rare causes include pancreaticobiliary disease, gastroparesis, celiac disease, lactose intolerance, and parasitic diseases, such as giardiasis. Patients who have no definite structural or biochemical explanation for their symptoms are considered to have functional dyspepsia ("non-ulcer" dyspepsia). There is a subset of patients in whom dyspepsia may coexist with a microbiologic and/or structural abnormality such as *Helicobacter pylori* gastritis or duodenitis, or the presence of gallstones, but a causal relationship between these abnormalities and dyspepsia may be unclear.

The patient's age is one of the important factors in tailoring the management of patients with dyspepsia, due to the very low probability of stomach cancer in younger patients (typically this cut-off is arbitrarily fixed at about 45–50 years of age). Thus, if an individual older than age 45 presents with new onset upper abdominal complaints, or patients younger than this age develop so called "alarm symptoms" (anemia, anorexia, weight loss, early satiety, dysphagia, and gastrointestinal bleeding either overt or occult), prompt endoscopic evaluation is required to detect the cause, prior to empirical therapy.

In a primary care setting, the patient's history is crucial in elucidating the cause of dyspepsia. Peptic ulcer disease is an important consideration in the differential diagnosis of dyspepsia, accounting for up to 25% of cases. Although it is impossible to distinguish gastric and duodenal ulcers by symptoms alone, the pain of both gastric and duodenal ulcers is typically epigastric, episodic, and often worse at night. Symptoms are often temporarily relieved with food or antacids in the case of duodenal ulcer; in contrast, food may precipitate gastric ulcer pain. Associated symptoms such as anorexia, nausea, or vomiting may point toward the diagnosis of a gastric ulcer or pyloric stenosis. Patients with gastric malignancy, which accounts for less than 2% of the cases of dyspepsia, may also present with similar symptoms.

Gastroesophageal reflux disease (GERD) may be the underlying disorder in 10% to 15% of patients with dyspepsia. Typical symptoms include heartburn or a retrosternal burning pain, or a feeling of regurgitation of food or of acid. However, about 20% of patients with GERD present with epigastric pain alone, thereby creating a diagnostic problem. If medications are responsible for dyspepsia, generally a temporal relationship can be established between medication intake and the onset of dyspeptic symptoms. Nonsteroidal anti-inflammatory drugs (NSAIDs) are the most common offending agents; other medications that cause dyspepsia are corticosteroids, iron preparations, digitalis, potassium supplements, bisphosphonates, niacin, and antibiotics, particularly erythromycin and ampicillin.

Functional or non-ulcer dyspepsia accounts for up to 60% of all cases of dyspepsia. Functional dyspepsia and PUD share many symptoms, thus making the distinction by history alone impossible. By definition, the cause of functional dyspepsia is obscure; the putative pathophysiologic abnormalities that have been proposed to cause or to be associated with functional dyspepsia are gastric acid hypersecretion, *H. pylori* infection, gastroduodenal dysmotility, visceral hyperalgesia, and psychological distress, including physical or sexual abuse. Although functional dyspepsia is a benign condition, it is the hardest to treat given the uncertain interplay between numerous pathogenic mechanisms.

Evaluation of Dyspepsia

Currently the best first test in the evaluation of dyspepsia is upper endoscopy. Barium meal radiographs are less sensitive and specific. However, in a young patient (age <45), in the absence of alarming symptoms, and after excluding other causes such as GERD and NSAID use by history, a "test and treat" strategy for *H. pylori* without endoscopy or radiography has been recommended. The justification for this approach is that among patients with uninvestigated dyspepsia who are *H. pylori* positive, a substantial number will have peptic ulcers and a few without ulcers may improve symptomatically following the eradication of *H. pylori*. Whether this strategy is suitable for affluent populations in the United States who have a very low prevalence of *H. pylori* is debatable because it may result in the diagnosis of almost as many false-positive *H. pylori* infections and lead to inappropriate eradication therapy. Furthermore, the cost benefits of the "test and treat" approach over one with early invasive testing remains unproved in practice. In other populations noninvasive testing for *H. pylori* either by serology or stool antigen test is reasonable. These tests are relatively less expensive compared to either upper endoscopy or indefinite empirical acid-suppressive therapy.

If symptoms persist after *H. pylori* eradication therapy or if empirical acid-suppressive therapy in *H. pylori*-negative patients fails, upper endoscopy should be undertaken. Ultrasonography is not recommended as a routine next step unless the history or biochemical tests are suggestive of pancreaticobiliary disease. In patients with diabetes or history suggestive of autonomic neuropathy, a gastric emptying scan (scintigraphy) may be considered to document gastroparesis. Even though functional dyspepsia should be considered a diagnosis of exclusion, clinicians should use their judgment on a case-by-case basis to limit the use of numerous invasive and expensive investigations whenever possible.

Management of Functional Dyspepsia

Once the cause of dyspepsia is established, management involves treating the underlying cause. The most challenging task is managing patients with functional dyspepsia. *H. pylori* eradication therapy for patients who do not have an ulcer may result in symptomatic improvement in a small minority (approximately in 15% of patients, at best) over placebo. However, most patients will remain symptomatic after eradication therapy, thus requiring other therapies.

Reassurance and explanation are important first steps in the management. Proving that the symptoms do not represent a malignancy may be sufficient. Patients should be educated to avoid precipitating agents, such as coffee, alcohol, smoking, NSAIDs, and spicy and fatty foods; this will help relieve symptoms in some patients. Exacerbating psychosocial factors including anxiety and depression should also be explored and treated appropriately. Pharmacologic therapy is not always required and if required, it should be individualized. No single drug has been clearly shown to be beneficial over the long term, and the results of pharmacologic therapy are disappointing overall.

First-line therapies usually involve a therapeutic trial of antisecretory agents such as H_2 receptor antagonists (H2RAs) or proton pump inhibitors (PPIs). A prokinetic agent such as metoclopramide (Reglan) 10 mg 1h after meals and at bedtime for 4 to 6 weeks may be a useful alternative. A drug holiday during therapy may help determine if the medication is still needed. The benefits of individual drugs should be weighed against the side-effect profile and cost. Metoclopramide, for example, is associated with neuropsychiatric

TABLE 1. **Classification of Gastritis**

Acute erosive and hemorrhagic gastropathy
Chronic gastritis
Helicobacter pylori gastritis (may be atrophic or non-atrophic)
Pernicious anemia–associated atrophic gastritis (type A gastritis or autoimmune gastritis)
Others: eosinophilic gastritis, infectious gastritis (cytomegalovirus or herpesvirus); granulomatous gastritis (Crohn's disease); and portal gastropathy.

complications and, therefore, cannot be recommended long term. Antidepressants such as amitryptiline (Elavil),* 50 mg at bedtime, or antispasmodics such as dicyclomine (Bentyl),* 10 to 20 mg every 8 hours, can be tried as a next step, but the results are marginal at best. Alternative therapies, such as acupuncture, cognitive behavioral therapy, and hypnotherapy have been anecdotally reported to be beneficial.

GASTRITIS

When the gastric mucosa is exposed to various insults, it may lead to epithelial damage and regeneration with minimal or no inflammation (gastropathy) or the epithelial damage may be associated with significant inflammation (gastritis). For an endoscopist, gastritis usually means petechiae, erosions, or erythema of the gastric mucosa. These endoscopic findings may not have a good correlation with the presence of inflammatory cells on biopsy. Strictly speaking, gastritis is a histopathologic diagnosis associated with the presence of inflammatory cells. Gastritis and gastropathy can be categorized according to the histologic features and the etiology (Table 1).

Acute Erosive and Hemorrhagic Gastropathy

The most common causes of acute erosive and hemorrhagic gastropathy include NSAIDs, alcohol, and stress due to critical illness. Clinically, the patient may present with nonspecific complaints such as epigastric pain, nausea, or vomiting, and occasionally with upper gastrointestinal bleeding alone. Upper endoscopy usually reveals erythema or erosions. Histologically, there is usually no or minimal inflammation, hence the term gastropathy, instead of gastritis. Stress gastropathy, most likely due to chronic gastric ischemia, may lead to gastric ulceration—usually small, multiple ulcers involving the proximal part of the stomach.

The management of symptomatic gastropathy as a result of NSAIDs or alcohol use involves minimizing or avoiding the offending agents or taking NSAIDs with food. A short-course of H2RAs or PPIs is recommended if the patients have persistent symptoms despite conservative measures. Long-term acid suppression therapy with PPIs may be necessary for patients thought to be at high risk of bleeding in whom chronic NSAID use is necessary. The development of cyclooxygenase (COX-2) selective NSAIDs has diminished but not eliminated clinically important gastroduodenal bleeding. Endoscopy is recommended only for patients with risk factors for developing an ulcer (see section on peptic ulcer disease). The majority of the critically ill hospitalized patients develop superficial erosions without leading to gastrointestinal bleeding, so that endoscopy is of no therapeutic benefit. Two risk factors that are associated with a high risk of bleeding are mechanical ventilation and a coagulopathy. In the absence of these two risk factors, the risk of significant bleeding is less than 0.1%. Preventing stress gastropathy and ulcers with the use of acid-suppression medications is strongly recommended in all critically ill patients, particularly if they have the previously mentioned risk factors. Intravenous H2RAs are generally used. The superiority of oral or intravenous PPIs over H2RAs in this setting has not been established.

Chronic *H. Pylori* Gastritis

H. pylori is a gram-negative spiral bacterium acquired in childhood that colonizes the gastric mucosa and usually causes an antral-predominant gastritis. In the developed world, infection is more prevalent in the elderly, in the poor, and in immigrants from high incidence regions such as Asia, Africa, and Central and South America.

Inflammation associated with chronic *H. pylori* colonization may be confined to the superficial mucosa or extend deeper into the gastric glands, leading, in some cases, to gastric atrophy (atrophic gastritis) and intestinal metaplasia of the gastric epithelium. The majority of all gastric and duodenal ulcers are caused by *H. pylori*; approximately 10% of all individuals with chronic gastritis due to *H. pylori* will eventually develop peptic ulcer disease. A more uncommon consequence of *H. pylori* infection is adenocarcinoma of the stomach, typically developing after many decades of infection and after histologic progression from atrophic gastritis, through intestinal metaplasia, and dysplasia. *H. pylori* infection is associated with a three- to sixfold increased risk of distal gastric cancer, leading to its designation by the World Health Organization as a carcinogen, and *H. pylori* is also a major risk factor for the relatively rare mucosa-associated lymphoid tissue (MALT) gastric B-cell lymphoma. (See section on peptic ulcer disease for detailed discussion of the diagnosis and management of *H. pylori* infection). Factors thought to be important determinants of individual clinical outcome following *H. pylori* infection include host genetics, nutritional and general health status, and specific *H. pylori* virulence genes.

Pernicious Anemia-Associated Atrophic Gastritis (Type A Gastritis or Autoimmune Gastritis)

This is an autoimmune disorder characterized by the presence of anti-parietal cell antibodies. The disease is more common in women and in people of Northern European descent. Parietal cell destruction in the gastric fundus leads to achlorhydria, and the impaired

*Not FDA approved for this indication.

intrinsic factor production results in vitamin B_{12} malabsorption leading to anemia and neurologic syndromes. Patients are at increased risk for developing carcinoid tumors (secondary to prolonged hypergastrinemia) and adenocarcinoma of the stomach. Treatment involves vitamin B_{12} supplementation. The utility of periodic endoscopic screening to detect gastric carcinoma or carcinoid tumors in these patients is controversial.

PEPTIC ULCER DISEASE

A peptic ulcer is a mucosal defect in the stomach or duodenum. As opposed to an erosion, which is a superficial lesion, an ulcer has perceivable depth extending into the submucosa. PUD is thought to occur when factors aggressive to the gastric mucosa dominate (such as *H. pylori*, gastric acid hypersecretion, and so on) or when mucosal defense mechanisms are impaired (by NSAIDs, for example) or both. The lifetime risk of PUD in the United States is approximately 10%, with a male to female ratio of 1.3:1 for a duodenal ulcer (DU) and 1:1 for a gastric ulcer (GU). DU occurs more commonly between ages 25 and 55, whereas GU affects a slightly older population (ages 40-70). NSAID use or *H. pylori* infection increases the peptic ulcer risk by about 20-fold. Cigarette smoking not only increases the ulcer risk (by twofold) but also retards ulcer healing and increases the risk of bleeding. Despite popular beliefs, alcohol and dietary factors have no established relation with the causation of ulcers or their healing. Psychological stress may play some role in idiopathic ulcers.

Etiology

Depending on their etiology, ulcers can be classified into four groups:

1. *H. pylori*-associated ulcers
2. NSAID-induced ulcers
3. Idiopathic (non-*H. pylori*, non-NSAID ulcers)
4. Zollinger-Ellison syndrome

Other less common causes include ulcers secondary to drugs other than NSAIDs (for example, potassium chloride, bisphosphonates), stress ulcers due to a critical illness, ulcers of Crohn's disease, and infectious causes (for example, cytomegalovirus ulcers in HIV patients, or herpes simplex virus).

H. pylori-*Associated Ulcers*

H. pylori infection is responsible for the majority of peptic ulcers. *H. pylori* is thought to be transmitted from person to person, probably via the fecal-oral route. The prevalence of *H. pylori* is between 20% and 50% in the Western world including the United States. However, *H. pylori* is much more prevalent in developing nations, affecting as many as 90% of the population. In the United States, the prevalence is higher in the elderly, probably reflecting the poor sanitary conditions that existed in the early part of the century, and is more common in African-Americans and in Hispanics. *H. pylori* is also more prevalent in people of low socioeconomic status, probably related to crowded childhood conditions.

Initial studies reported that *H. pylori* was present in about 90% of patients with duodenal ulcers and 60% of patients with gastric ulcer. More recent estimates show slightly lower prevalence of *H. pylori* in both DU and GU, probably reflecting the relative increase in NSAID-associated ulcer. Approximately 10% of all individuals infected with *H. pylori* develop peptic ulcer disease over their lifetime. The exact pathophysiologic mechanism(s) by which *H. pylori* causes either DU or GU and why only a minority of infected individuals will develop clinically overt disease is not known. Generally, DU is a disease of acid hypersecretion and GU is associated with states of low acid secretion. *H. pylori* can potentially cause both these secretory abnormalities. Gastric acid hypersecretion in DU occurs secondary to increased gastrin release by a healthy acid-secreting gastric corpus mucosa (Figure 1). In contrast, when the *H. pylori*–associated gastritis affects the proximal stomach too, this results in loss of gastric glands (atrophic gastritis) and hypochlorhydria with impaired mucosal defense leading to gastric ulceration and even gastric cancer.

NSAID-Induced Ulcers

NSAIDs are among the most prescribed medications in the United States. The incidence of ulcers in chronic NSAID users is approximately 15% to 20%. The risk of NSAID-induced ulcers increases dramatically with the presence of specific risk factors (particularly with age >60 years and a prior history of peptic ulcer), and also with high doses of NSAIDs and concurrent use of corticosteroids. NSAIDs cause gastric ulcers much more commonly than they cause duodenal ulcers. Up to 40%

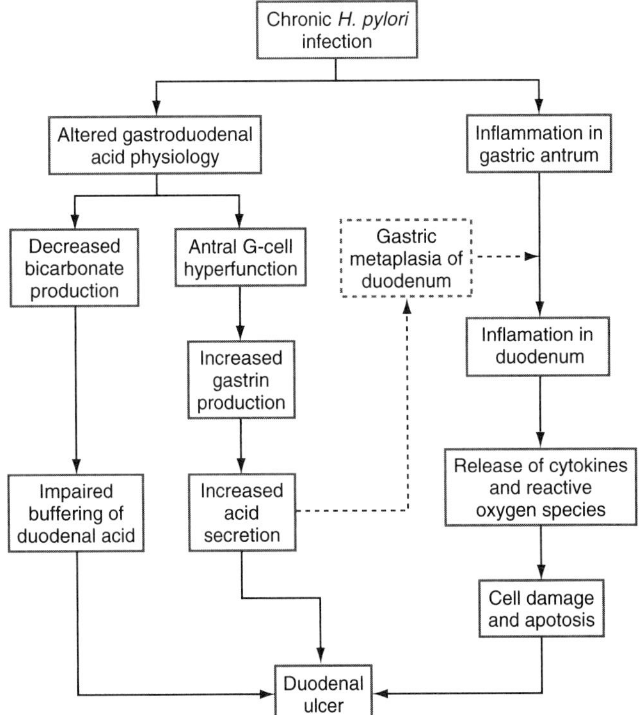

Figure 1. Proposed pathogenic mechanisms leading to *H. pylori*–induced duodenal ulcer.

of the NSAID ulcers are asymptomatic and patients commonly present with complications.

The most important mechanism by which NSAIDs cause ulcers is by indirectly decreasing prostaglandin production via the inhibition of the COX-1 enzyme. Prostaglandins are important in maintaining mucosal integrity by producing mucus, stimulating bicarbonate production, decreasing acid production, and maintaining mucosal blood flow. The analgesic and anti-inflammatory effects of NSAIDs result from the inhibition of the COX-2 isoenzyme. Non-selective NSAIDs cause inhibition of both COX-2, as well as COX-1, resulting in considerable gastrointestinal (GI) toxicity. The more recently developed selective COX-2 inhibitors (such as celecoxib [Celebrex], rofecoxib [Vioxx], and valdecoxib [Bextra], inhibit COX-2 to a much greater extent than COX-1 leading to their better GI safety profile. COX-2 inhibitors reduce the risk of gastroduodenal ulcers by 60% to 75% compared with nonselective NSAIDs.

*Idiopathic (Non-*H. pylori*, Non-NSAID) Ulcers*

There is a specific subgroup of patients who develop ulcers, in whom all the known etiologic factors are excluded. This subgroup should not be confused with patients with "unexplained" ulcers, where 60% of patients may have history of surreptitious NSAID use. Establishing the true incidence of idiopathic ulcers is also complicated by false-negative testing for *H. pylori*. The exact pathogenic mechanism that causes these idiopathic ulcers remains unknown. Genetic predisposition, defective mucosal defense mechanisms, and increased acid production have all been postulated.

Clinical Features

Clinical signs and symptoms are unreliable and are not specific enough to make a diagnosis of a peptic ulcer. Upper abdominal pain (dyspepsia) is present in over 80% of patients; however, only 25% of patients with dyspepsia have PUD. Pain is typically epigastric, described as burning in quality and nonradiating. Food or antacids may relieve DU pain, and nausea or anorexia may occur with GU. Nocturnal symptoms awaken two thirds of DU and one third of GU patients. Symptoms usually wax and wane over a period of months. The physical examination is usually normal—epigastric tenderness on palpation may be present but it is an unreliable sign with a positive predictive value of less than 50%. Stool test for occult blood is positive in one third of patients.

Diagnostic Work-Up

Routine laboratory studies are not helpful in establishing a diagnosis of PUD. Upper endoscopy is the gold standard in making a diagnosis of peptic ulcer. Endoscopy has the advantage of taking biopsies for the presence of *H. pylori* infection and in case of gastric ulcer, to rule out malignancy. However, endoscopy is relatively expensive and invasive. In the absence of alarm symptoms (see section on functional dyspepsia), double-contrast barium radiography may be a suitable second choice. If the barium radiograph shows an ulcer (gastric or duodenal), *H. pylori* must be tested for and treatment can be instituted with acid suppression therapy with or without antibiotics depending on the result. Gastric pH and fasting gastrin levels should be obtained only if there is clinical suspicion of a gastrinoma (see section on Zollinger-Ellison syndrome, later). For gastric ulcers, it is essential to repeat the endoscopy after 6 to 8 weeks of therapy to confirm the healing of the ulcer and re-biopsy if not healed, because 5% of gastric ulcers may be malignant.

Many tests are available to test for *H. pylori*. Testing for the presence of *H. pylori* can be made either by noninvasive or invasive methods (Table 2). An appropriate test should be chosen depending on the clinical situation. For example, testing for serologic antibodies against *H. pylori* may be appropriate for the initial testing for *H. pylori,* but it is not useful to check for eradication after therapy because it will not distinguish current active infection from prior infection that was treated (antibody levels fall slowly and unpredictably). Office-based qualitative antibody tests are cheaper than

TABLE 2. **Diagnostic Tests for *H. Pylori***

Diagnostic Test	Sensitivity (%)	Specificity (%)	Approximate cost in U.S. dollars*
Non-Invasive Tests			
Office-based finger-stick blood test	70-85	75-90	10-20
Serum antibody test	90-95	80-95	40-75
Urea breath test (^{14}C or ^{13}C)†	90-95	88-98	50-100
Stool antigen test‡	89-98	87-95	60
Invasive (Endoscopy-Based) Tests:			
Rapid urease test	80-90	95-100	10-20
Histology	92-95	98-99	150-250
Culture	60-98	100	100-200

*Cost of invasive testing does not include the cost of endoscopy.

†H2RA (H_2-receptor agonist) and PPI (proton pump inhibitor) should be held for 2 weeks prior to initial testing. To confirm eradication, the test should be done at least 4 weeks after completion of therapy.

‡H2RA and PPI should be held for 7 days prior to initial testing. To confirm eradication, the test should be done at least 4 weeks after completion of therapy.

antibody testing done in the laboratory but not as accurate, and have been largely superseded by stool antigen testing. Patients with alarm symptoms and all patients older than 45 years of age with dyspeptic symptoms should undergo endoscopy at which time *H. pylori* testing can be done by biopsy if an ulcer is found. Confirmation of the eradication of *H. pylori* should be considered after treating this infection in ulcer patients, by either the stool antigen test or the urea breath test depending on local resources. Confirmation of eradication by gastric biopsy is only recommended if endoscopy is performed for another reason, for example, to confirm healing of a gastric ulcer.

Differential Diagnosis

Functional dyspepsia is a major differential diagnostic consideration in all patients with upper abdominal pain (see section on functional dyspepsia). Other diseases that mimic the symptoms of PUD include gastric or pancreatic cancer, biliary colic, and mesenteric ischemia.

Treatment

Different classes of drugs are available to treat PUD (Table 3). Antacids heal ulcers and are cheap but are relatively ineffective, slow to produce healing, and have many side effects. Both PPIs and H2RAs block acid secretion, but PPIs inhibit >90% of the 24-acid output compared with 65% with H2RAs, hence PPIs heal the ulcer and relieve symptoms faster. Sucralfate (Carafate), has similar ulcer-healing rates as H2RAs. The mechanism of action of sucralfate is unknown; it probably coats the ulcer base thereby promoting ulcer healing and it may have other effects too. The frequent dosing schedule and large tablet size of sucralfate is not conducive to good compliance. Misoprostol is a prostaglandin analogue approved for preventing NSAID-induced ulcers. Compliance with misoprostol is also a problem particularly at high doses due to its gastrointestinal side effects of abdominal cramping and diarrhea.

H. pylori eradication is recommended in all ulcer patients who are *H. pylori* positive but should not be presumed to be present without a documented positive test. *H. pylori* eradication heals ulcers and reduces the ulcer recurrence dramatically, to less than 20% after 2 years. Selected *H. pylori* eradication regimens are summarized in Table 4. Confirmation of eradication is mandatory for complicated ulcers associated with bleeding, perforation, or obstruction and recommended in all cases with ulcers receiving *H. pylori* therapy. Treatment of idiopathic ulcers is difficult and often requires indefinite maintenance antisecretory therapy, particularly for complicated ulcers.

Prevention

Ulcer recurrence is frequent with continued use of NSAIDs or with persistent *H. pylori* infection. The incidence of antibiotic resistance to *H. pylori* is rising all over the world. In the United States, approximately 30% of *H. pylori* strains are now resistant to metronidazole (Flagyl) and 10% to 12% are resistant to clarithromycin (Biaxin), which decreases the cure rates by as much as 50% and 37%, respectively. If the patient has persistent symptoms after therapy, eradication failure should be strongly suspected and noninvasive testing for *H. pylori* should be performed. The value of testing *H. pylori* strains for their antibiotic sensitivity profiles is unproved. If the initial diagnosis of the ulcer was made by radiography, endoscopy is the next reasonable test. Drugs that have clearly shown to be superior to placebo in preventing NSAID-induced ulcers are PPIs and misoprostol (Cytotec).

TABLE 3. **Treatment Options for Peptic Ulcer***

PHARMACOLOGIC AGENT	ACTIVE ULCER (Gastric or Duodenal)†	PREVENTION OF NSAID-INDUCED ULCER RECURRENCE ‡
ANTI-SECRETORY AGENTS		
H_2-receptor antagonists (H2RA)		
Cimetidine (Tagamet)	400 mg bid or 800 mg qhs	Double the dose that is indicated for active ulcer§
Ranitidine (Zantac)	150 mg bid or 300 mg qhs	
Famotidine (Pepcid)	20 mg bid or 40 mg qhs	§
Nizatidine (Axid)	150 mg bid or 300 mg qhs	§
Proton pump inhibitors (PPI)		
Omeprazole (Prilosec)	20 mg qd	20 mg qd§
Lansoprazole (Prevacid)	30 mg qd	30 mg qd
Rabeprazole (Aciphex)	20 mg qd	20 mg qd§
Pantoprazole (Protonix)	40 mg qd	40 mg qd§
Esomeprazole (Nexium)	40 mg qd	40 mg qd§
MUCOSAL PROTECTANTS		
Sucralfate (Carafate)	1 gm qid	Not effective
Misoprostol (Cytotec)	200 μg qid	200 μg qid or 400 μg bid

*All patients should be tested for *Helicobacter pylori* and treated if positive.
†Duration of treatment for duodenal ulcer: 4 weeks with PPI and 6 weeks with H2RA. For gastric ulcer: 8 weeks with either PPI or H2RA.
‡Only lansoprazole and misoprostol are currently approved by the FDA for this indication.
§Not FDA approved for this indication.

TABLE 4. **Selected FDA-Approved *Helicobacter pylori* Eradication Regimens**

PPI* (omeprazole 20 mg or lansoprazole 30 mg) + amoxicillin 1 g + clarithromycin 500 mg	Each bid for 10 days
Esomeprazole* 40 mg qd + amoxicillin 1 g bid + clarithromycin 500 mg bid	For 10 days
PPI* (omeprazole 20 mg or lansoprazole 30 mg) + amoxicillin 1g + metronidazole 500 mg	Each bid for 10-14 days
Rabeprazole* 20 mg + amoxicillin 1 g + clarithromycin 500 mg	Each bid for 7 days
Bismuth subsalicylate 525 mg + metronidazole 250 mg + tetracycline 500 mg†	Each qid for 2 weeks with a H2RA for 4 weeks

*Although not yet approved by the FDA for this indication, pantoprazole can be substituted for other PPIs.
†For patients with penicillin allergy, use either this regimen or alternatively, PPI + clarithromycin + metronidazole.
Bid = two times daily; qid = four times daily; PPI = proton pump inhibitor.

Double the standard doses of H2RAs that are used for active ulcers are significantly better than placebo in preventing NSAID-induced gastroduodenal ulcers (see Table 3). PPIs are generally preferred over H2RAs given the simplicity of the dosing schedule. Alternatively, COX-2 inhibitors can be used instead of nonselective NSAIDs in patients with risk factors for developing an ulcer. However, if the patient is being treated for an active ulcer, COX-2 inhibitors should be held for 6 to 8 weeks if possible, as there are some concerns from experimental models that they might retard ulcer healing. The comparative cost-effectiveness of COX-2 inhibitors versus the use of nonselective NSAIDs in combination with a prophylactic antisecretory agent or misoprostol is not known, and the benefit of COX-2 inhibitors can be undermined by the concurrent use of aspirin in elderly patients. In this situation, prophylactic antiulcer agents should be considered, as should prophylactic *H. pylori* eradication in patients who will require long-term NSAIDs.

Complications

Hemorrhage

Gastrointestinal bleeding is the most common complication of PUD. Approximately 10% to 20% of ulcer patients develop significant gastrointestinal bleeding, with overall mortality up to 10%. Patients generally present with either melena or hematemesis. Endoscopy is indicated in all patients with clinically significant bleeding, both for diagnosis and therapy. High dose oral or intravenous PPIs should be instituted prior to endoscopy if upper gastrointestinal bleeding is suspected. All *H. pylori*–positive patients must have confirmation of eradication after therapy.

Perforation

Perforations occur in approximately 5% to 7% of ulcer patients. The incidence has not changed in spite of the decreasing prevalence of *H. pylori*, because the use of NSAIDs continues to increase. The decision whether to manage the perforation operatively or nonoperatively should be made on a case-by-case basis.

Obstruction

Duodenal bulb or pyloric channel ulcers may cause scarring and gastric outlet obstruction in approximately 2% of patients with PUD. Patients typically present with early satiety, vomiting, and weight loss. Management involves *H. pylori* eradication and acid suppression along with endoscopic dilation. Surgery is reserved for patients who do not respond to endoscopic therapy.

ZOLLINGER-ELLISON SYNDROME

Less than 1% of PUD is caused by Zollinger-Ellison syndrome (ZES). This syndrome results from a gastrin-producing neuroendocrine tumor (gastrinoma), two thirds of which are malignant. PUD is caused by increased acid production from very high serum gastrin levels. Most gastrinomas arise in the so-called gastrinoma triangle, bounded by the porta hepatis, neck of the pancreas, and the third portion of the duodenum. The pancreas and the duodenum are the two organs most commonly involved. Approximately one quarter of gastrinomas are part of the multiple endocrine neoplasia type 1 (MEN-1) syndrome, which is associated with parathyroid hyperplasia, pituitary tumors, and pancreatic endocrine tumors.

Gastrinomas commonly present between ages 30 and 50 years with a male-to-female ratio of 2 to 1. The clinical features include peptic ulcers (90%), diarrhea (60%), and GERD (20%), all of which are due to gastric acid hypersecretion. The majority of ulcers occur in the duodenal wall. ZES should be suspected if the ulcers are multiple, in unusual locations, refractory to treatment, or associated with diarrhea. The diagnosis is made by measuring fasting gastrin levels and gastric pH. If the gastrin levels are elevated to >1000 pg/mL in the right clinical setting, the diagnosis of ZES is established. Hypochlorhydria secondary to gastric atrophy from *H. pylori* or autoimmune gastritis, or due to acid suppression therapy by H2RAs and PPIs can also increase gastrin levels. Therefore, gastrin levels should be measured after H2RAs are held for 24 hours and PPIs for 1 week. The gastric pH should be measured to distinguish ZES from hypochlorhydria: gastric pH is less than 2 in ZES, whereas in achlorhydria secondary to gastric atrophy, gastric pH is greater than 2. Provocative tests, such as the secretin test, can also be used to diagnose gastrinoma. Intravenous administration of secretin may decrease or may slightly increase gastrin levels in normal patients and the patients with antral G-cell hyperplasia. In cases of gastrinoma, gastrin levels are significantly increased (more than 200 pg/mL) from the basal levels. Tumor localization can be made by somatostatin receptor scintigraphy (Octreoscan). Treatment involves medical therapy with a high dose PPI titrated against symptoms, gastric pH, and endoscopic findings. Surgical resection of isolated hepatic metastasis will decrease symptoms and prolong survival.

ACUTE AND CHRONIC VIRAL HEPATITIS

method of
RICHARD KENT ZIMMERMAN, M.D., M.P.H.
Department of Family Medicine and Clinical Epidemiology
University of Pittsburgh School of Medicine
Department of Behavioral and Community Health Sciences
Graduate School of Public Health
Pittsburgh, Pennsylvania

and

RICHARD D. CLOVER, M.D.
Office of the Dean
University of Louisville School of Public Health/Information Sciences
Louisville, Kentucky

Acute viral hepatitis is an infection of the liver. Symptoms range from none to fulminate hepatitis with jaundice that is potentially fatal. Although most persons recover, those with hepatitis from hepatitis B, C, or D viruses can develop chronic liver disease, cirrhosis, or hepatocellular carcinoma.

DIFFERENTIAL DIAGNOSES

Differential diagnoses for jaundice includes cirrhosis, toxic hepatitis (including hepatitis caused by ethanol), viral hepatitis, neonatal jaundice, obstructive biliary or pancreatic diseases, carcinomas (primary and metastatic), congenital disorders (e.g., Crigler-Najjar, Dubin-Johnson, and Rotor syndromes), drug toxicity, hemolytic disease, hemochromatosis, Wilson disease, and cholestatic jaundice of pregnancy. Diseases causing obstructive jaundice generally elevate lactate dehydrogenase (LDH) and alkaline phosphatase (ALP) out of proportion to the other liver enzymes and can be identified by imaging techniques such as ultrasound. Jaundice from alcoholic hepatitis generally results in the level of aspartate aminotransferase (AST) being twice the level of alanine transaminase (ALT).

The differential diagnosis of viral hepatitis includes hepatitis A, hepatitis B, hepatitis C, hepatitis D, hepatitis E, Epstein-Barr virus (EBV), and cytomegalovirus (Table 1). Although we focus on hepatitis A, B, and C in the initial work-up in the setting of chronic disease, we often order the following in chronic disease to make sure that treatable conditions are not missed: ferritin to evaluate for hemochromatosis and ceruloplasmin for Wilson disease.

HEPATITIS A

Disease Burden

Hepatitis A is one of the most common vaccine-preventable diseases in the United States. The reported incidence of hepatitis A is highest among children 5 to 14 years of age; approximately one third of reported cases involve children younger than 15 years of age. Many more children have unrecognized infection and can be the source of infection for others. Hepatitis A incidence varies by race/ethnicity, with the highest rates among American Indians/Alaskan Natives and the lowest rates among Asians; rates among Hispanics are higher than among non-Hispanics. These differences most likely reflect differences in the risk for infection related to factors such as socioeconomic levels, resultant living conditions, and more frequent contact with persons from countries where hepatitis A is endemic.

Epidemiology

Hepatitis A virus infection is acquired primarily by the fecal-oral route by either person-to-person contact or ingestion of contaminated food or water. Depending on conditions, the virus can be stable in the environment for months. On rare occasions, the virus has been transmitted by transfusion of blood or blood products.

The most frequently reported source of infection (12% to 26%) is either household or sexual contact with a person with hepatitis A. International travelers, especially to Mexico, account for an additional 4% to 6% of the infections. Only 2% to 3% of cases are associated with recognized food or waterborne disease outbreaks. Most persons with hepatitis A do not have an identified source for their infection.

Clinical Course

Hepatitis A virus is an RNA picornavirus that causes infections in humans after an incubation period of 28 days and can be either asymptomatic or symptomatic. The symptomatic illness classically has an abrupt onset of symptoms that include fever, nausea, anorexia, malaise, and jaundice. Most infections in children younger than 6 years of age are asymptomatic. In contrast, infections in adults are symptomatic, with 70% of adults developing jaundice. The illness is usually self-limited and lasts less than 2 months. However, an estimated 100 persons die as a result of acute liver failure resulting from hepatitis A each year. Although only 0.3% of all patients with acute hepatitis A develop fulminant hepatitis A, the rate is 1.8% among adults older than 50 years of age. Persons with chronic liver disease are at increased risk for fulminant hepatitis A.

During the acute illness, IgM class of antibody to hepatitis A (anti-HAV) develops and lasts for several months. IgG class of anti-HAV develops during recovery and lasts lifelong. IgG anti-HAV indicates immunity to infection.

TABLE 1. **Differential Diagnosis of Viral Hepatitis**

Virus	Primary Transmission Route(s)	Incubation Period	Epidemiology and Risk Factors
Hepatitis A virus	Fecal-oral, person-to-person contact, or ingestion of contaminated food	30 days average (range 15–50 days)	Household or sexual contact with an an infected person, day care centers, and common-source outbreaks from contaminated food
Hepatitis B virus	Sexual, blood, and other body fluids	120 days average (range 45–160 days)	Sexual promiscuity, male-to-male sexual practices, injection drug use, birth to an infected mother
Hepatitis C virus	Blood	Commonly 6–9 weeks (range 2 weeks–6 months)	Injection drug use, occupational exposure to blood, hemodialysis, transfusion, possibly sexual transmission
Hepatitis D virus	Blood, sexual, and other body fluids	2–8 weeks (from animal studies)	Requires active infection with HBV. Injection drug users and persons receiving clotting factor concentrates are at highest risk of infection.
Hepatitis E virus	Fecal-oral	26–42 days average (range 15–64 days)	No known cases originated in the United States. International travelers are the only high-risk group to date.
Epstein-Barr virus (EBV)	Oropharyngeal via saliva	4–6 weeks	Seroconversion by age 5 years in 50% of persons in United States. Children with an acutely infected sibling are at greater risk.
Cytomegalovirus (CMV-human herpes virus 5)	Intimate contact with infected secretions: sexual, perinatal, blood transfusion, and infected breast milk	About 3 to 8 weeks for transfusion-acquired CMV	Household or sexual contact with an infected person, male-to-male sexual practices, day care centers, perinatal transmission

Modified from Zimmerman RK, Ruben FL, Ahwesh ER: Hepatitis B virus infection, hepatitis B vaccine, and hepatitis B immune globulin. J Fam Pract 45:300;1997. Copyright Association of Teachers of Preventive Medicine; used with permission.

HEPATITIS B

Disease Burden

Hepatitis B virus (HBV) infection is a major health problem in the United States; 128,000 to 320,000 persons are infected annually (CDC, unpublished data). Approximately 6000 persons die annually of HBV-related complications of liver disease in the United States. Most of these deaths are in persons chronically infected with HBV (i.e., persons who test positive for hepatitis B surface antigen [HBsAg] for 6 months or more). Complications of chronic HBV infection include cirrhosis and primary hepatocellular carcinoma. About 150 persons in the United States die of fulminant hepatitis after acute infection. Infection is not uncommon, as seen by the 5% lifetime risk for acquiring hepatitis B virus. The number of persons chronically infected with HBV in the United States, each of whom is potentially infectious, is estimated at 1.25 million.

HBV infection, which can lead to hepatocellular carcinoma, is the second known leading cause of cancer worldwide.

Epidemiology

HBV can be contracted either from persons acutely or chronically infected with HBV. Transmission of HBV occurs primarily by blood exchange (e.g., via shared needles during injection drug use) and by sexual contact. Perinatal transmission from infected mothers during delivery is common when postexposure prophylactic measures are not used. The source of infection is not identified for 30% to 40% of hepatitis B cases. These cases may result from (1) underreporting of injection drug use and sexual activity, and (2) inapparent contamination of skin lesions or mucosal surfaces because HBsAg is found in, for example, impetigo lesions and saliva of persons chronically infected with HBV, and on toothbrush racks and coffee cups in their homes. Epidemiologic studies show that HBV is sometimes transmitted between preschool-age children. HBV does not appear to be transmitted by fecal-oral or airborne routes.

Measures to prevent spread of hepatitis B include vaccination, which will be discussed later, and universal precautions.

Importance of Age at HBV Infection on Development of Chronic Infection

Persons infected early in life are much more likely to become chronically infected than those infected during adulthood. Chronic HBV infection develops in 90% of those infected as infants, 30% to 60% of those infected before the age of 4 years, and 5% to 10% of those infected as adults. Up to 25% of infected infants will die of HBV-related chronic liver disease as adults. Although most acute infections in the United States occur in adulthood because of high-risk behaviors, 36% of all persons chronically infected in the United States contract HBV during early childhood.

Hepatitis B Antigens and Serologies

HBV is a DNA virus of the class *Hepadnaviridae*. The outer viral coat contains HBsAg, which is a marker of current infection and is present in both acute and chronic infections. HBsAg can be detected in the serum from 1 to 12 weeks (mean 30–60 days) after exposure to HBV. Persons can transmit HBV as long as HBsAg is present in their serum. The sensitivity and specificity of the tests for HBsAg are greater than 98%. The inner core contains hepatitis B core antigen (HBcAg), DNA, and hepatitis B e antigen (HBeAg).

HBcAg is found in liver tissue during acute or chronic infection. It is not detectable in serum by common laboratory techniques.

HBeAg is present during HBV replication and is a marker for high levels of infectivity. HBeAg is present early in acute infections and for variable periods in chronic infections.

Antibodies are produced against HBsAg (anti-HBs), HBcAg (anti-HBc), and HBeAg (anti-HBe).

Anti-HBs occurs after acute HBV infection with recovery and indicates immunity (Table 2). Anti-HBs can also develop in response to hepatitis B vaccination or be passively transferred by administration of hepatitis B immune globulin (HBIG).

The presence of anti-HBc indicates that the individual was infected with HBV at some time in the past; anti-HBc persists indefinitely both in persons who recovered from the infection and persons who are chronically infected. Anti-HBc does not develop following vaccination, so testing for anti-HBc is the best way to determine susceptibility in an unvaccinated person. The presence of IgM anti-HBc indicates acute or recent infection; IgM anti-HBc develops approximately 8 weeks after exposure to HBV (see Table 2).

Anti-HBe develops when HBsAg and HBeAg disappear and indicates that infectivity has diminished.

Diagnosis

The diagnosis of HBV infection is made by serologic testing. In acute infection, a test for HBsAg becomes positive between 1 and 12 weeks (mean 30–60 days) after exposure and remains positive for 3 months, on average. When tests to detect HBsAg become negative, the patient is said to have entered the "window" period, during which IgM anti-HBc, IgG anti-HBc, and anti-HBe can be detected in the blood, but HBsAg or anti-HBs cannot. Later, anti-HBs will appear. Tests to detect IgM anti-HBc become positive 3 to 5 weeks after HBsAg appears and before the onset of clinical symptoms; IgM anti-HBc remains detectable for 4 to 6 months after the onset of illness and is the best serologic marker of acute infection. Chronic infection (the carrier state) is defined by (1) the presence of HBsAg on at least two occasions, 6 months apart, or (2) positive test results for HBsAg and negative test results for IgM anti-HBc on a single specimen (see Table 2).

Clinical Description and Phases

Clinical signs and symptoms of acute hepatitis occur in about 50% of infected adults but in only 5% of infected preschool-age children. The onset of symptoms occurs months after exposure; the incubation period is 120 days on average (range 45–160 days). The clinical course of acute HBV infection has three phases: preicteric, icteric, and convalescent.

The preicteric phase occurs from onset of initial symptoms until the start of jaundice and typically lasts 3 to 10 days. Hepatic symptoms include anorexia, nausea, vomiting, and right upper-quadrant abdominal pain. Extrahepatic symptoms such as fever, malaise, rash, myalgia, and arthralgia may occur. Levels of ALT (SGPT) and AST, formerly known as serum glutamic-oxaloacetic transaminase, or SGOT, rise during the preicteric phase, followed by a rise in bilirubin level which leads to darkened urine 1 to 2 days before the icteric phase.

The icteric phase is heralded by jaundice and typically lasts 1 to 3 weeks. Gray-colored stools, hepatomegaly, hepatic tenderness, and sometimes splenomegaly may occur. ALT and AST levels usually peak in the icteric phase, and may be 400 to 4000 IU. Bilirubin levels also rise during the icteric phase, typically reaching 85 to 340 μmol/L (5 to 20 mg/dL) if the infected person has jaundice. In 1% to 2% of patients, the icteric phase leads to fulminant hepatitis, which has a 63% to 93% case-fatality rate.

The convalescent phase, which begins when jaundice disappears, is characterized by constitutional symptoms, such as malaise and fatigue, and may last for several months.

TABLE 2. **Interpretation of Laboratory Tests to Detect HBV Infection***

Patient Status	HBsAg	HBeAg	Total Anti-HBc	IgM Anti-HBc	Anti-HBs	Infectivity
Never infected	0	0	0	0	0	0
Early acute HBV infection	+	0	0	0	0	+
Acute HBV infection	+	+	+	+	0	+
Chronic HBV infection	+	+/0	+	0	0	+
Recovered from HBV	0	0	+	0	+	0
Vaccinated	0	0	0	0	+	0

Modified from Table 1 in Moyer LA, Mast EE: Hepatitis B: virology, epidemiology, disease, and prevention, and an overview of viral hepatitis. Am J Prev Med 10(Suppl):45-55; 1994. Public domain.

HBV, hepatitis B virus; 0, absent; +, present; +/0, variable presence.

Management of HBV Infection

Acute HBV infection is treated symptomatically. Certain contacts of infected persons should receive HBIG and hepatitis B vaccine.

Three treatments are available for chronic hepatitis B: (1) interferon, (2) lamivudine (Epivir-HBV), and (3) adefovir dipivoxil (Hepsera). Therapy with interferon alfa-2b (Intron A) stops viral replication in approximately 40% of cases and results in disappearance of HBsAg from the serum in 10% to 20% of treated persons. Other treatments include the nucleoside analogue lamivudine, which results in similar response rates. The combination of interferon and lamivudine may lead to a better response. The Food and Drug Administration approved adefovir dipivoxil in 2002. According to trials, more than half (53% to 64%) of patients receiving adefovir showed significant improvement in liver inflammation caused by HBV compared with 25% to 35% of patients receiving placebo. According to the literature, in HBeAg-positive patients, all three treatments have a response of about 70% during treatment, but it drops after treatment is stopped (e.g., 20% for interferon and 10% for lamivudine).

Persons with either acute or chronic infection should be counseled on (1) mechanisms of HBV transmission; (2) the need to inform contacts; (3) the importance of not donating blood, other body fluids, or tissues; (4) the importance of not sharing household articles that could be contaminated with blood; (5) the need to cover skin lesions to prevent the spread of HBV in blood and secretions; and (6) the importance of testing and vaccinating contacts.

HEPATITIS C

Disease Burden

Hepatitis C virus (HCV) is the most common reason for liver transplantation and causes an estimated 10,000 to 12,000 deaths each year. HCV infection is the most common chronic bloodborne infection in the United States, because an estimated 3.9 million (1.8%) Americans have been infected. Most of these are chronically infected and many may not be aware of this because they do not feel ill. Currently, HCV prevalence is highest in persons 40–59 years of age; within this group, the prevalence among African Americans is highest (6.1%). About 40% of chronic liver disease is related to HCV.

Epidemiology

HCV is caused by an RNA virus with six genotypes. About 70% to 75% of HCV infections in the United States are genotype 1.

HCV is transmitted primarily through infected blood, especially large or repeated percutaneous exposure. In the United States, common mechanisms include injection drug use, blood transfusion before 1993, and receipt before 1992 of clotting factors among hemophiliacs. Since 1994, risk for transfusion-transmitted HCV is too low to measure. Most newly acquired cases of HCV are due to injection drug use. Sexual transmission can occur but is uncommon. The risk of HCV from a needlestick is estimated at 2%; no treatment is currently recommended for accidental needlesticks. The risk of perinatal transmission is about 2% in anti-HCV positive women and 4% to 7% in women who are HCV RNA positive at delivery; no data exist on treatment.

Because of the mode of acquisition of HCV, many persons are also at risk for HIV.

Hepatitis C Serologies and Diagnosis

Third-generation enzyme immunoassays (EIA) have a sensitivity of >99% and a specificity of 99% in immunocompetent patients. It is positive in 50% to 70% of patients at the onset of symptoms in acute infection, rising to >90% after 3 months and >97% after 6 months. EIA cannot distinguish between acute, chronic, or resolved infection. False positives can occur in autoimmune disorders.

Before the third-generation EIA tests, supplemental antibody testing was conducted (e.g., recombinant strip immunoblot assay) to confirm the diagnosis. Given the high specificity of the third-generation tests and the availability of RNA assays, we no longer order supplemental antibody tests.

After a positive EIA, we confirm the diagnosis with a RNA assay. Qualitative HCV assays include reverse transcriptase—polymerase chain reaction (PCR) or transcription-mediated amplification. The specificity of PCR is >98% and it detects small amounts of RNA (e.g., 50 IU/mL). Some HCV-infected persons might have only intermittently RNA-positive tests in the setting of acute hepatitis C or end stage liver disease.

Quantitative HCV assays give the viral load and include quantitative PCR and branched DNA signal amplification assays. There is little correlation between the level of HCV RNA and disease progression. However, the viral load may help predict the likelihood of response to treatment or follow response to treatment. Quantitative assays may be less sensitive to very small amounts of RNA than the qualitative assays.

HCV genotype is helpful to predict responses to antiviral therapy. Persons infected with genotype 1 have much lower responses than those with other genotypes. Furthermore, the duration of therapy may vary by genotype; type 1 may require longer treatment.

ALT is insensitive to measure disease severity as the association between ALT level and histopathology is weak.

Liver biopsy provides the best information on fibrosis and shows other possible contributing etiologies including alcohol, iron, and steatosis. Furthermore, those with minimal or no fibrosis may decide to postpone therapy in light of its side effects. On the other hand, because genotypes 2 and 3 have a favorable response to therapy 80% of the time, it is not always necessary to perform a liver biopsy in these groups to make treatment decisions, as a National Institutes of Health (NIH) Consensus Conference noted.

Clinical Course

Acute infection is generally asymptomatic or mild and only one-quarter might have jaundice. ALT levels rise in an average of 4 to 12 weeks. Fulminant liver failure after acute infection is rare.

Most (60% to 85%) persons develop chronic infection. Most (60% to 70%) chronically infected persons have elevated ALT levels. A single normal ALT level does not exclude chronic infection and longer term evaluation is needed.

The course of chronic infection is insidious and slowly progressive over decades. Most studies have reported that cirrhosis develops in 10% to 15% of persons with chronic hepatitis C over a period of 20 to 30 years, varying by age at acquisition. After cirrhosis has occurred, the risk for hepatocellular carcinoma (HCC) increases. Other factors that increase the risk for cirrhosis include male gender, HIV, continued alcohol use, and concurrent chronic hepatitis B.

Management of Chronic HCV infection

In trials of pegylated interferon plus ribavirin (peginterferon alfa-2b [PEG-Intron]) (Rebetol) in previously untreated patients without decompensated cirrhosis, sustained viral response was 42% to 46% for genotype 1 and 76% to 82% for genotypes 2 and 3. According to the 2002 NIH Consensus Conference, recent data show that a 24-week course was as effective as a 48-week course for genotypes 2 and 3 but not for genotype 1. According to the conference, reduced ribavirin dosages of 800 mg daily can be used for genotypes 2 and 3 but standard dosages of 1000 mg to 1200 mg daily are recommended for genotype 1. Factors associated with response include genotype, lower baseline viral load, less fibrosis on biopsy, and lower body weight.

For genotype 1, early viral response, which is a decrease viral load of 2 logs at least at 12 weeks, is predictive of sustained viral response. Treatment can be discontinued at 12 weeks for those with genotype 1 who do not respond at 12 weeks because there is only a small chance of response with further therapy.

Treatment with interferon alfa-2b (Intron)* of acute hepatitis C has been done in small uncontrolled trials with good success.

Because of adverse effects, about 12% of patients discontinue pegylated interferon and ribavirin. Adverse effects include influenza-like symptoms, depression, anemia, and cytopenia. Depression can be treated with selective serotonin reuptake inhibitors, but we have had to stop interferon because of depression with suicidal ideation. Reduction in the dose of ribavirin can reduce anemia. Hemolysis from ribavirin has been reported in patients with renal insufficiency. Ribavirin is teratogenic; consequently, female patients should avoid becoming pregnant during therapy.

Antiviral therapy is recommended for adults with chronic hepatitis C who are at increased risk for progression to cirrhosis. These persons include anti-HCV–positive patients with persistently elevated ALT levels, detectable HCV RNA, or a liver biopsy that indicates either portal or bridging fibrosis or at least moderate degrees of inflammation and necrosis. Adults at low risk of progression to cirrhosis (i.e., no fibrosis), may elect periodic monitoring without interferon therapy or may choose to pursue therapy. Adults with liver failure are less likely to respond to interferon, and liver transplantation may be their best option. Treatment in children is experimental.

According to the NIH Consensus Conference, preliminary results show that 15% to 20% of those treated who failed to respond to standard interferon and ribavirin (Rebetron) therapy developed a sustained viral response on retreatment with peginterferon alfa-2b and ribavirin. Patients with advanced fibrosis or cirrhosis are at increased risk of liver failure and may wish to consider retreatment.

Because alcohol adversely affects response to treatment, use of alcohol should be strongly discouraged.

Screening for Hepatocellular Carcinoma

Screening for HCC is controversial. Alfa-fetoprotein tests have poor sensitivity and a high rate of false-positive results. Ultrasound is more sensitive but has false positives. More research is needed on screening for HCC. Because HCC is quite rare in the absence of cirrhosis, screening is not indicated in persons without cirrhosis.

HEPATITIS D

Hepatitis D virus (HDV), also called delta, is a defective RNA virus that requires HBV to replicate. HDV can either coinfect a person at the same time HBV is acquired or superinfect a person who is already HBV-infected. If coinfection occurs, the initial disease can be severe and may result in fulminant hepatitis, but chronic infection is unlikely. If superinfection occurs, chronic infection is likely, in which case most develop chronic liver disease. Transmission is primarily by injection drug use, although sexual transmission also occurs.

If coinfection occurs, both IgM and IgG antibody to HDV (anti-HDV) typically occur. After the infection resolves, anti-HDV eventually declines to levels that are not detectable with current tests. Tests for IgG anti-HDV are available in the United States.

If superinfection occurs, HDV RNA is present, HDAg is present, high titers of IgM HDV develop then drop, and high titers of IgG HDV develop and continue indefinitely.

HEPATITIS E

Hepatitis E virus (HEV) is enterically transmitted, usually from contaminated water. Although common worldwide, it is not often seen in the United States; cases may occur in travelers returning from overseas.

---

*Not FDA approved for this indication.

The incubation period is about 40 days. HEV does not cause chronic infection.

PREVENTION

Hepatitis A Vaccine

Rationale for Vaccination

Both licensed vaccines are highly immunogenic in persons older than 2 years of age. Protective antibody levels developed in 94% to 100% of people 1 month after the first dose and essentially 100% after the second dose. Available data indicate that hepatitis A vaccine (Havrix) is immunogenic in children younger than 2 years of age who do not have passively acquired maternal antibodies.

The efficacy of the hepatitis A vaccine is between 94% and 100%. Duration of protection has been evaluated in several studies; in both adults and children protection has been demonstrated for at least 6 to 8 years. Estimates of antibody persistence derived from kinetic models of antibody decline indicate that protection could persist for greater than 20 years.

Adverse Reactions

The most frequently reported side effects include soreness at the injection site, warmth at the injection site, and headache. Follow-up of longer than 5 years regarding adverse events from an estimated 65 million doses of hepatitis A vaccine administered worldwide did not find any serious adverse events among children or adults that could definitely be attributed to the vaccine.

Recommendations

The ACIP 1996 recommendations on the prevention of hepatitis A immunization focused primarily on vaccinating persons in groups shown to be at high risk for infection (e.g., travelers to countries with high or intermediate disease endemicity, men who have sex with men, injection drug users, persons with clotting-factor disorders), persons with chronic liver disease and children living in communities with high rates of disease. Outbreaks of HAV infection have occurred in injection drug users and homosexual males. For this reason, hepatitis A vaccine is recommended for injection drug users, users of orally or nasally administered street drugs who live in areas where epidemiologic data indicate a high incidence of hepatitis A infection, homosexual males, and bisexual males. Prevaccination testing is not indicated for adolescents but may be cost-effective in adults.

In October 1999, the ACIP added recommendations for routine vaccination of children in states, countries, or communities with rates that are twice the 1987–1997 national range or greater (i.e., >20 cases per 100,000 population). Consideration should be given to routine vaccination of children in states, countries, or communities with rates exceeding the 1987–1997 national average (i.e., >10 but <20 cases per 100,000 population). CDC has a map with hepatitis A rates at www.cdc.gov/ncidod/diseases/hepatitis/a/vax/index.htm.

Hepatitis B Vaccine

Rationale for Routine Hepatitis B Vaccination

Reasons to recommend routine infant vaccination against HBV include the following: (1) morbidity and mortality of HBV infection, especially when contracted in childhood; (2) transmission of HBV infection from child to child, although relatively infrequent, has been reported in schools, day care centers, and families and among playmates; (3) strategies focusing on immunization of high-risk persons have had little impact; (4) no risk factor for HBV infection can be identified in at least 30% of infected persons; (5) those who engage in high-risk behaviors (e.g., injection drug use), are not often compliant with the needed three-dose vaccination regimen; (6) many become infected soon after beginning such behaviors; and (7) routine infant hepatitis B vaccination is as cost-effective as other commonly used preventive measures.

The hepatitis B vaccines currently produced in the United States (Recombivax HB, Engerix-B) are manufactured by recombinant DNA technology using baker's yeast. Preexposure vaccination results in protective antibody levels in almost all infants and children (>95%). Efficacy (i.e., protection against HBV infection) is high (80% to 95%) for hepatitis B vaccines licensed in the United States when given to susceptible infants, children, and adults.

Underlying medical conditions associated with lower seroconversion include prematurity with low birth weight, immunosuppression, and renal failure. In comparison to full-term infants, premature infants with a birth weight less than 2 kg have lower seroconversion rates; the rates drop further if the birth weight is less than 1 kg. Therefore, hepatitis B vaccination should be delayed in preterm infants weighing less than 2 kg unless the infant is born to an HBsAg-positive mother.

Adverse Reactions

The most common adverse event after administration of hepatitis B vaccine is pain at the injection site, which occurs in 13% to 29% of adults and 3% to 9% of children. Mild, transient systemic adverse events such as fatigue and headache have been reported in 11% to 17% of adults and 8% to 18% of children. Temperature greater than 37.7° C has been reported in 1% to 6% of vaccinees.

Recommendations

The prevalence of HBV infection and its associated morbidity and mortality have led to the development of a comprehensive hepatitis B vaccination policy that includes recommendations for: (1) prevention of perinatal HBV infection, (2) routine infant vaccination, (3) catch-up vaccination of adolescents not previously vaccinated, (4) catch-up vaccination of young children at high risk for infection, and (5) preexposure vaccination of adults based on lifestyle or environmental, medical, and occupational situations that place them at risk, including health care workers, hemodialysis patients, household or sexual contacts of hepatitis B carriers, injection drug users, staff and residents of

TABLE 3. **Recommendations for Hepatitis B Prophylaxis for Percutaneous or Permucosal Exposure**

Exposed Person's Vaccination Status	Treatment when source is:		
	HBsAg Positive	**HBsAg Negative**	**Not Tested or Unknown**
Unvaccinated	HBIG × 1* and initiate hepatitis B vaccine	Initiate hepatitis B vaccine	Initiate hepatitis B vaccine
Previously vaccinated:			
1. Known responder	No treatment	No treatment	No treatment
2. Known nonresponder	HBIG × 2 or HBIG × 1 and initiate revaccination[†]	No treatment	If high-risk source, treat as if HBsAg positive
3. Response unknown	Test exposed for anti-HBs: 1. If inadequate,[‡] give HBIG × 1 and vaccine booster[§] 2. If adequate, no treatment	No treatment	Test exposed person for anti-HBs: 1. If inadequate,[‡] initiate vaccine booster dose and recheck titer in 1–2 months 2. If adequate, no treatment

Modified from Centers for Disease Control and Prevention: Updated US Public Health Service Guidelines for the Management of Occupational Exposures to HBV, HCV, and HIV and Recommendations for Postexposure Prophylaxis. MMWR 50 (RR-11):22;2001. Public domain.

HBsAg, hepatitis B surface antigen; HBIG, hepatitis B immune globulin; anti-HBs, antibody to HBsAg.

*HBIG dose, 0.06 mL/kg intramuscularly, within 24 hours of exposure.

[†]The option of giving one dose of HBIG and reinitiating the vaccine series is preferred for nonresponders who have not completed a second three-dose vaccine series. For persons who previously completed a second vaccine series but failed to respond, two doses of HBIG are preferred.

[‡]Adequate anti-HBs is 10 mIU/mL.

[§]Checking the response to vaccination is recommended at 1–2 months if HBIG was not given and after passive antibody is no longer detectable (e.g., 4–6 months) if HBIG was given.

institutions for developmentally disabled, at-risk public safety workers, recipients of clotting factors derived from plasma, persons with sexually transmitted diseases, prostitutes, homosexual or bisexual males, and persons with multiple sex partners in the previous 6 months.

Many (10% to 85%) infants born to mothers who are HBV carriers will become chronically infected with HBV themselves unless given postexposure prophylaxis including vaccination—and some of the infants so infected will die of chronic liver disease as adults. Therefore, infants born to women who are positive for HBsAg should receive at separate sites the first dose of hepatitis B vaccine and 0.5 mL of hepatitis B immune globulin (HBIG) within 12 hours of birth. This regimen is 75% to 95% effective in preventing chronic HBV infection. A second HBsAg test late in pregnancy is recommended for pregnant women who are at high risk for HBV infection (e.g., injection drug users, those with a recently diagnosed sexually transmitted disease, or those with multiple sex partners) and whose initial HBsAg test results are negative.

Postvaccination testing for anti-HBs is recommended only when the results will affect the individual subsequent medical care. Such persons include dialysis patients, infants born to HBsAg-positive mothers, sexual contacts of persons chronically infected with HBV, and health care workers at high risk of percutaneous or permucosal exposure to body fluids. Testing should be performed 1 to 2 months after completion of the vaccine series, with the exception of infants born to HBsAg-positive mothers, who should be tested at 9 to 15 months of age. An adequate antibody response to vaccination is 10 mIU/mL. Postvaccination testing is not indicated after routine vaccination of infants, children, adolescents, or persons at low risk of exposure (e.g., public safety workers and health care workers who do not have contact with patients or their body fluids). The protocol in Table 3 should be used for accidental needlestick injuries.

Revaccination is recommended for persons whose postvaccination level of anti-HBs is less than 10 mIU/mL. Such persons should receive three doses on a 0-, 1-, and 6-month schedule. Antibody testing should be conducted again 1 to 2 months after revaccination. Persons who do not respond after two series (six doses) of hepatitis B vaccine should be counseled about universal precautions and the need for HBIG if they are exposed. Also, testing such persons for HBsAg should be considered, because some may already be chronically infected. Hemodialysis and immunocompromised patients at risk for infection should have serological tests annually and should be given a booster dose when antibody levels decline to less than 10 mIU/mL.

MALABSORPTION

method of
RICHARD NEIL FEDORAK, M.D., and
CYRUS P. TAMBOLI, M.D.
University of Alberta
Edmonton, Alberta, Canada

Malabsorption syndrome is a term applied to any situation in which disease of the intestine adversely interferes with the extraction of energy and nutrients from orally ingested food. Malabsorption includes disorders of intraluminal mixing and digestion, in addition to disorders of intramural transport and absorption. It is thus conceptually useful to classify this syndrome into disorders causing impaired intraluminal digestion and those causing impaired intramural absorption (Table 1).

TABLE 1. **Classification of Malabsorption Syndromes**

Defective Intraluminal Digestion	Defective Intramural Absorption
Gastric Mixing Disorders	*Inadequate Absorptive Surface*
Postgastrectomy	Intestinal resection or bypass
Pancreatic Insufficiency	Mesenteric vascular disease with massive intestinal resection
Primary	Crohns's disease with multiple bowel resections
Cystic fibrosis	Jejunoileal bypass
Secondary	*Mucosal Absorptive Defects*
Chronic Pancreatitis	Biochemical or genetic abnormalities
Pancreatic carcinoma	Celiac disease
Pancreatic resection	Disaccharidase deficiency
Reduced Intestinal Bile Salt Concentration	Hypogammaglobulinemia
Liver and biliary disease	Abetalipoproteinemia
Hepatocellular disease	Hartnup disease
Cholestasis (intrahepatic or extrahepatic)	Cystinuria
Abnormal small-bowel bacterial proliferation	Monosaccharide malassimilation
Afferent loop stasis	Inflammatory or infiltrative disorders
Strictures	Crohn's disease
Fistulas	Amyloidosis
Ileocecal valve resection	Scleroderma
Blind loop(s)	Lymphoma
Multiple diverticula of the small bowel	Radiation enteritis
Hypomotility states (i.e., diabetes, scleroderma, intestinal pseudo-obstruction)	Eosinophilic enteritis
Hypochlorhydria	Tropical sprue
Interrupted enterohepatic circulation of bile salts	Infectious enteritis (e.g., salmonellosis)
Ileal surgical resection	Collagenous sprue
Ileal inflammatory disease (Crohn's disease)	Nonspecific ulcerative jejunoileitis
Primary bile acid malabsorption	Mastocytosis
Postcholecystectomy and truncal vagotomy	Dermatologic disorders (e.g., dermatitis herpetiformis)
Drugs (by sequestration or precepitation of bile salts)	Lymphatic obstruction
Neomycin	Intestinal lymphangiectasia
Calcium carbonate	Whipple's disease
Cholestryramine	Lymphoma

Although nonspecific treatments are available for the diarrheal symptoms associated with malabsorption, appropriate therapy and management of the malabsorption depends on the underlying physiologic defect being recognized and addressed. Because many diverse conditions (see Table 1) are capable of leading to clinical malabsorption, an understanding of pertinent intestinal physiology is useful to develop an appropriate therapeutic plan.

CARBOHYDRATE DIGESTION AND ABSORPTION

The orally ingested monosaccharide and disaccharide carbohydrates maltose, glucose, fructose, sucrose, and lactose are key sources of food energy. Starch is the only polysaccharide significantly utilized by humans. In the mouth, salivary α-amylase begins digesting starch, but it is rapidly inhibited in the acid milieu of the stomach. In the small intestine, pancreatic α-amylases continue to digest starch to produce oligosaccharides, maltose, maltotriose, glucose polymers, and α-limit dextrins. These molecules, along with ingested disaccharides, are subsequently further digested into monosaccharides by brush border disaccharidases, maltase, lactase, α-limit dextrinase, and sucrase-isomaltase into glucose, galactose, and fructose. All monosaccharides are then transported across the gastrointestinal epithelium via a series of active transporters located in the brush border.

From these physiologic considerations, carbohydrate malabsorption can occur in the following circumstances: (1) pancreatic insufficiency, (2) deficiencies of brush border disaccharidases (e.g., lactase deficiency), (3) generalized impairment of brush border and enterocyte function (i.e., celiac disease), and (4) loss of mucosal surface area (i.e., short-bowel syndrome).

Carbohydrate malabsorption leads to residual unhydrolyzed carbohydrates in the lumen of the intestine, which augments intraluminal fluid accumulation and diarrhea, by virtue of its osmotic effect. Furthermore, bacterial fermentation of malabsorbed carbohydrates that reach the colon produces short-chain fatty acids (which aggravate diarrhea) and hydrogen and carbon dioxide gases (which cause flatulence and bloating).

PROTEIN DIGESTION AND ABSORPTION

Pepsin, liberated from the stomach, is active and cleaves ingested proteins in the presence of an acidic pH. Once it enters the duodenum, gastric pepsin is rapidly inactivated by duodenal bicarbonate, and pancreatic proteases (trypsin, chymotrypsin, elastase, DNase, RNase, and carboxypeptidases A and B) and brush border dipeptidases complete the intraluminal protein digestion. The resultant individual amino acids are then transported across the enterocyte via sodium-dependent and sodium-independent amino acid and oligopeptide cotransporters.

From these physiologic considerations, protein malabsorption would be expected in diseases causing (1) pancreatic insufficiency, (2) generalized impaired enterocyte function (i.e., celiac disease), and (3) loss of mucosal surface area (i.e., short-bowel syndrome).

Protein malabsorption is much less common than carbohydrate or fat malabsorption. When protein malabsorption does occur, protein-losing enteropathy ensues, with subsequent hypoproteinemia and weight loss.

LIPID DIGESTION AND ABSORPTION

Although the process of fat digestion and absorption yields the highest caloric value per gram ingested, it is also the most complex and therefore vulnerable to dysfunction from a variety of causes. Lingual lipase can digest up to 30% of ingested lipids, whereas gastric lipase activity becomes significant only in the presence of pancreatic lipase insufficiency. The overall process of fat digestion and absorption consists of four distinct phases related to the respective functions of the pancreas, liver, intestinal mucosa, and lymphatics. Physiologically, these functions respectively involve (1) lipolysis of dietary triglyceride to fatty acid and β-monoglyceride; (2) micellar solubilization with bile acid; (3) uptake into the mucosal cell, with reesterification and assembly of the monoglyceride and fatty acid to form triglycerides, as well as chylomicron formation in the presence of cholesterol, cholesterol esters, phospholipids, and protein; and (4) delivery of chylomicrons in lymphatics to the body for utilization of fat.

From these physiologic considerations, malabsorption of fat caused by impaired lipolysis or micellar solubilization would be expected to occur in the following circumstances: (1) rapid gastric emptying and improper mixing, (2) altered duodenal pH, (3) pancreatic insufficiency, (4) cholestasis, and (5) an interrupted enterohepatic circulation. Fat malabsorption from impaired mucosal uptake, assembly, or delivery would be expected to occur after (1) generalized impaired enterocyte function, (2) failure of the repackaging process, (3) disorders of lymphatics, and (4) loss of mucosal surface area.

Failure to digest or absorb fat results in both fat malabsorption and a deficiency in fat-soluble vitamins. Loss of fat into the colon results in the hydroxylation of long-chain fatty acids into hydroxyl-fatty acids, which cause diarrhea by stimulating the colon to secrete fluid and by virtue of their osmotic effect.

HISTORY AND PHYSICAL EXAMINATION

A malabsorption syndrome may be suspected after a thorough medical history and physical examination. The patient may have one or more manifestations of the underlying disease or resultant nutrient deficiencies. These signs and symptoms are variable and can be subtle (Table 2). Classic textbook descriptions of florid nutrient deficiencies are rarely encountered in clinical practice in developed countries. Nevertheless, all patients with significant malabsorption have some degree of abdominal pain, bloating, diarrhea, flatulence, or weight loss. Increased delivery to the colon of osmotically active particles, especially carbohydrates and lipids, leads to colonic secretion of water and electrolytes and resultant chronic diarrhea. Fat malabsorption may cause foul-smelling, pale, greasy stools that are difficult to flush. Floating stools are caused by increased fecal gas content from increased bacterial fermentation of carbohydrates. The patient may complain of fatigue and weakness, often associated with anemia. Protein-calorie malnutrition may cause edema. Deficiencies of fat-soluble vitamins (A, D, E, and K) may be manifested as night blindness, bone pain and osteomalacia, neurologic symptoms, or easy bruising, respectively.

Skin and mucosal disorders, such as seborrheic dermatitis, hyperkeratosis, xerosis, cheilosis, and alopecia, are commonly caused by deficiency in one or more water-soluble vitamins, such as vitamin B_6, niacin, or vitamin C. Intensely pruritic erythematous papules over the extensor surfaces is typical of *dermatitis herpetiformis*, which is associated with gluten sensitivity in

TABLE 2. **Clinical Signs and Symptoms of Malabsorption**

Clinical Sign or Symptom	Deficient Nutrient
General	
Weight loss, decreased libido, anorexia, fatigue, amenorrhea	Protein-calorie
Skin, Hair, and Nails	
Psoriasiform rash, eczema	Zinc
Pallor	Folate, iron, vitamin B_{12}
Follicular hyperkeratosis	Vitamin A
Perifollicular petechiae	Vitamin C
Flaking dermatitis	Protein-calorie, niacin, riboflavin, zinc
Bruising	Vitamin K
Thick, dry skin	Linoleic acid
Pigmentation changes	Niacin, protein-calorie
Sparse thin hair, alopecia	Protein
Flat brittle nails, leukonychia	Iron, protein
Eyes	
Night blindness	Vitamin A
Xerosis, Bitot's spots	Vitamin A
Keratomalacia	Vitamin A
Corneal vascularization	Riboflavin
Mouth	
Glossitis	Riboflavin, niacin, folic acid
Tongue atrophy	Riboflavin, niacin, iron
Angular stomatitis	Riboflavin, iron
Cheilosis	Riboflavin
Hypogeusia	Zinc
Bleeding gums	Riboflavin, vitamin C
Scarlet, raw, fissured tongue	Niacin
Head and Neck	
Muscle wasting	Protein-calorie
Extremities	
Muscle wasting, edema	Protein-calorie
Neurologic	
Tetany	Calcium, magnesium
Paresthesias	Vitamin B_{12}, thiamine
Hyporeflexia, wristdrop/footdrop	Thiamine
Ataxia, proprioception defects	Vitamin B_{12}, folate
Dementia, disorientation	Niacin

10% to 20% of cases. Peripheral neuropathy occurs with cases of vitamin B_{12} deficiency and is manifested as loss of position or vibration sensation. A past medical history of previous abdominal surgery may suggest mixing disorders, pancreatic insufficiency, small-bowel bacterial overgrowth, bile salt wastage, or loss of intestinal mucosal surface area.

SYMPTOMATIC ANTIDIARRHEAL THERAPY

Effective therapy for malabsorption syndromes depends on identifying and treating the underlying disease, correcting nutritional imbalances, and providing symptomatic relief.

Oral Rehydration Therapy

Oral rehydration therapy is used to prevent dehydration and electrolyte loss. It works by enhancing sodium, and thus water, absorption through cotransport of sodium and glucose. Oral rehydration preparations should have a balanced sodium-to-glucose ratio (see Table 4). Solutions that have excess glucose may aggravate existing diarrhea as a consequence of their osmotic effect.

Hydrophilic Bulking Agents

Dietary fiber supplementation may be useful in the management of diarrhea. The ultimate effectiveness of a fiber depends not only on its water-holding capacity but also on its ability to hydrolyze fatty and bile acids, which, if not hydrolyzed, directly stimulate intestinal secretion. Bulking agents also increase chyme viscosity and thereby delay gastric emptying and reduce colonic transit times. Psyllium (5 to 7.5 g every 12 hours) is a hydrophilic agent that increases fecal water-holding capacity and may reduce diarrheal symptoms. Many psyllium-containing products are mixed with laxatives; these products must be avoided in patients with malabsorption and diarrhea.

Opioids

Opioids reduce diarrhea by decreasing intestinal secretion or promoting intestinal absorption, reducing intestinal motility, and increasing anal tone. Available opioids include naturally occurring preparations (paregoric and opium alkaloids) and synthetic preparations (codeine, diphenoxylate, and loperamide). These agents are very effective for symptomatic use in cases of acute and chronic diarrhea caused by malabsorption; however, side effects limit their acute use, and tolerance usually occurs with chronic use. Diphenoxylate (Lomotil) 5 mg initially and then 2.5 mg after each loose bowel movement to a maximum of 20 mg/d and loperamide (Imodium) 4 mg initially and then 2 mg after each loose bowel movement to a maximum of 16 mg/d have fewer central nervous system side effects than noted with other opioids. Diphenoxylate has been combined with atropine to limit its potential for abuse. Loperamide, which has the least number of side effects or abuse potential, is available without prescription. Codeine (30 to 60 mg every 4 hours as needed) is the most effective antidiarrheal opiate, but it also has the greatest side effect profile.

DEFECTIVE INTRALUMINAL DIGESTION

Gastric Mixing Disorders

Surgical alterations in gastric innervation, pyloric structure, and gastric capacity may have significant effects on nutrition. Nutritional disturbances and chronic weight loss occur predominantly in patients who have had a subtotal gastrectomy in the past. These patients may have disorders of calcium homeostasis or anemia secondary to iron and, less frequently, vitamin B_{12} deficiency, and they require appropriate nutritional supplementation. Extensive gastrectomy can also be associated with symptoms of a small gastric reservoir. Patients typically complain of early satiety and a sensation of epigastric postprandial discomfort, which can be prevented by eating small, frequent meals.

Pancreatic Insufficiency

Pancreatic insufficiency may be primary and due to cystic fibrosis or secondary and due to chronic pancreatitis, pancreatic resection, or, rarely, pancreatic carcinoma. Of these causes, chronic pancreatitis is by far the most common and leads to weight loss because of anorexia or because of fear that eating will initiate pain by activating the pancreatitis. Only after 90% of the exocrine secretory capacity of the pancreas is lost does chronic pancreatic exocrine insufficiency occur and result in malabsorption and weight loss. During pancreatic insufficiency, fat malabsorption is dominant, perhaps because of a limited capacity to up-regulate lipase production. Cystic fibrosis is a childhood equivalent of chronic pancreatic insufficiency, but the weight loss associated with this disease is probably caused as much by the anorexia of chronic infection as it is by the malabsorption induced by pancreatic enzyme and bile acid deficiencies.

Because of insufficient quantities of pancreatic enzyme in commercial oral supplements and because of acid pepsin inactivation of orally administered pancreatic enzymes, complete correction of the fat malabsorption resulting from pancreatic insufficiency is rarely accomplished. The postprandial delivery of pancreatic lipase is approximately 560,000 IU during the 4 hours after a meal. Malabsorption does not occur if approximately 5% (28,000 IU over a 4-hour period) is delivered to the duodenum with each meal. Pancreatic supplements are highly variable in enzyme activity (Table 3), with the lipase content ranging from 4000 to 25,000 IU per capsule. Therefore, it is important to know the lipase content of the preparation prescribed and to ensure that sufficient amounts (at least 28,000 IU per meal) are being delivered to the duodenum.

Another important factor to consider in the management of pancreatic insufficiency is acid and pepsin

TABLE 3. **Pancreatic Enzyme Preparations**

	Enzyme Content (Units per Capsule)			
Therapeutic Agent	**Type**	**Lipase**	**Amylase**	**Protease**
Cotazym	C	8000	30,000	30,000
Cotazym ECS-4	ECMS	4000	11,000	11,000
Cotazym ECS-8	ECMS	8000	30,000	30,000
Cotazym ECS-20	ECMS	20,000	55,000	55,000
Creon 10	ECMS	10,000	33,200	37,500
Creon 25	ECMS	25,000	74,700	62,500
Pancrease	ECMS	4000	20,000	25,000
Pancrease MT 4	ECMT	4000	12,000	12,000
Pancrease MT 10	ECMT	10,000	30,000	30,000
Pancrease MT 16	ECMT	16,000	48,000	48,000
Ultrase	ECMS	4500	20,000	25,000
Ultrase MT 12	ECMT	12,000	39,000	39,000
Ultrase MT 20	ECMT	20,000	65,000	65,000
Viokase	UCT	8000	30,000	30,000
Viokase	P	16,800	70,000	70,000
Zymase	ECMS	12,000	24,000	24,000

C = capsule; ECMS = enteric-coated microspheres encased in a cellulose capsule; ECMT = enteric-coated microtablets encased in a cellulose capsule; P = powder; UCT = uncoated tablet.

inactivation of orally administered pancreatic enzymes. Less than 8% of ingested lipase and less than 22% of ingested trypsin successfully passes through the stomach and remains active in the duodenum. Preventing acid peptic neutralization of enzyme supplements by coating capsules with acid-resistant and alkali-sensitive materials or by using antacids has resulted in little improvement in the delivery of lipase to the duodenum. Antacids increase gastric secretion, and dilution of enzyme concentrations below critical levels may explain the relative ineffectiveness of antacids. Enteric coating is effective only if pancreatic enzymes are delivered into the duodenum at the same time as ingested food and if adequate intraduodenal dissolution occurs.

Recently, pancreatic enzyme preparations coated with a pH-dependent polymer were developed to be stable at gastric pH (<4) and dissolve at a pH greater than 5 in the duodenum. This pH dissolution profile theoretically delivers pancreatic enzymes to the upper part of the small bowel intact. However, if gastric and duodenal pH remains low (<4) throughout the postprandial period, the enteric coat will not dissolve and the pancreatic enzyme supplement will traverse the upper gastrointestinal tract and not assist in digestion and absorption. A major criterion for determining the efficacy of enteric-coated enzyme preparations is the size of the microspheres. These microspheres influence the timing of enzyme delivery to the small intestine. It has been shown that microspheres with a diameter of approximately 1.4 mm appear to mix with chyme most thoroughly and are emptied from the stomach at the same rate as food.

Therefore, an ideal enteric-coated pancreatic enzyme capsule preparation should contain a high concentration of lipase to maximize fat digestion, be enteric coated to avoid destruction by gastric acid, and contain microspheres approximately 1.4 mm in diameter to allow efficient delivery of enzyme to the small bowel. In addition, H_2-receptor antagonists and proton pump inhibitors decrease acid production and pepsin activity and can be used to optimize pancreatic enzyme concentrations in the duodenum. Additional therapeutic maneuvers include smaller and more frequent meals, each with pancreatic enzyme replacement, and reduction of the amount of fat in the diet to 50 to 75 g/d.

Finally, deficiencies of the fat-soluble vitamins A, D, E, and K and the respective clinical signs of deficiency have all been demonstrated with pancreatic insufficiency. Supplemental vitamins should be provided. The water-soluble vitamins are readily absorbed, with the exception of B_{12}, the absorption of which depends on pancreatic enzymes to cleave B_{12} from R protein to allow B_{12} to be absorbed in the ileum. With adequate pancreatic enzyme replacement, supplemental B_{12} is usually unnecessary.

REDUCED INTESTINAL BILE SALT CONCENTRATION

Liver and Biliary Disease

Severe hepatocellular dysfunction and bile duct obstruction can cause steatorrhea. Indeed, the incidence of mild steatorrhea is 25% to 50% in patients with cirrhosis alone. Steatorrhea in these patients occurs as a consequence of inadequate micelle formation from bile salt insufficiency; however, secondary factors, including malnutrition, portal hypertension, bacterial overgrowth, and drugs (i.e., neomycin) may also play a role. In cases of both biliary obstruction and severe liver disease, nutrient malabsorption is not often a significant clinical problem, and the weight loss is usually multifactorial.

Abnormal Small-Bowel Bacterial Proliferation

Small-bowel bacterial overgrowth is a syndrome characterized by nutrient malabsorption associated with excessive numbers of bacteria in the small intestine. In addition to intraluminal bacterial metabolism, evidence indicates that bacteria-induced mucosal injury also results in the malabsorption of fats, carbohydrates, and proteins; however, there is no evidence that bacterial invasion into the mucosal wall is involved in the malabsorption process.

Bacterial deconjugation of bile acids is the primary mechanism for malabsorption of fats and fat-soluble vitamins during abnormal small-bowel bacterial proliferation. Normal fat absorption requires a critical concentration of conjugated bile acids for the assembly of mixed micelles. Bacterial deconjugation of bile acids by luminal bacteria, particularly anaerobic organisms, reduces the level of conjugated bile acids below the critical micellar concentration and leads to fat malabsorption. Clinical vitamin D, A, and E deficiencies can occur, but the synthesis of vitamin K by luminal bacteria accounts for the absence of coagulopathy in patients with bacterial overgrowth. In addition, deconjugated bile acids and bacteria-hydroxylated fatty acids have a direct toxic effect on the intestinal mucosa that results in further malabsorption of fats. Finally, both deconjugated bile acids and hydroxylated fatty acids are direct secretagogues that contribute to the development of rapid intestinal transit and diarrhea.

Bacterial overgrowth results in carbohydrate malabsorption secondary to its direct toxic effect on intestinal mucosa and the subsequent reduction of brush border disaccharidases and decreased uptake of monosaccharides. Lactase activity is the first to be reduced and is the last disaccharidase activity to recover after antibiotic therapy has been administered.

Hypoproteinemia is common in bacterial overgrowth, although severe protein malabsorption is rarely seen. Disruption of normal protein assimilation is caused by multiple factors: bacteria compete with the host for protein substrates, decreased amino acid and peptide uptake occurs as a result of mucosal injury, decreased levels of enterokinase impair the activation of pancreatic proteases, and finally, a protein-losing enteropathy can ensue.

The association of macrocytic anemia with bacterial overgrowth is the result of direct competition between the anaerobic intestinal flora and the host for vitamin B_{12}. When bacteria take up the vitamin, not only does it become unavailable to the host, but inactive metabolites are also produced that compete with normal vitamin B_{12} binding and absorption. Thiamine and nicotinamide are two other water-soluble vitamins that have been reported to be low in patients with bacterial overgrowth. Although iron deficiency anemia has not been clearly associated with bacterial overgrowth in humans, increased intestinal losses of iron and blood have been seen in severe cases. Mineral and trace element deficiencies have not been reported in patients with bacterial overgrowth.

Initial management of bacterial overgrowth consists of fluid and nutritional support, including the replacement of vitamin deficiencies. After diagnosing bacterial overgrowth, an attempt to identify an underlying cause should be made and surgical correction of anatomic causes of intestinal stasis considered. Bacterial overgrowth resulting from severe motility disorders is more difficult to manage. Prokinetic agents have been shown to normalize gastric motility in patients with motor disorders; however, their role in treating small intestinal bacterial overgrowth remains limited because of the absence of a potent small intestinal prokinetic agent.

Often, the underlying lesion is not correctable, and primary treatment is directed at suppressing the bacterial overgrowth with antibiotics. Numerous antibiotics have been reported to be effective, including tetracycline, ampicillin, erythromycin, clindamycin (Cleocin), ciprofloxacin (Cipro), metronidazole (Flagyl), and oral aminoglycosides. Many patients experience a remission after a single 7- to 10-day course of therapy with tetracycline or metronidazole. In patients with repeated recurrence of bacterial overgrowth, a repeating and rotating antibiotic regimen can be tried, such as 2 weeks of metronidazole followed by 2 weeks of ciprofloxacin.

Interrupted Enterohepatic Circulation of BileSalts

Three types of bile acid-induced malabsorption occur and can result from (1) severe disease, resection, or bypass of the distal ileum; (2) primary bile acid malabsorption; and (3) truncal vagotomy or cholecystectomy.

Ileal disease, resection, and bypass (i.e., Crohn's disease) permits dihydroxy bile salts to escape ileal absorption and enter the colon. If concentrations higher than 2 mmol/L are attained in the colon, diarrhea ensues as a consequence of a direct secretory effect of bile acids on the colon. Bile acid diarrhea must be differentiated from fatty acid diarrhea, which occurs if ileal disease or resection involves such a large segment of ileum (>100 cm) that hepatic synthesis cannot maintain an adequate intraluminal bile salt pool. Under these circumstances, steatorrhea ensues, and fatty acid-induced intestinal secretion complicates the picture. It is important to differentiate these two related syndromes because bile acid diarrhea responds to bile salt binders such as cholestyramine* (Questran) (4 gm every 12 hours) but the diarrhea of fatty acid malabsorption does not, and indeed, bile salt binders may worsen the symptoms. Therapy for fatty acid diarrhea is a low-fat diet supplemented with medium chain triglycerides (which are absorbed directly into the portal vein without the need for digestion) to prevent severe weight loss.

Primary bile acid malabsorption is characterized by excessive bile acid loss, which is responsive to cholestyramine but is not associated with histologic or macroscopic ileal disease. Increased fecal bile acids in patients with postcholecystectomy diarrhea suggest that cholecystectomy can lead to bile acid malabsorption syndromes. It is unclear why interruption of gallbladder storage would lead to increased bile acid malabsorption. Although many patients respond to cholestyramine, some do not, which raises the question of whether other pathophysiologic mechanisms are involved in this form of diarrhea. Neither primary bile acid malabsorption nor the postcholecystectomy syndrome results in significant enough bile loss to overwhelm the liver's ability to upregulate synthesis, and thus steatorrhea does not occur.

Drugs that Affect Digestion and Absorption

Drugs that interfere with nutrient absorption by direct interaction include tetracycline, which chelates calcium ions; cholestyramine, which binds to iron and vitamin B_{12}; and aluminum and magnesium hydroxide, which precipitate calcium and phosphate ions. Mucosal injury resulting in diminished nutrient absorption can occur with colchicine, neomycin, and methotrexate. Neomycin, 6 to 12 g/d, causes brush border damage by inhibiting enterocyte protein synthesis. Neomycin is also thought to impair micellar solubilization of bile salts, cholesterol, fatty acids, and fat-soluble vitamins by directly binding to bile salts. Methotrexate decreases the height of intestinal microvilli, as well as brush border membrane protein and lipid content. Drugs that produce histologic flattening in jejunal mucosa and that have been reported to cause fat malabsorption include methyldopa (Aldomet), allopurinol (Zyloprim), and mefenamic acid (Ponstel).

---

*Not FDA approved for this indication.

DEFECTIVE INTRAMURAL ABSORPTION

Inadequate Absorptive Surface

Short-bowel syndrome is a term that covers the symptoms and pathophysiologic disorders associated with a malabsorptive state resulting from the removal of a large portion of the small or large intestine. The extent of intestinal resection that will produce this syndrome varies from one person to another. In children, survival without enteral supplements or total parenteral nutrition is generally possible if more than 40 cm (i.e., 20% of normal length) of small intestine remains. In adults, survival without enteral or parenteral nutrition is generally possible if the residual length of small intestine is more than 150 cm (i.e., 25% of normal length). In general, if the ileocecal valve is removed, longer lengths of residual bowel may not prevent short-bowel syndrome.

Short-bowel syndrome refers only to a well-organized clinical pattern sometimes seen in patients with intestinal resection and is not necessarily related to the length of intestine removed. The clinical consequences of removing a portion of the small intestine are extremely variable and depend on a number of factors, including the extent of resection, site of resection, and subsequent adaptive processes.

Nutritional management of short-bowel syndrome is a dynamic process that follows the evolution of the clinical and adapted state of the bowel. Depending on the length of resection and the postsurgical adaptation, the process will result in one of four nutritional outcomes: maintenance of balanced nutritional status on a normal or modified oral diet, maintenance through the use of defined enteral formula diets, maintenance through enteral intake with parenteral electrolyte and fluid supplementation, or maintenance through total or partial parenteral nutrition supplemented by variable amounts of enteral intake. Whatever the source of nutrition, caloric intake should be increased slowly and progressively until it reaches a target of about 32 kcal/kg ideal body weight per day. This caloric intake goal, in general, will match the increased losses that result from inefficient and inadequate absorption.

Parenteral Therapy

In the immediate postoperative period, all patients with extensive small intestinal resection require total parenteral nutrition. As the amount of enteral nutrition is gradually increased, the duration and intensity of the parenteral nutrition infusion can be reduced. If more than 25% of a person's intestine remains, it should be possible for the patient to stop total parenteral nutrition completely.

Oral Therapy

A balanced solution containing carbohydrates and electrolytes can be given orally once stool output is less than 2 L daily. Clear fluid diets are not useful because they are inadequate in nutritional value; they are also severely hyperosmolar and likely to provoke osmotic diarrhea. Full fluid diets are also poorly tolerated because they contain lactose, and most patients with short-bowel syndrome are lactose intolerant. To optimize oral fluid and electrolyte absorption, a balanced oral replacement solution is necessary. A solution that contains an iso-osmotic sodium and glucose mixture takes advantage of the small intestinal sodium glucose cotransport carrier to enhance salt and water absorption (Table 4). Sport drinks such as Gatorade are too low in sodium to be of much use in patients with short-bowel syndrome.

Patients with more than 60 to 80 cm of small bowel should approach the reintroduction of oral feeding slowly until a normal or modified oral diet level is reached. Because gastric emptying is slower for solids, these patients should eat dry solids at a meal and take only isotonic fluids 1 hour later, because this regimen improves the absorption of nutrients. Diarrhea that occurs as a consequence of oral feeding can usually be managed by using an antidiarrheal agent, which should be taken on a regular basis 1 hour before meals and snacks. Waiting to take the antidiarrheal agent after the meal has started and the diarrhea has occurred is not effective.

Divalent cations, including calcium, magnesium, zinc, and copper, may bind to fatty acids in the stool, and excessive fecal losses of these minerals have been documented in patients with steatorrhea. Steatorrhea will also accentuate the malabsorption of fat-soluble vitamins (A, D, E, and K). Increased fecal fat losses also enhance dietary oxalate absorption, oxaluria, and renal stone formation. Recommendations based on dietary fat therefore need to be responsive to the individual patient's symptoms after bowel resection. In addition, it is important to balance the beneficial effects of fat restriction against the limitations on food palatability and caloric intake imposed by low-fat diets. A low-fat and low-oxalate diet, for instance, is likely to be completely unpalatable.

Medium chain triglycerides can be used as caloric supplements for patients with short-bowel syndrome. Medium chain triglycerides are hydrolyzed in the

TABLE 4. **Oral Replacement Solutions**

Solution	Glucose (mmol/L)	Sodium (mmol/L)	Potassium (mmol/L)	Chloride (mmol/L)	Base (mmol/L)	Osmolality (mmol/L)
WHO	111	90	20	80	30	331
Pedialyte	139	45	20	35	30	269
Gastrolyte	100	50	20	52	18	240
Gatorade	227	22	3	27	0	333

WHO = World Health Organization.

intestinal lumen to water-soluble components, which are absorbed in the absence of bile salts. Medium chain triglycerides have an unpleasant taste, however, and sometimes produce diarrhea because of their osmotic load in the proximal part of the small intestine (when given in a dose of more than 35 g/d) and thus do not provide essential fatty acids.

Enteral Therapy

Patients who cannot tolerate a normal oral diet and those with a short bowel (<60 to 80 cm) can often benefit from an enteral formula. If a chemically defined formula is used, it is important to control the rate of infusion to match osmotic inflow with osmolar absorption. Rates of full-strength infusion usually begin at 25 mL/h and gradually increase to 125 mL/h. The rate is modulated according to the tolerance displayed by the small intestine. If a polymeric formula is used, it should be lactose-free, because most patients with massive small intestinal resections do not have an adequate lactase reserve.

Vitamin and Mineral Supplementation

Enteral and parenteral solutions are supplemented with vitamins and minerals. As patients are weaned from these solutions and once the patient has stopped enteral or parenteral solutions completely, vitamin and mineral deficiencies may slowly occur because of inadequate intake (as the patient tries to prevent diarrhea), excess nutrient losses (from the short bowel), or a combination of both. Liquid vitamin and mineral oral supplementation regimens can be considered in some patients as they are weaned off parenterally supplied vitamins and minerals (Table 5). Liquid supplements are preferable to solid pills because hard outside matrices are often not dissolved during their rapid transit through a short bowel.

TABLE 5. **Sample Short-Bowel Oral Multivitamin/Mineral Routine**

ADEKs Multiple Vitamin
2 to 4 tablets daily (chewed or crushed throughly)
Each tablet contains vitamin A, 4000 IU; beta carotene, 3 mg; vitamin D, 400 IU; vitamin E, 150 IU; vitamin K, 0.15 mg; vitamin C, 60 mg; folic acid, 0.2 mg; thiamine, 1.2 mg; riboflavin, 1.3 mg; niacin, 10 mg; vitamin B_6, 1.5 mg; vitamin B_{12}, 12 μg; biotin, 50 μg; pantothenic acid, 10 mg; zinc, 7.5 mg
Calcium Gluconate Liquid
400 mg PO twice daily = 400 mg elemental calcium twice daily
Ferrous Sulphate Liquid
300 mg PO twice daily = 60 mg elemental iron twice daily
Osto-Forte (vitamin D_2) Capsule
50,000 IU once per week
Phosphate-Novartis (tablet dissolved)
500 mg PO twice daily = 500 mg elemental phosphorus twice daily
K-10 potassium Liquid
60 mL PO twice daily = 40 mEq KCl twice daily
Magnesium Glucoheptonate Liquid
30 mL PO twice daily = 150 mg magnesium twice daily

Mucosal Absorptive Defects

Celiac Disease

Celiac disease is treated with a gluten-free diet that involves avoiding all food products containing wheat, rye, barley, and oats. Because a gluten-free diet has a low roughage and fiber content, patients may require fiber supplementation. Specific nutrient deficiencies, including iron, folic acid, and calcium deficiency, should be corrected. It is important to note that many of the vitamin supplements contain gluten in the capsules, so a gluten-free vitamin pill needs to be identified for these patients.

Should the patient's symptoms persist or the jejunal biopsy findings remain grossly abnormal after 3 to 4 months of ingesting a gluten-free diet, the initial diagnosis should be questioned. However, the most common reason for inadequate response is a lack of patient compliance or inadvertent gluten ingestion. Corticosteroids can be used in cases of refractory sprue that does not respond to gluten withdrawal. The initial dose is 40 to 60 mg of prednisone daily, tapered off over a period of 1 to 2 months.

Disaccharidase Deficiency

The clinical symptoms associated with lactose or sucrose malabsorption are caused by low levels of the microvillus membrane disaccharidases required for their hydrolysis: lactase and sucrase-isomaltase, respectively. These reduced levels may be due to genetic alterations in expression of the enzymes or to reductions in enzyme activity as a consequence of intestinal injury. The clinical features and symptoms are those of malabsorption of carbohydrates.

Treatment of lactose intolerance includes (1) restriction of dietary lactose, (2) substitution of alternative nutrients to avoid reductions in energy and protein intake, (3) supplemental calcium intake, and (4) the use of commercially available enzyme substitutes. When lactose restriction is necessary, patients must be instructed to read labels of commercially prepared foods to identify hidden lactose. Calcium is supplemented in the form of calcium carbonate, 1000 mg/d. Commercially available lactase preparations are bacterial or yeast β-galactosidases. These products are not capable of completely hydrolyzing all dietary lactose, so patients must still restrict dietary lactose intake.

Isomaltase deficiency is a rare disorder caused by impaired synthesis of the intestinal enzyme sucrase-isomaltase. Patients are initially seen in childhood or, occasionally, adolescence. The primary approach to the treatment of sucrase-isomaltase deficiency is elimination or restriction of dietary sucrose.

Abetalipoproteinemia

After lipid digestion, fatty acids and monoglycerides are taken up by enterocytes and rearranged into apolipoprotein B–containing particles necessary for their transfer into the lymphatic circulation. Abetalipoproteinemia is an autosomal recessive disease characterized by the absence of apolipoprotein B.

Triglycerides cannot be packaged for transfer and thus accumulate in the cytoplasm of enterocytes. This accumulation of fat in enterocytes results in malabsorption of fat because the fat-engorged enterocytes are incapable of processing or transporting any more lipid.

Fat restriction, in particular long-chain fatty acids, alleviates the malabsorption. Medium-chain fatty acids can be used temporarily if severe malnutrition is present, but routine use should be avoided because it can worsen hepatic steatosis. The inability to form chylomicrons also leads to a deficiency in fat-soluble vitamins, and vitamin replacement therapy is necessary in all patients.

Lymphatic Obstruction

Intestinal Lymphangiectasia

Intestinal lymphangiectasia is a disease that can be either congenital or acquired in association with trauma, lymphoma, carcinoma, or Whipple's disease, and it causes protein-losing enteropathy and steatorrhea. It is the classic form of post-intramural obstruction malabsorption. The unique combination of malabsorption of fat, protein, and lymphocytes but normal absorption of carbohydrates relates to the obstructed lymphatic channels, which are the routes of absorption for fat, protein, and lymphocytes. Absorption of carbohydrates takes place by way of the portal circulation and remains unaffected. Treatment involves surgical repair of the underlying trauma or neoplasia.

Whipple's Disease

Whipple's disease represents infiltration of the intestine and lymphatics with *Tropheryma whippleii*. The histopathologic appearance of the small-bowel mucosa in Whipple's disease is diagnostic. The lamina propria is infiltrated by large foamy macrophages, which grossly distorts normal villous architecture and gives the villi a blunted, clublike appearance. The cytoplasm of these macrophages is filled with large periodic acid Schiff–positive glycoprotein granules. The lymphatic channels in the mucosa and submucosa are dilated, and fat droplets can be seen in the extracellular spaces within the lamina propria as a result of lymphatic obstruction by enlarged mesenteric lymph nodes. The gastrointestinal symptoms are thus those of clinical malabsorption. Similar histologic findings can be seen in any organ in the body, because Whipple's disease is a diffuse process. Given the concern with central nervous system involvement and relapses, it is reasonable to assume that all patients may have central nervous system involvement and to treat initially with an antibiotic that readily crosses the blood-brain barrier. Trimethoprim-sulfamethoxazole (Bactrim),* one double-strength tablet (trimethoprim, 160 mg; sulfamethoxazole, 800 mg) given twice daily for 1 year, is the best long-term option.

*Not FDA approved for this indication.

ACUTE PANCREATITIS

method of
GERARD V. ARANHA, M.D.
Hines VA Hospital
Loyola University Medical Center
Maywood, Illinois

Acute pancreatitis is an inflammation of the pancreas secondary to a variety of causes. The resulting inflammatory process results in the activation of a number of pancreatic proteolytic enzymes within the organ that can culminate in digestion of the organ itself. Most attacks of acute pancreatitis respond to medical management. However, in about 10% to 20% of patients, the severity of the inflammation can lead to life-threatening complications of infection with its attendant multisystem organ failure and death.

ETIOLOGY

The most common causes of acute pancreatitis are gallstones and alcohol abuse. It is to be noted that in the community and university hospital setting, the most frequent cause is usually gallstones rather than alcohol abuse. However, in the setting of the county hospital and the Veterans' Administration hospital systems, the etiology is the reverse. Other less common causes of pancreatitis include endoscopic retrograde cholangiopancreatography (ERCP), trauma, whether external or operative, and hyperlipidemia. Several medications have been implicated in the cause of pancreatitis, with the more common being azathioprine, valproic acid, thiazide diuretics, and drugs used against HIV. In addition, other etiologies include ischemia secondary to either hypotension or cardiopulmonary bypass surgery, viral disorders, abnormalities of the pancreatic duct and duodenum, hypercalcemia, scorpion venom, and a hereditary form related to germline mutations in the trypsinogen gene. In a certain number of cases, the cause of pancreatitis is unknown, and they are classified as idiopathic cases of acute pancreatitis (Table 1).

TABLE 1. **Causative Factors of Acute Pancreatitis**

Gallstones	Viral infection
Alcohol	Scorpion bites
Hyperlipidemia	Idiopathic
Hypercalcemia	Familial
ERCP	Tropical
Trauma:	Drugs:
Blunt	Azathioprine
Intraoperative	Mesalazine/sulfasalazine
Ischemia	Steroids
Pancreas divisum	Thiazide diuretics
Duodenal ulcer	Valproic acid
	Clonidine
	L-Asparaginase
	Sulfonamides
	Ethacrynic acid (Edecrin)

ERCP = endoscopic retrograde cholangiopancreatography.

PATHOGENESIS

In the past, numerous theories have been put forward as the cause of acute pancreatitis.

1. One theory hypothesized that because of the common channel between the bile duct and the pancreatic duct, obstruction of the channel and reflux of bile into the pancreatic duct activate the pancreatic enzymes. However, bile injected into the pancreatic duct in animal studies does not by itself activate pancreatic enzymes. Therefore, this theory does not hold water.
2. In another theory, it is thought that obstruction of the pancreatic duct leads to increased pressure in the duct with subsequent duct disruption and release of activated pancreatic enzymes. Once again, ligation of the pancreatic duct in animals results only in pancreatic edema, and thus this theory also remains unproved.
3. The third classic cause of pancreatitis was thought to be reflux of duodenal contents into the pancreatic duct. This theory has also been disproved because of the many patients who undergo ERCP and sphincterotomy—procedures that allow free reflux of duodenal contents into the pancreatic duct—but do not suffer recurrent acute pancreatitis.

Most specialists in pancreatic disease now believe that pancreatic enzymes exist within the acinar cell as inactive proenzymes (e.g., trypsinogen). When the exocrine pancreas is stimulated, most often by food, these proenzymes are released into the pancreatic duct. From there, the secretions enter the duodenum, where they interact with the duodenal enzyme enterokinase, which activates trypsinogen to trypsin. Trypsin then activates the other pancreatic proenzymes.

At present, it is thought that acute pancreatis results from death of the acinar cell with rupture, which leads to the release of activated digestive enzymes into the pancreas and subsequent autodigestion of the pancreas and surrounding tissues. It is still possible that the initial stimulus could be duct obstruction or reflux of bile or duodenal contents into the pancreas with resultant increased pressure in the duct, which by a mechanism yet to be delineated, leads to death of the acinar cell and release of the activated digestive enzymes. The role of alcohol, partial duct obstruction caused by gallstones, and ERCP in the activation of this process remains under investigation.

CLINICAL FEATURES AND DIAGNOSIS

Contrary to popular belief, a completely accurate method for the diagnosis of acute pancreatitis does not exist. Most patients with acute pancreatitis have severe and often persistent epigastric or upper abdominal pain that may radiate straight to the back or around the costal margin on both sides to the back. The attack is often related to the recent consumption of a large meal high in fat content or a large amount of alcohol. In addition, patients may get symptoms of nausea and vomiting. Physical examination may reveal a patient who appears dehydrated and as a result has tachycardia. Abdominal examination will often demonstrate distention, upper abdominal tenderness, and low or absent bowel sounds because patients with acute pancreatitis often have secondary reflex ileus of the small intestine. Elevated temperature, tachycardia, abdominal distention, ileus, and upper abdominal tenderness with a mass or fullness are more likely to be associated with a more severe form of acute pancreatitis.

It is important to remember that several other upper abdominal conditions may be manifested in a similar manner, such as acute cholecystitis, perforated gastric or duodenal ulcer, and small-bowel obstruction. Therefore, the diagnosis of acute pancreatitis sometimes becomes one of exclusion.

Laboratory investigation usually reveals an increased hematocrit if dehydration is present. On occasion, when the pancreatitis has been associated with severe hemorrhage, low hemoglobin is encountered. In uncomplicated acute pancreatitis, the white cell count is usually slightly above normal at 11,000/mm^3. Liver function tests are most often normal in uncomplicated pancreatitis, but transient elevations in serum bilirubin and alkaline phosphatase can be seen. These elevations are thought to be secondary to edema in the pancreatic head causing partial obstruction of the distal portion of the bile duct. It is often thought that serum amylase is an accurate predictor of acute pancreatitis, but in several series it has been shown that the sensitivity of serum amylase in diagnosing pancreatitis ranges from 55% to 80%. When patients with abdominal pain and hyperamylasemia were analyzed as a group, 70% of them were found to have pancreatitis because serum amylase is also elevated in other conditions such as perforated ulcer, gangrenous cholecystitis, and small-bowel obstruction with compromised bowel secondary to small-bowel ischemia or infarction. The level of serum amylase activity does not correlate with the severity of the pancreatitis. In studies it has been shown that the level of urinary amylase correlates best with the severity of pancreatitis. However, measurement of amylase in urine requires a 6- to 12-hour collection of urine for testing and is thus an impractical test. Peritoneal amylase is also a test that can be used to judge the severity of the pancreatitis, but aspirating fluid from a patient with a distended abdomen and distended bowel carries its own attendant risks and is therefore also impractical. Serum lipase activity often proves to be the most sensitive and specific test in the diagnosis of acute pancreatitis. Because serum lipase has a longer half-life than amylase does, it appears to be a better test for patients who are initially seen later in the course of the disease. It should be noted that serum lipase can be elevated in patients with cholecystitis and a perforated bowel. Sarr and colleagues stated that if a cutoff of three times the upper limit of normal serum lipase is used for the diagnosis of acute pancreatis, the sensitivity and specificity are close to 100%. Several other serum tests have been recommended to determine the severity and acuteness of pancreatitis. Warshaw and Lee proposed that increased RNase activity is an indicator of necrosis, but such an association awaits verification. Buchler and colleagues found that C-reactive protein levels higher than 10 mg/dL have greater than 90% accuracy in predicting severe necrotizing pancreatitis. Other serum tests such as α_1-antitrypsin and α_2-macroglobulin have also been claimed to accurately identify severe pancreatic infections, but these observations need confirmation.

Radiologic diagnosis of pancreatitis includes (1) a plain radiograph of the chest and abdomen, (2) ultrasonography, and (3) computed tomography (CT) of the abdomen. Plain radiographs of the chest may show pleural effusion, which is often due to irritation of the left diaphragm by pancreatitis and subsequent sympathetic effusion in the left pleural cavity. The abdominal plain film may show small-bowel ileus, a displaced stomach, and rarely, a sentinel loop of distended small bowel around the pancreas suggestive of local intestinal ileus. Ultrasonography can be difficult in a patient who has extensive small-bowel ileus. However, it is useful in determining whether gallstones or common duct stones are present.

The imaging modality most useful in the diagnosis of acute pancreatitis is CT. A CT scan in acute pancreatitis is useful in diagnosing the severity of the disease and in guiding future therapy. Findings on CT in acute pancreatitis may include pancreatic edema, a phlegmonous mass of inflamed pancreas and peripancreatic tissue, and a peripancreatic fluid collection. In addition, pancreatic abscesses and pancreatic necrosis may also be suspected from the CT scan. Furthermore, extension of the inflammation from the pancreas to other tissues, such as the retrocolic space, the perinephric space, and the mesentery of the small bowel and transverse colon, may also be seen. CT allows one to determine the vascular perfusion of the pancreas, and it should be performed during the arterial phase after an intravenous contrast-enhanced bolus is administered. This type of scan, also known as a dynamic CT scan, will reveal whether the pancreas is viable. A viable pancreas enhances as the contrast material flows to it, whereas lack of enhancement correlates with pancreatic necrosis. Sarr and associates stated that if more than 50% of the pancreas is nonperfused, the likelihood of pancreatic infection developing and subsequent surgical intervention is high.

ASSESSMENT OF THE SEVERITY OF DISEASE

As stated earlier, CT is a valuable imaging modality to assess the severity of acute pancreatitis. However, assessing the severity of the disease by clinical and laboratory examination has been the focus of investigation since the 1970s. In the mid-1970s, Ranson published his criteria for retrospectively and prospectively determining the severity of pancreatitis (Table 2). Eleven criteria were evaluated at admission or 48 hours after diagnosis. Patients with acute pancreatitis and one or two of Ranson's factors have a mortality of 1%, those with three to four risk factors have a mortality of 15%, and those with more than six risk factors have a mortality close to 100%.

TABLE 2. **Ranson Criteria**

AT ADMISSION
Age older than 55 y
White blood cell count >16,000/mm^3
Blood glucose >200 mg/dL
Serum lactate dehydrogenase >350 IU/L
Serum aspartate transaminase >250 r/dL
DURING THE INITIAL 48 HOURS
Hematocrit fall >10%
Blood urea nitrogen rise >5 mg/dL
Serum calcium <8 mg/dL
Arterial Po_2 <60 mm Hg
Base deficit >4 mEq/L
Estimated fluid sequestration >6 L

Since then, other clinical criteria have been published to assess the severity of pancreatitis, such as the Glasgow or IMRIE criteria and the Acute Physiology and Chronic Health Enquiry (APACHE II) criteria. The Glasgow or IMRIE criteria are a variation of the Ranson risk factors. The APACHE II system is based on an index of 12 physiologic variables, as well as the patient's age and history of major organ system abnormalities. This index is used widely in the critical care setting. It has been stated that the APACHE II score is more sensitive and specific than either the Ranson or Glasgow scale in predicting the severity of pancreatitis. It appears at present that if a multiple-factor scoring system is to be used, the best choice would be the APACHE II calculated at 24 hours. In this author's opinion, any patient with more than three Ranson criteria should be considered to have severe pancreatitis and be watched closely for the development of infected pancreatic necrosis. It is these patients with acute necrotizing pancreatitis in whom infected pancreatic necrosis might develop. Infected pancreatic necrosis accounts for the majority of the 20% of deaths that still occur after an attack of acute pancreatitis.

MEDICAL MANAGEMENT

Treatment of simple acute pancreatitis is medical management, which includes adequate fluid resuscitation and correction of the electrolyte imbalance. In addition, control of pain is essential. Further control of secretory stimulation of the pancreas with the use of a nasogastric tube and regulation of gastric pH with antacids and intravenous H_2 blockers or proton pump inhibitors may be necessary. With these measures, most patients with uncomplicated pancreatitis will have complete resolution of symptoms within 4 to 5 days. Antibiotics do not have any proven role in treating uncomplicated simple acute pancreatitis.

The 10% to 20% of patients with severe pancreatitis are an entirely different story. These patients have more than three Ranson criteria or an APACHE II score higher than 7. Such patients are best managed in the intensive care unit. In addition, because they need a large amount of fluid, their fluid requirements are best monitored with the use of a Swan-Ganz catheter, with which the amount of crystalloid and colloid given can be adequately monitored to maintain a proper hematocrit, circulating blood volume, and urine output. Renal failure from inadequate replacement of fluid in these patients is often a cause of their eventual demise. Patients with severe acute necrotizing pancreatitis may also have low calcium and magnesium levels, and it is important that these two ions be replaced in adequate quantity. Oral intake in these patients must definitely be withheld, and nasogastric suction is a necessity. In addition, a certain number of patients will require ventilatory support.

At present, no single specific drug can be used for acute necrotizing pancreatitis. In the past, studies involving aprotinin (Trasylol)* and glucagon* have shown no benefit. Similarly, somatostatin,† prostaglandins, low-molecular-weight dextrans, and free radical scavengers have yet to show a significant effect on the disease. More recently, clinical and experimental studies have suggested that platelet-activating factor antagonists and related anti-inflammatory cytokine agents may have a role. In limited trials, lexipafant (C-Lexin),* a platelet-activating factor antagonist, has reduced the severity of organ failure in patients with severe disease.

The use of antibiotics to prevent septic complications of acute pancreatitis is controversial. As stated earlier, the risk of infectious complications in patients with mild to moderate acute pancreatitis is very low, and prophylactic antibiotics should be avoided. However, patients with acute necrotizing pancreatitis, who are at intermediate to high risk for the development of infectious complications, may benefit from the use of prophylactic antibiotics such as imipenem, which penetrates pancreatic tissue. In addition, antifungal agents may be administered to patients with severe disease to decrease the incidence of superinfection in necrotic pancreatic tissue. Fungal agents such as fluconazole (Diflucan) may be used, among others.

It is generally thought that parenteral nutrition has no specific beneficial effect in the treatment of pancreatitis. Most often, in patients with simple uncomplicated pancreatitis, the attack subsides in 5 days and patients can go back to their old diet. However, in patients who have severe acute necrotizing pancreatitis and prolonged ileus, parenteral nutrition may be required until the ileus has subsided. If parenteral nutrition is chosen, the usual formulas to deliver adequate amounts of protein and carbohydrate should be used. Standard lipid solutions may also be used, but they should be avoided in patients with hypertriglyceridemia. Standard lipid solutions given parentally have not been shown to stimulate exocrine pancreatic secretion. Recently, there has been a trend in patients with severe acute pancreatitis to use alimental diets delivered distal to the ligament of Treitz, which may help maintain the gut mucosal barrier and minimize sepsis.

The value of peritoneal lavage in acute severe pancreatitis is controversial. The basis for the use of peritoneal lavage has been the removal of "toxins" and various metabolites from the peritoneal cavity to minimize their systemic absorption. Controlled trials have failed to show decreased mortality rates when peritoneal lavage is used or not. However, some evidence indicates that the incidence of cardiopulmonary complications in these patients is lessened. Therefore, it is thought that peritoneal lavage may be considered in selected patients who are deteriorating in the first several days of the onset of the disease in spite of all other adequate measures.

Endoscopic intervention is sometimes necessary in patients with acute severe pancreatitis, mainly those who are thought to have common duct stones that are being impacted at the ampulla. Such patients have elevated bilirubin and alkaline phosphatase levels, and they continue to show a continuous rise in serum amylase. Several randomized studies have demonstrated that in severe biliary pancreatitis, early endoscopic retrograde cholangiography without pancreatography, combined with endoscopic sphincterotomy and disimpaction of stones, may decrease the severity of attacks (Figure 1).

If infection is suspected in a patient with severe acute pancreatitis, percutaneous fine-needle aspiration of fluid may be performed, or infarcted pancreatic tissue may be demonstrated on CT. The material is sent for Gram stain and bacterial and fungal culture. If infection is thought to be present, in addition to necrosis, laparotomy and surgical débridement of the infected necrotic material are indicated (see Figure 1). Necrosis by itself that is not infected may not be an indication for surgery if the patient is in stable condition and responding to medical management.

SURGICAL MANAGEMENT

Close to 90% of patients with acute pancreatitis recover without any need for surgery. Surgery, however, will be necessary in certain patients. Patients with a mild to moderate degree of biliary pancreatitis will need to undergo laparoscopic cholecystectomy during the same admission after the pancreatitis and pain resolve (see Figure 1), usually within 4 days after admission. If at the time of surgery common duct stones are noted, they should also be removed. Alternatively, if common duct stones are observed at the time of laparoscopic cholecystectomy, they can be removed by postoperative ERCP and endoscopic sphincterotomy (see Figure 1). Patients with severe forms of biliary pancreatitis associated with a large inflammatory peripancreatic mass should have the cholecystectomy postponed until the peripancreatic reaction has resolved, which may take several months. However, in these patients, consideration may be given to early endoscopic sphincterotomy for the removal of stones to protect the patient from recurrent gallstone pancreatitis during the intervening period.

For patients with severe pancreatitis consisting of severe necrotizing pancreatitis and infected pancreatic necrosis, surgical intervention is necessary to

*Not FDA-approved for this indication.
†Not available in the United States.

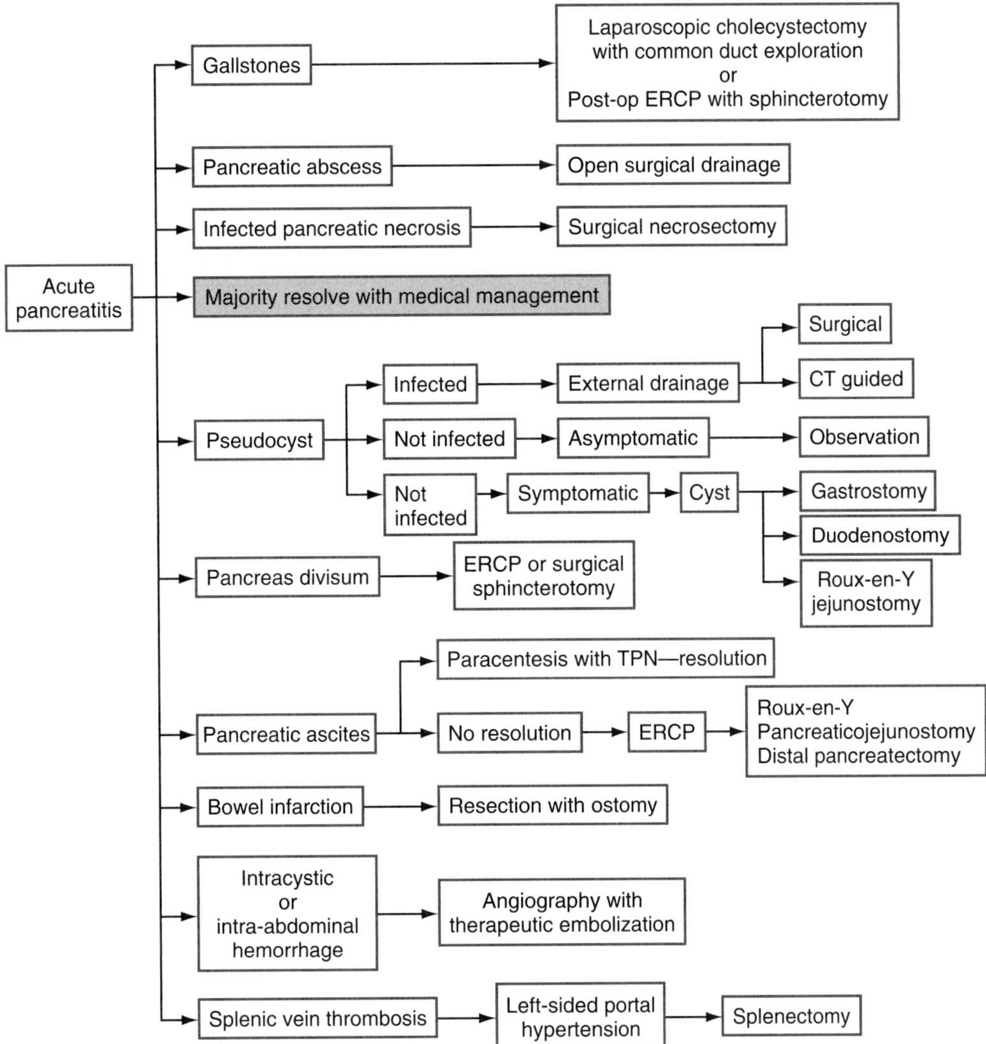

Figure 1. Surgical and therapeutic interventions for acute pancreatitis. CT = computed tomography; ERCP = endoscopic retrograde cholangiopancreatography; TPN = total parenteral nutrition.

remove the infected and devitalized pancreatic and peripancreatic tissue (see Figure 1). In addition, some patients require drainage of infected peripancreatic fluid collections (see Figure 1). The timing of surgery for patients with infected pancreatic necrosis is important. Most experienced pancreatic surgeons believe that it is preferable to delay surgical intervention in these patients until the second week.

At this point, the infected tissue is demarcated, and blunt dissection plus débridement of the tissue is safe and less likely to cause hemorrhagic complications (see Figure 1). If drainage of infected pancreatic necrosis become necessary, it is important to débride all dead tissue but preserve viable pancreatic tissue. Once the necrotic tissue has been removed, large drains are placed in the débrided area and brought out below the subcostal margin on both sides anteriorly. It is controversial whether closed or open drainage is the method of choice, but it is this author's preference to use conventional closed drainage with large-bore multiple drains. However, authorities generally agree about the necessity of draining infected pseudocysts or pancreatic abscesses. Both these entities should be drained by standard open surgical methods, although some infected pseudocysts can be drained under CT guidance (see Figure 1).

Surgery may also be required in patients who have recovered from an attack of acute pancreatitis but in whom pseudocysts later develop. Fluid collections occur in 50% to 60% of patients with acute pancreatitis. In the majority of circumstances, the fluid collections are absorbed spontaneously, and in only 5% of patients will fluid remain in the form of a pseudocyst. The pseudocysts in these patients may be symptomatic or asymptomatic. In symptomatic patients, abdominal pain and an inability to eat are often the initial symptoms. Once total parenteral nutrition is instituted, they are discharged and monitored for 6 weeks. At the end of the 6-week observation period, these patients are readmitted and evaluated by clinical and imaging modalities. If clinical improvement is seen and the patients are now pain free and can eat but imaging still shows the presence of a pseudocyst, they can be managed expectantly and monitored with serial CT scans until the cyst subsides (see Figure 1). In some cases, patients may need to be observed for up to a year before the cyst subsides. Patients who remain symptomatic after a 6-week period of observation may require drainage of the pseudocyst. Drainage is usually performed internally, and the cyst may be drained into the stomach via a cyst gastrostomy if the cyst is posterior to the stomach and adherent to it or with a Roux-en-Y cyst jejunostomy if the cyst is not adherent to the stomach but adherent to the mid-transverse mesocolon or is located in the body and tail of the pancreas. Alternatively, for cysts in the head of the pancreas, a cyst duodenostomy may be performed (see Figure 1). Pseudocysts may also be treated endoscopically and by radiographically guided drainage. In the literature it appears that endoscopic treatment can be used mainly for cysts that share a common wall with the posterior of the stomach or the duodenum. However, the results of endoscopically and radiologically drained pseudocysts are not as good as the results of surgically drained pseudocysts. Very rarely, cysts in the tail of the pancreas that are symptomatic require distal pancreatectomy (see Figure 1).

Surgery may be indicated for management of the complications of acute pancreatitis, including effects on surrounding organs. Intestinal infarction, particularly of the transverse colon, may result from thrombosis induced in the vessels of the transverse colon by the pancreatitis. This complication is usually manifested as sepsis, an abdominal mass, and gastrointestinal bleeding. Resection of the involved segments of bowel with proximal diversion (i.e., colostomy) is the treatment of choice. Massive intra-abdominal or gastrointestinal bleeding will occur occasionally in patients with acute pancreatitis. Causes can range from a ruptured peripancreatic aneurysm to stress ulcers or even splenic or portal vein thrombosis, and thus angiography is mandatory in these cases. In many instances, angiography with therapeutic embolization of bleeding vessels may be of great help in these acutely ill patients. Splenic vein thrombosis is relatively common in acute pancreatitis and may lead to left-sided portal hypertension with the development of transgastric varices. Splenectomy is curative in such cases (see Figure 1). Occlusion of the portal and superior mesenteric veins is unusual even in the most severe cases of pancreatitis.

Surgery is sometimes indicated for pancreatic ascites. In this case, a peripancreatic fluid collection ruptures into the peritoneal cavity. This complication is noted clinically by sudden abdominal distention in a patient with acute pancreatitis. Pancreatic ascites is treated by large-volume paracentesis, octreotide, and total parenteral nutrition. If this regimen does not control the situation, ERCP is indicated. If an area of ductal rupture and distal stricture is identified, a pancreatic duct stent may be placed to control the leak. Sometimes, unresolved pancreatic ascites will require surgical intervention. Because the site of leak in these patients is usually in the tail of the gland, distal pancreatectomy will be required (see Figure 1). At times the leak is in the body of the pancreas, in which case Roux-en-Y pancreaticojejunostomy can be performed (see Figure 1).

Finally, patients with acute pancreatitis may require surgery for pancreas divisum. In this condition the dorsal and ventral segments of the pancreas fail to fuse during embryologic development. This failure of fusion results in the duct in the body and tail of the pancreas draining into the duct of Santorini (minor papilla). Some patients with this anomaly have recurrent attacks of pancreatitis and will need therapeutic intervention. Such intervention may be in the form of endoscopic retrograde papillotomy of the minor papilla or open surgical sphincteroplasty of the minor papilla (see Figure 1).

CHRONIC PANCREATITIS

method of
DAVID B. ADAMS, M.D.
Medical University of South Carolina
Charleston, South Carolina

Hidden in the upper recesses of the retroperitoneum, the pancreas is an organ feared by surgeons and shunned by most physicians. Though vulnerable to chronic inflammation and fibrosis leading to pancreatic exocrine and endocrine insufficiency, chronic pancreatitis more commonly causes patient disability through intractable pain. The chronic upper abdominal pain associated with chronic pancreatitis poses a challenge to physicians and patients alike and requires a multidisciplinary team approach consisting of specialists from gastroenterology, radiology, anesthesia, pain medicine, and surgery.

Although postprandial pain located in the epigastrium and radiating into the intrascapular region is typical of chronic pancreatitis, multiple conditions may cause upper abdominal pain, and the pain of chronic pancreatitis varies in character, severity, and duration. Chronic fibrocalcific pancreatitis is the most common cause of pain in chronic pancreatitis and is usually associated with intraductal lithiasis and a dilated pancreatic duct. Chronic pancreatitis with nondilated ducts has become a more recognizable problem inasmuch as evaluation of patients with unexplained chronic abdominal pain has been improved with endoscopic ultrasonography, endoscopic retrograde cholangiopancreatography, pancreatic and biliary manometry, and magnetic resonance cholangiopancreatography. The most common cause of chronic pancreatitis is alcohol abuse. Though more frequently associated with acute pancreatitis, severe gallstone pancreatitis may produce chronic changes in the pancreas along with marked ductal abnormalities. Other causes of chronic pancreatitis that are becoming recognized with increasing frequency include pancreas divisum, sphincter of Oddi dysfunction, and familial pancreatitis. Additional well-known causes of chronic pancreatitis are hypertriglyceridemia, trauma, cystic fibrosis, and drug-related pancreatitis.

The chief indication for treatment of patients with chronic pancreatitis is intractable pain. The pain is typically located in the epigastrium and radiates posteriorly, and it is usually exacerbated by oral intake and associated with nausea. The mechanisms of pain in chronic pancreatitis are poorly understood, but the most popular hypothesis is that of ductal hypertension. After ductal obstruction develops downstream, patients with chronic pancreatitis continue to secrete fluid rich in enzymes and electrolytes, with subsequent build-up of high pressure in the pancreatic duct. Many patients, however, have no evidence of ductal obstruction and still have pain that is typical of chronic pancreatitis. Another possible cause of chronic pancreatitis pain is pancreatic and peripancreatic perineural inflammation. In patients with chronic pancreatitis, it has been observed that the splanchnic nerves in and around the pancreas become involved in a chronic inflammatory process associated with the infiltration of eosinophils and macrophages, which may provide an independent triggering mechanism for splanchnic pain receptors. It is not uncommon after total pancreatectomy for chronic pancreatitis to see patients have persistent pain that is typical of chronic pancreatitis. Another possible mechanism of pain is parenchymal hypertension, with the pain and chronic pancreatitis being attributed to a pancreatic compartment–type syndrome. In severe chronic pancreatitis, the pancreas is encased in a thick, fibrous inflammatory sheath. Intraparenchymal pressure may become elevated, and capillary blood flow may be impaired with the subsequent development of ischemia and pain. Excellent animal models of this hypothesis exist, but its application to human beings is speculative. The important issue is to remember that the pain mechanisms are not clearly understood and that routine laboratory and radiologic evaluation may fail to uncover evidence of chronic pancreatitis in patients who have chronic abdominal pain with a source verifiable by newer endoscopic and radiologic procedures.

The goals of therapy in the management of chronic pancreatitis are control of pain and preservation of the exocrine and endocrine function of the gland. This review focuses chiefly on surgical management of chronic pancreatitis with an optimistic view that in patients with favorable anatomic disorders, early surgery has the potential to prevent the development of a chronic visceral pain syndrome and preserve the endocrine and exocrine function of the gland. A number of patients, however, have no demonstrable anatomic disorders of the gland and need careful nonoperative management.

SURGICAL TREATMENT

Surgical treatment of chronic pancreatitis involves three strategies: (1) resection, (2) drainage procedures, and (3) splanchnic nerve block. A splanchnic nerve block can be performed in the operating room through an open abdomen or with minimally invasive techniques consisting of thoracoscopic resection of the greater and lesser splanchnic nerves. More commonly, splanchnic nerve ablation is performed chemically through a posterior approach under fluoroscopic control via techniques that have been developed by anesthesia pain specialists. Steroids and neurolytic agents can be instilled around the splanchnic nerves under endoscopic guidance as well, with endoscopic ultrasound used to direct transgastric injections. Though effective in cancer pain management where patient life expectancy is limited, splanchnic nerve blocks are of temporary duration and rarely provide long-term solutions to pain associated with chronic pancreatitis.

Current operative management of chronic pancreatitis includes longitudinal pancreaticojejunostomy (LPJ) (the Peustow procedure), pancreaticoduodenectomy (the Whipple procedure), local resection of the head of the pancreas along with LPJ (the Frey procedure), and duodenal-preserving resection of the head of the pancreas (the Beger procedure). LPJ is the mainstream therapy for chronic pancreatitis and has the advantages of an excellent success rate and low operative morbidity and mortality (Figure 1). Although success rates as high as 80% have been reported in the management of pain with LPJ, in a 6-year follow-up of 85 patients with chronic pancreatitis who underwent LPJ, 24% described their health status as good and 35% as fair. Many patients who considered their health status good continued to use alcohol, took narcotic analgesics for pain, and required insulin and enzyme supplementation. These data force to the surface the view that patients with chronic pancreatitis may have self-perceived good outcomes despite the development of exocrine and endocrine insufficiency and a need for narcotic analgesics. Hospital morbidity and mortality rates are low with LPJ and should be 5% or less. Small-bowel obstruction, gastrointestinal bleeding, pancreatic fistulas, and drain tract infection are complications reported after LPJ. Early postoperative mortality rates should approach 0%.

Patients with chronic pancreatitis frequently have other associated complications of chronic pancreatitis that require surgical attention, including the

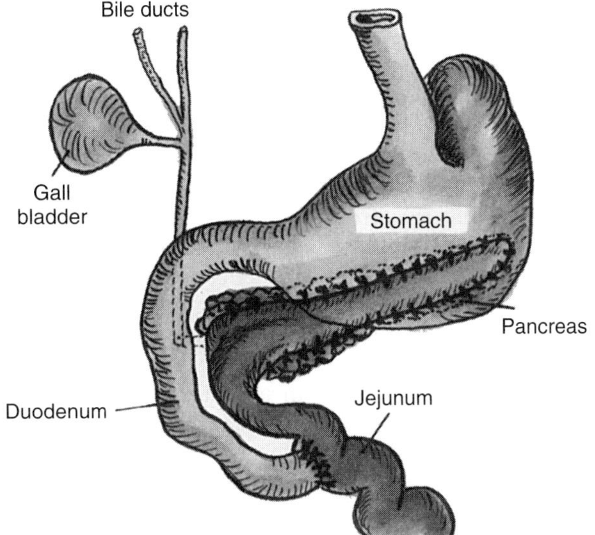

Figure 1. Peustow procedure.

development of a pancreatic pseudocyst, terminal biliary stenosis, splanchnic venous obstruction, pancreaticopleural fistulas, pancreatic ascites, pancreaticogastric fistulas, and pancreaticocolonic fistulas. In patients undergoing LPJ, pseudocysts can be readily managed with incorporation of the pseudocyst into the LPJ. Biliary stenosis is managed with choledochoduodenostomy. Patients who have splenic venous occlusion are treated with splenectomy. Internal pancreatic fistulas such as pancreaticopleural fistulas and pancreatic ascites are managed with LPJ alone. When fistulas exist between the pancreas and the stomach or colon, they can be managed with excision and closure of the fistula and LPJ.

Surgery for chronic pancreatitis is frequently palliative, particularly when associated with alcohol abuse. Long-term survival after LPJ approaches 75%. Mortality in this group of patients is related to the complications of continued alcohol abuse, as well as the complications of severe chronic pancreatitis. Not infrequently, patients are readmitted to the hospital for medical co-morbidities associated with chronic pancreatitis, including recurrent pancreatitis, drug and alcohol abuse, malnutrition, diabetes, cardiovascular disease, esophagitis, gastritis, psychiatric disorders, trauma, pneumonia, and anemia.

Patients who do well after LPJ are those who have a dilated pancreatic duct with evidence of ductal hypertension when the pancreatic duct is incised at the time of surgery. Many of these patients undergo preoperative endoscopic stenting. Relief of the pain with endoscopic stenting is a good sign that they will do well with the operation in terms of pain relief. However, endoscopic stenting is not a long-term solution because stent occlusion inevitably occurs.

A dilated pancreatic duct is one that measures greater than 7 mm in diameter on an endoscopic retrograde pancreatogram. The role of pancreaticojejunostomy in patients without dilated ducts has been a controversial issue. Some investigators report that most patients who undergo LPJ with nondilated ducts are pain free at long-term follow-up. However, others have noted that the vast majority of patients who undergo LPJ for narrow-duct disease require rehospitalization and continued narcotic analgesics for pain that is worse or similar to their preoperative pain. Most experts find that patients with nondilated pancreatic ducts and chronic pancreatitis are not good candidates for LPJ.

A 20-year history of outcome data has amassed for LPJ in the management of chronic pancreatitis, and success rates of up to 80% in terms of pain relief are reported, with follow-up periods ranging from 2 to 20 years. However, because many patients fail to achieve notable pain relief after LPJ, a variety of resection procedures have been used in an attempt to improve outcome in the surgical management of chronic pancreatitis. Failure of LPJ is ascribed to unsuccessful drainage of the head, and therefore attention has recently been directed toward the right side of the pancreas in an effort to improve drainage and relieve obstruction in the head of the pancreas. It is important to note that pancreatic cancer may coexist in patients who have an inflammatory mass in the head of the pancreas associated with biliary and pancreatic ductal obstruction, and resection of the head of the pancreas is the treatment of choice for carcinoma of the head of the pancreas, as well as for chronic pancreatitis associated with an inflammatory mass in the head. Normal expectations are that about 5% or less of patients undergoing surgery for chronic pancreatitis will be discovered to have an unexpected pancreatic malignancy.

The Whipple procedure has been used successfully in the management of severe complications of chronic pancreatitis (Figure 2), including problems such as pseudoaneurysm formation and hemorrhage from the gastroduodenal artery, obstruction of the splanchnic veins, and duodenal and biliary obstruction. This group of patients is formidable, and operating time, intensive care unit stay, and hospitalization can be prolonged. However, most of these patients are pain free throughout a long-term follow-up period. Beger has popularized an alternative approach to resection procedures for chronic pancreatitis that consists of a duodenum-preserving resection at the head of the pancreas. This technique involves preservation of the terminal bile duct and duodenum with an anastomosis performed between the jejunum and pancreas. In 128 patients who underwent this procedure, the mortality rate was less than 1%, 76% of the patients were pain free, and most remarkably, two thirds returned to work. In a randomized trial that compared duodenum-preserving pancreatic head resection with the Whipple procedure for chronic pancreatitis, the two procedures had similar morbidity and hospital stays, but 75% of those undergoing preservation of the duodenum were pain free as compared with 40% of those who underwent a pyloric-preserving Whipple resection. Though successful in Germany, this procedure has not been widely adopted in this country, and most surgeons continue to use either the classic Whipple resection or

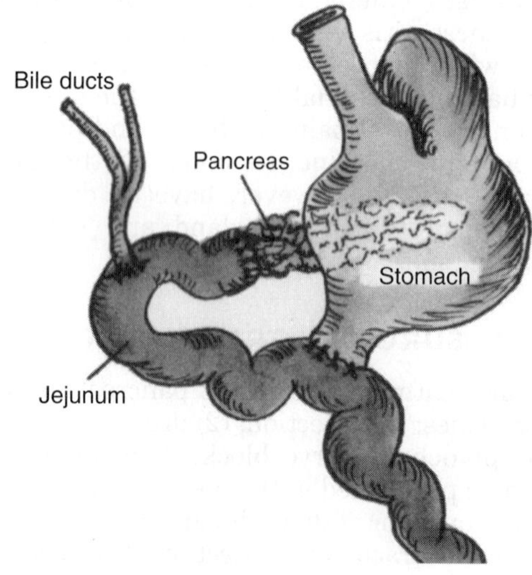

Figure 2. Whipple procedure.

the pyloric-preserving Whipple resection in managing chronic pancreatitis associated with a mass in the head of the pancreas. Because patients with chronic pancreatitis have chronically elevated creatine phosphokinase levels, a condition associated with impairment in gastric motility, pyloric resection frequently leads to improved gastric emptying after the Whipple procedure, and many experts shun the pyloric-preserving Whipple technique when operating for chronic pancreatitis.

Another approach to resection of the head of the pancreas is that popularized by Frey. He recommended excision of the pancreas overlying the ducts of Wirsung and Santorini and the duct of the uncinate in combination with LPJ. In the head of the pancreas, the anterior and posterior diameter is equal to the transverse diameter, and obstructed ducts in the head may not be well drained with LPJ. Frey believes that coring out the head of the pancreas and extending the LPJ into this head region improves the outcome. He has noted a zero mortality rate and a 22% complication rate with this procedure and reported that 34% of patients were pain free and 17 had minimal pain at follow-up.

An alternative approach to management of ductal lithiasis in the head combines intraoperative pancreatoscopy with electrohydraulic lithotripsy of pancreatic duct stones and LPJ. Clearance of intraductal stones in the head is successful with electrohydraulic lithotripsy and adds 45 minutes to the operative time. Transampullary passage of the pancreatoscope into the duodenum is usually possible. Early follow-up after this approach showed that 90% of patients viewed their health status as good or fair, with enzyme and insulin requirements being unchanged. This modality has been demonstrated in long-term follow-up to be safe and effective for the treatment of chronic calcific pancreatitis and may be shown to be a valuable alternative to the pancreatic resection procedures.

Patients who have nondilated pancreatic ducts associated with chronic pancreatitis have a less successful outcome after operative treatment than do those with dilated ducts, and decision making regarding the operative treatment plan is much more difficult. Nevertheless, many patients with severe, intractable pain and nondilated ducts can be helped with pancreatic ductal sphincteroplasty and resection procedures. Moreover, total pancreatectomy with auto-islet transplantation for the salvage of patients with narrow-duct disease who fail conventional operative therapy is currently enjoying enthusiastic interest.

Recommendations for the surgical management of pain with chronic pancreatitis are summarized in Table 1. In patients with dilated ducts and no stones, LPJ with possible local resection of the head of the pancreas or electrohydraulic lithotripsy is indicated. In patients with dilated pancreatic ducts and an inflammatory mass in the head of the pancreas, pancreaticoduodenectomy is the treatment of choice. In those who have nondilated ducts associated with sphincter of Oddi dysfunction or pancreas divisum, transduodenal major or minor duct sphincteroplasty can be undertaken. Frequently, many of these patients have undergone endoscopic sphincteroplasty, and the endoscopist may indicate that operative sphincteroplasty has the potential to overcome the anatomic obstacles that have precluded effective endoscopic sphincterotomy. However, in many instances, these patients have received the maximal benefit possible from sphincteroplasty and will be best served by pancreaticoduodenectomy.

TABLE 1. **Surgical Management of Chronic Pancreatitis**

Dilated ducts—no stones	LPJ +/− local resection of the head
Dilated ducts with stones	LPJ +/− electrohydraulic lithotripsy
Dilated ducts with an inflammatory mass in the head	Pancreaticoduodenectomy and distal LPJ
Nondilated ducts and pancreas divisum	Minor duct sphincteroplasty
Nondilated ducts and sphincter of Oddi dysfunction	Biliary sphincteroplasty and pancreatic duct septoplasty
Nondilated ducts and failure of sphincteroplasty	Pancreaticoduodenectomy
Nondilated ducts and failure of pancreaticoduodenectomy	Salvage total pancreatectomy with auto-islet transplantation

Abbreviation: LPJ = longitudinal pancreaticojejunostomy.

MEDICAL MANAGEMENT

In patients who fail operative treatment of chronic pancreatitis, many endoscopic, pharmacologic, and nutritional therapies are available (Table 2). Unfortunately, the mainstay of therapy in patients with the unremitting, severe visceral pain of chronic pancreatitis is long-acting narcotic analgesics. Management of pancreatitis pain with long-term narcotic analgesic treatment is avoided by most physicians because of fear that it will lead to addiction and drug abuse problems in patients who may already have severe psychosocial disturbances associated with alcohol abuse. Visceral pain is typically hard to manage with the techniques that are frequently used by anesthesia pain specialists in managing the somatic pain of orthopedic and neurologic disease. The use of long-acting narcotic analgesics in combination with short-acting narcotics for breakthrough pain is successful in keeping many patients out of emergency rooms and preventing hospitalization. An effective dose can be achieved, and when patients are using narcotics for pain relief, dosage and medications changes occur infrequently. In situations in which dosages are

TABLE 2. **Medical Management of Chronic Pancreatitis**

Low fat diet
Non-narcotic analgesics
Pancreatic enzymes
Octreotide acetate (Sandostatin)*
Narcotic analgesics
Jejunal enteral nutrition
Total parenteral nutrition

*Not FDA approved for this indication.

escalating or multiple problems with revision of narcotic formulations are being encountered, patients are most likely using narcotics for nonanalgesic purposes, and drug rehabilitation therapy is needed. To safely administer narcotic analgesics, it is necessary that the patient comply with strict guidelines, which includes signing of a narcotic contract (Table 3).

Pancreatic rest with total parenteral nutrition is successful in many patients in the short-term management of chronic pancreatitis pain, but infectious, nutritional, and vascular complications limit long-term use of this treatment. Enteral jejunal feeding is not associated with marked stimulation of the exocrine pancreas, and therefore placement of an endoscopic percutaneous gastrojejunal feeding tube frequently offers excellent nutrition and good pain relief in patients whose pancreatic pain is exacerbated by eating. Patients who have non–alcohol-related pancreatitis often have other motility disorders of the gastrointestinal tract that may make enteral nutrition difficult. Pancreatic enzyme supplementation is used in the belief that orally administrated enzymes will lead to feedback inhibition of pancreatic exocrine secretions and diminish intraductal pressure. Most patients with chronic pancreatitis who fail surgical therapy do not have notable pain relief with high-dose enzyme supplement therapy. Patients who have evidence of exocrine insufficiency along with weight loss and steatorrhea benefit most from enzyme supplementation.

The somatostatin analogue octreotide (Sandostatin)* has the potential to become an important therapy for treating abdominal pain unresponsive to other medical and surgical treatments. This synthetic hormone mimics the action of somatostatin, inhibits pancreatic exocrine secretions, and has been well studied in a multicenter trial of patients with chronic pancreatitis treated with a subcutaneous twice-daily dose. Recently, a long-acting formulation of octreotide has been developed, and a once-monthly intramuscular injection* offers promise for the long-term management of patients with chronic pancreatitis. By avoiding the necessity of twice-a-day subcutaneous injections, it has better patient acceptance and warrants further study.

Management of patients with chronic pancreatitis by minimally invasive endoscopic therapy has generated new interest and enthusiasm (Table 4). Patients who fail traditional medical therapy consisting of a

*Not FDA approved for this indication.

TABLE 3. **Opioid Drug Use for Chronic Nonmalignant Pain**

PATIENT-DOCTOR CONTRACT

1. **Background:** You have been diagnosed with a noncancerous chronic pain syndrome.
   In general, such conditions should not be treated with narcotic analgesics. Narcotics are relatively ineffective for this type of pain, and they can complicate treatment and slow rehabilitation. However, you have discussed this with your physician, and you desire narcotic therapy and understand and agree to the conditions of this contract.
2. **Risks:** Potential risks of using narcotics for pain include the following:
   a. *Physical dependence* (causing a withdrawal reaction if drugs are abruptly terminated)
   b. *Physical tolerance* (requiring progressively increasing doses to obtain relief)
   c. *Psychological addiction* (a behavioral change marked by drug craving and interference with psychological and social functioning)
   d. *Poorer outcome* of therapy/fewer functional improvements
   e. *Respiratory depression*
   f. *Psychological changes*
   g. *Constipation and/or nausea*
   h. *Fetal physical dependence* (if you are pregnant)
   i. *Decreased libido*
   j. *Incomplete and inadequate pain relief*
3. **Conditions:** You agree to the following:
   a. All other reasonable approaches to analgesia will be attempted before and along with narcotic therapy. You agree to try such things, which may include other non-narcotic medications, physical or occupational therapy, psychiatric evaluation, and behavior modification.
   b. A single physician will be responsible for writing all analgesic prescriptions. A designated alternative physician will be assigned in his/her absence.
   c. No attempt will be made to obtain analgesics from another treatment provider, a military or civilian health care facility, or the emergency room.
   d. Emergency room physicians may or may not treat an acute increase in your pain with a narcotic. They will not prescribe or dispense narcotics for you.
   e. No replacement medication will be given for lost or misplaced drugs.
   f. Increasing your own dose of narcotics will not be tolerated. The amount of medication prescribed must last until your next scheduled appointment.
   g. Breaking the terms of this contract could cause you to be disengaged from care at the Medical University of South Carolina.

PATIENT SIGNATURE ____________________

DOCTOR SIGNATURE ____________________

WITNESS SIGNATURE ____________________

DATE ____________________

From Portenoy RK: Opioids in nonmalignant pain. In Current Therapy of Pain. Philadelphia, CV. Mobsy, 1989.

TABLE 4. **Endoscopic Management of Chronic Pancreatitis**

Biliary and pancreatic sphincteroplasty and short-term stenting (sphincter of Oddi dysfunction)
Minor-duct sphincteroplasty and dominant-duct stenting (pancreas divisum)
Main duct stenting (dilated duct as a temporizing measures before durgery)
Endoscopic lithotripsy and stenting plus extraction of stones with a catheter technique and/or extracorporeal shock wave lithotripsy (dilated duct with intraductal lithiasis)
Endoscopic ultrasound-guided celiac plexus block
Percutaneous endoscopic gastrojejunal enteral nutrition

low-fat diet, common narcotic analgesics, avoidance of alcohol, and high-dose pancreatic enzyme therapy frequently benefit from the endoscopic therapy available at highly specialized centers. However, most patients who fail surgical therapy have undergone previous endoscopic therapy before their referral for surgical management. Endoscopic treatment includes relief of obstruction by placing stents or eliminating pancreatic duct stones, as well as endoscopic sphincterotomy for sphincter of Oddi dysfunction and pancreas divisum. Extracorporal shock wave lithotripsy has also been used in conjunction with endoscopic therapy. Endoscopic ultrasound and radiologically guided celiac plexus block and bilateral splanchnicectomy have been mentioned earlier as having a role in the management of patients with severe pain from chronic pancreatitis. This modality is most useful as a temporizing measure in those in whom operative treatment needs to be delayed. Permanent pain relief is unusual with this technique.

As with all new therapies, the subjective nature of the pain of chronic pancreatitis and the poor understanding of its pathophysiology are serious obstacles in studies directed at quantifying the effectiveness of different management strategies. No consensus has been reached regarding standards of care, and management of the pain associated with chronic pancreatitis remains very much an empirical discipline more akin to 19th than to 21st century medicine.

GASTROESOPHAGEAL REFLUX DISEASE

method of
MAJOR JOHN NAPIERKOWSKI, M.D., and
COLONEL ROY K. H. WONG, M.D.
Walter Reed Army Medical Center
Washington, District of Columbia

Gastroesophageal reflux disease (GERD) is the most common esophageal disorder, affecting both genders and all ages, races, and ethnicities to varying degrees. Up to 10% of adults experience heartburn daily, 20% weekly, and 40% monthly. GERD has been shown to have a more detrimental effect on emotional well-being than duodenal ulcer, menopause, mild angina, hypertension, or diabetes.

Of patients with heartburn three times per week, 60% to 70% have nonerosive reflux disease (NERD) and 30% to 40% have reflux esophagitis. Although heartburn is its classic feature, GERD can cause a broad array of symptoms and complications.

PATHOPHYSIOLOGY

Several mechanisms prevent esophageal injury from reflux: the antireflux barrier at the gastroesophageal junction, rapid neutralization and clearance of acidic refluxate, and esophageal mucosal integrity. Failure of these mechanisms can result in prolonged esophageal exposure to acid, pepsin, bile acids, and other gastroduodenal contents.

The lower esophageal sphincter (LES), the diaphragmatic crus, and the acute entry of the esophagus into the stomach (the angle of His) form the antireflux barrier. Disruptions of this mechanism, such as transient LES relaxations (tLESR), hypotensive LES pressures, and hiatal hernias (HH), can result in GERD. Causes of elevated intragastric pressures, such as delayed gastric emptying, also challenge the antireflux barrier, predisposing to GERD.

Once gastroduodenal contents enter the esophagus, rapid esophageal clearance, esophageal mucosal integrity, and buffering of the acidic contents prevent or minimize esophageal tissue injury. Esophageal dysmotility and HH impair esophageal clearance, epithelial disruption lowers the esophageal-injury threshold, and decreased bicarbonate-rich salivary secretion impairs the neutralization of acid.

Current evidence concerning the role of *Helicobacter pylori* in GERD is controversial with some data suggesting, if anything, a protective effect.

CLINICAL MANIFESTATIONS

Heartburn is the most common symptom of GERD and is characterized by a retrosternal burning discomfort extending from the epigastrium toward the throat. Regurgitation, another cardinal feature of GERD, represents the spontaneous, effortless reflux of gastric contents into the esophagus or pharynx, sometimes resulting in an "acidic taste." Many factors are known to predispose to GERD (see Table 3). Symptoms often occur after a meal, especially with exercise or recumbency. A subset of patients have "upright GERD" in which symptoms are more predominant while upright and often are associated with excessive belching. Dysphagia occurs in up to 30% of GERD patients and may be due to esophageal inflammation, stricture, malignancy, or peristaltic dysfunction. Less common symptoms of GERD include water brash (a sudden copious secretion of salty salivary fluid into the mouth), hiccups, and odynophagia. GERD can also be associated with epigastric burning, dyspepsia, indigestion, and nausea, which are typically more suggestive of peptic ulcer disease or biliary tract disease.

Additionally, 60% of noncardiac chest pain is caused by GERD. After the cardiac evaluation, empirical acid suppression is a cost-effective diagnostic and therapeutic approach.

Extraesophageal conditions associated with GERD (see Table 4) are increasingly recognized and are discussed subsequently.

DIAGNOSIS

A thorough history is the most important instrument in diagnosing GERD. Typical symptoms of heartburn and regurgitation are enough evidence for a trial of empirical therapy. Remission with a proton pump inhibitor (PPI) is as accurate as pH monitoring.

Several tests are available (Table 1). Besides an empirical trial of treatment, tests are usually performed for four reasons: (1) atypical symptoms; (2) chronic symptoms (for Barrett's screening); (3) refractory symptoms; and (4) alarm symptoms (dysphagia, odynophagia, bleeding, or weight loss). Endoscopy is usually the first choice because it offers versatility with direct visualization, biopsies, and sometimes treatment (e.g., stricture dilation). Typical symptoms combined with esophagitis on endoscopy are highly accurate for diagnosing GERD, but in most

TABLE 1. **Diagnostic Tests in GERD**

Test	Indication	Possible Findings	Comment
Empirical trial omeprazole (Prilosec) 40 mg PO bid or equivalent × 7 days	Diagnose GERD	Immediate symptom relief with >50% improvement in heartburn symptoms	Symptom relief with high-dose PPI is as accurate as any other test for GERD
Endoscopy	Chronic GERD	Barrett's esophagus, confirmed by mucosal biopsy	Only test for Barrett's esophagus
	Alarm symptoms (dysphagia, odynophagia, weight loss, bleeding)	Adenocarcinoma, strictures, esophagitis	Usually the first test for alarm symptoms
	GERD treatment nonresponse	Achalasia	Usually the first test for GERD treatment nonresponse; often done in conjunction with pH monitor
	Atypical GERD symptoms (e.g., noncardiac chest pain, extraesophageal symptoms, symptom overlap with other GI diseases)	Laryngitis, posterior pharyngeal erythema, infectious esophagitis, peptic ulcer disease	Often the first test (possibly after empirical therapy) for atypical symptoms; often done in conjunction with pH monitor
Barium contrast radiograph	*Alarm symptoms (dysphagia, odynophagia, weight loss, bleeding)	Mass, stricture, severe esophagitis	Most sensitive test for strictures
	*GERD treatment nonresponse	Achalasia	
	Document reflux of gastric contents and/or HH	Reflux, hiatal hernia	Physiologic and pathologic reflux are often indistinguishable Most sensitive test for HH
pH monitoring (standard 24-hour catheter)	GERD treatment nonresponse	Timing of acid reflux episode can be correlated to symptom diary	Usually performed as an adjunct to endoscopy
Bravo pH (catheter-free monitoring)	GERD treatment nonresponse	Timing of acid reflux episode can be correlated to symptoms diary	Clinical utility, safety not yet clear as it is not yet in widespread use; may offer less cumbersome, more accurate results
Dual pH monitoring (pH catheter with proximal and distal esophageal monitors)	Atypical GERD symptoms (noncardiac chest pain or extraesophageal symptoms)	Timing of acid reflux episode can be correlated to symptom diary; evidence of high reflux aids in diagnosis of extraesophageal symptoms	Usually performed as an adjunct to endoscopy
Esophageal manometry	Preoperative evaluation before anti-reflux surgery	Esophageal motility; poor motility helps guide surgical wrap Achalasia or other motor disorders contraindicate antireflux surgery	Most experts recommend EM prior to antireflux surgery (in addition to other testing)
	Assist placement of pH monitor	LES pressure and location	
Bernstein test	Noncardiac chest pain	Symptoms reproduction with intraesophageal acid infusion	Rarely performed test
Impedance testing	Possibly atypical symptoms (e.g., extraesophageal symptoms)	Nonacidic reflux	Undergoing studies; not in widespread clinical use
	GERD treatment nonresponse	Nonacidic reflux	

EM, esophageal manometry; GERD, gastroesophageal reflux disease; GI, gastrointestinal; LES, lower esophageal sphincter; PPI, proton pump inhibitor.
*Barium radiograph usually done if endoscopy cannot be performed for safety or availability reasons.

patients endoscopy is normal and, therefore, often cannot confirm the diagnosis.

Barium esophagram is most often used when endoscopy is unavailable or unsafe, or to document barium reflux. It is the most sensitive test for peptic strictures and HH, but it is less sensitive for esophagitis and early malignancy, and not useful for Barrett's esophagus.

pH monitoring is usually performed after endoscopy in the evaluation of atypical symptoms or when GERD symptoms are refractory to treatment. pH monitoring documents whether acid reflux is present, and it documents whether episodes of acid reflux correlate with symptoms. While it is a valuable test, its sensitivity and specificity are only about 85%, secondary to false-negative tests as patients may decrease caloric intake because of the uncomfortable nasal probe. A new catheter-free, endoscopically placed pH system may offer improved convenience and results, but further experience is needed to assess its clinical role.

Impedance testing is a catheter-based procedure used to detect nonacidic reflux. Its clinical use is being studied.

TREATMENT

Most patients who seek medical attention for GERD have had symptoms for 1 to 3 years and will continue to have chronic symptoms. Implementing lifestyle alterations to alleviate GERD is appropriate, but most patients require medications for relief. "Step-up therapy" involves initiating antacids or low potency antisecretory agents followed by increasing potency until relief is attained. "Step-down therapy" involves initiating therapy with a PPI, followed by titrating to a lower dose until minimum therapy is required to maintain remission.

Directly tailored medication regimens may be useful in some cases. In the few patients who have symptoms lasting less than 4 weeks, lifestyle alterations, usually combined with antacids or H2RAs, provide effective relief. Alginic acid (Gaviscon) may have a role, especially in patients who experience predominantly upright GERD. Many patients with NERD respond to on-demand therapy, whereas reflux esophagitis almost always requires maintenance therapy, usually with PPIs. For a summary of GERD treatment guidelines, see Table 2.

Lifestyle Modification

A number of nonpharmacologic steps can be taken to alleviate GERD symptoms (Table 3). Effective measures vary from person to person and are most reliably identified by patients on an individualized basis.

Medical Therapy

Antacids and Alginic Acid (Gaviscon)

For the treatment of mild, intermittent GERD symptoms, neutralizing antacids taken after meals and before bedtime are of clinical benefit when compared with placebo. Alginic acid (Gaviscon) forms a viscous layer on the gastric pool, creating a barrier to reflux and is most likely to benefit patients with upright GERD.

Histamine$_2$-Receptor Antagonists (H2RAs)

Only slight variations in efficacy exist between the available H2RAs (see Table 2). H2RAs have dose-dependent physiologic and clinical efficacy, and work by inhibiting histamine's stimulation of the parietal cell's acid production. They are more effective than neutralizing antacids in GERD, and when used in combination with antacids, relief of symptoms occurs more rapidly and lasts longer than when either class of medication is used alone. Some patients with GERD, especially those with reflux esophagitis, have persistent symptoms despite H2RAs, and require PPIs. Tachyphylaxis occurs with use of the H2RAs, and their ability to suppress meal-related gastric acid is limited. Nevertheless, H2RAs remain effective. While high dose PPIs will not inhibit nocturnal acid secretion, H2RAs can inhibit nocturnal acid secretion albeit for 2 to 4 weeks until tachyphylaxis occurs.

TABLE 2. **Treatment Strategies in GERD**

Indication	Treatment
All GERD patients	**Lifestyle alterations**
	Over-the-counter therapy
Intermittent, mild or moderate GERD of short duration	Antacids, alginic acid (Gaviscon), H2RAs
Mild–moderate nonerosive GERD	**H2RAs, prescription dose**
	famotidine (Pepcid) 20 mg bid
Unable to take PPI due to side effects or cost	ranitidine (Zantac) 150 mg bid
	cimetidine (Tagamet) 400 mg bid
	nizatidine (Axid) 150 mg bid
Inadequate response to H2RA	**PPI, standard dose**
	omeprazole (Prilosec) 20 mg qd
Intolerance of H2RA	esomeprazole (Nexium) 20 mg qd
	rabeprazole (Aciphex) 20 mg qd
	pantoprazole (Protonix) 40 mg qd
Erosive esophagitis	lansoprazole (Prevacid) 15 mg qd
Inadequate response to standard dose PPI	**PPI, standard dose bid**
Severe esophagitis	
Inadequate response to bid PPI	**PPI, high-dose**
7-day diagnostic test for GERD	**Consider adding nighttime H2RA**
Extraesophageal manifestations of GERD	
Intolerance to H2RAs and PPIs	**Prokinetics**
	bethanechol (Urecholine) 25 mg qid*
GERD associated with esophageal dysmotility	metoclopramide (Reglan) 10 mg qid
	cisapride (Propulsid) 10 mg qid
Esophagitis or severe GERD refractory to high-dose PPI, confirmed by pH monitoring	
GERD responsive to medical therapy, but long term medication undesirable due to side effects or cost	**Antireflux surgery**
Extraesophageal symptoms due to GERD proved by objective studies unresponsive to 3 to 6 mo of high-dose PPIs	

*Not FDA approved for this indication.

H2RAs are usually well tolerated and have a good safety profile. Ranitidine (Zantac) and cimetidine (Tagamet) are considered safe in pregnancy. Drug-to-drug interactions can occur with H2RAs because they are metabolized through the hepatic P450 enzyme system, which is important in the metabolism of many drugs.

Proton Pump Inhibitors

Regarding efficacy in heartburn relief, limited head-to-head comparisons suggest minimal variation among the available PPIs (see Table 2). PPIs have enhanced antisecretory activity because they affect the final common pathway of gastric acid production by poisoning activated proton pumps. Since peak PPI serum concentrations occur approximately 1 hour after administration, and because proton pumps are activated by food within 30 to 60 minutes of a meal, PPIs should be administered 30 to 60 minutes prior to a meal for maximal effect.

PPIs have demonstrated superior GERD symptom relief, effective esophagitis healing, good tolerability, and a long safety record. There have been no reported cases of carcinoids or gastric adenocarcinoma with over 10 years of PPI use. Side effects are infrequent and include diarrhea, nausea, and headache. Drug-to-drug interactions occur but are rare.

Prokinetic Agents

Bethanechol (Urecholine),* metoclopramide (Reglan), and cisapride (Propulsid) counteract some of the pathophysiologic abnormalities seen in GERD. They increase LES pressures, enhance esophageal peristalsis, and improve gastric emptying. They have a demonstrated clinical efficacy equivalent to H2RAs for mild to moderate esophagitis. However, because of significant side effects, these agents have not been favored in the treatment of GERD. Because of potential cardiac arrhythmias, cisapride (Propulsid) is only available by special request directly from the manufacturer.

Surgical Therapy

Laparoscopic Nissen fundoplication is the most commonly performed antireflux surgery in which an HH is reduced, the LES is fixed to the diaphragmatic

*Not FDA approved for this indication.

TABLE 3. **Lifestyle Recommendations to Alleviate GERD**

Recommendation	Rationale
Avoid reflux-inducing foods	Fatty foods decrease gastric emptying and decrease LES pressure Chocolate decreases LES pressure Peppermint decreases LES pressure Tomato-based foods induce HB as a direct effect on mucosa; GERD mechanism unclear Spicy foods induce HB as a direct effect on mucosa; GERD mechanism unclear
Avoid large meals	Large meals increase intragastric pressures
Avoid reflux-inducing beverages	Caffeine decreases LES pressure Alcohol decreases LES pressure Carbonated beverages increase intragastric pressure and induce belching Acidic beverages (red wine, citrus drinks, colas, coffee, and tomato juice) induce HB by direct contact effect on esophagus; GERD mechanism unclear
Avoid recumbency for 3 h after meals	Recumbency increases proximal intragastric pressure
Raise the head of the bed (use 6-8 inch blocks under the legs of the bed)	Recumbency increases proximal intragastric pressure
Avoid vigorous exercise after meals	Exercise increases intra-abdominal pressure and might compromise diaphragmatic portion of the antireflux barrier
Quit smoking	Smoking decreases salivation and decreases LES pressure
Lose weight if obese	Obesity increases intra-abdominal pressure
Avoid tight-fitting garments	Tight-fitting garments increase intra-abdominal pressure
Promote salivation with lozenges or gum	Saliva neutralizes acid, contains prostaglandin and EGF, which promote healing
Review medications	Examples of medications reducing LES pressure: Theophylline β-agonist inhalers Calcium channel antagonists Meperidine Anticholinergic medications Dopamine (Inotropin) Sildenafil (Viagra) Examples of medications potentially harmful to esophageal epithelium: Tetracycline NSAIDs Quinidine Potassium supplements Iron supplements Bisphosphonates

EGF, epidermal growth factor; GERD, gastroesophageal reflux disease; HB, heartburn; LES, lower esophageal sphincter.

crus, and the gastric fundus is "wrapped" around the gastroesophageal junction to form a barrier to reflux. Surgical therapy is directed at preventing acid and all gastroduodenal reflux, providing theoretical advantage over medical therapy.

Two randomized controlled studies comparing surgical therapy versus medical therapy have been performed. In the first, which preceded PPIs, surgery was more effective than H2RAs in healing esophagitis. The second study compared surgery to PPIs and demonstrated equivalent efficacy when PPIs could be titrated. At large referral centers, successful surgeries are reported to be as high as 92% to 97%, but at smaller community centers, success may be only 75%. Some series report that after 10 years, up to 60% of patients return to some form of medical therapy. Reported surgical morbidity ranges from 5% to 30% with the most common side effects being dysphagia, "gas-bloat syndrome," diarrhea, and nausea. Mortality estimates range from 0.5% to 0.2%.

Poor surgical outcomes are noted in patients who do not respond to PPIs, probably because many of these patients do not truly have GERD. Nevertheless, well documented reflux esophagitis that is refractory to PPIs is the best indication for antireflux surgery. Outside this very small cohort, the risk-benefit analysis favors medical therapy.

Endoscopic Therapies

Three endoscopic techniques for the treatment of GERD have been FDA approved for safety. The first technique employs radiofrequency ablation to injure the distal esophagus, which results in stenosis and possibly interference with tLESRs. The second technique involves endoscopic suturing of the distal esophagus to create a plication. The third technique involves the injection of a polymer into the region of the LES. Efficacy data in published studies appear promising but are short-term and not randomized controlled studies.

ESOPHAGEAL COMPLICATIONS OF GERD

Reflux Esophagitis

The most common abnormal finding in GERD is esophagitis, more often seen in men. Esophagitis ranges from nonerosive inflammation to deep or large confluent ulcerations of the distal esophagus. Reflux esophagitis can occasionally cause significant upper GI bleeding. Perforation and death are extremely rare but have been described with complications of reflux esophagitis.

Antacids, H2RAs, and prokinetics have unsatisfactory cure rates for esophagitis, but high dose PPIs can be expected to heal esophagitis in over 90%, usually within 8 to 12 weeks. However, 80% relapse within 6 months on PPI discontinuation. Even step-down therapy to H2RAs has been associated with high relapse rates. Evidence shows that maintenance dosing of PPIs at or near the healing dose is often needed.

Stricture

Peptic strictures complicate reflux esophagitis in 8% to 20% of cases. Strictures usually occur in the distal esophagus classically causing dysphagia and sometimes food impactions. Management is typically with endoscopic dilation procedures, and PPIs are usually effective in decreasing esophageal edema and preventing recurrent strictures.

Barrett's Esophagus and Adenocarcinoma

Approximately 10% of patients with chronic heartburn develop specialized intestinal metaplasia (SIM) of the esophagus, or Barrett's esophagus, which is a precursor for esophageal adenocarcinoma. The incidence of Barrett's adenocarcinoma has quadrupled over the past few decades, and the incidence of progression from Barrett's esophagus to adenocarcinoma is approximately 0.5% yearly. Men have a 10-fold risk for Barrett's compared to women, and whites have a 5- to 10-fold risk compared to non-whites. Although heartburn is a major risk factor for Barrett's, there are significantly more asymptomatic, undiagnosed Barrett's patients than are seen clinically, complicating Barrett's screening guidelines. In white males older than age 50 who have chronic heartburn, screening for Barrett's is widely recommended. When Barrett's is identified, surveillance endoscopies and biopsies are indicated.

EXTRA-ESOPHAGEAL MANIFESTATIONS OF GERD

Anatomic structures located above the esophagus are least resistant to gastroduodenal contents in comparison to the esophagus and stomach. Here, healing requires almost complete acid inhibition with high-dose PPIs and nighttime H2RAs for a period of 3 to 6 months.

Pulmonary Conditions

The association between GERD and asthma is well documented with up to 80% of asthmatics having GERD, and 40% having reflux esophagitis. Pulmonary symptoms may be mediated through a vagal reflex triggered by chemoreceptors in the esophagus; or pulmonary symptoms may result directly from microaspiration of refluxate.

Asthmatics who have heartburn (especially in association with asthma exacerbations) and asthmatics whose pulmonary symptoms are refractory to treatment should be evaluated and/or treated for GERD. pH monitoring combined with a symptom diary often provides useful diagnostic information in such cases. Many other pulmonary conditions have also been associated with GERD (Table 4).

Ear, Nose and Throat Conditions

A growing body of literature also demonstrates an association between GERD and ear, nose, and throat

TABLE 4. **Extraesophageal Conditions with Claimed or Proven Associations with Gastroesophageal Reflux Disease**

Pulmonary Conditions
- Cough
- Ashtma
- Chronic obstructive pulmonary disease (COPD)
- Chronic bronchitis
- Bronchiectasis
- Idiopathic pulmonary fibrosis (IPF)
- Sleep apnea
- Pneumonia

Oral Conditions
- Dental erosions
- Dental caries
- Oral leukoplakia

Ear, Nose, and Throat (ENT) Conditions
- Laryngitis
- Hoarseness
- Laryngomalacia
- Pachyderma laryngis
- Arytenoid fixation
- Paroxysmal laryngospasm
- Laryngeal cancer
- Vocal cord granuloma
- Vocal nodules
- Subglottic stenosis
- Pharyngitis
- Globus pharyngeus
- Sinusitis
- Otitis media

GERD, gastroesophageal reflux disease.

(ENT) disorders (see Table 4). The most prevalent symptom in the adult population is hoarseness. In the pediatric population, there is growing interest in the association between GERD and otitis media.

As with pulmonary symptoms, pH monitoring may provide useful information, and extended high-dose PPIs are often required.

TUMORS OF THE STOMACH

method of
JAMES O. PARK, M.D., and
MITCHELL C. POSNER, M.D.
University of Chicago Hospitals
Chicago, Illinois

Gastric tumors can be classified as benign or malignant, with hyperplastic polyps and adenocarcinomas accounting for the overwhelming majority within each category. Benign gastric tumors are of little clinical significance, except for the necessity of distinguishing them from malignant lesions. Although a wide variety of neoplastic entities can be encountered in the stomach, this review focuses on the more common and clinically pertinent tumors: adenomas, adenocarcinomas, lymphomas, carcinoid tumors, and stromal tumors.

ADENOMAS

Gastric polyps are divided into two categories based on their potential for malignant transformation: *hyperplastic* (no potential) and *adenomatous* (10% to 25% risk). Adenomas are benign pedunculated or sessile lesions lined by dysplastic, pseudostratified epithelium. The peak incidence is in the fifth to seventh decades of life, with a high prevalence in patients with familial adenomatous polyposis or Gardner's syndrome. Although adenomas can cause dyspepsia and hemorrhage, patients generally have few symptoms or physical findings, and a solitary, tubular or villous, antral lesion is usually found incidentally by barium study or endoscopy. Adenomas carry a distinct malignant potential that is proportional to size (significantly greater for polyps >2 cm), number, and degree of dysplasia. The presence of an adenoma also serves as a marker for increased risk of synchronous or metachronous carcinomas in the remaining gastric tissue.

Treatment

Adenomas are premalignant lesions that should be treated by polypectomy whenever clinically feasible. Pedunculated lesions are amenable to endoscopic removal, and this is sufficient therapy if no stalk invasion is found on histologic evaluation. Segmental resection is usually warranted for sessile lesions, or those with bleeding complications, and formal gastrectomy is recommended for invasive lesions, multiple polyposis, or multiple recurrent adenomas.

ADENOCARCINOMA

Incidence

Gastric adenocarcinoma, commonly referred to as *gastric carcinoma* or *stomach cancer*, accounts for 90% to 95% of all malignant tumors of the stomach. Worldwide, adenocarcinoma of the stomach remains the second most common cancer and cause of cancer death, with death rates measuring 50 to 78 per 100,000 in high-prevalence countries such as Costa Rica, Chile, Hungary, and Japan. The United States has seen a steady decrease in the incidence of gastric cancer over the past 6 decades, with intestinal-type antral tumors accounting for much of this decline. It is estimated that 13,400 men and 9,000 women in the United States alone will be diagnosed with stomach cancer in 2003, with 7,000 men and 5,100 women dying of the disease.

The incidence and mortality rate increase with advancing age, with a peak incidence in the sixth to seventh decades. Higher rates of gastric cancer are observed in African, Asian, and Hispanic Americans and in lower socioeconomic groups. Studies of migrants from areas of high (Japan) to low (United States) risk suggest that environmental exposure in early life may influence the risk of developing gastric cancer but that other factors may continually affect the predisposition to cancer.

Types

Two distinct histologic subtypes of gastric cancer—intestinal and diffuse—were described by Lauren in 1965. *Intestinal-type tumors* have a glandular structure, arise from areas of gastric atrophy or intestinal metaplasia, occur more commonly in older men, and represent the dominant histologic type in regions with epidemics of stomach cancer, suggesting an environmental origin. Ingestion of preserved foods containing nitrates and nitrites, cigarette smoking, and *Helicobacter pylori* infection are associated with an increased risk of developing intestinal-type cancer, whereas diets rich in fiber, beta carotene, and ascorbic acid are protective. A model for the pathogenesis of intestinal-type cancer proposes that chronic inflammation and atrophy of normal mucosa in association with hypochlorhydria or achlorhydria leads to subsequent bacterial overgrowth, resulting in chronic atrophic gastritis and free radical–induced mucosal injury by bacterial conversion of nitrates and nitrites to nitrosamines. Continued epithelial injury can cause metaplasia, dysplasia, carcinoma in situ, and, ultimately, invasive carcinoma. Previous partial gastrectomy and vagotomy for benign conditions, pernicious anemia, Ménétrier disease, and familial polyposis all contribute to an increased risk through this model sequence.

Diffuse-type tumors are more widespread throughout the mucosa, do not typically arise from precancerous lesions, occur more frequently in younger women, and represent the major subtype in endemic areas with a familial occurrence, suggesting a genetic origin. Although the overall decline in incidence of gastric cancer appears to reflect the reduction of the intestinal-type tumors, the diffuse subtype is seen with increasing frequency as the incidence of proximal gastric cancer has become more predominant in the past 15 to 20 years. This is a worrisome prospect because the diffuse-type lesions have a poorer prognosis, stage for stage. Many other classifications based on gross morphology and histologic differentiation exist, although none are independent prognostic indicators (Table 1).

TABLE 1. **Morphologic and Histologic Classifications of Gastric Adenocarcinoma**

Morphologic Categories
Fungating or polypoid
Ulcerating
Superficial spreading
Diffusely spreading (linitis plastica)
Borromann Classifiction
Type I: circumscribed, polypoid
Type II: ulcerated, with elevated borders
Type III: ulcerated, with partial infiltrtion
Type IV: diffusely infiltrative
Type V: unclassifiable
Ming Classification
Expanding-type tumors (favorable prognosis)
Infiltration tumors (poor prognosis)
World Health Organization Histologic Classification
Tumular
Papillary
Mucinous
Signet-ring cell
Broder's Histologic Grade
I (well differentiated) to IV (anaplastic)

Clinical Manifestations

Most patients with gastric cancer present with advanced disease. This reflects the insidious nature of the disease and the fact that symptoms of early gastric cancer are vague and nonspecific. Patients may have anorexia with weight loss, nausea and vomiting, early satiety and dysphagia, or epigastric discomfort. These symptoms may mimic those of benign gastric ulcer disease and may be either ignored or treated medically without further evaluation. Dysphagia occurs with tumors in the cardia with extension through the gastroesophageal junction. Early satiety is indicative of diffusely infiltrative tumor with loss of gastric wall distensibility. Persistent vomiting can occur with antral tumors obstructing the pylorus. Approximately 10% of patients present with signs of disseminated disease, including supraclavicular (Virchow) or axillary (Irish) nodes; periumbilical (Sister Mary Joseph node), ovarian (Krukenberg tumor), or pelvic (Blumer shelf) metastasis; jaundice, hepatomegaly, or ascites.

Diagnosis

A barium study or flexible upper endoscopy with tissue biopsy can be performed when gastric cancer is suspected. Double-contrast barium study is a sensitive, cost-effective test for detection of even small gastric lesions and is used for mass screening in Japan. Fiberoptic esophagogastroduodenoscopy is the diagnostic modality of choice for gastric cancer and should be performed in any patient with localized disease with anticipated surgical intervention. Accuracy of endoscopy is greater than 95% when biopsy samples are taken, and cytology obtained by fine-needle aspiration, lavage, or brushings yields a near 100% positive predictive value. Once a diagnosis is established, evaluation of the extent of disease involves clinical examination, routine blood tests (complete blood cell count, chemistries, liver profile), chest radiography, and abdominal and pelvic computed tomography. Endoscopic ultrasonography is a diagnostic adjunct that can provide highly accurate staging of the depth of primary tumor invasion and limited assessment of lymph node status. Laparoscopy and peritoneal lavage have been used as diagnostic tools to avoid open laparotomy and major resections in patients with disseminated disease not detectable by other modalities.

Staging

Depth of primary tumor penetration, presence of regional lymph node involvement, and spread to adjacent organs or distant sites remain the most important prognostic indicators for gastric cancer. Therefore, the American Joint Committee on Cancer (AJCC) staging classification, based on the TNM system, is currently used in the United States for staging of gastric cancer (Table 2). T stage has been demonstrated to be an independent prognostic indicator. *Early gastric cancer*, defined as disease confined to the mucosa or submucosa (Tis, T1) regardless of lymph node status, has a 5-year survival rate after resection of 70% to 95%, depending on the presence of nodal involvement. *Advanced gastric cancer* implies invasion of the muscularis propria, and these lesions are frequently associated with distant or contiguous spread, a higher stage, and poorer prognosis. Unfortunately, early gastric cancer represents only 10% to 15% of diagnosed cases in the United States. N stage is the single most significant determinant of recurrence and survival.

Treatment

Surgical resection remains the standard and only potentially curative therapy in localized gastric cancer. However, controversy persists regarding the extent of gastric resection (total versus subtotal gastrectomy), the extent of lymphadenectomy, and the role of adjuvant chemoradiotherapy. Retrospective Japanese series report survival rates of more than 95% with gastrectomy and perigastric lymphadenectomy for early gastric cancer. Gastric resection with regional lymphadenectomy is the treatment of choice for stage I, II, and III disease. Subtotal gastrectomy is the standard operative option for pyloric, antral, or body tumors. Subtotal resection provides survival equivalent to that of total gastrectomy if an adequate gross proximal margin is obtainable, with less associated morbidity. For proximal tumors involving the fundus or cardioesophageal junction, or for diffusely infiltrative lesions, total gastrectomy provides better functional results, with equivalent operative morbidity and mortality, when compared with proximal gastric resection. Standard regional lymphadenectomy involves removal of greater and lesser curvature perigastric lymph nodes.

TABLE 2. **American Joint Committee on Cancer Staging Classification for Gastric Adenocarcinoma**

Primary Tumor (T)

TX: Primary tumor cannot be assessed
T0: No evidence of primary tumor
Tis: Carcinoma in situ
T1: Invasion into lamina propria or submucosa
T2; Invasion into muscularis propria or subserosa
T3: Penetration of serosa without invasion of adjacent structures
T4: Invasion of adjacent structures

Regional Lymph Nodes (N)

The regional lymph nodes include perigastric nodes and nodes along the left gastric, common hepatic, splenic, and celiac arteries. Involvement of hepatoduodenal, retropancreatic, mesentric, and para-aortic nodes is classified as distant metastasis.
NX: Regional lymph nodes cannot be assessed
N0: No regional lymph node metastasis
N1: 1–6 metastatic regional lymph nodes
N2: 7–15 metastatic regional lymph nodes
N3: >15 metastatic regional lymph nodes

Distant Metastasis (M)

MX: Distant metastasis cannot be assessed
M0: No distant metastasis
M1: Distant metastasis

AJCC Clinical Stage Groupings

Stage 0: TisN0M0
Stage IA: T1N0M0
Stage IB: T1N1M0, T2N0M0
Stage II: T1N2M0, T2N1M0, T3N0M0
Stage IIIA: T2N2M0, T3N1M0, T4NB0M0
Stage IIIB: T3N2M0
Stage IV: Any TN3M0, T4N1M0, T4N2M0, Any N, Any NM1

Retrospective reports indicate that extended D2 lymphadenectomy for potentially curable gastric cancer can be performed safely, provides more staging information, and may result in improved survival compared with a more limited D1 resection. However, several more recent prospective randomized trials failed to demonstrate a survival advantage with D2 resections, bringing into question the therapeutic value of the routine application of D2 dissection. Routine prophylactic splenectomy is not advocated because it provides no survival benefit and leads to increased complications. Endoscopic treatment using cauterization, local injection, and laser therapy for protruding and depressed lesions without ulceration of less than 1 cm have been reported. Currently, these techniques are reserved for patients at high risk for conventional operations because of age or co-morbidities. Dysphagia due to tumors of the cardia may be relieved by endoscopic destruction of the lesion obstructing the gastric inlet or by endoscopic placement of stents.

Results of a recent randomized intergroup trial demonstrated improved disease-free and overall survival in stage II and III cancer patients receiving postoperative adjuvant chemoradiation therapy. Preoperative induction chemoradiation therapy is under investigation. All patients with stage IV disease should be considered for clinical trials. Although neither cure nor prolongation of life is achieved with chemotherapy, substantial palliation and occasional durable remissions are possible in select patients. Palliative radiation therapy may also alleviate bleeding, pain, and obstruction. There is little benefit in performing palliative total gastrectomy in patients with metastatic disease, and this procedure should be reserved for patients with uncontrollable bleeding or obstruction. Because survival is poor with all available single and multimodal treatment strategies, patients with recurrent gastric cancer should be considered candidates for phase I and II clinical trials.

LYMPHOMA

Incidence

Lymphoma is the second most common gastric malignancy after gastric adenocarcinoma, accounting for 3% to 5% of all malignant tumors of the stomach. More than 50% of patients with non-Hodgkin's lymphoma have gastrointestinal involvement. The stomach is the most common extranodal site involved, accounting for more than half of all primary gastrointestinal lymphomas. In the United States, the annual incidence is less than 1 in 100,000, although the numbers are increasing. More than 95% of gastric lymphomas are non-Hodgkin's lymphomas, and more than 90% are of intraepithelial B-cell origin, with 90% of the high-grade large cell type. Primary gastric lymphomas originate in the stomach without other solid organ or systemic involvement until very late in the disease course, whereas secondary lymphomas are systemic nodal lymphomas with secondary gastric involvement. The peak incidence is in the sixth decade of life, with a male predominance of 1.7:1. A fivefold increased risk is seen in patients with AIDS.

Clinical Manifestations

Less than 20% of cases present asymptomatically; however, the signs and symptoms are often nonspecific and difficult to distinguish from those of gastric adenocarcinoma. Symptoms of systemic lymphoma, namely, weight loss, fever, and night sweats, can be present in up to 40%. Complications including bleeding, obstruction, perforation, and fistulization are not uncommon; and findings such as massive splenomegaly and palpable peripheral adenopathy may indicate diffuse lymphoma. Mucosa-associated lymphoid tissue (MALT) tumors are low-grade monoclonal B-cell variants noted in the setting of chronic gastritis that are associated with *H. pylori* infection, with more than 90% seropositivity. Reports suggest that antibiotic eradication of the *H. pylori* may lead to tumor regression.

Diagnosis

The diagnosis of primary gastric lymphoma can be confirmed after exclusion of palpable peripheral lymphadenopathy and hepatosplenomegaly on examination, an abnormal peripheral blood smear, mediastinal adenopathy on chest radiography, and systemic involvement on imaging studies. Gastric lymphoma is difficult to distinguish from adenocarcinoma by contrast radiography or even endoscopy. Radiographically, primary gastric lymphoma presents as ulcers, enlarged folds, or multiple nodules, whereas a diffusely infiltrating lesion with the appearance of linitis plastica is more suggestive of secondary lymphoma. Ten percent to 20% of patients have completely normal results of an upper gastrointestinal series. Upper endoscopy with biopsy and cytologic evaluation, yielding an accuracy of nearly 90%, is usually required for diagnosis, although deep biopsies, occasionally full thickness, may be necessary. One distinguishing feature from adenocarcinoma is that peristalsis is often preserved in lymphoma.

Immunophenotyping by immunoperoxidase staining for lymphocyte markers may also be helpful in distinguishing malignant from benign disease. Endoscopic ultrasonography can define depth of tumor infiltration and abnormal perigastric lymph nodes with very high sensitivity and specificity and is a useful adjunct in diagnosis and staging. Computed tomography and magnetic resonance imaging are frequently used to detect distant metastases, including hepatic and splenic involvement.

Treatment

The Ann Arbor system is commonly used to stage primary gastric lymphoma (Table 3). Treatment of localized primary gastric lymphoma remains controversial because, unlike for other lymphocytic lymphomas, surgical resection has traditionally been recommended. For stage I and II disease limited to the stomach and regional nodes, attempted curative surgical resection followed by adjuvant radiation, chemotherapy, or both has been advocated. Postoperative radiation therapy for stage II disease has been shown to reduce local regional recurrence and improve 5-year survival. Therefore, radiation therapy has been advocated as an adjunct to surgery in patients with advanced but resectable disease, and combination chemotherapy and radiation therapy has been advocated in patients with unresectable disease or as second-line alternative therapy in poor surgical candidates.

Recent data suggest that nonoperative management with radiation and chemotherapy therapy alone may produce comparable outcomes to surgery in early-stage primary gastric lymphoma with preservation of the stomach. The main theoretical disadvantage of radiation or chemotherapy as a primary treatment modality is increased gastrointestinal complications, including bleeding or perforation, particularly in patients with advanced disease. These complications are rare, however. Patients with stage III and IV disease who present with complications of bleeding, obstruction, or perforation should also undergo attempted resection followed by adjuvant therapy. Patients without complications presenting with preoperative documentation of stage III or IV disease should be treated with radiation therapy and chemotherapy initially, and surgical resection should be reserved for persistent local disease of the stomach or for complications. For low-grade MALT lesions, data suggest that a trial of antibiotic eradication of *H. pylori* infection to induce regression of the tumor is warranted, although further follow-up is required to confirm its effectiveness.

CARCINOID TUMORS

Pathophysiology

Carcinoid tumors arise from enterochromaffin-like (ECL) cells of neural crest origin and are classified as

TABLE 3. **Ann Arbor Staging System for Lymphoma**

Stage I: involvement of a single lymph node region (I) or a single localized extralymphatic site (IE)
Stage II: involvement of two or more lymph node regions on the same side of the diaphragm (II) or with localized involvement of a single associated extralymphatic site (IIE)
Stage III: involvement of lymph node regions on both sides of the diaphragm (III) or with localized involvement of an extralymphatic site (IIIE), the spleen (IIIS), or both (IIIS + E)
Stage IV: disease that is diffusely spread throughout an extranodal site
The stages can be subclassified into A and B categories; the B designation is given to patients with constitutional symptoms of weight loss, fever, and night sweats

neuroendocrine or amine precursor uptake and decarboxylation (APUD) tumors. Although carcinoid tumors constitute 55% of all gut endocrine tumors, merely 2% to 3% of carcinoid tumors are found in the stomach, and these account for only 0.3% of all gastric tumors. The peak incidence is in the sixth to seventh decades, with a slight male predilection. Gastric carcinoids have been found in association with long-standing conditions of hypergastrinemia, such as pernicious anemia, atrophic gastritis, and Zollinger-Ellison syndrome with multiple endocrine neoplasia syndrome type 1.

Histologically, solid nests of small monotonous cells with rare mitoses and acinar or rosette formation are found in these tumors, located in the glandular base or submucosa. The benign or malignant nature of carcinoid tumors cannot be determined histologically; only the presence of metastases or invasion of adjacent structures is a true indicator of malignancy. Many carcinoid tumors are slow-growing indolent tumors that can be treated and often cured, especially in early stages. The occurrence of metastasis from carcinoid tumor relates directly to the size of the primary tumor (lesions <1 cm rarely, whereas lesions >2 cm frequently metastasize). Even when carcinoid tumors are malignant, however, they may be compatible with long-term survival, with an average time from the onset of symptoms to death from the disease of 8 years. The 5-year survival rate for carcinoid tumors approaches 100% with noninvasive tumors smaller than 2cm, 40% when the tumor diameter is more than 2cm, and 20% to 40% with hepatic metastases.

Clinical Manifestations

Carcinoid tumors secrete a variety of neuroendocrine peptides such as serotonin (manifested by elevated urinary 5-hydroxyindoleacetic acid), prostaglandins, kallikreins, catecholamines, somatostatin, and gastrin. Gastric carcinoid tumors are usually asymptomatic; however, they may cause chronic, intermittent abdominal pain or bleeding, suggesting partial obstruction or intussusception. Malignant carcinoid tumors induce fibrosis, which by fibrous adhesions may cause mechanical obstruction even when the primary tumor is small. Diarrhea, weight loss, and a palpable abdominal mass may also be present. Patients with carcinoid tumor are at increased risk for synchronous or metachronous second noncarcinoid GI malignancies. Malignant carcinoid syndrome (flush, diarrhea, bronchoconstriction, cardiac valvular lesions, arthropathy, and telangiectasia) is encountered in less than 10% of patients with gastric carcinoid tumors.

Diagnosis

Endoscopy and biopsy are valuable for diagnosing primary gastric carcinoid tumors. Positive argentaffin and argyrophil stains suggest the carcinoid tumor, and neurosecretory granules seen on electron microscopy are confirmatory. Computed tomography is valuable for demonstrating the mesenteric fibrosis and can evaluate tumor extension in the mesentery, the retroperitoneal space, and the liver. Somatostatin receptor localization techniques, measurement of plasma substance P, neurotensin, neuron-specific enolase, and chromogranins may aid in the diagnosis.

Treatment

Resection is the standard curative modality of localized disease, although gastric carcinoids tend to be less localized than those in other gastrointestinal sites. Gastric carcinoid tumors smaller than 1cm may be amenable to endoscopic excision. If the primary tumor is localized and all visible disease is resectable, 5-year survival rates are 70% to 90%. However, long-term follow-up is warranted because late recurrences do occur. Even if the regional disease is deemed unresectable or distant metastases are present, the disease is usually indolent, with median survivals of more than 2 years. Local complications, such as obstruction and intussusception, can be effectively palliated with either resection or bypass. In select patients with symptomatic hepatic lesions, resection or hepatic artery infusion of chemotherapeutic agents, combined with embolization with collagen, Gelfoam, or alcohol may provide palliation and decrease tumor bulk. The long-acting somatostatin analogue octreotide provides effective palliation in patients with carcinoid syndrome. Immunotherapy using low-dose interferon-α has been described with limited efficacy in controlling flushing and diarrhea. The prognosis for patients with recurring or relapsing disease is poor, and these patients should be considered for clinical trials. Attempts at re-resection of slow-growing tumors recurring in any single site can reduce tumor volume and provide long-term palliation.

MESENCHYMAL TUMORS

Incidence

Tumors of mesenchymal origin account for 1% to 3% of all gastric malignancies. The median age at diagnosis is 55, with a slight male predominance.

Pathophysiology

These stromal tumors were previously designated as smooth muscle tumors or as leiomyomas and leiomyosarcomas owing to the muscle marker staining that was observed. Most have a spindle cell histologic type and are of mesenchymal origin. Based on characteristic findings seen on electron microscopy and the indistinct cell line of origin with varying differentiation patterns, the term *gastrointestinal stromal tumor* (GIST) has been assigned to these tumors. Other less common tumors arising in the gastric mesenchyme include liposarcomas, fibrosarcomas, angiosarcomas, glomus tumors, and autonomic nerve tumors. Stromal tumors are indolent, slow-growing tumors found deep within the submucosa. Lesions smaller than 2 cm are generally clinically silent, whereas larger tumors have a tendency for ulceration and subsequent hemorrhage.

Clinical Manifestations and Diagnosis

Common symptoms include weight loss, abdominal pain, fullness, early satiety, gastrointestinal bleeding, and abdominal mass. The initial diagnosis is by contrast radiography or endoscopy, followed by assessment of metastatic involvement of the liver and lung using liver profile, chest radiography, and computed tomography. These studies often demonstrate smooth, lobulated, intraluminal lesions or highly invasive ulcers that are extraluminal. They are usually located antrally (25%) or corporally (40%). Primary tumor size and depth of primary invasion are important prognostic factors, with lesions bigger than 5cm in diameter being associated with poorer survival. Mitotic index is the most reliable predictor of malignancy, and lesions with more than 10 mitotic figures per 10 high-power fields have increased risk of metastasis.

Treatment

Currently, there are no definitive guidelines for the management of stromal tumors, and many centers treat these tumors based on experience with other soft tissue sarcomas. Two thirds of the lesions are resectable at presentation. Complete resection with a grossly normal margin, using wedge resection for small lesions and formal gastrectomy for more involved lesions, is recommended. Routine regional lymphadenectomy is not indicated because lymph node metastases are rare except by direct extension and studies have not shown survival benefit. The 5-year survival rates vary from 80% for low-grade lesions to 32% for high-grade lesions after resection. Intra-abdominal recurrence is quite common, with high mitotic index lesions recurring in up to 90% of cases within 5 years. This propensity for recurrence has prompted evaluation of radiation and chemotherapeutic adjunctive regimens. Because of the slow-growing nature of these tumors, long-term follow-up is required, including frequent abdominal computed tomography and consideration of re-resection if it is deemed feasible.

Patients with metastatic or unresectable GISTs may respond to imatinib mesylate (STI 571; Novartis Pharm.), which blocks the activity of KIT, a tyrosine kinase product of the proto-oncogene c-kit. This agent is currently being investigated in clinical trials.

TUMORS OF THE COLON AND RECTUM

method of
THEODORE JOHN SACLARIDES, M.D.
Rush Medical Center
Chicago, Illinois

When one considers both genders, colon and rectal cancer is the second most deadly malignant disease, after lung cancer. Approximately 150,000 new cases are diagnosed annually in the United States, and half of these patients may die of their disease. Approximately 60% to 70% of cases are sporadic, meaning that there are no identifiable predisposing conditions. Many of these cancers began as a benign, adenomatous polyp that, through a series of well-sequenced molecular changes, eventually transformed into an invasive cancer. Up to 30% of colorectal cancers occur in persons with a family history of this tumor in a first-degree relative; such a relationship confers an increased risk. Approximately 5% to 8% of cases result from inherited genetic defects such as familial adenomatous polyposis (FAP) or hereditary nonpolyposis colorectal cancer (HNPCC); with the former, the lifetime risk of colorectal cancer is 100%, and with the latter, it approaches 80%. The remaining cases are the result of inflammatory bowel disease, specifically ulcerative colitis. Patients with long-standing disease or involvement of the entire colon are especially at risk. Prior radiation to the pelvis and ureterosigmoidostomy for congenital bladder defects also confer an increased risk of colorectal cancer.

SCREENING

Screening strategies are designed for asymptomatic, low-risk persons, to detect adenomatous polyps and early, highly curable cancers. The presence of symptoms, such as bleeding, abdominal pain, or change in bowel habits, or a family history of colorectal cancer changes the approach from one of screening to surveillance. Surveillance is more likely to detect the condition being sought (cancer or polyps), and hence more invasive testing modalities are justified. Therefore, perhaps the first critical step is to determine a particular person's risk of colorectal cancer by inquiring into a personal history of the foregoing changes (e.g., bleeding) and into the family history with respect to cancer. *Low-risk* persons are those who lack symptoms and a personal or family history of colorectal cancer; approximately 2% of such individuals will develop colorectal cancer during their lifetime. *High-risk* persons are those with inflammatory bowel disease, FAP, and HNPCC; surveillance programs for these conditions are discussed shortly. *Intermediate-risk* persons have a personal history of colorectal polyps or cancer or a family history of colorectal cancer not as strong as one usually sees with FAP or HNPCC.

Screening for colorectal cancer should begin for the low-risk person at the age of 50 years. Although there are numerous ways to screen, avoidance of screening is not an option. Screening is more likely to detect cancers at an early stage at which the tumor is confined to the bowel wall and has not spread to regional lymph nodes or distant sites. Consequently, survival should be enhanced. The recommendations that follow are supported by reports from the American Cancer Society and the American Gastroenterological Association.

Fecal Occult Blood Test and Flexible Sigmoidoscopy

An annual fecal occult blood test alone reduces the mortality from colorectal cancer by 33% compared with controls. For at least 2 days before the test, dietary and medicinal restrictions should be observed. These include avoidance of red meat, turnips, horseradish, salicylates, and vitamin C. Two samples from three consecutive stools should be obtained, smeared on the guaiac-impregnated slides, stored at room temperature, and tested within 4 days. Rehydration increases the sensitivity to approximately 90%. A positive fecal occult blood test is indicated by a blue color after peroxide is added and is an indication for subsequent colonoscopy. In these instances, adenomas are found in 30% to 40% of cases and cancers in 10%.

Flexible sigmoidoscopy should be performed every 5 years, using the 60-cm instrument. This length permits examination of the entire sigmoid colon in virtually all patients, and if there is minimal sigmoid redundancy, the scope may actually reach the splenic flexure in some patients. Preparation for the test is performed with two small-volume enemas given 1 to 2 hours before. The addition of flexible sigmoidoscopy to the fecal occult blood test is complementary; small adenomas that are not bleeding and hence are likely to be missed by the fecal occult blood test may by found by sigmoidoscopy. Polyps larger than 1 cm found by sigmoidoscopy are an indication for colonoscopy; the likelihood of finding polyps more proximally in the colon approaches 30%.

Flexible Sigmoidoscopy and Air Contrast Barium Enema

This option is more invasive, but it is also more likely to detect lesions because complete visualization of the entire colon is possible in 90% to 95% of patients. Flexible sigmoidoscopy every 5 years is combined with an air contrast barium enema every 5 to 10 years. The combination of these two diagnostic entities is advised because overlapping loops of bowel in some patients may preclude precise radiographic assessment. An abnormal sigmoidoscopy or barium enema should be followed by colonoscopy.

Colonoscopy

The third option for the low-risk person is colonoscopy every 10 years. This time interval has been chosen because colorectal tumors are generally slow growing, and it takes 10 years for a colonic epithelial cell to evolve through hyperplasia, dysplasia, and in situ changes to an invasive cancer. This is the most invasive of the choices listed; however, many patients appreciate that the interval between tests is the longest of the three options, sedation is routinely given, and biopsy or removal of polyps or suspicious lesions is possible. Patient preparation is performed with either oral cathartics or nonabsorbable oral lavage solutions. If colonoscopy is normal, the next examination is in 10 years, as long as the patient does not experience a change in bowel habits or bleeding and does not have a change in family history. If a solitary polyp less than 1 cm is found and is completely removed, the next colonoscopy should be in 3 years. If a single polyp greater than 1 cm is found or if multiple polyps are found, follow-up colonoscopy should be performed in 1 year. If there is any concern about the adequacy of polyp removal, a follow-up examination within 6 months is prudent.

If cancer is found within an endoscopically removed polyp, a decision must be made whether polypectomy is sufficient treatment or whether surgical resection of the involved colonic segment and its accompanying mesenteric drainage is needed. The latter is chosen when there is a high likelihood of either persistent tumor at the original site or lymph node metastases. This determination is best made by close collaboration among the endoscopist, the surgeon, and the pathologist. Endoscopic polypectomy is sufficient treatment for a malignant polyp if the cancer is confined to the head of the *pedunculated* lesion, the margin of transection is uninvolved, there is no lymphovascular invasion, and the cancer is well differentiated. In most other instances, segmental colectomy is indicated, except for the patient who has serious co-morbid conditions that make the likelihood of surgical complications greater than any oncologic benefit derived from surgery. If cancer is found within an endoscopically removed *sessile* polyp, surgery is usually required even in the absence of any adverse prognostic features because there is no safety zone provided by a stalk, the lesion may not be completely removed, and assessment of the margins may not be possible if the lesion was removed in a piecemeal fashion.

SURVEILLANCE

The term *surveillance,* rather than screening, is used when underlying conditions place the patient at high risk of the condition being sought, which, in this instance, is colorectal cancer. Evaluating patients at risk must take into consideration that there is a reasonable chance that the chosen diagnostic test will yield a positive result. Therefore, the test must be sensitive and specific, and it must also provide an opportunity to obtain tissue for diagnosis and must be therapeutic as well. In this regard, colonoscopy is perhaps the best surveillance test. For the conditions described in the following sections, fecal occult blood testing with flexible sigmoidoscopy is not sufficient. Flexible sigmoidoscopy with air contrast barium enema can be considered if colonoscopy cannot be performed because of a tortuous colon.

Familial Colorectal Cancer

Familial colorectal cancer refers to clustering of colorectal cancer within a family, but the criteria for a dominantly inherited syndrome are not satisfied. The cause of familial colorectal cancer is not known, although it is thought to represent a combination of environmental and hereditary factors. As stated earlier, the low-risk person has a 2% likelihood of developing colorectal cancer. The risk increases to 1 in 17 if there is a first-degree relative of any age with colorectal cancer, 1 in 10 if the first-degree relative was less than 50 years old at the time of diagnosis, and 1 in 6 if there are two first-degree relatives at any age with colorectal cancer. Surveillance recommendations for unaffected, at-risk family members are as follows:

One first-degree relative more than 60 years old: low-risk screening, start at age 40 years
One first-degree relative less than 60 years old: colonoscopy at age 10 years less than the first-degree relative; repeat every 5 years
One first-degree relative plus another family member: same as above

These recommendations may change as our understanding of familial cancer evolves.

Familial Adenomatous Polyposis

Inherited as an autosomal dominant trait, FAP is estimated to occur in 1 of 7000 live births. Although FAP is responsible for only 1% of the entire colorectal cancer burden in this country, cancer is virtually guaranteed by the age 40 years if FAP is left untreated. Variants of FAP include Gardner's syndrome (osteomas, desmoid tumors, sebaceous cysts) and Turcot's syndrome (central nervous system tumors). The gene responsible for FAP was localized to the long arm of chromosome 5 and is known as the adenomatous polyposis coli (*APC*) gene. The protein product of this gene functions as a tumor suppressor; gene mutations cause a truncated protein product and resulting loss of tumor suppression. As a result, there is a propensity for epithelial neoplasia. The truncated protein product can be detected in a peripheral blood sample of an affected person and is used to direct further genetic sequencing and direct mutational analyses.

FAP should be suspected in any family in which successive generations have been affected with colon cancer at an early age. Regarding surveillance, the following clinical observations have helped to establish current guidelines. Colorectal polyps rarely develop before puberty and usually are not found in the proximal colon unless the rectum and sigmoid are involved. Colorectal cancer does not develop before the late teens, although anecdotal reports of cancer occurring in younger patients can be found. Surveillance of family members at risk is performed with either genetic or clinical (endoscopic) programs. The chief advantage of the former is that if genetic testing proves negative in an at-risk person, endoscopic screening can be avoided. If genetic testing is desired, consultation and counseling with a geneticist are considered essential and begin with obtaining a peripheral blood sample from a family member known to have FAP. This person is tested first because the specific mutation in the *APC* gene is shared by all affected people in a particular family. The protein truncation test is performed; there is an 80% likelihood of identifying the mutation. If the test does not identify a mutation in an affected person, genetic testing is not helpful, and at-risk family members should be enrolled in an endoscopic surveillance program. If the test identifies a mutation in an affected person, at-risk relatives can then be tested for the same mutation; this testing begins at puberty. If a mutation is identified in an at-risk family member, prompt endoscopic surveillance is instituted because penetrance is near 100%. If an at-risk relative does not share the same mutation in the *APC* gene, FAP has probably been excluded; however, concerns about false-negative results have led some investigators to advise repeating the genetic test in 2 to 3 years or to recommend flexible sigmoidoscopy at age 18, 25, and 35 years. If FAP has been excluded, screening recommendations for low-risk persons should be instituted.

Clinical surveillance for at-risk family members is performed with periodic flexible sigmoidoscopic examinations, beginning at puberty. Colonoscopy is not required. Endoscopic surveillance is recommended for at-risk persons who are known to have an *APC* mutation but have not shown phenotypic disease and for at-risk persons who have not undergone genetic testing for whatever reason. In this latter group, surveillance is paramount because their status is not known, and they have a 50% chance of having inherited the disease. Furthermore, detecting FAP only after symptoms (bleeding) have developed makes it more likely that cancer is present. Duodenal screening for polyps should begin by age 25 years; ampullary carcinoma is the second most common cancer in these patients.

Once there is phenotypic disease (colonic polyposis), surgical treatment is performed at the earliest convenience for the patient. The type of surgical procedure performed is determined in large part by how extensively the rectum is involved. If the rectum has 20 or fewer polyps, it can be spared. In these situations, the surgeon removes the abdominal portion of the colon and leaves its pelvic portion intact. An ileorectal anastomosis is performed; however, the rectal remnant must be watched with annual proctoscopy because of the 10% to 15% possibility of future rectal cancer. Many rectal polyps will regress spontaneously, and sulindac (Clinoril)* is also administered to control the rectum. If the rectum is heavily involved with polyps either at the onset or subsequently, the rectum cannot be saved. In this situation, the colon and rectum are removed, the anal canal and anal sphincter muscle are preserved, a neorectum is fashioned from the terminal ileum, and an anastomosis is constructed between the ileal reservoir and the anus. Fecal continence is less than perfect; however, the end result is far preferable to a permanent ileostomy, and there are few, if any, social, athletic, or sexual restrictions.

Hereditary Nonpolyposis Colorectal Cancer

Also inherited as an autosomal dominant disorder, HNPCC is associated with an 80% lifetime risk of developing colorectal cancer for those persons with the mutation. Affected persons are also at risk of developing extraintestinal malignant diseases including endometrial, ovarian, small bowel, renal, and gastric cancers. A detailed family history is essential and is all

*Not FDA-approved for this indication.

that is required to raise suspicion of this disease (see later). The following features also suggest HNPCC: early age of colorectal cancer (mean age, 44 years), proximal location within the colon (70% are proximal to the splenic flexure), high rate of synchronous or metachronous cancers (45% if the initial operation was less than a subtotal colectomy), and mucinous or poorly differentiated histologic features.

Family history criteria known as the Amsterdam criteria suggest the syndrome and have been dubbed the "3-2-1-0" rule. At least three relatives must have histologically confirmed colorectal cancer, one relative must be a first-degree relative of the other two. Colorectal cancer must involve at least two generations, and at least one case must involve someone less than 50 years of age. There should be no evidence of FAP. If these criteria are satisfied, a person must be considered at risk of HNPCC; however, many investigators have considered these criteria too strict, and some persons may escape detection for the following reasons. A kindred may not have an adequate number of relatives at risk to satisfy the Amsterdam criteria, or families may not be able to provide complete histories because of infertility issues, deaths from trauma or causes other than cancer, and lack of knowledge concerning all family members. Furthermore, the Amsterdam criteria do not take into consideration extraintestinal cancers. To circumnavigate these restraints and potentially identify more families at risk, the Bethesda criteria were established and include the following:

- Patients with colorectal cancer and a first-degree relative with colorectal cancer before the age of 45 years or an HNPCC-related cancer before age 45 years
- Patients with two HNPCC-related cancers
- Patients with poorly differentiated or right-sided cancers before age 45 years
- Patients with endometrial cancer before age 45 years
- Patients with a colorectal adenoma before age 40 years

HNPCC is caused by mutations to the genes that code for intranuclear proteins that correct errors in DNA replication, the DNA mismatch repair (MMR) system. These genetic sequences are located on chromosomes 2, 3, and 7. Five MMR genes have been identified: *hMLH1, hMSH2, hPMSS1, hPMS2,* and *hMSH2*. Approximately 90% of the mutations in HNPCC have been identified in *hMLH1* and *hMMSH2*. If errors in replication are not detected and repaired, segments of DNA with repetitive base sequences become unstable, a phenomenon known as *microsatellite instability*. This leads to dysfunction of oncogenes and tumor suppressor genes and results in carcinogenesis. Studies have shown that 75% to 95% of HNPCC tumors have microsatellite instability, in contrast to only 15% of sporadic cancers. Thus, the presence of microsatellite instability can be used as a potential marker for HNPCC and can be easily performed on resected specimens that have been fixed in paraffin.

Evaluation of at-risk relatives within a suspected HNPCC family can be performed with either clinical (endoscopic) or genetic testing. Regarding the former, colonoscopy is the test of choice and should begin at age 20 to 25 years or 10 years before the age of the youngest affected family member. The interval between examinations should be 2 years. The age at which intensive endoscopic surveillance should be discontinued is not well established. Approximately 10% of HNPCC cancers occur after the age of 60 years; therefore, frequent colonoscopy should be continued until co-morbid health conditions make such an approach unwarranted.

Genetic surveillance of at-risk family members is undertaken according to which criteria raised suspicion. If the Amsterdam criteria are satisfied, direct gene sequencing of an affected family member may be the first step, and one should first sequence the *hMLH1* and *hMSH2* genes. Once the exact mutation is known within a given family, at-risk relatives are tested for the same mutation with a peripheral blood sample. If the mutation is not present, HNPCC has not been inherited, and low-risk screening is instituted for that patient. Persons who test positive for the mutation have an 80% lifetime risk of developing colorectal cancer. Management of these patients may be with an endoscopic surveillance program, or it may be more aggressive, with prophylactic subtotal colectomy and ileorectal anastomosis. If suspicion was raised because of the Bethesda criteria, microsatellite instability testing on the affected relative's tumor may be performed as an initial screening test. If the tumor is microsatellite instability positive, then one may proceed with direct gene sequencing as outlined earlier. Consultation with an experienced geneticist or HNPCC registry is strongly encouraged, to streamline the testing along the most efficient pathway.

Once a cancer is found in a patient with HNPCC, surgical choices include segmental colectomy or subtotal colectomy with ileorectal anastomosis. The latter is perhaps the more sensible choice if one considers a metachronous cancer rate of 45% over the next 10 years. Of course, rectal surveillance must be instituted if an ileorectal anastomosis is performed. If rectal cancer is found and the patient has acceptable sphincter function, total proctocolectomy with an ileal pouch–anal anastomosis is the preferred operation.

One must not omit surveillance for extracolonic cancers. The lifetime risk of developing endometrial cancer is one third by age 70 years and is 10% for ovarian cancer, again by 70 years of age. Surveillance for endometrial cancer is performed with annual endometrial aspiration and transvaginal ultrasound beginning at age 25 to 35 years. Surveillance for ovarian cancer is performed with transvaginal ultrasound and serum CA 125 determinations annually beginning at the same age. Surveillance for small bowel, renal, and gastric cancers has not been well studied, and there are no universally accepted protocols.

Ulcerative Colitis

The association between *ulcerative colitis* and cancer has been known for quite some time. Some subgroups of patients with ulcerative colitis are at an especially high risk of cancer, and these include patients with total colonic involvement (pancolitis) and those with disease of long duration. The risk is increased approximately 1% to 2 % per year after 10 years of ulcerative colitis. Patients with primary sclerosing cholangitis are also at higher risk. Prevention of cancer requires removal of all mucosa at risk; such treatment would subject countless patients to radical surgery that may not be necessary. Surveillance programs have been promoted that are begun 8 years after the onset of pancolitis or 12 years after the onset of left-sided disease. Colonoscopy is performed every 1 to 2 years, with random biopsies every 10 cm. Biopsies are taken from flat mucosa that appears suspicious by nature of its color or nodular texture, from elevated or polypoid lesions, and from strictures. The presence of dysplasia is regarded by many as a precancerous marker and, consequently, an indication for colectomy. There are no convincing data, however, that colonoscopic surveillance programs reduce the mortality from colorectal cancer. If surgery is required for ulcerative colitis, total proctocolectomy with construction of an ileal reservoir and of an ileal pouch–anal anastomosis is considered the operation of choice for fit patients with normal sphincter function. The anal transition zone is preserved to enhance fecal continence. If the patient has colon cancer, this operation may still be performed; however, the operation is changed somewhat to include removal of the anal transition zone. If the patient has a middle to lower rectal cancer, the proctocolectomy should still be performed, although construction of the ileal pouch and anastomosis to the anus should be delayed pending completion of adjuvant pelvic radiation and/or chemotherapy.

SURGICAL CONSIDERATIONS FOR COLON CANCER

Once the diagnosis of colon cancer is made, the patient should be prepared for surgery. Co-morbid medical conditions should be addressed and optimized. Precautions should be taken for deep venous thrombosis prophylaxis, especially if the patient has a prior history of this disorder. If the patient has not lost a significant amount of weight and serum liver chemistry results are normal, most surgeons do not routinely obtain computed tomograms of the abdomen; however, the liver, all peritoneal surfaces, and the ovaries should be assessed intraoperatively. Bowel preparation is necessary to reduce the incidence of postoperative infections. This can be accomplished in various ways, but it generally involves a combination of cathartics, lavage solutions, and oral or intravenous antibiotics. The cathartic of choice is a hypertonic sodium phosphate laxative solution (Fleet) given the day before the operation. Caution should be exercised in patients with congestive heart failure, renal insufficiency, and hyperphosphatemia. Lavage solutions are nonabsorbable and do not cause fluid retention or shifts; however, the high volume (4 L) needed to cleanse the colon effectively may be intolerable for some patients. Likewise, oral antibiotics specific for anerobic and gram-negative pathogens may not be tolerated during bowel cleansing, and for this reason many surgeons use only intravenous antibiotics given shortly before the time of incision.

Laparoscopic colon surgery has become increasingly feasible and popular. Cited benefits include shorter hospital stay, faster return to preoperative functional status, less pain, fewer adhesions, and improved cosmesis. Concerns regarding laparoscopy include the ability to assess the extent of disease adequately (because palpation is not possible), whether a wide mesenteric clearance of potentially metastatic lymph nodes is possible, and whether recurrence of cancer in the wounds is increased. As laparoscopic techniques, laparoscopic instrumentation, and preoperative imaging studies have improved over the years, these concerns have been allayed for the most part. Laparoscopic colectomy for cancer remains a hotly debated topic, and studies thus far have shown that it probably provides oncologic results at least as good as those of conventional surgery. With insurance-driven concerns regarding costs, hospital stays have been reduced substantially, even for open surgery. If the patient has a large, bulky tumor that is fixed or invades adjacent structures, open surgery remains the technique of choice. Outcome studies have clearly shown that the most important factor in colon cancer surgery is the skill and experience of the surgeon, not whether laparoscopic or open surgery was performed.

After colectomy for cancer, follow-up is crucial; however, the most efficient means of doing so is controversial. The goal of a follow-up program is to detect local recurrence at its earliest and most curable stage. Recurrence of colorectal cancer is seen in approximately 40% of patients and is most likely to occur in the first 2 years. Therefore follow-up should be most intense during this period. At least two studies have shown that patients undergoing periodic history taking, physical examinations, and serum carcinoembryonic antigen determinations are more likely to have curative re-resections, improved 5-year survival rates after re-resection, and improved overall cumulative 5-year survival rates.

RECTAL CANCER

Rectal cancer has distinct differences from colon cancer. When similar stages are compared, rectal cancer is associated with higher recurrence rates. Patient-related concerns unique to rectal cancer include the fear of incontinence, permanent colostomies, and genitourinary dysfunction. The impact of the surgeon's expertise and skill on oncologic results and on the patient's gastrointestinal and genitourinary function and is even more pronounced compared with colon cancer.

The approach to the patient with rectal cancer must be individualized, taking into consideration the location of the tumor, the extent of local disease, the presence of metastatic disease, and the ability of the patient to tolerate a major pelvic operation. Three major advances since the early 1990s have had a major impact on the management of these patients: the use of endorectal ultrasound to stage local disease, the use of radiation and chemotherapy either preoperatively or postoperatively, and improved techniques of removing the regional lymphatic network and avoidance of a stoma.

Endorectal ultrasound is performed without sedation and with minimal discomfort. The probe is inserted transanally, and the tumor and rectal mesentery are examined to determine the depth of tumor penetration within the rectal wall and the presence of metastatic lymph nodes. Ultrasound is more accurate than computed tomography with respect to these issues and is certainly less expensive. Furthermore, ultrasound can be performed at the time of the initial consultation either in the office or at the patient's bedside in the hospital. If the lesion is confined to the superficial layers of the rectal wall and there are no suspicious lymph nodes, transanal excision may be considered if the lesion is accessible. In contrast, if the lesion has penetrated the full thickness of the wall, is adherent to or invading the prostate, seminal vesicles, or vagina, or has metastasized to neighboring lymph nodes, preoperative neoadjuvant radiation and chemotherapy should be considered.

Rectal cancer has become a multidisciplinary disease. Surgery alone is appropriate only for those lesions that have not penetrated beyond the muscularis propria or spread to lymph nodes. For lesions that have penetrated deeply or have spread to lymph nodes, a National Cancer Institute consensus statement was issued in 1991 declaring that the standard of care was to administer postoperative radiation and chemotherapy. Improved outcome was noted for patients so treated. Pioneers in the United States and abroad, however, began to administer radiation preoperatively and cited even better results, although many of these studies have been criticized for various reasons. Now the trend is to administer preoperative radiation and chemotherapy for lesions that, by ultrasound examination, have penetrated beyond the wall or have spread into lymph nodes. There are many theoretical advantages of giving radiation and chemotherapy before rather than after surgery; however, the details of this controversy are beyond the scope of this discussion. Perhaps the chief advantages are that such therapy is more effective if given before an operation, downstaging and improved resectability are noted, and gastrointestinal function is better because the radiated tissue is removed during surgery.

As stated previously, the skill and expertise of the surgeon are extremely critical. This has been proved in numerous outcomes studies in the United States and in Europe, including Scandinavia. Some of these studies looked at the technique of total mesorectal excision, which involves dissecting along proper fascial planes and sparing the autonomic nerves governing genitourinary function. When such a dissection is performed, lower local recurrence rates can be realized because of improved clearance of lymph node–bearing tissue within the pelvis. In addition, a surgeon skilled in the techniques of pelvic surgery is more adept at reconstructive procedures and avoidance of permanent colostomies.

SUMMARY

Colorectal cancer is a common malignant disease and is the second leading cause of cancer-related deaths in the United States. It is imperative that screening programs be instituted for patients when they reach 50 years of age. Such programs have been shown to reduce the mortality from colorectal cancer. It is also imperative that high-risk groups be identified, so proper surveillance programs can be followed. A family history will usually identify kindreds with FAP or HNPCC, and asymptomatic at-risk family members can then be enrolled in either clinical (endoscopic) or genetic surveillance programs. For these patients, consultation with a geneticist or registry physician is strongly encouraged. When surgery is required, it is essential that the patient be referred to a surgeon whose practice has a high volume of colorectal cancer cases. Better oncologic and functional results can then be anticipated.

INTESTINAL PARASITES

method of
J. DICK MACLEAN, M.D.
McGill University Centre for Tropical Diseases
Montreal General Hospital, Canada

and

THERESA W. GYORKOS, PH.D.
Department of Epidemiology and Biostatistics
McGill University, Montreal, Canada

THERAPEUTIC APPROACH

Intestinal parasites may be subdivided in several ways that orient the clinician searching for therapeutic options. One approach is taxonomic, dividing all parasites into protozoa, nematodes, cestodes, and trematodes (Table 1). Specific drugs often have a therapeutic impact on many parasites within the same taxonomic group (e.g., all trematodes except *Fasciola* respond to praziquantel).

A second approach divides all parasites based on their capacity to multiply in the intestine of the human host. All protozoa and some important nematodes (e.g., *Strongyloides* spp.) will do this. The therapeutic approach to parasites that multiply is eradication, whereas for the parasites that don't multiply, a reduction in their numbers may be sufficient.

Another important approach turns on the question of host immunocompetence or lack thereof. For parasites that produce increased pathology in the immunocompromised host (e.g., *Cryptosporidium, Isospora*, microsporidia, *Strongyloides*), special care in selecting the therapeutic agent and duration of therapy is required.

Last, community-based therapy has its own characteristics. In endemic areas, the choice of a community-based treatment strategy for intestinal helminth infections (i.e., whether systematic treatment, targeted treatment or selective treatment) depends on costs and

TABLE 1. **Taxonomic Divisions of Intestinal Parasites**

Protozoa	Nematodes	Cestodes	Trematodes	Coinfection in Endemic Areas
Balantidium	*Ancylostoma duodenale*	*Diphyllobothrium*	Intestinal trematodes	Nematodes
Blastocystis	*Ancylostoma caninum*	*Hymenolepis*	Liver trematodes	Schistosomiasis
Cryptosporidium	*Angiostrongylus*	*Taenia*	*Schistosoma*	
Cyclospora	*Anisakis*			
Dientamoeba	*Ascaris*			
Entamoeba	*Capillaria*			
Giardia	*Enterobius*			
Isospora	*Strongyloides*			
Microsporidium	*Trichinella*			
Nonpathogens	*Trichuris*			
	Trichostrongylus			

the magnitude of the prevalence and intensity of infection in the community.

Most drugs recommended here for parasite therapy are available commercially. Some recommendations are for uses not recommended by the Food and Drug Administration. Some agents manufactured abroad may be obtained by contacting the parasitic disease drug service of the Centers for Disease Control and Prevention (CDC) in Atlanta, Georgia (telephone: 404-639-3670). In Canada, restricted drugs can be obtained by approval of the Special Access Programme, Health Canada, Ottawa (telephone: 613-941-2108).

Recommended drugs and specific doses are listed in Table 2.

PROTOZOA

Balantidium coli

Found throughout the world, especially in swine-breeding regions, this large ciliate produces an ulcerative colitis. Clinical presentation can range from the asymptomatic to fulminant dysentery with fever. The diagnosis is made on stool microscopy or on colonic mucosal biopsy. Treatment is a tetracycline.

Blastocystis hominis

The significance of this frequently found organism (prevalence in up to 25% of stools of tropical travelers) is controversial. No anatomic pathology has been found. There have been anecdotal reports of resolution of diarrhea and gas when the organism is eradicated. Metronidazole (Flagyl), iodoquinol (Yodoxin), and paromomycin (Humatin) have been used with unimpressive results.

Cryptosporidium

This parasitic infection is a zoonosis found in a wide range of animals. It can easily contaminate inadequately treated municipal water supplies and can produce epidemics of diarrhea. It is also found infrequently as a cause of diarrhea in travelers. The illness presents as an acute enteritis, diarrhea with gas, without blood, mucus or fever and lasts 1–2 weeks in the immunocompetent host. It produces a chronic profuse wasting (malabsorption) diarrhea in severely immunocompromised HIV-infected patients.

Diagnosis may be made by stool microscopy (an acid-fast Kinyoun or fluorescent auramine-rhodamine stain), stool antigen capture testing, or small intestine biopsy.

There is no adequate treatment for *Cryptosporidium* infections. Almost all infections in the immunocompetent will resolve without treatment in 1–3 weeks. In the immunocompromised, in particular in those with CD4 counts below 100, treatment will involve supportive therapy (e.g., trials of less-than-ideal agents and adjustments of antiretroviral agents aimed at raising the CD4 count). Recent therapeutic agents include paromomycin, azithromycin (Zithromax), and nitazoxanide (Alinia).

Cyclospora

A small intestine infection found on all continents but most frequently in travelers to developing countries and, most recently, imported on raspberries from Central America, the epidemiology of this organism is poorly understood. The organism, producing an enteritis of diarrhea, cramps, and gas that can last several weeks, is diagnosed with stool microscopy using acid-fast stains (e.g., Kinyoun). Treatment with trimethoprim/sulfamethoxazole in the early days of infection appears to decrease the duration of symptoms.

Dientamoeba fragilis

This poorly understood organism is found in both travelers and nontravelers. As with *Giardia,* it is frequently found in stool examinations of the asymptomatic but has been associated with persistent watery diarrhea, gas, and cramps. Because there is no cyst form, this protozoan will disintegrate and go undiagnosed if stool is not collected directly into a preservative. Diagnosis is made by stool microscopy using standard laboratory stains (e.g., hematoxylin). The treatment of choice is iodoquinol* with less

*Not FDA approved for this indication.

TABLE 2. **Drugs for Parasitic Infections***

Infection		Drug	Adult Dosage	Pediatric Dosage
AMEBIASIS *(Entamoeba histolytica)*				
Asymptomatic				
Drug of choice:		Iodoquinol (Yodoxin)	650 mg tid × 20 d	30–40 mg/kg/d (max. 2 g) in 3 doses × 20 d
	OR	Paromomycin	25–35 mg/kg/d in 3 doses × 7 d	25–35 mg/kg/d in 3 doses × 7 d
Alternative:		Diloxanide furoate[1,2] (Humatin)[4]	500 mg tid × 10 d	20 mg/kg/d in 3 doses × 10 d
Mild to moderate intestinal disease[3]				
Drug of choice:[4]		Metronidazole (Flagyl)	500–750 mg tid × 7–10 d	35–50 mg/kg/d 3 doses × 7–10 d
	OR	Tinidazole[5,1]	2 g/d divided tid × 3 d	50 mg/kg (max. 2 g) qd × 3 d
Severe intestinal and extraintestinal disease[3]				
Drug of choice:		Metronidazole	750 mg tid × 7–10 d	35–50 mg/kg/d in 3 doses × 7–10 d
	OR	Tinidazole[5,1]	800 mg tid × 5 d	60 mg/kg/d (max. 2 g) × 5 d
ANCYLOSTOMA caninum *(Eosinophilic enterocolitis)*				
Drug of choice:		Albendazole[7] (Albenza)[1]	400 mg once	400 mg once
	OR	Mebendazole (Vermox)	100 mg bid × 3 d	100 mg bid × 3 d
	OR	Pyrantel pamoate[7,1] (Antiminth)	11 mg/kg (max. 1 g) × 3 d	11 mg/kg (max. 1 g) × 3 d
	OR	Endoscopic removal		
Ancylostoma duodenale, see Hookworm				
ANGIOSTRONGYLIASIS				
Angiostrongylus costaricensis				
Drug of choice:		See footnote 12		
ANISAKIASIS (Anisakis)				
Treatment of choice:		Surgical or endoscopic removal		
ASCARIASIS *(Ascaris lumbricoides, roundworm)*				
Drug of choice:		Albendazole[7,1]	400 mg once	400 mg once
	OR	Mebendaole	100 mg bid × 3 d or 500 mg once	100 mg bid × 3 d or 500 mg once
	OR	Pyrantel pamoate[7]	11 mg/kg once (max. 1 g)	11 mg/kg once (max. 1 g)
BALANTIDIASIS *(Balantidium coli)*				
Drug of choice:		Tetracycline[7,14,1]	500 mg qid × 10 d	40 mg/kg/d (max. 2 g) in 4 doses × 10 d
Alternative:		Metronidazole[7]	750 mg tid × 5 d	35–50 mg/kg/d in 3 doses × 5 d
		Iodoquinol[7]	650 mg tid × 20 d	40 mg/kg/d in 3 doses × 20 d
BLASTOCYSTIS *hominis* infection				
Drug of choice:		See footnote 16		
CAPILLARIASIS *(Capillaria philippinensis)*				
Drug of choice:		Mebendazole[7]	200 mg bid × 20 d	200 mg bid × 20 d
Alternatives		Albendazole[7,1]	400 mg daily × 10 d	400 mg daily × 10 d
Clonorchis sinensis, see Fluke infection				
CRYPTOSPORIDIOSIS *(Cryptosporidium)*				
Drug of choice:		See footnote 17		
CYCLOSPORA infection				
Drug of choice:[19]		Trimethoprim-sulfamethoxazole[7] (Bactrim)[1]	TMP 160 mg, SMX 800 mg bid × 7–10 d	TMP 5 mg/kg, SMX 25 mg/kg bid × 7–10 d
DIENTAMOEBA fragilis infection				
Drug of choice:		Iodoquinol[1] (Yodoxin)	650 mg tid × 20 d	30–40 mg/kg/d (max. 2g) in 3 doses × 20 d
	OR	Paromomycin[7] (Humatin)	25–35 mg/kg/d in 3 doses × 7 d	25–35 mg/kg/d in 3 doses × 7 d
	OR	Tetracycline[7,14]	500 mg qid × 10 d	40 mg/kg/d (max. 2g) in 4 doses × 10 d
	OR	Metronidazole[1]	500–750 mg tid × 10 d	20–40 mg/kg/d in 3 doses × 10 d
Diphyllobothrium latum, see Tapeworm infection				
Entamoeba histolytica, see Amebiasis				
ENTEROBIUS *vermicularis* (pinworm) infection				
Drug of choice:[21]		Pyrantel pamoate	11 mg/kg base once (max. 1 g); repeat in 2 weeks	11 mg/kg base once (max. 1 g); repeat in 2 weeks
	OR	Mebendazole	100 mg once; repeat in 2 weeks	100 mg once; repeat in 2 weeks
	OR	Albendazole[7,1]	400 mg once; repeat in 2 weeks	400 mg once; repeat in 2 weeks

Continued

TABLE 2. **Drugs for Parasitic Infections—cont'd**

Infection	Drug	Adult Dosage	Pediatric Dosage
Fasciola hepatica, see Fluke infection			
FLUKE, hermaphroditic, infection			
Clonorchis sinensis **(Chinese liver fluke)**			
Drug of choice:	Praziquantel (Biltricide)	75 mg/kg/d in 3 doses × 1 d	75 mg/kg/d in 3 doses × 1 d
OR	Albendazole[7,1]	10 mg/kg × 7 d	10 mg/kg × 7 d
Fasciola hepatica **(sheep liver fluke)**			
Drug of choice:[30]	Triclabendazole*[,1]	10 mg/kg once	10 mg/kg once
Alternative	Bithionol*[,1]	30–50 mg/kg × 10–15 doses	30–50 mg/kg on alternate days × 10–15 doses
Fasciolopsis buski, Heterophyes heterophyes, Metagonimus yokogawai **(intestinal flukes)**			
Drug of choice:	Praziquantel[7]	75 mg/kg/d in 3 doses × 1 d	75 mg/kg/d in 3 doses × 1 d
Metorchis conjunctus **(North American liver fluke)**[31]			
Drug of choice:	Praziquantel[7]	75 mg/kg/d in 3 doses × 1 d	75 mg/kg/d in 3 doses × 1 d
Nanophyetus salmincola			
Drug of choice:	Praziquantel[7]	60 mg/kg/d in 3 doses × 1 d	60 mg/kg/d in 3 doses × 1 d
Opisthorchis viverrini **(Southeast Asian liver fluke)**			
Drug of choice:	Praziquantel	75 mg/kg/d in 3 doses × 1 d	75 mg/kg/d in 3 doses × 1 d
GIARDIASIS *(Giardia lambia)*			
Drug of choice:	Metronidazole[7,1]	250 mg tid × 5 d	15 mg/kg/d in 3 doses × 5 d
Alternatives:[33]	Quinacrine[2]	100 mg tid × 5 d (max. 300 mg/d)	2 mg/kg tid × 5 d (max. 300 mg/d)
	Tinidazole [5,1]	2 g once	50 mg/kg once (max. 2 g)
	Furazolidone	100 mg qid × 7–10 d	6 mg/kg/d in 4 doses × 7–10 d
	Paromomycin[7,34,1]	25–35 mg/kg/d in 3 doses × 7 d	25–35 mg/kg/d in 3 doses × 7 d
HOOKWORM infection *(Ancylostoma duodenale, Necator americanus)*			
Drug of choice:	Albendazole[7,1]	400 mg once	400 mg once
OR	Mebendazole	100 mg bid × 3 d or 500 mg once	100 mg bid × 3 d or 500 mg once
OR	Pyrantel pamoate[7,1]	11 mg/kg (max. 1 g) × 3 d	11 mg/kg (max. 1 g) × 3 d
Hymenolepis nana, see Tapeworm infection			
ISOSPORIASIS *(Isospora belli)*			
Drug of choice:[37]	Trimethoprim-sulfamethoxazole[7,1]	160 mg TMP, 800 mg SMX bid × 10 d	TMP 5 mg/kg, SMX 25 mg/kg bid × 10 d
MICROSPORIDIOSIS			
Ocular *(Encephalitozoon hellem, Encephalitozoon cuniculi, Vittaforma cornease [Nosema corneum])*			
Drug of choice:	Albendazole[7] plus fumagillin[77*]	400 mg bid	
Intestinal *(Enterocytozoon bieneusi, Encephalitozoon [Septata intestinalis])*			
E. bieneusi[78]			
Drug of choice:	Fumagillin*	60 mg /d PO × 14 d	
E. intestinalis			
Drug of choice:	Albendazole[7,1]	400 mg bid × 21 d	
Disseminated *(E. hellem, E. cuniculi, E. intestinalis, Pleistophora* sp., *Trachipleistophora* sp. *and Brachiola vesicularum)*			
Drug of choice:[79]	Albendazole[7,1]	400 mg bid	
Necator americanus, see HOOKWORM infection			
Opisthorchis viverrini, see FLUKE infection			
Pinworm, see ENTEROBIUS			
Roundworm, see Ascariasis			
SCHISTOSOMIASIS *(Bilharziasis)*			
S. japonicum			
Drug of choice	Praziquantel (Biltricide)	60 mg/kg/d in 3 doses × 1 d	60 mg/kg/d in 3 doses × 1 d
S. mansoni			
Drug of choice:	Praziquantel	40 mg/kg/d in 2 doses × 1 d	40 mg/kg/d in 2 doses × 1 d
Alternative:	Oxamniquine[86] (Vansil)	15 mg/kg once[87]	20 mg/kg/d in 2 doses × 1 d[87]
S. mekongi			
Drug of choice:	Praziquantel	60 mg/kg/d in 3 doses × 1 d	60 mg/kg/d in 3 doses × 1 d
STRONGYLOIDIASIS *(Strongyloides stercoralis)*			
Drug of choice:[88]	Ivermectin	200 µg/kg/d × 1–2 d	200 µg/kg/d × 1–2 d
Alternative:	Thiabendazole	50 mg/kg/d in 2 doses (max. 3 g/d) × 2 d[89]	50 mg/kg/d in 2 doses (max. 3 g/d) × 2 d[89]
TAPEWORM infection – Adult (intestinal stage)			
Diphyllobothrium latum **(fish),** ***Taenia saginata*** **(beef),** ***Taenia solium*** **(pork),** ***Dipylidium caninum*** **(dog)**			
Drug of choice:	Praziquantel[7,1]	5–10 mg/kg once	5–10 mg/kg once

Continued

TABLE 2. **Drugs for Parasitic Infections—cont'd**

Infection	Drug	Adult Dosage	Pediatric Dosage
Alternative:	Niclosamide	2 g once	50 mg/kg once
Hymenolepis nana **(dwarf tapeworm)**			
Drug of choice:	Praziquantel[7,1]	25 mg/kg once	25 mg/kg once
–Larval (tissues stage)			
TRICHINOSIS (*Trichinella spiralis*)			
Drug of choice:	Steroids for severe symptoms **plus** mebendazole[7]	200–400 mg tid × 3 d, then 400–500 mg tid × 10 d	200–400 mg tid × 3 d, then 400–500 mg tid × 10 d
Alternative:	Albendazole[7]	400 mg bid × 8–14 d	400 mg bid × 8–14 d
TRICHOSTRONGYLUS *infection*			
Drug of choice:	Pyrantel pamoate[7]	11 mg/kg base once (max. 1 g)	11 mg/kg once (max. 1 gram)
Alternative:	Mebendazole[7,1]	100 mg bid × 3 d	100 mg bid × 3 d
OR	Albendazole[7,1]	400 mg once	400 mg once
TRICHURIASIS (*Trichuris trichiura,* whipworm)			
Drug of choice:	Mebendazole[1]	100 mg bid × 3 d or 500 mg once	100 mg bid × 3 d or 500 mg once
Alternative:	Albendazole[7,1]	400 mg × 3 d	400 mg × 3 d
Whipworm, See Trichuriasis			

*Adapted with special permission from The Medical Letter on Drugs and Therapeutics. The Medical Letter, Inc. New Rochelle, New York, April, 2002, pp. 1-12.

[1] Availability problems.

[2] The drug is not available commercially, but as a service can be compounded by Medical Center Pharmacy, New Haven, CT (203-688-6816) or Panorama Compounding Pharmacy 6744 Balboa Blvd, Van Nuys, CA 91406 (800-247-9767).

[3] Treatment should be followed by a course of iodoquinol or paromomycin in the dosage used to treat asymptomatic amebiasis.

[4] Nitazoxanide (an investigational drug in the U.S. manufactured by Romark Laboratories, Tampa, FL, 813-282-8544, www.romarklabs.com) 500 mg bid × 3 d is also effective for treatment of amebiasis (Rossignol JF et al: J Infect Dis 184:381, 2001)

[5] A nitro-imidazole similar to metronidazole, but not marketed in the U.S., tinidazole appears to be at least as effective as metronidzole and better tolerated. Ornidazole, a similar drug, is also used outside the U.S.

[7] An approved drug, but considered investigational for this condition by the U.S. Food and Drug Administration.

[12] Mebendazole has been used in experimental animals.

[14] Use of tetracyclines is contraindicated in pregnancy and in children younger than 8 years old.

[16] Clinical significance of these organisms is controversial, but metronidazole 750 mg tid × 10 d oriodoquinol 650 mg tid × 20 d has been reported to be effective (Stenzel DJ, Borenam PFL: Clin Microbiol Rev 9:563, 1996) Metronidazole resistance may be common (Haresh K, et al: Trop Med Int Health 4:274, 1999). Trimethoprim-sulfamethoxazole is an alternative regimen (Ok UZ et al: Am J Gastroenterol 94:3245, 1999)

[17] Three days of treatment with nitazoxanide (see footnote 4) may be useful for treating cryptosporidial diarrhea in immunocompetent patients. The recommended dose in adults is 500 mg bid, in children 4–11 years old, 200 mg bid, and in children 1–3 years old, 100 mg bid (Rossignol JA et al: J Infect Dis 184:103, 2001). A small randomized, double-blind trial in symptomatic HIV-infected patients found paromomycin similar to placebo (Hewitt RG et al: Clin Infect Dis 3:1084, 2000).

[19] HIV infected patients may need higher dosage and long-term maintenance. In case of cotrimoxazole intolerance, ciprofloxacin 500 mg bid × 7 d has been effective (Verdier R-I et al: Ann Intern Med 132:885, 2000).

[21] Since all family members are usually effected, treatment of the entire household is recommended.

[30] Unlike infections with other flukes, *Fasciola hepatica* infections may not respond to praziquantel. Triclabendazole, a veterinary fasciolide, may be safe and effective but data are limited (Graham CS et al: Clin Infect Dis 33:1, 2001). It is available from Victoria Pharmacy, Zurich, Switzerland, 41-1-211-24-32. It should be given with food for better absorption.

[31] MacLean JD et al: Lancet 347:154, 1996.

[33] In one study, nitazoxanide (see footnote 4) was as effective as metronidazole and has been used successfully in high doses to treat a case of *Giardia* resistant to metronidazole and albendazole (Ortiz JJ et al: Aliment Pharmacol Ther 15:1409, 2001; Abboud P et al: Clin Infect Dis 32:1792, 2001). Albendazole 400 mg daily × 120,000 U bid for 10 days may also be effective (A Hall, Q Nahar: Trans R Soc Trop Med Hyg 87:84, 1993; Dutta AK et al: Indian J Pediatr 61:689, 1994. Bacitracin zinc or bacitracindazole and quinacrine given for 3 weeks has been effective for a small number of refractory infections (Nash TE et al: Clin Infect Dis 33:22, 2001).

[34] Not absorbed; may be useful for treatment of giardiasis in pregnancy.

[37] Immunosuppressed patients: TMP/SMX qid × 10 d followed by bid × 3 weeks. In sulfonamide-sensitive patients, pyrimethamine 50-75 mg daily in divided doses has been effective. HIV-infected may need long-term maintenance. Ciprofloxacin 500 mg bid × 7 d also been effective (Verdier R-I et al: Ann Intern Med 132:885, 2000).

[77] Ocular lesions due to *E. hellem* in HIV-infected patients have responded to fumagillin eyedrops prepared from *Fumidil-B*, a commercial product (Mid-Continent Agrimarketing, Inc., Olathe, Kansas, 800-547-1392) used to control a microsporidial disease of honey bees (Diesenhouse MC: Am J Ophthalmol 115:293, 1993).For lesions due to *V. corneae*, topical therapy is generally not effective and keratoplasty may be required (Davis RM et al: Ophthalmology 97:953, 1990).

[78] Oral fumagillin (see footnote 77, Sanofi Recherche, Gentilly, France) has been effective in treating *E. bieneusi* (Molina J-M et al: AIDS 14:1341, 2000), but has been associated with thrombocytopenia. Highly active antiretroviral therapy (HAART) may lead to microbiologic and clinical response in HIV-infected patients with microsporidial diarrhea (Foudraine NA et al: AIDS 12:35, 1998; Carr A et al: Lancet 351:256, 1998). Octreotide *(Sandostatin)* has provided symptomatic relief in some patients with large volume diarrhea.

[79] Molina J-M et al: J Infect Dis 171:245, 1995. There is no established treatment for *Pleistophora.*

[86] Oxamniquine has been effective in some areas in which praziquantel is less effective (Stelma FF et al: J Infect Dis 176:304 1997;). Oxamniquine is contraindicated in pregnancy.

[87] In East Africa, the dose should be increased to 30 mg/kg, and in Egypt and South Africa to 30 mg/kg/d × 2 d. Some experts recommend 40–60 mg/kg over 2–3 days in all of Africa (Shekhar KC: Drugs 42:379, 1991).

[88] In immunocompromised patients or disseminated disease, it may be necessary to prolong or repeat therapy or use other agents. A veterinary parenteral formulation of ivermectin was used in one patient (Chiodini PL et al: Lancet 355:43, 2000).

[89] This dose is likely to be toxic and may have to be decreased.

[98] Sexual partners should be treated simultaneously. Metronidazole-resistant strains have been reported and should be treated with metronidazole 2–4 g/d × 7–14 d. Desensitization has been recommended for patients allergic to metronidazole (Pearlman MD et al: Am J Obstet Gynecol 174:934, 1996). High dose tinidazole has been used for the treatment of metronidazole-resistant trichomoniasis (Sobel JD et al: Clin Infect Dis 33:1341, 2001).

Continued

TABLE 2. **Drugs for Parasitic Infections—cont'd**

MANUFACTURERS OF SOME ANTIPARASITIC DRUGS

albendazole-Albenza (GlaxoSmithKline)
[§]artemether – Artenam (Arenco, Belgium)
[§]artesunate – (Guilin No. 1 Factory, People's Republic of China
atovaquone – *Mepron* (GlaxoSmithKline)
atovaquone proguanil- *Malarone* (GlaxoSmithKline)
bacitracin – many manufacturers
[§]bacitracin-zinc – (Apothekernes Laboratorium A.S., Oslo, Norway)
[§]benznidazole – *Rochagan* (Roche, Brazil)
[†]bithionol – *Bitin* (Tanabe, Japan)
chloroquine HCI and chloroquine phospate – *Aralen* (Sanofi), others
crotamiton – Eurax (Westwood-Squibb)
dapsone – (Jacobus)
[†]diethylcarbamazine citrate USP – (University of Iowa School of Pharmacy)
[§]diloxanide furoate – *Furamide* (Boots, United Kingdom)
[§]eflornithine (Difluoromethylornithine, DFMO) – *Ornidyl* (Aventis)
furazolidone – *Furoxone* (Roberts)
[§]halofantrine – *Halfan* (GlaxoSmithKline)
iodoquinol – *Yodoxin* (Glenwood), others
ivermectin – *Stromectol* (Merck)
malathion – *Ovide* (Medicis)
mebendazole – *Vermox* (McNeil)
mefloquine – *Lariam* (Roche)
[§]meglumine antimonate – *Glucantime* (Aventis, France)
[†]melarsoprol – *Mel-B* (Specia)
metronidazole – *Flagyl* (Searle), others
[§]miltefosine – (Zentaris)
[§]niclosamide – *Yomesan* (Bayer, Germany)
[†]nifurtimox – *Lampit* (Bayer, Germany)
*nitazonaxide – *Cryptaz* (Romark)
[§]ornidazole – *Tiberal* (Roche, France)
oxamniquine – *Vansil* (Pfizer)
paromomycin – *Humatin* (Monarch); Leshcutan (Teva Pharmaceutical Industries, Ltd., Israel; topical formulation not available in US)
pentamidine – isethionate – *Pentam 300, NebuPent* (Fujisawa)
permethrin – Nix (GlaxoSmithKline), Elimnate (Allergan)
praziquantel – *Biltricide* (Bayer)
primaquine phosphate USP
[§]proguanil – *paludrine* (Wyeth Ayerst, Canada; AstraZeneca, United Kingdom); in combination with atovaquone as *malarone* (GlaxoSmithKline)
[§]propamidine isethionate – *Brolene* (Aventis, Canada)
pyrantel pamoate – *Antiminth* (Pfizer)
pyrethrins and piperonyl butoxide – *RID* (Pfizer), others
pyrimethamine USP – *Daraprim* (GlaxoSmithKline)
[§]quinine dihydrochloride
quinine sulfate – many manufacturers
[†]sodium stibogluconate – *Pentostam* (GlaxoSmithKline, United Kingdom)
*spiramycin – *Rovamycine* (Aventis)
[†]suramin sodium – (Bayer, Germany)
thiabendazole – *Mintezol* (Merck)
[§]tinidazole – *Fasigyn* (Pfizer)
*triclabendazole – Egaten (Novartis, Switzerland)
trimetrexate – *Neutrexin* (US Bioscience)

*Available in the U.S. only from the manufacturer.
[§]Not available in the U.S.
[†]Available under an Investigational New Drug (IND) protocol from the CDC Drug Service, Centers for Disease Control and Prevention, Atlanta, GA 30333;404-639-3670 (evenings, weekends, or holidays: 404-639-2888).

effective alternatives being doxycycline (Vibramycin), paromomycin, and metronidazole.

Entamoeba histolytica

This protozoan of the large intestine can be the cause of a serious infection "amebiasis" in geographic regions with inadequate sanitary facilities. Clinical illness includes dysentery and extraintestinal infections, the large majority being liver abscesses. Asymptomatic carriers of *E. histolytica* are common.

The treatment of amebiasis has become complicated in the past decade, not for want of antiamebic drugs, but because of clinicians' inability to determine whether the patient has the pathogenic species *E. histolytica* deserving of treatment, or the nonpathogenic look-alike species, *E. dispar*, which does not merit treatment. Because the parasitology microscopist cannot distinguish the two species from each other, the laboratory will report the presence of *E. histolytica/dispar*. Unless hematophagous trophozoites are present (indicating *E. histolytica* infection), the decision to treat or not is in the clinician's hands. In some countries *E. histolytica/dispar* is in fact >90% *E. dispar*, whereas in some tropical countries up to 50% may be *E. histolytica*.

Four nonmicroscopic laboratory tests may separate *E. histolytica* from *E. dispar*. Two tools (PCR and enzymatic pattern analysis) are reference laboratory resources, not usually available to the clinician. The other two (amebic serology and stool antigen capture testing) may be available and useful but their sensitivity and specificity are problematic. Amebic serology is positive in 80% to 95% of symptomatic *E. histolytica* infections, but specificity in the clinical setting is poor because of persistence of antibodies after a resolved infection. Amebic antigen capture tests on stool appear sensitive and specific in heavy infections but may be insensitive in light-intensity infections, as are found at times in carriers.

Metronidazole is the treatment of choice for amebic liver abscess or amebic dysentery proven by biopsy or the presence of hematophagous trophozoites in the stool. This is followed by a luminal amebicide (e.g., diloxanide,* diodoquin) because the metronidazole may not reach high enough levels in the lumen of the colon to eliminate intraluminal ameba.

There are a number of more difficult therapeutic challenges. How to treat an asymptomatic carrier of, or a nondysenteric individual with, *E. histolytica/dispar* will depend on the diagnostic tools available.

1. A positive *E. histolytica* antigen capture test is sufficient assurance that *E. histolytica* is present, but neither a negative *E. histolytica* antigen capture test

*Not available in the United States.

nor a positive *E. dispar* antigen capture test is sufficient assurance that *E. histolytica* is not present.

2. Positive serology from a microscopically positive patient neither rules in nor rules out *E. histolytica*; it is only highly suggestive.

Until more sensitive and specific tools are available to differentiate *E. histolytica* from *E. dispar* the clinician is left to treat all *E. histolytica/dispar* as if they were pathogenic *E. histolytica*.

Giardia

A protozoan of the small intestine, *Giardia* is a zoonotic parasite found in most animals in the world. It is most frequently acquired by identifiable risk groups, such as North Americans who travel to developing countries, who drink contaminated freshwater (e.g., from lakes, ponds, recreational waters) in North America, or who attend day care centers. The illness, an acute gassy diarrhea without fever, an enteritis, often resolves in 1 to 2 weeks without treatment, but in a small but unknown percent, a chronic symptomatology occurs, which is most difficult to manage in IgA-deficient hosts. Asymptomatic carriers are not infrequent.

Treatment of asymptomatics—other than those who may be a source of infection to others (e.g. food handlers, daycare center employees)—may not be necessary.

Drug treatment for *Giardia* includes metronidazole, furazolidone (Furoxone), paromomycin, tinidazole, secnidazole, and quinacrine. Quinacrine can only be obtained with difficulty and some imidazoles (tinidazole, secnidazole) are available only outside of North America.

No drug is 100% effective. Increasing resistance to the standard dosage of metronidazole seems to be occurring, although poorly documented, so that doubling or even tripling the dosage of metronidazole may help. Alternatively, a combination of two anti-*Giardia* drugs may work.

The laboratory diagnosis of *Giardia* by microscopy of two or three stool specimens or antigen-capture testing has a sensitivity of less than 90%. *Giardia* is found only intermittently in the stool. Small bowel biopsies and duodenal aspirates are inefficient and also not terribly sensitive.

Isospora

An infection rarely seen in the immunocompetent traveler, *Isospora* has become increasingly recognized in AIDS patients, particularly those from the tropics. No nonhuman source of this parasite has been found. The illness, like *Cryptosporidium*, is a self-limited enteritis of several weeks' duration—unless in the immunocompromised, in whom the illness is a chronic wasting (malabsorption) enteritis.

Diagnosis is with standard stool microscopy, aided at times with a fluorescent auramine-rhodamine stain.

*Not FDA approved for this indication.

Treatment is trimethoprim/sulfamethoxazole (Bactrim),* or, in the sulfa-allergic, pyrimethamine (Daraprim).*

Microsporidia

A number of microsporidia, the most frequent being *Enterocytozoon bieneusi* and *Encephalitozoon intestinalis*, are associated with enteritis and at times biliary tree infections. These are rarely seen in immunocompetent individuals but almost always occur in the severely immunocompromised (CD4 <50). Of note, however, the prevalence of microsporidiosis in AIDS patients has fallen dramatically since the advent of combination antiretroviral therapy. Intestinal infections present with watery diarrhea, malabsorption, and dehydration. Biliary tree infections present with right upper quadrant pain and a rising alkaline phosphatase level.

Standard stool parasitology microscopy will not reveal microsporidia, whereas a modified trichrome stain will. Light microscopy of small intestine biopsies may reveal the 1-μm organism, but electron microscopy is far more sensitive and will also allow for the determination of the genus, useful in treatment decisions.

Treatment of *E. intestinalis* is albendazole (Albenza).* Absorption and presumably effectiveness is increased by taking the drug with a fatty meal. Treatment of *E. bieneusi* is more difficult. Albendazole is much less effective for this organism. Fumagillin (Fumidil-B),* a microsporidium-static agent, has shown some promise. Hydration and nutritional support (magnesium, potassium, calcium) are important with oral semielemental or parenteral nutrition. Currently the primary treatment of choice for symptomatic *E. bieneusi* infections is with combination antiretroviral agents.

Nonpathogens

Some laboratories will report these stool organisms and others will not. Reporting their presence may suggest a greater likelihood that a pathogen is present but missed. Clinical circumstances will determine whether repeated stool examinations are merited. The nonpathogens (*Entamoeba coli, Endolimax nana, Entamoeba hartmanni, Iodamoeba buetschlii, Entamoeba dispar, Trichomonas hominis, Chilomastix mesnili*) have not been associated with clinical illness and are not treated.

NEMATODES

Ancylostoma duodenale and *Necator americanus* (Hookworms)

Found worldwide in regions with inadequate sanitation facilities, these worms are acquired through skin contact with skin-penetrating larvae that arise

*Not FDA approved for this indication.

from eggs in feces deposited on the ground or used as fertilizer. Symptoms are rare except with heavy worm burdens, which result in an iron deficiency and protein deficiency caused by the blood-sucking habits of the adults attached to the small intestine mucosa. Stool microscopy for the characteristic eggs is a sensitive diagnostic tool after the 5-week incubation period. Treatment is mebendazole (Vermox) or albendazole* with a 90% eradication or worm burden reduction.

Ancylostoma caninum

This infection found in Queensland, Australia, produces aphthous ulcers and focal inflammation in the distal small intestine that persists for about a month and is associated with abdominal (epigastria, mid-and, right lower quadrant) pain at times mimicking an appendicitis. Stools for parasites are negative and peripheral eosinophilia is variable. Laparoscopy and serology appear to be the most sensitive diagnostic tools. Treatment is a benzimidazole (mebendazole,* albendazole*). Failure to respond suggests an alternative diagnosis.

Angiostrongylus costaricensis

A nematode of rodents with a slug intermediate host is found in Central and South America, where inadvertent consumption of slugs in salads or in water appears to be the source. The worm infects the ileocecal region producing abscesses and infarcts that can mimic appendicitis. With no eggs found in stools, the diagnosis depends on clinical suspicion induced by peripheral eosinophilia and ultrasounds. Treatment remains anecdotal, with reported benefits from the use of benzimidazoles (e.g., mebendazole*) and diethylcarbamazine.*

Anisakis simplex (Herringworm) and *Pseudoterranova decipiens* (Codworm)

These small nematodes in the flesh of seawater fish, if eaten raw, infect the consumer of these fish. *Anisakis* causes esophageal or gastric distress, whereas *Pseudoterranova* can penetrate the stomach or small intestine wall producing an abscesslike lesion with associated symptoms. No eggs are found in feces. The infection rarely involves more than one worm and is diagnosed endoscopically and treated with endoscopic or surgical removal.

Ascaris lumbricoides (Roundworm)

This foot-long roundworm is found worldwide but more frequently in warm climate locations lacking adequate sanitation. Transmission is fecal-oral, frequently via garden produce where human feces have been deposited, often intentionally as fertilizer. The diagnosis is made with the easy identification of a visible worm passed in the feces or by identification of the typical eggs by stool microscopy. The vast majority of infected persons are asymptomatic, those with symptoms having heavy worm burdens. Symptoms range from abdominal pain to those associated with small intestine obstruction. Heavy intensity new infections can produce cough or a pneumonitis (Loeffler syndrome) during lung passage. Rarely, *Ascaris* enter the biliary tree or pancreatic duct, or pass through postsurgery intestinal suture lines.

Present treatment is a benzimidazole such as mebendazole* or albendazole* or a number of earlier but equally effective nonabsorbable anthelminthics. The treatment of intestinal obstruction may require surgery and Loeffler syndrome, patience, and, at times, steroids. In persons with low to moderate worm burdens, mebendazole treatment will reduce or eliminate the worm burden by between 90% and 95%.

Capillaria philippinensis

A small intestine nematode that is found especially in the Philippines, *C. philippinensis* is acquired by eating uncooked freshwater fish. The worm buries itself in the small intestine mucosa and shares with *Strongyloides* the capacity to produce eggs and larvae that mature to adults without leaving the host (autoinfection). Diarrhea, abdominal pain, malabsorption, and weight loss can produce an impressive illness. Diagnosis is by stool microscopy. Treatment is with benzimidazoles.

Enterobius vermicularis (Pinworm)

An infection worldwide, this small roundworm of the colon produces a perianal itch in a small percentage of those infected. External dissemination and autoinfection is greatly enhanced by the worm's nightly deposition of eggs on the perianal skin. These eggs then contaminate the bedding and clothes and are ingested by the already-infected host or others in the immediate family. Diagnosis by stool microscopy is insensitive. Microscopic examination of transparent sticky pinworm paddles applied to the perianal skin before arising in the morning is sensitive. Pinworm treatment involves an antihelminthic (e.g., mebendazole) for the host and all immediate family members who possibly harbor the worm asymptomatically, and the cleaning of the egg-contaminated sleeping environment (vacuuming, changing sheets). Treatment repeated three times at two weekly intervals will eradicate adult pinworms that have developed since the previous treatment. Eggs are not killed by the drug.

Trichinella

Worldwide in distribution, the *Trichinella* parasite is acquired by eating uncooked meat (pork, bear, walrus) infected with long-living *Trichinella* larvae. Symptoms usually commence with upper abdominal pain, diarrhea,

*Not FDA approved for this indication.

*Not FDA approved for this indication.

eosinophilia, and mild fever as the larvae penetrate and mature in the small intestinal mucosa. The intestinal symptoms persist for up to a week, replaced with higher fevers, myalgia, and fatigue as the intestine-located adults produce blood-disseminating larvae. The early diarrheal phase may be greatly prolonged and unassociated with the larva dissemination-myalgia phase in partially immune individuals (e.g., in arctic regions). Diagnosis is based on raised creatine kinase, eosinophilia, muscle symptoms, and serology as the worms, eggs and larvae are rarely found in stool examinations. Treatment is steroids (e.g., prednisone 40–60 mg/d) and an anthelminthic (mebendazole,* albendazole*), which kills the intestine-dwelling adults. An absorbable anthelminthic alone, without prednisone, may, in killing some larvae, increase the host inflammatory response and should be limited to mild cases. The use of an anthelminthic during the incubation period appears to reduce the chance of developing the illness.

Trichuris (Whipworm)

A worldwide infection of the colon, with epidemiology similar to *Ascaris*, symptomatology (diarrhea, dysentery, anemia, prolapsed rectum) is rare except in the very small percentage with very heavy worm burdens. Diagnosis is made by seeing typical eggs on stool microscopy or, rarely, on seeing the small worms on colonoscopy or on the prolapsed rectum. Treatment is a benzimidazole (e.g., albendazole,* mebendazole), as for *Ascaris*, with equal success rates.

Trichostrongylus spp.

Small intestine roundworms found especially in sheep and goat-raising regions, they live partially buried in the intestinal mucosa. Symptoms are rare. Diagnosis is made by stool microscopy. Treatment is with benzimidazoles (e.g., albendazole,* mebendazole*).

Strongyloides stercoralis (Threadworm)

Found around the world in regions with inadequate sanitation facilities, this small worm lives buried in the small intestine mucosa. The worm is acquired through skin contact with skin-penetrating larvae from human feces deposited on the ground. An important characteristic of this worm is that some larvae may not be evacuated in the host's stool but infect the host via intestinal mucosa or perianal skin. The result is called autoinfection and can persist for life. Symptoms, often mild but not uncommon, include dyspepsia and intermittent urticaria or itchy linear lesions between the nipples and knees (cutaneous larva currens). Diarrhea is rare but possible in heavier worm burdens. In immunocompromised individuals, the larvae may leave the small intestine wall and disseminate (disseminated strongyloidiasis, hyperinfection) throughout the body in large numbers, carrying gram-negative bacteria from the intestine. The result is gram-negative peritonitis, pneumonitis, or meningitis with, at times, necrosis of the intestinal wall. Diagnosis of a standard case is difficult. Routine stool microscopy is less than 50% sensitive. Special cultures (Harada Mori, charcoal culture, agar plate) are better but still inadequate. Serology is the most sensitive (up to 90%) but cross reaction with other helminths complicates results. Diagnosis of hyperinfection is far easier (if thought of) as larvae are found in much larger numbers in stool and or sputum. Treatment of standard infections includes ivermectin or albendazole for 2 days. Hyperinfection may require days to weeks of treatment (ivermectin [Stromectol], combined at times with albendazole*) before *Strongyloides* are no longer found in stool or sputum.

*Not FDA approved for this indication.

CESTODES

Diphyllobothrium (Fish Tapeworm)

A worm genus of several species (e.g., *D. latum, D. dendriticum, D. pacificum*) and of worldwide distribution, it is acquired by eating raw freshwater fish. It lives in the small intestine producing infrequent symptoms. In northern Europe it can produce vitamin B_{12} deficiency. Diagnosis is by visualization of lengths of the tapeworm, or eggs in stool specimens. Eggs and segments may only be present intermittently in stool. Treatment is praziquantel* or niclosamide.*

Hymenolepis nana (Dwarf Tapeworm)

This small, half-centimeter tapeworm of the small intestine occurs worldwide, most frequently in children and institutions where fecal-oral spread is increased. Eggs can hatch and mature in the small intestine, with resultant increasing and heavy intensity worm burdens. Symptoms range from the asymptomatic to diarrhea, abdominal pains, and pruritus ani. Treatment is praziquantel* and the treatment of the whole family may be appropriate because of covert intrafamilial spread.

Taenia saginata (Beef Tapeworm), *Taenia solium* (Pork Tapeworm)

These tapeworms occur in areas where raw or undercooked beef or pork is consumed and meat inspection practices are inadequate. They live in the small intestine producing little symptomatology. The worms are diagnosed when visible segments are passed in stool or eggs are seen on stool microscopy. The eggs of the two species are indistinguishable microscopically. Speciation is accomplished by visualizing the uterine features in the proglottids (tapeworm segments). Treatment is praziquantel* or niclosamide.*

*Not FDA approved for this indication.

It is important to control fecal-oral contamination in *T. solium* (pork tapeworm) infections. *T. solium* eggs passed in stool, if ingested, hatch on contact with stomach acid and the larvae disseminate throughout the vascular system. The resultant cysts in most organs are asymptomatic but in brain or eye produce a range of severe pathologies called cysticercosis.

TREMATODES

Intestinal Flukes

Uncommon in the Americas, these flukes are mostly present in some tropical countries (e.g., Southeast Asia) where raw freshwater fish are consumed. On ingestion, the larvae (metacercaria) in the fish hatch and quickly become adults, living in the small intestine. They usually do not live longer than a year, are usually asymptomatic, but can produce diarrhea and abdominal symptomatology. The North American intestinal fluke *Nanophyetus salmincola,* found in West Coast raw salmon that has never been frozen, can produce persisting diarrhea. Treatment of the intestinal flukes is praziquantel.*

Liver Flukes (*Fasciola* spp., *Opisthorchis* spp., *Clonorchis, Metorchis*)

Examples found worldwide, these flukes are acquired by eating uncooked freshwater fish or freshwater plants. Ingested larva (metacercaria) hatch and pass through the small intestine wall and then liver capsule (*Fasciola*) or enter the biliary tree via the sphincter of Oddi (*Opisthorchis spp., Clonorchis, Metorchis*). This early active movement phase of the infection is associated with upper abdominal pain, fever, anorexia, and eosinophilia. Diagnosis is made by computed tomography of the liver or serology in *Fasciola*, and eggs in the stools of the others. Adults sooner (*Opisthorchis, Clonorchis, Metorchis*) or later (*Fasciola*) end up wedged in the biliary radicals and bile ducts, where they are asymptomatic or produce intermittent biliary symptomatology. Diagnosis is then made by serology and stool examination for eggs. Treatment is praziquantel for *Clonorchis, Opisthorchis,* and *Metorchis* and triclabendazole** for *Fasciola*.

Schistosoma spp.

Intestinal schistosome infections are acquired by larval penetration of skin in contact with fresh water in many tropical countries. *S. mansoni, S. japonicum, S. mekongi, S. intercalatum,* and other species live in colonic portal venules where they produce little pathology and no symptoms, but lay eggs that can die in submucosal locations or in the liver, producing granulomata with impact on the liver and colonic mucosa. Diagnosis is made by visualization of characteristic eggs on stool examination, on colonic mucosal or liver biopsy, or by ultrasound, suggesting the characteristic liver fibrosis and portal hypertension. Serology may be helpful. Stool eggs should be examined (flame cells) to determine whether the adult schistosomes are alive (dead eggs can be found for years after the adults have died). The same flame cell examination can be used to determine cure. Treatment is praziquantel.

*Not FDA approved for this indication.

**Investigational drug in the United States.

COMMUNITY-BASED THERAPY

Soil-Transmitted Nematodes (*Ascaris*, Hookworm, *Trichuris*) in Endemic Areas

Current World Health Organization (WHO) recommendations indicate that in communities where there is both a high prevalence (≥70%) and a high proportion of moderate to heavy infections (≥10%), based on stool surveys in schools, that there be targeted treatment of school-age children and systematic treatment of preschool children and women of childbearing age in mother and child care programs. In moderate prevalence (>50% but <70%) and low-intensity (<10%) situations, a similar strategy of treatment should be considered, although the frequency of treatment can be reduced. Last, where both prevalence and intensity are low (<50% and <10%, respectively), there need be only selective treatment. WHO recommends a choice of one of four drugs for these infections (albendazole,* levamisole,* mebendazole, or pyrantel pamoate); however, only albendazole and mebendazole are in a single-dose, single-tablet format, which greatly facilitates drug administration.

A rapid quantitative assessment of the prevalence and intensity of infection can be obtained with stool surveys in schools, using the Kato-Katz technique. Care should be taken to ensure that prevalence and intensity estimates are obtained from different geographic or ecologic zones that have been appropriately sampled before deciding on a treatment strategy. Implementing any type of community-based treatment strategy requires the active cooperation of the community itself (parents, leaders) and therefore information, education, and communication (IEC) activities should also be planned concurrently.

Intestinal Schistosomiasis (*S. mansoni*) in Endemic Areas

As with the community-based treatment of soil-transmitted nematodes, communities where intestinal schistosomiasis is endemic may also benefit from community-based treatment. An appreciation of the prevalence of infection from a school stool survey is sufficient to decide on an appropriate treatment strategy. WHO recommends that, where prevalence is high (≥50%), there be targeted treatment of school-age children (once annually) and other high-risk groups, and case treatment available to all. Where prevalence is moderate (≥10% but <50%), treatment should be

*Not FDA approved for this indication.

targeted to school-age children (once every 2 years) and case treatment should be available to all. Where prevalence is low (<10%), the recommended treatment strategy is targeted treatment of school-age children twice during primary school (once on entry and once on leaving) and case treatment available to all.

Praziquantel is the drug of choice for schistosomiasis. A standardized height pole for determining the number of praziquantel tablets for each person has been developed for sub-Saharan Africa, which eliminates the need to weigh individuals. Such height-standardized poles may be available in other countries.

Section 8
Metabolic Disease

DIABETES MELLITUS IN ADULTS

method of
WILLIAM C. DUCKWORTH, M.D.
VA Medical Center and University of Arizona
Phoenix, Arizona

The rapid increase in type 2 diabetes has led to the conclusion that a worldwide epidemic of this disease is occurring. Even in less developed countries, the number of patients with diabetes is increasing remarkably, although the total percentage of the population with this disease remains much lower than in the industrialized Western world. Undoubtedly, many factors are contributing to this increase, including increased recognition, increasing life span, and an increase in ethnic populations with higher prevalence rates, but clearly an overriding factor is increased obesity and reduced physical activity.

Several studies have now shown that even modest weight loss and increased physical activity can delay the onset of type 2 diabetes, thus emphasizing the necessity to focus on this preventive aspect in the total population, especially in individuals at risk for the disease. Pharmacologic therapy may also be valuable for high-risk individuals.

PATHOGENESIS

Type 2 diabetes is a heterogeneous disease with multiple abnormalities predisposing to the clinical syndrome. Most patients have an underlying genetic abnormality resulting in insulin resistance and progressive beta cell failure. It is likely that different genetic abnormalities in different populations can produce this combination of defects. Subpopulations of patients with clinical type 2 diabetes may have predominant abnormalities in insulin secretion with secondary defects in insulin action. This type is typified by the MODY (maturity-onset diabetes of youth) syndrome. Other rarer types of genetic abnormalities can also produce a picture consistent with type 2 diabetes, including receptor defects, insulin structural abnormalities, and others.

Ultimately, most patients with type 2 diabetes have a combination of insufficient insulin action and relative or absolute insulin deficiency. It is important to understand that insulin has multiple actions, not just effects on glucose uptake and metabolism. Insulin alters fat metabolism, protein turnover, and many enzymes and cellular processes. Even though the clinical focus is on glucose, it is likely that a significant number of type 2 patients have abnormalities in glucose levels secondary to other defects. In particular, abnormalities in fat metabolism, including both fat storage and fat oxidation, may be primary defects in many patients. Although this finding has implications for understanding the disease, the major clinical abnormalities at the onset of the syndrome are defects in glucose uptake and metabolism. Changes initially occur in insulin's action in muscle, with later alterations in hepatic glucose production and storage and defects in beta cell function. Progressive loss of beta cell function is a common feature of the disease.

For appropriate management of patients with type 2 diabetes, it is essential that the caregiver understand the underlying abnormalities and progressive nature of the disease. Different approaches to therapy must be used at each stage of the disease, with appropriate consideration of possible variations in pathogenesis.

GLUCOSE CONTROL

Microvascular Disease

The importance of glucose control in preventing or slowing progression of the microvascular complications of diabetes, including retinopathy, nephropathy, and neuropathy, is no longer in doubt. The Diabetes Control and Complications Trial (DCCT) established this fact in patients with type 1 diabetes, and the United Kingdom Prospective Diabetes Study (UKPDS), as well as several smaller trials such as the Kumamoto study, have confirmed the importance of glucose control in type 2 diabetes. Overall, one can expect an approximately 25% to 30% reduction in the development of microvascular complications for every 1% reduction in glycosylated hemoglobin (HbA_{1c}). This improvement is not an absolutely linear association because the benefit is greater with a reduction in higher HbA_{1c} levels and a lesser effect is seen at lower levels. Nevertheless, the benefit is clear at all levels of control, and thus the lowest possible HbA_{1c} level should be the goal for every patient. Completely normal HbA_{1c} levels are not possible in many patients, so realistic goals must be established, particularly in type 2 diabetes. Unacceptable hypoglycemia, other treatment side effects, life expectancy, quality of life, and patient acceptance may dictate alterations in individual patient goals.

Macrovascular Disease

Glucose control has not been proved to be a significant factor for prevention of macrovascular disease in patients with diabetes. Both the DCCT and the UKPDS showed nonsignificant reductions in myocardial infarction in the intensively treated group, but other studies have not shown this trend. One prospective, randomized trial (the VA Feasibility Study) actually showed a tendency for an increase in macrovascular events in intensively treated patients with established type 2 diabetes. This uncertainty has resulted in the initiation of two major prospective trials to determine the role of glucose control in preventing macrovascular disease in type 2 diabetes: the Veterans Affairs Diabetes Trial (VADT) and the National Institutes of Health Action to Control Cardiovascular Risk in Diabetes (ACCORD) trial, which are testing the hypothesis that intensive glucose control prevents major macrovascular endpoints. The VADT is a 20-site, 7-year study of 1700 patients with established type 2 diabetes with the defined aim of determining whether near-normal HbA_{1c} levels, compared with usual control in the VA population, alter the hard endpoint of macrovascular events. The ACCORD trial plans to study 10,000 patients but includes studies on lipid and blood pressure therapy in addition to glucose control. Both studies are currently in progress. Until information is available from these studies or from other sources, the only conclusion that can be reached is that the role of glucose control in macrovascular disease is uncertain.

What is established is that macrovascular disease in diabetes is strongly affected by lipid and blood pressure control. The current recommendation for management of low-density lipoprotein (LDL) cholesterol in patients with diabetes is to achieve levels less than 100 mg/dL, which reflects the conclusion that patients with diabetes, even those who have not had a previous macrovascular event, should be treated similar to nondiabetic individuals who have had a previous event. The recommendations also include controlling triglyceride levels and improving high-density lipoprotein (HDL) levels.

Blood pressure control is essential in patients with type 2 diabetes. The current recommendation is to achieve levels at or below 130/80 mm Hg. Treatment of blood pressure has been shown to not only decrease macrovascular events but also decrease microvascular complications, including retinopathy and nephropathy. It is essential that all patients with diabetes be intensively managed to achieve as nearly normal lipid and blood pressure levels as possible. Angiotensin-converting enzyme inhibitors and angiotensin II receptor blocker therapy may have additional benefits above and beyond blood pressure lowering, especially for nephropathy and perhaps macrovascular disease.

GLUCOSE MONITORING

Self-monitoring of blood glucose (SMBG) has been correctly recognized as one of the most important advances in the past 20 years in the care of patients with diabetes. Intensive control of blood glucose in type 1 diabetes is essentially impossible without SMBG. SMBG can also play an important role in the management of type 2 diabetes, but surprisingly, its precise role and importance remain uncertain and controversial. It is generally agreed that type 2 patients maintained with multiple insulin injections require SMBG, but in a typical patient taking oral agents or in a stable insulin program, consensus is lacking. Some of this confusion is due to results from various studies showing that in prospective, randomized trials, SMBG does not result in improved HbA_{1c} levels. In most of these trials, the patients have been randomized to either monitoring or not monitoring, without action on the results. In the few trials that have incorporated responses for the results, monitoring has been shown to be valuable. Even in short-term studies in which no action is taken, HbA_{1c} levels can improve, but this improvement is lost unless the data are incorporated into the overall patient care program. The dictum that unused data are useless is appropriate.

The following recommendation for SMBG in patients with type 2 diabetes is the author's opinion based on personal experience, literature data, and ongoing studies in which the author is involved. All patients should be given the means and the training to perform SMBG. All SMBG data should be reviewed by the caregiver and discussed with the patient at each visit. Patients should be encouraged to monitor blood glucose levels as appropriate for their condition. All suspected hypoglycemic episodes should be tested. Appropriate instructions regarding what constitutes true hypoglycemia should be given. Testing should also be done if symptoms of hyperglycemia occur or if an intercurrent illness is present.

For patients at their HbA_{1c} goal and stable with treatment, no other testing may be necessary, although intermittent testing to show the effect of dietary indiscretion or exercise may be instructive to the patient and encourage compliance. For patients who are stable with therapy (oral or oral plus standard insulin) and near their goal but needing reassessment, short-term intensive monitoring (e.g., three to four times daily for 1 week) may be more instructive than monitoring one to two times daily for 3 months. A study currently in progress is examining various approaches to establish the most effective and parsimonious SMBG regimen. Current data suggest that prelunch measurements are most likely to detect hypoglycemia and bedtime measurements most likely to predict hyperglycemia (i.e., elevated HbA_{1c} levels). It is possible that routine postprandial measurements may be more predictive of unacceptable hyperglycemia in reasonably well controlled patients.

DIET AND EXERCISE

Though trite, it is very true that diet and exercise are the foundation of all therapy for patients with type 2 diabetes and, in fact, for patients with glucose intolerance or those at high risk for diabetes. The current "epidemic" of type 2 diabetes, both in this country and around the world, is largely attributable to the increasing prevalence of obesity and to reductions in physical activity. Several studies, including the Diabetes Prevention Program, have shown remarkable decreases in progression from glucose intolerance to overt diabetes with relatively modest weight loss and increased physical activity. The primary goal for all obese patients, whether they be glucose intolerant or have overt type 2 diabetes, should be weight loss. Generally, weight loss is accomplished most effectively by instruction in appropriate diets by qualified nutritionists and continued support in this attempt by all members of the health care team. Long-term success is most often achieved by a relatively modest decrease in caloric intake sustained over the long term, that is, reducing caloric intake by 300 to 400 calories per day. Short-term, very low calorie diets, 400 to 800 total calories per day for 1 to 3 months, followed by a more modest restriction of 250 to 500 calories per day, may be quite useful in very obese individuals. Frequently, relatively small amounts of weight loss may result in striking improvement in glucose intolerance and hyperglycemia. Current recommendations from the American Diabetes Association (ADA) and other organizations are that the caloric distribution should be less than 30% total fat with less than 10% saturated fat, 10% to 20% protein, and 50% to 55% carbohydrates. Effort should be made to increase monounsaturated fat intake and fiber intake in these patients. This approach may result in secondary health benefits such as a reduction in cholesterol levels and risk for other diseases. Carbohydrate counting can be beneficial for many patients by drawing attention to intake and also by allowing adjustment of insulin therapy in patients taking multiple doses of short-acting insulin to reduce postprandial glucose levels.

Whenever possible, physical activity should be increased as tolerated. This activity should include regular planned exercise programs such as walking or other aerobic activity three to four times a week, with a goal of at least 30 to 40 minutes' duration at 60% maximal heart rate, calculated by subtracting age from 220. This objective will not be achievable initially in most patients, but it should gradually be approached. Resistance exercises have also been shown to be useful in patients with diabetes, and such exercises have attractions for many people, particularly younger patients. Alternating aerobic and resistance programs may confer benefit in reducing cardiovascular risk, as well as lowering glucose levels and increasing patient confidence and self-reliance. All exercise programs in patients at risk for cardiovascular disease should be planned with appropriate consultation by cardiologists, exercise physiologists, and other trained individuals. Supervised exercise programs are available in many locations. For patients with any complications or questions, exercise tolerance testing should be considered. In addition to planned exercise programs, patients should also be encouraged to increase daily physical activities by such simple means as increased walking during their routine daily activities. Examples would be parking at the end of the parking lot and walking to the mall, walking to the convenience store on the corner rather than driving, and walking up or down one flight of stairs rather than using the elevator. Severe complications such as peripheral neuropathy or vascular insufficiency, proliferative retinopathy, or foot lesions may restrict physical activity.

ORAL AGENTS

α-Glucosidase Inhibitors

α-Glucosidase inhibitors (AGIs) decrease the breakdown of carbohydrates in the intestine and thus delay absorption of glucose and decrease postprandial rises in glucose levels. Such an effect reduces the necessity for the impaired beta cell to secrete large amounts of insulin over a short period and may significantly improve glucose levels. These agents may be particularly useful in patients older than 60 to 65 years who have new-onset diabetes (aging pancreas syndrome).

Currently, two AGIs are approved for use in the United States, acarbose (Precose) and miglitol (Glyset). Dosages are given in Table 1, but it is recommended that therapy be initiated with a single 25-mg dose

TABLE 1. **Oral Agents Commonly Used**

	Starting Dose (mg)	Maximal Effective Dose (mg)
Sulfonylureas		
Glyburide (Micronase)	1.25–2.5 qd	15–20 qd
Glyburide (Glynase PresTabs)	1.5–3.0 qd	12 qd
Glipizide (Glucotrol)	2.5–5 qd	15–20 qd
Glipizide XL (Glucotrol XL)	2.5–5 qd	20 qd
Glimepiride (Amaryl)	1–2 qd	8 qd
Biguanides		
Metformin (Glucophage)	500 qd	2000 qd
Thiazolidinediones		
Rosiglitazone (Avandia)	2 qd	8 qd
Pioglitazone (Actos)	15 qd	45 qd
α-Glucosidase inhibitors		
Acarbose (Precose)	25 qd*	100 tid
Miglitol (Glyset)	25 qd*	100 tid
Meglitinides		
Repaglinide (Prandin)	0.5–1 qd*	8 qd
Nateglinide (Starlix)	60–120 qd*	120 qd

*Usually three times daily.

daily at the main meal with gradual increases to help offset the gastrointestinal (GI) side effects of these agents. The recommended approach is 25 mg of either agent before one meal a day, usually the evening meal, for 1 to 2 weeks with a gradual increase to administration before every meal and, subsequently, up to the maximal dose of 100 mg three times daily. With this approach, relatively few patients will find the side effects unacceptable.

The primary side effect of AGI therapy is flatulence, with occasionally some bloating and abdominal discomfort and rarely diarrhea. The other major but rare side effect is elevated liver function test (LFT) results. This effect is almost always reversible with discontinuation of the agent. AGIs should not be used in patients with intestinal disorders or a creatinine concentration over 2 mg/dL.

Hypoglycemia is not a side effect of AGIs, although it can occur when these agents are used in combination with an insulin secretagogue or with exogenous insulin. If hypoglycemia occurs under these conditions, treatment must be with either oral glucose tablets or intravenous glucose because anything other than monosaccharides may not be broken down in the gut and thus glucose will not be available for absorption. Lactose is an exception, and therefore milk might also be used for the treatment of hypoglycemia.

Sulfonylureas

Sulfonylureas (SUs) have been the mainstay of management of type 2 diabetes for over 40 years and, exclusive of insulin, were the only agents available in the United States until the early 1990s. Table 1 shows the most frequently used SUs currently available in this country. Glyburide (DiaBeta) is by far the most commonly used SU around the world. Its advantages of relatively low cost and potency are somewhat offset by the fact that while it is effective in most patients, it may produce hypoglycemia. This disadvantage is of particular importance in the elderly and is due, in part, to an increase in fasting insulin levels, as well as a long duration of action.

The other two commonly used agents are glipizide (Glucotrol), which has a lesser tendency to increase fasting insulin levels and causes a greater increase in postprandial insulin levels, and glimepiride (Amaryl), which has theoretical advantages in terms of nonpancreatic function. It also has a longer duration of action than glipizide and less tendency for hypoglycemia. Formulations of glyburide and glipizide with varying absorption properties are also available. Hard data showing advantages of one SU over another are sparse.

Other available SUs have no clear advantage and often have significant disadvantages. It is recommended that the practitioner choose among the three most commonly used agents with consideration of the individual patient. Typically, SU therapy is begun with the lowest effective dose (see Table 1) and increased every 1 to 2 weeks until therapeutic goals are attained or the maximal dose is reached. In practice, relatively little additional effect is seen for doses above 15 mg/d for glyburide and 20 mg/d for glipizide. In fact, in some patients, higher doses may be less effective.

The major side effect is hypoglycemia. Elderly patients and patients with renal disease are at greatest risk. SUs should be used cautiously or preferably not at all in patients with significant renal disease. Glimepiride is preferred in such patients if an SU is to be used.

Allergic reactions to SUs are relatively rare except in patients with allergies to sulfa. Other even less common problems include liver toxicity, GI disturbances, and drug interactions. Overall, except for hypoglycemia, this class of drugs is safe.

SU-induced hypoglycemia can be prolonged and severe. Patients requiring assistance in the emergency department should be admitted for observation because the long duration of action of these drugs may result in recurrent episodes.

Meglitinides

This relatively new, non-SU class of insulin secretagogues stimulates insulin secretion in a manner similar to the SUs, but with a very rapid onset and termination of action. Two agents are currently available, repaglinide (Prandin) and nateglinide (Starlix). They bind to the SU receptor but undergo very rapid dissociation and rapid turnover and must thus be taken immediately before or at the initiation of meals. Insulin is secreted in response to an elevation in glucose, with little or no response at normal glucose levels. Meglitinides clearly have important effects on postprandial glucose elevations, with lesser effects on fasting glucose.

Their pattern of action results in a lesser risk of hypoglycemia, especially prolonged or nocturnal events. This property makes them especially attractive for elderly patients or patients with predominantly postprandial hyperglycemia. They are also frequently useful in combination with insulin sensitizers, but they are ineffective in combination with SUs. These agents can be used in patients with significant renal disease because their metabolism is primarily hepatic.

Biguanides

Metformin (Glucophage) is the only member of this class currently available for clinical use. Phenformin was used previously, but its use was discontinued by the U.S. Food and Drug Administration (FDA) because of its tendency to produce lactic acidosis. Metformin was approved for use in the United States in the early 1990s after being available in Europe for more than 20 years. It has only rarely been associated with lactic acidosis, except in clinical situations such as renal insufficiency and congestive heart failure (CHF). It should not be used in patients with these conditions or in patients receiving contrast media for radiologic procedures. Despite semantic arguments, metformin can be considered an insulin sensitizer. Its primary effect is on the liver, with secondary effects on peripheral insulin-sensitive tissues such as muscle. In normal pharmacologic doses it does not produce hypoglycemia as a sole agent, although it can contribute to SU- or insulin-induced hypoglycemic effects. Metformin reduces insulin levels and insulin requirements in most patients with type 2 diabetes and in some insulin-resistant type 1 patients. In most insulin-resistant type 2 individuals, especially obese patients, metformin has become the drug of choice because of its multiple beneficial effects.

Weight gain is one of the most common side effects of glucose control in diabetes. Metformin therapy more frequently has a weight-maintaining or even weight-loss effect. Because obesity is a major factor in type 2 diabetes and even moderate weight loss can have beneficial effects, this property of metformin is an important advantage. The mechanism responsible for the weight loss is not clear, nor is the mechanism for weight gain with other therapy. One possible factor is the circulating insulin level, which is reduced by metformin and increased by SU or insulin therapy. Elevated insulin levels are associated with weight gain.

Elevated insulin levels have also been associated with an increased risk of atherosclerosis. Cause-effect relationships have not been established, but solid basic and theoretical considerations support a role for hyperinsulinemia in atherosclerotic heart disease. At the least, the reduction in peripheral insulin levels with metformin is a positive effect.

Metformin therapy is also the only glucose-lowering therapy that has been associated with a statistically significant decrease in macrovascular complications in type 2 patients. In the UKPDS, metformin treatment of newly diagnosed type 2 diabetes in obese individuals resulted in a significant reduction in myocardial infarction. The improvement was not clearly due to glucose lowering, however, because the HbA_{1c} difference was only 0.6% (compared with 0.9% in the major trial), and interpretation is difficult for several reasons, including the complicated design of the study, with multiple crossovers and combination therapy making it difficult to attribute effects to specific therapy. The issue is further obscured by the apparently deleterious effects of adding metformin to SU failures.

Nevertheless, the effects of metformin on insulin levels and weight gain and its additional beneficial effects on lipid-related cardiovascular risk factors may make this agent the preferred drug in insulin-resistant patients.

The major side effects include GI distress in newly treated patients and the potential for serious side effects (i.e., lactic acidosis) in those with renal or cardiac compromise.

To prevent these problems, patients with renal impairment, specifically, creatinine values over 1.6, or patients with a history of CHF should not be treated with this drug. To reduce GI complaints and increase patient acceptance, metformin should be started at a low dose to allow adaptation to the GI effects and only gradually increased. Many patients have no or minimal GI effects, but to reduce patient symptoms, the following is the suggested approach. Patients being started on metformin therapy should be given a single 500-mg dose before the evening meal for 3 to 5 days. If symptoms are present, it should be continued for up to 1 week. A second 500-mg dose should be added before the morning meal if no symptoms are present or if the patient has only minor GI complaints. Dosage levels can be increased as necessary after that, with changes made relative to the patient's symptoms or drug effectiveness. If done carefully, very few patients will be unable to tolerate this drug.

As with some SUs, doses lower than the maximum recommended (2550 mg) may be as or more effective. Doses over 1500 to 2000 mg are rarely indicated. Some anecdotal (and personal) experience has suggested that administration three times daily may have benefits over twice-daily dosing. If selected, 500 mg before meals three times daily or 500 mg with breakfast and lunch and 1000 mg at the evening meal is suggested. A long-acting preparation, metformin XL, is available; it offers patient convenience and may have reduced GI side effects. Again, however, some patients may benefit from twice-a-day administration rather than once daily.

Thiazolidinediones

The thiazolidinediones (TZDs) were developed as a true insulin sensitizer, and it increases the effect of insulin on peripheral tissues. These agents increase the effect of insulin on muscle and fat with secondary effects on the liver, and they directly address the primary defect in most patients with type 2 diabetes. The first representative of this class was troglitazone (Rezulin), which had important clinical effects on glucose levels in a significant proportion of patients with type 2 diabetes. This agent also had beneficial effects on lipid metabolism, lipid turnover, and vascular function. Unfortunately, troglitazone was associated with rare but serious side effects, including liver abnormalities and, in a few cases, hepatic failure leading to either death or liver transplantation. It has been withdrawn from the market.

Two newer agents are available, rosiglitazone (Avandia) and pioglitazone (Actos), that have not been implicated in serious hepatic effects but have been associated with LFT increases. Monitoring of LFTs every 2 months for the first year and subsequently "intermittently" is required. If LFTs increase to or above three times upper normal values, treatment with these TZDs should be stopped and the patient monitored carefully.

TZDs are PPAR-γ (peroxisome proliferator activating receptor-γ) agonists and have effects on the expression of multiple cellular proteins. The systems involved in their clinical benefit are not totally clear, but alterations in fat cell metabolism are prominent. TZDs may stimulate adipocyte differentiation, potentially leading to weight gain, but the increase in fat is the more metabolically benign peripheral fat tissue rather than the central adiposity associated with the metabolic syndrome (syndrome X).

The characteristics of TZDs are shown in Table 1. The usual approach to therapy is to begin with the recommended starting dose and monitor the effect of therapy for 3 to 6 weeks. Larger doses may be used with severely hyperglycemic (fasting blood glucose [FBG] >200) patients. Because of their mechanism of action, this period may be required to determine the clinical effects. Dosages may be increased as necessary, but two considerations are important. The full effect of any given dose may require 6 months or longer to be seen. Responsive patients may have remarkable decreases in HbA_{1c} levels, 2% to 3% or even more, especially if they start with greatly elevated levels (10% to 11% or higher). As monotherapy, TZDs do not produce hypoglycemia, but they may potentiate the effects of insulin or insulin secretagogues. Some patients will have little or no benefit from TZD therapy. The proportion varies in different populations, most likely reflecting the heterogeneity of type 2 diabetes. Patients already taking insulin may require reductions in dose or even cessation of insulin with TZD therapy.

The practical results of the foregoing are that monitoring of effectiveness is essential after beginning TZD therapy. TZD therapy should be stopped in nonresponders and alternative approaches used. In addition, obviously, the commonly used approach of "average expected reductions in HbA_{1c}" to evaluate drug usefulness is even less meaningful with TZDs than with other agents. As an extreme example, the average effect of 1.5% in population studies may be 0% in half the patients and 3% in the other half. Monitoring of effectiveness is thus essential with TZDs.

These agents are extremely useful in insulin-resistant type 2 patients, particularly the obese insulin-resistant group. TZDs are used, for the most part, as third-line therapy after an insulin secretagogue and metformin, but early use in patients with severe insulin resistance has many advantages. The primary barrier to more frequent and earlier use of TZDs is their cost, but a strong case for cost-effectiveness of these agents can be made in responsive patients.

As the use of these agents has increased, a major side effect of the current TZDs has become obvious and significant. They may cause or increase edema, particularly when used in combination with insulin. Although such edema occurs in a minority of patients, it can contribute to large increases in weight (20 to 40 lb or more over relatively short periods) and exacerbate or possibly precipitate CHF in some patients. The FDA has published precautionary statements about the combination of rosiglitazone and insulin. Even though head-to-head comparisons of pioglitazone and rosiglitazone are not available, it is likely that their effects are similar.

Practically speaking, TZDs should not be used in patients with advanced CHF (stage III or IV) and only with great caution in any CHF patient. All patients treated with TZDs should be monitored for weight gain, edema, and symptoms or signs of CHF. Minor edema may be treated with diuretics in patients who have achieved significant clinical benefit from TZD therapy, but these patients should receive close attention.

INSULIN THERAPY

As with oral agents, several new preparations of insulin with altered properties have been introduced over the past few years, including the rapidly absorbed analogues lispro and insulin aspart and the long-acting insulin preparation glargine. Table 2 lists the new as well as the older agents currently available for clinical use, along with some of their properties.

Most patients with type 2 diabetes will require insulin therapy for appropriate control at some point during their disease. Because type 2 diabetes is characterized by progressive loss of beta cell function, supplemental exogenous insulin is required by many patients (at least 50%) who have had the disease for a number of years. Insulin therapy may likewise be needed as temporary therapy during intercurrent illnesses such as severe trauma, stress, infection, and other medical events. Short-term insulin therapy may also be useful in some patients who are severely out of control to reduce glucose toxicity and restore, at least partially, both beta cell function and insulin action.

Many diabetologists now believe that insulin therapy should be used sparingly, with administration of only the amounts and types of insulin necessary to supplement other therapeutic approaches. Insulin therapy is not without problems, including hypoglycemia, weight gain, patient nonacceptance and thus inadequate compliance, and possible or theoretical disadvantages such as effects on blood pressure, vascular walls, and even atherosclerosis. The latter issue remains controversial, but one cannot totally

TABLE 2. **Insulin Preparations**

Type	Onset (h)	Peak (h)	Duration (h)
Short acting (e.g., Regular) (Humulin R, Novolin R)	0.5–1	2–4	4–6
Rapidly absorbed (lispro, aspart) (Humalog, NovoLog)	0.25–0.5	1–2	3–4
Intermediate acting (NPH, Lente) (Humulin N, Novolin H)	3–4	6–12	16–20
Long acting (Ultralente) (Humulin-U)	6–8	14–18	24
Daily (glargine) (Lantus)	Not applicable	None	24

ignore the available data that hyperinsulinemia and atherosclerotic heart disease may be related. The need for insulin therapy varies with individual patients and with the stage of the disease. Some patients initially have absolute insulin deficiency at or near the time of diagnosis of the disease, whereas others may not require insulin for many years. The former group may include patients with a variant of typical type 2 diabetes, such as individuals without the insulin resistance syndrome and patients with adult-onset autoimmune insulin deficiency (latent autoimmune diabetes of adults [LADA]). Type 2 syndromes with early insulin deficiency have been called type 1a by some people.

For the typical type 2 patient with diabetes, a single injection of insulin daily given at bedtime may suffice, either an intermediate-acting insulin or the long-acting glargine (Lantus). Fasting hyperglycemia resulting from increased overnight glucose output by the liver is a feature characteristic of progressive diabetes. Multiple insulin injections may also be required as the disease progresses or in individual patients earlier in the disease (e.g., LADA). These approaches may include intermediate insulin injections two or three times daily (or once-daily glargine) with multiple premeal short-acting insulin injections. The most common multiple-injection approach is NPH plus regular insulin before breakfast and before dinner. This author is not a fan of this approach because frequently the NPH given before dinner does not have sufficient duration of action to lower prebreakfast glucose levels without risking nocturnal hypoglycemia, but it must be stated that this combination can be effective in many individuals. Other approaches include NPH before breakfast and at bedtime with regular insulin given at the dinner meal, which is usually the largest of the day. A single injection of glargine with one or more premeal short-acting insulin injections is becoming increasingly popular. In the latter case, the trend is to use rapidly absorbed insulin such as lispro (Humalog) or aspart (NovoLog) for both theoretical and practical reasons.

INTEGRATED APPROACH TO THERAPY

The foundation of therapy for type 2 diabetes is diet and exercise. This statement is true for individuals at risk for development of the disease, those with glucose intolerance, and patients with diagnosed diabetes. The benefit for individuals with the metabolic syndrome ("prediabetes") and normal or mildly elevated glucose levels is a reduction in cardiovascular risk factors and delayed progression to overt diabetes. For patients with overt diabetes, the benefit is better control of hyperglycemia, reduced microvascular disease, reduced cardiovascular risk, and even potential reversion to a "prediabetes" condition. The importance of diet and exercise in all patients cannot be overemphasized.

Even in patients who adhere to diet and exercise programs, most will ultimately require pharmacologic therapy. Type 2 diabetes is characterized by dual defects, insulin resistance and insulin deficiency. It is both logical and practical to address both defects simultaneously. Monotherapy does not achieve therapeutic goals even initially in approximately 50% of patients, and by 3 years, the proportion increases to 60% to 80%. Delay in intensifying therapy results in prolonged hyperglycemia ("glucose toxicity") and increased difficulty in achieving control.

Given the dual defects, combination therapy, including an insulin sensitizer and an insulin secretagogue, offers the best opportunity to obtain early glucose control and maintain such control for a longer period (Table 3). Metformin or TZDs are the options for insulin sensitizers and SUs or meglitinides for secretagogues. Although strong theoretical arguments can be made for TZDs and meglitinides and ongoing studies may change the following recommendations, cost constraints make metformin plus a low dose of glyburide (2.5 to 5 mg), glipizide (5 to 10 mg), or glimepiride (1 to 2 mg) the usual regimen. A combination preparation (Glucovance) of glyburide plus metformin (2.5/500 or 5.0/500 mg, respectively) is available, and a glipizide-metformin preparation is also now available.

For patients with severe hyperglycemia (e.g., FBG >200), larger doses may be appropriate, but monitoring for hypoglycemia should be performed because rare patients may have a marked response. It is my preference to start with a low dose (e.g., 2.5 mg glyburide/500 mg metformin) for at least a few days, both to observe the patient and to decrease the GI effects of metformin, and then increase as required every 10 to 14 days. Other approaches are certainly acceptable as long as the patient is monitored. SMBG is an essential tool to evaluate progress.

TABLE 3. **Initial Therapy**

FBG	PPG	Treatment
<126	>200	AGIs, meglitinides; alternative: metformin, SU, TZD
126–140	>200	Metformin, TZD, SU; alternative: combination
141–200	200–300	Combination (metformin or TZD + SU or meglitinide)
201–300	>300	Combination oral (high dose) + exogenous insulin (hs NPH or glargine or multiple dose insulin may be temporarily needed)
>300		Multiple-dose exogenous insulin + combination oral. May reduce or stop insulin after control is achieved

Abbreviations: AGI = α-glucosidase inhibitor; FBG = fasting blood glucose; hs = at bedtime; PPG = postprandial glucose; SU = sulfonylurea; TZD = thiazoladinedione.

An alternative approach to a severely hyperglycemic patient (FBG >250) is to treat with insulin to obtain control (e.g., NPH insulin at bedtime) until fasting glucose levels are under 150 mg/dL and then stop the insulin with continued oral therapy.

For patients with mild hyperglycemia (FBG <140 and/or HbA_{1c} <7.0% to 7.5%), monotherapy may be useful, particularly in the elderly, those with primarily postprandial hyperglycemia, and patients motivated to comply with diet and exercise programs. For older patients and patients with postprandial hyperglycemia, AGIs or meglitinides may reduce the risk (e.g., hypoglycemia) and be clinically effective. In most other patients in this category, metformin or a TZD should be used. If goals are not achieved with low to moderate doses, a second agent should be added rather than simply increasing the dose of the original drug. Monitoring is essential.

If initial combination therapy does not achieve the treatment goals or if metformin is not tolerated (rare), a TZD can be substituted for metformin or added to the combination. The effectiveness of the TZD should be evaluated, while recognizing that a response may require 6 to 8 weeks. If no effect is seen, administration of the TZD should be stopped and other approaches used. Some patients do not respond to TZD therapy. LFTs every 2 months are required for the first year of therapy (Table 4).

Exogenous insulin therapy is necessary in most patients with type 2 diabetes, but oral therapy should not be stopped unless evidence of beta cell destruction (e.g., LADA) is noted. Insulin resistance is a constant feature of type 2 diabetes and should be treated at all stages of the disease. Stimulation of endogenous insulin secretion may have advantages (hepatic delivery, reduced peripheral insulin levels) over purely exogenous insulin delivery.

In most patients, exogenous insulin therapy should be initiated by bedtime administration of intermediate insulin. The goal is to reduce AM glucose levels by inhibiting hepatic glucose output. Doses are titrated until AM fasting goals are achieved. If daytime glucose or HbA_{1c} levels remain above goals, an AM dose of intermediate insulin can be added.

TABLE 4. **Failure to Achieve Goals of Therapy**

Treatment	Response
Monotherapy	Add sensitizer to secretagogues or AGI Add secretagogue to sensitizer
Combination therapy	Add TZD (triple therapy) or Add insulin (hs NPH or glargine) or If FBG acceptable, consider AGI
Oral + single insulin	Simplify oral therapy (e.g., discontinue ineffective TZD) and add multiple insulin injections (e.g., AM NPH to hs NPH, or short-acting ac insulin). Also, glargine may be substituted for hs NPH

Abbreviations: ac = before meals; AGI = α-glucosidase inhibitor; FBG= fasting blood glucose; hs = at bedtime; TZD = thiazoladinedione.

POSTPRANDIAL HYPERGLYCEMIA

The approach just presented is successful in most patients with type 2 diabetes. Combination therapy with oral agents plus intermediate- or long-acting insulin that restores fasting glucose to target levels also usually results in HbA_{1c} levels consistent with individual patient goals. In a minority of patients, HbA_{1c} may remain above goal even with this approach, especially in those seeking normal or near-normal levels. Although several explanations are possible, one recurrent issue is unacceptable postprandial hyperglycemia. Even though no consensus has been reached, many experienced professionals believe that postprandial hyperglycemia should be targeted for specific action when it exists. The primary approach is to add short-acting agents before each meal in patients with acceptable FBG to reduce postprandial excursions. Options include AGIs, meglitinides, and short-acting insulin (regular, lispro, or insulin aspart). Because many patients resist the inconvenience of adding short-acting insulin with each meal, it is frequently worthwhile to try oral agents. AGIs, if tolerated, may correct the problem in patients with relatively minor elevations in HbA_{1c}. A meglitinide can also be used in this situation if the patient is not taking an SU or if the SU therapy can be stopped. If these approaches do not work, the only option is to add short-acting insulin (regular, lispro, or insulin aspart) before one or more meals. The most common approach is to add short-acting insulin to the AM NPH dose. Though convenient, it rarely solves the problem. Usually, the need is greater with the evening meal, but SMBG can target individual needs and is essential for intensive control.

Finally, increasing interest is being shown in attempts to diagnose type 2 diabetes earlier when FBG is reasonably normal but postprandial hyperglycemia is present. Studies are in progress to examine this aspect more carefully, and currently, data are somewhat scarce, but it seems that either AGIs or meglitinides would be useful for this situation. Additionally, many elderly patients with recent onset of their diabetes and relatively normal FBG but unacceptable postprandial excursions may also be candidates for mealtime short-acting oral therapy.

TREATMENT GOALS

The goals of treatment in patients with type 2 diabetes are to restore the metabolic abnormalities to as nearly normal as possible. These goals for glucose control are given in Table 5 and are consistent with the recommendations of the ADA, although the ADA has recently eliminated the "action-suggested" category and some groups have adopted an HbA_{1c} goal of less than 6.5%. The ultimate purpose of these goals is to reduce morbidity, mortality, and patient care costs in individuals with diabetes. As always in medicine, general recommendations must be tailored to individual patients. Many factors may alter individual goals, some of which include reduced life expectancy; advanced complications, either microvascular or

TABLE 5. **Glycemic Targets**

Parameter	Normal	Goal	"Action Suggested"
Fasting (or preprandial) glucose	<110	<120	<80 or >140
Postprandial glucose	<140	<180	>180
Bedtime glucose	<120	100–140	<100 or >160
HbA_{1c} DCCT method	<6%	<7%	>8%

Glucose values are plasma values.
Abbreviation: DCCT = Diabetes Control and Complications Trial.

macrovascular; hypoglycemia unawareness or frequent unacceptable hypoglycemic episodes for any reason; and the inability or unwillingness of the patient to follow the required regimen. Ultimately, the issue is the benefit-risk ratio. It is becoming increasingly recognized that intensive management may include a reduction in quality of life that must be factored into individual therapy. As patients age, the benefit from intensive glucose on a relative basis decreases, and requirements for multiple drug therapy, frequent glucose monitoring, and the risk of drug side effects may make intensive therapy inappropriate for selected older, even healthy individuals. An overriding issue is the effect of glucose control on cardiovascular complications, and if reduction of hyperglycemia can be shown to reduce cardiovascular complications, greater emphasis on glucose control in the elderly would become more appropriate.

In patients with type 2 diabetes, management of associated metabolic abnormalities is essential. Space does not permit extensive discussion of these issues, but lipid and blood pressure control is even more important in patients with diabetes than in nondiabetic individuals. Current recommendations for blood pressure in patients with diabetes are levels less than 130/80 mm Hg and, for lipids, LDL levels less than 100, triglyceride levels less than 200, and HDL levels greater than 35. Appropriate management of lipid and blood pressure abnormalities is essential in the management of type 2 diabetes.

DIABETES MELLITUS IN CHILDREN AND ADOLESCENTS

method of
TANDY AYE, M.D., and
LYNNE L. LEVITSKY, M.D.
Pediatric Endocrine Unit
Massachusetts General Hospital
and Harvard Medical School
Boston, Massachusetts

The American Diabetes Association consensus statement on the classification of diabetes mellitus divides individuals with diabetes into three broad groups: type 1, type 2, and other specific types. Diabetes mellitus in the pediatric age group is usually type 1, caused by autoimmune beta cell destruction leading to insulin deficiency. However, in this past decade of epidemic obesity, there has been an increase in the occurrence of type 2 diabetes. Children with type 2 diabetes tend to be obese adolescents from susceptible genetic backgrounds who have insulin resistance as well as inappropriately low insulin release for the degree of insulin resistance. Rare children have maturity-onset diabetes of the young, autosomal dominant diabetes secondary to genetic defects of beta cell function. Some have diabetes secondary to pancreatic disease, endocrine disorders, medications, congenital infections, autoimmune disorders, or genetic syndromes. These children are treated like others with type 1 or type 2 diabetes depending upon the nature of their insulin response and degree of insulin resistance.

TYPE 1 DIABETES

Diagnosis

Children with type 1 diabetes may be asymptomatic with incidentally identified hyperglycemia, have symptomatic hyperglycemia, or have frank diabetic ketoacidosis. Polydipsia and polyuria because of hyperglycemia are often initial symptoms. Urinary frequency and enuresis are not uncommon in a previously toilet-trained child. Weight loss despite a ravenous appetite is frequently observed. Children who come to medical attention with these symptoms usually have glycosuria and hyperglycemia (blood glucose >200 mg/dL). Occasionally, intercurrent illness may elevate the blood sugar without a preceding history of polydipsia and polyuria. Diagnosis of diabetes is confirmed after recovery if the children meet standard glycemic criteria. Table 1 summarizes the criteria of the American Diabetes Association. Early identification of diabetes is important to prevent progression to ketoacidosis with dehydration, nausea, vomiting, respiratory decompensation, and change in mental status. The timeline of progression varies for each child from weeks to months and is usually more rapid in younger children.

Initial Evaluation

Clinical Evaluation

Initial clinical evaluation of the newly diagnosed child is important to determine immediate

TABLE 1. **Criteria for the Diagnosis of Diabetes Mellitus**

1. Symptoms of diabetes (polydipsia, polyuria, or unexplained weight loss) and any plasma glucose concentration ≥200 mg/dL (11.1 mmol/L)

or

2. Fasting (8 hours) plasma glucose ≥126 mg/dL (7.0 mmol/L)

or

3. 2-hour plasma glucose ≥ 200 mg/dL (11.1 mmol/L) during an oral glucose tolerance test (1.75 g/kg to maximum of 75 g glucose)

management. Evaluation should focus on degree of hydration, mental status, and normality of vital signs. Evidence of acidosis (Kussmaul respirations) and ketosis (acetone odor to breath) should be documented. Children who are asymptomatic (hyperglycemia only) require initiation of maintenance subcutaneous insulin therapy and an intensive educational process. Children with ketoacidosis require appropriate fluid replacement as well as insulin therapy. Treatment of ketoacidosis is discussed in the article on Diabetic Ketoacidosis that follows. In contrast to adults, ketoacidosis in children carries a risk for development of cerebral edema.

Laboratory

Diagnosis should be confirmed by the documentation of hyperglycemia (see Table 1). Measurement of electrolytes, calcium, phosphate, and magnesium and assessment of hydration with BUN and creatinine, as well as of the degree of acidosis by measurement of serum pH, and ketosis by measurement of urine or serum ketones establish the severity of biochemical illness and helps to govern initial therapy. Additional laboratory studies including a complete blood count and electrocardiogram are indicated in patients who present in ketoacidosis. The presence of anti-islet (IA2 and glutamic acid decarboxylase [GAD] antibodies) as well as insulin antibodies before treatment is strongly suggestive of type 1 diabetes mellitus. Glycosylated hemoglobin may be measured to establish a baseline value. Antithyroid antibodies and thyroid-stimulating hormone (TSH) levels can be useful because children with diabetes mellitus are at a greater risk of developing chronic lymphocytic thyroiditis. Screening may not be necessary before the age of 5–10 years unless there is an enlarged thyroid or symptoms of thyroid disease. Approximately 5% of children with type 1 diabetes will test positively for celiac disease. Screening for antiendomysial or tissue transglutaminase antibodies can be done at diagnosis or within a few months after diagnosis.

Treatment

Control of type 1 diabetes mellitus requires an educated patient and family and adequate tools to permit the child to achieve euglycemia. The components include insulin treatment, appropriate nutritional guidelines, glucose monitoring, and an educational program that teaches child and family to integrate diabetes management into a comfortable lifestyle.

Initiation of Insulin Therapy

Most children starting insulin therapy begin with at least a two injection per day insulin regimen. Each injection is a combination of a short-acting (regular or lispro [Humalog] or aspart [NovoLog]) and an intermediate-acting insulin (neutral protamine Hagedorn [NPH] Lente). Ultrashort-acting insulins (lispro, insulin aspart) are popular in pediatrics because they can be administered before, during, or immediately after a meal. Exogenous insulin administration is never physiologic, but this regimen largely relies for its success on continued endogenous insulin secretion at times during the day when insulin is necessary to control blood sugar and there is no insulin peak from the medication regimen. The initial insulin requirement ranges from 0.5 unit/kg per day in many young children to more than 1.0 unit/kg per day in adolescence. Initial insulin dosing is related to insulin sensitivity (increased in younger children and much decreased during adolescence), dietary carbohydrate intake, and residual endogenous insulin production. Available insulins are described in Table 2 and insulin management schemes are offered in Table 3.

Mealtime intake is less predictable for infants and toddlers and postmeal dosing with an ultrashort-acting insulin based upon carbohydrate intake helps

TABLE 2. **Insulin Preparations**

Insulin	Onset	Peak	Duration
Lispro (Humalog)	10–15 minutes	30–90 minutes	2+ hours
Aspart (NovoLog)	10–15 minutes	30–90 minutes	2+ hours
Regular	30–60 minutes	2–4 hours	6 hours
NPH	1–2 hours	4–6 hours	12–15 hours
Lente	1–2 hours	4–6 hours	12–15 hours
Ultralente	2–4 hours	6–14 hours	18–20 hours
Glargine (Lantus)*	1–2 hours	minimal	22–24 hours
70/30 NPH/Regular	30–60 minutes	3–8 hours	12–15 hours
75/25 NPH/lispro	10–15 minutes	30 minutes–8 hours	12–15 hours

*Insulin glargine cannot be mixed with other insulins.

TABLE 3. **Typical Insulin Administration Schedules**

Split mixed two injections/day		
Before breakfast	Before dinner	
45–55% NPH or Lente	15–25% NPH or Lente (Ultralente can be used to extend coverage until the morning)	
10–15% lispro, aspart, or Regular*	10–15% lispro, aspart, or Regular	
Split mixed three injections/day		
Before breakfast	Before dinner	Bedtime
50% NPH or Lente	15% NPH or Lente	15% NPH or Lente
10% lispro or aspart	10% lispro or aspart	
Basal insulin with supplemental insulin at meals		
Glargine insulin administered before bedtime	(40–50% of daily insulin)	
Before each meal	10–15% lispro or aspart administered depending on the carbohydrate content of the meal	

*Regular + lispro or aspart is sometimes given to prolong action.

to prevent hypoglycemic episodes. Sometimes a longer-acting basal insulin such as glargine (40% or less of total daily insulin) is chosen as the initial treatment in young children in order to facilitate management. Frequent blood glucose checks and appropriate administration of ultrashort-acting insulin protect children of this age from hypoglycemia while helping to maintain adequate glycemic control. For the same reasons, some parents will choose an insulin pump as a means of insulin administration in very young children.

Monitoring

A variety of glucose monitoring systems and strips are available. Smaller blood samples, faster meters, larger memory, and alternative sites of testing, such as the forearm, make the process easier. Blood glucose should be checked daily before each meal and at bedtime. Occasional nocturnal values are useful to avoid hypoglycemia. At times of insulin adjustment or intercurrent illnesses more frequent monitoring is required. Target blood glucose values should be 70 to 120 mg/dL before meals and 80 to 150 mg/dL 1 hour after meals. A record of the values and corresponding insulin doses helps to identify patterns and need for insulin dose adjustments.

Frequent or severe hypoglycemia or blood glucose greater than 200 mg/dL should provoke reassessment of insulin therapy and nutritional limits. Families need to check urine for ketones whenever the blood sugar is greater than 300 mg/dL or in times of illness. Ketonuria mandates more frequent blood sugar monitoring, additional doses of short-acting insulin, and increased fluid intake.

Nutrition

Nutritional counseling begins at the time of diagnosis. The classic approach is to provide an initial nutritional prescription based on caloric need with a distribution of carbohydrate (50%), protein (20%), and fat (30%) similar to a commonly recommended healthy diet. Complex carbohydrate and poly- and monounsaturated fat intake should be encouraged. This approach is relatively prescriptive. A more flexible management plan, used presently by most families who have the capacity to incorporate it into their lives, teaches estimation of carbohydrate to maintain glycemic control (carbohydrate counting).

The initial age-based caloric need can be estimated as: caloric intake = 1000 + 100 (age in years up to 12 years). The meal plan should be kept as close as possible to previous patterns. The eating habits, cultural practices, and special needs of the family need to be taken into consideration. Most children eat three meals a day, as well as a late afternoon snack and pre-bedtime snack. Younger children may take a midmorning snack as well. At the time of initial presentation, children have often lost weight, and over the next few weeks to a month, the caloric need may be much greater than expected. Guidelines for the content and timing of meals need to be established. Frequent visits with a nutritionist are indicated because of changing caloric needs for weight maintenance and growth.

When the family and child better understand the relationship between insulin, carbohydrate intake, and blood glucose, carbohydrate counting may be introduced. Frequent blood glucose determinations linked to carbohydrate counting and calculated injections of ultrashort-acting insulin increase flexibility in meal timing and content.

Physical Activity

Exercise is encouraged for healthy physical and emotional childhood development. Physical activity lowers blood sugar by enhancing glucose uptake in muscle and fat. The effects may be immediate or delayed. Some children need decreases in their intermediate or short-acting insulin following exercise. Others require extra food to prevent hypoglycemia. Management must be individualized.

Education

The Diabetes Control and Complications Trial proved that maintenance of nearly normal blood glucose levels substantially reduces the risk of long-term complications in people with diabetes. The challenge is to achieve such control. Regimens have become more complex as insulins with different timing of action and new delivery systems have become available.

All newly diagnosed children with diabetes who have ketoacidosis need to be hospitalized. However, a hyperglycemic child who does not have ketoacidosis can be maintained as an outpatient if the child is clinically stable; the family has adequate emotional, intellectual, and economic resources; and there is clinical support for the initiation of outpatient management.

Education of the child and family is a lifelong process. Immediate survival education includes mechanical training in insulin administration and blood glucose testing. Cognitive training must be allied with and closely follow the development of these mechanical skills. The family and child should understand the definition of diabetes, the necessity for blood glucose record keeping and interpretation, actions of different types of insulins, initial nutritional guidelines, and identification and treatment of hypoglycemia and hyperglycemia. The family also needs to be able to access a designated clinician member of the diabetes team. During the first week of diagnosis we instruct families to call daily with blood glucose values to plan insulin administration. Blood glucose values beyond established guidelines (usually less than 80 or greater than 250 mg/dL) require an immediate phone call to the clinician as well. The family and child then return to the outpatient department in 5 to 7 days to recheck skills, answer new questions, and revisit with other diabetes team members including a nutritionist, diabetes educator, and social worker or psychologist. The child is then seen again in 2 weeks, at 1 month, and then at 2- to 3-month intervals. Some families require a different educational regimen because of sociocultural or disorder-related issues.

In some institutions all newly diagnosed children with diabetes are admitted for a 2- to 3-day educational plan with the entire diabetes team. Upon discharge a similar follow-up schedule is established.

Additional Management Tools

Families should be given a prescription for glucagon to treat severe hypoglycemia and taught how to administer this agent. Glucagon is provided in 1 mg ready-to-mix vials. One half of each vial, or 0.5 mg, is adequate to treat severe hypoglycemia in most individuals. Children less than 5 years will respond nicely to 0.25 or 0.3 mg. If children use a glucose meter with the capacity to measure betahydroxybutyrate, then parents must learn to use the strips to measure serum ketones. For most children who are not using a meter with this capacity, dipsticks to measure urine ketones should be prescribed and their usage taught. Children younger than 10 years are particularly prone to viral illnesses with emesis. Some can become quite dehydrated, ketotic, or hypoglycemic as a result of such illness. It is our practice to prescribe suppositories containing promethazine (Phenergan) to be stored at home and used early in illness in such children to prevent the need for emergency room visits or hospitalizations. The parent is warned about the potential for rare extrapyramidal symptoms requiring treatment.

Long-Term Management

General Issues of Management

Children with type 1 diabetes should be seen at least every 3 months. At each visit, interval history and assessment of diabetes control should be the focus. The meter and the record book should be examined for glycemic control. Frequency and timing of hypoglycemia and hyperglycemia should be discussed. Wearing of emergency identification should be encouraged. On examination, blood pressure, growth, and pubertal status should be assessed. Thyroid enlargement, presence of lipohypertrophy or lipoatrophy, and sclerodactyly should be assessed. Fundi should be inspected at least yearly in older children and evaluation for sensory neuropathy using a standardized 10 g monofilament should be performed at least yearly in adolescents. Glycosylated hemoglobin levels should be obtained every 3 months. Values as close to normal as possible but less than 8% hemoglobin A_{1c} (mean blood glucose of 180 mg/dL) should be the goal for all children with diabetes. However, in young children, these goals may lead to severe hypoglycemia and should be tempered to match the individual. In children with an enlarged thyroid, symptoms of hypo- or hyperthyroidism, and in all children older than 10 years of age, TSH and thyroid antibodies should be obtained yearly. If thyroid antibodies are positive, the TSH should be measured at least annually. Total lipid panel, creatinine, and a random or overnight urine sample for microalbuminuria should be checked annually, particularly after puberty. Formal ophthalmologic examination should be requested yearly in pubertal patients and within 1 year of diagnosis in children older than age 10. Celiac disease can be associated with type 1 diabetes; any child with poor growth, anemia, or gastrointestinal symptoms should be evaluated. Screening for celiac disease with antiendomysial or tissue transglutaminase antibodies can be performed every 2 years.

Hypertension or microalbuminuria should be treated vigorously with angiotensin-converting enzyme (ACE) inhibitors. The usual first drug is lisinopril (Zestril)* in a dose of 5 mg daily. Dosing can be escalated until hypertension or microalbuminuria is controlled.

Accepted pediatric precepts of anticipatory guidance help the parent and child prepare for changes in diabetes control and management needs at different ages. Parents must remain intensively involved in

*Not FDA approved for this indication.

their child's diabetes management even during those early adolescent years when a major psychological task is separation from family. The balance between the participation of the child in diabetes management and maintenance of parental control is a delicate one. Children cannot be permitted full autonomy of diabetes care until the late teenage years. After the initial novelty of the equipment and attention from family and friends, children usually tire of daily monitoring and life restrictions. Peer pressure in adolescence can be a barrier to diabetes control. Issues of smoking, alcohol or other substance abuse, sexual activity, contraception, and pregnancy should be addressed at appropriate office visits. The role of smoking as a risk factor for long-term complications of diabetes should be stressed with child and family. If parents smoke, they should be encouraged to stop to provide an appropriate model for the child with diabetes. The necessity for impeccable glycemic control for healthy conception and pregnancy should be stressed to adolescent girls.

During adolescence there is a natural state of insulin resistance, and insulin requirements may increase. Weight gain may be a complication of increasing insulin dosage. Eating disorders are not uncommon. They should be considered in adolescents with erratic control and glycosylated hemoglobin levels higher than one should expect for the intensity of diabetes management. Omission of insulin can become a manifestation of an eating disorder.

The diagnosis of diabetes often burdens family lifestyle. Organization and vigilance necessary to manage the child may cause family conflicts and provoke marital discord. Family and individual counseling may become necessary. Finally, the pediatrician and pediatric diabetes team should facilitate the transition of the older adolescent to adult care providers.

Chronic Management of Insulin Therapy

After the initiation of insulin therapy, many children begin to regain some insulin-releasing capacity. Original insulin dosing may need to be lowered during the "honeymoon" or remission phase of diabetes. Families should be educated about the remission phase at the onset of diagnosis so that they understand that this temporary improvement does not mean the diabetes will disappear. Moreover, subsequent increased insulin need should not be viewed as a personal failure on the part of the child. Maintenance of euglycemia becomes more difficult after the remission phase. Frequent low blood glucose readings (<70 mg/dL) or high blood glucose levels (>150 mg/dL) should provoke reassessment of insulin therapy and nutritional management. Erratic control after the remission phase is often a sign that a change to a more intensive insulin regimen is necessary.

Intensification of Insulin Therapy

This may mean multiple insulin injections, greater attention to carbohydrate counting with the use of basal insulin such as glargine, and ultrashort-acting insulins with meals, or the use of the insulin pump.

Insulin pump therapy increases flexibility of diabetes management. Although it is particularly appealing to adolescents and their parents, pump therapy has been successful in infants and children of all ages. Pump technology has much improved in recent years. Pumps are about the size of pagers or cell phones and are worn on a belt or kept in a pocket. Insulin chambers or cartridges and subcutaneous catheters are changed every 2 to 3 days to maintain patency and prevent infection. Pumps use ultrashort-acting insulin (lispro or insulin aspart) infused in small, relatively frequent programmed boluses to provide basal insulin coverage, and calculated intermittent premeal boluses to cover carbohydrate intake. Alternative basal rates for different day and night periods are easily programmed. Insulin administration for meals is calculated much as it is for children receiving glargine insulin. A bolus insulin correction is made for blood glucose over 100 mg/dL. The correction is either determined empirically or based upon a correction factor (for ultrashort-acting insulin, 1800/total daily insulin dose = the decrease in blood glucose for each unit of insulin). Insulin administration for carbohydrate intake usually requires 1 unit for 20 to 30 grams in children younger than 5 years of age, 1 unit for 10 to 15 grams in preadolescents, and 1 unit for 8 to 10 grams during the insulin resistance of adolescence. Often, more insulin is necessary in the morning than later in the day. No commercially available pump "closes the loop" and infuses insulin based on blood sugar. The insulin pump presently is simply an insulin delivery device, requiring decision-making by parent and patient. The major disadvantage of insulin pump therapy is that the only insulin available to the patient is an ultrashort-acting preparation. Therefore, should there be failure of insulin administration for mechanical or other reasons, insulin-deficient ketoacidosis can develop within 4 to 6 hours. Frequent monitoring of blood glucose and ketones when indicated is therefore imperative. However, most studies have demonstrated glycemic improvement and ease of diabetes control with the introduction of an insulin pump. Waning of effect after years of use is related to decreased attention to blood glucose testing and insulin infusion, as with any other method of diabetes management.

Intensification of Glucose Monitoring

Two devices are presently available to offer a window into glycemic control not afforded by blood glucose monitoring even four to six times per day. A subcutaneous sensor (MiniMed) can be worn for 3 days at a time. The subcutaneously placed catheter sensor records blood glucose every 5 minutes. The information is then downloaded and is available to the physician. It is not designed to be used by the patient for moment-to-moment decision-making. A transcutaneous device, the GlucoWatch, can be worn for 12 to 15 hours at a time. It uses a disposable sensor pad and a reverse iontophoresis process to measure and report glucose every 10 minutes. Some patients report skin irritation with its use. Both devices are reasonably accurate and may provide additional feedback to the patient striving for excellent control.

TYPE 2 DIABETES MELLITUS

Diagnosis

Recent reports suggest that type 2 diabetes now represents 8% to 46% of all diabetes mellitus among children and adolescents. The percentage varies based on the age, ethnicity, and body composition of the child. Most but not all of the children are adolescents of African, Hispanic, Asian, and Native American descent. Typically there is a history of type 2 diabetes in one parent or another first- or second-degree relative. Obesity is the hallmark of the disease. Approximately 85% of the children have a body mass index greater than 27. Acanthosis nigricans, a skin condition characterized by hyperpigmentation and a velvety texture, is found in intertriginous areas in as many as 90% of the children. This is a marker of insulin resistance.

Children with type 2 diabetes usually have an indolent presentation. Some present with frank hyperglycemia and its symptoms. However, often glycosuria is found on a routine urinalysis and elevated blood glucose then confirms the diagnosis. Occasionally, the finding of acanthosis nigricans leads to a glucose tolerance test diagnosis (see Table 1). Type 2 diabetes is a product of insulin resistance and inadequate β-cell insulin secretion. Some obese young people with acanthosis nigricans remain euglycemic. Although they have a dysmetabolic syndrome, sufficient insulin secretion prevents the development of diabetes. In addition, not all children with type 2 diabetes have acanthosis nigricans as a physical marker of their hyperinsulinism.

Further laboratory work can help confirm the diagnosis of type 2 diabetes. Glycosylated hemoglobin values are elevated. Fasting insulin and C-peptide levels are elevated and autoantibodies to islet cells or insulin are usually negative. However, in some studies, up to 30% of young individuals with clinical type 2

TABLE 4. **Oral Hypoglycemics**

	Dose	Mechanism	Side Effects/Precautions
Biguanide			
Metformin (Glucophage)	500 mg bid to 1000 mg bid (500, 850, 1000 mg tablets)	Decreases hepatic glucose production Decreases intestinal glucose absorption Improves peripheral glucose uptake	GI disturbances, lactic acidosis Check creatinine, lactate, liver enzymes, stop before surgery, with illness, before use of IV contrast agents
Sulfonylureas			
Glipizide (Glucotrol)*	2.5–15 mg qd (scored 5 and 10 mg tablets)	Enhances beta cell insulin secretion	Hypoglycemia, GI disturbance, allergy, photosensitivity, metabolism and excretion slowed in hepatic and renal disease
Glyburide (DiaBeta, PresTab, Micronase)*	1.25–20 mg qd (1.25, 2.5, 5 mg tablets)		
Glimepiride (Amaryl)*	1–8 mg (1, 2, 4 mg tablets)		
Thiazolidinediones			
Rosiglitazone (Avandia)*	2–8 mg qd or 2–4 mg bid (2, 4, 8 mg tablets)	Peripheral insulin sensitizer	Edema, weight gain, abnormal liver transaminases, transient anemia; monitor liver function every other month
Pioglitazone (Actos)*	15–45 mg qd (15, 30, 45 mg tablets)		
Meglitinide analogues			
Repaglinide (Prandin)*	0.5–4 mg before meals (0.5, 1, 2 mg tablets)	Rapid beta cell depolarization and acute insulin release	Hypoglycemia, headache, GI disturbances, hepatic metabolism; increased risk of hypoglycemia in liver disease
Nateglinide (Starlix)*	60 mg to 120 mg before meals (60 and 120 mg tablets)		
α-Glucosidase inhibitors			
Acarbose (Precose)*	25–100 mg with meals (25, 50, 100 mg tablets)	Slows hydrolysis and absorption of carbohydrates	Transient GI disturbance because of carbohydrate malabsorption
Miglitol (Glyset)*	25–100 mg with meals (25, 50, 100 mg tablets)		

bid, twice per day; GI, gastrointestinal; IV, intravenous; qd, every day.

diabetes have positive islet antibodies. It is unclear whether they represent a slowly progressive form of type 1 diabetes or this is a response to islet destruction in type 2 diabetes.

The American Diabetes Association and the American Academy of Pediatrics recommend screening any child older than 10 years who is overweight or has signs of insulin resistance, a family history of type 2 diabetes mellitus or a genetically susceptible background. Recommended screening presently is a fasting plasma glucose level to be obtained every 2 years.

Treatment

There are no criteria for the most effective treatment of type 2 diabetes in the young. A National Institutes of Health–sponsored trial of various treatments including drugs and lifestyle change will be starting shortly and may eventually offer appropriate evidence-based guidance for treatment. From adult data, we infer that the most effective treatment is weight loss, exercise, and dietary change. Lifestyle changes, however, are most difficult to achieve and many children will require medication at the time of diagnosis.

In young people who present with marked hyperglycemia (blood glucose >300) or with ketoacidosis, insulin therapy is usually the initial drug of choice. Because these children are insulin-resistant, insulin doses may be much higher than those used in adolescents with type 1 diabetes. Treatment of diabetic ketoacidosis may require more than 0.1 unit/kg/hour of regular insulin. Children may need maintenance doses of more than 1 unit/kg of subcutaneous insulin per day. Various combinations of insulin with oral agents may be used. Insulin stimulates appetite. Therefore, often it is useful to combine it with one of the drugs that decreases insulin resistance so that the insulin dose can be maintained as low as possible. Insulin may be used at night to reduce nocturnal gluconeogenesis and morning glycemia without appreciably stimulating appetite. There are five classes of glucose-lowering oral agents that are used in adults and could be used in children. The only Food and Drug Administration–approved agent is metformin (Glucophage) and therefore it is commonly the first oral agent used. Available drugs are described in Table 4.

Our usual protocol is to start with metformin and titrate the dosing. If after 3 to 6 months of therapy euglycemia is not achieved, a second agent is added or insulin therapy is started. Lifestyle change is emphasized at each patient contact and we try to facilitate lifestyle change within a family as much as possible.

Long-term Management

Education and support should be offered at each visit and at least at three monthly intervals. Blood glucose monitoring should be done regularly, once or twice a day, at the initiation of any medication and with any dose adjustments. Glycosylated hemoglobin values should be obtained every 3 months. Yearly fasting lipid profiles and urine for microalbumin must be monitored. Dilated fundus examinations should be performed yearly. Blood pressure should be obtained, and careful neurologic examination and foot examination for neuropathy should be carried out at each visit. As in children with type 1 diabetes, ACE inhibitors are the drugs of choice to control blood pressure as well as treat microalbuminemia.

DIABETIC KETOACIDOSIS

method of
PATRICK J. BOYLE, M.D.
University of New Mexico Health Sciences Center
Albuquerque, New Mexico

One of the most dramatic presentations in medicine is that of the patient with *diabetic ketoacidosis* (DKA). The management of the disorder is one of the best examples of biochemistry in the human condition. Because of the infrequency with which most practitioners have the opportunity to care for either new or recurrent episodes of DKA in the patient with type 1 diabetes, the resolution of this metabolic emergency is handled with a myriad of methods. Approximately 1.25 million persons in the United States have type 1 diabetes, and the disease affects approximately 1 in 600 children. Most, but not all, of these children and young adults will present with DKA.

BIOCHEMISTRY

Two pivotal compounds, β-hydroxybutyrate and acetoacetate, are overproduced in the setting of DKA. Triglycerides are hydrolyzed to yield glycerol and free fatty acids. Through β oxidation of the free fatty acids in the mitochondria, ketone bodies are generated. Insulin is the single most potent regulator of lipolysis, a finding that supports the reasoning that insulin replacement is fundamental to the complete resolution of this acid-base disturbance. Measurement of these organic acids is not essential in the diagnosis or management of the disorder. Because of the molecular size of these anions, they are freely filterable by the kidney and appear in the urine. Ketone test stips included in most routine "dipstick" tests can detect only the α-ketoacid acetoacetate. Ketodiastix is a commercial product that can measure both organic acids in the urine. Because of the initial depletion of nicotinamide adenine dinucleotide (NAD) associated with this metabolic emergency, the usual patient has a great deal more β-hydroxybutyrate in the urine, so if one is using a test that measures primarily acetoacetate, the urine ketone test may appear only mildly positive.

Type 1 diabetes is characterized as a state of absolute insulin deficiency resulting from autoimmune destruction of the β cells. The plasma glucose concentration is the difference between liver glucose production and the clearance of glucose into peripheral tissues. The brain takes up glucose in an insulin-independent fashion, whereas muscle glucose uptake is driven by activation of a series of kinase phosphorylations ultimately leading to the mobilization of an intracellular pool of glucose transport proteins to the myocyte cell surface. The primary physiologic function of insulin is to suppress hepatic glucose production through a reduction in gluconeogenesis and glycogenolysis. However, rates of glucose clearance into muscle are impaired in the setting of insulin deficiency and contribute to the overall hyperglycemia. Additionally, because muscle primarily uses glucose for fuel, in the setting of insulin deficiency and lack of insulin-facilitated glucose transport and amino acid uptake, myocytes are forced to burn endogenous protein for fuel. Thus, part of the presentation in the patient with newly diagnosed diabetes or long-standing, poorly controlled type 1 diabetes is loss of muscle mass and weakness.

As the insulin concentration falls, the glucagon-insulin ratio rises, triggering a series of biochemical events that favor a rise in the systemic glucose concentration. The pentose phosphate shunt activity is decreased, and the concentration of fructose-2, 6-bisphosphate, a normal potent inhibitor of gluconeogenesis, is reduced. This leads to an increase in hepatic glucose production through new synthesis, as well as an increased rate of glycogen breakdown. Normally, insulin stimulates the enzymes responsible for the formation of uridine diphosphate glucose (UDPG) and subsequent conversion to glycogen. The concentrations of counterregulatory hormones (growth hormone, cortisol, and catecholamines) rise with the stress of the ketoacidemia and contribute to the activation of glycogenolysis and gluconeogenesis.

Without insulin, adipocytes have increased hormone-sensitive lipase activity. Thus, stored triglycerides are hydrolyzed to liberate free fatty acids and glycerol. Epinephrine and growth hormone also contribute to increased free fatty acid availability by increasing peripheral fat cell hydrolysis of triglyceride. Partially as a result of increased substrate availability, the mitochondrial rate of β oxidation increases. Additionally, however, production rises as a consequence of high glucagon levels stimulating the activity of carnitine acyl transferase in the mitochondria. Through this activation, there is an excessive shuttling of free fatty acids to the metabolic site of β oxidation, and the net rate of ketogenesis rises.

PHYSICAL AND CHEMICAL PRESENTATION

Physical examination findings in a patient in DKA are led by tachypnea. Often the inability to speak in full sentences over the telephone is a sign of significant acidemia. Because of the organic acidosis, there is an attempt toward restoring a normal acid-base status through the development of respiratory alkalosis. *Kussmaul's respiration* is the term used to describe the deep breathing regularly observed. Thus, the increase in tidal volume and a more rapid rate of respiration permit carbon dioxide (CO_2) to be blown off, causing the respiratory alkalosis.

Once the systemic glucose concentration exceeds the tubular capacity for glucose reclamation, approximately 180 mg/dL, glucose is cleared in the urine. Initially, this is a compensatory mechanism for clearing glucose from the plasma compartment, but as with all renally cleared solutes, water must also be cleared. Volume depletion ensues, and ultimately urine output declines as free water intake fails to keep up with urinary losses. Ketosis causes nausea, probably from central mechanisms, and this contributes to a decreased drive to drink. Vomiting is also common in patients in DKA, and it can contribute to fluid losses, bicarbonate loss from the upper gut, and dehydration. For unclear reasons, abdominal pain is a common presenting complaint in patients with DKA. The clinician must be vigilant in considering other common abdominal processes such as appendicitis or cholelithiasis (the risk of the latter is increased in patients with diabetes) as a cause of the abdominal pain.

DKA can have adverse neurologic outcomes. The oncotic pressure in the plasma favors the movement of water from various tissue compartments. The brain loses free water, and, in compensation, neurons are believed to generate idiogenic osmoles. These small proteins permit an equalization of the osmolality between the plasma and brain compartments. The idiogenic osmoles in the brain are slower to be cleared than the glucose molecules in the plasma compartment. Thus, as rehydration proceeds, fluid shifts into the brain to match the osmolality in the plasma compartment, and cerebral edema can be seen. Adults fortunately suffer limited rates of significant cerebral edema during the course of treatment of DKA. Overzealous hydration of smaller children or infants can precipitate critical brain edema, however, with its attendant risks.

Because of the volume contraction, the initial sodium and glucose concentrations are increased as a function of free water loss. Total body potassium depletion also occurs through urinary loss. However, as ketoacids accumulate, protons can be shifted intracellularly as a buffering mechanism. To maintain electrical neutrality, an exchange with potassium cations occurs for each proton shifted intracellularly. Thus, the presenting potassium concentration is generally elevated. However, as the acidosis resolves with insulin therapy, the total body potassium deficiency induced by the osmotic diuresis is unmasked, and potassium supplementation becomes essential.

INITIAL MANAGEMENT

The cornerstone of management of DKA is the administration of fluids and electrolytes. Because glucose is present in a rather fixed quantity in the vascular compartment, replacement of free water leads to a simple dilutional effect, and the glucose concentration can fall by as much as 50% with rehydration. Secondarily, renal blood flow is improved with volume expansion, and renal glucose clearance, which had fallen during the prerenal phase of the presentation, is reestablished. Thus, glycosuria is another mechanism for restoring normoglycemia. The plasma glucose concentration is simply the difference between rates of glucose production and glucose clearance. Insulin plays an important role in both parts of this equation. Insulin is the most potent inhibitor of hepatic glucose production, and the liver is the predominant site of most gluconeogenesis and glycogenolysis. Both of these metabolic methods for producing glucose are directly inhibited by insulin. In addition, insulin stimulates the glucose transport protein movement from the intracellular pool to the muscle and fat cell membranes. In adults with normal renal function, 1 to 3 L of normal saline can be safely given after the initial blood chemistry tests have been sent to the laboratory. After the initial fluid resuscitation, intravenous solutions should be changed to one half normal saline with potassium added. Conventionally, intravenous infusion rates after the switch in the intravenous fluid tonicity are around 150 mL/h, to maintain a diuresis of ketone bodies. Both the total amount of the initial normal saline and the subsequent half normal saline should be guided by restoration and maintenance of urine output. While the patient is still taking nothing orally, 5% dextrose may be given as part of the fluid replacement to help suppress starvation ketosis, which would otherwise contribute to the overall acidemia. I next discuss the administration of insulin during the acute phase of the illness.

Insulin is able to bind to plastic tubing used for intravenous infusions. Thus, the intravenous line must be primed with a sufficient amount of insulin to saturate binding sites on the polyethylene. At a concentration of 1 U of insulin in 10 mL of normal saline, binding site saturation is accomplished by wasting approximately 50 mL of the infusate. Many prominent sources recommend beginning insulin replacement with an intravenous bolus of 0.1 U/kg to saturate the insulin receptors on liver and muscle cells. The half-life of intravenous regular insulin is approximately 4 minutes. Thus, when an infusion is begun, a new steady-state plasma concentration is established within 20 minutes (five half-lives). Additional time is required to induce the postreceptor actions of insulin to reduce liver gluconeogenesis and glycogenolysis and to enhance muscle glucose uptake. Insulin infusions are generally begun at 0.05 U/kg/h. If a bolus is used, the recommendation is for 0.1 U/kg. However, given the short half-life, there is no clear-cut therapeutic advantage of using bolus insulin to saturate the receptors. Indeed, as mentioned earlier, boluses of insulin in the presence of hyperglycemia lead to significant shifts of potassium from the intravascular compartment to the tissue space. Theoretically, in the presence of a total body potassium deficit, using bolus insulin may contribute to acute hypokalemia and potential cardiac rhythm disturbances. We generally recommend that glucose concentrations be normalized no faster than 50 to 75 mg/dL/h, to minimize the likelihood of cerebral edema. Brain edema can occur with too rapid a normalization of systemic glucose concentration, but clinically significant cerebral edema is rare, except in small children.

The initial laboratory results have generally begun to return by the time the normal saline resuscitation has been completed. The diagnosis of DKA is confirmed by an increased anion gap [sodium − (chloride + potassium)], hyperglycemia, and the presence of ketones in the urine. Measurement of arterial blood gases should reveal a pH less than 7.35 and a partial pressure of CO_2 (P_{CO_2}) less than 40 mm Hg, findings documenting the compensatory respiratory alkalosis. P_{CO_2} values can often be very low to compensate for substantial organic acidosis. Subsequent laboratory evaluations should include electrolyte determinations at a frequency that will ensure adequate potassium replacement (approximately 2-hour intervals). Additionally, as the acidosis resolves, the anion gap will fall back toward normal, approximately 12. However, the bicarbonate concentration will remain low in the initial 48 hours of management. This nongap acidosis is largely the result of a hyperchloremia coming from the initial normal saline administration. This acid-base disturbance is quite analogous to excess chloride administration that can occur with total parenteral nutrition therapy. In the case of total parenteral nutrition, however, the solution is to add acetate to the total parenteral nutrition mixture. Acetate is not necessary for complete resolution of DKA. One additional factor that contributes to the nongap acidosis during the post-treatment phase is that saline is buffered to a pH of approximately 5.5. Generally between 36 and 48 hours, the bicarbonate concentration normalizes, whereas the anion gap remains normal. Giving potassium replacement as the phosphate salt rather than potassium chloride can minimize the total chloride load.

Potassium replacement cannot be given at a rate in excess of approximately 10 to 15 mEq/h. At such a rate, cardiac monitoring must occur to assess for prolongation of the QT interval and for ventricular dysrhythmias. The potassium deficit is commonly 80 to 120 mEq in DKA. The only condition that attenuates this need for potassium supplementation is coexistent renal insufficiency. In patients with significant diabetic nephropathy, potassium excretion is limited, and thus potassium replacement during the course of treatment must match. As mentioned earlier, as insulin administration begins and glucose clearance into muscle and fat is accelerated, potassium levels can be expected to fall. If potassium replacement is insufficient, substantial hypokalemia can be induced.

As glucose moves from the plasma compartment to any tissue, its metabolism is dependent on multiple phosphorylation steps. Thus, one would imagine that phosphate supplementation would accelerate the rate of recovery from DKA. In fact, phosphate supplementation is not essential for the normal recovery from DKA. The likely explanation is that the skeleton has an enormous capacity for supplying phosphate for the generation of ATP and biochemical catabolism of glucose.

The practitioner is also often tempted to administer sodium bicarbonate to accelerate the normalization of the acidosis. Bicarbonate anions combine with hydrogen cations to form carbonic acid, which, in turn, dissociates to CO_2 and water. Theoretically, the CO_2 would then be cleared through respiration. Unfortunately, CO_2 is also freely permeable across the blood-brain barrier, and once in the central nervous system, it induces paradoxical central nervous system acidosis. The net result is a reduction in central respiratory drive. Respiratory compensation for the organic acidosis from the ketoacid production is essential to prevent life-threatening acidosis. In general, for each 10 mm Hg fall in CO_2, there should be a rise in pH of approximately 0.1 U. Thus, if the pH is 7.3 with a P_{CO_2} of 10 mm Hg, an acute respiratory decompensation that elevates the P_{CO_2} to, say, 70 mm Hg would drop the pH to approximately 6.7. Perhaps this rather concerning fall in pH is what drives practitioners frequently to measure arterial blood gas values. Certainly, if the patient has underlying pulmonary disease, including pneumonia, a greater degree of concern must be exercised, and frequently arterial blood gas monitoring would be indicated. Conversely, in a young, otherwise healthy person without pulmonary disease, repeated arterial blood gas determinations are substantially less necessary.

UNDERLYING PATHOPHYSIOLOGY

Whereas the acute management of the acid-base disturbance and adequate attention to electrolyte imbalances are the focus of emergency management, the reason the patient initially developed DKA must be completely investigated (Table 1). If the presentation is the preliminary manifestation of type 1 diabetes, then the DKA is the result of incipient insulin deficiency. However, many patients who present with their first episode of DKA subsequently revert to a period of insulin independence, known as the "honeymoon period." Thus, at the time of the initial presentation, there is generally assumed to be roughly 20% of the β-cell mass left (80% having been destroyed by the autoimmune process). The development of DKA at the time of the first presentation of diabetes is often associated with another metabolic stress such as a viral upper respiratory or gastrointestinal infection that induces a state of relative insulin resistance. Normally, β cells compensate for such metabolic stresses, but with limited mass remaining in the presence of autoimmune destruction, the acute infection becomes the trigger for the first episode of DKA. In initial and subsequent presentations of DKA, other common infectious processes must be considered.

TABLE 1. **Causes of Diabetic Ketoacidosis**

First-time presentation with insulin deficiency
Infectious processes
  Viral upper respiratory infection or gastrointestinal infection
  Bacterial pneumonia, urinary tract infection, pyelonephritis, pelvic inflammatory disease
Vascular events
  Myocardial infarction, stroke, peripheral vascular occlusion
Pregnancy (normal or ectopic)
Inadequate insulin therapy

A complete physical examination must be performed to look for conditions such as sinus infections, otitis media, urinary tract infection, pneumonia, and abdominal processes such as appendicitis. Clouding the physical examination is the finding that abdominal pain and discomfort are common in DKA itself. Additionally, DKA induces a state of relative hypothermia. Thus, whereas a fever would normally lead the practitioner to consider an infectious process more strongly, a normal body temperature should trigger a heightened level of concern. Women must be evaluated for pelvic infections and pregnancy as a standard part of potential factors inducing DKA. The placenta produces hormonal factors that contribute to insulin resistance; thus, pregnancy (or ectopic pregnancy) can clearly cause a patient with established diabetes or a new diagnosis of diabetes to develop DKA. Therefore, in addition to standard electrolytes and arterial blood gas concentrations, a pregnancy test is essential in women. In older patients or in those with diabetes of sufficient duration to permit vasculopathy to have been established, myocardial infarction should be considered. Patients with diabetes are notorious for having limited pain in association with acute myocardial infarction. Finally, two uncommon but horrific infections must be mentioned.

In patients with long-standing low-grade acidosis associated with suboptimal insulin therapy, the metabolic stage is set to allow the growth of the fungus *Mucor. Mucor* requires iron in an oxidative state seen in chronic acidosis in order to flourish. *Mucor* mycosis is seen in the upper respiratory tract, most commonly in sinuses and the soft palate. Because the mycelia invade the microvasculature of these tissues, the infection induces thrombosis and tissue necrosis. The characteristic soft palate or turbinate color is therefore black as a result of tissue infarction. The early recognition of this condition is essential because therapy includes antifungal chemotherapy and aggressive surgical resection of the infected tissue.

The other rare infection seen in patients with poorly controlled diabetes is necrotizing fasciitis. The anaerobic *Streptococcus* associated with this fulminant infection generally starts as a bullous lesion in the perineum. As with *Mucor,* this infection requires aggressive débridement and antibiotic therapy. Both of these unusual infections invade adjacent tissues in a matter of minutes to hours. Thus, physical examination must include a complete assessment of the skin in the perianal and perineal regions and the epithelium of the nares and turbinates.

RESOLUTION OF TRANSITION TO SUBCUTANEOUS INSULIN REPLACEMENT

With normalization of the anion gap, and assuming the patient is no longer nauseated or has no contraindication to eating, subcutaneous insulin must be given. Because one cannot be certain that the patient will be able to hold down food, we generally recommend a dose of fast-acting insulin analogue (insulin lispro [Humalog] or insulin aspart [NovoLog]) approximately 15 to 20 minutes before the meal begins. The intravenous insulin should be stopped at the time of the meal, thus providing a crossover period from intravenous to subcutaneous therapy. The dose of the subcutaneous insulin is given as the sum of the number of units of insulin given over the last 4 hours plus 1 U of insulin for every 10 g of carbohydrates to be consumed (generally 40 to 50 g of starch would be served for an average meal). The usual intravenous insulin requirement as DKA is resolving is approximately 1.0 to 1.5 U/h. Therefore, the initial dose of subcutaneous insulin should be 8 to 10 U. If the patient does become nauseated and fails to eat or to hold down the first meal, then glucose supplementation to offset the dose of subcutaneous insulin can be given for a brief period. Given that the rapid-acting insulin analogues have a duration of action of less than 6 hours, additional subcutaneous insulin will be needed before the next scheduled meal.

With more of the population becoming overweight or obese, including 10% to 15% of all children, it is imperative to determine whether an overweight child with DKA has type 1 or type 2 diabetes. Type 1 diabetes is generally thought to occur only in children or teenagers; however, young to middle-aged adults can clearly develop type 1 diabetes. Therefore, one cannot stereotype type 1 diabetes as "juvenile onset." With the increasing numbers of overweight children, some will present with type 1 diabetes. Approximately 20% of patients with hyperosmolar "nonketotic" type 2 diabetes present with ketosis. This presentation may result from the patient not feeling well enough to eat during the days before admission owing to other illnesses. Starvation ketosis in conjunction with insulin resistance and type 2 diabetes cannot be distinguished clinically from full-blown type 1 DKA. Type 2 diabetes should be considered more likely in those patients who are overweight, have family histories of type 2 diabetes, and are more than 45 years of age. Overweight younger patients with DKA should be assumed to have type 1 diabetes until proven otherwise. Ultimately, type 1 can be differentiated from type 2 by measuring C-peptide concentration. Given that C-peptide is produced in molar concentrations equal to insulin in humans, and that commercial insulin administered to patients does not contain C-peptide, the concentration of C-peptide is a surrogate marker of β-cell mass. If the concentration is less than 0.6 ng/mL in the presence of hyperglycemia, then type 1 diabetes is favored. If the concentration is more than 4 ng/mL in the presence of hyperglycemia, then type 2 is favored. However, the gray zone between 0.6 and 4 ng/mL may indicate that the patient is on the way to developing type 1 diabetes but has not experienced sufficient autoimmune β-cell destruction to reduce C-peptide levels. Alternatively, patients with type 2 diabetes experience acute glucose toxicity in the islets, and this can limit the insulin response to hyperglycemia and can lead to spuriously low C-peptide concentrations that will rise after the systemic glucose concentration has been normalized for a time.

GOUT AND HYPERURICEMIA

method of
ANDREW E. THOMPSON, M.D., and
GRAHAM D. REID, M.B., Ch.B.
University of British Columbia
Vancouver, Canada

PURINE METABOLISM AND URIC ACID PRODUCTION

Uric acid is a product of the metabolism of purine nucleotides. The purine nucleotides adenosine monophosphate and guanosine monophosphate are important components needed for the formation of DNA molecules. The purines required to form these nucleotides are derived from three sources:

1. De novo synthesis catalyzed by the enzyme phosphoribosylpyrophosphate (PRPP) synthetase
2. Dietary sources
3. Recycling of purines catalyzed by the enzyme hypoxanthine-guanine phosphoribosyltransferase (HGPRT)

Through a series of reactions, purine nucleotides are metabolized to their respective purine bases. Catalyzed by the enzyme xanthine oxidase, the purine bases are then metabolized to xanthine and finally to uric acid (see Figure 1). Unfortunately, humans lack the enzyme uricase, which oxidizes uric acid to the highly soluble allantoin.

URIC ACID EXCRETION

Uric acid is excreted by the kidneys. It is freely filtered at the glomerulus, followed by an active transport process in the proximal tubule that results in reabsorption of more than 90% of the filtered load. Further downstream, in the proximal nephron, uric acid is secreted by a second active transport mechanism that accounts for a major portion of the uric acid excreted in urine. Finally, small amounts of uric acid undergo post-secretory tubular reabsorption. Figure 2 outlines the renal handling of uric acid.

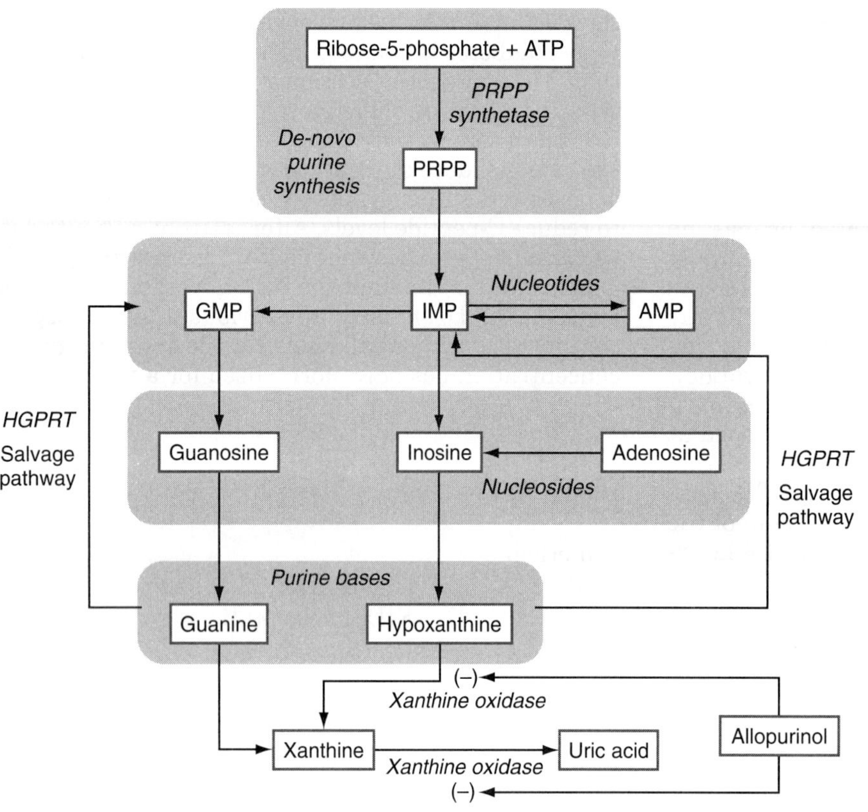

Figure 1. Production and metabolism of purine nucleotides. AMP, adenosine monophosphate; GMP, guanosine monophosphate; HGPRT, hypoxanthine-guanine phosphoribosyltransferase; IMP, inosine monophosphate; PRPP, phosphoribosylpyrophosphate.

ETIOLOGY OF HYPERURICEMIA

Hyperuricemia results from one of three possible mechanisms: overproduction of uric acid, underexcretion of uric acid, or a combination of both processes.

Overproduction of Uric Acid

Overproduction of uric acid is uncommon and occurs in only about 10% of patients with gout. Uric acid overproduction can result from an inherited enzyme abnormality, or it can be caused by an acquired uric acid load.

Enzyme Abnormality. Superactivity of the enzyme PRPP synthetase results in increased de novo synthesis of uric acid and subsequent hyperuricemia (see Figure 1). A partial or complete deficiency of HGPRT leads to a reduction in recycled purine bases and, consequently, hyperuricemia (see Figure 1). Both of these genetic enzyme abnormalities are X-linked, and patients have early adult-onset gout (age <30 years) and a high incidence of uric acid nephrolithiasis.

Acquired Urate Load. Increased cellular turnover can result in hyperuricemia by increasing the load of purine nucleotides. This condition is typically seen with malignant diseases, especially myeloproliferative

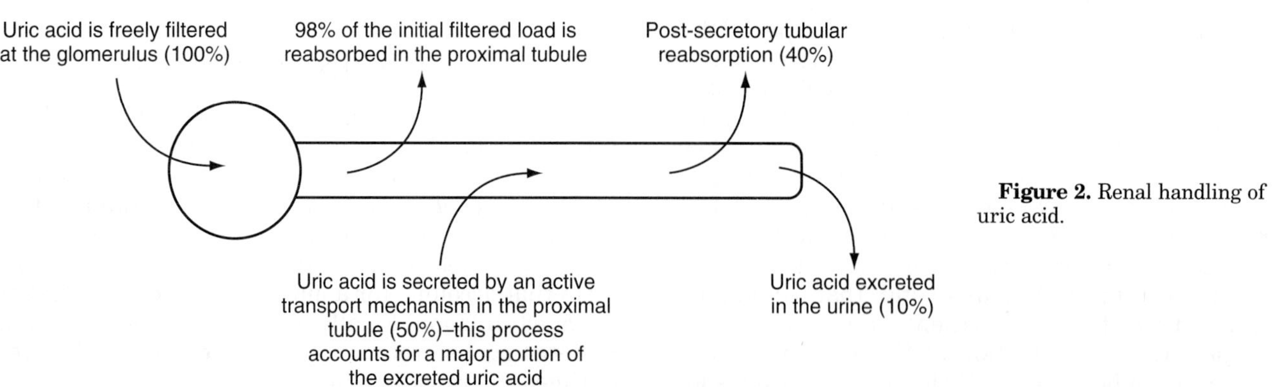

Figure 2. Renal handling of uric acid.

and lymphoproliferative disorders. It can also occur with nonmalignant diseases in which cellular turnover is increased, such as psoriasis and hemolytic anemia. A second mechanism of an increased urate load is through tissue breakdown with increased purine nucleotide catabolism. This mechanism is seen in the setting of tissue hypoxia and tumor lysis with chemotherapy, and it can be induced by drugs, specifically alcohol. Finally, increased purine ingestion can theoretically result in hyperuricemia.

Underexcretion of Uric Acid

Most patients (90%) with gout and hyperuricemia are underexcretors of uric acid. Over a wide range of filtered uric acid loads, the majority of patients with gout have a lower fractional excretion of uric acid than do those without gout. The differences in renal handling of uric acid between hyperuricemic and non-hyperuricemic subjects have not been completely determined. Hyperuricemia from underexcretion can be primary or result from any of the following secondary mechanisms:

Renal Disease. Any abnormality resulting in a reduction in the glomerular filtration rate can theoretically result in hyperuricemia. However, it is usually seen in the setting of chronic renal insufficiency.

Abnormal Metabolic States. Starvation, dehydration, diabetic ketoacidosis, and lactic acidosis can lead to hyperuricemia.

Drug Induced. Drugs that commonly impair the renal handling of uric acid and as a result cause hyperuricemia include thiazide diuretics, loop diuretics, ethanol, and low-dose salicylates. Less common medications include cyclosporine, ethambutol, pyrazinamide, and nicotinic acid. L-Dopa, theophylline, and didanosine (ddI, nucleoside analogue for the treatment of HIV) can also cause hyperuricemia, although the mechanisms are unknown.

Endocrinopathies. Hyperparathyroidism and hypothyroidism can give rise to hyperuricemia.

CLINICAL FEATURES, DIAGNOSIS, AND TREATMENT OF HYPERURICEMIA AND GOUT

Asymptomatic Hyperuricemia

Clinical Features. Asymptomatic hyperuricemia is the term applied to elevated serum uric acid levels in which symptomatic tissue deposition of uric acid has not occurred. The risk of gout developing increases with increasing hyperuricemia. Hyperuricemia is associated with but not necessarily causative of other conditions such as hypertension, hyperlipidemia, obesity, atherosclerosis, renal disease, renal calculi, and insulin resistance.

Diagnosis. Uric acid levels in males show a sharp increase at puberty and subsequently plateau. In females, uric acid levels remain low until menopause because of the enhanced effect of estrogen on renal urate clearance. After menopause, uric acid levels rise to levels to those comparable in men, and hyperuricemia in women is therefore typically seen after menopause. The diagnosis of hyperuricemia is made by detection of uric acid levels above the normal laboratory range.

Treatment. Although the risk of gout does increase with elevated uric acid levels, over 70% of patients with hyperuricemia will remain clinically asymptomatic. The long-term risks of urolithiasis, significant renal impairment, and coronary artery disease associated with hyperuricemia are very low, even with uric acid levels up to 6 SD above the normal mean. Hypertension is a much greater risk factor for renal impairment in this patient group than hyperuricemia. Based on the current available evidence, the potential benefits of treating asymptomatic hyperuricemia do not warrant incurring the potential risks associated with the treatment.

Acute Gout

Clinical Features. Acute gout defines the entity of uric acid crystal–induced joint synovitis. The first attack of acute gout typically occurs after 15 to 20 years of asymptomatic hyperuricemia. In men, attacks begin between the ages of 35 and 50 and, in women, usually 15 to 20 years after menopause. Acute gout is an inflammatory arthritis characterized by intense pain, swelling, and erythema of the affected joint or joints with resulting disability. This inflammatory response can be dramatic and often involves contiguous structures such as tendons (tenosynovitis) and soft tissue. The clinical picture of acute gout may be indistinguishable from septic arthritis with fever, leukocytosis, and an elevated sedimentation rate. Acute bacterial septic arthritis must always be considered in any episode of acute joint inflammation, and rare cases of coexisting gout and infection have been reported. Attacks may be precipitated by minimal trauma, acute illness (often seen in the hospital), surgery, excessive alcohol intake, or any insult that causes an increase in serum uric acid levels (i.e., starting or stopping allopurinol therapy). The typical attack reaches maximal intensity over a few hours and will usually resolve within a week to 10 days, although some episodes may be more gradual in onset, less severe, and persist for several weeks. Even if left untreated, the attack will eventually subside. About 80% of attacks involve a single joint (monoarthritis) and predominate in the lower extremity, and the first metatarsophalangeal and tarsal joints are classically affected. However, any joint can be afflicted, with the knees, wrists, elbows, metacarpophalangeal and proximal interphalangeal joints commonly being involved.

Diagnosis. The gold standard for the diagnosis of acute gout is identification of intracellular monosodium urate crystals in synovial fluid leukocytes. Hyperuricemia by itself is of little diagnostic value. Uric acid crystals appear as negatively birefringent when viewed under a polarizing microscope. This finding is very specific for the diagnosis of acute gout and has a sensitivity of 85% when synovial fluid can be obtained. When synovial fluid cannot be obtained, the diagnosis becomes presumptive and is based on the clinical findings and identification of risk factors, including previous episodes, excessive alcohol intake, obesity, family history, and medication use. Serum uric acid levels during an acute attack are not usually helpful because 40% of patients can have levels within normal limits. Furthermore, decreases in serum uric acid have been reported in the setting of acute gout. Other nonspecific laboratory findings during an acute attack include leukocytosis, thrombocytosis, and an elevated erythrocyte sedimentation rate. Commonly, joint radiographs in gout are completely normal apart from soft tissue swelling. This finding is true even for patients with recurrent attacks over many years.

Treatment of the Acute Attack. See Figure 3.

NONPHARMACOLOGIC

The application of ice and immobilization of an affected joint with a splint may provide a degree of symptom relief.

PHARMACOLOGIC

NONSTEROIDAL ANTI-INFLAMMATORY DRUGS. Nonsteroidal anti-inflammatory drugs (NSAIDs) are effective in reducing the acute inflammation of gout. In more than 90% of patients, complete resolution of the attack occurs within 5 to 8 days of initiation of therapy. If treatment is started immediately at the onset of symptoms, the inflammation may subside more promptly. Double-blind studies investigating the use of NSAIDs have shown no significant difference in efficacy, although traditionally indomethacin (Indocin), 50 to 75 mg orally three times daily*; naproxen (Naprosyn), 500 to 750 mg orally twice daily; and ibuprofen (Motrin, Advil),† 800 mg orally every 8 hours, have been used. NSAIDs should be used with great caution in patients with an increased risk of toxicity, such as those with previous or active peptic ulceration (with gastrointestinal hemorrhage), chronic renal failure, hypertension, congestive heart failure, inflammatory bowel disease, or systemic anticoagulation with warfarin or heparin. NSAIDs must be used with caution in elderly individuals (older than 65 years) because of a further increased risk of toxicity in this population. The cyclooxygenase-2 (COX-2) selective inhibitors celecoxib (Celebrex),† rofecoxib

*Exceeds dosage recommended by the manufacturer.
†Not FDA approved for this indication.

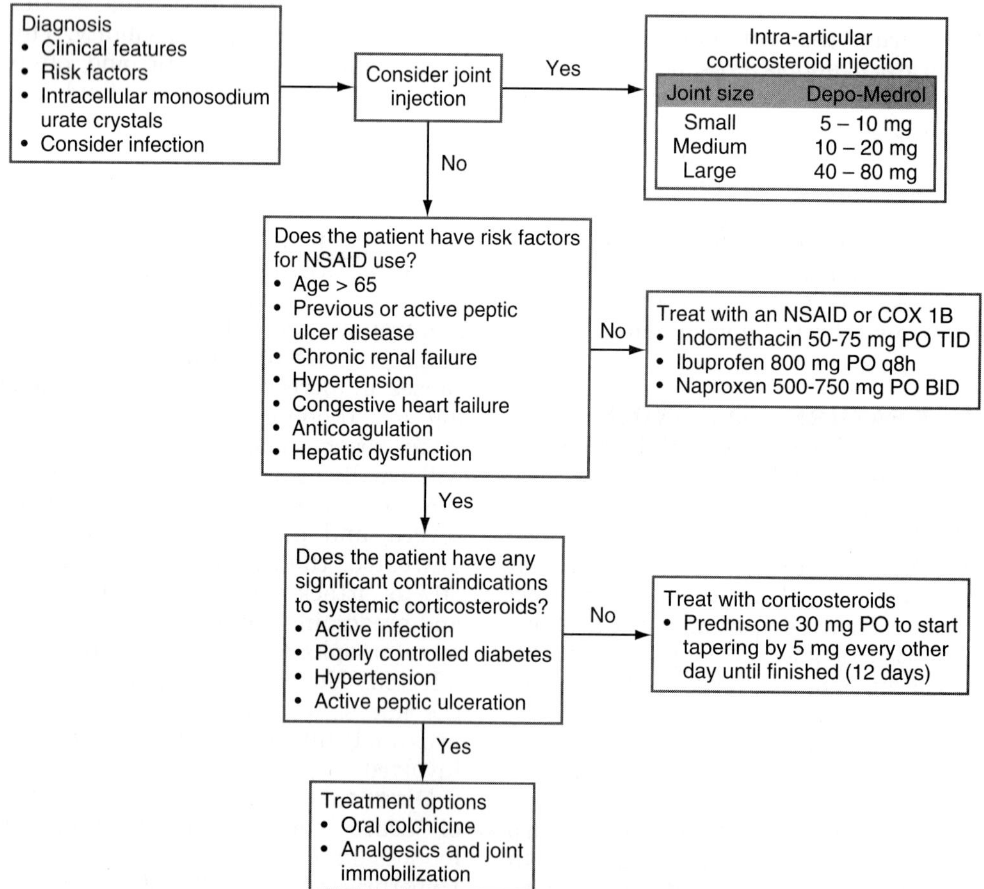

Figure 3. Algorithm for the treatment of an acute attack of gout. NSAID, nonsteroidal anti-inflammatory drug.

(Vioxx),† and valdecoxib (Bextra)† may be used during an episode of acute gout, although no randomized, controlled trials have been conducted. Another COX-2 selective agent, etoricoxib (Arcoxia),† 120 mg once daily, has been shown to be as effective as indomethacin, 50 mg three times daily.

COLCHICINE. Oral colchicine is an effective treatment for acute gout. In patients with normal renal function, doses of 0.6 mg every 6 to 8 hours on day 1, followed by colchicine, 0.6 mg twice daily, may be better tolerated than the traditional regimen of 0.6 mg orally every 1 to 2 hours. Colchicine is generally safe, although its use is frequently limited by abdominal cramps and diarrhea. Intravenous colchicine is potentially very dangerous and should be used with extreme caution, if ever.

CORTICOSTEROIDS. Intra-articular corticosteroids provide effective relief for acute gout. Intra-articular steroid injections are ideal for monoarticular attacks, especially in patients who may be at risk for toxicity with NSAIDs or colchicine. Methylprednisolone (Depo-Medrol) can be injected into the joint: 40 to 80 mg into a large joint, 20 to 40 mg into a medium-sized joint, and 10 mg into a small joint. Other intra-articular steroid preparations, including triamcinolone acetonide (Kenalog) and triamcinolone hexacetonide (Aristospan), may be used, but no comparative studies have been conducted. In a patient who refuses an injection or has polyarticular gout, systemic steroids can be very useful. As an example, one can start at 30 mg of prednisone per day and reduce the dose by 5 mg every other day, thereby tapering the therapy over a 12-day period. Intramuscular adrenocorticotropic hormone, 40 IU, has also been found to be a safe and effective alternative treatment.

Prevention of Future Gout. After the first episode of gout, patients may not have another for years. However, the recurrence rate is approximately 60% within the first year, about 80% by 2 years, and approximately 90% by 5 years. It is not appropriate to initiate long-term prophylactic therapy in patients with isolated intermittent episodes, except if extenuating circumstances are present. Dietary modifications, avoidance of alcohol and known precipitating medications, and increased fluid intake may be advised but rarely have a significant clinical impact. Indications for long-term prophylactic medications are as follows:

1. Recurrent acute episodes of gout affecting the patient's lifestyle
2. Patients at risk from complications of the treatment required for acute attacks
3. Patient acceptance of the need for compliance with lifelong pharmacologic therapy

Colchicine, allopurinol (Zyloprim), and the uricosuric agents sulfinpyrazone (Anturane) and probenecid (Benemid) are used for long-term prophylactic therapy, but they obviously have very different modes of action.

†Not FDA approved for this indication.

Colchicine, 0.6 mg orally daily to twice daily, will prevent acute attacks of gout, but of course it does nothing to prevent the continued buildup of total body uric acid stores. As such, its use is generally limited.

Allopurinol is frequently the most appropriate medication for patients requiring long-term preventive therapy. The goal of hypouricemic therapy with allopurinol is to lower serum uric acid to below the level at which uric acid precipitates within the joints. Allopurinol should not be started during an acute attack of gout because it may prolong the duration of the attack. The uric acid level should be reduced gradually by starting allopurinol at doses of 50 to 200 mg/d. The dose should be increased every 1 to 3 weeks until the serum uric acid level is about 300 μmol/L. Patients must be warned that on initiating therapy with allopurinol, the frequency of acute gout attacks may temporarily increase. As tissue stores are mobilized for excretion, the uric acid flux makes attacks more common ("mobilization gout"). It may take 3 to 4 months of the appropriate dosage of allopurinol before total body urate stores are depleted by continued uric acid excretion to a level at which acute attacks will not occur. During this time, colchicine or NSAIDs can be used prophylactically to reduce the frequency of these attacks; alternatively, each individual attack can be treated (see earlier).

Hypersensitivity reactions develop in approximately 2% of individuals receiving allopurinol, and 20% of these reactions are severe, some resulting in death. The clinical setting should be carefully considered before starting lifelong allopurinol therapy to ensure an appropriate benefit-to-risk balance.

Probenecid and sulfinpyrazone increase uric acid excretion by the kidney. If excretion exceeds production, total body uric acid stores will be depleted over time. These agents increase the risk of uric acid stone formation and are not effective in patients with significant renal impairment.

Chronic Tophaceous Gout

Clinical Features. Tophi are discrete collections of uric acid. Clinically apparent tophi may develop between 10 and 20 years after an initial attack if the hyperuricemia is left untreated. Tophi are most commonly found over the dorsal aspect of the fingers and toes (may be confused with osteoarthritic changes) and over the extensor surface of the forearms (olecranon bursa) and, less commonly, on the pinna of the ear. Chronic tophaceous gout is often seen in patients with an early age at the onset of recurrent gout, frequent attacks over many years, high serum uric acid values, and a predilection for upper extremity and polyarticular episodes. Joint inflammation in patients with chronic tophaceous gout may be less dramatic and more persistent and may mimic rheumatoid arthritis.

Diagnosis. The diagnosis is frequently based on a history of recurrent attacks of acute inflammation in joints typically affected by gout at increasing frequency over many years. Patients may initially be seen late in the course of chronic tophaceous gout with multiple and widespread tophi and chronic, persistent polyarticular joint inflammation. The classic radiographic changes are those of "punched out" lesions with overhanging margins adjacent to joints. These lucent areas are actually tophaceous deposits. Polarizing microscopic examination of material aspirated from tophi will reveal masses of urate crystals.

Treatment. The goal of pharmacologic treatment of chronic tophaceous gout is to lower the serum uric acid level, thereby creating a concentration gradient encouraging uric acid in tissues to move into the circulation. Again, the initial hypouricemic agent of choice is allopurinol, and administration and monitoring of treatment are identical to those used for preventing recurrent attacks of acute gout (described earlier).

Uric Acid and the Kidney

Uric acid may affect the kidney in three different ways:

1. Uric acid nephrolithiasis, or uric acid stone formation in the collecting tubules
2. Acute uric acid nephropathy
3. Urate nephropathy

The deposition of urate crystals in the renal interstitium results in a secondary chronic inflammatory response that can lead to chronic interstitial fibrosis and renal failure. Both uric acid nephrolithiasis and urate nephropathy are more common in patients with excessive uric acid production and excretion.

Uric Acid Nephrolithiasis

Only some patients with uric acid stones have an identifiable medical condition contributing to the stone formation. Such medical conditions include primary gout (10% to 20% have uric acid stones) and conditions predisposing to secondary gout, including myeloproliferative disorders and congenital metabolic enzyme defects, inflammatory bowel disease, diet-induced hyperuricemia, and renal hypouricemia (a defect in renal tubular reabsorption of uric acid). Patients with uric acid stones are generally older than those who form stones of other composition, but the clinical manifestations are similar.

Uric acid stones form in the setting of acidic urine (pH <5.5), which can be a clue to the diagnosis. Otherwise, 24-hour urine collections should be analyzed to evaluate for the presence of hyperuricosuria, hypercalciuria, hyperoxaluria, and hypocitraturia.

Adequate hydration (maintenance of urine output >2L/d) and urinary alkalinization (sodium bicarbonate, 650 mg orally three times daily), with a goal of achieving a pH of 6 to 6.5, are the cornerstones of medical management. Hydration and alkalinization can lead to the dissolution of uric acid stones and thus reduce the need for other invasive procedures. In patients who do not respond to the aforementioned measures or if concomitant hyperuricosuria is present, allopurinol may be used.

Acute Uric Acid Nephropathy

Acute uric acid nephropathy occurs in situations in which large amounts of uric acid are excreted in urine with resultant tubular obstruction from uric acid crystallization. This condition is most often seen with the tumor lysis syndrome after the administration of chemotherapy or radiation treatment. The diagnosis is suspected when acute renal failure develops in this setting and in association with hyperuricemia. Prevention is the best treatment of acute uric acid nephropathy. Pretreatment with allopurinol and fluid loading to maintain adequate urine output are necessary to prevent this problem.

Urate Nephropathy

Clinical Features. Urate nephropathy is rarely seen now because of early intervention. However, some patients have chronic renal insufficiency, a bland urine sediment, and hyperuricemia, which are findings compatible with urate nephropathy.

Treatment. Treatment consists of adequate hydration (maintenance of urine output >2 L/d) and the use of allopurinol as a hypouricemic agent.

HYPERLIPOPROTEINEMIAS

method of
CONRAD B. BLUM, M.D.
Columbia University College of Physicians and Surgeons
New York, New York

Elevations in plasma cholesterol and triglyceride levels are caused by increased levels of the plasma lipoproteins, the transport vehicles for the otherwise insoluble plasma lipids. Disorders of lipoprotein metabolism achieve their importance because of their clinical sequelae. Elevated levels of low-density lipoprotein (LDL) and low levels of high-density lipoprotein (HDL) increase the risk for development of atherosclerotic vascular disease, and high levels of partially degraded, very low density lipoprotein (VLDL) (termed remnant lipoproteins) are also atherogenic. Extremely high levels of the triglyceride-rich lipoproteins VLDL and chylomicrons can cause pancreatitis and xanthomatosis.

METABOLISM OF THE PLASMA LIPOPROTEINS

Four major classes of lipoproteins are found in plasma (Table 1). The lipoproteins are spherical particles with a core composed primarily of triglyceride or cholesteryl ester and a surface coat of unesterified

TABLE 1. **Major Classes of Plasma Lipoproteins**

Lipoprotein Class	Origin	Catabolism	Clinical Correlates of Elevation
Chylomicrons (>95% triglyceride)	Intestine	Lipoprotein lipase; remnants cleared by the liver	Pancreatitis Eruptive xanthomas Hepatosplenomegaly
VLDL (60% triglyceride)	Liver	Lipoprotein lipase, conversion to LDL	Glucose intolerance Hyperuricemia
LDL (50% cholesterol)	VLDL	LDL receptor	Atherosclerosis Corneal arcus Xanthelasma Tendinous xanthoma
HDL (50% protein, 25% cholesterol)	Liver and intestine	Selective cholesterol uptake by the liver	Decreased CHD risk (increased risk with low HDL)

Abbreviations: CHD = Coronary heart disease; HDL = high-density lipoprotein; LDL = low-density lipoprotein; VLDL = very low density lipoprotein.

cholesterol, phospholipid, and specific apolipoproteins. The various apoproteins function as detergents to solubilize the lipids in plasma; additionally, some act as recognition sites for cell surface receptors, and some are cofactors for enzymes involved in lipid metabolism.

Plasma lipoproteins contain varying amounts of all the lipids in plasma. LDL and HDL are rich in cholesterol and contain low levels of triglycerides. Normally, LDL is the major carrier of cholesterol in human plasma and accounts for approximately 70% of the total plasma cholesterol. Chylomicrons and VLDL are triglyceride rich. Chylomicrons are the transport vehicle for dietary triglyceride, whereas VLDL, secreted by the liver, is the transport vehicle for endogenous triglyceride. In the circulation, lipoprotein lipase hydrolyzes triglyceride in the core of VLDL and chylomicrons, yielding a smaller, shrunken remnant particle. The remnant lipoproteins are thought to be atherogenic. Chylomicron remnants are rapidly taken up by the liver. Most VLDL remnants undergo further conversion to form LDL particles.

Clearance of LDL from plasma occurs largely by a specific receptor-mediated process involving recognition of apo B-100, the sole apoprotein of LDL. Normally, this process accounts for two thirds of the clearance of LDL from plasma. Clearance of LDL via this mechanism is antiatherogenic. Another receptor, a scavenger receptor of macrophages, recognizes oxidized and other chemically altered forms of LDL. Clearance of LDL via the scavenger receptor pathway may contribute to the development of atherosclerotic plaque.

HDL particles have their origin both in the liver and in the intestine. Processes associated with the metabolic degradation of VLDL and chylomicrons further contribute to the formation of HDL. HDL concentrations in plasma are inversely related to the risk of coronary heart disease (CHD). The mechanism or mechanisms responsible for the inverse relationship between the HDL concentration and the risk of CHD include reverse cholesterol transport, the process by which HDL carries cholesterol from peripheral tissues to the liver. This process involves both the ABC-A1 cholesterol transporter in peripheral tissues and the scavenger receptor B1 (SR-B1) in the liver. Other mechanisms may also contribute to the inverse relationship between HDL levels and the risk of CHD, including (1) stimulation of prostacyclin synthesis by vascular endothelium, (2) HDL's capacity to act as a scavenger for polar surface active components released during lipolysis of triglyceride-rich lipoproteins, and (3) associations between low HDL levels and elevated concentrations of particularly atherogenic lipoproteins (e.g., VLDL remnants, chylomicron remnants, or small, dense LDL particles).

DIAGNOSIS OF THE HYPERLIPOPROTEINEMIAS

Although total plasma cholesterol and HDL cholesterol levels are not substantially altered by fasting or eating, assessment of plasma triglyceride levels requires a fasting blood sample. The usual method for determining LDL levels, with a calculation involving fasting triglyceride levels, also requires a fasting blood sample. However, LDL can be measured directly in nonfasting plasma with certain immunochemical or ultracentrifugal techniques. Acute injury or illness such as myocardial infarction or major surgery can lead to substantial reductions in LDL and HDL levels lasting as long as 2 to 3 months. Thus, blood samples for assessment of lipoprotein levels should be taken when the patient is in a metabolically steady state and taking the usual diet.

All the cholesterol in fasting plasma is normally found in VLDL, LDL, and HDL. Because the known composition of VLDL allows us to approximate its cholesterol content as one fifth the triglyceride level, LDL cholesterol is generally calculated as $C - Tg/5 - HDL$, where C is total plasma cholesterol, Tg is the fasting plasma triglyceride level, and HDL is the measured HDL cholesterol level. The approximation of VLDL cholesterol as one fifth the plasma triglyceride level loses its validity when chylomicrons are present (e.g., a nonfasting sample), when the plasma triglyceride level exceeds 400 mg/dL, and in rare patients with type III hyperlipoproteinemia (dysbetalipoproteinemia). Thus, in these circumstances, LDL cannot be approximated by this formula.

Because all the plasma lipoproteins contain cholesterol, hypercholesterolemia can be associated with elevation of any of the lipoprotein classes. However, a marked elevation in cholesterol with a normal triglyceride level generally indicates elevation of LDL and increased CHD risk. A lesser elevation of cholesterol with normal triglyceride levels can also be due to elevations of HDL, a circumstance associated with reduced CHD risk. A genetically determined elevation in LDL may be due to familial hypercholesterolemia (caused by defective or deficient LDL receptors), familial defective apoprotein B (caused by mutant apo B, which is poorly recognized by LDL receptors), familial combined hyperlipidemia (caused by increased secretion of apo B-100 in VLDL, the precursor of LDL), polygenic hypercholesterolemia (a heterogeneous group of imperfectly understood disorders), or the rare genetic conditions β-sitosterolemia and autosomal recessive hypercholesterolemia. Additionally, LDL levels may be elevated by diets high in cholesterol and saturated fats, obesity, hypothyroidism, diabetes mellitus, and nephrotic syndrome. Treatment with thiazide diuretics, glucocorticoids, sirolimus (Rapamune), or cyclosporine (Sandimmune) can also elevate LDL levels.

Elevations in VLDL and chylomicrons are manifested as hypertriglyceridemia in laboratory testing. Triglyceride levels are categorized by the Adult Treatment Panel III (ATP-III) of the National Cholesterol Education Program as normal (<150 mg/dL), borderline-high (150 to 199 mg/dL), high (200 to 499 mg/dL), and very high (≥500 mg/dL). Very high plasma triglyceride levels are generally due to elevations in VLDL and chylomicrons (type V hyperlipoproteinemia), and such high levels can cause pancreatitis and warrant drug therapy when nonpharmacologic measures are not sufficiently effective. One should attempt to reduce the fasting plasma triglyceride level to below 500 mg/dL, although such reductions are not always possible. Borderline-high and high triglyceride levels are most commonly associated with obesity and alcohol consumption. Triglyceride elevations in the range of 200 to 500 mg/dL can also occur as a result of treatment with estrogens, *cis*-retinoic acid, diuretics, β-blocking medications, sirolimus, and glucocorticoids. Additionally, borderline-high or high triglyceride levels can result from diabetes, uremia, nephrotic syndrome, or hypothyroidism. The risk of CHD is increased when hypertriglyceridemia occurs in association with diabetes and when it is due to either familial combined hyperlipidemia or type III hyperlipoproteinemia. In familial combined hyperlipidemia, elevated levels of cholesterol, triglyceride, or both are found in various members of the family. Rarely, hypertriglyceridemia is a consequence of familial type III hyperlipoproteinemia (dysbetalipoproteinemia). The pathogenesis of this very uncommon disease involves homozygosity for a mutation in apo E that renders it poorly recognizable to cell surface receptors. As a consequence, highly atherogenic remnants of VLDL and chylomicrons accumulate in plasma.

The most atherogenic lipoproteins are LDL, remnants of VLDL and chylomicrons, and lipoprotein (a). VLDL cholesterol is a useful surrogate measure of remnant lipoproteins. Thus, non-HDL cholesterol (total cholesterol − HDL cholesterol) reflects the cholesterol content of all of these atherogenic particles. For this reason, the ATP-III recognizes non-HDL cholesterol as a secondary target of treatment when fasting triglyceride levels are 200 mg/dL or higher. The primary target of treatment is LDL cholesterol.

TREATMENT OF ELEVATED LDL IN ADULTS

A large number of clinical trials have shown that decreasing LDL levels by dietary and pharmacologic measures reduces the risk for CHD in hypercholesterolemic patients. Furthermore, these trials show that cholesterol reduction decreases the frequency of fatal and nonfatal CHD events in patients who have already suffered an acute myocardial infarction. In these large studies, the risk of CHD fell by 2% for every 1% decrease in serum cholesterol levels. Angiographic studies have demonstrated that aggressive cholesterol reduction retards the growth of established atherosclerotic lesions and enhances the regression of these lesions, but a discrepancy has been noted between the substantial reductions in clinical events and the modest improvement in plaque size. This discrepancy is explained by changes in plaque composition (decreased lipid content and increased collagen in the fibrous cap), which have been documented in response to cholesterol reduction with the statin drugs. These observations provide the scientific underpinning for the current approach to treatment of elevated LDL levels.

The Adult Treatment Panel of the National Cholesterol Education Program has issued reports in 1988, 1993, and 2001 focusing on reduction of plasma levels of LDL, the major atherogenic lipoprotein. Current guidelines, as detailed in the 2001 report (the ATP-III report), focus on LDL cholesterol as the primary target of treatment. Plasma LDL cholesterol levels are categorized as optimal (<100 mg/dL), near optimal (100 to 130 mg/dL), borderline high (130 to 159 mg/dL), high (160 to 189 mg/dL), and very high (≥190 mg/dL). The approach taken calls for more aggressive therapy in those at higher risk (Table 2). Individuals are considered to be in one of three categories of CHD risk. Over 80% of deaths in persons who have survived a myocardial infarction are due to CHD. Therefore, the highest risk category includes those in whom CHD has already developed or those who have a 10-year CHD risk similar to that of patients with established CHD (>20%) (Table 3). These individuals are said to have "CHD-equivalent risk." An intermediate category of risk includes persons with at least two risk factors for CHD (other than elevated LDL cholesterol) (Table 4), which confers a 10-year CHD risk of 20% or less. A high HDL

TABLE 2. **LDL Levels: Initiation Treatment and Goals of Treatment for Adults**

Risk Category	LDL Goal (mg/dL)	LDL Level to Initiate TLC (mg/dL)	LDL Level to Initiate Drug Treatment (mg/dL)
CHD or 10-y CHD risk >20%	<100	≥100	≥130 (100–129: drug optional)*
≥2 Risk factors (10-y risk ≤20%)	<130	≥130	10-y Risk 10–20%: ≥130 10-y Risk <10%: ≥160
0–1 Risk factor	<160	≥160	≥190 (160–189: drug optional)

*Results of Heart Protection Study favor drug treatment in this group.
Abbreviations: CHD = coronary heart disease; LDL = low-density lipoprotein; TLC = therapeutic lifestyle change.

cholesterol level (≥60 mg/dL) is considered to be a negative risk factor for CHD and reduces the total number of risk factors present by one. The lowest risk category includes those with zero to one non-LDL risk factor; these individuals will usually have a 10-year CHD risk of less than 10%.

The ATP-III report provides an algorithm for calculating the 10-year risk for CHD (JAMA 285: 2486-2497, 2001). Additionally, a computerized spreadsheet (PC, Mac, or PDA) for calculating risk is available on the Internet (http://www.nhlbi.nih.gov).

Obesity is associated with an increased risk for CHD, but much of the increased risk of obese persons is due to other conditions that are secondary to obesity, including hypertension and low HDL cholesterol. Thus, although obesity should be earmarked for intervention, its presence is not used in determining the aggressiveness of LDL reduction. Similarly, physical inactivity is a target of intervention, but it is not used to determine the aggressiveness of LDL reduction. Treatment of obesity and increasing physical activity are particularly important in patients with the metabolic syndrome.

Before initiating intensive treatment of hyperlipoproteinemia by diet or medications, it is important to determine whether the lipoprotein disorder is secondary to another disease (e.g., hypothyroidism, nephrotic syndrome, diabetes mellitus) or to treatment with a medication. If so, attention to the primary cause may be the most appropriate treatment of the hyperlipoproteinemia.

Therapeutic Lifestyle Changes as Treatment of Elevated LDL Levels

Most patients with mild or moderate degrees of primary hypercholesterolemia from elevated LDL levels can be treated satisfactorily with therapeutic lifestyle changes; such therapy involves diet (reduction of cholesterol and saturated fats, addition of cholesterol-lowering plant stanols/sterols and soluble fiber), weight reduction for the overweight, and increased physical activity. Cholesterol-lowering medication is not needed for these individuals. The threshold for initiation of intensive therapy to reduce LDL cholesterol by therapeutic lifestyle changes or with drugs depends on an individual's overall risk for CHD (see Table 2).

Saturated fats and cholesterol in the diet suppress LDL receptor activity, thereby retarding clearance of LDL from plasma and elevating LDL levels in plasma. Obesity is associated with increased hepatic secretion of VLDL, the metabolic precursor of LDL. Furthermore, the addition of certain plant sterols and soluble fiber to the diet can reduce LDL. These principles underlie the specific recommendations for a therapeutic diet, as detailed in Table 5.

TABLE 3. **CHD Risk Equivalents**

Other clinical forms of atherosclerosis (peripheral arterial disease, abdominal aortic aneurysm, cerebrovascular disease)
Diabetes mellitus
Multiple risk factors conferring a 10-y risk of CHD >20%

Abbreviations: CHD = coronary heart disease.

Drug Therapy for Elevated LDL Levels

When LDL cholesterol is not satisfactorily controlled by dietary measures, the use of cholesterol-lowering medication should be considered. Nearly all patients with CHD or CHD risk equivalents will require cholesterol-lowering medication; those hospitalized for a major CHD event or procedure should be discharged with a prescription for a cholesterol-lowering drug if the admission LDL cholesterol level was 100 mg/dL or higher.

In patients without CHD, intensive dietary measures should usually be pursued for several months

TABLE 4. **Major CHD Risk Factors (Excluding LDL)**

Cigarette smoking
Hypertension (BP ≥140/90 or taking antihypertensive medication)
Low HDL cholesterol (<40 mg/d)*
FH of premature CHD
Male first-degree relative <55 y old
Female first-degree relative <65 y old
Age (men ≥45 y old; women ≥55 y old)

*HDL-C of ≥60 mg/dL is a negative risk factor (reduces the total count by one).
Abbreviations: BP = blood pressure; FH = family history; HDL = high-density lipoprotein; LDL = low-density lipoprotein.

TABLE 5. **Recommended Therapeutic Diet**

Nutrient	Recommended Intake
Saturated fat	<7% of total calories
Polyunsaturated fat	≤10% of total calories
Monounsaturated fat	<20% of total calories
Total fat	25–35% of total calories
Carbohydrate	50–60% of total calories
Fiber	20–30 g/d
Protein	15% of total calories
Cholesterol	<200 mg/d
Total calories	To achieve and maintain ideal weight

before considering cholesterol-lowering medication. However, it is appropriate to use medication sooner in those with CHD or a marked elevation in LDL cholesterol (≥190 mg/dL).

It is important to assess the changes in plasma lipoproteins and to monitor for potential adverse effects 6 to 12 weeks after initiating treatment with lipid-altering medications.

The major drugs for reduction of LDL cholesterol levels are inhibitors of 3-hydroxy-3-methylglutaryl coenzyme A reductase (the "statins"), bile acid sequestrants, ezetimibe, and nicotinic acid. The fibric acid derivatives (fenofibrate [Tricor], gemfibrozil [Lopid], and clofibrate [Atromid-S]) are less effective in reducing LDL cholesterol. The dosing and efficacy of these drugs are summarized in Table 6.

The Statins. The statins have become the mainstay of LDL-reducing therapy, and they are the most effective agents for reducing plasma LDL levels. Five of these drugs are now available: atorvastatin (Lipitor), fluvastatin (Lescol), lovastatin (Mevacor), pravastatin (Pravachol), and simvastatin (Zocor). Rosuvastatin (Crestor) is likely to be approved for use in the United States by the time this chapter is in print. During the summer of 2001, cerivastatin (Baycol) was withdrawn from the market because it caused acute myositis much more frequently (at least 10-fold) than did the other statins. The statins that remain available are extremely effective and well tolerated; they have an impressively low frequency of serious adverse effects.

The mechanism of action of these drugs depends on inhibition of the rate-limiting step in cholesterol biosynthesis and consequent stimulation of LDL receptor activity in hepatocytes. All these drugs are targeted to the liver by extensive first-pass hepatic extraction. Atorvastatin, lovastatin, and simvastatin undergo metabolism by cytochrome P450-3A4; fluvastatin is metabolized by cytochrome P450-2C9. The metabolism of pravastatin does not involve the cytochrome P450 system. With the maximal recommended dose, LDL reductions of 58% are found for atorvastatin, 34% for fluvastatin, 40% for lovastatin, 37% for pravastatin, and 46% for simvastatin. Small reductions in triglyceride levels and small increases in HDL cholesterol also occur.

TABLE 6. **Dosing and Efficacy of Lipid-Lowering Drugs**

Drugs	Initial Dose	Dose Range	Range of LDL Reduction (%)	Usual HDL Increase (%)
Bile Acid Sequestrants				
Cholestyramine (Questran, Questran Light, LoCholest, LoCholest Light, Prevalite)	4 g/d (1 scoop)	4–12 g bid	8–28	1–2
Colestipol (Colestid)	5 g/d (1 scoop)	5–15 g bid	8–28	1–2
Colesevelam (Welchol)	3.75 g/d (6 tablets)	4.375 g (7 tablets)	15–18	3
Fibric Acid Derivatives				
Fenofibrate (Tricor)	54–160 mg/d	54–160 mg/d	5–15*	10–20†
Gemfibrozil (Lopid)	600 mg bid	600 mg bid	5–15*	10–20†
Clofibrate (Atromid-S)	1 g bid	1 g bid	5–15*	10–20†
Inhibitor of Cholesterol Absorption				
Ezetimibe	10 mg/d	10 mg/d	18	3
Nicotinic Acid				
Immediate release (Niacor and others)	50 mg tid	500–2000 mg tid	5–25	20–50
Sustained release (Niaspan, SloNiacin, and others)	500 mg/d	1000–2000 mg/d	5–15	17–22
Statins				
Atorvastatin (Lipitor)	10 mg/d	10–80 mg/d	29–50	2–8
Fluvastatin (Lescol)	20–40 mg qpm	20–40 mg qpm, 40 mg bid; 80 mg (sustained release) daily	21–34	3–9
Lovastatin (Mevacor)	20 mg qpm	10–40 mg qpm, 40 mg bid	24–40	7–10
Lovastatin, extended release (Altocor)	20–60 mg qhs	10–60 mg qhs	25–42	3–8
Pravastatin (Pravachol)	20 mg qpm	10–80 mg qpm	18–37	5–15
Simvastatin (Zocor)	20 mg qpm	5–80 mg qpm	23–46	6–12

*The reduction in LDL is lessened by baseline hypertriglyceridemia; increases in LDL can occur in hypertriglyceridemic patients treated with fibric acid derivatives.

†The increase in HDL in response to fibrates is greatest in patients with baseline hypertriglyceridemia.

Abbreviations: HDL = high-density lipoprotein; LDL = low-density lipoprotein.

In clinical trials, these drugs have been shown to slow the angiographically assessed progression of coronary atherosclerosis. Additionally, they have reduced the incidence of clinical CHD events in patients with pre-existing CHD and in those without pre-existing CHD.

In the large clinical trials of statins, it has been calculated that essentially all the CHD reduction can be attributed to the observed reduction in LDL cholesterol resulting from statin treatment. However, the concept that the statins may prevent CHD events by means other than reduction of LDL has a theoretical basis. For instance, by reducing synthesis of the nonsterol products of mevalonate, the statins cause increased synthesis of nitric oxide synthase and thereby improve arterial vasodilatory function. The statins have also been shown to inhibit smooth muscle cell proliferation and stabilize plaque by increasing plaque collagen, and they have direct anti-inflammatory properties. The clinical importance of these so-called pleiotropic effects of the statins remains uncertain.

The statins are very well tolerated. The most important side effects are transaminase elevation (about 1% of patients) and acute myositis (about 0.1% of patients). These adverse effects are dose related. The risk of myositis is increased when the statins are used concomitantly with fibric acid derivatives (particularly gemfibrozil) or with cyclosporine. Additionally, the use of potent cytochrome P450-3A4 inhibitors such as macrolide antibiotics or azole antifungal agents will increase the risk of myositis with atorvastatin, lovastatin, or simvastatin. Theoretical considerations and animal experiments suggest that these drugs may be teratogenic; thus, they should not be used during pregnancy.

Bile Acid Sequestrants. The bile acid sequestrants cholestyramine (Questran, LoCholest, Prevalite), colestipol (Colestid), and colesevelam (Welchol) are anion exchange resins. They speed the clearance of LDL from plasma by increasing LDL receptor activity. As a consequence, plasma LDL levels can be reduced by 15% to 30%. The usual dose is 1 to 2 packets (or scoops) twice daily for cholestyramine or colestipol and 5 to 6 tablets daily for colesevelam. The bile acid sequestrants are particularly useful in combination regimens along with a statin or nicotinic acid. Because bile acid sequestrants act within the intestine and are not systemically absorbed, they are thought to be quite safe. The most common side effects are constipation, bloating, and abdominal pain. These side effects are much less frequent with colesevelam than with the other two bile acid sequestrants. These drugs interfere with the intestinal absorption of a variety of other medications; thus, other medications should not be given simultaneously with bile acid sequestrants. Bile acid sequestrants stimulate VLDL secretion, and they may thereby cause or exacerbate hypertriglyceridemia. Consequently, baseline hypertriglyceridemia is a relative contraindication to the use of a bile acid sequestrant.

Ezetimibe. Ezetimibe, a specific inhibitor of intestinal absorption of cholesterol and plant sterols, represents the newest class of lipid-lowering drugs. A consequence of reduced cholesterol absorption is a reduced hepatic cholesterol pool. This causes increased hepatic LDL receptor activity and accelerated clearance of LDL from plasma. Most of the cholesterol within the intestinal lumen is of biliary origin and not of dietary origin. Thus, blocking intestinal absorption of cholesterol with ezetimibe can be expected to reduce plasma levels of LDL even in patients with a zero-cholesterol diet. Systemic exposure to ezetimibe is very low, and this drug appears to be quite well tolerated. It has not yet been reported to cause significant adverse effects.

Ezetimibe reduces LDL cholesterol by about 18% and increases HDL cholesterol by about 3%. It has no significant effect on triglyceride levels. It has utility in monotherapy for patients who cannot tolerate statins, and it can be used in combination with statins.

Nicotinic Acid. Nicotinic acid (niacin) is a B vitamin, and in doses greatly exceeding those needed to prevent deficiency syndromes, it has a beneficial effect on plasma levels of VLDL, LDL, and HDL; additionally, nicotinic acid reduces the concentration of lipoprotein (a), a potentially atherogenic lipoprotein. Its primary action as a lipid-modifying medication involves a reduction in the secretion of VLDL, the metabolic precursor of LDL. In doses of 2 to 4.5 g daily, nicotinic acid typically reduces LDL cholesterol by 25%, reduces triglycerides by 50%, and increases HDL cholesterol by 25% to 50%. In angiographic trials, nicotinic acid has been shown to aid in limiting progression and enhancing regression of atherosclerosis.

Adverse effects prevent about one third of patients from taking nicotinic acid over the long term. Such side effects include cutaneous flushing, ichthyosis and itching, gastritis and peptic ulcer disease, hepatitis, hyperglycemia, and hyperuricemia. Flushing, which is prostaglandin-mediated, can be mitigated or abolished by aspirin taken 30 minutes before nicotinic acid. Sustained-release forms of nicotinic acid cause less flushing, but they are more likely to lead to hepatitis. A 15% to 20% elevation in plasma levels of homocysteine has recently been recognized as a side effect of nicotinic acid.

It has been suggested that a recently developed extended-release form of nicotinic acid (Niaspan) may be better tolerated and less hepatotoxic than previously available preparations. However, the literature on this agent has been inconclusive because of limited duration of follow-up, small sample size, and the use of relatively low doses of the extended-release preparation of nicotinic acid.

Fibric Acid Derivatives. The fibric acid derivatives fenofibrate, gemfibrozil, and clofibrate work by activating PPAR-α (peroxisome proliferator activating receptor-α). The main effects on plasma lipoproteins involve increased lipoprotein lipase activity, reduced synthesis of apo C-III (an inhibitor of lipoprotein lipase), and increased synthesis of the major HDL apoproteins (apo A-I and apo A-II). A physiologic consequence of the increased lipoprotein lipase activity is enhanced clearance of VLDL and remnant lipoproteins. The fibric acid drugs generally cause a modest reduction in LDL (about 10%) and a modest increase in HDL (also about 10%). In hypertriglyceridemic persons, these drugs often lead to an *increase* in LDL cholesterol levels.

The fibrates enhance the lithogenicity of bile and increase the frequency of biliary stone disease. The most common side effects of these drugs are gastrointestinal distress and decreased libido. When used in combination with a statin, the risk of myositis is increased.

In the Helsinki Heart Study, gemfibrozil caused a 34% reduction in the incidence of acute myocardial infarction and CHD death. In the Diabetes Atherosclerosis Intervention Study, in a diabetic patient population, fenofibrate caused a significant 40% reduction in the rate of progression of atherosclerosis.

The fibric acid derivatives are most useful in patients with hypertriglyceridemia in the setting of the metabolic syndrome. Obesity and insulin resistance underlie this syndrome, whose manifestations include hypertriglyceridemia, low HDL levels, a predominance of small dense LDL particles, and the presence of hypertension.

Combination Drug Therapy. Certain combinations of medications can be useful in treating markedly elevated LDL cholesterol levels. Combination therapy can maximize the reduction in LDL levels; it can also allow us to limit the dosage of individual LDL-reducing drugs, thus limiting side effects. For patients with elevations in both triglycerides and LDL, the addition of nicotinic acid or a fibric acid derivative to control triglyceride levels can allow the use of a bile acid sequestrant (otherwise precluded by hypertriglyceridemia) to help reduce LDL levels. The following are the most effective combinations for lowering LDL:

- A statin plus a bile acid sequestrant
- A statin plus nicotinic acid
- A statin plus ezetimibe
- Nicotinic acid plus a bile acid sequestrant
- A statin plus a bile acid sequestrant plus nicotinic acid

The combination of a fibric acid derivative with a statin should usually be avoided because of an increased risk of myopathy.

TREATMENT OF ELEVATIONS OF LDL IN CHILDREN

Children generally have lower levels of total and LDL cholesterol than adults do. Thus, the pediatric criteria for categorizing LDL cholesterol levels differ from the adult criteria. For children, acceptable LDL cholesterol is considered to be below 110 mg/dL; borderline LDL cholesterol, 110 to 129 mg/dL; and high LDL cholesterol, at least 130 mg/dL. For children 1 to 19 years of age, an LDL level of 130 mg/dL approximates the 95th percentile of the population distribution.

For pediatric populations, much debate has focused on the issue of when to screen for lipid disorders. Children should be tested if premature CHD has occurred in a parent or grandparent, if a parent has an elevated cholesterol level (>240 mg/dL), if the family history is not available, or if the child has at least two other risk factors for CHD.

Because of concern about the possible adverse effects of therapy given during periods of growth and development, the approach to treatment in children is much more conservative than in adults. No therapy whatsoever (not even diet) should be given to children younger than 2 years. For children at least 2 years of age, dietary therapy is warranted for borderline or high LDL cholesterol levels. In children who are at least 10 years old, drug therapy is recommended if LDL cholesterol remains above 190 mg/dL despite dietary measures; in those with two or more other risk factors for CHD, drug therapy is recommended when LDL cholesterol remains above 160 mg/dL despite diet.

The literature on the pediatric experience with statins is limited to one study involving 110 adolescents with heterozygous familial hypercholesterolemia treated with lovastatin and one study of 8 patients with homozygous familial hypercholesterolemia. Because of their safety, the bile acid sequestrants are the only cholesterol-lowering medications that are generally recommended for routine use in children. Other cholesterol-lowering drugs should be prescribed to children only after referral to a lipid specialist.

TREATMENT OF ELEVATIONS OF TRIGLYCERIDES

Nonpharmacologic therapy is advisable for nearly all patients with hypertriglyceridemia. Such therapy involves weight reduction for those who are overweight, exercise, and restriction of alcohol. In particular, when the hypertriglyceridemia is a component of the metabolic syndrome, therapeutic lifestyle changes are essential and especially effective. The ATP-III has suggested a diagnosis of metabolic syndrome when at least three of the following are present:

- Abdominal obesity (waist circumference >40 inches for men, >35 inches for women)
- Triglyceride level of 150 mg/dL or higher
- Low HDL cholesterol (<40 mg/dL for men, <50 mg/dL for women)
- Hypertension (systolic blood pressure ≥130 or diastolic blood pressure ≥85)
- Fasting glucose level of 110 mg/dL or higher

When elevations of triglycerides are due to a medication (e.g., estrogen) or to a specific disease, correction of the primary cause of the hypertriglyceridemia may be all that is necessary. When very high triglyceride levels (>500 mg/dL) persist despite these measures, drug therapy is warranted to prevent pancreatitis.

In patients with triglyceride levels of 200 mg/dL or higher, non-HDL cholesterol is a secondary target of therapy; LDL remains the primary target. Non-HDL cholesterol (total cholesterol minus HDL cholesterol) includes several atherogenic lipoproteins: LDL, VLDL remnants, some VLDL particles, and lipoprotein (a). The levels of non-HDL cholesterol for initiation of therapy and the goals of therapy are 30 mg/dL higher than the corresponding values for LDL cholesterol.

High (200 to 499 mg/dL) triglyceride levels that persist despite treatment with nonpharmacologic measures warrant consideration of triglyceride-lowering drugs in patients with established CHD, diabetes mellitus, type III hyperlipoproteinemia, familial combined hyperlipidemia, and the metabolic syndrome.

The most effective drugs for reducing triglyceride levels are nicotinic acid, fibric acid derivatives, and somatic fish oils. Because nicotinic acid has beneficial effects on VLDL, LDL, and HDL, it is the preferred agent when side effects do not preclude its use. Fibric acid derivatives often have the undesirable effect of raising LDL levels in hypertriglyceridemic patients. However, they do reduce triglyceride levels, and they raise HDL levels particularly well in the setting of hypertriglyceridemia.

Somatic fish oils contain large amounts of highly polyunsaturated omega-3 fatty acids. When given in large doses (9 to 16 g daily), they reduce hepatic secretion of VLDL. Fasting triglyceride levels can fall by over 50% in response to the fish oil. Unfortunately, therapeutic doses of fish oil also provide a significant burden of dietary calories (80 to 150 kcal daily). Additionally, treatment with fish oil can raise LDL levels.

TREATMENT OF LOW HDL LEVELS

In many epidemiologic studies, low HDL levels have been associated with increased risk for CHD. Furthermore, in several clinical trials that were designed to test the benefits of reducing LDL levels, small increases in HDL cholesterol have been independently associated with improved CHD risk. Additionally, in the VA HDL Intervention Trial, treatment with gemfibrozil caused a significant 22% reduction in the incidence of CHD; this therapy was associated with a 6% increase in HDL, a 31% reduction in triglycerides, and no significant change in LDL levels. Nonetheless, the base of knowledge supporting treatment to raise HDL levels is not as firm as that supporting treatment to reduce LDL levels. We can advise nearly everyone to pursue nonpharmacologic measures to raise HDL levels, including cessation of cigarette smoking, weight loss for the obese, and increased exercise. Furthermore, it is reasonable to attempt to avoid HDL-lowering medications in patients who already have low HDL levels. Such medications include androgenic and most progestational steroids, thiazide diuretics, β-blockers, and retinoids.

HDL levels can often be substantially increased by treatment with nicotinic acid and, in patients with hypertriglyceridemia, by treatment with fibric acid derivatives. Lesser increases in HDL levels (about 10%) occur when fibric acid drugs are used in normotriglyceridemic persons and in combination with statins.

In patients with low HDL levels, LDL cholesterol remains the primary target of therapy. In the AFCAPS-TexCAPS study, lovastatin caused a 36% reduction in the incidence of CHD in men and women with normal LDL cholesterol levels and below-average HDL levels. Thus, a statin would seem to be the drug of choice in patients with low HDL levels. When a statin is not tolerated or when combination drug therapy is needed to reduce LDL levels, a low HDL level may make nicotinic acid a particularly attractive choice.

For those who have hypertriglyceridemia and a low HDL level, non-HDL cholesterol is the secondary target of therapy.

Drug therapy designed specifically to raise low HDL levels (<40 mg/dL) may be considered in patients with established CHD and those with CHD risk equivalents. Isolated low HDL levels, in the absence of CHD or risk factors for CHD, often occur in vegetarian populations, whose CHD rates are low. Thus, a patient with isolated low HDL levels but without other CHD risk factors should not be given medication specifically for the purpose of raising HDL levels.

OBESITY

method of
SUPAWAN BURANAPIN, M.D., and
CAROLINE M. APOVIAN, M.D.
Boston University School of Medicine
Boston Medical Center
Boston, Massachusetts

Obesity refers to an excess of body fat. Currently, relative body weight is defined by the body mass index (BMI), calculated by dividing weight in kilograms by the square of the height in meters. The National Institutes of Health defines overweight as a BMI between 25 and 29.9 kg/m^2 and obesity as a BMI of greater than 30 kg/m^2. The National Health and Nutrition Examination Survey (NHANES) conducted from 1999 to 2000 indicated that an estimated 64% of U.S. adults are overweight or obese, based on a BMI greater than or equal to 25 kg/m^2. This represents an 8% increase in prevalence from the report of NHANES III (1988 to 1994). Most of this increase has been attributable to an increase in the obese category, with only a small increase in the prevalence of overweight. The age-adjusted prevalence of overweight and obesity among U.S. adults is 30% and 34%, respectively, but these prevalence rates are higher in some minority populations, especially non-Hispanic black women and Mexican American women.

BMI does not correlate well with distribution of body fat, which is an independent predictor of health risk. Therefore, the combination of BMI and body fat distribution is usually used to evaluate health risk from overweight and obesity. Central or abdominal obesity that reflects fat accumulation surrounding the visceral abdominal organs is associated with metabolic abnormalities including insulin resistance, glucose intolerance, dyslipidemia, and hypertension. A waist circumference of 40 inches (102 cm) or more in men or 35 inches (88 cm) or more in women defines central obesity. The waist circumference is particularly useful in patients categorized as normal or overweight by BMI.

ETIOLOGY

Obesity is the result of a failure in the regulatory system that balances total energy intake and total energy expenditure. It is the result of the interaction of genetic and environmental influences and is a complex multifactorial chronic disease. Genetic susceptibility can either play a major role in the pathogenesis of obesity or enhance susceptibility to its development. Occasionally, obesity may be the consequence of hypothalamic disease, hypothyroidism, Cushing's syndrome, or genetic diseases such as Prader-Willi syndrome, Alström's syndrome, and Laurence-Moon-Biedl syndrome. The genetic factors in obesity operate through susceptibility genes in a favorable environment. From 30% to 50% of the variability in total body fat stores is believed to be genetically determined. Environmental influences include an overall decrease in physical activity and overconsumption of highly calorie-dense foods. Environmental influences are more likely responsible for the current global energy imbalance and increasing prevalence of obesity rather than a change in genetic factors.

Since the 1970s, obesity research has focused on the identification of a mutant gene causing obesity and the potential roles of metabolic factors such as variations in energy expenditure and in patterns of fuel utilization. Studies using the monogenic and transgenic mutant models of obesity in rodents have identified proteins that regulate energy balance such as leptin (OB), the leptin receptor (OB-R), agouti-related protein (AGRP), neuropeptide Y (NPY), carboxypeptidase E (Cpe), pro-opiomelanocortin (POMC), galanin, α-melanocyte–stimulating hormone (α-MSH), melanocortin 4-receptor (MC4-R), and cocaine- and amphetamine-regulated transcript (CART). These models have contributed to the understanding of the complexity of regulatory mechanisms involved in energy balance. Information gleaned from this research has suggested new targets of drugs for treatment of obesity. The most intensively studied hormone related to obesity has been leptin, discovered in 1994. It is the protein product of the *ob* gene and is secreted from adipocytes. In rodent models, it is expressed primarily in white adipocyte tissue and functions as an afferent signal in a negative-feedback loop involved in the regulation of energy balance. Mutations of the *ob* gene in mice result in a syndrome of obesity, increased fat deposits, hyperglycemia, hyperinsulinemia, hypothermia, and impaired reproductive and thyroid function. The administration of recombinant leptin to leptin-deficient *ob/ob* mice as well as to normal lean and diet-related obese mice results in weight loss through decreased food intake and increased energy expenditure. In human beings, however, the expression of the *ob* gene is positively correlated with body fat and BMI. Leptin levels are high in most obese persons and decrease with weight loss. Because of this finding, it is believed that human obesity is associated with a leptin-resistant state.

HEALTH RISK AND CLASSIFICATION

The risk of morbidity and mortality from obesity is proportional to the degree of overweight as determined by BMI (Table 1). Obesity is associated with an increase in type 2 diabetes, hypertension, coronary heart disease, dyslipidemia, atherosclerosis, ischemic stroke, sleep apnea and respiratory problems, osteoarthritis, gallbladder disease, nonalcoholic steatohepatitis (fatty liver), stress incontinence, certain types of cancer (colon, endometrial, postmenopausal breast and prostate), and irregular menstrual cycles leading to infertility.

The National Institutes of Health recommend weight loss for obese and overweight persons with two

TABLE 1. **Classification of Overweight and Obesity by Body Mass Index, Waist Circumference, and Associated Disease Risk***

Weight Class	Body Mass Index (kg/m²)	Obesity Class	Disease Risk*/Waist Circumference *≤40 (men)/≤35 (women)*	*≤40 (men)/≤35 (women)*
Underweight	<18.5	—	—	—
Normal†	18.5–24.9	—	—	—
Overweight	25.0–29.9	—	Increased	High
Obese	30.0–34.9	I	High	Very high
	35.0–39.9	II	Very high	Very high
	≥40.0	III	Extremely high	Extremely high

*Risk for type 2 diabetes mellitus, hypertension, and cardiovascular disease.
†Increased waist circumference can be a marker for risk even in persons of normal weight.
Adapted from "Preventing and Managing the Global Epidemic of Obesity. Report of the World Health Organization Consultation of Obesity." WHO, Geneva, June 1996.

or more risk factors for obesity-related diseases. However, persons at lower risk should be counseled to make effective lifestyle changes to prevent any further weight gain.

EVALUATION AND ASSESSMENT

Patients should be evaluated and assessed for:

1. Anthropometrics, including height, weight, BMI, and waist circumference, to assess severity of obesity.
2. Medical history and physical examination to identify potential causes of obesity, obesity-related complications, and overall health status.
3. Family history of obesity and obesity-related diseases.
4. Current medications that may cause weight gain, including antipsychotics, antidepressants, mood stabilizers, anticonvulsants, steroids, insulin, and cyproheptadine.
5. Psychological, including screening for potential psychological barriers to treatment such as depression, anxiety, bipolar disorder, and eating disorders.
6. Nutritional information:

–Weight history, including age of onset of obesity, highest and lowest adult weights, patterns of weight gain and weight loss, and environmental triggers to weight gain or overeating.

–Diet history, including number and type of diets attempted, weight-loss medications both prescribed and over the counter, and success of previous weight-loss efforts.

–Current eating patterns, including 24-hour recall and meal patterns, nutrient density, and nutritional supplement use, as well as smoking and alcohol consumption history.

–Exercise history, including current and past exercise frequency, duration, and intensity, activities of daily living, and barriers to exercise, as well as attitudes toward physical activity.

–Motivation and readiness to lose weight, including reasons and motivations for weight loss, previous attempts at losing weight, family and friend support, understanding of risks and benefits, time availability, and potential barriers including financial limitations to the patient's ability to undergo permanent lifestyle change.

7. Laboratory tests, including complete blood count, blood glucose, electrolytes, liver function tests, thyroid function tests, and lipid panels, as well as a baseline electrocardiogram in patients older than 45 years (men) or 55 years (women) and in all high-risk patients.

TREATMENT

The goal of treatment is a weight loss of 5% to 10% of initial body weight in 6 months at a rate of approximately 1 to 2 lb/week and the maintenance of that weight loss through combined dietary change, increased physical activity, and lifestyle modification. Further weight loss can be considered after a period of weight maintenance. It is established that moderate weight loss (5% to 10% of initial weight) can significantly improve health problems and can decrease blood pressure as well as lipid and blood glucose levels.

Dietary Change

Low-Calorie Diets

The cornerstone of therapy for overweight and obesity is the low-calorie diet to control portion size and to decrease calorie intake to less than the energy expended. Balanced calorie-deficit diets providing 1000 to 1200 kcal/d for women and 1200 to 1500 kcal/d for men have been recommended to reduce intake by approximately 500 to 1000 kcal/d, to produce a weight loss of 1 to 2 lb/week. Diets should be low in saturated fat, with total fat intake less than 30% of total calories. Diets should also be low in simple sugars and refined carbohydrates, to reduce calorie intake further, but sufficient in protein to preserve muscle mass. Fruits and vegetables are recommended to provide fiber, vitamins, and minerals and to increase the volume of food ingested to help avoid feelings of deprivation and restriction. The U.S. Department of Agriculture's Food Guide Pyramid is widely used to educate patients regarding healthy eating and can be modified for safe weight loss by adhering to the lower limit of servings for each food group represented in the pyramid. Another approach is to follow the Acceptable Macronutrient Distribution Ranges (AMDR) (Dietary Reference Intakes for Energy, Carbohydrate, Fiber, Fat, Fatty Acids, Cholesterol, Protein, and Amino Acids [Macronutrients], National Academies Press, 2002), ranges of macronutrient intakes associated with reduced risk of chronic disease and providing sufficient essential nutrients. The Acceptable Macronutrient Distribution Ranges are as follows: for total fat intake, 20% to 35%; for carbohydrate, 45% to 65%; and for protein, 10% to 35% of total calories, with 10% of total calories from polyunsaturated fatty acids.

Very Low-Calorie Diets

Very low-calorie diets provide approximately 250 to 800 kcal/d and can be used in certain circumstances for rapid improvement of symptoms of sleep apnea, blood glucose levels, and blood pressure, for a psychological jump start, or in preparation for gastric bypass surgery in high-risk patients. This approach requires intensive medical monitoring as well as vitamin and mineral supplementation to meet recommended dietary allowances. Many medically supervised weight-management programs also use liquid meal replacements as well as the protein-sparing modified fast to provide very low-calorie diets to their patients. Patients who follow these diets should be monitored weekly by a team of physicians, dietitians, and/or physician assistants. Nonetheless, patients should be informed that although very low-calorie diets may promote greater weight loss than low-calorie diets initially, studies have shown that weight loss after 1 year is not significantly different.

Lifestyle Modification

Lack of physical activity is a contributor in the multifactorial pathogenesis of obesity. Increased physical activity is recommended not only to promote weight loss by increasing energy expended but also to improve mood, quality of life, and body composition, as well as to decrease the risk of disease. Regular exercise is also one of the best predictors of successful weight maintenance. The addition of moderate exercise to calorie restriction to promote weight loss has been demonstrated to preserve lean body mass, which is necessary to maintain resting metabolism. It has been shown that overweight and obese patients receive significant health benefits with daily physical activity, whether or not weight is lost. Overweight and obese men who achieve cardiorespiratory fitness have a lower all-cause and cardiovascular mortality risk than normal-weight sedentary persons. Unfit men have a higher risk of all-cause and cardiovascular mortality than fit men in all fat and fat-free mass categories. Metabolic parameters such as insulin, glucose, and lipid levels also improve with exercise alone. Therefore, increasing daily physical activity should be encouraged for weight loss, for weight maintenance, and for prevention and reduction of the risk of developing chronic diseases. Exercise should be initiated slowly and increased gradually to a goal of moderate-intensity exercise for at least 150 to 200 minutes/week.

Behavior modification is implemented in the treatment of obesity to help induce weight loss and to enhance weight maintenance by changing eating habits and exercise patterns. A typical program provides at least 16 weekly group lifestyle and behavior modification sessions that include self-monitoring of eating habits and physical activity, stress management, stimulus control, problem solving, contingency management, cognitive restructuring, and social support. These sessions are usually conducted by a dietitian or psychologist. A popular program used by many weight-management centers as a template for group sessions is Brownell and Wadden's LEARN Program for Weight Control (American Health Publishing, Dallas, TX, 1999).

Medication

Pharmacotherapy is appropriate for patients who have a BMI greater than or equal to 30, or greater than or equal to 27 with obesity-related medical conditions, as an adjunct to diet and exercise. Currently available medications can be classified into two groups: anorectic agents and malabsorptive agents.

Anorectic Agents

Anorectic agents suppress appetite or increase satiety, resulting in reduced food consumption. These medications work by increasing levels of serotonin, dopamine, norepinephrine, or a combination of these neurotransmitters in the nerve terminals of the hypothalamic feeding center in the brain.

NORADRENERGIC DRUGS

Noradrenergic drugs such as phentermine (Adipex-P), diethylpropion (Tenuate), phendimetrazine (Bontril PDM), and benzphetamine (Didrex) have been approved by the U.S. Food and Drug Administration (FDA) for short-term treatment of obesity (3 months or less). Phentermine has been the most prescribed drug in this class because of studies showing the efficacy of the popular drug combination "fen-phen." The mechanism of action of this class of drugs is suppression of appetite through an increase in norepinephrine levels centrally. Clinical trials have demonstrated that the combination of phentermine and a hypocaloric diet produces significantly more weight loss than a hypocaloric diet alone. Common side effects of phentermine are dry mouth, constipation, palpitations, increased heart rate and blood pressure, headache, and insomnia. Serious but uncommon side effects are chest pain, shortness of breath, skin rash, blurred vision, confusion or hallucinations, and uncontrolled body movements or seizures. The use of phentermine is contraindicated in patients with uncontrolled hypertension or cardiovascular diseases. Because the pharmacology and chemical structure of phentermine are closely related to those of amphetamines, phentermine may be physically and psychologically addictive. Therefore, patients with a history of drug abuse are not candidates for pharmacotherapy with phentermine. Phentermine should not be combined with monoamine oxidase inhibitors or tricyclic antidepressants because of the risk of sympathomimetic effects, especially hypertensive crisis. The usual dose of phentermine is 15 to 37.5 mg once daily before breakfast or 1 to 2 hours after breakfast.

SEROTONERGIC DRUGS

Serotonergic drugs act either by increasing the release of serotonin or by inhibiting its reuptake. Fenfluramine and dexfenfluramine were withdrawn from the United States market in 1997 because of their association with pulmonary hypertension and valvular heart disease. Selective serotonin reuptake inhibitors such as fluoxetine (Prozac)* and sertraline (Zoloft)* are indicated for depression and obsessive-compulsive disorder, but they have also produced some weight loss in patients treated. This initial weight loss has been shown to be transient, and, in fact, selective serotonin reuptake inhibitors tend to cause some weight gain in the long term.

SIBUTRAMINE

Sibutramine (Meridia) inhibits both norepinephrine and serotonin reuptake and weakly inhibits dopamine reuptake. The increase in norepinephrine and serotonin in the central nervous system leads to increased satiety and decreased food intake. Sibutramine use results in a peak in weight loss after 6 months that has been shown to be maintained for more than 1 year with continued use of the drug. It is approved by the FDA for weight loss and weight maintenance for up to 2 years in combination with diet control and behavioral modification. The initial starting dose is 10 mg

*Not FDA approved for this indication.

once daily in the morning. This can be increased to 15 mg/d after a 4-week interval with a less than 4-lb weight loss or decreased to 5 mg/d if patients cannot tolerate the 10-mg dose. Previous studies showed that subjects who followed a low-calorie diet with behavior modification and sibutramine, 10 to 15 mg, over a 6- to 12-month period produced and maintained a statistically and clinically significant greater weight loss (5% to 10% of pretreatment weight) than did subjects who received placebo with a low-calorie diet (1% to 4% weight loss). Metabolic parameters such as dyslipidemia, hyperuricemia, hyperglycemia, and hyperinsulinemia were also improved.

The most medically significant side effects of sibutramine are an increase in blood pressure and heart rate, although these are usually mild. Other common side effects are dry mouth, insomnia, headache, abdominal pain, constipation, and metallic taste. It is therefore recommended that patients have blood pressure and heart rate measured regularly while they are taking sibutramine. Sibutramine should not be used in combination with monoamine oxidase inhibitors because of the risk of increased norepinephrine activity leading to hypertensive crisis or excess serotonin activity resulting in serotonin syndrome. Patients who have poorly controlled hypertension, coronary artery disease, heart failure, arrhythmias, or stroke are not candidates for therapy with sibutramine.

Malabsorptive Agents (Agents That Decrease Fat Absorption): Orlistat

Orlistat (Xenical) acts locally in the gastrointestinal tract by binding to gastric, carboxylester, lipoprotein, and pancreatic lipases, the enzymes that are essential for digestion of long chain triglycerides, and causing these enzymes to become inactive. This change results in failure to hydrolyze dietary fat (triglycerides) into absorbable free fatty acids and monoacylglycerols. Orlistat's mechanism of action is complete in the gastrointestinal tract, and very little of the drug is absorbed systemically. Orlistat inhibits dietary fat absorption of up to 30% of fat calories ingested, thus reducing calorie and fat intake. The recommended dose is 120 mg three times a day with meals or up to 1 hour after meals. Randomized, placebo-controlled clinical trials showed that patients taking orlistat as an adjunct to a hypocaloric diet had significantly more weight loss than those on a hypocaloric diet alone in a 1-year period. With continued treatment for 2 years, orlistat also produced less weight regain as compared with placebo, and it also lowered total cholesterol, low-density lipoprotein, blood glucose, and blood pressure. Patients considering orlistat should be instructed regarding a well-balanced, hypocaloric diet with fat content limited to approximately 30% of total calories to prevent aggravating the gastrointestinal side effects of the drug. Because orlistat decreases the absorption of fat-soluble vitamins and beta carotene, patients should be informed to take a multivitamin containing fat-soluble vitamins at least 2 hours before or after taking orlistat. The adverse side effects of orlistat include oily spotting, abdominal pain, flatus with discharge, fecal urgency or incontinence, oily stool, and increased defecation, effects that are related to its pharmacologic action. These effects are usually mild to moderate and transient, and they can spontaneously resolve within a few weeks to 1 month. Treatment with orlistat is not related to an increased risk of gallstone formation based on current studies. Some patients may excrete excessive urinary oxalate on using orlistat; therefore, the drug should be used cautiously in patients with a history of hyperoxaluria or calcium oxalate stones. Contraindications for the use of orlistat are chronic malabsorption syndrome, cholestasis, and known hypersensitivity to orlistat or its components. Table 2 provides a summary of approved weight-loss medications.

Herbal and Dietary Supplements

Herbal and dietary supplements that claim to promote weight loss such as chitosan,* chromium, picolinate,* conjugated linoleic acid,* ephedra alkaloids* (ma huang), and *Garcinia cambogia** are very popular, but they are relatively unregulated, with proof of efficacy limited to small, uncontrolled trials. Herbal and dietary supplements should not be recommended or considered without caution because of insufficient data providing evidence of either safety or efficacy in terms of promoting weight loss. Well-designed studies of efficacy and safety are warranted

*Not FDA approved for this indication.

TABLE 2. **A Summary of Approved Weight-Loss Medications**

Medication	Dose	Action	Adverse Effects	Duration of Treatment
Phentermine (Adipex-P)	15, 30, 37.5 mg qd	Increased norepinephrine, suppression of appetite	Dry mouth, constipation, increased heart rate and blood pressure, restlessness, insomnia, potential for addiction	Short term, ≤3 mo
Sibutramine (Meridia)	5, 10, 15 mg Start with 10 mg qd Can increase or decrease as needed	Norepinephrine and serotonin reuptake inhibitor, early satiety	Increased blood pressure and heart rate, insomnia, dry mouth, constipation	Long term, ≤2 y
Orlistat (Xenical)	120 mg tid with meals or ≤1 h after meals	Inhibited gastric and pancreatic lipase, decreased fat absorption	Oily spotting, flatus with discharge, fecal urgency or incontinence, oily stool, increased defecation, decreased fat-soluble vitamin absorption	Long term, ≤2 y

to investigate herbal supplements for weight loss, and stricter regulation of dietary and herbal supplements for weight loss would be beneficial to both consumers and practitioners.

Medications Approved by the FDA for Indications Other Than Obesity

Medications approved by the FDA for indications other than obesity treatment that are currently undergoing clinical trials for weight-loss efficacy are: bupropion (Wellbutrin),* topiramate (Topamax),* and metformin (Glucophage).*

Bupropion (Wellbutrin) is a relatively weak inhibitor of the reuptake of norepinephrine, serotonin, and dopamine and is structurally related to diethylpropion. It has been used for depression and has been noted to produce small amounts of weight loss. Currently, trials are being conducted with sustained-release bupropion* for the treatment of obesity.

One of the side effects of using topiramate (Topamax)* as an antiepileptic or for affective disorder is weight loss from reduced food intake. Trials are ongoing for the safety and efficacy of topiramate in obese patients with and without eating disorders.

Metformin (Glucophage),* a hypoglycemic agent, not only decreases blood glucose by inhibiting glucose production and improves insulin sensitivity but also prevents weight gain or induces modest weight loss. It has been studied in obese nondiabetic adults and children to evaluate its efficacy and safety for weight loss and its effects on insulin resistance and related medical conditions.

Investigational Drugs

LEPTIN

A few children have been identified in the literature with leptin deficiency, which results in severe and early-onset obesity. Treatment with human recombinant leptin† in these patients has resulted in substantial weight loss and changes in body composition. A double-blind, placebo-controlled trial with high doses of recombinant leptin, up to 0.3 mg/kg, in obese leptin-sufficient adults for 4 to 24 weeks resulted in a modest dose-related weight loss in most, but not all, subjects. The only adverse events reported were pain and erythema at the injection sites. There are ongoing studies evaluating the efficacy of recombinant leptin in maintenance of weight loss as well as the efficacy and tolerability of different leptin formulations.

OTHER INVESTIGATIONAL MEDICATIONS

Other medications that are in clinical trials (phase III) to investigate weight-loss effects include the following:

1. Ciliary neurotrophic factor (Axokine): This agent can suppress food intake without triggering hunger signals or stress responses associated with food deprivation. Theoretically, the cessation of this treatment would not result in binge-eating or immediate weight regain.
2. Cannabinoid CB1 receptor antagonist (Rimonabant): This agent has resulted in reduced food consumption, especially of high-fat foods, and weight loss in clinical trials so far.
3. Other agents: A neuroactive cytokine, a peptide analogue of human growth hormone, and agonists of the β_3-adrenergic and cholecystokinin-A receptors are also being studied in ongoing clinical trials.

*Not FDA approved for this indication.
†Investigational drug in the United States.

Bariatric Surgery

Dietary change with and without behavior modification or drug therapy has an unacceptably high incidence of weight regain in the morbidly obese within 2 years of achieving maximal weight loss. Therefore, the National Institutes of Health recommend consideration of bariatric surgery in well-informed and motivated patients with a BMI greater than 40 in whom conventional treatment modalities have failed or in patients who have a BMI of 35 to 40 with multiple co-morbidities or severe lifestyle limitations, including cardiopulmonary risk factors, degenerative joint disease, sleep apnea, limited mobility, and inability to work. Surgery provides medically significant sustained weight loss for more than 5 years in most patients. Three types of gastric-restrictive operations are currently performed in the United States: the vertical-banded gastroplasty, gastric banding (lapband), and the Roux-en-Y gastric bypass. One malabsorptive operation is currently performed in the United States: the biliopancreatic bypass. The restrictive operations primarily limit the size of the functional stomach by partitioning the stomach and creating a very small gastric chamber for food storage. After the patient eats a small meal, this chamber is full, causing early satiety and compelling the patient to eat small amounts. A narrow outlet from the chamber to the rest of the stomach is designed to slow the passage of food from the chamber and thereby to prolong satiety and decrease snacking between meals. The vertical-banded gastroplasty can be performed laparoscopically or by an open surgical approach. The lapband is a laparoscopically placed band around the stomach pouch that can be adjusted as needed by injecting saline into a subcutaneous port. This procedure is currently undergoing FDA evaluation and is not yet approved for clinical use in the United States. The Roux-en-Y gastric bypass combines gastric restriction with subclinical malabsorption and can be performed laparoscopically or by an open surgical approach. It is the most effective weight-loss procedure in terms of percentage of weight loss and is considered the gold standard. The biliopancreatic bypass combines a modest amount of gastric restriction with intestinal malabsorption. The outcomes of these operations are assessed in terms of absolute

TABLE 3. **Outcome, Morbidity, and Mortality of Bariatric Surgery**

Procedure	Capacity of Gastric Pouch	Mean Excess Weight Loss*	Early Mortality Rate†	Early Morbidity Rate†	Complications
Vertical-banded gastroplasty	15-20 mL	60%	<10%	<1%	Stomal outlet stenosis, severe gastroesophageal reflux disease
Lapband	10-15 mL	Less consistent	Not applicable	Not applicable	High rate of stomal stenosis and erosion
Roux-en-Y gastric bypass	20-30 mL	65-75%	10%	≤1%	Deep venous thrombosis, pulmonary embolus, anastomotic leak, wound infection, incisional hernia, gallstones, iron and vitamin B_{12} deficiency, dumping syndrome
Biliopancreatic bypass	100-200 mL	75-80%	10-15%	1%	Anemia, fat-soluble vitamin deficiency, protein-calorie malnutrition

*Mean excess weight loss is defined as the difference between preoperative and ideal body weight.
†Early morbidity and mortality rates vary with patient's age, body mass index, and overall health. It is therefore recommended that patients lose at least 5% to 10% of their initial weight before undergoing surgery to lower the risk of perioperative complications.

weight loss and improvement in obesity-associated medical disorders and overall quality of life. Details of these four operations are summarized in Table 3.

Previous studies have demonstrated improvement or even resolution of obesity-related medical problems including improvement of diabetes mellitus, insulin resistance, hypertension, cardiovascular dysfunction, dyslipidemia, sleep apnea and the obesity hypoventilation syndrome, infertility, gastroesophageal reflux disease, hepatic steatohepatitis, osteoarthritis, and quality of life after successful bariatric surgery. Surgical patients should be monitored for complications and lifestyle adjustments throughout their lives.

SUMMARY

Obesity is a chronic, multifactorial disease that develops from the interaction of genetic and environmental factors. Effective treatments for obesity require a lifelong combination of diet modification, increased physical activity, and behavior therapy, with or without pharmacotherapy or bariatric surgery. Advances in our understanding of how and why obesity occurs will lead to more effective treatments, not only to develop safe and effective ways to lose weight but also to understand how to prevent obesity in high-risk patients.

SUGGESTED READINGS

Allison DB, Fontaine KR, Heshka S, et al: Alternative treatments for weight loss: A critical review. (Critical Reviews in Food Science and Nutrition) 41:1-28, 2001.

American Dietetic Association: Weight management. J Am Diet Assoc 102:1145-1155, 2002.

Anderson JW, Greenway F, Fujioka K, et al: Clinical trial using bupropion SR with a moderate-intensity lifestyle intervention. Obes Res 8:1S-88S, 2000.

Apovian C: The medical management of obesity and the role of pharmacotherapy: An update. Nutr Clin Pract 15:5-12, 2000.

Apovian C: Antiobesity drugs: Should they be used in the treatment of obesity? Nutr Clin Pract 13:251-256, 1998.

Ballinger A, Peikin SR: Orlistat: Its current status as an anti-obesity drug. Eur J Pharmacol 440:109-117, 2002.

Bray G: Obesity. In Fauci AS. (ed): Harrison's Principles of Internal Medicine, 14th ed. International Edition, McGraw-Hill, 1998, pp 454-462.

Brolin RE. Bariatric surgery and long-term control of morbid obesity. JAMA 288:2793-2797, 2002.

Brownell KD, Wadden TA: The LEARN Program of Weight Control: Special Medication Edition. Dallas, TX, American Health Publishing, 1999.

Campbell ML, Mathys ML: Pharmacologic options for the treatment of obesity. Am J Health Syst Pharm 58:1301-1308, 2001.

Davison MH, Hauptman J, DiGirolamo M, et al: Weight control and risk factor reduction in obese subjects treated for 2 years with orlistat: A randomized controlled trial. JAMA 281:235-242, 1999.

European Multicentre Orlistat Study Group: Randomized placebo-controlled trial of orlistat for weight loss and prevention of weight regain in obese patients. Lancet 352:167-172, 1998.

Flegal KM, Carroll MD, Ogden CL, Johnson CL: Prevalence and trends in obesity among US adults, 1999-2000. JAMA 288: 1723-1727, 2002.

Fontbonne A, Charles MA, Juhan-Vague I, et al: The effect of metformin on the metabolic abnormalities associated with upper-body fat distribution. Diabetes Care 19:920-926, 1996.

Fujioka K, Seaton TB, Rowe E, et al: Weight loss with sibutramine improves glycemic control and other metabolic parameters in obese patients with type 2 diabetes mellitus. Diabetes Obes Metab 2:175-187, 2000.

Grace GM: Gastric restrictive procedures for treating severe obesity. Am J Clin Nutr 55:556S-559S, 1992.

Hauptman J, Lucas C, Boldrin MN, et al: Orlistat in long-term treatment of obesity in primary care settings. Arch Fam Med 9:160-167, 2000.

Heymsfield SB, Greenberg AS, Fujioka K, et al: Recombinant leptin for weight loss in obese and lean adults: A randomized, controlled, dose-escalation trial. JAMA 282:1568-1575, 1999.

James WP, Astrup A, Finer N, et al: Effect of sibutramine on weight maintenance after weight loss: A randomized trial. Lancet 356:2119-2125, 2000.

Klaver J, Aronne LJ: Managing overweight and obesity in women. Clin Obs Gyn 45:1080-1088, 2002.

Kral JG, Sjostrom LV, Sullivan MBE: Assessment of quality of life before and after surgery. Am J Clin Nutr 55:611S-614S, 1992.

Langlois KJ, Forbes JA, Bell GW, et al: A double-blind clinical evaluation of the safety and efficacy of phentermine hydrochloride (Fastin) in the treatment of exogenous obesity. Curr Ther Res Clin Exp 16:289-296, 1974.

Lee CD, Blair SN, Jackson A: Cardiorespiratory fitness, body composition, and all-cause and cardiovascular disease mortality in men. Am J Clin Nutr 69:373-380, 1999.

Lee DW, Leinung MC, Arena MR, Grasso P: Leptin and the treatment of obesity: Its current status. Eur J Pharmacol 440:129-139, 2002.

Luque CA, Rey JA: The discovery and status of sibutramine as an anti-obesity drug. Eur J Pharmacol 440:119-128, 2002.

National Center for Health Statistics: Prevalence of overweight and obesity among adults: United States, 1999-2000. Health E-Stats. Hyattsville, MD: National Center for Health Statistics, 2002. (Accessed October 10, 2002 at *http://www.cdc.gov/nchs/products/pubs/pubd/hestats/obese/obese99.htm)*

National Institutes of Health: Gastrointestinal surgery for severe obesity: National Institutes of Health consensus development conference statement 1991. Am J Clin Nutr 55:615S-619S, 1992.

National Institutes of Health, National Heart, Lung, and Blood Institute: North American Association for the Study of Obesity: The Practical Guide to Identification, Evaluation, and Treatment of Overweight and Obesity in Adults. Bethesda, MD, National Institutes of Health, 2000.

National Task Force on the Prevention and Treatment of Obesity: Overweight, obesity and health risk. Arch Intern Med 160:898-904, 2000.

National Task Force on the Prevention and Treatment of Obesity: Long-term pharmacotherapy in the management of obesity. JAMA 276:1907-1915, 1996.

O'Leary JP: Gastrointestinal malabsorption procedures. Am J Clin Nutr 55:567S-570S, 1992.

Smith IG, Goulder MA: Randomized placebo-controlled trial of long-term treatment with sibutramine in mild to moderate obesity. J Fam Pract 50:505-512, 2001.

Smith U, Axelsen M, Hellebo-Johanson E, et al: Topiramate, a novel antiepileptic drug, reduces body weight and food intake in obesity. Obes Res 8:1S-10S, 2000.

Sugerman HJ, Kellum JM, Engle KM, et al: Gastric bypass for treating severe obesity. Am J Clin Nutr 55:560S-566S, 1992.

Trumbo P, Schlicker S, Yates AA, Poos M: Food and Nutrition Board of the Institute of Medicine, National Academies: Dietary reference intakes for energy, carbohydrate, fiber, fat, fatty acids, cholesterol, protein and amino acids. J Am Diet Assoc 102:1621-1630, 2002.

Wadden TA, Bartlett SJ, Foster GD, et al: Sertraline and relapse prevention training following treatment by very-low-calorie diet. Obes Res 7:363-369, 1999.

Wadden TA, Berkowitz RI, Sarwer DB, et al: Benefit of lifestyle modification in the pharmacologic treatment of obesity: A randomized trial. Arch Intern Med 161:218-227, 2001.

Weinsier RL, Hunter GR, Heini AF, et al: The etiology of obesity: Relative contribution of metabolic factors, diet, and physical activity. Am J Med 105:145-150, 1998.

Wirth A, Krause J: Long-term weight loss with sibutramine: A randomized controlled trial. JAMA 286:1331-1339, 2001.

Yanovski SZ, Yanovski JA: Drug therapy: Obesity. N Engl J Med 346:591-602, 2002.

VITAMIN K DEFICIENCY

method of
FRANK R. GREER, M.D., and
CAROL A. DIAMOND, M.D.
University of Wisconsin
Madison, Wisconsin

Vitamin K is a fat-soluble vitamin important for the formation of many vitamin K-dependent proteins including the plasma coagulation proteins (II, VII, IX, and X) and the plasma proteins C, S, and Z. Other vitamin K-dependent proteins are found in bone (osteocalcin and matrix Gla protein), kidney (nephrocalcin), spleen, lung, uterus, placenta, pancreas, thyroid, thymus, and testes. All of the known vitamin K-dependent proteins have in common gamma-carboxyglutamic acid (Gla), the unique amino acid formed by the postribosomal action of vitamin K-dependent carboxylase. Vitamin K is a necessary cofactor for the activity of this glutamyl carboxylase, located on the membrane of the endoplasmic reticulum. The Gla residues formed by the action of this carboxylase are located on the homologous amino-terminal domain of the protein, with a high degree of amino acid sequence identity common to all vitamin K-dependent proteins. They are required for the protein conformation that allows for calcium binding and the calcium-mediated interaction of these proteins with phospholipids.

The daily recommended intake for vitamin K is 1 μg per kg of body weight. The most important dietary form of this vitamin is Vitamin K_1 or phylloquinone. Green leafy vegetables are the best dietary source (50 to 800 μg per 100 g), but other foods contain significant amounts of vitamin K_1, including dairy products, meats, eggs, cereals, fruits, and other vegetables (1 to 50 μg/100 g). Although human milk is very low in vitamin K (2 μg/L), all infant formulas used in the United States have vitamin K_1 added (50 μg/L). Another potential source of vitamin K is the bacterial flora of the jejunum and ileum, which synthesize vitamin K_2 or menaquinone. The extent that this form of vitamin K can be utilized by humans is unclear, and it is even possible that menaquinone may be converted to phylloquinone, as has recently been shown in rodents. From 40% to 70% of dietary vitamin K is absorbed from the small intestine, and the absorption via chylomicrons and the lymphatic system is dependent on bile, pancreatic secretions, and dietary fat.

CLINICAL FEATURES

Vitamin K deficiency results in a coagulopathy. Specific signs of deficiency include bruising, epistaxis, bleeding from the gastrointestinal or genitourinary tract, menometrorrhagia, retroperitoneal bleeding, and intracranial hemorrhage (particularly in infants). Bleeding may follow trauma, needle punctures, or surgery.

ETIOLOGY

Vitamin K deficiency may result from decreased intake or fat malabsorption. Antibiotic inhibition of vitamin K_2 synthesis by intestinal bacteria may also be a factor. Prolonged total parenteral nutrition without supplemental vitamin K has also been reported to cause deficiency. Causes of fat malabsorption that may be associated with vitamin K deficiency include short bowel syndrome, biliary atresia, cholestatic jaundice, α_1-antitrypsin deficiency, pancreatic insufficiency (e.g., cystic fibrosis), and diseases of the small intestine (e.g., nontropical sprue or regional enteritis).

Therapy with vitamin K antagonists such as warfarin (Coumadin) may present as a coagulopathy identical to vitamin K deficiency. Warfarin is an active ingredient of some rodenticides, though superwarfarins (e.g., brodifacoum, difenacoum, chlorophacinone, bromadiolone, diphacenone, pindone, valone, flocoumafen, coumatetralyl) are now preferred as rodenticides due to warfarin resistance in rats. Poisoning with these rodenticides occurs accidentally or by attempted suicide. Poisoning has been observed after smoking a mixture of marijuana and d-CON, a rodenticide containing brodifacoum.

Vitamin K deficiency causes hemorrhagic disease in infants. This may occur as early as the first week of life or up to 3 months of age. The late form, with an incidence of one in many thousands, has the most significant mortality and morbidity. Because vitamin K crosses the placenta poorly, vitamin K levels are nearly undetectable in umbilical cord blood. Human milk is also very low in vitamin K, such that breast-fed infants are particularly at risk for hemorrhagic disease. A bleeding diathesis in newborns attributed to vitamin K deficiency has also been associated with maternal administration of anticonvulsants (e.g., phenobarbital, phenytoin [Dilantin], primidone [Mysoline]).

Beta-lactam antibiotics with an *N*-methyl-5-thiotetrazole side chain (cefamandole [Mandol], cefoperazone [Cefobid], and cephamycin [Mefoxin]) also contribute to the coagulopathy of vitamin K deficiency because they inhibit Gla synthesis in coagulation factors.

DIAGNOSIS

Prolongation of the prothrombin time (PT) and the activated partial thromboplastin time (aPTT) characterizes a deficiency of vitamin K. Values for platelet counts, plasma fibrinogen level, thrombin time, fibrinogen degradation products or fibrinogen split products, and D-dimer are normal. Vitamin K blood levels are not readily available. The diagnosis is confirmed by demonstration that vitamin K replacement restores PT and aPTT values to normal (within hours after parenteral vitamin K administration) (Table 1). Differential diagnosis includes disseminated intravascular coagulation and liver disease (see Table 1). PT and aPTT values in infants are notably higher than adult levels until at least 6 months of age.

Formulations of Vitamin K_1

Vitamin K_1 is available as a tablet (Mephyton, 5 mg) or a parenteral form for intramuscular or subcutaneous injection (AquaMEPHYTON, 10 mg/mL or 2.0 mg/mL). AquaMEPHYTON, when given intravenously, should be infused slowly at a rate of not more than 1 mg per minute to minimize adverse reactions, such as anaphylaxis and hypotension. It can be diluted (1 mg/mL) with a solution of 0.9% NaCl or 5% dextrose to facilitate the slow infusion rate.

TREATMENT

Parenteral vitamin K_1 should be given to patients with a suspected deficiency who show evidence of bleeding or extremely abnormal PT and aPTT values. The initial dose is 1.0 mg for newborn infants (0.3 to 0.5 mg for premature infants ≤1000 g weight), 2 to 3 mg for children up to 12 months of age, and 5 to 10 mg for ages 1 year to the mid-teens. The usual adult dose is 10 to 20 mg. Subcutaneous injection is preferred to the intramuscular route, which may result in hematoma formation. Slow intravenous infusion (5%/minute of the total dose diluted in saline or glucose) rarely causes hypotension or anaphylaxis. PT and aPTT should respond within 6 hours to a parenteral injection of vitamin K and within 24 hours of oral administration. When there is no response, another diagnosis should be considered.

For those poisoned with a superwarfarin preparation where rapid correction of coagulation status is necessary, the initial dose of vitamin K_1 in adults should be 10 mg given intravenously (5% of the total dose/minute diluted in saline or glucose), followed by a daily oral dose of 50 mg for weeks or months until superwarfarin is no longer detected in blood and normal measurements of PT and aPTT persist.

For those with vitamin K deficiency with extremely severe bleeding manifestations (e.g., intracranial hemorrhage in an infant), treatment includes not only vitamin K replacement but also fresh frozen plasma (10 to 20 mL per kg of body weight). Infusions of prothrombin-complex concentrates should be avoided because they carry a risk for thrombosis, especially in those patients who have associated liver disease. A risk of transmitting viral illnesses always exists whenever blood products are given.

TABLE 1. **Differential Diagnosis of Vitamin K Deficiency**

Test	Vitamin K Deficiency	Liver Disease	DIC
aPTT	Increased	Increased	Increased
PT	Increased	Increased	Increased
Platelets	Normal	Decreased	Decreased
Fibrinogen	Normal	Decreased	Decreased
D-dimer/FDP/FSP	Normal	Normal or Increased	Increased

aPTT, activated partial thromboplastin time; DIC, disseminated intravascular coagulation; FDP/FSP, fibrin degradation products/fibrin split products; PT, prothrombin time.

PREVENTION

All newborns should receive 1.0 mg of vitamin K_1 intramuscularly within the first hour after birth (0.3-0.5 mg for premature infants ≤1000 g birth weight). It has been recommended that pregnant women on anticonvulsants should receive 10 to 20 mg of vitamin K_1 daily for 2 to 3 weeks prior to delivery.

Patients with a decreased intake of vitamin K or malabsorption of the vitamin should receive prophylactic supplements. Prophylaxis is especially needed for severely ill patients in intensive care units who are not taking vitamin K and may be receiving prolonged antibiotic therapy. Prophylactic treatment with vitamin K_1 may be given orally in doses of 2.5 mg daily or 5.0 mg three times weekly or 10 mg subcutaneously once a week.

OSTEOPOROSIS

method of
STANLEY J. BIRGE, M.D.
Washington University School of Medicine
St. Louis, Missouri

Osteoporosis is a preventable disorder of the skeleton characterized by diminished bone strength that predisposes an individual to an increased risk of fracture. Both men and women of all races and ethnic groups are affected, although white postmenopausal women have the highest age-adjusted incidence of fracture. Osteoporotic fractures are a major cause of disability in older adults. The more common vertebral fractures cause disabling pain, disfiguring height loss, and an increased risk of death from pulmonary disease. Hip fracture is associated with the greatest disability and economic burden, estimated at $10 to $15 billion annually. Only a third of hip fracture patients regain their prefracture level of function, and half of those who do not will require nursing home placement.

PATHOGENESIS

The skeleton is constantly turning over through a process of osteoclastic bone resorption and osteoblastic bone formation. This process serves to replace old bone and accumulated microfatigue fractures with new bone on an average of every 2 years. Within each bone remodeling unit, resorption is coupled to formation, and no net change in bone mass results. After the third decade, the amount of new bone deposited becomes slightly less than the old bone removed by osteoclastic bone resorption, thereby resulting in a net loss of bone. Both men and women experience this age-related loss of bone. However, women experience an acceleration of this loss associated with the relatively abrupt loss of estrogens during the perimenopausal period. Men experience a more gradual decline in gonadal steroids over their life span and therefore experience a more gradual decline in bone mass. As a result of the conversion of testosterone to estradiol, men have approximately three times the level of estradiol as postmenopausal women of the same age.

TABLE 1. **Factors Contributing to Reduced Bone Mass**

Nonmodifiable	Modifiable
Advanced age	Smoking
Female sex	Low calcium intake
White/Asian race	Sedentary lifestyle
Family history of osteoporosis	Low body weight
Family history of hip fracture	Low vitamin D intake/sunlight exposure
Lactose intolerance	Stress/depression
Vitamin D resistance	

Multiple factors have been found to contribute to reduced bone mass (Table 1). Some of these factors are operational during the first 3 decades of life and affect peak bone mass, a critical determinant of bone mass later in life. Racial and sexual differences in bone mass and fracture incidence can be attributed to differences in peak bone mass. Although genetic factors exert a predominant role in the development of peak bone mass, physiologic, environmental, and modifiable lifestyle factors are also important. Risk factors for fracture include not only factors related to low bone mass but also factors related to falls, the geometry of the hip, the force of the impact (e.g., height), and the ability to absorb the impact of the fall (e.g., the age-related loss of muscle mass at the hip) (Table 2). After the age of 70, fall-related risk factors become the dominant determinant of hip fracture, an observation that has important implications in the prevention of hip fracture in the very old.

DIAGNOSIS

The diagnosis of osteoporosis begins with a history and physical examination to assess the risk for osteoporosis and fracture. A definitive diagnosis is based on assessment of bone mineral density (BMD), which accounts for about 70% of bone strength. Thus, bone density is an excellent predictor of fracture risk. Several different techniques are currently available to assess BMD at different skeletal sites. The gold standard is dual-energy x-ray absorptiometry (DEXA) of the hip and spine. Other less costly techniques are

TABLE 2. **Factors Contributing to the Risk of Fracture**

Increased height
Long hip axis
Lower extremity muscle weakness/atrophy
Poor visual acuity
Neurodegenerative disorders of the central nervous system
Age-related deterioration in postural stability
Medications affecting postural stability

TABLE 3. **Technologies for the Measurement of Bone Mineral Density**

Technique	Cost	Radiation Exposure	Precision (%)	Change (%) Required for Significance
Spine DEXA	+++	+	1.0	3
Hip DEXA	+++	+	1.5	4
Q-CT	++++	+++	3	8
Heel DEXA	+	+	2	5
Heel Ultrasound	+	0	4	11

Abbreviations: DEXA = dual-energy X-ray absorptiometry; Q-CT = quantitative computed tomography.

available to assess the BMD of peripheral sites such as the heel: portable DEXA and quantitative ultrasound technology (Table 3). The latter measurements are an excellent means of assessing hip fracture risk, though somewhat less effective than assessment of BMD by DEXA of the femoral head. These portable instruments have a role in screening populations for osteoporosis and fracture risk but are less helpful in monitoring therapy.

Criteria for the diagnosis of osteoporosis have been established by several groups, including the World Health Organization (WHO), which assesses BMD of the hip and spine relative to the peak BMD of the individual at these sites. Specifically, osteoporosis is defined as a BMD that is 2.5 standard deviations (SD) below the estimated peak BMD for that individual. Consequently, BMD is reported as the SD above or below the calculated peak BMD for the individual, or the "*t* score," as opposed to a "*z* score," or the SD from the average BMD of a sex- and age-matched control population. It is uncertain whether these criteria can be applied to other instruments measuring other sites.

WHO SHOULD BE EVALUATED?

The WHO and the National Osteoporosis Foundation have developed criteria to determine which individuals should undergo assessment of BMD (Table 4). Perhaps the most important group to be assessed is individuals who have experienced an osteoporotic fracture or a loss of height greater than 2 inches. Having had one osteoporotic fracture increases the risk of a subsequent fracture by 5- to 10-fold. In randomized clinical trials, this group is most likely to benefit from treatment.

TABLE 4. **Who Should Be Tested With Bone Densitometry?**

- All men and women older than 65 y
- All women younger than 65 y with risk factors for osteoporosis
- Men and postmenopausal women with an osteoporotic fracture
- Persons with a vertebral compression fracture or height loss >2 inches
- Persons receiving glucocorticoid therapy
- Persons with primary hyperparathyroidism
- Women considering therapy
- Persons being treated for osteoporosis (to monitor therapy)

However, less than 30% of patients with any fracture, as well as patients with a hip fracture, receive any therapy for osteoporosis. Patients with an increased risk for osteoporosis because of concurrent medical conditions, such as the initiation of long-term glucocorticoid therapy, anticonvulsant therapy, or surgical and medical gonadal ablation, are candidates for treatment and baseline assessment of BMD. More controversial is the screening of perimenopausal women. In women electing to initiate hormone replacement therapy, assessment of BMD would be of little value. However, obtaining a BMD measurement is very helpful in getting perimenopausal and postmenopausal women to initiate hormone replacement.

EVALUATION OF A PATIENT WITH LOW BONE MASS

The goal of evaluation of a patient with osteoporosis is to identify secondary causes of osteoporosis so that they may be treated (Table 5). A careful history will identify many of the modifiable and treatable factors contributing to the loss of bone mass. A limited biochemical evaluation is in order to detect medical conditions that may be contributing to the osteoporosis (Table 6). The single most important measure is 24-hour urinary excretion of calcium and creatinine on a known intake of calcium. With an 800- to 1200-mg calcium intake, the calcium-creatinine ratio (in milligrams) should be 0.15 to 0.25. Ratios in excess of 0.25 are consistent with states of increased bone turnover and resorption such as

TABLE 5. **Common Causes of Secondary Osteoporosis**

Endocrine	Chronic Drug Therapy
Hypogonadism	Corticosteroids
Hyperthyroidism	Thyroxine
Anorexia nervosa	Anticonvulsants
Type 1 diabetes mellitus	Loop diuretics
Hyperadrenocorticism	GRH antagonists
Nutritional	**Other**
Malabsorption syndromes	Hypercalciuria
Vitamin D deficiency	COPD
Calcium deficiency	Rheumatoid arthritis
Alcoholism	Organ transplantation

Abbreviations: COPD = chronic obstructive pulmonary disease; GRH = gonadotropin-releasing hormone.

TABLE 6. **Laboratory Evaluation of Osteoporosis for Exclusion of Secondary Causes**

Serum Chemistry Profile
Calcium
Phosphorus
CBC
25-Hydroxyvitamin D
Urine
24-h Urinary calcium/creatinine excretion
Albumin
Alkaline phosphatase
TSH
Total testosterone (men)

Abbreviations: CBC = complete blood count; TSH = thyroid stimulating hormone.

hyperparathyroidism, hyperthyroidism, renal calcium leak, and excessive intake of caffeine. Ratios less than 0.15 are consistent with malabsorption syndromes, secondary hyperparathyroidism, and vitamin D deficiency or resistance. Vitamin D resistance is an important diagnostic consideration in that it may affect up to 70% of patients with osteoporosis. It can be operationally defined as a low 24-hour urinary calcium-creatinine ratio in the presence of a normal serum 25-hydroxyvitamin D level. It is typically associated with thin, soft fingernails.

Biochemical markers of bone turnover are available and aggressively marketed. These markers provide useful information in population studies monitoring response to therapy, and they provide insight into the mechanism of the drug's action on bone. Because of the large measurement and physiologic variation in such assays, these markers have little clinical utility in monitoring an individual patient and are not a substitute in the diagnosis of osteoporosis.

SKELETAL MODALITIES OF TREATMENT

This past decade has seen the development of new drugs that have greatly expanded our options for the effective treatment of osteoporosis (Table 7). Treatment and prevention, however, begin by ensuring an adequate intake of calcium and vitamin D and promoting regular weight-bearing exercise. Clinical trials have demonstrated that calcium and vitamin D alone are capable of increasing bone density and reducing the incidence of spine and hip fractures. Nevertheless, calcium and vitamin D are not sufficient to prevent the accelerated loss of bone in perimenopause.

Calcium

In men and premenopausal women, 800 to 1000 mg of calcium is recommended. This requirement is increased to 1200 mg in postmenopausal women not receiving estrogen replacement and to 1500 mg in the elderly. The requirement can be achieved by increasing the consumption of dairy products, certain vegetables (broccoli), and, if necessary, calcium supplements. A simple method for calculating dietary calcium content assigns 300 mg to a dairy product–free diet and 300 mg for each serving (cup or slice) of dairy product. Calcium supplements come in many formulations, the most practical of which are calcium carbonate and calcium citrate. Little difference is seen in the absorption of these two salts if taken with meals. Calcium supplements should be taken in divided doses throughout the day and before bedtime. Some concern has been raised by unacceptable levels of lead contamination and the lack of bioavailability of some non–brand name products. Side effects include constipation and intestinal gas.

Vitamin D

The major source of vitamin D is sunlight exposure in younger adults and vitamin D–fortified milk, cereals, and soy products in older adults. The minimal daily requirement for vitamin D increases with age and menopause to 600 U, which in most cases requires supplementing the diet with a multivitamin containing 400 U of vitamin D. In many individuals with osteoporosis, this requirement may be as much as 10,000 to 20,000 U/d. In such individuals, a prescription is needed for vitamin D (Drisdol), which is supplied as 50,000 U of vitamin D per capsule. Because of the long half-life (22 days), vitamin D can be given monthly or weekly. The dose of vitamin D required is determined by increasing the dose every 3 months until a 24-hour urinary calcium-creatinine ratio between 0.15 and 0.20 is achieved. Vitamin D intake greater than 2000 U/d may cause hypercalciuria, hypercalcemia, and renal toxicity in patients without vitamin D resistance.

TABLE 7. **Drugs for the Treatment and Prevention of Osteoporosis**

Drug	Mechanism of Action	Cost	FDA-Approved		Relative Efficacy	
			Prevention	*Rx*	*Spine Fx*	*Hip Fx*
Hormone replacement	Antiresorptive	+	Yes	No	+++	+++
Raloxifene (Evista)	Antiresorptive	+++	Yes	Yes	+++	0
Alendronate (Fosamax) Risedronate (Actonel)	Antiresorptive	+++	Yes	Yes	+++	+++
Calcitonin (Miacalcin)	Antiresorptive	+++	No	Yes	+	0
Parathyroid hormone (Fortéo)	Anabolic	++++	No	Yes	++++	+++

Abbreviations: FDA = Food and Drug Administration; Fx = fracture; Rx = treatment.

Exercise

Bone formation and maintenance of skeletal mass are dependent on physical activity. In young and sedentary older adults, exercise modestly increases BMD. Despite their marginal effects on BMD, weight-bearing and resistance exercises are believed to be an important adjunct to the treatment and prevention of osteoporotic fractures. Clinical trials using exercise have demonstrated improved muscle strength and balance and a reduced risk of falls.

Hormone Replacement Therapy

The first line of approach to the pharmacologic prevention and treatment of osteoporosis is estrogen replacement. Estrogen replacement is also the most effective approach to the prevention of perimenopausal bone loss. In fertile perimenopausal women, estrogen is given in the form of birth control pills until menopause or an arbitrary age of 52, when therapy can be switched to one of the many forms of hormone replacement. In postmenopausal women at any age, estrogen is as effective as bisphosphonates in increasing bone mass. The Women's Health Initiative study demonstrates that postmenopausal estrogen is very effective in reducing the risk of hip and other osteoporotic fractures. However, its efficacy is lost 5 years after discontinuation of the hormone.

Adverse side effects include breast tenderness, a threefold increased risk of venous thromboembolic disease, a twofold increased risk of cholelithiasis, uterine bleeding, and endometrial cancer. In women with a uterus, estrogen is administered with a progestin to reduce the risk of endometrial cancer. Unfortunately, the addition of a progestin may increase the relatively small increased risk of breast cancer associated with estrogen replacement. Because of an increased incidence of breast cancer that becomes significant after 10 to 15 years of exposure to estrogen plus a progestin, the Food and Drug Administration (FDA) has advised that agents other than hormone therapy be considered for osteoporotic fracture prevention. However, the mortality from breast cancer actually decreases after 5 years of taking estrogen, a decrease that does not appear to be due to greater surveillance of estrogen users for breast cancer. The adverse effects of estrogen are dose-dependent, and therefore lower doses of estrogen equivalent to 0.3 and 0.45 mg of conjugated equine estrogens (Premarin) are being recommended for the treatment and prevention of osteoporosis.

Selective Estrogen Receptor Modulators

These drugs bind to the estrogen receptor but exert an antiestrogen effect on some tissues, including the breast and endometrium, while retaining estrogen activity on other tissues such as the skeleton. Raloxifene (Evista) is the first drug in this class approved for the treatment and prevention of osteoporosis. In the clinical registration trial, raloxifene, 60 mg daily, increased BMD by a third to half that observed with estrogen and bisphosphonates and decreased spinal fractures by the same amount as these agents. However, raloxifene had no effect on the prevention of hip fractures or other nonvertebral fractures.

Although raloxifene may reduce the incidence of breast cancer after short-term use, its use for more than 5 years raises some concern regarding a possible increased risk of breast cancer and mortality as seen with the similar drug tamoxifen. Because raloxifene causes hot flushes and muscle cramps in perimenopausal women, it is best initiated at least 3 years after the last menstrual period. Like estrogen, raloxifene increases the risk of thromboembolic disease.

Another example of this drug class is the plant-derived phytoestrogens such as soy phytoestrogens. At high doses, these agents increase bone mass in experimental animal models. Clinical trials in humans have been disappointing to date in demonstrating improvement in BMD and menopausal symptoms.

Calcitonin

Calcitonin (Miacalcin) nasal spray has only a modest effect on spine BMD, with less than half the patients treated showing an increase as compared with a greater than 90% response rate with estrogen and bisphosphonates. In the registration trial for nasal calcitonin, a significant reduction in the risk of vertebral fractures was observed at a dose of 200 IU but not at 100 or 400 IU. This trial had a 60% dropout rate. The major adverse effects were nasal mucosal irritation, flushing, and nausea. Because of the questionable efficacy and intolerance of this agent, its use is limited.

Bisphosphonates

Bisphosphonates are potent antiresorptive agents that increase BMD at the spine and hip comparable to the increase seen with estrogen. Randomized clinical trials with alendronate (Fosamax) and risedronate (Actonel) demonstrated a consistent 30% to 50% reduction in both vertebral and nonvertebral fractures, including hip fractures. Although clinical trials with etidronate (Didronel) demonstrated a reduction in vertebral fractures, these trials are limited, and as a result, this agent has not been approved by the FDA for the treatment of osteoporotic fractures. All three drugs must be given 30 to 60 minutes before breakfast on an empty stomach with an 8-oz glass of water while upright to facilitate passage into the stomach. The presence of food or medications will substantially reduce or abolish absorption of the drug. Once-a-week dosing with 70-mg and 30-mg tablets has greatly improved the acceptance and tolerance of alendronate and risedronate, respectively. The original drug in this class, etidronate, is given daily at 400 mg for 14 days every fourth month for up to 2 years. The addition of bisphosphonates to estrogen therapy provides little additional improvement in BMD, and no data are available on fracture outcomes. Alendronate and risedronate have been approved for the treatment of male osteoporosis and corticosteroid-induced osteoporosis. For the prevention of postmenopausal bone loss and steroid-induced bone loss, half the dose is recommended.

The major adverse side effect is esophagitis, which occurs in 10% to 15% of patients, and rarely, erosive esophagitis and stricture. Use of these agents should be avoided in patients unable to remain upright after dosing and before the first meal and in those with esophageal abnormalities that would delay tablet transit.

Parathyroid Hormone

Recombinant human parathyroid hormone (hPTH) has recently been approved for the treatment of osteoporosis. Its mechanism of action differs from that of other pharmacologic agents in that it stimulates bone formation and bone turnover. The hormone is administered as a daily subcutaneous injection. Clinical trials have demonstrated an increase in BMD of the spine and hip that is about 1.5 to 2.0 times greater than the increase seen with antiresorptive agents, an impressive 60% to 70% reduction in vertebral fractures, and a 50% reduction in nonvertebral fractures. These effects persisted for 18 months after discontinuation of treatment.

Adverse side effects are limited to nausea, headache, and hypercalcemia. Only 11% withdrew from the group receiving the highest dose, 40 mg, because of adverse drug effects as compared with 6% in the placebo group. Because of the high cost of treatment, parathyroid hormone will be targeted to individuals at greatest risk for fracture. One caveat is that parathyroid hormone is associated with postural instability and falls. It may be prudent to assess balance in frail elderly persons when initiating hPTH.

NONSKELETAL MODALITIES OF TREATMENT

After age 70, when 90% of hip fractures occur, nonskeletal age-related factors become an increasingly important determinant of the risk for hip fracture. A deterioration in postural stability because of multiple age-related factors increases the propensity for falls. Perhaps the most important factor in this regard are changes in the central nervous system causing postural instability. Both estrogen replacement and vitamin D appear to prevent or slow this age-related deterioration in postural stability. These two agents seem to be effective in the prevention of hip fracture in elderly populations. In contrast, the bisphosphonate risedronate was not effective in reducing hip fractures in women older than 80. Another age-related change is the loss of muscle mass around the head of the femur, an important factor in absorption of the energy of impact from a fall. External hip protectors have been developed to compensate for this loss of muscle mass, and several clinical trials have demonstrated their efficacy in the reduction of hip fracture risk in frail elderly populations. Exercise and modification of the environment are additional strategies for reducing the risk of falls.

SUMMARY

Osteoporosis is a preventable disorder, and new treatment modalities have been developed that significantly reduce an individual's risk for fracture. The greatest challenge is to identify those at risk for fracture so that effective treatment can be instituted.

PAGET'S DISEASE OF BONE

method of
STANLEY WALLACH, M.D.
American College of Nutrition
Clearwater, Florida

Paget's disease, as the second most common "metabolic bone disease," accounts for one to three million cases in the United States, based on radiographic studies of involved skeletal structures and/or an elevated blood level of bone-specific alkaline phosphatase. Although the original description of the condition by Sir James Paget in the 1870s was of a painful, deforming condition which he called osteitis deformans, more than 50% of afflicted individuals are asymptomatic, with focal involvement of mild to moderate degree in one or more nonstrategic bones. Among the remaining half of the involved population, there may be little deformity, and the pain pattern may be nonspecific, suggesting an arthritic rather than a skeletal condition. In perhaps 10% to 20% of Paget's disease patients a diagnosis can be made clinically based on physical findings of enlarged painful bones, and this tends to occur relatively late in the disease course, when the outcome of treatment may be more limited, although still worthwhile. The most commonly involved bones are the pelvis, skull, spine, femur, and tibia.

The evidence suggests that both genetic and environmental factors are involved in disease causation, although there has been heated controversy among the experts studying the problem. Several viruses of the Paramyxoviridae family have been incriminated as the arrays of inclusion bodies seen in the nuclei and cytoplasm of the grossly abnormal osteoclasts that drive the predominant bone resorption underlying disease evolution. Family and geographic clustering, supported by considerable genetic evidence, suggests that a gene on chromosome 18q may confer susceptibility to prolonged skeletal sequestration of the offending virus and/or its expression as pagetic lesions in the skeletal sites harboring the virus. The osteoblast, which is presumably uninfected, reacts to the extreme and unregulated osteoclast-induced bone resorption by equally chaotic bone formation superimposed on the bone resorption abnormality. The osteoclastic component is best measured by serum or urine levels of peptide fragments from the terminal ends of the bone collagen molecule, known as telopeptides. Telopeptides, liberated during bone breakdown, are not reutilized in the reactive new bone formation. The osteoblastic reaction is most easily measured by the serum level of bone-specific alkaline phosphatase, which is produced almost exclusively by the osteoblast.

The relationship of patient symptomatology to the amount of Paget's disease present is variable, but in general, those patients with longer courses and extensive, active foci of the disease have more pain, fractures, deformities, and neurologic abnormalities characteristic of the disease. The neurologic deficits are secondary to bone encroachment on, or reduced blood flow to, the brain, spinal cord, and dorsal root plexus. Peripheral neurologic abnormalities are most often due to a nonspecific peripheral neuropathy. The disease tends to advance slowly over the years, and a significant number of asymptomatic or mildly symptomatic patients eventually manifest sufficient clinical features to justify treatment. At the same time, true arthritic findings may develop due to either abnormal "wear and tear" on joint surfaces by the deformed pagetic bone constituting the joint or to direct subchondral excavation and cartilage destruction by the inflammatory component of the underlying pagetic bone. It is often difficult to distinguish true arthritic complications from the pseudoarthritic elements of the disease. Therefore, in designing treatment, if pain is an indication to start treatment, it should combine anti-pagetic and anti-arthritic drugs to "cover" both elements.

Whatever the inciting cause, the initial pathophysiology is the transformation of osteoclasts in discrete skeletal locations into abnormal bone-resorbing cells that digest bone rapidly and indiscriminately. These pagetic osteoclasts have an abnormal appearance and contain many more nuclei than normal osteoclasts. Combined with the equally disorganized and excessive osteoblastic response, a histologic picture consisting of a combination of abnormal bone loss and sclerotic bone of poor structural quality evolves. Affected bones are painful, thickened, and subject to deformation and pathologic fracture. Pagetic bone also contains a large capillary bed but with low pressure, thereby "stealing" blood flow from other organs. To compensate for this situation, when the amount of pagetic bone is large, cardiac output increases. Pagetic bones near skin surfaces (e.g., an affected tibia) are often warm to the touch because of the greatly increased blood flow. The sequential process of chaotic bone resorption and formation is repeated several times in affected bony areas as the process encroaches on previously unaffected adjacent bone. The rapidity of progression is variable. Over decades, most patients manifest elevated bone-specific alkaline phosphatase levels, serum and urine telopeptide levels, and increased radiotechnetium uptake on bone scans, indicating continuing disease activity.

DIAGNOSIS

The diagnosis of Paget's disease is usually not difficult if it is considered in the differential diagnosis when suggestive symptoms are present. An appropriate radiographic appearance and an elevated serum bone-specific alkaline phosphatase level are usually sufficient for diagnosis, although osteoblastic or mixed osteoblastic-osteolytic metastases from prostate, breast, and other carcinomas may rarely present a similar radiographic appearance. Bone scans define the extent of disease but should not be used in lieu of radiographs. It is important to take radiographs of all areas positive on bone scans to define the anatomy of the bony lesions. An isolated elevation of the serum bone-specific alkaline phosphatase is sometimes the only clinical finding because symptoms may be absent or so mild as to be ignored.

CLINICAL FEATURES

The most common clinical features of Paget's disease are summarized in Table 1. Orthopedic, rheumatologic, neurologic, ophthalmologic, otolaryngologic, and even cardiologic features can sometimes dominate the clinical picture and confuse the differential diagnosis. Pain is the most common presenting symptom and may be skeletal, muscular, or due to associated osteoarthritis. Headaches are frequently present with skull involvement even when there are no obvious neurologic abnormalities or head enlargement. Radicular pain indicates impingement of affected vertebral bodies on exiting spinal nerves.

TABLE 1. **Clinical Features of Paget's Disease**

Skeletal
Pain
Deformities
Fractures
Neoplastic conversion
Miscellaneous
Resorptive-sclerotic components
Increased bone vascularity
Neurologic
Cranial nerve deficits and syndromes
Medulla and cerebellum
Spinal cord and nerves
Miscellaneous
Steal syndromes
Peripheral neuropathies
Cardiovascular
Increased cardiac output
Generalized atherosclerosis
Cardiovascular calcification
Metabolic
Hypercalcemia, hypercalciuria, renal calculi
Primary hyperparathyroidism
Hyperuricemia, uric acid stones, gouty diathesis
Miscellaneous
Carpal/tarsal tunnel syndromes
Peyronie's disease

Deformities may take many forms, but anterior bowing of the long bones of the legs is the most common finding. Pagetic vertebrae are subject to compression and can cause kyphoscoliosis. When the pelvis is involved, the acetabular cups usually become osteoarthritic. As the underlying bone becomes structurally incompetent, pressure of the femoral heads may cause medial displacement of the acetabular cups, so-called *acetabular protrusion*. When the resorptive component of Paget's disease predominates, large areas of resorption may be present in the skull, so-called osteoporosis circumscripta. Similar advancing fronts of pagetic bone resorption may be seen in long bones and produce flame-shaped areas of demineralization. Behind such fronts, lunate areas of resorption may fail to undergo subsequent sclerosis and may remain as cyst-like areas devoid of structure. In some patients, cracks occur along the lateral aspects of sclerotic bones in the lower extremities. These fissure fractures, as well as the lunate areas of bone resorption, are subject to fracture with minimal trauma. Pagetic fractures can be catastrophic because of possible nonunion. Also, subsequent immobilization causes bone loss and predisposes to further fractures. Pagetic bone lesions undergo neoplastic transformation in approximately 1% of patients. Osteosarcomas or other types of sarcoma usually lead to death in 2 years or less.

Neurologic deficits sometimes dominate the clinical picture because of extensive Paget's disease of the skull and spine. The neurologic impairments arise from a combination of direct bony impingement on existing cranial and spinal nerves and on the spinal cord and from a pagetic steal of blood supply away from neurologic structures to surrounding pagetic bone sharing a common blood supply. Any cranial nerve can be impaired, but the auditory branch of the eighth cranial nerve is most commonly affected because the temporal bone encases the hearing apparatus. High-frequency sensorineural hearing loss occurs, similar to that of presbycusis but progressing at a more rapid rate. Visual problems can be caused by either optic nerve or oculomotor impairment. In addition, pagetic patients are susceptible to two retinal lesions, retinal mottled degeneration and angioid streaks. The lower cranial nerves and the medulla and cerebellum are particularly susceptible to damage when the posterior skull becomes so pagetic as to be flattened in the area of the foramen magnum, a condition known as "platybasia." Lower cranial nerve palsies, ataxia, and Valsalva maneuver–induced headaches characterize this neurologic syndrome, with the headaches resulting from partial obstruction of the aqueduct. When the aqueduct is completely obstructed, a hydrocephalus-dementia syndrome may occur.

Atherosclerosis and medial calcinosis are common in older pagetic patients. Subendocardial calcification, mitral annulus calcification, and calcific aortic stenosis also occur with increased frequency. However, the major cardiovascular feature of Paget's disease is the increased cardiac output required by the greatly increased blood flow through pagetic bones. Although this may ultimately result in left ventricular hypertrophy, overt congestive heart failure is rare except in patients with associated coronary artery disease sufficient to depress myocardial contractility.

Patients with Paget's disease are prone to defects in both calcium and uric acid metabolism. Approximately 5% of pagetic patients are hypercalcemic as a result of concomitant primary hyperparathyroidism. By contrast, an immobilization-related, nonparathyroid form of hypercalcemia, secondary to an imbalance between the rates of bone resorption and bone formation, is rare. Even in the absence of hypercalcemia, hypercalciuria, with or without calcium stone formation, can occur. Hyperuricemia, with or without gouty features or uric acid stone formation, is as common as abnormal calcium metabolism. The basis for these metabolic defects and their relation to the underlying Paget's disease are unclear.

Miscellaneous features of the disease include carpal/tarsal tunnel syndrome and Peyronie's disease. Their causal relationship to Paget's disease is also unknown.

TREATMENT

In addition to making the diagnosis of Paget's disease based on clinical, radiologic, and biochemical features, it is necessary to define the extent and anatomic location of the disease to ascertain its functional impact and the potential for complications. Many pagetic patients have moderate to severe symptomatology and need treatment. Table 2 outlines the features that are common indications for treatment. Pain that cannot be relieved by mild analgesics, nonsteroidal anti-inflammatory drugs, or COX-2 inhibitors is a prime indication for treatment. Radiologic evidence of extensive bone resorption that predisposes to fracture and neurologic deficits are also key indications for treatment. It is reasonable to treat patients with progressive visual or auditory defects. Treatment is effective in reducing bone blood flow and should be used before orthopedic surgery to reduce intra- and postoperative bleeding and thereby

TABLE 2. **Indications for Treatment of Paget's Disease**

Pain (unrelieved by analgesic, nonsteroidal anti-inflammatory, or COX-2 inhibitor drugs)
Excessive bone resorptive components
Neurologic deficits
Prolonged immobilization
Preparation for orthopedic surgery
Complications secondary to increased cardiac output
Extreme elevation of serum bone-specific alkaline phosphatase and/or serum/urine telopeptide levels

enhance healing. Prolonged immobilization secondary to fracture or surgery causes severe bone loss, and it is necessary to counteract this problem by starting treatment as early as possible. Treatment also normalizes elevated cardiac output, which benefits patients with abnormal cardiac function. Whether or not to treat patients with extreme elevations of the serum bone-specific alkaline phosphatase or telopeptide levels (i.e., 5 to 30 times normal), in the absence of other indications, is unclear but is probably defensible.

SPECIFIC AGENTS

Drug treatment of Paget's disease has been revolutionized by the development of the highly potent, so-called *third generation* bisphosphonates alendronate (Fosamax) and risedronate (Actonel). Along with a similar bisphosphonate, pamidronate (Aredia), which is used exclusively as an intravenous preparation, they are the treatments of choice for symptomatic Paget's disease. Three older drugs, synthetic salmon calcitonin (parenteral form, Miacalcin), disodium etidronate (Didronel), and plicamycin (Mithracin),* are still commercially available and can be used when none of the three advocated third-generation bisphosphonates is feasible. All these agents act by direct inhibition of the abnormally rapid osteoclastic bone resorption, but do so by different mechanisms. Control of the resorption rate permits more normal bone formation to occur, with more normal remodeling. Resorptive lesions improve, the increased vascularity of affected bone decreases, and bone mass of the enlarged bones decreases, allowing neurologic defects to improve. The biochemical abnormalities improve 30% to 70% as partial normalization of skeletal structure and metabolism ensues.

Alendronate (Fosamax)–Risedronate (Actonel)

These oral aminobisphosphonates (third generation) are highly effective suppressants of Paget's disease activity, reducing biochemical parameters more than 70% on average. In the doses used, they have very little inhibition of osteoblastic activity. Both agents need to be given daily, in the morning, on an empty stomach, with the patient remaining upright (sitting or standing) and fasting, except for copious tap water, for a minimum of 30 minutes, and preferably for an hour. The absorption rate is very low, less than 1% under most conditions, and the drugs may not be absorbed at all if admixed with food, other medications, or supplements. Risedronate appears to have more potency than alendronate because a smaller daily dose is given for a shorter period to achieve similar results. Once the therapeutic endpoint is achieved, i.e., relief of clinical features combined with maximum reduction in the abnormal biochemical parameters, periodic observation should be done and a new course of treatment should be given when clear evidence appears of a resumption of disease activity. This may occur within 6 to 12 months in many patients, but instances of prolonged remission after a single course of therapy have been noted.

The aminobisphosphonates are all intrinsically toxic to the distal esophagus and instances of severe heartburn, sometimes simulating anginal pain, have been reported. Fastidious attention to the administration of the drugs will lessen the frequency of the side effect. Nevertheless, patients with reflux disease, other esophageal or gastric problems, or difficulty swallowing pills may be unable to continue this form of treatment and will have to consider intravenous pamidronate or one of the other agents, parenteral salmon calcitonin, disodium etidronate, or plicamycin.*

*Not FDA approved for this indication.

Pamidronate (Aredia)

As an aminobisphosphonate, pamidronate also has low absorbability and an esophageal irritative effect when given orally. In the United States, it is available only as an intravenous preparation for intermittent treatment of acute hypercalcemia, Paget's disease, multiple myeloma, or osteolytic skeletal metastases. In Paget's disease, if sufficient drug is given to achieve a substantial remission of the clinical features and biochemical concomitants, the effects of treatment may last 6 months or longer before a repeat course is required. It is common for patients to experience malaise and low-grade fever during the first infusion of a course of treatment, but this is usually mild and not repeated on subsequent infusions. The pamidronate should be given by slow infusion to prevent acute impairment of renal function. Because of the potential for renal dysfunction, the aminobisphosphonates are relatively contraindicated in patients with prior renal insufficiency.

Disodium Etidronate (Didronel)

Etidronate, a first generation bisphosphonate, has been approved for Paget's disease for more than 20 years. It is a modulator of bone metabolism and inhibits bone formation and mineralization, as well as bone resorption. The major advantage of etidronate is its lower incidence of gastrointestinal side effects. However, approximately 10% to 20% of patients develop increased bone pain at the site of pagetic lesions. In these patients, the inhibiting effect of the drug on mineralization appears to predominate over its antiresorptive action, and a painful osteomalacia-like condition develops that requires discontinuation of the drug. The same complex dosing schedule is required as for other bisphosphonates.

*Not FDA approved for this indication.

Synthetic Salmon Calcitonin (Miacalcin Iniectable)

Synthetic salmon calcitonin (SCT) was the first antipagetic drug to receive approval and has been in routine use for more than 25 years. In most patients, the initial response is similar, regardless of whether 50 IU is injected subcutaneously three times a week or 100 IU daily. Because occasional secondary resistance to SCT due to neutralizing antibody production occurs, higher doses up to 200 IU daily are sometimes needed. The side effects of SCT, shown in Table 3, occur in 10% to 20% of patients, but are usually self-limited and undergo amelioration with continued treatment. Rarely, urticaria or severe nausea and vomiting may make it necessary to discontinue SCT.

Beneficial clinical and biochemical responses usually begin within weeks and are at a maximum within the first 12 months of treatment. An 18-month course of calcitonin treatment is advocated if an acceptable initial response is seen. In general, SCT should be used only if an aminobisphosphonate is contraindicated. However, it may be considered as the primary choice in patients with serious skeletal resorptive features or an acute fracture because of its additional analgesic action. Some physicians prefer SCT for neurologic complications because of the greater experience with SCT from initial research trials. Nasal spray SCT has some antipagetic activity but should not be used in preference to injectable SCT.

TABLE 3. **Specific Drugs for Paget's Disease**

Alendronate (Fosamax)

Dose: 40 mg daily, orally, on empty stomach
Duration: 6 mo
Side effects: Heartburn, nausea, vomiting, hoarseness, musculoskeletal pain, renal impairment, hypocalcemia
Drug resistance: Unknown

Risedronate (Actonel)

Dose: 30 mg daily, orally, on empty stomach
Duration: 2 mo
Side effects: Heartburn, nausea, vomiting, hoarseness, musculoskeletal pain, renal impairment, hypocalcemia
Drug resistance: Unknown

Pamidronate (Aredia)

Dose: 30-60 mg IV by slow infusion (2-4 hr)
Duration: 3-6 infusions given daily or every other day, depending on disease activity/patient response
Side effects: Fever, malaise, renal impairment, hypocalcemia
Drug resistance: Unknown

Disodium etidronate (Didronel)

Dose: 5-20 mg/kg daily, orally, on empty stomach
Duration: 6 mo (1-3 mo for 20 mg/kg dose)
Side effects: Increased bone pain, diarrhea, nausea, vomiting
Drug resistance
Primary: 15%
Secondary: 10-20%

Calcitonin

Synthetic salmon calcitonin (SCT) (Miacalcin injectable)
Dose: 50-100 IU, SC or IM, daily to three times / wk
Duration: 18 mo, with repeat courses as needed
Side effects: Metallic taste, anorexia, nausea, vomiting, nonspecific rash, urticaria, polyuria, diarrhea (rare)
Drug resistance
Primary: 15%
Secondary: 20%-30%

Plicamycin (Mithracin)*

Dose: 25 μg/kg, daily or every other day, by IV infusion
Duration: 9-10 infusions over 1½-3 wk period, with repeat courses as needed
Side effects: Anorexia, nausea, vomiting, abnormal hepatic and/or renal function, thrombocytopenia with gastrointestinal hemorrhage
Drug resistance: Unknown

*Not FDA approved for this indication.
IM, intramuscularly; IV, intravenously; SC, subcutaneously.

Plicamycin (Mithracin)*

Although this chemotherapeutic agent causes sufficient toxic damage to osteoclasts to produce a beneficial effect on Paget's disease, its concurrent toxicity to the gastrointestinal tract, liver, kidneys, and bone marrow indicate it should be reserved for patients who have become resistant to or have serious side effects from the bisphosphonates or SCT. It is not approved for this indication. Some patients should be hospitalized for a course of plicamycin, but others can take outpatient administration under special conditions.

Anti-Inflammatory Drugs

As noted earlier, osteoarthritis is a frequent concomitant of Paget's disease, and it is often difficult to differentiate the two on the basis of pain. It is often advisable to treat both conditions simultaneously to achieve optimal benefit with regard to pain and disability. In patients treated with one of the above agents and in whom there is a clear-cut response, as indicated by a declining serum bone-specific alkaline phosphatase level but an inadequate alleviation of the pain, the addition of a nonsteroidal anti-inflammatory agent or COX-2 inhibitor may make the difference between therapeutic success and failure.

*Not FDA approved for this indication.

TOTAL PARENTERAL NUTRITION IN ADULTS

method of
DARRYL T. HIYAMA, M.D.
David Geffen School of Medicine at the University of California, Los Angeles
Los Angeles, California

The concept of providing nutrition by intravenous infusion can be traced to the mid-1600s, when infusions of various nutrients were administered.

However, modern parenteral nutrition became technically feasible only after the development of subclavian vein cannulation in 1958, which eventually permitted the infusion of hypertonic solutions of glucose, amino acids, and fats into the central circulation. Since then, improvements have been made in the understanding and prevention of metabolic complications and in delivery techniques and systems, and there has been a relative explosion in disease-specific formulations for patients with organ failure or critical illness. Indeed, since the early 1990s, academic and commercial interest in producing a variety of enteral feeding products designed to enhance immunocompetence has been significant. Since the late 1980s, the use of enteral nutrition has been recognized to have numerous theoretical and practical advantages over the use of parenteral nutrition. In spite of this development, parenteral nutrition remains an essential component of nutritional support.

INDICATIONS

In spite of the intuitive impression that providing ill patients with intravenous nutrition should be beneficial, it has been difficult to demonstrate the clinical efficacy of parenteral nutrition for broad groups of patients. In part, this lack of conclusive evidence may result from the relatively small numbers of prospective, randomized, controlled clinical trials to evaluate nutritional support and parenteral nutrition. This fact is, of itself, remarkable considering the common use of nutritional support in current medical care. Further, in an era of evidence-based evaluation of medical therapies, many studies today focus on evaluating clinical outcomes such as length of hospital stay, nosocomial infections and other complications, and mortality. It is very likely that within the multitude of factors that influence such outcomes in any individual patient's care, the effect of nutrition may be overshadowed by other variables such as the primary illness, associated co-morbidities, and even age.

Scientific evidence suggests that specific subgroups of patients do derive measurable benefits from the use of nutritional support. Unfortunately, with the exception of the Veterans Administration Cooperative Study, most of the prospective, randomized, controlled clinical trials concerning the use of parenteral nutrition have involved relatively small numbers of patients. In turn, most of the subsequent studies concerning parenteral nutrition have relied on meta-analysis, a method that, of itself, has limitations. In 2001, a committee of the American Gastroenterological Association reported on a review of the available clinical trials evaluating the effects of parenteral nutrition in certain disease states and conditions including inflammatory bowel disease, acute pancreatitis, liver disease, renal failure, pulmonary disease, burns, AIDS, oncologic therapy, and critical illness. The conclusions of the committee are as follows: (1) in the *absence* of severe underlying malnutrition, withholding parenteral nutrition for up to 7 days is not harmful; (2) patients with short or inadequate bowel function are likely to benefit from parenteral nutrition because other modes of nutritional intake are not available; and (3) protein-sparing therapies appear to be efficacious for patients with hepatic encephalopathy, but not for those with renal failure.

Given the information available to date, certain recommendations regarding the general and specific indications for the use of parenteral nutrition can be made. Whenever the gastrointestinal tract is not viable, parenteral nutrition may be used, either as primary therapy or in a supportive role. In general, the use of parenteral nutrition is appropriate in the following circumstances:

1. A previously well-nourished patient who has been *without* nutrient intake for 7 days or more and in whom oral or enteral nutrition is not possible.
2. A previously well-nourished patient who is *expected* to be unable to eat for 7 days or more as a result of illness or the nature of medical therapy. This is especially pertinent to patients who become hypermetabolic because of multiple injuries, sepsis, severe acute pancreatitis, burns, and multiple organ dysfunction.
3. A patient with either clinical or biochemical evidence of *pre-existing* malnutrition. Studies have demonstrated that persons who have lost 10% or more of their usual body weight or who have serum albumin levels of less than 3 g/dL appear to be at increased risk of developing infectious and wound-healing complications.

Specific clinical situations in which evidence indicates that the use of parenteral nutrition has been shown to be of some clinical benefit are discussed later.

Short Bowel Syndrome

Before the introduction of parenteral nutrition, patients with short bowel syndrome rarely survived. Parenteral nutrition has been the most influential and dramatic development in the treatment of this condition. Early mortality has essentially been eliminated; however, the long-term use of parenteral nutrition is still associated with hepatic dysfunction and, on occasion, hepatic failure. In any patient who has anatomic or functional short gut syndrome, parenteral nutrition should be initiated early in the course of treatment. Simultaneously, when ileus has resolved, attempts should be made for the early institution of oral or enteral feedings to facilitate intestinal adaptation. The adaptation process requires several months; however, this process may enable many patients to eventually obtain most, if not all, of their nutrition by the enteral route. Those patients who have less than 60 cm of functioning small intestine, or 45 cm with an intact and competent ileocecal valve, will likely require lifelong parenteral nutrition support.

Acute Renal Failure

The use of parenteral nutrition in this setting is directed toward providing an energy source to avoid proteolysis and to minimize azotemia, while also reducing fluid administration to avoid hypervolemia. In the past, there was substantial interest in using protein restriction or in providing only essential amino acids during nutritional support in patients with renal failure, in the hopes of avoiding exacerbation of the azotemia. However, for patients with acute renal failure, good evidence demonstrates that the provision of a caloric source and of proteins is associated with fewer infectious complications and a greater likelihood of in-hospital survival, as opposed to providing a caloric source alone. Further, the evidence supporting the clinical benefit of using essential amino acids or the α-keto analogues as the nitrogen source is limited to a single early study. Therefore, for most patients in acute renal failure, a balanced standard parenteral nutrition formulation containing both glucose and essential and nonessential amino acids can be used while the azotemia is treated with hemodialysis. In the uncommon situation in which dialysis is not used, it may be possible to minimize azotemia and fluid overload for a limited time by using high-concentration dextrose solutions (dextrose 35%) with low-concentration amino acids (3.5%) in reduced volumes (1.5 L or less). In patients receiving hemodialysis, an option in providing parenteral nutrition is the use of intradialytic parenteral nutrition. Although this technique is more commonly applied to patients receiving chronic hemodialysis, it may be occasionally useful for patients with acute renal failure. Limited studies indicate that the technique is efficacious; patients have been documented to increase both their dry body weight and serum albumin levels when they receive parenteral nutrition with their dialysis treatment.

Hepatic Insufficiency

Patients with chronic liver failure commonly manifest moderate to severe malnutrition as a result of ascites, impaired protein synthesis, and altered protein and fat metabolism. Patients with acute liver failure may have similar metabolic derangements but are often hypermetabolic as well. In both chronic and acute liver failure, the levels of branched chain amino acids such as leucine and isoleucine are decreased in both the plasma and the cerebrospinal fluid. Simultaneously, the levels of aromatic amino acids are elevated. Prospective, randomized trials using branched chain amino acid–enriched parenteral formulations in patients with advanced liver failure demonstrated that patients can achieve a positive nitrogen balance and can experience a reduced incidence of encephalopathy when compared with using a standard amino acid formulation. In view of the expense of the branched chain amino acid–enriched formulations, the use of these products should be limited to patients who have pre-existing encephalopathy or who subsequently develop encephalopathy after a standard formulation is administered.

Acute Pancreatitis

There is good evidence to advise against the use of parenteral nutrition in patients with mild or moderate pancreatitis. Prospective trials of total parenteral nutrition support in such patients demonstrated a higher incidence of infectious complications, particularly catheter-related sepsis. However, in patients with severe pancreatitis, a delay in instituting total parenteral nutrition support is actually associated with a higher mortality and complication rate. Therefore, parenteral nutrition should be started early in the treatment of severe acute pancreatitis, within 24 to 48 hours of admission. The use of intravenous lipids in patients with acute pancreatitis has not been shown to exacerbate the disease as long as severe hyperlipidemia is not already present.

Critical Illness

The use of nutritional support within the first 48 hours after admission has been shown to improve survival and to reduce infectious complications and overall hospital length of stay in patients with burns, major abdominal trauma, and severe head injuries. If the gastrointestinal tract is available for use, enteral nutrition is preferred to parenteral nutrition because enteral feedings have been shown to reduce infectious complications, particularly pneumonia and intra-abdominal abscesses. Although branched chain amino acid–enriched parenteral formulations have been shown to improve nitrogen balance, with the exception of liver failure, no significant clinical benefit has been demonstrated with the use of these products in patients with critical illness.

Cancer

The indiscriminate use of parenteral nutrition in patients suffering from cancer cachexia is not advisable. Clearly, patients undergoing bone marrow transplantation benefit from the use of parenteral nutrition by gaining shorter hospitalization and better long-term survival. However, for patients with carcinoma, the abundance of evidence remains difficult to apply. Evidence suggests that the use of parenteral nutrition in patients with carcinoma who are receiving chemotherapy or radiation therapy may actually result in more infectious complications. However, the use of parenteral nutrition in severely malnourished patients undergoing surgery for gastrointestinal cancer is associated with fewer postoperative infectious complications and a reduced mortality rate. For the practitioner, a reasonable approach for patients with cancer is to use total parenteral nutrition if enteral nutrition is not feasible and the patient is actively receiving some form of antitumor therapy. It is advisable to monitor the patient's daily caloric intake closely to avoid overfeeding, a condition that may promote tumor growth.

Gastrointestinal-Cutaneous Fistulas

Fistulas that produce drainage or output of more than 500 mL/d should be initially treated with bowel rest and parenteral nutrition. Studies indicate that perhaps up to one third of fistulas may spontaneously close with this conservative form of treatment alone. The time required for this form of management is 6 to 12 weeks. If by the end of 12 weeks spontaneous closure has not occurred, then operative correction will likely be required.

Perioperative Nutritional Support

Numerous studies have investigated the use of parenteral nutrition in malnourished patients before they undergo a major surgical procedure. However, it has been remarkably difficult to demonstrate a clear-cut benefit of using preoperative parenteral nutrition in improving the outcomes for these patients. The available evidence consists of some small studies and the large Veterans Administration Cooperative Study. From this body of evidence, it seems that patients with mild or moderate degrees of malnutrition may actually have a higher risk of infectious complications when they are treated with preoperative parenteral nutrition and no improved overall outcome after operation. Only patients who are severely malnourished (i.e., serum albumin less than 2.5 g/dL, body weight loss greater than 10% of usual body weight) appear to benefit from the use of preoperative parenteral nutritional support. In this specific group of patients, the incidence of noninfectious complications, such as delayed wound healing, is reduced in the postoperative period by the use of preoperative parenteral nutrition. However, the time required for preoperative nutritional support may be 7 to 14 days. As noted earlier, postoperative nutritional support is appropriate for those patients who are not expected to resume oral feeding within 7 days or who demonstrated either clinical or biochemical evidence of malnutrition before their operations.

GUIDANCE IN THE ADMINISTRATION OF PARENTERAL NUTRITION

The principal issues in administering parenteral nutrition are:

1. Determination of caloric and protein needs.
2. Selection of a route of administration.
3. Initiation of therapy.
4. Monitoring for metabolic and infectious complications.

Determination of Caloric Needs

In general, healthy adults require approximately 25 kcal/kg/d, whereas adults with illnesses may require approximately 30 to 35 kcal/kg/d. For the individual patient, basal energy expenditure (BEE) should be calculated using the Harris-Benedict regression equations:

$$\text{BEE (male)} = 66.47 + (13.75 \times \text{body weight in kg}) + (5 \times \text{height in cm}) - (6.76 \times \text{age in years})$$

$$\text{BEE (female)} = 655.1 + (9.56 \times \text{body weight in kg}) + (1.85 \times \text{height in cm}) - (4.58 \times \text{age in years})$$

In turn, adjustments for physical activity and additional metabolic stress are made, depending on the clinical situation. The common factors used are as follows:

Bedridden patient, 1.2
Ambulatory, hospitalized patient, 1.3
Minor operation, 1.2
Skeletal trauma, 1.35
Sepsis, 1.6
Severe thermal injury, 2.1

The total caloric needs are therefore determined by the following equation:

$$\text{Total calories/d} = \text{BEE} \times \text{activity factor} \times \text{injury factor}$$

The calculated total caloric needs are less accurate in patients with critical illness. Often, the estimates may be accurate in only one third of patients. In the setting of critical illness, a calculation of total caloric needs may be used to initiate therapy. However, a more accurate method may be the use of bedside indirect calorimetry, if it is available. This technique allows for the determination of a resting energy expenditure from measurements of oxygen consumption and carbon dioxide production.

Glucose and Lipids

The two sources of calories in parenteral formulations are dextrose and fat. The maximal rate of hepatic oxidation of glucose is 5 mg/kg/min, or approximately 500 g/d for a 70-kg man. The daily dose of glucose varies according to the dextrose concentration of the formulation. Because the average patient usually receives approximately 2 to 2.5 L of parenteral nutrition per day, most total parenteral nutrition formulations contain a 25% to 28% dextrose concentration. Formulations containing higher dextrose concentrations may be used as part of an effort to reduce the volume of fluid administered, an approach that may be useful in patients with congestive heart failure or oliguric renal failure. Alternatively, formulations containing lower dextrose concentrations may be required for patients with glucose intolerance, as seen in diabetes mellitus or severe sepsis. When dextrose concentrations of 20% or less are used, the volume of fluid administered per day to meet the patient's caloric needs will be substantially increased.

Fat is both an energy source and a needed substrate for cell structure and immune function. In parenteral formulations, fat is present as emulsions of either safflower or soybean oil. A minimum of 4% to 6% of the total daily calories should be administered as fat to prevent essential fatty acid deficiency. In the United States, lipid emulsions are available in 250-mL aliquots of 2% lipid. Therefore, usually, 500 calories are provided each day as fat. Under certain circumstances, the percentage of calories provided as fat can be increased, with a concomitant reduction in glucose calories. Such an action may be useful in the setting of severe glucose intolerance, which is difficult to control with insulin administration, or in patients with ventilatory failure, in whom the reduction of carbon dioxide production is needed to ameliorate hypercarbia.

Determination of Protein Needs

Healthy adults require approximately 0.8 to 1.0 g protein/kg/day. In situations of metabolic stress, protein requirements increase dramatically as a result of a net increase in protein catabolism. Because there is no nonspecific storage form of protein, protein catabolism results in the loss of lean body mass, principally skeletal muscle. The resulting functional outcomes include reduced immune competence, poor wound healing, and the loss of skeletal muscle mass and strength. Therefore, the primary goal of nutritional support is to preserve lean body mass. In patients under metabolic stress, protein requirements increase to 1.5 to 2.0 g/kg/d. Patients with thermal injuries experience significant protein loss and may require 2 to 3 g/kg/d.

Modern parenteral nutrition formulations commonly contain amino acids in concentrations of 3% to 6% per liter resulting in average daily protein doses of 70 to 100 g/d for a 70-kg man. When parenteral nutrition is administered, attention should also be paid to the calorie-nitrogen ratio to ensure the provision of an adequate number of calories to facilitate protein synthesis and to minimize protein catabolism. In general, a ratio of 150 kcal/g of administered nitrogen (6.25 g protein = 1 g nitrogen) is recommended. In the setting of metabolic stress such as sepsis or injury, the protein needs exceed the caloric needs, and a lower ratio of 80:1 is recommended.

Selection of Route of Administration

Parenteral nutrition formulations may be infused by a peripheral or a central venous route. Peripheral parenteral nutrition is of limited value today because of its inherent limitations. Peripheral veins are susceptible to thrombophlebitis as a result of the irritant effect of the high-osmolarity nutrient solutions. Peripheral parenteral nutrition formulations have lower dextrose concentrations, usually 15%, to minimize the irritant effect. However, the volume of fluid required to administer an adequate number of calories is, in turn, markedly increased. In general, peripheral parenteral nutrition should be used if no practical central venous access is available and if the need for nutritional support is expected to be of very short duration.

Total parenteral nutrition infused into the central circulation is the preferred technique. Percutaneously placed subclavian or internal jugular central catheters are the most preferred types for central venous access, as opposed to femoral venous catheters, because the former sites are easier to keep free of infection. In our institution, peripherally inserted central catheters are frequently used as an alternative to subclavian or internal jugular catheters. Although these catheters are advantageous in terms of avoiding the potential complications of central venous catheter insertion, the incidence of thrombophlebitis remains relatively high.

Initiation of Therapy

Before the initiation of parenteral nutrition therapy, baseline laboratory studies should be obtained. These studies include complete blood count, serum electrolytes, blood urea nitrogen, serum glucose, creatinine, calcium, magnesium, phosphorus, albumin, prealbumin, alanine transaminase, aspartame transaminase, total bilirubin, alkaline phosphatase, and serum triglycerides.

Once the caloric and protein requirements have been determined as described earlier, a suitable formulation is selected. Most institutions have standard formulations from which a choice can be made. The use of standard formulations is more cost-effective for most hospital pharmacy departments because of the advantages of economies of scale. A formulation that will deliver the needed calories and protein in approximately 2 L of fluid is appropriate. When determining the electrolyte composition of the formulation, sodium should be provided at about 30 to 40 mEq/L or higher if warranted by the patient's serum electrolytes. The ratio of chloride to acetate is adjusted according to the patient's acid-base status. Potassium and phosphorus are provided in nominal amounts to account for existing deficiencies, or they are withheld if renal failure is present. Standard amounts of multivitamins (except vitamin K) and trace elements are added to the formulation. When therapy is initiated, insulin should not be added to the formulation. Instead, a regular insulin sliding scale dosage schedule should be provided for the patient, based on 6-hour fingerstick blood sugar determinations made as the formulation is being infused. Insulin should be administered with a goal of maintaining the blood glucose concentration at less than 200 mg/dL. After the first 24 to 48 hours of parenteral nutrition therapy, one half of the daily regular insulin dose that was required can be added to the formulation. A minimum of 20 U of regular insulin should be added per liter of formulation because insulin usually binds to the container and tubing material.

In our institution, the infusion is usually begun at a rate of 25 mL/h. It is advanced at increments of 25 mL/h at intervals of 8 hours until the target rate is achieved as long as the blood glucose levels remain at less than 200 mg/dL.

Monitoring of Metabolic Complications

Complications associated with parenteral nutrition therapy can be categorized as early (within 2 weeks of initiating therapy) and late (more than 12 weeks after initiating therapy) complications. Most early complications arise from disorders of glucose metabolism and electrolyte and acid-base abnormalities, whereas late complications are primarily manifestations of trace element deficiencies.

After the acquisition of baseline laboratory studies, fingerstick blood glucose determinations should be obtained every 6 hours, and blood glucose, serum sodium, potassium, chloride, bicarbonate, calcium, magnesium, phosphorus, and blood urea nitrogen values should be obtained daily until the target rate of infusion is achieved and the blood glucose and serum electrolytes have remained stable. Thereafter, the laboratory studies along with liver function studies, serum albumin, serum prealbumin, and complete blood count should be obtained twice weekly.

Early Complications

FLUID OVERLOAD

Patients at particular risk are elderly persons and patients with cardiac, renal, or hepatic failure. These patients may require the use of a higher dextrose concentration or an increase in lipid calories to decrease the volume of the infusate.

HYPERGLYCEMIA

Potential causes include too rapid advancement of the infusion rate, too high a dextrose concentration, and diabetes mellitus. The development of hyperglycemia later, after the patient's glucose levels had been stable, may be an early indication of occult infection or sepsis. The management of hyperglycemia includes adjustment of the infusion rate as described earlier. Regular insulin should be used to maintain blood glucose levels, whether it is administered subcutaneously or with the parenteral nutrition formulation. Occasionally, these initial maneuvers may be unsuccessful. In these situations, it may be necessary to reduce the dextrose concentration to 20% or less and to increase the proportion of calories provided as lipids.

HYPEROSMOLAR NONKETOTIC HYPERGLYCEMIC COMA

This relatively uncommon complication is more likely to occur in patients with adult-onset diabetes mellitus. It is characterized by severe hyperglycemia and dehydration but without ketoacidosis, and it is possibly precipitated by concomitant infection, poorly controlled hyperglycemia, or the hyperosmolar nature of parenteral nutrition. Despite the name, coma is present in only about 10% of cases. Central nervous system signs may range from drowsiness to frank obtundation. Clinical signs of dehydration are likely to be present. Laboratory studies demonstrate severe hyperglycemia (greater than 800 mg/dL), and serum osmolality is elevated as well (greater than 320 mOsm). Serum sodium levels may be either elevated or reduced. Immediate treatment should include aggressive hydration with 1 to 2 L of normal saline and discontinuation of the parenteral nutrition infusion. Insulin therapy is used for the hyperglycemia, with resumption of 5% dextrose infusion once the blood glucose level is less than 250 mg/dL.

HYPOKALEMIA, HYPOPHOSPHATEMIA, AND REFEEDING SYNDROME

Lowered potassium and phosphorus levels may result from hypervolemia and dilution or shifts from extracellular to intracellular compartments in response to hyperglycemia and insulin secretion. With patients who are severely malnourished, infusion of the high-dextrose solutions may result in significant sequestration of potassium and phosphorus in the intracellular compartment. These shifts may lead to arrhythmias, cardiac dysfunction, and neurologic symptoms. This so-called *refeeding syndrome* is most likely to occur within the first 2 weeks after nutritional support is initiated. Judicious and timely replacement of potassium, phosphorus, calcium, and magnesium is important.

CATHETER-RELATED SEPSIS

This complication actually may occur at any time during therapy, although it is most likely after the first 2 weeks. The diagnosis is confirmed by fever, leukocytosis, and positive blood cultures using specimens obtained through the catheter. Commonly, the organisms identified are *Staphylococcus epidermidis* or *S. aureus* or *Candida* species. A brief course of antibiotic therapy and catheter removal are usually very effective. The risk of developing catheter-related sepsis is highest with femoral vein catheters, followed by internal jugular and subclavian catheters. Multiple-lumen catheters have a greater risk of infection compared with dedicated single-lumen catheters. Cleansing of the catheter insertion site every 72 hours, preferably with chlorhexidine as opposed to iodophor, and the use of dry gauze and a semipermeable transparent dressing, to reduce moisture accumulation, are recommended. There is no evidence to support the use of prophylactic antibiotics.

Late Complications

TRACE ELEMENT DEFICIENCIES

Deficiencies of vitamins A, C, and B complex are uncommon because these vitamins are routinely added to formulations. Vitamin K and iron are not routinely added, and these should be supplemented if no dietary intake of these elements is available. Deficiencies of copper, selenium, molybdenum, and zinc may also occur, although these deficiencies are much less common. The osteopenia associated with the long-term use of parenteral nutrition is not related to a specific deficiency, but instead it probably results from the impairment of bone mineralization by aluminum, a contaminant of some of the formulation additives.

ASSOCIATED LIVER DISEASE

Prolonged use of parenteral nutrition is associated with certain hepatic abnormalities. Overfeeding of calories can result in fatty infiltration of the hepatic parenchyma, which may be manifested by mild to moderate elevation in serum hepatic transaminase levels. More problematic is the cholestasis and biliary sludge formation that may occur. Although the specific mechanism that causes this problem is yet to be elucidated, it is thought that the lack of stimulation to bile flow plays some role. Investigators have suggested that some enteral nutrition in association with parenteral nutrition may be beneficial to stimulate bile flow. The empirical use of ursodeoxycholic acid (Actigall)* to prevent bile stasis has also been advocated, although there is little scientific information to support this recommendation at this time.

*Not FDA approved for this indication.

PARENTERAL FLUID THERAPY FOR INFANTS AND CHILDREN

method of
KATHLEEN FRANCHEK-ROA, M.D.
Baylor College of Medicine
Houston, Texas

Dehydration and the need for parenteral fluid therapy are common in pediatric medicine. Infants and children are at risk for dehydration because (1) vomiting and diarrheal illnesses are common in young children; (2) infants and young children are dependent on others to meet their fluid requirements; (3) renal immaturity is present in infants; and (4) ill children sometimes refuse to drink enough fluid to maintain hydration, especially in the face of increased stressors such as fever.

The most common cause of dehydration in infants and children is infectious gastroenteritis. However, pediatric patients will commonly have gastrointestinal symptoms with illnesses unrelated to the gastrointestinal tract, such as pyelonephritis, otitis media, pneumonia, and metabolic diseases. Dehydration usually means loss of water, but this loss of water is generally accompanied by electrolyte disturbances. This article discusses the management of dehydration in children and infants older than 1 month, regardless of the etiology, and focuses on common electrolyte abnormalities in this patient population.

MAINTENANCE FLUID REQUIREMENTS

To understand rehydration therapy in dehydrated infants and children, it is necessary to understand the dynamics involved in fluid and electrolyte homeostasis in well children. Maintenance fluid requirements are determined by basal metabolism. Metabolism produces water, heat, and solute as byproducts. Heat is dissipated by water loss from the surface of the skin and via the respiratory tract during exhalation. This insensible water loss is electrolyte free and accounts for about 35% to 40% of the water loss. Solute wastes are excreted via urine, and this loss accounts for about 60% of fluid losses and all the electrolyte losses. These mechanisms help maintain homeostasis. Basal metabolic rates change for various ages and weights, and such change is not linear.

Maintenance fluid requirements are generally calculated by using the Holliday-Segar formula, which is based on energy expended (expressed as kilocalories). For all practical purposes, energy expended can be equated to fluid loss; for instance, 100 kcal expended is equal to 100 mL of fluid loss (Table 1). Some authorities argue that surface area is a more accurate way to calculate fluid requirements, especially in children weighing more than 10 to 20 kg. However, accurate determination of surface area requires a patient's weight and height and a table to calculate the value (see Table 2 for calculations used in the clinical setting for body surface area).

The maintenance requirement for sodium is 2 to 3 mEq/kg/d, and the potassium maintenance requirement is 1 to 2 mEq/kg/d.

EXAMPLE 1. CALCULATING FLUID AND ELECTROLYTE MAINTENANCE REQUIREMENTS. To calculate maintenance requirements for fluid and electrolytes in a 16-kg patient with the Holliday-Segar method, see Table 1:

$$\text{Maintenance fluids (mL)} = 1000 + 6(50) = 1300 \text{ mL/d}$$

$$\text{Sodium requirement} = 32\text{-}48 \text{ mEq/d}$$

$$\text{Potassium requirement} = 16\text{-}32 \text{ mEq/d}$$

TABLE 1. **Different Methods to Determine Maintenance Fluid Requirements Based on Weight or Surface Area**

Method 1*	
First 10 kg	100 mL/kg/d
10-20 kg	1000 mL + 50 mL/kg for each kg over 10
>20-80 kg	1500 mL + 20 mL/kg for each kg over 20
Method 2	
Because intravenous fluids are administered as mL/h, an easy way to calculate intravenous fluid rate for maintenance fluids is:	
First 10 kg	4 mL/kg/h
10-20 kg	40 mL/h + 2 mL/kg/h for each kg over 10
>20 kg	60 mL/h + 1 mL/kg/h for each kg over 20
Method 3	
<10 kg	100 mL/kg/d
>10 kg	1500 to 1600 mL/m²/d

*Holliday-Segar method from Holliday MG, Segar WE: The maintenance need for water in parenteral fluid therapy. Pediatrics 19:823-832, 1957.

TABLE 2. **Different Methods Used to Estimate Body Surface Area**

1. A quick way to calculate surface area using weight alone is: SA (m^2) = [wt (kg) × 4] + 7/[90 + wt (kg)]
2. To compute body surface area (m^2) using weight alone:

<5 kg	kg × 0.05 + 0.05
5-10 kg	kg × 0.04 + 0.1
10-20 kg	kg × 0.03 + 0.2
20-40 kg	kg × 0.02 + 0.4
>40 kg	kg × 0.01 + 0.8

3. Method to calculate surface area using height and weight:

$$m^2 = \sqrt{\frac{\text{Height(cm)} \times \text{Weight(kg)}}{3600}}$$

Reprinted, by permission, from Mosteller RD: Simplified calculation of body-surface area. N Engl J Med 317:1098, 1987

CLINICAL ASSESSMENT OF DEHYDRATION

When assessing an infant or child for dehydration, the estimation of the degree or severity of dehydration and the type of dehydration need to be determined. Dehydration is categorized according to severity (mild, moderate, or severe) and tonicity (isotonic, hypertonic, or hypotonic). Severity is determined by comparison with a recent premorbid weight (which is rarely available in clinical practice) or by the history and physical examination when a recent premorbid weight is not available. Tonicity is determined primarily by the serum sodium value.

Severity of Dehydration

Questions that should be addressed to caregivers to determine the severity of dehydration include a history of fever, vomiting and/or diarrhea, fluid intake, activity level, urine output, and underlying medical illnesses. The physical examination focuses on vital signs, mental status/activity level, anterior fontanelle, presence of tears with crying, sunken eyes, mucous membranes, capillary refill, and skin turgor (Table 3).

For infants, mild dehydration is estimated to be 5% of body weight and, in older children, 3% of body weight. Moderate dehydration is estimated to be about 10% of body weight in infants and 6% of body weight in older children. Severe dehydration as estimated by clinical examination suggests a fluid deficit of 15% of body weight in infants and 9% of body weight in older children (see Table 3).

Type of Dehydration

To assess the type of dehydration as isotonic, hypotonic, or hypertonic, the serum sodium value can be used because sodium is a major contributor to extracellular osmolality. In clinical practice, osmolarity and osmolality are used interchangeably because the density of water is 1 kg/L. Normal measured osmolality is 285 to 295 mOsm/kg serum water. Serum osmolality may be calculated as follows:

$$\text{Osmolality} = 2 \times \text{Plasma sodium (mEq/L)} + \text{Serum glucose}/18 + \text{BUN}/2.8$$

Extracellular sodium reflects the regulation of total body water in most clinical situations. Extracellular sodium regulation is controlled through the transcellular movement of water and renal handling of sodium.

In the clinical setting, determination of the tonicity of extracellular fluid is important because it dictates the *composition* of the rehydration fluid as well as the *rate* of rehydration. Hypernatremia is always associated with hyperosmolality. However, in patients with low serum sodium, it will be necessary to determine

TABLE 3. **Estimation of Dehydration**

Parameter	Mild Infant 5% Child 3%	Moderate Infant 10% Child 6%	Severe Infant 15% Child 9%
Heart rate*	NL	INC	INC
Respiratory rate*	NL	NL	INC
Blood pressure	NL	Orthostatic drop	Hypotensive
Skin turgor	NL	NL to slightly DEC	DEC
Eyes	NL	NL to sunken	Very sunken
Tears	NL	DEC	Absent
Mucous membranes	NL	Tacky	Dry
Capillary refill†	<2 s	2-3 s	>3 s
Fontanelle	NL	Slightly depressed	Sunken
Activity level	NL	NL to DEC	DEC
Urine output	NL to slightly DEC	DEC to none	None
Urine specific gravity‡	>1.020	>1.030	Maximal

*Heart rate and respiratory rate may be elevated if the child is febrile or agitated.
†Ambient temperature influences capillary refill.
‡The renal concentrating ability for infants (especially those younger than 3 months) is not yet mature; therefore, urine specific gravity in young infants may underestimate the degree of dehydration.
DEC, decreased; INC, increased; NL, normal.
Modified from Roberts KB: Fluid and electrolytes: Parenteral fluid therapy. Pediatr Rev 22:380-387, 2001.

whether the low value is associated with hypoosmolality. Therefore, determining both the sodium level and osmolality will help guide the physician in the institution of appropriate therapy.

Isonatremic Dehydration

In a dehydrated patient whose serum sodium level is normal (130 to 150 mEq/L), fluid loss is accompanied by concomitant electrolyte loss. These patients can be rehydrated fairly quickly (i.e., over a 24-hour period).

Hyponatremic Dehydration

True hyponatremic dehydration (serum sodium <130 mEq/L) is generally due to loss of more electrolytes than water or to parenteral administration of rehydration fluid that is low in sodium content. This type of dehydration is commonly seen in young children whose parents use only water, soda, or "rice water" to rehydrate their ill child.

If a patient with hyponatremic dehydration has no neurologic manifestations of low sodium, then after the patient has become hemodynamically stable and laboratory values have been obtained, the next step is to determine volume status (i.e., hypovolemia versus hypervolemia versus euvolemia) and osmolality. Determining the specific cause of hyponatremia is essential because it has important management implications. In our discussion, we are assuming that the patient is dehydrated, but it is important to briefly discuss other causes of hyponatremia that may not be accompanied by hypovolemia. An in-depth discussion of electrolyte abnormalities is beyond the scope of this article, but common situations will be discussed.

In the case of true hyponatremia in conjunction with *hypo*volemia, fluids need to be administered. In the case of hyponatremia in conjunction with *hyper*volemia, as seen in nephrotic syndrome, or in conjunction with *eu*volemia, as seen in the syndrome of inappropriate antidiuretic hormone secretion (SIADH), fluid restriction is the course of action. As illustrated, these types of patients need very different therapeutic approaches.

Serum sodium values less than 130 mEq/L can also be the result of "pseudohyponatremia," in which case the sodium level is normal but the measurement indicates a "low" sodium level. Causes of "pseudohyponatremia" include hyperglycemia, hyperlipidemia, and hyperproteinemia.

In cases of hyperlipidemia, the concentration of sodium is normal, but the sodium concentration (expressed as milliequivalents per liter) in whole plasma is decreased because water and salt are displaced as a result of the presence of lipids in plasma.

In patients with hyperglycemia, serum osmolality will be elevated but the measured serum sodium will be falsely low. Correction of serum glucose will correct the sodium level. The sodium level in patients with hyperglycemia can be estimated by adding 1.6 mEq of sodium for every 100-mg/dL increase in serum glucose, with normal serum glucose assumed to be 100 mg/dL.

As noted earlier, serum osmolality may be increased in the face of hyponatremia in patients with elevated blood glucose or blood urea nitrogen (BUN) levels. In this clinical situation, rapid fluid replacement could lead to severe neurologic events secondary to cerebral edema. This complication will be discussed in more detail in the next section on hypernatremic dehydration. To summarize, when assessing hyponatremia, serum osmolality will be important to determine.

Hypernatremic Dehydration

Hypernatremic dehydration, defined as a serum sodium level over 150 mEq/L, results from water loss in excess of electrolyte loss or from the exogenous intake of salt, which can occur when parents use soups with a high salt content to rehydrate their infant or child or when they improperly mix formula. Hypotonic fluid loss can occur in children with gastroenteritis, in those receiving diuretic therapy, in those with increased insensible loss, or because of the inability of the kidney to retain water. These situations occur if adequate free water is not provided. A strong thirst mechanism protects against the development of hypernatremia; however, in young and debilitated patients, the ability to self-administer fluids is compromised.

Hypernatremia is always associated with hyperosmolality. The degree of dehydration can be underestimated because of the shift of fluid from the intracellular space to the extracellular space to equalize the osmolality. This situation leads to cellular dehydration. The brain has a protective mechanism to prevent cerebral cellular dehydration by increasing the intracellular content of sodium, potassium, and amino acids and producing organic substances termed idiogenic osmoles. Maintaining the osmolality of the intracellular environment in the brain prevents movement of water out of the cells into the extracellular space. This change in intracellular osmoles is thought to be a fairly rapid process. The problem arises when the patient is provided parenteral fluids. The ability of the brain to extrude idiogenic osmoles is a slower process, and rapid fluid administration can lead to cerebral edema, seizures, or death.

LABORATORY EVALUATION

In most cases of mild dehydration, laboratory evaluation is not necessary, and the child can generally be rehydrated with oral solutions. In some cases of moderate dehydration and all cases of severe dehydration, assessment of the patient must include laboratory analysis. A brief discussion of the etiology of electrolyte abnormalities is included for further evaluation of dehydration in certain clinical situations.

Sodium. As mentioned previously, abnormal serum sodium levels dictate different approaches to therapy.

Potassium. Elevated potassium levels may indicate congenital adrenal hyperplasia, which may lead to dehydration secondary to vomiting. Elevated potassium levels may also be a sign of renal failure, in which case the elevated levels can be due to poor renal perfusion as a result of hypovolemia. Low serum levels of potassium may indicate potassium loss from vomiting and/or diarrhea or pyloric stenosis leading to dehydration secondary to vomiting.

Chloride. Low chloride levels, especially in the setting of hypokalemia and metabolic alkalosis, may indicate pyloric stenosis, which can lead to vomiting and dehydration.

Bicarbonate. Bicarbonate levels can be low as a result of diarrheal stools or lactic acidosis from poor perfusion and anaerobic metabolism. If a child is primarily vomiting, the bicarbonate level may be normal or high initially because of loss of acid in vomitus and contraction alkalosis, but it becomes low if the vomiting is prolonged, leading to hypovolemia and poor perfusion.

Glucose. Hypoglycemia may occur if the patient has had poor oral intake. Hyperglycemia may be present in diabetic ketoacidosis.

Blood Urea Nitrogen. BUN levels may be elevated secondary to prerenal azotemia. However, BUN may be low or show less of an elevation than expected if the patient's protein intake has decreased markedly, as seen during gastroenteritis or as a result of the decreased oral intake that occurs when a child is ill.

Creatinine. The creatinine level may be elevated secondary to prerenal azotemia or established acute renal failure.

Urine Specific Gravity. In patients with dehydration, urine specific gravity will be elevated because of the kidney's ability to conserve water and produce concentrated urine if the concentrating ability of the kidney is mature. Urine specific gravity will be dilute (i.e., <1.010) in the face of dehydration in patients with diabetes insipidus.

Urinalysis. Positive leukocyte esterase and nitrites may indicate a urinary tract infection. The presence of glucosuria may indicate diabetic ketoacidosis.

Electrolyte Analysis of Ongoing Fluid Loss. Analysis of continuous fluid losses can aid in further modification of the composition of parenteral fluids.

REHYDRATION THERAPY

When providing rehydration therapy to a dehydrated child or infant, the following components must be considered: (1) the hemodynamic state, (2) the degree of dehydration, (3) the composition of the replacement fluid, (4) the rate of rehydration, (5) the maintenance fluid requirement, and (6) ongoing fluid losses.

Initial Assessment—Evaluating for Signs of Shock

When evaluating a child for dehydration, the initial step involves rapid determination of the patient's hemodynamic status. If the patient is in hypovolemic shock, rapid administration of fluid needs to be initiated immediately. Blood is sent to the laboratory for the necessary evaluation as intravenous access is being obtained. The initial fluid to administer to restore intravascular volume quickly, *regardless of etiology or laboratory values*, is always normal saline (0.9% NS) or lactated Ringer's solution (LR). NS and LR are used as bolus fluids because they are isotonic when compared with plasma; therefore, intravascular volume can be restored quickly without fluid shifts (see Table 4). NS is used more frequently than LR to quickly restore intravascular volume in pediatric patients. Regardless of which isotonic fluid is used, the common dose for a bolus of fluid is 20 mL/kg administered by intravenous push if the patient is in shock or by infusion over a period of 30 to 60 minutes if the patient is stable.

After the initial bolus of fluids, the patient needs to be reassessed (i.e., heart rate, capillary perfusion, urine output, mental status) to ascertain the response to the initial attempt to restore intravascular volume. If no response or a minimal response to the initial bolus is seen, a second bolus of NS or LR is administered intravenously, the rate depending on the clinical status of the patient. The key to rehydrating a patient is continual reassessment. If a patient requires three or more fluid boluses (i.e., ≥60 mL/kg), other etiologies of shock should be considered, such as poor cardiac function, ongoing hemorrhage, or sepsis.

Degree of Dehydration

The most accurate way to calculate fluid loss is to have a recent premorbid weight and subtract the current weight. The weight difference in grams is equal to the fluid loss because 1 mL of water weighs 1 g; if this weight loss is acute, the loss of weight

TABLE 4. **Composition of Frequently Used Parenteral Solutions**

Electrolyte	Normal Saline	D5 0.5 NS	D5 0.2 NS	LR
Sodium (mEq/L)	155	75	35	130
Chloride (mEq/L)	155	75	35	109
Potassium (mEq/L)	—	—	—	4
Lactate (mEq/L)	—	—	—	28
Glucose (g/L)	—	50	50	—

D5 0.5 NS, 5% dextrose in 1/2 normal saline; D5 0.2 NS, 5% dextrose in ¼ normal saline; LR, lactated Ringer's solution; NS, normal saline.

Modified from Seigel NJ, Carpenter T, Gaudio KM: The pathophysiology of body fluids. In Oski FA (ed): Principles and Practices of Pediatrics, 2nd ed. Philadelphia, JB Lippincott, 1994, pp 60-79.

is attributed to fluid loss. Rarely in clinical practice is a recent premorbid weight available, however. Therefore, clinical assessment is most commonly used to gauge the severity of dehydration (see Table 3).

EXAMPLE 2: CALCULATING FLUID DEFICIT IN A DEHYDRATED PATIENT. In a 16-kg patient determined to be moderately dehydrated (6%), the fluid deficit is calculated as follows:

$$\text{Fluid deficit (L)} = \text{Weight (kg)} \times \text{\% Dehydrated (expressed in decimals)}$$

$$\text{Fluid deficit (L)} = (16)(0.06)$$

$$\text{Fluid deficit} = 0.960 \text{ L, or } 960 \text{ mL}$$

When calculating total replacement fluids, the fluid deficit, maintenance requirement for the patient, and the volume of bolus fluids given are included.

$$\text{Total replacement fluids} = \text{Fluid deficit} + \text{Maintenance fluids} - \text{Boluses given}$$

EXAMPLE 3: CALCULATING TOTAL REPLACEMENT FLUIDS IN A DEHYDRATED PATIENT. Our example of a child whose weight is 16 kg and who is estimated to be 6% dehydrated is used again:

$$\text{Fluid deficit} = 960 \text{ mL}$$

$$\text{Maintenance fluids}^* = 1000 + 50(6) = 1300$$

For boluses given, let us assume that one 20-mL/kg bolus was administered:

$$(16 \text{ kg})(20) = 320 \text{ mL}$$

$$\text{Total replacement fluids} = 960 \text{ mL} + 1300 \text{ mL} - 320 \text{ mL}$$

$$\text{Total replacement fluids} = 1940 \text{ mL}$$

It is important to realize that this number (i.e., total replacement fluids) represents one point in time. As a patient is rehydrated, the amount of fluid that is needed may change as the clinical course of the patient changes (e.g., ongoing fluid losses, able to take enteral fluids).

Composition of Replacement Fluids

In most clinical situations, the rehydration solution of choice is 5% dextrose in "half" normal saline (D5 0.5 NS) or in "quarter" normal saline (D5 0.2 NS) (See Table 4). Both of these solutions have been found to be relatively safe in most pediatric patients with dehydration. After the patient has been resuscitated and urine output has been established, the addition of 20 mEq KCl/L is appropriate. Exceptions to the recommended parenteral fluid composition are worth noting, such as in cases of severe hyponatremic or hypernatremic dehydration, for which the sodium concentration in the fluid may need to be altered; in diabetic ketoacidosis, for which dextrose may not be added initially; or in severe burn patients, in whom isotonic fluids may need to be continually administered. A detailed description of the treatment of these patients is beyond the scope of this article, but in the following paragraphs, some common specific clinical situations are discussed in which the parenteral fluid composition may need to be modified.

Hypokalemia. In cases of hypokalemia, the concentration of potassium in the replacement fluids can be increased, but this increase can limit the intravenous fluid rate. The type of access established—peripheral versus central venous access—also determines the concentration of potassium in the fluid. Potassium serum levels cannot be elevated quickly because potassium is primarily an intracellular ion. It is recommended that the rate of potassium infusion not exceed 0.2 to 0.3 mEq/kg/h without appropriate monitoring. It is important to note that correcting the acidosis can worsen the hypokalemia and hypocalcemia, so in these situations, correction of the potassium and calcium electrolytes should be done first before correcting the acidosis.

Severe Acidosis. Many pediatric patients who are dehydrated have some degree of acidosis as a result of metabolic acidosis or bicarbonate loss. Most cases of acidosis will resolve when the patient is rehydrated. However, in severe cases of acidosis, such as when the serum bicarbonate level is less than 10 mEq/L or arterial pH is below 7.2, rapid correction of the acidosis may need to be implemented. It is recommended that a bolus of bicarbonate be given to increase the serum bicarbonate level to about 15 mEq/L or the pH to no greater than 7.25. The starting dose is one third to one half the calculated extracellular bicarbonate deficit. The formula to calculate the bicarbonate deficit is as follows:

$$HCO_3 \text{ deficit (mEq)} = 0.5 \times \text{Weight (kg)} \times (\text{Desired } HCO_3 - \text{Measured } HCO_3)$$

EXAMPLE 4: CALCULATING BICARBONATE DEFICIT IN A PATIENT WITH METABOLIC ACIDOSIS SECONDARY TO DEHYDRATION. In our patient who weighs 16 kg and is 6% dehydrated with a serum bicarbonate value of 8 mEq/L, the bicarbonate deficit is calculated as follows:

$$HCO_3 \text{ (mEq)} = 0.5 \times 16 \times (15 - 8)$$

$$HCO_3 = 56 \text{ mEq}$$

*Using the Holliday-Segar formula—see Table 1.

It is important to keep in mind the following complications that can result from sodium bicarbonate ($NaHCO_3$) administration: hypernatremia, hyperosmolarity, rapid expansion of the extracellular fluid compartment, and increased lactate production. The production of CO_2 from the administration of sodium bicarbonate can actually *worsen* the acidosis if the patient has persistently poor tissue perfusion and/or hypoventilation. As mentioned previously, it should be kept in mind that correction of acidosis can worsen hypokalemia.

As stated earlier, most cases of mild to moderate acidosis correct themselves when the patient becomes rehydrated.

Hyponatremia. As discussed previously, most cases of hyponatremic dehydration can be treated with the aforementioned standard parenteral hydration fluids (D5 0.5 NS or D5 0.2 NS). However, in some cases of hyponatremia, it may be necessary to calculate the sodium deficit and modify the rehydration fluids accordingly. In patients with hyponatremia, serum sodium should be calculated so that the sodium level can be restored to 130 mEq/L while avoiding too rapid a change in serum sodium. To restore serum sodium to 130 mEq/L, the sodium deficit can be calculated as follows:

$$\text{Sodium deficit} = (\text{Sodium desired} - \text{Sodium actual}) \times 0.6 \times \text{Weight (kg)}$$

where 0.6 is the volume of distribution for sodium.

EXAMPLE 5: CALCULATION OF SODIUM DEFICIT IN A PATIENT WITH HYPONATREMIC, HYPO-OSMOLAR DEHYDRATION. In our patient who is 16 kg and estimated to be 6% dehydrated with a measured sodium level of 116 mEq/L, the sodium deficit is calculated as follows:

$$\text{Sodium deficit} = (130 - 116) \times 0.6 \times 16$$

$$\text{Sodium deficit} = 134 \text{ mEq}$$

$$\text{Sodium daily requirement} = 26\text{-}39 \text{ mEq/d (based on calorie expenditure)}$$

$$\text{Total sodium needed} = 160\text{-}173 \text{ mEq}$$

This patient received 50 mEq of sodium in the 320 mL bolus of normal saline. If the remaining fluids (1940 mL) were given as D5 0.2 NS, the patient would receive ~118 mEq of sodium in 24 hours. If the remaining fluids were given as D5 0.5 NS, the patient would receive ~195 mEq of sodium, which is closer to what the patient needs. Remember, potassium at 20 mEq/L needs to be added to the IV fluids once urine output is established.

Hypernatremia. In a patient who has hypernatremic dehydration, the composition of replacement fluids will need to take into consideration the free water deficit. The formula for calculating the free water deficit is as follows:

$$\text{Free water deficit (mL)} = 4 \text{ mL} \times \text{Weight (kg)} \times \text{Desired change in serum sodium}$$

or

$$\text{Free water deficit (L)} = 0.6 \times \text{Weight (kg)} \times \frac{P_{Na}}{Desired\,Na} - 1$$

EXAMPLE 6: CALCULATION OF FREE WATER DEFICIT IN A PATIENT WITH HYPERNATREMIC DEHYDRATION. In our patient who weighs 16 kg and is estimated to be 6% dehydrated with a serum sodium level of 160 mEq/L, the free water deficit is calculated as follows:

$$\text{Free water deficit} = 4 \text{ mL} \times 16 \times (160 - 150)$$

$$\text{Free water deficit} = 640 \text{ mL}$$

or

$$\text{Free water deficit} = 0.6 \times 16 \times [(160/150) - 1]$$

$$\text{Free water deficit} = 0.6 \times 16 \times 0.0666$$

$$\text{Free water deficit} = 0.640 \text{ L}$$

This patient still needs a maintenance sodium requirement that is 26 to 39 mEq/d. For this patient the maintenance fluid requirement is 1300 mL/d with an extra 640 mL of free water deficit. The free water deficit in this case is given over a 48-hour period (see the next section). This replacement could best be accomplished by administering D5 0.5 NS or D5 0.2 NS.

Rate of Fluid Rehydration

The next step in parenteral therapy is to determine how quickly the total replacement fluids can be administered. The rate of administration of parenteral fluids is determined by the serum sodium level or osmolality. Isotonic (or isonatremic) dehydration is defined as a serum sodium level between 130 and 150 mEq/L. If the serum sodium level is less than 130 mEq/L, the dehydration is considered to be hypotonic (or hyponatremic). Hypertonic (or hypernatremic) dehydration is defined as a serum sodium level greater than 150 mEq/L. Each will be discussed separately because the therapeutic approaches may need to be different.

Isonatremic Dehydration

Patients who are dehydrated and have normal serum sodium can be rehydrated fairly quickly—over a 24-hour period. Normally, half of the deficit and a third of the maintenance fluids can be given in the first 8 hours and then the remaining half of the deficit and two thirds of the maintenance given over the ensuing 16 hours.

EXAMPLE 7: RATE OF REHYDRATION IN A PATIENT WITH ISONATREMIC DEHYDRATION. In our patient who weighs 16 kg, is 6% dehydrated, and whose total volume of replacement fluids is 1940 mL, the rate of fluid administration is as follows:

Remaining deficit = 960 mL − 320 mL (bolus)
= 640 mL

Maintenance fluid = 1300 mL/d

The patient needs to receive half the deficit (640 mL/2 = 320 mL) and a third of the maintenance (1300/3 = ≈435 mL) over the first 8 hours (≈95 mL/h) and then the remainder of the deficit (320 mL) and two thirds of the maintenance (870 mL) over the next 16 hours (≈75 mL/h).

Hyponatremic Dehydration

In general, patients with hyponatremic dehydration can be treated as though they have isonatremic dehydration; that is, they can be rehydrated over a 24-hour period. If a patient has neurologic manifestations of hyponatremia, such as seizures, respiratory arrest, or decorticate posturing, rapid infusion of hypertonic (3%) saline is necessary. The rate of infusion should increase the serum sodium level by no more than 1 mEq/L/h and should not exceed 15 mEq/L/d.

It is also worth discussing a condition, albeit rare, that can result from rapid correction of hyponatremia: central pontine myelinolysis (CPM). CPM occurs in hyponatremic patients whose serum sodium is corrected rapidly. This condition is described as a demyelinating process that is generally observed in the pons but may involve other white matter areas of the brain. CPM is usually seen in patients with underlying disease, primarily liver disease, but a recent case report described a healthy child who had dehydration secondary to rotavirus gastroenteritis who developed CPM from rapid correction of hyponatremia.

In summary, with the aforementioned caveats in mind, rehydration of a patient with hyponatremic dehydration and no abnormal neurologic findings can be accomplished over a 24-hour period (the same as for a patient with isonatremic dehydration), and repeated clinical assessment and laboratory studies are used to guide the course of therapy. In most cases, rehydration will correct the sodium abnormality.

Hypernatremic Dehydration

No studies have determined the optimal rate of fluid rehydration in patients with hypernatremic dehydration. It is suggested that the optimal rate of change in sodium be no more than 10 mEq/d (i.e., 0.4 to 0.5 mEq/h). Clinical experience suggests that if the serum sodium level is between 150 and 165 mEq/L, replacement should be performed over a period of 48 hours. Unlike the situation with isonatremic and hyponatremic dehydration, the total replacement fluids are given at the same rate over a period of 48 hours (with the total replacement fluid calculation accounting for 2 days of maintenance fluids). If the serum sodium level is greater than 165 mEq/L, rehydration over a 72-hour period may be more appropriate.

EXAMPLE 8. CALCULATION OF PARENTERAL FLUID RATE IN A PATIENT WITH HYPERNATREMIC DEHYDRATION. In our patient who is 16 kg and estimated to be 6% dehydrated with a serum sodium level of 160 mEq/L, the rate of fluid rehydration is calculated as follows:

Maintenance fluids over *48 hours*
= [1000 + 50(6)] × 2 (for 48 hours)
= 2600 mL

Free water deficit (as calculated previously, see Example 6) = 640 mL

Total replacement fluids
= Maintenance fluids for 2 days
+ Free water deficit

Total replacement fluids = 2600 mL + 640 mL
= 3240 mL

Intravenous fluid rate = 3240/48 h ≅ 67 mL/h
(see Example 6 for the composition of fluids)

It is important to reiterate that boluses of NS (or LR) may be needed initially to stabilize the patient regardless of the sodium level. Frequent reassessment of the patient's clinical status and serum sodium levels cannot be overemphasized, especially in this clinical scenario.

Ongoing Fluid Losses

As mentioned previously, the initial assessment of a dehydrated patient is at one specific point in time. Once the patient has been resuscitated and stabilized and the deficit and maintenance fluids have been calculated and instituted, frequent reassessment of the patient's clinical status and serum electrolytes is necessary. Serum electrolytes should be reassessed every 6 to 12 hours, depending on the degree of abnormality, and after each electrolyte bolus. Ongoing losses as a result of vomiting, diarrhea, polyuria, or nasogastric aspirates need to be considered.

Gastric losses caused by vomiting or nasogastric aspirates should be replaced volume for volume with a solution that contains 140 to 155 mEq/L sodium, 15 mEq/L potassium, and 155 mEq/L chloride. Diarrheal losses can be measured in infants and young children by weighing the diaper and equating grams of diarrheal fluid with milliliters of fluid lost. These losses can also be corrected volume for volume with a solution composed of 40 mEq/L of sodium, potassium, bicarbonate, and chloride. Remember that the amount of potassium in the intravenous fluids limits the rate of administration.

ORAL REHYDRATION

No discussion of dehydration and fluid therapy in pediatric patients would be complete without discussing oral rehydration. The American Academy of Pediatrics has developed a practice guideline on the principles of oral fluid therapy. Oral rehydration therapy is the recommended mode of rehydration in children deemed to be mildly to moderately dehydrated. Even in a vomiting child, small amounts (i.e., 5 mL) of an appropriate oral rehydration solution (e.g., Pedialyte) given frequently (i.e., every 1 to 2 minutes) can successfully rehydrate a child. Though labor intensive, this technique can deliver 150 to 300 mL/h. Physiologically appropriate electrolyte solutions are the rehydration fluids of choice. Some of the commercially available sports drinks are not appropriate because they do not contain the correct electrolyte composition and are hyperosmolar as a result of their carbohydrate content. Use of these nonphysiologic fluids should be discouraged (see Table 5). Oral rehydration fluids that are hyperosmolar can worsen diarrhea and dehydration by drawing fluid into the gut and causing increased fluid losses. Parents need to be counseled on which oral fluids are appropriate.

If a child is judged to be mildly dehydrated, the child can be discharged from the clinic or emergency room with instructions on oral rehydration and signs of dehydration. Patients deemed to be moderately dehydrated may warrant observation in the clinic setting or emergency department to ensure that oral rehydration is tolerated and the deficit has been replaced before being discharged home. If the child is unable to tolerate the "PO challenge," parenteral fluid can be administered and oral rehydration attempted after the patient is stabilized. Oral rehydration has no role in a child considered to be severely dehydrated.

SUMMARY

To conclude, the important aspects of dehydration and parenteral therapy in pediatric patients are summarized in the following list. See Figures 1 and 2 for algorithms to be used for assessing and managing dehydration in pediatric patients and Table 6 for a summary of the formulas used in this article.

1. Infants and children are at risk for dehydration for numerous reasons, among them the facts that vomiting and diarrheal illnesses are common in the first years of life, infants and children become dehydrated from illnesses other than those related to the gastrointestinal tract, and infants and young children are unable to meet their own fluid requirements.
2. The degree of dehydration in a patient who is hypernatremic may be underestimated because of the intracellular loss of fluid that occurs to maintain extracellular osmolality.
3. When assessing a patient in shock, rapid administration of intravascular isotonic fluids must be instituted, regardless of the serum sodium level.
4. The etiology of the dehydration must be determined after the patient is resuscitated to guide further therapeutic interventions.
5. Hyponatremic and isonatremic dehydration can usually be managed similarly while keeping in mind the rare occurrence of CPM if severe hyponatremia is corrected too rapidly.
6. Hyponatremic dehydration is usually accompanied by hypo-osmolality. However, hyperglycemia presents with hyponatremia and hyperosmolality, and it needs to be considered when calculating the rate of rehydration to prevent cerebral edema.
7. Hypernatremic dehydration needs to be corrected slowly to prevent cerebral edema.
8. The recommended route of fluid rehydration in mild to moderately dehydrated pediatric patients is oral. Parenteral fluid administration is recommended

TABLE 5. **Commercially Available Fluids Used for Oral Rehydration**

Fluid	Carbohydrate (mmol/L)	Sodium (mmol/L)	Potassium (mmol/L)	Base HCO_2 (Citrate or Bicarbonate) (mmol/L)	Osmolality
Infalyte	70	50	25	30	200
Pedialyte	140	45	20	30	250
Rehydralyte	140	75	20	30	310
WHO*	111	90	20	30	310
Cola†	700	2	0	13	750
Apple juice†	690	5	32	0	730
Chicken broth†	0	250	8	0	500
Sports drinks†	255	20	3	3	330

*World Health Organization oral rehydration solution.
†Liquids *not recommended* for oral rehydration therapy.
Modified from American Academy of Pediatrics: The management of acute gastroenteritis in young children. Pediatrics 97:424-435, 1996.

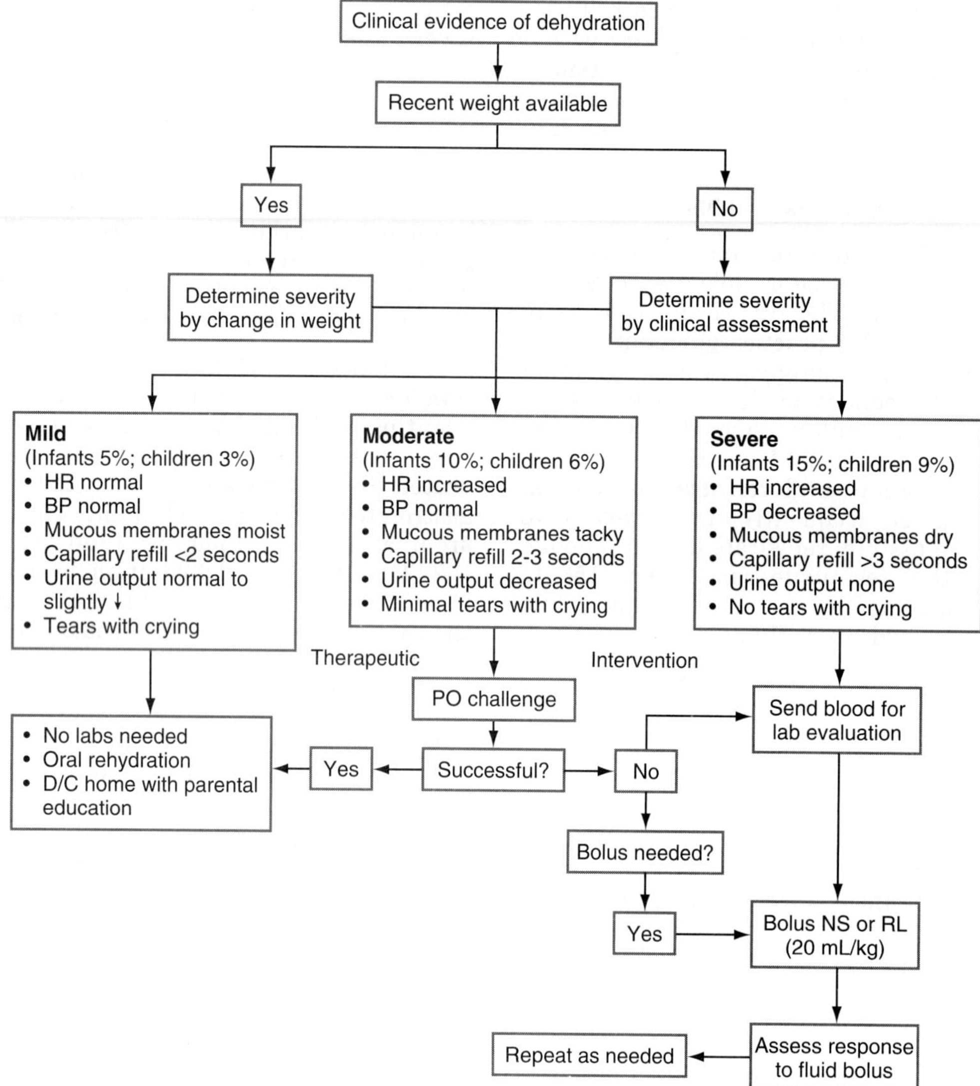

Figure 1. Algorithm for initial assessment of dehydration in pediatric patients. BP, blood pressure; D/C, discharge; HR, heart rate; NS, normal saline; PO, oral; RL, lactated Ringer's solution.

TABLE 6. **Summary of Formulas Used in Treating Patients with Dehydration**

1. Osmolality = 2 × Plasma sodium (mEq/L) + Serum glucose/18 + BUN/2.8
2. Estimating the correct serum sodium level in hyperglycemia:
   Corrected serum sodium value = Serum sodium level + 1.6 mEq (each 100-mg/dL increase in serum glucose)*
3. Bolus fluids = 20 mL × Weight (kg)
4. Fluid deficit (L) = Weight (kg) × % Dehydrated
5. Total replacement fluids = Fluid deficit + Maintenance fluids − Boluses given
6. HCO_3 deficit (mEq) = 0.5 × Weight (kg) × (Desired HCO_3 − Measured HCO_3)
7. To restore serum sodium to 130 mEq/L, the sodium deficit can be calculated as follows:
   Sodium deficit (mEq) = (Sodium desired − Sodium actual) × 0.6† × Weight (kg)
8. Free water deficit (mL) = 4 mL × Weight (kg) × (Desired change in serum sodium), *or*
   $$\text{Free water deficit (L)} = 0.6 \times \text{Weight (kg)} \times \frac{P_{Na}}{\text{Desired Na}} - 1$$

*Normal serum glucose is assumed to be 100 mg/dL.
†The volume of distribution for sodium is 0.6.
BUN, blood urea nitrogen.

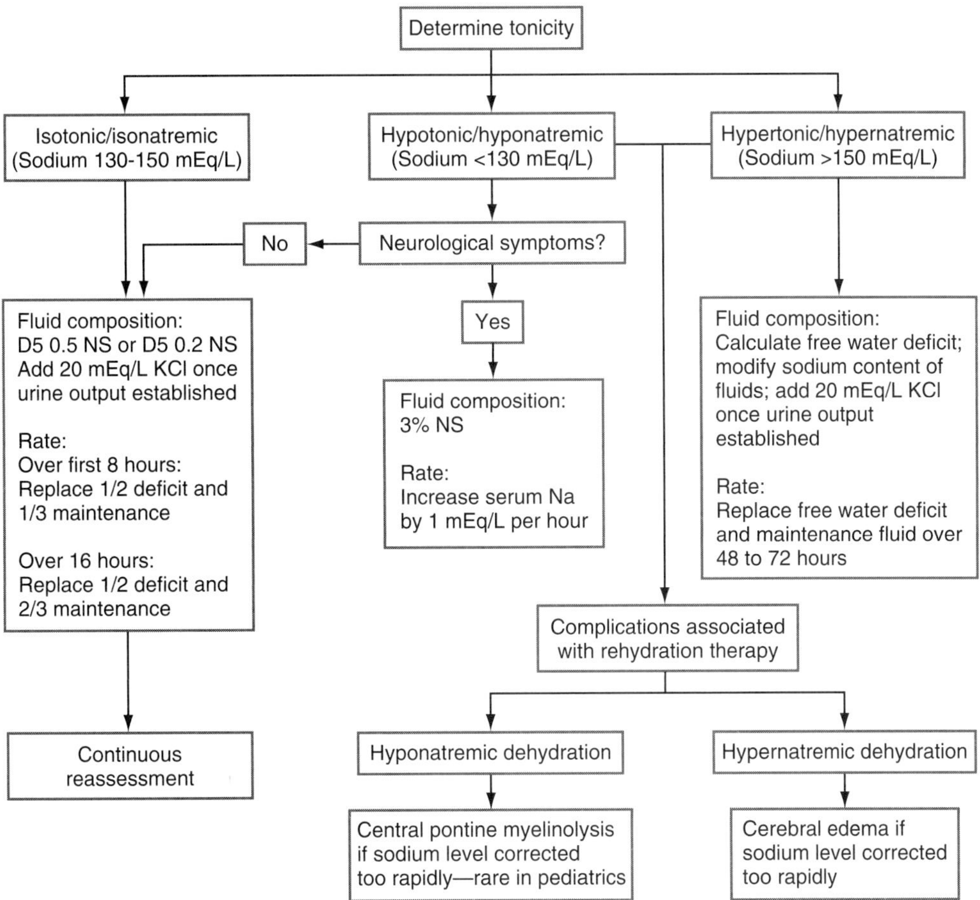

Figure 2. Algorithm for rehydration in pediatric patients. D5, 5% dextrose; 0.5 NS, one-half normal saline; 0.2 NS, one-quarter normal saline.

in severely dehydrated children and those who fail a "PO challenge."

9. Last but not least, continual reassessment of the patient and laboratory values must be ongoing to ensure that the therapeutic approach is appropriate.

ACKNOWLEDGMENT

I would like to thank Rita Sheth, M.D., for her editorial comments.

Section 9

The Endocrine System

ACROMEGALY

method of
WILLIAM F. YOUNG, Jr., M.D., M.Sc.
Mayo Medical School
Rochester, Minnesota

Chronic growth hormone (GH) excess from a GH-producing pituitary tumor results in the clinical syndrome *acromegaly*. If untreated, this syndrome is associated with increased morbidity and mortality. Although the annual incidence is estimated to be only three people per 1 million population, GH-secreting pituitary adenomas are the second most common hormone-secreting pituitary tumor. Ectopic neoplasms that produce GH or GH-releasing hormone (GHRH) are rare (<1%) causes of acromegaly. The effects of the chronic GH excess include acral and soft tissue overgrowth, progressive dental malocclusion, degenerative arthritis related to chondral and synovial tissue overgrowth within joints, low-pitched sonorous voice, excessive sweating and oily skin, perineural hypertrophy leading to nerve entrapment (e.g., carpal tunnel syndrome), eustachian tube obstruction leading to recurrent serous otitis media, proximal muscle weakness, carbohydrate intolerance, hypertension, colonic neoplasia, and cardiac dysfunction. The mass effects of GH-producing pituitary macroadenomas (>10 mm) are similar to those of other pituitary macroadenomas. They include visual field defects, oculomotor pareses, headaches, and pituitary insufficiency.

DIAGNOSTIC EVALUATION

The patient with acromegaly has a characteristic appearance with coarsening of facial features, prognathism, frontal bossing, spade-like hands, and wide feet. Often there is a history of progressive increase in shoe, glove, ring, or hat size. These changes may occur slowly and may go unrecognized by the patient, family, and physician. Comparison with earlier photographs of the patient is helpful in confirming the clinical suspicion of acromegaly.

High plasma GH levels are not diagnostic of acromegaly. Basal plasma GH levels are increased in patients with poorly controlled diabetes mellitus, chronic hepatic or renal failure, or conditions characterized by protein-calorie malnutrition such as anorexia nervosa. The diagnosis of acromegaly depends on two criteria: a GH level that is not suppressed to less than 1 micrograms per liter after an oral glucose load (75 to 100 grams) and an increased (based on normal range adjusted for age and sex) serum concentration of insulin-like growth factor 1 (IGF-1, a GH-dependent growth factor responsible for many of the effects of GH and previously known as somatomedin C). Serum IGF-1 levels are rarely falsely positive. IGF-1 levels do rise in pregnancy two- to threefold above the upper limit of gender and age-adjusted normals. The laboratory assessment of acromegaly is supplemented with magnetic resonance imaging of the pituitary and with visual field examination by quantitative perimetry. If imaging of the pituitary fails to detect an adenoma, then plasma GHRH concentration and computed imaging of the chest and abdomen are indicated in search of an ectopic GHRH-producing tumor (e.g., pancreatic neoplasm, small cell lung tumor).

TREATMENT

Treatment is indicated for all patients with signs and symptoms of acromegaly and biochemical confirmation. The goals of treatment are to prevent the long-term consequences of GH excess, to remove the intrasellar mass, and to preserve normal pituitary tissue and function. Treatment options include surgery, irradiation, and medical therapy. Surgery is the treatment of choice and should be supplemented, if necessary, with irradiation or pharmacotherapy or both. The criteria for cure are: (1) clinical remission, (2) normal suppression of the GH level by oral administration of glucose, and (3) a normal serum IGF-1 concentration.

Surgical Therapy

Transsphenoidal adenectomy by an experienced neurosurgeon is the only treatment option that has the potential for providing a permanent cure. If diagnostic imaging studies are negative, serum GHRH should be obtained to exclude an ectopic GHRH-secreting neoplasm. In those patients with normal blood GHRH concentrations and normal sellar MRI, transsphenoidal surgery is indicated for a presumed GH-secreting microadenoma (≤10 mm). Selective adenectomy of a GH-secreting microadenoma with preservation of surrounding normal pituitary tissue is routinely possible. Potential complications of transsphenoidal surgery include anterior pituitary insufficiency, transient or permanent diabetes insipidus, cerebrospinal fluid rhinorrhea, meningitis, loss of vision, and hemorrhage. All patients are given glucocorticoids perioperatively, and endogenous glucocorticoid production is assessed before dismissal; the typical hospital stay is 2 days. The mortality is approximately 0.4%. The cure rate after transsphenoidal surgery is approximately 80% for microadenomas and 30% for macroadenomas. The recurrence rate after apparent surgical cure is less than 10%.

In many patients with GH-secreting macroadenomas, transsphenoidal surgery is primarily a debulking procedure before radiation therapy. Radiation therapy is indicated if biochemical evidence of acromegaly persists postoperatively, and it is usually initiated 1 to 3 months postoperatively. The transcranial surgical approach occasionally is necessary for debulking a massive macroadenoma with marked suprasellar extension. This approach is associated with a longer hospital stay and increased morbidity.

For the rare patient with an ectopic GHRH-producing neoplasm, surgical removal usually results in return of the blood GH level to normal and regression of acromegaly.

Radiation Therapy

Radiation therapy is typically reserved for those patients who have failed surgical treatment. When conventional radiation therapy, administered with a linear accelerator (4500 to 5000 cGy given over a period of 6 weeks), is used as the initial treatment, GH levels of less than 5 micrograms per liter are found in 20% of patients at 2 years, in 40% by 5 years, and in 70% by 10 years. Unfortunately the irradiation affects the normal pituitary cells as well as the adenomatous tissue. Various degrees of hypopituitarism (e.g., hypogonadism, hypothyroidism, and secondary adrenal insufficiency) are present in at least 50% of the patients 10 years after irradiation. Other potential side effects include hair loss, damage to the optic nerves, brain necrosis, and radiation-induced neoplasia.

Most clinical neuroendocrinology centers favor gamma-knife stereotactic radiotherapy over conventional radiation therapy because: (1) the mean time to normalization of GH and IGF-1 levels is much quicker (≈ 1.5 years), (2) the target selectivity of gamma-knife stereotactic radiotherapy may result in fewer long-term side effects compared to conventional radiation therapy, and (3) gamma-knife stereotactic radiotherapy can be administered in 1 day versus 25 days for conventional radiation therapy. The only factors that preclude gamma-knife stereotactic radiotherapy are very large tumors and adenoma proximity to the optic chiasm.

Because of the temporal lag between the treatment and the return of GH and IGF-1 levels to normal and the high incidence of hypopituitarism, radiation therapy should be considered to be adjunctive and reserved for patients with persistently high GH levels after transsphenoidal surgery.

Medical Therapy

Medical therapy is typically used to normalize GH and IGF-1 levels in patients who: (1) are not cured with surgery, (2) are not good surgical candidates, (3) have cavernous sinus invasion and no chance for surgical cure, or (4) refuse surgery.

An analogue of somatostatin, octreotide (Sandostatin), is the drug of choice to treat residual autonomous GH hypersecretion following transsphenoidal surgery. When given subcutaneously three times daily, octreotide brings GH and IGF-1 levels to normal in approximately 65% of patients. Decreased pituitary tumor size, documented by MRI, occurs in approximately 30% of patients. For convenience and more consistent drug levels, long-acting octreotide (Sandostatin LAR Depot) may be administered every 28 days in depot intramuscular injections (10, 20, or 30 mg per injection). Most patients treated with octreotide will experience transitory loose stools for the first week of therapy. Octreotide therapy may affect insulin requirements in insulin-treated diabetics. Almost half of acromegalic patients on long-term octreotide therapy develop either asymptomatic gallstones or gallbladder sludge.

Growth hormone-receptor antagonists are a new class of pharmaceuticals that was approved by the Food and Drug Administration in 2003. Pegvisomant (Somavert),* is a 191 amino acid GH analogue that blocks the action of GH and thus prevents the production of IGF-1. In initial studies, pegvisomant was administered in a single daily subcutaneous dose and the IGF-1 normalization rate was greater than 90%. Pegvisomant should be used in those patients who do not normalize IGF-1 with octreotide therapy.

MONITORING OF TREATMENT RESULTS

Frequently, after complete removal of a GH-secreting pituitary adenoma but before dismissal from the hospital, patients note that their fingers feel less stiff and that the hyperhidrosis has disappeared. The GH response to an oral glucose load and the IGF-1 level 6 weeks postoperatively determine whether the patient may be considered to have a short-term cure. Screening for the status of other pituitary hormones is done at this time (e.g., blood analyses for cortisol, free thyroxine, testosterone, or estradiol, and urinalysis for fasting-state osmolality). These studies and visual field examination by quantitative perimetry are repeated 3 and 12 months postoperatively. MRI of the pituitary is done 12 months after the operation for microadenomas and at 3 and 12 months for macroadenomas.

If all studies give normal results 1 year postoperatively, a long-term cure is probable; an annual general medical examination, measurement of basal GH and IGF-1 values, and a visual field examination are

*Not FDA approved for this indication.

needed. Steroid coverage for stress is indicated for 1 year postoperatively, regardless of glucocorticoid levels. If glucocorticoid or posterior pituitary insufficiency is identified, these patients should carry identification indicating that they need additional corticosteroids or vasopressin (Pitressin), in the event of an accident or serious illness. A bracelet or necklace may be obtained from the Medic Alert Foundation.

After successful surgical treatment, there is a marked regression of the soft tissue excess but the bone changes are permanent. After the soft tissue changes have stabilized, combined oral and plastic surgery may be indicated (e.g., mandibular osteotomies, recession of the supraorbital ridges, rhinoplasties, and reduction of tongue size). Disabling hypertrophic osteoarthropathy of the hip may require total hip replacement.

The annual follow-up program for patients who have radiation therapy includes assessing the GH response to an oral glucose load, determination of the IGF-1 level, MRI of the sella, visual field examination, and surveillance for anterior and posterior pituitary insufficiency. If pituitary target gland deficiencies are identified, the secondary nature of these deficiencies should be confirmed, and replacement therapy should be started (see chapter on hypopituitarism). In the interval before the radiation therapy affects the autonomous GH secretion, pharmacologic therapy is begun and is continued if found to be effective. The pharmacologic agent is then withdrawn for 4 weeks annually to see if the radiation therapy returned the GH and IGF-1 values to normal; if not, the pharmacologic treatment is continued for another year.

ASSOCIATED CONDITIONS

A GH-secreting pituitary tumor may be part of multiple endocrine neoplasia type I (pituitary tumor, pancreatic tumor, and primary hyperparathyroidism) or the Carney complex (spotty facial pigmentation, myxomas of the heart and skin, primary pigmented nodular adrenal dysplasia, testicular Sertoli cell tumors, mammary myxoid tumors, schwannomas, and GH-secreting pituitary adenomas). Hypertension and impaired glucose tolerance are commonly associated with acromegaly and are frequently relieved or cured with effective treatment. Acromegaly is associated with an increased incidence of neoplastic lesions (e.g., adenomatous colonic polyps and carcinoma) and cardiovascular disease, and these patients should have periodic general medical examinations. Obstructive sleep apnea is a very frequent complication of acromegaly, and all patients should be tested for this disorder.

ADRENOCORTICAL INSUFFICIENCY

method of
JOSEPH M. HUGHES, M.D.
Columbia University
Bassett Healthcare
Cooperstown, New York

Adrenocortical insufficiency, also referred to as Addison's disease, is an uncommon endocrine disorder. The presentation may vary from the nonspecific symptoms of anorexia, nausea, and weight loss to the dramatic hypotensive crisis. The original description by Thomas Addison in 1849 was of a patient with adrenocortical destruction, and the term Addison's disease typically is reserved for those with primary adrenocortical failure. The challenge for the clinician is to establish not only the diagnosis but also the etiology. Patients may present with either primary adrenocortical failure or secondary adrenal insufficiency, disruption of hypothalamic/pituitary function. The long-term treatment with glucocorticoids and mineralocorticoids is effective but differs depending on the etiology. Finally, special attention must be given to the unique problem of patients with potential adrenal insufficiency from chronic pharmacologic doses of glucocorticoids.

CLINICAL PRESENTATION

As noted previously, the presenting symptoms are often nonspecific, which frequently delays the diagnosis. The clinician often thinks of adrenal insufficiency presenting in crisis with vomiting, diarrhea, dehydration, and life-threatening hypotension. However, most patients have had a chronic course with symptoms present for a prolonged period. The prominent ones are anorexia, weight loss, fatigue, nausea, diarrhea, and abdominal pain. The symptoms, when associated with physical findings and laboratory clues, should prompt evaluation.

There may be a paucity of findings on physical exam. The clinician may be struck when reviewing the vital signs by weight loss and hypotension, particularly orthostatic. Examination of the skin may help to distinguish primary from secondary causes. The patients with primary causes, from increased plasma corticotropin (ACTH) levels and the subsequent stimulation of melanocytes, are described with bronzing of the skin and also increased pigmentation of the buccal mucosa, gingiva, palmar creases, scars, and pressure points (e.g., the elbows). A further clue to the etiology may be the finding of vitiligo, which is associated with autoimmune adrenalitis.

There are characteristic findings on routine laboratory testing, electrolytes, blood urea nitrogen, glucose, creatinine, and hematology profile, which further suggest the diagnosis to the clinician. The most common is hyponatremia, which is seen in both primary and secondary forms, even though the etiology is different. In secondary causes, antidiuretic hormone excess has been proposed as an explanation, whereas in primary causes—because of the destruction of the adrenal cortex—there is aldosterone deficiency. The finding of hyperkalemia from hypoaldosteronism often prompts the investigation for adrenal insufficiency and is specific for primary adrenal insufficiency. Azotemia develops because of dehydration. Hypercalcemia is reported. Hypoglycemia is uncommon and is most often seen with secondary forms. The complete blood count may demonstrate eosinophilia in up to 20% of patients. Less common findings are anemia and neutropenia.

EVALUATION

The diagnosis can usually be made by three tests: random cortisol levels, plasma ACTH levels, and the synthetic corticotropin stimulation test. The random cortisol can be a helpful test as a first step. A value less than the lower limits of normal may be diagnostic and provide enough data to initiate therapy in patients with clinical signs and known pathology; for example, a hypothalamic/pituitary lesion. The converse is also true. The random cortisol level greater than 20 μg/dL, unless the patient's presentation is highly suspicious for adrenal insufficiency, makes the diagnosis unlikely. It is important to remember that patients with adrenal insufficiency may have a random cortisol level in the laboratory's normal range and require further testing to establish the diagnosis.

The rapid synthetic corticotropin stimulation test is the principal investigation for the diagnosis of adrenal insufficiency. Synthetic tetracosactin (Synanthem,* Cortrosyn) is the 1 to 24 amino acid sequence of human ACTH. The traditional dose has been 250 μg given either intravenously or intramuscularly. Plasma cortisol levels are measured at time 0, 30, and 60 minutes and can be drawn at any time during the day. Various criteria have been used to determine a normal response. Typically baseline, peak, and the delta from baseline to peak levels have been used. However, careful study by different authors has shown that a peak level at any time greater than 20 μg/dL is a normal response. Levels less than these indicate adrenal insufficiency, but do not distinguish between primary and secondary failure.

There has been a great deal of discussion recently about the recommended dose of tetracosactin (Cortrosyn). There is agreement that the standard dose, 250 μg, delivers pharmacologic concentrations. Newer protocols have advocated using 1 μg, a more physiologic concentration. The hypothesis is that the low-dose protocol would allow the diagnosis of borderline/mild cases of adrenal insufficiency. Previously, when only the high dose test was used, some patients with normal tests became adrenally insufficient, especially during times of extreme stress. This is a concern, especially when the etiology is secondary adrenal insufficiency. At our hospital we have performed both tests, and our experience shows normal patients having inadequate stimulation with the low-dose test. Our protocol is to use the high-dose test almost exclusively, except in the special situation where one expects possible borderline secondary adrenal insufficiency.

The clinician is simultaneously diagnosing and establishing the etiology. The now-accurate measurement of plasma ACTH levels has proven to be very helpful in distinguishing primary from secondary failure. In primary failure, the pituitary is intact and one anticipates elevated ACTH levels, typically greater than 100 pg/mL. ACTH levels should be low with secondary failure. However, the concentrations may also be in the normal range.

After determining that the patient has either primary or secondary insufficiency, radiologic studies provide important information. With primary failure, the computed tomography scan may show atrophied adrenals in autoimmune adrenalitis. Enlarged glands with high-density areas or calcification suggest hemorrhage, granulomatous disease, or neoplasm. The magnetic resonance scan of the hypothalamic/pituitary region in patients with secondary insufficiency is often diagnostic.

Infrequently, other studies can be helpful when the diagnosis of adrenal insufficiency or the etiology is in question. The gold standard test for diagnosing secondary adrenal insufficiency is the insulin tolerance test. Because the patient must become hypoglycemic and it has been implicated in fatalities (albeit rarely), the test is best performed by those familiar with the protocol. There have been several prolonged ACTH protocols used to distinguish primary from secondary insufficiency. Finally, because corticotropin-releasing hormone (CRH) has been available for testing, measuring ACTH levels after CRH localizes secondary insufficiency to either a lesion in the hypothalamus or pituitary.

ETIOLOGY

After the diagnosis of primary adrenal insufficiency has been established, the clinician is confronted by multiple possible etiologies (Table 1). The most common in 80% to 90% of patients is autoimmune adrenalitis, which is often associated with other autoimmune diseases (Table 2). These should be searched for and may be present at the time of diagnosis or may appear months or years later. The diagnosis of autoimmune adrenalitis may be the first finding in a patient with an autoimmune polyendocrine syndrome. Tuberculosis has been reported as the second most common cause. Finally, although rare,

TABLE 1. **Causes of Primary Adrenal Insufficiency**

Autoimmune
Infectious—Tuberculosis, histoplasmosis, blastomycosis, coccidiomycosis, cryptococcosis, HIV, cytomegalovirus
Hemorrhage—Sepsis, anticoagulation
Metastatic disease—Lung, breast
Drugs—Ketoconazole, aminoglutethimide
Infiltrative diseases—Sarcoid, hemachromatosis, amyloidosis
Familial—Adrenoleukodystrophy, adrenomyeloneuropathy, familial glucocorticoid deficiency

*Not FDA approved for this indication.

TABLE 2. **Associated Autoimmune Disease With Adrenal Insufficiency**

Thyroid disease—Hashimoto thyroiditis or Graves' disease
Type 1 diabetes mellitus
Pernicious anemia
Primary ovarian or testicular failure
Vitiligo
Gastrointestinal—Celiac disease, inflammatory bowel disease, chronic hepatitis
Rheumatologic—Sjögren syndrome
Alopecia
Neurologic—Multiple sclerosis
Hypoparathyroidism
Chronic candidiasis

the young male presenting with adrenal insufficiency should make one consider adrenoleukodystrophy or adrenomyeloneuropathy.

Secondary adrenal insufficiency may also be from a number of diseases (Table 3), but is most commonly from chronic glucocorticoid therapy, pituitary tumors, or iatrogenic causes. It is important to remember that radiation-induced adrenal failure may present 5 or more years after therapy. When the patient is found to have secondary adrenal insufficiency, other hypothalamic/pituitary hormonal deficiencies should be sought, because isolated ACTH deficiency is rare.

TREATMENT

When considering the treatment of adrenal insufficiency one must understand the management of adrenal crisis, long-term glucocorticoid and mineralocorticoid therapy, and stress dose glucocorticoids at the time of acute illness.

In adrenal crisis, the goal is to reverse the hypovolemia with normal saline, 2 to 3 liters infused rapidly, and to administer parenteral glucocorticoids. The choice of glucocorticoid is critical. If the diagnosis of adrenal insufficiency has not been established and diagnostic testing is required, then 4 mg of dexamethasone (Decadron) IV should be given every 12 hours. Dexamethasone does not interfere with the cortisol assay. Consequently, as the patient is receiving dexamethasone, corticotropin stimulation testing can be performed. Preferably, the ACTH level is obtained and the corticotropin stimulation tests are performed close to the time of initiation of therapy. If the diagnosis and etiology of adrenal insufficiency is known, then either dexamethasone or hydrocortisone (Hydrocortone)

TABLE 3. **Causes of Secondary Adrenal Insufficiency**

Steroid therapy
Iatrogenic—Pituitary or adrenal adenoma surgery, radiation therapy
Pituitary tumors, adenoma, craniopharyngioma, Rathke cleft cyst
Infiltrative—Sarcoid
Pituitary infarction
Lymphocytic or granulomatous hypophysitis
Isolated ACTH deficiency
Metastasis
Tuberculosis

100 mg IV every 6 to 8 hours can be used. Intravenous glucocorticoid on a tapering dose may be required for several days until oral replacement therapy is begun. Mineralocorticoids are not required in the acute management. When the patient is stable, oral therapy is initiated.

All patients with adrenal insufficiency require glucocorticoids. I usually prescribe hydrocortisone (Hydrocortone). Even though the plasma concentrations rise and fall rapidly after oral administration, most patients respond well to single morning dose and at times a second early afternoon dose. Individualizing the dose is important to prevent long-term complications from overreplacement. I have found the calculation, 12 mg/m^2/day, helpful in determining the dose of hydrocortisone. For example, if the total daily calculated dose is 25 mg, then 20 mg could be given in the morning and 5 mg in the early afternoon. Long term, the patient may find that only the morning dose is required. Some experts prescribe the longer acting preparations prednisone or dexamethasone (Decadron). The rationale is a more prolonged pharmacologic effect as opposed to that seen with hydrocortisone or cortisone acetate. The usual doses are 5 mg for prednisone and 0.5 mg for dexamethasone. Because of the prolonged action and an attempt to mimic the circadian rhythm, these medications are given in the morning or at bedtime. Patients with primary adrenal failure, because of destruction of the adrenal cortex, are unable to produce aldosterone. Because the renin/angiotensin/aldosterone system is intact in patients with secondary adrenal insufficiency, aldosterone is infrequently required. Mineralocorticoid is prescribed as fludrocortisone (Florinef). The usual dose is 0.1 mg/d. The patient should obtain a medical alert bracelet and be instructed in stress dose steroid at the time of acute illness. For example, the patient doubles or triples the dose of glucocorticoids for 3 days with a febrile illness. There is no need to taper the dose. If the patient has vomiting or profuse diarrhea, then the patient should be instructed to seek emergency care. Some patients are capable of giving intramuscular glucocorticoids (Decadron, Hydrocortone) at home in an attempt to prevent the need for an emergency department visit. For outpatients having procedures, giving 50 to 100 mg of hydrocortisone IV before, and then converting to oral stress doses, is appropriate. The adrenal cortex is also a source of androgens. In patients, especially women, with decreased libido and persistent fatigue, dehydroepiandrosterone 25 to 50 mg daily may be added.

After glucocorticoids and mineralocorticoids have been prescribed, the clinician constantly monitors the adequacy of the treatment. There is equal concern for insufficient as well as excessive doses, particularly glucocorticoids. Through the history, the clinician learns about symptoms of low-grade adrenal insufficiency, particularly fatigue and orthostatic hypotension. On exam, one looks for evidence of Cushing syndrome, particularly weight gain, striae, and facial plethora indicating possible overreplacement. Osteoporosis is always a concern. On laboratory testing, the sodium and potassium levels, and plasma renin or plasma renin activity levels should be normal if the patient is receiving adequate doses of fludrocortisone.

ADRENAL SUPPRESSION AND CHRONIC GLUCOCORTICOID THERAPY

Chronic glucocorticoid (prednisone) therapy causes secondary adrenal insufficiency. There is generalized consensus about the doses and duration of prednisone therapy that cause suppression. If prednisone at doses greater than 20 mg per day for more than 3 weeks is prescribed, then the dose of prednisone should be tapered. Also, patients that have required prednisone at doses greater than 5 mg daily for months to years are presumed to be suppressed. If there is a question about the integrity of the hypothalamic/pituitary/adrenal axis in patients on 5 mg or less per day of prednisone, then a corticotropin stimulation test can be helpful. After establishing suppression, then a prolonged taper is required, because 6 to 12 months are required for the axis to recover.

The tapering of prednisone must be gradual, especially after the 5 mg dose is reached. An approach to the patient on high-dose prednisone is to decrease the dose by 5 to 10 mg increments every 2 weeks until reaching the 20 mg dose. Afterward, the dose should be adjusted by 5 mg or less again every 2 weeks until the 5 mg dose is established. At that point, decreasing the dose by 1 mg per month is a conservative approach. After the patient reaches the 1 or 2 mg per day dose, a corticotropin stimulation test can be helpful. Also, a fasting cortisol before the dose of prednisone greater than 10 ng/dL usually predicts normal adrenal function. Often the limitation in tapering prednisone is the activity of the underlying disease, not the integrity of the hypothalamic/pituitary/adrenal axis. Stress dose steroids for major illness, surgery, or trauma should be provided for the first year after successfully stopping prednisone.

CUSHING'S SYNDROME

method of
KATHRYN G. SCHUFF, M.D.
Oregon Health and Science University
Portland, Oregon

Cushing's syndrome refers to the pathologic manifestations of excess glucocorticoid hormone. Classically described signs include central obesity, moon facies, purple striae, and muscle wasting (Table 1); however, the findings are usually more subtle, and extensive overlap can be demonstrated with more common syndromes such as polycystic ovary syndrome, insulin resistance syndrome, and depression. Because of this overlap, practitioners must have a low threshold for considering the diagnosis and initiating evaluation, but they must also recognize that most patients tested

TABLE 1. **Signs and Symptoms of Cushing's Syndrome (in Order of Decreasing Likelihood Ratio for Predicting the Presence of Cushing's Syndrome)**

Osteoporosis, unexplained
Weakness
Ecchymoses
Hypokalemia ($K^+ < 3.6$)
Central obesity
Plethora
Diastolic blood pressure ≥105 mm Hg
Red or violaceous striae
Acne
Pitting edema
Hirsutism
Oligomenorrhea
Abnormal glucose tolerance
Generalized obesity

will not have true Cushing's syndrome. In addition, because of the rarity of the syndrome (previously quoted at seven per million population, but more recently estimated to affect up to 4% of obese diabetics), mass screening is not recommended because even with highly accurate screening tests, screening would generate thousands of false-positive results for every patient with true Cushing's syndrome identified.

We recommend evaluating patients who have multiple symptoms or progression of symptoms over time (e.g., by comparing old photographs) and patients with symptoms more specific for Cushing's syndrome: proximal muscle weakness, spontaneous ecchymoses, hypokalemia, unexplained osteopenia, abnormal fat distribution (centripetal, supraclavicular), unusual weight gain, difficult-to-control hypertension (especially in younger patients), and growth retardation and obesity (in children).

DIAGNOSTIC EVALUATION

Etiologies of Cushing's Syndrome, the Pseudo-Cushing's State, and Preclinical Cushing's Syndrome

The pathologic etiologies of Cushing's syndrome are varied (Table 2), but they have the common final pathway of glucocorticoid excess. Mild hypercortisolemia caused by other illnesses is not pathologic, but rather referred to as the pseudo-Cushing's state, and it must be excluded from true Cushing's syndrome. Preclinical (or subclinical) Cushing's syndrome is a recently described entity consisting of mild hypothalamic-pituitary axis (HPA) abnormalities (but not diagnostic of Cushing's syndrome) in patients with incidentally discovered adrenal abnormalities. Etiologies of true Cushing's syndrome include exogenous glucocorticoid administration and endogenous glucocorticoid production from a variety of tumors.

Exogenous Glucocorticoid Use

Cushing's syndrome from exogenous glucocorticoids is the most common etiology and is usually obvious. Identification of an exogenous source of glucocorticoids

TABLE 2. **Etiologies of Cushing's Syndrome, Preclinical Cushing's Syndrome, and the Pseudo-Cushing's State**

Pseudo-Cushing's state
- Acute/chronic medical illness
- Psychiatric illness
- Alcoholism

Preclinical (subclinical) Cushing's syndrome
- Adrenal adenoma (incidentaloma)

Cushing's syndrome
- Exogenous glucocorticoid use
  - Oral glucocorticoids (prednisone, dexamethasone, hydrocortisone)
  - Inhaled glucocorticoids (rare)
  - Topical glucocorticoids
  - Injected glucocorticoids
    - Articular and periarticular
    - Intramuscular (for allergic or rheumatologic conditions)

Endogenous glucocorticoid production
- ACTH-dependent
  - Pituitary corticotroph adenoma
  - Pituitary corticotroph hyperplasia (possibly caused by ectopic CRH)
  - Ectopic ACTH syndrome
    - Oat cell lung carcinoma
    - Foregut carcinoid tumors (bronchial, thymic, splenic)
    - Pheochromocytoma
    - Medullary thyroids carcinoma
    - Islet cell tumors
- ACTH-independent
  - Adrenal adenoma
  - Adrenal carcinoma
  - Rare: micronodular hyperplasia
    - Macronodular hyperplasia
      - Ectopic receptor expression (gastic inhibitory peptide—food responsive, interleukin-1, luteinizing hormone, vasopressin, β-adrenergic)
    - Pigmented micronodular hyperplasia (Carney complex)
    - Adrenal rests
    - McCune-Albright (activating mutations)

CRH = corticotropin-releasing hormone; ACTH = adrenocorticotropic hormone.

can sometimes be difficult either because the patient does not identify the glucocorticoid as a "drug" or the significance of the glucocorticoid use is not recognized because of its route of administration. Particular problems occur with triamcinolone because variation in its rate of metabolism can result in persistent drug levels for months. High-performance liquid chromatography (HPLC) for detection of synthetic steroids is sometimes helpful in these cases. Finally, the diagnosis can be very difficult in patients who are taking the drug surreptitiously, especially if hydrocortisone, prednisone, or prednisolone are taken, which cross-react in the "cortisol" assay. Collection of laboratory specimens in a monitored environment and subsequent confrontation of the patient are difficult, but often necessary.

Endogenous Cushing's Syndrome

Once the question of endogenous Cushing's syndrome has been raised, either because of clinical features or as part of the evaluation of an incidental adrenal mass, the diagnostic evaluation as outlined in Figure 1 focuses on answering three questions in stepwise fashion: (1) Does the patient have Cushing's syndrome? (2) Is the Cushing's syndrome adrenocorticotropic hormone (ACTH) dependent or ACTH independent? (3) Is the ACTH-dependent syndrome caused by a pituitary adenoma or the ectopic ACTH syndrome?

Step 1: Diagnosing Cushing's Syndrome

Pseudo-Cushing's States

Documenting Cushing's syndrome requires demonstration of pathologic hypercortisolemia. One of the most difficult and important tasks is exclusion of mild hypercortisolemia and other abnormalities of the HPA axis that are not pathologic, but rather secondary to other medical and psychiatric illnesses. These conditions are referred to as pseudo-Cushing's states or pseudo-Cushing's syndrome (see Table 2). Clinical manifestations of hypercortisolism are not usually present (except in the case of alcoholism), and the hypercortisolemia resolves with treatment of the underlying condition. Therefore, it is important to not evaluate the patient while acutely ill (e.g., hospitalized) and with careful consideration for conditions that can cause the pseudo-Cushing state. In addition, some biochemical tests help make this distinction.

Dexamethasone Suppression Versus 24-Hour Urinary Free Cortisol

The two most common tests used to demonstrate hypercortisolemia are the overnight dexamethasone suppression test and measurement of 24-hour urinary free cortisol excretion. The dexamethasone suppression test is simple to perform and involves administering 1 mg of dexamethasone at midnight and obtaining a serum cortisol level at 8 AM the next morning. A normal result is suppression of serum cortisol to less than 5 μg/dL. False-positive results can occur in women who are pregnant or taking oral contraceptives or in patients taking medications that accelerate dexamethasone metabolism: rifampin (Rifadin), phenytoin (Dilantin), phenobarbital, and primidone (Mysoline), as well as alcohol. The possibility of a false-positive result can be investigated by determining a simultaneous dexamethasone level. Measurement of 24-hour cortisol excretion requires patient compliance with the 24-hour urine collection; high urine volumes and carbamazepine (Tegretol) (in the HPLC assay) can cause false-positive results. Both tests offer high sensitivity, and a normal dexamethasone suppression test essentially excludes a diagnosis of Cushing's syndrome, as do three or four normal 24-hour urinary free cortisol determinations. However, the overnight dexamethasone suppression test suffers from imperfect specificity and a significant number of false-positive results in patients with other medical conditions. Therefore, a positive dexamethasone suppression test requires confirmation by measurement of 24-hour cortisol excretion.

In patients with clear hypercortisolemia (24-hour urinary free cortisol greater than 300 μg/d in a nonhospitalized patient), the diagnosis of Cushing's syndrome is confirmed. However, a number of patients

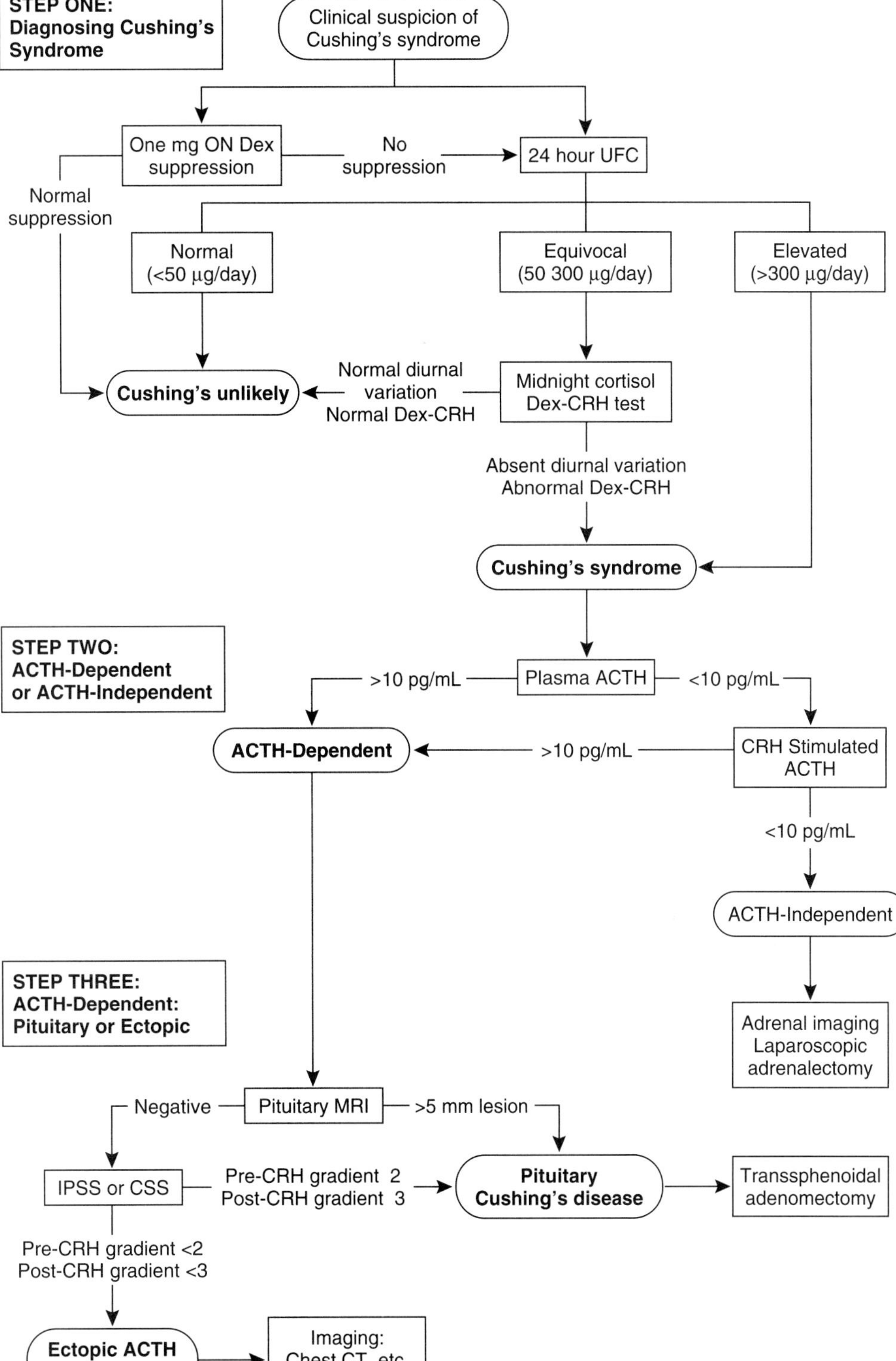

Figure 1. Algorithm for the diagnosis of Cushing's syndrome. *Abbreviations:* ACTH = adrenocorticotropic hormone; CRH = corticotropin-releasing hormone; CSS = cavernous sinus sampling; CT = computed tomography; Dex = dexamethasone suppressed; IPSS = inferior petrosal sinus sampling; MRI = magnetic resonance imaging; ON = overnight; UFC = urinary free cortisol.

with true Cushing's syndrome have more mild hypercortisolemia, and further evaluation is required to distinguish them from patients with pseudo-Cushing's states. Two tests that are useful in this regard are assessment of diurnal cortisol rhythm and the dexamethasone-suppressed corticotropin-releasing hormone (Dex-CRH) stimulation test.

Diurnal Variation

One of the features of Cushing's syndrome is abrogation of the diurnal rhythm in cortisol secretion, which can be evaluated by measuring a midnight sleeping cortisol level. This technique obviously requires either hospitalization and drawing blood for a cortisol level from an indwelling catheter or, alternatively, assessment of a salivary cortisol level, which correlates with serum free cortisol levels. Unfortunately, many salivary cortisol determinations currently suffer from lack of reproducibility and sensitivity. Midnight serum cortisol levels are less than 7.5 μg/dL in normal subjects and most patients with pseudo-Cushing's states, except those with severe depression.

Dex-CRH Test

The Dex-CRH test uses a higher dose of dexamethasone to exclude false-positive results seen in the 1-mg test; because this dose will also suppress some pituitary adenomas, it takes advantage of the relative over-responsiveness of these tumors to CRH to improve this problem with sensitivity. In this test, 0.5 mg of dexamethasone is given orally every 6 hours for 48 hours, followed by a 100-μg (or 1-μg/kg) ovine CRH (Acthrel) stimulation test at 8:00 AM. Failure of cortisol to be suppressed to less than 1.4 μg/dL and to remain suppressed after CRH stimulation confirms a diagnosis of Cushing's syndrome and appears to be efficacious in distinguishing Cushing's syndrome from the pseudo-Cushing state.

Preclinical Cushing's Syndrome

A phenomenon of modern technologic intervention is identification of "incidental" adrenal masses in a significant percentage of patients. Careful evaluation of such patients has led to the recognition of preclinical or subclinical Cushing's syndrome. Evaluation of multiple aspects of the HPA axis reveals subtle abnormalities consistent with autonomous glucocorticoid function in 5% to 20% of patients. Diagnostic criteria vary but include an abnormal dexamethasone suppression test in addition to one other criterion of abnormal HPA axis function: lower ACTH levels, a blunted ACTH or cortisol response to CRH, or loss of normal diurnal rhythm. In addition, the finding of unilateral uptake on iodocholesterol scans (at baseline or after dexamethasone suppression) may be useful not only in diagnosis but also in predicting adrenal insufficiency after unilateral adrenalectomy. Therapy for preclinical Cushing's syndrome is also controversial. Because of the higher prevalence of hypertension, diabetes, and obesity in these patients than in controls and because of improvements in these parameters after surgery, many authors recommend adrenalectomy if any of these features are present.

Step 2: ACTH-Dependent or ACTH-Independent Disease

ACTH-independent Cushing's syndrome accounts for about 20% of cases of endogenous Cushing's syndrome (see Table 2) and is most commonly due to benign adrenal adenomas (60% of ACTH-independent cases) and malignant adrenal carcinomas (40%). The remainder of causes are rare; the Carney complex (mesenchymal tumors, or myxomas, of the heart, skin, breast; pigmented skin lesions: lentigines and blue nevi, multiple pigmented adrenocortical nodules, and other functional endocrine tumors) is important to distinguish because of its familial inheritance and the risk of sudden death from the associated cardiac myxomas.

A plasma ACTH level less than 10 pg/mL defines ACTH-independent disease. However, because ACTH secretion may be episodic, a low random level should be confirmed by measurement after administration of 100 μg (or 1 μg/kg) of ovine CRH. Once ACTH-independent disease is diagnosed, we recommend evaluation with adrenal computed tomography (CT) to localize the adrenal lesion.

Step 3: ACTH-Dependent Disease: Pituitary or Ectopic

Most cases of endogenous Cushing's syndrome are ACTH dependent (80% of cases), and the most common etiology is a benign pituitary corticotroph adenoma, which accounts for 85% to 90% of ACTH-dependent cases and is the most common cause of endogenous Cushing's syndrome overall. Rarely, only corticotroph hyperplasia is found pathologically, and it should prompt evaluation for ectopic CRH production. The ectopic ACTH syndrome (10% to 15% of ACTH-dependent cases) is sometimes obvious because of lung carcinoma (50% of ectopic cases). More difficult to diagnose is the occult ectopic variety, which is most commonly caused by foregut carcinoids (35% of ectopic cases), usually bronchial and other neuroendocrine tumors (see Table 2 for details).

A variety of biochemical tests have been proposed to distinguish pituitary Cushing's disease from the ectopic ACTH syndrome, including the low-dose–high-dose dexamethasone suppression test, CRH stimulation tests, and desmopressin and metyrapone testing. Unfortunately, all lack adequate sensitivity and specificity and serve only to minimally increase the post-test probability over the 85% to 90% pretest probability of a pituitary lesion. Therefore, we recommend against any biochemical testing for this differential diagnosis.

Instead, once ACTH-dependent disease has been confirmed with an ACTH level greater than 10 pg/mL, we recommend performing a pituitary magnetic resonance imaging (MRI) scan and, if a definite lesion larger than 5 mm is seen, proceeding with pituitary surgery. The likelihood of a patient having both the occult ectopic ACTH syndrome and a pituitary "incidentaloma" is sufficiently small that false-positive results are minimized. However, the sensitivity is poor, and more than half the patients with Cushing's disease will have a negative MRI and require additional evaluation.

Inferior petrosal or cavernous sinus sampling is significantly more accurate than biochemical testing and, though invasive, has been shown to be safe when performed by experienced personnel. The procedure involves simultaneous bilateral sampling for ACTH levels from either the petrosal or cavernous sinuses before and after administration of 100 μg (or 1 μg/kg) of ovine CRH. Demonstrating an ACTH gradient greater than 2 in the petrosal or cavernous sinus as compared with the periphery at baseline or greater than 3 after ovine CRH indicates a pituitary source. This procedure also provides information regarding the intrapituitary location of tumors to help guide surgical therapy if a lateralization (side-to-side) ratio greater than 1.4 is found. High accuracy requires excellent catheter position. The accuracy of lateralization is also affected by the symmetry of flow through the cavernous and petrosal sinuses.

If a petrosal or cavernous-peripheral gradient is not observed, thus suggesting the ectopic ACTH syndrome, imaging should be undertaken, starting with chest CT and then proceeding to neck, abdomen, and pelvic CT. Octreotide scanning is sometimes helpful but does not usually identify lesions not already seen on CT scanning. Positron emission tomography is useful in medullary thyroid carcinoma, but this diagnosis is generally obvious and experience is not yet extensive with other tumors. Often, lesions are not identified immediately, but found on serial examinations performed every 6 to 12 months.

Caveats in the Diagnostic Evaluation

A stepwise approach to these questions is critical because the premise of many of the recommended tests is that the evaluation is being done on a specific "category" of patients, such as patients proven to have Cushing's syndrome or patients proven to have ACTH-dependent disease. Proceeding in the evaluation without clearly classifying the patient at each step can result in misdirected testing, misdiagnoses, and even inappropriate therapy. For example, an AM ACTH level of 20 pg/mL in a patient who actually did not have Cushing's syndrome would incorrectly suggest ACTH-dependent disease, or lack of an ACTH gradient during inferior petrosal sinus sampling because of low ACTH levels in ACTH-independent disease would misdirect evaluation for the ectopic ACTH syndrome. Likewise, because of the significant incidence of pituitary and adrenal "incidentalomas" and the common finding of nodular adrenal disease in late pituitary Cushing's syndrome, it is critical to define a biochemical diagnosis before imaging procedures. One final caveat that applies to every step of the evaluation is that the patient must be hypercortisolemic at the time of any evaluation. Cyclic Cushing's syndrome or periodic hormonogenesis occurs in approximately 15% of cases and can be very confusing. In addition, medications used to lower cortisol levels must be stopped at least 4 weeks before any evaluation.

THERAPEUTIC INTERVENTION

Exogenous Glucocorticoid Use

Although the diagnosis is usually straightforward, management of Cushing's syndrome resulting from exogenous glucocorticoids is difficult because of the beneficial effect of glucocorticoids in managing the underlying disease. This benefit is often the limiting factor in attempts to taper or discontinue the glucocorticoid. Alternate-day regimens may have some benefit in allowing HPA axis recovery, but slow tapers are still usually required. Patients should wear MedicAlert bracelets and receive stress doses of glucocorticoids as discussed elsewhere for adrenal insufficiency.

Endogenous Cushing's Syndrome

Once the etiology of endogenous Cushing's syndrome is defined, the intervention in almost every etiology is surgical excision of the offending tumor. The exception is lung carcinomas; whatever modality of therapy is appropriate for the carcinoma usually also treats Cushing's syndrome resulting from ectopic ACTH secretion.

Pituitary Surgery

Selective adenomectomy via a trans-sphenoidal approach is the procedure of choice for all pituitary lesions except those with extensive cavernous sinus involvement, where a transfrontal approach may be indicated. Exploration of the gland should be initiated on the side indicated by inferior petrosal or cavernous sinus sampling or MRI, but the contralateral side of the gland should be included if typical tumor is not encountered. A number of centers use intraoperative ultrasound to try to improve localization of the adenoma. If tumor is not identified on either side, we advocate hemihypophysectomy of the side predicted to contain the tumor because such tumors can be tiny and are semiliquid and often "lost" during suctioning.

Adrenal Surgery

Unilateral adrenalectomy is the treatment of choice for unilateral adrenal adenomas or carcinomas and is curative for adenomas. Treatment of carcinomas is difficult, with metastases present in up to 30% at the time of diagnosis and a median survival of only 12 to 14 months. Bilateral adrenalectomy is indicated to cure hypercortisolemia if trans-sphenoidal surgery for pituitary Cushing's disease is not curative, in the ectopic ACTH syndrome if the ectopic source remains occult, and in the rare cases of bilateral nodular hyperplasia. Laparoscopic adrenalectomy, either unilateral or bilateral, depending on the disease, has essentially replaced open adrenalectomy in many institutions because of significantly shortened postoperative recovery and hospital stay and decreased acute and chronic pain. In experienced hands, conversion to an open procedure occurs in a small number of patients, overall mortality is low, operative times are only slightly longer, and morbidity is similar to that of an open procedure. Exceptions include patients with adrenal carcinoma, massive adrenal lesions (>6 to 10 cm, depending on the experience of the surgeon), or other factors that preclude laparoscopic surgery such as coagulopathy or previous surgery or trauma in the area.

Postoperative Management

Postoperative management of all patients with Cushing's syndrome includes perioperative "stress" doses of hydrocortisone, 100 mg intravenously or orally every 8 hours for 1 day, with tapering to slightly higher than replacement doses, usually hydrocortisone, 20 mg twice daily orally by discharge. An AM cortisol level less than 2 μg/dL on the second postoperative day after withholding hydrocortisone for 24 hours is highly predictive of surgical cure. Hydrocortisone is tapered as tolerated. Patients successfully cured by surgery will experience secondary adrenal insufficiency for up to 18 months postoperatively and need reassurance that the symptoms that they are experiencing as their hydrocortisone is tapered are an encouraging sign of their cure. Periodic AM cortisol levels and low-dose (1 μg) cosyntropin (Cortrosyn) stimulation testing will demonstrate gradual recovery of the HPA axis. Patients will require stress doses of steroids for surgeries or severe medical illnesses and should wear a MedicAlert bracelet until recovery of their HPA axis is documented. Patients undergoing unilateral adrenalectomy do not usually require mineralocorticoid replacement. After bilateral adrenalectomy, fludrocortisone (Florinef), 0.1 mg orally daily to twice daily, is titrated as discussed elsewhere for primary adrenal insufficiency.

Patient undergoing pituitary surgery need careful monitoring for abnormalities of vasopressin secretion, both diabetes insipidus and the syndrome of inappropriate antidiuretic hormone secretion. These conditions can occur several days postoperatively, after the patient has been discharged. All patients undergoing pituitary surgery also need testing of pituitary function (thyroid, gonadal, and growth hormone axes) at a 6-week postoperative visit.

Management of Patients Not Cured by Pituitary Surgery

Although trans-sphenoidal adenomectomy is fairly efficacious in the management of these tumors, a number of patients are not cured by surgery, particularly if the tumor is a macroadenoma or demonstrates invasion. Depending on the initial operative findings, patients may be offered a second trans-sphenoidal exploration, possibly including hemihypophysectomy if that was not performed during the first surgery. If a second surgery is not indicated or not successful or the patient declines, consideration should be given to pituitary irradiation and/or bilateral adrenalectomy. Radiosurgery, either by gamma knife or linear accelerator, is very efficacious in curing patients with Cushing's disease. When compared with conventional fractionated radiotherapy, targeted radiosurgery appears to offers a faster cure, a theoretically lower risk of cognitive effects and vision loss, but probably similar rates of eventual hypopituitarism. Proton beam therapy is also efficacious, but less commonly used. Cure of Cushing's syndrome occurs over a period of several months to years. Control of hypercortisolemia by bilateral adrenalectomy or medical therapy is required until cure is achieved. The risk of Nelson's syndrome, rapid growth of a pituitary tumor after removal of negative cortisol feedback (such as with bilateral adrenalectomy), may be lessened with pituitary irradiation.

Medical Management of Cushing's Syndrome

Several agents are available to control the hypercortisolemia of Cushing's syndrome. Indications for medical therapy include preoperative preparation (e.g., to assist in the management of severe hypertension or psychosis) and control of hypercortisolism while awaiting the effects of pituitary irradiation or localization and therapy for occult ectopic ACTH secretion. The most commonly used agent is ketoconazole (Nizoral),* which inhibits a number of steroidogenic enzymes involved in cortisol biosynthesis. Typical doses range from 200 to 1200 mg/d. Its use is limited by hepatotoxicity, which occurs in 15% of patients but is usually reversible within 3 months of discontinuing the medication. Metyrapone (Metopirone) blocks the final step in cortisol synthesis and is very efficacious; however, some tachyphylaxis occurs, and it is not currently readily available. Aminoglutethimide (Cytadren) inhibits the initial step in cortisol synthesis and is fairly effective, but it is not well tolerated. Mitotane (*o,p′*-DDD) (Lysodren) is an enzyme inhibitor that also causes adrenolysis. It has significant side effects, including dramatic increases in low-density lipoprotein cholesterol. Centrally acting agents that decrease ACTH secretion include cyproheptadine,* which is not very effective and not well tolerated, and bromocriptine (Parlodel),* which also has a poor response rate. Mifepristone (RU-486) (Mifeprex)* is a progesterone and glucocorticoid receptor antagonist used to block the action of cortisol. It is very efficacious in reversing acute symptoms; however, because it does not reduce cortisol levels, dosage titration must be done on clinical grounds and is often difficult. Unfortunately, none of these medications have favorable enough efficacy or side effect profiles to be considered first-line or definitive therapy and, instead, are temporizing measures until definitive therapy is undertaken.

*Not FDA approved for this indication.

DIABETES INSIPIDUS

method of
GERTRUDE S. LEFAVOUR, M.D.
UMDNJ Robert Wood Johnson Medical School
New Brunswick, New Jersey

Diabetes insipidus (DI) is a clinical disorder of water metabolism characterized by the excretion of large volumes (>50 mL/kg with ad lib intake) of dilute urine (osmolality <300 mOsm/kg) and the excessive urinary loss of solute-free water. The antidiuretic hormone, arginine vasopressin (AVP), synthesized in the hypothalamus and stored in the posterior pituitary gland, is the primary regulator of water excretion causing water channels called aquaporin 2 to be inserted into the luminal membrane of the collecting duct, permitting water movement into cells. Normally with small increases (1% to 2%) in body fluid osmolality above 280 to 285 mOsm/kg, AVP secretion increases linearly and steeply, causing maximal urinary concentration (1200 mOsm/kg). In addition to osmotic stimuli for AVP release, it is released nonosmotically with large decreases (>7% to 10%) in blood volume. DI may be divided into central DI (CDI) resulting from inadequate production of AVP and thus responsive to hormone replacement, nephrogenic DI (NDI) due to lack of renal responsiveness to AVP, and accelerated metabolism of AVP in pregnancy due to release of vasopressinases from the placenta which rapidly degrade vasopressin and oxytocin. CDI or NDI is seen in partial or complete forms. The most common etiologies are listed in Table 1.

Clinical Manifestations

The majority of patients with DI maintain water balance and present with a serum sodium in the upper range of normal because thirst mechanisms are intact, and hyperosmolality is the most potent stimulus for thirst. The most common presenting symptoms of DI are thirst (frequently craving iced or very cold water), polyuria, and nocturia. Other symptoms include incontinence or enuresis and fatigue from inadequate sleep due to nocturia. Urine output ranges from 3 to 18 L/day. Patients with CDI usually have an abrupt onset of symptoms, whereas the onset of symptoms is more gradual in NDI. When thirst is intact, physical exam is unrevealing, and serum sodium, and osmolality are usually normal or at the upper limit of normal. A low urinary osmolality or urine-specific gravity on laboratory testing may be the only abnormality. If the hypothalamic disorder producing CDI also produces hypodipsia, the patient is at risk of severe hypernatremia. In cases of CDI associated with trauma or surgery, a typical triphasic response is common. An initial polyuric phase within 24 hours and lasting up to 5 days, due to inhibition of AVP release from the hypothalamic injury, is followed by an antidiuretic phase when stored hormone is released. During this second phase, the patient is at risk of hyponatremia if water intake is excessive. Permanent DI may then occur, although it is transient in up to 60% of postoperative cases.

TABLE 1. **Causes of Diabetes Insipidus**

Central DI (CDI)

Idiopathic
Trauma, neurosurgery
Tumor—primary, metastatic
Infiltrative—Langerhans' cell histiocytosis, sarcoidosis, Wegener's syndrome
Familial—autosomal-dominant, autosomal-recessive, X-linked recessive
Hypoxic or ischemic encephalopathy
Infection

Nephrogenic DI (NDI)

Drugs—lithium, demeclocycline, cidofovir, foscarnet, amphotericin B, aminoglycosides, cisplatin, rifampin
Metabolic—hypokalemia, hypercalcemia
Urinary tract obstruction
Familial—X-linked, autosomal recessive
Amyloidosis, Sjögren's syndrome
Sickle cell disease or trait
Chronic tubulointerstitial renal disease

Pregnancy-Related DI

Pre-existing central or nephrogenic DI
Occurring during pregnancy—vasopressin-responsive, vasopressin-resistant and DDAVP-sensitive, vasopressin- and DDAVP-resistant
Transient DI and fatty liver of pregnancy
Post-partum—associated with Sheehan's syndrome

CDI, central diabetes insipidus; DI, diabetes insipidus; NDI, nephrogenic diabetes insipidus.

Diagnosis

DI must be distinguished from other causes of polyuria including solute diuresis and disorders of thirst. In the latter, polyuria is secondary to the intake of large quantities of water. In addition, polyuria must be distinguished from more common complaints of frequency or nocturia in which the total urine volume is not increased.

Clues to the presence of CDI include the abrupt onset of marked polyuria, particularly after cranial surgery, head trauma, shock, or ischemia and a preference for iced water. Malignancy with hypercalcemia, prolonged lithium use, chronic hypokalemia, or urinary tract obstruction suggest NDI. A family history of DI suggests inherited forms of the disease. Nocturia is usually minimal or absent in psychogenic polydipsia. A solute diuresis is suggested from the recent administration of mannitol, radiocontrast, excessive saline, high protein feedings, or the finding of persistently elevated glucoses.

The initial step in a patient complaining of polyuria is its documentation by the collection of a 24-hour urine specimen for volume, osmolality, and creatinine. A volume of greater than 3 L and a dilute osmolality (<150 to 300 mOsm/kg) is compatible with DI. A spot urine osmolality of less than 150 mOsm/kg is less reliable than that measured on a 24-hour sample. Urine osmolality in a solute diuresis will be hypertonic to plasma (300 to 500 mOsm/kg) and in a mixed water and solute diuresis will be mildly hypotonic (150 to 300 mOsm/kg). Occasionally a volume-depleted patient with DI may show a mildly concentrated urine. Blood studies should include the measurement of electrolytes, blood urea nitrogen (BUN), creatinine, glucose, osmolality, and calcium.

Once DI is confirmed, the type must be determined for proper treatment. In classic cases, the diagnosis will be obvious and further testing is not needed. If the serum sodium is elevated or at the upper limit of normal with a low urine osmolality (or specific gravity less than 1.003), the diagnosis is DI rather than primary polydipsia, and measurement of plasma AVP or a test dose of desmopressin (DDAVP) or aqueous vasopressin (Pitressin) will distinguish central from nephrogenic causes. Serum levels of AVP during pregnancy are not recommended since degradation may occur in vitro, and women should be tested with DDAVP, which, as mentioned, is resistant to vasopressinases. Since most patients with DI allowed access to water do not present with hypertonic dehydration, further testing is frequently necessary. Standard water deprivation testing alone is usually adequate but measuring AVP levels with water deprivation testing may be helpful. Occasionally, particularly with psychiatric patients who do not cooperate with standard water deprivation testing, an osmotic stimulus to AVP secretion can be substituted by the infusion of hypertonic saline at 0.1 mL/kg/minute for no more than 2 hours with measurement of plasma AVP before and after infusion.

Water deprivation testing must be done under careful supervision to avoid rapid dehydration and hypertonicity in patients with severe DI. This testing can be done in the outpatient setting, but ad lib fluid intake must be allowed until 2 hours before beginning the test. Baseline measurements of weight, serum and urine osmolalities, and serum sodium are obtained, then all fluids are withheld. Measurements of body weight and urine osmolality hourly with serum measurements of sodium and osmolality every 2 hours are taken until 3% of body weight is lost, or urine osmolality varies by less than 30 mOsm/kg over 2 to 3 hours despite rising serum osmolality or serum osmolality greater than 295. At this point 5 units of aqueous vasopressin (Pitressin) subcutaneously or 10 μg of desmopressin (DDAVP) by nasal insufflation is administered with measurements of urine osmolality at 30, 60, and 120 minutes.

The normal response to fluid restriction is a two- to fourfold rise in U_{osm} unchanged after exogenous AVP because endogenous AVP effect is maximal when serum osmolality reaches 295 to 300 mOsm/kg. With complete DI, U_{osm} remains low, increasing at least 50% (usually 100% to 800%) following AVP administration with a decrease in urine flow. In partial central DI, U_{osm} usually rises to greater than 300 with fluid restriction with a subnormal response to administered AVP (9% to 50%). In nephrogenic DI some increase (up to 45%) in U_{osm} is observed during water restriction without further change after AVP administration, and the urine remains hypotonic. Polydipsic patients increase urine osmolality to 500 or greater during water restriction and demonstrate no further change with AVP. This subnormal response is due to medullary washout or down-regulation of AVP release from prolonged polydipsia and polyuria. Occasionally it is difficult to distinguish between partial CDI and polydipsia even with measurement of AVP levels. When this occurs, a *closely supervised* 2 to 3 day trial of desmopressin (DDAVP) may be tried; however, the patient must be tested frequently to detect hyponatremia because thirst may not abate. Finally, an MRI should be performed in patients with newly diagnosed central DI or primary polydipsia. In normal patients, a bright signal from the posterior pituitary on T1-weighted images is seen that is absent in central DI; however, the incidence of false-positive and false-negative scans is too high to use MRI alone to diagnose CDI.

Treatment

A treatment plan to control polyuria can be formulated once a diagnosis of DI has been established. If thirst mechanisms are intact and there is no acute illness present, patients will usually be normonatremic and in normal water balance. If the patient is hypernatremic, then water deficits must first be corrected.

Water deficit can be estimated from the patient's current serum sodium, a normal serum sodium (140 mEq/L), and current total body water (TBW) estimated as 60% of body weight. If losses are purely due to water without solute as in DI then:

$$(\mathrm{Na}^+) \times \mathrm{TBW}_{\mathrm{current}} = 140 \times \mathrm{TBW}_{\mathrm{usual}}$$

Water deficit may then be estimated by the formula:

$$\text{Water deficit} = 0.6 \times (\text{body weight [kg]}) \times (([\mathrm{Na}^+]/140) - 1)$$

This value gives an *estimate* of the positive water balance needed to return the serum sodium to 140 mEq/L and does not include ongoing losses. In chronic hypernatremia, the rate of correction that is usually thought to be safe to avoid cerebral edema is 0.5 mEq/L/hour.

For stable patients with central DI, the initial aim of therapy is the allowance of adequate sleep by decreasing nocturia. The synthetic analogue of AVP, desmopressin (DDAVP), is administered once or twice a day by nasal spray or nasal insufflation in an initial dose of 5 μg at bedtime. The usual maintenance dose is 5 to 20 μg once or twice daily. Oral preparations with 5% to 10% of the potency of the nasal preparation are available, although less widely used. The starting dose is 0.05 mg at bedtime with the usual daily dose ranging from 0.1 to 0.8 mg in divided doses. Absorption is decreased by food, although the effect is not usually clinically significant. Occasionally parenteral desmopressin (DDAVP) at 1 to 2 μg intravenously or subcutaneously once or twice daily is preferable in postoperative patients or very young children. The minimal dose to control symptoms is used in order to avoid possible hyponatremia, and patients must be advised to drink only when thirsty. In hospitalized patients with DI or the acute onset of DI from trauma, ischemia or surgery, the use of parenteral aqueous vasopressin (Pitressin) is preferable because the duration of action (4 to 6 hours) is short. Doses of 5 to 10 units can be given just as polyuria returns. In hospitalized patients with DI, inappropriate use of intravenous saline causing conversion of a water diuresis to a mixed water and electrolyte diuresis must be avoided. The ability to metabolize glucose may be exceeded if large volumes of dextrose in water (up to 500 to 1000 mL/hour) are given to keep up with urinary losses before starting AVP. In this case an AVP-resistant osmotic diuresis with marked hyperglycemia can develop. Drugs, such as the oral hypoglycemic chlorpropamide (Diabinese),* 125 to 500 mg daily, clofibrate (Atromid S)* 500 mg four times a day), carbamazepine (Tegretol),* 100 to 300 mg twice daily, hydrochlorothiazide (HydroDIURIL) 25 to 50 mg daily, amiloride (Midamor),* 10 to 20 mg daily, or indomethacin (Indocin),* 50 to 150 mg daily, have been used to augment the action of desmopressin (DDAVP) in complete CDI and may be effective alone in partial CDI. Serious side effects, as well as lack of FDA indications for CDI, limit their role. During pregnancy, desmopressin (DDAVP) is the only effective treatment and is safe, although the dosage required is usually somewhat greater. Therapy for transient DI of pregnancy should be discontinued as soon as DI resolves post partum.

Nephrogenic DI does not respond to desmopressin (DDAVP), clofibrate (Atromid S), chlorpropamide (Diabinese), or carbamazepine (Tegretol). Most patients with NDI have only partial resistance to AVP and some response to pharmacologic doses of desmopressin (DDAVP), but the cost is usually prohibitive. The first step in treating NDI should be an attempt to correct the underlying disorder, such as hypercalcemia, or to discontinue an offending drug, such as lithium. This may cause resolution of DI. If the cause cannot be eliminated or if DI is permanent (for example, from lithium), thiazide diuretics such as hydrochlorothiazide (HydroDIURIL) 25 to 100 mg daily and salt restriction to cause mild volume depletion and increased proximal tubular reabsorption with decreased distal delivery are the mainstays of therapy. Amiloride (Midamor),* a potassium sparing diuretic, in a dose of 10 to 20 mg daily can be additive to thiazide diuretics and is used in lithium-induced reversible NDI because it helps block lithium uptake by the distal nephron. NSAIDs, such as indomethacin (Indocin),* 50 to 150 mg daily, inhibit prostaglandin synthesis and increase concentrating ability by removing the antagonistic action of prostaglandins on AVP. The use of NSAIDs with thiazide diuretics may be additive, but renal function must be monitored to avoid toxicity. Additionally, a low protein, low sodium diet to decrease urinary solute excretion can significantly reduce the daily urine volume. To illustrate, if urinary solute is 900 mOsm/day and maximum urine osmolality is 150 mOsm/kg, urine output will be 6 L/day (900/150 = 6). If urine solute can be decreased to 500 mOsm/day by sodium and protein restriction, urine output will decrease significantly to 3.3 L/day.

*Not FDA approved for this indication.

HYPERPARATHYROIDISM AND HYPOPARATHYROIDISM

method of
DAVID J. HOSKING, M.D.
City Hospital
Nottingham, United Kingdom

Hypercalcemia and hypocalcemia are commonly detected as a result of routine autoanalyzer screening. Problems most commonly arise because of difficulties with the diagnosis of the cause of the abnormality rather than from issues of management, which are usually straightforward.

HYPERPARATHYROIDISM

Primary hyperparathyroidism is a relatively common problem (about 1:1000 over the age of 50 years are affected in out-patient surveys) and is often detected coincidentally from biochemical tests performed for other conditions. Most patients are asymptomatic or show nonspecific clinical features and will be treated conservatively, but recent improvements in parathyroid imaging and the advent of minimally invasive surgery have led to a re-evaluation of the management of this condition.

Clinical Features and Evaluation of Disease Activity

Most students remember the symptoms of hyperparathyroidism as "stones, bones, and abdominal groans" but about one half the patients will be asymptomatic, although this needs to be defined objectively by appropriate investigation. Following restoration of normocalcemia by parathyroidectomy, many patients will recognize that they had experienced nonspecific complaints such as weakness, lethargy, abdominal discomfort, and constipation preoperatively.

The importance of the clinical symptoms is that together with the level of serum calcium, they determine the need for parathyroidectomy. The most important symptoms are those centered on PTH target organ dysfunction, and include enlarging renal calculi, nephrocalcinosis or renal impairment, any episode of acute pancreatitis, and significant bone disease. Clinical parathyroid bone disease is rare, but these patients tend to lose cortical bone and dual energy x-ray densitometry (DXA), particularly at the hip, is an important way of defining the skeletal impact of excess PTH. A pragmatic approach to the need for parathyroidectomy would be to use interventional criteria similar to those for osteoporosis in the non-hyperparathyroid population such as a T score less than −2.5 together with age and other relevant risk factors. Because many patients are elderly, a Z score less than −2 would be a reasonable indication of the degree of bone loss, independent of the effects of aging. Other less certain indications include hypercalciuria (>10 mmol/day) and neuropsychiatric symptoms,

TABLE 1. **Common Causes of Hypercalcemia**

Hyperparathyroidism
Malignancy
Chronic renal failure
Milk alkali syndrome
Familial hypocalciuric hyperparathyroidism
Sarcoidosis
Vitamin D intoxication
Chronic lithium therapy
High turnover bone disease with immobilization

such as depression, confusion, and dementia. Some patients will fail to comply with conservative treatment or choose surgical versus conservative treatment.

The level of serum calcium at which parathyroidectomy is indicated in an otherwise asymptomatic patient is uncertain but is generally taken, somewhat arbitrarily, as a value above 3.0 mmol/L. This degree of hypercalcemia will be accompanied by impaired water reabsorption by the kidney leading to an increased risk of dehydration, an acute hypercalcemic crisis, and renal failure with cardiovascular collapse.

Measurement of PTH is critical to the confirmation of parathyroid overactivity and exclusion of other common causes of hypercalcemia that are usually associated with suppressed PTH secretion (Table 1). Most commercial assays measure both intact 1-84 PTH and a large N-terminal 7-84 PTH fragment with the result that although 90% of patients will have a clearly raised value, some will have a PTH in the upper half of the reference range. This is consistent with the diagnosis of hyperparathyroidism because a normal value is inappropriate in the presence of a raised calcium value. Measurement of two consecutive 24-hour urines for creatinine and calcium is essential to exclude the uncommon condition of familial hypocalciuric hyperparathyroidism, where the urinary calcium-to-creatinine clearance is less than 0.01 with a PTH that is often normal but may be raised in 5% to 10% of cases. The importance of this investigation is that the hyperparathyroidism is due to a cell defect and does not respond to a localized parathyroidectomy.

There have been substantial advances in parathyroid imaging in the last few years, largely driven by the interest in minimally invasive surgery where accurate localization of a parathyroid adenoma is essential. Dual isotope subtraction scanning using ^{99m}Technetium-sestamibi has 90% sensitivity and almost 99% specificity for a solitary parathyroid adenoma but performs less well where there is multiglandular disease. Parathyroid imaging is an important investigation in patients with failed or recurrent hyperparathyroidism, but it is uncertain whether it is needed in previously untreated cases where an experienced parathyroid surgeon has a better than 90% probability of finding the adenoma, particularly if it is small.

Differential Diagnosis

Separation of hyperparathyroidism from the other causes of hypercalcemia requires a careful history and physical examination combined with appropriate biochemical and radiologic investigations. Malignancy is often detected by these methods, although a small PTHrP-secreting tumor, usually of squamous origin in the head or neck, can cause diagnostic problems because both clinically and pathophysiologically it can mimic primary hyperparathyroidism but can be identified by the combination of a suppressed PTH with a raised PTHrP. Chronic renal failure with tertiary hyperparathyroidism or overtreatment with hydroxylated vitamin D metabolites should not present problems of diagnosis, but milk alkali syndrome requires more scrutiny because patients may deny the self-medication. Here the critical test is to demonstrate the presence of a metabolic alkalosis (raised bicarbonate) in the presence of renal failure (which would normally be accompanied by a metabolic acidosis). There may be clinical or radiologic evidence of sarcoidosis, but together with vitamin D intoxication, it is one of the few causes of hypercalcemia that responds to glucocorticoid therapy (prednisolone 40 mg/d). Chronic lithium (Eskalith) therapy may be accompanied by mild hypercalcemia, which may regress if the mental state permits drug withdrawal but some patients develop primary hyperparathyroidism. Pagets disease or severe thyrotoxicosis may rarely be accompanied by hypercalcemia if the patient becomes immobile, but the underlying disease will usually be obvious.

Treatment

Surgical parathyroidectomy is currently the only definitive treatment for hyperparathyroidism, although many patients will be managed conservatively. The serum calcium should be measured on the day before surgery to confirm that it is still at a level requiring treatment. A bilateral neck exploration is the standard approach but because about 90% of patients will have a single adenoma, many surgeons will perform a unilateral exploration if they identify a normal parathyroid on the side of the adenoma. A bilateral approach is needed for failed or recurrent hyperparathyroidism or where there is the possibility of hyperplasia. Minimally invasive parathyroidectomy through a small (<4 cm) incision, often under local anesthesia, as a day case is an emerging technique but is critically dependent on careful case selection and parathyroid imaging. Patients with parathyroid hyperplasia, multiglandular disease, and abnormal neck anatomy are not suited for this technique, and in some studies this has excluded 33% to 75%. Up to 70% of patients will develop transient hypoparathyroidism on the first postoperative day but mild hypocalcemia (2.0 to 2.2 mmol/L) does not require treatment and patients usually recover within a week. Patients with significant parathyroid bone disease may develop more severe, symptomatic hypocalcemia due to a transient uncoupling of bone formation and resorption (hungry bone syndrome) which may last 6 to 8 weeks. Treatment consists of calcitriol (Rocaltrol), 1 to 2 μg daily with calcium supplements 1 to 2 g/d and a high calcium diet. Permanent hypoparathyroidism is rare in experienced hands but is more common after re-exploration for resistant or recurrent disease.

TABLE 2. **Common Causes of Hypoparathyroidism**

Postsurgical damage
Hypomagnesemia—alcohol excess, thiazides, severe diarrhea
Parathyroid infiltration/damage
  iron or copper overload
  metastatic disease
  ^{131}I
Genetic syndromes
  failure of parathyroid gland development
  pseudohypoparathyroidism
Idiopathic parathyroid failure

Conservative treatment of primary hyperparathyroidism involves regular monitoring of serum calcium, creatinine, and blood pressure (every 6 months), PTH and 24-hour urine calcium (every 12 months) and DXA (every 2 to 3 years) until bone mineral density is stable or the rate of loss can be established. Abdominal radiography and/or ultrasound will also be required to evaluate renal calculi with a frequency that will be determined on clinical grounds. Osteoporosis and renal calculi should be treated on the same basis and with the same drugs as for the non-hyperparathyroid patient.

HYPOPARATHYROIDISM

Clinical Features

Although some patients will present with symptoms of hypocalcemia, the majority will be detected as a result of routine screening. Paresthesias of the finger tips, toes, or around the mouth are typical as is carpopedal spasm, although this is seen much more commonly in normocalcemic individuals with a respiratory alkalosis due to hysterical hyperventilation. Epileptic seizures can occur and these can be either tonic-clonic seizures or partial seizures where consciousness is altered but not lost. Psychosis, laryngeal spasm, and extrapyramidal movement disorders are rare and all the symptoms seem to depend on the rate of change of serum calcium rather than upon its absolute level. As will be discussed in the next section, it is also important to look for evidence of the primary conditions which may cause parathyroid failure (Table 2).

Diagnosis

The first step is to review the history (Figure 1) looking particularly for evidence of previous thyroid surgery, significant alcohol excess, or bone pain. Hypocalcemia occurs as an early event after surgery for hyperparathyroidism as a consequence of persistent, and usually increased, bone formation at a time when bone resorption is low due to the rapid reduction in PTH (the hungry bone syndrome). It may also occur after thyroidectomy where thyrotoxicosis has only recently been controlled and bone turnover is still high. More commonly, hypoparathyroidism develops as a late feature of thyroid surgery as a result of progressive scarring and presumably progressive ischemia of the parathyroid glands. Patients who have had repeat thyroidectomies are particularly at risk for this complication. Hypocalcemia is a serious complication of acute pancreatitis and, if severe, indicates a bad prognosis but rarely causes diagnostic difficulties. Magnesium deficiency leads to reversible (functional) parathyroid failure and is most common in alcoholics, as a complication of severe diarrhea and complicating some diuretic (thiazide) and cytotoxic (cisplatin) therapy. It is a predominantly intracellular ion and serum levels are an unreliable guide to deficiency, which has to be confirmed by retention (>50% over 24 hours) of an intravenous magnesium load (0.1 mmol/kg).

Bone pain does not occur in hypoparathyroidism and its presence usually indicates osteomalacia, which is particularly common in the elderly and those with poor diets and insufficient sunlight exposure. Much less commonly severe hypocalcemia may complicate sclerotic metastases from carcinoma of the prostate or breast and, very rarely, multiple myeloma. It may also occur as a transient phenomenon as lytic metastases heal with chemotherapy.

The clinical history and examination will usually give clues to the underlying cause of the hypocalcemia but the next step is to send blood for serum phosphate, creatinine, alkaline phosphatase and magnesium (Figure 2). Fasting samples are best because hypophosphatemia may be masked by the postprandial rise in phosphate and it is also cost effective to include liver function tests in this request if there is a question of alcoholism or malignancy because this will be critical in the interpretation of the alkaline phosphatase. If renal failure seems likely then urea and electrolytes need to be included as well as a hematology request for a full blood count because this will detect the

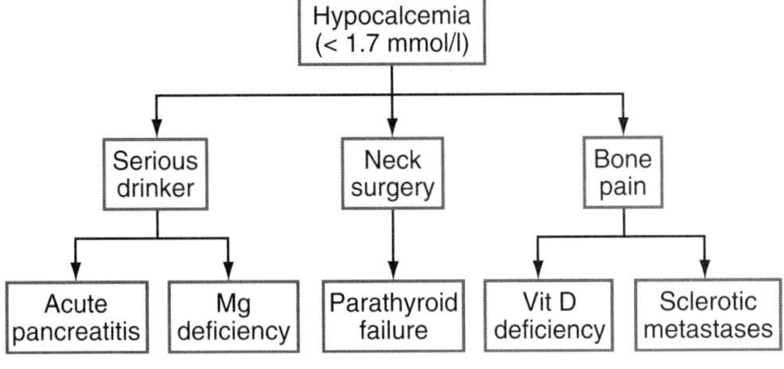

Figure 1. Diagnosis.

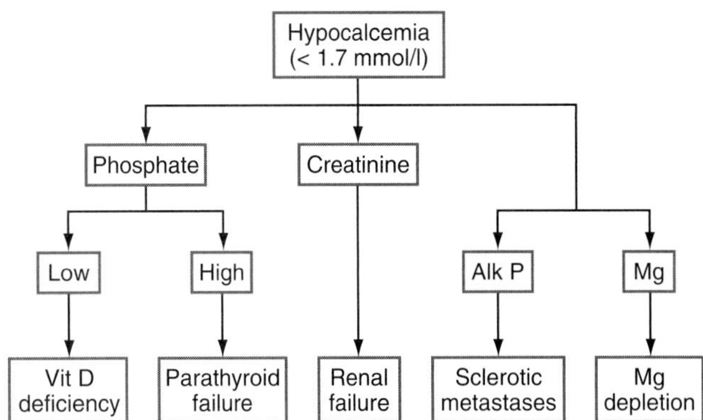

Figure 2. Biochemistry.

normochromic normocytic anemia of chronic renal failure or the macrocytosis of (current) heavy alcohol consumption, liver disease, and hypothyroidism. The other important request is for a serum PTH which will be high in vitamin D deficiency, renal failure, and sclerotic metastases but low in parathyroid failure and magnesium deficiency. Further investigation, such as skeletal radiology (pseudofractures of osteomalacia or evidence of sclerotic metastases) or hospital referral will depend on the results of the initial tests. The biochemistry of hypoparathyroidism in the presence of a raised PTH suggests the rare condition of pseudohypoparathyroidism due to end organ resistance and these patients may show features of Albrights Hereditary Osteodystrophy (short stature, short metacarpals, truncal obesity, and basal ganglia calcification). Patients with sclerotic metastases will usually, but not always, show clinical evidence of the underlying tumor, have bone pain, and a low serum phosphate level. A strong suspicion of hypomagnesemia requires confirmation by a magnesium retention test.

Treatment

Hypocalcemia never responds to treatment with oral calcium because without vitamin D it will not be absorbed from the upper small bowel (Figure 3). Active calcium transport in hypoparathyroidism can be corrected with calcitriol or alfacalcidol (1 μg daily) although this latter preparation requires hepatic 25 hydroxylation and this may be impaired in magnesium deficiency. Net calcium absorption can then be increased to the level required to maintain normocalcemia by the addition of calcium supplements (1 to 1.5 g/d in divided doses). The advantage of using a combination of low-dose vitamin D metabolites with calcium supplementation is that the level of serum calcium depends on a high net calcium absorption and, if hypercalcemia develops, it responds quickly to a reduction in calcium intake. Hypoparathyroid patients need a high throughput of calcium to compensate for the lack of PTH-regulated distal renal tubular calcium reabsorption, which means that they have a high urinary calcium excretion when normocalcemic. However, renal stone disease is uncommon under these circumstances. Where there is concern about hypercalciuria, it is worth adding a thiazide diuretic (bendroflumethiazide [Naturetin],* 2.5 to 5 mg/d), which may limit distal renal tubular calcium loss and maintain normocalcemia at a lower urinary calcium level. Older patients can often be controlled with low-dose calcitriol without calcium supplements because the age-related decline in glomerular filtration rate limits renal calcium excretion.

An alternative approach is to use high doses of vitamin D alone but calcitriol and alfacalcidol† stimulate bone turnover and if hypercalcemia develops, it may resolve more slowly because of the skeletal contribution to extracellular fluid calcium. Resolution can be speeded up by treatment with prednisolone 10 mg every 8 hours.

All types of hypoparathyroidism respond equally well to calcitriol and calcium supplementation, but the more severe the hypocalcemia then the longer it will take to achieve normocalcemia, although even the most severely affected patients can be expected to respond within one week. In the presence of severe symptomatic hypocalcemia a more rapid response can be achieved by covering the first 2 to 3 days of oral treatment with a calcium infusion (100 mL 10% calcium gluconate in 1 L of 5% dextrose over 24 hours). This is unlikely to cause hypercalcemia because the labile pool of calcium in bone will be depleted and this will take up the infused calcium. As the serum calcium rises, the filtered load will increase and renal excretion will limit the development of hypercalcemia.

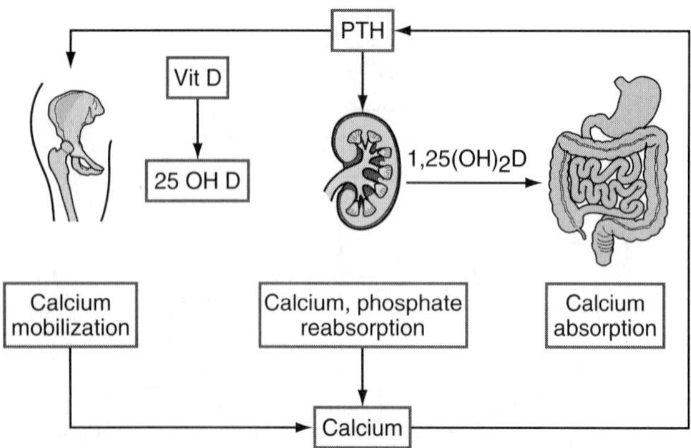

Figure 3. PTH-Vitamin D endocrine system.

*Not FDA approved for this indication.
†Not available in the United States.

PRIMARY ALDOSTERONISM

method of
MICHAEL STOWASSER, M.B.B.S., PH.D.
Hypertension Unit
University of Queensland Department of Medicine
Princess Alexandra Hospital
Brisbane, Australia

Once considered rare, primary aldosteronism (PAL) is now thought to be the most common potentially curable and specifically treatable form of hypertension, possibly accounting for 5% to 10% of hypertensives. This change in perspective followed improvements in screening methods, and recognition that most patients with PAL lack hypokalemia and many have plasma aldosterone levels that lie within the normal range. Reliable detection and optimal management requires that (1) the diagnosis is considered in all hypertensives; (2) samples are collected under standardized conditions of diet, posture, and time of day; (3) medications known to alter volume-dependent hormone levels are avoided or their effects taken into account; and (4) reliable methods are used to confirm PAL and determine the subtype.

PATHOGENESIS

By definition, aldosterone production in PAL is excessive to the body's requirements and relatively autonomous of its normal chronic regulator, renin-angiotensin II (AII). This results in excessive sodium reabsorption via amiloride-sensitive epithelial sodium channels within the distal nephron (leading to hypertension), and continues in the face of renin-AII suppression. Urinary loss of potassium, exchanged for sodium at the distal nephron, may eventually result in hypokalemia if severe and prolonged enough.

Pathologic expression of PAL is highly variable, with different histologic subtypes frequently coexisting in the one patient. The most common is adrenal cortical hyperplasia (diffuse or nodular), followed by solitary adenoma (often associated with hyperplasia of zona glomerulosa), and adrenocortical carcinoma is rare. Adrenal venous sampling (AVS) studies have shown that autonomous aldosterone production may be bilateral or even contralateral to the side of an apparently solitary adrenal nodule, or unilateral in patients with bilateral hyperplasia. From a management point of view, it is more important to differentiate subtypes based on their functional (rather than pathologic) characteristics (as described in the following sections).

A dominantly inherited and glucocorticoid-remediable variety of PAL (familial hyperaldosteronism type I, FH-I) is caused by a "hybrid gene" mutation composed of 5′ sequences derived from the 11β-hydroxylase gene (*CYP11B1*) and 3′ sequences derived from the aldosterone synthase gene (*CYP11B2*). The "hybrid gene" encodes an enzyme that synthesizes aldosterone. Unlike *CYP11B2*, however, it is regulated by ACTH and not AII by virtue of its ACTH-responsive *CYP11B1* regulatory sequences. Aldosterone production in FH-I is therefore regulated by ACTH rather than by AII, and is therefore glucocorticoid-suppressible. Unlike *CYP11B2*, the "hybrid gene" is expressed not only in zona glomerulosa, but also in zona fasciculata, where cortisol is available as a substrate for its gene product activity; this probably explains excessive production of 18-hydroxy- and 18-oxo-cortisol ("hybrid steroids") in FH-I.

A second, more common familial variety of PAL (FH-II) is neither glucocorticoid-remediable nor associated with the "hybrid gene," and is clinically, biochemically and morphologically indistinguishable from apparently sporadic PAL. Its genetic bases remain uncertain, but in one affected family a genome-wide search revealed linkage with a locus in chromosome 7p22.

Although morbidity in PAL mainly results from hypertension, recent experimental and clinical evidence suggests that aldosterone excess can bring about adverse cardiovascular sequelae (remodeling and fibrosis) independently of its hypertensive effects, possibly by acting directly on myocardial or vascular cells or indirectly through other mediators (e.g., AII, endothelin and plasminogen activation inhibitor type 1). In animal studies, both aldosterone excess and a high salt intake appear to be necessary for induction of cardiac fibrosis. Coronary vasculitis appears to be an early manifestation.

CLINICAL FEATURES

Hypertension in PAL may be mild or severe. In FH-I, hypertension is frequently of early onset and may be severe enough to cause early death, usually from hemorrhagic stroke. Family screening in FH-I and FH-II has revealed highly diverse phenotypes with some patients being normotensive, suggesting that PAL may evolve through a preclinical phase. Most patients with PAL are normokalemic. When hypokalemia does occur, it may be associated with nocturia, polyuria, muscle weakness, muscle cramps, or palpitations.

SCREENING

Measurement of the plasma aldosterone to plasma renin activity (PRA) ratio (ARR) is widely regarded as being the most reliable available means of screening for PAL. However, false positive results occur in patients receiving β-adrenoceptor blocking agents, α-methyldopa, and clonidine, patients with renal impairment and in the elderly. False negatives may be encountered among patients with PAL who are hypokalemic or in the presence of severe dietary salt restriction, renovascular hypertension, or malignant hypertension, and in patients taking diuretics (including spironolactone), dihydropyridine calcium channel antagonists, or AII receptor antagonists. Angiotensin-converting enzyme (ACE) inhibitors appear much less capable of stimulating PRA in patients with PAL than in those without, but still have the potential to cause false negative ratios.

Because plasma potassium is a powerful chronic regulator of aldosterone production, hypokalemia may be associated with false negative ratios and should be corrected before screening. Sensitivity of the ARR is improved if patients maintain a liberal dietary salt intake before testing, and by collecting samples midmorning (approximately 9–10 AM) from seated patients who have been ambulant for at least 2 hours. It is advisable to cease diuretics (including spironolactone) for at least 4 weeks, and β-adrenoreceptor blockers, α-methyldopa, clonidine, dihydropyridine-type calcium channel antagonists, ACE inhibitors, and AII-receptor antagonists for at least 2 weeks before testing, if possible, substituting when necessary with other agents (such as hydralazine [Apresoline], prazosin [Minipress], or slow-release forms of verapamil [Calan SR]) that have a lesser effect on the ratio.

Useful information can sometimes be obtained even when patients are still taking medications known to interfere. A raised ARR in a patient taking a diuretic, dihydropyridine calcium channel blocker, ACE inhibitor, or AII receptor antagonist is strongly suggestive of PAL, whereas a normal ARR in a patient taking a β-adrenoceptor blocker would make the diagnosis highly unlikely.

An ARR greater than 30 (plasma aldosterone in ng/100 mL, PRA in ng/mL/h) is suggestive of PAL and is highly specific. Others regard a ratio of >20 in combination with a plasma aldosterone concentration of >15 ng/dL as a positive screen for PAL, but this approach has the potential to miss patients with lower plasma aldosterone levels.

CONFIRMING THE DIAGNOSIS

Fludrocortisone (Florinef) suppression testing (FST) is generally considered the most reliable means of confirming PAL. Within the Greenslopes and Princess Alexandra Hospital Hypertension Units (GHHU and PAHHU), failure of upright (1000 h) plasma aldosterone to suppress to less than 6 ng/100 mL at the conclusion of 4 days of administration of a high sodium diet, slow-release sodium chloride (Slow Na, 30 mmoles thrice daily with meals), and fludrocortisone acetate (0.1 mg every 6 hours) is regarded as diagnostic, provided that on day 4 (1) upright PRA is suppressed (<1 ng/mL/h); (2) plasma cortisol levels are lower at 1000 h than at 0700 h, thereby excluding an acute ACTH rise that may have prevented aldosterone suppression; and (3) plasma potassium is in the normal range, achieved by giving sufficient slow-release potassium chloride* 6 hourly to keep levels (measured 3–4 times daily) close to 4.0 mmol/L.

At the Mayo Clinic, a 24-h urinary aldosterone level of more than 12 μg/d on the third day of oral salt loading (sufficient to achieve a urine sodium excretion of more than 200 mmole/day, with enough potassium supplementation to maintain normokalemia) is regarded as diagnostic.

Other groups measure plasma aldosterone at the conclusion of an intravenous infusion of 0.9% saline (usually 2 L over 4 hours). Levels regarded as diagnostic for PAL have varied from >5 to >10 ng/100 mL. This approach requires only a brief outpatient visit, but, in the GHHU's experience, lacks sensitivity for detection of PAL (including surgically curable forms).

DIFFERENTIATING THE SUBTYPES

Genetic testing of peripheral blood for the "hybrid gene" is diagnostic for FH-I, and is performed on all patients with positive FST at GHHU and PAHHU. Demonstration of marked, sustained plasma aldosterone suppression during 4 days administration of dexamethasone* (0.5 mg 6 hourly) is strongly suggestive of the diagnosis. The presence of adrenal mass lesions on computed tomography (CT) scanning does not exclude FH-I. Elevated levels of "hybrid steroids," although highly sensitive for FH-I, are not specific, occurring in most patients with the AII-unresponsive variety of aldosterone-producing adenoma (APA).

For patients without FH-I, optimal management relies on the differentiation of those in whom autonomous aldosterone production is confined to one adrenal (consistent with APA), in which case unilateral adrenalectomy would be expected to substantially improve or cure hypertension, from those with bilateral production (consistent with bilateral adrenal hyperplasia [BAH]). Adrenal CT lacks reliability as it misses many APAs yet may demonstrate nonfunctioning nodules in the contralateral gland and apparently unilateral lesions in patients with BAH. Responsiveness of aldosterone to upright posture or AII infusion occurs in most patients with BAH, but also in those with AII-responsive APA, which makes up more than 50% of APAs removed at GHHU and PAHHU. Both BAH and AII-responsive APA are associated with normal "hybrid steroid" levels. For these reasons, AVS, with comparison of adrenal with peripheral venous aldosterone:cortisol ratios, is the only dependable way to differentiate bilateral from unilateral PAL, and at GHHU and PAHHU is performed on all patients with positive FST (other than those with FH-I).

Adrenal CT is useful for detecting large (>2.5 cm) mass lesions that may warrant removal based on malignant potential.

TREATMENT

In FH-I, hypertension is readily controlled by giving glucocorticoids in low doses (e.g., 0.125–0.5 mg of dexamethasone* per day), which do not cause Cushingoid side effects. Complete suppression of ACTH-regulated aldosterone production is not usually necessary. Family screening by genetic testing should be undertaken to identify affected relatives.

For patients who lateralize on AVS, unilateral adrenalectomy (now performed laparoscopically with faster recovery than the open approach) results in cure of hypertension in 50%–60% and improvement in the remainder. Time taken to achieve maximal blood pressure (BP) response varies markedly (from a few days to over 12 months), and determines the rate at which antihypertensive drugs may be gradually withdrawn.

At GHHU and PAHHU, patients undergo FST 1 to 3 months postoperatively to assess the remaining adrenal for autonomy of aldosterone production. All patients lateralizing preoperatively on AVS have shown either biochemical cure (70%) of PAL or improvement (30%) on postoperative FST. Patients with positive FST and residual hypertension demonstrate excellent responses to small doses of amiloride (Midamor)* or spironolactone (Aldactone).

For patients demonstrating bilateral aldosterone production on AVS, treatment with aldosterone antagonists usually brings about substantial improvement in hypertension control, although generally not as gratifying as the BP response to unilateral adrenalectomy in patients who lateralize. Only small doses of spironolactone (12.5–25 mg twice daily) or amiloride (2.5–7.5 mg twice daily) are required for optimal therapeutic effect, starting with the lowest dose and waiting several weeks before increasing. Even at these low doses, side effects relating to actions on sex steroid

*Not FDA approved for this indication.

*Not FDA approved for this indication.

receptors (gynecomastia, menstrual irregularities, and reduced libido) can occur in patients taking spironolactone. The recent availability of a more selective aldosterone antagonist (eplerenone [Inspra])* therefore represents an important potential therapeutic advance, but clinical experience in PAL remains limited. Aldosterone antagonists must be used with caution in patients with impaired renal function. In such patients, concurrent administration of a potassium-wasting diuretic in low dosage can be used to avoid hyperkalemia, monitoring potassium and creatinine levels carefully.

*Not FDA approved for this indication.

HYPOPITUITARISM

method of
ROSHANAK MONZAVI, M.D.
Fellow, Division of Pediatric Endocrinology, Diabetes, and Metabolism
Keck School of Medicine, University of Southern California

and

MITCHELL E. GEFFNER, M.D.
Division of Pediatric Endocrinology, Diabetes, and Metabolism
Keck School of Medicine, University of Southern California

Hypopituitarism is a rare condition that refers to a decrease or absence of function of two or more hormones produced by the pituitary gland. When all pituitary hormone production is deficient or decreased, the term *panhypopituitarism* is applied.

Anatomy

The pituitary gland is located below the optic chiasm and is attached to the hypothalamus above by a thin stalk. The anterior portion of the pituitary, the adenohypophysis, is derived from the Rathke pouch and receives regulatory signals from the hypothalamus through the portal system, resulting in the production of growth hormone (GH), thyroid-stimulating hormone (TSH), adrenocorticotropic hormone (ACTH), luteinizing hormone (LH), follicle-stimulating hormone (FSH), and prolactin. The posterior portion of the pituitary, the neurohypophysis, receives neural signals via axons that originate in the hypothalamus, and is responsible for the production of antidiuretic hormone (ADH) and oxytocin.

Etiology

Hypopituitarism is a rare condition, resulting from either congenital or acquired etiologies, that occurs in between 1 and 1.5 per 100,000 individuals. Congenital hypopituitarism, which usually presents in early childhood, may occur as a result of birth trauma, in association with midline anatomic defects such as optic nerve hypoplasia (with or without absence of the septum pellucidum), or secondary to mutations of genes that encode for various pituitary transcription factors. Acquired hypopituitarism in either children or adults may result from tumors, hydrocephalus, or other mass effect, radiation or surgery to the head, trauma, vascular abnormalities, infiltrative disease, and infarction or hemorrhage. Whereas in children hypopituitarism usually results from primary hypothalamic disease or dysfunction, new-onset hypopituitarism in adults may stem from either pituitary or hypothalamic pathology.

PRESENTATION, DIAGNOSIS, AND TREATMENT OF HYPOPITUITARISM IN ADULTS

When hypopituitarism is caused by an acute process such as infarction or hemorrhage, it may produce sudden headache, hypotension, collapse, and may even be life-threatening. However, in most cases (e.g., when caused by tumor, surgery, radiation, or trauma), the onset of hypopituitarism is insidious and symptoms may be non-specific, such as fatigue, lack of sense of well-being, and weight gain. Symptoms are, by and large, related to which hormonal deficiencies are present. Each hormone deficiency will be discussed in the context of clinical presentation, diagnosis, and treatment (Tables 1 and 2).

Growth Hormone Deficiency

Adults with GH deficiency (GHD) present with unfavorable body composition, including reduced lean body mass and increased fat mass, especially in the abdominal area; elevated serum cholesterol, and decreased bone mineral density (BMD) (Table 1). Functional correlates of this presentation include decreased muscle strength and exercise tolerance, and impaired sense of well-being. GHD is present in almost all cases of "idiopathic" and organic hypopituitarism in both children and adults, but may present in childhood as an isolated and idiopathic deficiency; however, this latter entity appears to be frequently overdiagnosed. The existence of the syndrome of idiopathic, isolated GHD in adults has yet to be convincingly shown and, in most cases under consideration, low stimulated GH levels appear to be secondary to associated obesity as opposed to true GHD.

Diagnosis of adult GHD requires GH provocative testing after an overnight fast. As suggested previously, GH stimulation is required in patients previously diagnosed with childhood-onset, idiopathic, isolated GHD; recent studies suggest that as many as 67% of these individuals will retest as normal. However, in adults with previously documented childhood-onset GHD, in the setting of multiple pituitary hormone deficiencies or a radiologic abnormality involving the sella or suprasellar region, retesting for adult GHD is

TABLE 1. **Diagnosis and Treatment of Growth Hormone Deficiency**

Hormone Deficiency	Common Diagnostic Modalities	Treatment
Growth Hormone (GH)	GH stimulation tests: Insulin tolerance test (ITT): IV Regular insulin bolus at 0.05–0.1 unit/kg (use lower dose when there is higher index of suspicion for GHD). Measure plasma glucose (bedside and in laboratory) and serum GH levels at 0, 15, 30, 45, 60, and 90 min (some investigators will also obtain a 15-min sample, as "high" baseline GH values, which reflect detection of a random spontaneous secretory burst, may preclude further increase in response to pharmacologic provocation and make test results difficult to interpret). The test can be terminated by administration of oral or IV glucose if serious hypoglycemia occurs or is imminent; the results will still be valid as long as adequate hypoglycemia was attained. GHRH/arginine: GHRH as Geref Diagnostic by IV bolus at 1 µg/kg (maximum 100 µg) and l-arginine HCl (10%) at 0.5 g/kg (maximum 30 g) by IV infusion over 30 min; measure serum GH levels every 15 min for 90 min. Arginine (alone): as above Glucagon: 0.5–1 mg given IM or SQ; measure serum GH levels every 30 min for 4 hours.	Somatropin (Genotropin, Humatrope, Norditropin, Nutropin, and Saizen in the United States) Dose: 0.15–0.3 mg SC daily; maximum: 1 mg/d.

TABLE 2. **Diagnosis and Treatment of Other Pituitary Hormone Deficiencies**

Luteinizing hormone (LH) Follicle-stimulating hormone (FSH)	Random serum LH and FSH Random serum testosterone in men Random serum estradiol in women GnRH (Factrel) stimulation test: 100 µg IV GnRH as bolus; measure serum LH and FSH levels at 0, 20, 40, 60, and 90 min; measure estradiol or testosterone at baseline.	**Women:** Combination estrogen and progesterone therapy; multiple single and combined hormone therapy formulations are available, including estrogen and progesterone derivatives in oral contraceptives. **Men:** Testosterone: Intramuscular depot form [testosterone enanthate (Delatestryl) or testosterone cypionate (Andro-Cyp, DepAndro, and Depotest)]; dose: 50–400 mg IM every 2–4 weeks Topical patch (Testoderm and Androderm); dose: 4-mg or 6-mg patch daily Topical gel (AndroGel); dose: 5G packet (= 5 mg) daily
Thyroid-stimulating hormone (TSH)	Serum-free T_4 and TSH TRH (Thypinone) stimulation test: IV TRH bolus of 200–500 µg; measure serum TSH at 0, 20, and 60 min Serum TSH measurements every 30 min between 23:00–02:00 to detect twofold nocturnal physiologic surge	Levo-thyroxine (Synthroid, Levothroid, and Levoxyl) Dose: 75-200 µg PO daily
Adrenocorticotropic hormone (ACTH)	ITT: See above under GH; measure serum cortisol in addition to GH at 0 and 60 min. CRH stimulation test: CRH (Acthrel) 1 µg/kg; measure plasma ACTH and serum cortisol levels at 0, 15, 30, 45, and 60 min Short ACTH stimulation test: synthetic ACTH 1-24 (Cortrosyn) 250 µg IV bolus; measure serum cortisol levels at 0 and 60 min Short low-dose ACTH stimulation test: ACTH 1-24 (Cortrosyn) at 1 µg IV bolus; measure serum cortisol levels at 0 and 60 min Long ACTH test: ACTH 1-24 (Cortrosyn) 250 µg by IV infusion over 8–12 hr on 3 consecutive days; measure urine 17-OHCS and creatinine before and on days 1, 2, and 3	Hydrocortisone (Cortef) Dose: 20–30 mg/d divided in two ([2/3] in AM, [1/3] in PM) or three doses ([1/2], [1/4], [1/4]) per day Alternatives: prednisone, dexamethasone
Antidiuretic hormone (ADH)	Water deprivation test: 8 hr of water deprivation followed by 10 µg intranasal or 2 µg IM DDAVP; multiple measurements of serum and urine osmolalities during and after water deprivation test	Desmopressin (DDAVP) Oral: 50–1000 µg/d Intranasal: 5–60 µg/d Subcutaneous: 2–4 µg/d Usually given in divided doses

probably not necessary, because persistence of GHD into adulthood occurs in >90% of these cases.

In adults, the insulin tolerance test (ITT) is the gold standard for evaluation of GHD. A stimulated serum GH level of >5 μg/L is considered normal, and a level of <3 μg/L is considered diagnostic of severe GHD by the Growth Hormone Research Society (GHRS) and of <5 μg/L by the U.S. Food and Drug Administration. The ITT is contraindicated in patients with electrocardiographic evidence or a history of ischemic heart disease, and in patients with a known seizure disorder. Alternative testing protocols in adults employ the combination of arginine and GH-releasing hormone (GHRH), or, less often, arginine or glucagon as single agents. Cut-offs to define GHD using these other agents are currently being developed and may be higher than those used with the ITT, depending on the potency of the stimulus. Although potentially useful in children, measurement of the serum levels of the GH surrogates, IGF-I and IGFBP-3, alone is not reliable in diagnosing GHD in adults. However, normal levels of IGF-I and IGFBP-3 mitigate against a diagnosis of GHD in obese adults despite their expected low GH response to pharmacologic stimulation.

The treatment for GHD is synthetic human GH, somatropin (Genotropin, Humatrope, Norditropin, Nutropin, and Saizen in the United States). The recommended starting dose for treatment of adult GHD, as per the GHRS, is 0.15–0.3 mg/d given by subcutaneous (SC) injection with a 31-gauge needle. This dose can be increased gradually based on clinical and biochemical response, typically not exceeding 1.0 mg/d. Treatment efficacy may be monitored by measuring IGF-I and IGFBP-3, the latter being less useful in adults than in children. Side effects of GH seen in adults include fluid retention, mild arthralgias, and insulin resistance. There is no evidence that GH therapy in adults increases cancer risk. However, active malignancy remains a contraindication for GH therapy. Other contraindications include benign intracranial hypertension, proliferative or preproliferative diabetic retinopathy, and pregnancy.

Gonadotropin Deficiency

Hypothalamic gonadotropin-releasing hormone (GnRH) or pituitary gonadotropin (LH or FSH) deficiency may occur as an isolated entity; as part of a constellation of findings, such as occurs in Kallmann syndrome (with associated absent or reduced sense of smell) or in conjunction with multiple other hormone deficiencies (Table 2). After GH, LH and FSH are the most commonly deficient pituitary hormones in adults with hypopituitarism. Men with hypogonadotropic hypogonadism have decreased libido, erectile dysfunction, diminished facial and body hair, gynecomastia, and soft testes, especially if the problem is longstanding. Affected women have irregular menses or amenorrhea, hot flashes, decreased libido, and vaginal dryness. Both men and women may also develop osteopenia if their gonadotropin deficiency is longstanding and if appropriate hormone replacement is not provided.

Random measurements of serum LH and FSH, as well as an estrogen level in women and a testosterone level in men, are usually sufficient diagnostic measures to evaluate gonadotropin deficiency in adults with hypopituitarism. Occasionally, intravenous administration of synthetic GnRH (gonadorelin [Factrel]) is employed in an attempt to distinguish hypothalamic from pituitary etiologies, with the rationale being that, with hypothalamic disease, LH and FSH levels will rise, whereas this will not occur with pituitary disease. Unfortunately, the response may also be blunted with longstanding hypothalamic disease because the pituitary needs endogenous GnRH priming to remain responsive to exogenous stimulation. More certain differentiation may require repeated pulses of exogenous GnRH. Knowledge of the specific etiology does not affect initial sex-steroid replacement, but may influence the choice of therapeutic regimen for fertility therapy. In women, target-organ response, such as endometrial thickness determined by pelvic ultrasound and a progesterone withdrawal test to induce menstrual bleeding, may also be useful diagnostic strategies.

Treatment in women consists of cyclical estrogen and progesterone therapy, until at least 50 years of age. This length of therapy may be influenced by other factors, such as bone mineral density (BMD). The estrogen is important for maintenance of BMD, vaginal lubrication, youthful skin, and normal breast architecture. The progesterone component allows for induction of menses and provides uterine protection against the potential cancer-causing effects of long-term unopposed estrogen. If a woman has had a hysterectomy, estrogen therapy alone is adequate. The long-term safety of female hormone replacement therapy is uncertain. If there is clear evidence of osteoporosis or severe osteopenia, calcium, vitamin D, or antiresorptive agents, such as bisphosphonates, may be useful treatment adjuncts. Men typically receive testosterone replacement therapy intramuscularly as testosterone enanthate (Delatestryl) or testosterone cypionate (Andro-Cyp, DepAndro, and Depotest) or topically by patch (Testoderm and Androderm) or gel (AndroGel). With the cutaneous preparations, serum testosterone levels need to be followed to assure values within the reference range. For both men and women, induction of fertility will require further therapy with synthetic or recombinant gonadotropins, human chorionic gonadotropin, or GnRH (by pump) under the supervision of a specialist with expertise in the area of reproductive endocrinology.

Central Hypothyroidism

Deficiency in hypothalamic thyrotropin-releasing hormone (TRH) or pituitary TSH results in central hypothyroidism. Unlike GHD, which can occur as an isolated entity, TSH deficiency is almost always part of a more global hypopituitarism resulting from pituitary or hypothalamic damage, and is usually preceded by, or associated with, GH and gonadotropin deficiencies (see Table 2). Clinical manifestations of central hypothyroidism in adults are similar to those of primary hypothyroidism, albeit generally milder. These include, but are not limited to, fatigue, muscle aches, weight gain, cold intolerance, constipation, bradycardia, and prolonged deep tendon reflexes.

Diagnosis is based on a low serum free thyroxine (fT_4) level, with a low, normal, or slightly increased serum TSH level. This aberrant TSH measurement may be an artifact because of its immunoactivity in the laboratory assay. If, as a result, the diagnosis of central hypothyroidism remains problematic, a TRH (Thypinone) stimulation test has traditionally been the next approach. In this test, the peak TSH response normally occurs at 20 minutes. In patients with pituitary hypothyroidism, the TSH response will be significantly blunted throughout the test, whereas, in patients with hypothalamic hypopituitarism, the peak TSH response is typically exaggerated and delayed, occurring at 60 minutes. Unfortunately, TRH is currently not being manufactured. An alternative method to diagnose central hypothyroidism involves measurement of serial TSH levels at nighttime, preferably every 30 minutes between 2300 and 0200, to determine if the normal nocturnal TSH surge takes place. Lack of a twofold increase of TSH during this period suggests the presence of central hypothyroidism.

Treatment consists of levo-thyroxine (Synthroid, Levothroid, and Levoxyl) replacement, which typically requires smaller doses than are necessary to treat patients with primary hypothyroidism. In adults, a mean dose of 125 μg/d (range, 75–200 μg/d) is usually sufficient to restore normal thyroid function. The adequacy of treatment is monitored by serial measurements of fT_4; because the cause of the hypothyroidism is central, serum TSH levels are not helpful.

ACTH Deficiency

Deficiency of either hypothalamic corticotropin-releasing hormone (CRH) or pituitary ACTH causes underproduction of cortisol by the adrenocortical zonas fasciculata and reticularis (see Table 2). Unlike the more complete primary variant, central adrenal insufficiency typically has a milder phenotype, in which there may be no clinical manifestations during normal daily living or only mild and nonspecific symptoms, such as fatigue, weakness, headache, and anorexia. However, under stressful conditions, such as surgery, trauma, or serious illness, cortisol deficiency, regardless of cause, may lead to vomiting, dehydration, hypotension, shock, and even death.

To diagnose central adrenal insufficiency, measurement of a random plasma ACTH or serum cortisol level, or a 24-hour urine-free cortisol level is typically not useful. Although an elevated fasting serum cortisol level at 0800 may be helpful to rule out the disorder, a low random cortisol level does not automatically secure the diagnosis. Therefore, definitive diagnosis of CRH or ACTH deficiency requires stimulation testing. The ITT, as described previously, is a very useful test for definitive assessment of cortisol production. Alternative diagnostic modalities include the CRH and ACTH stimulation tests. The interpretation of the CRH (Acthrel) test is similar to that of the GnRH test, recognizing that multiple doses may need to be given to ensure that lack of ACTH and cortisol responsiveness truly reflects pituitary disease rather than lack of endogenous hypothalamic priming. However, the CRH test is not commonly employed for this purpose. The ACTH protocols include short and long and high- and low-dose variants. In the most commonly employed version (at least until recently), the short ACTH test, 250 μg of synthetic ACTH 1-24 (Cortrosyn), with similar activity to native ACTH, is given intravenously with blood draws at 0 and 60 minutes. A normal response is characterized by a rise in serum cortisol by >10 μg/dL over baseline *and* a 1-hour level >18 μg/dL. Because the adrenal gland requires prior ACTH exposure for a normal cortisol response to ACTH, this test provides a reasonable estimate of endogenous ACTH secretion. It is safer and faster than is the ITT, but it is not as reliable if ACTH deficiency has not been longstanding or if ACTH reserve has been affected by prior exogenous cortisol therapy. A longer ACTH stimulation test can be done, with 8- to 12-hour infusions of Cortrosyn on 3 consecutive days, in which 24-hour urine 17-hydroxycorticosteroids (17-OHCS) and creatinine are measured on the day before and on each treatment day. A normal response is a three- to five-fold increase of 17-OHCS over baseline. Recently, a refined version of the short ACTH stimulation test has been developed in which only 1 μg of Cortrosyn, a much more physiologic provocation, is administered. The degree of concordance of the results from the low-dose ACTH stimulation test with those of the ITT remains the subject of investigation. Metyrapone,* an inhibitor of 11-hydroxylase deficiency, had been used to assess the integrity of the hypothalamic-pituitary-adrenal axis, but this agent is no longer being manufactured.

Treatment for CRH or ACTH deficiency involves administration of replacement glucocorticoid at a maintenance dose and taking into account incomplete oral absorption. Using the physiologic glucocorticoid, hydrocortisone (Cortef), a standard adult dose is 20–30 mg/d given in either two or three doses per day, with the morning dose being higher than the other dose(s). The typical distributions of doses are $\frac{2}{3}$ and $\frac{1}{3}$ or $\frac{1}{2}$, $\frac{1}{4}$, and $\frac{1}{4}$, with the twice- and thrice-daily regimens, respectively. Longer-acting synthetic glucocorticoids, such as prednisone and dexamethasone, may be substituted recognizing their fourfold and approximately 50-fold greater potencies over hydrocortisone when calculating their respective dosages. Mineralocorticoid replacement is not required, because aldosterone production is regulated by the renin-angiotensin system, and, hence, is not affected by disturbed hypothalamic-pituitary function. Patients must be taught to increase their glucocorticoid dose by two- to threefold in the setting of a serious illness or trauma. If an affected individual becomes very sick or is not tolerating medication by mouth, hydrocortisone

*Not available in the United States.

injections (which should be available in the home and the administration of which has previously been taught to a family member or partner) must be given and the patient seen immediately by a healthcare professional. Patients with all forms of adrenal insufficiency are strongly encouraged to wear a Medic-Alert bracelet and to carry an information card.

Prolactin Deficiency or Excess

Prolactin deficiency is very rare and, if present, does not need to be treated—although in females, it may have some effect on lactation, but little if any effect on ovarian function. Prolactin excess is more common secondary to loss of its normal predominantly inhibitory regulation because of damage to the hypothalamus or the hypothalamic-pituitary stalk. However, this excess is usually very mild and presents with no symptoms or only mild galactorrhea, which does not require treatment.

ADH Deficiency

Although anterior pituitary dysfunction is more common, posterior pituitary disturbances may also be present in adults with hypopituitarism (see Table 2). When ADH deficiency is present, there will be symptoms of central diabetes insipidus (DI), including polyuria and polydipsia. DI can be transient after head trauma or surgery, or it may be permanent. The diagnosis is made based on the results of a formal water deprivation test, in which the patient is fasted for a period of up to 8 hours while undergoing sequential measurements of body weight, vital signs, and serum and urine osmolalities. Once the 8 hours have passed or if the patient loses 5% of his or her body weight first, the test is terminated by administering 10 µg of intranasal DDAVP (see the following section) or 2 µg of intramuscular vasopressin, followed by measurements of serum and urine osmolalities 30 minutes later. A high and persistent urine output, along with a low urine osmolality in the presence of a high serum osmolality during the water deprivation phase, followed by reduction in urine output and normalization of the osmolalities in response to DDAVP, strongly suggests the presence of central DI. Treatment is with desmopressin (DDAVP) or 1-desamino-8-d-arginine vasopressin, the biochemical manipulations of which prolong its action and diminish its vasoconstrictive properties compared with native arginine vasopressin, given in divided doses either orally (50–1000 µg/d), intranasally (5–60 µg/d), or subcutaneously (2–4 µg/d). Some cases of postsurgical DI spontaneously remit up to 6 months after the operative procedure.

Oxytocin Deficiency

Another hormone released by the posterior pituitary is oxytocin, the two major actions of which are stimulation of uterine contractions at parturition and smooth muscle contractions in the mammary gland during infant suckling. It is not clear if there are any effects of human oxytocin deficiency, although some studies have shown impaired lactation, but not parturition, in oxytocin-deficient mice.

SUMMARY

Hypopituitarism is a treatable condition in which affected patients should be able to have a normal life if appropriate hormone replacement therapy is given. After adequate hormone replacement is established, doses tend to remain stable, but long-term follow-up is necessary to monitor the efficacy and safety of these hormones, most of which will be required for the remainder of the patient's life. Follow-up with an endocrinologist is mandatory for the purposes of future medication dose adjustments, ongoing monitoring for efficacy and safety of the replaced hormones, and to address any special circumstances that arise, such as desire for fertility and management of intercurrent stress, illness, or surgery.

HYPERPROLACTINEMIA

method of
MARK E. MOLITCH, M.D.
Northwestern University Feinberg School of Medicine
Chicago, Illinois

PRETREATMENT EVALUATION

Manifestations of Hyperprolactinemia

The presence of even minute amounts of milk expressible from one or both breasts that persists for more than one year after cessation of breast-feeding or its occurrence in the absence of pregnancy generally is taken as a definition of inappropriate lactation. Prolactin (PRL) levels are abnormal in about 5% to 10% of women with galactorrhea.

Hyperprolactinemia suppresses the pulsatile secretion of gonadotropin releasing hormone, causing anovulation. About 10% of women with amenorrhea alone and 75% of women with galactorrhea-oligo/amenorrhea are found to have hyperprolactinemia.

Infertility also may be a presenting symptom and is invariable when gonadotropin levels are suppressed. Of women presenting with infertility, 10% to 20% are found to have hyperprolactinemia.

Chronic hyperprolactinemia in males results in decreased testosterone levels causing impotence and decreased libido in over 90% of cases. Galactorrhea in men has been reported in 10% to 20% of cases.

Hyperprolactinemic, hypogonadal patients have a decreased bone mineral density, and correction of the hyperprolactinemia usually results in an increase in bone mass. Hyperprolactinemic women who are not amenorrheic and hypoestrogenemic have normal bone mineral density.

PRL-secreting macroadenomas (>10 mm in diameter) may also cause mass effects such as hypopituitarism, visual field disturbance, and cranial nerve palsies, depending on the extrasellar extent of the tumor.

Diagnostic Evaluation

Because PRL is secreted episodically, when levels are borderline several samples may need to be obtained to determine whether sustained hyperprolactinemia exists. A number of conditions and medications can cause hyperprolactinemia (Table 1). Most of these can be ruled out on the basis of a careful history and physical examination and routine chemistry and thyroid blood tests. Pregnancy must always be excluded. The most difficult distinction lies in the differentiation between hypothalamic and pituitary disease. PRL levels less than about 250 ng/mL can be due to any cause. Levels greater than about 250 ng/mL are seen only in patients with prolactinomas or in patients with renal failure.

When there is no obvious cause of the hyperprolactinemia from routine screening, a radiologic evaluation of the hypothalamic-pituitary area is mandatory to exclude a mass lesion. *This includes patients with mild PRL elevations.* Magnetic resonance imaging (MRI) provides considerably more anatomic detail than computed tomography (CT). It is very important to distinguish between a large nonsecreting tumor causing modest PRL elevations (usually <250 ng/mL) from a PRL-secreting macroadenoma (PRL levels usually >250 ng/mL), as the therapy is quite different. Because MRI and CT are now able to detect incidental nonsecreting tumors, cysts, infarcts, and so on, the finding of a "microprolactinoma" on scan in a patient with elevated PRL levels may not always be a true positive finding.

Paradoxically, some patients with large PRL-secreting macroadenomas discovered because of mass effects may have what appear to be normal or only slightly elevated PRL levels when, in fact, they actually have very high PRL levels. This may occur with two-site immunoradiometric assays (IRMA) or chemiluminometric (ICMA) assays and is due to the "hook effect," in which very high amounts of the hormone saturate the two antibodies used. To avoid this conundrum, the PRL should always be remeasured at 1:100 dilution in patients with macroadenomas and normal to modestly elevated PRL levels, because PRL levels in samples with the "hook effect" will then increase dramatically if the tumor is a prolactinoma.

Patients found to have macroadenomas, hypothalamic disease, or empty sellae should have an evaluation of the sufficiency of their other anterior and posterior pituitary hormones. Visual field testing is necessary only in patients whose tumors abut the optic chiasm, as visualized on MRI scan.

TABLE 1. **Differential Diagnosis of Hyperprolactinemia**

Pituitary Disease	**Other**
Prolactinomas	Pregnancy
Acromegaly	Hypothyroidism
"Empty sella syndrome"	Renal failure
Lymphocytic hypophysitis	Cirrhosis
Cushing's disease	Pseudocyesis
Pituitary stalk section	Ectopic
Hypothalamic Disease	**Idiopathic Medications**
Craniopharyngioma	Phenothiazines
Meningioma	Butyrophenones
Dysgerminoma	Monoamine oxidase inhibitors
Clinically nonfunctioning pituitary adenoma	Tricyclic antidepressants
Other tumors	Reserpine
Sarcoidosis	Methyldopa
Langerhans' cell histiocytosis	Metoclopramide
Neuraxis irradiation	Atypical antipsychotics
Vascular	Verapamil
	Cocaine
Neurogenic	Serotonin reuptake inhibitors
Chest wall lesions	Protease inhibitors (?)
Spinal cord lesions	
Breast stimulation	

TREATMENT

Idiopathic Hyperprolactinemia

Women in this category may require treatment because they wish to decrease troublesome galactorrhea, to resume normal cycling, to restore libido and normal estrogen status, or to become pregnant. In the woman with menses and without bothersome galactorrhea, reassurance may be all that is necessary. In the amenorrheic woman with estrogen deficiency, with its risk of osteoporosis, treatment consists of either lowering PRL levels with a dopamine agonist or estrogen/progesterone replacement. The latter has not been shown to cause the appearance of a tumor. When fertility is an issue, bromocriptine is necessary.

Bromocriptine is the usual dopamine agonist used when fertility is desired because it has the most extensive safety and efficacy profile. Otherwise, cabergoline is preferable because of greater efficacy and fewer adverse effects. Side effects of bromocriptine can be minimized by starting with the low dose of 1.25 mg daily with a snack at bedtime. The dose is gradually increased over a few weeks to 2.5 mg twice daily and PRL levels checked 1 month later; if PRL levels are not normal, then the dose is gradually increased. Most patients respond within 1 to 2 months if they are going to respond. Doses higher than 7.5 mg per day of bromocriptine are usually not necessary except in some patients with very large tumors. Psychotic reactions and exacerbation of preexisting schizophrenia have been reported rarely. Bromocriptine can also be given intravaginally to reduce nausea.

Pergolide (Permax), another dopamine agonist, has been approved by the United States Food and Drug Administration only for the treatment of Parkinson's disease, but there is considerable, well-documented experience with its use in prolactinoma patients.* Hyperprolactinemia can be controlled with single

*Not FDA approved for this indication.

daily doses of 50 to 150 μg and pergolide is comparable to bromocriptine with respect to tolerance and efficacy. Some patients who do not respond to bromocriptine do so to pergolide and vice-versa. No safety data are available for pergolide during pregnancy. Recently, cardiac valvular abnormalities have been reported in a small number of patients. Therefore, some caution is needed in using this drug.

Cabergoline (Dostinex), has a very long half-life and can be given orally once weekly. It is more efficacious than bromocriptine and pergolide and causes substantially fewer side effects in doses of 0.5 to 3.0 mg weekly.[†]

Prolactinomas

Observation

The indications for therapy in patients with prolactinomas may be divided into two categories: effects of tumor size and effects of hyperprolactinemia. In about 95% of patients, microprolactinomas do not enlarge over a 4- to 6-year period of observation. It is very unlikely for a prolactinoma to grow significantly with no increase in PRL levels and scans, after the initial one, are carried out only if PRL levels rise. A microadenoma that is documented to be growing demands therapy for the size change alone, as it may be one of the 5% that will grow to be a macroadenoma.

The presence of a macroadenoma already indicates a propensity for growth and should be treated. Local or diffuse invasion or compression of adjacent structures, such as the stalk or optic chiasm, are additional indications for therapy.

Other indications for therapy are relative, being due to the hyperprolactinemia itself. These include decreased libido, menstrual dysfunction, galactorrhea, infertility, hirsutism, impotence, and premature osteoporosis. The ability to follow a patient closely with PRL levels, MRI scans, and estimations of bone mineral density and fairly precise estimates of the efficacy of various modes of therapy (see later) allow a highly individualized way of following patients and selecting the proper timing and mode of therapy. For most patients, medical therapy with dopamine agonists is preferred as initial therapy.

Surgery

In experienced neurosurgical hands, about 70% to 80% of patients with microadenomas and 25% to 30% with macroadenomas can have their PRL levels normalized by transsphenoidal surgery. However, there is about a 20% recurrence rate of hyperprolactinemia, bringing the ultimate cure rate to as low as 50% to 60% for microadenomas and 10% to 20% for macroadenomas. For virtually all of these recurrences, the recurrence is that of hyperprolactinemia and not documented radiologic evidence of tumor regrowth.

The mortality rate from surgery for microadenomas is 0.27% and for macroadenomas is 0.95%, whereas the major morbidity rate for microadenomas is 0.4% and for macroadenomas is 6.5%. Transient diabetes insipidus is quite common with surgery but permanent diabetes insipidus occurs in only about 1% of surgeries on macroadenomas. Surgery involving craniotomy is much more hazardous.

Radiotherapy

Because of the excellent therapeutic responses to transsphenoidal surgery and medical therapy (see later), radiotherapy is generally not considered to be a primary mode of treatment for prolactinomas, causing normalization of PRL levels in only about one third of patients from 2 to 14 years of age. Radiotherapy is best reserved as adjunctive therapy for those patients with enlarging lesions who have not responded to either medical or surgical treatment. Newer, focused, stereotactic forms of radiotherapy ("gamma knife" or linear accelerator) cause a more rapid response. However, the major side effect of all forms of radiotherapy is hypopituitarism, occurring in more than 50% of patients over time.

Medical therapy

BROMOCRIPTINE

Bromocriptine (Parlodel), is able to normalize prolactin levels or effect return of ovulatory menses in 60% to 80% of patients. There is considerable interindividual variability in sensitivity to the drug. The dose must be started low and gradually increased to reduce side effects (see earlier). In most cases, bromocriptine needs to be continued to maintain PRL levels near normal with concomitant resolution of galactorrhea and amenorrhea or impotence. No ill effects have been found with long-term use.

Macroadenoma size reduction also occurs in response to bromocriptine, more than 75% of patients having some tumor size decrease. About 40% to 50% have a greater than 50% reduction in tumor size, 25% to 30% have a 25% to 50% reduction in tumor size, 10% to 15% have a less than 25% reduction, and 10% to 20% have no evidence of any reduction in tumor size. The time course of tumor size reduction is variable. Some patients may experience extremely rapid decreases in tumor size, significant changes in visual fields being noted within 24 to 72 hours, and significant changes noted on scan within 2 weeks. In others, little change may be noted at 6 weeks, but scanning again at 6 to 12 months may show significant changes. A progressive decrease is often noted over several years. Visual fields may be expected to improve in 80% to 90% of patients with significant visual field abnormalities.

The extent of tumor size reduction does not correlate with basal PRL levels, nadir PRL levels achieved, the percent fall in PRL, or whether PRL levels reached normal. Some patients have excellent reduction of PRL levels to normal but only modest changes in tumor size, whereas others have persistent hyperprolactinemia

[†]Exceeds dosage recommended by the manufacturer.

(although >75% suppression from basal values) with complete disappearance of tumor. A reduction in PRL levels always precedes any detectable change in tumor size and PRL nonresponders are also tumor-size nonresponders. Once maximum size reduction is achieved, the dose of bromocriptine can often be gradually reduced, following PRL levels and only discontinuing the drug if there are no increases in PRL levels or tumor size on just 2.5 mg per day. Although some tumors expand rapidly when bromocriptine is discontinued in a patient with a macroadenoma that has become reduced in size, this is not usually the case with long-term therapy. About 10% to 20% of patients can maintain normal PRL levels after stopping treatment and 70% to 80% with marked tumor-size reduction will not experience tumor re-expansion with stopping therapy.

Reduction in tumor size may also cause improvement in other pituitary function. Normalization of testosterone levels may not occur for 6 to 12 months, however. When the prolactinoma is present prepubertally, improved pituitary function allows resumption of normal growth and pubertal development.

One concerning problem is the tumor that initially shrinks in response to bromocriptine and then enlarges. This is usually due to noncompliance, which is further worsened by the tendency for the patient and physician to resume the full dose, instead of gradually restarting. This tends to make side effects worse, further exacerbating the noncompliance. Although extremely rare, tumors that continue to enlarge while being treated with bromocriptine may turn out to be carcinomas.

PERGOLIDE

Pergolide (Permax) has similar efficacy in reducing tumor size with somewhat better tolerance. Some patients may respond to pergolide who did not respond to cabergoline.

CABERGOLINE

Cabergoline (Dostinex) is more efficacious than either bromocriptine or pergolide with respect to normalization of PRL levels and tumor size reduction. For patients without prior treatment, over 90% will have a greater than 50% reduction in tumor size. More than one half of patients who do not respond adequately to bromocriptine will respond well to cabergoline. This greater efficacy is also accompanied by fewer side effects. Nearly two thirds of patients can maintain normal PRL levels without tumor enlargement after the drug has been stopped after 4 or more years of therapy. Many patients respond well to once-weekly dosing although others may need twice-weekly dosing.

Rare patients respond to dopamine agonists with a stepwise reduction in PRL levels with stepwise increases in drug dosage. In these cases, the dose of drug can continue to be increased as long as hormone levels continue to fall. The maximum drug dosage recommended in the package insert is 2 mg/week[†] but larger doses have been used in several studies, and patients with Parkinson's disease often require much higher doses and have few adverse effects.

[†]Exceeds dosage recommended by the manufacturer.

ESTROGEN REPLACEMENT THERAPY

Limited data suggest that estrogen replacement therapy* may correct the estrogen deficiency in patients with microadenomas without stimulating tumor growth. However, PRL levels should be monitored carefully in patients receiving estrogens alone to detect the rare patient that may have an estrogen-responsive tumor that may enlarge. Patients with macroadenomas generally require dopamine agonists for control of tumor size and would rarely be candidates for estrogen replacement alone.

Recommendations

Medical therapy with dopamine agonists has high efficacy and tolerability and appears to be the primary treatment of choice. This is particularly true for macroadenomas, in which dopamine agonists usually cause appreciable tumor shrinkage along with normalization of PRL levels, whereas surgery rarely offers a cure. Unless fertility is the primary reason for treatment, cabergoline is generally preferred because of its better efficacy and fewer adverse effects.

PREGNANCY

Effects of Dopamine Agonists on the Developing Fetus

As a general principle, it is advised that fetal exposure to bromocriptine be limited to as short a period as possible. Mechanical contraception should be used until the first two to three cycles have occurred, so that an intermenstrual interval can be established and a woman will know when she has missed a menstrual period. Thus, bromocriptine can be stopped after being given for only about 3 to 4 weeks of gestation. When used in this fashion, bromocriptine has not been found to cause any increase in spontaneous abortions, ectopic pregnancies, trophoblastic disease, multiple pregnancies, or congenital malformations. Long-term follow-up studies of children whose mothers took bromocriptine in this fashion have shown no ill effects. At the time of this writing, the safety data on cabergoline use in this fashion are very limited and so it cannot be recommended for women whose primary indication is to become pregnant.

Effect of Pregnancy on Prolactinoma Size

Estrogens have a marked stimulatory effect on PRL synthesis and secretion, and the hormonal milieu of pregnancy can stimulate lactotroph cell hyperplasia and prolactinoma growth. However, review of data of women who became pregnant shows that the risk of significant, symptomatic enlargement of microadenomas is

*Not FDA approved for this indication.

only 1.4% and of macroadenomas is 26.2%. In comparison, of women with macroadenomas treated with prior surgery and/or irradiation, the risk of significant tumor enlargement is only 3%. Bromocriptine has been used successfully during pregnancy to reduce symptomatic tumor enlargement in a number of cases. No ill effects on the infant were observed in these cases. The use of prophylactic bromocriptine throughout the pregnancy likely prevents tumor regrowth during the pregnancy in most cases, but no formal studies have been carried out.

Recommendations for Management

For the hyperprolactinemic woman with a microadenoma or a macroadenoma that is intrasellar or extends infrasellarly, bromocriptine is preferred as the primary treatment for such patients because of its efficacy in restoring ovulation and very low (1.4%) risk of clinically serious tumor enlargement. Bromocriptine is stopped when pregnancy is diagnosed and the patient is carefully followed throughout gestation. PRL levels do not always rise during pregnancy in women with prolactinomas, as they do in normal women. PRL levels may also not rise with tumor enlargement. Therefore, periodic checking of PRL levels is of no benefit. Because of the low incidence of tumor enlargement, routine, periodic visual field testing is not cost effective. Visual field testing and MRI scanning (without gadolinium) are performed only in patients who become symptomatic.

In a woman with a larger macroadenoma that may have suprasellar extension, there is a 26% risk of clinically serious tumor enlargement during pregnancy when only bromocriptine is used. There is no clear-cut answer as to the best therapeutic approach and this has to be a highly individualized decision that the patient has to make after a clear, documented discussion of the various therapeutic alternatives. One approach is to use just bromocriptine to allow ovulation, discontinue it when pregnancy is documented, and then observe the patient carefully for evidence of tumor growth. A second approach, that of prepregnancy transsphenoidal surgical debulking of the tumor, greatly reduces, but does not eliminate the risk of, serious tumor enlargement. After surgical debulking, bromocriptine is usually required to restore normal PRL levels and allow ovulation. A third approach, that of giving bromocriptine continuously throughout gestation, has been advocated. At this point, however, data regarding the effects of continuous bromocriptine therapy on the developing fetus are still quite meager, and such therapy cannot be recommended without reservation. Should pregnancy at an advanced stage be discovered in a woman taking bromocriptine or even cabergoline, the data that exist are reassuring and would not justify therapeutic abortion. For patients with macroadenomas who were treated with bromocriptine alone or after surgery, careful follow-up with monthly visual field testing is warranted. Repeat MRI scanning (without gadolinium) is reserved for patients with symptoms of tumor enlargement, evidence of a developing visual field defect, or both.

Should symptomatic tumor enlargement occur with any of these approaches, reinstitution of bromocriptine is less harmful to the mother and child than surgery. Any type of surgery during pregnancy results in a 1.5-fold increase in fetal loss in the first trimester and a fivefold increase in fetal loss in the second trimester, although there is no risk of congenital malformations from such surgery. Thus, bromocriptine reinstitution would appear to be preferable to surgical decompression. Such medical therapy must be very closely monitored, however, and transsphenoidal surgery or delivery (if the pregnancy is far enough advanced) should be performed if there is no response to bromocriptine and vision is progressively worsening.

HYPOTHYROIDISM

method of
STEPHANIE A. FISH, M.D., and
SUSAN J. MANDEL, M.D., M.P.H.
University of Pennsylvania School of Medicine
Philadelphia, Pennsylvania

Hypothyroidism is the physiologic state of thyroid hormone deficiency caused most frequently by thyroid gland failure and less commonly by hypothalamic/pituitary dysfunction or tissue resistance to thyroid hormone. Hypothyroidism affects up to 15% of adult women and 8% of adult men in North America, with an increasing incidence as people age. Table 1 lists the many causes of hypothyroidism.

ETIOLOGY

Primary Hypothyroidism. Primary thyroid gland failure accounts for nearly 99% of cases of hypothyroidism. The most common cause of primary hypothyroidism in iodine-sufficient areas such as North America is chronic autoimmune (Hashimoto's) thyroiditis; although worldwide, iodine deficiency remains the most common cause of hypothyroidism and affects over 200 million people. More than 90% of patients with Hashimoto's thyroiditis have positive antithyroid peroxidase (TPO) antibodies. Most patients with Hashimoto's thyroiditis have symmetrical thyroid enlargement, but the thyroid gland may atrophy as the patient ages. Hypothyroidism may occur after treatment of hyperthyroidism by either radioiodine ablation or surgical removal of the thyroid gland. Thyroidectomy for benign or malignant nodular thyroid disease may also result in hypothyroidism. External radiation therapy of the neck can cause hypothyroidism with a dose-dependent effect and a gradual onset. Iodine excess can lead to hypothyroidism in patients with underlying autoimmune thyroid disease by inhibiting iodine organification and thyroid hormone synthesis. Certain medications used to treat nonthyroid conditions can

TABLE 1. **Etiologies of Hypothyroidism**

Primary Hypothyroidism

Hashimoto's (chronic lymphocytic, autoimmune) thyroiditis
Iatrogenic causes
- Radioactive iodine therapy for hyperthyroidism
- Post-thyroidectomy
- External radiation therapy to the neck for benign or malignant conditions

Medications that interfere with normal thyroid function
- Antithyroid drugs (propylthiouracil [PTU], methimazole [Tapazole], perchlorate)
- Lithium, interferon alfa, interleukin-2
- Iodine excess (supersaturated solution of potassium iodide [SSKI], povidone-iodine, radiocontrast materials)
- Amiodarone

Congenital (1 in 3000 live births, most commonly caused by dysgenesis of the thyroid)
Endemic goiter from iodine deficiency (rare in North America, more common in central Asia and central Africa)
Infiltrative diseases
- Amyloidosis
- Hemochromatosis
- Lymphoma
- Fibrous (Riedel's) thyroiditis

Central Hypothyroidism

TSH deficiency from pituitary disease
- Postpartum infarction (Sheehan's syndrome)
- Tumors (pituitary adenoma, craniopharyngioma, meningioma, glioma, metastasis)
- Infiltrative diseases (hemochromatosis, histiocytosis X)
- Granulomatous disease (sarcoidosis, tuberculosis)
- Hypophysitis
- Trauma (surgery, external radiation therapy to the pituitary or brain, head injury)

TRH deficiency from hypothalamic disease
- Tumor (craniopharyngioma)
- External radiation therapy to the brain

Transient Hypothyroidism

Painless (lymphocytic) thyroiditis
Postpartum thyroiditis
Subacute (viral, granulomatous) thyroiditis

Peripheral Resistance to Thyroid Hormone

TRH, thyrotropin-releasing hormone; TSH, thyroid-stimulating hormone.

cause hypothyroidism, including lithium carbonate, amiodarone (Cordarone), interferon alfa, and interleukin-2. Less common causes of hypothyroidism include infiltrative diseases such as amyloidosis and hemochromatosis. Congenital hypothyroidism, usually caused by dysgenesis of the thyroid gland, affects 1 in 3000 live births in the United States, and all infants born in this country are screened for this disorder at birth.

Central Hypothyroidism. Central hypothyroidism accounts for less than 1% of all cases of hypothyroidism. Secondary hypothyroidism is caused by thyroid-stimulating hormone (TSH) deficiency, and tertiary hypothyroidism is caused by thyrotropin-releasing hormone deficiency. Secondary hypothyroidism can result from any of the causes of hypopituitarism, most often a pituitary adenoma. Other causes of secondary hypothyroidism include postpartum pituitary necrosis (Sheehan's syndrome), trauma, hypophysitis, and infiltrative diseases such as histiocytosis X and sarcoidosis. Patients who have received whole-brain radiation therapy for cranial neoplasms or leukemia are at risk for central hypothyroidism.

Transient Hypothyroidism. Transient hypothyroidism may occur in the setting of either subacute or autoimmune thyroiditis. Initially, transient hyperthyroidism develops and lasts 4 to 12 weeks as stored thyroid hormone from the inflamed gland is released, followed by transient hypothyroidism lasting 2 to 16 weeks because of an impairment in hormone synthesis by thyroid follicular cells; recovery of thyroid function generally follows. Lymphocytic (painless or postpartum) thyroiditis is an autoimmune disorder, and subacute granulomatous (DeQuervain's) thyroiditis is viral in etiology. Approximately 10% of patients with thyroiditis will remain hypothyroid permanently.

DIAGNOSIS

The signs and symptoms of hypothyroidism are nonspecific and vary according to the magnitude of thyroid hormone deficiency and the acuteness with which the deficiency develops. The most common symptoms include fatigue, weight gain, cold intolerance, and constipation. The most common signs include bradycardia, muscle weakness, fluid retention, and a delayed relaxation phase of the deep tendon reflexes.

Because of the variable and nonspecific manifestations of hypothyroidism, the diagnosis relies on laboratory testing. Primary hypothyroidism is characterized by a high serum TSH concentration and a low serum free thyroxine (T_4) concentration. Secondary hypothyroidism is defined by a low or low-normal serum free T_4 concentration and a serum TSH concentration that is not appropriately elevated. Patients in whom central hypothyroidism is diagnosed should be evaluated for adrenocortical, gonadal, growth hormone, and posterior pituitary dysfunction.

Subclinical Hypothyroidism. Subclinical hypothyroidism is biochemically characterized by a high serum TSH level in the presence of a normal serum free T_4 concentration. It is a common condition that affects up to 15% of women and 8% of men older than 60 years. Studies have shown that 5% of patients with subclinical hypothyroidism and positive anti-TPO antibodies annually progress to overt hypothyroidism with frankly low serum thyroid hormone levels. In the past, subclinical hypothyroidism was thought to be asymptomatic. However, in multiple randomized prospective trials, many patients who receive therapy for subclinical hypothyroidism experience improvement in the results of psychometric testing, standardized symptom scores, myocardial contractility, and serum lipoprotein profiles.

Screening. Given the prevalence of hypothyroidism and the availability of an inexpensive screening test in the form of the TSH assay, attention has focused on developing optimal screening programs for the general adult population. The cost-effectiveness of periodic screening has been investigated by using a computer simulation model, and such screening compares favorably with other generally accepted prevention programs such as mammography in women older than 40 years. The American Thyroid Association recommends screening with a serum TSH measurement every 5 years in adults older than 35 years.

TREATMENT

The thyroid gland synthesizes both T_4 and triiodothyronine (T_3). However, most circulating T_3 (80%) is produced by deiodination of T_4 predominantly in the liver. Serum T_4 is tightly bound to several serum binding proteins, including thyroid-binding globulin (TBG), which allows T_4 to have a long half-life in plasma (6 to 7 days). In contrast, serum T_3 is less avidly bound to serum proteins and has a shorter plasma half-life (1 day). T_3 is preferentially bound by nuclear thyroid hormone receptors and initiates the molecular events associated with thyroid hormone action. The administration of oral levothyroxine sodium (LT_4) replacement therapy results in very stable serum T_4 concentrations throughout the day with physiologic peripheral deiodination of T_4 to T_3. If T_3 is administered orally, wide fluctuations in serum T_3 concentrations occur throughout the day. Therefore, LT_4 is the preferred therapy for hypothyroidism. Table 2 lists the currently available thyroid hormone preparations.

The goal of LT_4 therapy for hypothyroid patients is to restore the euthyroid state. The average daily replacement dose of LT_4 in adults is approximately 1.6 µg/kg body weight. Young, healthy patients can be started on full replacement doses of LT_4. However, for patients older than 55 years and those with known coronary artery disease, a lower dose (25 µg/d) should be initiated and gradually titrated (12.5- to 25-µg increments) to full replacement.

The serum TSH level is the principal guide for monitoring LT_4 therapy in patients with primary hypothyroidism with a target range of 0.5 to 2.0 µIU/mL. The target serum TSH concentration is lower in patients with thyroid cancer, and the TSH should be suppressed to serum levels between 0.05 and 0.2 µIU/mL. The serum TSH concentration is not an accurate measure of the adequacy of LT_4 therapy in patients with central hypothyroidism. Instead, clinical symptoms and the serum free T_4 level must be monitored and kept in the upper half of the normal range.

Because of the long half-life of serum T_4, it takes 6 weeks for a steady state to be achieved after initiation or adjustment of LT_4 therapy, and serum TSH levels should be measured at that time. The LT_4 dose should be adjusted and serum TSH levels measured 6 weeks later until the TSH is normalized. Successful LT_4 treatment should reverse the symptoms and signs of hypothyroidism, although some neuromuscular and psychological symptoms may not disappear for several months after normalization of serum TSH levels. This delay in resolution of some hypothyroid symptoms should be discussed with patients at the initiation of LT_4 therapy so that they have a realistic expectation of the therapeutic effect. After identification of the proper LT_4 maintenance dose, the serum TSH level should be monitored 3 months later and then yearly. If the brand of LT_4 is changed, serum TSH must be measured again 6 weeks later because the LT_4 brands are not interchangeable. Table 3 lists some of the common situations and drugs that may necessitate a change in LT_4 dosage.

As noted earlier, the thyroid gland does secrete some T_3, the biologically active hormone. In a recent study with a limited number of patients, combined LT_4 and T_3 therapy was reported to produce small improvements in cognitive function, mood, and physical symptoms when compared with LT_4 therapy alone. However, T_3 therapy needs to be used cautiously because it causes wide fluctuations in serum T_3 concentrations throughout the day as a result of its rapid gastrointestinal absorption and relatively short serum half-life. Until further studies with larger numbers of patients confirm these findings, we recommend treating hypothyroidism with LT_4 alone.

In patients with central hypothyroidism, the possibility of other hormonal deficiencies needs to be addressed because administration of LT_4 to patients with unsuspected and untreated secondary adrenal insufficiency can precipitate an acute adrenal crisis.

No side effects are seen with appropriate LT_4 therapy because LT_4 is an identical synthetic product of a hormone normally present in serum. The only "side effects" occur if patients are either undertreated or overtreated with thyroid hormone. Some patients are allergic to the dyes or fillers in various preparations, and these patients should be treated with multiples of the 50-µg tablet, which is white and does not contain any dye.

TABLE 2. **Thyroid Hormone Preparations**

Generic Name	Brand Name(s)	Available Dosages
Levothyroxine sodium (LT_4)	Levothroid Levoxyl Synthroid Unithroid	25, 50, 75, 100, 112, 125, 137,* 150, 175, 200, and 300 µg
Liothyronine sodium (T_3)	Cytomel	5, 25, and 50 µg
Liotrix (T_4 and T_3)	Thyrolar	1U = 50 µg T_4 and 12.5 µg T_3; available in 1/4, 1/2, 1.0, 2.0, and 3.0 U
Thyroid USP (LT_4 and T_3)	Armour Thyroid	60 mg (1 grain [gr]) = 38 µg T_4 and 9 µg T_3; available in 15 mg (1/4 gr), 30 mg (1/2 gr), 60 mg (1 gr), 90 mg (1.5 gr), 120 mg (2 gr), 180 mg (3 gr), 240 mg (4 gr), and 300 mg (5 gr)

*Not available in Unithroid brand.

TABLE 3. **Conditions Requiring Adjustment of the Levothyroxine in Patients With Hypothyroidism**

Increased LT_4 Dose Required

Impaired LT_4 absorption

Gastrointestinal disorders—Crohn's disease, celiac disease
Drugs/supplements—vitamins with iron, iron supplements, bile acid sequestrants, sucralfate, calcium carbonate
Diet—soy, high fiber products

Increased LT_4 metabolism

Drugs—phenobarbital, phenytoin, carbamazepine, rifampin
Hemangiomas—increased activity of type 3 deiodinase

Blocked conversion of T_4 to T_3

Amiodarone
Selenium deficiency

Pregnancy

Estrogen therapy

Decreased Dose Required

Androgen therapy

Decreased clearance of LT_4

Aging

Low TBG levels

Nephrotic syndrome

LT_4, levothyroxine; TBG, thyroxine-binding globulin; T_3, triiodothyronine.

SPECIAL SITUATIONS

Pregnancy. Hypothyroid women who receive LT_4 replacement generally require a 25% to 40% dosage increase during pregnancy. Hypothyroid women should be instructed to take LT_4 and iron-containing prenatal vitamins and iron supplements at different times to ensure optimal LT_4 absorption. A serum TSH level should be measured as soon as a hypothyroid woman becomes pregnant because an increase in the LT_4 dosage may be needed as early as 5 to 6 weeks' gestation. A recent study has indicated that inadequately treated maternal hypothyroidism may be associated with decreased IQ scores in the child. Maternal serum TSH levels should be monitored throughout the pregnancy, with adjustment of the LT_4 dosage to maintain a normal serum TSH concentration. After delivery, the LT_4 dose should be decreased to the prepregnancy level and a serum TSH concentration measured 6 weeks later.

Surgery and Other Procedures. Surgery is well tolerated in appropriately treated hypothyroid patients. However, even in patients with untreated or inadequately treated hypothyroidism, studies have reported few adverse effects of surgery and general anesthesia. These patients do have a higher incidence of perioperative and postoperative ileus, hypotension, and hyponatremia. They are also less likely to have a fever with a postoperative infection and have increased sensitivity to anesthesia and narcotic pain medications. Urgent surgery, routine outpatient procedures, and angioplasty should not be postponed in hypothyroid patients. However, elective surgery can be delayed until the euthyroid state is restored.

Myxedema. Myxedema coma is severe hypothyroidism leading to decreased mental status, hypothermia, hypotension, bradycardia, hyponatremia, hypoglycemia, and hypoventilation. It is a medical emergency with a mortality rate approaching 80%. Initial therapy for myxedema coma consists of glucocorticoids for the possibility of concomitant undiagnosed adrenal insufficiency and high doses of thyroid hormone (both LT_4 and T_3 have been used). Supportive measures include mechanical ventilation, fluid replacement, and correction of hyponatremia and hypothermia. In addition, an underlying stress such as infection or gastrointestinal bleeding is often present and must be treated.

Transient Hypothyroidism. For patients with transient hypothyroidism caused by autoimmune or subacute thyroiditis, the exact time for discontinuation of LT_4 therapy may be difficult to determine. The hypothyroid phase of this disease can last up to 6 months when it is due to postpartum or autoimmune thyroiditis and may be shorter in viral thyroiditis. Therefore, for patients suspected to be in the hypothyroid phase of thyroiditis, we recommend continuation of LT_4 therapy to normalize the serum TSH level for 6 months. Afterward, the LT_4 dose should be decreased by 50% with measurement of serum TSH and free T_4 levels 4 to 6 weeks later. If these values are normal, the LT_4 may be discontinued and thyroid function can be reassessed in another 6 weeks.

Patients Taking Levothyroxine for Unclear Reasons. Frequently, patients may be treated with LT_4 without any documentation of hypothyroidism. To assess whether LT_4 therapy is truly needed, we recommend decreasing the LT_4 dose by 50% and rechecking serum TSH and free T_4 levels in 4 to 6 weeks. A recent study has indicated that patients with symptoms of hypothyroidism and normal thyroid function had no symptomatic improvement with LT_4 therapy when compared with placebo therapy.

HYPERTHYROIDISM

Method of
VICTOR M. MONTORI, M.D., M.SC., and
HOSSEIN GHARIB, M.D.
Mayo Clinic
Rochester, Minnesota

Thyrotoxicosis is a combination of symptoms and signs in patients with excessive levels of the thyroid hormones thyroxine (T_4) and/or triiodothyronine (T_3). Hyperthyroidism refers to thyrotoxicosis due to overproduction of these hormones by the thyroid gland. Diagnosis is clinical and should always be supported by thyroid function tests and sometimes by radioisotope studies. Treatment can be symptomatic and supportive or definitive with the use of antithyroid medications, radioactive iodine, or surgery. Treatment of hyperthyroidism should preferably be conducted in consultation with an endocrinologist.

DIAGNOSIS

History and Physical Examination

The clinical presentation in young patients ranges from no symptoms and a suppressed sensitive (third-generation) serum TSH level (<0.1 mU/L) to overt or clinical hyperthyroidism. The latter includes symptoms associated with increased adrenergic tone and resting energy expenditure, and to other hormonal effects. Symptoms related to an increased adrenergic tone include: nervousness, tremor, hyperreflexia, increased stool frequency, palpitations, diaphoresis, lid retraction, lid lag, irritability, insomnia, headaches, muscle weakness, and widened pulse pressure with elevation of the systolic blood pressure. Those related to increased energy expenditure include: heat intolerance, warm and moist skin, and unintentional weight loss without anorexia. In elderly patients the presentation may be subtle with atrial fibrillation, weight loss, weakness, and depression.

Patients with Graves' disease often have a goiter, may present with hyperthyroidism alone, or with one or more signs of eye and skin involvement. The goiter is usually diffuse and may have an overlying bruit. Signs of ophthalmopathy include proptosis, lid lag, lid retraction, and impaired extraocular muscle function. Signs of dermopathy include onycholysis, acropachy, and pretibial myxedema with peau d'orange skin changes on the anterior shins.

Patients with granulomatous (DeQuervain's) thyroiditis may have a history of recent viral infection, neck pain, and present with a tender goiter. Patients with silent (painless) thyroiditis may present in the post-partum period and have no anterior neck pain.

Patients with exogenous thyrotoxicosis may have no goiter. Those with iodine-induced thyrotoxicosis may have a history of recent exposure to iodinated contrast material (recent angiogram, urogram, or computed tomography scan) and a multinodular goiter.

Laboratory Evaluation

Diagnosis is established by sensitive TSH and thyroid hormones measurements. The first step is to determine if the patient has hyperthyroidism. An undetectable sensitive (third-generation) serum TSH level (<0.1 mU/L) is usually the first indicator of thyroid hormone excess. However, in patients with symptoms of hyperthyroidism, the sensitive TSH alone is insufficient and total T_3 and free T_4 levels should also be measured. With some exceptions (secondary hypothyroidism associated with low T_3 and T_4 levels; nonthyroidal illness; amiodarone use; glucocorticoid therapy; subclinical hyperthyroidism due to mild or early thyroid disease; or excessive thyroid hormone replacement), patients will also have elevated T_3 and/or T_4 levels. Hyperthyroid patients with measurable TSH levels may have pituitary TSH hypersecretion (Table 1).

The second step is to determine the etiology of hyperthyroidism. For this purpose, radioactive iodine (RAI) uptake and scanning are helpful (Table 2).

TABLE 1. **Causes of Hyperthyroidism**

Common	Uncommon
Autonomous activity	Pituitary TSH hypersecretion
Graves' disease	Ectopic thyroid tissue (HCG)
Toxic adenoma	Metastatic follicular thyroid cancer
Plummer's disease	Struma ovarii
Hormonal discharge	
Granulomatous thyroiditis	
Lymphocytic thyroiditis	

Patients taking thyroid hormones, for replacement or suppressive therapy, may have subclinical or overt hyperthyroidism due to overtreatment. Thyrotoxicosis may also occur when patients unknowingly take over-the-counter "nutraceuticals" containing thyroid hormone extracts or surreptitiously take thyroid hormone for weight loss or other purposes. In both cases, patients usually do not have a goiter and the thyroid uptake is low (<3%; normal 24-hour ^{131}I uptake is 6% to 29%).

In all age groups, Graves' disease is the most common cause of hyperthyroidism. Graves' disease is an autoimmune disease in which thyrotropin receptor stimulating antibodies stimulate thyroid gland growth, thyroid hormone synthesis and release. The most important differential diagnosis is with thyroiditis (through disruption of the thyroid follicles and release of preformed thyroid hormones) and toxic nodular disease (multinodular goiter or toxic adenoma). We have listed some clinical findings associated with Graves' disease, in particular those resulting from infiltrative eye and skin disease. Graves' disease is associated with increased thyroid hormone production and, thus, is associated with high-normal (in spite of suppressed TSH levels) or increased ^{131}I uptake (>29%). Although TSH receptor antibodies are present in almost all patients with Graves' disease, we measure them only in cases of diagnostic uncertainty.

Thyroiditis may be indistinguishable from Graves' disease in the absence of extrathyroidal manifestations of the latter. In contrast to Graves' disease, thyroiditis is associated with low ^{131}I uptake (<3%). Additionally, patients with granulomatous thyroiditis may have anterior neck pain and elevated sedimentation rate. Patients with transient lymphocytic thyroiditis may have a painless goiter, family history of autoimmune disease, and anti-thyroperoxidase (TPO) antibodies.

Toxic multinodular goiters (Plummer's disease) are more frequent in the elderly and may be difficult

TABLE 2. **Low Radioiodine Uptake (RAIU) and Hyperthyroidism**

Thyroiditis
Graves' disease with iodine overload
Iodine-induced thyrotoxicosis
Exogenous thyrotoxicosis
Ectopic thyroid tissue

to diagnose. Patients usually present with large multinodular glands, but in some patients the goiter could be substernal. Elderly patients may present with cardiac arrhythmias, weight loss, and fatigue rather than with the classic thyrotoxic findings. Patients with multinodular goiter may develop thyrotoxicosis after iodine exposure, e.g., following contrast injection for radiologic procedure. The RAI uptake is typically normal or slightly elevated with heterogeneous distribution on the thyroid scan.

THERAPY

Graves' Disease

Once diagnosis is established, we present patients with the following treatment options: antithyroid drugs (ATDs), ^{131}I therapy, or surgery (Table 3).

Thionamides are antithyroid drugs that inhibit the synthesis of thyroid hormones with gradual decrease in the concentrations of T_3 and T_4 over weeks of treatment. Remission of Graves' disease may coincide with treatment with these medications. ATDs are more effective in achieving long-term remission in patients with mild hyperthyroidism, with small goiters, and with very low or undetectable titers of thyrotrophin-receptor stimulating antibodies. We start propylthiouracil (PTU) at doses of 100 to 150 mg orally every 8 hours or methimazole (Tapazole) at doses of 10 to 40 mg orally once daily. The dose is increased after 3 to 4 weeks if no benefit is evident. In each patient, we find the lowest dose that maintains euthyroidism and we keep patients on this dose for 18 months. This is the time frame associated with optimal relapse prevention. With this strategy 20% to 50% of patients achieve long-term remission. If the patient has a recurrence (usually 3 to 6 months after discontinuation), we offer RAI or surgery. These medications can cause mild allergic reactions or major side effects (hepatitis, polyarthritis, thrombocytopenia, and agranulocytosis). We ask patients to discontinue the drug and to contact their primary care doctors or the emergency room if they develop a sore throat or any significant febrile illness. ATDs require close monitoring of thyroid function during initiation, maintenance, and discontinuation to ascertain recurrence of hyperthyroidism. In our practice, very few patients opt for this approach and often prefer other forms of therapy. Nonetheless, PTU is the treatment of choice for Graves' disease during pregnancy and lactation.

RAI therapy has been used for over 50 years and is very effective and safe. We aim to make patients hypothyroid. Because of this approach, very few patients require a second dose. The dose is estimated from goiter size and RAI uptake using the following formula:

$$\frac{100\text{–}200\ \mu\text{Ci} \times \text{thyroid gland weight [g]}}{\text{RAI uptake \%}}$$

The usual dose is 10 to 20 mCi. We offer this treatment immediately after diagnosis without pretreatment with ATDs. In adult women we require a negative pregnancy test to proceed unless the patient has had tubal ligation or hysterectomy, or has reached menopause. We inform patients of the precautions needed following RAI treatment. Some patients may experience a short-lived exacerbation of thyroid symptoms or anterior neck pain following ^{131}I treatment. Serum TSH is checked 6 to 8 weeks after treatment and monthly thereafter. When the TSH begins to rise, we start levothyroxine (Synthroid), identify the dose that will achieve a normal TSH (0.5 to 3.0 mU/L), and continue this treatment for life with yearly TSH monitoring. Smokers with significant ophthalmopathy appear at some poorly-defined risk of worsening ophthalmopathy following ^{131}I treatment. In these patients, in addition to smoking cessation interventions, we offer corticosteroids (prednisone 0.5 mg/kg for 1 week followed by a 2-week taper) to decrease the risk of worsening ophthalmopathy.

Near-total or bilateral subtotal thyroidectomy represents an effective treatment that resolves the thyrotoxic symptoms, usually resulting in postoperative hypothyroidism requiring life-long levothyroxine replacement. Thyroidectomy is an effective option in patients with amiodarone-induced thyrotoxicosis that requires immediate relief of their thyrotoxic symptoms, in those with large goiters especially those with compressive symptoms, in patients with suspicious nodules, in patients with contraindications to ^{131}I (pregnancy) or ATDs, and in patients preferring definitive treatment without radiation. Surgical morbidity is lower in centers with better surgical experience. As a result, hypoparathyroidism, vocal cord dysfunction due to recurrent laryngeal nerve injury, infection, and hematoma are rare complications.

For patients with symptomatic thyrotoxicosis awaiting definitive treatment, ATDs, beta-blockers, and stable iodine may provide temporary symptom relief. In our practice, we use either once daily, long-acting propranolol (Inderal LA), 80 mg/d, or atenolol (Tenormin), 50 mg/d. Beta-blockers provide faster relief than ATDs and are particularly useful in the preoperative period. Intravenous propranolol (Inderal) and esmolol (Brevibloc) can be used in critically ill patients or in the perioperative setting. Stable iodine (see Table 3) decreases the release of glandular hormones and is effective for 7 to 10 days. Lugol's solution (8 mg iodide per drop) given as 5 drops three times per day or saturated solution of potassium iodide (SSKI, 40 mg iodide per drop) given as 1 drop three times per day can also be used in severe thyrotoxicosis and in the preparation of patients for surgery (in combination with β-blockers).

TABLE 3. **Treatment Options**

Thionamides
Radioactive iodine (^{131}I)
Stable iodine (^{127}I)
Thyroidectomy
Other: β-blockers, lithium

Toxic Multinodular Goiter (Plummer's Disease)

In our experience, RAI or thyroidectomy represents effective treatment choices for Plummer's disease. If the RAI uptake is high and/or the patient is not a good surgical candidate, a high dose (30 mCi) of ^{131}I is administered with follow-up measurements of TSH and T_4 levels. RAI treatment is associated with a 20% chance of recurrence, in which case patients can receive a second ^{131}I dose or opt for thyroidectomy. These patients should not be offered iodide preoperatively because of risk of exacerbating the thyrotoxicosis.

Toxic Adenoma

For young patients and patients with a small (<4 cm) toxic nodule, our first choice of treatment is a single dose of 20 to 40 mCi ^{131}I. Treatment results in hypothyroidism in 10% to 20% of cases and in nodule disappearance in almost 50% of cases. For older patients or patients with larger nodules we consider surgery.

Thyroiditis

For patients with subacute thyroiditis, treatment is supportive with β-blockers and analgesics. In patients with amiodarone-induced thyroiditis, discontinuation of amiodarone, and treatment with β-blockade, and potassium perchlorate* may be useful. ATDs are ineffective in thyroiditis, given that symptoms are due to release of preformed thyroid hormones.

Pregnancy

Thyrotoxicosis during pregnancy is almost always due to Graves' disease and improves as the pregnancy proceeds. We use PTU as the ATD of choice in this setting, keeping T_4 levels in the upper limits of normal in pregnancy. Mothers may experience an exacerbation of the thyrotoxicosis after delivery. The newborn may have transient thyroid dysfunction if exposed to ATDs or transient neonatal hyperthyroidism due to passage of thyroid receptor antibodies through the placenta. Beta-blockers have been used during pregnancy. Post-partum thyroiditis is usually autoimmune and requires supportive therapy as described earlier.

*Not FDA approved for this indication.

THYROID CANCER

method of
KAREN R. BORMAN, M.D.
University of Mississippi Medical Center
Jackson, Mississippi

Thyroid cancer is the most common endocrine malignancy. About 18,000 new cases and 1200 cancer-related deaths occur annually in the United States. Tumors can be characterized by cell of origin (Table 1). Papillary and follicular lesions are frequently considered together as differentiated thyroid cancer (DTC) and stage-for-stage have very similar prognoses. Optimal management of thyroid cancer presents multiple challenges. The natural history ranges from preventable through genetic detection in infancy (e.g., heritable medullary cancer) to nearly uniformly fatal despite aggressive intervention (e.g., anaplastic carcinoma). Most thyroid cancers present as thyroid nodules, yet most nodules are not cancers. Relatively few tumors recur but recurrences often presage death from thyroid cancer. Long-term survival is common but does not guarantee cure. Finally, virtually no class A evidence exists to guide clinical decision-making due to the low incidence, the generally indolent behavior, and the prolonged natural history of thyroid malignancy.

DIAGNOSIS AND INITIAL STAGING

In the vast majority of thyroid cancers, patients present with a solitary nodule or dominant palpable nodules, but only about 5% of thyroid nodules are malignant. Microscopic familial MTC may be detected through genetic screening or provocative calcitonin testing of kindred members, whereas lymphoma may cause diffuse thyromegaly. History and physical examination are poor predictors of thyroid malignancy; only about 15% of nodules thought to be clearly malignant clinically prove to be so when resected. Features that do strongly suggest malignancy and that should usually lead to excision are personal history of neck irradiation, family history of thyroid cancer or of multiple endocrine neoplasia (MEN)-associated endocrinopathies (hyperparathyroidism and pheochromocytoma), and synchronous cervical lymphadenopathy without obvious benign origin. Increased likelihood of fine needle aspiration (FNA) sampling error in large (>4 cm) lesions should generally lead to excision. Large cysts (>4 cm) and cysts that recur after aspiration merit resection.

FNA is the single most reliable, efficient, and cost-effective initial diagnostic test for thyroid cancer. Radionuclide scintigraphy and ultrasonography cannot confidently identify or exclude malignancy. Ultrasound guidance for thyroid FNA is helpful when nodules are small, deep, or otherwise difficult to define. Aspiration should be repeated when inadequate material is obtained; repeatedly inadequate aspirations should lead to excision. Suspicious, indeterminate, and frankly malignant aspirates mandate resection. Follicular aspirates are variably classed as suspicious or indeterminate, because the differentiation of follicular carcinoma from follicular adenoma requires histopathologic demonstration of capsular or vascular invasion and is not possible by FNA cytology. Medullary thyroid cancer (MTC) can be diagnosed confidently by FNA using stains for calcitonin, amyloid, and carcinoembryonic antigen (CEA); not all MTC lesions stain positive for all markers. Overlap of FNA findings between thyroid lymphoma and Hashimoto's thyroiditis may

TABLE 1. **Thyroid Cancers by Cell of Origin**

Type	Cell Origin	Frequency %	10-Year Survival %
Papillary	Follicular	80	>90
Follicular	Follicular	10	80
Hürthle cell	Follicular oxyphil	1	70
Anaplastic	Follicular	1-2	<2
Medullary	Parafollicular ("C")	5	40
Lymphoma	B-lymphocytes	1	45
Metastases	Primary tumor	Rare	Determined by primary

require core needle biopsy or, rarely, excision for resolution.

Initial, preoperative staging in many cases is limited to a chest radiograph. Radioiodine scintigraphy has no utility for patients with intact thyroids. Chest radiograph abnormalities are further evaluated by anatomic imaging (chest computed tomography [CT] scan without contrast and magnetic resonance imaging [MRI]; CT contrast contains iodine that may interfere with postoperative radioiodine scanning and therapy). All patients with vocal complaints or who have had prior cervical operations should undergo laryngoscopy to document the functional status of the recurrent laryngeal nerves. An anatomic imaging study of the neck and superior mediastinum should be performed on every patient with vocal complaints, with symptoms referable to the trachea or esophagus, or with palpable cervical lymphadenopathy. MTC presenting as a palpable nodule is associated with a high risk of disseminated disease, warranting chest CT, hepatic MRI, and radionuclide technetium bone scan. Cervical and mediastinal anatomic imaging is appropriate after an FNA diagnosis of anaplastic cancer or lymphoma. Abdominal CT scan and bone marrow aspiration are added to thyroid lymphoma staging when chemotherapy would otherwise be withheld. Technetium scintigraphy and alkaline phosphatase determination are utilized for evaluation of thyroid cancer patients with focal bone pain. Abnormal results are correlated with plain radiographs; metastatic bone lesions from both follicular and parafollicular origin thyroid cancers are typically osteolytic. Central neurologic symptoms or signs should prompt head CT scan without contrast or MRI. Spine MRI is valuable in the rare case of peripheral neurologic findings of spinal cord compression. When FNA discloses cancer metastatic to the thyroid, preoperative staging is determined by the natural history of the primary tumor. Kidney, breast, melanoma, and lung cancers are the most common sources of thyroid metastases.

Preoperative hormonal testing is histology driven. Preoperative serum thyroglobulin (Tg) will identify the 5% to 10% of DTC that do not secrete Tg, sparing the latter patients the expense of serial postoperative surveillance Tg levels. Tg levels must always be accompanied by simultaneous antithyroglobulin antibody testing (anti-Tg Ab) for proper interpretation. When anti Tg Ab are present, Tg levels should not be used to make treatment decisions. Basal (unstimulated) calcitonin and CEA levels are indicated in all patients with MTC. Stimulated calcitonin levels are appropriate for patients with normal basal levels. Calcitonin stimulation is ideally accomplished with both calcium and pentagastrin as secretagogues but diminishing commercial availability of pentagastrin has led to predominance of calcium-based testing. Uncomfortable flushing and nausea may occur with stimulated calcitonin release. All MTC patients should be screened for pheochromocytoma before any cervical exploration. Seemingly sporadic MTC may instead represent the index case of an MEN kindred (5% to 10% of "sporadic" MTC cases). While the presenting lesion of MEN2A and 2B is nearly always MTC, pheochromocytoma also affects 25% to 50% of such patients. Undiagnosed pheochromocytoma can cause intraoperative death during thyroidectomy. Screening has traditionally been accomplished via 24-hour urine testing for catecholamines and for their metabolites. Newer data suggest that normal serum metanephrine levels efficiently and cost-effectively exclude pheochromocytoma so that more cumbersome urine testing can be reserved for patients with elevated blood catechol levels. Pheochromocytomas associated with MEN2A and 2B are almost never extra-adrenal, and so they are readily localized by adrenal MRI (or CT without contrast). Serum calcium and parathyroid hormone levels are measured when MEN2A is known or strongly suspected. Finally, genetic counseling and DNA testing (RET proto-oncogene analysis) should be strongly considered in all MTC patients to detect unsuspected familial MTC.

PRIMARY SURGICAL TREATMENT

The appropriate extent of thyroidectomy for thyroid cancer remains somewhat controversial, especially for intermediate-sized DTC. Lobectomy is the complete removal of one thyroid lobe and isthmus, while near-total thyroidectomy is ipsilateral total lobectomy plus at least 90% contralateral lobectomy. Intermediate resections are termed *subtotal*. Total thyroidectomy attempts to leave no gross thyroid tissue; however, scintigraphic evidence of small areas of residual tissue is common. In clinical practice, total and near-total thyroidectomy are essentially interchangeable for DTC. The minimum operation for any thyroid cancer is complete lobectomy on the side of the malignancy. Lobectomy is sufficient operative treatment for so-called "occult" papillary thyroid cancer that is less than 1 cm in diameter, is confined to the thyroid, and is not an

Table 2. **Potential High-Risk Features of Differentiated Thyroid Carcinoma**

Papillary cancer (includes mixed papillary-follicular, follicular variant of papillary)

Age/Gender: men >40 yr, women >50 yr
History of cervical irradiation, especially in childhood or adolescence
Palpable contralateral lobe abnormalities
Primary tumor diameter >4 cm
Tall cell, columnar, or insular histology
Extrathyroidal (extracapsular) extension
Distant metastases

Follicular cancer (includes Hürthle cell cancer)

Oxyphil (Hürthle, oncocytic) or insular histology
Primary tumor diameter >4 cm
Angioinvasion
Major capsular invasion
DNA aneuploidy
Nodal or distant metastases

unfavorable histologic subtype (Table 2). Lobectomy is also adequate resection for low-risk follicular cancer with no angio-invasion and minimal capsular invasion (see Table 2). Ipsilateral lobectomy plus contralateral subtotal lobectomy or near-total thyroidectomy is the appropriate procedure for papillary cancer with high-risk features (see Table 2). The choice between the two procedures is largely governed by local patient anatomy and surgeon experience; some thyroid tissue may be purposefully left in situ to protect a recurrent laryngeal nerve or a superior parathyroid gland. The same two procedures are appropriate for follicular or Hürthle cell cancers with angio-invasion or major capsular invasion. If Hürthle cell cancer is known preoperatively, total resection should be attempted because these lesions are usually not radioiodine sensitive. Any thyroid remnant left behind by subtotal or near-total resection for DTC should be of a size to allow single-dose ablation with radioactive iodine (RAI), facilitating postoperative surveillance with Tg levels and whole-body iodine scanning. For lesions more extensive than occult, but without clearly unfavorable features (see Table 2), unilateral or bilateral resection is chosen based on patient and surgeon factors (e.g., co-morbid conditions limiting life expectancy, adverse local anatomy, limited neck endocrine operative experience). When only lobectomy is performed and permanent pathology discloses unexpected unfavorable prognostic features (see Table 2), prompt "completion thyroidectomy" (at least subtotal and preferably near-total contralateral lobectomy) should be undertaken.

Total thyroidectomy is performed for the rare anaplastic tumor that is confined to the thyroid and should be part of a multimodality treatment plan. Debulking of extensive anaplastic cancers may aid in control of local symptoms, but sacrifice of functioning recurrent laryngeal nerves or resection of adjacent viscera is seldom, if ever, indicated. Tracheostomy may be considered for impending airway obstruction. Lobectomy suffices for a unilateral metastasis to the thyroid; bilateral resections are reserved for bilateral metastases. Thyroid lymphoma is treated by at least a generous biopsy for permanent histopathology and cell markers; more extensive resection (debulking) may enhance the response to multimodality therapy, particularly of non-MALT lymphomas. Nerves and other vital structures should not be sacrificed nor should adjacent viscera be resected. MTC is treated at a minimum by near-total thyroidectomy because postoperative RAI is ineffective for residual tumor; total thyroidectomy is preferred.

Complications of thyroidectomy include early postoperative bleeding with airway compromise necessitating urgent reoperation, injury to the recurrent laryngeal nerve (hoarseness when unilateral and acute airway obstruction when bilateral), injury to the external branch of the superior laryngeal nerve (vocal fatigue, diminished volume, and altered range), and hypoparathyroidism (transient or permanent). Re-exploration for hemorrhage should follow less than 1% of thyroidectomies. Permanent nerve and parathyroid injury rates should each be less than 2% for bilateral resections.

The extent of lymphadenectomy for DTC is even more controversial than the type of thyroid resection because the presence of involved nodes correlates poorly with overall survival as long as the primary tumor is intrathyroidal. Prophylactic lymphadenectomy has little if any role. Ipsilateral modified radical or selective neck dissection is performed for preoperatively palpable lateral adenopathy or for grossly positive nodes identified intraoperatively. Central neck dissection is similarly performed for palpable or grossly positive anterior nodes. Nodes should be very carefully evaluated intraoperatively for lesions with unfavorable prognostic features (see Table 2). Central neck and upper mediastinal dissection is always performed for MTC, with the addition of ipsilateral modified radical neck dissection if the MTC is palpable. Contralateral modified neck dissection is added for palpable familial MTC.

Nerve injury and hypoparathyroidism rates increase with lymphadenectomy. Pneumothorax, lymph leak (thoracic duct injury) and Horner's syndrome (sympathetic ganglion injury) may occur with mediastinal or lateral dissections. Wound complications (e.g., bleeding, infection, and flap necrosis) also increase with more extensive lymphadenectomy.

POSTOPERATIVE THYROXINE SUPPRESSION

Virtually all patients who have undergone more than lobectomy for thyroid cancer of any type will require thyroxine (T_4) (Synthroid) replacement to be chemically and clinically euthyroid. "Suppression" refers to the intentional administration of thyroxine to reduce thyroid stimulating hormone (TSH) levels as a cytostatic or adjuvant treatment for DTC. Suppression significantly improves relapse-free survival for DTC and is clearly indicated, but the degree of suppression is debated. Control and prevention

TABLE 3. **TSH Suppression Target Levels by DTC Tumor Stage**

Tumor Stage*	Target TSH Level (mU/L)
T_1 N0 M0	Lower 1/2 normal range
$T_{2\text{-}3}$ N0 M0	0.1-0.5
$T_{2\text{-}3}$ N1 M0	0.05-0.1
T_4 or M1	<0.05

*All T and N1 stages are pathologic stages, other stages may be clinical or pathologic.

M, metastases; N, nodes; T, tumor; TSH, thyroid stimulating hormone.

of tumor must be balanced against potential risks of accelerated bone loss and cardiac irritability. The degree of TSH suppression can be reduced after 5 to 10 years of disease-free survival. Suggested target TSH levels by tumor stage are provided in Table 3.

POSTOPERATIVE RADIOIODINE

Postoperative therapeutic uses of RAI include remnant ablation, adjuvant therapy, and treatment of metastases. RAI is used for DTC but not other tumor types. Most papillary and follicular cancers will take up RAI; Hürthle cell metastases typically do not. Remnant ablation refers to the intentional administration of RAI to destroy any residual normal thyroid tissue after bilateral resection. The dose of RAI required varies with the volume of residual thyroid but treatment can often be accomplished as an outpatient (<30 millicuries) after near-total thyroidectomy. Remnant ablation facilitates postoperative surveillance with Tg levels and whole body scans (see later). Therefore, remnant ablation should be strongly considered at least for patients with DTC and high-risk prognostic features portending increased recurrence rates (see Table 2). Adjuvant RAI refers to the planned administration of larger, "therapeutic" doses to patients in whom all gross DTC has been resected but who are deemed at particularly high-risk for residual microscopic disease and/or recurrence (e.g., extrathyroidal invasion by primary tumor and extracapsular extension by tumor in lymph nodes). Treatment of DTC metastases utilizes large doses and is performed on an inpatient basis. RAI is most effective for thyroid bed and pulmonary micrometastases, is of limited efficacy for cervical nodal metastases, and is ineffective for bone and pulmonary macrometastases. RAI potential complications include salivary gland dysfunction, leukopenia, ovarian failure, and oligospermia (Table 4). Lifetime cumulative maximal RAI dose for adults is 800 to 1000 millicuries. All postoperative uses of RAI require careful patient preparation (see later).

TABLE 4. **Complications of Radioiodine Therapy**

Acute and Intermediate (within 3 months of RAI treatment)

Painful thyroid remnant or metastases
Dysphagia
Dose-dependent sialadenitis
Transient leukopenia or thrombocytopenia
Transient, dose-dependent anosmia or diminished sense of taste
Transient alopecia

Long-term (>3 months after RAI treatment)

Reduced salivary gland function
Chronic or recurrent conjunctivitis
Complete xerostomia
Increased frequency of influenza
Transient (women <30 years) or permanent (women >30 years) ovarian failure
Transient or persistent oligospermia

Potential but rarely reported (1% or less)

Bone marrow suppression
Aplastic anemia
Leukemia
Bladder cancer
Pulmonary fibrosis

RAI, radioiodine.

SURVEILLANCE FOR RECURRENCES

The ideal postoperative surveillance beyond history and physical examination for DTC patients consists of serial Tg levels and whole-body iodine scans. Tg levels and scans are helpful for surveillance only for patients rendered athyroid by surgery, RAI, or the combination thereof. Surveillance scans (and RAI treatment if indicated) are done annually until two successive scans are negative and then at 5-year intervals in the absence of signs and symptoms or rising Tg levels. Tg levels are most sensitive in thyroprival patients but are more conveniently measured on thyroxine; attention to the normal range of the laboratory performing the Tg assay is crucial for optimal interpretation. Tg levels are measured every 6 months for 3 years, then annually for life if persistently normal. MTC patients are followed with calcitonin and CEA levels rather than with Tg levels. Intensive surveillance beyond 5 disease-free years is unnecessary in known sporadic MTC cases (RET proto-oncogene testing is negative) if basal and stimulated CT results are normal. Interval rescreening for pheochromocytoma and hyperparathyroidism is appropriate for MTC patients if genetic testing is positive or has not been performed. Neck ultrasonography is useful for patients with Hürthle cell cancers, with locally advanced non-Hürthle DTC (primary tumor >4 cm or positive cervical nodes), and with MTC. Cervical sonography is performed annually for 3 years, then at lengthening (2 to 5 year) intervals. Plain chest radiographs should be performed annually for all thyroid cancer patients. Surveillance after resection of a thyroid lymphoma or metastasis is individualized based on the cell origin, stage, and natural history of the primary tumor.

TREATMENT OF RECURRENCES

Hürthle cell cancers that recur in the neck (thyroid bed or nodes) are best treated by reoperation if complete resection is possible without sacrifice of vital structures because these cancers are usually RAI resistant. Maximal thyroxine suppression is given postoperatively; external beam radiotherapy (XRT) may be added for residual disease or extracapsular nodal extension. Little information is available to guide treatment of unresectable Hürthle tumors; XRT may provide some palliation. For non-Hürthle DTC, thyroid bed recurrences are treated with RAI and maximal thyroxine suppression. Cervical nodal metastases are best treated by reoperation followed by RAI and maximal thyroxine suppression. Resectable bone metastases from DTC (including Hürthle cell tumor) should be removed; unresectable lesions are treated with XRT. RAI is given for the occasional bone metastasis with significant isotope uptake. Pulmonary micrometastases are treated with RAI. Macrometastases are resected whenever possible followed by maximal thyroxine suppression; postoperative RAI is added for non-Hürthle DTC. Unresectable lesions are palliated with RAI (non-Hürthle) or XRT (Hürthle).

RAI, XRT, and chemotherapy have little efficacy for MTC, so that operative treatment of recurrences is more aggressive than for DTC. Neck MCT recurrences are treated by reoperation whenever technically feasible; extensive cervical operations should be preceded by laparoscopy and intraoperative sonography to detect miliary liver metastases. MRI is superior to CT for anatomic imaging of MTC. Postoperative cervical XRT may enhance local control. Resectable bone or liver metastases should be excised if morbidity can be limited. XRT is used for unresectable bone metastases. Octreotide (Sandostatin)* may palliate symptomatic hypercalcitoninemia.

SPECIAL CONSIDERATIONS

Asymptomatic Elevations of Tumor Markers

Management of asymptomatic DTC patients with elevated Tg levels but negative whole body scans is problematic. Cervical ultrasonography with sonogram-guided FNA of abnormalities is the most specific and likely helpful test. Chest CT and alkaline phosphatase levels are done in sonogram-negative patients; abnormal alkaline phosphatase should prompt bone scan. Empirical therapeutic dose RAI may be indicated for patients with negative imaging and normal alkaline phosphatase, particularly for patients younger than 45 years of age and with Tg levels greater than 10 while on thyroxine (or >40 after thyroxine withdrawal). Because the natural history of DTC is indolent and prolonged, the morbidity of any empirical treatment must be minimal to be justifiable (see Table 4).

Asymptomatic MTC patients with elevated calcitonin levels also present management challenges. MIBG or octreotide scans may help identify metastases but cannot entirely exclude them. Cervical reoperations with extensive microdissection will clear hypercalcitoninemia in about 25% of cases. Pulmonary and hepatic micrometastases are the common causes of persistent or recurrent calcitonin elevations. Laparoscopy and intraoperative sonography to detect miliary liver metastases should precede neck reoperation. Thoracoscopy with apical wedge lung biopsy may also be informative. Empirical cervical XRT may aid local control and decrease calcitonin levels if reoperation is not feasible; XRT also may be used adjuvantly after reoperation. Long-term survival with hypercalcitoninemia is well documented.

Preparation for Radioiodine

Maximal uptake of RAI is achieved when TSH is greater than 30; higher TSH levels may further increase efficacy. This thyroprival state can be achieved through withholding of thyroid hormone or through administration of recombinant human TSH (Thyrogen) (rhTSH). T_4 (Synthroid) must be withheld for 5 to 6 weeks; T_3 (Cytomel) must be withdrawn for just 1 to 2 weeks and patients often better tolerate this preparation method. Patients can now remain on replacement T_4 and receive two intramuscular injections of rhTSH followed by RAI whole-body scan and Tg measurement at 48 hours after the second rhTSH dose. RAI administration and Tg assay must be promptly performed since rhTSH is rapidly cleared by the euthyroid patient and TSH levels quickly decline. There are anecdotal reports of rhTSH preparation for therapeutic RAI but rhTSH is not yet FDA approved for this indication.

Familial Medullary Thyroid Cancer

Heritable MTC accounts for about 20% of MTC and is invariably multicentric. It occurs as the index endocrine lesion of MEN2A and MEN2B and as the only lesion of familial non-MEN MTC (FMTC). All familial forms of MTC have been linked to the RET proto-oncogene on chromosome 11 although to varying codons, and they demonstrate varying virulence. RET proto-oncogene testing is done on peripheral blood lymphocyte DNA and can be performed at birth. Over 90% of gene carriers will develop MTC, while gene-negative patients will not and do not require serial screening for MEN endocrinopathies. MEN2B is the most virulent of the heritable forms and total thyroidectomy plus central neck lymphadenectomy should be performed in the first year of life. MTC associated with MEN2A is of intermediate aggressiveness and children who are gene positive should undergo total thyroidectomy and central neck dissection at about 5 years of age. FMTC is the most indolent of heritable MTC variants but therapy similar to MEN2A is warranted because FMTC cannot always be crisply distinguished prospectively from FMTC. If heritable MTC is not discovered until a thyroid mass is palpable, then bilateral modified radical neck dissections are added to total thyroidectomy and central neck dissection.

Pediatric and Reproductive Issues

Over 90% of DTC lesions occurring in patients under 21 years are papillary. Extrathyroidal extension and positive cervical nodes are common. Distant metastases

*Not FDA approved for this indication.

are present in about 25% of patients at presentation and nearly always include pulmonary metastases. Despite the prevalence of what are poor prognostic features in adults, disease progression is slow and long-term survival is the norm for children with DTC. Survival is not clearly improved by remnant ablation or adjuvant RAI. Preoperative neck and chest CT scans are indicated whenever cervical adenopathy is palpable to define the extent of adenopathy for primary resection. Because of the frequency of distant disease, near-total thyroidectomy with central neck dissection (plus ipsilateral modified radical neck dissection for palpable or intraoperatively detected positive lateral nodes) should be strongly considered for all but small, clearly intrathyroidal lesions. Hypoparathyroidism can be minimized by liberal performance of parathyroid autotransplantation, by leaving a contralateral small superior pole thyroid remnant, and by surgeon experience. Metastases should be resected whenever possible without undue morbidity. Unresectable metastatic disease often responds completely to RAI, but the risks of RAI must be weighed carefully against the indolent behavior of metastases in children. Overall survival for thyroid cancer in patients younger than 21 years of age exceeds 90% at 15 years, despite more advanced disease stage at diagnosis. Children, especially females, treated with cervical XRT for nonthyroidal childhood malignancies (e.g., Hodgkin's disease and neuroblastoma) have a substantially increased risk of subsequent DTC, with a peak incidence at 15 to 20 years after XRT. Thyroid cancer is typically multicentric and development of a thyroid nodule after XRT should be treated by near-total thyroidectomy.

In females, RAI therapy does not change the fertility rate, the rate of stillbirths or premature births, or the risk of carcinogenesis in offspring. The rate of spontaneous abortions does increase transiently after RAI, and conception should be avoided for 12 months after each dose of RAI. Males may experience oligospermia that is most often transient (see Table 4).

FUTURE DIRECTIONS

Because of the low frequency, often-indolent course, and prolonged natural history of DTC, class A evidence obtained through randomized, controlled clinical trials likely will remain limited. The even greater rarity of MTC and anaplastic thyroid cancers will similarly restrict even multicenter trials. The role of FDG-PET scans in the diagnosis and treatment of all types of thyroid cancer is being explored. Presently the limit of detection by PET scan is a minimal tissue mass of >1.5 cm, limiting its utility. Trials of radiofrequency ablation for unresectable disease of all thyroid histologic types are underway. Whether rhTSH (Thyrogen) is equivalent to thyroid hormone withdrawal in raising TSH levels for maximal uptake of therapeutic doses of RAI by DTC is under active study. Standardized Tg assays would facilitate the postoperative surveillance of DTC patients and could markedly reduce the need for whole-body RAI scans. Tamoxifen (Novadex), retinoids, anti-TSH receptor agents, and SSTR5 receptor analogues could prove useful for RAI-resistant DTC. Work is ongoing with octreotide-based scans and with SPECT using RAI-MIBG and anti-CEA antibodies coupled to RAI for better imaging of thyroid cancers. Dissemination of information about MTC and widespread availability of RET proto-oncogene testing should lead to even better outcomes of heritable MTC. Cytotoxic antibodies coupled to tumor markers (Tg for DTC and calcitonin and CEA for MTC) could help address the patient with rising tumor marker levels but negative imaging. More effective chemotherapeutic drugs are needed for anaplastic cancer.

PHEOCHROMOCYTOMA

method of
GRAEME EISENHOFER, PH.D.
National Institutes of Health
Bethesda, Maryland
and
WILLIAM MUIR MANGER, M.D., PH.D.
New York University Medical Center
New York, New York

PRESENTATION AND DIAGNOSIS

Pheochromocytoma is a treacherous neuroendocrine tumor, which, if not recognized and properly treated, will eventually almost invariably cause devastating cardiovascular complications and death. Of seminal importance for the clinician is to think of this rare tumor in the differential diagnosis of sustained or paroxysmal hypertension—especially if there are any manifestations that may be caused by excess circulating catecholamines. Occasionally a patient may be asymptomatic and normotensive, particularly if the tumor is familial or discovered as an adrenal incidentaloma.

Symptoms and Signs

The presence of pheochromocytoma is usually indicated by signs and symptoms that reflect the physiologic effects of catecholamines released by the tumor (Table 1). Hypertension is the most common sign and it can be sustained or paroxysmal. Symptoms include headache, palpitations, diaphoresis, pallor, dyspnea, nausea, attacks of anxiety, and generalized weakness. Although headache, palpitations, and sweating are nonspecific symptoms, their presence with hypertension should arouse immediate suspicion of the tumor. Signs and symptoms that occur in paroxysms reflect episodic catecholamine hypersecretion. Paroxysmal attacks usually last less than an hour with intervals between attacks varying widely and as infrequently as once every few months. These attacks are usually accompanied by pronounced but transient signs and symptoms, whereas manifestations are usually less pronounced when hypertension is sustained.

TABLE 1. **Clinical Symptoms and Signs of Sporadic and Hereditary Pheochromocytoma**

		Sporadic (n = 76)	Hereditary	
			VHL (n = 33)	MEN 2 (n = 20)
Hypertension	>95	18	40	
Sustained	50	15	10	
Paroxysmal	>45	3	30	
Manifestations	**Sustained Hypertension (n = 39)**	**Paroxysmal Hypertension (n = 37)**	**VHL (n = 33)**	**MEN 2 (n = 20)**
Headache	72	92	24	35
Diaphoresis	69	65	18	35
Palpitations or tachycardia	51	73	18	35
Anxiety or nervousness	28	60	15	25
Nausea	26	43	6	10
Tiredness or fatigue	15	38	6	10
Faintness or lightheadedness	3	11	9	10
Constipation	13	0	10	0

Numbers reflect approximate percents of patients exhibiting signs and symptoms. In sporadic pheochromocytoma, manifestations are shown separately for patients with sustained and paroxysmal hypertension. Data for hereditary pheochromocytoma are from patients in whom the tumor was detected by routine screening.

Prevalence

Pheochromocytomas are rare, occurring in less than 0.05% of patients with both systolic and diastolic hypertension. However, due to the high prevalence of hypertension and the wide spectrum of symptoms produced by pheochromocytoma, many of which occur in other clinical conditions, pheochromocytomas must be considered in many patients with and without hypertension.

Hereditary Pheochromocytoma

Most pheochromocytomas are sporadic, but perhaps as many as 20% of these tumors occur in several familial tumor syndromes.

Adrenal pheochromocytomas in multiple endocrine neoplasia type 2 (MEN 2a or 2b) result from mutations of the *ret proto-oncogene* on chromosome 10q11.2. There is often coexistence of medullary thyroid cancer (MTC) or C-cell hyperplasia and parathyroid adenoma or hyperplasia in MEN 2a; in MEN 2b, MTC or C-cell hyperplasia, mucosal neuromas, thickened corneal nerves, alimentary tract ganglioneuromatosis, and a marfanoid habitus often coexist but hyperparathyroidism is rare.

In von Hippel-Lindau syndrome (VHL), family-specific mutations of the *VHL tumor suppressor gene* on chromosome 3p25-26 determine the varied clinical presentation of tumors, including retinal angiomas, central nervous system hemangioblastomas, pheochromocytomas, and tumors in the kidneys, pancreas, and epididymides.

Familial paragangliomas (some catecholamine-producing) occur secondary to mutations of genes for several succinate dehydrogenase enzymes on chromosomes 11q23, 11q13.1, and 1q21. In addition to paragangliomas, this familial condition also includes a predisposition to adrenal pheochromocytomas.

Neurofibromatosis type 1, due to mutations on chromosome 17q11.2, is the most common familial condition coexisting with pheochromocytoma, which occurs in about 1% of patients with these mutations.

When pheochromocytomas are found by routine screening in MEN 2 or VHL, the patient is often normotensive and asymptomatic. Thus, testing for pheochromocytomas in these patients should not depend on presentation of signs and symptoms, but should be carried out periodically as part of a routine screening and surveillance plan.

A hereditary basis should be considered in all patients with pheochromocytoma and in their relatives, where genetic testing may be indicated. Calcitonin, serotonin, and prostaglandins may be released from MTC and cause severe diarrhea. Hypercalcitonemia suggests MTC or C-cell hyperplasia. Treatment of these conditions should be delayed until after pheochromocytoma removal.

Malignant Pheochromocytoma

Although mostly benign, about 10% to 15% of pheochromocytomas are malignant. Diagnosis of malignant pheochromocytoma is not possible based on histopathologic features, but instead requires evidence of metastatic lesions (e.g., in liver, lungs, lymphatic nodes, and bones). Metastases can occur more than 20 years after removal of an apparently benign solitary tumor. Therefore, all pheochromocytomas should be considered to have the potential for malignancy.

Biochemical Diagnosis

Biochemical evidence of excessive catecholamine production is crucial for diagnosis of pheochromocytoma. This is usually achieved from measurements of catecholamines and metabolites of catecholamines in urine or plasma (Table 2).

Colorimetric assays of catecholamines, total metanephrines, and vanillylmandelic acid (VMA) have now largely been superseded by high performance liquid

TABLE 2. **Biochemical Markers for Diagnosis of Pheochromocytoma**

Biochemical Test (assay method)	Tumor Unlikely	Tumor Possible	Tumor Likely
Urine Tests			
Catecholamines (HPLC)			
Norepinephrine (μg/24 h)	<80	>80 and <300	>300
Epinephrine (μg/24 h)	<20	>20 and <50	>50
Fractionated normetanephrine and metanephrine (HPLC)			
Normetanephrine (μg/24 h)	<500	>500 and <1400	>1400
Metanephrine (μg/24 h)	<200	>200 and <1000	>1000
Total metanephrines (spectrophotometry)			
Sum of NMN and MN (mg/24 h)	<1	>1 and <2	>2
Vanillymandelic acid (spectrophotometry)			
VMA (mg/24 h)	<6.0	>6 and <12	>12
Blood Tests			
Catecholamines (HPLC)			
Norepinephrine (pg/mL)	<500	>500 and <2000	>2000
Epinephrine (pg/mL)	<80	>80 and <400	>300
Free normetanephrine and metanephrine (HPLC)			
Normetanephrine (pg/mL)	<110	>110 and <400	>400
Metanephrine (pg/mL)	<60	>60 and <150	>150

chromatographic (HPLC) assays that allow diagnostically more sensitive separate (fractionated) measurements of norepinephrine and epinephrine or their respective O-methylated metabolites, normetanephrine, and metanephrine. The latter can be measured in either the free forms or the much higher deconjugated forms (i.e., free plus sulfate-conjugated metabolites).

Pheochromocytomas continuously produce free normetanephrine and metanephrine by a process that is independent of catecholamine release. Measurements of plasma-free normetanephrine and metanephrine therefore provide a more sensitive test for diagnosis of pheochromocytoma than measurements of plasma or urinary catecholamines, particularly in patients where tumors secrete catecholamines episodically or in low amounts.

The high diagnostic sensitivity of measurements of plasma-free or urinary-fractionated normetanephrine and metanephrine (Table 3) makes these tests the most suitable choice for the initial workup of a patient with suspected pheochromocytoma. Negative results by these tests virtually exclude pheochromocytoma, whereas negative results by other tests do not.

Increases in plasma-free or urinary-fractionated metanephrines (i.e., normetanephrine and metanephrine) are usually high enough to conclusively establish the presence of most cases of pheochromocytoma. However, where increases are of smaller magnitude, false-positive results remain difficult to distinguish from true-positive results and additional biochemical testing is necessary. This is more of a problem for measurements of the urinary-fractionated than of plasma-free normetanephrine and metanephrine. The latter test provides better confirmation and excludes the tumor in more patients than the former test.

Tumor Localization

Magnetic resonance imaging (MRI) and computed tomography (CT) are the most appropriate imaging modalities for initial localization of pheochromocytoma. CT has good sensitivity (>95%) for detection of adrenal tumors, particularly those larger than 1 cm. MRI has similar sensitivity for detecting adrenal tumors, but is superior to CT for detecting extra-adrenal tumors. Other advantages of MRI include good anatomic resolution, avoidance of radiation exposure, and a characteristic high signal intensity of pheochromocytomas by T2-weighted imaging. This latter characteristic makes MRI more specific than CT for identifying pheochromocytomas.

TABLE 3. **Sensitivity and Specificity of Biochemical Tests for Diagnosis of Pheochromocytoma**

Biochemical Test	Sensitivity (%) (n = 214)	Specificity (%) (n = 644)
Plasma-free normetanephrine and metanephrine	99	89
Plasma norepinephrine and epinephrine	84	81
Urinary-fractionated normetanephrine and metanephrine	97	69
Urinary norepinephrine and epinephrine	86	88
Urinary total metanephrines	77	93
Urinary vanillylmandelic acid	64	95

Positive identification of an adrenal mass as a pheochromocytoma can be accurately achieved using ^{131}I-metaiodobenzylguanidine (^{131}I-MIBG) scintigraphy. The high specificity of the agent is a consequence of its active uptake and storage by pheochromocytoma tumor cells. The agent is also useful for detecting extra-adrenal tumors and is recommended for identifying presence of metastases before surgery is considered. However, due to limited sensitivity (70%-85%), a negative ^{131}I-MIBG scan does not exclude pheochromocytoma. Single photon emission computed tomography with ^{123}I-MIBG offers improved sensitivity. Other promising methods for localizing pheochromocytoma include positron emission tomography utilizing ^{11}C-hydroxyephedrine, ^{18}F-6-fluorodopa, and ^{18}F-6-fluorodopamine, the latter 90% sensitive.

In rare cases, where imaging studies are all negative, but where suspicion of a pheochromocytoma remains high, vena caval sampling may be useful for localizing the source of high circulating levels of catecholamines or free metanephrines.

MANAGEMENT

Preoperative Management

Cure for pheochromocytoma requires total surgical removal. Endotracheal intubation, anesthesia, and surgical manipulation of the tumor can provoke massive release of catecholamines with potentially fatal consequences. It is therefore imperative that patients with pheochromocytoma be appropriately prepared for surgery.

The goal for preoperative management of patients with pheochromocytic hypertension is relaxation of the constricted vasculature, expansion of the reduced plasma volume, and normalization of blood pressure for about 2 weeks before operation. Returning blood volume to normal minimizes the possibility of shock resulting from sudden diffuse vasodilation at the time of tumor removal.

Phenoxybenzamine (Dibenzyline), an α-adrenoceptor blocker, is most commonly used for preoperative control of blood pressure. The drug is administered orally at a dose of 10 to 20 mg two to three times daily for 2 weeks before surgery. At some centers, a supplemental dose (0.5 to 1.0 mg/kg) is administered at midnight before surgery, in which case appropriate safeguards are required to avoid orthostatic hypotension. Intravenous fluids may be administered if there is concern that blood volume has not been adequately replaced.

Alternatives to phenoxybenzamine for preoperative blockade of catecholamine-induced vasoconstriction include calcium channel blockers and selective α_1-adrenoceptor blocking agents, such as terazosin (Hytrin)* and doxazosin (Cardura)*. Compared to phenoxybenzamine, these drugs have advantages of fewer side effects and are less likely to cause false-positive elevations of plasma and urinary levels of norepinephrine and norepinephrine metabolites.

A β-adrenoceptor blocker may be used for preoperative control of arrhythmias, tachycardia, or angina. However, loss of β-adrenoceptor-mediated vasodilation in a patient with unopposed catecholamine-induced vasoconstriction can result in dangerous increases in blood pressure. *Therefore, β-adrenoceptor blockers should never be employed without first blocking α-adrenoceptor-mediated vasoconstriction.* The combined α- and β-adrenoceptor blocker, labetalol (Normodyne),* does not provide a useful solution due to more potent effects on β- than α-adrenoceptors, which in a patient with pheochromocytoma may lead to severe hypertension. Additionally, the drug can interfere with some biochemical diagnostic tests, and MIBG localization studies.

Alpha-methyl-*para*-tyrosine (metyrosine, Demser), at a dose of 250 to 500 mg three to four times daily, provides a useful adjunct to the above drugs for preoperative management in patients with highly active tumors where blood pressure remains poorly controlled. Metyrosine inhibits tyrosine hydroxylase, the rate-limiting enzyme in catecholamine biosynthesis, thereby decreasing the ability of the tumor to secrete catecholamines and increase blood pressure.

Surgery and Intraoperative Management

Induction of anesthesia and surgical removal of pheochromocytoma may cause considerable cardiovascular instability, even after appropriate preoperative control of blood pressure. Sedation with benzodiazepines or barbiturates can be useful, particularly in patients with anxiety or in those prone to panic. In addition to standard anesthetic monitoring, an arterial line is required for blood pressure monitoring.

Induction of anesthesia requires use of sedative hypnotics, opioids, and muscle relaxants that have minimal effects on catecholamine release or cardiovascular stability. Atropine should also be avoided due to the possibility of severe tachycardia. Morphine, fentanyl/droperidol (Innovar)†, and droperidol (Inapsine) should be avoided, because they may release tumor catecholamines and cause hypertension. Phenothiazines may cause hypotension and should also be avoided. Intubation should be carried out after administration of muscle relaxants while monitoring arterial pressure and ECG. A central line for central venous pressure monitoring and administration of drugs for cardiovascular control is placed after intubation. Anesthesia is usually maintained using the volatile anesthetic, isoflurane.

The laparoscopic approach for tumor removal is now largely replacing laparotomy as the method of choice for surgical resection of most abdominal pheochromocytomas. Laparoscopic surgery for pheochromocytoma is a difficult and demanding task requiring an

*Not FDA approved for this indication.

*Not FDA approved for this indication.
†Not available in the United States.

experienced surgeon and a team of specialists. In such a setting, operative times, blood loss, and complications are similar by both open and laparoscopic approaches, but advantages of the latter include less postoperative pain, a shortened hospital stay and convalescent period, and improved cosmetic result. Some hemodynamic instability can occur during insufflation of the abdominal cavity with carbon dioxide, a reaction most likely due to effects of increased intra-abdominal pressure on the tumor. Any subsequent release of catecholamines from the tumor into the circulation, particularly during manipulation of the mass, is best limited by clamping the venous drainage of the tumor. Once dissected free, removal of the tumor without fragmentation and spillage is facilitated using a laparoscopic bag.

Maintenance of cardiovascular stability is a challenge for the anesthetist that requires availability of specific drugs. Because episodes of cardiovascular instability can be extreme, rapid, and unexpected, with hypertension alternating with hypotension, these agents should ideally be quick acting and have short durations of effect. Intravenous phentolamine (Regitine) and nitroprusside (Nitropress), provide effective short-term control of intraoperative hypertension; the latter agent has an advantage of a shorter duration of action. Control of arrhythmias can be achieved using lidocaine or the short-acting β-adrenoceptor blocker, esmolol (Brevibloc). Propranolol (Inderal) and metoprolol (Lopressor) can also be used, but have longer durations of action. Profound hypotension can be a problem, particularly at the time of venous clamping and tumor isolation. This is most appropriately corrected using intravenous fluids, with pressor agents, such as phenylephrine, if needed.

Pheochromocytomas of the chest, neck, and urinary bladder require special surgical procedures; otherwise, management is similar to that of abdominal tumors. Pheochromocytomas discovered during early pregnancy should be removed. Otherwise, pregnancy may be carried to term under careful management, with a cesarean section required to avoid the stress of labor and vaginal delivery.

In patients with hereditary pheochromocytoma there is a high probability that both adrenals harbor or will eventually develop pheochromocytomas. Complete surgical removal of both adrenals has, therefore, been advocated as a prophylactic cure in such patients. Lack of adrenal cortical function, however, requires steroid replacement therapy and is associated with significant morbidity. Partial adrenalectomies are, therefore, now often recommended. In such situations the benefits of preserving adrenocortical function should be weighed against the risk of further disease.

Postoperative Care and Follow-up

Although a few patients remain hypertensive in the immediate postoperative period, most require treatment for hypotension, which is best remedied by administration of fluids. Hypoglycemia in the period immediately after tumor removal is another problem that is best prevented by infusion of 5% dextrose started immediately after tumor removal and continuing for several hours thereafter. Postoperative hypoglycemia is transient, whereas low blood pressure and orthostatic hypotension may persist for up to a day or more after surgery and require care with assumption of sitting or upright posture. Hypertension may result from fluid overload, insufficient analgesia, urinary retention, or residual disease. Close postoperative monitoring should continue until the patient's condition stabilizes.

Despite successful surgery, about 25% of patients with previous high blood pressure remain hypertensive. Completeness of tumor resection should be confirmed about 6 weeks after surgery by biochemical testing and a return of abnormally elevated test results to normal. Five year postsurgical survival for patients with sporadic pheochromocytoma who have no evidence of metastatic disease is about 95%. However, 5% to 10% of patients operated for pheochromocytoma develop recurrent disease. Due to this relatively high risk, biochemical testing should continue at yearly intervals throughout life, irrespective of the presence of signs and symptoms.

Metastatic Pheochromocytoma

There is currently no effective cure for malignant pheochromocytoma and therapy is generally directed at controlling blood pressure and symptomatology. Most treatments are palliative, but in some cases may reduce tumor burden and significantly prolong survival.

Alpha- and β-adrenoceptor blockers provide the accepted method for controlling symptoms and treating high blood pressure. Levels of circulating norepinephrine in patients with extensive disease can be extraordinarily high. In such patients considerations should be given to the potentially cytotoxic effects of catecholamines on the myocardium. Inhibition of catecholamine synthesis with metyrosine can be especially useful in patients with high circulating levels of catecholamines. A cardioselective β-adrenoceptor blocker may also be useful for protecting the myocardium.

Surgery in patients with metastatic pheochromocytoma is rarely appropriate or useful. Exceptions include cases where debulking of a large primary mass may be useful for reducing very high levels of catecholamines. Surgery may also be appropriate for lesions in acutely life-threatening or debilitating anatomic locations. In such situations radiotherapy, radiofrequency ablation, and embolization may offer alternative treatments, but only after appropriate medical blockade.

Chemotherapy with a combination of cyclophosphamide (Cytoxan),* vincristine (Vincasar PFS),* and dacarbazine (DTIC-Dome)* provides partial remission and improvement of symptoms in up to 50% of patients with malignant pheochromocytoma. Radionuclide therapy using high doses of ^{131}I-MIBG

*Not FDA approved for this indication.

provides an alternative palliative therapy that can also be effective in temporarily reducing tumor burden and symptoms.

Without treatment the 5 year survival of patients with malignant pheochromocytoma is generally less than 50%. However, the course can be highly variable with some patients living 20 or more years after identification of metastases.

THYROIDITIS

method of
ULLA FELDT-RASMUSSEN, M.D., and
AASE KROGH RASMUSSEN, M.D.
National University Hospital, Rigshospitalet
Copenhagen, Denmark

Thyroiditis is an inflammatory condition of the thyroid gland of various etiologies and pathogenesis. It is important to distinguish between thyroiditis and other causes of thyroid dysfunction and goiter because treatment strategies are different. Thyroiditis may be clinically characterized by thyrotoxicosis, euthyroidism, or myxedema. The hyperthyroidism is not due to overproduction of thyroid hormone, but to destruction of the follicular structure and release of preformed hormone from the colloid into the bloodstream. It may be associated with pain and/or tenderness over the thyroid gland and may sometimes manifest systemic symptoms with fever and elevated erythrocyte sedimentation rate (ESR).

Thyroiditis can be classified in different ways, such as related to debut (acute, subacute, and chronic), course (transitory or permanent) or to etiology (infectious, autoimmune, and drug-induced). The prevalence of autoimmune thyroiditis depends on the iodine intake in a population; e.g., non-postpartum silent thyroiditis is almost absent in countries of low iodine intake. Presence of thyroid autoantibodies may serve as a diagnostic aid (Table 1). Thyroperoxidase autoantibodies (anti-TPO) are most often present in Hashimoto's, atrophic, silent, and postpartum thyroiditis while thyrotropin (TSH) receptor antibodies (TRAb) can distinguish between postpartum thyroiditis and postpartum debut of Graves' disease.

ACUTE SUPPURATIVE THYROIDITIS

Bacterial infection of the thyroid gland is very rare in developed countries and is often caused by pyogenic bacteria, but also miliary tuberculosis, fungi, and *Pneumocystis carinii* in HIV-infected individuals may be causative agents. In clinically acute thyroiditis, patients present with fever and a tender thyroid mass. The most important differential diagnoses are subacute DeQuervain's thyroiditis, thyroid carcinoma, and bleeding into a cyst. Ultrasound is valuable in the diagnosis, and the treatment consists of drainage and appropriate antibiotic drugs.

SUBACUTE THYROIDITIS

This condition usually results in a transitory hyperthyroid phase followed by a temporary hypothyroidism and finally restitution. In some of the disease variants only one of these phases is seen. It can be classified in two clinical forms: Subacute granulomatous DeQuervain's thyroiditis, which appears to be a viral infection of the thyroid gland; and silent or painless thyroiditis, which is autoimmune of nature and in countries with relatively low iodine intake almost entirely seen with debut 3 to 6 months post partum, postpartum thyroiditis. Antithyroid drugs are irrelevant for treatment of the hyperthyroid phase and symptomatic therapy with β-blockers (such as propranolol [Inderal],* 40 to 120 mg/d) may be used. The hypothyroid phase is treated with levothyroxine [Synthroid, Eltroxin],† e.g., 50 to 150 μg/d and it is important to try to withdraw therapy after 2 to 4 months. Permanent hypothyroidism is not uncommon in autoimmune thyroiditis (silent and postpartum) but very rare after DeQuervain's thyroiditis (Table 2).

DeQuervain's Thyroiditis

This is a rare condition associated with a specific tissue type B35 and thought to be of viral nature. It is characterized by severe tenderness of the gland, fever, malaise, and elevated ESR. It is often misdiagnosed as throat angina due to the fever and massive pain, but is easily diagnosed by palpation of the thyroid gland, absence of signs of throat infection, biochemical evidence of hyperthyroidism, and subsequent demonstration of a low radioiodine or ^{99m}Technetium (Tc) uptake and very high ESR (often >100 mm/hour). The disease may start unilaterally or bilaterally and, in most patients, the subacute phase lasts 2 to 4 months. The hypothyroid phase often starts after 2 to 4 months and may last for an additional 2 to 7 months. Symptoms in the initial phase can be ameliorated by anti-inflammatory drugs such as acetylsalicylic acid [aspirin]* and nonsteroidal anti-inflammatory drugs (a large variety of these exist, and none has been demonstrated superior) or in more severe cases, prednisolone (30 to 60 mg/d). The pain and tenderness of the thyroid gland will usually be relieved in 24 to 48 hours. The treatment should be tapered over weeks to months depending on the ESR and symptoms.

Silent (Painless) Thyroiditis

This condition is a painless variant of subacute thyroiditis without tenderness of the gland or elevated ESR. It is histopathologically different from subacute DeQuervain's thyroiditis and has a histology rather similar to that of Hashimoto's thyroiditis; it is often considered a variant of this chronic thyroiditis and is also associated with presence of thyroid autoantibodies, in particular anti-TPO and anti-Tg. Goiter may or may

*Not FDA approved for this indication.
†Not available in the United States.

TABLE 1. **Diagnostic Use of Anti-Thyroid Autoantibodies in Different Thyroid Diseases**

Thyroid Disease	Anti-TPO	Anti-Tg	TRAb
Hashimoto's thyroiditis	+	(+)	–
Atrophic thyroiditis	+	(+)	–
Silent thyroiditis	+	(+)	–
Postpartum thyroiditis	+	(+)	–
Graves' disease	–	–	+
Postpartum debut of Graves' disease	(+)	(+)	+
Thyroid carcinoma	–	+	–
Neonatal hypothyroidism	+	+	+
Pregnancy with previous or present Graves' disease	–	–	+
Nontoxic diffuse or nodular goiter	–	–	–
Toxic nodular goiter	–	–	–

+ = diagnostic/prognostic value; (+) = Doubtful diagnostic value; – = No diagnostic value in clinical routine.

Anti-Tg, antithyroglobulin antibodies; anti-TPO, antithyroperoxidase antibodies; TRAb, anti-TSH-receptor antibodies, thyroid stimulating or blocking antibodies.

not be present and permanent hypothyroidism more often develops than in DeQuervain's thyroiditis (see Table 2). The diagnosis rests on demonstration of hyperthyroidism combined with low radioiodine or ^{99m}Tc uptake and should thus be distinguished from iodine contamination (usually iodine-containing contrast media, medications, or naturally high iodine intake such as from seaweed). The hyperthyroid phase usually does not require treatment but symptoms may be relieved by β-blockers and the hypothyroid phase by levothyroxine.

Postpartum Thyroiditis

This autoimmune thyroiditis occurs 2 to 6 months post partum in predisposed women, i.e., the majority have positive anti-TPO and/or anti-Tg already before pregnancy (see Table 1). Development of symptomatic disease is associated with an autoimmune exacerbation in the postpartum period. The condition is seen in 5% to 9% of all pregnancies, and is more prevalent in women with type 1 diabetes (up to 25%). The presence of the autoantibodies in the woman's serum is predictive of the disease because 30% to 50% of autoantibody-positive women develop postpartum thyroiditis with increasing likelihood the higher the anti-TPO level. There is a high recurrence rate in subsequent pregnancies and permanent hypothyroidism is not rare (see Table 2). The hyperthyroid phase is often overlooked and the symptoms are mild. If, however, the woman presents to the physician in the hyperthyroid phase, it is important to distinguish between postpartum thyroiditis and postpartum debut of Graves' disease or other causes of thyrotoxicosis. The differential diagnosis is most conveniently and rapidly made by ^{99m}Tc-scintigraphy, which demonstrates no uptake. This procedure can even be performed during breast-feeding (unlike radioiodine uptake). Presence of anti-TPO or TRAb may also be of differential diagnostic aid (see Table 1), but it must be kept in mind that a high

TABLE 2. **Comparison Between Characteristics of Subacute DeQuervain's Thyroiditis and Silent Thyroiditis (Including Postpartum Thyroiditis)**

	DeQuervain's Thyroiditis	Silent Thyroiditis
Age at debut	20-60 years	5-93 years; males 30-60 years; postpartum women
Sex ratio (F/M)	5:1	2:1
Etiology	Viral	Autoimmune
Pathology	Follicular destruction and inflammation	Lymphocytic infiltration
Painful goiter	Yes	No
Fever and malaise	Yes	No
Sedimentation rate	Elevated	Normal
Reduced ^{131}I-uptake	Yes	Yes
Ultrasound	Hypoechogenic	Hypoechogenic
Treatment of hyperthyroidism	Steroids, acetylsalicylic acid, NSAID	None, symptomatic β-blocker
HLA-haplotype	B35 high risk	DR3 low risk
TSH receptor antibodies	<40%	Rarely
Anti-TPO- and Tg-antibodies	Sometimes	Very often
Permanent hypothyroidism	Very rarely	Sometimes

Anti-Tg, antithyroglobulin antibodies; anti-TPO, antithyroperoxidase antibodies.

proportion of patients with Graves' disease also have anti-TPO antibodies. If β-blockers are necessary, breast-feeding should be discouraged. The hypothyroid phase occurs in median 19 weeks post partum and often requires treatment with levothyroxine. Permanent hypothyroidism is seen in 25% to 30% while the remaining patients are fully restituted within one year after delivery (see Table 2). These women are, however, at risk of later development of hypothyroidism and should be followed with measurement of thyroid function approximately every two years.

CHRONIC THYROIDITIS

This is an autoimmune disease with lymphocytic infiltration of the thyroid and often high levels of anti-TPO and/or anti-Tg (see Table 1). Most cases of chronic thyroiditis are due to Hashimoto's (with goiter) or atrophic (without goiter) thyroiditis, but rarely a fibrous variant, Riedel's thyroiditis, can be seen. Patients with Hashimoto's thyroiditis may have a very large goiter, sometimes even tender during the active inflammatory phase of the autoimmunity. During this active phase, the patient may experience relapsing episodes of destructive hyperthyroidism. The goiter, which is usually firm on palpation, may also grow rapidly due to active inflammation and elevated TSH and the most important differential diagnoses are, in these cases, thyroid carcinoma, subacute de Quervain's thyroiditis, acute suppurative thyroiditis, and bleeding into a cyst. Most often, however, the disease develops during years or even decades and patients present with various degrees of hypothyroidism from mild forms (so-called *subclinical hypothyroidism*) to more severe symptomatic cases. The mild forms are characterized by elevated TSH with normal peripheral thyroid hormones and it is somewhat controversial whether these patients should be treated. Recent evidence has demonstrated that even mild hypothyroidism may be detrimental for both cognitive brain function and the heart, indicating that these patients should start treatment with levothyroxine earlier than previously anticipated. It is even discussed if patients with TSH levels in the high normal range, in view of the logarithmic distribution of serum TSH values, should be treated. The longer the period of developing hypothyroidism, the older the patient and the more severe the hypothyroidism, the more slowly should levothyroxine therapy be initiated. In young patients a dose of 50 or 100 μg/d can be started, whereas elderly patients should start on 25 or 50 μg every second day. In patients with ischemic heart disease it may be necessary to initiate therapy during cardiac monitoring, and in severe cases the patient may have to be surgically treated for ischemic heart disease before levothyroxine can be started. The dose should be titrated upward during monitoring of the clinical symptoms (heart rhythm and ischemia) every 2 to 4 weeks. Measurement of thyroid function need not be performed before several months after initiating therapy. The aim is normalization of the TSH level to below mean of the reference range without suppression and with normalized free thyroxine concentration. Once a stable therapy has been obtained, TSH and free thyroxine should be monitored once a year. In cases of instability, noncompliance or changed bowel absorption should be considered. Combination treatment with triiodothyronine has been suggested but available evidence is still too sparse for this to be recommended. During pregnancy it is often necessary to increase the dose of levothyroxine by 30% to 50%. Considering the detrimental effect of low thyroid hormones in the mother on the development of the fetal brain, close monitoring during pregnancy is recommended. Measurement of serum TSH levels is not sufficient because patients may become overtly biochemically hypothyroid with a low free thyroxine long before TSH levels start to increase.

DRUG-INDUCED THYROIDITIS

Several drugs have been demonstrated to induce thyroid dysfunction, in some cases due to thyroiditis (Table 3). Amiodarone (Cordarone), is a frequently prescribed iodine containing antiarrhythmic, which in approximately 24% of patients induces either hyper- or hypothyroidism. The type 2 variant is a destructive cytotoxic thyroiditis that should be treated with prednisolone (40 mg/d). It is difficult to distinguish from the type 1 iodine-induced variant because both have low radioiodine uptake due to the iodine load from amiodarone. Measurement of serum interleukin-6 has been shown to be helpful, but is not used in routine clinical practice. Like most other destructive types of thyroiditis, hypothyroidism may subsequently develop with a need for levothyroxine therapy. Type 1 may develop into hypothyroidism, but the mechanism is different (iodine induced). Abnormalities in

TABLE 3. **Drugs Inducing Thyroiditis and Thyroid Dysfunction**

Drug	Cause of Thyroid Dysfunction	Treatment
Amiodarone type 1	Iodine-induced	Antithyroid drugs, potassium perchlorate, thyroidectomy
Amiodarone type 2	Destructive thyroiditis	Prednisolone
Lithium type 1	Antithyroid blocking effect	Levothyroxine
Lithium type 2	Autoimmune thyroiditis	Levothyroxine
Interferon α	Autoimmune thyroiditis	β-blocker, levothyroxine
Interleukin-2	Autoimmune thyroiditis	β-blocker, levothyroxine
Radioiodine	Destruction by radiation	Prednisolone

thyroid function are also often seen after initiating lithium therapy. Most of these patients do not develop thyroiditis, but a proportion of them have an autoimmune thyroiditis with anti-TPO antibodies and hypothyroidism. The condition may resolve if the medication is discontinued. Radioiodine therapy is frequently used for treatment of hyperthyroidism and/or goiter. Most patients display a transient elevation of thyroid hormones 2 to 4 weeks after therapy, but in some rare cases there is a more severe destructive type of thyroiditis, with hyperthyroidism. It can be treated with prednisolone but antithyroid drugs are useless. Treatment with immune-modulating drugs such as interferon alfa or interleukin-2 may result in an autoimmune thyroid reaction resembling silent thyroiditis. Diagnosis and treatment is also similar to this.

Section 10

The Urogenital Tract

URINARY TRACT INFECTIONS IN MALES

method of
FLORIAN M.E. WAGENLEHNER, M.D., PH.D.,
and
KURT G. NABER, M.D., PH.D.
Hospital St. Elisabeth
Straubing, Germany

Bacterial infections of the urinary tract in males increase with age from 0.03% in schoolboys to 20% in men older than 70 years of age. In the premature infant period there is an elevated risk of developing a urinary tract infection (UTI) in 4% to 25%. Recurrent UTIs in male children are mainly seen in the first two years of age.

Bacterial UTI in adult men is rare, when compared with women in the same age group. Only when subvesical obstruction in men becomes more prevalent with age, associated UTIs also increase.

Bacterial infections of the urinary tract cover kidney infections as well as infections of the draining urinary system. For the clinical approach, UTIs can be classified into uncomplicated UTIs and UTIs with complicating factors (complicated UTIs).

UNCOMPLICATED URINARY TRACT INFECTION

Uncomplicated UTIs in otherwise healthy males are rare due to the longer urethra and (apparently) to urethral immune globulin A (IgA) production. Nevertheless in the cases where uncomplicated UTIs are present, this is possibly due to specific pathogenic properties of infecting strains or special sexual practices in males. However, UTI in males should always be investigated for complicating factors.

Diagnosis

Symptoms in cystitis are mainly dysuria and can be confounded with urethritis. Therefore, exact microbiologic investigations have to be conducted. Pathogens causing uncomplicated cystitis or pyelonephritis in males are essentially the same as in the female population, and consist mainly of *Escherichia coli* and *Staphylococcus saprophyticus* or group B streptococci. Whereas urethritis is caused by distinct pathogens, such as *Neisseria gonorrhoeae*, *Chlamydia trachomatis*, *Ureaplasma urealyticum, Mycoplasma hominis,* and *Mycoplasma genitalium*. Usually pathogens in cystitis can equal 10^5/mL urine or more. Nevertheless smaller numbers in a clean-catch specimen should also be regarded as pathogenic. Concomitantly, there have to be greater than or equal to 8 polymorphonuclear leucocytes per high power (×1000) microscopic field in the urinalysis. The prostate may be involved in acute cystitis as well.

Men with urethritis might have a discharge on examination. Complications of urethritis can be epididymo-orchitis, reactive arthritis, or Reiter's syndrome. Diagnosis is made by a Gram-stained urethral smear containing greater than or equal to 5 polymorphonuclear leukocytes per high power (×1000) microscopic field, and/or the identification of greater than or equal to 10 polymorphonuclear leukocytes per high

TABLE 1. **Shift in the Bacterial Spectrum of Complicated Urinary Tract Infections from 1983 to 2001***

Species	1983 %	1990 %	1996 %	1998 %	2000 %	2001 %
Escherichia coli	35.2	21.8	32.0	27.2	30.7	31.5
Proteus spp.	12.7	6.1	7.8	5.8	7.0	8.9
Klebsiella spp.	6.8	5.4	7.8	6.5	10.0	7.4
Pseudomonas spp.	5.1	12.0	7.8	12.0	10.9	7.2
Other gram-negatives	7.6	4.8	9.3	9.2	8.8	7.5
Enterococcus spp.	16.0	29.3	19.9	22.0	21.9	23.2
Staphylococcus spp.	16.5	20.6	15.4	17.3	10.7	14.3
Total (n)	393	441	354	382	488	517

*Urologic Clinic, St. Elisabeth Clinic, Straubing, Germany.

power (×1000) microscopic field on a Gram-stained preparation from a first-pass urine specimen after not having passed urine for 4 hours. Mere microscopy of the Gram stain for Gram-negative diplococci has sensitivity of greater than 90% to exclude gonorrhea. Additionally culture, amplified antigen detection tests, or nucleic acid amplification tests should be performed on all samples. The most sensitive test for diagnosis of chlamydia is nucleic acid amplification of smears or first voided morning urine, with a sensitivity of 70% to 95% and a specificity of 97% to 99%.

Treatment

As empiric treatment of uncomplicated cystitis in adult men, fluoroquinolones should be favored because of their improved effectiveness. Possible agents could be ciprofloxacin (Cipro) 500 mg twice daily, levofloxacin (Levaquin) 500 mg or gatifloxacin (Tequin) 400 mg once daily. Duration of therapy should be 7 days (see Table 2). Short-term therapy, such as for acute cystitis in women, is not established in men.

Treatment for gonorrheal urethritis should also be in concordance with local resistance rates. In any case treatment should be instigated at the patient's first visit. Recommended single dose regimens are: Ciprofloxacin 500 mg, Ofloxacin 400 mg, or alternatively, ceftriaxone (Rocephin) 250 mg intramuscularly (IM), spectinomycin (Trobicin) 2 g IM, cefixime (Suprax) 400 mg or amoxicillin 3 g plus probenecid 1 g (only if local penicillin resistance is <5%). Additionally treatment for non-gonorrheal urethritis should be carried out, employing one of the following agents: Doxycycline (Vibramycin) 100 mg, twice a day for 7 days, azithromycin (Zithromax) 1 g orally in a

Table 2. **Recommendations for Empiric Antibiotic Therapy of UTI**

Diagnosis	Frequent Pathogens	Calculated Initial Therapy	Duration of Therapy
Cystitis uncomplicated	*Escherichia coli* *Klebsiella* spp. *Proteus* spp. *Staphylococcus*	Fluoroquinolone* Fosfomycin tromethamine (Monurol) Alternatively: Aminoglycoside	7 days (only in males)
Pyelonephritis acute, uncomplicated	*Escherichia coli* *Proteus* spp. *Klebsiella* spp. Other enterobacteria staphylococci	Fluoroquinolone* 2nd generation Cephalosporin Alternatively: Aminopenicillin/BLI Aminoglycoside	7-10 days
Urethritis	*Neisseria gonorrhoeae*	Ciprofloxacin (Cipro) Ofloxacin Ceftriaxone (Rocephin) Spectinomycin (Trobicin) Cefixime (Suprax) Amoxicillin + Probenecid	Single dose
Urethritis	Nongonococcal	Doxycycline (Vibramycin) Azithromycin (Zithromax) Erythromycin Ofloxacin Roxithromycin Clarithromycin	7 days Single dose 7 days Single dose 7 days 7 days
UTI complicated nosocomial UTI Pyelonephritis acute, complicated	*Escherichia coli* *Enterococci* *Pseudomonas* spp. Staphylococci *Klebsiella* spp. *Proteus spp.* *Enterobacter* spp. other enterobacteria *(Candida* spp.*)*	Fluoroquinolone* Aminopenicillin/BLI 2nd generation cephalosporin 3rd generation cephalosporin When initial therapy fails: *Pseudomonas* active Acylaminopenicillin/BLI 3rd generation cephalosporin Carbapenem In *Candida*: Fluconazole (Diflucan) Amphotericin B (Fungizone)	3-5 days until after defervescence respectively treatment of complicating factors
Urosepsis	*Escherichia coli* other enterobacteria after urologic procedures multiresistant pathogens: *Pseudomonas* spp. *Proteus* spp. *Serratia* spp. *Enterobacter* spp.	3rd generation cephalosporin ± Aminoglycoside Fluoroquinolone* Pseudomonas active Acylaminopenicillin/BLI Carbapenem	3-5 days until after defervescence, respectively; treatment of complicating factors

BLI, β-lactamase inhibitor
*Fluoroquinolone with sufficient urinary concentration, not for use in children.

single dose, or alternatively, erythromycin 500 mg, 4 times a day for 7 days, ofloxacin 200 mg orally twice a day for 7 days, roxithromycin 150 mg orally twice a day for 7 days, or clarithromycin 250 mg orally twice a day for 7 days (see Table 2). Treatment of partners in urethritis is important.

COMPLICATED UTI

Complicated UTIs are found in males much more frequently than uncomplicated UTIs, and complicating factors should be meticulously investigated. The antimicrobial spectrum in complicated UTIs is much broader than in uncomplicated UTIs (Table 1). In early childhood congenital factors such as uretero-renal reflux, urethral valves, phimosis, or congenital neurologic disorders have to be thought of, whereas in later age acquired factors, such as HIV infection, diabetes mellitus, or acquired neurologic disorders or urine transport disturbances are more frequent. A significant portion of UTI in early childhood are febrile (>101.3°F) or develop into febrile UTI and have to be treated with great care. An effective antibiotic therapy has to be initiated within the first 24 to 48 hours. The frequency of UTIs in association with primary uretero-renal reflux in males declines markedly after 2 years of age. UTIs in association with significant obstructive disease are even more prone to cause renal damage, above all, in the case of subvesical obstruction in males, such as urethral valve disease. *Proteus* spp. is a rare cause of UTI in children, however it can be observed in 1- to 2-year-old boys with phimosis and obstructed urinary flow. It is then frequently associated with infection stones in the urogenital tract.

Complicated UTI in adult males can be due to a variety of causes. With increasing patient age the risk of catheterization for an underlying urologic disease (i.e., prostatic hyperplasia) increases.

Other causes include immunosuppressive disorders, such as HIV infection. About 20% of patients infected with HIV experience at least one episode of UTI during their disease, depending on the CD^4-cell count. Patients infected with HIV-1 and a CD^4-cell count less than 200 mm^3 are at increased risk for bacteriuria. However, only 60% of infections are symptomatic. The risk for the acquisition of a UTI is also determined by the length of hospitalization.

Treatment

Only certain antibiotic substances can be used for treatment of UTI. The antibiotic must possess the adequate pharmacodynamic and pharmacokinetic prerequisites, i.e., high renal, unmetabolized clearance, with good antibacterial activity, both in acidic and alkaline urine. Because, in the treatment of nosocomial UTI more resistant, frequently multiresistant isolates must be considered, antibiotic therapy should be, at best, in accordance with susceptibility testing or the antibiotic cover must be broadened. Multiple substances are available (Table 2): First through fourth-generation cephalosporins, ureidopenicillins, with or without β-lactamase inhibitors, monobactams, and carbapenems. For empirical therapy of severe UTI, for example pending urosepsis, broad-spectrum antibiotics should be used, (i.e., broad spectrum penicillins with β-lactamase inhibitors, third- and fourth-generation cephalosporins, fluoroquinolones, and carbapenems) (see Table 2). Possible synergism with aminoglycosides, which block protein synthesis and thus block the forming of toxins or virulence factors, might be useful for initial therapy, if side effects are considered. In order to decrease the selection pressure for resistant pathogens, suitable antibiotics from different classes should be used. Antibiotic prophylaxis is indicated if recurrent UTIs pose the hazard of renal damage.

But, in all cases of complicated UTI, the complicating factors must be diagnosed and treated efficiently in addition to antibiotic therapy.

BACTERIAL INFECTIONS OF THE URINARY TRACT IN WOMEN

method of
PATRICIA D. BROWN, M.D., and
JACK D. SOBEL, M.D.
Wayne State University School of Medicine
Detroit, Michigan

Urinary tract infection (UTI) is common in women and accounts for more than 7 million physician visits annually in the United States. It is estimated that 50% of women will have at least one episode of acute cystitis at some point during adulthood. A number of risk factors for UTI are recognized, including diabetes mellitus, catheterization, instrumentation, and structural or functional abnormalities of the urinary tract; however, most women with UTI have none of these predisposing factors. Epidemiologic studies have demonstrated a strong association between vaginal intercourse and the risk of UTI in young women. In addition, studies have suggested an independent association between the risk of UTI and the contraceptive method used in sexually active women. The use of a diaphragm with spermicide has been associated with a higher risk of infection. This contraceptive method has been shown to increase rates of vaginal colonization with uropathogenic organisms and decrease rates of colonization with lactobacilli. Few data are available regarding the relative risk of UTI in association with other methods of contraception.

The pathogenesis of UTI in women is almost always ascending infection from organisms that originate from the fecal flora. Hematogenous infection can occur but is exceedingly rare. Uropathogens first colonize the vaginal introitus and urethra and may then gain entry into the bladder. Bacterial virulence factors and host factors are important in the progression from colonization to symptomatic infection of the bladder (lower tract infection or cystitis). Once organisms gain entry into the bladder, the infection may ascend further, via the ureter, to the kidney (upper tract infection or pyelonephritis). Although local host factors such as vesicoureteral reflux may increase the risk of pyelonephritis, most otherwise healthy women with upper tract infection do not have any demonstrable structural or functional abnormality of the urinary tract.

UTI can be further categorized as complicated and uncomplicated. Factors associated with complicated UTI are outlined in Table 1.

The microbiology of UTI is very predictable. Most infections are caused by *Escherichia coli. Staphylococcus saprophyticus* is an important pathogen in young, sexually active women with cystitis and may account for up to 20% of infections in this group. Complicated or nosocomially acquired infections may be due to *Klebsiella, Proteus, Enterobacter, Pseudomonas,* or *Enterococcus.*

CLINICAL FINDINGS AND DIAGNOSIS

Patients with acute cystitis have complaints of dysuria, urgency, frequency, and hesitancy, often with suprapubic or lower abdominal pain. Hematuria may be present; though often alarming to the patient, hematuria does not portend a poor prognosis or suggest a complicated infection. The presence of hematuria can help distinguish UTI from vaginitis or urethritis in women with dysuria. Although low-grade fever may occur, temperature elevations in excess of 38°C should raise the suspicion of pyelonephritis. Risk factors for occult upper tract infection include the presence of symptoms for more than 7 days, as well as any of the conditions listed in Table 1. In addition, it has been shown that up to one third of patients evaluated in urban emergency departments with acute cystitis may have occult pyelonephritis.

Once suspected from the clinical findings, the diagnosis of UTI can be confirmed by microscopic examination of a clean-catch midstream urine sample. The sample should be centrifuged at 2000 rpm for 5 minutes and examined under high power for the presence of bacteria and leukocytes (white blood cells [WBCs]). The presence of one or more bacteria per high-power field (HPF) has a sensitivity of 90% to 95% and a specificity of 80% to 90% for the detection of significant bacteriuria. The presence of significant pyuria, defined as more than 5 WBCs per HPF, has a sensitivity of 80% to 90%, but the specificity is variable (30% to 80%). When microscopic examination of urine is not available, biochemical tests in the form of a rapid dipstick may be used to detect the presence of bacteriuria and pyuria. The dipstick method relies on the detection of nitrites produced by certain bacteria from dietary nitrates. Although the specificity of nitrite detection is 92% to 99%, its sensitivity is poor; some uropathogens (e.g., *Enterococcus, Pseudomonas*) do not produce nitrites, and urine must be retained in the bladder for several hours for nitrites to be detectable. The rapid dipstick method may also be used to detect leukocyte esterase liberated by WBCs in the urine. The sensitivity and specificity of the leukocyte esterase test are 75% to 96% and 94% to 98%, respectively.

Urine culture remains the gold standard for the diagnosis of UTI. Isolation of 10^5 or more colony-forming units (CFU) per milliliter of bacteria from a properly collected urine sample is considered significant bacteriuria. However, it has been shown that up to 50% of women with UTI may have counts lower than this, and counts as low as 10^2 CFU/mL may be sufficient to confirm the diagnosis of UTI in a symptomatic woman. Because the microbiology of acute uncomplicated cystitis is so predictable and because short-course antibiotic therapy is frequently used, pretherapy urine culture is not considered cost-effective. Urine culture should be obtained in patients who fail to respond to therapy, those in whom symptoms recur shortly after the completion of therapy, and women with complicated UTI.

The differential diagnosis of acute cystitis in women includes the acute urethral (frequency-dysuria) syndrome and vaginitis. The acute urethral syndrome may be caused by *Chlamydia trachomatis, Neisseria gonorrhoeae,* or herpes simplex virus. *Candida* or *Trichomonas* vaginitis may be manifested as dysuria, so a careful history of gynecologic symptoms should be obtained in women with suspected UTI and a pelvic examination performed when appropriate. In patients primarily with urinary frequency, interstitial or radiation cystitis, urethral stenosis, cystocele or prolapse, or neurologic causes of detrusor muscle instability should be considered.

TABLE 1. **Factors Associated With Complicated Urinary Tract Infection**

Factors
Obstruction (bladder outlet obstruction, uterine prolapse, stones, tumor, congenital abnormalities)
Foreign body (catheter, stent)
Postvoid residual greater than 100 mL (neurologic disease, medications)
Vesicoureteral reflux
Recent invasive urologic procedure
Renal transplant
Azotemia
Ileal loop
Immunosuppression
Diabetes mellitus
Pregnancy
Nosocomial infection

TREATMENT OF ACUTE CYSTITIS

As discussed earlier, nonpregnant adult women with acute uncomplicated cystitis may be treated empirically without obtaining a urine culture. Urine microscopy or a dipstick should be used whenever possible to support the clinical diagnosis of UTI. Trimethoprim-sulfamethoxazole (TMP-SMZ; Bactrim or Septra) should be given as one double-strength tablet twice daily for 3 days. Single-dose therapy has been studied but is associated with high relapse rates. Three-day therapy has been shown to achieve cure rates comparable to those of longer courses of treatment and is as well tolerated as single-dose therapy. During the past decade, a number of reports have shown that the prevalence of resistance to TMP-SMZ in uropathogenic *E. coli* is increasing, which has led some experts to recommend that this antimicrobial not be used for empirical therapy in communities where the prevalence of resistance exceeds 10% to 20%. Because culture is not routinely performed in women with acute uncomplicated cystitis, most providers lack access to data regarding the prevalence of TMP-SMZ resistance in their local community. Because TMP-SMZ achieves very high concentrations in the urine, some have questioned the clinical implications of in vitro resistance. However, several recent studies have shown that women infected with a TMP-SMZ–resistant isolate who are treated with this agent are more likely to experience clinical failure as compared with women infected with a TMP-SMZ–susceptible isolate. At the present time, it is our recommendation that TMP-SMZ remain first-line therapy for acute uncomplicated cystitis. Clinicians need to be aware of the issue of emerging resistance and consider the possibility of resistance when evaluating a patient who fails to respond to initial empirical therapy. Although the risk factors for infection with a TMP-SMZ–resistant uropathogen are at present poorly defined, several studies have suggested that a history of recent antibiotic use is important. Clinicians may want to consider alternative therapy for women who have taken TMP-SMZ in the several weeks preceding the diagnosis of UTI.

Fluoroquinolones can be used for the treatment of acute uncomplicated cystitis in patients who are allergic to TMP-SMZ, and they are effective as short-course (3-day) therapy. Norfloxacin (Noroxin), ciprofloxacin (Cipro), ofloxacin (Floxin) and levofloxacin (Levaquin) are effective, though expensive alternatives to TMP-SMZ. Uropathogenic *E. coli* have generally remained susceptible to nitrofurantoin (Macobid); however, cure rates with 3-day therapy are inferior to those achieved by TMP-SMZ or fluoroquinolones, so more prolonged (7-day) courses of therapy are required. Although nitrofurantoin has been associated with a diverse array of toxicities, short-course therapy is safe and associated with few side effects. Fosfomycin tromethamine (Monurol) is approved in the United States for the treatment of acute uncomplicated cystitis. A 3-g single dose achieves therapeutic concentrations in the urine for 1 to 3 days. Even as a single dose, it is a more expensive alternative than 3 days of TMP-SMZ or 7 days of nitrofurantoin.

Patients who fail to respond to empirical short-course therapy should have urine obtained for culture and susceptibility testing, with further treatment guided by these results. An initial response to short-course therapy followed by a prompt recurrence of symptoms is suggestive of occult pyelonephritis. Cultures should also be performed in these women, and they should receive 2 weeks of antibiotic therapy, with treatment adjusted if necessary based on culture results. Nitrofurantoin should not be used for the treatment of suspected pyelonephritis.

Failure of short-course therapy in a sexually active young woman should suggest the possibility of urethritis from *Chlamydia*, especially if sterile pyuria is documented. In these cases, a 7-day course of doxycycline should be considered. Short-course therapy should not be used for the treatment of elderly women with acute cystitis; a 7-day course of therapy is preferred. A suggested management strategy for acute cystitis is outlined in Figure 1.

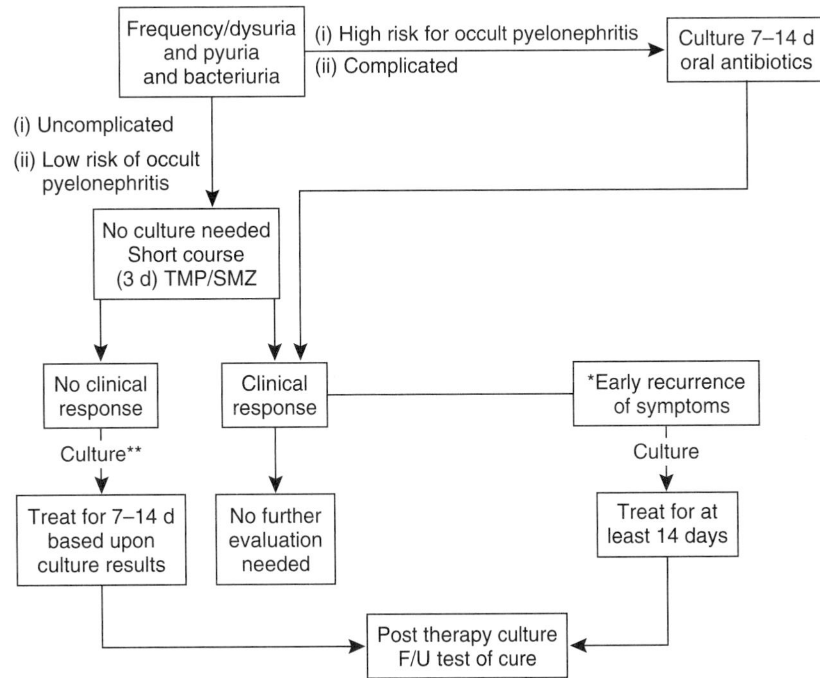

Figure 1. Suggested management strategy for acute cystitis.

RECURRENT URINARY TRACT INFECTION

Frequent, recurrent UTI (more than two episodes of infection per year) will develop in approximately one quarter of women with an episode of acute cystitis. Women with recurrent UTI tend to have reinfection rather than relapse. Strategies that can be used to manage recurrent UTI include continuous low-dose prophylaxis, postcoital prophylaxis (single-dose therapy taken within 2 hours of intercourse), and self-start therapy. Trimethoprim (Proloprim), TMP-SMZ, norfloxacin, and nitrofurantoin have been shown to be effective as prophylaxis. In postmenopausal women with frequent recurrent UTI, the use of estrogen replacement therapy, either oral or intravaginal, has been shown in several studies to be effective in preventing recurrent infections.

ASYMPTOMATIC BACTERIURIA

Asymptomatic bacteriuria is defined as the presence of 10^5 CFU/mL or more of the same organism in two separate clean-catch urine specimens in the absence of urinary tract symptoms. The prevalence of asymptomatic bacteriuria in nonpregnant women younger than 65 years is 3% to 6%. In elderly women, the prevalence of asymptomatic bacteriuria may be as high as 50%. In young women, sexual intercourse and the use of a diaphragm with spermicide have been shown to be risk factors for asymptomatic bacteriuria, just as they are for symptomatic UTI. Asymptomatic bacteriuria has never been shown to lead to renal damage in the absence of pre-existing anatomic abnormalities or obstruction of the urinary tract, and no benefit is gained from treatment, including the treatment of elderly, catheterized, or diabetic patients. The one exception is in pregnancy, where the prevalence of asymptomatic bacteriuria is 3% to 15%. In pregnant women with asymptomatic bacteriuria, the risk of pyelonephritis during the pregnancy is 20% to 40% versus 1% to 2% in pregnant women without asymptomatic infection. Pyelonephritis during pregnancy is associated with preterm labor and low-birth-weight infants. Accordingly, all pregnant women should be screened with a urine culture during early pregnancy, and those with significant bacteriuria should be treated with 7 days of antimicrobial therapy guided by culture and susceptibility results. Nitrofurantoin is considered first-line therapy for pregnant women; cephalosporins or amoxicillin may be used for susceptible isolates. TMP-SMZ and amoxicillin-clavulanate (Augmentin) are considered second-line agents; fluoroquinolones are not recommended for use during pregnancy. Successful treatment should be documented by repeat urine culture 1 to 2 weeks after the conclusion of therapy. These patients should have repeat urine culture every 4 to 6 weeks for the remainder of the pregnancy.

INVESTIGATIONAL STUDIES

Diagnostic imaging, urodynamic studies, and cystoscopy are rarely indicated in women with acute uncomplicated UTI. If stones or obstruction are suspected, excretory urography (intravenous pyelography) can be used; however, renal ultrasound with plain abdominal films is now considered an acceptable alternative. Diagnostic imaging is also indicated to exclude a suppurative complication of pyelonephritis in patients who fail to respond to appropriate therapy for upper tract infection. Precontrast and postcontrast computed axial tomography is considered the imaging modality of choice in this setting. Prospective studies have shown that less than 5% of women with cystitis have a correctable structural or functional abnormality of the urinary tract. Urologic investigation should be restricted to women with frequent, recurrent infections whose condition cannot be controlled with antibiotic prophylaxis strategies.

BACTERIAL INFECTIONS OF THE URINARY TRACT IN GIRLS

method of
ANTOINE E. KHOURY, M.D., FRCSC, FAAP,
and
K. AFSHAR, M.D., FRCSC
University of Toronto
Hospital for Sick Children
Toronto, Ontario, Canada

In addressing urinary tract infection (UTI) in girls, we will discuss issues ranging from asymptomatic bacteriuria to pyelonephritis. To prevent permanent renal damage, recognition of risk factors is essential. A structured approach to the diagnosis and management of UTI in girls is presented.

EPIDEMIOLOGY

In the first year of life, UTI is more common in boys than girls, but starting at the second year of life, the incidence of bacteriuria increases in girls. In school-aged children, UTI is two to three times more common in girls. A shorter urethral length and a higher incidence of voiding dysfunction (VD) are probably contributing factors.

CLASSIFICATION OF URINARY TRACT INFECTIONS

UTI may be classified according to manifestations, location, and other criteria. Noncomplicated UTIs are characterized by lower urinary tract symptoms, absence of systemic findings, and a normal urinary tract. Complicated UTIs are associated with fever, flank pain, systemic illness, or a known anatomic or functional problem. In children younger than 5 years, these clinical symptoms and signs are not accurate, and children should be approached as though they have a complicated UTI until proved otherwise.

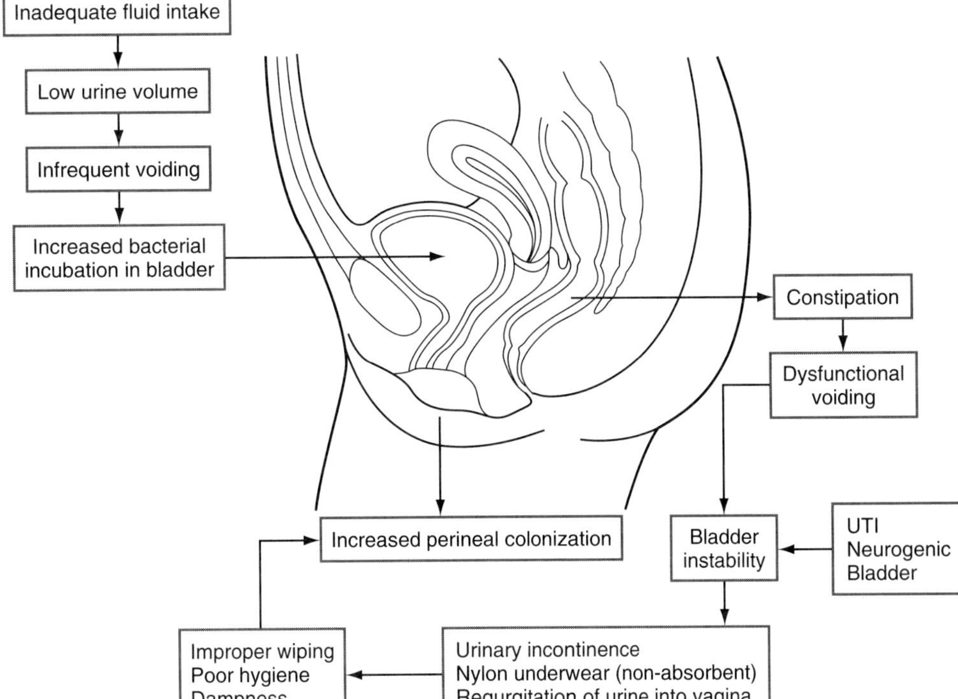

Figure 1. Pathogenesis of urinary tract infection (UTI) in girls.

ETIOLOGY

Gram-negative enteric bacteria are the most common organisms, with *Escherichia coli* being the most prevalent species. Enterococci and coagulase-negative staphylococci are the most common gram-positive bacteria causing UTI.

PATHOGENESIS

Understanding the pathogenesis of UTI has important therapeutic implications. Periurethral colonization by enteric organisms followed by ascending infection of the urinary tract is the most common means of bacterial access. Figure 1 highlights various host factors facilitating the access of organisms to the urinary tract and initiating the process of adhesion and invasion of the bladder wall. Urinary stasis leads to increased incubation time, which allows bacteria to overcome host resistance. Functional disorders of voiding and constipation have been identified as significant predisposing factors. Vesicoureteral reflux (VUR) facilitates involvement of the upper tract and pyelonephritis (Table 1).

DIAGNOSIS

History and Physical Examination

In neonates and infants, the symptoms are nonspecific, with fever being the most common. Lethargy, irritability, poor feeding, diarrhea, abdominal distention, and jaundice are other potential manifestations. In older children, abdominal pain and lower urinary tract symptoms such as dysuria, urgency, frequency, and incontinence may be identified. A history of holding maneuvers (leg crossing, squatting, etc.), daytime or nighttime incontinence, and constipation point toward DV. A history of a previous UTI and a family history of urinary tract abnormalities such as VUR should be obtained.

Abdominal examination may reveal flank or suprapubic tenderness. A palpable bladder may indicate an emptying problem. A palpable mass may represent stool in the colon, a sign of severe constipation. Examination of the genitalia may reveal signs of local irritation secondary to incontinence. Labial adhesions, vaginal discharge, and signs of sexual abuse should be noted.

TABLE 1. **Factors Affecting the Incidence and Severity of Urinary Tract Infection**

Bacterial Factors	Host Factors
P-fimbriae adhesion	Age
Rapid doubling time	Gender
Cell wall porins to prevent lysis	Voiding dysfunction
Capsular antigens to prevent phagocytosis	Constipation
Cellular toxins such as hemolysins	Anatomic abnormalities (vesicoureteral reflux, obstruction, neurogenic bladder, etc.)
Aerobactin to accumulate iron	Genetic factors (P1 blood group)
Ability to colonize the bowel and lower urinary tract	Immature immune system
	Low urinary IgA
	Eradication of normal flora by medications
	Lack of breast-feeding
	Sexual activity

TABLE 2. **Recommendations for Antimicrobial Therapy**

Drug	Treatment Dosage	Prophylaxis Dosage
Nitrofurantoin (Macrodantin)	5-7 mg/kg/d q6h	1-2 mg/kg/d
Cotrimoxazole (Septra)*	8-10 mg/kg/d q12h	2-3 mg/kg/d
Amoxicillin (Amoxil)	20-40 mg/kg/d q8h	20 mg/kg/d
Cephalexin (Keflex)	25-100 mg/kg/d q6h	20 mg/kg/d
Ceftriaxone (Rocephin) (IV)	75 mg/kg/d q24h	
Ampicillin (IV)	100 mg/kg/d q6h	
Gentamicin (Garamycin) (IV)	7.5 mg/kg/d q8h	
Tobramycin (Nebcin) (IV)	5-7.5 mg/kg/d q8h	

*Dosage based on trimethoprim component.
Modified from McKenna PH: Urinary Tract Infection in Girls. *In* Rakel RE, Bope ET (eds): Conn's Current Therapy 2002. Philadelphia, WB Saunders, 2002.

The sacral area should be examined for signs of spinal dysraphism, such as a hair patch or skin dimples.

Urinalysis and Urine Culture

A common problem in the diagnosis of UTI is a false-positive urine culture as a result of poor specimen collection technique. The gold standard for the diagnosis of UTI is quantitative urine culture, but at least 24 hours is required for such culture. Urinalysis may be of value for initial screening. Four components of the urinalysis are important: (1) during microscopic examination for white blood cells (WBCs), more than 10 WBCs per high-power field in the sediment is considered pyuria; (2) the presence of bacteria in the sediment represents at least 30,000 bacteria per milliliter of urine; (3) leukocyte esterase produced by the breakdown of WBCs in urine can be detected by dipstick; and (4) conversion of nitrates to nitrites by bacteria is also identified by dipstick. Although no individual test is as accurate as urine culture, a combination of tests is helpful in diagnosing UTI. For example, when urine microscopy for bacteria, nitrites, and WBC esterase are positive, the sensitivity for UTI is 100%. Conversely, when all three are negative, the negative predictive value approaches 100%.

Urine culture results should be interpreted in the context of other information, such as the method of collection and the patient's symptoms and age. A positive culture from a bag specimen is more likely to be due to contamination by skin flora. A bag specimen culture is only reliable when it is negative. A midstream

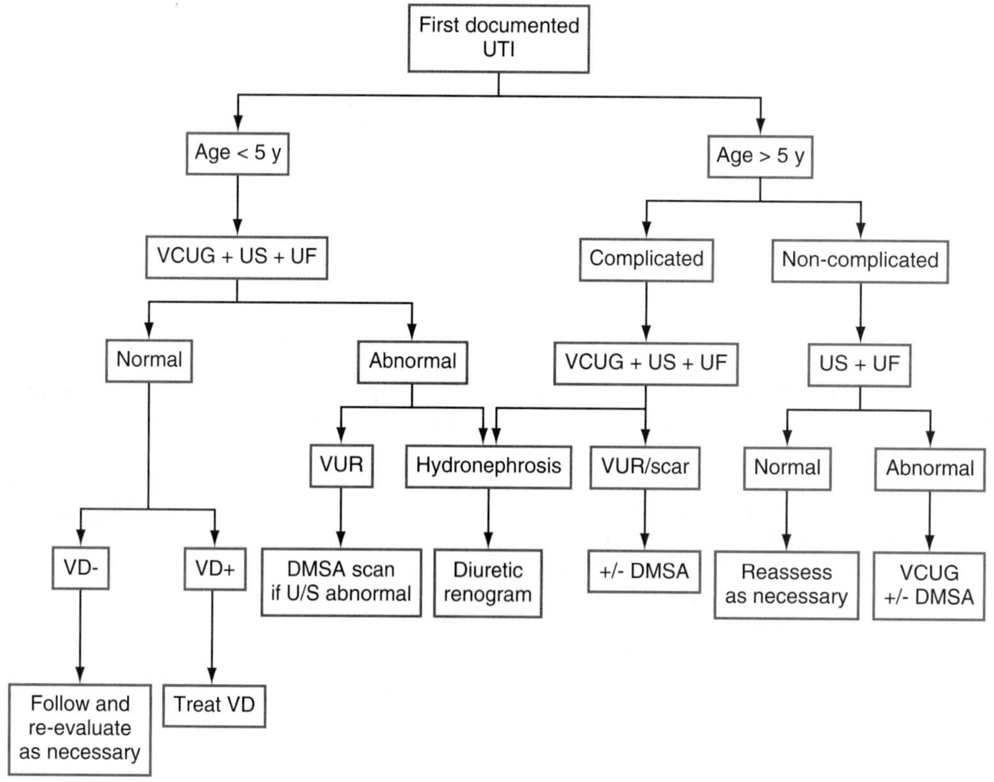

Figure 2. Investigation of urinary tract infection (UTI) in girls.

voided specimen is reliable in toilet-trained girls, especially if associated with significant pyuria. In a younger child, catheterization with a No. 5 French feeding tube or suprapubic aspiration is preferable. We do not recommend regular cultures in asymptomatic children.

Diagnostic Imaging

Every child with a well-documented UTI should be investigated. The goal of imaging is to identify risk factors for recurrence and renal damage. Such factors include, but are not limited to VUR (present in 21% to 57% of cases) and urinary obstruction. In a girl younger than 5 years with documented UTI, ultrasound of the urinary tract and a voiding cystourethrogram (VCUG) are recommended. Ultrasound evaluates the size and shape of the kidneys and provides information about the parenchyma and the collecting system. It can also identify dilated ureters. Bladder wall thickness and postvoid residual are assessed. VCUG detects VUR and evaluates the bladder wall and urethra. We recommend imaging studies after the first episode of infection because a high percentage of girls will have recurrent

TABLE 3. **Management of Voiding Dysfunction and Constipation**

Voiding Dysfunction	Constipation
Educate the family (pamphlets, Internet*)	Increase fluid intake
Increase fluid intake (1.5-2 L/d)	Oral agents:
Timed voiding (every 2-3 h)	Diet: fiber
Double void if postvoid residual is high	Fiber: psyllium (Metamucil)
General hygiene (e.g., wipe from front to back)	Stimulant: senna (Senokot)
Dietary changes (e.g., avoid caffeine)	Hyperosmolar agent: MiraLax lactulose
Establish a reward system—avoid punishment	Salts: milk of magnesia
Follow progress with a voiding diary	Lubricants: mineral oil
Consider pelvic muscle retraining and biofeedback therapy	Enemas
	Lubricant: mineral oil, Fleet
	Stimulant: bisacodyl
	Do not use phenolphthalein in children
	A moderate- to high-dose stimulant may be needed in severe cases, but it should be used short-term
	In severe cases, initial clean up may be achieved faster by using an enema or oral MiraLax

*For further information, please visit http://www.yourchildshealth.echn.ca/kids.htm.

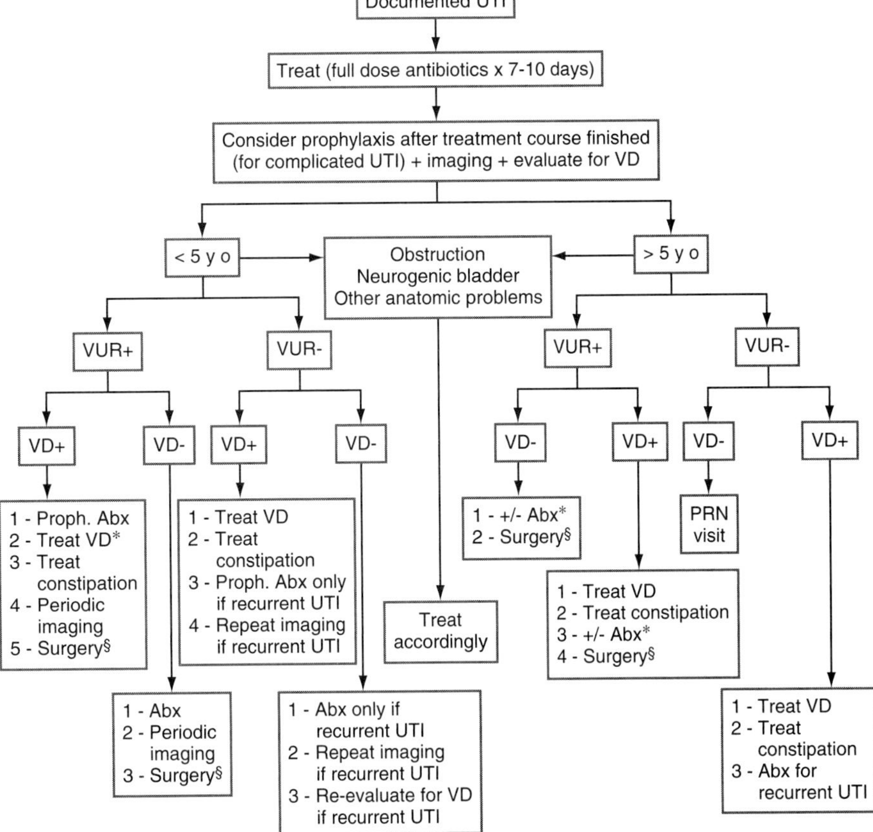

Figure 3. Management of urinary tract infection (UTI) in girls.

infection in the next years, the yield of the studies is high, and the consequences of not detecting these abnormalities, though uncommon, are serious. For example, 17% of cases of prepubertal UTI result in renal scars, 10% to 20% of which lead to hypertension and, rarely, end-stage renal disease. If the girl is older than 5 years at the initial evaluation, only ultrasound is performed initially. Further studies are dependent on the ultrasound result and the clinical situation.

Other studies are ordered according to the history and results of the physical examination and preliminary imaging. A plain radiograph of the abdomen may show calculi, stool load, and abnormalities of the spine. A dimercaptosuccinic acid (DMSA) nuclear scan evaluates the renal cortex for scarring and differential function. A diuretic nuclear renogram is used to assess obstruction. Intravenous pyelography is rarely performed. Full urodynamic studies, which are invasive, are indicated only in patients with severe anatomic or functional disorders.

A voiding diary, noninvasive uroflowmetry, and determination of the postvoid residual by ultrasound, with or without patch electromyography, can provide useful information about micturition. Cystoscopy and urethral dilation have no role in the diagnosis of UTI in these girls. Our approach is shown in Figure 2.

MANAGEMENT

The goal of management is to treat the acute infection and prevent recurrence and renal damage.

Table 2 summarizes the recommendations for antibiotic therapy. Empirical treatment starts with antibiotics effective against gram-negative organisms, which can later be changed according to culture results. Co-trimoxazole (Septra) is a good initial choice because it decreases the vaginal flora. The sulfa component is not safe in neonates, so trimethoprim (Proloprim) or ampicillin may be used in this group. Nitrofurantoin (Macrodantin) is effective only in urine and cannot eliminate bacteria in tissue. Most of the aforementioned medications have minimal effect on enteric flora, which lowers the incidence of drug resistance. Septic patients require intravenous treatment with ampicillin and gentamicin (Garamycin) or third-generation cephalosporins. Prophylactic antibiotics (daily low dose) include co-trimoxazole, nitrofurantoin, or cephalexin (Keflex). Prophylaxis is used in patients younger than 5 years with VUR or in those in whom conservative management has failed to prevent recurrent UTI.

Management of VD is of paramount importance. Our approach includes a bladder-retraining program entailing increased fluid intake, timed voiding every 2 to 3 hours, general hygienic measures, and aggressive treatment of constipation, as shown in Table 3. More sophisticated methods involving computer games to achieve behavioral changes have been used with success.

VUR is closely related to UTI and VD. Treatment of VD and prophylactic antibiotics are required in the majority of cases. Surgical correction of VUR is indicated for breakthrough infections or progressive renal damage. Surgery in the face of untreated VD is ill advised. Our approach is summarized in Figure 3.

Management of UTI in girls is evolving. Differentiating complicated from noncomplicated infection and considering the age at initial evaluation are helpful in management. Identification of risk factors is essential to prevent serious consequences. Some issues still await better clarification by prospective studies, such as the role of antibiotics in patients older than 5 years.

CHILDHOOD ENURESIS

method of
MARK P. CAIN, M.D.
Indiana University School of Medicine
James Whitcomb Riley Hospital for Children
Indianapolis, Indiana

Enuresis, or inappropriate wetting, is one of the more common diagnoses referred to a pediatric urology specialist. It is found in 5% to 10% of school-aged children, and can be a source of significant distress for both the child and parents. A great deal of interest has been focused toward childhood voiding disorders. As with many medical problems, the field has become more complex with changes in terminology as the specific etiology of the many underlying problems is understood. There are multiple potential causes of childhood incontinence, including anatomic, neuropathologic, and functional disorders. The majority of the children presenting with daytime and nighttime wetting will present with functional voiding abnormalities, and this discussion will focus primarily on the otherwise healthy child that presents with day or nighttime urinary incontinence. Unlike the child that presents with urinary tract infection, most of these children do not require complex radiographic or invasive bladder studies.

NORMAL BLADDER FUNCTION

To understand the abnormalities of urinary control, it is best to first start with a brief description of the normal development of urinary continence. The functional anatomy of the bladder is simple—a low pressure storage reservoir that is surrounded with smooth muscle; a "static" internal sphincter mechanism that passively holds urine; and a more complex external sphincter mechanism that has both smooth and skeletal muscle and is under voluntary control. During normal voiding, the detrusor muscle surrounding the bladder contracts, with reflex relaxation of the internal sphincter. The external sphincter complex should remain relaxed during micturition. Voiding can be postponed by increasing the tone in the external sphincter complex, which will in turn (eventually) suppress the detrusor contraction.

The newborn and young child will empty the bladder reflexively 20 or more times a day. The bladder contraction is modulated by a spinal cord reflex that responds to stretching in the bladder wall, resulting in complete and efficient bladder emptying. With increasing age, the bladder capacity increases (approximately one ounce per year, with a rough estimate of bladder capacity equaling age + 2 = bladder capacity in ounces). With further development there is inhibition of the spinal micturitional reflex, and recognition of bladder filling. Initial bladder control is usually associated with some degree of urgency behavior, but most children master voluntary control between 2 and 3 years of age. Complete urine and stool continence develops with nocturnal bowel control first, followed by daytime bowel control, daytime urinary control, and finally nocturnal urinary control. From a very simplified perspective, urinary control is obtained when there is low pressure filling of an adequate capacity bladder that can be emptied with a detrusor contraction associated with complete relaxation of the sphincter complex. Abnormalities in any of these variables may lead to incontinence.

Many children who present with daytime urgency incontinence will be "busy" children that will rely on the external voluntary sphincter to suppress bladder contraction. The bladder contractions eventually become more forceful and result in urgency dribbling and damp pants. This is very typical of the child during early toilet training, but can become problematic if the child continues to depend on this dyssynergic bladder function because it leads to continual increased muscle activity in the perineal muscles, leading to worsening dysfunctional voiding and constipation. The converse can also be true, with constipation due to painful stooling leading to stool withholding and constipation, with secondary urinary symptoms. This is now commonly referred to as "dysfunctional elimination syndrome," and it involves abnormalities in both bladder and bowel elimination.

EVALUATION

History

Characterization of urinary incontinence is key to separating the more common functional voiding disorders from neuropathic or anatomic problems. Classic patients with an anatomic abnormality leading to incontinence will usually present with continual urinary leakage their entire life, often with no recognition of when the leakage occurs. These patients are best evaluated with ultrasound imaging of the kidneys and bladder to identify the anatomic problem. Children with functional disorders will often have a variable period of successful toilet training followed by progressive incontinence, and some will present with a history of recurrent urinary infections as well. It is imperative to have the parents involved in the process of evaluating the history, as many will be unaware of the child's habits and in this circumstance a voiding diary will be useful to document the voiding and stooling history and to engage the parents. The patient history will frequently help differentiate the cause of urinary leakage—whether it is due to an overactive bladder, infrequent voiding, or a neuroanatomic problem. Some of the key elements of the history are as follows:

Onset of incontinence—At what age was the child toilet trained? Did the child have a long period of continence after toilet training? Were there any other circumstances associated with the onset of incontinence (medical or social)?

Severity of incontinence—Does the child wet through the clothing, or just stain the undergarments? Does it occur daily? If it is nighttime wetting only, how many times does the child wet the bed in an average week?

Patterns associated with incontinence—Does the child exhibit micturitional posturing (squatting, crossing legs, and so on) prior to wetting? Does the child wet immediately after voiding on the toilet (suggesting vaginal reflux of urine)? Does the child wet after holding urine for an extended period of time?

Voiding history—Does the child have daytime urgency? How frequently does the child void during the day (every 10 to 15 minutes or 2 to 3 times daily)? Does the child have an interrupted stream suggesting obstruction? Is the urinary stream deflected? Is there pain associated with voiding? Is there ever blood in the urine? Is there a history of urinary tract infection? Is there a history of infrequent, or hard stools, or a problem with encopresis?

The family history is also important to elicit because nocturnal enuresis has a strong genetic component, and some believe that the age of resolution in the family is predictive of when the child might expect to outgrow the condition.

Other important factors are a history of urologic or nephrologic disorders, such as posterior urethral valves, vesicoureteral reflux, or nephrogenic diabetes insipidus that may impair urinary concentrating ability. A history of previous urologic surgery may also impair urinary control. All of these patients would be good candidates for early referral to a urologist.

Physical Examination

The physical examination for voiding disorders can be tailored to exclude a limited number of associated findings. The abdomen should be examined for the presence of constipation or palpable masses. The back should be carefully examined to exclude abnormalities of the gluteal crease or evidence of a sacral dimple that may suggest underlying spinal cord pathology. The anal sphincter tone should be evaluated, and if a neurologic abnormality is suspected, the anal wink assessed. The perineal examination will sometimes demonstrate excoriation and/or fecal soiling that will correlate to the severity of urine/stool leakage. The genitalia in girls should be examined to exclude labial adhesions that may cause urine to pool in the vagina, and to ensure that a subtle abnormality of the urethra or vagina was not overlooked when the child was younger. In males, the urethral meatus should be evaluated to rule out narrowing or inflammation. Because circumcision is becoming less routine, the uncircumcised penis should be fully evaluated to make sure the foreskin is retractable, and does not allow pooling of urine due to phimosis. A simple neurologic examination assessing gait, reflexes, and evidence of high foot arches will exclude significant neurologic sources.

Laboratory/Radiographic Evaluation

Children with mild daytime or nighttime symptoms who have no history of urinary tract infection and have a normal examination should be evaluated with a urinalysis to rule out medical renal disorders or urinary tract infection. No other workup is necessary unless they are refractory to standard therapy. Patients with more complicated voiding disorders, the presence of significant encopresis, a history of urinary tract infection, or a neurologic abnormality should undergo evaluation with a renal and bladder ultrasound, voiding cystourethrogram with abdominal film (KUB) and lumbosacral spine film, urinalysis, and urine culture. More complex evaluation with spinal magnetic resonance imaging (MRI) is pursued in patients with very abnormal physical examination of the lower spine, or with an abnormality on the plain film of the spine. Occult spina bifida of one or two lumbar vertebrae is a common finding, and has minimal clinical ramifications. Bladder evaluation with urodynamics is an invasive test that is not routinely performed, but can be helpful in patients that are refractory to standard therapy, or who have a suspected neurologic lesion.

Many urologists have the capability to perform ultrasound examination inexpensively in the office, and in this scenario a post-void bladder ultrasound can be very helpful to evaluate the patient's ability to empty the bladder.

MANAGEMENT

Engaging the child and the family in the treatment plan is key. In general, children with daytime incontinence will have either: (1) a failure to store urine (usually due to an overactive bladder with uninhibited contractions), (2) failure to empty their bladder (urinary retention), or (3) a combination of both. Each of these abnormalities requires specific treatment. It is also important to identify even subtle constipation because failure to address this in the treatment plan will often lead to failure or recurrence of symptoms.

DAYTIME (DIURNAL) ENURESIS

The classic patient presents with periodic urgency with micturitional posturing (squatting on the heel, dancing, holding groin, and so on) with or without recurrent lower urinary tract infections. The urinary stream may be interrupted due to the poor ability to relax the external sphincter complex. Functional bladder capacity is usually diminished.

Initial measures are focused toward developing a timed voiding schedule (every 2 hours, prior to the uninhibited bladder contraction), good perineal hygiene, and dietary changes to include high fiber foods. If this is not successful, then anticholinergic medication is added, either oxybutinin (Ditropan),* or tolterodine (Detrol).* Both are available in immediate release tablets given two or three times daily, or in extended release tablets. The advantage of the extended release tablet is a significant reduction in the common side effects including constipation, facial flushing, and dry mouth. If constipation is a factor, this can be treated with mineral oil, polyethylene glycol (Miralax), lactulose (Cephalac) or Senokot. Low-dose suppressive antibiotics are also initiated for patients with a history of frequent urinary tract infection. This should be continued until the underlying risk factor for infection has been corrected.

Children that are refractory to therapy should be evaluated with a bladder ultrasound to ensure that they are emptying their bladder. Poor emptying due to chronic increased tone in the external sphincter complex can be treated with biofeedback training, but requires skilled nursing personnel. More recently, selective α-adrenergic inhibitors such as doxazosin (Cardura),* have been used in the pediatric population to improve bladder emptying.

Young girls with post-void dribbling in their underpants are usually vaginal voiders, and the incontinence is due to trapping urine in the vagina, which then leaks out after the patient stands up. This can be managed by either having the child sit backwards on the toilet, or spreading the legs widely apart when voiding.

INFREQUENT VOIDING

Children with infrequent voiding and daytime wetting are best managed with a strictly timed voiding schedule. These patients often have chronically overdistended, large bladders with poor sensation during filling. Urinary tract infection and constipation are common in these patients. In extreme conditions, when therapy as listed earlier is unsuccessful, a trial of intermittent catheterization may be necessary.

NOCTURNAL ENURESIS

Nighttime wetting is a very common condition in the school-aged child, with approximately 15% to 20% of children having occasional nocturnal wetting. This is usually attributed to a maturational delay of the ability to subconsciously suppress the micturition reflex. Spontaneous resolution occurs in 15% each year. The condition is benign from a medical standpoint,

*Not FDA approved for this indication.

but can cause significant psychological distress in some children. A decision to treat should be based on the child and family's motivation.

The evaluation and history are identical to the patient presenting with daytime wetting. Ten percent to 15% of children with nocturnal enuresis will also have daytime accidents, and in this group of patients, it is critical to address the small functional bladder capacity first, as this will limit the success of therapy directed solely to nighttime wetting.

Treatment options are directed toward the underlying factors that can lead to wetting: duration and depth of sleep, amount of urine produced overnight, and functional bladder capacity. Wetting occurs whenever the duration of sleep allows enough urine to be produced to overwhelm the bladder capacity, leading to a reflex contraction and a wet bed. The majority of these patients are very deep sleepers and will not wake even after the accident.

Initial measures should include evening fluid restrictions, and motivational therapy based on praise and positive rewards. The child cannot control the enuresis, and should not be punished for failure. Conditioning therapy, usually with an alarm system, is effective in approximately 50%, and provides the only sustained long term "cure" of any of the therapies. This is labor intensive for both child and parent because it requires the child to be awakened and taken to the bathroom to empty the remainder of his/her bladder whenever the alarm sounds. On average 3 to 4 months of continual use of the alarm is necessary for the child to achieve success.

The commonly used medications for nighttime wetting are tricyclic antidepressants imipramine (Tofranil), and desmopressin acetate (DDAVP). In patients with daytime symptoms of enuresis and small functional bladder capacity, the long-acting anticholinergics (Detrol LA,* Ditropan XL*) provide a significant increase in the bladder capacity, and can be started as initial therapy or as combination therapy with other medications for nocturnal enuresis.

Imipramine (Tofranil) has several mechanisms of action that are beneficial for nighttime wetting. It acts centrally to allow easier arousal for deep sleepers, has weak anticholinergic actions that relax the bladder, and tightens the bladder sphincter. Dosing should be tapered starting at 25 mg, and can be increased to 50 mg/d for preadolescents, and up to 75 mg/d for adolescents. Side effects can be profound in some patients, including insomnia, weight loss, anxiety, and personality changes. Fatal overdosage has been reported secondary to irreversible cardiac arrhythmia.

Desmopressin acetate (DDAVP) is a synthetic analogue of vasopressin, a potent antidiuretic. It is currently marketed as a 0.2 mg tablet, and can be used in doses of 0.1 to 0.6 mg/d, usually titrating the dose upward by one tablet per week. The drug is given 30 to 60 minutes prior to bedtime, and should be combined with fluid restriction in the evening. Side effects have been uncommon, occurring in less than 1%. Seizures have been reported secondary to hyponatremia, and some clinicians will avoid the medication in patients with a history of seizure disorders. Improvement in number of wet nights per week can be seen in 50% to 70% of patients, and combining DDAVP with either the bed alarm or long-acting anticholinergics will increase the success.

*Not FDA approved for this indication.

URINARY INCONTINENCE

method of
DEBORAH BARTHOLOMEW, M.D.
Ohio State University College of Medicine and Public Health
Columbus, Ohio

Aging of the population will require that primary care physicians have knowledge about the evaluation and treatment of urinary incontinence. It is thought to affect at least 20% of the adult population at some point in their life. Though more common in women, this disability increases in both sexes with advancing age. Its effect on quality of life can be severe, with social isolation and withdrawal; the cost of treatment is estimated to be in the billions of dollars. Incontinence is frequently the primary reason for nursing home admission. Patients are often embarrassed or reluctant to raise the issue because they erroneously attribute their problem to an expected consequence of aging. It is important to ask patients specifically about incontinence in as much as the vast majority of patients can be helped without referral to a specialist. An overview of urinary incontinence is presented along with a simplified workup and directed therapeutic options.

ETIOLOGY OF INCONTINENCE

Incontinence is simply defined as involuntary urine loss that is considered problematic and can be objectively demonstrated. *Reversible* causes of incontinence must be excluded. Helpful mnemonics include DIAPPERS (delirium, infection, atrophy, pharmaceuticals, psychological, excessive output, restricted mobility, and stool impaction) and DRIP (delirium, restricted mobility, retention, infection, impaction, pharmaceuticals, polyuria). Medications that can affect continence are listed in Table 1. Discussion with caretakers can be enlightening. Frequently, a simple bedside commode or a change in the timing of a medication is all that is needed. Urinalysis or an office urine dipstick test for nitrates, blood, and leukocyte esterase is a necessary first step in evaluation.

Functional incontinence implies that the urinary tract is normal but that restrictions in mobility or cognition impede effective toileting. Education of caregivers in the techniques of prompted or scheduled voiding may help decrease the frequency of incontinent episodes.

Urge incontinence, also known as detrusor instability or overactive bladder syndrome, is urine loss

TABLE 1. **Drug Side Effects**

Medication	Effect	Example
Diuretics	Frequency, urgency, polyuria	Furosemide (Lasix), hydrochlorothiazide
Anticholinergics	Retention, overflow incontinence, fecal impaction	Antihistamines, tricyclic antidepressants
Calcium channel blockers	Retention, overflow incontinence	Verapamil (Calan)
α-Adrenergic blockers	Stress incontinence	Prazosin (Minipress)
β-Adrenergic agonists	Retention	Terbutaline (Brethine)
Psychotropics	Retention, overflow incontinence	Perphenazine (Trilafon), haloperidol (Haldol)
Narcotics, sedatives	Retention, fecal impaction, loss of voluntary control	Meperidine (Demerol)
α-Adrenergic agonists	Retention	Pseudoephedrine (Sudafed)
β-Adrenergic antagonists	Retention	Propranolol (Inderal)
Central antihypertensives	Stress incontinence	Methyldopa (Aldomet), reserpine

associated with a strong urge to void. The volume lost is usually large, and the patient has considerable difficulty stopping the leakage. It is most often due to inappropriate detrusor contractions, which can be precipitated by the sound of running water or by movement, or the contractions can be spontaneous. The degree of severity ranges from an inability to delay urination when the bladder is full to almost constant urgency with frequent small-volume voiding, decreased capacity, and multiple incontinent episodes. Urge incontinence increases with age and with loss of estrogen in women. When a definite neurologic etiology is present, the term *detrusor hyperreflexia* can be applied. Examples of causes of detrusor hyperreflexia include dementia, multiple sclerosis, Parkinson's disease, stroke, and spinal cord injury. Any obstruction of the bladder neck can result in an overactive bladder. Benign prostatic hypertrophy in men is a classic example. Iatrogenic causes such as surgical overcorrection during retropubic urethropexy can result in retention and high postvoid residuals, as well as detrusor instability with new-onset urge incontinence.

Sensory urgency with or without incontinence occurs in the absence of inappropriate bladder motor activity and characterizes the urethral syndrome and interstitial cystitis. Patients experience strong urgency and often urinate small volumes hourly. Chlamydial urethritis should be excluded by culture of the urethra. Urethral instability and urine loss result from a drop in urethral pressure without bladder contractions.

Genuine stress incontinence is more common in women and is usually the result of hypermobility of the bladder neck associated with pelvic floor relaxation. The pelvic floor is composed of the levator ani muscle, whose function in maintaining continence is dependent on both fascial attachments and neuromuscular function. Vaginal delivery is often the culprit behind the pelvic floor disruption, but pudendal nerve injury is also recognized as an important contributor to incontinence. Urinary loss occurs immediately after any stress associated with an increase in abdominal pressure that exceeds urethral pressure (e.g., cough, sneeze, or the Valsalva maneuver). The loss is immediate and usually of small volume, but the amount can vary with the severity. Other symptoms and signs of pelvic floor relaxation are often present, such as uterine or vaginal vault prolapse and difficulty evacuating stool. Patients can frequently learn to contract their pelvic floor muscles (the Kegel maneuver) in anticipation of stress to prevent urine loss. A subset of genuine stress incontinence is intrinsic sphincter deficiency. The urethra may or may not be hypermobile, but it is unable to generate the appropriate resistance to overcome any detrusor pressure. The resulting incontinence is severe and may be constant. Patients may leak urine at night and with simple movement. *Mixed incontinence* includes varying degrees of overactive bladder and genuine stress incontinence.

Overflow incontinence may result from any obstruction at the level of the bladder neck or urethra, or it may be due to an inability of the bladder to effectively empty with an adequate contraction. Aging does account for some degree of detrusor decompensation. Iatrogenic causes include overzealous correction during incontinence surgery, which is fortunately usually transient. Benign prostatic hyperplasia results in elevated postvoid residuals and, if severe, overflow incontinence. Patients who have undergone radical prostatectomy may experience incontinence because of problems of denervation, loss of the bladder neck, and detrusor instability. It is rare to have prolonged urinary difficulty after routine prostatectomy. Significant pelvic prolapse can lead to urethral kinking. Diabetic neuropathy may result in sensory and motor nerve damage with subsequent hyporeflexia or areflexia of the bladder and overflow incontinence. These patients lose the sensation of bladder filling and then cannot generate an adequate contraction to effectively empty the bladder. Urinary tract infection, reflux, and renal damage can result.

Extraurethral causes of incontinence should not be forgotten. Ectopic ureters are usually diagnosed in childhood. In patients with a history of inflammatory bowel disease, diverticulitis, malignancy, pelvic surgery, or irradiation, a fistula may develop between the bladder, urethra, and/or ureter and the vagina or skin. The urine loss is usually constant and severe. Malignancy, either primary or recurrent, must always be excluded as the cause of the fistula. Urethral diverticula can result in postvoid dribbling.

Psychogenic causes are rare and may require detailed interviews, observation, and testing.

EVALUATION OF INCONTINENCE

A detailed history is essential to look for any precipitating or exacerbating factors and to help establish the severity and lifestyle effects. Useful questions include inquiries regarding the use of protective barrier devices such as pads/diapers, limitations on activities, the presence of nocturia and enuresis, and any sensation of uncontrollable urge preceding the urine loss. Previous surgical and medical therapies tried, as well as a detailed obstetric history, are important to obtain. Many providers use a questionnaire to gather information before the appointment.

Paradoxically, it is well established that the history is a poor tool to distinguish genuine stress incontinence from urge incontinence. Symptoms often overlap and are not exclusive to either condition. Therapy is markedly different, and distinction is therefore critical. An absolutely essential component of the evaluation is the requirement that the examiner reproduce the patient's symptoms objectively, which is not always an easy task in the clinical setting. Without such reproduction, therapeutic attempts are subject to fail. A voiding diary or urolog (Table 2) can be a useful tool. Patients are asked to measure the amounts voided and the quantity and type of liquids ingested over a 24-hour period. All incontinent episodes are recorded along with any urge symptoms or precipitating activities. Such record keeping is best done for 2 to 3 days that are typical of the patient's normal activities. It is prudent to complete the log during a workday and over a weekend. This simple diary can lend insight into the severity of the incontinence and guide further testing. It can also guide therapeutic intervention by uncovering dysfunctional habits such as bolus drinking of large volumes of bladder irritants. The 32-oz soda so prevalent in our fast-food culture is a classic example. Women have also been conditioned to believe that ingesting large volumes of fluid may help with weight loss. Other irritants include caffeinated beverages and alcohol. Intake should be limited to 2 L/d, with minimal caffeine and carbonated beverages. After behavior modification, the voiding log can be used to monitor therapeutic results.

Further evaluation is then performed as indicated. Urinary tract infection must always be excluded by culture. A simple dipstick evaluation of the urine must be accomplished before any urethral instrumentation. Microscopic or gross hematuria requires referral for cystourethroscopy to exclude bladder neoplasia, especially in smokers. Attempts are then made to reproduce the patient's symptoms. Various provocative maneuvers can be performed with the patient standing over a towel or by directly observing the urethral meatus in the dorsal position. The patient should have a comfortably full bladder. Coughing, the Valsalva maneuver, heel bouncing, and running water are used as stimuli, with direct observation of any urine loss. If these techniques are not successful, they can be repeated after filling the bladder with 300 mL of sterile water. If demonstrable urinary loss is still not apparent, phenazopyridine (Pyridium)* may be prescribed. The patient is then asked to wear a pad while performing normal activities. Orange staining of the pad will confirm urinary leakage. Simple observation of gait and agility will lend insight into functional barriers. The neurologic examination can be brief, with knee jerk, sensory examination of the lower extremities and perineum, and observation of the bulbocavernosus reflex and anal wink. The goal is to test for gross sensory or motor impairment and to ensure the integrity of the sacral segments S2-4. A complete pelvic examination is performed with attention to any defects in support. Reduction of the vaginal vault or of uterine prolapse must be accomplished and can be performed by placing the bottom blade of a bivalve speculum into the vagina, reducing the prolapse, and securing the blade to the patient's buttocks with tape. Unless this maneuver is accomplished, incontinence may be masked by urethral kinking. A sterile, cotton-tipped applicator is lubricated, placed into the bladder, and slowly withdrawn until slight resistance is encountered at the bladder neck. The angle with the horizontal is noted. The patient is then asked to cough or perform a Valsalva maneuver, and the change in the angle to the horizontal is noted. A hypermobile urethra is defined as greater than a 30-degree angle at rest or a change of greater than 30 degrees. A bimanual examination is performed to detect any pelvic

*Not FDA approved for this indication.

TABLE 2. **Voiding Diary/Urolog**

Time	Amount/Type of Intake (mL) (cc)	Amount Urinated (mL) (cc)	Activity	Leak Volume	Urge Present With Leak (Y or N)
Morning					
Afternoon					
Evening					
Night					
Totals					

Example

Time	Amount/Type of Intake (mL) (cc)	Amount Urinated (mL) (cc)	Activity	Leak Volume	Urge Present With Leak (Y or N)
6:45 AM		550 mL	Awakening		
7:00	2 cups coffee 2 beers		Turned on faucet	Large	Y

masses. A complete rectal examination, including assessment of prostate size and nodularity, is performed in men. Rectal sphincter tone and fecal impaction are noted.

Bladder function during the storage phase should be investigated, especially if the possibility of an overactive bladder exists. Simple office urodynamic studies can be accomplished with minimal equipment. A urinary catheter, Toumy syringe with the piston removed, and sterile water dyed with methylene blue are all that is needed. The patient is catheterized and the catheter attached to the Toumy syringe. The bladder is filled with aliquots of 50 mL of sterile, blue, room temperature water with the syringe held at the level of the symphysis pubis. The study can be done in the dorsal lithotomy or standing position. The volume at first sensation, first desire to void, urgency, and maximal capacity is recorded. Provocative maneuvers such as coughing, running water, and heel bouncing are performed. Any rise in the meniscus of the fluid in the syringe is presumed to be due to bladder contraction, provided that the patient is not using any abdominal muscles. The patient is asked to try to suppress the contraction. Urgency associated with this contraction or loss of urine is diagnostic. Though lacking sensitivity, this technique is an acceptable, easy method for making the diagnosis of overactive bladder or detrusor instability. During a normal filling phase, no rise in bladder pressure should occur. An overactive bladder is diagnosed by objective demonstration of a contraction either spontaneously or with provocation during the filling phase while the patient is attempting to suppress the contraction. Simple uroflowmetry can be performed with the aid of a stopwatch and a graduated urine collection device that fits in the toilet to assess the voiding phase of bladder function. The patient is asked to void normally. Either the patient or the examiner can time the void. A normal result requires at minimum a 150-mL void at a flow rate greater than 20 mL/s. A postvoid residual is immediately obtained with straight catheterization. Normal residuals should not exceed 50 to 100 mL.

The decision regarding who should be referred for more complex urodynamic testing is really based on a few premises. Any patient in whom the symptoms cannot be reproduced in the office setting requires referral. Microscopic hematuria, especially in smokers, requires further testing with cystourethroscopy to exclude bladder cancer. Patients who have undergone previous surgery for incontinence or who have had radical surgery for malignancy or radiotherapy require multichannel urodynamic testing. Extremes of age and medically complicated patients such as diabetics benefit from more detailed testing. Patients with mixed symptoms may also benefit. Severe incontinence suggestive of intrinsic sphincter deficiency requires assessment of urethral closure pressure by urethral profilometry.

THERAPY FOR INCONTINENCE

Prompted or scheduled voiding can be of assistance in improving *functional incontinence.* Eliminating infection and fecal impaction may result in a complete cure. Frequently, either changing medications or the timing of diuretics will result in improvement in quality of life. Elimination of bladder irritants such as caffeine and carbonated and acidic beverages is useful in both urge and stress incontinence. Bladder retraining with an emphasis on voiding spaced every 2 to 3 hours is helpful in both stress and urge incontinence. Either a motivated caregiver or a dedicated nurse or physical therapist can improve the quality of life in most elderly patients.

Improving muscle strength and function through the use of pelvic floor exercises can improve control in patients with *genuine stress incontinence.* An effective squeeze must be demonstrated by the patient with the examiner's finger in the vagina to ensure that the appropriate muscles are being used. Patients should do 10 repetitions with the contraction held for 10 seconds four times a day for 2 months. Weighted vaginal cones provide feedback to the patient that the appropriate muscles are being exercised and provide muscle strengthening with graduated weights. Physical therapists trained in pelvic floor rehabilitation use biofeedback and electrical stimulation with excellent results, both for genuine stress incontinence and for overactive bladder. Several companies have developed portable biofeedback and electrical stimulation units that can be used in the office or at home. Extracorporeal magnetic resonance therapy for bladder retraining has recently been approved by the U.S. Food and Drug Administration. For patients with mild genuine stress incontinence associated with exercise, insertion of a large tampon may elevate the bladder neck enough to restore continence. Devices are available that occlude the urethra (Impress Soft Patch, Fem-Assist). Various pessaries are now available to insert vaginally and elevate the bladder neck (Introl Bladder Neck Support, Incontinence Dish). The only pharmacologic therapy helpful in genuine stress incontinence is the use of estrogen either orally or vaginally. Mild genuine stress incontinence may respond to over-the-counter remedies containing the α-adrenergic agent pseudoephedrine. The gold standard of surgical therapy has been retropubic urethropexy, with long-term cure rates in excess of 80%. This procedure is superior to needle urethropexy and vaginal cystocele repair. Other options available include tension-free vaginal tape and primary pubovaginal sling urethropexy. For the subcategory of intrinsic sphincter deficiency, periurethral injections of bulking agents are used when the urethra is fixed and a sling or tension-free vaginal tape when the urethra is hypermobile. Injections are also useful for postprostatectomy incontinence.

The obvious cure for obstructive *overflow incontinence* is to relieve the source of obstruction. Frequently, time alone will be all that is needed in postsurgical cases. The patient may be taught clean intermittent self-catheterization until normal voiding function returns. Prophylactic antibiotics are not necessary. Urethrolysis is reserved for recalcitrant postoperative retention. α-Adrenergic antagonists and

5α-reductase inhibitors may be useful in men with benign prostatic hypertrophy.

No good pharmacologic therapy is available to restore effective bladder contractions. End-organ damage from diabetes or denervation injuries from procedures such as radical prostatectomy may require lifelong self-catheterization and strict voiding schedules. The goal is to avoid ureteral reflux and further renal damage.

An *overactive bladder* is never treated surgically. The mainstay of therapy for this condition has been anticholinergic medication (Table 3). The most common side effects are blurred vision, constipation, and dry mouth. Newer longer-acting anticholinergics are now available with fewer side effects. Uncontrolled narrow-angle glaucoma is a definite contraindication to their use. Relief of obstruction, such as benign prostatic hypertrophy, is often all that is needed to resolve associated urge symptoms. Likewise, in mixed incontinence, or genuine stress incontinence surgery results in relief of the urge incontinence in more than half of patients. Estrogen therapy, either systemic or local, is also useful for urge symptoms. In patients who appear to have pure urge incontinence by history and examination, an anticholinergic medication may be tried empirically, with urodynamic testing reserved for those who fail. Excellent results are usually obtained with a combination of bladder-retraining techniques and pharmacologic therapy. Electrical stimulation therapy is a useful adjunctive tool. For severe, recalcitrant cases, the Interstim sacral nerve stimulation system (Medtronics) is now approved for use.

TABLE 3. **Pharmacologic Therapy for Incontinence**

Class	Drug	Dose	Indications	Cautions
Estrogen replacement therapy	Oral conjugated estrogens (Premarin)	0.625–1.25 mg/d	Genuine stress incontinence	Add progestin if uterus present
	Estradiol vaginal ring (Estring)	3 mo	Urge incontinence	
	Vaginal estradiol cream (Estrace)	2 g/d vaginally for 2 wk then 1 g twice a wk		
α-Adrenergic agonist	Pseudoephedrine (Sudafed)*	15–30 mg PO bid	Genuine stress incontinence	Avoid in hypertensives Dry mouth Sedation
Tricyclic antidepressants (α-adrenergic and anticholinergic)	Imipramine HCl (Tofranil)*	25 mg qd–75 mg bid	Urge incontinence Mixed incontinence	Caution in the elderly Cardiac and anticholinergic effects Orthostatic hypotension Avoid with MAO inhibitors, glaucoma
Anticholinergics (antispasmodic and anticholinergic)	Oxbutymin (Ditropan) Ditropan XL Tolterodine tartrate (Detrol) Detrol LA	2.5–5 mg PO bid–tid 5, 10, or 15 mg qd 1–2 mg PO bid 2–4 mg qd	Urge incontinence	Avoid with MAO inhibitors, glaucoma Same as tricyclics

*Not FDA approved for this indication.
MAO, monoamine oxidase.

EPIDIDYMITIS

method of
EUGENE MINEVICH, M.D., and
CURTIS A. SHELDON, M.D.
University of Cincinnati
Cincinnati, Ohio

Acute epididymitis is an inflammation or infection of the epididymis. It is frequently observed by urologists, emergency medicine practitioners, and primary care physicians and accounts for approximately 600,000 medical visits per year. Acute epididymitis most commonly occurs in patients aged 15 to 30 years and patients older than 60 years of age. Most commonly it involves the entire epididymis and sometimes the vas deferens (*deferentitis*) or even spermatic cord (*funiculitis*). It can be bilateral in 5% to 10% of the patients. When infection is severe and it extends to the adjacent testicle the diagnosis of *epididymo-orchitis* is appropriate. *Chronic epididymitis* refers to epididymal pain and inflammation lasting more than six months.

PATHOPHYSIOLOGY

Acute bacterial epididymitis is usually caused by a retrograde spread of infection from the urinary tract. Obstructive urethral pathology, instrumentation, indwelling catheters, bacterial prostatitis, and urethritis are common risk factors for acute epididymitis. Aside from sexually transmitted gonococcal or chlamydial infection, the most common bacterial etiologic agent is *Escherichia coli*. Unusual systemic infections such as tuberculosis or systemic fungal infections occasionally result in blood-borne infection of epididymis. Cytomegalovirus epididymitis has been seen in immunocompromised patients.

Chemical epididymitis may be induced by urethro-vaso-epididymal reflux of sterile urine during Valsalva's maneuver or strenuous exertion. Obstruction of the prostate (benign prostate hypertrophy) or urethra (stricture in adults, meatal stenosis or posterior urethral valves in children) creates a predisposition for reflux that normally does not occur. Ectopic ureter is a frequent cause of recurrent epididymitis in children. The antiarrhythmic drug amiodarone (Cordarone) is known to cause an inflammation usually in the head of the epididymis, and can occur in as many as 3% to 11% of patients on the drug. Trauma to the scrotum can be a precipitating event for *traumatic epididymitis.*

CLINICAL PRESENTATION AND LABORATORY EVALUATION

The patient usually presents with gradual onset of scrotal pain and swelling on the affected side of the scrotum. Fever and chills occur in only 25% of patients with acute epididymitis. Patients may have noticed dysuria, frequency, and urgency several days prior to scrotal manifestation. In the presence of urethritis urethral discharge may precede acute epididymitis by more than 30 days or may not occur at all. Physical examination will reveal swelling, induration, and exquisite tenderness of the affected epididymis. Erythema and different degrees of scrotal cellulitis may be present. Elevation of the affected hemiscrotum may relieve the pain of epididymitis (Prehn's sign) as opposed to testicular torsion, in which pain is often exacerbated by further elevation. A reactive inflammatory hydrocele is frequent with advanced epididymo-orchitis, which makes a scrotal examination difficult.

Urinalysis findings in patients with epididymitis are positive for pyuria or bacteriuria in only 25% of patients. Midstream urine culture as well as culture and Gram stain of urethral discharge can help to guide therapy. In protracted cases appropriate cultures and skin tests should be obtained if tuberculosis is suspected. In systemically ill patients, a white blood cell count and blood culture are appropriate. Radiologic and endoscopic evaluation of the urinary tract may be required in children and adults with suspected structural abnormalities.

DIFFERENTIAL DIAGNOSIS

The major concern, especially in prepubertal boys, is distinguishing acute epididymitis from testicular torsion. Torsion of the testicle is a surgical emergency because it causes strangulation of gonadal blood supply with subsequent testicular necrosis and atrophy if unrelieved. Testicular salvage is likely if the duration of torsion is less than 6 to 8 hours. If physical examination is unable to distinguish acute epididymitis from testicular torsion, scrotal color Doppler ultrasound or radionuclide scan can be performed. If testicular torsion is clinically suspected, an immediate surgical scrotal exploration is indicated. A negative exploration of the scrotum is more acceptable than the loss of a testis that might have been salvaged.

Testicular tumor should be included in the differential diagnosis for patients presenting with a painless palpable scrotal mass. Similarly, persistent swelling after a course of antibiotics for presumed epididymo-orchitis is an indication for further evaluation. Scrotal ultrasound is usually definitive in visualizing an intratesticular mass. Tumor markers (α-fetoprotein and β-HCG) are helpful for initial evaluation and for follow-up. Testis biopsy is indicated if testicular tumor cannot be ruled out.

TREATMENT

The management of epididymitis includes bed rest and scrotal elevation. This reduces vascular engorgement and contributes to the relief of discomfort and resolution of the inflammatory response. Additional pain control can be provided with analgesics or narcotics. Antibiotic therapy in all cases should be governed by the results of cultures if possible. Empirical antibiotic therapy with trimethoprim-sulfamethoxazole (Bactrim, Septra)* or a fluoroquinolone (Cipro, Levaquin),* in patients with nonspecific epididymitis is usually indicated for 2 weeks. Systemic illness warrants hospitalization and coverage with intravenous antibiotics. In young men, in whom sexually transmitted infection is most likely, treatment with ceftriaxone (Rocephin)* and doxycycline (Vibramycin)* for 10 days should be initiated. A single dose of azithromycin (Zithromax)* is an alternative to doxycycline, which may circumvent compliance problems.

When scrotal abscess or pyocele is suspected, scrotal ultrasound is often confirmatory and may lead to earlier exploration and a shorter hospitalization. Epididymectomy is reserved for the rare patient with refractory pain secondary to chronic or recurrent epididymitis. Such men should be cautioned that 25% of patients will not experience relief after surgery.

*Not FDA approved for this indication.

PRIMARY GLOMERULAR DISEASES

method of
BRAD H. ROVIN, M.D., FACP
The Ohio State University College of Medicine and Public Health
Columbus, Ohio

Glomerular diseases have a wide spectrum of clinical manifestations, from asymptomatic urinary abnormalities to severe kidney failure requiring dialysis or transplantation. Treatment of glomerulopathies may be divided into immunosuppressive therapies that interrupt the pathophysiologic mechanisms of glomerular injury, and adjunctive therapies designed to slow the tendency toward progressive kidney failure that is often seen after renal injury, especially in patients with hypertension, persistent proteinuria, and loss of nephron mass. This chapter focuses on primary glomerulopathies, which are diseases confined primarily to the kidney. *Primary glomerulopathies* include minimal change nephrotic syndrome, membranoproliferative glomerulonephritis, and IgA nephropathy. *Secondary glomerulopathies* occur when glomeruli are injured during a systemic disease that usually affects multiple organs. Examples of systemic disorders that can target the kidneys are diabetes mellitus and systemic lupus erythematosus. Treatment of secondary glomerulopathies is directed toward the systemic process.

DIAGNOSIS OF GLOMERULAR DISEASE

A diagnosis of glomerular disease should be entertained in patients with hematuria, proteinuria, or an abnormal urinary sediment showing dysmorphic red blood cells, erythrocyte casts, leukocytes in the absence of bacteria, or leukocyte casts. Urinary protein should be quantified with a 24-hour urine collection, or by determining the ratio of urine protein to creatinine in a spot urine sample. This ratio estimates the grams of urine protein excreted in 24 hours. Although less accurate than a 24-hour collection because of diurnal variations in urine protein excretion, the urine protein:creatinine ratio can be obtained easily and rapidly, and is a reasonable initial approximation of protein loss. Urine protein should also be characterized by urine protein immunoelectrophoresis. This will help localize the source of proteinuria to the glomerular compartment (low- and high-molecular-weight proteins) or the tubulointerstitial compartment (mainly low-molecular-weight proteins), and can alert the clinician to multiple myeloma if monoclonal light chains are present. Although nonglomerular processes (e.g., interstitial nephritis) may result in urinary abnormalities similar to glomerulonephritis, proteinuria in excess of 2 grams per day, consisting of both low- and high-molecular weight proteins (albumin or larger), is almost always indicative of a glomerulopathy. In severe glomerular injury, proteinuria can exceed 3.5 grams in 24 hours. This degree of proteinuria is termed *nephrotic range* proteinuria, and is often associated with systemic manifestations, such as hypoalbuminemia, hyperlipidemia with lipiduria, edema, hypercoagulability, protein malnutrition, and increased susceptibility to infection that comprise the nephrotic syndrome. In addition to urine studies, serologic studies such as antinuclear antibody (ANA), antineutrophil cytoplasmic autoantibody (ANCA), hepatitis profile, or HIV status may be helpful in reaching a specific diagnosis. For most primary glomerulopathies, however, a kidney biopsy is needed to establish a definitive diagnosis. The kidney biopsy also conveys prognostic and therapeutic information. For example, a biopsy showing severe glomerular sclerosis or interstitial fibrosis may suggest a poor outcome, despite therapy. Such findings should decrease enthusiasm for aggressive and potentially toxic immunosuppressive therapy.

THERAPEUTIC OPTIONS IN GLOMERULAR DISEASE

Because the pathogenesis of most primary glomerular diseases appears to have an immune basis, immunosuppression forms the foundation of specific treatment. Additionally, several adjunctive therapies directed at complications of glomerular disease, such as proteinuria and hypertension, have been shown to protect the kidneys from the progressive deterioration of kidney function that is often seen even after resolution of the initiating immune process. A general approach to immunosuppression and preservation of kidney function will be outlined first, followed by the application of these regimens to specific glomerular diseases.

Immunosuppression

Corticosteroids

Corticosteroids are both immunosuppressive and anti-inflammatory. Immunosuppression, including attenuation of lymphocyte responses to antigen and reduction of pro-inflammatory cytokine production, generally occurs with prolonged dosing of up to 1 mg/kg/d of prednisone. Higher doses are primarily used acutely to reduce inflammation through effects on lymphocyte viability, leukocyte trafficking, granulocyte degranulation, and capillary permeability. As outlined in Table 1, a number of steroid protocols that vary mainly in duration and intensity are used to treat glomerular diseases. While all protocols provide immunosuppression, intensive therapy (see Table 1) offers potent anti-inflammatory effects that are especially useful in severe glomerular diseases that rapidly progress to kidney failure. These glomerulopathies are generally characterized by considerable inflammation and distortion of glomerular architecture (e.g., necrosis and crescents). These steroid schedules should not be viewed as invariant, but can be modified based on clinical manifestations and overall response to therapy. For example, patients who demonstrate rapid improvement may tolerate an accelerated taper. Conversely, if relapse occurs during the taper, steroids can be recycled to a higher level dictated by the severity of the relapse.

Drugs that induce the hepatic cytochrome P-450 system, such as phenytoin (Dilantin), phenobarbital, carbamazepine (Tegretol), and rifampin (Rifadin), increase the metabolism of glucocorticoids. To compensate, the prednisone dose has to be approximately doubled.

Alkylating Agents

For situations in which steroid resistance is encountered, or for treatment of severe glomerular disease, an alkylating agent such as cyclophosphamide (Cytoxan),* or chlorambucil (Leukeran),* is often required. Cyclophosphamide may be given intravenously or orally. I prefer oral cyclophosphamide because it is efficacious, convenient to administer, readily titrated according to peripheral leukocyte counts, and cost effective. The initial daily dosage is 1.5 to 2 mg/kg ideal body weight/day (maximum, 150 mg/d). Duration of therapy depends on the disease, but the frequency of delayed malignancies (bladder and hematologic) is increased after the equivalent of 1 year of daily oral therapy. Therapy beyond 6 months

*Not FDA approved for this indication.

TABLE 1. **Corticosteroid Protocols Commonly Used in the Treatment of Glomerular Disease**

Regimen	Initial Therapy[1] Dose	Initial Therapy[1] Duration	Tapering Protocol Dose	Tapering Protocol Duration
Standard therapy	1 mg/kg/d[2,3]	6-8 wks	1.6 mg/kg qod	4 wks
Rapid taper			1.2 mg/kg qod	4 wks
			0.8 mg/kg qod	4 wks
			0.4 mg/kg qod	4 wks then stop
Standard therapy	1 mg/kg/d	6-8 wks	1.6 mg/kg qod	4 wks
Slow taper			1.2 mg/kg qod	4 wks
			1.0 mg/kg qod	4 wks
			0.8 mg/kg qod	4 wks
			0.6 mg/kg qod	4 wks
			0.4 mg/kg qod	4 wks
			0.2 mg/kg qod	4 wks then stop
Intensive therapy[4]	Methylprednisolone (Solumedrol) IV, 500-1000 mg	3 days[5]		
	60 mg/d (<80 kg)	4 wks[6]	50 mg/d[7]	Wk 5
	80 mg/d (>80 kg)		40 mg/d	Wk 6
			30 mg/d	Wk 7
Begin alternate day taper				
			30/25 mg/d	Wk 8
			30/20 mg/d	Wk 9
			30/15 mg/d	Wk 10
			30/10 mg/d	Wk 11
			30/5 mg/d	Wk 12
			30/0 mg/d	Wk 13
			20-25 mg qod	Wks 14-15 Maintain until wk 52; then withdraw slowly as tolerated

[1]Doses given are for oral prednisone unless otherwise indicated, and are based on ideal body weight for adults. Decrease initial dose by 25% for elderly patients.
[2]Maximum oral prednisone dose for any regimen is 80 mg/d.
[3]Use 2 divided doses when prednisone exceeds 50 mg/d.
[4]Intensive therapy is associated with a high risk of infection and should be reserved for carefully selected patients.
[5]Do not use beyond 3 days because of high risk of infection. IV steroids can be skipped, depending on disease severity.
[6]Patients who are responding well may be able to reduce this to 2 wks and accelerate the taper.
[7]Patients who started on 80 mg/d should reduce dose to 60 mg/d during wk 5 and 40 mg/d during wk 6.
IV, intravenously; qod, every other day.

should thus be carefully considered. To avoid acute bladder toxicity, patients are encouraged to take extra fluid (at meals and bedtime) to achieve at least 2 liters of daily urine output during therapy. Leukocyte count should be monitored weekly, and if the neutrophil count falls below 2000 cells per mm^3, cyclophosphamide should be withheld until the neutrophil count rises above this level. Cyclophosphamide can then be restarted at one half to two thirds of the previous dose. In situations where intravenous administration is desirable, such as poor patient compliance, the usual dose of cyclophosphamide is 750 mg/M^2 body surface area, given every 4 weeks for a duration of 6 months. To avoid irreversible gonadal failure, gonadal function may be suppressed during treatment using leuprolide beginning 4 weeks before cyclophosphamide, and continuing every 4 to 6 weeks, for not more than 6 months. The initial dose of cyclophosphamide should be reduced by 25% in patients with renal insufficiency and a serum creatinine greater than 2.

Chlorambucil* is an alternative to cyclophosphamide without bladder toxicity. Oral chlorambucil is given in doses of 0.15-0.2 mg/kg ideal body weight/day (maximum, 14 mg/d). Duration of therapy depends on the disease being treated. Leukocyte counts should be monitored and, if severe leukopenia occurs, the dose of chlorambucil should be adjusted as for cyclophosphamide.

*Not FDA approved for this indication.

Antimetabolites

When long-term administration of a cytotoxic agent is required, or for maintenance of remission after completing alkylating agent therapy, oral azathioprine* (Imuran) at a dose of 1 to 2 mg/kg ideal body weight/day can be used. Experience with solid organ transplantation indicates that this drug may be safely administered for years. In addition, azathioprine has been used in pregnant patients. Leukopenia is the major side effect of azathioprine, so leukocyte counts should be monitored and the dose adjusted according to the white cell count. The dose of azathioprine must be decreased by 50% during concomitant allopurinol (Zyloprim) administration.

Mycophenolate mofetil* (CellCept) is receiving increasing attention as a cytotoxic agent that is safer than cyclophosphamide and more effective than

*Not FDA approved for this indication.

azathioprine. It may have a role not only in maintenance therapy after alkylating agent-induced remission, but also as primary therapy in some glomerulopathies. Mycophenolate mofetil is used orally in doses of 0.25 to 1.0 gram twice a day. It can cause leukopenia and thrombocytopenia requiring dose adjustment. Gastrointestinal side effects (nausea, diarrhea) are generally not limiting at the doses used to treat glomerular disease.

Calcineurin Inhibitors

Although mainly used in transplantation immunosuppression, cyclosporine* (Neoral, Sandimmune) has also found utility in the treatment of primary glomerular disease, especially after other therapies have failed. Unfortunately many glomerular diseases relapse quickly when cyclosporine is discontinued. Cyclosporine (3.5 to 5 mg/kg ideal body weight/day) is given in two divided doses, and usually continued until complete remission has been maintained for 6 to 12 months. It is prudent to taper the cyclosporine dose by 25% every 2 months to determine the lowest dose needed to maintain remission. To minimize nephrotoxicity, trough blood levels should be monitored by radioimmunoassay. Drugs that block the cytochrome P-450 system (e.g., erythromycin, clarithromycin [Biaxin], verapamil [Calan], diltiazem [Cardizem], amlodipine [Norvasc], fluconazole [Diflucan], ketoconazole [Nizoral]) can increase the level of cyclosporine, so concomitant administration requires dose reduction. Conversely, drugs that induce the P-450 system enhance the metabolism of cyclosporine, and may require the dose to be increased.

Kidney Protective/Antiprogression Therapy

The complications of glomerular disease, including increased intra-glomerular pressure, systemic hypertension, proteinuria, and hyperlipidemia have been implicated in causing kidney damage along with the primary process affecting the glomeruli. These same complicating factors also contribute to the progressive decline in kidney function often seen once a critical number of nephrons are lost, even if the primary process is no longer active. Treatments directed at lowering blood pressure, urine protein losses, and serum lipids protect the kidneys and favorably modify the risk of progressive nephropathy. In glomerular diseases that are poorly responsive to immunosuppressive therapy, antiprogression therapy is the mainstay of treatment. In addition to the therapies recommended below, there is some evidence that lifestyle modifications, including cessation of tobacco use and weight reduction (if obese) may also benefit kidney health.

Blood Pressure Control

Strict blood pressure control is effective in slowing progressive kidney disease in patients with glomerulonephritis, proteinuria, and renal insufficiency. Systolic blood pressure correlates better with kidney disease progression than with diastolic pressure, and should be maintained in the 120 to 129 mm Hg range, or lower if tolerated. Ideally, diastolic blood pressure should be around 75 mm Hg. Certain antihypertensive medications may confer additional renal protection beyond that associated simply with systemic blood pressure control. In this regard, angiotensin-converting enzyme inhibitors (ACEi) should be part of the antihypertensive regimen, if possible, because they favorably affect glomerular hemodynamics and are antiproteinuric and antifibrotic. ACEi with the high affinity for tissue ACE (e.g., ramipril [Altace]) may be particularly efficacious for kidney protection. The amount of ACEi needed to achieve renal protection is small (e.g., enalapril [Vasotec], 5 mg/d), and it is not yet known whether larger doses are more renoprotective. Angiotensin type I receptor blockers (ARBs) have been shown to be renoprotective in the glomerulopathy associated with type II diabetes, and are expected to have similar effects in primary glomerular diseases. ARBs are recommended in patients who do not tolerate ACEi. The theoretical benefits and risks of combining ACEi and ARBs therapy are under investigation. Beta-blockers and long-acting nondihydropyridine calcium channel blockers (verapamil [Calan] and diltiazem [Cardizem]) also appear to have antiproteinuric-kidney protective effects. These agents may be used in conjunction with an ACE inhibitor or an ARB. Dihydropyridine calcium channel blockers, while excellent antihypertensive medications, do not attenuate, and may even worsen, proteinuria and renal function. A dihydropyridine should be used in patients with kidney disease only if absolutely necessary for blood pressure control. The undesirable renal effects of dihydropyridine calcium channel blockers may be partially mitigated by the concomitant use of an ACEi or ARB.

Diet

The antiproteinuric effects of the medications discussed above can be abolished in patients with a high salt intake. Sodium must be restricted to 2 to 2.5 g/d, unless renal salt wasting is present. This also helps control edema in nephrotic patients. Sodium intake is readily assessed by measuring the urinary sodium content of a patient's 24-hour urine submitted for evaluation of proteinuria.

Although counter-intuitive, high protein diets can actually make proteinuria worse in hypoalbuminemic patients. In contrast, dietary protein restriction may slow progressive renal disease, improve serum albumin, and reduce proteinuria in nephrotic individuals. Patients with moderate renal insufficiency (in general, a serum creatinine level of <3 mg/dL) who are not acutely ill or catabolic should restrict daily dietary protein to 0.7 to 0.8 g/kg of ideal body weight. In advanced renal insufficiency (in general, a serum creatinine level of >3 mg/dL), protein intake should be reduced to 0.6 g/kg/d. These diets must have adequate calories, and more than 50% of the protein should be of high biologic value. Consultation with a dietitian is appropriate. Patients with heavy proteinuria should modify their protein restriction

*Not FDA approved for this indication.

by adding 1 gram of dietary protein for every gram of protein lost in the urine.

Hyperlipidemia is a common problem encountered in nephrotic patients that may contribute to progressive renal damage. This is often difficult to control in patients who remain nephrotic, and usually requires both dietary and pharmacologic intervention. Hydroxymethylglutaryl-coenzyme A reductase inhibitors are recommended for hyperlipidemic patients with glomerular disease and sustained heavy proteinuria.

SPECIFIC GLOMERULOPATHIES

Minimal Change Disease

Minimal change disease (MCD) accounts for 85% of idiopathic childhood nephrotic syndrome, but only approximately 15% of adult nephrotic syndrome. Long-term prognosis is good, with few patients progressing to chronic renal failure. Patients typically present with nephrotic syndrome. Urinary sediment tends to be bland, with evidence of lipiduria (oval fat bodies and fatty casts) and occasionally red blood cells or erythrocyte casts. Diagnosis is made by renal biopsy, which shows normal glomeruli by light microscopy, no immune deposits by immunofluorescence, but glomerular epithelial foot process fusion by electron microscopy. Systemic diseases (Hodgkin's lymphoma) and drugs (nonsteroidal anti-inflammatory drugs) may cause glomerular lesions similar to those of MCD. MCD is usually very responsive to therapy with corticosteroids. Although progression to renal failure is rare and spontaneous remission occurs, patients should be treated with prednisone to induce remission and avoid complications of the nephrotic syndrome. Treatment for adults should be initiated with *standard* prednisone therapy (see Table 1) until complete remission (urine protein <500 mg/d) occurs, or for 6 weeks (whichever comes first). If remission occurs, prednisone is tapered according to the rapid taper schedule. By 6 weeks if there is only a partial response (proteinuria >0.5 but <3 g/d), prednisone should be decreased according to the slow taper protocol. Most patients (80% to 90%) achieve remission with this initial therapy. If prednisone is poorly tolerated or there is no response to therapy after 3 to 4 months, patients may be switched to an alkylating agent (plus 10 mg prednisone/day) for 8 to 12 weeks. This should induce remission in 80% of steroid-resistant patients.

MCD has a high incidence (75%) of relapse (proteinuria >3 g/d). The first relapse should be treated with prednisone, but patients who relapse frequently or cannot be tapered off prednisone need treatment with an alkylating agent for 8 to 12 weeks. No more than two courses of alkylating agent therapy are indicated in the treatment of MCD.

Patients who do not respond to steroids or alkylating agents should be treated with kidney protective therapy, and cyclosporine (Sandimmune)* can be considered. If the patient does not have a significant reduction in proteinuria after 4 months of cyclosporine, it should be stopped.

*Not FDA approved for this indication.

Focal Segmental Glomerulosclerosis

Focal segmental glomerulosclerosis (FSGS) initially causes glomerular scarring that involves only a segment of the glomerulus, and does not involve all glomeruli (focal). This histologic pattern is common, and may be seen in the advanced stages of other kidney diseases such as reflux nephropathy, human immunodeficiency virus (HIV) nephropathy, hypertensive nephrosclerosis, obesity-related nephropathy, and heroin-abuse nephropathy. Exclusion of other conditions supports a diagnosis of primary FSGS. FSGS is a common form of idiopathic nephrotic syndrome in adults, does not usually spontaneously remit, is difficult to treat, and, in the setting of nephrotic syndrome, often progresses to kidney failure unless a complete or partial remission of proteinuria can be achieved with therapy. If chosen appropriately, approximately 30% of nephrotic patients may respond to corticosteroid therapy. Ideally, patients should have a serum creatinine less than 2.5 mg/dL and a renal biopsy showing less than 25% interstitial fibrosis. Standard prednisone therapy (see Table 1) should be used for up to 8 weeks. If complete remission occurs, prednisone may be tapered according to the rapid taper schedule; if partial remission is achieved consider a slow steroid taper (see Table 1). In our experience patients who respond to steroids tend to show some improvement within 2 months of high-dose therapy. If there is no response by 2 months, we discontinue high-dose steroids. At this point, treatment decisions become difficult and long-term results tend to be less satisfactory. All patients with steroid-unresponsive FSGS should be treated with kidney protective therapy, and may be considered for cyclosporine, which has shown efficacy in FSGS.

Membranous Glomerulopathy

Idiopathic membranous glomerulopathy (MGN) is an important cause of nephrotic syndrome in adults, especially in people older than 50 years of age. Clinical presentation is similar to that of MCD and FSGS, although the development of proteinuria can be more insidious. Microscopic hematuria is common. Kidney biopsy, required for the diagnosis, demonstrates immune deposits in the glomerular basement membrane (GBM). Formation of new GBM around these immune deposits causes thickening of the GBM. A variety of systemic processes may result in MGN, including systemic lupus erythematosus (SLE), adenocarcinoma (lung, colon, breast, prostate), viral infections (HIV, hepatitis B, C, or G), and drugs (captopril [Capoten], gold salts, penicillamine [Cuprimine]). These conditions should be excluded before instituting therapy for idiopathic MGN.

Studies to determine the best treatment of MGN have been hampered by its natural history. MGN is indolent, has a high rate of spontaneous remission

(20% to 30%) and relapse, but can progress to chronic renal insufficiency (20% to 25%). All patients should be considered for kidney protective therapy. The use of specific immunosuppressive therapy is reserved for patients with risk factors for progressive renal deterioration. The factors most strongly associated with progressive MGN are persistent heavy proteinuria (>8 g/d for >6 months), elevated serum creatinine, and greater than 20% interstitial fibrosis on renal biopsy. Moderate risk factors for progression are male sex, uncontrolled hypertension, and age older than 50 years.

Patients at risk for progression should be treated with a combination of prednisone and an alkylating agent. This regimen consists of daily oral prednisone (0.5 mg/kg ideal body weight/d) for 1 month, followed by an alkylating agent for 1 month. A low dose of prednisone (10 mg/d) is continued during the alkylating agent month. This cycle is repeated twice to complete 6 months of therapy. The effects of therapy may be delayed, and no decision regarding success should be made for 3 to 6 months after completion of initial therapy. If remission is achieved carefully follow the patient for relapse of proteinuria and retreat once with a second round of alternating steroid and cytotoxic therapy as outlined above. Patients in partial remission should be continued on kidney protective therapy. Therapeutic failures may be tried on cyclosporine or azathioprine for 1 year. Mycophenolate mofetil (Cellcept)* has also shown promise in treating patients with persistent MGN. Of the many etiologies of nephrotic syndrome, MGN with heavy proteinuria is particularly associated with a thrombotic tendency, and thus the prophylactic use of low-dose aspirin (81 mg/d) seems reasonable.

Membranoproliferative Glomerulonephritis

Idiopathic membranoproliferative glomerulonephritis (MPGN) occurs as one of three histologic variants. In general, these nephritides show increased cellularity and matrix in the glomerular mesangium, and thickening of glomerular capillary walls. Patients with MPGN are usually young (<30 years of age) and present with hematuria and proteinuria that can be in the nephrotic range. Urine sediment is more active (casts and cells) than in the previously discussed nephrotic glomerulopathies. Secondary MPGN is more common than primary MPGN in adults, and may be seen with infections (hepatitis B and C), cryoglobulinemia, chronic lymphocytic leukemia, and B cell lymphoma. Hepatitis C has been increasingly implicated as a cause of MPGN. The prognosis of patients with primary MPGN and nephrotic syndrome is poor; 50% have renal failure within 10 years of diagnosis. Despite several trials, no clear therapy has emerged for adults with idiopathic MPGN, in contrast to children who appear to benefit from alternate-day steroid therapy. Patients with renal insufficiency or proteinuria should receive kidney protective therapy.

*Not FDA approved for this indication.

IgA Nephritis

IgA nephritis (IgAN) is the most common form of glomerulonephritis in the world. It is characterized by microscopic or gross hematuria, especially in association with a mucosal infection. The urine sediment may be nephritic with erythrocyte casts and moderate proteinuria, or patients may have nephrotic-range proteinuria. Prognosis is fair but the disease can slowly progress, and 20% to 30% of patients reach end-stage renal disease over time (up to 2 decades). Biopsy demonstrates mesangial expansion and proliferation with mesangial deposition of IgA. IgAN may also show rapid progression to renal failure with two distinct morphologic patterns on biopsy. Some patients with acute renal failure develop glomerular crescents and necrosis, whereas others demonstrate mainly tubulointerstitial damage with acute tubular necrosis and erythrocytes in tubules, often in association with a disease exacerbation characterized by macroscopic hematuria. Mesangial IgA deposition can also be seen in chronic liver disease, chronic infection with methicillin-resistant *Staphylococcus aureus*, HIV, inflammatory bowel disease, Henoch-Schönlein purpura (possibly a systemic form of IgA nephritis), and SLE.

The variable natural history of idiopathic IgAN necessitates a variety of approaches to therapy. Patients with low levels of proteinuria (between 0.5 and 1 g/d) and preserved renal function should be followed closely and considered for renal protective therapy. Risk factors for renal functional decline are uncontrolled hypertension, persistent proteinuria (>1 g/d), renal insufficiency at diagnosis, and glomerular or tubulointerstitial sclerosis on biopsy. Kidney protective therapy should be instituted for high-risk patients. It is prudent to avoid or minimize situations that stimulate the mucosal immune system (i.e., limit contact with people who have upper respiratory infections or gastroenteritis). Although immunosuppressive therapy has not shown consistent benefit, patients with heavy proteinuria (>3 g/d) and preserved renal function may have attenuation of proteinuria with a 6-month (at least) course of prednisone, starting with 1 mg/kg/d on alternate days for 8 weeks followed by a gradual taper. Patients with renal insufficiency seem to derive fewer benefits from steroids. Because of the immunomodulating effects of omega-3 fatty acids, fish oil supplementation (Max EPA,* 6 grams twice daily), has been used to treat progressive IgAN. Although fish oil is relatively safe, results of therapy have been mixed. For patients with IgAN who have acute renal failure and severe crescentic GN, intensive prednisone therapy plus oral cyclophosphamide (Cytoxan)* may be of benefit. In this situation it is important to identify patients with acute renal failure due to tubulointerstitial damage, as this usually resolves without treatment and does not warrant intense immunosuppression. Some patients with IgAN may thus require re-biopsy to aid in treatment decisions.

*Not FDA approved for this indication.

Rapidly Progressive Glomerulonephritis

Rapidly progressive glomerulonephritis (RPGN) is a clinical syndrome in which renal insufficiency (>50% decrease in function) occurs quickly (<3 months) because of a glomerulopathy. Biopsy, which is essential for the diagnosis, often reveals cellular glomerular crescents or necrosis. There may be other, more disease-specific findings on biopsy, such as linear glomerular basement membrane (GBM) immunoglobulin deposition in anti-GBM antibody disease. RPGN can complicate many of the nephropathies already discussed (e.g., MPGN, IgAN, and MGN). Idiopathic RPGN is usually divided into anti-GBM antibody disease, immune-complex disease, and pauci-immune glomerulonephritis (which shows few immune deposits on biopsy). RPGN may be considered a renal-limited form of a systemic process: anti-GBM disease (a limited form of Goodpasture's syndrome); immune-complex disease (a limited form of autoimmune disease such as SLE); or pauci-immune glomerulonephritis (a limited form of Wegener's granulomatosis). Pauci-immune glomerulonephritis, which is more common than the other types of RPGN, is typically associated with the presence of anti-neutrophil cytoplasmic antibodies (ANCA) in the serum. Treatment of these renal-limited diseases is similar to treatment of their systemic counterparts. Other systemic conditions must be excluded before starting the intense immunosuppression required to treat idiopathic RPGN. These include infection, drug hypersensitivity, and malignancy. If RPGN is suspected a kidney biopsy must be performed *urgently* and treatment started as soon as possible to improve chances of kidney survival.

Anti-GBM antibody disease should be treated with intensive prednisone therapy (see Table 1) plus 8 to 12 weeks of cyclophosphamide (Cytoxan)* and 10 to 14 sessions of daily plasmapheresis to remove circulating anti-GBM antibodies. After completing cyclophosphamide, azathioprine (Imuran)* or mycophenolate mofetil (Cellcept)* may be considered for 1 year to maintain remission, although relapse is infrequent in anti-GBM disease. Anti-GBM patients who present with kidney failure requiring dialysis have a poor prognosis and rarely recover kidney function, so intense immunosuppression may not be indicated in such cases. Pauci-immune RPGN is also treated with intensive prednisone therapy plus cyclophosphamide, but cyclophosphamide is given for 4 to 6 months rather than 8 to 12 weeks. Cyclophosphamide should be followed by maintenance azathioprine (or mycophenolate) for 1 year, because of the high frequency of relapse. Patients with pauci-immune RPGN who require dialysis at presentation may also benefit from early plasmapheresis. Idiopathic immune-complex RPGN is treated with intensive prednisone therapy, 8 weeks of cyclophosphamide, and maintenance immunosuppression to complete 1 year of total therapy.

If no renal response is seen by 8 to 10 weeks, remission of the RPGN is unlikely, and it is appropriate to taper and discontinue therapy. Relapse may occur in any type of RPGN, but is especially common in pauci-immune disease and should be treated aggressively using the same guidelines as for initial therapy.

*Not FDA approved for this indication.

PYELONEPHRITIS

method of
NAYEF EL-DAHER, M.D., PH.D.
Park Ridge Hospital
Rochester, New York

Acute pyelonephritis is defined as the acute inflammatory process of the renal parenchyma, caused by microbial agents. Most commonly, it is caused by a bacterial infection from gram-negative organisms. This infection is more difficult to treat compared with a bladder infection, which is usually a superficial infection of the mucosa of the urinary bladder (cystitis).

ETIOLOGY

The most common organisms causing community-acquired acute pyelonephritis are gram-negative bacilli. *Escherichia coli* is the most common gram-negative organism causing acute pyelonephritis, accounting for more than 80% of all cases of acute pyelonephritis. Other gram-negative organisms include *Proteus*, *Klebsiella* and *Pseudomonas* species. Among the gram-positive organisms causing acute pyelonephritis are the *Staphylococcus* species (*Staphylococcus aureus* and *Staphylococcus*-coagulase negative organisms) and enterococci, including vancomycin-resistant enterococci (VRE). The most common organisms causing acute pyelonephritis in hospitalized patients are the gram-negative organisms including *E. coli, Proteus, Klebsiella, Enterobacter,* and *Pseudomonas* species. Among the gram-positive organisms, staphylococci and enterococci are more often isolated. Anaerobic organisms are rarely a pathogen in urinary tract infections, in general. *Staphylococcus saprophyticus* tends to cause acute cystitis in young, sexually active females and rarely causes acute pyelonephritis.

PATHOGENESIS OF URINARY TRACT INFECTION

Urinary tract infections are caused as a result of an interaction between bacterial virulent factors and the host defense mechanisms. There are two possible routes by which bacteria can invade and spread within the urinary tract. The first one is the ascending route and the second is the hematogenous route.

Ascending Route

The lower urinary tract (urethra) is usually colonized with bacteria, most commonly gram-negative rods. Any compromise on the host defense (either by instrumentation, obstruction, minor trauma) results in pushing the organism from the distal urethra into the bladder, causing a local inflammation of the superficial mucosa. Subsequently, this infection can be spread upward to involve the ureter and the renal parenchyma. The fact that urinary tract infections are far more common in females than in males supports this theory. The female urethra is shorter and wider compared to that of a male, making contamination more likely. It has been documented that an organism causing urinary tract infections in women colonized the vaginal introitus and the peri-urethral areas before causing a urinary tract infection. Colonization is usually achieved by adhesive properties of the organisms (adhesins). The adhesins of uropathogenic *E. coli* exist as either pili or as outer membrane proteins.

The Second Route

This is the hematogenous route. Hematogenous spread can cause acute pyelonephritis by seeding the renal parenchyma causing diffuse pyelonephritis with micro- or macro-abscesses. The most common organisms causing this type of acute pyelonephritis are almost always gram-positive (staphylococci and enterococci) as a complication of persistent bacteremia or endocarditis.

EPIDEMIOLOGY

Women are most frequently affected by urinary tract infections and acute pyelonephritis. Acute pyelonephritis can be uncomplicated or complicated. Uncomplicated pyelonephritis occurred in a young woman who lacked any evidence of structural, functional, or any co-morbidity that increased the risk of having a urinary tract infection (Table 1). Complicated pyelonephritis usually occurs as a result of acute pyelonephritis in an immunocompromised host or in the presence of multiple complicating factors (obstruction, immunosuppression, diabetes mellitus, pregnancy, sickle cell anemia, and so on).

CLINICAL PRESENTATION

The classical clinical manifestation of a patient with acute pyelonephritis includes fever, chills, flank pain, and frequently lower urinary tract symptoms (e.g., frequency, urgency and painful micturition). A wide spectrum of illness is encountered in patients with acute pyelonephritis ranging from mild illness to severe life-threatening infection with sepsis and septic shock. This spectrum of presentation depends on multiple factors (bacterial and host factors). Only a minority of patients with acute pyelonephritis develop complications, such as intrarenal abscess and/or sepsis or septic shock. In general, a severe manifestation usually is associated with an immunocompromised status in patients with multiple co-morbidities infected by a multiple drug-resistant organism (MDR). Other less frequent symptoms usually include sweats, headache, nausea, vomiting, malaise, abdominal pain, generalized weakness, and dehydration.

TABLE 1. **Complicating Factors in Urinary Tract Infection (Pyelonephritis)**

Obstruction (foreign body, catheter, stone, etc.)
Urinary tract functional and structural abnormality
Immunosuppression—"drug-induced," HIV, malignancy, renal transplant
Co-morbidity—diabetes mellitus, pregnancy, sickle cell anemia
Pyelonephritis caused by multi-drug resistance (MDR) organism, e.g., oxacillin-resistant *Staphylococcus aureus* (ORSA)
Others—Surgically created *ileal* loop, male sex

DIAGNOSIS

Preferred methods for urine collection include: midstream clean catch, catheterization, and suprapubic aspiration.

Urine analysis, culture, and sensitivity of the causative agents are the cornerstones for the diagnosis of acute pyelonephritis. It should be emphasized that the finding of pyuria is non-specific and a patient with pyuria may or may not have infection. However, the vast majority of symptomatic patients with acute pyelonephritis have pyuria. Microscopic hematuria is usually seen in acute urinary tract infection, mainly hemorrhagic cystitis, but is rarely seen in acute pyelonephritis. The presence of hematuria usually suggests the presence of calculi, tumor, vasculitis, and others. White cell casts in the presence of the acute infectious disease process usually provides strong evidence of acute pyelonephritis. One of the most useful parameters in urine analysis is the presence of bacteria (bacteriuria). The presence of significant bacteria ($>10^5$/mL) on un-spun urine indicates the presence of urinary tract infection.

Urine and blood cultures should be considered on every patient presenting with clinical pictures suggestive of acute pyelonephritis. Urine and blood cultures preferably should be done before initiating any antibiotic treatment. Positive blood cultures in the proper clinical setting will confirm the diagnosis of acute pyelonephritis.

MANAGEMENT

Uncomplicated pyelonephritis usually responds to appropriate antibiotic treatment plus hydration in 24 to 48 hours. Usually the patient will experience defervescence and white count will normalize. For those patients, switching intravenous antibiotic into oral medication to be continued for 14 to 21 days is appropriate. Follow-up urine culture is not indicated routinely. Follow-up urine culture is required within 1 to 2 weeks of completion of therapy in a pregnant woman, in children, and in patients with recurrent, symptomatic pyelonephritis.

Patients who fail to respond to intravenous antibiotics and hydration (e.g., continue to have fever and repeated positive blood cultures), need further investigation to explore the possibility of complicating pyelonephritis. Those patients should have computed tomography scan (CT) or perhaps an intravenous pyelography examination to exclude the possibility of urinary obstruction, or intrarenal or perinephric abscess formation.

Quick intervention to correct any urinary obstruction is vital. Urology evaluation for possible removal of renal stone and/or tumor or relieving the pressure by an urgent urostomy is vital in the management of acute pyelonephritis. When intravenous antimicrobial therapy fails to treat a patient with acute pyelonephritis due to abscess formation, percutaneous drainage with culture and sensitivity should be tried. Selecting antimicrobial agent or agents with good activity against the causative organisms with good renal tissue penetration is highly indicated under these circumstances (trimethoprim-sulfamethoxazole [Bactrim] and/or fluoroquinolones). Almost all renal abscesses less than 5 cm in diameter could be treated medically with no surgical intervention. Renal abscesses more than 5 cm in diameter need surgical drainage; percutaneous drainage usually gives an excellent outcome. Nephrectomy is only indicated for treatment of severe life-threatening emphysematous pyelonephritis and in patients with diffuse severely damaged renal parenchyma.

Acute uncomplicated pyelonephritis (mild to moderate) responds well to oral antimicrobial agents. Oral antimicrobial agents currently recommended include trimethoprim-sulfamethoxazole (Bactrim), 800 to 160 mg twice a day, first-generation cephalosporins (Keflex), 500 mg four times a day, amoxicillin/clavulanate (Augmentin), 875 mg twice a day, and fluoroquinolones (e.g., ofloxacin [Floxin], 400 mg twice a day, and ciprofloxacin [Cipro], 500 mg twice a day).

In hospitalized patients with severe complicated pyelonephritis, parenteral therapy should be used. Empirical treatment includes a wide selection of antimicrobial agents: Fluoroquinolones (Cipro 400 mg every 12 hours, Floxin 400 mg every 12 hours), third- and fourth-generation cephalosporins (ceftriaxone [Rocephin] 1 g every 24 hours, ceftazidime [Cefizox] 2 g every 8 hours, cefepime [Maxipime] 2 g every 12 hours), ampicillin-sulbactam combination (Unasyn), 3 g every 6 hours, ticarcillin/clavulanate combination, 3.1 g every 4 to 6 hours. All empirical antibiotic treatment should be changed or modified according to culture result and sensitivity. Parenteral antibiotic should be switched to an oral agent once a clinical response has occurred (patient is asymptomatic, white blood cells normalized, and no fever or chills).

TRAUMA TO THE GENITOURINARY TRACT

method of
RICHARD A. SANTUCCI, M.D., and
THEODORE D. BARBER, M.D.
Wayne State University School of Medicine
Detroit, Michigan

Although medical innovations such as modern antibiotics have continued to increase the life expectancy of humans, morbidity and mortality secondary to trauma remain a significant international health problem. In the United States, trauma remains the leading cause of death in individuals younger than 45 years of age.

Approximately 10% of all major trauma victims will have a genitourinary (GU) injury. When assessing a patient for possible GU trauma, as with assessment of all trauma victims, initial evaluation should proceed according to the ABCDE mnemonic (*A*irway, *B*reathing, *C*irculation, *D*isability, *E*xposure), with an AMPLE history (*A*llergies, *M*edication, *P*ast medical history, *L*ast meal, *E*vents surrounding injury) obtained if the patient is verbal. It should be noted that female trauma victims require a thorough vaginal exam, as female GU injuries can be subtle in their presentation. Additionally, it is important that the evaluating physician understands the mechanism of injury, as this knowledge will guide subsequent treatments. In patients sustaining penetrating trauma by gunshot or knife wound, attention needs to be given to the trajectory of the projectile when assessing for GU involvement. Additionally, in the case of gunshot wounds, knowledge of the characteristics of the weapon used are a valuable asset, as tissue damage with high velocity weapons (e.g., rifles) is much greater than that seen with low velocity weapons (e.g., handguns). Assessment of GU trauma requires judicious use of laboratory tests (including urinalysis), radiologic imaging, and consultation with a urologist in those patients thought likely to require surgical intervention.

Although an exhaustive discussion of the diagnosis and treatment of GU trauma is beyond the scope of this review, it is our hope that this article will provide an adequate blueprint to guide primary care physicians in the evaluation and initial treatment of trauma patients with GU tract injury.

RENAL INJURIES

Of all injuries to the GU tract, renal injury is the most common, affecting up to 10% of all seriously injured patients. Hematuria provides the best indicator of traumatic GU injury, although it should be noted that some major injuries may occur in the absence of hematuria. In up to one third of renovascular injuries, for example, hematuria is absent. When assessing for GU bleeding, it is recommended that the first aliquot of urine be used, as later samples may be diluted secondary to diuresis of intravenous fluids used in resuscitation. Contrast-enhanced computed tomography (CT) plays a vital role in injury assessment (Figure 1). While not all patients with renal injury require imaging, indications for imaging include: blunt trauma with gross hematuria or patients with microscopic hematuria and shock (systolic blood pressure [SBP] < 90), penetrating injuries with any degree of hematuria, and children with any findings suggestive of renal injury. Should a patient require emergent surgical exploration, "single shot" intraoperative excretory pyelography may be performed in lieu of CT.

Trauma centers increasingly rely on newer, fast spiral CT to assess injury (Figure 2). These rapid studies, however, do not provide adequate time for contrast to fill the renal parenchyma and collecting

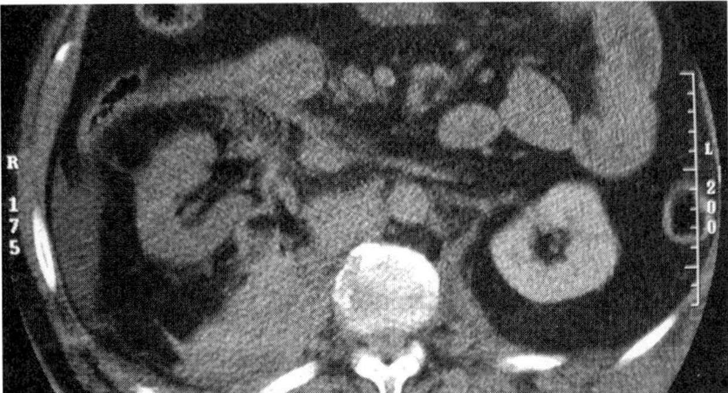

Figure 1. Grade IV renal injury (arterial thrombosis) manifesting as subtle lack of perfusion to the right kidney.

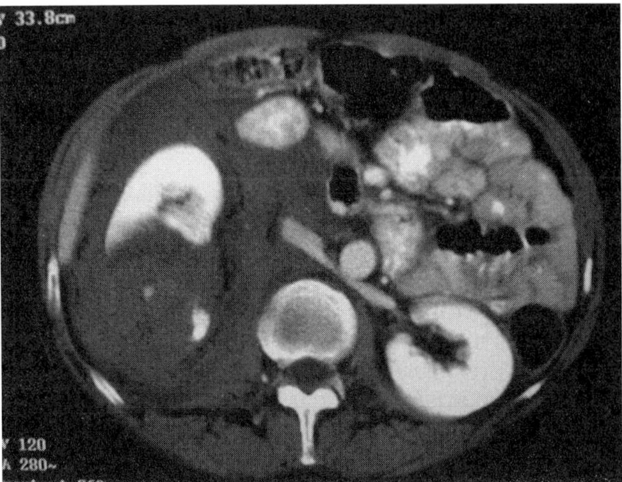

Figure 2. Grade IV renal injury (parenchymal disruption that extends into the collecting system).

system and care must be taken to obtain both immediate and delayed images 10 minutes after contrast injection. Ultrasound cannot clearly identify parenchymal, vascular, or collecting system injuries and should not be used. The degree of renal injury should be graded according to the American Academy for the Surgery of Trauma (AAST) guidelines (Table 1). Significant injuries requiring surgical exploration occur in only 2% of blunt renal trauma cases, but surgical exploration is needed in the majority of gunshot wounds to the body. Grade I-III injuries are most likely able to be managed nonoperatively with a regimen of hospital admission and bed rest until resolution of gross hematuria. Although grades IV and V more often require exploration, they, too, can often be conservatively managed in properly selected and monitored patients. Absolute indications for surgical exploration include: persistent renal bleeding (>2 units/day) and pulsatile perirenal hematoma (indicating renovascular avulsion). Relative indications for exploration include: urine extravasation and a devitalized segment, bilateral renal artery thrombosis, and renovascular injury in a solitary kidney. On occasion, complications from renal trauma are seen after resolution of the acute injury. In patients with persistent urinary extravasation, an internal ureteral stent may be placed which typically corrects the urinoma. Delayed gross hematuria is best treated by a return to bed rest, whereas massive hematuria or retroperitoneal hemorrhage requires either urgent angiographic embolization or speedy surgical exploration. In the case of abscess formation, percutaneous drainage with later surgical drainage for nonresponders is the preferred method of management.

URETERAL INJURIES

Ureteral injuries constitute less than 1% of all urologic trauma, but they are often associated with a significant degree of morbidity and even mortality. Patients with traumatic ureteral injuries often have significant associated injuries. It is important to note that although hematuria is a hallmark for GU injury, as many as 45% of patients with ureteral injury fail to demonstrate this finding. The delayed appreciation of ureteral injury is associated with fever, leukocytosis, and peritonitis, but findings including anuria, urinary leakage from the wound, and hydronephrosis should also raise suspicion of ureteral injury.

Should ureteral injury be suspected, it is recommended that an abdominal and pelvic CT with contrast be performed. It is imperative that delayed images be obtained in order to allow contrast to extravasate from

TABLE 1. **AAST Organ Injury Severity Scale for the Kidney**

*GRADE	Type	Description
I	Contusion	Microscopic or gross hematuria, urologic studies normal
	Hematoma	Subcapsular, nonexpanding without parenchymal laceration
II	Hematoma	Nonexpanding perirenal hematoma confirmed to renal retroperitoneum
	Laceration	<1.0 cm parenchymal depth of renal cortex without urinary extravasation
III	Laceration	>1.0 cm parenchymal depth of renal cortex without collecting system rupture or urinary extravasation
IV	Laceration	Parenchymal laceration extending through renal cortex, medulla, and collecting system
	Vascular	Main renal artery or vein injury with contained hemorrhage
V	Laceration	Completely shattered kidney
	Vascular	Avulsion of renal hilum which devascularizes kidney

*Advance one grade for bilateral injuries up to grade III.
AAST, American Academy for Surgery of Trauma.

the ureters, providing the optimal chance to visualize any injury. If time, or the extent of injury do not allow for a CT to be performed, an intraoperative "one-shot" intravenous pyelogram may be obtained instead (2 mg/kg IV contrast given 10 minutes before flat plate abdominal x-ray).

Once a ureteral injury is suspected, it is critical that a urologist be consulted for further management. Given the tenuous blood supply to the ureters, surgical intervention is often required. Although contusions secondary to blunt trauma are the most "minor" of ureteral injuries, healing of the injury is frequently associated with stricture or breakdown. In the case of penetrating injuries from gunshot wound, extensive débridement is frequently required as microvascular damage has been found 2 cm proximal and distal to the point of transection. Finally, in those individuals whose other injuries make primary ureteral repair at the time of injury impossible, the ureter may be ligated, a percutaneous nephrostomy tube placed, and a secondary reanastomosis performed when the patient has stabilized.

BLADDER INJURIES

With its protected, retropubic location, blunt bladder injuries are usually found in association with other severe injuries, such as pelvic fracture. Up to 10% of cases of traumatic pelvic fracture are associated with bladder rupture. When assessing for bladder injury, it is also critical to check for urethral injury.

Bladder injuries are classified as either intraperitoneal or extraperitoneal. Injury should be suspected in the presence of gross hematuria, failure of urethral catheter to return urine, and absence of voiding. Delay in diagnosis will result in patients with peritoneal irritation, sepsis, and blood urea nitrogen measurements that are elevated out of proportion to the creatinine (because of peritoneal absorption of urea in the urine). Diagnosis is confirmed either via retrograde cystography (plain abdominal x-ray obtained after at least 350 cc of contrast have been infused into the bladder by gravity) (Figure 3) or CT scan of the pelvis (following infusion of 350 cc of contrast diluted 1:6 to assure optimal CT quality) (Figures 4 and 5).

Once diagnosed, treatment for each type of injury varies. Intraperitoneal bladder ruptures require surgical closure for several reasons: these ruptures are often much larger than suggested by radiologic imaging (average size 6 cm), they are associated with persistent urinary leakage when conservative management is attempted, and persistent urinary leakage causes peritonitis which may be fatal. In the case of extraperitoneal rupture, conservative treatment is possible although surgical intervention may be required in the case of bony fragments projecting into the bladder, during open repair of associated pelvic fractures (in order to prevent hardware contamination with spilled urine), and surgical repair of other associated injuries. Typically, a catheter is left in place for 10 to 14 days after which time cystography is repeated and if no extravasation is found, the catheter is removed. In addition to catheter placement for extraperitoneal bladder ruptures, it is recommended that antibiotic prophylaxis be instituted on the day of injury and continued until 3 days after the catheter is removed. Intraperitoneal bladder ruptures require that antibiotics be administered only for 3 days perioperatively.

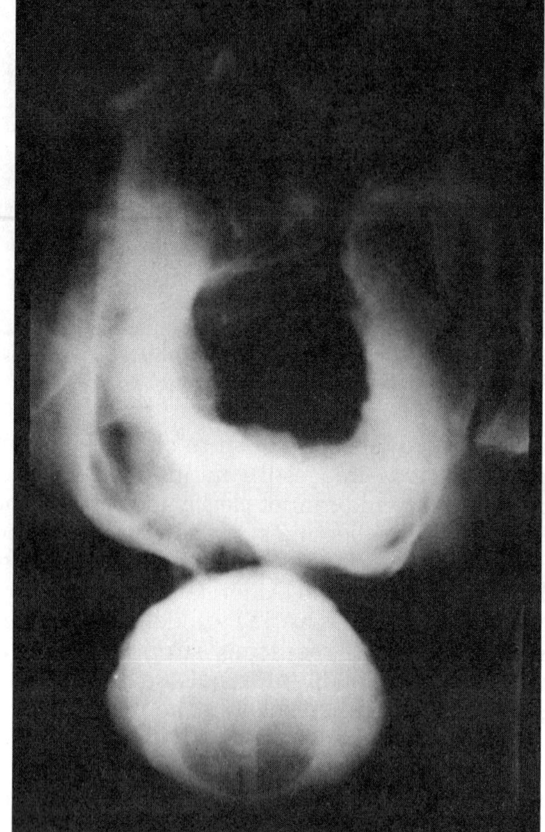

Figure 3. Plain cystogram showing an intraperitoneal bladder rupture.

URETHRAL INJURIES

Posterior urethral injuries are overwhelmingly associated with bilateral pubic rami fractures, and bladder rupture is found in a significant number of

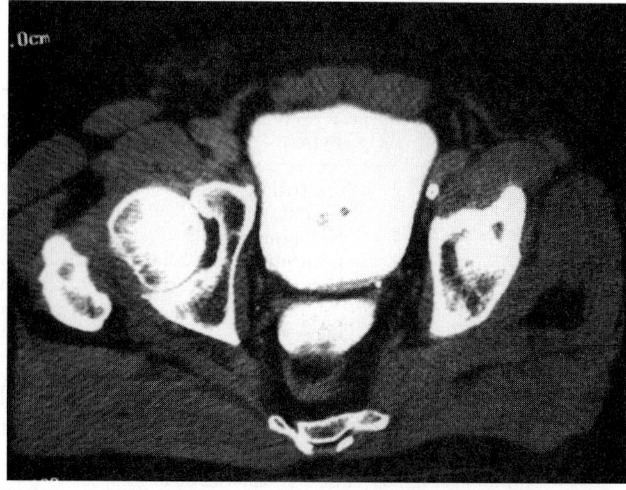

Figure 4. CT cystogram showing intraperitoneal bladder rupture.

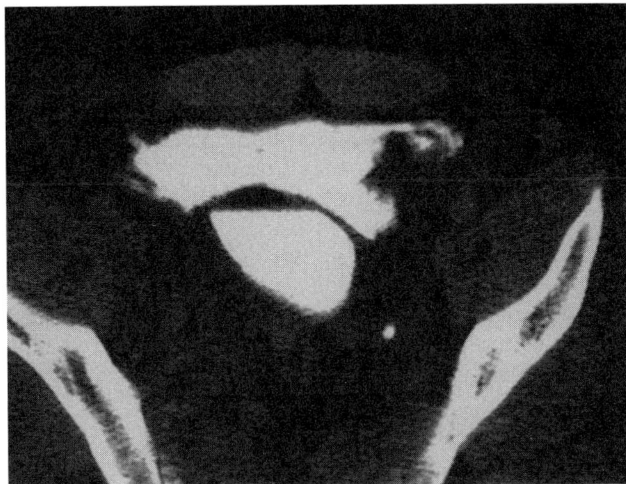

Figure 5. CT cystogram showing extraperitoneal bladder rupture.

these patients. Classically, urethral disruption is associated with the triad of blood at the urethral meatus, inability to urinate, and (in men) a high riding mobile prostate, although these findings are present in less than 50% of patients. While much has been made of the finding of "high-riding" prostate, this sign is unreliable, as the pelvic hematoma often found in cases of urethral injury obscures the contour of the prostate.

Once urethral disruption is suspected, an immediate retrograde urethrogram should be performed (Figure 6). If this fails, the patient requires surgical placement of a formal suprapubic catheter or attempt at endoscopic placement of a urinary catheter. Alternatively, a single, gentle attempt may be made by the urologist to place a urethral catheter prior to suprapubic catheter placement. Open primary realignment for urethral injury is not recommended because it is associated with an unacceptably high incidence of intraoperative blood loss, and postoperative impotence and incontinence. Whether urethral catheterization is achieved via retrograde placement or by intraoperative means using a combination of cystoscopic and fluoroscopic guidance, it is recommended that the catheter remain in place for 6 weeks, at which time either a voiding cystourethrogram or pericatheter retrograde urethrogram is obtained. If no extravasation is seen, the catheter may then be removed.

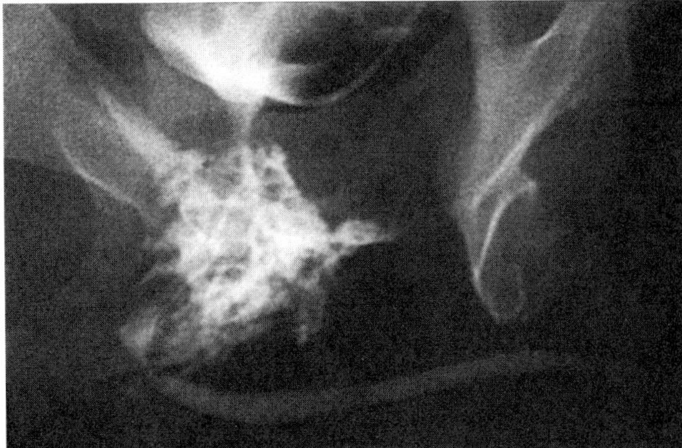

Figure 6. Retrograde urethrogram showing urethral disruption.

Anterior urethral injuries are rare, most often isolated, and largely involve the bulbar urethra. In contrast to the treatment for posterior urethral injuries, primary surgical repair is recommended for both low velocity gunshot wounds and lacerations. High velocity gunshot wounds, devastating shotgun wounds, and severe blunt crush injuries all require urinary diversion via suprapubic catheterization and delayed reconstruction because these injuries are associated with a large amount of tissue damage.

EXTERNAL GENITAL TRAUMA IN MALES

Penile injuries may be divided into three main categories: amputation, soft tissue injury, such as penile fracture, and penetrating injury. The most common cause of penile amputation is a result of self-mutilation, frequently in patients with a history of psychiatric illness. If possible, the severed portion of the penis should be retrieved and an attempt made at reimplantation. Should either the severed portion of the penis not be found or be unable to be reimplanted, operative débridement and formalization of the penile stump will be necessary.

Penile fracture typically presents with a classic history of the patient sustaining an acute bend of the erect penis followed by a popping sound and immediate detumescence. On physical examination, penile swelling and ecchymosis are nearly always present. It is important for the examining physician to be alert to the possibility of associated urethral injury. Should urethral injury be suspected, a retrograde urethrogram should be performed. Once penile fracture has been diagnosed and urethral injury assessed, immediate repair of the fractured corpora is recommended. Any associated urethral injury may be repaired at the time of corporal repair by spatulated reanastomosis and silicone catheter drainage.

Isolated penile soft tissue injuries are rare. As with any skin wound, initial treatment of a penile soft tissue wound involves irrigation, débridement of necrotic tissue, and use of appropriate antimicrobial agents. Although clean, uninfected wounds may be closed primarily after irrigation/débridement, old or infected wounds should be treated with wet to dry dressing changes and antimicrobial prophylaxis against suspected pathogens. Should the amount of skin lost from the penis be too excessive to allow primary closure, non-meshed, split-thickness skin grafts may be used for coverage.

In the case of the unfortunate patient who catches his penis in his trouser zipper, following local anesthetic penile block, a single attempt should be made to open the zipper. If this fails a pair of metal snips may be used to cut the zipper slider, or a pair of surgical clamps used to pull the zipper apart tooth by tooth.

Management of penetrating penile injuries combines treatment modalities for both penile fracture and soft tissue injury. As in the case of penile fracture, primary closure of any corporal disruption is recommended.

Once the corpora has been repaired, the skin wound should be treated as any other penile soft tissue injury. Should injury to deep structures (e.g., posterior urethra) exist, a staged repair with placement of a suprapubic tube may be necessary.

The testicles are surrounded by the tough tunica albuginea and as a result, a significant amount of force is required to cause tunical rupture. However, up to 50% of patients who suffer a direct blow to the testicle will have testicular rupture. In addition, the intratesticular parenchymal blood vessels are delicate and rupture easily, causing hematoma formation. The diagnosis of testicular rupture is complicated by the fact that there are no specific symptoms indicative of testicular rupture. Diagnosis is best made by thorough physical examination (aided by a local anesthetic cord block if necessary) and judicious use of ultrasound imaging.

Treatment for testicular injury is guided by a low threshold for surgical exploration. Any patient with an equivocal physical examination, hematocele, intratesticular hematoma, or rupture of the tunica albuginea should undergo exploration. Hematoma evacuation and débridement of devitalized testicular tissue helps to prevent later need for orchiectomy, preserve testicular hormonal production, and preserve spermatogenesis.

PROSTATITIS

method of
BURKE A. CUNHA, M.D.
Winthrop-University Hospital
Mineola, New York
State University of New York School of Medicine
Stony Brook, New York

Prostatitis is the most common urinary tract infection in adult men. The term prostatitis represents a variety of clinical syndromes that describe infection of the prostate.

Prostatitis may be classified as acute or chronic bacterial prostatitis. Chronic nonbacterial prostatitis, as well as a variety of inflammatory states related to the prostate, are the noninfectious counterparts of prostatitis. These states have been classified by the National Institutes of Health (Table 1).

ACUTE BACTERIAL PROSTATITIS

Clinical Presentation

Acute bacterial prostatitis is an acute inflammation of the prostate due to common uropathogens. The pathogenesis of prostatitis is unclear. Clinical presentation is that of an acute urinary tract infection. The patient usually presents with high fevers accompanied by chills, and may or may not develop urinary retention. Rectal exam reveals an exquisitely diffusely tender prostate. Bacteremia often accompanies acute bacterial prostatitis, and the organism isolated from the blood is the same as from the urine.

Antimicrobial Therapy

The first consideration in the selection of an antimicrobial for acute bacterial prostatitis is selecting an appropriate spectrum. The spectrum of the antibiotic that is appropriate for the treatment of acute bacterial prostatitis is one that is active against the common aerobic gram-negative bacillary uropathogens, e.g., *Escherichia coli*. Group D streptococci (enterococci, and other organisms, and other less common gram-negative pathogens may also cause acute bacterial prostatitis). *Staphylococcus aureus* or *Pseudomonas aeruginosa* are also uncommon causes of acute prostatitis and usually follow recent urologic instrumentation because these organisms are not uropathogens. Therefore, coverage should be directed against the common aerobic coliform bacteria that are the usual uropathogens. Pathogens in acute bacterial prostatitis are readily culturable from the urine, and therapy may be modified depending on results of urine culture/susceptibility testing.

In acute bacterial prostatitis, the prostate is inflamed, accounting for its exquisite tenderness on palpation. Inflammatory mediators, e.g., cytokines, cause increased capillary permeability, which permit the entrance of nearly all antimicrobials into the parenchyma of the inflamed prostate. The inflammation of the gland permits antimicrobials, which normally would not be able to penetrate the prostate, to enter the parenchyma of the prostate. For the reason given, in acute bacterial prostatitis, tissue penetration is not a therapeutic consideration as it is in chronic bacterial prostatitis.

The duration of treatment in acute bacterial prostatitis remains controversial. Short courses of therapy

TABLE 1. **National Institutes of Health Classification and Definition of Prostatitis**

Category	Syndrome	Definition
I	Acute bacterial prostatitis	Acute infection of the prostate
II	Chronic bacterial prostatitis	Recurrent infection of the prostate
III	Chronic nonbacterial prostatitis/chronic pelvic pain syndrome (CPPS)	No demonstrable infection
IIIa	Inflammatory CPPS	Semen, expressed prostatic secretions (EPS), or voided bladder urine–3 (VB3) reveals white blood cells (WBCs)
IIIb	Noninflammatory CPPS	Semen, EPS, and VB3 do not demonstrate WBCs
IV	Asymptomatic inflammatory prostatitis	No subjective symptoms, but WBCs are found in prostatic secretions or in prostate tissue during an evaluation for other disorders.

range from 7 to 10 days, in which symptoms resolve using an antimicrobial with the appropriate spectrum regardless of its pharmacokinetic characteristics. Others prefer a longer course of therapy, i.e., 2 to 4 weeks, to prevent treatment failures/subsequent chronic bacterial prostatitis. The extended approach is preferred because the initial episode is the best chance to eradicate the infection from the gland. If the patient is admitted to the hospital, initial antibiotic therapy may be given intravenously or orally. Patients with acute bacterial prostatitis who are less ill may be treated orally as outpatients. Patients who are initially started on intravenous therapy should be switched to an equivalent oral antibiotic as soon as there is clinical improvement, which is usually within 72 hours, and the remainder of therapy completed with an oral agent in the hospital/outpatient setting. Various antibiotic options are available (Table 2).

Patients with acute bacterial prostatitis should not be instrumented during infection. Complications of acute bacterial prostatitis include prostatic abscess or subsequent chronic bacterial prostatitis. For these reasons, patients with acute bacterial prostatitis should have follow-up after treatment to ensure the infection has been eradicated. Patients who develop a prostatic abscess usually require surgical drainage in addition to appropriate antimicrobial therapy.

CHRONIC BACTERIAL PROSTATITIS

Clinical Presentation

Most patients with chronic bacterial prostatitis give a history of antecedent episode(s) of acute bacterial prostatitis. Patients with chronic bacterial prostatitis have less impressive physical findings than patients with acute bacterial prostatitis, and their symptoms are more variable. Some patients with chronic bacterial prostatitis are asymptomatic or minimally symptomatic and the diagnosis is made by urine culture and physical examination. On examination the prostate is usually boggy and not exquisitely tender as with acute bacterial prostatitis. Patients with chronic bacterial prostatitis often present with recurrent urinary tract infections. Urinary tract infections in men are uncommon and recurrent infections should suggest chronic bacterial prostatitis. Alternately, adult men with infected stones (bladder or renal), structural urologic abnormality, or infected prostatic calculi may present with recurrent urinary tract infection. Fever, if present, is low grade in contrast to acute bacterial prostatitis where temperatures often exceed 102°F.

Antimicrobial Therapy

The treatment of chronic bacterial prostatitis rests on not only selecting an agent active against the

TABLE 2. **Antimicrobial Therapy of Acute Bacterial Prostatitis**

Organism	Antibiotic	Usual IV Dose*	IV → PO Switch or PO Therapy	Duration[†]
Escherichia coli				
	Aztreonam (Azactam)	2 g (IV) q8hr	Doxycycline (Vibramycin) 100 mg (PO) q12hr	2-4 weeks
	or		or	
	Ceftriaxone (Rocephin)	1 g (IV) q24hr	ciprofloxacin 500 mg (PO) q12hr	2-4 weeks
	or		or	
	Ciprofloxacin (Cipro)	400 mg (IV) q24hr	gatifloxacin 400 mg (PO) q24hr	2-4 weeks
	or		or	
	Gatifloxacin (Tequin)	400 mg (IV) q24hr	levofloxacin 500 mg (PO) q24hr	2-4 weeks
	or			
	Levofloxacin (Levaquin)	500 mg (IV) q24hr		2-4 weeks
Enterobacter faecalis (non-VRE)[‡]	Ampicillin/sulbactam (Unasyn)	1.5 g (IV) q6hr	amoxicillin 1 g (PO) q8hr	2-4 weeks
			or	
			TMP-SMX (Bactrim) 1 DS (PO) q12hr	2-4 weeks
(VRE)	Linezolid (Zyvox)	600 mg IV q12h	600 mg PO q12h	2-4 weeks
	Doxycycline (Vibramycin)	100 mg IV q12h	100 mg PO q12h	2-4 weeks
Staphylococcus aureus (methicillin susceptible)				
or				
Pseudomonas aeruginosa				
	Cefepime (Maxipime)	2 g (IV) q12hr		
	or			
	Meropenem (Merrem)	1 g (IV) q8hr		
	or			
	Piperacillin/tazobactam (Zosyn)	4.5 g (IV) q8hr		

*Adult with normal renal function.
[†]A total duration of therapy, i.e., IV alone, IV → PO, PO alone.
[‡]VRE, Vancomycin-resistant enterococci.

TABLE 3. **Antibiotic Therapy of Chronic Bacterial Prostatitis**

Organisms	Usual Oral Dose	Duration
Escherichia coli/coliforms	Trimethoprim (Proloprim) 100 mg (PO) q12hr	1-3 months
	or	
	TMP-SMX (Bactrim) 1 dose (PO) q12hr	1-3 months
	or	
	Doxycycline (Vibramycin) 100 mg (PO) q12hr	1-3 months
	or	
	amoxicillin 1 g (PO) q12hr	1-3 months
	or	
	Ciprofloxacin (Cipro) 500 mg PO q12h	1-3 months
	or	
	Gatifloxacin (Tequin) 400 mg (PO) q24hr	1-3 months
	or	
	Levofloxacin (Levaquin) 500 mg (PO) q24hr	1-3 months
Enterococcus faecalis (non-VRE)*	amoxicillin 1 g (PO) q8hr	1-3 months
	or	
	TMP-SMX 1 dose (PO) q12hr	1-3 months
(VRE)	Doxycycline 100 mg (PO) q12h	1-3 months
Staphylococcus aureus (methicillin susceptible)	ciprofloxacin 500 mg (PO) q12hr	1-3 months
or	or	or
Pseudomonas aeruginosa	gatifloxacin 400 mg (PO) q24hr	1-3 months
	or	
	levofloxacin 500 mg (PO) q24hr	1-3 months

*VRE, Vancomycin-resistant enterococci.

causative pathogen, but also on selecting an agent that will penetrate the minimally inflamed prostate. Because the same pathogens that cause chronic bacterial prostatitis also cause acute bacterial prostatitis, spectrum considerations in selecting an antimicrobial agent are the same. However, the critical factor in the treatment of chronic bacterial prostatitis is selecting an agent that penetrates into the prostate in the absence of inflammation.

The prostate is a multi-septate gland with a lipid-rich parenchyma. Therefore, antimicrobials with certain physiochemical characteristics are able to penetrate the prostate in the absence of inflammatory mediators. The most important physiochemical characteristics that predict antibiotic penetration into the prostate are lipid solubility and ionization potential. The antibiotics that penetrate well into the noninflamed prostate include clindamycin, trimethoprim-sulfamethoxazole, doxycycline, and fluoroquinolones. In general, ß-lactam antibiotics do not penetrate well into the noninflamed prostate parenchyma. Several antimicrobial regimens are useful in treating chronic bacterial prostatitis (Table 3).

The duration of therapy for chronic bacterial prostatitis is 1 to 3 months. I favor 3 months, to increase the probability that the pathogens are totally eliminated from the prostate parenchyma. Patients not responding to 3 months of appropriate antimicrobial therapy with an agent that penetrates the noninflamed prostate should be suspected of having infected prostatic calculi until proven otherwise. The majority of adult men have micro-prostatic calcifications, but only a minority become infected. However, in patients with chronic bacterial prostatitis, infection of microscopic calculi is suggested by a recurrence of infection after an adequate duration of treatment, i.e., 3 months. The best way to treat such patients is by transurethral resection of the prostate (TURP) to eliminate the infected calculi. Fortunately, this is rarely necessary as a last resort. The more common causes of therapeutic failure in treating a chronic bacterial prostatitis is in using an agent that does not adequately penetrate the noninflamed prostate or not treating the infection for sufficient duration.

NONBACTERIAL PROSTATITIS

There are a variety of noninfected prostatic syndromes that present with prostate symptoms but have no infectious component. These inflammatory conditions do not require antimicrobial therapy and for that reason are not discussed here. Patients with inflammatory prostatic symptoms should be differentiated from patients with chronic bacterial prostatitis, for which antimicrobial therapy is essential in treatment.

BENIGN PROSTATIC HYPERPLASIA

method of
JOHN KEFER PH.D., and
JOHN S. WHEELER M.D.
Loyola University Medical Center
Maywood, Illinois

EPIDEMIOLOGY

Benign prostatic hyperplasia (BPH) is one of the most common medical conditions in older males. Age and normal androgenic function are two of the more well established risk factors for this condition.

Whereas BPH is rare before the age of forty, the prevalence of histologic BPH at autopsy is 50% by 60 years of age, and 90% by 85 years of age. Approximately 40% of males 70 years of age or older, will have lower urinary tract symptoms consistent with BPH, and as the U.S. population ages, the prevalence continues to increase. Symptomatically, approximately 25% of 55-year-old men experience decreased urinary flow rate and other symptoms of BPH. By 75 years of age, this increases to 50%. Age, however, is not a causative factor of BPH. Although the risk for development of symptoms from BPH doubles for each decade of life between 60 and 90 years of age, it is important to note that clinical symptoms of the individual patient do not necessarily progress with age.

Normal androgenic function is also required for development of BPH, and both androgenic and estrogenic hormonal stimulation can induce prostatic hypertrophy. Other factors, such as race, sexual activity, smoking, socioeconomic status, vasectomy, alcohol intake, and diet have not been conclusively demonstrated to be involved in development of BPH.

PATHOPHYSIOLOGY

The pathophysiology of BPH is poorly understood because there is no direct correlation between prostatic glandular enlargement and symptomatology of BPH. Because the condition is rare in those younger than 40 years of age and does not develop in castrated men, it is accepted that BPH development requires aging and functional testes for androgen production. BPH is thought to originate in the transitional zone of the prostate, which surrounds the prostatic urethra between the bladder neck and the verumontanum. There are two main components involved in the development of BPH; a static and a dynamic component. The static component relates to proliferation of epithelial cells and stromal cells in the prostatic transitional zone (TZ). BPH occurs when the transitional zone enlarges, usually evident as median or lateral lobe hypertrophy. There is evidence that proliferation of the epithelial cell component is regulated through inhibitory paracrine signaling from the prostatic stromal cell component. Proliferation of transitional zone tissue has been shown to be induced by testosterone and its biologically active conversion product, dihydrotestosterone. Conversion of testosterone to dihydrotestosterone occurs by the enzyme 5α-reductase. Two forms of this enzyme have been described, type 1 and type 2. Type 5α-reductase contributes to circulating levels of dihydrotestosterone and is present in liver, skin, and other organs. Type 2 5α-reductase is present in urogenital tissues, localized to both the epithelial and stromal component of developing and adult prostates. Individuals lacking 5α-reductase type 2 do not develop genitalia and prostates.

Whereas the static component relates to epithelial and stromal transitional zone proliferation, the dynamic component is related to the prostatic smooth muscle. High concentrations of α_1-adrenergic receptors occur in the prostatic capsule and bladder neck. An increase in tone of the smooth muscle tissues is responsible for increased urethral resistance and pressure. Pharmacologic blockade with α_1-antagonists blocks prostatic smooth muscle contraction and decreases urethral resistance and pressure, subsequently relaxing the dynamic component of BPH.

SYMPTOMS

The diagnosis of BPH is presumptive, based on the symptomatology of the patient. These symptoms, commonly referred to as lower urinary tract symptoms (LUTS) are not specific for BPH. LUTS includes frequency, retention, intermittency, decreased force of stream (FOS), straining, urgency, and nocturia. Individuals with LUTS should be carefully assessed to determine the cause, to confirm diagnosis of BPH, and to exclude other bladder and prostate pathologic processes. It is important to note that a prostate of normal size on digital rectal examination (DRE) does not rule out a diagnosis of BPH because palpable prostate size does not correlate with degree of obstruction or severity of LUTS. However, the odds of having moderate to severe symptoms are five times higher for men with enlarged prostates versus those with normal prostates.

Symptoms of BPH are difficult to assess and quantify, yet they are the key to proper diagnosis and treatment of BPH. Because the vast majority of procedures performed for BPH are to provide symptomatic relief, it is necessary to quantify the level of interference in the quality of life of the patient. Assessment of interference on quality of life can be reliably accomplished using the well-validated AUA Symptom Score (International Prostate Symptom Score; IPSS) (Table 1). Symptoms based on overall score are classified as mild (0 to 7), moderate (8 to 19), and severe (20 to 35). The subjective impact of these symptoms on overall quality of life must also be taken into account. The patient with a severe-range AUA score may feel the symptoms are less bothersome than a patient with a lower AUA score, and this subjective impact on quality of life can direct therapeutic options.

DIAGNOSIS

Diagnosis of BPH relies on an accurate medical history eliciting the specific voiding complaints, as

TABLE 1. **AUA Symptom Score**

LUTS	None	1 in 5	<50%	50%	>50%	Always
Retention	0	1	2	3	4	5
Frequency	0	1	2	3	4	5
Intermittency	0	1	2	3	4	5
Urge	0	1	2	3	4	5
Decreased force of stream	0	1	2	3	4	5
Straining	0	1	2	3	4	5
Nocturia	0	1	2	3	4	5
Total						
QOL						

AUA = American Urological Association; LUTS = lower urinary tract symptoms; > = greater than; < = less than; QOL = quality of life.

well as quantification of these symptoms using an IPSS. Other possible causes of LUTS also must be ruled out, including UTI, urolithiasis, diabetes, urethral stricture, overactive bladder secondary to neurologic or other causes, congestive heart failure, or prostate/bladder cancer. Medications that can exacerbate obstructive symptoms include: tricyclic antidepressants, anticholinergic agents, diuretics, narcotics, and first generation antihistamines and decongestants. Physical examination should include DRE for prostatic abnormalities, such as palpable nodules, induration or irregularities of malignancy, or infection. On DRE, while the transitional zone is the area of the prostate involved in BPH, only the posterior lobes of the prostate are palpable. Abdominal examination may detect a suprapubic or low abdominal mass in a patient with BPH-induced retention. The AUA recommends all men older than age 50 receive an annual prostate-specific antigen (PSA) serum level to screen for prostate cancer. In African American males or men with a family history of prostate cancer in a first-degree relative, PSA screening should begin at 40 years of age or younger. The normal range for PSA is up to 4.0 ng/mL. Other valuable laboratory data include: urinalysis to rule out infection or hematuria, a serum creatinine level to determine renal function, and urine cytologic studies if irritative voiding symptoms are present. More sophisticated studies, such as urinary flow rate, postvoid residual, and pressure flow urodynamic studies are appropriate for evaluation of men with more severe symptoms (IPSS > 8), or with more complex co-morbidities. These tests are often used to determine baseline function prior to initiation of therapy, or to determine subsequent response to therapy. In patients who fail medical therapy, urodynamic pressure-flow studies and cystoscopy may be appropriate to evaluate the need for operative intervention, and to rule out other urologic pathologies. Cystoscopy is also reserved for situations in which invasive treatment is strongly considered. If watchful waiting or noninvasive therapies are appropriate, invasive diagnostic tests are usually not necessary.

TREATMENT

Watchful Waiting

Indications for treatment of BPH rely, in large part, on the subjective nature of the symptoms. For the majority of patients with BPH, symptoms are not severe or bothersome enough to warrant long-term medical or surgical intervention. Advising the patient toward lifestyle modification, such as minimizing evening fluid intake, avoiding caffeine, and avoiding decongestants, anticholinergics and other medications that impair voiding often provides effective resolution of symptoms. In a study of 556 men with moderate symptoms of BPH comparing outcomes following transurethral resection of the prostate (TURP) versus watchful waiting over 3 years, 8% of men randomized to TURP and 17% of men with watchful waiting failed treatment. Treatment failure with watchful waiting was mostly due to high postvoid residuals and significant increases in IPSS symptoms. Patients who respond poorly to watchful waiting have multiple medical and surgical options for treatment of BPH.

α-Adrenergic Blocking Agents

α-adrenergic antagonists have been shown in numerous randomized placebo-controlled trials to be safe and effective in the treatment of BPH. The most commonly prescribed α-adrenergic blockers appear to have similar safety profiles and clinical efficacy. Terazosin (Hytrin) and Doxazosin (Cardura) were the first α-antagonists available for treatment of BPH; however, these drugs also have vasoactive effects, and orthostatic hypotension was a significant concern, requiring careful dose titration. Tamsulosin (Flomax) is a unique α-blocker, which does not induce orthostatic hypotension, and so does not require dose titration. Overall, the most common side effects include headaches, dizziness, asthenia, and drowsiness. Sexual side effects are limited to retrograde ejaculation.

5α-Reductase Inhibition

Finasteride (Proscar) is a type II 5α-reductase inhibitor that blocks conversion of testosterone to dihydrotestosterone, the androgen involved in development of BPH. Finasteride represents the paradigm for androgen suppression of BPH and is emphasized here. Finasteride has its greatest therapeutic effect in men with prostates greater than 40 grams, and treatment for 6 months or more is usually required for a clinical response. The first randomized, multicenter, double-blind, placebo-controlled trial investigating the efficacy of finasteride demonstrated significant improvement in maximum flow rate and decreased prostatic volume. Since then, further studies have confirmed these findings. The longest duration randomized, double-blinded, placebo-controlled study confirmed the symptom improvement and decrease in prostate volume demonstrated in previous studies on finasteride, and it also demonstrated a reduced risk of acute urinary retention and surgical intervention with finasteride use.

Finasteride has also been demonstrated to reduce BPH-associated hematuria. It is effective as adjuvant therapy, following other treatments, and as neoadjuvant therapy prior to minimally invasive therapy. Adverse effects include decreased libido, ejaculatory dysfunction, and gynecomastia. In the patient being monitored for prostate cancer with prostate-specific antigen testing, finasteride therapy must be taken into account when interpreting PSA values; finasteride has been shown to decrease PSA value by 50%, leading to a false-negative PSA test result.

PHYTOTHERAPY

Phytotherapeutic agents are increasing in popularity in the treatment of BPH. Commonly prescribed in

Europe for treatment of BPH-associated LUTS, these agents are increasingly self-prescribed by patients in the United States. Because of increasing availability and growing public interest in herbal remedies, between 30% to 90% of patients seen by urologists for LUTS/BPH are taking some form of phytotherapy for BPH. These herbal preparations claim to benefit "the health of the prostate and bladder," however, the mechanism of these therapies is poorly established. Of greater concern is that the bioavailability, safety and efficacy profile, and dose of these preparations are highly variable and impossible to compare across products, leading to potential toxicity or drug-to-drug interactions. The origins of the extracts most commonly used in "prostate health pills" include South African star grass,* saw palmetto,* African plum tree,* stinging nettle,* and rye pollen,*. Zinc,* tofu,* selenium,* vitamin E,* and amino acids* are also frequently included.

Saw palmetto extract is the most popular phytotherapeutic agent. The mechanism of action is unknown. It is most commonly thought to inhibit 5α-reductase; however, many other mechanisms have been proposed. A recent meta-analysis of numerous randomized trials using saw palmetto described a mild to moderate improvement in flow and LUTS; however, because of small study sample, variable products, short treatment times, and variable outcomes, these study conclusions are difficult to interpret.

African plum is used commonly in France, and has been shown to have several in vitro effects, such as antiestrogen effects, leukotriene blockade, and inhibition of fibroblast growth factors. The beneficial effects of this extract may be through a protective effect on the bladder. Rabbits, given African plum extract and subjected to partial bladder outlet obstruction, demonstrated protective effects on bladder mass, compliance, and contractility. However, the in vivo effects in humans are not known. Studies in human subjects have been limited, and currently no conclusions can be made regarding the efficacy of the extract.

South African star grass has been shown in vitro to increase plasminogen activators, as well as to stimulate release of transforming growth factor-β (TGF-β), an inducer of apoptosis. These in vitro effects have not been shown to occur in vivo, and have not been demonstrated to be clinically relevant. A meta-analysis of four clinical trials of South African star grass extract, β-sitosterol, concluded that β-sitosterol improved urologic symptoms and flow rates in men. However, the long-term effectiveness and safety profile of this compound are unknown. These results are nonetheless encouraging, and if duplicated, may demonstrate a role of β-sitosterol in medical management of BPH/LUTS.

Stinging nettle, used in Germany for treatment of LUTS/BPH, and rye pollen are both thought to improve the health of the prostate. However, both lack strong clinical data indicating therapeutic benefit. The evidence regarding efficacy and safety in phytotherapy is difficult to interpret and these studies should be viewed cautiously.

In general, there is no standard of care for management of patients using phytotherapeutic agents. Patients should be cautioned that doses, efficacy, side effects, and drug interactions with phytotherapy are unknown. For the patient refusing traditional medical therapy of α-blockers and finasteride, phytotherapy may be attempted as long as the patient understands the limitations of these agents. If retention, UTI, calculi, or decreased renal function occurs, phytotherapy should be discouraged, and more aggressive medical and surgical management should be undertaken.

MINIMALLY INVASIVE THERAPIES

The most commonly employed surgical procedure, and the gold standard for BPH, is transurethral resection of the prostate (TURP), involving endoscopic resection of the obstructive component of the prostate. TURP is highly effective, improving symptoms in 88% to 95% of patients. The most frequent complications of the procedure are: inability to void postoperatively, clot retention, incontinence, impotence, and retrograde ejaculation. A number of new, minimally invasive therapies have been developed to reduce the complications associated with TURP, as well as to provide alternatives for the unfavorable surgical candidate. Most minimally invasive therapies use energy, such as radio waves, laser, ultrasound, microwaves, or electrical current. Transurethral incision of the prostate (TUIP), involves endoscopic placement of one to two incisions into the prostate and capsule to reduce urethral constriction. This procedure is highly effective on prostate glands less than 30 grams and is well-documented and safe, with comparable efficacy to TURP in well-selected patients. TUIP is associated with a 78% to 83% change of symptom improvement. Because TUIP is associated with fewer retrograde ejaculations, less morbidity, and a reoperation rate of less than 1% in 10 years, this procedure is the treatment of choice for small gland BPH in men concerned with fertility and ejaculation.

Transurethral needle ablation (TUNA) is a process whereby low level energy is transferred by radio frequency to the prostate, creating a well-defined necrotic lesion within the prostatic parenchyma, while preserving the urethral mucosa. A cystoscope-like catheter with two needles set at 90 degrees from each other ablates tissue in 3 to 5 minutes when needles reach temperatures of 80 to 100 degrees Fahrenheit. Urethral and rectal temperatures are also vigorously monitored as the device adjusts. Preliminary studies show an increase in peak flow and a decrease in symptom score following TUNA, with no major complications. Transient urinary retention is reported in 10% to 40% of patients. In a prospective study, TURP was superior to TUNA in increasing flow rates, but demonstrated comparable improved symptoms at 1 year postoperatively.

*Not FDA approved for this indication.

Interstitial laser coagulation (ILC) uses a similar principle to TUNA, but introduces a laser fiber directly into the prostate through the urethra. The energy delivery spares the urethral mucosa and results in prostatic parenchymal tissue coagulation. After 1 year, improvement in symptoms and increased peak urinary flow was 60% to 65%. Disadvantages are prolonged catheterization (18 days, average), and retrograde ejaculation. Visual laser ablation of the prostate (VLAP) is a similar technique, but is performed using a side-firing Nd:YAG laser fiber. Several prospective randomized trials of TURP versus VLAP demonstrated similar results, showing equivalent improvements in symptom scores and increases in flow rates. Significant disadvantages of VLAP are due to urethral mucosa ablation by direct laser coagulation. Urinary retention, requiring prolonged postoperative catheterization, irritative LUTS symptoms of 2 to 6 weeks average duration, and retrograde ejaculation occur in more than one third of patients undergoing VLAP.

Transurethral microinvasive thermotherapy (TUMT) heats prostatic transitional zone tissue to 42 degrees Celsius, inducing tissue damage. Thermotherapy preferentially destroys smooth muscle by coagulative necrosis, while water-conductive cooling of the urethral mucosa preserves periurethral tissues. Although prospective studies indicate that TURP produces more pronounced urinary improvements versus TUMT, thermotherapy consistently improves symptom scores by 75% and increased peak flow rates by 75%. Furthermore, TUMT is a procedure done under local anesthesia. Retrograde ejaculation and urinary retention with prolonged catheterization occurs in greater than one third of patients.

BPH is an extremely common disease in aging males. Physicians have many therapeutic options available for treating BPH, including watchful waiting, medical therapy, TURP, and a broad range of minimally invasive surgeries. Decisions toward proper therapeutic regimen depend in large part on patient symptom scores. Men with low symptom scores without bother are appropriately managed through watchful waiting. As scores increase, more aggressive management is appropriate. The efficacy of medical therapy has reduced the frequency of invasive therapy; however, the patient who fails medical therapy has a broad range of therapeutic options for minimally invasive therapy for BPH.

ERECTILE DYSFUNCTION

method of
EDWARD D. KIM, M.D.
University of Tennessee Medical Center
Knoxville, Tennessee

Significant advances in the recognition and treatment of erectile dysfunction (ED), previously known as impotence, have been made in the last decade. Defined as the consistent inability to get or maintain an erection suitable for intercourse, it is estimated that 18 to 20 million men in the United States are affected. Difficulties with erections increase with aging, as demonstrated by a recent study that showed a greater than 60% prevalence in men in their 60s and a greater than 80% prevalence in men in their 70s. The evaluation of ED should be cost-effective and start with a history and physical examination. Etiologies may be hormonal, psychological, vasculogenic, or neurogenic. Most men will not have a reversible cause of their ED, however.

ERECTILE PHYSIOLOGY

As a result of sexual stimulation, the parasympathetic-mediated cavernous nerves originating from S2-S4 release nitric oxide (NO), which stimulates the formation of cyclic guanosine monophosphate (cGMP) (Figure 1). This cGMP is directly responsible for corporal smooth muscle relaxation, which enables increased arterial dilation and inflow. The erectile

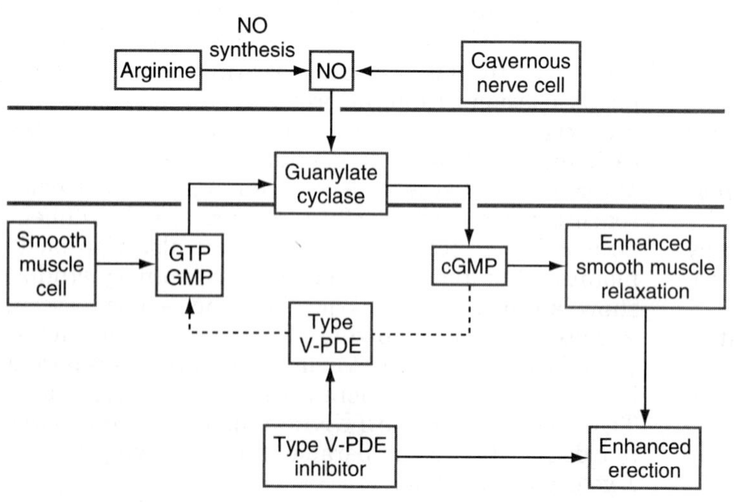

Figure 1. The biochemical process involved in erections and the mechanism of action of sildenafil citrate. The cavernous nerves (S2-S4) innervate the penis and release nitric oxide (NO). NO stimulates the production of cGMP in the smooth muscle cells of the penis. cGMP is directly responsible for increasing smooth muscle relaxation, which leads to increased arterial inflow and an erection. When cGMP is metabolized by type V-phosphodiesterase (PDE), the penis undergoes detumescence. Sildenafil (Viagra) inhibits type V-PDE and increases the available cGMP, thereby leading to an enhanced erection.

tissue of the penis is composed of the paired corpora cavernosa and the corpus spongiosum. The arterial supply to the penis is derived from branches of the internal pudendal artery. As the corporal bodies fill with blood, the draining venules between the external sinusoids and the tunica albuginea become compressed, thereby trapping the blood within the penis. Detumescence is initiated by the degradation of cGMP, a process that is enzymatically mediated by type V-phosphodiesterase (PDE).

EVALUATION OF ERECTILE DYSFUNCTION CAUSES

ED starts to appear in men in their 40s. In most practices, the majority of ED is secondary to organic causes related to endothelial dysfunction such as diabetes, hypertension, atherosclerotic heart disease (Table 1), and a variety of medications (Table 2). Anti-hypertensive medications often cause a decline in potency because of their desired effect in reducing systemic blood pressure, resulting in a decrease in perfusion pressure to the penis.

Most men will not have a reversible cause. Endocrine disorders may be treatable with hormone replacement with subsequent restoration of potency. However, hypogonadism is the direct cause of ED in only 8% to 16% of men. Low or borderline low testosterone levels are the most common endocrine abnormalities detected and should prompt further hormonal evaluation with a serum follicle stimulating hormone (FSH), luteinizing hormone (LH), and prolactin. The age-related decline starting in the fifth decade of life in bioavailable testosterone is known as androgen deficiency in aging men (ADAM) or andropause. Testosterone replacement therapies are most appropriate for men with clearly documented hypogonadism resulting in decreased libido, and for carefully selected men with hypogonadism and decreased quality of erections. Chronic smokers have a greater incidence of penile vascular insufficiency as a result of arterial insufficiency. Nicotine is likely the mediator responsible for both acute and chronic effects of smoking.

Regardless of the organic cause of ED, one cannot minimize the psychosocial disorders that may both cause and result from this disorder:

- Depression
- Esteem issues, coping mechanisms
- Partner relationships, past and present
- Altered social or occupational role
- History of abuse or trauma
- Anxiety; fear of failure

TABLE 1. **Organic Risk Factors for Erectile Dysfunction**

Vascular disease	Diabetes mellitus
Hypertension	Hypogonadism
Smoking	Hyperlipidemia
Alcohol use	Surgery or trauma to pelvis or spine
Peyronie's disease	Neurologic disease
Medications	

TABLE 2. **Common Medications and Substances Associated With Erectile Dysfunction**

Alcohol	Clofibrate
Antiandrogens	Estrogens
Anticholinergics	H_2 blockers
Antidepressants	Ketoconazole (Nizoral)
Antihypertensives (sympatholytics)	Marijuana
	Narcotics
β-blockers	Psychotropic drugs
Cigarettes and tobacco	Phenothiazines
Cocaine	Spironolactone (Aldactone)

HISTORY

The history remains one of the most important diagnostic tools for elucidating the cause of ED. Questions related to concurrent illnesses, previous surgery, medications, tobacco and alcohol use, stress levels, and a thorough review of systems are essential. The partner's contributions to relationship type and history, events surrounding the onset of problems, pre- and post-problem sexual interaction, expectations of treatment outcome, and the partner's own sexual desires are extremely important and informative. It is most important to determine the real nature of the problem—to discover whether the patient is having problems with loss of desire for sex, premature ejaculation, retrograde ejaculation, delayed orgasms, or ED. Once it is established that ED is the problem, then it is important to determine its duration and degree.

PHYSICAL EXAMINATION

The examination should have emphasis on the penis, testes, and lower extremity circulation, and prostate. Significant testicular atrophy could signify hypogonadism. While stretched, the penis should be examined for plaques suggestive of Peyronie's disease. Foreskin cracking and frenular irritations, suggestive of chronic balanitis, are usually exacerbated during erection and can cause sufficient discomfort to dissuade one from continuing intercourse. Obese patients may have compromised functional penile length, rather than penile shrinkage.

LABORATORY EVALUATION

The evaluation should be cost-effective and individualized based on the clinical index of suspicion. A screening total testosterone level and urinalysis, which may detect previously undiagnosed diabetes, are advisable (Table 3). Hypercholesterolemia is a common finding on lipid profile testing. A screening PSA is helpful, because prostate cancer and ED occur in the same age groups. Advanced testing with nocturnal penile tumescence testing and/or duplex ultrasonographic evaluation of the penile arterial blood flow is occasionally indicated for younger men in search of a reversible cause. These tests are not necessary for most patients as the treatment choices are unchanged.

TABLE 3. **Suggested Laboratory Testing**

Primary	Serum total testosterone Urinalysis
Secondary	Serum chemistries, CBC Free testosterone, prolactin, LH PSA
Tertiary	Penile duplex ultrasonography Nocturnal penile tumescence testing Dynamic infusion cavernosometry and cavernosography Biothesiometry

TREATMENT

In the late 1970s and early 1980s, the only dependable treatment for impotent men whose problems were not hormonally related was the implantation of a penile prosthesis. Now, sildenafil citrate (Viagra) has become the first-line treatment choice for the majority of men (Figure 2). Other treatments include intracavernous injections, vacuum constriction devices, MUSE, and penile prostheses.

Sildenafil Citrate (Viagra)

Sildenafil, introduced in April 1998, is the first effective oral pill for the treatment of ED and it functions as a selective inhibitor of cyclic guanosine monophosphate (cGMP)-specific type V-phosphodiesterase (PDE) (see Figure 1). By inhibiting type V-PDE, Viagra causes increased smooth muscle relaxation, inflow of blood into the corpus cavernosum, and thus improved erections, but does not itself produce an erection. Sexual excitation and stimulation must be present for Viagra to have an effect.

Sildenafil is most commonly prescribed at 50 and 100 mg. The effect is dose-dependent with up to 80% to 85% of men having improved erections. The patient should be instructed to take Viagra about 1 to 2 hours prior to sexual activity for peak effect. While most men will respond favorably to the first several doses, late responders may require 7 to 8 administrations for best results. Efficacy has been demonstrated across a wide range of etiologies, including hypertension, coronary artery disease, diabetes mellitus, depression, peripheral vascular disease, psychogenic, radical prostatectomy, and spinal cord injury.

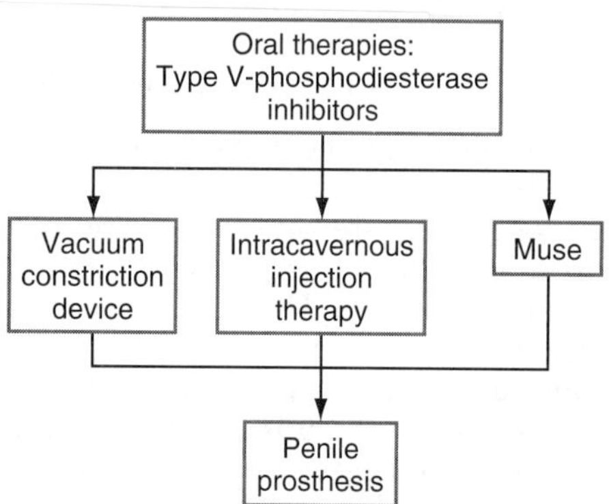

Figure 2. Algorithm for the treatment of organic erectile dysfunction. Sildenafil citrate has become the first-line treatment since its introduction in 1998. Intracavernous injection therapies, vacuum constriction devices, and alprostadil (Muse) represent minimally invasive second-line treatment choices.

The major contraindication is the concomitant use of nitrates, because of the potentiation of hypotensive effects of nitrates. Viagra should be used with caution in men with cardiac disease, because increased sexual activity may increase the aerobic requirements of the myocardium. The risk is underdiagnosed or inadequately treated cardiac disease in a patient undertaking sexual activity, not the medication itself. The mild vasodilatory effect of sildenafil may actually exert a cardioprotective effect. An exercise stress test can predict which men with suspected cardiac disease would experience angina during intercourse.

With a half-life ($t_{1/2}$) of 4 hours, the side effects tend to be short-lived and generally mild. The most common side effects include mild headache, dyspepsia, and flushing, which are seen in 7% to 16% of men in a dose-dependent fashion. An unusual side effect in about 3% of men is a short-lived visual blue haze as a result of cross-reactivity with type V-PDE in the retina. Discontinuation rates from side effects of 2.5% are equal to the placebo group.

Intracavernous Injection Therapy

Intracavernous injection therapy is a minimally invasive and effective second-line therapy that involves the direct injection of vasoactive medications into the corporal bodies of the penis, thereby stimulating and simulating the natural erectile physiology. The dose is adjusted so that the erection may spontaneously resolve after approximately one hour. Commonly used medications are prostaglandin E_1 (PGE_1; Caverject), papaverine, and phentolamine (Regitine).*

The principal steps involved are: (1) preparation of the syringe (1cc, 29 gauge, 1/2 inch needle); (2) selection and preparation of the site for injection; (3) injection; and (4) compression of the injected site. Maximum erection is achieved within 10 to 15 minutes. Absolute contraindications include treatment with monoamine oxidase (MAO) inhibitors, known hypersensitivity to one of the components, and a propensity toward secondary forms of priapism (sickle cell disease, multiple myeloma, leukemia). Relative contraindications include anticoagulant therapy, poor manual dexterity, and morbid obesity. Priapism (0.3% incidence) can damage the intracorporal tissue when present for more than 4 to 6 hours. Prolonged and frequent use of injection therapy may result in the development of a Peyronie's-like tunical plaque, most likely representing a local reaction to repetitive injections, in approximately 5% of patients.

Vacuum Constriction Devices

Vacuum constriction devices are effective, noninvasive, second-line therapies that involve external penile appliances that generate a negative pressure on the penis, thus creating an erection. The tumescence is maintained by the placement of a constriction band at

*Not FDA approved for this indication.

the penile base. The mechanism of erection is different than with intracavernous injection therapy because little smooth muscle relaxation is induced. The physiologic state created consists of venous stasis and eventually decreased arterial inflow. The primary advantage is that firm erections are possible in up to 98% of men. The disadvantages are its cumbersome use with lack of spontaneity and the lack of rigidity proximal to the constriction band, leading to a "hinge" effect. Long-term compliance rates are often less than 50%. The side effects are uncommon, but may include penile irritation, a temporary decrease in penile sensation, decreased antegrade ejaculation, and bruising with small petechiae formation.

Muse

MUSE is an FDA-approved alternative representing intraurethrally administered alprostadil (PGE_1). After urinating, the applicator is inserted into the urethra. The onset to erection is 7 minutes. In a multicenter, placebo-controlled study involving 996 men, 65.9% had erections judged to be "sufficient" for intercourse during in-office testing. Of those men who responded in the clinic, 64.9% were able to have intercourse at least once during home application. The main advantage is the avoidance of needles and ease of application. Because of the small, but significant risk of hypotension (3.3%), it is recommended that initial testing be performed in the office. Drawbacks include its cost of $20 to $25 and relative lack of efficacy in producing rigid erections. Other adverse effects included penile and perineal discomfort, minor urethral trauma, and hypotension.

Penile Prosthesis

The penile prosthesis represents a surgical form of treatment. It is highly advisable that the patient first try and fail or dislike the first and second-line therapies prior to prosthesis placement. Penile prostheses may be malleable (bendable) or inflatable. Most men prefer the inflatable prosthesis because of the ability to vary its rigidity. The malleable prosthesis is preferable when the patient has poor manual dexterity or has a spinal cord injury and needs a prosthesis for better condom catheter use. The commonly implanted inflatable prostheses are either two- or three-piece (penile cylinders, reservoir, pump) systems.

The primary advantages are the relative spontaneity compared to other treatment methods, applicability and effectiveness for all types of organic dysfunction, and high patient satisfaction. Complications, as with any other surgery, include bleeding, infection, and the risks of anesthesia. These problems are relatively uncommon and are minimized with meticulous intraoperative hemostasis and by the use of intravenous antibiotics prior to and after surgery. Men are also advised about perceived decrease in penile size, mechanical malfunction, the inability to effectively use newer treatments in development, and erosion.

Treatment of Hypogonadism

If the testosterone level is normal, additional supplementation will not improve sexual function and in fact may be deleterious because it inhibits the patient's own production of the hormone. Replacement therapy can be treated effectively with intramuscular testosterone (Depo-Testosterone) (200 mg every other week), patches (Testoderm) (5 mg/d), or topical gels (Androgel 1%) (5 mg/d). Testosterone levels should be monitored during therapy.

Ineffective Therapies

Yohimbine,* a tree bark extract, was used extensively as an oral therapy for ED prior to the introduction of Viagra. The proposed mechanism of action was increased blood flow to the penis mediated by a poorly defined adrenergic blockade. High-dose, blinded, placebo-controlled studies fail to document the benefit of yohimbine. Arterial bypass procedures are rarely indicated and are considered experimental given the small caliber of the penile arteries, the diffuse nature of the atherosclerosis, and the extent of end-organ dysfunction. Similarly, venous ligation surgery is generally ineffective for men with veno-occlusive dysfunction.

The Near Future

Further oral therapies may be available in the United States by late 2003. Most promising are the second generation of type V-PDE inhibitors, including tadalafil citrate (Cialis)† and vardenafil citrate (Nuviva),† both having similar efficacy with Viagra. In early 2002, these agents had received conditional approval from the U.S. Food and Drug Administration, pending additional data. Tadalafil has a $t_{1/2}$ of 17.5 hours, thereby providing efficacy for up to 36 hours. Vardenafil citrate has a similar $t_{1/2}$ to Viagra, but potentially with fewer side effects because of increased type V-PDE selectivity.

Sublingual apomorphine (Uprima),† available in a 3 mg dose in Europe since 2001, is a dopamine agonist that functions as a centrally acting initiator of erections. Improvements in erections have been observed in approximately 50% to 60% of men using 4 to 6 mg doses with an onset to erection in 10 to 14 minutes. Concern over syncope (0.4% at 4 mg dose) may delay its FDA approval. Oral phentolamine† is a corporal smooth muscle relaxant that may improve the quality of an erection. Available internationally for 5 years, 40% to 60% of men reported improved erections at a 40 to 60 mg dose. Human trials were suspended by the FDA in August 1999 because of concern about its carcinogenic potential in rats.

The topical route using papaverine, minoxidil, and PGE_1 has also been tested, but difficulty in penetrating the thick tunica covering the corporal smooth muscle is a problem. The most promising of these agents is a topical PGE-1 gel applied to the glans and meatus.

The evaluation and treatment of ED are now easily accomplished, in large part because of more successful forms of therapy. Advances in the understanding of the physiology of erections have enabled these more effective treatments, of which oral agents are the most promising.

*Not FDA approved for this indication.

†Not yet approved for use in the United States.

ACUTE RENAL FAILURE

method of
JAMES W. LEWIS, M.D.
Riverside Nephrology Associates, Inc.
Columbus, Ohio

Acute renal (kidney) failure represents a constellation of medical problems, i.e., increase in nitrogenous wastes (blood urea nitrogen and creatinine), derangement of acid-base milieu, and electrolyte abnormalities (specifically affecting sodium, potassium, calcium, and phosphorus regulation). Acute renal failure is the cause of 1% to 5% of routine hospital admissions and 30% of intensive care admissions. The prognosis depends on the underlying cause: surgical patients have a 40% to 80% mortality. Mortality among patients with medical causes for their acute renal failure is less than 25%.

Diagnosis

The diagnosis is frequently based on both the urine volume and the rise in the blood urea nitrogen (BUN) and creatinine. Oliguria is defined as urine output of less than 400 mL/d. Anuria is defined as less than 100 mL/d. A rise in the creatinine serially is the other measure of acute kidney failure (AKF). A creatinine level can rise from 0.5 mg/dL per day to 1.5 mg/dL per day. Patients in a hypercatabolic state can have a rise in creatinine between 1 to 2 mg/dL per day, while most oliguric patients will have a rise in creatinine of 1 mg/dL per day. Older and smaller patients will have a rise in creatinine of only 0.5 mg/dL per day. The rise in creatinine and persistent oliguria are the hallmarks of acute kidney failure.

Two other caveats are important. The BUN will rise normally 10 mg/dL per day in a patient with acute kidney failure, but the BUN can rise more rapidly if gastrointestinal bleeding is occurring, the patient is receiving corticosteroids, or the patient is in a hypercatabolic state. The BUN will rise more slowly if the patient is consuming little protein in his or her diet. The other caveat is that not all patients are oliguric. Some of the patients with acute kidney failure are transiently oliguric and then make 1 L of urine per day or be even more polyuric (up to 4 L per day).

PRERENAL AZOTEMIA

Acute kidney failure is frequently divided into three categories: prerenal azotemia, intrinsic disease, and obstructive azotemia.

Prerenal azotemia is the most common variety and constitutes 50% of all the cases of acute kidney failure. In prerenal azotemia, the integrity of the renal parenchyma is maintained and the kidney's ability to concentrate and dilute remains intact. The natural history of prerenal azotemia is that the renal function frequently reverts to normal within 24 to 72 hours with intervention. The physiology of prerenal azotemia represents a decrease in the glomerular filtration rate resulting from a decrease in renal perfusion pressure and intense renal vasoconstriction or possibly both of these phenomena. Laboratory data best describes and distinguishes prerenal azotemia from parenchymal injury and obstructive azotemia. Because the kidney maintains its ability to concentrate and dilute, the urine sodium is low (usually less than 20 mEq on a spot urine), and the fractional excretion of urine is less than 1. The urine sodium is measured routinely in the laboratory and the fractional excretion of sodium is calculated by dividing the urine/serum sodium by the urine/serum creatinine and multiplying that number by 100. Also, the urine sediment remains bland, usually without sediment. Hyaline casts can occur in this situation, but it is felt that the hyaline casts are not diagnostic of any true injury to the kidney (Table 1).

Prerenal causes of acute kidney failure in the hospital setting are usually (in order of frequency) congestive heart failure, excessive loss of fluid either from gastrointestinal loss, diuretics, or third spacing of fluids in the abdominal cavity. Three more frequently occurring causes are discussed because of the high usage of these drugs and compounds. These include nonsteroidals, angiotensin-converting enzyme inhibitors in overly diuresed individuals, and radiocontrast agents. These particular causes can also fall into the intermediate category of acute kidney failure because there is a prerenal component that can transform into an acute intrinsic injury. Thus, prerenal azotemia can predispose to intrinsic injury.

Nonsteroidal Anti-Inflammatory Drugs (NSAIDs)

Nonsteroidal anti-inflammatory drugs (NSAIDs) inhibit prostaglandin-mediated afferent arteriolar vasodilation in the glomerulus. Prostaglandin I_2, called prostacyclin, prostaglandin E_2, and prostaglandin D_2 diminish vascular resistance resulting in dilatation of the vascular bed leading to a redistribution of blood flow from the renal cortex to the juxtamedullary portion of the kidney. The prostaglandins are necessary for preglomerular capillary vasodilation. NSAIDs tend to decrease this blood flow and cause medullary ischemia. Predisposing factors for this to occur are congestive heart failure, chronic renal failure, and hypovolemia. The picture that is produced is usually an acute elevation of the BUN and creatinine, elevation of the potassium, and salt and water retention.

Therapy in this situation includes: (1) identifying in the history that the patient is taking prescribed or over-the-counter NSAIDs; (2) discontinuation of these drugs, (3) returning the patient to a euvolemic state, (4) correcting the potassium with sodium polystyrene sulfonate (Kayexalate) 30 g orally frequently with 50 to 100 mL of sorbitol, a sodium polystyrene sulfonate (Kayexalate) enema of 50 g retained for 1 hour and then cleared with a tap water enema, and (5) correcting the diet to lower the potassium. The natural history is reversibility, but it can take 5 to 10 days.

TABLE 1. **Laboratory Evaluation in Kidney Failure**

Test	Prerenal	Intrinsic	Postrenal
BUN/Creatinine	>20	10-20	10-20
Urine osmolality	>350	≤ 300	>400 early, ≤ 300 later
U_{Na} (mEq/L)	<20	>30	<20 early, >40 later
FE_{Na}	<1	>2-3	<1 early, >3 later
Urine microscopic evaluation	Normal hyaline casts	ATN: dark granular casts, renal epithelial cells GN: dysmorphic RBCs, RBC casts; WBCs AIN: eosinophils, WBC, WBC casts	Normal

AIN, allergic interstitial nephritis; ATN, acute tubular necrosis; FE_{Na}, fractional excretion of sodium; GN, glomerulonephritis; U_{Na}, urine sodium.

Radiocontrast-Mediated Kidney Dysfunction

The natural history of radiocontrast-mediated kidney dysfunction (RCKD) is that it will usually occur within 24 to 48 hours after the dye for a CT scan or an arteriogram is given. The patient can become oliguric within this period of time, but the phenomenon frequently clears in 3 to 10 days, and usually in a shorter period of time. In other cases, the effect can lead to persistent oliguria and there can be a requirement for dialysis. Predisposing factors include dehydration, presence of diabetes mellitus, chronic kidney disease, older aged individuals, and large volume of contrast. The kidney dysfunction occurs via a vasoconstriction mechanism and, with this renal hypoperfusion, intratubular precipitation and ongoing generation of free oxygen radicals occur.

Therapy needs to be initiated before the dye is given. This includes: (1) hydration with 0.45% saline or 0.9% normal saline at 75 mL/hour for 8 hours before the dye is given (closely assessing the fluid balance in patients with congestive heart failure), (2) low molecular weight dye, (3) acetylcysteine (Mucomyst)* in a dose of 600 mg twice daily, and (4) use of fenoldopam mesylate (Corlopam)* in a dose of 0.01 to 0.05 μg/kg/minute intravenously for 3 hours before the procedure. The acetylcysteine (Mucomyst) study used a limited number of patients. Fenoldopam mesylate (Corlopam) still has mixed reviews regarding its results.

Angiotensin-Converting Enzyme Inhibitors

Angiotensin-converting enzyme (ACE) inhibitors are widely used for the treatment of hypertension, congestive heart failure, and diabetic nephropathy. Acute kidney failure may occur in conditions in which angiotensin plays a pivotal role in glomerular filtration rate. This is especially known to happen in patients who have bilateral renal artery stenosis or unilateral stenosis of the renal artery with the contralateral kidney atrophic. The ACE inhibitor affects the ability of the glomerular efferent arteriole to vasoconstrict. Volume depletion, usually brought on by aggressive diuresis or significant vomiting or diarrhea in association with an ACE inhibitor, can also produce acute kidney failure. The patient will develop a nonoliguric acute kidney failure and frequently have hyperkalemia; this will be reversible in a few days, once the ACE inhibitor is removed and the patient is returned to a euvolemic state.

Therapy includes: (1) identifying that the patient is taking an ACE inhibitor, (2) discontinuation of the ACE inhibitor, (3) returning the patient to a euvolemic state, and (4) assessing the potassium status and using sodium polystyrene sulfonate (Kayexalate) if necessary.

Cocaine

Cocaine can induce kidney dysfunction through different pathways. The initial effect of cocaine is vasoconstriction of both afferent and efferent arterioles. This is frequently slow to resolve and may take 7 to 14 days. Cocaine has also been associated with rhabdomyolysis and malignant hypertension. The natural history depends on the pathway. If rhabdomyolysis occurs, kidney injury will probably be prolonged, and the problems of oliguria, rapid rise in creatinine and potassium, and changes in calcium and phosphate will occur. If the vasoconstrictive model occurs, renal dysfunction is slow to worsen and slow to resolve. If malignant hypertension occurs, the renal dysfunction progresses on a slower basis and the main problem is hypertension. Therapy includes: (1) identification that cocaine has been used, (2) discontinuation of the cocaine, (3) hydration, (4) monitoring the electrolytes and acid-base disturbance, and (5) closely assessing the blood pressure and beginning therapy when indicated.

Therapy for Prerenal Azotemia

Therapy for prerenal azotemia has been described above in individual situations, but it is important to repeat this for the following reasons: (1) the history gives valid preliminary data, especially in regard to home medications for arthritis, blood pressure control, and use of recreational drugs; (2) physical examination helps make the decision regarding fluids and how freely fluids can be given, especially in regard to the presence of volume depletion (that can be ascertained by blood pressure and pulse in the supine and upright positions), as well as the presence of a third heart sound on cardiac examination and rales on pulmonary examination; (3) urine sodium and fractional

*Not FDA approved for this indication.

excretion of sodium; (4) urine sediment looking for the absence of significant cells or casts; (5) ultrasound of the kidneys to exclude obstruction; (6) fluids, depending on what kind of fluid is lost (upper gastrointestinal looses need isotonic fluid; skin losses are usually replaced by hypotonic fluids; if the patient is hypertensive, then isotonic fluid needs to be given first) (Table 2).

ACUTE KIDNEY FAILURE WITH INTRINSIC INJURY

Acute kidney failure with intrinsic injury has the worst prognosis with mortality varying between 40% to 80%. The diversity in etiology of acute renal failure with intrinsic injury is wide. Although acute tubular necrosis (ATN) is frequently associated with intrinsic injury, there is a long list of causes that includes the large blood vessels, small blood vessels, glomeruli, interstitium, and the tubules. The clinical course varies depending on the cause of the acute kidney failure (Table 3).

Vascular Causes of Intrinsic Acute Kidney Failure

The incidence of renal failure due to large vessel disease (bilateral renal artery stenoses) or smaller vessel disease (atheroembolic disease or scleroderma) is rising because of the aging of the population and the associated frequency of significant vascular disease in the abdominal aorta. The presence of bilateral renal artery stenosis is frequently diagnosed at the time of cardiac catheterization in the population with significant coronary disease or in the presence of oliguria when a patient is receiving an angiotensin-converting enzyme (ACE) inhibitor or angiotensin receptor blocker (ARB) and has bilateral renal artery stenosis. The urine sediment in this situation is bland, and the diagnostic test is the renal arteriogram. Although surgery has been the cornerstone of therapy for many years, the aged individual frequently necessitates a more conservative approach with angioplasty and stenting procedures as opposed to surgery. Atheroembolic disease is frequently seen in patients that have recently undergone intravascular stents or have abdominal aortic aneurysms. The urine sediment again is frequently bland, but the patient can have eosinophilia and hypocomplementemia; and livedo reticularis, blue toe syndrome, and cutaneous infarcts are seen on physical examination.

Therapy depends on the situation, but the renal arteriography with angioplasty and stenting for renal artery stenosis has become the intervention of choice. The alternative therapy is to observe the patient and, if necessary, begin dialysis. There is no therapy for atheroembolic disease. Fluid balance, monitoring electrolytes, and acid-base balance are the cornerstones of therapy.

TABLE 2. **Intravascular Volume Depletion**

Reduced cardiac output
Congestive heart failure
Pericardial effusion
Intravascular fluid loss
Hemorrhage
Renal fluid losses (excessive diuresis from diuretics, osmotic diuretics)
GI losses (vomiting, diarrhea)
Skin and mucus membranes (burn) loss
"Third space" losses (pancreatitis)
Systemic vasodilation
Sepsis
Antihypertensives
Renal vasoconstriction
Pharmacologic agents
Nonsteroidal anti-inflammatory drugs (NSAIDs)
Angiotensin-converting enzyme inhibitors
Radiocontrast (intravenous dye)

Glomerulonephritis

Acute glomerulonephritis is often associated with systemic disease, especially the presence of vasculitis, lupus erythematosus, postinfectious disease, and hepatitis. The urine sediment frequently reveals red blood cell casts, red blood cells, granular casts, and proteinuria. Thrombotic thrombocytopenic purpura/hemolytic uremic syndrome (TTP/HUS) involves small vessels, as do malignant hypertension and postpartum acute renal failure. In these cases, the urine sediment may be bland or normal because the patient has ischemia to the glomerulus. The diagnosis of most glomerulonephritides and TTP/HUS are dependent both on blood tests (ANCA, ANA, anti-DNA, antiglomerular basement membrane antibody, platelet count, and presence of schizocytes on peripheral smear) and the clinical scenario. Therapy depends on the glomerular changes on kidney biopsy. Therapy can include prednisone,* cyclophosphamide (Cytoxan),* and plasmapheresis. Renal function can deteriorate and dialysis may be necessary (see Table 4).

Interstitial Disease

The most common cause in the category of interstitial disease is acute interstitial nephritis. The histologic finding is marked edema of the interstitium and focal or diffuse infiltration with the presence of lymphocytes, macrophages, eosinophils, and polymorphonuclear leukocytes. The two most common scenarios are acute allergic interstitial nephritis and acute bacterial pyelonephritis. The acute allergic interstitial nephritis (AIN) is usually associated with antibiotics such as β-lactams, methicillin, rifampin (Rifadin), sulfonamides, and ciprofloxacin (Cipro). The diagnostic test is eosinophilia and urinary eosinophilia frequently associated with fever and rash. Pyelonephritis is a clinical syndrome associated with a urinary tract infection, fever, and toxicity. Other drugs that can cause these scenarios are diuretics, NSAIDs, and anticonvulsants.

---

*Not FDA approved for this indication.

TABLE 3. **Confirming Differential Diagnoses for Major Causes of Intrinsic Acute Kidney Failure**[1]

Diagnosis	Typical Urinalysis	Some Confirmatory Tests
Diseases Involving Large Renal Vessels		
Renal artery thrombosis	Occasionally RBCs	Elevated lactate dehydrogenase with normal transaminases, renal arteriogram
Atheroembolism	Often normal; eosinophiluria, rarely casts	Eosinophilia, hypocomplementemia, skin biopsy, renal biopsy
Renal vein thrombosis	Proteinuria, hematuria	Inferior venacavogram and selective renal venogram; Doppler flow studies; MRI
Diseases of Small Vessels and Glomeruli		
Glomerulonephritis or vasculitis	RBC casts or granular casts; RBCs; WBCs; mild proteinuria	Low C3, antineutrophil antibodies, antiglomerular basement membrane antibodies; antistreptolysin O, antiDNA, cryoglobulins, renal biopsy
HUS or TTP	May be normal; RBCs, mild proteinuria; granular casts	Anemia, thrombocytopenia, schistocytes on blood smear; increased lactase dehydrogenase; renal biopsy
Malignant hypertension	RBCs; RBC casts; proteinuria	LVH by echocardiography or electrocardiography; resolution of ARF with control of blood pressure
ARF-Mediated by Ischemia or Toxins		
Ischemia/intrinsic tubular damage	Muddy brown granular or tubule epithelial cell casts; $FE_{Na} > 1\%$; $U_{Na} > 20$ mEq/L; SG = 1.010	Clinical assessment and urinalysis
Exogenous toxins	Muddy brown granular or tubule epithelial cell casts; $FE_{Na} > 1\%$; $U_{Na} > 20$ mEq/L; SG = 1.010	Clinical assessment and urinalysis
Endogenous toxins:		
Possible rhabdomyolysis (seizures, coma, trauma, ETOH abuse)	Urine supernatant tests positive for heme	Hyperkalemia, hyperphosphatemia, hypocalcemia, increased circulating myoglobin, creatine kinase MM, uric acid
Possible hemolysis (blood transfusion)	Urine supernatant pink and positive for heme	Hyperkalemia, hyperphosphatemia, hypocalcemia, hyperuricemia; pink plasma positive for hemoglobin
Possible tumor lysis (recent chemotherapy), myeloma (bone pain), ethylene glycol ingestion	Urate crystals, dipstick negative proteinuria, oxalate crystals, respectively	Hyperuricemia, hyperkalemia, hyperphosphatemia (for tumor lysis) circulating or urinary monoclonal spike (for myeloma); toxicology screen, acidosis, osmolal gap (ethylene glycol)
Acute Diseases of the Tubulointerstitium		
Allergic interstitial nephritis	WBC casts, WBCs (frequently eosinophiluria), RBCs; proteinuria	Systemic eosinophilia, skin biopsy of rash area (leukocytoclastic vasculitis), renal biopsy
Acute bilateral pyelonephritis	Leukocytes, proteinuria, RBCs, bacteria	Urine and blood cultures

ARF, Acute renal failure; ETOH, ethyl alcohol; FE_{Na}, fractional excretion of sodium; LVH, left ventricular hypertrophy; RBC, red blood cell; SG, specific gravity; U_{Na}, urine sodium; WBC, white blood cell.

[1]From Brenner BM: Brenner & Rector's The Kidney, 6th ed. Philadelphia, WB Saunders, 2000, p 1229.

Therapy is to: (1) identify the drug that the patient was taking either at home or in the hospital; (2) discontinue the drug; (3) monitor the BUN/creatinine, potassium, and acid-base disturbance (the natural history is usually short-lived, 5 to 10 days); (4) use prednisone for AIN and antibiotics for pyelonephritis.

Tubular Disorders

The most common cause of hospital-acquired acute kidney failure is tubular injury, frequently called acute tubular necrosis (ATN). As mentioned, there is an intermediate syndrome in which prerenal azotemia is manifested as a continuum and the prerenal azotemia eventually becomes ATN. This is seen in tubular injury, hepatorenal syndrome, radiocontrast-mediated kidney dysfunction, and NSAID use.

The physiologic course involves a fall in the glomerular filtration rate (GFR) because of a fall in the renal blood flow (RBF) with, then, a disruption in tubular epithelium and backleak of glomerular filtrate and obstructed urine flow. The injury pattern can last from 1 to 30 days and eventually recovery occurs with regeneration of the renal parenchymal cells. The diagnosis is confirmed by: (1) clinical picture with rising BUN/creatinine levels; (2) urine sodium greater than 30 mEq and a fractional excretion of sodium greater than 2; and (3) a urine sediment revealing dark granular (muddy brown) casts. Five percent of the group that develop ATN do not recover.

TABLE 4. **Therapy for Acute Renal Failure in Systemic and Vascular Diseases**

Disease	Therapy
Acute post-streptococcal glomerulonephritis	No specific therapy
Rapidly progressive glomerulonephritis (Goodpasture's syndrome)	Pulse methylprednisolone (Solu-Medrol)* 1 g IV for 3 d and cyclophosphamide (Cytoxan)* 1-3 mg/kg/d; plasmapheresis, 4 L/d for 1-3 wk
Systemic lupus erythematosus	Prednisone 1-2 mg/kg/d; cyclophosphamide (Cytoxan)* 0.5 g/m² IV × 12 mo
Subacute bacterial endocarditis	Antibiotics
Large vessel polyarteritis	Prednisone 1-2 mg/kg/d; cyclophosphamide (Cytoxan)* 1-3 mg/kg/d; or both
Microscopic polyangiitis (P-ANCA positive)	Prednisone 1-2 mg/kg/d; cyclophosphamide (Cytoxan)* 1-3 mg/kg/d; or both
Henoch-Schönlein purpura	No specific therapy
Wegener's granulomatosis	Pulse methylprednisolone 1 g IV for 3d; cyclophosphamide (Cytoxan)* 1-3 mg/kg/d
Malignant hypertension	Intensive care unit monitoring; IV antihypertensives; dialysis, if required
HUS/TTP (hemolytic-uremic syndrome/ thrombotic thrombocytopenic purpura)	Plasmapheresis

*Not FDA approved for this indication.
IV = intravenously.

COMPLICATIONS OF ACUTE KIDNEY FAILURE

Hyperkalemia

Hyperkalemia is potentially the most life-threatening complication of acute kidney failure. The serum potassium can worsen because of both oliguria and metabolic acidosis. Mild hyperkalemia (less than 6.0 mEq/L) can be managed by adjusting the enteral diet or total parenteral nutrition. There are no changes in the electrocardiogram (ECG) when the potassium is below 6 mEq/L. If the potassium rises to 6.5 mEq/L or above, ECG changes can occur because of the underlying cardiac milieu or because of the potassium itself. The ECG changes at this point are minimal or show peaking of the T-waves. The next change occurs when the potassium rises to 7.0 to 7.5 mEq/L. At this point the ECG can show prolongation of the P-R interval or dampening of the P wave. When the potassium rises above 7.5 to 8.0 mEq/L, the QRS can widen and the ECG can show signs of a sine wave. Clinical characteristics only begin when the potassium is above 7.5 to 8.0 mEq/L. The characteristics are usually weakness, hyporeflexia, and ascending paralysis. Patients with associated cardiac disease can have bradyarrhythmia or other cardiac arrhythmias.

Therapy for hyperkalemia includes: (1) calcium gluconate 10% at 10 to 30 mL, which has an onset in 1 to 3 minutes and clears in 5 to 10 minutes; (2) intravenous dextrose (one vial of 50 g) with regular insulin 5 to 10 units intravenously, onset is within 15 to 30 minutes; (3) sodium bicarbonate, which has an effect in 15 to 30 minutes; (4) albuterol sulfate (Albuterol)* (20 mg/ 4 mL in a nebulizer) that has an onset in 10 to 30 minutes; and (5) oral sodium polystyrene sulfonate (Kayexalate) (15 to 30 g) with 70% sorbitol (50 to 70 mL) or sodium polystyrene sulfonate (Kayexalate) enema (50 g) that is retained for 1 hour and then cleared with a tap water enema. This works in 1 to 2 hours.

Metabolic Acidosis

Metabolic acidosis doesn't usually require treatment unless the patient has a dropping bicarbonate or the pH of the blood is below 7.2. When the pH is below 7.2, the cardiac output will drop and the patient can develop congestive heart failure.

Therapy can include: (1) one to two vials of sodium bicarbonate 7.5% (one vial equals 44 mEq of sodium bicarbonate) given intermittently depending on the pH or serum bicarbonate; (2) dextrose 5% in 1 liter of water with 3 ampules of sodium bicarbonate in a 500-ml solution; and (3) 3% and 5% sodium bicarbonate (however, this is a hypertonic solution and hypernatremia will usually occur).

Hyponatremia

Excessive water or hypotonic fluid intake is the frequent reason for hyponatremia in the patient with acute renal failure. The treatment is to correct the hyponatremia by: (1) utilizing isotonic fluid, especially if the patient is hypovolemic, and (2) fluid restriction if the patient is volume overloaded.

Hypocalcemia/Hyperphosphatemia

Mild hyperphosphatemia (5 to 10 mg/dL) is a common consequence of acute kidney failure. The phosphorus can be higher, especially in hypercatabolic states or if the total parenteral nutrition is high in phosphorus. Hypercatabolic states include rhabdomyolysis or sepsis. With hyperphosphatemia, there is a concomitant decrease in calcium. The calcium can also be reduced because of associated low protein stores. The hypocalcemia rarely causes symptoms because of the associated acidosis seen in patients with acute kidney failure. Hyperphosphatemia can be corrected by: (1) reducing the phosphorus in the parenteral nutrition; or (2) using calcium acetate (PhosLo) to bind the phosphorus in the gut. Calcium can be corrected (assuming the calcium is accurate, taking the serum albumin into account) with more calcium in the parenteral nutrition. Intravenous calcium is short-lived and thus is usually not used.

Malnutrition

Nitrogen balance is usually negative in acute kidney failure, especially in parenchymal injury associated

*Not FDA approved for this indication.

with surgery or systemic inflammatory response syndrome (SIRS). Factors that contribute to this negative nitrogen balance include poor calorie intake, infection, surgery, acidosis, and uremia. Nutritional supplementation is quite important in this situation. Hyperalimentation and parenteral nutrition have not consistently shown a benefit, however, 1 to 1.5 g/kg of high-biologic value protein along with appropriate carbohydrate and lipid is deemed acceptable. Enteral feeding is equally acceptable depending on the function of the gastrointestinal tract. Therapy is either with enteral or parenteral nutrition with appropriate kcal/kg with associated high biologic-value protein.

Treatment includes fluids. This is the major issue in patients who have acute intrinsic kidney failure. The patient may require fluid or may require restriction of fluid.

In an ICU setting, central venous catheter monitoring is quite informative: both central venous pressure (CVP) and pulmonary capillary wedge pressure (PCWP) are important. A low CVP or a low PCWP suggests that the patient's fluid balance is hypovolemic. In the presence of a low CVP or low pulmonary artery pressure, the patient with acute intrinsic kidney failure may respond to fluid administration because the patient could be hypovolemic. The other possibility, based on the clinical setting and the CVP or PCWP, is that the patient is "third spacing" fluid, and the pulmonary artery pressure will not rise when that occurs. The usual fluid utilized in this situation is 0.9% saline. If the hemoglobin is not above 10, packed red blood cells can be used to try to raise the central venous pressure or the pulmonary artery pressure to maximize the intravascular space.

When the patient is not in an ICU setting, then fluid assessment is made by both blood pressure and pulse in both the supine and sitting positions. This is the simplest way to assess the fluid balance.

1. The patient may remain oliguric regardless if fluid is given. When orthostatic, the patient would require fluid just to stabilize the intravascular space. The appropriate clinical finding is the cardiac and pulmonary examination, assessing for the presence of a third heart sound or basilar or bibasilar rales. If either of these is present, the patient probably will not tolerate much in the way of fluid. If these physical findings are not present and if the patient has orthostasis, then fluid can be tried with monitoring of the pulmonary and cardiac status.

2. Diuretics: Potent loop diuretics, specifically furosemide (Lasix) and torsemide (Demadex), have been used to convert patients from oliguric acute kidney failure with intrinsic injury to the polyuric state. Polyuric renal failure has a lower morbidity and mortality than does oliguric kidney failure. Polyuria changes the natural history of the disease; moreover, it is easier to manage a patient in a polyuric renal state than the patient that remains oliguric. Furosemide (Lasix) is the appropriate medication in this case, and it can be given in doses of 40 to 160 mg intravenously every 6 hours. Mannitol can also be used, but it can increase the intravascular space and it predisposes patients to fluid overload.

3. Renal dose dopamine hydrochloride: Dopamine hydrochloride in doses of 1.0 to 3.0 μg/kg per minute has been used in the past for acute kidney failure. Dopamine hydrochloride is a selective renovasodilator that elicits natriuresis and increases urine output in animal studies. In human studies, the data is equivocal. At this point, the general literature suggests that this drug is of minimal significance, but it can be used for raising blood pressure. Its effect in improving renal function is quite marginal. The major risk is tachyarrhythmias that can occur in the form of tachycardia, supraventricular tachycardia, and ventricular arrhythmia.

Adjustment of Drug Dosage

Patients who have acute kidney failure frequently require adjustments in drug dosages for impairment of kidney function. These drugs include antibiotics, digoxin, and drugs indicated for ulcer therapy.

Dialysis

Indications to start dialysis in acute renal failure are not specific. The usual indications are: (1) oliguria with less than 400 mL of urine output per day and the perception that the patient is fluid overloaded; (2) pulmonary edema that is not responsive to conservative diuretic management; (3) hyperkalemia with the serum potassium rising above 6.0 to 6.5 mEq/L, (4) symptomatic uremia as manifested by encephalopathy and pericarditis; and (5) metabolic acidosis with a decreasing bicarbonate in the presence of acidemia.

The delivered dose of dialysis for acute renal failure may be higher than in the chronic stable dialysis patient. A temporary dialysis catheter, either through the femoral vein, the jugular vein, or the subclavian vein, is placed. Data suggest that bioincompatible dialysis membranes may improve mortality. This data suggests that these patients will have a better outcome. The frequency of dialysis is difficult to assess. It frequently depends on the fluid status, the presence or absence of hyperkalemia, metabolic acidosis, and the blood pressure. The mortality in these populations is quite high, but again it depends on the underlying cause of the renal failure.

In continuous veno-venohemodialysis (CVVHD), a patient is dialyzed continuously through one of the catheters. This is especially effective in patients who are hypotensive and require significant fluid removal. Preliminary studies published to assess the benefit of intermittent hemodialysis versus CVVHD have shown little difference. The principal benefit of the CVVHD is the fluid removal and easier management of hypotension while the patient is on dialysis.

Acute Peritoneal Dialysis

Acute peritoneal dialysis is the third option in the dialysis regimen. It initially requires a catheter to be placed in the abdomen and is most frequently performed by a surgeon. A rigid peritoneal dialysis catheter can also be placed by a physician trained in this technique.

The exchanges are standard 2 L peritoneal dialysis solution, and the retention of the fluid is usually 1 to 4 hours. The fluid is drained after that time and another 2 L peritoneal dialysis solution is instilled. The peritoneal fluids are 1.5%, 2.5%, and 4.25% solutions. The major risk is in the placement of the catheter because a ruptured bowel can occur. The benefit is stabilization of blood pressure. Peritoneal dialysis is also quite effective in the pediatric population.

OBSTRUCTIVE (POSTRENAL) FAILURE

Postrenal azotemia usually occurs from an obstruction at the prostate in men and in the ureters in women. The most common occurrence is in older males with enlarged prostate causing prostatic obstruction or ureteral obstruction from extension of prostate cancer into the periureteral areas. The initial evaluation is done by ultrasonography, which is informative in 80% of the cases. The ultrasound is occasionally noninformative because the patient is dehydrated and the obstruction won't be easily identified. CT scanning is the alternative method of evaluation, and it is especially informative when it is done using "stone protocol" with very fine cuts in the CT scanning technique. The diagnosis is made based on the urine sediment, urine sodium, and the ultrasound or CT scan. The therapy is most frequently a Foley catheter or suprapubic tube. If obstruction is still present, then either unilateral or bilateral nephrostomy tubes are placed. This is a multidisciplinary approach that frequently requires collaboration by the nephrologist, urologist, and radiologist.

CHRONIC KIDNEY FAILURE

method of
ANTHONY J. BLEYER, M.D.
Wake Forest University School of Medicine
Winston-Salem, North Carolina

Chronic kidney failure is an arbitrary term that refers to a loss of kidney function at some time in the past or present. Chronic kidney failure is frequently regarded as slowly progressive over time, but this is not necessarily so. Some patients may have chronic kidney failure that is not progressing, or its progress may have been stopped with appropriate treatment. Examples of chronic kidney failure include diabetic nephropathy, hypertensive nephrosclerosis, polycystic kidney disease, and kidney failure after surgical removal of kidney tissue due to malignancy.

Measurement of Kidney Function

The glomerular filtration rate (GFR) is used as a marker of kidney failure, although this is only one aspect of kidney function. At present, we do not have an inexpensive, simple, accurate test to measure kidney function. We, therefore, rely on the serum creatinine and several equations derived from this to estimate glomerular filtration rate. Figure 1 shows the Cockroft-Gault formula. In epidemiologic studies, this equation has not been found to be a very precise predictor of GFR. However, for the individual patient in clinical practice, this equation does give us a reasonable estimation of GFR. It is important to not simply rely on the serum creatinine, because the GFR varies widely for the same serum creatinine for patients of different ages, gender, and weight. Unfortunately, the Cockroft-Gault formula does underestimate GFR in African-Americans, and the Modification of Diet in Renal Disease (MDRD) formula may be preferable (see Figure 1).

Following the reciprocal serum creatinine over time is also a good measurement of kidney function. In steady state, the GFR is approximately equal to the creatinine clearance, which equals creatinine production/serum creatinine. One can assume that creatinine production stays relatively stable over time. Therefore, following the change in 1/serum creatinine is proportional to following the GFR. Figure 2 shows a reciprocal graph on which the reciprocal creatinine can be followed over time. For many patients the change in GFR (and therefore reciprocal serum creatinine) will be linear over time. Abrupt changes in GFR can be identified by deviations from linearity on the graph. Following the reciprocal serum creatinine is only reliable once the serum creatinine rises above 2 mg/dL. For copies of this graph or for a copy of this graph with international units, please email the following address: ableyer@wfubmc.edu

As one can see, if the decline in renal function is linear, a change in the serum creatinine from 1 mg/dL to 2 mg/dL takes approximately the same time as a change from 2 mg/dL to 4 mg/dL, or 4 mg/dL to 8 mg/dL. Therefore, as kidney function worsens, the serum creatinine will tend to rise more rapidly. It is important to appreciate the acceleration in the rise of serum creatinine, so that one does not wait too long prior to referring the patient for transplant evaluation or consideration of dialysis.

Table 1 provides an overview of the stages of kidney failure. Management of patients with preserved GFR includes treatment of the underlying disease and treatment of co-morbid conditions. As the GFR declines, treatment of associated conditions and preparation for dialysis becomes more important.

$$\text{Creatinine clearance (mL/min)} = [(140 - \text{age}) \times \text{weight (kg)}] \div [\text{serum creatinine (mg/dL)} \times 72]$$

Figure 1. Cockroft-Gault formula. Multiply result by 0.85 if female. From Cockroft DW, Gault MH: Predication of creatinine clearance from serum creatinine. Nephron 16:31-41, 1976. Abbreviated MDRD formula: GFR (mL/min/1.73 m^2) = 186 × (serum creatinine)$^{-1.154}$ × (age)$^{-0.203}$ × (0.742 if female) × (1.21 if African-American). From National Kidney Foundation, Kidney Disease Outcomes Quality Initiative: Clinical Practice Guidelines for Chronic Kidney Disease: Evaluation, Classification, and Stratification. Am J Kidney Dis 39 (Suppl 1):S85, 2002.

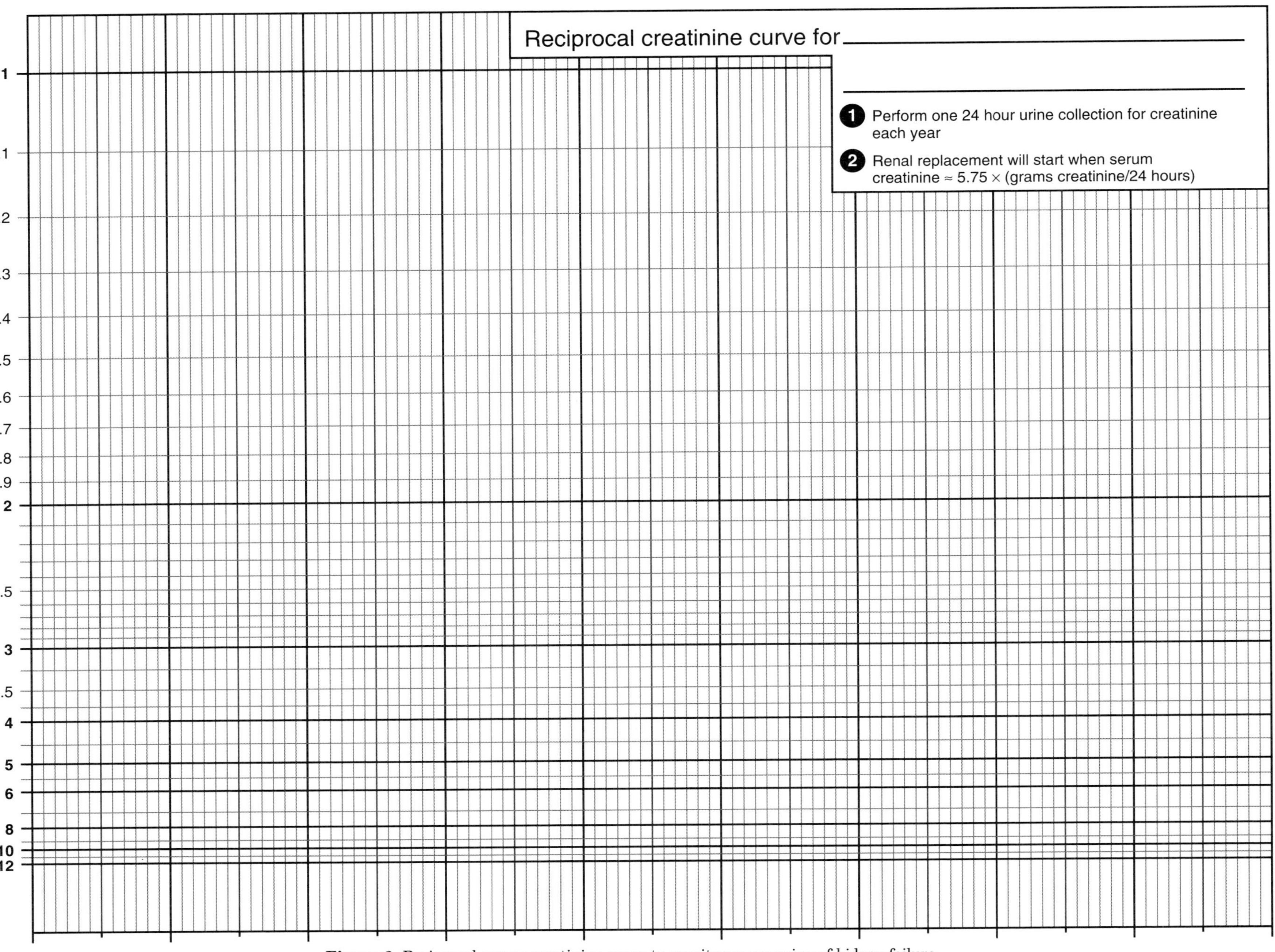

Figure 2. Reciprocal serum creatinine curve to monitor progression of kidney failure.

TABLE 1. **National Kidney Foundation Stratification of Chronic Kidney Disease**

Stage	Description	GFR (mL/min)	Action
	At increased risk	≥90 (with risk factors for chronic kidney disease)	Screening, chronic kidney disease risk reduction
1	Kidney damage with normal or increased GFR	≥90	Diagnosis and treatment, treatment of co-morbid conditions, slowing progression, cardiovascular disease risk reduction
2	Kidney damage with mildly decreased GFR	60-89	Estimating progression
3	Moderately decreased GFR	30-59	Evaluating and treating complications
4	Severely decreased GFR	15-29	Preparation for kidney replacement therapy
5	Kidney failure	<15	Renal replacement therapy (if uremia present)

Source: National Kidney Foundation, Kidney Disease Outcomes Quality Initiative: Clinical Practice Guidelines for Chronic Kidney Disease: Evaluation, Classification, and Stratification. American Journal of Kidney Diseases Volume 39, Supplement 1, February 2002.

Identification of the Cause of Kidney Failure

It is important to be certain of the cause of kidney failure. Renal artery stenosis, vasculitis, and several types of glomerulonephritis are examples of treatable conditions. For all these conditions, treatment should begin early. If the physician has any uncertainty regarding the cause of renal insufficiency, the patient should be referred to a nephrologist for definitive diagnosis. Conditions such as critical renal artery stenosis are not uncommon in diabetics and may be mistaken for diabetic nephropathy. Patients with human immunodeficiency virus (HIV) infection may be incorrectly assumed to have HIV nephropathy when they may have a treatable crescentic glomerulonephritis. In many cases, a one time evaluation for ascertainment of renal diagnosis by a nephrologist may be all that is required, with subsequent follow-up provided by the primary care physician.

TREATMENT OF SPECIFIC ASPECTS OF CHRONIC KIDNEY FAILURE

Hypertension

Treatment of hypertension is vitally important to the patient with chronic kidney failure. The physician must be extremely motivated to treat blood pressure and to lower it to a level at least less than 140/90 mm Hg. Newer recommendations even suggest lowering of the blood pressure to levels less than 130/85 mm Hg in patients with kidney failure to prevent progression of disease. It is inexcusable to tolerate a high blood pressure because the patient has kidney failure. In reality, tighter control is warranted in the patient with kidney failure. The physician must break down every barrier that prevents good blood pressure control. Barriers include medication cost, noncompliance due to side effects, and simple lack of patient motivation. Good blood pressure control should be obtained over the course of several months. This usually involves at least monthly visits. It may be easier for patients to call with their blood pressure readings every several weeks and adjust dosages over the telephone. Patients with chronic renal failure will likely need several agents to control their blood pressure. The physician should start with one agent, increase the dosage to the maximum recommended or maximum tolerated dosage, and then add another agent. If blood pressure cannot be controlled, the patient should be referred to a nephrologist or cardiologist who can attain control. Tight control will delay progression of kidney disease. In addition, tight control will prevent target organ damage in other organs. Patients with chronic kidney failure are at markedly increased risk of left ventricular hypertrophy and hypertrophic cardiomyopathy. Treatment of hypertension can prevent this complication even when kidney failure progresses. Even though a patient may be progressing inexorably to dialysis, treatment of hypertension remains important to prevent cardiovascular complications and to make the patient the best possible candidate for kidney transplantation.

Agents of Choice

Angiotensin-converting enzyme (ACE) inhibitors or angiotensin II receptor blockers are the agents of choice for the treatment of hypertension. These agents have been found to delay the progression of kidney disease in diabetic nephropathy and other kidney diseases as well. These agents delay progression of kidney disease by mechanisms in addition to blood pressure control. However, usage of ACE inhibitors can be difficult in patients with chronic kidney failure. ACE inhibitors are associated with the development of hyperkalemia, and some kidney failure patients—especially diabetic patients—may have pre-existing hyperkalemia. There are several methods that may be used to prevent the development of hyperkalemia. First, the patient should be instructed in a 2 gram potassium diet if hyperkalemia is likely to be a problem (see later). Patients should avoid salt substitutes high in potassium. Second, a diuretic may be used to both control blood pressure and increase urinary potassium losses. This should not be a potassium-sparing diuretic, and patients should be told not to increase potassium in their diet when taking the diuretic—a frequent warning placed on prescription bottles. Third, if the patient is acidemic, sodium bicarbonate should be started as treatment (see later). Fourth, the angiotensin II receptor blockers may cause hyperkalemia less often than ACE inhibitors.

Serum potassium and serum creatinine is frequently checked one week after starting ACE inhibitors in patients with chronic kidney failure to make sure the serum potassium does not rise and that kidney function remains stable.

ACE inhibitors may cause a rise in the serum creatinine, as they may be associated with a decline in glomerular pressure with a mild decline in GFR when first used. If the serum creatinine rises markedly, a diagnostic study should be obtained to rule out renal artery stenosis. Patients on ACE inhibitors should be warned to avoid becoming pregnant. If they have concomitant kidney failure, they should also avoid use of nonsteroidal agents. Congestive heart failure, renal artery stenosis, usage of nonsteroidal agents, and volume depletion also reduce renal perfusion. If these conditions occur in the setting of ACE inhibition, acute kidney failure may develop. If a transient rise in serum creatinine occurs due to a combination of the above factors, it may be appropriate to stop the ACE inhibitor for a short time and then restart it with close follow-up.

Diuretics

Most patients with chronic kidney failure will not have their blood pressure controlled without the use of a diuretic. Even patients without edema have been found to have increased total body salt and water in clinical studies. Furosemide (Lasix) is traditionally used in chronic kidney failure because hydrochlorothiazide is less likely to be effective. Control of dietary sodium is also important. (see later). The appropriate dosage of furosemide is dependent on the level of kidney function. A starting dosage of 20 mg of furosemide per day in patients with only a mild decrease in GFR is appropriate. Weights should be followed, and the dosage should be increased as needed.

The use of other agents is likely to be required as well. Diltiazem (Cardizem) and verapamil (Calan) have been shown to decrease proteinuria and are likely renoprotective. Dihydropyridine calcium channel blockers (such as nifedipine [Procardia], felodipine [Plendil], and amlodipine [Norvasc]) have not been proven to be as renoprotective. A difficulty arises if blood pressure still is elevated on the calcium channel blocker and the patient requires a β-blocker. Patients may develop A-V nodal blockade and symptomatic bradycardia if receiving both a β-blocker and diltiazem or verapamil. For this reason, many chronic kidney failure patients will ultimately need a β-blocker and a dihydropyridine calcium blocker in addition to an ACE inhibitor and diuretic.

Chronic kidney failure patients may require the use of numerous medications to control blood pressure. If blood pressure cannot be controlled, referral to a nephrologist or cardiologist is paramount.

Anemia

A decline in hemoglobin levels is not uncommon, even in patients with a serum creatinine less than 2 mg/dL. Uremia results in decreased red blood cell survival, as well as decreased red blood cell production. Patients with renal failure are also at risk of anemia due to GI bleeding, iron deficiency from poor dietary intake, and B_{12} and folate deficiency. However, the decline in hemoglobin is usually the result of erythropoietin deficiency. Unfortunately, erythropoietin levels are not clinically useful at this time, and erythropoietin therapy is started empirically in patients with decreased GFR.

It is important to rule out iron deficiency, gastrointestinal blood loss, and vitamin B_{12} and folate deficiency prior to starting erythropoietin. Iron deficiency is particularly common and important to treat, because patients with iron deficiency will be resistant to erythropoietin. Iron studies should be obtained and oral iron given if the ferritin is less than 100 ng/mL or the iron saturation is less than 20% and the ferritin level is not greater than 500 ng/mL. Oral iron will likely be needed as the hemoglobin rises in these patients with administration of erythropoietin. Intravenous iron should be considered if the patient cannot tolerate oral iron, or if iron stores do not replete after a reasonable period of time. There is a small risk of anaphylaxis with various iron preparations, and caution must be used in their administration. Iron studies should be obtained monthly.

The use of erythropoietin increases red blood cell production and results in a marked improvement in quality of life in patients with kidney failure. Use of erythropoietin in chronic kidney failure patients is valuable, but cumbersome.

There are several choices for erythropoietin administration. These include Epogen, ProCrit, and Aranesp (novel erythropoiesis stimulating protein). ProCrit and Epogen are standard erythropoietin preparations, with ProCrit being used more commonly in chronic kidney failure. Aranesp is a hyperglycosylated analogue of erythropoietin with a longer half-life. Aranesp may require dosing only once every two weeks, while Procrit or Epogen require at least weekly dosing. All forms of erythropoietin are expensive, and reimbursement policies cause difficulty in their usage in chronic kidney failure patients. The cost of these medications will be several hundred dollars per month. While the medications may be reimbursed by the patient's insurance, many patients will have to buy them and wait for reimbursement to occur. Most patients do not have the money for the up-front cost of these agents. Sometimes the physician's office or clinic will buy the medication and attempt to obtain reimbursement. However, many physicians do not want to go through the cumbersome process of obtaining reimbursement. For this reason, many patients will ultimately receive erythropoietin from a nephrologist who deals with this problem commonly and is familiar with the dosage adjustment strategies. Erythropoietin therapy usually is initiated when the hemoglobin concentration falls to less than 10 g/dL, or the patient has symptomatic anemia. The goal is to keep the hemoglobin level between 11 and 12 g/dL. If the hemoglobin level rises above 12 g/dL, the cost of erythropoietin may not be reimbursed. Hemoglobin levels are checked every two weeks initially and then monthly. Dosage must be monitored closely to prevent polycythemia or persistent anemia.

Smoking

Smoking has been associated with increased rate of loss of kidney function in patients with kidney disease, in normal elderly patients, and in other populations. Stopping smoking is profoundly important in the patient with kidney failure, and the specter of dialysis may provide the inducement to some patients to stop smoking.

Blood Glucose Control

Strict control of diabetes has been found to be effective in delaying progression of kidney failure in patients with early diabetic nephropathy, but advantages of strict control in patients with more advanced kidney failure have not been shown. Obviously, good control of blood glucose levels should be maintained. However, it is important to note that diabetic patients with chronic kidney failure are at risk for hypoglycemia (see later) and should be monitored closely.

Nutrition

Proper nutritional management of the chronic kidney failure patient is somewhat complex. The most important principle is that the patient remain well nourished. As kidney failure progresses, the patient's nutritional status worsens and protein intake decreases. Patients lose weight and muscle mass. The earliest symptom of uremia is frequently anorexia, and one of the earliest signs is weight loss. For this reason, careful attention to appetite is important, and other causes of anorexia (diabetic gastroparesis or peptic ulcer disease) should be dealt with aggressively. Use of nutritional supplements may be important. If weight loss progresses and kidney function is marginal, consideration of renal replacement therapy must take place.

How much protein should the patient consume? The Modification of Diet in Renal Disease Study recently showed little benefit for a very low protein diet in the prevention of kidney disease progression. Despite frequent consultation with dietitians, patients on the low protein diets were more likely to lose muscle mass than controls. However, excessive protein intake is likely to increase serum phosphate and blood urea nitrogen and should be avoided. An 0.8 to 1 gm/kg protein diet is reasonable. If patients are young and have slowly progressive disease, one may consider the usage of a low protein diet. However, this needs to be carried out by a nephrologist with special interest in this area in conjunction with intensive care by a dietitian.

Obesity is a problem in many patients with chronic kidney failure, and controlled weight loss is important. Weight loss may prevent progression of disease and is frequently required if the patient is to become a kidney transplant recipient.

Drug Dosage Adjustment

Drug dosage adjustment is very important in patients with kidney failure. It is important to consult the Physician's Desk Reference or another appropriate guide and review all of the patient's medications.

There are several very important medications that must be discussed. First of all, metformin (Glucophage) should not be used in patients with chronic kidney failure. It can cause a severe, deadly lactic acidosis. Its use should be stopped as soon as there is evidence of kidney failure. Allopurinol (Zyloprim) dosage should be decreased because increased levels of the metabolite oxypurinol may develop in kidney failure.

It is extremely important that the dosage of insulin and other hypoglycemic medications be monitored closely. The kidney normally metabolizes insulin and other hypoglycemic agents. In addition, the kidney is a major site of gluconeogenesis. As kidney failure develops, insulin half-life is prolonged, renal gluconeogenesis is impaired, and patients frequently develop a poor appetite. These factors can all contribute to the development of hypoglycemia. Therefore, blood sugars should be monitored closely, with the likelihood that medication dosages will require a reduction. Many patients will not alert their physician when blood sugar drops, and this can result in repeated episodes of hypoglycemia.

For the most part, nonsteroidal anti-inflammatory agents should be used sparingly in patients with kidney failure. Many of these patients will be taking ACE inhibitors and diuretics, and the addition of a nonsteroidal can lower intraglomerular pressure and result in acute kidney failure and hyperkalemia. Antacids such as Maalox, Milk of Magnesia, and Mylanta should be avoided because of the risk of hypermagnesemia. Intravenous contrast should be avoided.

Renal Osteodystrophy

The serum phosphorus characteristically rises above the normal range only in the last several months prior to the onset of dialysis. However, abnormalities in calcium phosphate metabolism frequently begin well before this. The physician must be especially attentive to patients who have a long duration of renal failure and acidemia. Such patients would include patients with a history of reflux nephropathy. Long-term renal failure with acidemia is likely to accelerate and accentuate the changes of renal osteodystrophy.

The use of calcium carbonate (for example, Tums or Os Cal) or calcium acetate (PhosLo) with meals can help to prevent phosphate absorption and prevent the development of renal osteodystrophy. However, recently it has become apparent that renal failure patients have increased vascular calcifications, and that calcium-containing medications may contribute to this. There are no prospective trials in chronic renal failure to guide us as to the best treatment at this time. Many nephrologists recommend that patients take one 500 mg calcium carbonate tablet with each meal when the glomerular filtration rate decreases to the 30 to 40 mL/minute range. At this time, it is prudent to check an intact parathyroid hormone level, and consider increasing the calcium dosage if the PTH level is elevated greater than 1.5 to two times the upper limit of normal. One might consider using calcium acetate instead of calcium carbonate if the patient is concomitantly receiving an agent that neutralizes gastric pH, because calcium carbonate may not dissolve in neutral gastric secretions. Sevelamer (Renagel)* is a calcium-free phosphate binder. Its use in chronic renal failure has not yet been established, but it may be an agent of choice in this condition in the future. If the patient is found to have an elevated intact PTH level, measurement of serum 1,25 dihydroxy vitamin D levels should be performed. If the level is low, treatment with calcitriol (Rocaltrol) starting at a dose of 0.25 μg/d may be beneficial. Treatment of acidemia is also important in preventing renal osteodystrophy.

Acidosis

Acidosis may develop as a result of kidney failure, or as a result of tubulo-interstitial disease. Acidemia causes a decrease in appetite, worsens hyperkalemia, and negatively affects bone metabolism. For these reasons, acidosis should be avoided. Addition of calcium carbonate or calcium acetate will help to neutralize the normal daily acid load and have positive effects on renal osteodystrophy. These agents should be considered first and dosed at meal time to maximize phosphate-binding effects. If acidosis persists, sodium bicarbonate tablets or sodium citrate (Bicitra) should be tried. It is important to remember that both these agents result in a sodium load, and diuretic dosage may need to be increased. The normal individual produces about 1 mEq/kg acid each day, so up to 70 mEq of sodium bicarbonate may be required to improve the serum bicarbonate level. Careful titration of the dosage and monitoring of serum bicarbonate levels will be required. Sodium bicarbonate tablets contain 650 mg (7.7 mEq), and Bicitra contains 1 mEq/mL sodium citrate. Alkali therapy can be started with approximately 30 mEq/d and titrated upward.

Hyperkalemia

Hyperkalemia is not uncommon in patients with chronic kidney failure. Hyperkalemia is especially common in diabetic patients, who frequently have a type IV renal tubular acidosis. Patient education regarding foods high in potassium is of primary importance. A patient education sheet on high-potassium foods can be obtained on the Internet at http://www.kidney.org/general/ atoz/content/potassium.html, a site sponsored by the National Kidney Foundation. Foods that are high in potassium include tomatoes, avocadoes, bananas, oranges, prunes, raisins, and potatoes. Usage of diuretics in hypertensive or edematous patients will help to decrease serum potassium concentration as well as treat acidemia. Sodium polystyrene sulfonate (Kayexalate) may also be used if hyperkalemia is problematic and cannot be controlled by the previously described measures. Alone, sodium polystyrene sulfonate causes constipation, and it is therefore often prepared in a 70% sorbitol solution. A dosage of 30 grams of sodium polystyrene sulfonate several times per week can usually control resistant hyperkalemia. If the sodium polystyrene sulfonate in sorbitol causes diarrhea, the patient can be prescribed sodium polystyrene sulfonate powder.

Edema

Edema tends to worsen as the glomerular filtration rate declines. The dosage of diuretic required to treat edema will frequently be higher than that used in the treatment of hypertension. Furosemide (Lasix) is commonly used as the initial agent in the treatment of edema. Starting dosage may be 20 or 40 mg orally each day. Over time, the dosage may need to be increased up to 160 mg orally twice per day. If Lasix alone is ineffective, metolazone (Zaroxolyn) may be added. The following practical guidelines have been quite useful to the author: (1) The patient should weigh herself or himself daily. Increases in weight over a short period of time are likely due to salt and water retention. Patients are instructed to call the office if their weight increases by more than 3 to 5 pounds. If they are edematous at presentation, one should aim for a fluid loss of 1 to 2 pounds per day until their edema-free weight is reached. If the patient is carefully following his or her weight, development of anasarca and pulmonary edema can frequently be avoided. (2) The patients should also be alert to symptoms of dizziness and volume depletion. Most patients will be taking an ACE inhibitor as well, and a drop in the blood pressure can decrease glomerular perfusion, resulting in acute kidney failure. (3) Edema may remain a persistent problem, especially in patients with the nephrotic syndrome. Restriction of salt in the diet is especially important. Patients with edema should be maintained on a 2 gram sodium diet. In the edematous patient, diuretic dosage may be inadequate or dietary sodium intake problematic. To determine this, obtain a 24-hour urine collection while the patient is in a steady state (i.e., weight is stable over several days). If the urinary sodium is much greater than 2 grams (87 mEq), advocate salt restriction. If urinary sodium is less than 2 grams, increase diuretic usage.

Gout

With worsening kidney function, the patient's ability to excrete uric acid may decrease. Patients with pre-existing gout may have a worsening of their condition. Diuretics will increase proximal tubular reabsorption of uric acid, further increasing serum uric acid concentration. Treatment of acute exacerbations of gout become more difficult. Usage of nonsteroidal anti-inflammatory medications is likely to

*Not FDA approved for this indication.

result in worsening kidney function and, in general, should be avoided. A prednisone taper is likely to be beneficial acutely, and colchicine may also be beneficial in the short term. When patients develop an attack of gout, one should consider whether allopurinol (Zyloprim) will be needed to prevent further attacks. Allopurinol should be started only after any acute gout attacks have entirely resolved. Initiation of allopurinol therapy can cause an acute gout attack. The patient should be warned regarding this and told to continue with the allopurinol. The dosage of allopurinol should be titrated up slowly, and is about one half the normal dosage in renal failure.

Smooth Transition

Despite all efforts, some patients will develop progressive kidney failure. The primary goal in these patients is to provide a seamless transition to renal replacement therapy. A new paradigm has developed in this area. Previously, nephrologists would have patients wait until they were nauseated and extremely ill prior to starting dialysis. Now we realize that adapting to renal replacement therapy is one of the biggest challenges these patients will have in their life. These patients should therefore be given the opportunity to be in the best possible physical condition at the time they face this great stress. Previously, dialysis would start for most patients at a BUN of approximately 100. Today, patients start dialysis when their estimated GFR falls to less than 10 mL/min. This can occur at blood urea nitrogen levels of 70 mg/dL and at serum creatinine values less than 4 mg/dL. Prior to reaching a GFR of 10 mL/minute, patients should be informed as to the different types of renal replacement therapy; they should be referred for transplantation evaluation; and they should have a fistula placed if they are opting for hemodialysis. Referral to a nephrologist should occur at a point no later than when the GFR falls to less than 25 mL/minute, so that appropriate management and treatment of end-stage renal disease can be started.

In the past, renal replacement therapy was considered primarily in healthy, younger patients with isolated kidney disease. These patients could remain relatively healthy, despite extremely poor kidney function. Today many patients are elderly and diabetic. Due to multisystem disease, these patients do not tolerate uremia well. Weight loss, which occurs during uremia may be reversed in younger individuals, but elderly patients do not recover totally from the nutritional depletion experienced prior to dialysis. For this reason, extreme vigilance is required in the elderly patient who is being followed, and earlier referral for evaluation for dialysis is frequently needed.

It is also most helpful and most appropriate for the primary care doctor to initiate a discussion with elderly patients as to whether they wish to receive dialysis, and to be supportive if they do not desire renal replacement therapy. Dialysis is an extremely arduous procedure, and many elderly patients have trouble tolerating it. It is appropriate for elderly, debilitated patients, frequently residing in nursing homes or who suffer from dementia, to not undergo dialysis and receive comfort care. Some patients may opt for a limited trial of dialysis to see how they tolerate treatment.

Referral for transplantation evaluation should occur at about 1 year prior to when the patient is anticipated to require renal replacement therapy, probably at a GFR between 30 and 40 mL/min. Transplant evaluations frequently do not occur rapidly, and delays may occur in the evaluation and workup of potential recipients. If the patient is to have a cadaveric transplant, the patient may be on the waiting list up to 3 to 4 years. It is important to note that graft survival for patients is better if they undergo transplantation prior to requiring dialysis. Simply accepting the notion of transplantation may take some patients a year or longer.

If patients do not have a potential living donor for transplantation, they will have to consider hemodialysis or peritoneal dialysis. The major advantage of peritoneal dialysis is that patients have the independence and freedom to provide their own therapy; the major disadvantage of peritoneal dialysis is that patients must be responsible and capable to perform their own dialysis treatments. Peritoneal dialysis is a good first therapeutic option for patients with kidney failure, because it is likely better in preserving residual kidney function. Also, the remaining residual kidney function makes the performance of peritoneal dialysis easier. In addition, patients are usually more independent and in better health when they first develop kidney failure. For this reason, peritoneal dialysis is a good option at this time point for many.

Hemodialysis is also a good option for renal replacement therapy, especially in the more debilitated patient. Hemodialysis is more successful when a fistula is used for treatment. Fistulas are connections between a native artery and vein, and may take more than six months to develop. For this reason, it is very important for the patient to have a nephrologist referral about 1 year prior to starting dialysis, so that fistula placement and transplantation referral can be explored. The patient should tour the dialysis center at that time and make a decision regarding peritoneal dialysis or hemodialysis.

In summary, there are three major paradigms in the treatment of chronic renal failure. First, steps must be taken to prevent progression of disease. These include hypertension control, blood sugar control, cessation of smoking, and possibly, weight loss. Second, steps must be taken to preserve the patient's overall health. These include treatment of hypertension, anemia, prevention of renal osteodystrophy, and correct dosage of medications. Third, the physician must attempt to provide a seamless transition to the start of renal replacement therapy. Successful management of the patient requires careful attention to all three of these areas and will be of great benefit to the patient.

MALIGNANT TUMORS OF THE UROGENITAL TRACT

method of
OFER YOSSEPOWITCH, M.D., and
GUIDO DALBAGNI, M.D., F.A.C.S.
Memorial Sloan-Kettering Cancer Center
New York, New York

In the following chapter, the four most common urogenital malignancies, prostate, bladder, renal, and testicular cancer, are outlined. The chapter provides a concise description of the epidemiology, clinical diagnoses, and established treatment paradigms.

PROSTATE CANCER

Prostate cancer, the most commonly diagnosed cancer and the second leading cause of cancer-related death in men in the United States, accounts for approximately 180,000 new cases and 37,000 deaths annually. The widespread use of the prostate-specific antigen (PSA) assay, beginning in the early 1990s, has triggered a stage migration in which the majority of patients with newly diagnosed prostate cancer present with clinically localized disease. Management of localized prostate cancer includes expectant management (watchful waiting), radical prostatectomy, and radiotherapy (external beam radiation or interstitial brachytherapy). Metastatic disease is generally treated with androgen ablation and chemotherapeutic regimens.

Watchful Waiting

Recognizing the high prevalence of prostate cancer in the population, the morbidity associated with local treatment options, and that some cancers would not affect an individual's quality-adjusted life expectancy has led to the concept of deferred therapy, otherwise known as watchful waiting. Watchful waiting is based on close surveillance of patients through serum PSA levels and digital rectal examination, while acknowledging that the cancer may progress within the gland but that the opportunity for curative local treatment is not lost. Case selection criteria have not been standardized, but, in general, watchful waiting is reserved for men with low grade (Gleason score equals 6) tumors involving a small percentage of biopsy cores, and with a short (less than 10 years) life expectancy. However, recent prospective randomized comparative trials have demonstrated a disease-specific survival benefit in radical surgery over watchful waiting in an unselected population cohort.

Radical Prostatectomy

Radical prostatectomy is a major treatment alternative for localized prostate cancer. A better understanding of the anatomy of the prostate has allowed urologists to achieve complete resection of the tumor with a clear margin of resection and better control of bleeding, and to preserve the sphincter mechanism and the neurovascular bundles, which are important for recovery of urinary and sexual functions. The procedure is most commonly performed through a lower abdominal (retropubic) approach or a less popular perineal approach. Recently, a laparoscopic surgical approach has been introduced. In contemporary series using this approach, hospital stays are short, perioperative mortality is lower than 0.5%, and serious complications, such as rectal injury, deep vein thrombosis, and embolic events, are rare.

The risk of incontinence following radical prostatectomy varies from 5% to 30% and is dependent on the level of experience of the surgeon, as well as the definition of incontinence. Time may also play a role, because full recovery may not occur for weeks or months after the procedure. Likewise, recovery of erectile function varies widely among patients (30% to 70% in different series) and is directly influenced by the patient's age, quality of erections before the operation, and the ability of the surgeon to preserve adequately the neurovascular bundle. Most men are impotent immediately following the procedure, with gradual recovery of function expected within 6 to 12 months.

Radical prostatectomy has been shown to confer long-term cancer-specific survival in numerous studies. Serum PSA levels should become undetectable following removal of the entire prostatic tissue. Thus, a detectable PSA after a radical prostatectomy is usually the result of recurrent disease. The probability of freedom from PSA ("biochemical") recurrence is used as an intermediate endpoint in most series. This varies according to initial clinical stage, biopsy Gleason score, and preoperative PSA level, and can be better predicted by analyzing the pathologic specimen. When the disease is confined to the organ and has not extended into the periprostatic fatty tissue, 95% and 90% of the patients remain free of progression at 5 and 10 years, respectively. Extension into the periprostatic soft tissues or the seminal vesicles decreases the probability of freedom from progression to 75% and 45% at 5 years, respectively. Noteworthy is the fact that the median time from PSA recurrence to overt clinical metastases has been reported to be 8 years. No long-term clinical benefit has been demonstrated for preoperative hormonal therapy, despite an apparent reduction in the number of positive surgical margins in several comparative trials.

Radiation Therapy

Radiation therapy can be delivered externally, internally, by implantation of radioactive sources into the gland itself, or by a combination of both. In general, outcomes with external beam therapy in clinically organ-confined prostate cancer are reported to be similar to those obtained with radical surgery. For patients with locally advanced disease, results are less favorable, with 30% to 40% reported to relapse locally by the tenth year following treatment with standard doses.

Current conventional techniques use simulators and CT scans of the pelvis to determine the location, shape, and energy distribution both to the target volume and to the surrounding organs. Conventional techniques are fairly well tolerated, though rectal morbidity (discomfort, tenesmus, and diarrhea) and irritative urinary symptoms (frequency, urgency, dysuria, and nocturia) may occur in 40% to 60% of patients. Erectile function tends to diminish gradually with time, rendering only 50% of the patients potent at 7 years after irradiation.

More contemporary approaches use three-dimensional conformal radiation therapy (3D-CRT) techniques with sophisticated computer-generated treatment plans to deliver an increased radiation dose to the prostate with less morbidity to the surrounding normal organs. A significant reduction in both acute and late radiation morbidity, with a concomitant feasible escalation in radiation doses, has been demonstrated. Preradiation and postradiation, hormonal therapy combined with radiotherapy, versus radiotherapy alone, has been shown to offer a survival advantage in patients with locally advanced disease.

Interstitial brachytherapy is based on infiltrating the tumor tissue with radioactive seeds, thus avoiding the inevitable exponential decay in radiation energy as a function of distance. Overall, the procedure is well tolerated and is reported to have a therapeutic effect similar to surgery or external irradiation. Most practicing urologists tend to reserve this treatment option for tumors with good prognostic features. They exclude patients who had previously undergone transurethral prostatectomy. Side effects are mainly urinary urgency and frequency, and dysuria. Occasional proctitis is observed, and impotence to some degree has also been reported.

Metastatic Prostate Cancer

A distinct group of patients include individuals with no evidence of metastases but who have a rising PSA following watchful waiting or local therapy. For these patients, it is imperative to determine whether the rising PSA is a result of local recurrence (and thus additional local therapy might be curative), or evidence of distant micrometastases. Several algorithms have been advocated to resolve this clinical dilemma, including prediction by the clinical-pathologic features of the primary cancer, time to PSA recurrence, and the PSA doubling time. The use of imaging studies such as CT, MRI, or bone scans is often uninformative, and biopsy of the prostate, for those who had previously received radiation, or biopsy of the urethrovesical anastomosis, for those who had undergone radical prostatectomy, might be misleading. For patients with a rising PSA following radiation therapy, a salvage radical prostatectomy might be considered if there is no evidence of distant metastases, if the cancer was amenable to extirpative surgery before radiation, and if a transrectal prostate biopsy has demonstrated residual cancer. Morbidity from this procedure is quite high. For patients with an elevated PSA following prostatectomy, radiation therapy is recommended if the PSA level does not exceed 1 to 2 ng/mL and if the PSA level after the surgery was undetectable (indicating that a disease-free status was attained).

Metastatic prostate cancer generally involves the bone and may cause bone pain, epidural cord compression, pathologic fractures, and anemia resulting from myelophthisis. As prostate cancer growth is largely dependent on the presence of androgens, their removal or blockade is the mainstay of treatment for patients with advanced disease. The following techniques are available to achieve androgen deprivation in the target cells: (1) surgical castration (bilateral orchiectomy), (2) medical castration (estrogens, long acting GnRH agonists or antagonists), and (3) androgen blockade in the target cells (steroidal antiandrogens and pure antiandrogens). Inhibitors of adrenal androgens synthesis, such as ketoconazole (Nizoral),* or aminoglutethimide (Cytadren),* are used as second-line treatment.

Long acting GnRH analogues, such as leuprolide acetate (Lupron) or goserelin acetate (Zoladex), act by downregulating the secretion of LH and FSH from the hypophysis; but these induce an initial rise in serum LH and testosterone, which may result in a clinical flare of the disease. As such, these agents are contraindicated in patients with significant obstructive symptoms or spinal metastases with imminent cord compression. The flare can be prevented by pretreatment with antiandrogens. The use of estrogens, such as diethylstilbestrol (Stilphostrol), has been abandoned in the United States because of their cardiovascular toxicity; yet their use is still prevalent in Europe, particularly in Scandinavian countries. Pure (or nonsteroidal) antiandrogens, which include flutamide (Eulexin), bicalutamide (Casodex), and, less commonly, nilutamide (Nilandron), act by blocking the androgen receptor at the target organ but at the same time induce a temporary and limited rise in LH and testosterone levels. Side effects include gynecomastia, fatigue, disturbed liver function tests, and, most significantly, diarrhea. Steroidal antiandrogens, such as cyproterone acetate (Androcur),† lower the plasma LH and testosterone levels, and have been reported to induce fewer side effects.

Many physicians recommend hormonal therapy for PSA elevation, though it is not clear whether such an approach confers any survival benefit over initiation of hormonal treatment only at overt clinical metastases. Likewise, the role of complete androgen blockade (surgical or medical castration and an antiandrogen) has been questioned. A recent large meta-analysis indicated no survival advantage over castration alone. It is also not clear whether the class of antiandrogen influences outcome. For patients who progress on hormonal therapy, a discontinuation of treatment is required to evaluate for a withdrawal response. Paradoxically, the

*Not FDA approved for this indication.
†Not available in the United States.

discontinuation often includes clinical improvement. This has yet to be completely understood.

BLADDER CANCER

Bladder cancer is the fourth most common cancer in men and the seventh most common in women with an annual incidence of approximately 55,000 new cases and a mortality rate of 12,500 deaths per year. The disease is three times more prevalent in men, primarily seen at 65 years or older, and rarely diagnosed before the age of 40. Cigarette smoking constitutes the major risk factor, increasing the hazards of developing urothelial cancer two- to fourfold relative to the nonsmoking population. The risk persists for 10 years or longer following cessation of smoking. Other associated risk factors include aniline dyes, chronic phenacetin abuse, and cyclophosphamide (Cytoxan) exposure. Transitional cell carcinoma is the most prevalent histologic subtype, comprising 90% to 95% of the tumors in Western countries. Exposure to *Schistosoma haematobium* (bilharziasis) and chronic bladder irritation in the presence of an indwelling catheter or calculi have been associated with an increased risk of developing squamous cell carcinoma of the bladder.

Painless gross hematuria is the most common presenting symptom occurring in 80% to 90% of the patients with bladder tumors. Irritative urinary symptoms such as urinary frequency, urgency, or dysuria are less frequently seen, and are more common in patients with carcinoma in situ (CIS). Documentation of hematuria in individuals older than 40 years of age requires a thorough evaluation of the urinary tract with bladder cystoscopy, a urine cytologic examination for malignant cells, and imaging of the kidneys and ureters using intravenous pyelogram or CT-urography scan to rule out coexisting upper tract tumors. Other noninvasive urine assays have been developed to assist in the diagnosis of bladder cancer, but, thus far, none has been proved to be as efficient as cystoscopy.

In general, bladder cancer is stratified into three major categories, each with a distinct biologic behavior. These include non–muscle-invasive tumors (confined to the mucosa and submucosa), muscle-invasive tumors (invading the muscularis propria layer), and metastatic disease. At presentation, 75% of tumors are non–muscle-invasive, 20% are invasive, and up to 5% have *de novo* metastases. Carcinoma in situ (CIS) is a high-grade flat lesion confined to the mucosa but considered a precursor of the lethal muscle-invasive subtype.

Transurethral resection (TUR) of the tumor remains the mainstay of diagnosis and treatment. An accurate pathologic assessment based on the TUR specimen should distinguish between tumors confined to the mucosa (stage Ta), those invading the lamina propria but still non-muscle invasive (stage T1), and those invading the muscle layer (T2). A bimanual examination under anesthesia and a CT scan are used to assess for the possibility of extravesical and metastatic disease. Further treatment is based on disease extent, and is determined by the stage and grade of the tumor.

Non–Muscle-Invasive Tumors

Although Ta, T1 and Tis tumors are under the same category, the global term of "superficial bladder cancer" is imprecise when the different natural history and progression potential for each of these subtypes are considered. Thus, non–muscle-invasive tumor is a better term. TUR is usually effective in completely eradicating the disease, however, 30% to 80% of the patients develop recurrent disease within 5 years, and an additional 20% will experience stage progression. Intravesical therapy is used as an adjunctive therapy to endoscopic resection, aiming at reducing the risk of disease recurrence and progression. Intravesical chemotherapy (thiotepa, doxorubicin [Adriamycin], mitomycin C [Mutamycin],* epirubicin [Ellence]*) has a minimal impact on recurrence and no effect on progression. Administration of the immune modulator bacillus Calmette-Guerin (BCG) (Tice BCG) has been shown to delay time to progression and is considered the gold standard for carcinoma *in situ*. Patients with persistent carcinoma *in situ* or T1 tumors shortly following treatment with BCG should be considered candidates for cystectomy.

Muscle-Invasive Disease

Once a tumor involves the detrusor muscle, the standard treatment is removal of the entire bladder and urinary diversion. For solitary, well-defined T2 lesions, bladder-sparing approaches, including transurethral resection alone or combined with chemoradiation, should be contemplated if the patient refuses surgery. In males, radical cystectomy involves removal of the pelvic lymph nodes, bladder, prostate, and seminal vesicles, whereas in females, the resection also includes removal of the uterus, fallopian tubes, ovaries, and vagina. Urinary reconstruction includes an ileal conduit diversion to the skin, or a low-pressure internal reservoir using a detubularized bowel segment, which is anastomosed to the skin (continent cutaneous diversion) or to the retained urethra (orthotopic neobladder). The 5-year survival rate varies inversely with the depth of invasion and lymph node status: 70%, 50%, and 35% of the patients with organ-confined (T2), extravesical (T3), and lymph node-positive disease, respectively, are expected to be free of disease at 5 years.

Metastatic Disease

Patients with metastatic disease include those whose tumor has recurred after definitive local treatment and those who present with metastases. Urothelial cancer is generally considered a chemotherapy-sensitive neoplasm, with a number of chemotherapeutic agents proven effective as single agents. Yet, because of incomplete and short-term response, combination multidrug regimens have been used to improve response rates and durability. The traditional MVAC (methotrexate, vinblastine [Velban], doxorubicin [Adriamycin], and cisplatin [Platinol]) have been recently supplanted by other regimens, such as paclitaxel (Taxol)*, carboplatin (Paraplatin), gemcitabine (Gemzar)*, and cisplatin (Platinol), which have been shown to confer similar or higher response rates with significant reduction in the profile of side effects. Long-term survival may be obtained in 10% to 15% of patients with metastatic disease. Patients with adverse features, such as visceral involvement, impaired performance status, or bone metastases, are rarely cured. In these cases, median survival rarely exceeds 6 months. Radiation therapy is reserved for patients who are deemed unfit candidates or who are reluctant to undergo cystectomy.

RENAL CANCER

Renal cell carcinoma (RCC) accounts for 3% of all adult malignancies. Every year, approximately 30,000 new cases of RCC are diagnosed, and 12,000 patients die of the disease. Risk factors include cigarette smoking, obesity, and acquired cystic disease resulting in end-stage renal failure. Although the majority of cases are sporadic, several familial syndromes have been associated with renal cancer, including von Hippel Lindau (VHL) syndrome, tuberous sclerosis, and congenital polycystic kidney disease.

Renal cancer is no longer considered a unidimensional entity. A contemporary classification system (the "Heidelberg" classification) for renal cortical tumors defines several major categories, namely conventional (clear cell) carcinoma, papillary carcinoma, and chromophobe carcinoma. These different subtypes display distinct cytogenetic abnormalities and histopathologic features, and a differing metastatic potential. Other relatively rare forms include collecting duct (Bellini) carcinoma and medullary carcinoma. The latter tend to afflict younger patients and are very aggressive tumors. Benign cortical lesions, such as oncocytoma and renal cell adenoma, are often clinically indistinguishable from the malignant subtypes.

The clinical presentation of renal cancer has evolved over recent years because of the widespread use of radiologic imaging, including abdominal ultrasound and CT scans. The classic triad of hematuria, flank pain, and abdominal mass indicating a large mass is rarely encountered, and most patients are diagnosed with incidentally detected small renal masses. Thus, stage migration has occurred, contributing to an increased use of nephron-sparing surgery (partial nephrectomy) and an improved 5-year survival rate. The standard evaluation of patients with suspected renal cell tumors includes a CT scan of the abdomen and pelvis, a chest radiograph, and urine cytology for centrally located lesions. A CT of the chest is warranted only if metastases are suspected from the chest radiograph. This avoids false-positive findings, which may influence the approach to the primary tumor. Doppler ultrasound or MRI is indicated for patients with suspected invasion of the renal vein or inferior vena cava by a tumor thrombus.

*Not FDA approved for this indication.

Treatment

The standard treatment of renal cortical tumors has also evolved over the last two decades. The traditional radical nephrectomy (removal of the kidney and Gerota's fascia, including the ipsilateral adrenal and the perihilar lymph nodes) is considered the gold standard for all renal tumors. Numerous studies have demonstrated that partial nephrectomy is as effective in providing local tumor control for renal tumors 4 cm and possibly larger. Therefore, nephron-sparing surgery, previously indicated on a mandatory basis for patients with a single kidney or bilateral tumors, is now broadly applied for patients with small masses and a normal contralateral kidney. For larger tumors, ipsilateral adrenalectomy is indicated only if the tumor involves the upper pole of the kidney, or if the CT scan displays conspicuous adrenal abnormalities. For patients with a tumor thrombus extending into the cava or right atrium, an aggressive surgical approach to remove the entire disease is warranted. There is no therapeutic role for regional lymph node dissection, and there are no data to support the use of adjuvant chemotherapy, radiotherapy, or immunotherapy, following successful surgical extirpation. Recently, total nephrectomies and a select group of partial nephrectomies have been performed laparoscopically.

Metastatic Disease

Metastatic renal cell carcinoma is associated with a dismal prognosis. Unfortunately, approximately one third of the patients with RCC exhibit metastases at the time of initial presentation, and an additional one third develop distant metastases after removal of the kidney. Results with the use of hormonal therapy, chemotherapy, and radiation therapy have been generally disappointing, and immunomodulation by interleukin-2 (Proleukin) or interferon-α (PEG-Intron),* represents the only encouraging pathway for treatment of metastatic RCC. The overall response rate in several large series has been approximately 15%, however in fewer than 5% was the response durable. Patients are more likely to exhibit a favorable clinical response to immunotherapy if they have good performance status, have undergone a cytoreductive nephrectomy, exhibit nonbulky pulmonary metastases as opposed to other visceral sites or bones, and have no constitutional symptoms.

TESTICULAR CANCER

Primary germ cell tumors (GCTs) of the testis, which constitute 95% of all testicular neoplasms, are the most common solid tumor in men between the ages of 20 and 35 years. Because more than 90% of all newly diagnosed patients and about 80% of patients with metastatic disease will be cured, management of testicular cancer has become a model for the successful multidisciplinary approach to solid tumors. Associated risk factors include undescended testis

*Not FDA approved for this indication.

(in particular, abdominal cryptorchidism), testicular feminization syndrome, and Kleinfelter's syndrome.

A painless and firm testicular mass in the aforementioned age group is pathognomonic for a testicular malignancy. Often, patients present with testicular swelling and discomfort, and have been managed with antibiotics for prolonged periods. This results in a significant delay in accurate diagnosis, which is associated with a more advanced stage and a possible worse outcome. Metastatic disease may manifest as back pain resulting from bulky retroperitoneal disease, dyspnea due to pulmonary metastases, and gynecomastia as a consequence of elevated β-human chorionic gonadotropin (HCG) levels. Ultrasound examination of the testis is the imaging modality of choice, with a high sensitivity and specificity. Whenever an intratesticular hypoechoic mass is diagnosed, inguinal radical orchiectomy should be performed. Scrotal orchiectomy or other trans-scrotal biopsies should be categorically discouraged to avoid tumor spread by additional pathways other than the retroperitoneal lymph nodes. Based on pathologic assessment of the orchiectomy specimen, along with the levels of serum markers (α-fetoprotein, β-HCG and lactate dehydrogenase), GCTs are divided into two major categories: seminomatous and nonseminomatous tumors. The latter include embryonal carcinoma, choriocarcinoma, yolk sac tumor, and the more differentiated variant, teratoma. Staging evaluation of GCT includes determination of serum markers before and after removal of the testis and a CT scan of the chest, abdomen, and pelvis to assess for retroperitoneal, mediastinal, or visceral metastases. Clinical stage I is defined by no evidence of disease following orchiectomy, stage II by metastasis confined to the retroperitoneal lymph nodes (further subcategorized to IIa, IIb, and IIc according to tumor extent), and stage III by metastasis above the diaphragm. Of note, testicular cancer is the only urologic malignancy in which tumor markers have been incorporated into the staging system (stage I is designated for patients with a normal CT scan and elevated markers).

TREATMENT

Paradigms are based on tumor pathology and clinical staging as depicted earlier.

Nonseminoma

Stage I can be managed by rigorous surveillance protocols that include periodic physical examination, tumor marker evaluation, and frequent imaging with chest radiographs and CT scans. Patient compliance is essential for surveillance to be successful. A second treatment option for clinical stage I is regional retroperitoneal lymph node dissection (RPLND). A nerve-sparing procedure should be performed, including identification and dissection of individual nerve fibers along the ipsilateral sympathetic trunk, to avoid potential impairment of ejaculation. If vascular invasion is present in the primary tumor, or if the tumor extends into the tunica, spermatic cord, or scrotum, RPLND is preferred over surveillance. Either approach should cure more than 95% of patients.

Patients with clinical stage II are managed according to the extent of disease. Limited disease (stage IIa) is usually managed by RPLND, whereas larger (>3 cm) retroperitoneal lymph nodes are treated with up-front chemotherapy consisting of cisplatin (Platinol), bleomycin (Blenoxane), and etoposide (VP-16 [VePesid]).

Seminoma

Inguinal orchiectomy followed by retroperitoneal radiation therapy cures about 98% of patients with stage I seminoma. Surveillance has been suggested but is generally not recommended because of an increased risk of late relapse (more than 2 years following orchiectomy). Nonbulky retroperitoneal disease (stage IIa and IIb) is also treated with radiation therapy.

Advanced Germ Cell Tumors

Regardless of histology, patients with stage IIc or III are treated with chemotherapy. A complete response has been noted in 60% of patients, and an additional 10% to 20% become disease-free following surgical removal of residual disease. Postchemotherapy surgery is an integral part of therapy. It is indicated for any residual radiographic abnormalities if the primary histology was nonseminoma, and for masses larger than 3 cm if the primary histology was seminoma.

URETHRAL STRICTURE

method of
KRISTIAN R. NOVAKOVIC, M.D., and
ROBERT C. FLANIGAN, M.D.
Loyola University Medical Center and Hines VA Hospital
Maywood, Illinois

ANATOMY

The male urethra is generally divided into four sections: the prostatic, membranous, bulbar, and penile urethra. The anterior urethra describes the bulbar and penile segments of the urethra distal to the perineal membrane. The posterior urethra includes the prostatic and membranous portions. The corpus spongiosum surrounds the anterior urethra throughout its length. It lies within a groove between the paired corpora cavernosa on the ventral surface of the penis. A separate fascial sheath surrounds the corpus spongiosum making it easy to separate from the overlying corpora cavernosa. This ease of separation facilitates surgical repair of the urethra. Anterior urethral strictures may result from injury to the urethral epithelium and/or surrounding corpus spongiosum. The injury often initiates a scarring process that causes progressive narrowing of the urethral lumen. Occasionally the scarring extends to involve adjacent tissues. Posterior urethral strictures are typically confined to the urethra itself, and are characterized by a more localized fibrotic process that can lead to complete obliteration of the urethral lumen. This discussion will focus on the etiology, clinical presentation, evaluation, and treatment options for male urethral stricture disease.

ETIOLOGY

Trauma causes the majority of anterior urethral strictures as well as many posterior strictures. Straddle injuries, in particular, commonly involve the anterior urethra, whereas pelvic fracture can lead to posterior injury and even total urethral disruption. Iatrogenic injuries secondary to urologic procedures are not uncommon. Posterior urethral strictures can form following radical prostatectomy or transurethral resection of the prostate (TURP). Anterior strictures may result from aggressive instrumentation of the urethra. The severity of these urethral injuries may not be readily apparent, and symptoms may not appear for some time following the injury.

Inflammatory processes remain an important, although infrequent cause of urethral stricture. Today, gonococcal urethritis seldom progresses to urethral stricture formation with appropriate and timely antibiotic therapy, thus emphasizing the need for prompt diagnosis and treatment. Other causes of urethritis such as *Chlamydia* and *Ureaplasma urealyticum* may progress to urethral stricture although there is little data on stricture formation associated with these infections. Balanitis xerotica obliterans (BXO), or lichen sclerosis of the glans penis, is an inflammatory process of uncertain etiology that often causes phimosis and meatal stenosis. The process can spread proximally to the penile urethra causing anterior urethral stricture. Inflammatory strictures typically trigger a more extensive injury resulting in longer strictures that are more complicated to manage.

Strictures have also been associated with urethral ischemia, which can occur when cardiopulmonary bypass is employed for cardiovascular procedures. Urethral carcinoma should always be considered as a potential cause of urethral stricture and, finally, congenital urethral strictures do exist but are exceedingly rare.

EVALUATION

The typical presentation of urethral stricture is that of obstructive voiding symptoms. Patients primarily complain of diminished urinary stream. Frequently, the symptoms have progressed slowly over a period of time and many patients tolerate significant obstruction before seeking treatment. Strictures may also present with urinary tract infections, epididymitis, or prostatitis. High urethral pressures proximal to a stricture can initiate urethral bleeding. In severe circumstances, a periurethral abscess may develop. Acute urinary retention is an infrequent presentation of stricture.

A careful history will often elicit the probable cause of the stricture. The patient should be questioned regarding any previous pelvic trauma and any history of sexually transmitted disease (STD), especially recurrent episodes. Physical exam can provide qualitative information about the extent of the scarring process. In the case of BXO, the foreskin is thickened and sclerotic. The glans demonstrates fibrosis and is often whitish in appearance with multiple fissures, ulcerations, and meatal stenosis. Urine should be sent for analysis along with appropriate urethral culture if STD is suspected.

Patients suspected of having a urethral stricture should be referred to a urologist. For the non-urologist, gentle urethral catheterization, especially in patients with acute urinary retention, should be attempted using a well-lubricated catheter. An experienced physician may dilate the urethral stricture using filiform and followers or urethral sounds. Today urethral catheterization in stricture patients is often attempted under direct vision (using a flexible endoscope) with placement of a guidewire across the stricture into the bladder. Dilation is carried out using a sequential dilating system over the wire, and placement of a council tip Foley catheter over the guidewire. Sequential dilation is much safer when a wire is in place.

It is important to determine the extent of the lesion, as well as its exact location, in order to develop a sound treatment plan. Often the scarring process will involve tissues proximal and distal to the obvious stricture. Failure to fully characterize the extent of the lesion may lead to unsuccessful treatment. Evaluation of strictures often begins with radiographic assessment using a retrograde urethrogram. The images demonstrate the caliber of the urethra and approximate length and location of the stricture. When possible, a voiding cystourethrogram can be combined with the retrograde study to further clarify the proximal urethral anatomy. In some cases, more proximal strictures may become apparent using the combined technique. Ultrasound can also help delineate the depth and extent of periurethral spongiofibrosis associated with anterior urethral strictures. In addition, it can provide information on the length of urethra involved. Ultrasound is, therefore, a potential alternative to retrograde urethrography but is probably more useful as an adjunct. Finally, endoscopic evaluation of the urethra is important to visualize healthy urethra proximal and distal to the stricture.

TREATMENT

There are multiple treatment options for urethral strictures ranging from simple dilation to open excision and graft placement. Thorough evaluation of the stricture preoperatively will help determine which procedure has the best chance for success. A treatment plan that maximizes the chances of long-term success should be advocated.

Dilation is the mainstay in the treatment of urethral strictures. Anterior strictures with minimal spongiofibrosis often are cured with simple dilation, while some posterior strictures also respond. Patients who are not surgical candidates can sometimes be managed with recurrent dilation including self-dilation to prevent recurrent stricture formation. The key to successful dilation is to minimize additional trauma. Tearing the stricture leads to further, sometimes more severe scarring and recurrent stricture. Balloon-dilating catheters may be a less traumatic way to dilate strictures. If more traditional sequential dilation is employed, successive dilation over a period of time is more effective than complete dilation during a single session.

Internal urethrotomy describes a procedure whereby the stricture is incised, causing it to spread apart and, therefore, increase urethral diameter. The urethra then heals by secondary epithelialization. This procedure can be employed for management of both anterior and posterior strictures. The success of the procedure depends on the rate of epithelialization. If the process occurs slowly, the natural contraction of the wound edges may limit the effectiveness of the procedure. Internal urethrotomy is now performed under direct vision (direct vision internal urethrotomy or DVIU). Traditionally the anterior urethra is incised at the 12 o'clock position to avoid the urethral vasculature. However, anatomically, the anterior urethra has a fairly thin covering of corpus spongiosum at this position, especially in the bulbar urethra. Because the goal of internal urethrotomy is to incise through the depth of the stricture, there is potential to incise into the corpora cavernosa leading to significant hemorrhage. Should this occur with more distal strictures, there is a risk of erectile dysfunction relating to the cavernosal injury. Alternative incisions at 3 and 9 o'clock may also provide a satisfactory result. It is generally agreed that short anterior strictures less than 1.5 cm and with minimal spongiofibrosis may respond well to DVIU.

Posterior strictures can also be managed with internal urethrotomy, however, the risk of damage to the urethral sphincter mechanism is quite high. Traumatic membranous urethral strictures that are not completely obliterative may also be treated with internal urethrotomy. Treatment of post prostatectomy strictures, in our experience, is best handled usually with dilation procedures to minimize subsequent sphincter incompetence. Internal urethrotomy may also be employed when the stricture is located only at the bladder neck urethral junction.

The most common complication from internal urethrotomy is recurrence. If unsuccessful, repeat procedures generally do not increase the success rates and should be eschewed in favor of open urethral reconstruction.

Urethral stents are another option available for the treatment of urethral stricture. They are used in conjunction with urethral dilation or internal urethrotomy and are designed to prevent post-procedural wound contraction and narrowing of the urethral lumen. Placement of the stent is of paramount importance. The stents are most useful for short strictures in the bulbar urethra. More proximal placement can interfere with the urethral sphincter mechanism causing incontinence, and placement too close to the bladder neck can lead to bladder stone formation. More distal placement has been associated with pain during intercourse or simply when sitting. Younger patients are less likely to tolerate urethral stents, regardless of careful placement. Other problems include restricture, which often occurs either proximal or distal to the limit of the original stent. This can be treated with an additional, overlapping stent in some cases, however, if strictures remain refractory, a complicated, multistage urethral repair is necessary.

Open urethral reconstruction is increasingly viewed as the most definitive procedure in urethral stricture repair. A multitude of techniques exist ranging from simple excision and reanastomosis to complicated fasciocutaneous flaps and free-tissue grafting. Again, the key to determining which procedure to choose is accurate characterization of the urethral stricture.

When possible, excision of the stricture and primary anastomosis is the procedure of choice. The procedure is best suited to more proximal strictures of the bulbar urethra and posterior urethra where the ease of urethral mobilization facilitates the repair. Strictures of 1 to 2 cm in length are easily managed while lengths of up to 4 cm have also been repaired in this fashion. The keys to success are complete excision of the area of fibrosis and creation of a widely spatulated, tension-free anastomosis. Using this technique with more distal penile urethral strictures almost inevitably causes ventral penile curvature with erection. Hence, for distal urethral strictures, this procedure should only be offered to those patients who are not concerned with sexual function. In appropriately chosen patients, success rates greater than 95% have been reported.

When primary excision and anastomosis is not a viable option, for example, in patients with longer bulbar strictures, a form of urethral substitution is performed. Substitution can occur in the form of a flap or graft. There are four general graft types: full thickness skin graft, split thickness skin graft, bladder epithelial graft, and buccal mucosal graft. Recently a trend toward the use of buccal mucosal grafts has emerged. Buccal mucosa is easy to harvest and manipulate. Its use is especially valuable for treatment of strictures caused by BXO where healthy penile skin may not be available. Several techniques for graft placement have been described. Although still controversial, it is generally agreed that tabularized grafts should be avoided in favor of onlay procedures that minimize the tissues requiring neovascularization. Success rates of better than 90% have been reported in several series.

Flaps are perhaps the most versatile techniques for urethral stricture repair and can be used throughout the anterior urethra. Whereas a graft requires the generation of a new vascular supply, flaps are positioned with their blood supply intact. Islands of penile or scrotal skin can be mobilized on a vascular pedicle and transferred to repair the urethral defect created after incision of the urethral stricture. In uncircumsized males, excess penile skin for use in flap reconstruction is plentiful, however, circumsized males rarely lack sufficient skin for creating a pedicle flap. Onlay repairs, again, are significantly more successful than tabularized flaps. Skin used in the flap must be hairless and free from inflammatory conditions such as BXO.

FUTURE DIRECTIONS

Emerging techniques in tissue engineering may offer additional options for urethral substitution in reconstruction. Already, acellular collagen matrices derived from bladder have been used in urethral construction. These matrices facilitate native urethral regeneration and have been successful in several cases. Further research in this area may provide repair options for even the most complicated stricture in cases where adequate native tissues may not be available.

Urethral strictures often present a complex problem in urologic management. Thorough evaluation helps guide the therapeutic approach with the best chance for long term success.

RENAL CALCULI

method of
MARGARET S. PEARLE, M.D., PH.D.
Department of Urology
The University of Texas Southwestern Medical Center
Dallas, Texas

Nephrolithiasis is a common disorder, with an approximate incidence of 0.4% to 1% and a prevalence of 5% to 12%. Although not all stones are symptomatic, even asymptomatic calyceal stones carry a 50% risk of becoming symptomatic within 5 years of diagnosis. Unfortunately, those who have experienced a stone are not immune from recurrence; nearly 50% of first-time stoneformers will develop another stone within 5 years. Given the magnitude of the disease, it is not surprising that the total annual cost of evaluation and treatment of nephrolithiasis in the United States has been estimated at nearly $2 billion.

Advances in the surgical management of nephrolithiasis have rendered virtually all urinary tract stones amenable to minimally invasive treatment. However, at the same time, diagnostic protocols and medical treatment regimens have been refined and simplified and are highly effective in preventing stone recurrence. Thus, despite the ease with which stones can now be treated surgically, the cornerstone of stone management remains prevention.

DEMOGRAPHICS AND EPIDEMIOLOGY

The incidence of stone disease peaks in the third to fifth decade of life, with many patients experiencing their first stone in their early 20s. Males are affected more commonly than females by a ratio of 2 or 3 to 1, and Caucasians have a higher incidence of stone disease than African Americans. Interestingly, the gender predilection in favor of men observed in the Caucasian population is reversed in African Americans, in whom there is a female predominance.

THE ACUTE STONE EVENT

Signs and Symptoms

Nonobstructing stones in the kidney rarely cause significant symptoms; however, stones obstructing the ureteropelvic junction or ureter may cause a constellation of symptoms known as renal colic that are characterized by acute pain originating in the flank and radiating around to the lower abdomen, groin or testicle (labia) (Figure 1). The pain is often paroxysmal, lasting a few minutes or more at a time, and is often associated with nausea and vomiting. Unlike the patient with peritonitis, the patient with renal colic characteristically is unable to lie or sit still and often paces the floor or writhes in pain.

The location of the pain may reflect the location of the stone. Flank and upper abdominal pain are usually associated with stones in the proximal and mid ureter. However, distal ureteral stones are typically associated with irritative voiding symptoms, such as frequency and urgency, as well as lower abdominal or flank pain.

History

Typical symptoms of renal colic are highly suggestive of a stone. In addition, a family history of stones or underlying medical conditions associated with stone disease such as chronic diarrhea, gout, recurrent urinary tract infections, or bone disease may raise the suspicion of a stone. Patients should be also questioned about kidney disease, renal anomalies, or systemic illnesses that affect kidney function such as diabetes or a solitary kidney that could impact the choice of diagnostic tests or the need for urgent intervention.

Physical Examination

On physical examination, nonspecific signs such as tachycardia and hypertension may accompany pain. Although a low grade fever (<100°F) is not uncommon with uninfected, obstructing stones, temperatures above 100°F should alert the clinician to the possibility of obstructive pyelonephritis, a clinical emergency. The remainder of the physical examination is remarkable only for flank or abdominal tenderness in the region overlying the stone. Peritoneal signs are distinctly uncommon and if present should prompt consideration of an acute abdomen. Occasionally, testicular pain may constitute the predominate symptom of a ureteral stone; careful examination of the testicles should distinguish a renal from primary gonadal etiology.

Laboratory Evaluation

Laboratory evaluation should include a white blood cell count and differential, hemoglobin, blood urea nitrogen, creatinine, potassium and bicarbonate. Mild leukocytosis (10,000 to 15,000/mm^3) is a common finding in patients with obstructing stones because of demargination of white blood cells in response to stress. However, a white blood cell count higher than 15,000/mm^3 is suggestive of infection and if present in

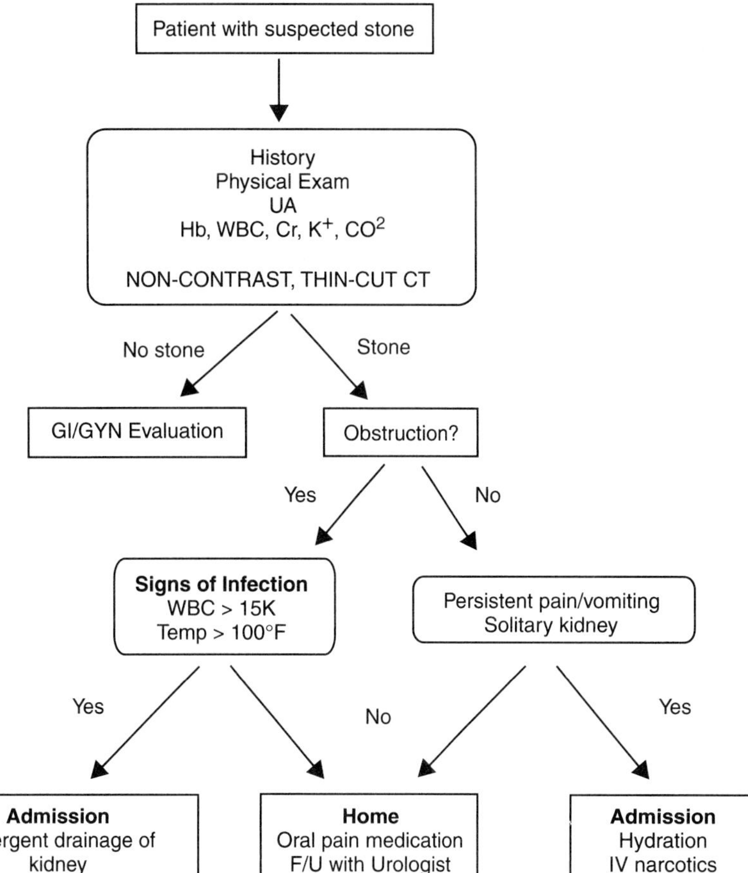

Figure 1. Algorithm for management of the acute stone event.

association with obstruction should raise suspicion of obstructive pyelonephritis, which requires prompt drainage of the collecting system.

An elevated creatinine may reflect dehydration, bilateral obstruction, or unilateral obstruction in the face of renal insufficiency. Renal insufficiency should preclude the use of nephrotoxic agents, including intravenous contrast for radiographic imaging. Serum electrolytes can identify metabolic disturbances, such as acidosis or hyperkalemia that may accompany obstruction.

The urinalysis also provides useful diagnostic information. Although the finding of red blood cells in the urine is suggestive of urinary tract stones, microhematuria may be absent in 10% to 25% of patients experiencing an acute stone event and thus should not exclude the diagnosis of a stone. Although white blood cells in the urine may represent inflammation resulting from the stone, significant pyuria may indicate infection. Other urine parameters, such as pH and the presence of crystals, are not critical in the acute management of the stone, but may suggest the etiology and type of stone disease: uric acid stones for pH <5.5 and struvite stones for pH >7.

Radiographic Imaging

The imaging study of choice in the setting of acute flank pain is non-enhanced, thin-cut (5 mm), helical computed tomography (Figure 2). With this modality, overlapping images are acquired rapidly (within a single breath-hold) without the need for intravenous contrast. Helical CT has been shown in randomized trials to be more sensitive than intravenous urography for detecting ureteral calculi. In addition, CT will reliably identify stones of all compositions including radiolucent uric acid stones, with the exception of indinavir stones. However, a plain abdominal radiograph (KUB) should also be obtained so that if the stone is visible on plain film, a simple KUB may be used for follow-up, obviating the need for repeat CT.

The use of noncontrast CT in the acute setting does not preclude the subsequent need for contrast imaging. For surgical intervention or follow-up, contrast imaging such as an intravenous urogram is recommended to verify ipsilateral renal function, to assess the degree of obstruction and to delineate renal and ureteral anatomy.

Management

The initial goal of treatment in the acute setting is to provide prompt pain relief. Narcotic analgesics such as morphine sulfate or meperidine (Demerol) have traditionally provided excellent pain control. Intravenous nonsteroidal analgesics such as ketorolac (Toradol) are also effective but should be used with caution because of reported cases of acute renal failure. Agents aimed at reducing ureteral peristalsis and facilitating

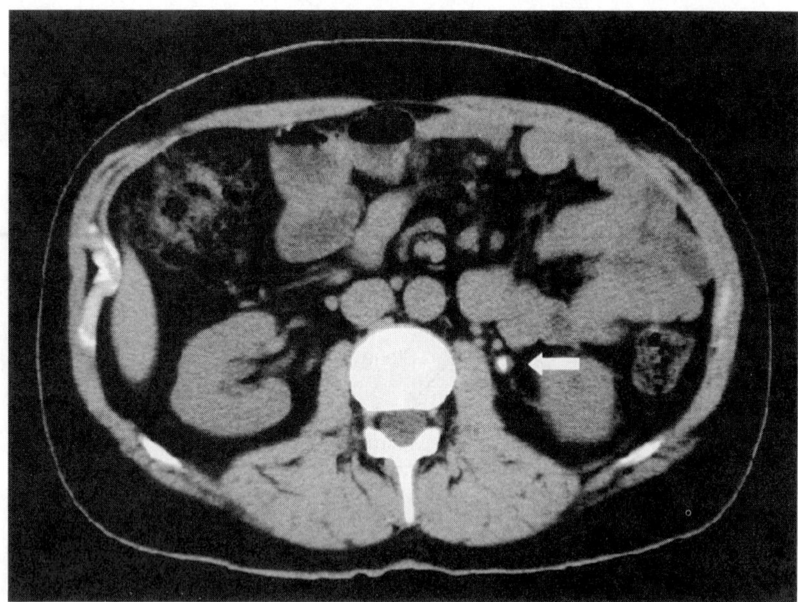

Figure 2. Nonenhanced helical computed tomography image of a left proximal ureter stone. Note tissue density around stone representing ureter *(arrow)*.

stone passage, such as steroids and calcium channel blockers, have shown promise in clinical trials.

The indications for hospitalization include failure to maintain adequate pain relief with oral analgesics, inability to retain oral fluids, solitary or functionally solitary kidney and clinical signs of infection. For the patient with an obstructing stone and clinical signs of infection (temperature >100°F or leukocytosis >15,000/mm^3), urgent decompression of the collection system with a nephrostomy tube or ureteral stent is mandated to prevent life-threatening sepsis.

Most ureteral calculi will pass spontaneously without the need for surgical intervention. The likelihood of spontaneous passage depends on a number of factors including the size and location of the stone. Small stones located in the distal ureter have a high likelihood of spontaneous passage while larger stones in the proximal ureter are less likely to pass. For stones <4 mm, 4–6 mm, and >6 mm, the probability of spontaneous passage regardless of location in the ureter is estimated at 57%, 35%, and <8%, respectively, according to natural history studies in the literature.

SURGICAL MANAGEMENT

Surgical intervention is necessary for ureteral stones that fail to or are unlikely to pass spontaneously, and for renal calculi associated with persistent pain, obstruction, location in the renal pelvis where the potential for obstruction is high, associated infection or loss of renal function, and branched, or staghorn calculi. The treatment of asymptomatic calyceal calculi is controversial; some advocate treatment of all stones because of the ease of treatment, whereas others recommend observation and medical management.

The choice of surgical therapy depends on the size, location, and composition of the stone, renal, or ureteral anatomy and patient characteristics. Options include shock wave lithotripsy, ureteroscopy, percutaneous nephrostolithotomy, and, in rare cases, open or laparoscopic stone removal.

Shock Wave Lithotripsy

Shock wave lithotripsy (SWL) is a noninvasive treatment based on the principles of acoustical physics. Using ultrasound or fluoroscopic imaging, the stone is positioned at the focal point of the shock waves, and repeated firing fragments it into pieces that pass with the urine over time.

SWL is the most common surgical modality for the treatment of renal and ureteral stones. Performed on an outpatient basis, SWL is associated with a high success rate and low morbidity for small to moderate sized renal and ureteral calculi. Complications are most commonly related to obstruction from passing stone fragments.

The success of SWL depends on the size, location, and composition of the stone. Stones in the lower pole of the kidney may fragment well but are less likely to clear than stones elsewhere in the kidney. Likewise, calcium oxalate monohydrate and calcium phosphate stones fragment less efficiently than calcium oxalate dihydrate or struvite stones, and cystine stones are relatively shock wave–resistant.

Ureteroscopy

Most ureteral and some renal calculi can be successfully treated via small caliber flexible or semirigid ureteroscopes in conjunction with small intracorporeal lithotripsy devices that are passed through the working channel of the endoscope to fragment the stone into spontaneously passable-size fragments. Like SWL, ureteroscopy is an outpatient procedure associated with a high success rate and low complication rate consisting primarily of ureteral perforation and stricture formation. Ureteroscopy is a useful modality for patients who fail SWL or when SWL or a percutaneous approach is contraindicated, such as patients with uncorrected bleeding abnormalities.

Percutaneous Nephrostolithotomy

A percutaneous endoscopic approach is indicated for large or complex renal calculi or for stones that have failed SWL or ureteroscopy. Percutaneous nephrostolithotomy (PCNL) involves passage of a large caliber endoscope through a sheath inserted percutaneously through the flank directly into the collecting system. Smaller stones are retrieved intact, whereas large renal stone burdens are efficiently fragmented and removed without relying on passage of large volumes of stone fragments through the ureter. PCNL requires general anesthesia and usually involves a 1- to 2-day hospital stay. The most common complications associated with PCNL are bleeding (4% to 5% transfusion rate) and access-related injuries such as hydrothorax. Stone free rates of 70% to 100% can be expected for unselected stones and >90% for non–staghorn calculi.

Open and Laparoscopic Stone Removal

Laparoscopic or open stone removal is reserved as a salvage procedure for endoscopic or SWL failures, and should rarely, if ever, be required as first-line treatment except in cases of complex anatomic abnormalities that require simultaneous correction.

MEDICAL EVALUATION AND MANAGEMENT

Despite the ease with which stones can be treated surgically, the need for effective diagnostic protocols and medical treatment regimens remains undiminished. Surgical stone removal fails to change the natural history of stone disease; thus, patients at high risk of recurrence should be targeted for medical evaluation and treatment.

Patient Selection

Few question the need for evaluation and medical management of patients with active, recurrent stone disease. However, the need to evaluate the first-time stoneformer is controversial. First-time stoneformers at high risk of recurrence, such as those with a strong family history of stone disease or underlying medical risk factors, may benefit from evaluation and medical therapy. For first-time stoneformers without clear-cut risk, a trial of simple conservative dietary measures (high fluid intake, modest salt and animal protein restriction, limited oxalate-rich foods) may be warranted.

Metabolic Evaluation

A metabolic evaluation includes a thorough history, serum chemistries and intact parathyroid hormone (PTH), urinalysis, stone analysis, plain abdominal radiograph, and one or more 24-hour urine collections. A careful history should elicit underlying medical risk factors, such as chronic diarrhea resulting from intestinal disease or surgery (bowel resection, pancreatic insufficiency, ulcerative colitis, Crohn disease), recurrent urinary tract infections, nephrocalcinosis, gout, bone disease, or hyperthyroidism as well as use of stone-provoking medications such as calcium supplements, vitamin D, acetazolamide (Diamox) (a carbonic anhydrase inhibitor that induces metabolic acidosis), and vitamin C. A dietary history should identify environmental risk factors such as dehydration, salt abuse, high calcium or oxalate intake, and excess animal protein intake.

A basic serum chemistry profile, including creatinine, potassium, bicarbonate, phosphorus, uric acid and intact PTH, will identify systemic abnormalities such as hyperuricemia, hyperparathyroidism (elevated calcium and PTH, low phosphorus) and distal renal tubular acidosis (low bicarbonate and potassium, high chloride). Urinalysis might reveal the hexagonal crystals of cystine stones or coffin-lid crystals of struvite stones. The stone composition may imply the associated metabolic derangement for uric acid, cystine, or struvite stones but is less specific for calcium stones. Last, a KUB may show nephrocalcinosis suggesting renal tubular acidosis or medullary sponge kidney.

A 24-hour urine collection is subjected to a variety of biochemical assays to identify metabolic and environmental risk factors. Although most laboratories can perform individual specified assays, a variety of commercial kits are available to facilitate urine collection and processing through a centralized laboratory that performs a standardized battery of biochemical assays and physicochemical measurements.

Urine is analyzed for total volume, pH, creatinine, calcium, sodium, oxalate, citrate, uric acid, potassium, magnesium, phosphorus, and sulfate. Assessment of urine creatinine level determines the adequacy of the urine collection; for women, 24-hour urine creatinine should be 18–20 mg/kg and for men 20–22 mg/kg.

In some cases, it is advantageous to analyze a second 24-hour urine specimen after a week of dietary restriction (low calcium, sodium, and oxalate) to identify correctable environmental or dietary risk factors. In addition, a fast and load test whereby a fasting 2-hour urine is obtained followed by a 4-hour urine collected after ingestion of a 1 gram calcium load distinguishes among the various etiologies of hypercalciuria.

Diagnosis and Treatment

Calcium stones are associated with a variety of pathophysiologic abnormalities including hypercalciuria, hyperuricosuria, hypocitraturia, hyperoxaluria, and low urine pH. In contrast, uric acid, cystine and struvite stones have a single associated metabolic abnormality (Table 1). Treatment is directed at correcting the underlying metabolic derangements and eliminating environmental risk factors with diet and medication.

TABLE 1. **Metabolic Abnormalities, Diagnostic Criteria, and Treatment Regimens**

Condition	Metabolic/ Environmental Defect	Associated Stone Composition	Diagnostic Criteria		Treatment	
			Blood	*Urine*	*Intervention*	*Physiologic Action*
Hypercalciuria						
Absorptive	↑GI Ca absorption	Calcium oxalate, calcium phosphate	Nl Ca, Nl PTH	↑Ca	Thiazides + potassium citrate (Urocit-K)	↓urinary Ca, ↑urinary citrate
Renal	Impaired renal Ca reabsorption	Calcium oxalate, calcium phosphate	Nl Ca, ↑PTH	↑Ca	Thiazides + potassium citrate	↓urinary Ca, ↑urinary citrate
Resorptive	Primary hyperparathyroidism	Calcium phosphate	↑Ca, ↓Phos, ↑PTH	↑Ca	Parathyroidectomy	Normalizes serum PTH and Ca
Hyperuricosuria	Dietary purine excess, uric acid overproduction, increased renal uric acid excretion	Calcium oxalate, uric acid	—	↑uric acid	Purine restriction, allopurinol (Zyloprim)	↓urinary uric acid
Hypocitraturia	GI alkali loss, hypokalemia, distal renal tubular acidosis, idiopathic	Calcium oxalate, calcium phosphate	—	↓citrate	Potassium citrate	↑urinary citrate
Hyperoxaluria						
Primary	Oxalate overproduction	Calcium oxalate	—	↑oxalate	Pyridoxine (vitamin B6), ↓dietary oxalate, liver-kidney transplant	↓urinary oxalate
Dietary	↑dietary oxalate	Calcium oxalate	—	↑oxalate	↓dietary oxalate	↓urinary oxalate
Enteric	↑intestinal oxalate absorption	Calcium oxalate	—	↑oxalate, ↓Ca, ↓pH	↓dietary oxalate, calcium citrate (Citracal), potassium citrate	↓urinary oxalate, ↑pH, ↑urinary citrate
Low urine pH	Metabolic acidosis, idiopathic	Uric acid, calcium oxalate	—	↓pH	Potassium citrate	↑urinary citrate
Cystinuria	Impaired renal cystine reabsorption	Cystine	—	↑cystine	Potassium citrate, tiopronin (Thiola)	↑pH, ↓urinary cystine
Infection stones	Infection with urease-producing bacteria	Struvite	—	↑pH	acetohydroxamic acid (Lithostat), antibiotics, surgical stone removal	Inhibits urease, treats infection, removes infectious source

Hypercalciuria

Hypercalciuria is the end result of a variety of metabolic disorders. Absorptive hypercalciuria (AH), the most common form of hypercalciuria, is due to intestinal overabsorption of calcium, which leads to suppression of PTH and increased renal calcium excretion. AH is classified as type I or type II based on the urinary response to a low calcium diet; AH is correctable with a low calcium intake in type II but not type I AH. AH is characterized by normal serum calcium and PTH, high urine calcium, normal or high fasting urine calcium, and increased urine calcium after an oral calcium load.

Renal hypercalciuria (RH) is due to impaired renal tubular calcium absorption resulting in renal calcium loss and secondary hyperparathyroidism. RH is characterized by normal serum calcium, elevated urine calcium, and high fasting urine calcium.

AH II may be treated with dietary calcium restriction in patients with adequate bone mineral density. For more severe forms of AH II and for AH I and RH, thiazide diuretics (hydrochlorothiazide 25–50 mg daily) or indapamide (Lozol) (1.25–2.5 mg daily) constitute the primary treatment. Thiazides directly stimulate calcium reabsorption in the distal tubule and indirectly stimulate reabsorption in the proximal tubule. Because thiazides induce hypokalemia and hypocitraturia, the addition of a potassium citrate supplement is advisable. Because sodium enhances urinary calcium excretion, limitation of dietary salt is also advisable.

Primary hyperparathyroidism, the most common form of resorptive hypercalciuria, is due to excessive PTH secretion from a parathyroid adenoma that leads to bone resorption and increased synthesis of 1,25-$(OH)_2D$. Primary hyperparathyroidism is characterized by hypercalcemia, hypophosphatemia, inappropriately high serum PTH, and hypercalciuria. Primary hyperparathyroidism is treated with surgical removal of the adenoma-containing parathyroid gland.

Hyperuricosuria

Hyperuricosuria is a risk factor for both uric acid and calcium oxalate stones and is most commonly the result of purine overindulgence. At low pH (<5.5), the poorly soluble undissociated form of uric acid precipitates to form uric acid stones. At pH >5.5, monosodium urate predominates and promotes calcium oxalate stone formation by providing a nidus for calcium oxalate crystallization. Although restriction of animal protein may normalize urinary uric acid, the addition of allopurinol (Zyloprim) (300 mg daily), a xanthine oxidase inhibitor that prevents uric acid production, may be necessary in some cases.

Hypocitraturia

Citrate inhibits calcium stone formation by complexing with calcium and reducing urinary saturation of calcium salts and also by directly inhibiting calcium oxalate and calcium phosphate crystal growth. Urinary citrate excretion is determined by acid-base balance: acidosis inhibits citrate excretion while alkalosis promotes it. A variety of conditions affecting acid-base balance are associated with hypocitraturia, including chronic diarrheal syndrome, renal tubular acidosis, thiazide use, and idiopathic hypocitraturia. Potassium citrate (Urocit-K) therapy (40–60 mEq daily in three divided doses) restores normal urinary citrate, raises urine pH, and lowers urinary saturation of calcium salts.

Hyperoxaluria

Hyperoxaluria is caused by high substrate availability (vitamin C, oxalate-rich foods such as brewed tea, chocolate, nuts, dark green leafy vegetables), increased oxalate production (primary hyperoxalosis), or increased intestinal oxalate absorption (enteric hyperoxaluria). Enteric hyperoxaluria is the most common etiology of hyperoxaluria and is due to intestinal disease or resection. In these states, poorly absorbed fatty acids and bile salts complex with calcium, thereby preventing calcium oxalate complexation and increasing oxalate availability for reabsorption. Bile salts may also directly increase colonic permeability to oxalate, further increasing urinary oxalate. Chronic diarrheal states are additionally associated with low urine volume resulting from dehydration and low urine pH and hypocitraturia as a result of metabolic acidosis.

Treatment of enteric hyperoxaluria is aimed at correcting acidosis and preventing dehydration. Potassium citrate therapy increases urine pH and normalizes urine citrate. Limitation of dietary oxalate, and in severe cases, addition of a calcium supplement, will reduce intestinal oxalate absorption and subsequently lower urinary oxalate excretion. For primary oxalosis, dietary oxalate restriction and pyridoxine (vitamin B6), which favors an alternate metabolic pathway reducing oxalate production, may be beneficial. In severe cases, liver-kidney transplant is necessary.

Low Urine pH

Low urine pH (<5.5) is typically associated with uric stones, but may also predispose to calcium oxalate stone formation. Treatment is aimed at raising urine pH (potassium citrate) and normalizing urinary uric acid (limiting purine-rich foods or allopurinol), thereby preventing further stone formation and potentially resulting in dissolution of existing uric acid stones.

Cystinuria

Cystinuria is an inherited metabolic defect in the intestinal and renal transport of dibasic amino acids (cystine, ornithine, lysine, and arginine) leading to excessive urinary cystine excretion. Cystine stone formation is a consequence of the poor solubility of cystine in urine (250 mg/L), which in part is determined by urine pH. High fluid intake is essential for reducing urinary cystine concentration, but because cystine solubility increases with increasing urine pH, the addition of potassium citrate may further reduce urine cystine concentration. When fluid and alkali therapy fail, the addition of a chelating agent, such as

D-penicillamine (Cuprimine) or alpha mercaptopropionyglycine (Thiola) will further reduce urine cystine by forming a more soluble cysteine-sulfhydryl complex.

Infection Stones

Chronic infection with urea-splitting organisms leads to the formation of magnesium ammonium phosphate (struvite) stones often in combination with calcium phosphate (apatite) stones. Urease catalyzes the hydrolysis of urea to ammonium, producing an alkaline urine that promotes the crystallization of magnesium, ammonium, and phosphate. The most common urease-producing organisms are *Proteus*, *Pseudomonas*, and *Klebsiella*. Treatment of struvite stones requires complete stone removal and eradication of infection because the stone harbors bacteria that are inaccessible to systemic antibiotics. In some cases, initiation of a urease inhibitor (acetohydroxamic acid, or Lithostat, 250 mg three times daily) is indicated for severe disease.

Section 11

The Sexually Transmitted Diseases

CHANCROID

method of
RICHARD STEEN, P.A., M.P.H.
Family Health International
Arlington, Virginia

Chancroid is caused by the gram-negative bacillus *Haemophilus ducreyi*, a fragile organism that thrives under conditions of commercial sex and male non-circumcision, especially where access to condoms and antibiotics is limited. With no nonhuman reservoir, chancroid has disappeared from many regions over the past century as such conditions have become less common. In remaining endemic areas of Africa, Asia, and the Caribbean, genital ulcers are among the most common sexually transmitted infection (STI) syndromes seen, and chancroid is a major etiologic agent. In non-endemic areas, chancroid outbreaks have been linked to commercial sex and crack cocaine use.

Chancroid is an important cofactor in heterosexual HIV transmission. Male circumcision is highly protective against both *H. ducreyi* and HIV infection, and the interaction of chancroid and HIV infection accounts for at least part of the HIV-protective effect of circumcision. Topical hygiene—simple washing with soap and water within a few hours of sexual exposure—effectively reduces risk of chancroid infection.

Most patients with chancroid report direct contact with a sex worker or a partner with direct contact, and outbreaks typically show high male-to-female ratios. *H. ducreyi* has a short duration of infectivity and requires high rates of partner change (estimated 15 to 20 sex partners per year) to spread within a population. Control measures that reach core groups with high rates of partner change are effective in controlling outbreaks.

Chancroid causes superficial ulcerations, often with suppurant inguinal lymphadenopathy. Classically, chancroid is differentiated from syphilis by the soft, irregular borders of the ulcerations (soft chancres), which are painful. Atypical presentations are common, however, especially with HIV co-infection. Most infections are symptomatic, but vaginal ulcers may be inapparent in women. *H. ducreyi* is fastidious and difficult to culture. Polymerase chain reaction (PCR) testing may be available from referral laboratories. Because of the difficulty of establishing a reliable etiologic diagnosis, initial syndrome management—including treatment for both chancroid and syphilis—should be provided for all genital ulcers that are not clearly herpetic.

TREATMENT

There are several highly effective treatment options for chancroid. Single dose regimens include azithromycin 1 g orally or ceftriaxone 250 mg intramuscularly. Equally effective is erythromycin base 500 mg orally 3 to 4 times a day for 7 days or ciprofloxacin 500 mg orally twice a day for 3 days. Healing may be slower in individuals with HIV infection and treatment may need to be extended.

Fluctuant lymph nodes should be aspirated though a large-bore needle inserted through adjacent healthy skin. Excision should be avoided, as spontaneous or iatrogenic rupture of buboes is associated with delayed healing and fistula formation. Patients should be reviewed weekly until ulcers have completely resolved. Repeat aspiration is often necessary and provides considerable symptomatic relief.

Suspected cases of chancroid should be reported to the local health department. Contact tracing and presumptive epidemiologic treatment of contacts has been effective in containing recent outbreaks in North America. Because of the close association between chancroid and HIV, anyone with suspected chancroid should be strongly encouraged to undergo counseling and voluntary HIV testing.

GONORRHEA

method of
ANNE ROMPALO, M.D.
Johns Hopkins University School of Medicine
Baltimore, Maryland

EPIDEMIOLOGY

Although the incident rates of gonococcal infections in the United States have been declining steadily since the 1980s, gonorrhea is still a significant public health problem in the United States. Over 600,000 new cases of gonorrhea are reported annually, but reported cases underestimate the incidence. It is currently estimated that private clinicians, as opposed to public health clinics, report over one half of gonorrhea cases and state health departments are currently notified of 64% to 80% of gonorrhea cases identified in medical care organizations.

Gonorrhea rates vary with geography and demographics. Highest U.S. rates are reported from the South, but in the West, increasing rates are reported among men having sex with men. Gonorrhea rates peak in men ages 20 to 24 years and in women ages 15 to 19 years. Currently there are disproportionately high rates among African-Americans, and Hispanic and Native Americans compared to whites and Asians. Behaviors that increase the risk of acquiring gonorrhea include multiple or new sex partners, inconsistent condom use, illicit drug use, and exchange of sex for money or drugs.

Transmission is more efficient from an infected male to a female partner during vaginal intercourse, and the rate is approximately 50% to 70% per sexual contact. Infected women transmit gonorrhea to the urethra of their male partners at 20% per vaginal intercourse episode, and this rate increases to 60% to 80% after four or more exposures. Transmission by rectal or oral intercourse has not been quantified but appears to be efficient.

MICROBIOLOGY

Neisseria gonorrhoeae is a gram-negative diplococcus that infects mucus-secreting epithelial cells. It is oxidase-positive, nonmotile, does not form spores, divides by binary fission every 20 to 30 minutes, and utilizes glucose. It grows best on selective media, such as Thayer-Martin medium. Because it does not tolerate drying, specimens collected for culture are best plated immediately and incubated at 36°C in a 3% to 5% CO_2 environment. Nucleic acid amplification tests are now available that have excellent sensitivity and specificity and allow less invasive collection of specimens for adequate test performance (Table 1).

TABLE 1. **Performance of Tests for Diagnosis of Gonorrhea**

Diagnostic Method	% Sensitivity	% Specificity
Culture	80–95	100
Gram Stain		
Males-symptomatic	90–95	95–100
Males-asymptomatic	50–70	95–100
Females	50–70	95–100
Hybridization (Pace 2)	92.1–96.4	98.8–99.1
Ligase chain reaction	96.7–98.6	99.7–99.9
Polymerase Chain Reaction (COBAS)		
Cervical	92.4	99.5
Female urine	64.8	99.8
Male urine (symptomatic)	94.1	99.9
Strand Displacement Amplification		
Cervical	96.6	98–100
Female urine	84.9–98.5	99.3–100
Male urethral	97.9	91.9–100
Male urine	99.2	92.5–100
Transcriptional Mediated Amplification		
Cervical	91.3	98.7
Female urine		99.3
Male urine	97.1	99.2
Male urethral	98.8	98.2%

CLINICAL MANIFESTATIONS

Gonorrhea attaches to different types of epithelial cells via a number of different structures on its surface. *N. gonorrhoeae* has the ability to alter its surface structures, particularly pilin, lipo-oligosaccharide antigens, and less frequently protein 1 antigens, which help it evade the host response. It is ingested by the cell and can cause asymptomatic or symptomatic infection.

Men with urethral gonorrhea can develop overt, symptomatic urethritis within 2 to 7 days after inoculation. Symptoms may include purulent urethral discharge often accompanied by dysuria. On physical examination the discharge may appear mucopurulent, but often it can be clear or cloudy. Asymptomatic infection does occur and may be more common than previously believed owing to the availability of urine screening tests. Asymptomatic infection has been linked to specific gonococcal phenotypes and represents a reservoir that perpetuates transmission from men to women.

Complications of gonococcal infections are rare in men but may include epididymitis, inguinal lymphadenitis, penile edema, periurethral abscess or fistula, accessory or Tyson's gland infection, balanitis, and urethral stricture. Males with epididymitis can present with unilateral testicular pain and testicular swelling, which is usually associated with overt or subclinical urethritis.

Genital infection among women occurs as symptomatic disease far less frequently than among men. Women may have gonococcal cervicitis and report symptoms in only 50% of cases. Symptoms may occur within 10 days of infection, but the exact incubation period remains unclear. When symptoms occur they may be nonspecific and include abnormal vaginal discharge, intermenstrual bleeding, dysuria, lower abdominal pain, or dyspareunia. On physical examination, the cervix may appear edematous with mucopurulent or purulent discharge and easily induced friability.

As with men, women can develop urethritis and 40% to 90% of women with cervical gonococcal infection have urethral co-infection. Women with total abdominal hysterectomies can develop urethral infections after sexual exposure to an infected partner. Symptoms may include dysuria, although most infections are asymptomatic. Accessory gland infections can also occur involving Skene's or Bartholin's glands.

Often the infection is unilateral, and occlusion of the duct of the gland may result in abscess formation.

Pelvic inflammatory disease (PID) refers to an ascending infection to the endometrium and/or fallopian tubes. Symptoms include lower abdominal pain, discharge, dyspareunia, intermenstrual bleeding, and fever. However, silent or asymptomatic PID can occur. The clinical diagnosis of PID is imprecise, but exam findings include uterine tenderness, adnexal tenderness, or cervical motion tenderness. Cervicitis may or may not be present. Long-term sequelae of PID include chronic pelvic pain, tubal infertility, or ectopic pregnancy.

Both men and women may develop anorectal gonococcal infection if they engage in receptive anal intercourse. In 35% to 50% of women with gonococcal cervicitis who do not acknowledge rectal sexual contact, however, the rectal mucosa may be co-infected. This may be a result of perineal contamination with infected cervical secretions. Most rectal gonorrhea cases are asymptomatic, but occasional severe proctitis may result. Symptoms, if present, include anal irritation, painful defecation, constipation, rectal bleeding and/or discharge, and tenesmus. Evaluation with an anoscope is recommended with symptomatic patients and signs of infection may include purulent discharge, erythema, or easily induced bleeding as well as normal mucosa.

Pharyngeal gonococcal infection is most often asymptomatic, and exudative pharyngitis is rare.

Disseminated gonococcal infection (DGI) occurs infrequently, in only 0.5% to 3% of cases. Gonococcal strains that are resistant to killing by normal human serum have a propensity to produce bacteremia. DGI occurs more frequently in women and often within 7 days of menses. Clinical manifestations include skin lesions, arthralgias, tenosynovitis, arthritis, hepatitis, myocarditis, and rarely, endocarditis and meningitis. Typical skin lesions are acrally distributed and sparse, and they appear as pustular lesions on an erythematous base. Synovial cultures are positive in only 50% of septic arthritis cases.

DIAGNOSIS

Table 1 presents the sensitivities and specificities for nonculture tests for the diagnosis of gonococcal infections at different sites. If Gram staining is available, however, it is the most rapid and inexpensive method. In men presenting with symptomatic gonococcal urethritis, the Gram stain will show gram-negative intracellular diplococci in over 95% of urethral exudates. Cervical Gram stains have sensitivities of approximately 50% but specificities of 95%. Specimens for rectal Gram stain are best collected via anoscopy, with a reported sensitivity of about 80%.

Culture, unlike nonculture techniques, can be used for any anatomic site, and is the test of choice in medicolegal situations. Culture should be used if antibiotic susceptibility is in question. Although the emergence of quinolone-resistant gonorrhea is still low in the United States, with the exception of Hawaii and California, culture should be taken in patients who have symptoms that persist after treatment is completed, and any gonococci that are isolated should be tested for antimicrobial susceptibility.

TREATMENT

The 2002 Centers for Disease Control and Prevention Sexually Transmitted Disease Treatment Guidelines recommendation for the treatment of uncomplicated gonococcal infections in adults is summarized in Table 2. To be considered as a recommended treatment for uncomplicated gonorrhea, an antimicrobial regimen should cure >95% of urogenital infections. It is important to note that quinolones are now approved for treatment of uncomplicated gonococcal infection in children who weigh more than 45 kilograms. Also, ofloxacin is no longer recommended for treatment of uncomplicated pharyngeal gonorrhea because it does not reliably cure greater than 90% of these infections. The recent discontinuation of cefixime production has limited oral treatment options for urogenital and pharyngeal gonorrhea.

TABLE 2. **2002 Recommendations for Uncomplicated Genital, Rectal, and Pharyngeal Infection in Adults and Adolescents***

Ceftriaxone (Rocephin)[1]	125 mg	IM	Once or
Ofloxacin (Floxin)[2]	400 mg	PO	Once or
Ciprofloxacin (Cipro)[2]	500 mg	PO	Once or
Levofloxacin (Levaquin)[2]	250 mg	PO	Once
PLUS (for treatment of chlamydial infection—if Chlamydia infection not ruled out)[4]			
Azithromycin (Zithromax)[3]	1.0 g	PO	Once or
Doxycycline (Vibramycin)[2]	100 mg	PO	bid × 7 days
Recommended Initial Regimen for Disseminated Gonococcal Infection			
Ceftriaxone (Rocephin)	1 g IM or IV		q24h or
Alternate Regimens			
Cefotaxime (Claforan)	1 g IV		q8h or
Ceftizoxime (Cefizox)	1 g IV		q8h or
Ciprofloxacin (Cipro)	400 mg IV		q12h or
Ofloxacin (Floxin)	400 mg IV		q12h or
Levofloxacin (Levaquin)	250 mg IV		q24h or
Spectinomycin (Trobicin)	2 gs IM		q12h
Recommended Oral Regimen After Improvement			
Ciprofloxacin (Cipro)	500 mg PO		bid or
Ofloxacin (Floxin)	400 mg PO		bid or
Levofloxacin (Levaquin)	500 mg PO		qd

[1]If penicillin-allergic, consider potential cephalosporin cross-reactivity (3%–5%).

[2]Contraindicated in pregnancy and in children. Not recommended for infections acquired in Asia or the Pacific, including Hawaii.

[3]Safety and efficacy in pregnancy not established. Not recommended for gonococcal treatment. Azithromycin 2.0 g dose is effective for uncomplicated gonococcal infection but is expensive and causes gastrointestinal distress too often to be recommended.

[4]If co-infection rate is high and sensitive chlamydia tests not available, or patient is unlikely to return for chlamydia treatment.

*Adapted from the 2002 CDC STD Treatment Guidelines.

Bid, twice daily; IM, intramuscularly; IV, intravenously; PO, by mouth; q, every.

Alternative regimens for uncomplicated gonococcal infections of the cervix, urethra, and rectum include spectinomycin 2 grams in a single intramuscular dose. This is useful for treatment of patients who cannot tolerate cephalosporins and quinolones, but if spectinomycin is used, pharyngeal cultures should be performed because cure rates of spectinomycin for pharyngeal gonococcal infections are 53%. Ceftriaxone or spectinomycin remain the recommended options for treating urogenital gonorrhea in pregnant women.

Gonococcal infections acquired in Hawaii, California, Asia, the Pacific, or other areas with increased prevalence of fluoroquinolone resistance should be treated with ceftriaxone 125 mg IM. Other third-generation cephalosporins may be considered, depending on sensitivity testing. However, several alternative oral cephalosporin regimens for the treatment of uncomplicated gonococcal urogenital infections have been evaluated but not recommended by the CDC because they have not met the efficacy criteria, have undocumented or unacceptable efficacy for treating pharyngeal infection, or because of safety concerns. Azithromycin 2 g, in a single dose, has 99.2% efficacy for urogenital infections and 100% efficacy for pharyngeal infections. However, gastrointestinal intolerance is a significant side effect and the 500 mg tablet formulation may be better tolerated. Azithromycin in the 1 g single dose is insufficiently effective and is not recommended.

Patients treated for uncomplicated gonococcal infections need not return for a test of cure. However, patients who refrain from any sexual activity and have persistent symptoms should be evaluated by culture for *N. gonorrhoeae*, and any gonococci isolated should be tested for antimicrobial susceptibility to investigate the possibility of fluoroquinolone resistance.

Patients should refer anyone with whom they have had sexual contact within the previous 60 days for diagnosis and treatment of *N. gonorrhoeae* and *Chlamydia trachomatis*. Patients with gonorrhea should avoid sexual intercourse until therapy is completed and until they and their sex partners have been treated and no longer have symptoms.

NONGONOCOCCAL URETHRITIS

method of
JOHN A. MATA, M.D.
LSU Health Science Center
Shreveport, Louisiana

Nongonococcal urethritis (NGU) is a sexually transmitted disease syndrome with several etiologic causes, and it surpasses gonococcal urethritis (GU) in incidence. The most important and clinically dangerous pathogen is still *Chlamydia trachomatis*. The prevalence of *C. trachomatis* isolated from the urethra (15% to 55%) is declining, but identification is important because the organism can be isolated from 30% to 60% of female partners of men with NGU. The management of urethritis, therefore, mandates that an effort be made to treat the patient's sexual partner promptly. Other etiologic causes of nonchlamydial NGU include *Ureaplasma urealyticum*, *Mycoplasma genitalium*, *Trichomonas vaginalis*, herpes simplex virus, and cytomegalovirus. The prevalence of *M. genitalium* is increasing, especially in persistent or recurrent cases of NGU. The risk of urethritis increases as the number of sexual contacts increases, and infection may occur after a single episode of intercourse with an infected partner in up to 20% of cases. The disease may also be transmitted through oral/anal sex with an infected partner. Asymptomatic infection may occur in up to 50% of the contacts of women with chlamydial cervical infection. Urethritis in homosexual males is more likely to be gonococcal than nongonococcal. Young men of higher socioeconomic status are more often affected by NGU than GU. There is no proof that alcohol, caffeinated beverages, or urethral stripping cause urethritis. Smoking and circumcision may be independent risk factors for development of NGU.

DIAGNOSIS

The usual incubation period for NGU is 7 to 28 days, but longer periods do occur. The urethra is the most common site of infection in all men. Urethritis may be manifested by urethral discharge, dysuria, or urethral itching. Compared to GU the discharge in NGU is often scant and clear or whitish and the dysuria mild to moderate or absent. NGU is diagnosed when Gram-negative intracellular diploccocci are *not* identified on a urethral smear. Urethritis can be confirmed by documenting any of the following signs:

- Urethral discharge—mucoid or purulent
- Gram stain of urethral secretions demonstrating greater than 5 white blood cells (WBCs) per oil immersion field
- Positive leukocyte esterase test on first-void urine or microscopic examination of urine sediment demonstrating greater than 10 WBCs per high powered field

Endourethral swab cultures for *C. trachomatis* may be employed when available. The specimen is taken 2 to 4 mm inside the urethra and placed in special transport media. Nucleic acid amplification tests now enable detection of *N. gonorrhoeae* and *C. trachomatis* on all specimens. The tests are more sensitive than the culture techniques for *C. trachomatis* and are now the preferred method for detection. Empiric treatment of symptoms without documentation of urethritis is recommended for high-risk patients or those unlikely to return for follow-up. Such patients are treated for both gonorrhea and chlamydia. Partners of patients treated empirically should also be evaluated and treated.

TREATMENT

Because NGU is caused by varied organisms that respond differently to treatment, results of therapy are inconsistent. Table 1 lists a current recommended

TABLE 1. **Treatment of Nongonococcal Urethritis**

Azithromycin (Zithromax) 1 g PO in a single dose
Doxycycline (Vibramycin) 100 mg PO bid × 7 days
Erythromycin base (E-Mycin, ERYC, E-Base) 500 mg PO qid × 7 days
Erythromycin ethylsuccinate (EES) 800 mg PO qid × 7 days
Ofloxacin (Floxin) 300 mg PO bid × 7 days
Levofloxacin (Levaquin) 500 mg PO daily × 7 days

Bid, twice daily; PO, by mouth.

antibiotic regimen. Treatment should begin soon after diagnosis. In fact, single dose regimens are becoming more popular and ensure immediate compliance. *T. vaginalis* infection should be treated with metronidazole (Flagyl). Patients are instructed to return to the office or clinic for follow-up if symptoms persist or recur after therapy. Patients are instructed to abstain from sexual activity for one week and refer all sex partners within the preceding 60 days for evaluation and treatment.

Persistent or Recurrent Urethritis

Patients with recurrent symptoms and signs of urethritis should be re-evaluated. Objective signs of persistent urethritis should be sought prior to antibiotic treatment. Patients initially cured only to have symptoms return shortly after exposure to a sexual partner may be treated with a recommended regimen again. Partner referral is again emphasized. An intraurethral culture is sent and a urine specimen is examined again for evidence of *T. vaginalis*. Tetracycline-resistant *U. urealyticum* may be a cause of treatment failure. Urologic workup may be indicated in those patients failing a second treatment course. Male patients may have a urethral stricture or chronic prostatitis. If the patient was compliant and re-exposure is ruled out, treatment with metronidazole (Flagyl) 2 g orally in a single dose plus erythromycin base (E-Base) 500 mg orally four times a day for 7 days is recommended. Complications in men with chlamydia-negative urethritis are unusual but emotional problems including guilt, depression, and fear of loss of sexual function are not uncommon. Epididymitis or nonbacterial prostatitis may result but generally do not cause severe physical problems. Because *C. trachomatis* is a major source of morbidity, it is crucial to eradicate this pathogen. Untreated male contacts with GU or chlamydial NGU are a major source of infection for pelvic inflammatory disease (PID) in women. Approximately 20% of women with chlamydial lower genital tract infection will develop PID. Treatment of male contacts decreases the rate of further infection and slows the sexually transmitted disease cycle.

GRANULOMA INGUINALE (Donovanosis)

method of
NANCY J. ANDERSON, M.D., and
AGNIESZKA NIEMEYER, M.D.
Loma Linda University
Loma Linda, California

Granuloma inguinale, or donovanosis, is a chronic, slowly progressive infection causing granulomatous ulceration of the genital, perineal, and inguinal skin. It is extremely rare in the United States, but is still endemic in certain tropical and subtropical areas, such as New Guinea, India, the Caribbean, South Africa, Brazil, and among aborigines in Australia. The causative organism, *Calymmatobacterium granulomatis,* is a gram-negative obligate intracellular bacillus that is serologically related to *Klebsiella* species.

After an incubation period of 1 to 12 weeks (most commonly 2 weeks), single or multiple subcutaneous nodules or papules develop at the site of inoculation, which later erode to form painless ulcerations with clean, friable bases and distinct rolled margins. Lesions may become confluent and without treatment may cause progressive mutilation and destruction of local tissue. Autoinoculation is a common feature, producing lesions on adjacent skin, termed "kissing" lesions. Unless bacterial superinfection develops, true inguinal lymphadenopathy does not occur in donovanosis. However, inguinal enlargement (pseudobuboes) may occur as a result of subcutaneous granulomas. Systemic symptoms are uncommon. Both sexual and nonsexual modes (rare) of transmission have been reported. Contact with infective exudates is probably responsible for transmission to sexually inactive persons.

Complications of chronic granuloma inguinale infection include: phimosis, urethral stenosis, scarring, fibrosis, fistulas, and lymphatic obstruction, with genital edema and possible elephantiasis. Prolonged ulceration may lead to development of squamous cell carcinoma of the region.

Granuloma inguinale has a variety of presentations. The most characteristic include:

1. Ulcerovegetative, or ulcerogranulomatous form, the most common form. Characterized by large, extensive, nonindurated ulcerations with beefy-red, friable granulation tissue that bleeds easily
2. Nodular form with soft, red nodules and plaques that eventually ulcerate
3. Hypertrophic, or verrucous form, consisting of large, dry, vegetating masses that clinically resemble condyloma acuminatum
4. Sclerotic, or cicatricial form, the rare form of the disease. Characterized by dry, nonbleeding ulcer that expands into plaque and bandlike scarring of the genitalia. Because of the constrictive nature of this variant, associated lymphedema may occur.

The causative agent of donovanosis is difficult to culture, and diagnosis requires direct visualization of bipolar-staining (safety pin–shaped) intracytoplasmic inclusion bodies, called Donovan bodies, on tissue crush preparation or biopsy. Polymerase chain reaction has been used successfully to identify the organism, but this technique is not readily available.

TREATMENT

Recommended (CDC 2002) first line treatment includes one of the following:

- **Doxycycline** (Vibramycin, Doryx, Monodox) 100 mg orally twice a day
- **Trimethoprim-sulfamethoxazole** (Bactrim DS, Septra DS)* 160 mg/800 mg tablet orally twice a day

Alternative regimens include one of the following:

- **Ciprofloxacin** (Cipro)* 750 mg orally twice a day
- **Erythromycin** base (E-Mycin, Ery-Tab, Eryc)* 500 mg orally four times a day
- **Azithromycin** (Zithromax)* 1 g orally once per week

The treatment should be continued for at least 3 weeks or until all lesions have completely healed. Addition of aminoglycoside (e.g., gentamycin 1 mg/kg intravenously every 8 hours) to the above regimens has been recommended by some specialists for complicated cases. Surgical intervention may be necessary to correct scarring and fibrosis resulting from long-standing disease. Pregnant women should be treated with the erythromycin regimen and consideration should be given to the addition of a parenteral aminoglycoside. Azithromycin may prove to be useful in pregnant women but published data are lacking. Patients with granuloma inguinale and HIV infection should receive the same regimens as those who are HIV negative; parenteral aminoglycoside should be strongly considered.

*Not FDA approved for this indication.

LYMPHOGRANULOMA VENEREUM

method of
NANCY J. ANDERSON M.D., and
AGNIESZKA NIEMEYER M.D.
Loma Linda University
Loma Linda, California

Lymphogranuloma venereum (LGV) is an uncommon, systemic, sexually transmitted disease caused by the L1, L2, or L3 serotypes of the obligate intracellular organism, *Chlamydia trachomatis*. The disease is epidemic in parts of Africa, Asia, and South America but uncommon in the United States. Acute disease is more commonly seen in men, whereas women mostly present with late complications of the disease.

The course of the disease in LGV consists of three separate stages. The first stage starts after the incubation period of 3 to 30 days as a small, painless, eroded papule or pustule on the genital or rectal mucous membranes. The lesion typically heals within 1 week and goes unnoticed by the affected person. The second stage begins within 2 to 6 weeks later and consists of unilateral, painful inguinal and/or femoral lymph nodes. These painful lymph nodes, known as buboes, may become fluctuant and rupture or may develop into hard, nonsuppurative masses. The affected lymph nodes are often situated above and below Paupart's ligament, giving rise to the "grove" sign. In women the deep pelvic lymph nodes may be involved, which may produce symptoms of lower abdominal or back pain. In the second stage, systemic symptoms such as fever, chills, malaise, and arthralgia are common. Systemic spread of *C. trachomatis* may lead to arthritis, pneumonitis, hepatitis, and rarely, to pulmonary infection, cardiac involvement, aseptic meningitis, or ocular inflammatory disease. The third stage of untreated LGV consists of various combinations of anogenital fistulas, rectal strictures, perirectal abscesses, chronic perineal lymphatic obstruction, fibrosis, and genital elephantiasis. Rarely, adenocarcinoma has been reported as a complication of long-standing LGV disease.

The diagnosis of LGV is made by clinical presentation and by complement-fixation test titer of 1:64 or greater. Although serologic testing is only genus specific, complement-fixation titers from other chlamydial infections are rarely over 1:16. Immunofluorescent testing and polymerase chain reaction analysis has been used for diagnosis of LGV, but these methods are not readily available.

TREATMENT

The treatment recommended by the Centers for Disease Control and Prevention (2002) is doxycycline (Vibramycin, Doryx, Monodox) 100 mg orally twice a day. Alternative treatment, which is preferred for pregnant women, is erythromycin base (E-Mycin, Ery-Tab, Eryc) 500 mg orally four times a day. Treatment should be given for 21 days or until lesions are healed. Some STD specialists believe that azithromycin (Zithromax)* 1.0 g orally once weekly for 3 weeks is likely effective, but clinical data are lacking. Fluctuant lymph nodes should be aspirated to prevent tissue breakdown and the formation of chronic draining sinuses. In patients with strictures and fistulas, reconstructive surgery may be necessary. Persons with LGV and HIV infection should receive the same regimens as those who are HIV-negative. Prolonged therapy may be required.

Persons who had sexual contact with a patient who has LGV within 30 days before the onset of the patient's symptoms should be examined and tested for evidence of chlamydial infection and treated. Patients with LGV should be screened for other sexually transmitted diseases and should receive counseling and serologic testing for HIV.

*Not FDA approved for this indication.

SYPHILIS

method of
CHARLES HICKS, M.D.
Duke University Medical Center
Durham, North Carolina

Syphilis is an infection caused by the spirochete *Treponema pallidum,* and it may have both acute and chronic manifestations. The clinical expression of syphilis is notoriously protean, and in any one individual it occurs in different stages over time. The vast majority of cases are transmitted sexually, although it may also be transmitted vertically from an infected woman to her newborn child. Early syphilis is a reportable infection in the United States, and therefore statistics on the incidence of new infection are relatively accurate. In the late 1980s and early 1990s, a mini-epidemic of early syphilis occurred and ultimately produced case rates that were higher than at any time since the introduction of penicillin. The number of cases peaked in 1990 (20.3 cases per 100,000 population) and has fallen consistently since then, with an all-time low of 2.5 cases per 100,000 people noted in 1999. New cases of syphilis have been concentrated in a relatively small number of counties, a feature that led to hope that eradication of syphilis might be feasible. Unfortunately, recent outbreaks in a variety of different populations suggest that eradication is probably unlikely.

CLINICAL MANIFESTATIONS

Syphilis is classically divided into stages based on clinical manifestations and time from acquisition of the organism. The initial stage is referred to as primary syphilis and represents local infection at the site of inoculation of the organism. After an average incubation period of 2 to 3 weeks, a papule appears at this site of inoculation and is typically painless. The papule soon ulcerates to produce the classic chancre of primary syphilis, a 1- to 2-cm ulcer with a raised, indurated margin. Regional lymphadenopathy may be present. Chancres heal spontaneously within 3 to 6 weeks even in the absence of treatment. Because the ulcer is painless, many patients do not seek medical attention, thereby enhancing the likelihood of transmission.

Although a chancre is an initial local infection with *T. pallidum,* syphilis becomes systemic very quickly. Widespread dissemination of the spirochete occurs during the primary stage of the infection. Weeks to a few months later, a systemic illness that represents secondary syphilis will develop in approximately 25% of individuals with untreated infection. Patients with secondary syphilis may not have a history of a preceding chancre because the primary infection may have been asymptomatic or gone unnoticed. Secondary syphilis can produce a wide variety of symptoms, including a generalized rash (often involving the palms and soles), fever, generalized lymphadenopathy, malaise, patchy alopecia, aseptic meningitis, and uveitis, among others. It is this wide array of manifestations that has given syphilis its reputation as the "great imitator."

If syphilis is not diagnosed during this period, the infection may become clinically quiescent, a property referred to as latency. Latent syphilis refers to the period during which patients infected with *T. pallidum* have no symptoms but have infection demonstrable by serologic testing. Based on the likelihood of spontaneous clinical mucocutaneous relapse, this period has classically been separated into two categories: early latent and late latent syphilis. Patients in the early latent period are believed to be potentially infectious, in contrast to late latency, when transmission is no longer probable.

Because of data suggesting that a response to therapy during latent syphilis may require differing approaches, the U.S. Public Health Service (USPHS) has modified this definition by categorizing early latent syphilis as infection of 1 year's duration or less. All other cases are referred to as late latent syphilis or latent syphilis of unknown duration. The USPHS recommends a longer duration of therapy for patients with late latent syphilis based on the notion that the biology of the spirochete evolves over time. In late latent syphilis, *T. pallidum* is thought to have a slower metabolism and a more prolonged dividing time, thus requiring a longer duration of therapy.

Late or tertiary syphilis is defined as the stages of syphilis that occur after primary and secondary or latent syphilis. It typically involves the central nervous system (CNS), cardiovascular system, or the skin and subcutaneous tissues. Late syphilis can arise as early as 1 year after initial infection or up to 25 to 30 years later.

DIAGNOSIS

Irrespective of its stage, the diagnosis of syphilis is complicated by the fact that the organism cannot be cultivated in vitro. Thus, indirect methods of diagnosis are required. The chancre of primary syphilis is best diagnosed by darkfield microscopy, whereas later stages of syphilis are usually diagnosed by serologic testing (VDRL [Venereal Disease Research Laboratory] or RPR [rapid plasma reagin]). Serologic tests are also useful in assessing response to treatment. The diagnosis of neurosyphilis is made by examination of cerebrospinal fluid (CSF). A reactive CSF VDRL is diagnostic of neurosyphilis, but in some cases, the diagnosis is based on an otherwise unexplained CSF pleocytosis in the setting of reactive serum syphilis serology.

TREATMENT

Treatment of syphilis requires prolonged courses of antibiotics because *T. pallidum* divides slowly, an average of one doubling in vivo per day. The organism remains highly sensitive to penicillin, and no resistance has been reported to date, although sensitivity tests are rarely performed because the organism cannot be cultivated in vitro. Long-acting depot penicillin preparations have proved very successful in treating the early and late stages of syphilis. A single dose of benzathine penicillin G (Bicillin L-A), 2.4 million U intramuscularly (IM), provides low but persistent serum levels of penicillin and is standard therapy for all forms of early syphilis, by which is meant infection of less than 1 year's duration. For patients with latent syphilis, a single dose of benzathine penicillin as therapy is therefore only appropriate when it is possible to document that the patient had nonreactive serologic findings of syphilis within the past year or if it can be well documented that the patient had a chancre of primary syphilis within the past year. Otherwise, the condition should be referred to as latent syphilis of unknown duration, for which three doses of benzathine penicillin are recommended (see later). Some authorities suggest that a second dose of benzathine penicillin given 1 week after the first improves the likelihood of a serologic response in patients with early syphilis, but such an effect has not been proved.

A small number of patients do not respond to this approach, as indicated by failure of serum VDRL titers to decrease at least fourfold over a 6- to 12-month follow-up period. In some cases, this failure may be due to reinfection. Such serologic treatment failures are managed by giving another course of benzathine penicillin and making sure that all sexual contacts are also treated.

Alternative treatments for patients with early syphilis who are allergic to penicillin include azithromycin (Zithromax),* 1 g given as a single dose, doxycycline, 100 mg orally (PO) twice daily for 14 days, or ceftriaxone (Rocephin),* 1 g IM daily for 10 days, but these regimens are less well studied. Pregnant patients allergic to penicillin should be advised to undergo desensitization and then receive standard penicillin treatment.

Patients with late syphilis or with latent syphilis of uncertain duration require more prolonged courses of therapy. In this setting, benzathine penicillin G remains the treatment of choice for most cases and is given at a dose of 2.4 million U IM once weekly for three doses. This therapy provides low but persistent serum levels of penicillin and is standard for all forms of late syphilis other than neurosyphilis.

*Not FDA approved for this indication.

Patients with late syphilis who are allergic to penicillin may be treated with doxycycline, 100 mg PO twice daily for 28 days, but few data on efficacy in this setting are available. Ceftriaxone, 1 g/d intravenously (IV) or IM for 10 to 14 days may also be effective, but data are limited.

Proper management of patients with proven or suspected neurosyphilis can be challenging. Early data from the 1950s suggested that benzathine penicillin might be successful in treating neurosyphilis, but two considerations have caused a revision in the initial recommendation for its use in patients with neurosyphilis. First, it is well known that administration of benzathine penicillin results in no measurable CSF levels of penicillin, and thus there is theoretical cause to worry that benzathine penicillin might not be effective in CNS infection. Second, a number of cases have been reported in which symptomatic neurosyphilis subsequently developed in those with early syphilis who were treated with benzathine penicillin. In some instances, viable *T. pallidum* organisms were demonstrated in CSF after therapy. Consequently, treatment has evolved to a shift toward the use of aqueous penicillin G, 3 to 4 million U IV every 4 hours for 10 to 14 days, for clinically manifested neurosyphilis. The same regimen is also suggested for patients strongly suspected of having late CNS syphilis because of a compatible clinical syndrome, reactive serum syphilis serology, and CSF pleocytosis, even when the CSF VDRL is nonreactive. If patients with neurosyphilis are allergic to penicillin, desensitization to penicillin (preferred) or the use of ceftriaxone,* 1 g/d IV for 10 to 14 days, is suggested.

Patients treated for neurosyphilis should have serum VDRL titers measured at 3 and 6 months and then at 6-month intervals for 2 years. Serum VDRL titers should fall at least fourfold within a year. Repeat neurologic examinations and CSF analysis

*Not FDA approved for this indication.

TABLE 1. **Recommended Treatment Regimens for Syphilis**

Type of Syphilis	Treatment of Choice	Alternative Treatment
Primary, secondary, early latent syphilis	Benzathine penicillin, 2.4 million U IM as 1 dose	Azithromycin (Zithromax)*, 1 g PO as 1 dose, *or* Doxycycline, 100 mg PO bid for 14 d, *or* Ceftriazone (Rocephin)* 1 g IM qd for 10 d
Late latent, cardiovascular, or gummatous syphilis	Benzathine penicillin, 2.4 million U IM weekly for 3 doses	Doxycycline 100 mg PO bid for 28 d, *or* Ceftriaxone*, 1 g IM or IV qd for 10–14 d
Neurosyphilis	Aqueous penicillin G, 3–4 million U IV q4h for 10–14 d	Penicillin desensitization *or* Ceftriaxone,* 1 g IV qd for 10–14 d
Syphilis in pregnancy	As listed above	If penicillin-allergic, desensitize
Congenital syphilis	Aqueous penicillin G, 50,000 U/kg IV q12h for 7 d, then q8h for 3 d to complete 10 d of therapy	If penicillin-allergic, desensitize

*Not FDA approved for this indication.

may also be used to determine the adequacy of treatment. CSF cell counts and protein should decrease over a 3-month period. Rising serum VDRL or worsening CSF parameters are indications for retreatment. Retreatment ordinarily requires 14 days of IV aqueous penicillin G. No evidence has indicated that longer courses of treatment or the use of different antibiotics changes the outcome.

Management of syphilis in pregnancy and congenital syphilis requires special expertise. Dosing in neonates must account for altered metabolism in the first days of life. Penicillin should be used in virtually all such cases (Table 1). Consultation with experts experienced in the management of congenital syphilis is recommended. Table 1 summarizes the treatment recommendations for persons with syphilis.

Section 12
Diseases of Allergy

ANAPHYLAXIS AND SERUM SICKNESS

method of
DENNIS K. LEDFORD, M.D.
*University of South Florida College of Medicine
Joy McCann Culverhouse Airway Disease
Research Center and the
James A. Haley V.A. Hospital
Tampa, Florida*

ANAPHYLAXIS

Definitions and Causes

Anaphylaxis is a systemic syndrome with variable mechanisms and clinical presentations. There is no universally accepted clinical definition. The clinical manifestations result from the release of mast cell and/or basophil-associated mediators. The severity is variable but often life threatening. The cause of death in anaphylaxis is usually either airway obstruction or cardiovascular collapse with intractable shock. The manifestations are shown in Figure 1. Urticaria and angioedema are the most frequent clinical manifestations, reported in approximately 90% of affected subjects (Table 1).

The causes of mast cell or basophil mediator release are variable, but IgE-dependent mechanisms are often assumed, i.e., specific IgE on the surface of mast cells or basophils binds to an allergen, such as a drug or food, triggering release of mediators. Some authors use the term anaphylactoid to describe anaphylaxis without evidence of specific IgE. An example of an anaphylactoid reaction is a radiocontrast reaction. The clinical features are indistinguishable from anaphylaxis but the cause of mediator release is a physical effect of radiocontrast media, most likely osmolarity or ionic strength. Another example of non-IgE dependent anaphylaxis is a blood transfusion reaction in which complement is activated without specific IgE recognition of antigens in the blood. In this article, the term *anaphylaxis* will be used to refer to both anaphylaxis and anaphylactoid reactions because the treatments are identical. Agents responsible for anaphylaxis are listed in Table 2.

Diagnosis

Anaphylaxis is often apparent because the episode is rapid in onset and incapacitating. If anaphylaxis is suspected, assessment of the cardiovascular system, particularly documentation of blood pressure and pulse, followed by evaluation of the respiratory tract is essential. Documentation of the cardiovascular and respiratory examinations is particularly important as anaphylactic death is usually due to cardiovascular or respiratory failure. Cutaneous features are almost invariably present; therefore a careful skin examination is useful. Generalized urticaria associated with anxiety or hyperventilation syndrome, globus hystericus, laryngospasm, or vasovagal reactions are commonly confused with anaphylaxis. Vasovagal reactions are usually characterized by diaphoresis and cool, clammy skin coupled with bradycardia. Anaphylaxis, in contrast, is usually associated with erythematous skin and tachycardia, although bradycardia rarely occurs. Brachycardia is common in subjects receiving β-blocker therapy prior to the onset of anaphylaxis. The differential diagnosis of anaphylaxis is summarized in Table 3. Rapid recognition of anaphylaxis is essential because the prognosis improves with prompt intervention.

Laboratory diagnosis is generally of limited value because treatment must be initiated while awaiting test results, but confirmation may be of value in post-event assessment. Blood or urine histamine measurements are generally not helpful owing to the short half-life of histamine. Plasma histamine is increased for approximately 30 to 60 minutes after onset of anaphylaxis. A mast cell proteinase, tryptase, has a longer half-life. Tryptase concentrations peak 1 to $1^1/_2$ hours after onset of anaphylaxis, and detectable tryptase persists for 5 hours or more. Measuring serum tryptase concentrations and specific IgE to a suspected cause (such as a penicillin or insect venom) may be of value in confirming suspected anaphylaxis as a cause of death.

Recurrent and Persistent Anaphylaxis

Anaphylaxis is an acute syndrome and generally resolves within one to two hours. Biphasic anaphylaxis, with recurrences 8 to 12 hours after the initial event, occurs in 5% to 20% of affected individuals. The timing of the recurrence is similar to the late-phase response described with mast cell degranulation following allergen challenge of the respiratory tract or skin. The manifestations of biphasic anaphylaxis are identical to acute anaphylaxis. There are no

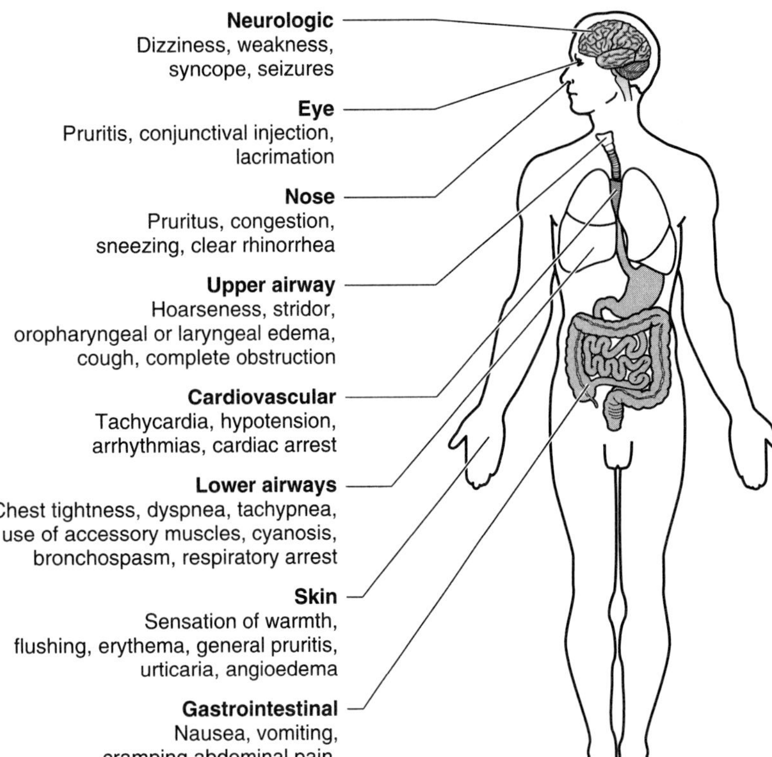

Figure 1. The manifestations of anaphylaxis.

distinguishing features that predict the likelihood of biphasic anaphylaxis, with the exception of one report describing that initial episodes in biphasic anaphylaxis, compared to uniphasic anaphylaxis, require larger dosages of epinephrine for symptom control. Prolonged anaphylaxis, lasting from 5 to 32 hours, also occurs. The frequency of prolonged anaphylaxis is highly variable according to the literature, varying from less than 1% to approximately 25%. The prevalence probably approximates the lower figure. The possibilities of biphasic and prolonged anaphylaxis should be considered when affected subjects are being discharged from observation. Observation of treated subjects for up to 24 hours may be indicated to recognize delayed or persistent symptoms and minimize risk. Administration of systemic glucocorticosteroid

TABLE 1. **Frequency of Occurrence of Signs and Symptoms of Anaphylaxis**

Signs/Symptoms	Prevalence %
Urticaria and angioedema	85–90
Dyspnea, wheeze	40–50
Dizziness, syncope, hypotension	30–35
Nausea, vomiting, diarrhea, cramping, abdominal pain	30–35
Flush	45–50
Upper airway edema (angioedema)	50–69
Headache	15
Rhinitis	15–20
Substernal pain	6
Itch without rash	5
Seizure	1–2

TABLE 2. **Agents That Cause or Are Associated with Anaphylaxis**

IgE Dependent

Foods (particularly peanut, tree nut, fish, shellfish, seeds)
Medications
Insect venoms
Latex
Allergen vaccines (immunotherapy)
Hormones
Animal or human proteins
Coloring agents derived from animals (e.g., carmine)
Enzymes
Polysaccharides
Exercise following ingestion of specific food or medications
Protamine (used to reverse anticoagulation following surgery)

Non-IgE Dependent

Radiocontrast media
Angiotensin-converting enzyme inhibitor therapy with renal dialysis
Ethylene oxide exposure via gas adsorbed to dialysis tubing
Opioids
Muscle relaxants (may be IgE dependent)
Idiopathic
Exercise
Physical factors (cold, heat)
Nonsteroidal anti-inflammatory drugs

Complement Mediated

Intravenous immunoglobulin
Dextran
Blood transfusion reactions
Renal dialysis

TABLE 3. **Differential Diagnosis of Anaphylaxis**

Vasodepressor or Vasovagal Reactions
Flush Syndromes
Carcinoid
Postmenopausal
Chlorpropamide (Diabinese) and alcohol
Medullary carcinoma of thyroid
Autonomic epilepsy
Restaurant Syndromes
Monosodium glutamate ingestion
Metabisulfite ingestion or inhalation
Scrombroidosis (increased histamine in fish due to spoilage)
Other Forms of Shock
Hemorrhagic
Cardiogenic
Endotoxic or septic
Excess Endogenous Production of Histamine
Systemic mastocytosis
Urticaria pigmentosa (cutaneous mastocytosis)
Basophilic leukemia
Acute promyelocytic leukemia (tretinoin treatment)
Functional Syndromes
Panic attacks
Hyperventilation syndrome
Munchausen's stridor
Vocal cord dysfunction syndrome
Globus hystericus
Somatoform disorder
Miscellaneous
Hereditary angioedema
Urticarial vasculitis
Pheochromocytoma
Episodic angioedema with eosinophilia
Seizure
Stroke
Red man syndrome following vancomycin (Vancocin) administration
Capillary leak syndrome

therapy during the initial episode may minimize the likelihood of biphasic or persistent anaphylaxis.

Treatment

Treatment of anaphylaxis is optimized by prompt recognition of the syndrome, because survival correlates with time between onset of symptoms and administration of epinephrine (Figure 2). Antihistamine therapy, either oral or parenteral, is not life-saving. Therefore, the first priority is assessment of the probability of anaphylaxis and, if anaphylaxis is suspected, administration of intramuscular (IM) epinephrine 1:1000 0.05–0.5 mL (0.01 mg/kg in children; maximum dose, 0.3 mg). Intramuscular administration of epinephrine, compared to subcutaneous administration, results in more rapid and greater concentration of plasma epinephrine. The preferable site of administration is the lateral thigh in adults because the depth of the subcutaneous fat is generally less than in other sites such as the deltoid. The affected subject should be closely observed and frequently reassessed with repeat administration of epinephrine every 5 minutes if necessary. In the event of rapid onset of severe hypotension, intravenous (IV) epinephrine is an option. This may be prepared by mixing 0.1–0.3 mL 1:1000 aqueous epinephrine in 10 mL of normal saline and infusing by slow push over several minutes. Another consideration in a desperate situation would be to place 0.1 ml of 1:1000 aqueous epinephrine in a syringe, aspirate 0.9 mL of blood via an IV access and inject the mixture over several minutes.* IV epinephrine has resulted in death from ventricular arrhythmia, but the decision to employ this therapy is based upon risk assessment of shock.

The airway should be assessed while the cardiovascular manifestations are treated. Oxygen should be administration at 4 to 8 L/minute. Angioedema of the upper airway may necessitate early oral-tracheal or naso-tracheal intubation, prior to swelling of sufficient severity to obstruct the airway. Tracheostomy may be necessary if angioedema obstructs the upper airway. More commonly, wheezing develops and should be treated aggressively, both with epinephrine and nebulized albuterol (Ventolin, Proventil) 2.5 to 5 mg in 3 mL saline. Levalbuterol (Xopenex) 0.63–1.25 mg in unit dose ampules may be considered if tachyarrhythmia is a concern following parenteral epinephrine. IV aminophylline,* 5 mg/kg over 30 minutes, is another consideration for intractable wheezing. Aminophylline is associated with significant risk of toxicity, and dosage should be adjusted for prior theophylline therapy. There are no data justifying the use of oral leukotriene therapy in acute anaphylaxis, but there is a rationale for its use. Leukotrienes are produced and released by mast cells and basophils following activation. Oral leukotriene therapy is associated with a minimal bronchodilation during the first few hours after administration. Leuktotrienes cause intravascular leakage, potentially contributing to the vascular volume depletion and hypotension of anaphylaxis. Finally there are minimal or no side-effects associated with administration of one oral dose of montelukast (Singular)* 10 mg or zafirlukast (Accolate)* 10 to 20 mg.

If hypotension does not respond to the initial therapy, large-bore venous access should be established with administration of several liters of colloid as rapidly as possible. The large volume of colloid is necessary because of intravascular volume depletion due to vascular leakage. Antihistamine therapy, both H1-inhibitors such as diphenhydramine (Benadryl), 50 mg or 5 mg/kg in children, and H2-inhibitors such as ranitidine (Zantac),* 50 mg in adults and 1 mg/kg in children, is helpful but not life saving. Antihistamine therapy may minimize hypotension. Vasopressor therapy, such as dopamine (Intropin) 400 mg in 500 mL of 5% dextrose in water administered at a rate of 2 to 20 μg/kg/minute, is indicated for hypotension refractory to IV colloid and epinephrine. Subjects treated with β-blocker therapy are particularly at risk for intractable hypotension during anaphylaxis. In this situation, IV glucagon* may be of value, this therapy

*Not FDA approved for this indication.

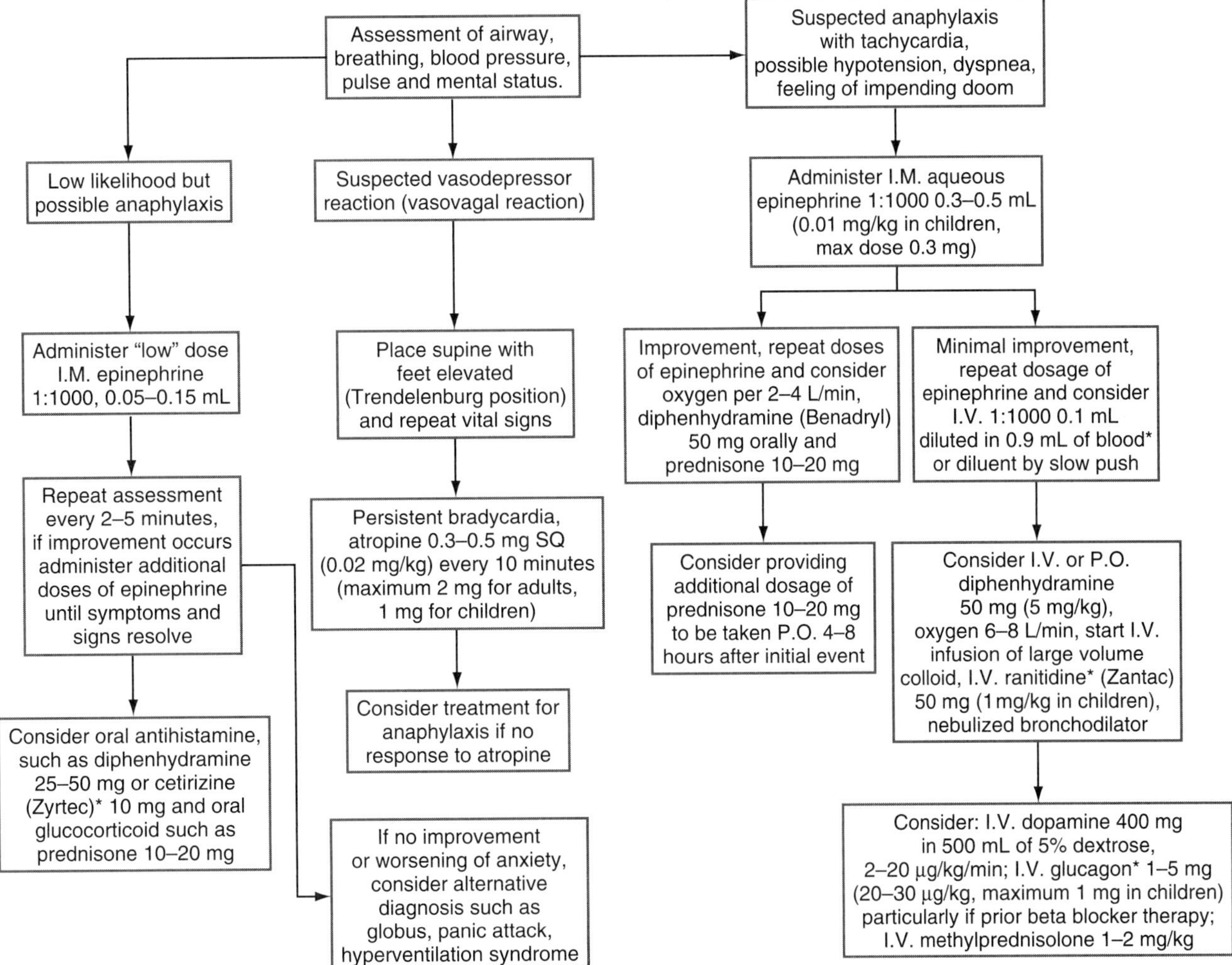

Figure 2. Treatment of anaphylaxis.

increases cyclic AMP through a mechanism not dependent on the β-receptor. One to 5 mg of glucagon is administered over 5 minutes, followed by an infusion of 5 to 15 μg/minute. The dosage in children is 20 to 30 μg/kg to a maximum of 1 mg. IV glucagon often results in nausea with risk for vomiting and aspiration.

Oral or IV glucocorticosteroid therapy is not helpful for the management of acute anaphylaxis. Glucocorticosteroid therapy may be useful in minimizing biphasic or persistent anaphylaxis. Therefore, oral prednisone 20 to 50 mg (0.5–1 mg/kg) or IV methylprednisolone (Solumedrol) 1 to 2 mg/kg is reasonable. Subjects discharged from observation after immediate response to treatment may benefit from an additional dose of oral prednisone to be administered 4 to 8 hours after the initial event. This additional glucocorticosteroid may minimize delayed reactions.

Some authors have recommended administering small doses of epinephrine at the site of a sting or medication injection responsible for anaphylaxis. The rationale is to reduce blood flow to the site of allergen deposition and delay absorption. No studies have confirmed that this is beneficial, but the practice is reasonable. Tourniquets applied between the heart and the source of allergen, such as insect venom in an extremity, have also been suggested. Care should be taken not to cause ischemia of the affected area.

Identification of the cause of anaphylaxis is essential to prevent future episodes. Testing, particularly by the skin test method, should be delayed for 4 to 6 weeks because the tests are falsely negative immediately following anaphylaxis. In vitro testing (CAP assay or RAST) is another consideration, particularly with food allergens. Skin testing with peanut or other highly potent food allergens or latex in allergic subjects may result in anaphylaxis. For these allergens, in vitro testing is preferred initially. Medical warning bracelets or necklaces are recommended to facilitate future recognition of sensitivity. Epinephrine should be prescribed for self-treatment of subsequent episodes. Autoinjectors, such as EpiPen 0.3 mg or EpiPen Jr 0.15 mg, facilitate rapid administration by affected subjects.

SERUM SICKNESS

Definitions and Etiology

Serum sickness and *serum sickness–like disorder* are terms used inconsistently. The pathophysiologic syndrome described by these terms is the constellation of symptoms and findings described to occur five to twelve days after therapeutic use of foreign proteins. Historically these proteins were used as antitoxins, as in the treatment of diphtheria with horse serum. The majority of current cases are due to antibiotics, although animal-derived antisera are still used for treatment of snake bites, spider bites, and scorpion stings. Animal antisera are also used in immunomodulator therapy such as antilymphocyte globulin to control renal transplant rejection. Potential causes of serum sickness are listed in Table 4.

The histologic appearance of affected blood vessels in serum sickness is that of hypersensitivity vasculitis. This process usually affects postcapillary venules with immune complex deposition, complement activation, and leukocytoclastic vasculitis. The endogenous production of large quantities of antigen and specific antibody occurs in some cases of chronic hepatitis C, hepatitis B, subacute bacterial endocarditis, systemic lupus erythematosus, and rheumatoid arthritis.

TABLE 4. **Therapeutic Agents That May Cause Serum Sickness**

Proteins from Other Species	
Antitoxins	
Antivenins	
Hormones	
Monoclonal antibodies	
Streptokinase (Streptase)	
Antibiotics	
Acyclovir (Zovirax)	Streptomycin
Cephalosporins	Sulfonamide
Ciprofloxacin (Cipro)	Tetracycline
Chloramphenicol (Chloromycetin)	Trimethoprim-sulfamethoxazole (Bactrim)
Griseofulvin (Fulvicin)	Zidovudine (Retrovir)
Isoniazid (Nydrazid)	
Lincomycins (Lincocin)	
Metronidazole (Flagyl)	
Penicillins	
Other Drugs	
Acetylsalicyclic acid (Aspirin)	Hydantoins
Allopurinol (Zyloprim)	Hydrochlorothiazide
Amitriptyline (Elavil)	Ibuprofen (Motrin)
Barbiturates	Indomethacin (Indocin)
Captopril (Capoten)	Iron dextran (InFeD)
Carbamazepine (Tegretol)	Methimazole (Tapazole)
Cimetidine (Tagamet)	Phenylbutazone*
Colchicine	Procarbazine (Matulane)
Cyclophosphamide (Cytoxan)	Propranolol (Inderal)
Diltiazem (Cardizem)	Spironolactone (Aldactone)
Fluoxetine (Prozac)	Tamoxifen (Nolvadex)
Furosemide	Thiouracil (Propylthiouracil)
Gold salts	Trazodone (Desyrel)
Heparin	Warfarin (Coumadin)

*Not available in the United States.

The differential diagnosis of serum sickness includes causes of hypersensitivity vasculitis.

Clinical Manifestations

Onset of symptoms and signs usually is 7 to 10 days after antigen exposure, typically following a relatively large amount of antigen. Thus, IV infusion or tissue injection is more likely to result in serum sickness as compared with oral administration. The latent period may be as short as 2 to 7 days with a secondary antigen exposure or longer than 2 weeks with a long-acting drug such as benzathine penicillin. Fever, 39°C, or higher, is the most frequent sign and generally is present at the onset of the syndrome. Dermatologic manifestations occur in more than 90% of cases. These include urticaria, palpable purpura, and morbilliform eruptions. The findings of serum sickness following antithymocyte globulin have been carefully documented in the literature. A characteristic skin manifestation in these cases is the palmar-plantar sign, an erythematous, serpiginous lesion occurring at the juncture of the palmar or plantar skin with the dorsal skin of the hands or feet. Arthralgias, myalgias, and arthritis occur variably, with reports of less than 10% of affected subjects to 60% to 70%. Affected joints in decreasing order of frequency are knees, ankles, shoulders, wrists, lower thoracic and cervical spine, and temporomandibular joints. Renal abnormalities occur in more than 50% of subjects. Findings include microscopic hematuria, hyaline casts, hemoglobinuria, mild proteinuria, and transient increases of serum creatinine. Red blood cell casts, renal failure, or nephrotic syndrome are not typical. Other manifestations of serum sickness include lymphadenopathy, polyserositis, abdominal pain, nausea and vomiting, diarrhea, occult GI bleeding, dyspnea, and wheezing.

Laboratory abnormalities in serum sickness include elevation of acute phase reactants, such as erythrocyte sedimentation rate and C-reactive protein, leukopenia or leukocytosis, thrombocytopenia, positive immune complex assays, decrease in serum complement, abnormal urinalysis, positive rheumatoid factor, and transient elevation of liver enzymes. None of these laboratory tests are particularly sensitive or specific. A skin biopsy may be of value in confirming the diagnosis. Identification of a monoclonal protein, antineutrophil cytoplasmic antibody (ANCA), or pauci-immune vasculitis (lack of immune complex deposition) should prompt a search for an alternative diagnosis.

Treatment

Elimination of the causal drug or source of antigen results in resolution in more than 90% of cases. If the drug or antiserum is lifesaving, the serum sickness syndrome may be treated and the causal agent continued. Increased amount of the causal antigen increases the likelihood of more severe serum sickness. Therefore, minimizing dosage may permit continued therapy without inordinate risk. Specific antibiotic or antiviral therapy is the primary treatment for serum sickness related to infection, such as subacute bacterial endocarditis or chronic active hepatitis.

The symptoms of serum sickness may be relieved with a variety of treatments, but pharmaceutical therapy rarely affects the final outcome. Antihistamines are useful in controlling urticaria or pruritus associated with morbilliform eruptions. Nonsteroidal anti-inflammatory drugs alleviate fever, joint inflammation, and myalgias. Parenteral or oral glucocorticosteroid therapy effectively minimizes symptoms and signs and is a consideration for severe disease, particularly if the urinary sediment is abnormal or renal function is impaired. Suggested dosage is 0.5 to 2 mg/kg/d of prednisone or equivalent for 5 to 10 days. Glucocorticosteroid therapy does not prevent serum sickness; therefore, pretreatment in high risk situations is not indicated. Reports in the medical literature describe limited or questionable benefits from a variety of additional drugs. These include oral dapsone* 25 to 100 mg/d, pentoxifylline (Trental)* 400 mg three times daily, and colchicine* 0.5 mg twice daily. Immunosuppressive therapy is not indicated except for severe renal insufficiency. Significant renal impairment suggests an alternative diagnosis, such as microscopic polyarteritis.

Subjects with a history of serum sickness are at increased risk of more rapid, severe disease if the causal agent is reintroduced. Every effort should be made to avoid repeat exposure.

*Not FDA approved for this indication.

ASTHMA IN ADOLESCENTS AND ADULTS

method of
KRZYSZTOF KOWAL, M.D.
Brigham and Women's Hospital
Boston, Massachusetts

and

LAWRENCE DUBUSKE, M.D.
University Medical School of Bialystok
Bialystok, Poland

Bronchial asthma affects more than 17 million Americans. Asthma can appear at any age, but most patients experience asthma before they are 30 years old. Despite great effort in attempting to apply more effective treatment of asthma, the prevalence as well as mortality caused by this chronic disease has been increasing. In this article, several essential issues concerning the diagnosis and treatment of bronchial asthma are discussed to facilitate better cooperation between general practitioners and allergy specialists to achieve optimal patient care.

Bronchial asthma is an inflammatory disease of the airways that is clinically characterized by attacks of breathlessness, coughing, and wheezing. Airway obstruction and bronchial hyper-reactivity underlie this clinical syndrome. Not only constriction of bronchial smooth muscle but also edema of bronchial mucosa and increased mucus production are responsible for the increased airway resistance. Several histologic changes are found in the bronchial wall of asthmatic patients: desquamation of bronchial epithelium; infiltration of the mucosa with inflammatory cells, including activated T cells and eosinophils; and in chronic, advanced disease, basement membrane thickening with collagen deposition. The latter changes are irreversible and may be responsible for loss of the ability of the constricted airways to fully respond to bronchodilatory treatment.

EVALUATION

Appropriate management of asthma requires proper evaluation, including correct diagnosis and staging of the severity of the disease and determination of the factors precipitating bronchospasm.

Diagnosis

The diagnosis of asthma is often made on the basis of a typical history that includes attacks of abrupt dyspnea with a dry, nonproductive cough and wheezing. Symptoms are not exacerbated during exercise, although in patients with exercise-induced bronchoconstriction, they usually appear 5 to 10 minutes after exercise. In many patients, asthma attacks occur at night, usually between 3 and 6 AM. One of the characteristic features of bronchial asthma is its reversibility, which occurs spontaneously or after treatment. Accordingly, at the time of physical examination in a physician's office, no abnormalities might be found. Similarly, lung function test results that are within normal limits do not exclude the diagnosis. Spirometry is considered the gold standard for both diagnosis and evaluation of the severity of bronchial asthma, as well as determination of response to medication. The parameter that is most useful in evaluating asthma patients is forced expiratory volume within the first second (FEV_1). In disciplined patients, serial measurement of the peak expiratory flow rate (PEFR) with a portable peak flowmeter may provide an objective determination of lung function, especially when exposure to certain substances is considered to be a precipitating factor, as occurs with occupational asthma. Asthma should always be differentiated from other upper and lower respiratory diseases, including laryngeal dysfunction and infiltrative lung disease. In older patients, especially smokers, cardiac failure, chronic obstructive pulmonary disease, and airway tumors should always be considered in the differential diagnosis.

Classification of Asthma Severity

According to the guidelines of the American Academy of Allergy, Asthma, and Immunology, asthma management should be adjusted to the severity of the disease. Classification criteria are based on patient symptoms and include the frequency of asthma attacks and nocturnal symptoms, as well as objective measures of lung function, including FEV_1 (Table 1). This evaluation is restricted to nontreated patients. For patients already receiving therapy for asthma, a good alternative for assessing the severity of disease is to record the frequency of bronchodilator use, the daily dosage of inhaled corticosteroids, or the requirement for oral corticosteroids.

Precipitating Factors

Bronchoconstriction can be induced by a broad spectrum of specific and nonspecific factors, including allergens, respiratory tract infections, gastroesophageal reflux, drugs, SO_2, and cold air.

Allergens. Aeroallergens are responsible for most cases of allergen-induced bronchoconstriction, with food allergens only rarely inducing asthma attacks in adults. In asthmatic patients, the allergens most frequently precipitating bronchoconstriction are dust mites, mold, cockroaches, and animal dander. Moreover, sensitization to dust mite allergens during childhood positively correlates with the development of asthma later in life. In certain occupations, allergen exposure may be related to the workplace. Exposure to seasonal allergens is also associated with an increase in airway responsiveness. Currently, the most reliable approach for evaluating the role of individual allergens in the asthmatic process consists of a carefully taken history, physical examination, and skin prick testing using the aeroallergens most commonly encountered in the geographic area or workplace. In patients who cannot be tested by skin prick, the use of in vitro blood tests to search for the presence of IgE antibodies to a screening panel of aeroallergen is a good alternative. Identification of allergens that are crucial for the development of asthma symptoms is necessary for effective allergen avoidance and for formulation of specific immunotherapy.

Respiratory Tract Infections. Both upper and lower respiratory tract infections in asthma patients have been shown to be among the most common causes of asthma exacerbation, and the exacerbation is often reflected as a progressive increase in asthma symptom intensity, decrease in FEV_1, and increase in bronchial reactivity to nonspecific agents. With time, untreated respiratory tract infections may be associated with significant impairment in lung function and the subsequent necessity for hospital admission or even intensive care treatment. Even mild upper respiratory tract symptoms such as rhinorrhea may precede severe asthma exacerbation. Moreover, other more subtle symptoms may indicate the presence of infection, such as frontal headaches connected with sinusitis, which may induce loss of control of asthma symptoms. Among infectious agents, rhinoviruses have been shown to be the most commonly associated with asthma exacerbation. More than a hundred distinct antigen serotypes of these viruses have been identified, thus making the possibility of an effective vaccine highly improbable.

Gastroesophageal Reflux. Aspiration of microparticles within the acidic contents of the stomach can result in a persistent cough even in otherwise healthy persons. These irritants can trigger severe bronchoconstriction in asthma patients. Moreover, if not treated, gastroesophageal reflux may precipitate asthma attacks that are resistant to the action of anti-inflammatory medications such as inhaled corticosteroids. Interestingly, β_2-agonists, theophylline (Slo-Phyllin), and anticholinergics aggravate gastroesophageal reflux. Therefore, all patients who report heartburn or regurgitation should be evaluated for the presence of gastroesophageal reflux.

Foods and Additives. In adults, food is rarely involved in IgE-mediated bronchoconstriction. Most of the reported asthma attacks associated with food ingestion are caused by food preservatives such as sodium metabisulfate. Up to 10% of asthma patients react with bronchospasm to the ingestion of sulfite,

TABLE 1. **Classification of Asthma Severity**

	Clinical Features Before Treatment		
Asthma Severity	***Symptom Severity***	***Nighttime Symptoms***	***Lung Function Parameters***
Severe persistent	Continual symptoms Limited physical activity Frequent exacerbations	Frequent	FEV_1 or PEFR ≤60% of predicted PEFR variability >30%
Moderate persistent	Daily symptoms Exacerbations ≥2 times/wk	>1 time/wk	FEV_1 or PEFR between 60% and 80% of predicted PEFR variability >30%
Mild persistent	Symptoms >2 times/wk but <1 time/d	>2 times/mo	FEV_1 or PEFR ≥80% of predicted PEFR variability 20–30%
Mild intermittent	Symptoms ≤2 times/wk Asymptomatic between exacerbations	≤2 times/mo	FEV_1 or PEFR ≥80% of predicted PEFR variability <20%

Abbreviations: FEV_1, forced expiratory volume in the first second; PEFR, peak expiratory flow rate.

which is often used as a preservative in wine, beer, dried fruit, and salad bars.

Drugs. Practically any drug can induce allergic reactions, including bronchoconstriction. Aspirin and other nonsteroidal anti-inflammatory drugs are the most common asthma-precipitating medications. Especially in patients with nasal polyps, asthma associated with severe bronchospasm can often occur on exposure to nonsteroidal anti-inflammatory drugs. Other drugs that relatively commonly induce or exacerbate bronchoconstriction in asthma patients are β-adrenergic blockers. Angiotensin-converting enzyme inhibitors can induce coughing, sometimes associated with upper airway angioedema.

Nonspecific Stimuli. Several chemical substances such as SO_2 can induce bronchospasm via nonspecific irritation of bronchial receptors. Similarly, abnormal constriction of airways in response to histamine and methacholine is characteristic of bronchial asthma. These substances are commonly used in nonspecific bronchial provocation tests to evaluate the degree of airway reactivity. In addition, physical stimuli such as exercise and inhalation of cold, dry air often trigger bronchospasm in asthma patients.

MANAGEMENT

Management of asthma patients consists of three approaches: (1) the most important—avoidance of precipitating factors, (2) pharmacotherapy, and (3) specific immunotherapy. A stepwise approach to asthma treatment is recommended. With the understanding that asthma is a chronic disease, it is essential to precisely adjust therapy according to the severity of the asthma to achieve optimal control of the disease and to minimize the risk of any adverse effects of medications.

Allergen Avoidance

To cost-effectively manage asthma, allergen avoidance measures should be undertaken after definitive recognition of an allergen as a factor precipitating asthma attacks. Usually, skin prick testing or detection of allergen-specific IgE in the blood of asthma patients in combination with a typical history is essential for evaluation of the role of individual allergens in triggering bronchoconstriction.

House Dust Mites. Dust mites are the allergens most commonly associated with an allergic asthmatic reaction. Dust mites require a warm humid climate for optimal reproductive conditions, whereas at humidity below 50%, they have reduced survival. Typically, dry, mountain regions are practically free of dust mites. The main reservoirs for dust mites in the home are pillows, mattresses, bedding, and carpeting. Encasing mattresses and pillows with dust-impermeable covers and washing bedding weekly in hot water (>130°F), as well as reduction of indoor humidity to below 50%, are essential to significantly decrease exposure to dust mite allergen. It is also advisable to remove carpets and all upholstered furniture from the bedroom. The efficacy of acarides, which kill mites, and tannic acid sprays, which denature mite proteins, is limited by the need for frequent treatment of carpets and furniture. HEPA (high-efficiency particulate air) filters are of little value in reducing dust mite exposure because the dust mite allergens are locally, not widely, disseminated in the atmosphere. HEPA filters may, however, assist in removing cat and dog dander allergens from the home atmosphere.

Animal Allergens. The only effective measure for reducing exposure to animal dander is to remove the animals from the house, followed by intensive cleaning of the entire home environment. It has been shown that after removal of a cat from a house, even after intensive cleaning of the home, cat allergen can be detected in the environment for longer than 10 years after removal of the cat.

Mold. Investigation of potential mold exposure is especially advocated for inhabitants of old houses. A search for mold sources, especially in the basement, under sinks, in the shower stall, in the kitchen, and on walls and ceilings, is recommended. Mold elimination depends on reducing indoor humidity to below 50% to significantly reduce exposure to these allergens. Air conditioners and humidifiers may be an important source of mold allergens.

Cockroaches. Uncovered or exposed food or garbage in the house attracts cockroaches. If cockroach infestation is suspected, poison bait or traps may be used, although the best results can be achieved by commercial exterminators. Exposure to cockroach dander can occur in offices and businesses.

Other Allergens. For patients with asthma exacerbations during the pollen season, systematic review of weather forecasts, as well as pollen counts, may assist in allergen avoidance. On days with high pollen exposure, such as warm, sunny, breezy days, it may be advisable to remain indoors or in an environment with air conditioning or HEPA filtration. Similarly, for patients sensitive to smog or cold air, it is necessary to monitor weather forecasts and to keep relatively constant temperature and humidity in the home.

Pharmacotherapy

Bronchial asthma is a chronic disease. Once diagnosed, asthma should be treated in most patients as a lifetime condition. Therapeutic agents that influence the course of asthma are called control or maintenance medications. They should be used on a regular, everyday basis. Reliever medications are used "on demand" and are designed to provide quick relief whenever an asthma attack occurs. A stepwise approach to asthma treatment is recommended by the National Asthma Education and Prevention Program (NAEPP). In this approach, dosages of individual medications have to be finely tuned to the severity of the disease so that maximal benefit is achieved at minimal risk for the development of adverse medication effects. Therapy for most patients should be started at higher doses to maintain control of symptoms and to decrease bronchial hyper-reactivity and suppress airway inflammation. Subsequently, dosages are carefully tapered (step-down approach) to a minimal effective maintenance dose. If the disease progresses such that the maintenance medication is not sufficient to control the disease process, an increase in the dosage of control medications or the introduction of another maintenance medication is recommended. In practice, this step-up approach is recommended when increased symptoms, reduced ability to perform everyday tasks, or increased use of reliever medications occurs or when a gradual reduction in lung function parameters is noted.

Maintenance Therapy

Maintenance therapy includes inhaled and (if necessary) oral corticosteroids, long acting β_2-agonists, leukotriene modifiers, cromolyn (Intal), nedocromil (Tilade), and theophylline. These drugs should be taken on an everyday basis indefinitely. Every effort has been made to improve the efficacy and safety of these agents. Several new pharmaceuticals are currently under investigation, including anti-IgE and anticytokine agents (Table 2).

Inhaled Corticosteroids. Corticosteroids are the most potent anti-inflammatory medications used in bronchial asthma therapy. They improve lung function and decrease bronchial hyper-responsiveness. Topical application of corticosteroids directly to the airways significantly diminishes their adverse effects, especially the irreversible adverse effects associated with prolonged corticosteroid therapy. The effect of inhaled corticosteroids becomes clinically recognizable after approximately 1 week, whereas the maximal effect is generally seen after 4 to 8 weeks of continuous therapy. Patients usually experience fewer asthma attacks, disappearance or reduction of nocturnal symptoms, reduced need for inhaled β_2-agonists, and decreased diurnal PEFR variability. After establishing the diagnosis of bronchial asthma, the earlier inhaled corticosteroids are introduced for treatment, the greater the beneficial effect that can be achieved. Most inhaled corticosteroid preparations are effective when administered twice daily, but in many patients, asthma control can be achieved with single daily dosing. In general, it is the total daily dosage of inhaled corticosteroids rather than the frequency of administration that is crucial for a therapeutic effect. Most inhaled corticosteroids are available in the United States as metered-dose inhalers, although budesonide (Pulmicort) is delivered via a dry powder inhaler and fluticasone (Flovent) is available both as a metered-dose inhaler and as a dry powder inhaler.

Adverse side effects induced by inhaled corticosteroids can be divided into two groups: local, which are frequent but not usually serious, and systemic, which are infrequent but can be serious and irreversible. Oral candidiasis, dysphonia, and hoarseness are the most common local adverse effects. They may occur in up to 30% of patients, but this percentage can

TABLE 2. **Maintenance Therapy for Asthma**

	Long-Term Control	Quick Relief
Step 4: severe persistent	Daily medications: High dose ICS, *and* Long-acting bronchodilator (long-acting β_2-agonist or sustained-release theophylline [Theo-Dur]) A leukotriene modifier may be considered, *and* if required Oral corticosteroids	Short-acting bronchodilator: inhaled β_2-agonist as needed for symptoms
Step 3: moderate persistent	Daily medications: Either medium-dose ICS *or* low- to medium-dose ICS, *plus* Long-acting bronchodilator (long-acting β_2-agonist or sustained-release theophylline [Theo-Dur]) A leukotriene modifier may be considered If needed, medium to high-dose ICS and long-acting bronchodilator, especially for nighttime symptoms	Short-acting bronchodilator: inhaled β_2-agonist as needed for symptoms
Step 2: mild persistent	One daily medication: Either low-dose ICS, *or* Cromolyn (Intal) or nedocromil (Tilade) Sustained-release theophylline (Theo-Dur) as an alternative A leukotriene modifier may be considered	Short-acting bronchodilator: inhaled β_2-agonist as needed for symptoms
Step 1: intermittent	No daily medication	Short-acting bronchodilator: inhaled β_2-agonist as needed for symptoms
	Step-down Review treatment every 1–6 mos; gradual stepwise reduction in treatment may be possible	Step-up If control is not maintained consider a step-up

Abbreviation: ICS, inhaled corticosteroid.

be significantly reduced by using spacers and oral rinsing after each inhalation. Reflex coughing, which is dependent on the method of administration rather than the preparation itself, may occur in patients using metered-dose inhalers. Coughing can be prevented by using spacers or occasionally by premedication with β_2-agonists.

Most important systemic side effects, including adrenal suppression, osteoporosis, growth suppression, and cataracts, are relatively rare. All the newer inhaled corticosteroids are extensively metabolized by the liver, thereby reducing the swallowed portion of the drug that reaches the systemic circulation. Beclomethasone (Vanceril or Beclovent) is an exception because its first-pass hepatic metabolism is relatively low, so the swallowed part of the drug can be responsible for systemic effects. The adverse effects of corticosteroids are dose dependent. To achieve optimal control of asthma, the dosage of inhaled corticosteroids should be tapered to the lowest dose that is still effective. Tapering of corticosteroids should be careful and slow. Usually, the dose reduction should be performed step by step. To decrease the dose 50%, it is typically necessary to maintain the patient at the original dose for at least 6 to 8 weeks, assuming that an exacerbation of asthma does not occur during the initial maintenance period.

Cromolyn and Nedocromil. The main action of cromolyn and nedocromil is stabilization of mast cells and subsequent prevention of mediator release on exposure to provoking agents. Both cromolyn sodium and nedocromil are delivered by inhalation, and even though their action is characterized by mild efficacy, their safety profiles are excellent, with no systemic toxicity. These characteristics make them perfect candidates as first-line therapy for mild asthma in children and adolescents. Moreover, they can be recommended for use "as needed" in the treatment of patients with episodic asthma before anticipated exposure to bronchospasm-triggering factors, such as before exercise in exercise-induced asthma or before casual animal exposure in dander-triggered asthma. An additive effect of combination therapy with these agents and inhaled corticosteroids has been suggested by some authors, although evidence for potential steroid sparing is fragmentary. Therefore, it seems reasonable to try cromones as first-line maintenance therapy alone or in combination with low-dose inhaled steroids in those at high risk for corticosteroid-induced adverse effects, such as adolescents and postmenopausal women. The potential drawback of both cromolyn and nedocromil is the necessity to use them four times a day, which, especially in young, active, and nonregimented patients, may result in low compliance.

Leukotriene Modifiers. The leukotriene modifiers used for asthma treatment can interfere with leukotriene synthesis either by inhibiting 5-lipoxygenase, which is the main mechanism of action of zileuton (Zyflo), or by directly blocking the leukotriene D_4 receptor, which is the main target of zafirlukast (Accolate) and montelukast (Singulair). All three medications improve symptoms and pulmonary function and reduce the need for quick-relief bronchodilators. According to recommendations of the NAEPP, they should be used for the treatment of mild persistent asthma as an alternative to low-dose inhaled corticosteroids. The percentage of patients who respond to leukotriene modifiers is less than those who respond to inhaled corticosteroids. Leukotriene receptor antagonists give a smaller magnitude of benefit with respect to improvement in FEV_1 or PEFR than inhaled corticosteroids do. The maximal benefit achieved with leukotriene receptor antagonists is often noted in the first week of therapy, considerably faster than the case with inhaled corticosteroids. Data on leukotriene receptor antagonists regarding suppression of inflammation in asthma and reduction of disease progression are much less than for inhaled corticosteroids.

Combination treatment with a leukotriene receptor antagonist and an inhaled corticosteroid has been shown to have an additive effect in improving patient symptoms and lung function parameters, as well as in protection against allergen-induced bronchoconstriction. The addition of montelukast or zafirlukast to an existing high-dose inhaled corticosteroid regimen may allow dose reduction of the inhaled corticosteroid with maintenance of lung function. Montelukast (10 mg) and zafirlukast (20 mg) are administered orally once or twice daily, respectively. Zileuton (600-mg tablets) has to be taken four times a day. Approximately 3% of patients receiving zileuton have increased hepatic enzyme levels, most frequently occurring during the first 3 months of therapy, so it is recommended that alanine transaminase levels be evaluated before, once a month during the first 3 months, and every 3 months thereafter. The use of zafirlukast and montelukast has been reported in patients with Churg-Strauss syndrome, although it seems that corticosteroid withdrawal, in patients receiving these medications, rather than the leukotriene receptor antagonist was responsible for the clinical appearance of this syndrome. Several drug interactions, most importantly with warfarin (Coumadin) and theophylline, have been reported for zileuton and zafirlukast. Moreover, it must be remembered that zafirlukast should not be ingested with meals because food significantly decreases absorption of this medication.

Long-Acting β_2-Agonists. Both inhaled and oral long-acting β_2-agonists are available as adjunctive therapy for asthma. Salmeterol (Serevent) is an inhaled bronchodilator, whereas albuterol (Proventil Repetabs) is an oral bronchodilator formulated as a sustained-release tablet. Both medications provide prolonged (approximately 12 hours) bronchodilation, improvement in symptoms and lung function, and protection against factors triggering bronchospasm, which make them especially useful in the treatment of nocturnal symptoms. Salmeterol may allow a reduction in the maintenance inhaled corticosteroid dose, although it should be remembered that neither salmeterol nor albuterol can be used as a single agent for the treatment of persistent asthma. Moreover, these drugs do not provide prompt relief during an acute asthma attack and should therefore not be used instead of short-acting β_2-agonists such as inhaled albuterol to treat acute bronchospasm. Nevertheless, salmeterol twice daily has been shown to improve the therapeutic outcome of severe asthma attacks when added to a standard regimen that includes nebulization with high-dose short-acting β_2-agonists. The addition of salmeterol to an existing regimen of moderate-dose inhaled corticosteroid has been shown to be more effective in improving lung function than either the addition of montelukast or doubling the dose of inhaled corticosteroids. Several systemic side effects such as tachycardia, palpitations, anxiety, and muscle tremor are relatively common with any β_2-agonist treatment. Interestingly, these adverse effects may diminish within 2 weeks of treatment, but the bronchodilatory action is sustained. In general, inhaled long-acting β_2-agonists are associated with fewer adverse effects than oral sustained-release albuterol is, and the incidence of adverse effects can be even further reduced by the application of inhalation chambers and mouth washing after each inhalation. Long-acting β_2-agonists should be used very carefully in patients with cardiovascular problems, as well as in older patients. Recently, the combination of an inhaled long-acting β_2-agonist (salmeterol) and a corticosteroid (fluticasone) was introduced as a dry powder delivery system (Advair Diskus). It is recommended that one inhalation be taken twice daily with either of three fixed-dosage formats: salmeterol, 50 μg, plus either 100 μg fluticasone, 250 μg fluticasone, or 500 μg fluticasone. Although convenience is enhanced with this fixed-dosage combination therapy, the ability to titrate the dose of the inhaled corticosteroid is eliminated. Some recent evidence suggests that combination therapy with salmeterol and fluticasone may enhance the efficacy of fluticasone by increasing the translocation of fluticasone to the nucleus, thereby increasing its ultimate clinical effect. The relevance of this phenomenon remains to be proved.

Theophylline. Theophylline has several advantages in the treatment of bronchial asthma. Theophylline preparations are inexpensive, and many formulations are available, including continuous-release preparations that permit maintenance of a relatively constant plasma level of the drug. Moreover, several mechanisms participate in the overall beneficial effect of methylxanthines in asthma treatment. Theophylline is a strong bronchodilator, but it also has some anti-inflammatory effect. Theophylline is, however, not recommended by the NAEPP as the first line of monotherapy in bronchial asthma treatment. Theophylline stimulates respiration and improves contraction of respiratory muscles and mucociliary clearance, which makes it a particularly attractive medication for the treatment of nocturnal symptoms. Sustained-release theophylline (Theo-Dur) once daily in the evening improves asthma symptoms and lung function during the night, but it is also associated with less nocturnal oxygen desaturation than treatment with long-acting β-agonists is. Unfortunately, therapy with theophylline is limited by its narrow therapeutic range and a significant number of adverse effects, including nausea, headache, tremor, agitation, and sleeplessness. Furthermore, several factors, including age, smoking, febrile illness, and diet, can significantly influence the absorption and bioavailability of theophylline. Moreover, a significant number of drugs influence the metabolism of theophylline and result in either suboptimal or toxic blood concentrations. It is recommended that blood levels of theophylline be measured to maintain concentrations between 5 and 15 μg/mL during maintenance therapy. Special attention should be paid while prescribing theophylline for patients with cardiac disease.

Oral Corticosteroids. Asthma can usually be well controlled with inhaled corticosteroids, often in combination with long-acting β_2-agonists, theophylline, and/or leukotriene receptor antagonists. Relatively few patients truly need chronic therapy with oral corticosteroids. For such patients, the lowest possible dose should be given, preferably as one single dose on an alternate-day schedule. Short-acting oral corticosteroids are recommended to diminish the suppressive effect on adrenal function. Parenteral therapy with intramuscular corticosteroids for the treatment of chronic asthma should be avoided because of both toxicity and lack of the ability to adjust the corticosteroid dosage (Table 3).

Other Medications. Several immunosuppressive drugs, including methotrexate (Rheumatrex), cyclosporine (Neoral), intravenous immune globulin (Gamimune N), dapsone, and hydroxychloroquine (Plaquenil), have been studied in an attempt to permit a reduction in the oral corticosteroid dose in steroid-dependent asthmatics or for corticosteroid-resistant asthma. Unfortunately, these agents are associated with a high rate of toxicity and, for some, very modest efficacy, which is unacceptable in bronchial asthma treatment. Recently, promising effects have been obtained with inhaled lidocaine,* although this approach should still be considered experimental. The use of monoclonal antibodies to IgE receptor has recently been shown to allow a reduction in the oral corticosteroid dose, along with improvement in asthma symptoms and lung function, but without evidence of significant systemic adverse effects.

Quick-Relief Medications

Acute exacerbation of asthma symptoms with deterioration in lung function despite regular and appropriate use of maintenance therapy is an indication for quick-relief medications. Short-acting β_2-agonists, ipratropium bromide (Atrovent), or a brief course of oral corticosteroids should be considered for such patients.

Short-Acting β_2-Agonists. Several short-acting β_2-agonists are available, including albuterol (Proventil or Ventolin), pirbuterol (Maxair), and metaproterenol (Alupent). They cause prompt bronchodilation, usually within 5 to 10 minutes after inhalation. They are recommended as the therapy of

*Investigational drug in the United States.

TABLE 3. **Corticosteroids for the Treatment of Asthma**

Generic Name	Brand Name	Dosage Form	Dose		
			Low	*Medium*	*High*
Beclomethasone dipropionate	Beclovent, Vanceril	MDI 42 μg/puff 84 μg/puff	2–8 puffs/d 1–4 puffs/d	8–16 puffs/d 4–8 puffs/d	>16 puffs/d >8 puffs/d Max: 0.84 mg/d
Budesonide	Pulmicort Turbuhaler	DPI 200 μg/puff	2 puffs/d	4 puffs/d	8 puffs/d Max: 1.6 mg/d
Flunisolide	AeroBid	MDI 250 μg/puff	2–3 puffs/d	4–5 puffs/d	>5 puffs/d Max: 2 mg/d
Fluticasone propionate	Flovent	MDI 44 μg/puff 110 μg/puff 220 μg/puff	2–4 puffs/d — —	4–10 puffs/d 2–4 puffs/d 1–2 puffs/d	— >4 puffs/d >2 puffs/d Max: 0.88 mg/d
	Flovent Rotadisk	DPI 50 μg/puff 100 μg/puff 250 μg/puff	2–4 puffs/d 1–2 puffs/d —	— 2–4 puffs/d 1–2 puffs/d	— >4 puffs/d >2 puffs/d Max: 1 mg/d
Triamcinolone acetate	Azmacort	MDI 100 μg/puff	4–8 puffs/d	8–12 puffs/d	12 puffs/d Max: 1.6 mg/d

Abbreviations: DPI, dry powder inhaler; MDI, meter-dose inhaler.

choice for the treatment of acute asthma attacks. If the asthma attacks are mild and occur only intermittently, short-acting β_2-agonists are recommended on an "as needed" basis. For exercise-induced asthma, premedication with a short-acting β_2-agonist 15 minutes before planned exercise is advocated. It should be emphasized that for mild persistent asthma, monotherapy with β_2-agonists has not been shown to improve control of the disease. Nevertheless, short-acting β_2-agonists should be used for relief of acute symptoms in asthma patients unless otherwise contraindicated.

Anticholinergics. The main advantage of ipratropium bromide is the absence of serious adverse effects. The medication is not as effective in the treatment of acute asthma attacks, but it has an excellent safety profile and is a good alternative, especially for older patients, as well as those with cardiac disease. The bronchodilation provided by ipratropium is additive to that of inhaled β_2-agonists during asthma exacerbations. A combination of ipratropium and albuterol is available as a metered-dose inhaler (Combivent).

Oral Corticosteroids. Acute asthma exacerbations, especially moderate to severe exacerbation or attacks precipitated by viral infections, should be treated with brief courses of oral corticosteroids. In contrast to inhaled corticosteroids, oral corticosteroid therapy promptly reverses resistance to the bronchodilatory action of inhaled β_2-agonists, which often occurs during asthma exacerbations. It is recommended that a short (<10 days) course of prednisone or methylprednisolone (Medrol) be used. No tapering is necessary after a short course (<6 days) of oral corticosteroids.

ALLERGEN IMMUNOTHERAPY

In patients with allergic asthma, avoidance of allergen exposure is an important therapeutic approach. Unfortunately, many aeroallergens that precipitate asthma attacks, including house dust mites and pollen, are difficult or even impossible to avoid. Allergen-specific immunotherapy (SIT) has been shown to be clinically effective in the treatment of allergic rhinitis. In patients with bronchial asthma, especially those suffering from both allergic rhinitis and asthma, SIT has been efficacious in achieving significant improvement in lung function. SIT consists of serial subcutaneous injections of increasing doses of a relevant allergen to provide immunologic tolerance to this antigen. Both the efficacy and the prevalence of adverse effects are dose dependent, so SIT should be initiated only by skilled allergists to avoid serious adverse effects or suboptimal, ineffective treatment. Several allergens, including birch, grass, and ragweed pollen, house dust mites, and cat dander, have been extensively studied as factors precipitating asthma. It has been shown that these allergens can be effectively used in SIT to reduce asthma symptoms.

Before a patient is treated by SIT, it is necessary to demonstrate that the asthma symptoms are related to the individual allergen exposure, as well as to prove that an IgE-mediated reaction is involved in the pathogenesis of the symptoms. To fulfill the latter condition, skin prick testing should be performed with clinically relevant allergens or an assessment made to determine the presence of allergen-specific IgE in the blood by using allergen-specific IgE assays.

Although SIT is not recommended for all asthma patients, it should be considered in allergen-induced asthma patients when (1) it is difficult to control the asthma symptoms with pharmacotherapy and allergen avoidance, (2) the patient is at risk for the development of serious adverse effects from pharmacotherapy, and (3) the symptoms are present at least 4 months a year. It has been shown that better clinical improvement can be obtained with SIT in younger patients or when instituted earlier in the course of the disease. SIT is particularly cost-effective when used to modify the natural history of the disease in young patients before irreversible changes have developed.

Initial symptom improvement may require 6 to 12 months of SIT, although to achieve long-lasting improvement, SIT should be continued for at least 3 to 5 years. Local and systemic adverse effects can occur during SIT. Serious adverse effects include anaphylactic shock, which can occur during dose advancement, during periods of high allergen exposure, or during allergic rhinitis or asthma exacerbations. Anaphylaxis occurs in less than 1% of all injections, but the risk of a life-threatening anaphylactic reaction is always present, even during maintenance dosing, so SIT should be administered in facilities equipped to treat anaphylaxis. Most of the serious side effects take place within the first 30 minutes after SIT injection. Half an hour's observation after each injection in an office equipped to treat anaphylaxis, including the availability of injectable epinephrine, is a must.

The use of SIT has several contraindications, the most important of which is the absence of clinically relevant allergen sensitization. Careful and precise selection of patients is a prerequisite for successful SIT. Uncontrolled asthma, significant cardiovascular or systemic disease, and immunologic disturbances are also contraindications to SIT. Pregnancy is considered to be a relative contraindication. Initiation of immunotherapy during pregnancy is contraindicated, although maintenance treatment is allowed. Finally, patient collaboration is essential. Those who are not disciplined to come for injections on a prolonged basis are not candidates for SIT.

ASTHMA IN CHILDREN

method of
ANAND C. PATEL, M.D., and
LEONARD B. BACHARIER, M.D.
Department of Pediatrics
Division of Allergy and Pulmonary Medicine
Washington University School of Medicine and
St. Louis Children's Hospital
St. Louis, Missouri

Asthma is the most common chronic disease of childhood, affecting nearly 5 million children younger than age 18. In 1998, asthma accounted for nearly 6 million outpatient visits, more than 850,000 emergency department visits, more than 174,000 hospitalizations (more than any other disease in children), and 246 deaths, resulting in health care costs in excess of $3 billion. Asthma also accounts for more than 10 million missed school days a year. The prevalence of asthma in children increased 55% from 1980–1996, peaking at 8.2% of children ages 5 to 14 in 1995, and currently stands at approximately 6%.

In recognition of the significant cost to both patients and society that asthma exerts, the National Heart, Lung, and Blood Institute's National Asthma Education and Prevention Program (NAEPP) convened the first Expert Panel on asthma in 1989. The resulting guidelines, first released in 1991, and updated twice, most recently in 2002 (available at http://www.nhlbi.nih.gov/guidelines/asthma/index.htm), reflect and have prompted a change in the way asthma is viewed and treated. First and foremost, the guidelines focus on the recognition of asthma as an inflammatory disease of the airways and the consequent use of preventive anti-inflammatory medications, rather than on treatment of symptoms and acute exacerbations. The guidelines also provide a stepwise, severity-based model for medical management of asthma, emphasize the critical role of the patient and patient education, and highlight the importance of identification and avoidance of asthma triggers.

In this article, we review the evaluation and management of asthma in children, with a focus on the severity-based asthma therapy. In addition, we discuss topics that, in our experience, are important considerations particular to asthma in children.

DEFINITION, PATHOGENESIS, AND PATHOPHYSIOLOGY

Our understanding of asthma has progressed substantially over the last 20 years. Asthma is a multifactorial illness characterized by chronic and potentially progressive airway inflammation, which is associated with a state of airway hyperreactivity. Airway hyperreactivity is thought to be related to a combination of factors—allergic sensitization to specific allergens, increased smooth muscle mass, alterations in β-adrenergic receptor function, and in the specific case of aspirin sensitive asthma, abnormalities of the arachidonic acid pathways. The hyperreactive airway responds to a variety of stimuli through bronchoconstriction; mucus hypersecretion leading to mucus plugging; and airway edema, all of which contribute to airflow obstruction. By definition, the resulting airflow obstruction is at least partially reversible, and in the presence of either known or unknown stimuli, worsens episodically. However, the inflammation is chronic and long-term, appears to result in permanent changes in the airway (a process called airway remodeling), the significance and prevalence of which are not yet completely elucidated, but may be a factor in the progressive decline in lung function seen in asthmatics. Host factors felt to contribute to the development of asthma and to asthma severity include atopy, allergen exposure, rhinitis, sinusitis, viral infection, and gastroesophageal reflux. Environmental factors include tobacco smoke exposure (both passive and active), air pollution, psychologic factors (including stress), socioeconomic status, adherence, obesity, diet, exercise, and drugs (including aspirin [ASA] and nonsteroidal anti-inflammatory drugs).

Given the reversibility of the bronchoconstriction, asthma therapy in the past focused on relief of bronchoconstriction using bronchodilators. However, this approach did not address the underlying airway inflammation. Emerging evidence suggests that ongoing airway inflammation can lead to progressive changes in the airways of asthmatics, a process termed *airway remodeling*. Airway remodeling may be responsible for the progressive decline in forced expiratory volume in 1 second (FEV_1) of asthmatics through life, and is evident even among children with mild to moderate asthma. Baseline data from the Childhood Asthma Management Program (CAMP) cohort demonstrated that longer duration of asthma before entry into CAMP was associated with lower levels of lung function (FEV_1 and FEV_1/forced vital capacity [FVC] ratio) in children with mild to moderate asthma ages 5–12 years, independent of levels of atopy, presence of household allergens, and prior use of anti-inflammatory medications.

Wheezing in childhood is common, with nearly 50% of children experiencing at least one wheezing episode during the first 6 years of life. However, most of these children do not go on to develop chronic asthma. These are the children who appear to "outgrow their wheezing." The Tucson Children's Respiratory Study has generated a metric, the Asthma Predictive Index (API), which can assist in predicting course of wheezing in children who wheeze before age three. To have a positive API, a child must wheeze before age 3, and have either one of two major criteria, or two of three minor criteria (Table 1). Children who wheezed frequently before age 3 and had a positive API at age 3 years were 4 to 10 times more likely to have active asthma between ages 6 and 13 than children with a negative API. Even children with only one wheezing episode before age 3 were 2.6 to 5.5 times more likely to have persistent asthma if their API was positive. Thus this index can be used to guide caregivers and clinicians as to the likely course of a child's wheezing.

Other studies suggest that asthma symptoms can remit in adolescence only to return again in adulthood. In general, the amount of wheezing in early adolescence serves as a predictor of severity in early adult years, with the majority of those wheezing at age 14 continuing to wheeze at age 28. However, despite a resolution of symptoms in adolescence, many children with asthma in childhood continue to have measurable airflow obstruction on pulmonary function testing or bronchial hyperreactivity as young adults. This remission of symptoms appears to be due to an increase in airway caliber secondary to normal growth in adolescence leading to higher reserve airflow capacity such that even when diminished by the bronchoconstriction, the airway is large enough for flow to proceed without significant reduction. Persistence of childhood airway disease into adulthood is concerning because of the observed development of chronic airflow obstruction, with loss of bronchodilator response and a decline in FEV_1 over time greater in adults with asthma than in asymptomatic peers. These findings suggest that asthma, even uncomplicated by cigarette smoking, may be a precursor of a chronic obstructive pulmonary disease (COPD)-like syndrome in adults. Thus, although not known with any certainty, it seems possible that optimal treatment of childhood asthma with careful attention to both symptoms and levels of pulmonary function can improve the outcome of asthma in adulthood and decrease the possibility of development of COPD.

TABLE 1. **Asthma Predictive Index Criteria**

Major	Minor
Physician-diagnosed parental asthma	Physician-diagnosed allergic rhinitis
Physician-diagnosed eczema	Wheezing apart from colds
	Blood eosinophilia (≥4%)

Adapted from Castro-Rodriguez JA, et al: A clinical index to define risk of asthma in young children with recurrent wheezing. Am J Resp Crit Care Med 162; 1403:2000.

DIAGNOSIS

Asthma most commonly presents as wheezing, with or without cough. Cough-only presentations, termed cough-variant asthma, also exist but are less frequent. Other common presenting complaints include shortness of breath (either with or without exertion), chest tightness, and air hunger. Given the frequency with which these symptoms appear in children, it is critical to differentiate between other causes of wheeze or cough, and asthma. In younger children, wheezing is often a sign of an acute infection (classically, viral infections including bronchiolitis), or congenital anomaly in contrast to older children, where wheezing is most likely to be seen in the context of asthma. Thus, the index of suspicion for other causes of wheezing should be higher in children under age 5. Table 2 lists some conditions that can cause symptoms similar to asthma, and should be considered both in the setting of new onset symptoms and in the case of a sudden change in severity of an asthma patient's course.

TABLE 2. **Differential Diagnosis of Persistent or Recurrent Cough or Wheezing in Children**

- Extrinsic airway compression, including:
  - Vascular rings
  - Primary or metastatic malignancies in the mediastinum
  - Mediastinal lymphadenopathy secondary to infections or malignancy
- Intrinsic causes of airway narrowing or partial obstruction, including:
  - Airway tumor
  - Bronchogenic cyst
- Stridor mistaken for wheezing, with numerous causes, including:
  - Tracheomalacia, bronchomalacia, or laryngomalacia
  - Subglottic stenosis
  - Craniofacial abnormalities (i.e., choanal atresia or stenosis)
  - Upper airway foreign body
  - Tracheal webs
- Vocal cord dysfunction
- Foreign body aspiration
- Congenital heart disease
- Gastroesophageal reflux
- Rhinitis and/or sinusitis
- Cystic fibrosis
- Bronchiectasis
- Primary ciliary dyskinesia
- Asthma

EVALUATION

History

As with every patient, obtaining a complete and accurate history is critical in the evaluation of the child with recurrent episodes of cough or wheeze. Questions should cover the nature, frequency, and severity of symptoms; triggering factors; and response, or equally importantly, lack thereof to previously used therapies.

Age of onset of symptoms is likewise an important consideration, as 80% of asthmatics have first symptoms before age 5. Thus a 14-year-old presenting for the first time with wheezing and no prior history of symptoms should prompt a careful workup for other causes before asthma is diagnosed.

History should also include a review of predisposing factors such as genetics (family history of asthma or allergic disease) and environmental factors and a review of other medical conditions that are known to be associated with asthma, such as allergies, rhinitis, sinusitis, eczema, and gastroesophageal reflux. Finally, and perhaps most challenging, is obtaining history of psychosocial factors that can, in and of themselves, provoke symptoms, mimic symptoms, and interfere with adherence to the management plan.

Physical Examination

The physical examination of an asymptomatic asthmatic child is generally normal. In more severe disease, one may find an increased anteroposterior (AP) diameter of the chest. During exacerbations, one may find expiratory wheezes, a prolonged expiratory phase, and poor or absent air movement. Although present in some adult asthmatics, nasal polyps must prompt an evaluation for cystic fibrosis, because cystic fibrosis remains the most common cause of nasal polyps in children. Given the variability in the exam of the child with asthma, the exam should focus on assuring the absence of findings suggestive of other diseases, such as the presence of crackles, digital clubbing, and hypoxemia, as well as to uncover factors that worsen disease, including nasal and sinus disease.

Pulmonary Function Tests

With the help of well-trained and experienced pulmonary function technicians, children as young as 4 to 5 years of age are often capable of performing spirometry. Spirometry measures usually obtained include FVC, FEV_1, the ratio of FEV_1/FVC, as well as other measures of airflow including the forced expiratory flow between 25% and 75% of FVC (FEF_{25-75}). Although FEV_1 is included in the NAEPP guidelines as one gauge of measuring severity, most children with asthma have FEV_1 within the normal range (FEV_1 82% to 118% predicted). The FEV_1/FVC ratio, a measure of airflow obstruction, may be more sensitive in identifying airflow abnormalities in children.

Airway reactivity is a feature of asthma and is often assessed as the percent change in airflow (FEV_1) after administration of bronchodilator. Thus bronchodilator response judged by spirometry before and after bronchodilator is a helpful tool in determining whether or not a patient has bronchodilator-responsive obstruction, consistent with asthma, or fixed obstruction consistent with other disease states. A 12% increase in FEV_1 is considered a significant bronchodilator response, an increase that is above and beyond that seen in nonasthmatics. However, not all children with asthma demonstrate a significant change in FEV_1 after bronchodilator administration. Absence of a response to bronchodilator should not exclude asthma as a diagnosis, as other stimuli (see the following section) may be required to demonstrate airway reactivity.

Spirometry also provides both inspiratory and expiratory flow-volume loops, which are helpful in detecting other types of airflow obstruction. A fixed airway obstruction, such as a mediastinal mass resulting in extrinsic airway compression, will cause abnormalities of both the inspiratory and expiratory loops. Abnormalities of the inspiratory loop with a normal expiratory loop are suggestive of extrathoracic obstruction, such as is seen with vocal cord dysfunction. The variable intrathoracic obstruction seen in asthma generally creates abnormalities on the expiratory loop, but when severe enough can also affect the inspiratory loop.

Other tests of pulmonary function can be helpful when a patient is difficult to diagnose or manage, such as lung volumes and diffusing capacity of carbon monoxide (DLCO). Total lung capacity should be normal, with air trapping often seen on the basis of an increased residual volume to total lung capacity ratio (RV/TLC). DLCO is normal in asthma, and abnormalities should prompt further investigation for interstitial lung diseases.

Laboratory Evaluation

Asthma remains a clinical diagnosis. However, laboratory evaluation can be helpful in distinguishing asthma from other diseases. Measurement of serum immunoglobulins (IgG, IgA, and IgM) may help in differentiating between asthma and a humoral immunodeficiency in a child with recurrent lower respiratory tract infections. Any child with any combination of recurrent pneumonias, chronic cough, poor growth/failure to thrive, exam findings of crackles, digital clubbing, or nasal polyposis should undergo a sweat chloride determination to exclude cystic fibrosis. Similarly, a child with recurrent otitis media, sinusitis, and bronchiectasis should undergo biopsy for evaluation of ciliary function and ultrastructure in order to evaluate for primary ciliary dyskinesia. In potentially exposed patients, a tuberculin skin test will help to exclude mycobacterial infection.

Allergy Testing

All children with persistent asthma should be evaluated for allergic sensitization, either via skin testing or by in vitro determination of allergen-specific IgE (such as the CAP-RAST system), as identification of allergic sensitization allows the clinician to instruct the family on allergen avoidance and control measures that may aid in asthma control. Positive skin tests to foods, especially eggs, may predict a greater risk of persistent asthma in younger children. However, in evaluating young children, one must remember that while allergic sensitization is detectable in infancy, negative allergy skin testing or CAP-RAST testing in early childhood does not preclude the development of allergic sensitization later in childhood.

Radiology

A chest radiograph (AP and lateral views) aids significantly in excluding other disease entities. Findings such as bronchiectasis, foreign bodies, and congenital abnormalities may be completely invisible to clinical exam, but when found are important and lead toward consideration of other diagnoses. The chest radiograph of an asthmatic, on the other hand, is often normal, but may show hyperexpansion/flattened diaphragms, peribronchial cuffing, increased AP diameter, and areas of atelectasis.

Challenge Testing

Although the diagnosis of asthma can usually be made on the basis of history, physical examination, spirometry before and after bronchodilator treatment, and confirmed by tracking of symptom response to treatment, patients with atypical presentations, poor response to asthma medications, or lack of a response to bronchodilator during spirometry can be difficult to firmly diagnose. Because asthma contains a component of bronchial hyperreactivity, challenging the airway with an agent known to provoke bronchoconstriction may be helpful in evaluating such patients. Challenges can either be tailored to the specific patient's trigger—for example, cold air or exercise challenges, or nonspecific bronchoconstricting stimuli, such as methacholine. Negative bronchial challenges should prompt evaluation of other possible diagnoses. When performed in an experienced laboratory, these challenges are safe and can provide diagnostic clarification.

Bronchoscopy

Bronchoscopy is never necessary for the diagnosis of asthma. However, when airway structure or tissue abnormalities are suspected, or when patients with severe disease fail to respond to therapy, bronchoscopy can be helpful. Direct visualization may find airway abnormalities such as aberrant tracheal bronchi, intrinsic mass or foreign body obstruction, complicating factors such as bronchomalacia, or vascular rings. Bronchoalveolar lavage fluid can be helpful in quantifying airway inflammation (eosinophilia/neutrophilia), aspiration (lipid-laden macrophages), or occult infection.

CLASSIFICATION OF ASTHMA SEVERITY

Once a diagnosis of asthma is established, one must determine the severity of the patient's disease in order to approach treatment per the NAEPP guidelines. Although the guidelines provide FEV_1 and peak expiratory flow (PEF) criteria for severity classification, the high percentage of asthmatic children with FEV_1 values in the normal range suggest that these should be used cautiously in children. Rather, it appears that symptom frequency and medication use are more sensitive indicators of disease state and should be chief considerations in classifying a patient's disease severity. Classification not only helps to guide initial management but also provides a way to assess improvement and improves asthma care delivery.

The current NAEPP guidelines classify asthma as either intermittent or persistent, with mild, moderate, and severe forms of persistent disease (Table 3). Three major features of asthma—daytime symptom frequency, nighttime symptom frequency, and interference with exercise/activity further define levels of severity before institution of controller therapy. Asthma is considered to be persistent if symptoms occur more

TABLE 3. **Classification of Asthma Severity**

Severity	Symptoms	Nighttime Symptoms
Intermittent	Symptoms ≤2 times/week Asymptomatic and normal PEF between exacerbations Exacerbations brief (from a few hours to a few days); intensity may vary	≤2 times per month
Mild persistent	Symptoms >2 times/week but <1 time/day Exacerbations may affect activity	3–4 times per month
Moderate persistent	Daily symptoms Daily use of inhaled short-acting β_2-agonist Exacerbations affect activity Exacerbations >2 times/week; may last days	5–9 times per month
Severe persistent	Continual symptoms Limited physical activity Frequent exacerbations	≥10 times per month

Note: Patient is assigned the highest level of severity for which he or she meets any single criterion.

Adapted from National Institutes of Health National Heart, Lung, and Blood Institute. National Asthma Education and Prevention Program Expert Panel Report II: Guidelines for the diagnosis and management of asthma. Publication No. 97-4051A. Bethesda, MD: US Department of Health and Human Services, 1997.

often than twice per week or if nighttime symptoms occur more often than twice per month, or if exacerbations begin to affect activity. Nighttime symptoms are a particularly important marker of more severe and uncontrolled disease.

MANAGEMENT

After the patient has been diagnosed with asthma of a defined severity, management decisions can be made based upon the NAEPP algorithm. Although pharmacologic interventions are an important piece of management, to be successful, asthma management must include interventions for all of the contributing factors. Thus if a patient has allergic sensitization to aeroallergens, allergen exposure must be minimized. Exposure to environmental irritants such as tobacco smoke must similarly be minimized. Comorbid medical conditions that are known to complicate asthma, such as sinusitis and gastroesophageal reflux, must be treated independently. Contributing psychosocial stressors should also be addressed.

However, without the active understanding and participation of patients and their caregivers, asthma cannot be optimally managed. Thus, along with treating the asthma and comorbidities, patient and caregiver education and support are essential.

GOALS OF ASTHMA MANAGEMENT

Without predefined, clear goals, patients, caregivers, and clinicians alike can easily be frustrated by asthma management. Goals allow all involved to see when things are going well, and when they are not—what is acceptable, and what should cause concern. The NAEPP guidelines provide a set of goals of therapy, with a focus on reducing symptoms and, thus quick-reliever medication use (Table 4). With appropriate management and follow-up, most asthmatics are able to attain these goals.

TABLE 4. **Goals of Asthma Therapy**

Minimal or no chronic symptoms day or night
Minimal or no exacerbations
No limitations on activities; no school/parent's work missed
Minimal use of short-acting inhaled β_2-agonist
Minimal or no adverse effects from medications
Normal lung function

Adapted from National Institutes of Health National Heart, Lung, and Blood Institute. National Asthma Education and Prevention Program Expert Panel Report II: Guidelines for the diagnosis and management of asthma. Publication No. 97-4051A. Bethesda, MD: US Department of Health and Human Services, 1997.

ASTHMA PHARMACOTHERAPY

Until recently, asthma therapy was focused on the relief of bronchoconstriction. Agents such as theophylline (Theolair, others) and the β-adrenergic agonists were the primary agents used and effectively improved the acute airway obstruction through bronchodilator activity. However, with an increased understanding of asthma as an inflammatory process, newer treatment paradigms have focused on treating this persistent inflammation in order to prevent bronchospasm. Thus we have arrived at the current state, with two general classes of medications, quick reliever medications and controller medications. Controller medications are used to treat the underlying persistent inflammation (Table 5), whereas quick reliever medications are used to treat acute symptoms and exacerbations (Table 6).

TABLE 5. **Controller Medications**

Class	Agents	Mechanism/Comments
Inhaled corticosteroids (ICS)	Budesonide (Pulmicort), flunisolide (AeroBid), fluticasone (Flovent), triamcinolone (Azmacort), beclomethasone (QVAR, Vanceril, Beclovent)	Directly anti-inflammatory through inhibition of lymphocyte activity and cytokine secretion.
Long-acting β_2-adrenergic agonists (LABA)	Formoterol (Foradil), salmeterol (Serevent)	Acts through β_2-adrenergic receptors to relax airway smooth muscles, resulting in bronchodilation.
Combination therapy (ICS + LABA)	Fluticasone/salmeterol (Advair), budesonide/formoterol (Symbicort)*	Single dry powder inhalers containing both ICS and LABA. Significantly easier to use, providing a potential adherence benefit. First-line agents in treatment of moderate to severe persistent asthma in patients older than age 5.
Leukotriene modifiers	Montelukast (Singulair), zafirlukast (Accolate), zileuton (Zyflo)	Antagonize the production (Zileuton) or effect (Montelukast, Zafirlukast) of the cysteinyl-leukotrienes (LT C4/D4/E4), which mediate bronchoconstriction, mucus secretion, and other components of asthma.
Methylxanthines	Theophylline	Phosphodiesterase inhibitor. Exact mechanism of action in asthma unclear. Therapeutic levels generally 5–15 μg/mL.
Systemic corticosteroids	Prednisone, prednisolone (Orapred), methylprednisolone (Solu-Medrol)	Directly anti-inflammatory through inhibition of lymphocyte activity and cytokine secretion. Significant systemic side effects when used for extended periods.

*Not available in the United States.

TABLE 6. **Quick Reliever Medications**

Class	Agents	Mechanism
Short acting β_2-adrenergic agonists	Albuterol (Ventolin, Proventil), pirbuterol (Maxair), levalbuterol (Xopenex), bitolterol (Tornalate), terbutaline (Brethine), metaproterenol (Alupent)	Acts through β_2-adrenoceptors to relax airway smooth muscles, resulting in bronchodilation. Rapid onset of action.
Anticholinergic agents	Ipratropium (Atrovent), atropine*	Relax airway smooth muscle through inhibition of parasympathetic nervous system input. Second-line agent, often used in combination with albuterol during severe acute exacerbation.
Systemic corticosteroids	Methylprednisolone (Solu-Medrol), prednisolone (Orapred), prednisone	Directly anti-inflammatory through inhibition of lymphocyte activity and cytokine secretion. Beneficial within 4 hours of administration, limited side effects with 5–10 day course.

*Not FDA approved for this indication.

These medications form the armamentarium available for asthma management. Based upon the currently available evidence and opinion of the Expert Panel, algorithms using these medications for severity-specific treatment of asthma are outlined in Table 7 for children older than age 5 and in Table 8 for children ages 5 and younger. Beyond this, as of the 2002 update of the guidelines, a special indication for the use of inhaled corticosteroids in young children has been added. Based on the previously discussed results from the Tucson Children's Respiratory Study, the Expert Panel recommends that any child age 5 or younger who has had had more than three episodes of wheezing in the past year that lasted more than 1 day and affected sleep and who have either one major or two minor API criteria (see Table 1) should be strongly considered as a candidate for controller therapy, preferably inhaled corticosteroids.

CONTROLLER MEDICATIONS

Inhaled Corticosteroids

The focus of long-term controller therapy is on inhaled corticosteroids (ICS). Studies in adults have demonstrated that ICS therapy leads to significant improvement in asthma control as reflected by reductions in asthma symptoms, exacerbation rates, hospitalizations, asthma death, quality of life, and airway hyperreactivity.

In children, convincing data are provided by the CAMP trial, which involved treating 1041 children with mild to moderate asthma with either placebo, inhaled nedocromil (Tilade), or inhaled budesonide (Pulmicort) for 4.3 years. In this trial, children who received ICS had significant improvements in airway hyperresponsiveness, fewer asthma symptoms, less albuterol (Ventolin) use, longer times until need for

TABLE 7. **Severity-based Asthma Therapy for Children Older Than 5 Years of Age**

Severity	Preferred Treatment	Alternative Treatments (Listed Alphabetically)	If Needed
Intermittent	No daily medication needed		Severe exacerbations may occur, separated by long periods of no symptoms. A course of systemic corticosteroids is recommended.
Mild persistent	Low-dose ICS	Cromolyn (Intal), LTM, nedocromil (Tilade) *or* sustained release theophylline (Theobid, others) (level 5–15 μg/mL)	
Moderate persistent	Low-to-medium dose ICS *and* LABA	Increased ICS within medium dose range *or* low- to medium-dose ICS and either LTM or theophylline	Particularly in patients with recurring severe exacerbations Preferred treatment Increased ICS within medium dose range and add LABA Alternative treatment (listed alphabetically)
Severe persistent	High-dose ICS *and* LABA		Increased ICS within medium dose range and add either LTM or theophylline *and*, if needed Corticosteroid tablets or syrup (2 mg/kg/d, generally not exceeding 60 mg/d).

ICS, inhaled corticosteroid; LABA, long-acting inhaled β_2-agonist; LTM, leukotriene modifier.

All patients: Short-acting bronchodilator: 2–4 puffs short acting inhaled β_2-agonists as needed for symptoms. Use of short-acting inhaled β_2-agonists on a daily basis, or increasing use, indicates the need to initiate or increase long-term control therapy ("step up").

Adapted from National Institutes of Health National Heart, Lung, and Blood Institute. Executive Summary of the NAEPP Expert Panel Report—Guidelines for the Diagnosis and Management of Asthma—Update on Selected Topics 2002. Bethesda, MD: NIH Publication No. 02-5075; 2002.

TABLE 8. **Severity-based Asthma Therapy for Children 5 Years of Age and Younger**

Severity	Preferred Treatment	Alternative Treatments (Listed Alphabetically)	If Needed
Intermittent	No daily medication needed		Severe exacerbations may occur, separated by long periods of no symptoms. A course of systemic corticosteroids is recommended.
Mild persistent	Low-dose ICS (with nebulizer or MDI with holding chamber with or without face mask or DPI)	Cromolyn *or* LTM	
Moderate persistent	Low-to-medium dose ICS *and* LABA *or* Medium-dose ICS	Low-dose ICS *and* either LTM *or* theophylline	Particularly in patients with recurring severe exacerbations Preferred treatment Medium-dose ICS *and* LABA Alternative treatment Medium dose ICS and either LTM or theophylline
Severe persistent	High-dose ICS *and* LABA		*and*, if needed Corticosteroid tablets or syrup (2 mg/kg/d, generally not exceeding 60 mg/d).

ICS, inhaled corticosteroid; LABA, long-acting inhaled β_2-agonist; LTM, leukotriene modifier; MDI, metered-dose inhaler; DPI, dry powder inhaler.

All patients: Short-acting bronchodilator: 2–4 puffs short acting inhaled β_2-agonists as needed for symptoms. Use of short-acting inhaled β_2-agonists on a daily basis, or increasing use, indicates the need to initiate or increase long-term control therapy ("step-up").

Adapted from National Institutes of Health National Heart, Lung, and Blood Institute. Executive Summary of the NAEPP Expert Panel Report—Guidelines for the Diagnosis and Management of Asthma—Update on Selected Topics 2002. Bethesda, MD: NIH Publication No. 02-5075; 2002.

oral corticosteroids for an asthma exacerbation, fewer courses of oral corticosteroids, fewer urgent care visits and hospitalizations, and less need for supplemental ICS as a result of poor asthma control.

Although the clinical benefits are significant, concern over their potential side effects merits consideration. In general, ICS are well-tolerated, but potential side effects of ICS include effects on skeletal growth and bone density, alteration of the hypothalamic-pituitary-adrenal axis, and local side effects (i.e., oral candidiasis and hoarseness). In particular, growth is a major concern of caregivers, clinicians, and older patients. However, although several clinical trials have noted a small decrease in growth initially (≈1 cm in the first year of therapy, which does not appear to be additive or progressive), several studies suggest that final adult height is not affected.

Thus given the significant morbidity and mortality associated with asthma, and in weighing the significant benefits of ICS therapy against the minimal risks, the NAEPP places ICS as first-line therapy in all patients with persistent asthma. ICS dosing is based on asthma severity, and is outlined in Table 9.

Leukotriene Modifiers

The cysteinyl leukotrienes (LTC4/LTD4/LTE4) are produced by eosinophils and mast cells, and mediate many processes involved in asthma, including mucus secretion, bronchoconstriction, and increased vascular permeability. By modifying these activities, either through inhibiting leukotriene synthesis at 5-lipooxygenase (zileuton [Zyflo]), or by blocking binding at leukotriene receptor 1 (zafirlukast [Accolate], montelukast [Singulair]), leukotriene modifiers (LTMs) selectively attenuate a portion of the inflammatory component of asthma. Clinical trials in both children and adults have shown these agents to be both safe and effective in reducing asthma symptoms and in improving lung function. In addition, montelukast has been shown to have a specific effect on exercise-induced bronchospasm. However, the data in adults show greater improvements in lung function and symptom reduction with ICS over LTM, and thus these LTM agents should be considered as an alternative to ICS as monotherapy in mild persistent asthma, and as an adjunct to ICS therapy in patients with more severe asthma.

Long-acting β_2-agonists

Given that the main goal of asthma treatment is treatment of the underlying inflammation, it is not surprising that long-acting β_2-agonists (LABAs) are not recommended for monotherapy of persistent asthma, and may in fact be detrimental if used in this role. However, these agents are important in providing sustained bronchodilation, and when combined with anti-inflammatory therapy, provide improved asthma symptom control. Studies in adult asthma patients uncontrolled on low-dose ICS monotherapy have shown that adding a LABA to a low-dose ICS is superior to doubling the ICS dose. Addition of LABA may also allow for a reduction in ICS dose, potentially very important in children where the growth effects of high-dose ICS is a concern. Despite the lack of clinical trial data in children, the compelling evidence of the efficacy of ICS plus LABA therapy in adults has led to the recommendation for the use of a combination of ICS and LABAs as preferred therapy in children 5 years of age and older with moderate to severe persistent asthma.

TABLE 9. **Estimated Comparative Daily Dosages for Inhaled Corticosteroids**

	Low Daily Dose		Medium Daily Dose		High Daily Dose	
Drug	*Adult*	*Child**	*Adult*	*Child**	*Adult*	*Child**
Beclomethasone CFC (Beclovent, Vanceril) 42 or 84 μg/puff	168–504 μg	84–336 μg	504–840 μg	336–672 μg	>840 μg	>672 μg
Beclomethasone HFA (QVAR)40 or 80 μg/puff	80–240 μg	80–160 μg	240–480 μg	160–320 μg	>480 μg	>320 μg
Budesonide DPI (Pulmicort) 200 μg/inhalation	200–600 μg	200–400 μg	600–1200 μg	400–800 μg	>1200 μg	>800 μg
Inhalation suspension for nebulization (child dose)		0.5 mg		1.0 mg		2.0 mg
Flunisolide (AeroBid) 250 μg/puff	500–1000 μg	500–750 μg	1000–2000 μg	1,000–1,250 μg	>2,000 μg	>1250 μg
Fluticasone (Flovent) MDI: 44, 110, or 200 μg/puff	88–264 μg	88–176 μg	264–640 μg	176–440 μg	>660 μg	>440 μg
DPI: 50, 100, or 250 μg/inhalation	100–300 μg	100–200 μg	300–600 μg	200–400 μg	>600 μg	>400 μg
Triamcinolone acetonide (Azmacort) 100 μg/puff	400–1000 μg	400–800 μg	1,000–2,000 μg	800–1200 μg	>2,000 μg	>1200 μg

*Children ≤12 years of age.

Adapted from National Asthma Education and Prevention Program Expert Panel Report—Guidelines for the Diagnosis and Management of Asthma—Update on Selected Topics 2002. J Allergy Clin Immunol 110:S214;2002.

Other Controller Medications

Cromolyn (Intal) and nedocromil (Tilade) are well-tolerated agents that exert anti-inflammatory activity through unknown mechanisms. They are not as potent as ICS, and are thus considered only as alternatives to ICS in children with mild persistent asthma. However, these agents are effective in the prevention of exercise induced asthma and are occasionally used with or without short-acting β agonists in that setting.

Theophylline (Theolair, others) has been a mainstay of treatment for more than 50 years, exerting its proven benefits on pulmonary function and asthma symptoms through an unknown mechanism. Though a methylxanthine in structure, and a phosphodiesterase inhibitor in function, theophylline has a number of effects not explained by these properties, including bronchodilation, stimulation of respiration centrally, and anti-inflammatory activity. However, it has a relatively narrow therapeutic range, the potential for significant side effects (including headache, emesis, nausea, tachycardia, anorexia), multiple drug interactions (including many antiseizure medications, macrolide antibiotics, and ciprofloxacin [Cipro]), and requires monitoring of levels. Theophylline is now reserved for use in combination with other agents in moderate to severe persistent asthma, and it may be particularly effective in those patients with significant nocturnal symptoms.

MONITORING AND REASSESSMENT

After asthma therapy has been initiated, monitoring and reassessment are needed to determine the level of asthma control achieved, and attainment of the goals of therapy. Monitoring should be individual to each patient, but consistent. In general, options for monitoring include assessment of symptom frequency and severity and medication use, with or without the use of peak flow monitoring. Studies on asthma monitoring have shown no clear benefit to the use of peak flow monitoring; however, moderate or severe persistent asthmatics, especially those with poor perception of symptoms, may benefit from regular peak flow monitoring. Also, in patients who have a well-established baseline peak flow, peak flow monitoring during symptoms can be helpful in guiding intervention.

Another important component of monitoring is pulmonary function testing. Because one of the goals of asthma therapy is normal lung function, monitoring of lung function objectively by spirometry is appropriate, especially in moderate or severe persistent asthmatics, and in those who have poor symptom perception. With appropriate asthma therapy, FEV_1 or FEV_1/FVC ratio should improve, and ideally normalize.

Improvement in PFTs is also positive feedback for the patient and caregivers, who can be given a quantitative result of their efforts in asthma therapy. For asthma patients with poor symptom perception, PFTs may provide the only reliable monitoring tool and can be helpful in directing therapy in this difficult to manage group of patients. Also, spirometry can detect the presence of vocal cord dysfunction in the setting of well-documented, appropriately treated asthma. Detecting this entity and treating it appropriately can prevent unnecessary and frustrating changes in medication aimed at treating a nonasthma airflow obstruction component that is both a common mimic and comorbidity of asthma.

Pre- and postbronchodilator spirometry can also be helpful in finding patients who have significant reactivity (as measured by the difference in FEV_1 before

TABLE 10. **Asthma Severity Monitoring Questionnaire**

Numbers 1–7 to be completed by patient/parent at each physician office visit. Please fill in ONE circle for EACH question, that BEST describes your/your child's asthma. *EXAMPLE:* ●

1. How often have you/your child had a cough, wheeze, shortness of breath, or chest tightness during the past MONTH?	○ 2 or fewer times per *week*	○ 3-6 times per *week*	○ daily	○ continously
2. How often have you/your child awakened from sleep because of coughing, wheezing, shortness of breath, or chest tightness in the past MONTH?	○ 2 or fewer time per month	○ 3-4 times per month	○ 5-9 times per month	○ 10 or more times per month
3. In the past MONTH, how often have you/your child had cough, wheeze, shortness of breath, or chest tightness while exercising or playing?	○ 2 or fewer times per month	○ 3-4 times per month	○ 5-9 times per month	○ 10 or more times per month
4. How often doses asthma keep you/your child from doing what you/the child want?	○ 2 or fewer times per month	○ 3-4 times per month	○ 5-9 times per month	○ 10 or more times per month

5. Think about all activities that you/your child did during the past MONTH. How much were you bothered by your asthma

○ not bothered at all ○ hardly bothered at all ○ bothered a little ○ somewhat bothered ○ quite bothered ○ very bothered ○ extremely bothered

6. How many days of school have you/your child missed due to asthma in the last MONTH? ☐☐ days ○ do not attend school

7. How many days of work have you/your child missed due to asthma in the last MONTH? ☐☐ days ○ do not work

and after bronchodilator therapy) even on controller medications. Finding highly reactive patients can be helpful in treating them with agents more targeted towards their bronchoreactivity such as the LABAs or theophylline. This may allow these patients to have better symptom control or attenuate the severity of their exacerbations.

In our experience, asthma symptom severity and frequency, and thus the degree of symptom control, can be quickly assessed by use of a short, focused questionnaire. The questionnaire should cover not only symptoms, which can be underreported, especially if disease has been severe but not diagnosed, but also activity limitation and days of school/work lost. Although not symptoms per se, missed days of school/work and activity limitation, if present, indicate that the goals of asthma therapy have not been met. Another useful way to get at symptoms is to ask what, if anything, the patient or caregiver notices when the patient misses medications. A set of questions used in our clinic can be found in Table 10. These questions, along with a 1-month history of short-acting β-agonist use, systemic corticosteroid use, emergency department visits, and hospitalizations provide a complete picture of the patient's current asthma status.

Depending upon the level of symptom control, it may be possible to either reduce medications after asthma is well controlled or increase medications if it is not. The NAEPP guidelines refer to this process as "step down" for reduction in therapy and "step up" for increases in therapy.

On reassessment, if a patient's symptoms are controlled, current treatment can be continued, or a step-down can be undertaken. If, on the other hand, a patient's symptoms are not controlled with appropriate therapy, several factors should be considered before a step-up is made. First, the medications should be reviewed, and in children, special attention should be paid to medication delivery device (with or without holding chamber, dry powder inhaler (DPI), or nebulizer) technique. Incorrect technique can lead to some or all of the medication being lost rather than delivered to the lungs and can be misinterpreted as nonadherence. Second, one should consider common comorbid conditions such as gastroesophageal reflux and sinusitis. If these are present, treatment of the comorbidity can provide greater relief than a step-up. If consideration of these factors yields no other explanation for the lack of symptom control, a step-up may be required.

The Global Initiative for Asthma provides an algorithm for reassessment of severity in patients who are receiving controller therapy (Table 11). Once the asthma is classified, one can return to the guidelines and treat per the new level of severity (see Tables 7 and 8), stepping up or down as indicated.

ENABLING CAREGIVERS TO DETECT AND MANAGE ACUTE ASTHMA EPISODES—THE ASTHMA ACTION PLAN

Even in the setting of well-controlled asthma, acute asthma exacerbations will occur, often in the setting of a viral respiratory tract infection. However, given the right set of tools, the patient and caregiver can effectively manage most exacerbations at home. To do this, patients and caregivers must be provided not only with quick reliever medications, but with a clear, written plan for detecting and appropriately managing worsening asthma symptoms. This Asthma Action Plan (AAP) is the central component for home asthma management.

In our experience, a simple three-tiered action plan based on a traffic light analogy combines ease of use, comprehensibility, and flexibility in response depending on symptom severity. In the first tier is the patient's daily therapy, given regardless of any change in symptoms, the "green zone." Green zone medications may include daily controller medications

TABLE 11. **Algorithm for Reassessing Asthma Severity Based on Current Treatment and Symptoms While Treated**

	Current Treatment Step		
	Step 1: Mild Intermittent	*Step 2: Mild Persistent*	*Step 3: Moderate Persistent*
Symptoms on Current Therapy	***Reassessed Asthma Severity***		
STEP 1: MILD INTERMITTENT			
Symptoms ≤2 times per week Asymptomatic and normal PEF between exacerbations Exacerbations brief (from a few hours to a few days); intensity may vary Nighttime symptoms ≤2 times per month	Intermittent	Mild persistent	Moderate persistent
STEP 2: MILD PERSISTENT			
Symptoms >2 times/week but <1 time/day Exacerbations may affect activity Nighttime symptoms 3–4 times per month	Mild persistent	Moderate persistent	Severe persistent
STEP 3: MODERATE PERSISTENT			
Daily symptoms Daily short-acting β_2-agonist use Exacerbations affect activity Exacerbations >2 times/week; may last days Nighttime symptoms 5–9 times per month	Moderate persistent	Severe persistent	Severe persistent
STEP 4: SEVERE PERSISTENT			
Continual symptoms Limited physical activity Frequent exacerbations Nighttime symptoms ≥10 times per month	Severe persistent	Severe persistent	Severe persistent

Adapted from National Institutes of Health National Heart, Lung, and Blood Institute. Global Initiative for Asthma—Global Strategy for Asthma Management and Prevention. Bethesda, MD: NIH Publication No. 02-3659, 2002.

(e.g. ICS), as well as medications for preventing exercise-induced asthma (i.e., pre-exercise use of short-acting β-agonists or cromolyn/nedocromil). At the first sign of symptoms (cough, wheeze, chest tightness, or decrease to below 80% of personal best peak flow; or in younger children, with the acquisition of any viral infection, especially in children known to worsen significantly with even the most minor upper respiratory infection), the caregiver should be taught to go to the next tier, the "yellow zone."

In the "yellow zone," the patient should receive an inhaled short-acting β_2-adrenergic agonist, which may be repeated up to three times in the first hour. Another common "yellow zone" intervention is doubling the ICS dose (or adding ICS if not already used), although the evidence for this maneuver is not conclusive. Over the next several days, the patient should be watched closely, with particular attention paid to the occurrence of nocturnal awakenings. Inhaled short-acting β_2-adrenergic agonists should be used as needed. Increased ICS use should be continued for 7 to 10 days after baseline status is achieved to control the increased inflammation produced during the exacerbation. If this increased "yellow zone" therapy is not successful in improving symptoms significantly or in restoring peak flows to >80% of personal best, systemic corticosteroids may be needed. If the caregiver reaches this point, the clinician should be contacted, and systemic corticosteroids started if judged necessary.

Symptoms may progress beyond the "yellow zone" rapidly, with response to short-acting β_2-agonist therapy lasting 2 hours or less, developing respiratory distress, significant retractions, inability to complete sentences, or acrocyanosis. If this happens, the caregiver should move to the "red zone." In this zone, the patient should receive short-acting β_2-agonist therapy as in the "yellow zone," along with initiation of systemic corticosteroids, and seeking immediate medical attention (i.e., EMS). Availability of oral corticosteroids at home allow for administration based upon physician advice or AAP, and may prevent further symptom progression, the need for emergency department care or hospital admission. By helping the caregiver discern between exacerbations which are significant but manageable at home, and those that require immediate outside assistance, the AAP empowers caregivers, resulting in better home care, and will likely lead to fewer emergency department visits and hospitalizations.

Management of childhood asthma requires that the clinician, caregiver, and patient all share the "goals of asthma therapy" and work together to achieve those goals.

Achieving the goals requires a combination of several interventions beyond appropriate, guideline-based therapy, including empowering the caregiver and patient to deal with acute exacerbations, monitoring of symptoms and medication use at home, and regular follow-up to continuously reassess asthma control and optimize therapy. To accomplish this, communication between clinician and caregiver is essential, including continuous education and review of asthma care components. When applied successfully, this approach can lead to asthma control in nearly all patients.

ALLERGIC RHINITIS CAUSED BY INHALANT FACTORS

method of
JAMES N. BARANIUK, M.D.
Georgetown University
Washington, DC

Allergic rhinoconjunctivitis is the most common manifestation of atopy. Its prevalence has risen to approximately 20% of the American population, and it is one of the leading causes of visits to physicians. The direct cost was well over the 1996 estimate of $2.6 billion (based on government statistics), with industry estimates showing that loratadine alone had sales rise to nearly $2.5 billion dollars per year. These costs do not include self-medication. The indirect cost is even larger because allergic rhinitis is a major cause of days lost from work for both workers with allergic rhinitis and parents who must stay home to care for sick children with allergic rhinitis or complications and co-morbid conditions such as sinusitis, otitis media, and asthma. Allergic rhinitis is present in at least 80% of asthma patients, especially children. Studies show that it may be difficult to control asthma unless the nasal inflammation is also controlled.

HOW THE NOSE RUNS

It is easiest to understand the nefarious subtleties of allergic rhinitis and its treatment by knowing how the nose works. I have developed a reductionist approach that divides the nasal mucosa into four nearly independent compartments (Figure 1). First, the nasal cavity is enclosed in a bony box. Unlike bronchi or the supraglottic region, no external elastic or muscular force will increase nasal patency. Instead, the thickness of the mucosa regulates the volume of the nasal airspace and thus nasal airflow. Mucosal thickness is determined by the degree of filling of the deep venous sinusoids (top of Figure 1), which dilate in inflammation and thicken the mucosa. A thickened mucosa impinges on the nasal airspace volume and thereby results in obstruction and increased nasal airflow resistance. Sympathetic nerves constrict the arteriovenous anastomoses that supply these vessels and cause them to collapse. This mechanism accounts for the nasal patency that develops during exercise, for example. Oral α_1-adrenergic (pseudoephedrine [Sudafed]) and topical α_2-adrenergic (oxymetazoline [Afrin], xylometazoline [Otrivin]) agonists are effective nasal decongestants. Conversely, the absence of sympathetic tone, as in Horner's syndrome, leads to default vasodilation and nasal obstruction.

Histamine and other mediators released from mast cells during the immediate phase of the allergic reaction contract the endothelial cells of the superficial postcapillary venules (right side of Figure 1). Hydrostatic pressure causes the plasma to be rapidly

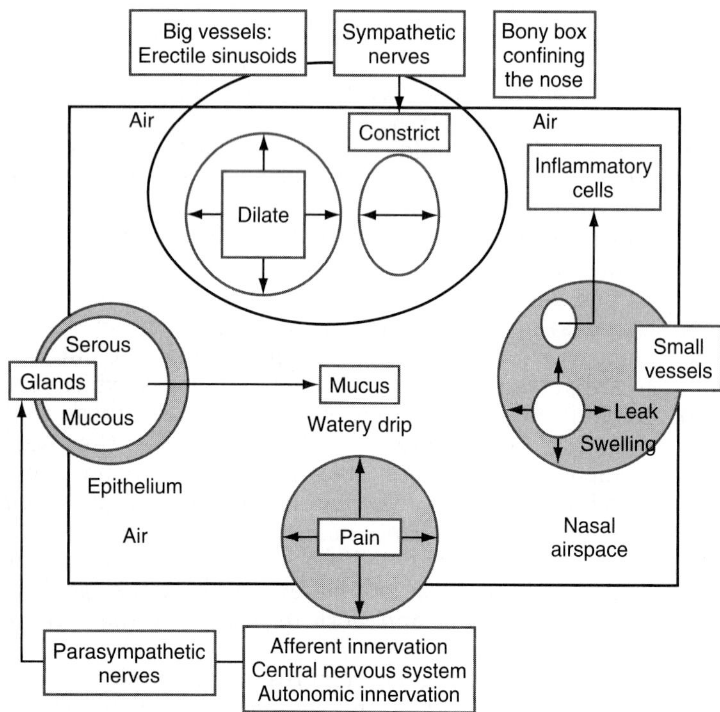

Figure 1. How the nose runs.

extravasated and forces the interstitial fluid through the epithelial tight junctions to form the watery rhinorrhea of allergic rhinitis. Histamine, cysteinyl leukotrienes, cytokines, and other mediators activate endothelial cells so that their surface expression of selectins and integrin adhesion molecules (e.g., the vascular cell adhesion molecule VCAM-1) is increased and eosinophils, basophils, neutrophils, TH_2 lymphocytes, and potentially hematopoietic progenitor cells bind tightly and become flattened against the endothelial wall. Drugs are now under development to selectively block the adhesion of specific leukocyte subsets. When "second signals" for chemotaxis are also present, such as eotaxin, RANTES and other cytokines, leukocytes will pass through the endothelium and form a perivascular infiltrate. Epithelial cell chemokine secretion (e.g., eotaxin, granulocyte-macrophage colony-stimulating factor [GM-CSF]) will induce mucosal mast cells to secrete tryptase and eosinophils into the epithelium and nasal lumen. Topically applied nasal steroids potently reduce these two cell populations.

Histamine stimulates H_1 receptors on very slowly conducting, nonmyelinated, type C "itch"-specific nerves that convey this sensation through a unique spinal cord and thalamic pathway to autonomic regulatory centers in the brainstem and higher centers in the central nervous system (bottom of Figure 1). Blockage of H_1 receptors on itch nerves and contraction of the endothelial cells that regulate vascular leak are two of the most important functions of antihistamines. Itch nerves form the afferent limb of systemic reflexes such as the sneeze, allergic salute (using the palm of the hand to rub the nose in an upward direction), and nasal parasympathetic responses. These cholinergic reflexes induce exocytosis of glandular secretions (left of Figure 1) that combine with plasma to form highly viscous, mucinous coagulant masses that can also obstruct nasal airflow and potentially sinus orifices. These reflexes are the basis for using anticholinergic drugs for rhinitis. Because of ciliary stasis, allergic subjects must sneeze and blow their nose to clear the mucus from nasal passages. Such airflow obstruction can lead to nocturnal sleep disturbances. This glutinous, bungee cord–like macromolecular matrix is also a mediator-rich milieu that can pass retrogradely to irritate the nasopharynx, pharynx, and supraglottic region and cause nausea once it is finally swallowed. Components of this reductionist rhinitis model also form the mechanistic bases of other forms of rhinitis, and this overlap can make the differential diagnosis a challenge to navigate (see Tables 1 and 2).

ONTOGENY OF ALLERGIC RHINITIS

Sensitization generates allergen-specific TH_2 lymphocytes with their characteristic sets of cytokines: interleukin-4 (IL-4), IL-5, IL-9, IL-10, IL-13, and potentially others (Figure 2). IL-4 and IL-13 share some receptor proteins and have similar actions. They promote heavy chain switching of B cells to allergen-specific IgE production and mast cell maturation and inhibit potentially competitive TH_1 lymphocyte genesis. IL-5 is a potent chemoattractant and growth factor for eosinophils.

Sensitization may occur in utero as a result of elevations in umbilical cord total IgE and antigen-specific IgE. Infants, immigrants, and allergic subjects who move to a new location generally require about two to

TABLE 1. **Differential Diagnosis of Inflammatory Rhinosinusitis Based on Potential Pathogenic Mechanisms and the Predominant Infiltrating Cellular Components**

Eosinophil Predominant	Neutrophil Predominant	Complex Infiltrates
Allergic rhinitis	Infectious rhinitis	Common cold syndromes
Intermittent	Acute bacterial sinusitis	Granulomatous and vasculitic diseases
Perennial	Acute infectious exacerbations of chronic sinusitis	Wegener's granulomatosis
Food allergy with rhinitis	Nasal polyps in cystic fibrosis	Malignant midline granuloma
Allergic fungal sinusitis	HIV/AIDS-related infectious rhinosinusitis	Sarcoidosis
Occupational rhinitis with eosinophilia	Humoral immunodeficiency	Granulomatous infections
IgE mediated	IgA, IgE, IgG subclass and other deficiencies	Tuberculosis
Non–IgE mediated	Common variable	Leprosy
Nonallergic rhinitis with eosinophilia syndrome (NARES)	Hypogammaglobulinemia	Syphilis
Blood eosinophilia with nonallergic rhinitis and eosinophilia syndrome (BENARS)	Young's syndrome of sinopulmonary disease, azoospermia, and nasal polyps	Autoimmune disorders
Chronic eosinophilic sinusitis syndromes (CESS)	Kartagener's syndrome of bronchiectasis, chronic sinusitis, nasal polyps, and immotile cilia	Relapsing polychondritis
Nasal polyps with eosinophilia	Foreign body with infection	Systemic lupus erythematosus
Aspirin/NSAID sensitivity	Corrosive occupational rhinitis	Sjögren's syndrome
Triad asthma		Atrophic rhinitis
Asthma		Postoperative
Sinusitis		Senile rhinitis
Nasal polyps		Oxena
Churg-Strauss syndrome with eosinophilic granuloma		Klebsiella rhinitis
Eosinophilic granuloma		Basophilic/metachromatic rhinitis
		Goblet or squamous cell metaplasia without leukocyte infiltration secondary to exposure to smoke, pollutants, or other toxicants

TABLE 2. **Differential Diagnosis of Noninflammatory Rhinosinusitis Based on Potential Pathogenic Mechanisms**

Structural Anomalies	Hormonal	Neural Dysfunction	Other
Deviated septum Hypertrophic turbinates (mechanism undefined) Ostiomeatal complex (OMC) anatomic variants Concha bullosa Haller's cells Paradoxic curvature of the middle turbinate Choanal atresia Tumors Benign Neoplastic Adenoidal hypertrophy with potential recurrent infections Complications of excessive surgical excision of mucosa Fracture of cribriform plate Cerebrospinal rhinorrhea (high glucose) Hypertrophy of fleshy components of anterior nasal valve Rhinophyma Foreign body	Pregnancy (estrogen and progesterone) Hypothyroidism Acromegaly	Absent sympathetic function (absent vasoconstriction) Horner's syndrome Hyperactive cholinergic parasympathetic function (excessive mucus exocytosis) Cholinergic rhinitis Vidian neurectomy effects Loss of parasympathetic and sympathetic innervation Food/nocifer-activated cholinergic reflex–mediated rhinitis Gustatory rhinitis, "salsa sniffles" Cold dry air–induced rhinorrhea, "ski bunny rhinitis" Antihypertensive agents β-Adrenergic antagonists α-Adrenergic antagonists Reserpine Rhinitis medicamentosa Chronic topical α-adrenergic agonist abuse Cocaine abuse Nociceptive rhinitis/irritant rhinitis with increased nociceptive nerve sensitivity to weather changes, perfume, tobacco smoke, and other inhalants Bright light–induced nasal congestion	Idiopathic "vasomotor rhinitis" Perennial, nonallergic, noninfectious rhinitis Nasal hyperresponsiveness to mediators Histamine Methacholine Endothelin Bradykinin Nonallergic rhinitis of chronic fatigue syndrome (CFS), fibromyalgia, and allied syndromes displaying hyperalgesia Side effects of eyedrops delivered via nasolacrimal ducts Ketorolac (Acular) in acetylsalicylic acid (ASA)/nonsteroidal anti-inflammatory drug (NSAID) sensitivity Glaucoma medications

three seasons of exposure before new sensitivities develop. Pollen counts, geographically significant allergens, and durations of seasons are available at websites such as www.aaaai.org. Typically, trees begin to pollinate in late winter to early spring, with heavy production by birch, oak, maple, mountain cedar, and mulberry in different regions. Grass pollen typically follows, but it may have a season lasting a couple of months in Canada to year-round in Florida. The types of weeds and the duration of their pollination seasons vary by geographic region. Ragweed is important on the East Coast, whereas *Salsola* (Russian thistle) is important in the high plains. Fungal spores such as *Alternaria* are found in all climates, including the desert. In general, counts are highest in regions with high humidity and mild climates and negligible when the ground is covered by snow or ice. Fungi are also important indoor allergens that arise from dank, previously flooded basements, bathrooms, condensation on windows, kitchens, and humid areas with poor air circulation. Cockroaches, dog and cat dander (skin and salivary proteins), and dust mite (*Dermatophagoides farinae, Dermatophagoides pteronyssinus*, and others in tropical regions) feces are especially important indoor allergens. Dust mites do not live on skin, but stay in the warm and humid environment of pillows, mattresses, and box springs. They have an essential ecologic niche in that they consume the kilograms of skin scales that we desquamate nightly and rub into our bedding. Without them, we could have accumulations of 1 to 1.5 ft of skin scales in our bedrooms. As we roll about in bed or have pillow fights, the dust mites and their fecal packets become airborne and spread throughout the house only to settle on high shelves, curtains, furniture, and carpets. A telling historical feature is that allergic people rarely vacuum because the dust that is stirred up will cause fits of itching, sneezing, and coughing. Schools are another prime location to find bounties of allergen; the sticky dander is carried to school by pet owners, where it joins cockroach salivary and other proteins as part of the institutional house dust.

IgE circulates in low concentrations and is rapidly and tightly bound to mast cells by their high-affinity receptors (FcεRI). With re-exposure, the allergenic protein diffuses to the mucosal mast cells, binds IgE molecules, and cross-links their receptors. Granules are hydrated and release preformed histamine, tryptase, kininogenase, many other enzymes, and heparin. Arachidonic acid is released and metabolized into prostaglandin D_2 (PGD_2) and the cysteinyl leukotrienes C_4, D_4, and E_4. As noted in Figure 1, histamine (H_1 receptors), leukotrienes (cysteinyl leukotriene receptors 1 and 2 [CTL1 and CTL2]), PGD_2, bradykinin, and other factors act redundantly on the postcapillary venule endothelium to cause vascular leak and up-regulation of adhesion molecules. H_1 receptors stimulate the itch nerves and recruit cholinergic glandular secretion. These events constitute

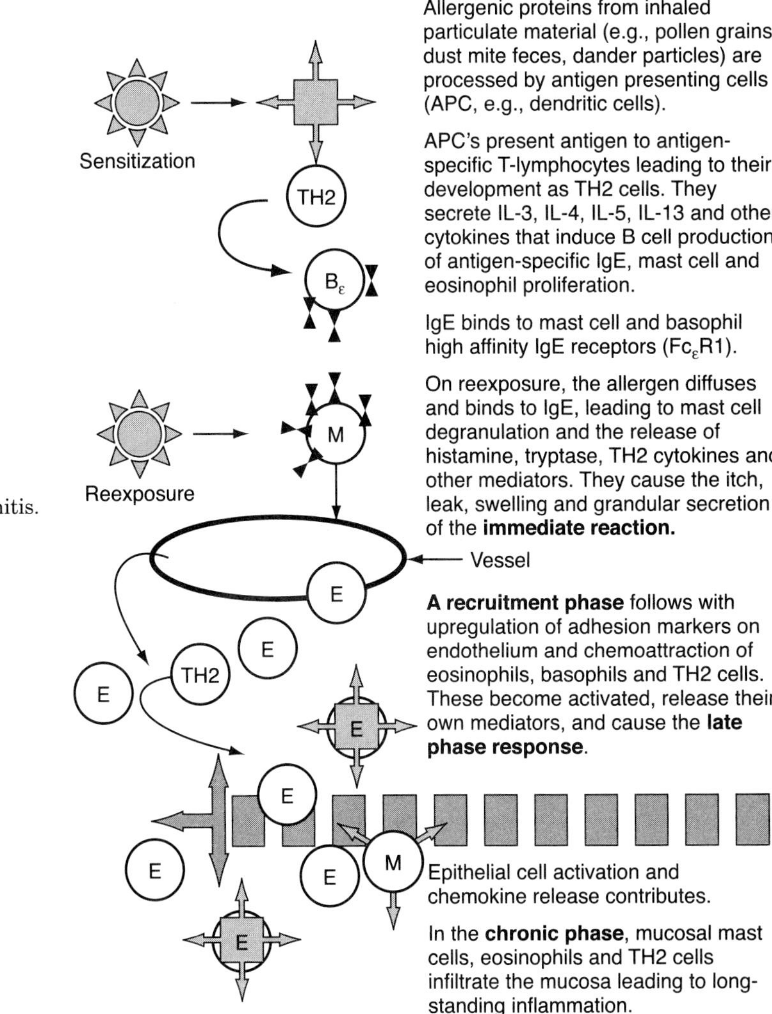

Sensitization
TH2
B_ε
Allergenic proteins from inhaled particulate material (e.g., pollen grains, dust mite feces, dander particles) are processed by antigen presenting cells (APC, e.g., dendritic cells).
APC's present antigen to antigen-specific T-lymphocytes leading to their development as TH2 cells. They secrete IL-3, IL-4, IL-5, IL-13 and other cytokines that induce B cell production of antigen-specific IgE, mast cell and eosinophil proliferation.
IgE binds to mast cell and basophil high affinity IgE receptors ($Fc_\varepsilon R1$).
Reexposure
M
On reexposure, the allergen diffuses and binds to IgE, leading to mast cell degranulation and the release of histamine, tryptase, TH2 cytokines and other mediators. They cause the itch, leak, swelling and grandular secretion of the **immediate reaction.**
Vessel
E
TH2
A recruitment phase follows with upregulation of adhesion markers on endothelium and chemoattraction of eosinophils, basophils and TH2 cells. These become activated, release their own mediators, and cause the **late phase response**.
Epithelial cell activation and chemokine release contributes.
In the **chronic phase**, mucosal mast cells, eosinophils and TH2 cells infiltrate the mucosa leading to long-standing inflammation.

Figure 2. Ontogeny of allergic rhinitis.

the immediate allergic reaction. Mast cells also release TH_2 cytokines, which promote atopic inflammation; transforming growth factor-β (TGF-β), which activates fibroblasts and induces the deposition of collagen; and the endogenous pyrogens IL-1β, IL-6, and tumor necrosis factor-α (TNF-α). Uptake of these factors through the superficial fenestrated capillaries may permit systemic circulation of these proteins with effects on bone marrow (eosinophilopoiesis) and central nervous system centers such as the hypothalamus and limbic system. These effects include malaise, forgetfulness, problems with acquisition of new learning, and other systemic acute phase response effects of "hay fever" and allergic fatigue syndrome.

After limited exposure, such as brief exposure to cat allergen, mediators of the immediate phase are rapidly degraded and symptoms may end. However, the chemokines and activated endothelial cells combine to recruit circulating leukocytes to the mucosa during the 4- to 6-hour "recruitment phase." Once a sufficient population of activated eosinophils, basophils, and TH_2 lymphocytes has accumulated, they release their own mediators, including strongly alkaline eosinophilic proteins, halide free radicals (eosinophil peroxidase), histamine, cysteinyl leukotrienes, and TH_2 cytokines. These mediators set off the "late phase response." Continued activation of the immediate-late phase cycle leads to chronic allergic mucosal inflammation, with tryptase-secreting mucosal mast cells, eosinophils, activated endothelium and epithelium, and antigen-specific TH_2 cells releasing their cytokines and mediators. The duration of the antigen exposure and its intensity will determine the severity of the inflammation and the relative balance of symptoms between an immediate phase response consisting of itchy, swollen, watery rhinorrhea and more late phase effects such as swelling, congestion, malaise, and a thick mucinous discharge. These variations in symptoms are important historical clues for making the diagnosis.

DIAGNOSIS AND DIFFERENTIAL DIAGNOSIS OF ALLERGIC RHINITIS

The diagnosis of allergic rhinitis can be derived from the pathophysiologic principles just outlined. Itchy and watery eyes, nose, and palate, sneezing, and nasal obstruction that develops on exposure to seasonal allergens, temporary exposure to high concentrations of dander or dust mites (e.g., vacuuming), or reproducible, stereotypic responses to occupational protein exposure (e.g., baker's rhinitis caused by dust mites in flour) are fairly straightforward. Reduction or elimination of symptoms by avoiding such exposure and the presence of a positive family or personal history of other atopic diseases such as atopic dermatitis, asthma, or food allergy also strengthen the diagnosis.

Sensations such as nasal congestion, fullness, obstruction to airflow, and even mucus hypersecretion when exposed to strong odors, perfumes, gasoline, changes in barometric pressure or humidity, and ingestion of wine or beer are present in about half of allergic rhinitis subjects. However, this syndrome of irritant rhinitis is due to nonallergic mechanisms. Neural hyperresponsiveness is the most likely explanation. Neurotropic cytokines released during allergic inflammation may up-regulate the afferent and efferent pathways and cause this overlap of allergic and nonallergic rhinitis. These irritant rhinitis symptoms are also present in 10% to 15% of the population without atopy. These patients may have been treated with multiple antihistamines or even long courses of antibiotics for presumed sinusitis without success when in fact they have nonallergic rhinitis. Contemplation of the presence (see Table 1) or absence (see Table 2) of inflammatory cells and specific symptom complexes provides a more logical approach to this surprisingly large differential diagnosis.

Physical signs such as the "classic" edematous ("boggy"), enlarged ("swollen"), pale to violaceous mucosa with watery discharge are found in about a third of cases, particularly those with severe acute rhinitis. Another third may have a red mucosa with thick strands of mucus bridging the adjacent turbinates, and another third may have minimal clinical findings. Venous stasis accounts for the "allergic shiners" beneath the eyes. A transverse crease across the lower third of the nose is a result of the allergic salute. Edematous eyelids with prominent skin creases (Dennie's lines), conjunctival injection, and edema are also common because allergic conjunctivitis may predate and be more severe than the allergic rhinitis symptoms. Persistent nasal obstruction with mouth breathing can lead to hypognathia, mandibular deformity, bite abnormalities, and hypertelorism.

CONFIRMATORY TESTING

Once a presumptive diagnosis of allergic rhinitis is made, an allergist will confirm the diagnosis by allergy skin testing. Skin tests assess the presence of allergen-specific IgE on the surface of cutaneous mast cells. Drops of standardized extracts are placed on the skin, and a tiny puncture or scratch is made through the epidermis to allow the extract to penetrate the stratum corneum to the dermal mast cells. The number and types of extracts tested depend on the diversity of local allergenic flora and household fauna. Cross-linking of IgE leads to mast cell degranulation with histamine release. Histamine stimulates the itch nerves. They are highly branched in the dermis and release calcitonin gene–related peptide (CGRP) and other neuropeptides by the axon response mechanism. CGRP causes a ring of erythema ("flare") by dilating the spiral arterioles and permitting red, hot, oxygenated blood to rise to the superficial plexus of vessels. Histamine also causes local edema ("wheal") by the mechanisms outlined earlier. The size of these reactions is graded on a 0 to 4+ scale after 15 minutes. If these tests are negative but atopy is still strongly presumed to be present, intradermal allergen injections are performed. Again, the wheal and flare reaction is measured after 15 minutes. In both cases, histamine is included as a positive control to determine whether subjects have antihistamines in their system that would cause a false-negative response. A glycerol negative control is included to detect dermographism. Nasal provocation tests have been used in Europe, but they are very time-consuming because only one allergen can be tested per visit. Blood can also be drawn for radioallergosorbent tests (RASTs), enzyme-linked assays (EIAs), and other in vitro measurements of allergen-specific circulating serum IgE. These tests can be performed in patients taking antihistamines, but they can be negative or equivocal when skin tests are positive. In vitro testing for allergen-specific IgG is an unproven test of atopy and should not be performed.

Measuring total serum IgE is of limited benefit because one treats the patient, not the laboratory value. It is useful when IgE is absent and the patient has nonallergic rhinitis symptoms, negative skin test results, or potential partial humoral immunodeficiency or when IgE levels are very high, as may occur in atopic dermatitis, allergic bronchopulmonary aspergillosis, or hyper-IgE syndrome. Eosinophil counts are generally in the upper normal to mildly elevated (<12%) range, but they may be elevated in other eosinophilic nasal disorders (see Table 1).

APPROACH TO THERAPY

The true prevalence of allergic rhinitis is not known because many patients self-diagnose and self-prescribe antihistamines, decongestants, or more recently, the mast cell stabilizer cromolyn (NasalCrom). Many of these subjects have symptoms that are not sufficiently severe to prompt a doctor's visit, are not noticeably impaired at work or other activities, or have no access to health care. Over-the-counter antihistamines were generally sedating until the recent switch of loratadine (Claritin) from prescription status (Table 3). Many subjects have claimed that they were not sedated while using these drugs, but driving simulation and other tests indicate that they were as incapacitated as though they had had one drink of alcohol, except that they were not aware of their impairment. Manufacturers' instructions indicate that these medications should not be taken if driving or operating heavy equipment, but unfortunately, these instructions are generally disregarded. It is not known how many traffic or work site accidents may be due to the use of sedating antihistamines.

TABLE 3. **Histamine H_1 Receptor Antagonists**

Generic Name	Trade Name	Formulation	Usual Dose	Sedation
OVER-THE-COUNTER ANTIHISTAMINES				
Azatadine*	Optimine	Tab: 1 mg	>11 y: 1 mg bid	Yes
Brompheniramine*	Dimetane	Elixir: 2 mg/5 mL Tab: 4, 8, 12 mg	0.35 mg/kg/24 h in 3–4 doses; 4 mg q4–6h, 8–12 mg bid	Yes
Chlorpheniramine	Chlor-Trimeton	Tab: 4, 8, 12 mg	4 mg q4h, 8 mg q8h; 12 mg bid	Yes
Clemastine	Tavist	Syrup: 0.67 mg/5 mL Tab: 1.34, 2.68 mg	0.67–1.34 mg bid; 1.34 mg q4–6h,[†] 2.68 mg bid	Yes
Diphenhydramine	Benadryl	Syrup: 12.5 mg/5 mL Chewable: 12.5 mg Caps: 12.5, 25 mg	5 mg/kg/24 h in 3–4 doses	Yes
Hydroxyzine	Atarax, Vistaril (Rx only)	Syrup: 10, 25 mg/5 mL Tab: 10, 25, 50, 100 mg	2 mg/kg/24 h in 3–4 doses; 25-50 mg q4–6h	Yes
Loratadine	Claritin	Syrup: 5 mg/5 mL Tab: 10 mg Reditab: 10 mg	2–5 y: 5 mg qd >5 y: 10 mg qd	No[‡]
	Claritin-D 12 Hour	Tab: 10 mg loratadine + 120 mg pseudoephedrine	1 Tab bid	
	Claritin-D 24 Hour	Tab: 10 mg loratadine + 240 mg pseudoephedrine	1 Tab qd	
PRESCRIPTION ANTIHISTAMINES				
Azelastine	Astelin	Nasal solution 0.1%, 137 μg/spray	5–11 y: 1 spray/nostril bid>11 y: 2 spray/nostril bid	12%[§]
Cetirizine	Zyrtec	Syrup: 5 mg/5 mL Tab: 5, 10 mg	2–5 y: ½–1 tsp qd 6–11 y: 1–2 tsp qd >11 y: 10 mg qd	14%[§]
Cyproheptadine	Periactin	Syrup: 2 mg/5 mL Tab: 4 mg	0.25 mg/kg/24 h in 3–4 doses; 4 mg q4–6h	Yes
Desloratadine	Clarinex	Tab: 5 mg	5 mg qd	No[‡]
Fexofenadine	Allegra	Caps: 60 mg Tab: 30, 60, 180 mg	6–11 y: 30 mg bid >11 y: 60 mg bid; 180 mg qd	No
	Allegra-D	Tab: 60 mg fexofenadine + 120 mg pseudoephedrine	>11 y: 1 Tab bid	
Promethazine	Phenergan	Syrup: 6.25, 25 mg/5 mL Supp: 12.5, 25, 50 mg Tab: 12.5, 25, 50 mg	0.5 mg/kg/24 h bid; 12.5–50 mg tid	Yes

*Not available as a single ingredient in the United States.
[†]Exceeds dosage recommended by the manufacturer.
[‡]Sedation occurs at higher doses of loratadine and its active metabolite desloratadine.
[§]Azelastine and cetirizine cause more drowsiness than fexofenadine does, especially if used at higher than the recommended doses. Cetirizine is recommended for use at night.

If allergic symptoms or sedation is excessive or if patients respond to direct-to-consumer advertising and thus want a specific prescription treatment, they will generally see their primary care physician. The physician should review the nasal, ocular, other allergic, and family histories and examine the eyes, nose, tympanic membranes, pharynx, chest, and skin for evidence of atopic disease. The time course and severity of symptoms help in classification. "Mild intermittent" allergic rhinitis lasts for less than 4 weeks. This condition is treated with a nonsedating antihistamine or intranasal corticosteroid. Cromolyn may be used, but with the understanding that it is a prophylactic medication that must be taken before allergen exposure. If significant ocular symptoms do not respond to the antihistamine, levocabastine (Livostin), the mast cell stabilizer cromolyn (Opticrom), acetaminophen (Panadol), or nonsteroidal anti-inflammatory (ketorolac [Acular]) eyedrops are indicated. α-Adrenergic agonists constrict vessels but do not ameliorate the underlying disease process.

Persistent rhinitis with symptoms lasting longer than 4 weeks can be due to indoor allergens or prolonged pollen seasons such as the Florida grass season. Intranasal corticosteroids are clearly the best option because these drugs are generally beneficial within 1 to 3 days, block cytokine production, decimate mucosal mast cell and eosinophil populations, and return the epithelium to normal function (Table 4). Higher than standard starting doses may be required

TABLE 4. **Intranasal Glucocorticoid Agents**

Generic and Trade Names	Formulation	Dose per Puff	Dose/U	Age	Usual Starting Dose
BECLOMETHASONE					
Beconase	Aerosol*	42 µg	200	6–11 y	1 spray/nostril bid
Vancenase Pockethaler				>11 y	
				6–11 y	2 sprays/nostril bid
Beconase AQ and	Aqueous†	42 µg	200	>11 y	
Vancenase AQ				>11 y	1 spray/nostril bid
Vancenase AQ 84 µg	Aqueous	84 µg	120		2 sprays/nostril bid
					2 sprays/nostril bid
BUDESONIDE					
Rhinocort	Aerosol	32 µg	200	>5 y	4 sprays/nostril qd
Rhinocort Aqua	Aqueous	32 µg	120	>5 y	1 spray/nostril qd-bid
FLUNISOLIDE					
Nasalide	Aqueous	25 µg	200	6–13 y	1 spray/nostril tid
Nasarel				>13 y	2 sprays/nostril bid
FLUTICASONE					
Flonase	Aqueous	50 µg	120	4–11 y	1 spray/nostril qd
				>11 y	2 sprays/nostril qd
MOMETASONE					
Nasonex	Aqueous	50 µg	120	3–11 y	1 spray/nostril qd
				>11 y	2 sprays/nostril qd
TRIAMCINOLONE					
Nasocort	Aerosol	55 µg	100	>5 y	2 sprays/nostril qd
Nasocort AQ	Aqueous	55 µg	120	6–11 y	1 spray/nostril qd
				>11 y	2 sprays/nostril qd

*Aerosols are solutions in fluorocarbon-pressurized canisters that must be shaken before use and have a forceful spray velocity.
†Aqueous solutions are dispensed in pump spray bottles as a liquid spritz.

to get the inflammation under control. The dose can be gradually tapered as symptoms become alleviated. It is unclear how low you can go with the dose because some studies indicate that "prn" use is sufficient once the allergic inflammation abates and the symptoms are well controlled. The dose may be preventively increased before a pollen season or period of intense allergen exposure (e.g., visiting a house with multiple pets). This boost will provide prophylactic protection and prevent the inflammatory cascade from ever becoming established. A nonsedating antihistamine can be added for excessive itching or nasal discharge symptoms. Ocular symptoms should be treated topically as outlined earlier.

ROLE OF THE ALLERGY CONSULTANT

Rhinitis can be a surprisingly frustrating condition to treat and may require consultation with both an allergist and an otorhinolaryngologist. Shifting from one antihistamine or intranasal steroid to another will not work if the patient uses them intermittently and only after periods of severe symptoms. Apparent treatment failures and other factors listed in Figure 3 are reasons for referring patients to a board-certified allergist-immunologist for confirmation of the diagnosis, evaluation of the differential diagnosis (see Tables 1 and 2), selection of an optimal treatment regimen, and intensive patient education about avoidance measures and correct use of medications.

For example, many people spray nasal steroids against the nasal septum and flex their head downward. Steroids are vasoconstrictors and, when sprayed onto the septum with a pressurized delivery device, may compromise blood flow to the avascular nasal cartilage. Septal perforation could result. However, many of these cases may have been complicated by cocaine abuse. A more satisfactory method is to shake the spray bottle, tilt the head slightly forward and laterally, and use the opposite hand to direct the spray into the nostril by aiming toward the outer canthus or ear. The subject should sniff gently to pull the liquid up toward the middle meatus between the inferior and middle turbinates, where the maxillary and other sinuses drain. It may be necessary to pull the nostril open and sniff to prevent the drug from dripping out of the nostril. If the head is tilted backward, the drug will drain down the oropharynx and be lost. I tell my patients to "flush a $10 bill down the toilet because that is what they have done with their medicine." This approach focuses their attention on learning the correct technique and may improve compliance. They should not spray twice into one nostril and then immediately move to the opposite one because it will be very difficult to effectively coat the nasal cavity with even a very adhesive (thixotropic) drug preparation. Parents may have to assist their children with the delivery device.

The most consistent problem with intranasal steroids has been minor epistaxis or blood staining of

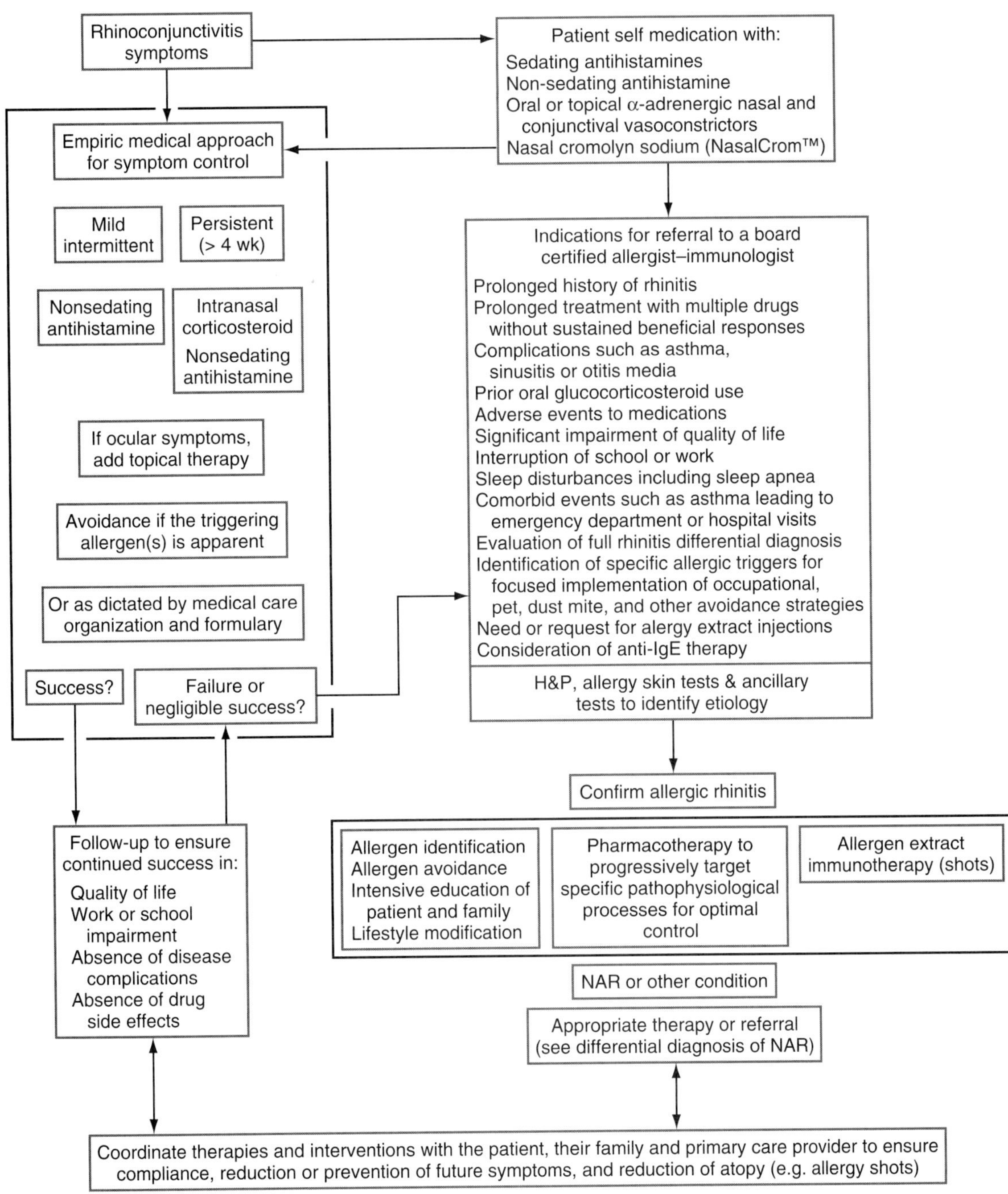

Figure 3. Allergic rhinitis diagnosis and treatment algorithm. H&P, history and physical examination; NAR, nonallergic rhinitis.

mucus. The bleeding can originate from Kiesselbach's plexus or the turbinate surface that receives the most intense spray. Bleeding is also a part of severe allergic rhinitis. Excessive mucus can be carried anteriorly by ciliary motion, then dry, adhere, and contract on the epithelial surface. Removal of this crust can lacerate the superficial lamina propria and lead to bleeding.

The steroid can be discontinued for several days and replaced with saline nasal sprays. Vaseline, Nose-Better gel, or other protective products can be placed in the nostril with the little finger or a cotton-tipped applicator to lubricate the epithelial surface. The anticholinergic agent ipratropium bromide (Atrovent Nasal Spray, 0.3% or 0.6%, 1 to 2 puffs as needed up to 8 puffs per day) may be useful to reduce the glandular exocytosis of mucins. Vasoconstrictors such as oral pseudoephedrine (30 to 60 mg) or topical oxymetazoline or xylometazoline (2 sprays of a 0.5% solution per nostril bid) are not a good alternative because they will vasoconstrict, but prolonged use (>3 days) may lead to rebound vasodilation and *rhinitis medicamentosa*. This effect is controversial, however, because some investigators find no rebound phenomena after 30 continuous days of use.

The cysteinyl leukotriene (CTL1) receptor antagonist montelukast (Singulair), 10 mg/d, has been approved by the FDA for rhinitis. This claim is based on a small, but statistically significant improvement in symptom scores when compared with placebo and loratadine. No studies of objective measures of nasal mucosal swelling, such as nasal airflow resistance, have been conducted to support these subjective claims. The magnitude of the benefit may be comparable to that of histamine H_2 antagonists, which were briefly popular because some studies showed that they reduced histamine-induced vasodilation in some vascular beds.

Other therapies of potential value include humanized antibodies to circulating IgE (Xolair).* This drug can be dosed to reduce IgE concentrations to negligible levels. This treatment has exceptional potential as an adjunct to allergen extract therapy (see later). Humanized antibodies to IL-5 very effectively eradicated eosinophilia, but they did not change bronchial hyperresponsiveness during a short trial in asthmatics. This product may be beneficial in other eosinophilic processes (see Table 1) but has not been tested extensively.

PATIENT EDUCATION

A critical area where an allergist can assist is in patient education about avoidance measures. Everyone who is skin tested should be given specific avoidance advice. If they are sensitive to pollens, they should have written instructions with specific dates for them to start prophylactic intranasal steroid therapy. If they exercise outdoors, they should run or perform outdoor activities early in the morning before the peak of pollen release. Pollen begins to be released as the dew dries on allergen plant flowers in midmorning. Face masks with high-efficiency particulate air (HEPA) filters are effective in screening pollen, fungal spores, dander, and dust mite feces from inhaled air. Indoors, electrostatic furnace filters that can be washed monthly are very effective at trapping circulating allergens and particulate matter. HEPA filters can be placed in bedrooms about 3 ft off the ground to clean the air without stirring up carpet or floor dust. Animals must be kept out of the bedroom because they are often found sleeping on the head of a mouth-breathing allergic child. If the pet cannot be given away to a good home, sequestering them to another part of the house will be a partial solution. Animal dander can be washed from pets weekly, but it can be a challenge to institute this practice in older pets. Allergic parents should be counseled before buying a kitten or puppy that may become their child's worst allergenic nightmare. Cockroach sensitivity requires a thorough examination for these pests in the home and fumigation if even a single one is found. It is not possible to eradicate dust mites. Instead, they can be contained by putting synthetic or woven encasings on pillows, mattresses, and box springs, which will trap them where they live. Sheets and other bedding should be washed in hot (>130°F) water to kill the mites and denature their fecal proteins. Stuffed toys are stuffed with dust mites and should also be removed from the bedroom. Washable "hypoallergenic" stuffed toys are now available. Favorite stuffed toys can be put in a clear plastic bag and stored on a high shelf so that children can see their friend but not suffocate in the plastic. Bare floors are preferred over carpets because the former are easier to keep clean. Throw rugs that can be regularly washed are acceptable. Medications should be used before exposure so that mast cells are stabilized before IgE-mediated degranulation, histamine receptors are blocked before histamine is released, and steroids can enter mucosal cells to counter the onset of proinflammatory changes that follow mast cell degranulation.

ALLERGY SHOTS

Allergy shots (allergen immunotherapy) have been effective therapy for allergic conjunctivitis (about an 80% success rate), rhinitis (60% to 70%), and atopic asthma (50%) for nearly a century. They remain the only therapy that can permanently eliminate allergen-specific allergic reactions. Over 20 placebo-controlled trials have shown improvement with single allergens such as grass, cat, *Alternaria,* and dust mites. Allergy shots fell from favor because they were used excessively and inappropriately in an era when no alternatives were available and because of the introduction of glucocorticoids, β-adrenergic agents, and nonsedating antihistamines as medical therapy for atopic asthma and rhinitis. It is now clear that asthmatics who are older than 50 years, have a forced expiratory volume in 1 second (FEV_1) of less than 60%, or have fixed obstruction (e.g., chronic obstructive pulmonary disease [COPD]) do not benefit as do younger subjects with purely atopic disease. Re-evaluation of these studies has indicated that children who received allergy shots for allergic rhinitis had a lower prevalence of asthma, thus suggesting that the "allergic march" from mild to more severe disease could be halted by this therapy. Standard practice now is to give allergy shots to patients who prefer this intermittent, natural therapy over daily medication, patients who have unacceptable side effects with standard therapy, and those with concomitant severe rhinitis and mild asthma. With the development of novel therapies, these standards may need re-evaluation.

To formulate an allergen extract, the allergist examines the skin test results and compounds a mixture of extracts that are relevant to the patient's seasonal and perennial exposure and sensitivity. Extract quality has improved as a result of international standardization efforts. Subcutaneous injections begin with tiny doses because larger ones would induce anaphylaxis. During this build-up phase, each subsequent dose is raised incrementally at weekly intervals until a dose about 1000 times more concentrated can be tolerated. Caution must be used because the injections may initially build up IgE responses and induce large local wheal and flare reactions or, if systemically absorbed, induce asthma, laryngeal edema, anaphylaxis, and

*Investigational drug in the United States.

rarely, death. Therefore, shots must be given only in a medical facility equipped for resuscitation and treatment of these conditions. The build-up phase may take 4 to 9 months, depending on the patient's sensitivity, reactions, and rate of dose elevation. Once the maintenance dose is tolerated, injections are given at 2- to 4-week intervals to complete 3 years of therapy. The goal is to cumulatively administer approximately 10 to 20 μg of the principal individual allergenic proteins from each extract. At some point during the maintenance phase, the concentration of allergen-specific IgE begins to decrease. At the end of 2 years, TH_1 lymphocytes have been found to be infiltrating the nasal mucosa. TH_1 lymphocytes mediate delayed-type (granulomatous) hypersensitivity, secrete interferon-γ, and stimulate macrophages to secrete IL-12. These cytokines can antagonize the sensitization of TH_2 lymphocytes and may induce TH_2 cell tolerance (the inability of TH_2 cells to respond to allergens) or even TH_2 cell apoptosis. Recent developments to improve allergen shot therapy include the potential use of humanized anti-IgE to reduce the risk of anaphylaxis and shorten the build-up phase; "rush desensitization," in which the build-up phase is accelerated by the administration of extracts at, for example, 15-minute intervals so that the maintenance dose is reached within 1 to 3 days; assessment of oral, sublingual, and nasal routes of administration; and the addition of novel adjuvants such as covalent linkage of bacterial CpG nucleotide sequences to the allergens to enhance the still mysterious immune modulation that brings success to this therapy.

ALLERGIC REACTIONS TO DRUGS

method of
MICHAEL J. RIEDER, M.D., PH.D., FAAP, FRCPC, FRCP (GLASGOW)
Division of Clinical Pharmacology
Biotherapeutics Research Group
Child Health Research Institute,
Robarts Research Institute
Departments of Paediatrics, Physiology & Pharmacology and Medicine
University of Western Ontario
London, Ontario, Canada

SCOPE OF THE PROBLEM

The era of specific therapy, which began with the landmark observations of Fleming and Dömagk in 1928 and 1935, has provided clinicians with the ability to provide cure or control for many common and important diseases, as illustrated by the other chapters of this book. However, these benefits have not been without risks, with one of the major risks being the risk of adverse drug reactions. Adverse drug reactions (ADRs) are undesired effects of drugs that can arise as a predictable consequence of the pharmacology of the drug or as an unpredicted consequence related to variables such as the genetic background of the patient or an altered immune response.

The importance of ADRs relates to their frequency, severity, and burden on the health care system. ADRs are among the top six causes of death in North America, and, in addition to being a source of considerable morbidity and mortality, the economic costs of adverse drug reactions is in the billions. As an illustration, it is estimated that there are 90,000 to 100,000 deaths a year in the United States from adverse drug events. Given that the usual incidence of ADRs during a course of therapy is 5%, and as complex therapy and common infections including HIV infection appear to increase this risk, evaluation and management of adverse drug events is an important skill set for all physicians.

CLASSIFICATION OF ADRs

There are several classification schemes for ADRs, some of which are more detailed than others, but the basic tenet of most of these schemes is that ADRs can be considered to be predictable (or type A—augmented) or unpredictable (type B—bizarre). Predictable drug reactions are predicated on the drug's pharmacology, are dose-dependent, and are often self-limited, whereas unpredictable ADRs cannot be predicted *a priori* on the basis of the drug's pharmacology, are not dose-dependent, and often are more severe than predictable reactions (Table 1).

The most common types of ADRs are predictable adverse drug reactions (roughly 80% of adverse reactions), but the most severe adverse drug reactions, notably those associated with mortality, are unpredictable adverse drug reactions. As an illustration, every day in the United States, one or two people die of penicillin allergy, one of the most common forms of drug allergy.

RISK FACTORS FOR ADRs

There are some well-described risk factors for adverse drug reactions that can be broadly grouped into four major areas. The first consideration is history, in that a personal history of having an ADR to a drug is a risk factor for ADRs to other drugs. As well, we have found that it appears that having a family history of having ADRs increases the risk of having an ADR. It is important to note that ADRs to specific

TABLE 1. **Classification of Adverse Drug Reactions**

Predictable	**Unpredictable**
Side effects	Intolerance
Interactions	Allergic-pseudoallergic
Toxicity	Idiosyncratic
Characteristics	
Common	Uncommon
Often self-limited	Significant morbidity and mortality
Usually dose-related	No obvious dose relationship

drugs and germane to drug allergic responses to specific drugs and other antigens are not inherited.

Another risk factor for ADRs relates to polypharmacy. Not unsurprisingly, the more medications a patient takes, the higher the risk for an ADR. This is probably due to a combination of factors. First, there is the simple additive issue—if there is a 5% risk of an ADR to one drug, it is likely that there will higher rates when we use more than one drug. Second, patients taking many medications are likely to have more complex disease and may have impairment of drug clearance, as detailed below. Also, polypharmacy is more common at the extremes of age, as noted in the following sections. A third area related to risk factors for ADRs is related to impairment of the organs of drug clearance (conventionally the liver and kidney), which can occur as a result of development immaturity (in the very young), senescence (in the extreme elderly), or disease. Thus being at the extreme of age is also a risk factor.

Finally, for reasons that remain obscure, female gender is a risk factor for ADRs. This is seen even after adjustments are made for the fact that there are drug classes that are more commonly used in men than women and vice versa.

DRUG ALLERGY

The term "drug allergy" is frequently used in association with ADRs, but in fact drug allergy accounts for a distinct minority of overall adverse drug reactions. That being said, as noted previously, drug allergy is represented disproportionally among fatal and severe ADRs. As well, although drug allergy represents perhaps at most 10% of ADRs, it is increasingly clear that the immune system is involved in up to 40% of upredictable ADRs, most notably in the case of idiosyncratic ADRs that appear to occur in genetically vulnerable subsets of the population.

Drug allergy can be distinguished from other types of unpredictable ADRs by timing, symptom development, and response to rechallenge. The timing of development of symptoms is an important clue in the diagnostic evaluation of a possible drug allergy. Drug allergy that manifests as anaphylaxis usually occurs within minutes to hours of exposure, whereas urticarial reactions and bronchospasm typically occur within hours of exposure. In the case of serum sickness–like reactions, which are not classically considered drug allergy but appear quite clearly to be immune-mediated, the usual time course is development of symptoms 10 to 21 days after starting therapy. The classic theory of drug allergy requires priming of the immune system, and thus drug allergy would not be anticipated on first exposure to a drug. The response to rechallenge is typically amplified in the case of drug allergy, although the caveat is some idiosyncratic ADRs initiated by bioactivation of drugs to reactive intermediates and then probably mediated by the immune system (such as aromatic anticonvulsant hypersensitivity), although not drug allergy as currently understood, may be markedly more severe on rechallenge than with the initial exposure.

THE CLINICAL APPROACH TO A SUSPECTED ADVERSE DRUG REACTION

The approach to untoward events associated with therapy is primarily clinical, and laboratory evaluations are, in the main, unhelpful in the differential diagnosis of possible ADRs. The diagnosis of an ADR is almost entirely made on the basis of careful clinical evaluation. The clinical approach to an untoward effect related to therapy starts with careful history and physical examination. History needs to focus on the details of drug exposure, including determining indications for therapy, time of drug exposure, timing of the development of symptoms, previous drug exposure, other exposures, and other health issues. As an illustration, symptoms such as rash can be due to a variety of etiologies, including infection, and thus a rash that began before antimicrobial therapy was started is unlikely to be due to drug allergy. The time course can also be valuable if the drug has been discontinued (i.e., did symptoms improve when drug therapy was stopped?). A caveat that must be remembered is that, although drug allergy usually resolves shortly after drug therapy is stopped, other ADRs that appear to be mediated by the immune system, such as serum sickness–like reactions, often continue to develop for days despite discontinuation of therapy. The history should be conducted with care, notably in avoiding the use of leading questions. A tenet to be remembered is that, when bad things happen during treatment, patients tend to blame the drug and doctors tend to blame the disease. The truth often lies somewhere in between.

Physical examination is crucial in determining the precise nature of untoward events associated with drug therapy, particularly when these events have a cutaneous component. Although not universally true, some cutaneous manifestations are more typical of ADRs, especially drug allergy, than others. As an example, urticarial rashes (although potentially due to many causes) are more likely to be attributable to drug allergy than would, for example, a pustular eruption. Physical examination may also be important in determining if therapy has achieved the desired goal, which will be an important consideration in planning management.

At this point, the clinician must review the differential diagnosis to decide if the untoward signs and symptoms associated with therapy are in fact an ADR or if they may be due to other etiologies. In making this critical decision, clinicians may need the assistance of expert consultation as well as colleagues in drug information. Given the rapidly expanding number of new therapeutic agents, it is highly likely that the clinician may be faced with a drug or combination of drugs with which he or she is unfamiliar. Given this situation, clinicians should take advantage of the many sources of drug information now available, including drug information pharmacists, regional drug information services, and online electronic database resources such as PubMed.

After weighing the clinical data and considering the possible etiologies, the clinician must determine if untoward events associated with therapy are likely to represent an ADR, and what type of ADR these events represent. The clinician must then formulate a management plan as to how to deal with the ADR as well as with the initial diagnosis for which therapy had been prescribed. Therapy for drug allergy will be considered in the following sections. This usually includes the prompt discontinuation of therapy with the drug in question. If the disorder for which therapy had been originally prescribed has resolved (such as an infection that has been cured), then no further therapy for the original problem may be necessary. On the other hand, if the original problem has not been resolved and better control is deemed necessary (as in the case of epilepsy with frequent seizures), then it will be necessary to return to the treatment plan and review therapeutic options. In the case of predictable ADRs such as side effects, it may be possible to treat through the ADR, in the expectation that symptoms of the ADR are usually mild and usually will resolve with continuing therapy. This has been well established in the case of HIV infection, in which treating through ADRs to antiretroviral therapy is commonly used given the importance of controlling viral burden in improving the health of people living with HIV infection. In the face of unpredictable ADRs such as drug allergy or idiosyncratic drug reactions, however, continuing therapy may be associated with a significant risk of severe morbidity or even mortality. In this case, consideration must be given to alternate therapy, although efficacy may be less than desired and the patient may be at risk for other toxicities.

After the diagnosis has been made and the treatment plan has been decided upon, it is important to communicate this information clearly to the patient, where appropriate (as in the case of children or the developmentally challenged) the patient's family, and to other health care providers involved in the patient's care. Information that needs to be conveyed includes the decision as to whether an ADR occurred and the nature of the ADR, what potential impact this has on future therapy, what other agents may need to be avoided or used with caution, and what the therapeutic plan is, both for the ADR and for the original diagnosis. Drug-allergic patients must always understand what they are allergic to and which drugs and drug families which that they must avoid. Clear and forthright communication of these issues is important in providing safe therapy, in improving compliance, and in helping to sustain the doctor-patient relationship. Compliance is a key determinant of therapy, and work by us and others has demonstrated that patient awareness of and agreement with management planning is important in compliance with treatment. An often poorly acknowledged but nonetheless real issue is that patient confidence in the therapeutic planning of the physician is probably affected by the development of an ADR, and to re-establish an effective working relationship in which patient and physician can find common ground in management planning, candor is essential.

As noted previously, there needs to be communication with other health care providers involved in the patient's care, notably given the multidisciplinary care often required for medically complex patients—the very patients most at risk for ADRs. Finally, there may need to be communication with drug regulatory agencies, especially for unusual ADRs and for ADRs to new drugs, especially when these ADRS are very severe. In the process of drug approval, the majority of drugs are clinically evaluated in less than 10,000 and often less than 5,000 patients. The rate of severe drug hypersensitivity to many drugs is in the range of 1 per 2,000 to 1 per 20,000. Thus it is highly unlikely that a severe drug hypersensitivity would be detected in premarketing testing, and the role of the clinician in postmarketing surveillance is crucial. Indeed, essentially all of the severe drug hypersensitivities—such as sulfonamide-induced erythema multiforme, anticonvulsant-associated Stevens-Johnson syndrome, and halothane hepatitis—have been described by astute clinicians who have noted unusual symptoms in association with drug exposure and who carefully analyzed these untoward events and determined that they most likely represented an ADR. In the case where a clinician suspects an ADR, notably to a newly introduced drug or if the ADR is of an unusual or very severe nature, the clinician should report his or her suspicion to the appropriate drug regulatory agency, such as the MedWatch program managed by the Food and Drug Administration.

Confirmation of the ADR should be conducted if possible, but there are very few agents for which confirmatory testing is available.

THERAPY OF DRUG ALLERGY AND IMMUNE MEDIATED ADRS

The first consideration in management of drug allergy and immune mediated ADRs is whether the drug should be discontinued or whether to treat through the symptoms of the adverse event. Because this type of ADR often worsens with continuing therapy, it would be unusual not to stop therapy with the offending drug. The therapy of drug allergy, in common with the therapy of most ADRs, is largely supportive and there are few specific therapies that are effective. Therapy to some extent is predicated on the nature of the allergic response. In the case of classic drug allergy, drug-specific IgE modulates a response that can include urticaria, bronchospasm, and angioedema.

Anaphylaxis is the most severe manifestation of drug allergy and must be considered a medical emergency. Treatment starts with the ABCs—ensuring a patent airway, that the patient is breathing, and that there is adequate circulation. Oxygen and intravenous fluids are two agents that should be given to every patient who presents with anaphylaxis. Epinephrine is commonly used in the therapy of anaphylaxis

TABLE 2. **Therapy of Anaphylaxis**

1. Establish a patent Airway
2. Ensure that the patient is Breathing and that there is adequate air exchange
3. Ensure that the patient has adequate Circulation (rate, rhythm, blood pressure and microcirculation)
4. Administer oxygen
5. Start an intravenous line with normal saline
6. Administer epinephrine
7. Administer β_2-agonist or antihistamine as needed for control of bronchospasm or urticaria. The use of these agents should *not* be construed to be suitable replacements for epinephrine in the acute management of anaphylaxis
8. Monitor the patient closely—up to 25% of patients who experience an episode of anaphylaxis may have a rebound episode within the first few hours after treatment

(Table 2) and can be life-saving. The use of β_2-agonists for bronchospasm is important, and the best delivery route is by aerosol unless the patient has such severe airway compromise that effective ventilation is not possible. In this case, it may be necessary to give β_2-agonists by the intravenous route, switching to the aerosol route when the patient's ventilation improves. Corticosteroids are frequently administered to patients undergoing anaphylaxis, and although there is little literature to support this approach it is widely used. In this case, a dose of prednisone or methylprednisolone (Solu-Medrol) in the range of 1–2 mg/kg is often given as an initial dose and then followed by a 5-day course of therapy.

Management of urticaria is largely symptomatic and antihistamines are commonly used to reduce patient discomfort. Although anecdotal, by report conventional antihistamines may be somewhat more effective for this indication than H_1 selective agents. Management of bronchospasm includes the use of β_2-agonists such as albuterol (Proventil) as well as oxygen if necessary. The preferential method of delivery for β_2-agonists, as noted previously, is via aerosol. The management of angioedema in the absence of anaphylaxis is somewhat controversial, and although antihistamines are commonly used, there is little evidence that they are of benefit.

In the case of ADRs that appear to be mediated by the immune system, optimal therapy is somewhat less clear. Antihistamines, nonsteroidal anti-inflammatory drugs (NSAIDs), and brief courses of corticosteroids have all been used for the therapy of serum sickness–like reactions, with no evidence of efficacy. Use of these agents, notably the antihistamines and NSAIDs, may provide symptomatic relief. In the case of more severe ADRs believed to have an immune component, such as drug-induced Stevens-Johnson syndrome, there is no uniformly accepted therapy beyond the provision of excellent supportive care and avoiding infection. A variety of therapies, including pulse doses of corticosteroids or intravenous immunoglobulin, has been reported in case reports or small series. Given the complex nature of these ADRs and the uncertainty with respect to optimal therapy, consideration should be made for consultation with clinicians expert in the management of hypersensitivity and immune-mediated ADRs.

CONFIRMATORY TESTING FOR DRUG ALLERGY

As noted previously, there are few confirmatory tests available for drug allergy or ADRs that appear to be mediated by the immune system (Table 3). The most useful test in common clinical practice is penicillin skin testing, which for IgE-mediated penicillin allergy has greater than 95% sensitivity and specificity. However, it should be noted that these excellent results are only obtained if the antigens tested include both the major determinants and the minor determinant mixture. Testing in the absence of the minor determinant mixture is associated with a high false-negative rate, in the range of 35%. Thus, unless the complete antigen mixture is available, it would be unwise to conduct skin testing. As well, the personnel conducting the testing must be expert in

TABLE 3. **Confirmatory Testing for Suspected Adverse Drug Reactions**

Test	Role
Skin testing	Extremely useful for a limited number of drugs (penicillin, local anesthetics). Requires supply of suitable antigen (see text) and expertise with the technique; should only be conducted in settings where equipment and expertise in resuscitation is readily available
Patch testing	Useful for study of T-cell responses. Requires expertise in administering the test, and false negatives are very common (60% to 70% false negative)
Detection of specific antibody	Clinical utility not clearly demonstrated; many drugs produce an antibody response but antibody-disease correlation remains elusive in most cases. Certain specific assays (RAST to penicillin) are useful but not markedly more than alternate forms of testing (e.g., skin testing)
In vitro cytotoxicity assay	Useful for a limited number of drugs (sulfonamides, aromatic anticonvulsants); requires special expertise and very expensive
Lymphocyte transformation assay	Useful for studies of T-cell responses. Requires special expertise and false negatives are very common (60% to 70% false negative)
ELISPOT assay	Sensitive assay for detection of specific immune signaling responses; large number of cells needed, special expertise needed, precise correlation with ADRs is unclear
Rechallenge	Remains gold standard of determining if therapy will be tolerated or if an adverse event will occur; has to the patient and thus must be done in controlled circumstances by personnel expert in conducting rechallenges

skin testing and must have ready access to expertise and equipment for resuscitation.

There are a number of laboratory tests which have been used to evaluate drug allergy, but with few exceptions the role of these tests in the evaluation of possible ADRs remains unclear. In the case of penicillin-specific RAST testing, although testing is useful it is no better than penicillin skin testing, and because penicillin skin testing involves a direct challenge to the patient, the role of RAST testing remains controversial. In the hands of a small cadre of experts patch testing, lymphocyte transformation tests, and in vitro cytotoxicity assays have provided interesting information of mechanistic significance in understanding how some ADRs mediated by immunity may evolve, but these tests have not made the transition into methods that can be used routinely in clinical care. The development of pharmacogenomic techniques to evaluate possible ADRs offers promise, but given the current state of our knowledge with respect to phenotype-genotype correlations and ADRs it is likely that it will be some time before the full potential of the Human Genome Project affects the clinical evaluation of possible drug allergy.

As noted, the gold standard remains rechallenge. There are two possible roles for rechallenge. In the setting in which an ADR is almost certainly the result of a particular drug, there is little clinical utility and considerable ethical concern with respect to re-exposing the patient to the drug in question. However, it may be useful to conduct a challenge to determine if the patient can tolerate therapy with alternate agents, notably when there is an ongoing need for treatment. Alternately, if the untoward events are viewed as being unlikely to be due to an ADR, notably in a setting in which there is a therapeutic advantage for the patient to be able to take a particular drug, then rechallenge may be useful in confirming that the adverse events associated with therapy were not related to the drug in question and that future therapy would be a reasonable therapeutic option.

In either case, the patient and family as appropriate must clearly understand what the goal of rechallenge is and what the results of the rechallenge will mean for the patient. Rechallenge often starts with use of a small fraction of the therapeutic dose (for example, 1/10th of the desired therapeutic dose) followed by dose escalation if the rechallenge is tolerated. Rechallenge should only be performed by personnel expert in the technique and only in settings with ready access to equipment for and personal expertise in resuscitation.

THERAPEUTIC IMPLICATIONS OF MECHANISTIC STUDIES

Over the past decade, there have been a number of studies exploring the mechanism(s) of drug allergy and of ADRs that appear to be mediated by the immune system. In the case of drug allergy, it is increasingly clear that drug allergy is a more dynamic process than previously believed, and that there are patients who develop and who then lose drug allergies. It is also clear that, across the developed world, drug allergy and allergic disease in general is steadily increasing in incidence.

With respect to ADRs that appear to be mediated by the immune system, it is increasingly clear that many of these ADRs occur among special subsets of patients, either due to genetics or disease, and that bioactivation of a parent drug to a reactive metabolite that results in an immune response is an important component of severe ADRs to these agents. It also appears that, at least for some of these reactions, alteration in T-cell response from humoral to cell-mediated responses may be a key event in the immune modulation of these reactions, and that this may result from the effect(s) of reactive metabolites on specific signaling pathways involved in T-cell activation and cell signaling, including the Jak and Stat kinases or *Fas*-mediated pathways.

IMPORTANCE OF DRUG ALLERGY TO THE PRACTICING CLINICIAN

Drug allergy and ADRs mediated by the immune system include some of the most severe and life-threatening adverse reactions seen in clinical practice. Clinicians must have a high index of suspicion and remain vigilant when treating the patients under their care with any drug and must have an organized, focused approach to the diagnosis and management of suspected drug allergy.

ALLERGIC REACTIONS TO INSECT STINGS

method of
DAVID F. GRAFT, M.D.
Park Nicollet Clinic
Minneapolis, Minnesota

The normal response to an insect sting is transient redness, pain, and itching at the sting site. A large local reaction occurs in 10% of people and consists of swelling greater than 5 cm in diameter that persists for longer than 24 hours. For example, a sting on the hand may produce swelling of the hand and entire forearm.

Systemic allergic reactions resulting from stings by insects of the order Hymenoptera (honeybees, yellow jackets, hornets, wasps, and imported fire ants) affect 1% of the U.S. population and may be mild, with only cutaneous symptoms (pruritus, urticaria, angioedema), or more severe, with potentially life-threatening symptoms (laryngeal edema, bronchospasm, hypotension). Approximately 50 deaths per year are attributed to insect stings in the United States. Only one or two occur in children; the number of deaths increases gradually with age and reaches 10 deaths per year for each 10 years of life for persons aged 40 to 49, 50 to 59, and 60 to 69 years. The true incidence of insect sting–related fatalities may be even higher because sudden deaths on the golf course or at poolside may be mistakenly ascribed to heart attacks or strokes. Patients with insect sting hypersensitivity often alter their lifestyles, work patterns, and leisure activities to avoid future stings.

ACUTE MANAGEMENT

Treatment recommendations for large local reactions include antihistamines, the application of ice packs, and elevation of the affected limb. A short course of prednisone (0.5 to 1 mg/kg/d for 5 days), especially if initiated immediately after the sting, may be the best therapy for massive local reactions. Sting sites should be kept clean; imported fire ant stings are especially easily infected.

Patients with anaphylaxis require careful observation. An intramuscular (preferred) or subcutaneous injection of epinephrine (1:1000) at a dose of 0.3 to 0.5 mL (in children, 0.01 mL/kg; maximum, 0.3 mL) is the cornerstone of management and is often sufficient to terminate a reaction. Patients with a history of cardiac disease warrant careful monitoring. The epinephrine may be repeated in 10 to 15 minutes if necessary. An oral antihistamine such as diphenhydramine hydrochloride (Benadryl), 12.5 to 50 mg, is also usually given. It may lessen urticaria or other cutaneous symptoms, but in more serious or progressive reactions, its use should not delay the administration of epinephrine. Diphenhydramine hydrochloride may also be administered parenterally (50 mg in adults every 4 hours; 5 mg/kg/d in divided doses every 4 to 6 hours [maximum, 50 mg per dose] in children) for more serious reactions.

Inhaled sympathomimetic agents such as albuterol (Proventil) may decrease bronchoconstriction but do not address other systemic manifestations such as shock. Theophylline may be helpful if bronchoconstriction persists after the administration of epinephrine. Severe reactions often necessitate treatment with oxygen, H_2 antihistamines such as cimetidine (Tagamet),* volume expanders, and pressor agents. Corticosteroids such as prednisone (0.5 to 1 mg/kg/d) are commonly used, but their delayed onset of action (4 to 6 hours) limits their effectiveness in the early stages of treatment. Intubation or tracheostomy is indicated for severe upper airway edema that does not respond to therapy. Allergic reactions are generally more severe in patients who take β-blocking drugs. Furthermore, reactions in these patients may be more difficult to treat because β-blockers impede the response to epinephrine and other sympathomimetic medications. Glucagon,* 1 to 5 mg given over a period of several minutes intravenously, may be helpful in this clinical situation.

Systemic reactions commencing more than several hours after a sting are generally mild, and most are easily managed with oral antihistamines and observation. On occasion, anaphylaxis may be prolonged or biphasic. Close observation and continued treatment are essential in these situations. The administration of corticosteroids as early in treatment as feasible may help diminish later symptoms.

*Not FDA approved for this indication.

DECREASING FUTURE REACTIONS

Preventing Stings

Future stings can be avoided by taking commonsense precautions to significantly reduce exposure. Because many stings in children occur when they step on a bee, shoes should always be worn outside. Hives and nests around the home should be exterminated. Good sanitation should be practiced because garbage and outdoor food, especially canned drinks, attract yellow jackets. Perfumes and dark or floral-patterned clothing should be avoided.

Emergency Epinephrine

To encourage prompt treatment, epinephrine is available in emergency kits for self-administration (Table 1). These kits are used by insect sting–allergic people immediately after the sting to "buy time" to get to a medical facility. The Ana-Kit contains a preloaded syringe that can deliver two 0.3-mL doses of epinephrine. Incremental doses may also be given. Physicians who prescribe this kit must provide thorough instructions and must be confident that the patient can perform the injection procedure. These kits can be confusing to nonmedical personnel, and some patients have a tremendous fear of needles. The EpiPen (0.3 mg of epinephrine) and EpiPen Jr. (0.15 mg of epinephrine) offer a concealed needle and a pressure-sensitive spring-loaded injection device, which makes them suitable for patients and families who are uncomfortable with the injection process. Aerosolized epinephrine may also be used to achieve therapeutic levels of epinephrine in plasma and may be especially helpful for laryngeal edema and bronchospasm. Patients who are receiving maintenance injections of venom immunotherapy are advised that emergency self-treatment will probably not be required. However,

TABLE 1. **Epinephrine Injection Kits for Emergency Self-Treatment of Systemic Reactions to Insect Stings**

Injection Kit	Dosage
EpiPen*	Delivers 0.3 mL of a 1:1000 solution (0.3 mg epinephrine)
EpiPen Jr.*	Delivers 0.3 mL of a 1:2000 solution (0.15 mg epinephrine)
Ana-Kit†	Delivers 2 doses of 0.3 mL of a 1:1000 solution (total, 0.6 mg epinephrine)

*The EpiPen and EpiPen Jr. are spring-loaded automatic injectors distributed by Dey Laboratories, Port Washington, NY.

†Ana-Kit is capable of delivering fractional doses and is distributed by Hollister-Stier Laboratories, Spokane, WA.

From Graft DF: Insect stings. *In* Gellis SS, Kagan BM (eds): Current Pediatric Therapy. Philadelphia, WB Saunders, 1990.

they should have the kit available if they are far from medical facilities. Wearing of a MedicAlert bracelet or medallion (Medic Alert Foundation International, 2323 Colorado Avenue, Turlock, CA 95382) is also advised.

Venom Immunotherapy

The clinical history is the key to determining the need for venom immunotherapy (Table 2). A careful history discloses the type, degree, and time course of the symptoms and often reveals the culprit insect. A patient who has experienced a sting-induced systemic reaction should be referred to an allergist, who will perform skin tests with dilute solutions of honeybee, yellow jacket, yellow hornet, white-faced hornet, and *Polistes* wasp venom. Radioallergosorbent testing (RAST) cannot replace venom skin testing but may provide additional information. Whole-body extract materials were used before 1979 to diagnose and treat insect allergy, but they were shown to be ineffective, and venom supplanted their use. To date, fire ant venom has been available only in small research quantities. Fortunately, the fire ant whole-body extract seems more potent than those previously available for other Hymenoptera species and has been successfully used for skin testing and treatment.

Adults with systemic reactions (generalized urticaria, angioedema, bronchospasm, laryngeal edema, or hypertension) and positive venom skin test results commence venom immunotherapy. Children with more severe reactions and positive venom skin test results are also given venom immunotherapy. Because the recurrence rate in children with a history of milder reactions (limited to the skin, i.e., urticaria) is only 10%, venom treatment is not required. Patients with large local reactions do not generally start venom injections because of their low risk of systemic reactions. A recent report described patients with systemic reactions and negative venom skin test results who still reacted again on subsequent stings. The authors suggested evaluation by RAST and repeat venom skin tests. These patients should practice sting avoidance measures and be prepared to treat reactions with antihistamines, epinephrine, and other medications.

Increasing amounts of venom (or whole-body extracts for fire ant sensitivity) are given weekly for several months until the patient can tolerate a venom dose equivalent to one or more insect stings. Venom injections are given every 4 weeks during the first year of treatment, and then the interval can be extended to 6 weeks. Venom therapy is highly effective, with 97% of patients protected from reactions to subsequent stings (the risk of an allergic reaction for untreated insect sting–allergic persons is probably about 60%). Disadvantages of venom treatment include cost and systemic and local reactions to the injections. No long-term side effects have been reported. Patients should be informed of the possible risks and closely observed for 30 minutes or more after each injection. Injections should be administered only in settings where adequate means of treating systemic reactions are available.

In about 25% of patients, negative skin test results develop after 3 to 5 years of treatment, and these patients may be able to discontinue therapy. Furthermore, a 5-year course of venom injections is probably sufficient for most patients, with those who have very severe reactions being the major exceptions. A position paper on discontinuation of venom immunotherapy was recently published by the American Academy of Allergy Asthma and Immunology in the *Journal of Allergy and Clinical Immunology*.

TABLE 2. **Selection of Patients for Venom Immunotherapy**

Sting Reaction	Skin Test/ RAST	Venom Immunotherapy
Systemic, non–life-threatening (child): immediate, generalized, confined to the skin (urticaria, angioedema, erythema, pruritus)	+ or –	No*
Systemic, life-threatening (child): immediate, generalized, may involve cutaneous symptoms but also has respiratory (laryngeal edema or bronchospasm) or cardiovascular symptoms (hypotension/shock)	+	Yes
Systemic (adult)	+	Yes
Systemic	–	No
Large local (>2 inches [5 cm] in diameter; >24 h)	+ or –	No*
Normal (<2 inches [5 cm] in diameter; <24 h)	+ or –	No

*Exceptions are sometimes made.
Abbreviation: RAST, radioallergosorbent test.
From Graft DF: Insect stings. *In* Gellis SS, Kagan BM (eds): Current Pediatric Therapy, Philadelphia, WB Saunders, 1990.

Section 13

Diseases of the Skin

ACNE VULGARIS AND ROSACEA

method of
OTTER Q. ASPEN, M.D., and
ROBERT S. STERN, M.D.
Department of Dermatology
Beth Israel Deaconess Medical Center
Harvard Medical School
Boston, Massachusetts

Sometime between 11 and 30 years of age, most people develop acne. The condition varies greatly in severity and duration among persons. In women, acne often persists and may worsen after age 30. Acne vulgaris is a hormonally driven disorder of the pilosebaceous unit.

For both diagnosis and to guide therapy, it is helpful to categorize acne lesions as either noninflammatory or inflammatory. Comedones are the noninflammatory and often the initial lesion of acne. Clinically, two types of comedones are seen: (1) the open, or "blackhead," appearing as a dilated pore filled with darkly colored keratinous material, and (2) the closed, or "whitehead," which is a small, flesh-colored to white papule. The inflammatory lesions of acne are papules and pustules in the most common form, and nodules and cysts in more severe disease. The pathogenesis of acne is thought to consist of (1) androgen stimulation of sebum production, (2) obstruction of the sebaceous follicle outlet by keratin plugs, (3) colonization of the subsequently trapped sebum and keratin by *Propionibacterium acnes*, and (4) an inflammatory reaction to the materials, bacteria, and bacterial products.

COMEDONAL ACNE

Particularly among younger patients or among mature women using topical preparations (cosmetics), facial acne often consists primarily of comedones; few inflammatory lesions may be present. For these patients, topical treatments, particularly topical retinoids, are often sufficient.

Benzoyl Peroxide

For all types of mild acne, benzoyl peroxide from 2.5% to 10% is potentially useful and often sufficient. It is a mainstay of the initial treatment of mild to moderate acne, either as monotherapy or as part of combination therapy with oral or other topical agents. It is available over the counter and in many inexpensive formulations, including washes, lotions, and gels. Used once a day, it is usually well tolerated, but irritation can be a problem. Even after more than 40 years, benzoyl peroxide remains the "gold standard" in the therapy of mild to moderate acne.

Retinoids

When benzoyl peroxide is not sufficient, topical retinoids are often effective as a single-agent therapy in comedonal acne, or in combination with other agents in patients with mild to moderate inflammatory acne, particularly if comedones are present. Substantial clinical improvement generally requires 6 to 12 weeks of treatment. Maximum improvement usually occurs in 3 to 4 months.

Initial worsening of acne and local irritation are the principal drawbacks to topical retinoid use. Irritation is greatest initially, but usually is sufficiently mild to not require treatment. If desired, a noncomedogenic moisturizing lotion may be suggested. Some patients with histories of eczema may find topical retinoids too irritating even with moisturization. There are three topical retinoids available: tretinoin (Retin-A), adapalene gel (Differin), and tazarotene gel (Tazorac). Although claims of greater efficacy or equivalent with less irritation are made, these are not well founded. Branded and newer topical retinoids cost 50% to 150% more than generic tretinoin and are not proven superior. Therefore, we begin with topical tretinoin cream 0.025%, and adjusting the dose depending on response and tolerability. Sun protection and avoiding pregnancy (on theoretical grounds only) are recommended.

INFLAMMATORY ACNE

Acne varies greatly from a few papules and pustules to multiple cysts. Therapy should be tailored according to the extent, number, and distribution of lesions; the extent to which the patient is bothered by their disease; and by the tendency to scar. There is a wide misperception that acne is caused by patients not keeping their skin clean, so addressing this concern and advising not to wash too frequently, which may exacerbate the irritation seen with topical agents, is also important.

MILD TO MODERATE ACNE

For most types of acne, a sequential approach to therapy is recommended. The most common form of acne is mild to moderate acne that includes papules, pustules, and a mild to moderate comedonal component. For these patients, my initial recommendation is usually benzoyl peroxide plus a topical antibiotic, either erythromycin (Erycette, Erygel) or clindamycin (Cleocin T), each used once a day. There is little evidence demonstrating superiority of one topical aminoglycoside over another. Combination preparations (benzoyl peroxide plus aminoglycoside in a single agent) are associated with more irritation and greater cost than using the two preparations separately. If the patient has a relatively heavy comedonal component, consider switching either the benzoyl peroxide or the topical antibiotic to a topical retinoid.

MODERATE TO SEVERE ACNE

If inflammatory acne is widespread or the lesions are large, initial therapy with oral as well as topical agents is often recommended. Studies have shown that initiation of therapy consisting of both topical agents and systemic antibiotics on the *initial visit* is cost effective when compared with trials of isolated topical therapies and then progression to the combined approach. The analysis holds true even when factoring in the increases in side effects experienced by patients on systemic antibiotics.

The usual first oral agent added to the regimen is tetracycline or a tetracycline derivative. For some women who experience acne that changes in severity with their menstrual cycle, addition of the oral contraceptive pills (OCP) Triphasil may be useful. For women already using OCPs, consider switching to a less androgenic version than that already in use. OCPs in common usage with the lowest androgen activity contain the synthetic progestin norgestimate (Ortho Tri-Cyclen).

Oral Antibiotics

Tetracycline 500 mg twice daily is a commonly used approach, and relatively effective and inexpensive. The most frequent toxicities are nausea, diarrhea, photosensitivity, and candidal vaginitis in women. Other tetracyclines commonly used include: doxycycline (Doryx, Vibramycin) 50–100 mg twice daily every day, which is also inexpensive and can be taken with meals with better gastrointestinal tolerance, but has great photosensitivity (with twice-daily dosing); and minocycline (Minocin Oral) 50–100 mg twice per day every day, which is effective, but significantly more expensive and has a risk of vestibular side effects and hypersensitivity reactions that may be severe. Erythromycin 250–500 mg twice daily is an inexpensive alternative if tetracyclines are ineffective or not tolerated, but its use is associated with frequent gastrointestinal disturbance and is probably less effective than tetracycline. Finally, trimethoprim-sulfamethoxazole (Bactrim)* may be used if other antibiotics fail. It has significant risk of adverse effects with prolonged use and is a frequent cause of allergic reactions, which may be severe. There is little evidence for efficacy of many other antibiotics, including the penicillins and cephalosporins.

Hormonal Therapy

Inhibiting androgen-driven increases in sebum production is the theory behind these treatments. One approach is to prescribe OCPs to women with moderate acne, which serve to inhibit 5α-reductase and increase the amount of circulating sex hormone binding globulin. However, most women with acne do not have abnormal levels of androgens for their age. Currently, levonorgestrel-ethinyl estradiol (Triphasil) is the only contraceptive approved for acne therapy.

Another anti-androgen sometimes used in women is spironolactone (Aldactone),* which decreases ovarian production of testosterone and binds to testosterone receptors. A common starting dose is 100 mg every day. Studies support the long-term safety of this treatment, although side effects (menstrual irregularities, mild central nervous system symptoms, breast tenderness) are common in early treatment. Concomitant use of an OCP helps control menstrual irregularities and prevents pregnancy, which should be avoided while using spironolactone.

Isotretinoin (Accutane)

Isotretinoin has revolutionized the treatment of severe inflammatory and nodulocystic acne, but its potential toxicity limits its use to those with severe disease not responsive to or intolerant of other therapies. Isotretinoin inhibits sebaceous gland differentiation, alters keratinization in the follicle, and has some anti-inflammatory activity. Its mechanism of action is, however, unknown.

Dosing varies by the individual, typically about 1.0 mg/kg/d for 20 weeks. For patients with extensive truncal involvement, doses of up to 2.0 mg/kg/d may be used. Patients often worsen in the first months of therapy, and subsequent improvement often continues after the 20-week course of therapy is completed. Remissions average about 18 months. Depending on relapse severity, treatment with conventional therapies including oral antibiotics may be sufficient. Retreatment may be required and is usually at least as effective as the initial therapies. Multiple treatments may increase the risk of bone changes, including hyperostosis.

The known and reputed side effects of isotretinoin use are many, and in some cases quite serious. Because of this, a physician must obtain a special qualification permit to prescribe isotretinoin. Of the known risks of isotretinoin use, teratogenicity (major fetal abnormalities, spontaneous abortion, premature births, and low IQ scores of surviving infants) is of

*Not FDA approved for this indication.

particular concern. *Pregnancy and the risk of becoming pregnant are absolute contraindications for use.* Female patients considering isotretinoin therapy of childbearing potential should start an OCP regimen 1 month before, for the duration of, and for 1 month after use. Food and Drug Administration regulations and manufacturer recommendations stipulate very specific testing and precautions to avoid pregnancy. No damage to male reproductive ability has been demonstrated.

Elevated cholesterol and triglyceride levels are common side effects of initial isotretinoin use. However, those patients with hypercholesterolemia during treatment have been shown to be the same with elevated cholesterol before treatment, and the significance of the elevated triglycerides continues to be debated.

Depression is another common concern among patients, and has been widely publicized in the media. Studies have failed to demonstrate any statistically significant increase in incidence or severity of depression or other psychiatric disorders in users of isotretinoin. Although the weight of evidence at this time fails to establish a link, studies performed so far lack the power needed to exclude the possibility of an occasional idiosyncratic reaction.

Other serious but less frequent toxicities include pseudotumor cerebri, myalgias with significant elevations of creatine kinase, hepatitis, a serum sickness–like reaction vasculitis with severely inflamed lesions, and pyogenic granuloma–like lesions in a few patients treated for nodulocystic acne. Less serious but more common complaints consist of dry skin, lips, eyes, and thinning of hair (usually regrows after treatment). It is common to see epistaxis and flares of atopic dermatitis particularly in winter months.

Acne fulminans is a rare complication of severe acne manifesting as sudden onset cystic acne with suppuration and ulceration, malaise, fatigue, fever, generalized arthralgias, leukocytosis, and an elevated erythrocyte sedimentation rate (ESR). It is unpredictable and not preventable. Current protocol is oral prednisolone* 0.5-1.0 mg/kg/d for 4 to 6 weeks followed by a taper to zero.

Rosacea is a disorder of sebaceous glands plus hyperresponsive superficial facial vasculature. It is characterized by papules and pustules on a background of erythema and telangiectasia of facial skin. It generally affects middle-age patients, and there is usually a long history of episodic flushing in response to increases in skin temperature (drinking hot liquids, eating spicy foods, exposure to sun or heat) or ingestion of alcohol. The process tends to affect mainly the middle third of the face, from forehead to chin. Comedones are not typically present. Some patients with rosacea develop rhinophyma (enlarged sebaceous glands and thickened skin on the nose). Telangiectasias may become prominent, and are permanent unless destroyed. Antibiotics are useful for the initial component.

*Not FDA approved for this indication.

Topical Therapy

Topical clindamycin and erythromycin are useful and inexpensive. Topical metronidazole (MetroGel) is as effective for rosacea, but expensive. Topical antibiotics are applied twice daily for several months and then tapered. Effective and well-tolerated therapy for the flushing associated with rosacea is not available. Tretinoin and benzoyl peroxide preparations may aggravate the erythema and are usually not used.

Systemic Therapy

Systemic antibiotics are effective in treating rosacea, as well as the keratitis or blepharitis that may accompany the condition. Tetracycline or erythromycin 250 mg twice daily is often effective initially. After the first month, the dosage can often be lowered and ultimately discontinued. Recurrences are common, and repeated courses of antibiotics may be needed.

Surgical Therapy

Medical treatment has a limited effect on erythema and no impact on telangiectasias. Rhinophyma may be treated with dermabrasion, curettage, or laser therapy. Telangiectasias can be treated with laser therapy.

In conclusion, there are many treatments available for acne vulgaris and rosacea. To decide what therapy is initially appropriate, it is necessary to assess the severity of the disease in the patient, the impact of the disease on the well being of the patient, and to judge the potential benefits and risks associated with any treatment. The intermittent and sometimes chronic nature of these diseases necessitates good follow-up of patients and recognition on the part of the physician that adjustments may have to be made to any given regimen of treatment.

HAIR DISORDERS

method of
DIRK M. ELSTON, M.D.
*Departments of Dermatology and Pathology
Geisinger Medical Center
Danville, Pennsylvania*

Effective management of hair disorders depends upon accurate diagnosis. History and physical examination together with a few inexpensive blood tests will establish the cause in most cases of nonscarring alopecia. Scalp biopsies are generally essential for the accurate diagnosis of scarring alopecia. The evaluation of hair loss should be performed in an efficient and cost-effective manner. Broad panels of blood tests are costly and seldom of benefit.

The initial steps in the evaluation are to determine if the hair loss is scarring versus nonscarring and patchy versus diffuse. Nonscarring alopecia preserves the follicular openings (ostia). Patchy alopecia may present with circumscribed areas of complete hair loss, or localized areas of hair thinning. The following sections will lead you through the evaluation of the most common hair disorders.

The most common forms of *nonscarring* alopecia are trichodystrophy (shaft fracture), pattern alopecia, telogen effluvium, tinea, and alopecia areata. When evaluating a patient with nonscarring hair loss, one must determine if the hair is breaking or is shedding at the root. Examine the scalp. If patches of short hairs are noted, hair breakage is likely. Collected hairs can be examined microscopically. A hair shed at the root will end with a nonpigmented blunt bulb. A hair shaft that is frayed or loses pigment and tapers at the proximal end is a sign of shaft fracture.

SHAFT FRACTURE/TRICHORRHEXIS NODOSA

Shaft fracture is generally related to an inherited or acquired defect in the hair shaft—a trichodystrophy. The most common form of trichodystrophy is trichorrhexis nodosa. It is common in African-American patients and is a sign of overprocessed hair. Trichorrhexis nodosa is characterized by a frayed node along the hair shaft that resembles two broom sticks pushed together. Patients with trichorrhexis nodosa can be reassured that their scalp and hair follicles are healthy, although the hair shafts are damaged. They should adopt gentle hair care practices to reduce shaft fracture while healthier hair regrows. A reduced frequency of hair relaxing by an experienced professional is generally adequate to allow for gradual regrowth of normal hair shafts.

Some inherited trichodystrophies are associated with genetic syndromes, and an accurate diagnosis is essential. The accurate diagnosis of a trichodystrophy is established by microscopic examination of involved hair shafts by an experienced clinician or dermatopathologist.

PATTERN ALOPECIA

Pattern alopecia presents with central hair thinning. In males, vertex thinning is generally accompanied by recession in the area of the temples. Balding in men is mediated by dihydrotestosterone (DHT). Men with pattern alopecia may be treated with topical 5% minoxidil (Rogaine Extra Strength for Men) or oral finasteride (Propecia), 1 mg daily. Oral finasteride inhibits the enzyme 5-α reductase, and inhibits the formation of DHT. Finasteride treatment is generally well-tolerated, although occasional patients experience impotence. Impotence is typically reversible when the drug is stopped. Minoxidil's mode of action is to lengthen the duration of anagen and produce a longer, and somewhat thicker, hair fiber.

In women, the pathogenesis of pattern alopecia is complex, and finasteride is of no benefit to the majority of women with pattern alopecia. The frontal hairline is usually preserved, but the part is distinctly wider anteriorly. Women with temporal hair recession may be more likely to respond to finasteride,* whereas women with a preserved frontal hairline are not likely to benefit from finasteride. Women with a preserved frontal hairline may be treated with topical 2% minoxidil (Rogaine), but are not likely to derive greater benefit from the more expensive 5% formulation (Rogaine Extra Strength for Men). Antiandrogens, such as spironolactone (Aldactone)* 100 mg twice daily may also be useful in the setting of female pattern alopecia. In women of childbearing potential, spironolactone is generally used in conjunction with an oral contraceptive. Side effects include urinary frequency, nausea, irregular periods, and the potential for potassium retention.

Women with pattern alopecia should also be evaluated for causes of telogen effluvium (see the following section). Telogen effluvium is common, and often accelerates the course of pattern alopecia. The presence of active shedding of hairs at the root, together with central thinning and a preserved frontal hair line and wide anterior part, suggest pattern alopecia with a superimposed telogen effluvium. Central thinning with a wide anterior part, in the absence of significant increased shedding, suggests pattern alopecia alone.

Women with virilization require an endocrine evaluation. A total testosterone and DHEA-S screen for ovarian and adrenal tumors. History and physical examination are sufficient to identify or exclude polycystic ovarian syndrome (PCOS). The diagnosis of PCOS requires clinical evidence of androgen excess (such as hirsutism), together with historical evidence of anovulation (periods more than 40 days apart or fewer than nine periods per year). Patients with PCOS are at increased risk for heart disease and possibly uterine cancer. Their risk factors should be addressed medically. Check serum lipids! They are the single most important lab test in patients with PCOS. Hormonal cycling can be useful to prevent endometrial hyperplasia and reduce the risk of cancer.

Patients with PCOS often have mildly increased testosterone and may have increased prolactin levels. Only 50% have an elevated luteinizing hormone/follicle-stimulating hormone ratio. Hormonal studies only rarely affect management in patients with PCOS. Serum lipids do affect management, and lipid studies should always be ordered.

TELOGEN EFFLUVIUM

Telogen effluvium is characterized by active shedding of hairs with a nonpigmented clublike bulb. A gentle pull on a large tuft of hair generally results in the easy extraction of numerous club hairs.

An average adult has approximately 100,000 scalp hairs. At any given time, 90% of these are in the active growth, or anagen, phase. Approximately 10% are normally in the resting, or telogen, phase. Telogen hairs rest for 3 to 5 months, and then are shed to make way for a new anagen hair. During times of stress, the body converts large numbers of hairs to telogen phase. The larger the telogen conversion, the

*Not FDA approved for this indication.

TABLE 1. **Newer Oral Antifungal Agents for Tinea Capitis**

Antifungal Agent	Dose	Usual Duration of Therapy
Fluconazole (Diflucan)*	5–6 mg/kg/d	20 days
Itraconazole (Sporanox)*	3–5 mg/kg/d	4 weeks (6 weeks for *Microsporum canis* infections)
	5 mg/kg/d	1 week, repeatedly monthly until cured (allows therapy to be adjusted to clinical response)
Terbinafine (Lamisil)*	Patient <20 kg: 62.5 mg/d Patient 20–40 kg: 125 mg/d Patient >40 kg: 250 mg/d	2–4 weeks (generally ineffective against *Microsporum canis*)

*Not FDA approved for this indication.

more significant the shedding will be 3 to 5 months later.

Generalized telogen effluvium commonly occurs 3 to 5 months after a major surgery, pregnancy, or crash diet. Prolonged generalized telogen effluvium may also be related to nutritional deficiency or thyroid disorder. Patients should be questioned about dietary habits, use of vitamins or supplements, and frequency of meat consumption. Heavy periods or other sources of blood loss may result in nutritional deficiency. Iron is a critical nutrient for hair growth, and serves as a good screen for nutritional status. A blood count is an inadequate screen, as the body will manufacture blood at the expense of hair. Serum iron, total iron binding capacity (TIBC), iron saturation, and ferritin should be determined. A low serum ferritin is always a sign of iron deficiency. A normal ferritin does not exclude iron deficiency, because ferritin behaves as an acute phase reactant, and is elevated in inflammatory states. Iron deficient males and postmenopausal women must always be examined for sources of blood loss.

A careful history and physical examination may suggest signs of thyroid disease. A thyroid-stimulating hormone (TSH) test is generally an adequate screen for thyroid disease in a patient with suggestive signs or symptoms.

Generalized telogen effluvium can also result from a papulosquamous disorder of the scalp, such as seborrheic dermatitis or psoriasis. Patchy telogen effluvium is usually associated with an inflammatory papulosquamous scalp condition. In these areas, anagen hairs convert to telogen, and are then shed. The scalp is usually red or scaly. These conditions may be treated with selenium sulfide (Selsun), coal tar (T-gel and others) or zinc pyrithione shampoo (Head and Shoulders and others), and a topical corticosteroid preparation such as triamcinolone (Kenalog) spray or clobetasol (Olux) foam. African American patients often prefer an oil-based product, such as fluocinolone in peanut oil (Derma-Smoothe).

TINEA

Tinea capitis can present as a circumscribed boggy and purulent kerion, as an alopecic patch with black dots, or as patchy alopecia with minimal scale. Widespread patchy hair thinning with seborrheic-like scale in an African-American child should always raise the suspicion of tinea. Culture is slow, so a timely diagnosis commonly depends upon a properly performed potassium hydroxide (KOH) examination. Kerion lesions will have the lowest yield on KOH examination, but a short broken hair within a kerion pustule may demonstrate fungal spores. Black dot and "seborrheic" tinea are best diagnosed by rubbing the scalp with a moist gauze pad. The short broken hairs that adhere to the gauze provide the best yield of fungal spores. On KOH examination, the short broken hairs will contain chains of large spherelike spores. The chains are entirely confined to the interior of the hair fiber in most cases of tinea.

Topical agents are only used as adjunctive treatments in the management of tinea capitis. Either 2.5% selenium sulfide (Selsun)* shampoo or 2% ketoconazole (Nizoral)* shampoo can be used to reduce the burden of spores and decrease contagion. Cure depends upon oral antifungal agents. For a child, griseofulvin (Grifulvin V) suspension can be used in twice daily doses of 5 to 15 mg/kg/d given with a fatty meal, whole milk, or ice cream. At least 2 months of therapy is generally required. Griseofulvin may cause a nagging headache, which typically responds to a reduction in dose. Treatment for at least 2 weeks beyond clinical cure with negative cultures is reasonable because of the high rate of recurrence. Asymptomatic siblings and natural bristle brushes are common sources of reinfection.

Newer antifungal agents, including fluconazole (Diflucan), itraconazole (Sporanox), and terbinafine (Lamisil)* in doses noted in Table 1 have been used in various dosage schedules to treat tinea capitis. Such off-label uses are likely to increase, because pill forms of griseofulvin are difficult to obtain.

ALOPECIA AREATA

Alopecia areata generally presents with circumscribed smooth areas of hair loss. The scalp appears normal or slightly pink. Short fractured exclamation point hairs may be noted at the periphery of an active patch, and easily extractable hairs from the edge of the lesion will demonstrate a nonpigmented tapered fracture instead of a normal hair bulb. Alopecia areata affects pigmented scalp hairs. Gray or white hair is rarely affected. Patients with salt-and-pepper hair can develop white hair "overnight" as a result of alopecia areata.

Alopecia totalis involves the entire scalp. Alopecia universalis involves the entire body. A diffuse form of alopecia areata exists that may mimic pattern alopecia

*Not FDA approved for this indication.

or telogen effluvium. Clues to the correct diagnosis include the presence of nail pitting, tapered hair fractures, and a history of periodic regrowth.

Alopecia areata is autoimmune in etiology, and is sometimes associated with other autoimmune disorders such as vitiligo, diabetes mellitus, and thyroid disease. A TSH or fasting blood sugar is only indicated if signs or symptoms of thyroid disease or diabetes are present.

In questionable cases, a biopsy is useful for confirmation. Histologically, alopecia areata is characterized by follicular miniaturization, a peribulbar lymphoid infiltrate that may contain eosinophils, and pigment incontinence from the hair bulb. These histologic features may also be seen in syphilis. Clinical features of syphilis and alopecia areata may show significant overlap. Patients should be examined for other signs of syphilis, such as a papulosquamous rash on the trunk, lesions of the palms and soles, and pink to gray mucous patches. Serologic testing for syphilis should be considered, especially in adults with new patches of hair loss.

Circumscribed areas of alopecia areata may occasionally respond to daily applications of potent topical corticosteroid preparations, but the response to injected corticosteroids is more rapid and much more reliable. Triamcinolone (Kenalog, 3–10 mg/mL) is injected intradermally with a 30-gauge needle. A response is generally noted within 1 month. Injections are repeated monthly until the regrowth is self-sustaining. If eyebrows are injected, a lower concentration of 3–5 mg/mL is generally used. Attention must be paid to the total dose of injectable steroid, because systemic absorption occurs.

Widespread alopecia areata may be treated with topical corticosteroid preparations such as betamethasone dipropionate (Diprosone)* lotion, fluocinonide (Lidex)* solution, or clobetasol (Olux)* foam. Clobetasol is a class I corticosteroid, and should generally not be used continuously for periods of more than 2 weeks. After the first 2 weeks, it can be applied on weekends, whereas a less potent corticosteroid is applied daily during the remainder of the week. In young children, milder preparations such as betamethasone valerate (Betatrex) lotion are often more suitable for long-term use on the scalp.

Refractory alopecia areata may respond to oral corticosteroids, but the response is often temporary, and the risks must be weighed against the benefits of hair regrowth. In general, a 1- to 2-month trial of prednisone* is reasonable in cases of widespread, rapidly progressive alopecia areata. A tapered dosage schedule, beginning with 1 mg/kg/d is reasonable. Topical corticosteroid therapy should be started when the dose falls below 0.3 mg/kg/d. Oral cyclosporine,* in doses of 2–5 mg/kg/d can be effective, but the response is temporary, and potential side effects limit the desirability of treatment with cyclosporine (Sandimmune). Unfortunately, topical cyclosporine is ineffective. Newer topical macrolides are more active topically, and are being studied in the setting of alopecia areata.

*Not FDA approved for this indication.

Topical immunotherapy with DNCB, diphencyprone,† and squaric acid dibutyl ester† are also being studied. Topical or systemic PUVA (psoralen with ultraviolet A)* therapy and topical minoxidil (Rogaine)* are alternatives in refractory cases.

Children and adults with alopecia areata may suffer social isolation as a result of their hair loss. The Alopecia Areata Foundation is an excellent source of support and information for patients with this disorder. Every year, the American Academy of Dermatology hosts Camp Discovery, a summer camp for children with significant skin disorders. Some socially withdrawn children with alopecia areata find the camp a life-changing experience.

SCARRING ALOPECIA

During the active, evolving stage of hair loss, patches of alopecia commonly appear red and inflamed at the base of the hair shaft. Sometimes crops of pustules are noted. Hairs are often grouped into tufts, resembling doll's hair. During the active inflammatory phase, intact anagen hairs with a pigmented bulb are often easily extracted from the involved areas. Inflamed areas gradually evolve into smooth, hairless patches with no follicular ostia. Although some types of cicatricial alopecia result in rapid hair loss, slow progression of hair loss is more common. The slowly progressive nature of scarring alopecia often leads to inappropriate therapeutic complacency. Scarring alopecia must be treated aggressively to prevent the gradual progression to large areas of permanent scarring.

Inflammatory alopecia is often a manifestation of lupus erythematosus, lichen planus of the scalp, or folliculitis decalvans (recurrent suppurative folliculitis related to staphylococci). Skin biopsies are generally required to establish the diagnosis and to guide treatment. The biopsies should be evaluated by someone with special expertise in hair disorders. Therapy is generally difficult and prolonged, and most patients with scarring alopecia should be referred to an expert in the field.

*Not FDA approved for this indication.
†Not yet approved for use in the United States.

CANCER OF THE SKIN

method of
TATYANA R. HUMPHREYS, M.D.
Cutaneous Surgery
Thomas Jefferson University
Philadelphia, Pennsylvania

Skin cancer is the most common malignancy in humans and accounts for one third of newly diagnosed cancers. Approximately one in five Americans will be diagnosed with skin cancer in their lifetime and more than 1 million cases are diagnosed each year. Because the incidence of skin cancer is increasing each year, the primary care physician needs to be familiar with clinical presentation, treatment options, and prevention. This article addresses the most common primary skin cancers: basal cell carcinoma (BCC) and squamous cell carcinoma (SCC).

BCC accounts for 75% of nonmelanoma skin cancers. The vast majority (99%) occurs in Caucasians. BCC typically occurs on sun-exposed areas on the head and neck, with the nose being the most common site (30%). SCC is the second most common skin cancer. It accounts for 20% of nonmelanoma skin cancers. It occurs most commonly in Caucasians but is more common than BCC in non-Caucasians. Eighty percent occur on the head, neck, or hands, which are sites of chronic sun exposure.

Ultraviolet radiation (UVR), especially UVB, is a well-established cause of nonmelanoma skin cancer. UVR affects the skin both through direct DNA mutation with oncogene activation and the suppression of local immune responses. UV-induced mutations of the p53 tumor suppressor gene prevent apoptosis of damaged cells, leading to the development of SCC. Other environmental causes of nonmelanoma skin cancer include therapeutic radiation exposure, arsenic ingestion, and chemical carcinogens such as industrial hydrocarbons and soot. Certain subtypes of human papillomavirus (HPV 6, 11, 16, 18) have also been linked to the development of SCC, especially in immunosuppressed patients. Transplant patients on immunosuppressant drugs frequently demonstrate increased occurrence, accelerated development, and more frequent metastasis of SCC. Specific genetic syndromes such as basal cell nevus syndrome and xeroderma pigmentosum are characterized by the early development of skin cancer.

CLINICAL FEATURES

There are three distinct clinical types of BCC: superficial multifocal, nodular, and infiltrating or morpheaform. The superficial multifocal variety presents as a flat erythematous plaque with slightly elevated borders. The nodular type is typically a smooth translucent papule with telangiectasia. Nodular BCCs may often ulcerate and become pigmented causing them to be mistaken for nevi or melanoma. The morpheaform or sclerosing type has a subtle scarlike appearance with ill-defined borders.

As with BCC, SCC can have many different clinical manifestations. Bowen's disease (SCC in situ) presents as a red scaling macule or plaque. Invasive SCC typically looks like a firm red papule or nodule that may be covered with keratotic debris. The keratoacanthoma is a clinical subtype of SCC that is characterized by a central keratotic plug and a history of sudden onset and rapid growth. Keratoacanthomas may occasionally involute spontaneously but should still be treated as other SCCs because their biologic behavior is not always benign or predictable. SCC of the mucous membranes may present as an area of chronic irritation, erosion, or leukoplakia.

TREATMENT AND PROGNOSIS

Factors that influence the choice of treatment modality include location of the tumor, depth of invasion, histology, and pre-existing medical conditions. A summary of treatment options appears in Table 1. Although BCCs typically do not have any biologic potential for metastasis and grow very slowly, they may result in significant local tissue destruction and even disfigurement if left untreated. Cutaneous SCC carries an average 2% to 4% risk of metastasis on nonmucosal skin. Factors associated with a higher risk of metastasis are summarized in Table 2. Lymph node evaluation before surgery is important for staging. The presence of palpable adenopathy preoperatively warrants further evaluation and referral to a qualified head and neck surgeon who may recommend fine-needle aspirate of enlarged regional nodes and additional imaging studies.

Destructive Therapy

Destructive therapies include electrodesiccation/curettage and cryotherapy with liquid nitrogen. These techniques are most appropriate for nonfacial nodular or superficial BCC and SCC in situ because they may result in a hypopigmented scar. Destructive therapy is contraindicated for infiltrating BCCs and invasive SCCs because there is an unacceptable risk of recurrence and no histologic confirmation of adequate treatment margins. Initial curettage helps delineate the clinical margins of the lesion. Typical cryotherapy regimens used are a subsequent 30-second freeze for superficial BCC or SCC in situ and two 30-second freeze periods with an intervening thaw period for nodular BCC. The use of cryotherapy for skin cancer should ideally be performed with the of thermocoupling electrodes to ensure adequate freezing, unless the practitioner is experienced in this technique. The area

TABLE 1. **Treatment Options for Nonmelanoma Skin Cancer**

Modality	Contraindication
Destruction	
Cryotherapy	Invasive squamous cell carcinoma, infiltrating basal cell carcinoma
ED&C	Tumors meeting Mohs' criteria (see Table 3)
Laser	
Photodynamic	
Excision	Tumors meeting Mohs' criteria (see Table 3)
Mohs' micrographic surgery	Poor surgical candidate Unresectable tumor
Radiation	Patients younger than 40 years of age
Chemotherapy (topical)	Invasive squamous cell carcinoma, infiltrating basal cell carcinoma
5-Fluorouracil (Efudex)	Tumors meeting Mohs' criteria (see Table 3)
Imiquimod (Aldara)*	

*Not FDA approved for this indication.
ED&C, electrodesiccation and curettage.

TABLE 2. **High-Risk Squamous Cell Carcinoma**

Location on the ears, lip
Size >2.0 cm
Depth >4 mm
Perineural invasion
Poorly differentiated histology

of treatment should encompass 4 mm beyond the clinical borders of the lesions. If electrodesiccation and curettage (ED&C) is employed, then three cycles are usually performed. The risk of recurrence with these methods of destruction is approximately 5% to 10%. It is the author's opinion that cryotherapy yields better cosmesis because of its relative specificity for cellular destruction and sparing of noncellular dermal matrix components.

Superficial skin cancers may be ablated using the carbon dioxide or erbium:yttrium-aluminum-garnet lasers. Photodynamic therapy is an alternative for multiple or numerous skin cancers and employs the use of an oral or topical photosensitizing agent followed by exposure to visible light that results in tumor destruction. Limited availability and photosensitivity restrict the use of this technique.

Excision

Conventional surgical excision offers histologic confirmation of margin of selected tumors and a slightly lower recurrence rate than destructive therapy. For BCC, excision should be performed with 3 to 4 mm of clinically normal skin beyond the curetted tumor. Excision with 4- to 6-mm margins is the recommended treatment for invasive SCC. Cure rates for excision are approximately 95%.

Mohs' Micrographic Surgery

A specialized technique known as Mohs' micrographic surgery, named after Dr. Frederick Mohs, was developed for treatment of certain skin cancers that are likely to recur with other usual types of treatment. The indications for Mohs' surgery are summarized in Table 3. SCCs at greater risk for metastasis (Table 3) should be treated with Mohs' micrographic surgery. When Mohs' surgery is performed, the skin cancer is removed with 1- to 2-mm margins. Frozen sections are then prepared so that both the deep and lateral margins can be completely visualized on a continuous horizontal plane and microscopic examination performed intraoperatively. Residual tumor is localized and mapped. Additional tissue layers are removed where residual tumor is found until margins are clear. The result is complete tumor removal with sparing of surrounding normal tissue. The cure rate is typically 98% to 99% for primary tumors (recurrence rate 1% to 2%).

TABLE 3. **Indications for Mohs' Micrographic Surgery for Nonmelanoma Skin Cancer**

Recurrent skin cancer
Ill-defined clinical borders
Critical anatomic location necessitating tissue sparing
Location at risk for recurrence (nose, ears)
Infiltrative histology
Size >2.0 cm

Radiation

Radiation therapy is generally appropriate for patients who are poor surgical candidates or when surgical resection would result in excessive morbidity. Radiation is delivered over 4 to 6 weeks for a typical total of 4000 to 6000 cGy. The need for multiple visits over the course of several months makes it less time and cost effective than other modalities. Because of skin changes associated with radiation and increased risk of a secondary malignancy, it is not the treatment of choice for patients younger than 40 years of age. Prophylactic radiation may also be indicated postoperatively for aggressive SCC at significant risk for metastasis or tumors that exhibit perineural invasion.

Topical Chemotherapy

Topical chemotherapeutic agents such as 5-fluorouracil (Efudex) can be effective for superficial multifocal BCC and SCC in situ but are contraindicated for invasive tumors. Application of 5-FU once daily for 3 to 4 weeks generates a marked local inflammatory response and tumor necrosis. The principal disadvantage is patient discomfort that may compromise compliance. Topical 5-FU may also cause superficial resolution of the lesion that can camouflage persistent dermal tumor. It is therefore recommended primarily for treatment of actinic keratoses.

Imiquimod cream (Aldara)* is a topical biologic response modifier that locally upregulates interferon-α production. It is currently Food and Drug Administration (FDA) approved for the treatment of genital warts. Preliminary clinical studies have confirmed its efficacy in clearing small nodular BCCs less than 1.0 cm in size when used daily for 6 to 12 weeks. Erythema, oozing, crusting, and bleeding are expected reactions after several weeks of therapy. The therapeutic efficacy is around 80%. FDA approval has not yet been granted for this indication.

Systemic Chemoprophylaxis

The use of oral isotretinoin (Accutane)* can decrease the rate of skin cancer development in high-risk patients (organ transplant recipients, basal cell nevus syndrome patients). A typical daily dose of 1 mg/kg will suppress new tumor development but a rebound phenomenon can occur upon cessation. Typical side effects such as dry eyes, dry mouth, dry skin, headache, and laboratory abnormalities (increased liver function tests [LFTs], cholesterol, and

*Not FDA approved for this indication.

triglycerides) may limit patient tolerability. This is not an FDA-approved indication.

Cox 2 inhibitors* retard carcinogenesis and may emerge as effective oral prophylaxis for skin cancer. Clinical trials are currently in progress. Other potential experimental agents include a variety of oral and topical antioxidants such as vitamin E and green tea.

*Not FDA approved for this indication.

CUTANEOUS T CELL LYMPHOMA

method of
STANFORD I. LAMBERG, M.D.
The Johns Hopkins Medical Institutions
Baltimore, Maryland

Cutaneous T cell lymphoma (CTCL), which includes mycosis fungoides (MF) and its variant Sézary syndrome (SS), is a malignancy of thymus-derived helper lymphocytes, usually $CD4^+$ in phenotype. Males are affected twice as often as females, and the races are affected equally. The average age at onset is 55 years, although cases in young adults and even children do occur. Additional variants, distinguished by clinical features and immunophenotyping, have differing courses, prognoses, and responses to therapy. This group includes pagetoid reticulosis (Woringer-Kolopp disease), a solitary patch that often responds to localized radiation and has a good prognosis; lymphomatoid papulosis, self-healing, recurrent papules, usually $CD30^+$ (Ki-1), that evolve into or are already lymphoma in about 10% to 20%; and large T cell lymphomas, either $CD30^+$ or $CD30^-$, with or without clinical lesions of MF.

DIAGNOSIS

In most cases, CTCL begins with subtle lesions that are only clinically and pathologically suggestive of the disease. Most patients with CTCL have pruritus; itching is especially severe in those with SS.

In the so-called premycotic phase, the eruption often resembles a common benign disorder such as psoriasis or atopic eczema. Other more distinctive patterns include poikiloderma atrophicans vasculare, characterized by patches of telangiectasia, atrophy, and pigmentation resembling radiation dermatitis; alopecia mucinosa, or patchy hair loss associated with an inflammatory and mucinous infiltrate within and around hair follicles; and large-plaque parapsoriasis, usually seen as scaly, pink to dusky, sometimes slightly infiltrated patches. When MF is more advanced, individual plaques become thickened, reddish brown, flat, annular, or serpiginous. In SS, erythroderma is the hallmark and is accompanied by thickened facial features, enlarged lymph nodes, and large numbers of circulating atypical lymphocytes. Histologic sections of skin obtained by biopsy usually show numerous atypical lymphocytes with convoluted nuclei near and within the epidermis, as well as clusters within the epidermis (Pautrier's microabscesses).

Molecular techniques and immunophenotyping have become important tools to confirm a suspected pathologic diagnosis and to estimate prognosis. Their role in selecting the best therapy is being examined. Demonstration of dominant clonality in skin, lymph nodes, and blood, particularly of the T cell receptor gene, is strong evidence of malignancy, even in early-stage lesions. Most cases of MF/SS are predominantly $CD4^+$, in comparison to the population of $CD8^+$ cells, and numbers of $CD7^+$ cells are often decreased.

STAGING

The TNM (tumor-node-metastasis) classification system, modified for CTCL, is most commonly used to describe the extent of disease (Table 1). The presence or absence of features that have been found to be associated with a differing clinical course and prognosis should first be determined. These findings can then be used to stage the disease (Table 2). The only clinical variables found to be significantly associated with survival in patients with CTCL are the extent of T (skin) and N (peripheral lymph node enlargement) involvement. A peripheral lymph node biopsy is not generally obtained in patients with early patch/plaque disease, especially if the nodes are not palpable, because such lymph nodes are rarely positive or show only dermatopathic lymphadenitis by light microscopy. Histologically proven lymph node involvement, as well as extracutaneous lymphoma in blood (B) or viscera (M), indicates further shortening of survival and may affect treatment selection.

Tests recommended for evaluation and staging of patients with CTCL are listed in Table 3. A distinction is made in Table 3 between tests known to have prognostic significance and can therefore be justified as routine and those more suitable if the patient is enrolled in a research protocol. For example, computed axial tomographic scans, which are nearly always negative, even in advanced disease, are not justifiable as a routine evaluation procedure in patients with early-stage disease.

TREATMENT

Optimal therapy for CTCL has not yet been established (Table 4). Long remissions and possible cures have been claimed in patients with early disease, but present modes of treatment are not curative in patients with visceral involvement. A National Cancer Institute (NCI) study confirmed the widely held impression that late-stage patients with extensive plaques, tumors, or erythroderma do more poorly when treated aggressively, usually because of increased susceptibility to superinfection. The NCI study left unanswered the controversy over aggressive (multimodal topical and systemic) therapy versus conservative (topical modality) therapy in patients with early patch/plaque disease.

TABLE 1. **TNM Classification for Cutaneous T Cell Lymphoma (Mycosis Fungoides/Sézary Syndrome)***

Skin (T)	
T0	Clinically and/or histologically suspicious lesions
T1	Limited plaques, papules, or eczematous patches covering <10% of skin surface
T2	Limited plaques, papules, or eczematous patches covering ≥10% of skin surface
T3	Tumors (≥1)
T4	Generalized erythroderma
Lymph Nodes (N)	
N0	No clinically abnormal peripheral lymph nodes; pathologic findings not CTCL
N1	Clinically abnormal peripheral lymph nodes; pathologic findings not CTCL
N2	No clinically abnormal peripheral lymph nodes; pathologic findings positive for CTCL
N3	Clinically abnormal peripheral lymph nodes; pathologic findings positive for CTCL
Peripheral Blood (B)	
B0	Atypical circulating cells not present (<5%)
B1	Atypical circulating cells not present (≥5%)
Visceral Organ (M)	
M0	No visceral organ involvement
M1	Visceral involvement (must have pathologic confirmation)

*Peripheral blood involvement (B) has not been incorporated into the staging classification for this disorder.

Abbreviation: CTCL, cutaneous T cell lymphoma.

Modified from Bunn PA Jr, Lamberg SI: Report of the Committee on staging and Classification of Cutaneous T-Cell Lymphoma. Cancer Treat Rep 63:725–728, 1979.

Too few patients were enrolled in this group to provide meaningful data.

Development of optimal schedules for present therapies and investigation of new forms of therapy cannot occur unless patients with CTCL are entered into ongoing treatment protocols. Information on studies in progress can be obtained by calling the Cancer Information Service, NCI, Bethesda, MD, at 1-800-4CANCER or from the NCI Web site, http://www.cancer.gov/search/clinical_trials/.

General Measures

Pruritus is a common, sometimes overwhelming problem for patients with CTCL. Moderate relief may be gained by the use of systemic antihistamines such as hydroxyzine (Atarax), 25 mg orally every 4 hours as needed, topical emollients such as Eucerin, or topical corticosteroids such as betamethasone, fluocinonide, or triamcinolone in either cream or ointment form applied as needed or overnight under plastic wrap occlusion.

TABLE 2. **Staging Classifications for Cutaneous T Cell Lymphoma**

Stage	Skin	Lymph Nodes	Visceral Involvement
IA	T1	N0	M0
IB	T2	N0	M0
IIA	T1,T2	N1	M0
IIB	T3	N0, N1	M0
III	T4	N0, N1	M0
IVA	T1–T4	N2, N3	M0
IVB	T1–T4	N0–N3	M1

Modified from Lamberg SI, Bunn PA Jr: Cutaneous T-cell lymphomas: Summary of the Mycosis Fungoides Cooperative Group–National Cancer Institute Workshop. Arch Dermatol 115:1103–1105, 1979.

TABLE 3. **Recommended Evaluation Procedures**

	Routine	Investigational
History and physical examination	X	
Skin biopsy	X	
Complete blood count, serum tests, renal function tests, uric acid, serum calcium	X	
Peripheral smear to determine the absolute lymphocyte count and percentage of Sézary cells	X	
Chest radiograph	X	
Scans and/or biopsies of organs when history or physical examination suggests abnormalities	X	
Lymph node biopsy	X	X
Liver biopsy	(see text)	X
Bone marrow biopsy		X
Abdominal ultrasound/computed tomography	X	

At present, topical therapy is used in patients with disease considered to be confined to the skin, and systemic therapy is used for disease proven to involve the viscera, including the lymph nodes and blood. Total skin electron beam (TSEB) radiotherapy is the most aggressive of the topical options. It is also the most likely to induce remissions and even "cures."

Specific Measures

Photochemotherapy

PUVA, long-wavelength ultraviolet light (UVA) combined with oral psoralen, suppresses early thin lesions in most cases, especially if the pathology is only "suspicious" for CTCL. Indeed, some of these patients may remain clear after a course of therapy, but they may have parapsoriasis en plaque rather than CTCL. Control of patients with thickened MF plaques or tumors with definite CTCL pathology is unlikely with this therapy alone. Such patients require frequent maintenance light treatments to maintain control along with other modalities.

Topical Mechlorethamine

Topical application of mechlorethamine (nitrogen mustard [HN_2], Mustargen) can yield excellent response rates (60% to 90%). About 10% of patients remain clear after therapy is stopped, but such patients have early-stage disease with questionable histologic evidence of CTCL. For thicker plaques and definite histologic evidence of CTCL, sustained remission usually requires continued use of the agent. Although no bone marrow suppression or other systemic toxicity is associated with topical HN_2, epidermal neoplasms appear at a several-fold higher rate

TABLE 4. **Comparison of Treatment Options**

	Advantages	Disadvantages
Topical steroids	Symptomatic relief Defer more definitive Rx to observe the course	Alter skin pathology Questionable long-term benefit No effect on infiltrated plaques
PUVA	Skin clearing in early disease Side effects are minimal	May only mask skin disease Defers more definitive therapy High relapse rate without maintenance No effect on thick plaques or tumors Associated with other late skin cancers
Mechlorethamine (HN_2, Mustargen)	Ease of use at home 10% long-term remission of early MF	"Cure" rate is low High rate of allergic reactions No effect on thick plaques or tumors
Carmustine (BCNU, BiCNU)	Ease of use at home Response rate like that of topical HN_2 Low rate of allergic contact dermatitis	Potential bone marrow suppression Telangiectasia, pigmentation, skin tenderness
Bexarotene gel (Targretin)	Ease of use at home Not carcinogenic	May be irritating to skin Expensive
Electron beam	High long-term disease-free rates One course of therapy	Significant cutaneous side effects Expensive Limited availability
Systemic chemotherapy	May maintain remissions Sometimes induces remissions Palliation of late stage	Significant side effects Complete response is unlikely Increases susceptibility to infection
Bexarotene (Targretin)	Benefits 30% Single daily dose Side effects similar to those of other retinoids	Increases triglycerides and decreases TSH and T_4 Expensive
Interferons	May salvage late-stage disease Adjuvant with other modalities	Significant side effects Expensive IM dosage required
Photopheresis	May be effective in Sézary syndrome Minimal side effects	Limited availability Only response with high peripheral counts
Ontak (denileuken diftitox) (denileuken diftitox)	May salvage late-stage disease (10%–35%)	Significant systemic reactions in all Only for patients with CD25 expression

Abbreviations: MF, mycosis fungoides; PUVA, psoralen plus ultraviolet A; T_4, thyroxine; TSH, thyroid-stimulating hormone.

than expected. About a third of users eventually become allergic to the agent.

Instructions. Advise the patient to pry off the metal cap of a 10-mg vial of Mustargen* and mix the contents in 1 to 2 oz of water just before use. Suggest use of the medication in a shower or tub before bedtime. Tell the patient to apply the entire volume from head to toe with a 2-inch nylon brush, with a small amount reserved to be further diluted for painting in the intertriginous areas. The patient may add a teaspoonful of glycerin to the solution if the skin is dry and itchy. On arising, patients should bathe and may apply an emollient such as Eucerin.

Nitrogen mustard may also be used in ointment form (five to nine 10-mg vials of Mustargen dissolved in a small amount of absolute or 95% ethanol and mixed into a pound of Aquaphor). The aqueous form may be used to induce remission and the ointment form for maintenance, particularly in patients who experience excessive dryness from the liquid form. No efficacy studies comparing the preparations have been conducted, however.

Treatment is carried out daily until complete clearing, which may take several months to a year or even longer. Once clear, therapy should be continued for 6 to 24 months, perhaps at a decreased frequency, and then discontinued. Many patients clear except for one or a few patches; such patients often require continuous therapy to maintain control. Some patients become allergic. About half can be desensitized by graded increases of diluted HN_2, generally managed by dermatologists who have previous experience with the agent.

*This use of this agent is not listed in the manufacturer's official directive.

Topical Carmustine

Though less frequently used than HN_2, topical carmustine (BCNU)* is an effective alternative. It is particularly useful in patients who became allergic to HN_2 and still have early-stage disease. Local irritation and persistent telangiectases usually develop, however. Because the drug is absorbed, patients have a risk of reversible bone marrow depression with decreased leukocytes and platelets, usually delayed for 6 weeks after use.

Instructions. Supply the patient with a stock solution by prescribing a 100-mg vial of BCNU dissolved in 50 mL of absolute or 95% ethanol to be stored at home in the refrigerator. Advise the patient to add 5 mL of the stock to about 60 mL of water and paint the solution on the entire body once daily, as with HN_2. Because of the potential for bone marrow suppression, treatment should continue for only 6 to 8 weeks. If the response is incomplete, this course can be followed immediately by treating individual lesions with the

*Not FDA approved for this indication. This use of this agent is not listed in the manufacturer's official directive.

undiluted alcoholic stock solution up to twice daily (up to 70 mg or 35 mL/wk). Alternatively, after a 6-week rest period, the patient can be retreated with twice the concentration (10 mL stock per 60 mL water) for another 6 to 8 weeks. The cycle of treatment may be repeated as necessary to suppress visible lesions.

Complete blood counts, including platelet counts, should be obtained every 2 to 4 weeks during and for 6 weeks after total body and intensive local applications.

Total Skin Electron Beam Radiotherapy

MF is radiosensitive, and conventional orthovoltage radiation therapy has been used for decades. TSEB radiation has a distinct advantage over orthovoltage radiation. The penetration of electrons, being particles, can be controlled to reach depths as shallow as a few millimeters, whereas orthovoltage radiation passes deeply into tissues. A large surface dose can thus be given with electron beam radiotherapy without deep tissue injury or bone marrow suppression.

Most patients in early stages will achieve a complete remission, and up to a third will remain clear and, perhaps, cured. TSEB radiotherapy is also useful for later stage disease but must be combined with adjuvant chemotherapy, such as topical HN_2 or low-dose methotrexate, to maintain clearing because recurrence is common. In late stages, TSEB radiotherapy is less useful because the palliation is only temporary.

Therapy is usually fractionated over a period of 6 to 10 weeks to a total of about 3000 to 3600 cGy. All portions of the body must be treated; a higher recurrence rate has been found in patients who elect scalp shielding to prevent loss of scalp hair. Acute side effects, which usually subside in a month, include skin edema, erythema, and fissuring. Hair, nails, and sweat gland function usually return in 3 to 6 months. The treatment is costly ($5000 to $10,000). Most large cities now have medical centers capable of TSEB radiotherapy.

Interferons

Interferons, especially recombinant interferon alfa-2a (Roferon-A)* and gamma-1b (Actimmune),* are proving useful as primary treatment in early-stage CTCL and in combination with radiation, retinoids, or PUVA in later stages. Most patients have an objective response, and up to 20% appear to undergo full remission. Although low doses, 3 million U three times a week, can be tried, especially as an adjuvant, many patients require the maximal tolerated dose for maximal response, 15 to 50 million U/d or every other day given intramuscularly or subcutaneously. Fever and a flulike illness develop for a few days, and most patients have persistent fatigue and anorexia. The degree of leukopenia is the dose-limiting side effect, but recovery is rapid and systemic infections are rare. Intralesional interferon is also useful for individual tumors.

*Not FDA approved for this indication.

Systemic Chemotherapy

Chemotherapeutic agents that have been effective in some cases include methotrexate, fludarabine (Fludara), deoxycoformycin (pentostatin), CHOP (cyclophosphamide [Cytoxan], hydroxydaunomycin [Adriamycin], Oncovin [vincristine], and prednisone), and EPOCH (etoposide,* prednisone, Oncovin, cyclophosphamide, and hydroxydaunomycin [doxorubicin]). Two newer agents approved by the Food and Drug Administration (FDA) for use in CTCL are bexarotene (see Retinoids) and denileuken diftitox (see Interleukin-2 Fusion Toxin).

Retinoids

Bexarotene (Targretin) for oral and topical use has been approved by the FDA for the treatment of CTCL refractory to at least one previous course of systemic therapy. The therapeutic oral dose is 300 mg/m^2/day, a level at which about a third of patients achieve at least a partial response. For a 70-kg, 6-ft person, the surface area is about 2 m^2. Therefore, eight 75-mg capsules per day are required. The medication is expensive, about $1500 for 100 capsules, or about $120 per day for a person this size. Side effects are significant. They often include quite high lipid levels that require systemic agents for control; central hypothyroidism; and the signs and symptoms of retinoid therapy that may be seen with etretinate and isotretinoin, including headache, dry skin, leukopenia, pruritus, and nausea. Liver function tests should be performed at baseline; after weeks 1, 2, 4; and once stable, at 8-week intervals. Thyroid function tests should be obtained at baseline and then monitored to watch for decreases in thyroid-stimulating hormone and thyroxine levels. Blood lipid levels, especially triglycerides, should be determined at baseline, weekly until the lipid response is established, and then at 8-week intervals. Alterations, especially if triglyceride levels are greater than 400 mg/dL, should be controlled with antilipemic therapy (not gemfibrozil) and dose reduction. White blood cell counts and differential should be obtained at baseline and at intervals.

Bexarotene gel is initially applied once every other day for the first week, with application frequency increased at weekly intervals to once, twice, three times, and up to four times a day, depending on individual lesion tolerance. Most patients require many weeks of treatment before a response is evident. The medication is expensive, about $1000 for a 60-g tube.

Interleukin-2 Fusion Toxin

Denileuken diftitox (Ontak) is the product of the fusion of sequences of interleukin-2 (IL-2) with amino acid sequences of diphtheria toxin fragments. The combination directs the cytocidal action of diphtheria toxin to cells that express the IL-2 receptor. To qualify for treatment, at least 20% of the cells in skin lesions must be positive for CD25, the α chain of the IL-2 receptor. The drug is administered at 9 to 18 μg/kg/d

*Not FDA approved for this indication.

intravenously for 5 consecutive days and repeated every 3 weeks. The major side effects are a flulike syndrome, which occurs in most patients, and capillary leak syndrome, seen in 10%.

Extracorporeal Photopheresis

Extracorporeal photochemotherapy holds promise for the treatment of patients with significant numbers of circulating atypical lymphocytes. In this procedure, the patient's centrifugally separated white blood cells are exposed to UVA in the presence of psoralen and then infused back into the patient. Whether because of a direct cytotoxic effect on the lymphocytes or because of an additional anti-idiotype antibody reaction induced by lymphocyte damage, a substantial reduction in the number of circulating atypical cells is seen in most patients. Furthermore, skin lesions often improve, presumably because of movement of atypical cells from the skin into the circulation, where they can be targeted. Side effects are minimal, but the treatment, given in the hospital over a period of 1 to 2 days monthly, is expensive and not widely available. Adjuvant therapy with interferons may improve the response rate. Although trials continue, extracorporeal photopheresis has been approved by the FDA for the treatment of CTCL.

Treatment by Stage

Early MF Apparently Confined to the Skin: T1 and N (Any) or T2 and N0-N1 (M0)

Ninety percent of patients with limited patch-stage disease do not progress beyond this stage. Because most patients receive some form of therapy, it is unclear whether it is the treatment or the natural history of the disease that confers the good prognosis in patients in this group. Data from the Mycosis Fungoides Cooperative Group (MFCG) show 5-year survival rates decreased to 83% in comparison to insurance data for what was expected for persons without MF of the same age and sex. Therapies are generally skin directed, either PUVA, topical nitrogen mustard, or more aggressively, TSEB radiotherapy.

Later Stage MF with Poorer Prognostic Signs, Though Apparently Confined to the Skin: T2 and N2 or T3 (M0)(B0)

Curative therapy cannot yet be achieved in patients with this extent of disease. Sustained remissions may occur with topical therapy in combination with systemic therapy, especially interferon-α, the retinoid bexarotene, or oral methotrexate (25 to 50 mg/wk in a single weekly dose). Generally, some form of radiation therapy (orthovoltage and/or electron beam) helps induce clearing of thick plaques or tumors, and an additional topical or systemic therapy is used in an attempt to maintain the remission. Maintenance topical therapy may be HN_2, PUVA, BCNU, or bexarotene gel. Five-year survival rates are reduced in this group of patients to 64% (MFCG data) and 73% (1999 Stanford data).

Late-Stage CTCL with Visceral Involvement, Failure of Previous Therapy, or Sézary Syndrome

Treatment in this stage is palliative. Because aggressive systemic chemotherapy may shorten the survival of patients with late-stage disease by increasing the chance of sepsis, safer chemotherapeutic agents are immunomodulators such as interferons, retinoids, and extracorporeal photopheresis. Denileuken diftitox and the systemic agents fludarabine and deoxycoformycin are alternatives. Five-year survival rates are reduced in tumor stage T3 patients to 50%, to 35% in SS (stage T4) patients (MFCG data), and, if extracutaneous involvement is present (stage M1), to less than 20% (2001 Stanford data).

PAPULOSQUAMOUS ERUPTIONS

method of
DAVID C. GORSULOWSKY, M.D.
Stanford University School of Medicine
Stanford, California
University of California at San Francisco and Veterans Affairs Medical Center
San Francisco, California

and

MATTHEW H. KANZLER, M.D.
Santa Clara Valley Medical Center
San Jose, California and Stanford University School of Medicine
Stanford, California

Papulosquamous eruptions are those that are palpable and scaly. They may or may not appear to be inflammatory in nature. We shall describe the clinical appearance of the common conditions, followed by a summary of treatment goals and modalities.

SEBORRHEIC DERMATITIS

Seborrheic dermatitis is the most common papulosquamous eruption. Although it may occur at any age, it is most common during infancy or after adolescence. Although excessive sebum production was originally suspected as the cause, this is probably not important. Causative factors may include androgenic hormones and anxiety, although no firm evidence exists. The yeast *Pityrosporon orbiculare* plays a role in at least some cases.

The condition shows moderately erythematous plaques with overlying fine white to yellow coarse scales. Occasionally, scale without underlying inflammation leads patients to complain of "dry skin." Seborrheic dermatitis most often affects the nasolabial folds, eyelids, eyebrows, scalp (Figure 1), and outer ear areas. Other sites include the sternal, axillary, and groin areas. Patients experience mild to moderate pruritus.

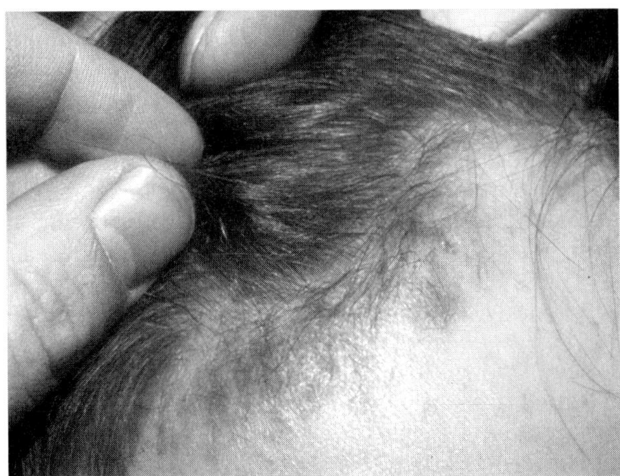

Figure 1. Seborrheic dermatitis of the scalp.

Seborrheic dermatitis, especially when severe, may be a presenting sign of immunodeficiency (e.g., AIDS), or of neurologic disease. In these cases, the dermatitis is usually severe and resistant to treatment.

Therapy

The goal of therapy in seborrheic dermatitis is to control the underlying inflammation and to remove scales. For facial involvement, very mild topical corticosteroid therapy is the first therapy, and generally should not exceed 2.5% hydrocortisone in potency. For resistant cases, one may compound 2% precipitated sulfur with hydrocortisone. The scalp responds most often to nightly corticosteroid solutions, lotions, gels, or foams (e.g., Synalar solution, Lidex solution or gel, Cordran lotion, Olux foam).

For longer term therapy, especially with scalp involvement, one should employ shampoos containing selenium sulfide (e.g., Selsun), zinc pyrithione (Head & Shoulders 1%, DHS Zinc 2%), salicylic acid, or tar. Generally, these are nonprescription preparations; however, some prescription shampoos contain corticosteroids (e.g., fluocinolone [Capex]). The patient should shampoo three to five times weekly, applying the shampoo and rinsing 5 to 10 minutes later. The patient may desire a conditioner after the medicated shampoo, because these preparations tend to dry the hair. Mineral oil or products containing salicylic acid may help remove thicker scales, as can products containing peanut oil, such as Derma-Smoothe F/S.

Topical antifungal agents, such as ketoconazole (Nizoral) cream (2%) or econazole (Spectazole) cream are effective in some patients with seborrheic dermatitis. This effect is probably the result of these drugs' activity against *P. orbiculare*. The advantage of topical antifungal agents is their lack of atrophogenic properties (such properties may be associated with long-term corticosteroid therapy). However, the antifungal medications are more effective as maintenance agents after initial control of inflammation.

The care provider should remind patients of the recurrent nature of the condition. Topical emollients are of no benefit.

TINEA CORPORIS

Dermatophyte infection of the epidermis is termed tinea corporis when on the trunk or proximal extremities. Other terms such as tinea cruris, pedis, manum, and facei refer to the same type of infection in other respective locations.

Tinea presents with erythematous plaques exhibiting peripheral white scale. This configuration is the reason tinea is sometimes called ringworm. A microscopic preparation in potassium hydroxide (KOH) can quickly identify fungal elements. The confirmatory test is a culture, which takes 2 to 4 weeks to identify the organism.

An eruption of crural plaques, especially when moist, is often mistakenly diagnosed as tinea cruris. This distinct eruption, called intertrigo, is maceration, a result of warmth and occlusion.

Therapy

Because of the drastic difference between treatments of intertrigo and tinea, establishment of the diagnosis is necessary before initiating therapy. The physician should treat intertrigo with drying agents (e.g., powder), a mild corticosteroid preparation (preferably in a lotion), and lowering of local temperature.

One can treat localized tinea with topical antifungal preparations, including butenafine (Mentax) cream, econazole (Spectazole) cream, terbinafine (Lamisil) cream, and oxiconazole (Oxistat) cream or lotion. Extensive eruptions respond to terbinafine (Lamisil), 250 mg by mouth daily for 7 days.

Because tinea cruris depends on moisture for persistent infection, dryness is a goal. Zeasorb or other absorbent powders are effective agents.

PSORIASIS

Psoriasis, affecting 1% to 3% of the population, exhibits a chronic relapsing course. It is inherited in some cases and then is associated with certain antigens of the major histocompatibility complex. Its onset may be at any age, but a new presentation after the fourth decade may presage immunosuppressed states.

Environmental and iatrogenic factors are important. Psoriasis may appear in areas of local trauma, the so-called Koebner phenomenon. Upper respiratory infections often precede psoriasis of the guttate or papular form. Medications, including lithium and β-adrenergic blockers, as well as some nonsteroidal anti-inflammatory drugs (especially indomethacin), can exacerbate psoriasis. Anxiety plays a role in exacerbation as well.

Characteristic lesions are well-demarcated erythematous plaques with overlying silvery-white to gray scales. These plaques often involve extensor surfaces

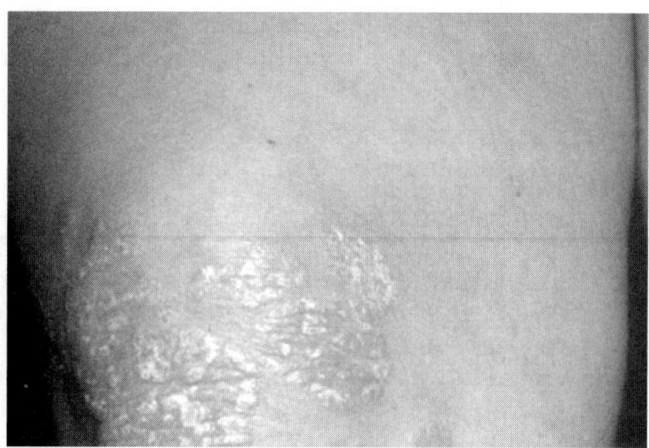

Figure 2.

such as elbow and knee areas (Figure 2). They may also involve the scalp, trunk, intertriginous areas, or other locations. Nail findings include pits, oil spot discoloration, distal onycholysis (separation of the nail plate from the bed), and subungual debris.

If psoriasis is present, one condition helping to confirm the diagnosis is psoriatic arthritis. Fifteen to 25% of patients may exhibit this seronegative condition, many of whom have clinical features identical with rheumatoid arthritis.

Several variants of psoriasis exist. Generalized erythroderma may be associated with an acute flare and may be accompanied by fever or other systemic signs, often mimicking septicemia. Guttate psoriasis appears with 0.5- to 1.0-cm papules and may follow an upper respiratory infection. Pustular psoriasis exhibits numerous small, sterile pustules overlying erythematous plaques, localized to the palms and soles (palmoplantar pustulosis), or generalized.

Other inflammatory conditions (e.g., atopic dermatitis) may resemble psoriasis. It is important to differentiate these conditions, however, because treatments such as systemic corticosteroids, which may improve atopic dermatitis, may cause a severe flare of psoriasis upon their withdrawal.

Therapy

Topical corticosteroids are the first line of outpatient therapy for psoriasis. Table 1 lists some of these medications, arranged by potency. Bases that are more occlusive, such as ointments, provide increased potency, compared with lesser occlusive bases, such as creams and lotions. Patients usually prefer cream and lotion bases, however, since these are more elegant (i.e., they penetrate rapidly).

Once-daily application of corticosteroids is proven as effective as multiple applications. This obviously can save financial resources.

To increase potency of the medication, the patient may occlude resistant lesions with plastic wrap after the corticosteroid, or use corticosteroid-impregnated (e.g., Cordran) tape. However, because this may increase the atrophogenic properties of the preparation, occlusion should typically be used for only a few days. Patients should be monitored closely for development of side effects, including folliculitis, skin atrophy, telangiectasia, and striae. The highest potency corticosteroids can even cause hypothalamic-pituitary-adrenal axis suppression.

The choice of a particular preparation depends on several factors, including the site of treatment, patient preference, resistance to therapy, and monetary cost. If a patient is sensitive to preservatives, an ointment base may be appropriate, because it usually contains fewer of such chemicals. The super-potent corticosteroid preparations listed in group I of Table 1 are indicated only for resistant lesions in thick-skinned areas. The physician should not allow unlimited or prolonged courses with these agents. In intertriginous areas, penetration and absorption are increased; here, the physician should choose creams and lotions with lower potency. Patients with lesions in hair-bearing areas typically desire medications in lotion, solution, or foam bases.

Thick or scaly lesions may require keratolytic agents such as salicylic acid (2% to 20%), urea (2% to 40%), or lactic acid (6% to 12%), especially necessary in hyperkeratotic lesions of the palms and soles. Some

TABLE 1. **Some Common Corticosteroid Preparations**

Group	Generic Name	Brand Name
I	Clobetasol propionate	Temovate, Olux
(super-potent)	Halobetasol propionate	Ultravate
II	Fluocinonide	Lidex
(potent)	Betamethasone dipropionate	Diprolene AF
III	Fluticasone propionate	Cutivate ointment
	Triamcinolone acetonide	Aristocort A ointment
IV	Fluocinolone acetonide	Synalar
(mid-strength)	Triamcinolone acetonide	Aristocort A cream
V	Hydrocortisone butyrate	Locoid
	Fluticasone propionate	Cutivate cream
VI	Desonide	DesOwen
	Alclometasone dipropionate	Aclovate
VII	Hydrocortisone	Hytone
(mild)	Hydrocortisone	Pramosone

commonly available preparations are Keralyt gel (6% salicylic acid), Lac-Hydrin cream (12% ammonium lactate), and Carmol 40 (40% urea).

Crude coal tar (1% to 5%) or liquor carbonis detergens (5% to 10%) may effectively treat large, thick plaques. Tar preparations are effective alone, or combined with corticosteroids. Patients usually prefer to use them at bedtime, due to their messy character and their odor. Anthralin (Anthra-Derm) (a vegetable-derived tar) preparations are effective in concentrations of 0.1% to 3.0%. Patients apply these medications for 10 to 30 minutes (stronger concentrations), or overnight (weaker concentrations), and then wash them off. The disadvantages of anthralin are irritation of normal skin and staining of normal skin and environmental objects. Therefore, the patient should apply anthralin strictly to lesions. The advantage of tar-based preparations is their usefulness for long-term therapy and in inducing longer lasting remissions than corticosteroid preparations.

Newer preparations include calcipotriene (Dovonex) and tazarotene (Tazorac), derivatives of vitamins D and A, respectively. Studies show that they are as effective as corticosteroids in controlled conditions. However, in clinical practice they may be most useful as adjunctive therapy. Because their mechanisms of action differ from corticosteroids, combination therapy often produces superior results when compared with monotherapy.

For patients with extensive involvement, acute and long-term management with ultraviolet B or ultraviolet A phototherapy may be the most effective and appropriate treatment. When combined with psoralen (PUVA therapy), ultraviolet A can be very effective. However, the practitioner must be very familiar with dosing of the light, frequency of treatments, and side effects such as pruritus, erythema, and blisters. Long-term side effects of PUVA therapy include cataracts and skin cancer. Typically, patients should not use non-medical sources of ultraviolet light, such as tanning booths.

Unresponsive patients may require other systemic agents. However, only those physicians familiar with their use should prescribe these potent medications. Methotrexate (Rheumatrex), at a dosage of 5 to 25 mg once weekly, is a well-established therapy for widespread psoriasis, especially for long-term treatment. Methotrexate can cause hepatic dysfunction, requiring periodic liver biopsies to detect drug-induced fibrosis. Other agents such as sulfasalazine (Azulfidine),* cyclosporine (Neoral), and hydroxyurea* (Hydrea) are other effective agents for extensive eruptions. Acitretin (Soriatane), at a dosage of 25 to 50 mg/d, alone or in combination with PUVA, is especially effective in the treatment of generalized erythrodermic or pustular psoriasis.

Important adjunctive treatments include liberal use of emollient preparations. In addition, patients should avoid hot water, other irritants, scratching, and removal of scales, which may produce the Koebner phenomenon.

*Not FDA approved for this indication.

LICHEN PLANUS

Lichen planus (LP) is an eruption of violaceous polygonal papules of the flexor surfaces (Figure 3), genitalia, and mucous membranes. It is occasionally associated with hepatitis C, and newly diagnosed patients should receive screening for this infection. The lesions frequently resolve within 1 to 2 years. Pruritus may be severe and intractable.

Characteristically, fine, white lacelike lines overlie the violaceous papules of LP. These are Wickham's striae, and are pathognomonic of the condition. Oral and genital lesions typically are lacy white plaques on the buccal mucosa or glans penis, respectively. However, they may present as painful erosions or ulcers.

Therapy

Topical or intralesional corticosteroids* are only moderately effective in treating lichen planus. Tacrolimus (Protopic)* ointment may improve mucous membrane lesions. For extensive or eruptive forms of the condition, the physician should consider phototherapy. Severely pruritic patients may require antipruritic lotions or oral antihistamines (topical antihistamines are common causes of allergic reactions).

PITYRIASIS ROSEA

Pityriasis rosea (PR) is a pruritic exanthem that occasionally follows an upper respiratory or other infection by 1 to 4 weeks. Despite the finding of virus-like particles in lesions, researchers have been unable to prove the viral etiology of PR. A single 2- to 3-cm lesion, the herald patch, may signal the onset. Lesions of PR are oval, pink to erythematous 1- to 1.5-cm plaques, with circinate fine white scale. Most commonly, they are configured in a "fir tree" distribution on the trunk (Figure 4). However, inverse PR may involve the axillary or groin areas.

PR may mimic secondary syphilis lesions. However, PR typically is confined to the trunk and proximal extremities. When the eruption involves the palms or soles, serologic testing for syphilis may be indicated.

*Not FDA approved for this indication.

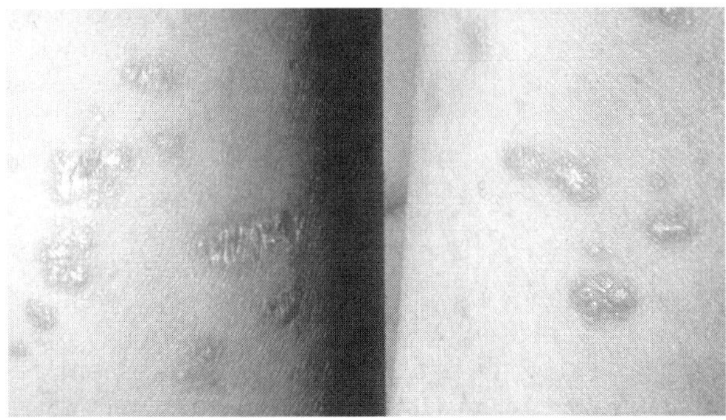

Figure 3. Lichen planus.

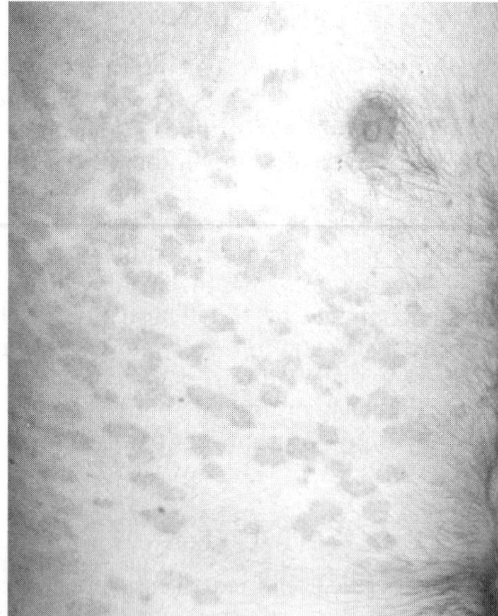

Figure 4. Pityriasis rosea.

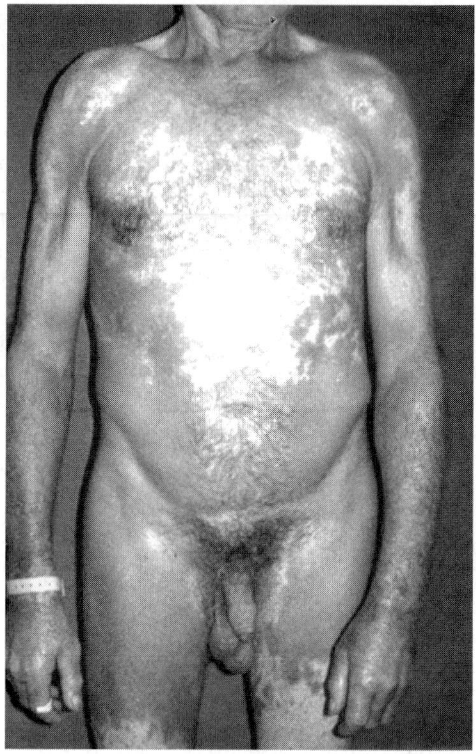

Figure 5. Pityriasis rubra pilaris.

Therapy

Because the condition is noncontagious and temporal, the physician should reassure patients that the condition resolves within 6 to 12 weeks. Some cases respond to a 2-week course of oral erythromycin.* Mild topical corticosteroid preparations* (e.g., Pramosone 2.5% lotion [includes a topical anesthetic]) may reduce pruritus.

PITYRIASIS RUBRA PILARIS

Pityriasis rubra pilaris (PRP) is characterized by large salmon-colored to erythematous plaques with fine adherent scale (Figure 5). Initially, patients present with perifollicular papules. Subsequently, there are patches of uninvolved skin located within these plaques, so-called "islands of sparing." Marked hyperkeratosis of the palms and soles and severe scalp involvement are characteristic. Many patients' eruptions progress to generalized erythroderma.

Therapy

Because topical corticosteroids are not effective, PRP usually requires systemic therapy with methotrexate* or acitretin.* Most cases resolve within 1 to 2 years, but PRP may last for several years or a lifetime.

MYCOSIS FUNGOIDES AND PARAPSORIASIS

Mycosis fungoides (MF), a cutaneous T cell lymphoma, may present as a papulosquamous eruption during its early stages. Large or small erythematous to violaceous plaques may exhibit fine scale and be located anywhere on the body.

Parapsoriasis exhibits small or large, oval erythematous plaques on the trunk. Some dermatologists consider large-plaque parapsoriasis to be a precursor of mycosis fungoides. Small-plaque parapsoriasis generally exhibits a benign, though stubborn, chronic course. Biopsy is necessary to differentiate benign and malignant conditions. Because MF can progress to internal involvement and death, complete workup and close follow-up are necessary.

Therapy

The physician may choose to not treat parapsoriasis, because it is asymptomatic. However, it may respond to topical corticosteroid preparations or phototherapy. For treatment of cutaneous or systemic MF, see the chapter on cutaneous T cell lymphoma.

*Not FDA approved for this indication.

CONNECTIVE TISSUE DISEASES

method of
JEFFREY P. CALLEN, M.D.
Division of Dermatology
University of Louisville School of Medicine
Louisville, Kentucky

This chapter will concentrate on treatment of the cutaneous manifestations of the three most commonly encountered collagen vascular diseases—lupus erythematosus, dermatomyositis, and scleroderma. Treatment of the systemic manifestations is beyond the scope of this chapter; however, a discussion of the interrelationship between the skin and systemic disease is pertinent to the discussion of evaluation and treatment of the cutaneous disease and will be briefly discussed.

LUPUS ERYTHEMATOSUS

Patients with lupus erythematosus may manifest a variety of skin lesions, including those that have a "specific" histopathology characterized by inflammation at the interface of the epidermis and dermis and those skin lesions that might occur in other conditions as well as lupus erythematosus. This discussion will focus on treatment of the patient with an interface dermatitis, primarily the most common subsets of discoid lupus erythematosus (DLE) and subacute cutaneous lupus erythematosus (SCLE). Before therapy, a thorough evaluation is needed.

The goals of management of the patient with DLE or SCLE are to improve the patient's appearance and to prevent the development of deforming scars, atrophy, or dyspigmentation. In addition, the majority of patients with chronic cutaneous LE (CCLE) or SCLE have disease that primarily affects their skin and may be reassured that their prognosis is relatively benign.

A complete list of the patient's medications will assist in the exclusion of drug-induced cutaneous LE. The most common drugs that have been reported to induce or exacerbate cutaneous LE, primarily SCLE, are hydrochlorothiazide, antihypertensive agents, and terbinafine. Also, patients who smoke may have more severe clinical disease than nonsmokers.

Cosmetic problems are often of major importance for the patient with cutaneous LE. Dyspigmentation may follow both DLE and SCLE and may be effectively hidden by agents such as Covermark or Dermablend. Scarred lesions may be excised if they are inactive; however, the possibility of reactivation resulting from manipulation exists.

Photosensitivity is generally prevalent in patients with cutaneous LE. From 57% to 73% of patients with SLE have a history of photosensitivity, whereas those with SCLE report photosensitivity of 70% to 90% and those patients with DLE are estimated at 50%. The action spectrum has been defined by photoprovocation testing and includes ultraviolet (UV) A, UVB, and occasionally visible light. Phototesting does not reproduce lesions in all or even a majority of patients and should be reserved for investigations or in individual circumstances where it is necessary for workers compensation or other medical legal circumstances.

Sunscreens are a cornerstone of therapy. The ideal sunscreen would be broad in its spectrum and water resistant. Unfortunately, no sunscreen is able to block all UV radiation that might exacerbate cutaneous LE in any patient; therefore, patients should also be encouraged to alter their sun-related behavior and to use sunprotective measures including sun-protective clothing. It is my recommendation that the patient apply a high SPF, broad-spectrum sunscreen daily. It is possible that by the time this chapter is published a new sunscreen containing Mexoryl XL† and Mexoryl SL† will be available in the United States. The addition of these two chemicals has been tested in LE patients and forms the most effective sunscreens to date.

Topical corticosteroids are usually prescribed for patients with cutaneous LE. An appropriate topical corticosteroid is selected for the area of the body being treated as well as the type of lesions that are present. Facial lesions should be treated with low- to midpotency agents such as 2.5% hydrocortisone,* desonide (DesOwen),* alclometasone (Aclovate),* or hydrocortisone valerate.* Lesions on the trunk and arms may be treated with midpotency agents such as triamcinolone acetonide (Kenalog),* or betamethasone valerate (Luxiq).* Lesions on the palms or soles and hypertrophic lesions often require superpotent corticosteroids such as clobetasol (Temovate)* or halobetasol (Ultravate).* Patients prefer creams over ointments; however, the ointments may be more potent and possibly are more effective. For lesions on hairy areas, most patients prefer a lotion or foam. The prescribing physician should consider the total amount of corticosteroid that the patient applies, as it is possible to cause hypothalamic-pituitary-adrenal axis suppression with use of even as little as 2 ounces per day of the superpotent corticosteroids.

Several other topical agents might be of use in individual patients with cutaneous LE. However, none of these agents have been tested in any systematic manner. Retinoids, specifically tretinoin (Retin-A),* might be effective and have primarily been utilized in patients with DLE and hypertrophic LE. Tazarotene (Tazorac,* a topical retinoid) might also be used. Topical application of calcipotriene (Dovonex)* might also be useful for cutaneous LE. Another nonsteroidal agent that might be considered in the future would be tacrolimus ointment (Protopic)* or pimecrolimus cream (Elidel).* Finally, because it is known that systemically administered interferon is effective for cutaneous LE, it might be helpful to apply imiquimod (Aldara)* to individual lesions.

Intralesional injections of corticosteroids are often effective in patients with lesions that are refractory to topical corticosteroids. Small amounts of triamcinolone acetonide may be injected with a 30-gauge needle into multiple areas. I use a concentration of 3 mg/mL when injecting skin lesions. These injections are often very effective in control of the lesions but do not prevent the development of new lesions. The potential for cutaneous atrophy or dyspigmentation similar to that seen with the disease should be discussed with the patient; however, in most cases an experienced dermatologist is able to inject without a great risk. Also, as noted with topical corticosteroids, the total dose of intralesional corticosteroids should be noted. Alternative agents for intralesional injection have not been well tested.

*Not FDA approved for this indication.
†Not available in the United States.

When existing lesions are not controlled with topical agents or intralesional corticosteroids, systemic therapy is often indicated. The first line therapy is the use of an antimalarial drug. Antimalarials seem to work less well in patients who smoke. The antimalarial that I prefer is hydroxychloroquine sulfate (Plaquenil). This drug is used in doses of 200 mg orally once or twice per day, or in a dose of <6.5 mg/kg/day. The onset of action of the antimalarial agents is roughly 4 to 8 weeks and for this reason some physicians have advocated higher initial loading doses. Hydroxychloroquine is also of benefit to the joint symptoms and malaise that may accompany cutaneous LE. Hydroxychloroquine is less toxic, but also less effective than chloroquine phosphate (Aralen),* which is used in doses of 250–500 mg/day.‡ Thus patients who fail to fully respond to hydroxychloroquine may be switched to chloroquine; however, I believe that these two agents should not be used together because of my concern that ophthalmologic toxicity may be enhanced. Another antimalarial, quinacrine HCl (Atabrine),† may add benefit to either hydroxychloroquine or chloroquine and is not associated with ophthalmologic toxicity. This agent is not readily available, but several compounding pharmacies in the United States have it available.

Antimalarial drugs may cause nausea, diarrhea, myopathy, cardiomyopathy, or psychosis. Cutaneous eruptions have also been reported with antimalarial drugs; in addition, generalized or localized pruritus, a lichenoid drug eruption, or dyspigmentation of the hair, nails, and mucous membranes may occur in patients treated with these agents. Hematologic toxicity may occur and may be manifest late in the course of therapy. Hematologic toxicity appears to be more common with quinacrine than the other antimalarials. Fortunately, the frequency of these side effects with antimalarials is relatively uncommon with the exception of the gastrointestinal side effects.

Ocular toxicity, including irreversible retinopathy, has been reported with chloroquine and hydroxychloroquine, but not with quinacrine. Ophthalmologic toxicity is probably dose related, and may also be related to duration of therapy. If detected early, these changes most often do not progress if the drug is stopped. Although there are other ocular changes including blurring of the vision and corneal deposition of the antimalarial, these are reversible upon cessation of the drug. Ophthalmologic evaluation, preferably by a physician familiar with these agents, should be performed at baseline or shortly after initiation of therapy and then periodically (e.g., every 6–12 months).

In difficult cases, multiple other approaches have been advocated for the treatment of cutaneous LE. In general, low-dose systemic corticosteroids (<1 mg of prednisone* per day or its equivalent) are rarely effective for DLE, and only partially effective for SCLE lesions. Corticosteroids are effective for the acute lesions of photosensitivity, the malar rash, or for vasculitic lesions that may complicate LE. The chronic use of oral or intramuscular corticosteroids for patients with cutaneous disease should be avoided.

Dapsone,* given in doses of 25 to 200 mg daily, has been useful for patients with vasculitic lesions that may accompany LE, SCLE lesions, bullous LE, and oral ulcerations. A variety of other antibiotics have been used in small case series or open-label studies for the treatment of cutaneous LE including cefuroxime axetil (Ceftil)* and sulfasalazine (Azulfidine).*

Auranofin (Ridaura),* an oral form of gold, has been used for cutaneous LE. Complete remission occurs in a minority of patients, about 15%, whereas a partial response has been noted in about two thirds of those treated. Auranofin is begun at a dose of 3 mg per day; after 1 week, the dose may be raised to twice daily if the patient experiences no problem with nausea, diarrhea, or headache. I have treated patients with as high as 3 mg three times per day without difficulty. Monitoring with regular complete blood counts and urinalysis is suggested.

Thalidomide (Thalomid)* has recently become more available and is being used for patients with cutaneous LE with some regularity. Its mechanism of action is believed to involve decrease in inflammatory mediators, particularly tumor necrosis factor-α (TNF-α) and Fas-ligand. Induction with 100 to 300 mg daily at bedtime results in improvement in 90% of the patients who are able to tolerate the drug. Toxicity commonly associated with thalidomide use includes drowsiness, headache, weight gain, amenorrhea, and dizziness. Drowsiness and dizziness may persist during the following day. Neuropathy, usually sensory, may limit the ability of patients to continue thalidomide on a long-term basis. Neuropathy may be reversible, but there are patients whose neuropathy has progressed despite stopping the drug. Whether nerve conduction studies should be performed at the onset of therapy and periodically is not known. Thalidomide is a potent teratogen and accordingly the drug manufacturer has developed a program to prevent the chance of pregnancy in patients exposed to the drug. The program requires the prescribing physician and the pharmacy to register with the company and that the patient take extra precautions in taking the drug. No more than a 1-month supply may be prescribed at any one time. Unfortunately the response to thalidomide is not durable in most patients; therefore, long-term, low-dose maintenance therapy may be necessary.

Oral retinoids are effective in many patients who have failed previous less toxic therapies. Isotretinoin (Accutane)* and acitretin (Soriatane)* have both been used in doses similar to those used for acne vulgaris or psoriasis respectively. The response is not durable and after short courses the patient will still need further suppressive therapy. These agents are particularly helpful in patients with hypertrophic lesions, or those with lesions on the palms or soles. These patients are monitored for lipid abnormalities, liver enzyme elevations, and cytopenias. In addition, these agents

*Not FDA approved for this indication.
†Not available in the United States.
‡Exceeds dosage recommended by manufacturer.

*Not FDA approved for this indication.

are teratogenic and should not be used in potentially pregnant women. If the clinician decides to use these in women of childbearing age, pregnancy prevention counseling should take place at each visit and pregnancy prevention methods should be provided to the patient.

Several cytotoxic agents have been reported to be beneficial for the control of cutaneous LE lesions. Azathioprine (Imuran)* has perhaps had the greatest number of reports, but methotrexate (Rheumatrex)* and mycophenolate mofetil (CellCept)* have also been reported to benefit patients with "recalcitrant" disease.

High-dose intravenous immune globulin* has been used in several patients. One gram/kg/d for 2 consecutive days monthly was administered to these patients who had failed multiple previous therapies. There was an excellent result in 4 of the 10 patients, but response is short-lived. Toxicity is minimal, but this therapy is extremely expensive.

The use of cytokine therapy has been reported. I predict that there will be additional reports of newer agents that are available and are just beginning to be tested for some dermatologic indications, as well as others that are not currently on the market. Because thalidomide may be effective through its effects on TNF-α, it might be possible that infliximab (Remicade)* or etanercept (Enbrel)* might also prove to be of benefit to patients with cutaneous LE. However, several patients have developed subacute cutaneous LE while on etanercept and both drugs are associated with the development of antinuclear antibodies in a subset of patients. Therefore their use should be with great caution.

DERMATOMYOSITIS

Dermatomyositis (DM) is a rare disorder of unknown etiology. A set of criteria to aid in the diagnosis and classification of DM and polymyositis (PM) were first proposed in 1975 by Bohan and Peter. Four of the five criteria are related to the muscle disease: (1) progressive proximal symmetrical weakness, (2) elevated muscles enzymes, (3) an abnormal electromyogram, (4) an abnormal muscle biopsy, and (5) the presence of compatible cutaneous disease. Subsequently, it has been recognized that there are many patients with compatible cutaneous disease that do not have initial manifestations of their muscles as defined by clinical weakness and elevated enzymes. This subset is termed amyopathic DM (ADM). Additionally there are patients in whom the myopathy resolves while the skin disease continues; these patients have been termed postmyopathic dermatomyositis. Some patients with DM, primarily older adults, have an associated malignancy.

In the patient with amyopathic dermatomyositis, the prognosis is good in the absence of malignancy. For patients with muscle disease, the prognosis depends upon the severity of the muscle disease, the presence of lung disease, esophageal dysfunction, or malignancy.

*Not FDA approved for this indication.

Children and adolescents with DM often develop calcinosis that can result in disability or discomfort.

Treatment provides control of the muscle inflammation and results in a return to normal function of the patient who might otherwise become disabled from the weakness. The skin disease is often symptomatic and is cosmetically displeasing; therefore, the goal of therapy is to relieve the symptoms and improve the patient's self-image and ability to interact with other people. Some patients with DM have an associated malignancy, and treatment of the malignancy might in some patients result in a control of the disease process. In children with DM treatments are aimed also at the prevention of calcinosis, or when the calcinosis occurs at its eradication.

Systemic corticosteroids are a first-line therapy for the DM patient with muscle disease. Relatively high doses, 1–2 mg/kg/d of prednisone* are generally suggested. In addition, the early use of a corticosteroid-sparing agent is often proposed with methotrexate* or azathioprine (Imuran)* being the most frequently suggested agents. Well-controlled, randomized trials are lacking for this disease. Many of the studies have included patients with malignancy-associated myositis, a condition that is believed to respond less well than DM.

Skin disease is treated in a similar manner to cutaneous lupus erythematosus with slight modifications. I usually use 1% hydrocortisone ointment for the cutaneous lesions of DM except in the scalp, where I use either a corticosteroid foam or lotion. Recently, several reports have suggested that topical tacrolimus (Protopic) ointment* or pimecrolimus (Elidel) cream* might be effective for some patients. In addition, many patients complain that their lesions are exceedingly dry; therefore, topical applications of ointments containing petrolatum are helpful.

In patients who fail to respond to topical therapy or to the administration of corticosteroids for their systemic disease, there are several alternative approaches. Antimalarial agents, hydroxychloroquine (Plaquenil),* chloroquine (Aralen),* or quinacrine (Atabrine)* have been successfully used as "steroid-sparing" therapies. However, about one third of the patients with DM will develop an adverse drug reaction to these agents. The eruption is usually self-limiting, but in most cases it is extremely pruritic. I believe that at the onset of therapy the patient should be warned of this possibility. In patients that fail to respond, I usually next prescribe oral methotrexate* and gradually advance the dose to tolerance or to 35 to 40 mg per week. The response when seen occurs about 6 to 8 weeks after the "full" dose of the methotrexate is achieved. Another immunomodulatory agent that is effective is mycophenolate mofetil (CellCept).* This agent is administered orally in a dose of 1.5 gm twice daily. I have not found that agents such as thalidomide,* dapsone,* retinoids, azathioprine,* or cyclosporine (Neoral)* are effective in the limited number of patients I have treated.

*Not FDA approved for this indication.

Biologic agents may have a future use in this disease. Intravenous immune globulin* 1 gm/kg/d on 2 consecutive days each month is often effective for both the skin lesions and for the muscle disease. This therapy has been tested in a controlled trial. Recently several anecdotes have suggested that the TNF-α inhibitors infliximab (Remicade)* or etanercept (Enbrel)* might be useful, but because these agents regularly induce antinuclear antibodies and in some patients induce lupus-like disease, I have been hesitant to recommend their use in dermatomyositis until a controlled trial can be performed. Last, a drug in development that is a humanized antibody directed at C5 has shown promise in early phase 2 studies. Whether other agents that affect T cells such as alefacept† or efaluzimab† will be effective for DM-associated skin disease needs to be studied.

SCLERODERMA

Scleroderma refers to hardening of the skin. It can be part of a process localized to the skin or may be part of a systemic process known as progressive systemic sclerosis. It appears that these two disorders are distinct and that few, if any, patients with localized scleroderma will develop systemic sclerosis. In this discussion I will limit my remarks to patients with localized scleroderma.

There are several variants of localized scleroderma. Plaque-type morphea is perhaps the most common variant and is manifest as a localized induration of the skin. Sometimes there is hyperpigmentation. In some patients there are surface changes that include a cigarette paperlike epidermal atrophy with a rough surface and small indentations known as "dells." These patients have overlapping features with lichen sclerosus et atrophicus. Linear scleroderma (morphea) most often occurs on the extremities, or on the face. On the face it is often referred to as "en coup de sabre." Some of these patients have deep tissue involvement and a resulting facial hemiatrophy known as Parry-Romberg syndrome. The relationship between linear scleroderma and the Parry-Romberg syndrome is controversial. Rarely patients will develop generalized plaques of morphea or deep lesions known as morphea profunda. Several other variants are rare, but have been reported including bullous morphea, keloidal morphea, and pansclerotic morphea. Last, there are some patients with atrophy and hyperpigmentation of the skin known as the atrophoderma of Pasini and Perini. Whether this entity belongs in the localized scleroderma spectrum is controversial.

There are no tests that confirm the diagnosis of morphea, but it is reasonable to perform a skin biopsy, which usually reveals homogenization of collagen bundles. In the early inflammatory stage, there is often a perivascular lymphohistiocytic infiltrate in the reticular dermis and the fibrous trabeculae of subcutaneous tissues. Numerous plasma cells may also be present. The dermis is typically edematous, with collagen bundle swelling in lower reticular dermis. In the late sclerotic stage, the inflammatory infiltrate usually becomes absent. Collagen bundles become thick, dense, homogenous, and eosinophilic, with collagen changes extending to the upper dermis and possibly also involving the panniculus, fascia, and muscle. Hair follicles, sweat glands, and subcutaneous fat are progressively lost as collagenous material accumulates.

*Not FDA approved for this indication.

†Not available in the United States.

Evaluation of the patient will occasionally reveal an eosinophilia, a positive antinuclear antibody, positive anti–single-stranded DNA antibodies, and positive antihistone antibodies. Patients with these abnormalities may well have a more prolonged course of their disease.

Because most patients have a benign course, the first step in management is to reassure the patient and family that the process is benign and often self-limited. For patients with surface changes suggestive of lichen sclerosus, the use of potent to superpotent topical corticosteroids is usually effective. In addition patients in the "early" inflammatory stage may also improve with topical corticosteroids therapy. Several open-label studies have documented improvement in localize scleroderma with the use of topically applied calcipotriene (Dovonex)* ointment. Most often this therapy is used under occlusion. In Europe the use of UVA1 light has been reported to be effective, but this therapy is not widely available in the United States. Its use in both low and high doses has been reported to be beneficial clinically, but in addition there are data that demonstrated a decrease in the tissue collagen with an increase in collagenase in patients responding to therapy. Although a topical vitamin D derivative is useful, the data on the use of oral vitamin D are at best mixed and I have abandoned its use because of concerns that calcium metabolism might be affected. Therapy with methotrexate alone or in combination with corticosteroids has been useful, but I have been unable to notice an effect in the small number of patients whom I have treated.

*Not FDA approved for this indication.

CUTANEOUS VASCULITIS

method of
MICHELLE T. PELLE, M.D., and
VICTORIA P. WERTH, M.D.
University of Pennsylvania School of Medicine
Philadelphia, Pennsylvania

In 1866, Kussmaul and Maier reported autopsy findings from a 27-year-old man with "periarteritis nodosa." For years after that first description, vasculitis was perceived as a single disease entity. Today, the term encompasses many syndromes, but there remains no universal system for its classification. One approach focuses on the caliber of the vessels involved (i.e., small, medium or large). In many of the cutaneous

TABLE 1. **Classification of Vasculitis Based on the Size of Involved Blood Vessels**

Small-Vessel Vasculitides
Immune complex-associated
Leukocytoclastic vasculitis
Connective tissue disorders*
Drug-induced vasculitis
Paraneoplastic vasculitis
Infection-associated
Henoch-Schönlein purpura
Urticarial vasculitis
Cryoglobulinemia*
Erythema elevatum diutinum
Pauci-immune (ANCA)-associated
Wegener's granulomatosis*
Churg-Strauss syndrome*
Microscopic polyangiitis*
Miscellaneous small-vessel vasculitides
Behçet's disease†
Inflammatory bowel disease
Sarcoidosis
Medium-Vessel Vasculitides
Classic polyarteritis nodosa*
Cutaneous polyarteritis nodosa*
Rheumatoid vasculitis*
Kawasaki disease
Buerger's disease

*Overlap of small and medium-sized vessels may occur.
†May involve small, medium, and large blood vessels.
ANCA, antineutrophil cytoplasmic antibodies.

vasculitides, small- and medium-vessel involvement frequently overlaps (Table 1).

IMMUNE COMPLEX–MEDIATED SMALL-VESSEL VASCULITIDES

Leukocytoclastic vasculitis (LCV), also referred to as hypersensitivity angiitis or necrotizing vasculitis, most commonly manifests as palpable purpura below the knees. Petechial, erythematous papular, nodular, and ulcerative eruptions may also occur in a variable skin distribution and lesions tend to appear in crops. Drugs are a common cause (Table 2), but LCV may also occur in association with connective tissue disease (CTD), malignancy, and infection. A full one third to one half of cases have no identifiable cause. Postcapillary venules and muscular arterioles within the papillary and reticular dermis are predominantly affected.

Direct immunofluorescence (DIF) is a particularly helpful diagnostic test to differentiate the variants of immune complex vasculitis. LCV is characterized by mixed deposition of IgM, IgG, and complement around dermal vessels. If CTD is present, an *in vivo* antinuclear antibody may be visible.

TABLE 2. **Drug Classes Associated With Cutaneous Vasculitis**

Antibacterials	Antihypertensives
Antivirals	Anticoagulants
Antifungals	Antineoplastics
Vaccines	Hematopoietic growth factors
Interferons	Nonsteroidal anti-inflammatories
Antithyroid agents	Leukotriene inhibitors
Anticonvulsants	Psychoactive agents
Antiarrhythmics	Sympathomimetics/drugs of abuse
Diuretics	TNF inhibitors

Henoch-Schönlein purpura (HSP, IgA vasculitis) occurs more commonly in children than in adults. Purpura and/or nonpurpuric papules and plaques are distributed over the lower extremities and abdomen. HSP is characterized by intense perivascular deposition of IgA on DIF. Fever and joint symptoms are typical. HSP is classically described as a tetrad of cutaneous vasculitis, arthritis, glomerulonephritis, and ileitis, but severe systemic disease is uncommon. Refractory cases of HSP in adults may signal underlying IgA paraproteinemia. In such cases, livedo reticularis may indicate involvement of medium-sized vessels. Low serum C3, leukopenia, and thrombocytopenia have been associated with severe HSP nephritis.

Urticarial vasculitis (UV) is characterized by urticarial papules that persist more than 24 hours and heal with purpura. Lesions affect the trunk and proximal extremities and are often accompanied by a burning sensation. Urticarial vasculitis may be self-limited (normocomplementemic) or resemble systemic lupus (hypocomplementemic urticarial vasculitis syndrome, HUV). HUV shows striking IgG deposition on DIF around blood vessels and along the basement membrane zone (lupus band). UV has also been associated with hepatitis C infection and with visceral and hematologic malignancies and lymphoma.

Cryoglobulinemic vasculitis (CV) occurs mostly in types II and III cryoglobulinemia. Recurrent crops of purpura (palpable and nonpalpable) occur diffusely on the extremities and trunk. Serum C4 levels may be disproportionately low (normal C3). Luminal thrombi are common, and immune complex deposition occurs around both small and medium dermal vessels. CV is highly associated with active hepatitis C virus (HCV) infection. The definitive test to establish *active* HCV infection is detection of HCV RNA by polymerase chain reaction. CV may also be complicated by renal disease and/or mononeuritis multiplex.

A complete history and physical examination will dictate the extent of the systemic workup required. A complete blood count with differential, platelets, serum creatinine, blood urea nitrogen, urinalysis, liver enzymes, bilirubin, and stool sample for occult blood will help to identify if there is systemic vasculitis. Eosinophilia, while helpful if present, occurs in only 20% of drug-induced vasculitis (DIV) cases when they are confined to the skin (compared to 80% of systemic DIV). New or worsening leg edema may signal renal involvement. Pulmonary, renal, gastrointestinal and/or musculoskeletal symptoms should prompt further workup for antineutrophil cytoplasmic antibodies (ANCA)–associated vasculitis, malignancy, dysproteinemia, and connective tissue disease. Monitoring for proteinuria and elevated serum creatinine should be continued for at least 6 months, because renal involvement can be delayed.

Abscess, bacteremia, endocarditis, and meningitis may be infectious triggers of vasculitis. Organisms with the propensity to cause LCV include chronic streptococcal infections, meningococcus, hepatitis B and C, cytomegalovirus, Rocky Mountain spotted fever, mycoplasma, syphilis, and fungal pathogens. Opportunistic mimickers of vasculitis must not be forgotten, especially in the presence of cutaneous ulceration or disease refractory to immunosuppressive therapy. The atypical mycobacteria are an insidious example.

Oral corticosteroids* are the mainstay of therapy if there is systemic involvement, excluding immune complex vasculitides of infectious origin. Corticosteroids (prednisone) should be initiated early (1 mg/kg/day) and tapered slowly over 1 to 2 months, depending on disease severity. Osteoporosis prevention is begun concomitantly, with a regimen that includes daily calcium supplementation and an oral bisphosphonate dosed once weekly. In milder cases of LCV, dapsone and/or colchicine* may constitute adequate therapy or expedite steroid tapering. Antihistamines provide relief of burning symptoms or pruritus. Antimalarial agents may be useful in urticarial vasculitis. When there is refractory cutaneous vasculitis or steroid-unresponsive systemic vasculitis, immunosuppressive therapy (azathioprine [Imuran]* or mycophenolate [CellCept]*) is required in addition to corticosteroids to control the disease process and enable corticosteroid tapering. Intra-venous immunoglobulin has been successful in some severe cases of gastrointestinal HSP. Cyclophos-phamide* is reserved for systemic and/or deeply ulcerative (larger vessel) refractory cases. Pulsed cyclophosphamide is preferable to continuous oral dosing to minimize long-term side effects (hemorrhagic cystitis, bladder cancer, and lymphoproliferative malignancies).

PAUCI-IMMUNE SMALL-VESSEL VASCULITIDES

Wegener's granulomatosis (WG) may occur as a necrotizing small-vessel vasculitis, resembling LCV, or as a medium-vessel vasculitis, in which case ulcerative lesions may develop that resemble pyoderma gangrenosum. Antineutrophil cytoplasmic antibodies in a cytoplasmic pattern (c-ANCA) are positive in 75% to 80% of cases. A perinuclear ANCA pattern (p-ANCA) is present in 10% to 15%. Histology reveals necrotizing and granulomatous vasculitis. Skin changes may precede systemic involvement. Paranasal, pulmonary, renal, and neurologic disease occur most commonly. Saddle nose deformity may develop after long-standing disease.

Churg-Strauss syndrome (CSS) occurs in three phases. Asthma and allergic rhinitis may be present for months to years before the onset of eosinophilia. Ultimately, an eosinophilic and granulomatous vasculitis evolves, with a predilection for the lungs and peripheral nerves (mononeuritis multiplex and/or polyneuropathy). In nearly one half of cases, CSS involves the myocardium, often with fatal consequences. Nodular and papulonecrotic skin lesions occur mainly over the extensor elbows. CSS patients can develop a migratory, seropositive arthritis of large joints, which may resemble rheumatoid arthritis. c-ANCA occurs in 25% to 30% of patients and the same percentage is positive for p-ANCA.

*Not FDA approved for this indication.

WG and CSS patients frequently have aggressive underlying systemic disease. They require prompt immunosuppressive therapy in combination with oral corticosteroids. All cases are unique, but a general approach can be outlined. Pulsed or oral cyclophosphamide is initially utilized to bring the disease under control, typically over a 3-month duration, with gradual tapering of corticosteroids. Patients are then switched to an alternative maintenance drug (azathioprine,* mycophenolate,* or methotrexate*) to minimize long-term cyclophosphamide sequelae. In WG, hematuria should prompt a dose increase or a return to cyclophosphamide. Unfortunately, neither ANCA nor eosinophilia provide reliable markers of disease activity, although ANCAs are now felt to play a pathogenic role. Because upper respiratory infections trigger relapse of pauci-immune vasculitis, prophylaxis with trimethoprim-sulfamethoxazole (Bactrim*) for up to 2 years is recommended. A high index of suspicion for opportunistic infections should be maintained in these patients. Recently, attention has been focused on the unmasking or provoking of CSS by leukotriene inhibitors. Other drugs known to induce ANCA-positive vasculitis are hydralazine and propylthiouracil.

Behçet's disease mostly occurs as a lymphocytic small-vessel vasculitis and is characterized clinically by severe oral and genital aphthae, pathergy, and eye abnormalities. Behçet's disease represents the only cutaneous vasculitis that affects small, medium, and large vessels, including veins. In Behçet's small-vessel vasculitis, pustular lesions develop and resemble folliculitis. When medium vessels are involved, nodular lesions resemble erythema nodosum (EN), but in contrast to EN, they may ulcerate and scar. Bruits can be heard in the presence of large-vessel disease. Vasculitis is not demonstrated in the orogenital ulcers of Behçet's disease. Successful remissions have been achieved with dapsone (plus colchicine), azathioprine (Imuran), and cyclosporine (Neoral). Rapid remission can be achieved with thalidomide* (100 mg/d) in appropriate patients.

MEDIUM-VESSEL VASCULITIDES

Cutaneous polyarteritis nodosa (PAN) affects the muscular arteries of the skin and spares veins. In classic PAN, there may be comorbid gastrointestinal ischemia, severe mononeuritis multiplex, and congestive heart failure. Skin findings include livedo reticularis of the lower extremities and tender, sometimes ulcerative, nodules. This combination of nodular and livedoid vasculitis is quite specific for PAN. Healing may evolve to atrophic stellate scars resembling *atrophie blanche*. PAN limited to the skin is often controlled with dapsone* or methotrexate* alone, but steroids may be needed occasionally. Dependent edema should be avoided in these patients because it often triggers flares of PAN.

*Not FDA approved for this indication.

Rheumatoid vasculitis (RV) typically presents as acral (distal extremity) purpura progressing to ulceration. It most often occurs in burned-out rheumatoid patients with inactive, seropositive joint disease following years of immunosuppression. However, it can complicate early disease. Dapsone* can be effective, but combination prednisone with immunosuppressives, sometimes pulsed cyclophosphamide,* can be required, because RV can be hard to bring under control.

Buerger's disease (thromboangiitis obliterans) occurs in tobacco smokers and is characterized by digital arteriolar vasculitis and vasospasm resulting in digital infarction. Prompt smoking cessation is mandatory to stop progression. The disease affects both light and heavy smokers. Aggressive wound care and vasodilators can prevent digital amputations.

*Not FDA approved for this indication.

DISEASES OF THE NAILS

method of
ANTONELLA TOSTI, M.D., and
MASSIMILIANO PAZZAGLIA, M.D
University of Bologna
Bologna, Italy

The nail unit consists of four specialized epithelia: the nail matrix, the nail bed, the proximal nail fold, and the hyponychium. The nail matrix is a germinative epithelial structure that gives rise to a fully keratinized multilayered sheet of cornified cells known as the nail plate. In longitudinal sections, the nail matrix consists of a proximal and a distal region, which respectively, produce the dorsal and ventral nail plate. Nail plate corneocytes are tightly connected by desmosomes and complex digitations.

The nail plate is a rectangular, translucent, and transparent structure that appears pink because of the vessels of the underlying nail bed. The proximal part of the nail plate of the fingernails show a whitish, half-moon shaped area, the lunula, that corresponds to the visible portion of the distal nail matrix. The shape of the lunula determines the shape of the free edge of the plate. The nail plate is firmly attached to nail bed, which partially contributes to nail formation along its length. The longitudinal orientation of the capillary vessels in the nail bed explains the linear pattern of the nail bed hemorrhages. Proximally and laterally, the nail plate is surrounded by the nail folds. The horny layer of the proximal nail fold forms the cuticle, which intimately adheres to the underlying nail plate and prevents its separation from the proximal nail fold. Distally the nail bed continues with the hyponychium, which marks the separation of the nail plate from the digit. The nail plate grows continuously and uniformly throughout life. Average nail growth is faster in fingernails (3 mm per month) than in toenails (1 to 1.5 mm per month). Replacement of a fingernail usually requires about 6 months, replacement of a toenail 12 to 18 months.

BRITTLE NAILS

Nail brittleness causes several clinical symptoms including splitting, softening, lamellar exfoliation, and onychorrhexis.

Nail brittleness is often precipitated or worsened by exposure to environmental factors that dehydrate the nails, such as detergents and solvents. The condition is more common in middle-aged women because the lipid content of the nails is under hormonal control and it decreases after menopause.

Systemic Therapy:

Biotin* 2.5 to 5 mg/d for at least 6 months. Iron supplementation should be given if ferritin levels are below 10 μg/mL.

Topical Therapy:

Application of hydrophilic petrolatum (Aquaphor)* on wet nails at bedtime helps to retain the moisture in the nail plate. Nails should be rehydrated with repeated application of moisturizers containing lactic acid, urea, phospholipids, hyaluronic acid, α-hydroxy acids, and proteoglycans.

ACUTE PARONYCHIA

Acute paronychia is most commonly precipitated by a minor trauma and is generally caused by *Staphylococcus aureus*, although other bacteria and herpes simplex can be responsible in some cases. The affected digit is painful and shows erythema, swelling, and pus formation.

Whenever possible cultures should be taken and the abscess should be drained to avoid matrix compression and damage. Treatment of bacterial infections includes local medications with antiseptics and systemic antibiotics in accordance with the results of cultures.

In acute paronychia due to herpes simplex treatment with acyclovir (Zovirax)* 15 mg/kg/d is indicated for 5 days.

CHRONIC PARONYCHIA

Chronic paronychia is variety of contact dermatitis that affects the proximal nail fold. It is most often caused by irritants but may also be due to immediate or delayed allergy. Immediate hypersensitivity to food ingredients is common in food handlers. Clinically, the proximal and lateral nail folds show mild erythema and swelling. The cuticle is lost and the ventral portion of the proximal nail fold becomes separated from the nail plate. With time the nail fold retracts and becomes thickened and rounded.

Secondary colonization by bacteria and fungi, especially *Candida* species is common and may cause self-limited episodes of painful acute inflammation with pus formation. The presence of *Pseudomonas aeruginosa* produces green discoloration of the nail.

Beau's lines and onychomadesis may occur as a consequence of nail matrix damage. Management and

*Not FDA approved for this indication.

prognosis of the disease are very similar to those of contact dermatitis, and definitive cure of chronic paronychia is quite uncommon. The best treatment associates a high potency topical steroid (clobetasol propionate† 0.05% [Temovate] ointment) at bedtime with a topical antifungal in the morning to contrast secondary microbial colonization. Systemic steroids (methylprednisolone* 20 mg/day) can be prescribed in severe cases to obtain fast relief of inflammation and pain. Systemic antifungals are not useful and chronic paronychia should not be misdiagnosed as *Candida* onychomycosis. Acute exacerbation of chronic paronychia does not necessitate antibiotic treatment.

ONYCHOLYSIS

Onycholysis describes the detachment of the nail plate from the nail bed. Most commonly onycholysis originates from the central or lateral portion of the nail plate free margin, and progresses proximally. The onycholytic area looks whitish because of the presence of air under the detached nail plate. It may occasionally show a greenish or brown discoloration due to colonization of the onycholytic space by chromogenic bacteria (*Pseudomonas aeruginosa*), molds, or yeasts. Onycholysis may be idiopathic or represent a symptom of numerous diseases such as psoriasis, onychomycosis, contact dermatitis, and drug reactions. Photo-onycholysis is precipitated by ultraviolet exposure and is most commonly caused by drugs; it is often painful and originates in the central portion of the nail plate. The pathogenesis of idiopathic onycholysis is still unknown but an impairment in the nail bed keratinization has been suggested. A waterborne environment facilitates the development of this condition, which is much more frequent in housewives.

The detached nails should be cut away and this should be repeated until the nail plate grows attached. A symptomatic treatment with a topical antiseptic solution (thymol 4% in chloroform)† or a topical imidazole derivative (Spectazole 1% cream)* can be prescribed. Pseudomonas colonization can be treated with sodium hypochlorite solution (Dakin's solution) or 2% acetic acid. Gentamicin cream* can be alternatively used after removal of the onycholytic nail plate.

ONYCHOMYCOSIS

The term onychomycosis describes the infection of the nail by fungus. Although most cases of onychomycosis result from a dermatophytic invasion of the nail, onychomycosis due to nondermatophytic fungi is becoming more common worldwide. *Candida* onychomycosis is a very uncommon condition that occurs only in immunocompromised patients, such as patients with chronic cutaneous candidiasis or HIV infection.

Treatment of onychomycosis depends on the responsible fungi, the type of onychomycosis, the number of affected nails, the age of the patient, and the medications in use. Choice of treatment should, therefore, take into account possible drug interactions. Because differential diagnosis of onychomycosis includes a large number of different diseases, treatment should be started only when the diagnosis is confirmed by a positive microscopy and/or culture.

Onychomycosis Due to Dermatophytes

The affected digit (most commonly a toenail) shows subungual hyperkeratosis with onycholysis (distal subungual onychomycosis); proximal leukonychia (proximal subungual onychomycosis); or superficial friable leukonychia (white, superficial onychomycosis exclusively affects toenail).

Topical Treatment

White, superficial onychomycosis and distal subungual onychomycosis are limited to the distal nail (should not normally affect the lunula) of a few digits.

1. Amorolfine 5% nail lacquer† once or twice a week
2. Ciclopirox 8% nail lacquer (Penlac) once a day

Treatment should last for 6 to 12 months.

Systemic Treatment

For proximal subungual onychomycosis and distal subungual onychomycosis involving several digits:

1. Terbinafine (Lamisil) 250 mg daily. Treatment duration is 2 months for fingernails and 3 months for toenails.
2. Itraconazole (Sporanox) pulse therapy: 400 mg daily for one week a month. Treatment duration is 2 months for fingernails and 3 months for toenails. The drug should be administered with a meal to optimize absorption.
3. Fluconazole (Diflucan)* 150 or 300 mg weekly for 6 months up to 1 year.

Systemic treatment with terbinafine or itraconazole produces mycologic cure in more than 90% of fingernail infections and in about 60% to 80% of toenail infections. These success rates can be increased by associating a topical treatment with an antifungal nail lacquer.

Recurrences and reinfection are not uncommon (up to 20% of cured patients). They may possibly be prevented by the regular application of topical antifungals on the previously affected nails, soles, and toe webs.

Onychomycosis Due to Non-Dermatophytes

Toenails are usually affected and most commonly show proximal subungual onychomycosis (PSO) or distal subungual onychomycosis (DSO) associated with periungual inflammation.

Onychomycosis due to non-dermatophytic molds generally responds poorly to systemic treatment. Chemical or surgical avulsion of the affected nail greatly increases chances of cure.

PSO or DSO due to *Scopulariopsis brevicaulis*, *Fusarium* species and *Acremonium* species respond better to topical than to systemic therapy.

*Not FDA approved for this indication.
†Not available in the United States.

*Not FDA approved for this indication.
†Not available in the United States.

Topical Treatment

1. Amorolfine 5% nail lacquer,† once or twice a week.
2. Ciclopirox 8% nail lacquer (Penlac), once a day for 8 to 12 months.
3. Terbinafine (Lamisil) cream, once a day for 8 to 12 months, after chemical nail avulsion using 40% urea in petrolatum.

Systemic Treatment

Nail infections due to *Aspergillus* species

1. Itraconazole (Sporanox), 400 mg/d for 1 week a month for 3 months.
2. Terbinafine (Lamisil), 250 mg/d for 3 months.

Cure of the onychomycosis may require a longer treatment than that of dermatophyte onychomycosis.

Onychomycosis Due to Candida Species

Onychomycosis due to *Candida* species is a sign of immunodepression most commonly affecting fingernails.

Systemic Treatment

1. Itraconazole (Sporanox), 400 mg/d for 1 week a month for 3 months.
2. Terbinafine (Lamisil), 250 mg/d for 3 months.
3. Fluconazole (Diflucan),* 150 or 300 mg weekly for 6 months up to 1 year.

Topical Treatment

1. Amorolfine 5% nail lacquer,† once or twice a week.
2. Ciclopirox 8% nail lacquer (Penlac), once a day for 8 to 12 months.

Both can be useful to prevent recurrences.

Candida onychomycosis usually responds very well to treatment. Recurrences are frequent because this type of infection affects immunocompromised patients.

NAIL PSORIASIS

Treatment of nail psoriasis is often disappointing, and only rarely lives up to patients' expectations. Nail psoriasis is often precipitated and aggravated by traumas (Koebner's phenomenon) and does not improve with sun exposure and often worsens during summer. Choice of treatment depends on localization of the disease in the nail apparatus. In nail matrix psoriasis, the affected nails show irregular pitting and/or diffuse nail plate surface abnormalities. Nail bed psoriasis produces subungual hyperkeratosis, onycholysis, and reddish discoloration of the nail bed.

Topical Treatment

Topical treatment is useful in nail bed hyperkeratosis due to nail bed psoriasis, after removal of the onycholytic nail plate.

*Not FDA approved for this indication.
†Not available in the United States.

1. Tazarotene (Tazorac)* gel with or without occlusion.
2. Topical calcipotriol (Dovonex) * twice a day

Topical treatment should last for several months.

Intralesional Treatment

Intralesional steroids are useful in nail matrix and nail bed psoriasis. However, this treatment is painful and may be complicated by local side effects (subungual hematoma, reversible atrophy, and hypopigmentation).

Triamcinolone acetonide (Kenalog R) 2.5 mg/mL, at a dose of 0.2 to 0.5 mL per nail, should be injected through the nail folds or the hyponychium using a 25-gauge needle. Injections should be repeated monthly for 5 to 6 months.

Systemic Treatment

Acitretin (Soriatane),* 0.3 to 0.5 mg/kg/d can be utilized in severe nail matrix psoriasis with nail plate crumbling involving several or all nails. The drug is contraindicated in women who may become pregnant if unprotected by valid contraceptive for at least 3 years.

When nail psoriasis is associated with skin or joint psoriasis, methotrexate (Rheumatrex) or cyclosporine (Neoral) can be successfully utilized.

PUSTULAR PSORIASIS

Pustular psoriasis produces relapsing inflammatory or pustular lesions of the nails and periungual skin; the condition is most commonly limited to one digit (Hallopeau's acrodermatitis).

The distal portion of the digit may be swollen and erythematous and patients complain of intense pain. Recurrent pustular flares may produce a definitive atrophy of the nail matrix with absence of the nail plate. Bone resorption can occasionally occur.

Treatment

1. Acitretin (Soriatane), 0.5 mg/kg/d produces immediate clearing of the inflammatory changes in the great majority of patients. It is the treatment of choice when the disease affects several nails and in long-lasting cases (see systemic treatment of psoriasis for contraindications).
2. Topical calcipotriene (Dovonex), twice a day, is the best option for pustular psoriasis limited to one or two nails and is also very useful as maintenance therapy after interruption of retinoids.

LICHEN PLANUS

Specific nail involvement occurs in about 10% of patients with lichen planus and permanent damage of at least one nail occurs in approximately 4% of patients. Most commonly the nail changes consist of thinning, longitudinal ridging, and distal splitting of the nail plate. Definitive destruction of the nail matrix is responsible for pterygium and onychoatrophy.

Treatment is mandatory to avoid nail scarring. Dorsal pterygium is irreversible.

*Not FDA approved for this indication.

Systemic steroids are effective in treating nail lichen planus and prevent destruction of the nail matrix. Intramuscular triamcinolone acetonide (Kenalog),* 0.5 mg/kg every month for 2 to 3 months, usually produces recovery of the nail abnormalities. This therapy has also been successfully utilized in children with nail lichen planus. Intralesional injections of triamcinolone acetonide (as for nail psoriasis) represent a possible though painful alternative when the disease is limited to a few fingernails. Mild relapses are frequently observed, but recurrences are usually responsive to therapy.

YELLOW NAIL SYNDROME

This term describes the association of slowly growing yellow nails with primary lymphedema and respiratory tract involvement. Nails are pale yellow to yellow-green in color, thickened, opaque and excessively curved from side to side. The cuticle is absent and onycholysis is frequent. The nail changes may improve spontaneously or after resolution of the associated systemic disease.

Oral vitamin E at dosages of 600 to 1200* IU daily for 6 to 18 months may induce complete clearing of the nail changes.

Pulse therapy with itraconazole (Sporanox) 400 mg/daily for 1 week a month for 4 to 6 months may resolve the nail changes in about 25% of patients. The drug probably acts by increasing nail growth.

INGROWN NAILS

Ingrown nails are a common complaint, which most commonly affects the great toe of young adults. Hyperhidrosis, congenital malalignment, improper cutting of toenails, as well as unsatisfactory footwear, all contribute to the development of this painful condition. The condition starts when spicules breaking off from the lateral edge of the nail plate penetrate into the tissues of lateral nail fold. In this phase the inflammatory reaction produces pain, redness, and swelling. Treatment is conservative with extraction of the embedded spicula and introduction of a package of nonabsorbent cotton (soaked in a disinfectant) under the corner of the nail to prevent further penetration of the lateral nail fold. This medication should be replaced daily.

In advanced stages the lateral edge of the nail plate is enclosed in an overgrowth of granulation tissue that with time may become epithelialized. Although application of high potency steroids or cryosurgery may reduce the granulation tissue, chemical (phenol) matricectomy is the treatment of choice.

MYXOID CYSTS

Myxoid cysts are a common benign tumor of the nail unit, most frequently affecting elderly women.

Cysts localized in the proximal nail fold may compress the nail matrix and produce longitudinal depression or grooves in the nail plate. The cysts frequently communicate with the distal phalangeal joint through a tract that pumps synovial fluid into the cysts.

Treatments of myxoid cysts include surgical excision, intralesional injections of triamcinolone acetonide (Kenalog 3 to 5 mg/mL) or sclerosing agents (3% solution of sodium tetradecylsulfate)† after evacuation of the cyst content with a sterile needle. Cryosurgery (two 30-second freezes) is effective but painful and associated with considerable morbidity. Unfortunately recurrence rates are high in all of the available treatments, and cysts frequently recur even after surgery if the tract leading from the cyst to the joint capsule is not dissected.

*Not FDA approved for this indication.

†Not available in the United States.

KELOIDS

method of
BRIAN BERMAN, M.D., Ph.D., and
VAREE POOCHAREON, B.S.
University of Miami School of Medicine
Miami, Florida

Keloids are exaggerated scars consisting of excessively dense, fibrous tissue growing in all directions, resulting in a prominent protrusion above the skin. Keloids may occur after all types of cutaneous trauma, sometimes appearing years after an initial wound, and going on to persist for years, extending beyond the boundaries of the original wound and prone to recur following excision. Though keloids may form in any location, they are most commonly located on the chest, shoulders, upper arms, back, and head and neck areas, including the earlobes (most often resulting from an earlobe piercing). Size and shape of keloids vary, and though most lesions are round or oval, they may have irregular or clawlike borders, with consistency ranging from doughy soft to rubbery hard. Early keloids are often erythematous, becoming pale with age. These scars most commonly appear among more pigmented persons, especially African Americans, and often arise between the ages of 10 and 30 years, although they may occur at any age in all patients, without gender predisposition. Although patients tend to present with solitary or few lesions, multiple lesions may occur, for example, with acne or varicella. Keloid patients often seek medical attention for pain, tenderness, pruritus, and burning associated with their lesions, as well as for cosmetic purposes, because keloids can be disfiguring and psychologically distressing. Histologically, keloids are characterized by large, broad bundles of pink collagen in a whorl-like arrangement, embedded in an amorphous ground substance with little elastic tissue present. Local metabolic activity, mast cells, eosinophils, lymphocytes, and plasma cells are all increased.

PATHOPHYSIOLOGY

A variety of abnormal cellular and immunologic characteristics are associated with keloid formation. Keloidal fibroblasts produce abnormal amounts of extracellular matrix (ECM) and high levels of plasminogen inhibitor, resulting in inferior breakdown of fibrin. Macrophages release fibroblast-activating cytokines, such as platelet-derived growth factor (PDGF) and transforming growth factor-β (TGF-β), which activates ECM production. Lower wound levels of interleukin-1 (IL-1) that normally promote collagenase activity may also result in ECM accumulation. There is reduced tissue oxygen concentration in keloids, perhaps due to occlusion of the excess microvessels grown, higher tissue metabolic rate, or reduced oxygen diffusion to the wound space, which stimulates fibroblasts to proliferate and produce collagen. Collagen synthesis in keloids can continue for years, possibly due to overexpression of the insulin-like growth factor (IGF) signal transduction pathway (shown to increase expression of type I and III procollagen) and IGF-I receptors on fibroblasts. In normal wound healing, interferon-α (IFN-α) down-regulates collagen synthesis; IFN-γ reduces collagenase activity; IFN-α, -β, and -γ inhibit production of collagen; and IFN-α and -β reduce fibroblast production of glycosaminoglycans (GAGs), which form a scaffold for collagen deposition. Reductions of IFN-α, IFN-γ, and tumor necrosis factor-α (TNF-α) concentrations have all been found in keloids. Keloid fibroblasts may also undergo apoptosis, or programmed cell death, at lower rates than that of normal scar fibroblasts, and mutations in p53 are believed to predispose cells to hyperproliferation.

TREATMENT

The treatment of keloids is still a formidable challenge, despite the range of therapeutic options available. No single therapy has been shown to be superior, and size, location, depth, patient age, and past response to treatment greatly influence the type of therapy chosen.

Surgical Excision

The aim of surgical excision is to remove the bulk of the keloid, replacing it with a narrower, more cosmetically acceptable scar. As a monotherapy, excisional surgery yields a 45% to 100% recurrence rate and should rarely be used because the procedure effectively wounds the keloid-prone patient once more. Combination with other postoperative modalities, such as silicone sheeting, irradiation, intralesional corticosteroids and interferon, results in lower recurrence rates. Surgeons are recommended to apply basic soft tissue handling techniques, closing with minimal tension and using buried sutures when necessary for layered closure.

Corticosteroids

The mainstay of keloid therapy has been intralesional corticosteroid injections, thought to alter fibroblast proliferation and production of inflammatory mediators, as well as to down-regulate collagen gene expression within the keloid. As a monotherapy, corticosteroids can soften and flatten scars to a limited extent, providing mostly symptomatic relief at the risk of significant injection pain, atrophy, pigment alteration, and formation of telangiectases with repeated injections. Corticosteroids are usually injected into various areas of the keloid, repeated at intervals of 6 to 8 weeks. When combined with surgical excision, the majority of studies show less than 50% recurrence of keloids.

Silicone Dressings

Silicone dressings, due to their benign nature, have been favored in certain cases amenable to application of sheeting, with improvement reported in scar volume, firmness, tenderness, and pruritus. Antikeloidal effects, however, may result from a combination of occlusion and hydration rather than from the effect of silicone.

Compression

The mechanism of compression therapy for keloids is unclear, but improvement may result from the reduction in collagen fiber cohesiveness. Patients treated with all manner of compression therapies, including button compression, pressure earrings, pressure-gradient devices, and nonsilicone occlusive sheeting have shown improvement in previous studies, with reductions in keloid height, tenderness, and pruritus.

Cryotherapy

Cryosurgical media, such as liquid nitrogen, can affect the microvasculature and cause cell damage via intracellular crystals, leading to tissue anoxia and a variable response. This form of treatment may also be painful, requiring repetition every 20 to 30 days, and is potentially inappropriate in patients with darker skin because of the risk of hypopigmentation due to destruction of melanocytes.

Radiation

Radiation therapy destroys fibroblasts from both normal and keloidal skin, affecting ECM gene expression as well. This modality is rarely used as monotherapy, and is far more successful in preventing recurrence when combined with surgical excision. Radiation is mainly reserved for scars resistant to other therapies, and although few case reports describe the development of malignancy following radiation therapy for keloids, caution is advised when treating areas around the breasts and thyroid and in treating young children.

Laser Therapy

Lasers can burn, coagulate, or evaporate keloid tissue in such a way as to minimize scar contraction when compared to scalpel wounds. Although both carbon dioxide and argon lasers showed early promise, neither are frequently used, as recurrence rates reach almost 100% when used as a monotherapy. The neodymium:yttrium-aluminum-garnet laser is used on the basis that collagen deposition can be inhibited, but with mostly anecdotal reports of its effects. The 585-nm flashlamp-pumped pulsed-dye laser, however, has been shown to be effective in reducing subjective symptoms such as pruritus, erythema, and height of keloids, with improvement in 57% to 83% of the cases.

Interferon

Interferons, with their antiviral and antiproliferative properties, have been shown to enhance keloidal collagenase activity, reduce synthesis of collagen and GAGs, and induce apoptosis. Antifibrotic effects of different interferon subtypes showed variable impact on reducing keloid size or recurrence when used alone or as an adjuvant. As a monotherapy, intralesional interferon-α2b (IFN-α2b)(Intron A)* has been shown to be largely ineffective, but works better as an adjuvant to surgical excision or laser therapy, with recurrence rates lower than surgical procedures alone. Interferon therapy is commonly associated with low-grade fever, flu-like illness for 48 to 72 hours after injection, and pain on injection.

Imiquimod

Imiquimod (Aldara),* is an immune response modifier that indirectly acts to stimulate cell-mediated immune pathways, inducing local synthesis and release of IFN-α, IFN-γ, TNF-α, and IL-1, -6, -8, and -12. Surgical excision of keloids, followed by 2 months of once-daily topical application of imiquimod 5% cream beginning the day of the surgery, resulted in lower recurrence rates than for surgery alone. Local skin reactions such as mild eczema and erythema may occur, but further study with longer follow-up periods and larger sample sizes is recommended.

CONCLUSION

Prevention and patient education is absolutely paramount in keloid therapy. Proposals for prevention include avoidance of nonessential cosmetic surgery, piercings, and tattoos in keloid-forming patients, as well as careful handling of tissue during surgical procedures. Treatments are generally chosen on a patient-to-patient basis, and although no universally effective method of treating keloids exists, polytherapy is generally favored over monotherapy, especially when surgery is considered. A variety of biologic and pharmacologic agents targeted at the abnormal immunologic responses in keloid formation have been examined (not presented here), though there are limited clinical studies to support their efficacy. Further controlled studies with larger patient populations, longer follow-up periods, and more uniform standards of evaluation are recommended for all possible treatment options for keloids, and hopefully will, at the very least, improve the quality of life for many symptomatic keloid patients.

*Not FDA approved for this indication.

CUTANEOUS WARTS

method of
TAMI DE ARAUJO, M.D., and
BRIAN BERMAN, M.D., PH.D.
University of Miami School of Medicine
Miami, Florida

Cutaneous warts are common, benign epithelial tumors caused by infection with human papillomavirus (HPV). In addition to warts being classified according to their location (e.g., oral, palmar, plantar, genital) and their morphology, different types of HPV have been associated with specific types of warts (Table 1).

Warts are most commonly found in children and adolescents and reach a prevalence of up to 20% in

TABLE 1. **Clinical Characteristics of Cutaneous Warts and Their Associated HPV Subtype**

Common warts, or *verruca vulgaris,* are characterized by a firm, keratotic papule with an irregular, spiked surface. The "black dots" often found after paring this type of wart represent thrombosed, dilated dermal capillaries within the lesion. They are localized mainly on the hands, thus the name "hands warts"; however, they may appear elsewhere on the skin. Filiform warts are manifested as tall and thin projections, localized more often on the face and scalp. **HPV types 1, 2, 4, 57**

Flat warts, or *verruca plana,* are flat, usually small (2–4 mm) lesions with irregular borders and smooth or slightly scaly surfaces; they are often multiple and sometimes grouped and confluent. These warts are found most frequently on the dorsa of the hands and the face, especially on the chin, cheeks, and forehead. **HPV types 3, 10**

Plantar warts are small punctate depressions on the soles or more typical keratotic surface with a collar of thickened keratin. **HPV types 1, 2, 4, 57**

Intermediate warts have features of common and flat warts. **HPV types 2, 3, 10, 28**

Gential warts can occur as small flesh-colored papules to large cauliflower-like lesions and are discussed elsewhere in this book. **HPV types 6, 11**

Myrmecia are deep, painful keratotic plaques that resemble calluses. These lesions are common in teenagers and are preferentially located on the pressure points of the foot. Differentiation from calluses can de made by the absence of dermatoglyphics in plantar warts. **HPV type 1**

Mosaic warts occur when plamar or plantar warts coalesce into large plaques. **HPV type 2**

Oral warts are manifested as small white papules on the oral mucosa. **HPV types 6, 11, 32**

Epidermodysplasia verruciformis is an autosomal dominantly inherited disorder associated with the presence of multiple flat warts and squamous cell carcinomas on the skin. **HPV types 5, 8**

Verrucous carcinoma is an unusual variant of squamous cell carcinoma found most commonly on the foot, but also in the oral cavity (oral florid papillomatosis) and genital area (giant condyloma of Buschke and Löwenstein). **HPV type 16**

Abbreviation: HPV, human papillomaviurs.

these groups. There seems to be no difference in incidence between the sexes. The disease is transmitted from person to person and to a lesser degree by contaminated fomites.

Intact cell-mediated immunity is required for the body's ability to control HPV infection, and indeed, immunosuppressed patients are particularly susceptible to the development of warts. Warts in these patients are usually resistant to treatment, found in greater numbers, and have a higher chance of malignant conversion than those found in immunocompetent patients.

The diagnosis of warts is usually based on clinical examination alone. On histologic examination, the presence of acanthosis and papillomatosis in the epidermis, hyperkeratosis, and parakeratosis with elongated rete ridges is suggestive of a wart. Southern blot hybridization analysis can be performed for identification of the viral etiology and for typing. Among the benign warts, however, the causative HPV genotype does not appear to have any impact on the efficacy of the different treatment modalities.

TREATMENT

Before initiating therapy, the patient should understand that warts can spontaneously resolve and that even though many options are available, no single treatment has a 100% success rate. When considering a treatment modality, not only its efficacy but also the recurrence rate for that particular modality should be taken into account (Table 2).

Additionally, the choice of treatment should take into consideration the location of the lesions, the disability caused by them (pain, interference with function, cosmetic embarrassment), and the age and immune state of the host.

Destructive Methods

Patient Applied

Keratolytics. Salicylic acid is a keratolytic that acts by slowly destroying the virus-infected epidermis, and the resulting mild irritation may also stimulate an immune response. It can be applied by the patient at home and requires daily application for a period of weeks to months. Many preparations are commercially available, including adhesive plasters, pads, solutions, or gels in either a flexible or acrylic collodion. The plasters and pads contain 40% salicylic acid and should be held in place with tape. Solutions and gels of salicylic acid and lactic acid are commonly used as well. These preparations can be particularly effective in young patients who cannot tolerate other treatment modalities or as an adjunct to therapy in adults. Before the application of wart paints, excess keratin should be removed by paring the lesion with either a scalpel blade or a pumice stone. Soaking the area in warm water may facilitate penetration of the treatment agent into the skin. Cure rates for common and plantar warts have varied between 70% and 80%.

TABLE 2. **Recurrence Rates for Different Treatments of Warts**

Cryotherapy	25%–39%
Curettage and cautery	25%
Surgical excision	19%–22%
CO_2 laser	6%–49%

Physician Applied

Cryotherapy. Liquid nitrogen (−196°C) applied by a physician, either by a spray canister or a cotton-tipped applicator, is a common and effective therapy for most cutaneous warts. Cure rates between 40% and 82% have been reported. Cryotherapy may have an effect on wart clearance either by simple necrotic destruction of HPV-infected keratinocytes or possibly by inducing local inflammation conducive to the development of an effective cell-mediated response.

Before initiating cryotherapy, paring of thick lesions should be performed. Liquid nitrogen can then be applied to a wart in two freezing cycles of approximately 10 to 60 seconds, depending on the size and location of the lesion. The area frozen should include a 1- to 2-mm rim of normal surrounding tissue. It has been suggested, however, that the HPV genome can be found as far as 1 cm beyond the lesion, thereby leading to recurrence of the wart around the site where cryotherapy was performed. This therapy can be repeated every 1 to 3 weeks until resolution of the lesions is achieved.

Short-term side effects include blistering, pain, and erythema at the site of treatment. Depigmentation and scarring may occur, and onychodystrophy can follow treatment of periungual warts. Caution must be used when freezing lesions over tendons and in patients with poor circulation.

Cantharidin. Cantharidin is an extract of the green blister beetle that causes focal destruction of the epidermis and blistering, so it should be avoided on the face. It is administered topically as a 0.7% collodion solution after paring the wart with a blade, and the area is then occluded for up to 1 week. Treatment is repeated every 1 to 4 weeks, depending on the size and location of the wart. The major advantage is that cantharidin is painless when applied, thus making it a good alternative for children. It should be applied by the physician and washed off 6 to 8 hours later.

Chemical Agents. Irritant chemicals such as bichloroacetic acid solution and trichloroacetic acid solution in concentrations of up to 50% may also be used for the treatment of warts. These agents act by destroying and peeling off the infected keratinocytes and may cause painful reactions at the site of application. Clearance rates vary between 25% and 86%. They find greater use in patients with a small number of warts on moist surfaces, particularly the plantar and genital areas.

Curettage and Cautery. Surgical removal of warts can be achieved by curettage or blunt dissection, followed by cautery. This method may be particularly useful for filiform warts located on the face and extremities. Scarring is usual after these procedures, and recurrence is seen in up to 30% of cases, thus making this therapeutic modality a poor choice.

Lasers. Carbon dioxide, pulsed dye, and erbium: YAG lasers have all been used in the treatment of recalcitrant viral warts, but none have proved superior to conventional therapy in long-term follow-up studies. Concern about viral spread from the laser plume and the cost of treatment are limiting factors.

Immunomodulating Agents

Patient Applied

Imiquimod 5% Cream (Aldara).* This new locally applied immune response modifier induces local release of cytokines, including interferon-α, tumor necrosis factor-α, interferon-γ, and interleukin-12, by peripheral mononuclear blood cells and lymphocytes. It is currently approved by the Food and Drug Administration for the treatment of genital and perianal warts, although several reports describe successful use in the treatment of common flat and plantar warts. Side effects include itching, mild erythema, and a burning sensation at the treatment site.

Cimetidine (Tagamet).* Cimetidine has a weak immunomodulatory effect and has been recommended for the treatment of warts. It may act as an immunomodulating agent at high doses by inhibiting supressor T cell function while increasing lymphocyte proliferation, thereby enhancing cell-mediated immune responses. Even though open-label trials have suggested efficacy, controlled trials have not shown any advantage over placebo.

Physician Applied

Dinitrochlorobenzene (DNCB),* Squaric Acid Dibutylester (SADBE), and Diphencyprone (DCP). These agents have all been used to induce a delayed hypersensitivity reaction for the treatment of warts. DNCB has mutagenic properties, and therefore SADBE and DCP have been used as alternative sensitizers. Clearance rates with DCP and SADBE have varied between 8% and 86% in several reports. Patients are first sensitized with a 2% to 3% solution of SADBE or DCP in acetone applied to a 1-cm-diameter area of the inner part of the arm with a cotton-tipped applicator. Several applications 10 to 14 days apart may be necessary until local erythema and vesiculation are observed. Once sensitization is achieved, the patient's warts can be treated with a diluted solution of the substance (0.03% to 6%) at weekly intervals until clearance is obtained. Side effects include localized dermatitis and irritation. Drawbacks of this treatment are that some patients cannot be sensitized whereas others get troublesome eczematous reactions.

***Candida* or Mumps Antigens.** These agents were injected into common warts in one pilot study and shown to be as effective as cryotherapy for the clearance of cutaneous warts. Interestingly, patients treated with *Candida* or mumps antigen injections showed resolution of anatomically distinct, untreated warts, thus suggesting induction of HPV immunity in these patients.

*Not FDA approved for this indication.

Antimitotic Therapy

Patient Applied

Retinoids. Retinoids act by disrupting epidermal growth and differentiation, with a consequent reduction in the bulk of the wart. Both oral and topical preparations have shown some success in the treatment of warts. Facial warts should not be treated with wart paint because of the risk of severe irritation and scarring, but they might benefit from treatment with topical retinoids. Topical tretinoin 0.05% cream (Retin-A) applied daily produced 85% clearance rates as compared with 32% in the placebo group in a randomized controlled trial. Oral retinoids* have been helpful, especially in immunocompromised patients; however, the warts tend to recur once use of the drug is stopped. Side effects include abnormal liver enzyme levels, elevated triglycerides, teratogenicity, and xerosis.

Physician Applied

Bleomycin (Blenoxane). Intralesional bleomycin* in a single dose of 250 to 1000 U/mL has been used to treat warts that have failed to respond to other modalities of treatment. Response rates have varied from 75% to 100% for hand warts and 50% to 70% for plantar lesions. Pain both on application and afterward is the main limiting factor, and topical or injected anesthesia is often needed. Side effects include tissue necrosis, scarring, nail loss, and Raynaud's phenomenon at the injection site. Bleomycin should not be used in pregnant women because of the risk of significant systemic absorption after intralesional administration.

5-Fluouracil. 5-Fluouracil* destroys cells by inhibiting DNA and RNA synthesis. Topically applied 1% fluorouracil cream (Fluoroplex)* has been demonstrated to be especially useful for the treatment of plantar warts, with reported clearance rates of 70% to 92%. It can be used alone or in combination with topical tretinoin. Local irritation and erythema are common side effects.

Other Treatments

Many other treatment modalities have been used for the treatment of viral warts, though with insufficient data regarding efficacy. Such modalities include photodynamic therapy (PDT) with topical 20% aminolevulinic acid (ALA) (Levulan Kerastick)* followed by irradiation with red light (ALA-PDT), topical cidofovir,* hypnosis, homeopathy, and local heat treatment.

Immunosuppressed Patients

Warts in immunosuppressed individuals are less likely to resolve spontaneously and are more resistant

*Not FDA approved for this indication.

to treatment, so the use of more aggressive modalities such as bleomycin (Blenoxane) injection and oral retinoids may be necessary. Cryotherapy, salicylic acid–containing preparations, and sensitizers such as DCP and SADBE have been used alone or in combined regimens, but results are frequently unsatisfactory.

Successful treatment of generalized HPV infection in a patient with a primary immunodeficiency has been achieved with the use of granulocyte-macrophage colony-stimulating factor and interferon-γ immunotherapy. Imiquimod 5% cream has also been used to treat facial warts in an HIV-infected individual, with subsequent clearance of the lesions. A recent report demonstrated resolution of recalcitrant hand warts with potent antiretroviral therapy (containing a protease inhibitor). Interestingly, oral warts appear to increase sixfold when this therapeutic regimen is used.

ANOGENITAL WARTS

method of
GEO VON KROGH, M.D., PH.D.
Karolinska Hospital
Stockholm, Sweden

Human papillomavirus (HPV) is the most heterogeneous of human viruses, with 200 genetic types identified by DNA hybridization. Genital HPV infections are sexually transmitted. In 90% of patients, anogenital warts ("condylomas") are caused by the "low-risk" HPV types 6 and 11, and 0.5% to 1% of persons 15 to 40 years old are affected. Condylomas are not associated with an increased risk of cervical cancer, but co-vary epidemiologically with "high-risk" HPV infections (types 16/18, etc.) that may induce cervical intraepithelial neoplasia. Females in Sweden are encouraged to undergo Papanicolaou smear testing according to national health policy.

MORPHOLOGY

Condylomas are multifocal and polymorphic, with three major types: acuminate, papular, and flat warts. *Acuminate warts* are pathognomonic "cauliflower-like" growths predominating on moist and thin epithelium; they exhibit punctuated and/or loop-like dermal vessels. *Papular* and *flat* lesions are associated with differential diagnostic problems because they lack the typical surface irregularities of warts and are often reddish brown, grayish white, or pigmented.

Preputial cavity warts commonly develop in uncircumcised men, whereas penile shaft warts are more common in circumcised men. Vulvar warts frequently develop in females. The vagina/cervix is concurrently afflicted in 25% of cases. Warts involve the urinary meatal lip in 10% to 28% of males and 5% of females; in 95% of cases only the distal 10 to 25 mm of the urethra is affected. Warts also occur in the pubic, groin, and perianal areas and sometimes grow up to the dentate line of the anorectal junction when receptive anal sex has been practiced.

TABLE 1. **Bowenoid Papulosis Versus Bowen's Disease**

Clinical Features	Bowenoid Papulosis	Bowen's Disease
Patient age	25–35 y	≥40 y
Lesion features		
Number	1–15 occasionally up to 30 plaques	Solitary, multiple or plaques
Color	Reddish brown	Reddish brown to bright red
	Grayish white	Grayish white
	Ashen gray or brownish black	Ashen gray to brownish black
	Mucosa colored	
Surface	Smooth velvety or peeling	Irregular moist, dry, or peeling Sometimes erosive
Size	2–10 occasionally up to 35 mm	≥10–15 mm

Pigmented, brownish red, and lichenoid lesions may be an indication of intraepithelial neoplasia, including the entities *bowenoid papulosis* and *Bowen's disease* (Table 1). Routine biopsy is not needed for newly developed acuminate warts but is recommended in atypical cases, if warts are resistant to treatment, in patients older than 35 to 40 years, and in immunosuppressed patients. In patients with cervical lesions, histopathologic assessment of a biopsy specimen obtained during colposcopy is mandatory (gynecology).

The *Buschke-Löwenstein "giant condyloma"* is a rare variant of HPV type 6/11 in which semi-malignant plaques invade the underlying dermal structures (subcutaneous fat, urethra, and rectum).

SYMPTOMS

Most patients have no physical symptoms, but psychosexual distress often influences libido, mood, and emotions. Some lesions bleed, itch, burn, or are associated with fluctuating intermittent episodes of vulvovaginitis, balanoposthitis, and/or dyspareunia.

THERAPY

No therapeutic "recipe" exists for all patients; most modalities achieve clearance within 1 to 6 months, but relapses occur for months or years in 20% to 30% of patients because of failure of immune recognition (Table 2). The choice of therapy depends on a combination of factors: the number of warts, the

TABLE 2. **Comparison of Therapies for Genital Warts**

Modality	Cure Rates (%)	Recurrence Rates (%)
Podophyllotoxin (Condylox)	11–86	17–38
Imiquimod (Aldara)	40–80	13–23
Trichloroacetic acid (TCA)	70–80	36
Surgery	70–80	20–30

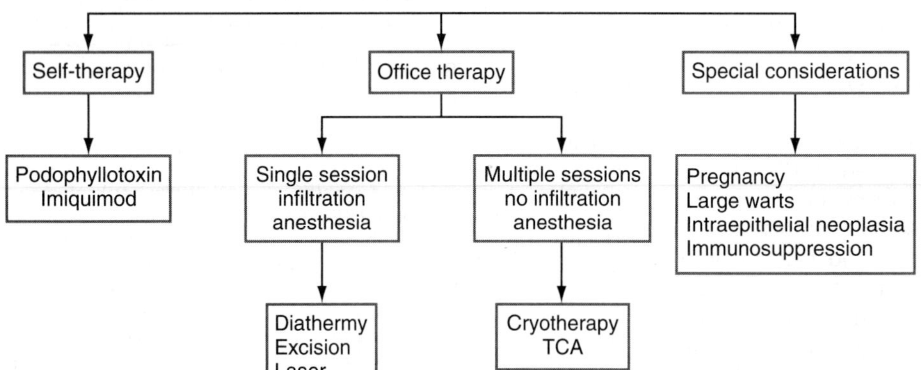

Figure 1. Suggested algorithm for treatment of external condylomas. TCA, trichloroacetic acid.

anatomic site, wart morphology, and patient preference (Figure 1). Podophyllin and flurouracil* are no longer recommended because of low efficacy and toxicity problems. Psychosexual counseling and a supportive attitude are important elements of proper therapy. Periods of coital rest during therapy may minimize side effects such as burning and pain.

Home Therapy

Podophyllotoxin Solution, Cream, or Gel

Podophyllotoxin, a purified extract of the podophyllum plant, binds to cellular microtubules and inhibits mitotic division of condyloma cells. A tinted 0.5% solution registered in Europe (Wartec,** Warticon**) is convenient for penile warts; the foreskin is retracted and the solution containing patent blue as a color indicator for optimal compliance is applied to each wart area with a specially designed plastic applicator or cotton-wool swabs. A 0.5% gel (Condylox) is registered in the United States, and in Europe and Asia, a 0.15% cream (Wartec,** Warticon**) is available to be rubbed into vulvar warts with the index finger, with the assistance of a hand-held mirror and a good light source. Podophyllotoxin is applied in one or several cycles (courses) twice daily, interrupted by 4 to 7 drug-free days. Warts that react become necrotic 4 to 5 days after initial application, and the shallow ulceration left behind heals within a few days. Half the patients experience transient burning, tenderness, and erythema. The clearance rate is as high as 86% on thin mucosa and as low as 11% on dry skin. Recurrence rates in various studies range from 17% to 38%. Women of childbearing age must be informed that they must either use proper contraceptives or abstain from penetrative sexual activity during therapy cycles. Podophyllotoxin is contraindicated during pregnancy.

Imiquimod Cream

Imiquimod (Aldara) is an immune response modulator that induces the local production of interferons and recruitment of immune cells. Imiquimod 5% cream, supplied in single-use sachets, is applied in the evening three times per week for a maximum of 16 weeks. A therapeutic response develops more slowly than with podophyllotoxin (mean, 7 to 8; range, 2 to 16 weeks). Total wart clearance occurs in less than half the cases, but 70% to 90% of patients have significant improvement. In U.S. studies, clearance rates were higher for females (77%) than for circumcised males (40%). In European studies involving uncircumcised males, its efficacy was 62% after 13 weeks of therapy. Recurrence rates after imiquimod therapy are 13% to 23%, somewhat lower than those reported with other modalities.

Mild to moderate erythema, erosions, and tenderness develop in two thirds of patients. Erosions causing discontinuation of therapy are rare when a drug-free rest period of a week or so is recommended. The safety of imiquimod during pregnancy has not been established.

Office Procedures

Trichloroacetic Acid

Trichloroacetic acid (TCA, 80% to 90% solution), a caustic corrosive cellular agent, is applied with a cotton-tipped applicator at weekly intervals. Care and experience are required because deep ulcers may develop. Response rates are 70% to 80% after one to four office visits, but the warts recur in up to 36%. An intense burning sensation may be experienced for up to 10 minutes after application. TCA can be used safely during pregnancy.

Surgery

The method of choice depends on the distribution of warts and the clinical skill and experience of the physician. Epithelial depigmentation often follows.

Local lidocaine/prilocaine (EMLA) cream, which exerts an anesthetic effect within 10 to 15 minutes, reduces the discomfort of infiltration anesthesia by needle stick. *Infiltration anesthesia* with 5 to 10 mg/mL of lidocaine (Xylocaine) separates lesions and facilitates accurate removal and sparing of uninvolved skin bridges for re-epithelization. The use of adrenaline as an adjuvant is contraindicated on the penis. Extensive anal warts are best removed under *general anesthesia* by a proctologist. In children and sensitive patients, general anesthesia may be preferred for surgical procedures.

Scissors excision is feasible for exophytic warts, with the assistance of diathermy to control hemostasis

*Not FDA approved for this indication.
**Not available in the United States.

and facilitate destruction of surrounding lesions. *Diathermy* and *CO_2 lasers* produce identical results and are performed with surgical masks/smoke evacuators.

Extensive foreskin warts are sometimes best managed by *circumcision.*

Cryosurgery causes epidermal necrosis and dermal capillary injury. Clinic treatment is usually performed weekly. A "halo" is established a few millimeters around the lesion, and freezing is continued for 20 seconds. A freeze, thaw, freeze technique should be used. Open application of liquid N_2 may be accomplished with a spray device or directly with a swab. Closed systems use CO_2, N_2O, or N_2 applied through a cryoprobe.

Situations for Special Consideration

- Intra-anal (anal canal) warts: TCA, electrosurgery, and laser.
- Vaginal warts: TCA, electrosurgery, and laser.
- Cervical warts: excisional biopsy, cryotherapy, electrosurgery, or laser.
- Meatal warts: cryosurgery, diathermy, and laser. Caution: adhesions/stenosis may occur.
- Warts may be large in early pregnancy but often regress spontaneously after delivery. The risk of laryngeal papillomatosis developing in the infant is 1 in 400. It has not, however, been proved that treatment diminishes this risk. Symptomatic and conservative treatment with TCA or surgery is recommended. Rarely, cesarean section is indicated because of blockage of the vaginal outlet.
- HIV infection and organ transplantation have been associated with an increase in multicentric, refractory condylomas.

MELANOCYTIC NEVI

method of
DANIEL A. SMITH, M.D., and
CLIFTON R. WHITE, Jr., M.D.
Oregon Health & Science University
Portland, Oregon

The term nevus (plural, nevi) is used for a variety of melanocytic and nonmelanocytic skin conditions. Although a number of nonmelanocytic pigmented lesions (e.g., epidermal nevus) and hamartomatous lesions (e.g., sebaceous nevus) are referred to as nevi, this discussion will focus on melanocytic nevi, which are defined histologically by nests (collections or theques) of melanocytes and a benign architectural pattern. The lay term for a melanocytic nevus is *mole.*

EPIDEMIOLOGY

Melanocytic nevi are very common in the general population, with increased prevalence associated with lighter skin color. Most nevi are acquired during late childhood, adolescence, and early adulthood. A small number are present at birth (approximately 1% of newborns). The number of nevi in an individual progressively declines after the third decade of life. No gender predilection exists. Both genetic and environmental factors influence the development of nevi. Patients with numerous nevi often have phenotypically similar family members. Ultraviolet light exposure is thought to increase the number of nevi that develop in an individual, and studies suggest that regular sunscreen use may decrease the number of acquired melanocytic nevi.

CLINICAL PRESENTATIONS

Melanocytic nevi have diverse clinical presentations. Congenital nevi are divided arbitrarily into small (<1.5 cm), medium (1.5 to 20 cm) and large/giant (>20 cm) categories based on greatest diameter. Congenital nevi may have numerous terminal hairs (hypertrichosis). Over time, many congenital nevi become more elevated and develop a more palpable surface texture and darker pigmentation. Congenital nevi grow in proportion to the individual. The risk of melanoma developing in a congenital nevus is controversial; there is some consensus that large/giant congenital nevi carry a slightly higher risk of malignant transformation than small and medium congenital nevi.

Common acquired melanocytic nevi are classified into three basic categories according to the location of the melanocytic nests in histologic specimens (Table 1). These histologic categories often correlate with clinical presentation. Junctional nevi contain nests of melanocytes limited to the dermal-epidermal junction. Clinically, junctional nevi present as brown to dark-brown, well-circumscribed, symmetrical, small (<1 cm) macules (flat surface).

Compound nevi are characterized by nests of melanocytes along the dermal-epidermal junction and in the dermis. Compound nevi present clinically as brown, well-circumscribed, symmetrical, small (<1 cm) papules (raised surface). Intradermal nevi have nests of melanocytes confined to the dermis. Intradermal nevi present as light-brown to flesh-colored, well-circumscribed, symmetrical, small (<1 cm) papules (raised surface). Some compound and intradermal nevi may be dome-shaped or pedunculated and may be mistaken for skin tags (acrochordons).

Many clinical variations of common acquired nevi are recognized and often are designated with specific names. Blue nevus is a type of intradermal melanocytic nevus with a blue or blue-gray clinical hue resulting from pigment deposition deeper in the dermis. Blue nevi are most common on the scalp, sacral area, and dorsal hands and feet.

Halo nevus is a melanocytic nevus surrounded by a zone or halo of depigmentation. The central nevus often undergoes complete involution over time. Halo nevi result from an immune response to melanocytes in the nevus.

Nevus spilus (speckled lentiginous nevus) consists of a larger tan macule or patch (flat), within which are smaller brown macules or papules (flat or raised). The

TABLE 1. **Clinical and Histological Characteristics of Common Acquired Melanocytic Nevi**

Characteristic	Junctional Nevus	Compound Nevus	Intradermal Nevus
Color	Brown to dark brown	Brown	Flesh-colored or pink
Surface	Flat (macule)	Raised (papule)	Raised (papule)
Melanocyte location	Dermoepidermal junction	Dermoepidermal junction and dermis	Dermis

tan areas demonstrate increased single melanocytes histologically (lentiginous), while the smaller brown areas may show increased single melanocytes, a junctional nevus, or a compound nevus.

Spitz nevus (spindled and epithelioid cell nevus) most often presents as a red, dome-shaped papule. Spitz nevi are more common in children and often are found on the head and neck. Spitz nevi can be very difficult to distinguish from melanoma histologically; therefore, it is important to provide an adequate biopsy sample for histologic examination.

One type of melanocytic nevus described by Clark (dysplastic nevus, atypical nevus) often exhibits one or more of the following features: asymmetry (in color or shape), border irregularity, color variation, and diameter greater than 6 mm. The acronym ABCD is used to remember these features (Table 2). On occasion, it may be difficult to distinguish clinically between atypical nevi and melanoma; biopsy and histologic examination often are required.

Recurrent nevi (incompletely excised nevi that subsequently repigment) can be a particularly difficult diagnostic problem. Patients with these lesions often present with pigmentation in the scar from the prior partial removal of a nevus. Recurrent nevi often are irregular clinically and histologically and may be very difficult to differentiate from melanoma.

EVALUATION

Examination of patients with pigmented lesions should be performed in good light and should be complete. Importantly, one should examine the scalp, axillae, buttocks, genitalia, oral mucosa, palms, and soles in addition to areas that have regular or intermittent sun exposure. Many clinicians find a magnifying glass helpful in the evaluation of melanocytic nevi. Patients with many nevi or with atypical nevi may be photographed for comparison at future examinations.

Dermoscopy (dermatoscopy, epiluminescence microscopy) is the examination of pigmented lesions using a hand-held magnifier (usually 10×) with or without oil interface. Lesions are evaluated on a variety of morphologic criteria with the goal of improving clinical diagnostic accuracy. In the hands of experienced users in defined research protocols, dermoscopy has been shown to increase diagnostic accuracy for pigmented lesions. It is not yet clear how dermoscopy affects clinical decision-making.

Many melanocytic nevi require histologic examination to rule out melanoma. Indications for biopsy include: atypical features (see Table 2); recent growth or changes in a pre-existing nevus; new nevi in older patients; ulceration; bleeding; pruritus; or pain (Table 3).

TABLE 2. **Characteristics of Some Nevi and Many Melanomas: The "ABCDs" of Pigmented Lesions**

Asymmetry of color or shape
Border irregularity
Color variation
Diameter greater than 6 mm

TREATMENT OPTIONS

Most melanocytic nevi are asymptomatic, unchanging, and benign in appearance. These do not require treatment, although patients often request removal of benign-appearing nevi for cosmetic reasons. Counseling patients about scarring before removing a nevus for cosmetic reasons is prudent. All excised nevi should be examined histologically, regardless of clinical appearance.

There are several methods for removal and/or biopsy of melanocytic nevi. Several factors should be considered in the selection of method: adequacy of specimen for histologic examination, healing time, and cosmetic result.

Punch Biopsy/Excision

This procedure requires a circular cutting instrument (punch) with a diameter ranging from 2 to 8 mm. The punch is applied to the skin and rotated with downward pressure. The specimen then is grasped gently at the edge with forceps and is transected at the base with scissors. The defect generally is closed with one or two sutures. Rather than suturing smaller punch biopsies, some clinicians allow defects to heal by secondary intention. The punch biopsy is simple to perform, heals rapidly, generally has good cosmetic result, and allows histologic examination of the full thickness of the lesion. However, selecting a punch diameter 2 to 3 mm greater than the diameter of the lesion to be excised is critical in order to provide an adequate specimen for histologic

TABLE 3. **Indications for Treatment of Melanocytic Nevi**

Symptomatic nevus (pain, pruritus, ulceration, and bleeding)
Changing nevus
Recurrent nevus
Atypical nevus
New nevus in an older patient
Cosmetic concerns

examination. Many of the features distinguishing a nevus from melanoma occur at the periphery of the lesion and can be evaluated only with an adequate specimen. Sutures from punch biopsies generally are removed after 5 to 7 days on the face, and 12 to 14 days on the trunk and extremities.

Shave Biopsy/Excision

The shave biopsy is performed with a scalpel (generally a no. 15 blade) or a straight razor blade. While a superficial shave procedure often is used to biopsy suspected neoplasms, such as basal cell or squamous cell carcinomas, it is not recommended generally for biopsy of melanocytic neoplasms. The superficial shave technique often transects the base of the lesion, preventing measurement of thickness in melanomas and increasing the possibility of recurrent nevi.

A variation of the shave biopsy is the "saucerization" technique. This is performed by first excising the lesion with the scalpel initially directed downward at a 45-degree angle to the skin and by then completing the removal with a similar angle directed upward. A 1–2 mm margin of normal skin is taken around the lesion. The depth of the excision is the deep dermis, leaving a defect with a "saucer-shaped" silhouette. This technique provides an excellent specimen for histologic examination. Cosmetic results are very good on the trunk and proximal extremities. Disadvantages of this technique include the need for more extended wound care, longer healing time, and larger scar.

Elliptical Excision

The elliptical excision removes the pigmented lesion with a variable margin of clinically normal skin. The ellipse is designed with a length-to-width ratio of approximately 3:1. The depth of the excision extends into the subcutaneous fat. Smaller defects may be closed with simple interrupted sutures, whereas larger defects generally are closed with buried absorbable sutures and superficial nylon sutures. The elliptical excision provides an excellent specimen for histologic examination, has a good cosmetic result, and heals rapidly. Disadvantages of this technique include additional time required to perform the procedure and a longer scar.

Incisional Biopsy

The incisional biopsy technique is used to sample a suspicious pigmented lesion that is too large to excise easily in the outpatient clinic setting. The incisional biopsy generally is performed with a scalpel and may be in the form of an ellipse (closed with sutures) or a modified "saucerization" procedure. In either case, a part of the lesion including a small portion of adjacent clinically nonpigmented skin is removed for histologic examination; management is based on histologic diagnosis.

MELANOMA

method of
ALLAN C. HALPERN, M.D.
Memorial Sloan-Kettering Cancer Center
New York, New York

Malignant melanoma can arise in melanocytes of the skin, mucosa, and eye. Cutaneous melanoma is the most common form of the disease. Because the other types of melanoma entail somewhat different clinical considerations, this chapter will specifically address the subject of cutaneous melanoma.

EPIDEMIOLOGY

The incidence of melanoma has increased dramatically since the 1980s with an associated, albeit less precipitous, increase in mortality. Although some of the increase in incidence may be related to length-time bias associated with increased detection pressure, rising mortality rates and current population demographics portend significant increases in the melanoma patient population over the decades to come. Melanoma is primarily a disease of the white population, but it does occur in all racial/ethnic groups. Among whites, the strongest risk factor for melanoma is nevi (moles). Patients with increased numbers of common nevi and those with any dysplastic (clinically atypical) nevi are at greater risk. Those with light colored hair, eyes, and skin who tend to burn or freckle rather than tan are also at increased risk. Approximately 5% of melanomas occur in the setting familial melanoma. In a subset of these melanoma-prone families, melanoma risk segregates with the presence of large numbers of dysplastic nevi. Affected members of these families have a lifetime melanoma risk that approaches 100%.

ETIOLOGY

Sunlight is the primary environmental exposure associated with melanoma. The specific wavelengths, timing, and dosimetry of ultraviolet radiation that cause melanoma have not been elucidated and likely vary by histiogenic type. Lentigo maligna melanoma, occurring in chronically sun-exposed areas, is associated with chronic cumulative sun exposure. Superficial spreading melanoma, the most common type, is associated with intense intermittent sun exposure. Acral lentiginous melanoma of the palms and soles is unlikely to be ultraviolet mediated. In approximately one third of familial melanoma families, germline mutations of the P16 (CDKN2) or CDK4 genes segregate with the disease. These high penetrance/low prevalence germline mutations do not appear to play a significant role in melanoma susceptibility in the population at large. On the other hand, high prevalence/low penetrance germline mutations in pigmentation genes such as the melanocortin receptor gene may play a major role in melanoma susceptibility in the general population.

PREVENTION

Current efforts in melanoma prevention focus on sun protection beginning in early childhood and continuing throughout life. Recognition of potential causative roles for both UVA and UVB in melanoma forms the basis for recommendations against all intentional UV-induced tanning. Conflicting data on the utility of sunscreen for melanoma prevention has been a source of controversy. In common practice, sunscreens are often used in lieu of sun-protective clothing and in conjunction with sun-seeking behaviors. Current recommendations emphasize the avoidance of intentional sun exposure and tanning, the use of sun-protective clothing, and the use of a double application of SPF 30 or higher broad-spectrum sunscreen to areas not readily covered with clothing.

Screening/Surveillance

Early detection remains the most effective strategy for reducing melanoma mortality. Improved public education in the warning signs of melanoma and increased rates of skin self-examination hold the greatest promise in this regard. Formal clinical trials of the utility of melanoma screening are lacking. The potential utility of screening programs for identifying high-risk individuals and educating the public in self-detection are self-evident. Inclusion of complete skin examinations and solicitation of a history of changing skin lesions during routine medical care has the greatest potential to enhance case finding in clinical practice. Patients with a personal history of melanoma, family history of melanoma, many nevi, or dysplastic nevi may benefit from routine dermatologic evaluation. For patients with many atypical nevi, the acquisition of baseline whole body photography can facilitate the recognition of new or changing lesions during patient self-examination and professional follow-up.

DIAGNOSIS

Presenting as pigmented lesions on the surface of the skin, the majority of melanomas are first detected by patients or their friends and relatives. Recent public education campaigns emphasizing the ABCD signs of early melanoma (Asymmetry, Border irregularity, Color variegation, and Diameter >5 mm) have led to increased public awareness and self-referral to physicians. The most sensitive sign of melanoma is a change in the color, shape, or size of a pigmented lesion over the course of months. Another important clinical sign is the presence of a pigmented lesion that stands out as distinctly different in appearance than the remainder of a patient's moles. Patients with the relatively rare amelanotic variant of melanoma present with a pink lesion that typically defies diagnosis until a more advanced stage.

The clinical diagnosis of melanoma relies on visual inspection. The key to effective diagnosis is the performance of a complete cutaneous examination that permits identification of lesions in hidden anatomic sights, as well as comparison among an individual's multiple lesions. Dermoscopy, a form of skin surface microscopy, is being increasingly utilized as an aid to diagnosis. The recent availability of dermoscopy tutorials with sizable image archives has facilitated the diffusion of the technique into dermatologic practice. Automated systems employing image analysis of dermoscopic and spectroscopic images are being developed as aids to diagnosis.

Definitive diagnosis of melanoma requires a biopsy. Excisional biopsy is the preferred method. Incisional biopsy runs the risk of misdiagnosis due to sampling error and precludes definitive assessment of prognostic factors. Incisional biopsy may, however, be indicated for large lesions and lesions occurring in surgically sensitive anatomic sites.

PROGNOSIS/STAGING

The American Joint Commission on Cancer (AJCC) staging system for melanoma has undergone several iterations (Table 1). Increased internet access to stage-specific data that fails to distinguish between these iterations is a common source of confusion for patients and physicians alike. Another common, and often alarming, source of confusion for patients is the distinction between Clark level and stage, both of which are indicated by Roman numerals. Recent changes to the current AJCC staging classification include an emphasis on micrometastasis identified by sentinel node biopsy and an emphasis on the prognostic importance of ulceration of the primary. The TNM classification on which staging is predicated has also

TABLE 1. **New AJCC Stage Groupings for Cutaneous Melanoma**

Stage	Definition	5-Year Survival Rate, % ± SE
IA	≤1 mm; no ulceration (Clark level II/III)	95.3 ± 0.4
IB	≤1 mm with ulceration or (Clark level IV/V)	90.9 ± 1.0
	1.01–2 mm; no ulceration	89.0 ± 0.7
IIA	1.01–2 mm with ulceration	77.4 ± 1.7
	2.01–4 mm; no ulceration	78.7 ± 1.2
IIB	2.01–4 mm with ulceration	63.0 ± 1.5
	>4 mm; no ulceration	67.4 ± 2.4
IIC	>4 mm with ulceration	45.1 ± 1.9
IIIA	Single micronode; no ulceration	69.5 ± 3.7
	2 to 3 micronodes; no ulceration	63.3 ± 5.6
IIIB	1 to 3 macronodes or in-transit metastatsis; no ulcer	52.8 ± 4.1
	1 to 3 micronodes; with ulceration	46.3 ± 5.5
IIIC	1 to 3 macronodes; with ulceration	29.0 ± 5.1
	≥4 nodes, matted, or nodes plus in-transit metastasis	26.7 ± 2.5
IV	Distant skin, subcutaneous, nodal, or lung metastasis	18.8 ± 3.0
	All visceral metastases or elevated LDH with metastasis	9.5 ± 1.1

AJCCS, American Joint Committee on Cancer Staging; LDH, lactate dehydrogenase.
From Journal of Clinical Oncology, 19:3635–3648, 2001.

TABLE 2. **New TNM Classification**

Tumor Classification	Thickness	Ulceration
T0	MIS	N/A
T1	<1 mm	a. W/O and Clark level II/III b. with and/or Clark level IV/V
T2	1–2 mm	a. W/O b. with
T3	2–4	a. W/O b. with
T4	>4	a. W/O b. with
Node Classification	**No. of Metastatic Nodes**	**Type Nodal Metastasis**
N1	1 node	a. micrometastatic b. macrometastatic
N2	2–3 nodes	a. micrometastatic b. macrometastatic
N3	4 or more, or matted, or in transit + nodes	

MIS, melanoma in situ; N, nodes; NA, not applicable; T, tumor(s); W/O, without.

From Journal of Clinical Oncology, 19:3635–3648, 2001.

been modified. Among the changes has been a transition to integer breakpoints for Breslow tumor thickness and a reliance on the number of metastatic lymph nodes rather than their gross dimensions. These changes have resulted in improved prognostic stratification at the expense of increased complexity (Table 2).

TREATMENT

There has been a recent proliferation of sometimes conflicting "evidence-based" guidelines for the management of melanoma. While these offer welcome reviews of the literature and present the opinions of expert clinicians, our current state of knowledge precludes a cookbook approach to patient care. The constellation of a patient's medical condition, the details of their melanoma, and their personal lifestyle and therapeutic preferences should form the basis of appropriate decision-making.

Treatment of the Primary Site

The cornerstone of therapy for primary melanoma is definitive excision with a margin of clinically uninvolved skin. Proposed margins are outlined in Table 3. In recent years, sentinel lymph node biopsy (SLNB) has become common practice for melanomas greater than 1 mm in thickness and for thinner melanomas

TABLE 3. **Recommended Excision Margins**

Thickness	Margin
In situ	0.5–0.8 cm
0–1 mm	1.0 cm
1–2 mm	1–2 cm
>2 mm	2 cm

with high risk attributes (i.e., Clark's level IV or V, the presence of ulceration, or extensive dermal regression). SLNB entails preoperative lymphoscintigraphy and intraoperative use of a vital blue dye and radiocolloid tracer to identify the draining sentinel (first) node for the melanoma primary site. Routine histology, immunochemistry, and polymerase chain reaction (PCR) have been used to evaluate the sentinel node for presence of melanoma. While several groups including the World Health Organization have suggested that SLNB is standard care for primary melanomas greater than 1 mm, it remains a procedure of unproven clinical utility. The potential utility of the procedure relates to improved survival, improved prognostic stratification permitting informed decisions regarding adjuvant therapy, and improved control of regional metastatic disease. Two ongoing multicenter trials, the Multicenter Selective Lymphadenectomy Trial and the Sunbelt Melanoma Trial, are designed to address the clinical utility of this procedure. Until the data from these trials are available, decisions regarding sentinel node biopsies should be individualized. A major consideration in this regard is the patient's preference regarding adjuvant therapy.

Local/Regional Disease

Patients with regional lymph node metastases are treated with therapeutic lymphadenectomy followed by consideration of adjuvant therapy. Patients with local/in-transit metastases are treated with surgical excision, laser therapy, or intralesional immunotherapy. Isolated limb perfusion has not been shown to impact overall survival, but can be highly effective palliative therapy for extensive local or regional limb metastases.

Adjuvant Therapy

High-dose interferon alpha-2B (Intron A) is an FDA-approved adjuvant therapy for stage III melanoma. There is relatively consistent data suggesting that interferon is an active agent in this disease. In two of three Eastern Cooperative Oncology Group (ECOG) trials (ECOG 1684, ECOG 1694) there was a statistically significant difference in disease-specific survival in patients treated with 1 year of high-dose interferon. A third ECOG trial (ECOG 1690) failed to demonstrate a similar difference. The extent of the effect of adjuvant interferon therapy on all cause mortality, relative to the toxicity of the therapy, has led to varied adoption of this therapy among oncologists. In the absence of a well tolerated, clearly efficacious adjuvant therapy, patients with stage III disease should be offered the opportunity to participate in clinical trials of the varied adjuvant vaccine protocols currently being evaluated.

Distant Metastatic Disease

Single agent chemotherapy with dacarbazine (DTIC) remains the mainstay of therapy for distant metastatic disease. Multiple drug chemotherapy regimens have been extensively studied and have failed to demonstrate clear-cut superiority over this single drug regimen. Other agents with single agent activity include cisplatin (Platinol-AQ),* carmustine (BiCNU),* paclitaxel (Taxol),* docetaxel (Taxotere),* and temozolomide (Temodar).* Temozolomide is an oral form of dacarbazine with greater central nervous system penetrance. The addition of immunotherapies (interferon-α and interleukin-2) to chemotherapy has been termed *biochemotherapy*. This highly toxic regimen has been associated with high response rates but an unclear impact on overall survival. In the absence of highly effective therapies, patients with stage IV disease should be offered the opportunity to participate in clinical trials of experimental therapies.

LABORATORY EVALUATION AND FOLLOW-UP

Initial and periodic evaluation of all melanoma patients should include a complete history, extensive review of systems, and a problem-orientated physical examination including complete skin examination and lymph node evaluation. Routine radiologic imaging is not indicated in patients with stage I or II disease. Radiologic and nuclear imaging techniques (e.g., positron emission tomography) are useful in the evaluation and management of patients with stage III and IV disease. Lifelong skin surveillance for additional primary lesions is indicated for all melanoma survivors.

*Not FDA approved for this indication.

PREMALIGNANT LESIONS

method of
VICTOR A. NEEL, M.D., PH.D, and
ARTHUR J. SOBER, M.D.
Harvard Medical School
Massachusetts General Hospital
Boston, Massachusetts

SKIN CANCER PRECURSORS

Tumors that arise in the skin account for more than 10,000 deaths in the United States each year. Familiarity with the morphologic aspects of the precursors of these malignancies can avert both mortality and deforming surgery. However, the line between a precursor of a skin cancer and the actual skin cancer is not always clear and not every precursor lesion proceeds to tumor formation. As we learn more about the molecular biology of the tumors, we will be more able to predict the outcome of an individual lesion. Until that time, the thoughtful application of epidemiologic studies will have to guide the clinician's assessment of the risk of any benign lesion becoming malignant.

This review will limit itself to precursors of the three most common skin cancers: basal cell carcinoma, squamous cell carcinoma, and melanoma. These three entities account for more than 96% of all malignancies originating in the skin.

Precursors to Basal Cell Carcinoma

Basal cell carcinoma (BCC) is the most common neoplasm in man and almost one in three Americans will develop at least one of these tumors in their lifetime. Although mortality due to BCC is fleetingly rare, the tumors can create devastating cosmetic and functional deficits if left untreated or partially treated. BCC belongs in a spectrum of neoplasms derived from primordial keratinocytes in the hair follicle. Abnormalities in the PATCHED tumor suppressor signal cascade are thought to underlie the development of most BCCs.

The great majority of BCCs arise in the absence of precursor lesions, but one common growth, the nevus sebaceous, frequently gives rise to BCC. Nevus sebaceous is a congenital pilosebaceous hamartoma usually found on the head. At birth, it appears as a circumscribed, yellowish plaque. Dependent on endogenous sex hormones for growth, the lesion is quiescent until the second decade when it thickens and often becomes verrucous. In addition to BCC, other benign adnexal tumors may develop in these lesions, the most common of which is syringocystadenoma papilliferum. Current estimates of the frequency of BCCs arising in nevus sebaceous is about 7%, although this has recently been called into question by a group suggesting that many of the BCCs that were originally diagnosed were actually a less malignant relative of BCC called *trichoblastoma*.

The management of nevus sebaceous depends on the size and location. As with many precursor lesions of the skin, careful and periodic clinical evaluation is an acceptable option. However, many practitioners and patients feel uncomfortable waiting for a malignancy to develop and prefer prophylactic removal. This is usually deferred until the patient is old enough to undergo surgery with local anesthetic.

Precursors to Squamous Cell Carcinoma

Squamous cell carcinoma (SCC), unlike BCC, can be an aggressive tumor and may metastasize, accounting for approximately one fourth of the skin cancer deaths. Therefore, it is imperative to detect and treat these tumors early. The precursors of SCCs have different presentations depending on their etiology and location. For instance, the ingestion of arsenical compounds produces premalignant scaly spicules on the palms and soles termed "arsenical keratoses," while patients with an inherited immunodeficiency called epidermodysplasia verruciformis present with a tinea versicolor–like eruption on the trunk. In addition, some common chronic skin conditions, such as oral lichen planus or lichen sclerosis et atrophicus of the vulva, can evolve into SCC.

Actinic Keratosis

By far the most common precursor to SCC is actinic keratosis (AK), an ultraviolet light–induced pink plaque with adherent scale. Some variants contain pigment and can be confused with a melanocytic lesion. Aberrant behavior or expression of the p53 tumor suppressor has been detected in many of these premalignancies. Because of this observation, some authors contend that actinic keratoses are evolving malignancies rather than precursors. However, the majority of AKs (greater than 90%), do not progress to invasive SCC. Nonetheless, many fair skinned individuals have many discrete lesions, so the overall risk of developing SCC can be high in patients with diffuse solar damage.

Local destruction, topical chemotherapeutics, and photodynamic therapy are currently employed for the treatment of AKs. Physical destruction with liquid nitrogen is quick and effective if the number of lesions is small and the lesions are well-circumscribed. Infrequently, however, this modality can cause hypopigmentation or scarring. The use of 5% 5-fluoruracil (Efudex) twice a day for 3 weeks or 0.5% 5-flurouracil (Carac) once a day for 2 to 4 weeks is an effective therapy for diffuse lesions. Patients must be told to expect considerable crusting and some discomfort. Another topical agent, imiquimod (Aldara),* has also been reported to be effective in treating actinic keratoses. It apparently works by stimulating local production of several antitumor cytokines, including interferon. Patients apply the topical cream three times a week for 6 to 12 weeks, depending on the response. Photodynamic therapy with the topical photosensitizer aminolevulinic acid can treat a large number of lesions in a single in-office session and is a valuable tool in patients unwilling or unable to self-treat with topical therapy. With all of these methods, close follow-up is essential because lesions that do not respond completely may represent early invasive SCC. These resistant lesions should be biopsied.

Human Papilloma Virus (HPV)-Induced Premalignancies

Oncogenic variants of HPV have been implicated in several cutaneous malignancies. These viruses produce proteins that interfere with the cellular gatekeeping proteins p53 and Rb, leading to unchecked cellular divisions and decreased rates of apoptosis in transformed cells. The HPV 16 variant has been frequently associated with a condition known as bowenoid papulosis. A largely indolent and symptomless condition arising most commonly on the penis in young men, the lesions of bowenoid papulosis consist of clusters of fleshy pigmented papules. Although spontaneous regression has been documented, conservative removal is the mainstay of treatment.

HPV variants 5 and 8 have been associated with SCC in the rare genetic syndrome epidermodysplasia verruciformis. Patients with this inherited defect in cell-mediated immunity develop excessive numbers of plane warts and distinctive confluent, reddish brown collections of truncal lesions that simulate tinea versicolor clinically. Careful follow-up is important in these cases because one in four patients develops invasive SCC.

Another important group of patients requiring vigilant monitoring for the development of SCC is the organ transplant patients on immunosuppressants. By the end of the fifth year on transplantation medication, more than 90% of patients have warts, largely in sun-exposed areas. Over time, this population of patients develops numerous verrucous plaques resembling the lesions seen in patients with epidermodysplasia verruciformis. It is prudent to treat SCC lesions in transplant patients aggressively because many succumb to metastatic SCC.

Chronic Conditions Associated With SCC

There are several common dermatologic conditions that occasionally have been linked to the development of SCC. These include genital lichen sclerosus et atrophicus, oral lichen planus, erythema ab igne, and burn scars. Of these, burn scars are the most serious. SCC developing in these lesions, the so-called *Marjolin's ulcer*, has a 40% rate of metastasis. With all of these conditions, routine surveillance of an informed patient represents the best method for early detection and treatment.

PRECURSORS TO MALIGNANT MELANOMA

Of all the controversies in dermatology, none has been more heatedly debated than whether cutaneous melanoma has a histologically definable precursor. While melanoma is occasionally associated with both congenital nevi and "dysplastic" nevi, it must be remembered that 50% to 80% of melanomas appear to arise without obvious precursors. Recent studies have found that mutations in the B-raf oncogene are found in 60% to 80% of melanomas; however, at least as many clinically benign nevi show similarly high rates of mutation at this locus.

Congenital melanocytic nevi are classified according to their size at birth: small (<1.5 cm), medium (>1.5 and <20 cm) and large (>20 cm). Only the large, or giant, nevi have been definitively associated with an elevated rate of malignant transformation, with a lifetime risk of cutaneous melanoma of about 10%. Leptomeningeal melanoma is also occasionally found in patients with giant nevi, particularly of the "bathing-suit" (truncal) distribution. The management of congenital nevi is controversial, but with small lesions close follow-up is a reasonable approach, if excision would be cosmetically or functionally distressing. Unfortunately, giant nevi, with a higher rate of transformation, are often unresectable and because of the deep origin of the primary tumor, early detection is almost impossible. Serial photography and sequential partial excisions may be of help to monitor and treat these very difficult lesions. There is no

*Not FDA approved for this indication.

uniform agreement on the management of giant congenital nevi.

While an individual acquired nevus has an extremely low transformation rate, patients with numerous "benign" lesions appear to have an increased risk of developing melanoma. The relative risk of developing melanoma in a patient with less than 25 nevi is 1.6, whereas a patient with more than 100 nevi has a relative risk of 9.8. Multiple, bland-appearing nevi should alert the clinician to an increased risk of melanoma and identify patients in whom close surveillance may be beneficial.

The management of "dysplastic" or clinically atypical melanocytic nevi provokes heated debate among pigmented lesion experts. While the inherent malignant potential of any particular nevus is uncertain, the presence of multiple atypical nevi is nearly uniformly accepted as a marker for patients with an increased risk of developing melanoma. Approximately one in four melanomas develop in association with an atypical nevus. Atypical nevi differ from benign acquired nevi in their larger size, asymmetric borders, color variegation, and their "atypical" histologic appearance. The use of the "ABCD" rule for diagnosing melanoma will often identify clinically atypical nevi as clinically suspicious. Indeed, patients with more that ten atypical lesions have a 12-fold increased risk of developing melanoma. Some families with dysplastic nevi and familial melanoma carry a mutation in genes regulating p16, a tumor suppressor gene important in controlling the cell cycle. Patients in these families have a very high rate of developing one or more melanomas and should be monitored closely.

In the management of patients with atypical nevi, family history, previous history of melanoma, and the number of atypical nevi are useful in determining frequency of follow-up. Patients are usually followed at 6 to 12 month intervals and are advised to return sooner for the evaluation of interval changes. The use of standard photography or digital imaging devices to track changes in lesions can obviate multiple and sometimes unnecessary surgical procedures. Any lesions that are noted by the patient or the clinician to be changing require prompt evaluation and possible biopsy.

BACTERIAL DISEASES OF THE SKIN

method of
FREDERIC W. STEARNS, M.D.
University of Oklahoma College of Medicine
Tulsa, Oklahoma

Bacterial skin infections account for approximately 17% of all dermatology visits and 18% of all pediatric clinic visits. People in the United States have an estimated five million skin infections annually. Familiarity with bacterial skin infections, their predisposing factors, complications, and postinfection sequelae can alleviate immediate suffering, decrease contagion, and, in extreme cases, prevent loss of limbs and death.

The skin is the body's initial defensive line against the surrounding swarm of all environmental pathogens, including bacteria, viruses, and fungi. Initial evaluation of a suspected infection must include a search for a "portal of entry" that defeats the skin's normal barrier function. These portals can be penetrating wounds, burns, diseases that change skin surfaces, or changes in the skin's normal flora. Psoriasis, Darier's disease, and atopic dermatitis, for example, are typically colonized with *Staphylococcus aureus* rather than the more benign *Staphylococcus epidermidis*. Diseases such as HIV and diabetes mellitus, chemotherapy for malignant and nonmalignant conditions, and inherited problems, such as Job's syndrome, decrease host resistance and make bacterial infections more likely.

FOLLICULITIS

Hair follicle structures are particularly susceptible to bacterial infection. *S. aureus* and *Streptococcus pyogenes* are the most common organisms involved. Yellow pustules grouped in areas shaved or scratched lead to the diagnosis, and shaving, sweating, or scratching cause the lesions to spread. Tender truncal lesions are seen with hot tub exposure ("hot tub folliculitis"); these are usually caused by *Pseudomonas aeruginosa* or *Pseudomonas cepacia*. Acne that responds initially to systemic antibiotics but becomes resistant can be superinfected with gram-negative organisms, producing a "gram-negative folliculitis."

Treatment

Local measures are essential to clear superficial folliculitis. Lubrication in shaved or abraded areas, treatment of pruritus, and topical antibiotics can be effective. Topical antibacterials such as povidone-iodine (Betadine),* mupirocin (Bactroban), clindamycin (Cleocin-T),* and erythromycin (Akne-mycin)* are helpful. Resistant cases frequently require systemic β-lactamase-resistant antibiotics or minocycline (Dynacin) if the involved organism is methicillin-resistant. Hot-tub folliculitis resolves spontaneously in 1 to 2 weeks, but only if the tub is disinfected. Gram-negative folliculitis in acne patients responds well to isotretinoin (Accutane).*

FURUNCLES AND CARBUNCLES

Painful, tender, erythematous nodules called *furuncles* are a deeper infection of the hair-follicle structure. Further extension of this process produces carbuncles, multiple lesions interconnected to form multiloculated abscesses. Most deeper lesions occur in areas with heat, sweat, and friction: axillae, perineum, buttocks, and inframammary regions. The thick skin of the neck produces many carbuncles.

*Not FDA approved for this indication.

Treatment

Large lesions require incision and drainage, and appropriate systemic antibiotics are required. Frequently, a traditional 7 to 10 day course of antibiotics will be inadequate for clearing and lesions recur. Warm compresses to encourage spontaneous drainage are always appropriate. Recurrent axillary and groin lesions that do not respond to treatment may be hidradenitis suppurativum, an inflammatory problem of sweat glands that produces nonfollicular subcutaneous abscesses that may or may not have bacterial involvement. Antibiotics are usually tried along with incision and drainage to control hidradenitis, but sometimes entire involved areas have to be excised.

IMPETIGO/PYODERMA/ECTHYMA

Impetigo is a common, communicable disease. It is the most common skin infection seen in children. Organisms involved are *S. aureus*, *S. pyogenes*, or a Staph/Strep mixture. Flaccid, thin-walled blisters that rupture to form moist, slightly crusted erosions are seen in the bullous (Tilbury-Fox) impetigo variant that accounts for 30% of impetigo cases overall. These are frequently annular in appearance and are associated with phage group II *Staphylococcus* producing a toxin that creates the bullae. Seventy percent of impetigo cases are moist, erythematous erosions covered with a thick, honey-colored crust. While most nonbullous impetigo is caused by *S. aureus*, the number where both *S. aureus* and *S. pyogenes* are cultured is increasing. The face, extremities, and groin are particularly involved and antecedent trauma (abrasions, insect bites, burns, chicken pox, molluscum, and atopic dermatitis) predispose to subsequent infection. Complications include pneumonia, septicemia, glomerulonephritis, septic arthritis, osteomyelitis, and necrotizing fasciitis.

A particular interest is *S. pyoderma* caused by strains containing M protein groups (2, 40, 53, 55–57, and 60) that are associated with acute, poststreptococcal glomerulonephritis. These strains are different from strains producing acute streptococcal pharyngitis and do not incite acute rheumatic fever. Glomerular disease particularly affects children under 10 years of age, occurs within 3 weeks of the skin infection, and does not seem to be inhibited by antibiotics.

Peculiar, persistent perianal erythema was initially described in pediatric patients and is now found in adults as well. It is associated with *S. pyogenes* and responds to appropriate antibiotic therapy. Certain individuals can be asymptomatic "carriers" of *S. pyogenes*. Nasal and pharyngeal carriage is most common, but vaginal, rectal, gastrointestinal, and fingernail carriage also occur. Epidemiologists investigating operating room infection clusters have to culture extensively to locate the source.

The causative organisms of impetigo also produce ecthyma, a clinical variant typically affecting immunocompromised individuals. These lesions are painful rather than pruritic, depressed ("punched out"), and require systemic treatment to resolve.

Treatment

Treatment of underlying skin problem (e.g., dermatitis), gentle removal of crusts, warm compresses, and gentle, frequent cleansing are essential. Topical antibiotics such as mupirocin (Bactroban), clindamycin (Cleocin-T),* and erythromycin (Akne-mycin),* frequently resolve limited areas of involvement. Frequent application (3 to 4 times a day), extended treatment (at least 1week after clinical clearing), and treatment of the surrounding area improve results. I frequently treat both the nose and the fingernails because their colonization leads to recurrent infection. *S. aureus* now has some strains that are resistant to mupirocin and erythromycin, but these drugs continue to be effective for streptococcus. Ecthyma, carrier states, and diffuse impetigo require systemic antibiotics. Beta-lactamase resistant antibiotics such as amoxicillin-clavulanate potassium (Augmentin), azithromycin (Zithromax), clarithromycin (Biaxin), erythromycin (E-Mycin), cephalexin (Keflex), and dicloxacillin (Dynapen) should be used. Macrolide resistance increases year-by-year, so erythromycin, azithromycin, and clarithromycin should be used only when indicated by penicillin/cephalosporin allergy. Methicillin-resistant staphylococcus will sometimes respond well to minocycline (Dynacin), and clindamycin (Cleocin) has good tissue penetration.

ERYSIPELAS AND CELLULITIS

The incidence of erysipelas and cellulitis is increasing. Erysipelas affects superficial skin layers and is red, raised, and tender. The face was classically involved, but 85% of cases now appear on the feet and legs. Cellulitis affects subcutaneous tissues but a clear-cut clinical differentiation between erysipelas and cellulitis is frequently difficult. Local signs of infection are accompanied frequently by fever and leukocytosis, but blood cultures are positive in only 5% of cases. Lymphangitis and lymphadenitis are common. A search should be made for a portal of entry, such as toe-web tinea, puncture wounds, burns, abrasions, eczema, psoriasis, or stasis dermatitis. Facial erysipelas can follow streptococcal upper respiratory infections.

Beta-hemolytic streptococcus causes the majority of these infections, with group A being the most common but groups B, C, and G also being isolated. *S. aureus* is less common. A variety of other gram-positive organisms have been cultured, including *S. epidermidis*, *Streptococcus iniae* (a fish pathogen), *S. pneumoniae*, *Erysipelothrix rhusiopathiae*, *Pneumococcus*, *Clostridia*, and gram-negative organisms such as *Haemophilus influenzae*, *Pseudomonas*, *Aeromonas*, *Legionella*, *Moraxella*, and *Helicobacter cinaedi*. A bluish-purple facial induration in a child following an upper respiratory infection suggests

*Not FDA approved for this indication.

H. influenzae infection and prompt treatment can prevent *H. influenzae* meningitis. Antibiotics specific to cultured organisms are essential, but culture of needle aspirates and tissue produce only a disappointing 20% organism recovery.

Treatment

Acute treatment should cover β-hemolytic streptococcus and *S. aureus*, changing antibiotics when culture results indicate. *H. influenzae* infection should be considered in children because it might make amoxicillin-clavulanate (Augmentin) the drug of choice. These patients are systemically ill and frequently need fluid and electrolyte monitoring. Surgical débridement or incision and drainage of loculated areas may be required. Systemic conditions such as diabetes, malnutrition, and alcoholism, as well as local factors affecting skin surface integrity and perfusion, should be addressed. Portals of entry need to be closed. Long-term treatment is the rule: organisms can "hide" in sclerosed lymphatics, poorly perfused tissue, and implants. Vaccination, when available, is important.

PARONYCHIAS AND FELONS

Paronychias and felons are the most common hand infections, representing approximately one third of total hand infections. Paronychias involve the lateral soft-tissue fold surrounding fingernails and toenails. Felons are subcutaneous abscesses of the distal pulp of the fingertip (not all fingertip abscesses are felons). Both can be caused by penetrating trauma (splinters, cuts, abrasions) while paronychias frequently involve removal or disruption of the cuticle by manipulation or for cosmesis. *S. aureus* is the most common organism but some felons have opportunistic gram-negative organisms or mixed organisms as well. Chronic paronychia can be occupational in people doing "wet work," such as bartenders, dairy farmers, dishwashers, and housewives. It involves *Candida albicans* in 95% of cases.

Treatment

Appropriate antistaphylococcal systemic antibiotics should be used for acute cases. Restoring normal cuticles can prevent acute paronychias from becoming chronic and will prevent *Candida* from colonizing and flourishing in the proximal nail fold. Quite specific instructions on manicuring and pedicuring should be given and artificial nails usually have to be removed. Colorless Castellani's paint* or 5% thymol in chloroform* used around the nail margins can produce an environment unsuitable for *Candida* and gram-negative organisms and long-term oral nystatin cuts down on the source for reseeding damaged areas.

*Not FDA approved for this indication.

TOXIC EPIDERMAL NECROLYSIS

Toxic epidermal necrolysis can be induced by medications or by a toxin produced by *S. aureus*, phage group II. The skin becomes tender, particularly in intertriginous areas, then develops erythema, resembling scarlatina. Bullae develop in 1 to 2 days that drain and desquamate. Pathologists can frequently differentiate between drug-induced and staphylococcal necrolysis on a skin biopsy. Children and debilitated patients are more likely to have the "staphylococcal scalded skin syndrome."

Treatment

Beta-lactamase resistant antistaphylococcal antibiotics should be given systemically. Depending on the levels of toxin produced, significant areas of skin can be lost, leading to fluid and electrolyte problems and loss of skin barrier and temperature control functions. Treatment is similar to that for burn patients. Because of the superficial split in the skin, surprisingly little scarring results. Differentiation between infection and drug etiology is important because readministration of a causative drug will reproduce the disease.

FOURNIER'S GANGRENE/ NECROTIZING FASCIITIS

Mixed bacterial infections of the skin have been described involving various organisms. Streptococcal gangrene involves group A β-hemolytic streptococcus with or without other organisms. Other infections have one or more anaerobes (e.g., *Peptostreptococcus* and *Bacteroides*) with a facultative species (nongroup A *Streptococcus*, *Enterobacter*, *Proteus*, and so on). The clinical picture is the same: damaged tissue, acute onset, high fever, severe toxicity, rapid progression with superficial and deep tissue destruction leading to septicemia and, frequently, death. There can be a deceptive period of localized swelling but the course is rapid once begun. This infection has been popularized as "flesh-eating bacteria" in the press.

Treatment

Prompt surgical intervention, aggressive antibiotic therapy, and medical support can be lifesaving. Mortality and morbidity are high, and it pays to have multiple disciplines involved in the management of these complex infections.

VIRAL DISEASES OF THE SKIN

method of
GISELA TORRES, M.D.
*University of Texas Medical Branch
Center for Clinical Studies
Houston, Texas*

and

STEPHEN K. TYRING, M.D., PH.D., M.B.A.
*University of Texas Medical Branch
Center for Clinical Studies
Houston, Texas and
Galveston, Texas*

ENTEROVIRUS/COXSACKIEVIRUS

Enteroviruses are the most common cause of viral exanthems in children during the summer and fall and they are transmitted via the fecal-oral route. These infections have a variety of nonspecific mucocutaneous manifestations. Two distinct syndromes, herpangina and hand-foot-mouth disease (HFMD), have been best described. A variety of coxsackievirus strains, most commonly A 16, and enterovirus 71 are associated with HFMD. This disease typically affects young children, but may occur at any age. Fever and malaise precede the onset of mucocutaneous lesions classically in the mouth, hands, and feet, although not all of the sites are always involved. The lesions, especially those in the oral mucosa, become papular, then vesicular with an erythematous halo, and ultimately ulcerate, often causing pain with eating and swallowing. More widespread macular and papular lesions may occur and lymphadenopathy is often associated. The disease is usually self-limited and resolves in 1 to 2 weeks, although rare cardiopulmonary complications or meningoencephalitis can occur. Diagnosis is clinical, but can be confirmed by polymerase chain reaction (PCR), and treatment is supportive.

Herpangina, also caused by coxsackieviruses and other enteroviruses, is transmitted through the same route as HFMD and can occur in epidemics during the summer. It affects young children and they present with sudden onset of fever, malaise, and pharyngitis. Small gray-white vesicles with surrounding erythema develop on the posterior oropharynx and eventually ulcerate. Symptoms resolve in 1 to 2 weeks without sequelae and only supportive treatment is needed. Rare complications are similar to those for HFMD.

HERPES SIMPLEX VIRUS TYPES 1 AND 2

Best known for their clinical manifestations of herpes labialis and herpes genitalis, herpes simplex virus (HSV)-1 and HSV-2 are the etiologic agents of several mucocutaneous diseases (Table 1). HSV is transmitted via direct contact between an infected person shedding the virus or their secretions and the mucosal surfaces or abraded skin of a susceptible individual. The virus travels from the initial site of infection to the dorsal root ganglion, where it remains dormant. Various stimuli, such as ultraviolet light, extremes of temperature, trauma, or stress, may precipitate viral replication and cause recurrent clinical outbreaks. Primary infection, as well as recurrent episodes of viral shedding/infection, may be clinically apparent or occur asymptomatically.

Cold sores and fever blisters (herpes labialis) are commonly caused by type 1 HSV. Oral lesions rarely occur from type 2 HSV, usually acquired through oro-genital contact. Approximately 80% to 90% of the population is seropositive for HSV-1, but only 30% to 40% of those have clinically apparent outbreaks. Primary herpes labialis often occurs in childhood and is usually asymptomatic. When symptoms occur, fever is followed by sore throat, edema, and painful vesicular eruptions on the lips, gingiva, palate, or tongue. These lesions progress to ulcerations that last 2 to 3 weeks. Submandibular or cervical lymphadenopathy may be present. Recurrent outbreaks are often preceded by a prodrome of pain, burning, itching, or tingling. Localized papular or vesicular lesions develop and eventually ulcerate or crust. Symptoms of untreated recurrences last approximately 7 to 10 days. Treatment of herpes labialis consists of topical or oral antiviral medications. This can be done episodically or as chronic suppressive therapy (if needed owing to frequency or severity of outbreaks or infection in an immunocompromised patient) (Table 2).

Herpes whitlow, vesicular outbreaks in the digits, is commonly due to infection with type 1 and usually occurs in children due to thumb sucking. Occurrence in dental and medical health care workers has decreased secondary to use of gloves and universal precautions. HSV in the digits due to type 2 infection is increasingly recognized probably owing to digital-genital contact. Herpes gladiatorum is also usually due to HSV-1 and is seen as papular or vesicular eruptions in the torso of athletes in sports involving close physical contact (classically, wrestling). Eczema herpeticum is another variant of HSV infection that

TABLE 1. **Common Mucocutaneous and Visceral Infections With Herpes Simplex Virus**

Disease	Most Commonly Associated HSV Serotype
Herpes labialis (cold sores/fever blisters)	HSV-1
Gingivostomatitis	HSV-1
Herpes gladiatorum (torso of athletes)	HSV-1
Herpes whitlow (hands and digits)	HSV-1 or 2
Herpetic keratoconjunctivitis	HSV-1
Eczema herpeticum/Kaposi's varicelliform	HSV-1
Erythema multiforme	HSV-1 or 2
Herpes folliculitis	HSV-1
Lumbosacral herpes	HSV-1 or 2
Disseminated herpes (in immunocompromised hosts)	HSV-1 or 2
Herpes genitalis	HSV-2 (30% of primary is HSV-1)
Neonatal herpes	HSV-2
Herpes encephalitis	HSV-1

TABLE 2. **Treatment of HSV Infections**

Herpes Labialis	
Episodic topical	1% penciclovir cream (Denavir) every 2 hours while awake for 5 days (avoid use in mucous membranes)
	10% doconasol cream (Abreva) 5 times daily for 5–10 days
	5% acyclovir ointment (Zovirax topical) 5 times daily for 5 days
Episodic oral	Acyclovir (Zovirax) 400 mg tid daily for 5 days*
	Famciclovir (Famvir) 500 mg tid for 5 days*
	Valacyclovir (Valtrex) 500 mg bid for 5 days* or
	2 gm BID for 1 day at the very first sign of symptoms/prodrome
Chronic suppression	Acyclovir (Zovirax) 400 mg bid*
	Famciclovir (Famvir) 250 mg bid*
	Valacyclovir (Valtrex) 500 mg qd*
Herpes Genitalis	
Primary infection	Acyclovir (Zovirax) 200 mg 5 times daily for 10 days or 400 mg tid for 10 days*
	Famciclovir (Famvir) 250 mg tid for 10 days*
	Valacyclovir (Valtrex) 1000 mg bid for 10 days*
Episodic topical	5% acyclovir ointment/cream (Zovirax topical) 5 times daily for 5 days*
Episodic oral (for recurrent infections)	Acyclovir (Zovirax) 400 mg tid for 5 days*
	Famciclovir (Famvir) 125 mg bid for 5 days*
	Valacyclovir (Valtrex) 500 mg bid for 3 days
Chronic suppression	Acyclovir (Zovirax) 400 mg bid*
	Famciclovir (Famvir) 250 mg bid*
	Valacyclovir (Valtrex) 500 mg qd for patients with <10 outbreaks/yr and 1000 mg qd for patients with 10 or more outbreaks/yr
Immunocompromised	
Limited cutaneous disease	5% acyclovir ointment/cream (Zovirax topical) 6 times daily for 10 days
Recurrent uncomplicated herpes labialis or genitalis	Acyclovir (Zovirax) 400 mg tid for 10 days
	Famciclovir (Famvir) 500 mg bid for 7 days*
	Valacyclovir (Valtrex) 500 to 1000 mg bid for 7 days*
Mucocutaneous or disseminated infection	Acyclovir IV 5mg/kg every 8 hours for 7 days if >12 years-old and for children 12 years old or younger, 250 mg/m^2 every 8 hours for 7 Days
Acyclovir-resistant HSV	Foscarnet IV 40 mg/kg every 8–10 hours for 10–21 days
	1% Cidofovir compounded cream/gel qid* (not FDA approved, but recommended by the CDC for localized acyclovir-resistant HSV)
Neonatal HSV	Intravenous acyclovir (Zovirax) 10 mg/kg given every 8 hours for 14 days

*Not FDA approved for this indication.
BID, two times daily; TID, three times daily.

commonly develops in patients with atopic dermatitis, burns, or other ulcerative or inflammatory skin conditions. This condition may be localized or disseminated in the skin and can occur at any age, although children are more commonly affected. HSV has been shown to be the most common identifiable cause of erythema multiforme; toxic epidermal necrolysis can also occur in association with recurrent HSV infections. Oral antiviral medications, acyclovir (Zovirax),* valacyclovir (Valtrex),* and famciclovir (Famvir),* may be used (off label) as therapy for these conditions and chronic suppressive therapy could also be considered depending on the severity of the condition, frequency, and the age and immune status of the patient. No current specific treatment guidelines for the above HSV infections are available, but the same doses as for treatment of herpes genitalis are commonly used in practice.

Infection with herpes simplex virus-2 is rapidly rising with an estimated seroprevalence of 20% to 23% in the United States and up to 40% worldwide. Genital herpes (GH) is usually caused by HSV-2 infection via sexual contact and occasionally by HSV-1 infection from oro-genital contact. A true primary episode of GH occurs 2 days to 2 weeks after exposure to the virus and has the most severe clinical manifestations, possibly leading to systemic complications such as aseptic meningitis, which occurs in up to 25% of women. Symptoms of primary GH last 2 to 3 weeks on average. Painful vesicular lesions in the external genitalia, vagina, perineum, buttocks, and cervix of women and in the penis, anus, and perineum of men are often associated with fever, swelling, inguinal lymphadenopathy, dysuria, vaginal/penile discharge, and generalized malaise. Many individuals are exposed to HSV-2 but do not experience a clinical episode with their primary infection; their virus lies latent for months to years and up to one half of seropositive individuals do not have a clinical outbreak. The initial clinical episode of genital HSV in those patients previously exposed, as well as the recurrent outbreaks, are not as severe as true primary infections and are often preceded by prodromes of pain, itching, tingling, or burning.

HSV shedding is greatest during clinically evident outbreaks; however, transmission from seropositive individuals to their seronegative partners frequently occurs during asymptomatic shedding periods. Barrier

*Not FDA approved for this indication.

methods are not completely satisfactory in preventing transmission of GH because transmission can occur to and from uncovered skin and mucosa or if the integrity of the barrier is compromised.

Treatment of GH generally consists of episodic courses of oral acyclovir, its more bioavailable pro-drug, valacyclovir, or famciclovir (see Table 2). Chronic suppressive therapy with these medications has been shown to decrease HSV asymptomatic shedding and, in a recent study, chronic valacyclovir therapy was shown to significantly decrease HSV transmission to susceptible partners of HSV-2 positive individuals. Genital HSV suppression should be considered in immunocompromised patients and patients with frequent and/or severe outbreaks. Other reasons to consider suppressive therapy are the gender and HSV serostatus of partners and possibility of pregnancy in a female partner. Commercially available topical treatment for GH is much less efficacious than oral therapy. A topical immune response modifier gel, resiquimod,[‡] has been shown to delay recurrences of GH in phase II clinical trials and is currently undergoing phase III studies. Different types of HSV vaccines have also been under investigation for the treatment and prevention of GH. A prophylactic HSV-2 vaccine was recently shown to confer protection against the virus in women that were serologically negative for both HSV types. It did not, however, prevent HSV infection in men, and is undergoing further clinical studies.

Disseminated HSV infection can occur in pregnancy and in immunocompromised individuals. Atypical presentations of HSV occur in these patients and can be a diagnostic challenge. Cutaneous and/or visceral dissemination should be treated promptly with intravenous acyclovir. Acyclovir-resistant HSV strains are not uncommon in the immunocompromised patient with recurrent HSV infections. Intravenous foscarnet (Foscavir) or cidofovir (Vistide)* may be used in these cases (see Table 2). HSV in the newborn can range from localized skin, mucosal, or eye infections to encephalitis and disseminated infection. About 75% to 80% of HSV infections in neonates are acquired peripartum, but *in utero* and postpartum transmission also occurs. The likelihood of transmission from mother to infant depends on factors, such as the type of genital infection at time of delivery, duration of rupture of membranes, type of delivery, and presence or absence of transplacental antibodies. Detection and typing of HSV can be done through viral culture of untreated lesions, or by direct fluorescence antigen assays. Tzanck smears can be performed in the office, but findings are not specific for the type of herpesvirus. Several HSV-1 and -2 serologic assays are used for detection of antibodies against these viruses. ELISA assays and a rapid HSV-2 POCKit test are commercially available; Western blot is available for research only. HSV DNA detection is performed in specific instances by PCR.

*Not FDA approved for this indication.
‡Investigational drug in the United States.

VARICELLA ZOSTER VIRUS

Primary infection with varicella zoster virus (VZV) causes chickenpox. Chickenpox can occur at any age, but is more common in young children, affecting 90% of children worldwide. Primary VZV (human herpesvirus 3) develops after exposure to contaminated secretions or respiratory droplets, or contact with skin lesions of an infected individual. An incubation period occurs for 2 weeks after exposure, during which time the virus replicates and spreads from the upper respiratory mucosa to the lymph nodes, blood, and internal organs. A prodrome of headache, fever, malaise, and gastrointestinal symptoms can occur several days before the onset of a pruritic, erythematous macular rash that starts on the head and spreads caudally to the trunk and proximal extremities. The rash then progresses to papules and vesicles and eventually may form pustules; it crusts after 2 to 3 weeks. Complications of primary VZV infection are most common at the extremes of age. These range from bacterial superinfection of the skin to meningoencephalitis, neurologic complications, and VZV pneumonia. Reye's syndrome can occur in infected children treated with aspirin. Immunocompromised individuals have a higher rate of complications, and VZV in pregnant women can result in devastating fetal complications.

Primary VZV (chickenpox) should be managed both symptomatically, and with systemic antivirals within 48 hours of rash onset (see Table 3). Seronegative pregnant women, newborns, and immunocompromised patients with a known VZV exposure should receive prophylaxis within 96 hours of exposure with varicella zoster immunoglobulin (VZIG). Despite administration of VZIG, over one third of exposed patients will still develop clinical varicella. A live, attenuated VZV vaccine (Oka strain) has been shown to be 71% to 91% effective in preventing disease altogether and 95% to 100% in preventing severe primary disease.

Approximately 20% of individuals infected with VZV will have a recurrence of the infection, known as herpes zoster or shingles. During primary VZV infection, the virus spreads from the sensory nerve endings to the dorsal root ganglion, where it remains latent. Reactivation of the virus occurs secondary to an unknown stimulus, and the virus replicates and travels down the sensory nerve. The inflammatory response in the nerve and ganglion often results in significant pain. A vesicular rash in the dermatomal distribution of the nerve follows the prodromal neuralgia and may be associated with fever and flu-like symptoms. The vesicular eruption crusts in approximately 2 weeks, but residual pain usually remains. The pain may persist for months to years after all signs of skin infection are resolved. This condition is known as post-herpetic neuralgia (PHN) and is a common complication in people over 50 years of age. Other complications of herpes zoster may include bacterial superinfection, ocular complications, Ramsey-Hunt syndrome (facial palsy and lesions in the external and middle ear due to involvement of the facial or auditory nerves), nerve palsies, and visceral

TABLE 3. **Treatment of Varicella Zoster Virus**

Chickenpox	
Immunocompetent children	Oral acyclovir (Zovirax) 20 mg/kg 4 times daily for 5 days
Immunocompromised children	500 mg/m^2 IV every 8 hr for 7–10 days
Immunocompetent adults	Oral acyclovir (Zovirax) 800 mg 5 times daily for 7 days Valacyclovir (Valtrex) 1000 mg tid for 7 days* Famciclovir (Famvir) 500 mg tid for 7 days*
Immunocompromised adults	IV acyclovir (Zovirax) 10 mg/kg q8 hr for 7 to 10 days
Shingles	
Immunocompetent or **uncomplicated** immunocompromised patients	Acyclovir (Zovirax) 800 mg 5 times daily for 7 days Valacyclovir (Valtrex) 1000 mg tid for 7 days Famciclovir (Famvir) 500 mg tid for 7 days
Immunocompromised (**complicated**)	IV acyclovir (Zovirax) 10 mg/kg every 8 hr for 7 days
Prophylaxis	
Newborns, seronegative pregnant women, and immunocompromised	VZIG 125 U/10 kg IM within 96 hr of exposure
VZV vaccine (Oka strain)	Single dose if between 12 months to 12 years of age Two doses given 4–8 wks apart if older than 13 years

IM, intramuscularly; IV, intravenously; tid, three times daily.
*Not FDA approved for this indication.

or CNS dissemination. Shingles only recurs in 5% of patients. Dissemination and recurrence of shingles are not uncommon in the immunosuppressed. Patients with herpes zoster can transmit VZV to individuals not previously exposed to the virus or the vaccine or to those severely immunocompromised that come in direct contact with the skin lesions; chickenpox, not shingles, would develop in these patients. Both primary VZV and herpes zoster are usually diagnosed clinically. If needed, laboratory tests including Tzanck smears, serology, viral culture, PCR, and direct immunofluorescence are available.

Treatment of shingles should be initiated within 72 hours of the development of vesicles. Oral analgesics and antipruritics are used along with antiviral medications (see Table 3). Steroids in addition to antivirals have not shown greater benefit than antivirals alone in the treatment of acute shingles. In a recent study, VZV vaccine given to bone marrow transplant patients was shown to be effective in preventing shingles. Clinical trials are underway to determine if the vaccine would also be protective against herpes zoster in the general population. Available treatment of PHN is outlined in Table 4, although none of these modalities are completely effective. The use of gabapentin (Neurontin)* in combination with one of the antiviral drugs during the acute phase may be neuroprotective and reduce the incidence of PHN.

EPSTEIN-BARR VIRUS

Epstein-Barr virus (EBV) is transmitted via an infected person's body fluids, usually saliva. EBV (herpesvirus 4) infects the epithelial cells of the oropharynx and eventually enters a latent phase. Serologic testing is the ideal method of diagnosis of EBV. Detection of heterophile antibodies can be done in a rapid test (monospot), which is most sensitive in older children and adults, and between the second and twelfth weeks after infection. If the monospot is negative or a definitive diagnosis is needed, titers of IgG and IgM against the viral capsid antigen and of IgG

*Not FDA approved for this indication.

TABLE 4. **Treatment of Postherpetic Neuralgia**

Topical treatments (skin must be completely healed)	Topical anesthetics: lidocaine cream,* gel,* or patch, EMLA cream* Capsaicin cream applied every 4 hours
Analgesics	Narcotic and non-narcotic analgesics
Anticonvulsants	Gabapentin (Neurontin) 300 mg qd gradually increased up to 1200 mg tid as tolerated
Tricyclic antidepressants	Amitryptyline 10–25 mg qd increased gradually to up to 75 mg qd* Maprotiline (Ludiomil)* Desipramine (Norpramin)*
Steroids	Intrathecal methylprednisolone* is only steroid treatment that has shown significant success in trials
Sympathetic nerve blocks	
Transcutaneous electrical stimulation	
Acupuncture	

*Not FDA approved for this indication.
tid, three times daily; qd, every day.

against EBV nuclear antigens (EBNA) can be done. The antibodies against EBNA are especially helpful in determining the stage of infection (if present, primary infection occurred over 1 month previously).

Infectious mononucleosis is the most common clinical manifestation of primary EBV infection. It usually presents with fever, pharyngitis/sore throat, malaise, splenomegaly, and lymphadenopathy that occur after an incubation period of 21 to 50 days. Multiple other gastrointestinal, rheumatologic, and generalized signs and symptoms can be associated. Cutaneous manifestations include an erythematous exanthem involving the trunk and proximal extremities that may spread to the face and distal extremities. Mucosal petechial and purpuric lesions develop in one fourth of these patients. If penicillin derivatives (classically ampicillin) are given to patients with infectious mononucleosis, the majority will develop a pruritic macular rash within 10 days of taking the medication. The lesions develop in the extensor surfaces and generalize over the trunk and extremities, including palms and soles, eventually progressing to desquamation. This reaction should not be labeled as an allergic reaction to penicillin.

Erythema multiforme, erythema nodosum, and a variety of other dermatologic manifestations have been associated with EBV. In children who have been immunized while having primary EBV infection, infantile papular acrodermatitis can occur. Because infectious mononucleosis is mostly a self-limited infection, treatment consists of supportive measures. Corticosteroids and antiviral agents have been studied, but neither class individually or in combination improves the clinical course of the infection.

EBV has been associated with several malignancies and lymphoproliferative disorders. EBV-associated angiocentric cutaneous lymphoma and subcutaneous lymphoma can manifest with papules, nodules, ulcers, bullae, or panniculitis. EBV, however, is not associated with adult cutaneous T cell lymphoma (mycosis fungoides). Immunocompromised individuals, especially those coinfected with HIV and EBV, commonly develop oral hairy leukoplakia. Adherent white plaques are classically found in the lateral borders of the tongue, although they may spread to the ventral or dorsal tongue and, rarely, to the buccal mucosa. The lesions are painless and have not been found to be precancerous. Various therapeutic agents are available, although treatment is usually not necessary (Table 5). Lesions tend to recur after treatment is discontinued.

TABLE 5. **Treatment of Oral Hairy Leukoplakia**

Topical	Tretinoin* Podophyllin resin 25%* Trichloroacetic acid*
Oral	Acyclovir (Zovirax) 800 mg five times daily for 7–14 days* Valacyclovir (Valtrex) 1000 mg tid for 7–14 days* Famciclovir (Famvir) 500 mg tid for 7–14 days*
Cryotherapy	
Surgical excision	

*Not FDA approved for this indication.
tid, three times daily.

CYTOMEGALOVIRUS

Transmission of cytomegalovirus (CMV) occurs via body fluids and infection is nearly ubiquitous in adults. CMV (herpesvirus 5) infection is usually asymptomatic in immunocompetent individuals and mucocutaneous manifestations are rare, though primary CMV infection can cause a mononucleosis-like picture. Newborns and immunocompromised patients, however, are at risk to develop significant clinical disease. CMV infection is part of the TORCH syndrome (toxoplasmosis, other infections, rubella, CMV, and HSV) in newborns and is the most common congenital viral infection and infectious cause of deafness and mental retardation in the United States. Infected babies may display a "blueberry-muffin" appearance due to purpuric skin lesions secondary to persistent dermal hematopoiesis and can have hepatic and CNS complications. In immunocompromised individuals, CMV may cause a variety of cutaneous lesions ranging from a morbilliform rash to ulcers and can disseminate. In HIV positive patients, perineal CMV ulcerations are common and CMV retinitis may occur in patients with low CD4 counts. Viral cultures from urine or saliva, CMV antigen detection, and serologic and PCR assays are used for diagnosis. Anti-CMV antivirals have FDA approval for treatment of CMV retinitis, but are used off label for other symptomatic CMV infections (Table 6). CMV immunoglobulin is used in some transplant recipients as prophylaxis against severe disease.

HUMAN HERPESVIRUSES 6 AND 7

The majority of adults are seropositive for human herpesvirus 6 (HHV 6) because infection is acquired in early childhood. HHV 6 rarely causes clinical symptoms, but is known to be the etiologic agent of roseola infantum, also known as exanthem subitum or sixth disease. Exanthem subitum typically occurs in children 6 months to 3 years of age. High fever, occurring approximately 10 days after exposure and lasting 3 to 5 days, is followed by the development of rose/pink colored macules and papules over the trunk and neck. The disease is typically self-limited and rarely results

TABLE 6. **Treatment of CMV Retinitis***

Ganciclovir (Cytovene)	1000 mg PO tid or 500 mg PO 6 times daily
Valganciclovir (Valcyte)	Start 900 mg PO bid, then qd for 3 weeks
Foscarnet (Foscavir)	60 mg/kg to 120 mg/kg IV qd for 2–3 weeks
Cidofovir (Vistide)	5 mg/kg IV q week for 2 weeks
Fomivirsen	Intravitreal injection

*Renal Adjustment Needed for Patients With Creatinine Clearance <30.
bid, two times a day; PO, by mouth; qd, every day; qid, four times daily.

TABLE 7. **Common Skin Diseases Caused by Viral Infection**

Virus	Disease Classically Associated
Human Papillomaviruses	Genital warts (condyloma acuminatum), verruca vulgaris, plantar warts, verruca plana
Human Herpesviruses	
HSV-1	Herpes labialis, herpes whitlow, herpes gladiatorum
HSV-2	Herpes genitalis, TORCH syndrome
VZV	Chickenpox, herpes zoster
EBV	Infectious mononucleosis
CMV	"Blueberry muffin baby" (TORCH Syndrome)
HHV 6	Exanthem subitum
HHV 7	Exanthem subitum
HHV 8	Kaposi's sarcoma
Enterovirus/Coxsackievirus	Hand-foot-mouth disease, herpangina
Parvovirus B19	Erythema infectiosum, papular purpuric hands and gloves syndrome
Poxviruses	Molluscum contagiosum, smallpox, human orf, milker's nodules
Rubella togavirus	Rubella (German measles), "Blueberry muffin baby" (TORCH syndrome)
Rubeola	Measles

Abbreviations: bid, two times a day; PO, by mouth; qd, every day; qid, four times daily.

in complications, such as febrile seizures and meningoencephalitis. Seriously ill patients have been treated with anti-CMV antiviral medications. Human herpes virus 7 (HHV 7) has been associated with some cases of roseola infantum and pityriasis rosea, but is otherwise not known to cause clinical disease (Table 7).

HUMAN HERPESVIRUS 8

Previously known as Kaposi-associated herpes virus, human herpesvirus 8 (HHV 8), is the causative agent of Kaposi's sarcoma (KS), a malignancy of vascular endothelial origin. Classic KS occurs in immunocompetent men of Mediterranean or Jewish descent and in people from tropical Africa. KS also develops in the immunocompromised, especially in patients with HIV/AIDS. The modes of HHV 8 transmission remain controversial, but transmission by sexual contact, especially anal intercourse, and mother-to-child transmission are known to occur. Classic KS is typically benign and manifests as violaceous or brown to dark blue macules or plaques in the extremities. KS in AIDS and other immunocompromised patients typically starts as red or violaceous macules, plaques, and nodules on the trunk and face and in mucosal surfaces. The lesions are associated with pain and easy bleeding, and gastrointestinal and pulmonary involvement or lymphatic dissemination can occur. Treatment of KS depends on the type of lesion and extent of disease. In HIV-positive patients, highly active antiretroviral therapy (HAART) may be the best treatment. Limited disease may be treated with cryotherapy, laser therapy, topical alitretinoin (Panretin 0.1% gel), intralesional chemotherapy, radiotherapy, electrodessication, or excision. Systemic interferon-α (IntronA, Roferon-A), paclitaxel (Taxol), doxorubicin (Adriamycin), daunorubicin, vinblastine (Velban), bleomycin (Blenoxane),* and retinoic acid have been used for systemic disease.

*Not FDA approved for this indication.

PARVOVIRUS B19

Parvovirus B19 is the cause of erythema infectiosum or fifth disease, typically occurring in school-aged children. It is transmitted through aerosolized droplets or via vertical transmission from mother to fetus. In children, 1 to 2 weeks after exposure, low-grade fever, malaise, and upper respiratory symptoms develop. A characteristic rash then arises, consisting of brightly erythematous patches and mild edema over the cheeks ("slapped cheek" appearance) that fade over a 4-day period and are followed by pink macules and papules over the trunk, neck, and extremities. Cough, pharyngitis, gastrointestinal symptoms, and conjunctivitis may be associated. Diagnosis is mainly clinical, but serologic detection of antibodies and PCR for DNA are available for confirmation. In adults, parvovirus B19 infection is usually asymptomatic; however, it may present with arthralgias and a rare pruritic macular rash in the extremities. Another rare manifestation is the papular pruritic gloves and socks syndrome (PPGSS). Patients with this disease present with fatigue and fever and rapidly progressive erythema of the hands and feet associated with swelling, tenderness, and pruritus. Complications of parvovirus B19 infection are rare, but it may cause meningoencephalitis and transient aplastic crises in immunosuppressed anemic individuals and in those with chronic hemolytic anemia. Infection in pregnant women can have devastating effects, such as fetal hydrops and demise. Treatment of diseases associated with this virus is only supportive. Individuals at risk should avoid contact with sick children and those known to be infected with the virus.

POXVIRUSES

Smallpox, also known as variola, is the most serious of the poxvirus-caused illnesses and has been eradicated by worldwide vaccination with vaccinia virus. However, new concerns have stemmed from the possibility of this virus being used as a biologic weapon, especially because it is fatal in up to one third of cases. The smallpox virus is transmitted via respiratory particles. Prodrome of fever, malaise, headache, and backache precedes the onset of a rash that starts in the mouth, palms, and soles and spreads to the extremities and trunk centrifugally. Macules and papules develop into vesicular and pustular lesions that eventually crust. Gastrointestinal and cardiopulmonary involvement can occur and hemorrhagic lesions, a variant of the disease, are associated with almost 100% mortality. Respiratory and contact isolation must be enforced immediately if smallpox is suspected. Treatment is primarily supportive and antivirals, such as cidofivir, have been shown to work only in vitro. Postexposure vaccination may be effective and should be done as soon as possible.

Molluscum contagiosum (MCV) is the most common poxvirus infection, transmitted via skin-to-skin or sexual contact. There are two identified strains of MCV, but they are clinically indistinguishable. Small, firm, umbilicated papules develop on the skin 2 to 8 weeks after exposure. The lesions are typically in the axillae, body folds, and genitalia. In patients with atopic dermatitis and immunocompromised patients, molluscum can spread extensively, especially in HIV-positive individuals. Diagnosis is clinical, but PCR and histologic examination of cellular material can be useful. Molluscum contagiosum, if untreated, will eventually go into remission in healthy individuals. Many patients opt for treatment, however. Removal of the lesions can be achieved surgically, with curettage, cryosurgery, laser therapy, tape stripping, and liquid nitrogen freezing. Topical treatments include cantharidin,† podophyllin,* salicylic* and lactic acids,* iodine,* and tretinoin,* among others. Imiquimod 5% (Aldara)* cream has been successful in several patients, including those who are HIV positive. Oral cimetidine (Tagamet),* 40 mg/kg/d and, in HIV patients, intravenous or topical cidofovir,* (2 mg/kg/wk IV or 3% cream) have been effective.

Human orf, or contagious ecthyma, is caused by a poxvirus transmitted from sheep or goats to humans. After a short incubation period, the disease goes through six stages where papular skin lesions develop and eventually turn into nodules, crust, and shed. Fever, regional lymphadenopathy, and lymphangitis can be associated. The disease is self-contained, lasting approximately 1 month and there is no specific treatment. Milker's nodules is another disease caused by a poxvirus present in cows and transmitted to humans by direct contact. The lesions are similar to those in orf and the disease has a similar progression. Diagnosis of these diseases can be confirmed via culture, immunofluorescence, or biopsy.

RUBELLA

Rubella (German measles), is caused by a togavirus and is a common disease of childhood, but may occur in adults. It can be prevented by immunization with MMR (measles, mumps, rubella) vaccine, which is typically given at 12 to 15 months of age for the first dose and at 4 to 6 years of age for the second dose. The vaccine may be given in children as young as 6 months of age in the context of an outbreak and it should be avoided in pregnant women. The virus is transmitted via respiratory droplets or by in-utero transmission. After an incubation period of approximately 15 days, a prodrome of fever, headache, coryza, conjunctivitis, and lymphadenopathy occurs. Petechiae may develop in the palate and pink-to-red macules and papules appear on the face and neck and spread caudally to the trunk and extremities. The exanthem fades after 3 to 4 days. Complications are uncommon and include thrombocytopenic purpura, arthralgias, and CNS complications. Treatment is supportive. Neonatal infection is part of the TORCH syndrome and can result in several congenital abnormalities including heart defects, deafness, cataracts, and mental retardation. Rubella is diagnosed by serologic assays and pregnant women should be tested during the first trimester.

RUBEOLA VIRUS

Measles is another disease preventable by immunization with MMR vaccine and is caused by rubeola virus (measles), a paramyxovirus. The virus is acquired through inhalation of contaminated aerosolized droplets. The disease typically occurs in children and begins with a prodrome of high fever, cough, coryza, conjunctivitis, and periorbital edema about 1 to 2 weeks after exposure. Koplik's spots, blue-white papules with an erythematous base, develop on the oral mucosa and erythematous macules and papules develop in the skin of the face and neck and subsequently spread to the trunk and extremities. Gastrointestinal symptoms and generalized lymphadenopathy are often associated with the disease. Uncomplicated measles resolves in about 10 days. Otitis media is the most common complication. It may also lead to encephalitis, hepatic and gastrointestinal involvement, and pneumonia. Prevention via vaccination should be emphasized, because no effective therapy is available for measles. Treatment is supportive and antibiotics are indicated only when secondary bacterial infections occur. In young infants and immunocompromised individuals with a known exposure to the rubeola virus, administration of intravenous immunoglobulin may prevent or ameliorate the disease.

---

*Not FDA approved for this indication.
†Not available in the United States.

PARASITIC DISEASES OF THE SKIN

method of
H.L. GREENBERG, M.D., and
HARRY SHARATA, M.D., PH.D.
University of Wisconsin
Madison, Wisconsin

In treating parasitic diseases of the skin, it is important to have a high index of suspicion and to obtain a complete history, including recent travel (Table 1). Diagnoses are made through specialized laboratory studies. A continually updated resource for treatment is available at the Centers for Disease Control (CDC) website www.cdc.gov/travel/diseases.htm.

PROTOZOAL INFECTIONS

Protozoal infections have a life cycle that includes trophozoite (motile) and cyst (nonmotile) forms.

Amebiasis

Cutaneous amebiasis is usually seen in developing countries and is caused by a single celled organism, *Entamoeba histolytica.* The lesion of amebiasis is often painful, nonspecific, irregular, and ulcerated. Because of its appearance, cutaneous amebiasis may be confused with syphilis and infectious granulomas. There may also be associated adenopathy, and untreated persons may develop worsening infection or experience spread to internal organs. This organism is transmitted through fecal-oral contact. Cutaneous amebiasis may result from anal intercourse in an asymptomatic host, those with amebic dysentery, or from an abscess located in the anogenital region including the penis, perineum, buttock, or abdomen. Trophozoites may be identified in the ulcer or from stool studies. Treatment includes metronidazole (Flagyl), 750 mg by mouth (PO) twice daily (bid) for 7 to 10 days for extraintestinal disease, followed by iodoquinol (Yodoxin), 650 mg PO three times daily (tid) for 20 days for an intestinal source.

Leishmaniasis

Cutaneous leishmaniasis is transmitted by an infected sand fly bite and patients present with sores of different sizes and shapes with raised edges and a central crater, which may be painful. Treatment includes sodium stibogluconate (Pentostam),* 20 mg (pentavalent antimony)/kg/d intravenously (IV) or intramuscularly (IM) for 20 to 28 days, available as an Investigational New Drug (IND) from the Centers for Disease Control and Prevention (CDC).

Trypanosomiasis

There are three different trypanosomes: *Trypanosoma brucei* variants (*Trypanosoma gambiense* and *Trypanosoma rhodesiense*) and *Trypanosoma cruzi.* The two disease forms of the trypanosomes, Chagas' disease and African sleeping sickness, are discussed subsequently.

Chagas' disease is caused by *T. cruzi,* and is found in Texas, Mexico, Central and South America; transmission is by the reduviid (kissing) bug. Initial infection may be inapparent on the skin or may show a boardlike erythematous induration with a subcutaneous nodule (chagoma). Romaña's sign is seen if the bite is near the eye, yielding eyelid edema and conjunctivitis. Systemic involvement can lead to central nervous system (CNS) disease, dilated cardiomyopathy, megaesophagus, and megacolon. Diagnosis is based on hematologic examination (motile trypomastigotes). Alternatively, a diagnostic challenge, whereby the patient is exposed to hungry reduviid bugs, which will later be sacrificed and examined for trypomastigotes, may be performed. Early treatment relieves parasitemia in 2 days with symptomatic improvement in 3 to 10 days and the prevention of systemic sequelae. Treatment efficacy is reduced with visceral involvement. Nifurtimox (Lampit),* available through the CDC Parasitic Drug Service, is dosed at 8 to 10 mg/kg/d PO (in divided doses) four times daily for 120 days.

African sleeping sickness, East and West, are caused by *T. rhodesiense* and *T. gambiense,* respectively and are found mostly in Africa. Transmission occurs through an infected tsetse fly bite. A painful chancre (red, erythematous nodule) surrounded by a white halo measuring 1 to 3 cm, develops at the bite site 50% of the time, usually within 4 to 5 days. Posterior cervical adenopathy (Winterbottom's sign) may develop in association with the nodule. As parasitemia develops, the patient may demonstrate fevers, generalized pruritic eruptions with erythematous annular plaques, and symmetrical adenopathy. Transient edema of eyelids, palms, and soles occurs within weeks to months. Early treatment is essential to prevent CNS involvement including personality changes, slurred speech, seizure, confusion, and sleeping abnormalities. Treatment for *Trypanosoma* infection varies depending on the species; the disease is fatal (within months to years) if not treated. For *T. brucei* or *T. gambiense,* first-line therapy is eflornithine (Ornidyl),* available from the World Health Organization (WHO), dosed at 100 mg/kg IV every 6 hours for 14 days, followed by 75 mg/kg/d PO for 21 to 30 days. *The commercially available topical formulation should not be used to treat trypanosomal disease.* Suramin sodium (Antrypol),* available from the CDC Parasitic Drug Service, is used to treat both *T. brucei gambiense* and *T. rhodesiense.* Suramin sodium dosage is 0.2 g IV test dose, followed by 20 mg/kg (maximum dose 1 g) IV on days 1, 3, 7, 14, and 21.

HELMINTHS

Ancylostoma braziliense

Ancylostoma braziliense is the causative agent of cutaneous larva migrans, or creeping eruption.

*Not FDA approved for this indication.

TABLE 1. **Cutaneous Parasites and Their Treatment**

Class	Disease Name	Geographic Distribution	Causative Organism	Recommended Treatment
Protozoa	Cutaneous Amebiasis	Developing countries	*Entamoeba histolytica*	Metronidazole (Flagyl)* 750 mg PO tid × 7–10 d
	Leishmaniasis	Africa, Asia, Middle East, Central and South America	*Leishmania* species	Sodium stibogluconate (Pentostam)* 20 mg/kg/d IV or IM × 20–28 d.
	Chagas'	Central and South America	*Trypanosoma cruzi*	Nifurtimox (Lampit)* 8–10 mg/kg/d PO, qid in divided doses × 120 d
	African sleeping sickness	Africa	*Trypanosoma brucei*	Eflornithine (Ornidyl)* 100 mg per kg IV, q6h × 14 d
Helminths	Cutaneous larva migrans	Worldwide	*Ancylostoma braziliense*	Albendazole (Albenza)* 400 mg PO × 1 d
			Strongyloides stercoralis	Ivermectin (Stromectol) 200 µg/kg PO × 1–2 d
	Dracunculiasis	Rural Africa, Yemen	*Dracunculus medinensis*	Surgical removal, metronidazole (Flagyl)* 250 mg tid × 10 d
	Loiasis	Africa	*Loa loa*	Diethylcarbamazine (Hetrazan)* 9 mg/kg/d PO in 3 divided doses × 21 d
	Elephantiasis, lymphatic filariasis	Asia, Africa, Caribbean, South America	*Wuchereria bancrofti* and *Brugia* species	Diethylcarbamazine* 6 mg/kg/d PO in 3 divided doses × 6–12 d
	River blindness	Africa and Latin America	*Onchocerca volvulus*	Ivermectin 150 µg/kg PO q6–12 mo
Arthropoda	Scabies	Worldwide	*Sarcoptes scabiei*	5% permethrin (Elimite) cream +/– Ivermectin 200 µg/kg PO × 1 dose
	Body lice	Worldwide	*Pediculus humanus*	Symptomatic, clean clothing
	Pubic and head lice, crabs.	Worldwide	*Pediculus pubis and P. capitus*	5% permethrin (Elimite), repeat in 1 wk
	Chiggers, tungiasis	Central and South America, Africa	*Tunga penetrans*	Flea removal, symptomatic Rx
	Myiasis	Worldwide	*Dermatobia hominis*/botfly	Surgical removal, topical therapies

*Not FDA approved for this indication.
IV, intravenously; PO, by mouth; q, every; qid, four times daily; tid, three times daily.

Hookworm larvae (*Ancylostoma*) from contaminated dog or cat feces residing in the soil, beach, or other sandy areas penetrate the feet and other contact areas of the skin, causing typical lesions. Patients may present initially with an erythematous papule that develops into a wandering, lower epidermal serpiginous tract that can be intensely pruritic in a matter of hours. Associated excoriations from pruritus may become secondarily infected. Once present, the larvae progress 1 to 2 cm a day; another cutaneous larva migrans, *Strongyloides stercoralis,* may progress up to 10 cm a day. Diagnosis is usually clinical; however, a "wet prep" of the tissue may show larvae on microscopy. Whereas the larvae may naturally die in weeks, treatment with albendazole (Albenza),* 400 mg PO for 1 day is effective for *Ancylostoma.*[‡] An alternative therapy is mebendazole (Vermox), 500 mg PO for 1 day or 100 mg PO twice daily (bid) for 3 days.

*Not FDA approved for this indication.
[‡]Investigational drug in the United States.

Treatment of *Strongyloides* infection involves ivermectin (Stromectol), 200 µg/kg/d PO for 1 to 2 days, or thiabendazole 25 mg/kg/d PO bid for 2 days. Application of liquid nitrogen may be used to treat the advancing burrow area.

Infection prevention includes minimizing exposure through protective means including shoes and beach towels. Pet owners should have suspected pets examined and remove fecal matter from areas where human exposure is likely.

Dracunculiasis

Dracunculiasis occurs once the human host drinks water with microscopic water fleas infected with the larvae of *Dracunculus medinensis*. The larvae are released from the fleas in the intestine, where they mate and develop into worms that travel to and rest in the subcutaneous skin. Within 1 year a blister forms over the now pregnant female worm (now some 70 to 120 cm in length). Once exposed to water, the blister ruptures and the worm releases its larvae.

Surgical removal is considered definitive treatment and involves delicately winding the now mature Guinea worm around a small stick as it emerges through the skin. Care is taken to remove the whole worm as residual parasite can lead to inflammation. Metronidazole (Flagyl),* 250 mg PO tid for 10 days may be used as adjunctive therapy. Living in an area with good water treatment will prevent infection. Currently, infection is confined to rural African countries and Yemen.

Filarial Diseases

Filarial diseases include infection with *loa loa* (loiasis), *Onchocerca volvulus* (onchocerciasis), *Wuchereria bancrofti* (filariasis), and *Wuchereria brugia* or *(Wuchereria) malayi* (filariasis). Diagnosis is the same in filarial cases and involves a hematologic examination of thick and thin blood sample smears for the presence of microfilariae. Because microfilariae concentrate in the peripheral capillaries, blood draws through finger sticks are recommended. Antigen detection using an immunoassay for filarial antigens may be used for identification, as may an antibody test. However, because of antigenic cross-reactivity and lifelong postexposure positivity, it may not be possible to distinguish between past and current infection.

Loiasis

The filarial parasite *L. loa* causes migratory angioedema, which lasts from hours to days, and results in localized areas of swelling in the arms, legs, face, and trunk called *Calabar swellings*. In some cases, infection with *L. loa* will have subconjunctival migration of the adult worm visible as a raised serpiginous lesion in the scleral conjunctiva. Transmission occurs via the *Chrysops* fly bite. Treatment is the same as with other filarial diseases and involves diethylcarbamazine (Hetrazan),* 50 mg PO on day 1 followed by 9 mg/kg/d PO in three divided doses for 21 days. Encephalopathy has been observed with this medication, and is thought to be a reaction to the release of parasite antigens from microfilarial destruction.

Lymphatic Filariasis

Lymphatic channel obstruction by microfilarial migration of *W. bancrofti* or *B. malayi* leads to elephantiasis. Mosquitoes pass larvae to the human host; adult worms, measuring 8 to 10 cm, block lymphatics and produce microfilariae. Physical symptoms include massively enlarged extremities with occasional ulcers and sterile abscess formation. Like other filarial diseases, microfilariae are visible in blood samples. Treatment is with diethylcarbamazine (Hetrazan),* 6 mg/kg/d PO in three divided doses for 6 to 14 days. Ivermectin* 200 μg/kg PO for 1 dose can be used.

Onchocerciasis

Onchocerca volvulus is a filarial parasite transmitted by the blackfly (genus *Simulium*). Infection is seen in Africa and Latin America, adjacent to rivers where the blackfly larvae develop. The adult worm parasite resides in the subcutaneous tissue where a localized pruritic nodule develops. Adult worms produce millions of microfilariae that spread throughout the subcutaneous tissue and skin yielding an early maculopapular eruption with an asymmetrical distribution. Later, the eruption becomes hyperpigmented, with loss of skin elasticity, mottling, and atrophy. When infestation is great, there may be microfilariae deposition in the anterior chamber and other areas of the eye leading to chronic inflammation and vision loss, better known as *river blindness*. Treatment is ivermectin (Stromectol), 150 μg/kg PO every 6 to 12 months until free from disease. Unfortunately, ivermectin is only active against the microfilariae because adult worms are resistant to this therapy.

Schistosomiasis

The three main *Schistosoma* species infecting humans are *Schistosoma haematobium, Schistosoma japonicum,* and *Schistosoma mansoni*.

Cutaneous schistosomiasis is known as *cercarial dermatitis* or *swimmer's itch*. Patients present after skin exposure to water contaminated with larvae (cercariae) from snails or waterfowl. Typically the patient will experience an itching, prickly sensation within minutes of cercariae penetration, sparing covered areas. Within 24 hours, red papules develop and may coalesce into blisters that last 5 to 7 days. This presentation is an allergic reaction, because infection with the nonhuman species of *Schistosoma* is self-limited and does not require specific treatment. Symptomatic treatment with oral antihistamines and topical steroids are all that is needed. Human schistosomiasis is treated with praziquantel (Biltricide), 20 mg/kg two to three times in 1 day.

Seabather's eruption is a closely related cercarial dermatitis occurring in salt water and demonstrating an eruption, confined to the swimsuit area, of pruritic, crusted papules within hours of bathing that resolve in several days. Treatment is the same as for cutaneous schistosomiasis.

ARTHROPODA

Scabies

Scabies is a common disease caused by a mite, *Sarcoptes scabiei* (var. *hominis*) (Megnin, 1880). The infestation is usually related to poor hygiene, but is commonly seen in nursing homes, hospital wards, schools, and other close quarters. Transmission may occur through sexual contact and in areas of mite infestation including plush furniture, bedding, carpet, and clothes. Mite survival away from a host

*Not FDA approved for this indication.

may last as long as 3 days. Vacuuming and discarding the used bag is essential. Scabies mites are small, with females measuring 0.4 × 0.3 mm, and males are half that size. Preferential sites of infestation include soft, hairless body parts including intergluteal folds, interdigital webs, genitalia, flexor wrist surface, lower abdomen, and axilla. Infants may have palmoplantar and scalp involvement. Immunosuppressed, debilitated, or institutionalized patients may have a severe and chronic infestation. In Norwegian scabies, numerous mites infest hands, feet, genitalia, and auricles leading to prominent hyperkeratosis and crusting.

The mite lives in subcorneal burrows a few millimeters long and often attach to a vesicle at the blind end. Identification of the mite is obtained by pricking the vesicle with a blade, smearing the contents onto a glass slide, adding a drop of 25% KOH, waiting 10 minutes, and then covering with a cover slip. Gentle heating over a flame helps dissolve keratin and release the mite. A chain of dark brown feces (scybala) or egg shells with or without larva are diagnostic (even if the mite is missed). Superficial shave biopsy demonstrates the tissue reaction typical of an insect bite (i.e., patchy lymphocytic infiltrate with eosinophils).

Adults should be treated from the neck down; infants can be treated from the scalp down. Preferred topical therapy is with 5% permethrin (Elimite) topical cream left on for 8 to 10 hours to be repeated in 1 week. An alternative therapy is Crotamiton 10% topical (Eurax) repeated in 24 hours, (safety and effectiveness in children not established; treatment in pregnancy is category C). Lindane 1% cream left on 8 to 12 hours is also effective therapy, but has a slight risk of CNS toxicity and seizure; treatment in pregnancy is category B. Patients who are immunocompromised or who fail to resolve may use ivermectin (Stromectol), 200 μg/kg PO for one dose.

Post-scabetic itch may be treated with topical steroids, such as triamcinolone or hydrocortisone. Persistent post-scabetic nodules may occur within a year of the original treatment and may be treated with triamcinolone 5 to 10 mg/mL intralesional injection or high-potency topical steroids (e.g., clobetasol [Temovate]) 0.05% ointment or cream bid as needed. Animal scabies are transient bites that manifest as allergic reactions and are not true infestations. Antihistamines and topical steroids may be used to treat both post-scabetic itch and animal scabies.

Pediculosis

Lice are ectoparasites; their only hosts are humans. Lice begin as nits (eggs) cemented to the hair base, becoming nymphs on the hair shaft and growing into adults on the distal hair shaft over a 2- to 3-week period. The louse feeds on blood several times daily. The typical louse bite yields a pruritic red macule with central hemorrhage. There are three types of human lice discussed subsequently: *Phthirus pubis*, *Pediculus humanus* (var. *capitis*, and *corporis*).

Pediculosis Corporis

Body lice are longer than head and pubic lice. They are seen more commonly in people who wear the same clothing daily, i.e., the homeless, refugees, and soldiers in wartime. Patients may have a wide variety of presentation from papuloerythematous eruptions to urticarial lesions. Involved areas include the buttocks and trunk. Severe cases may have bloody streaks with crusts secondary to deep excoriations. The lice and eggs are not found on the skin itself, but rather in the clothing, often in the seams. After bathing with soap and water, corticosteroid ointments and oral antihistamines may be used to control pruritus. All clothes and bedding will require laundering as detailed later. Incineration of heavily infested clothing may be necessary.

Pediculosis Pubis

Crab lice are broad, crablike, slow-moving organisms infesting the pubic, axillary, eyebrow, and eyelash hair. These organisms are typically transmitted through sexual contact, and workup of other sexually transmitted diseases may be indicated. Patients usually present with intense pruritus, eczematous change, excoriations, and secondary infection of "crabs." Bruise-like blue patches (maculae caeruleae) may be found on the trunk.

Pediculosis Humanus Capitis

Head lice are most commonly seen in children, usually schoolgirls who share combs or brushes. Lice may be confused with dandruff or hair products, such as hairspray. Typically, the occipital scalp shows the most involvement, followed by the posterior and lateral scalp; lesions may extend down the nape of the neck to the upper shoulders in those with longer hair. Pruritus, scalp excoriations, and broken papules are almost always present, and secondary impetigo may occur. Those in close association with the affected patient should also be treated.

Pediculosis Therapy

Permethrin 5% cream (Elimite) or 1% over-the-counter (Nix) should be applied as a shampoo or lotion and rinsed after 10 minutes with water. Repeat dosing may be needed to kill new progeny in 1 week.

Lindane (Kwell) 1% shampoo is second-line therapy for pediculosis. It is applied to dry hair for 4 minutes, worked into a lather, and rinsed off. A repeat treatment in 1 week may be necessary. There is potential for seizure if toxic amounts of drug are used.

Eyelash involvement is treated with mechanical removal and petrolatum to the eyelashes three to five times daily for 1 week. Alternatively, physiostigmine (Eserine)* 0.25% ophthalmic ointment has been used and is applied three to five times a day for 3 days.

After initial topical therapy, it is important to remove residual nits with a comb/tweezer combination because nits may be viable for up to 1 month.

*Not FDA approved for this indication.

All clothing and bedding that has been in contact with the affected individual is laundered in hot water with detergent, and placed in a hot dryer for at least 20 minutes. Dry cleaning is an acceptable alternative. Items that are plush and not washable should be sealed in plastic for at least 2 weeks prior to usage. Affected contacts need treatment.

Tungiasis

Tungiasis commonly known as *chiggers* or *jiggers* is due to flea infestation with (*Tunga penetrans*) or the sand flea. In this disease the female flea will penetrate the skin, lay eggs, and produce larvae over a 2- to 3-week period. Development of a painful, necrotic papule or vesicle ensues with a black, necrotic crust. Treatment is flea removal.

Myiasis

Myiasis is caused by the larvae of the human botfly known as *Dermatobia hominis*. The larvae burrow deep into the skin and the cutaneous reaction is an erythematous papule with central pore. Occasionally the larvae will protrude through the pore. Petroleum jelly or raw bacon/pork fat are placed over the pore enticing the larvae out. Surgical removal is curative.

FUNGAL DISEASES OF THE SKIN

method of
BARRY S. ZINGMAN, M.D.
Montefiore Medical Center
Bronx, New York

Fungal infections of the skin, hair, and nails are some of the most common infections worldwide, with special prominence in children, the elderly, men, and immunocompromised hosts such as those with diabetes, cancer, or HIV infection. Generally, such superficial fungal infections are caused by dermatophytes from the *Trichophyton, Microsporum*, and *Epidermophyton* genera, but less frequently infection may be due to nondermatophyte fungi such as *Candida* or *Malassezia (Pityrosporum)* species.

The diagnosis of superficial fungal infections is usually straightforward and based on suggestive clinical characteristics and response to empirical treatment. In unclear or recalcitrant cases, confirmation of the diagnosis can be attempted by a potassium hydroxide (KOH) preparation or histologic examination of scrapings, examination of scrapings under Wood's light, or culture. These methods are insensitive, however, because fungal elements are sometimes difficult to detect by microscopy, and tinea species grow poorly on routine culture media. Growth of dermatophytes is best performed on specific mycologic media at laboratories experienced in fungal isolation. However, depending on the particular fungal disease, the optimal site to obtain scrapings varies and affects the yield on culture.

The differential diagnosis depends on the location of the suspected fungal infection and specific clinical characteristics. Most commonly, discrimination must be made from eczema, contact dermatitis, acneiform eruptions, folliculitis of other cause, skin maceration, psoriasis, lichen planus, and trauma.

TINEA PEDIS

Tinea pedis (also called "athlete's foot") is most commonly caused by *Trichophyton rubrum*, spread by contact with infected desquamated skin, and prevalent in postpubescent males. Infection may be asymptomatic or cause various degrees of interdigital itching and cracking, erythema, scaling (occasionally causing an extensive "moccasin sole" appearance, one manifestation of "dry-type" tinea pedis), and rarely, blisters. The disease can become extensive in immunocompromised patients, especially those with AIDS.

TINEA CRURIS

Tinea cruris (also called "jock itch") is most commonly caused by *T. rubrum* or *Epidermophyton floccosum*. Occurring more frequently during the summer months, tinea cruris is characterized by unilateral or bilateral medial thigh and/or scrotal redness, itching, and scaling, generally with a sharp border and occasionally with papules and pustules near the leading edge. No satellite lesions are present as with candidiasis of the skin.

TINEA CORPORIS

Also called ringworm, tinea corporis is now relatively infrequent in the United States and is more commonly seen in tropical parts of the world. However, cases still occur in this country, especially in the homeless, HIV-infected persons, and inner-city children. Typical cases are caused by *T. rubrum* and appear round, well demarcated, and scaly, with central clearing and little inflammation. Lesions may be hyperpigmented in darker skinned individuals. Less commonly, infection is derived from animal sources such as cows, dogs, and cats and is caused by *Trichophyton verrucosum* or *Microsporum canis*. Animal-associated species tend to cause a more nodular and inflammatory form of tinea corporis that is especially seen in children. Kerions are characteristic large pustular lesions caused by these dermatophytes.

TINEA MANUUM

Tinea infection of the hand usually involves only a single palm, and concurrent foot infection is typical. The appearance is that of a diffuse, dry, scaly eruption, similar to the "moccasin sole" form of tinea pedis. *T. rubrum* is the most frequent cause.

TINEA FACIEI AND TINEA BARBAE

Tinea infections of the face (tinea faciei), though typically caused by *T. rubrum*, appear different from infections by this organism at other sites. Lesions may be follicular, pruritic, and mildly red, with inexact margins. Highly inflamed and pustular lesions of the neck and beard (tinea barbae) are caused by the animal dermatophytes *T. verrucosum* or *Trichophyton mentagrophytes*, thereby being similar to tinea corporis lesions caused by these dermatophytes, and they are mainly an occupational illness.

TINEA CAPITIS

Tinea capitis (scalp ringworm) is principally a disease of children. After puberty, changes in the fatty acid content of sebum are believed to inhibit dermatophyte growth and lead to a dramatic decline in incidence of the disease. Large geographic variation occurs in the overall incidence, as well as the causative genera and species, but most infections are due to *Trichophyton* species. Characteristic features of tinea capitis include mild to severe scaling, itching, hair loss, erythema, and sometimes pustules or kerions. Ectothrix infections have dermatophyte arthrospores forming on the outside of the hair shaft and cause hair breakage just above the surface of the scalp. In endothrix infections, arthrospores form within the hair shaft, so hair breakage occurs at the skin surface. Favus is a particularly severe form of tinea capitis caused by *Trichophyton schoenleinii* in which a thick inflammatory crust forms on the scalp and hair follicles. It may lead to scarring and permanent alopecia if untreated.

ONYCHOMYCOSIS

Onychomycosis, or fungal infection of the nails (also called tinea unguium), usually occurs in the setting of chronic dermatophyte infection of adjacent skin. The disease is common in elderly, diabetic, and

TABLE 1. **Treatments of Choice for Fungal Infections of the Skin, Hair, and Nails**

Infection	Preferred Agents/Regimens	Alternative Agents/ Regimens*	Adjunctive Treatments/Comments
Tinea pedis	Topical azole[†] or terbinafine (Lamisil)	Azole powder or PO,[‡] terbinafine, natifine (Naftin) powder	Improve foot hygiene; Whitfield's ointment may be applied for extensive disease; oral agents may be more effective for "dry-type" disease
Tinea cruris	Topical azole	Azole powder or PO, terbinafine	
Tinea corporis	Topical or PO azole	Terbinafine	Minimum treatment for 4–6 wk; PO if > 1–2 lesions or large areas of skin involvement
Tinea manuum	Topical or PO azole	Terbinafine	
Tinea faciei	PO azole or PO terbinafine		
Tinea barbae	PO azole or PO terbinafine		
Tinea capitis	Griseofulvin (Fulvicin) ultramicrosize PO (children), itraconazole (Sporanox) PO, terbinafine PO, fluconazole (Diflucan) PO		Selenium sulfide (Selsun) or ketoconazole (Nizoral) shampoo is used only as an adjunct to oral therapy
Onychomycosis	Pulse itraconazole PO,[§] daily terbinafine PO	Daily itraconazole PO, pulse terbinafine, PO[‖] ciclopirox (Penlac) nail lacquer	Prolonged therapy needed (3–6 mo); topical therapy is usually ineffective alone, although success has been shown with some regimens, including combined oral plus topical treatments; fingernails respond better than toenails; culture of deep specimens may help guide therapy; débridement or nail removal may be needed
Tinea versicolor	PO azole, selenium sulfide shampoo or lotion, ketoconazole shampoo	Azole or terbinafine	Recurrence common; hypopigmentation may persist despite treatment
Candidiasis	Topical azole or nystatin	PO or IV azole, amphotericin B (Fungizone)	Improve underlying cause such as moisture, diabetes

*All treatments are topical except as noted.
[†]Topical azoles include clotrimazole (Lotrimin), econazole, ketoconazole, miconazole, oxiconazole, and tioconazole.
[‡]PO azoles include ketoconazole, fluconazole, and itraconazole.
[§]Itraconazole pulse therapy: 200 mg PO twice daily for 1 week of the month, repeated for 3 to 4 consecutive months.
[‖]Terbinafine pulse therapy: 500 mg/d PO for 1 week of the month, repeated for 3 to 4 consecutive months.
IV, intravenously; PO, by mouth.

immunocompromised individuals, but it also occurs frequently in those without predisposing conditions. Various forms of onychomycosis may occur, but the most common begins at the distal and lateral subungual margins of the nail, may extend to involve the whole nail, and is caused by *T. rubrum*. Affected nails are typically thickened and raised, with white or yellow discoloration and various degrees of cracking. Nail growth may be impaired, and at times the nail dislodges spontaneously or with minor pressure. Candidiasis of the nails almost exclusively involves the fingernails, sometimes inoculated by nail biting, and it is usually less extensive than typical dermatophytic infection.

TINEA (PITYRIASIS) VERSICOLOR

Tinea versicolor is not a true tinea infection because it is caused by lipophilic skin commensals of the *Malassezia* genus, most commonly *Malassezia furfur*. This common infection is characterized by hypopigmented or hyperpigmented macules of the trunk or proximal ends of the extremities, sometimes with scaling. The diagnosis is usually clinical, but it can be confirmed by a scraping that demonstrates numerous round yeasts with short hyphae. After treatment, the pigmentation changes may persist for weeks or months, often until subsequent sun exposure.

CANDIDIASIS

Candida species are normal colonizers of the mouth and vagina, but especially in settings such as antibiotic exposure, dry mouth, excessive skin moisture, extremes of age, and immunocompromise, they can cause disease on the skin and mucosal surfaces. In the mouth or vagina, candidiasis is suggested by white plaques, cheesy exudates, and erythema. Candidiasis of the mouth can also be manifested in other forms such as erythematous plaques, angular cheilitis, acute or chronic atrophic lesions (the latter in the setting of dentures), or chronic hypertrophic plaques. Candidiasis of the skin most commonly occurs in moist or occluded areas such as the groin, buttocks (especially under diapers), and axilla, but it can involve any area, including the nails (described earlier). "Satellite lesions" help differentiate skin candidiasis from tinea or other conditions.

TREATMENT

See Table 1.

DISEASES OF THE MOUTH

method of
FRANK C. POWELL, M.D., and
SHARAREH AHMADI, M.B., MRCPI
Regional Centre of Dermatology
Mater Misericordiae Hospital
Dublin, Ireland

Diseases of the mouth can be a source of misery for both patients and physicians who are unfamiliar with the approach to examination of this area. They may represent a localized anomaly of limited significance or the presentation of potentially life-threatening multisystem disease. Evaluation of a patient with oral lesions requires a systematic approach with resources to appropriate investigations in certain circumstances. Many oral lesions can be diagnosed by obtaining a full history, including family history, drug ingestion, symptoms of concurrent systemic disease, and careful clinical examination carried out in good lighting of the mouth, lips, surrounding skin, and draining lymph nodes. A general physical examination is necessary if an oral presentation of systemic disease is suspected. Occasionally a biopsy is required to provide histologic solution to more difficult problems.

This article should enable physicians to approach the diagnosis and management of the common lesions, which affect the lips, oral cavity, and tongue, with a degree of confidence. Access to an atlas of oral lesions is essential to those whose experience is limited in this area.

DISORDERS OF THE LIPS

Cheilitis

Cheilitis is the term applied to any inflammatory condition involving the lips.

Drug-Induced Cheilitis

Retinoids, such as etretinate*,† and isotretinoin,* cause dryness and cracking of the lips in most patients. The mechanism of this pharmacologic effect is unknown, but is dose related. Patients should be instructed to apply frequent greasy lubricants.

Infective Cheilitis

Recurrent herpes labialis is a common cause of blisters at the mucocutaneous junction. Itchy papules progress to vesicles, pustules, and finally crusts. They occasionally become infected with *Staphylococcus* or *Streptococcus*, resulting in impetiginized lesions. Acyclovir 5%* cream should be applied five times daily at the first sign of infection and fusidic acid 2% cream† added in the latter stages if impetiginization is suspected.

Herpes zoster and papillomaviruses also affect the lips, which is the most common extragenital site for

*Not FDA approved for this indication.
†Not available in the United States.

primary syphilitic lesions. In males these tend to occur on the upper lip and in females on the lower lip. In secondary syphilis, moist, flat, warty lesions (condylomata lata) may appear at the mucocutaneous junctions and commissures.

Actinic Cheilitis

This premalignant condition tends to primarily affect the protuberant lower lip of adults who have had prolonged sun exposure. It is manifested by hyperkeratosis and desquamation. As the condition become more established, crusting, erosions, and intermittent bleeding occurs. Biopsy may be necessary to evaluate the degree of dysplasia. Treatment with 5% fluorouracil (Efudex),* topical tretinoin (Retin-A),* CO_2 laser, or 5% imiquimod (Aldara)* cream can be effective in clearing lesions of actinic cheilitis, but discomfort and local irritation will be experienced with many of these products. If ulceration or any infiltration suggestive of invasive tumor is detected, surgical excision is the treatment of choice.

Angular Cheilitis

Angular cheilitis (perleche) are recurrent painful fissures at the commissures of the lips with surrounding erythema and scaling from which *Candida albicans*, *Staphylococcus aureus,* or streptococci may be cultured. Perleche may result from mechanical irritation (dentures), nutritional deficiency, or overfolding of the lips, which promotes accumulation of saliva, and erosion of intact skin facilitating the growth of bacteria and yeast in these areas. It is most often seen in the elderly or the immunocompromised patient.

Treatment may require new dentures, miconazole nitrate 2% cream (Monistat),* and fusidic acid 2% cream*,† applied locally. Plastic surgical correction of overfolding skin may be necessary in some cases.

Exfoliative Cheilitis

Exfoliative cheilitis is characterized by scaling, erythema, and desquamation of the keratinized labial surface and vermilion border due to repetitive biting, picking, or licking of the lips. In adult patients, underlying psychiatric disturbance or personality disorder may be suspected.

Granulomatous Cheilitis

This is a rare, chronic, soft-to-firm nontender swelling of one or both lips, which shows granulomatous changes on histology. Extraintestinal Crohn's disease and sarcoidosis should be considered in the differential diagnosis. The granulomatous changes may be confined to the lips (Miescher's cheilitis) or be associated with scrotal tongue and recurrent facial palsy (Melkersson-Rosenthal syndrome). The swelling may eventually become permanent. This condition is poorly responsive to therapy. Injection of 1 mL (10 mg) of triamcinolone* into the affected lips, repeated every 4 to 6 months may help. This may be combined with surgical reduction (cheiloplasty).

*Not FDA approved for this indication.
†Not available in the United States.

Contact Cheilitis

This acute weeping dermatitis of the lips is due to irritant or allergic contact factors. Lipstick may be responsible, and following sensitization, their further use is contraindicated. When the dermatitis extends beyond the lips into the oral cavity, toothpaste and mouthwashes should be suspected. Topical triamcinolone acetonide* 0.1% in emollient oral paste is useful to treat the dermatitis on the labial and mucosal surfaces.

Tumors

Benign Tumors

Benign tumors of the lips are relatively common and should be recognized easily by the examining physician.

Mucocele. A labial mucosal cyst presents as a raised, soft dome-shaped lesion on the lower lip with a slight bluish tinge. They are usually asymptomatic, originate from minor salivary glands or their ducts, and can occur at any age. They appear abruptly, increase in size rapidly, and tend to be persistent. Simple excision is usually curative, and allows confirmation of the benign nature of one of the commonest cysts of oral soft tissue.

Fordyce Spots. These represent ectopic sebaceous glands and appear as small, discrete white-to-yellow papules. They commonly occur at the commissures of the lips and on the anterior buccal mucosa. They are asymptomatic and require no treatment.

Malignant Tumors

Squamous Cell Carcinoma. This is the commonest malignancy to affect the lip and usually arises in an area of actinic damage. Tobacco smoking is also a major risk factor. Like actinic cheilitis, it is more common in men with outdoor activity and mainly affects the lower lip. Surgical excision following early diagnosis is the preferred mode of therapy because these lesions can metastasize early.

Lentigo Maligna. This is melanoma in situ. It may occur on the labial surface. The lesion requires total surgical excision with long-term follow-up.

Melanoma. This is usually darkish brown to black in tumor, but amelanotic lesions have been reported. It is rare and has a poor prognosis. Lesions are usually asymptomatic in the early stages, and bleeding may be the first sign. The typical sites of involvement include the lips and gingiva. Asians appear more predisposed to this malignancy than do whites.

Vascular Tumors

Venous lake. This appears as a small, bluish purple, soft swelling, usually on the lower lip of elderly people. The lesion blanches on prolonged pressure. It may

*Not FDA approved for this indication.

bleed after trauma and is treated with electrocautery, argon laser, or surgical excision.

Telangiectasia. These may occur sporadically, or be seen in hereditary hemorrhagic telangiectasia, and in acquired disorders such as the CREST syndrome, chronic liver disease, pregnancy, and post irradiation. If required for cosmetic reasons cauterization or laser therapy is effective.

Pigmentation

Ephelides are sun-induced freckles, which occur most frequently in childhood, and tend to reduce in number with age. They are usually multiple, uniform light tan color, less than 1 cm in size with regular outline. They appear and darken with sun exposure and tend to fade in its absence. No treatment is required.

Solar lentigos are more common in older individuals and persist indefinitely. They range in size from 2 mm to 2 cm and are usually tan to dark brown in color. Variation in color or irregularity of outline should raise the suspicion of lentigo maligna and is an indication for histologic evaluation. Nonsun-exposed lentigos may be the component of the LEOPARD, LAMB, CARNEY or NAME syndromes.

Nevi may be found on the keratinized epithelium of the lip, the buccal mucosa, and the hard and soft palates.

Labial melanotic macules are common small, discrete, macular areas of hyperpigmentation ranging from tan to dark brown in color. They may be irregular in outline and can enlarge up to 1 cm in diameter. They mainly affect the lower lip and typically present between the ages of 35 and 42 years. The etiology is unclear, but there may be a genetic predisposition. Malignancy has not been reported to develop in these lesions, but establishing the diagnosis may require a skin biopsy.

DISORDERS OF THE ORAL CAVITY

Stomatitis Medicamentosa

This is a drug eruption affecting the oral mucous membranes, which may represent an idiosyncratic reaction or a toxic or pharmacologic effect. Cytotoxic agents, such as methotrexate (Rheumatrex), may cause ulcerative stomatitis (most marked at sites of trauma). The tendency to develop diphenylhydantoin gingival hyperplasia can be reduced by meticulous oral hygiene, but the fibrotic enlargement may require surgical excision. Gold, penicillamine, and sulfonylureas may cause a lichenoid stomatitis. Pharmacologic reactions to drugs include: xerostoma with antihistamines and anticholinergics and hemorrhage with anticoagulants. Elimination of the suspected agent is often sufficient in management.

Stomatitis Nicotina

Stomatitis nicotina causes a grayish-white, wrinkled hard palate with papular swellings, resulting from enlargement of the palatal mucous glands and dilation of their ducts. They are seen in some heavy smokers and cessation of smoking leads to gradual resolution. No local therapy is required.

Herpes Gingivostomatitis

Herpes simplex virus (HSV) infection is a common infection affecting the oral mucosa. In general, HSV-1 causes primary herpetic stomatitis (and secondary infection of recurrent herpes labialis). Oral infection with HSV-2 may be sexually transmitted in saliva. The incubation period is 3 to 7 days. Many infections with HSV occur in childhood, and are subclinical. Symptomatic patients present with malaise, anorexia, fever, cervical lymphadenopathy, and diffuse, purple, boggy gingivitis, with multiple vesicles followed by erosion of the oral mucosa and gingiva. Stomatitis generally resolves in 7 to 10 days, but the virus may remain latent in the trigeminal ganglion. Reactivation can occur following sun exposure, trauma, or immunosuppression. Cytologic smear (Tzanck's preparation) is diagnostic of HSV if large, multinucleated, giant cells are seen. In mild cases, treatment with hydration, analgesics, and antimicrobial mouth washes (e.g., chlorhexidine gluconate 0.2% solution [Peridex]) is sufficient. Topical lidocaine may ease discomfort. In severe cases and in immunocompromized patients, acyclovir (Zovirax), 200 mg five times daily for adults (half dose for children, and double dose for immunocompromized patients) is used for primary infection and prophylactic antiviral drug therapy such as acyclovir, 400 mg twice daily may suppress frequent recurrent infection.

Herpes Zoster (Shingles)

Mouth ulcers are seen if shingles affect the maxillary or mandibular divisions of the trigeminal nerve. The initial symptoms are paresthesia and severe pain, which may simulate toothache. After 2 to 3 days vesicles with an erythematous base appear in crops along the affected dermatome. Ulcers appear on the site of the mucosa affected, and resolve spontaneously. Postherpetic neuralgia can be distressing. Treatment with acyclovir (800 mg five times daily for 7 to 10 days), valacyclovir (Valtrex) (1 g three times daily for 7 days), or famciclovir (Famvir) (500 mg three times daily for 7 days) is helpful if initiated early in the process. Tricyclic antidepressants, such as nortriptyline (Pamelor)* (10 to 25 mg at night) or gabapentin (Neurontin)* (300 mg 3×/d), have been used for postherpetic neuralgia.

Other Viral Infections

Epstein-Barr virus (EBV) appears in the saliva of patients with infectious mononucleosis and causes palate petechiae and white exudates on edematous tonsils with nonspecific oral ulceration. Oral hairy leukoplakia is seen in severe immunodeficiency, especially HIV infection, as a consequence of

*Not FDA approved for this indication.

opportunistic infection with EBV. Generally, the condition does not require treatment, but zidovudine (Retrovir)* or acyclovir* (800 mg four times daily) may also be useful, if symptomatic or very florid. Lesions usually recur when treatment is discontinued. Cytomegalovirus may also rarely cause oral ulceration. Herpangina is a self-limiting condition of young children caused by coxsackievirus, manifested by ulcers predominantly on the soft palate. Hand-foot-and-mouth disease is caused by coxsackie A virus. Any area of the mouth (especially the palate) may be involved with vesiculopustules, which superficially ulcerate. The condition is self-limiting. Condyloma acuminatum, verruca vulgaris, and human papillomavirus infection can also affect the oral mucosa and patients present with oral warts.

Candida

Candida albicans is a normal inhabitant of the oral cavity. However, when the patient's mucosal tissue resistance and immune responsiveness is reduced (chronic disease, cancer, diabetes, pregnancy, immunosuppressive or radiation therapy, broad-spectrum antibiotics, and oral contraceptives), it can become a significant pathogen invading the mucosa. The clinical features are creamy, milk-curd exudates on a bright erythematous base, which leaves a raw surface when scraped for culture specimen. In debilitated patients, oral candidiasis may give rise to a generalized erythematous atrophic mucosal inflammation. Chronic candidiasis in denture wearers causes a patchy inflammation of the palatal mucosa with a burning sensation of the roof of the mouth. Hyperplastic lesions may be mistaken for leukoplakia or tumors. Treatment with 1 mL of nystatin (Mycostatin) oral suspension four times daily or ketoconazole (Nizoral) 2% cream four times daily may be helpful. Systemic fluconazole (Diflucan) (100 mg daily for 7 to 10 days), or itraconazole (Sporanox) (200 mg daily for 7 to 10 days) has proved beneficial in many patients with persistent infection, despite topical therapy.

Acute Necrotizing Gingivitis (Vincent's Disease)

This is an acute onset of gingival soreness, bleeding, and halitosis caused by a mixed (mainly anaerobic) flora consisting of fusiform bacteria and spirochetes. Fatigue, stress, smoking, or immune defects are the main predisposing factors. The mouth ulceration is usually restricted to the interdental papillae. There may be pyrexia and malaise and cervical lymphadenopathy. Management is supportive with improvement of oral hygiene. Regular cleansing with chlorhexidine gluconate 0.2% solution mouthwash and soft toothbrush is very effective. Oral metronidazole (Flagyl),* 200 mg three times daily for 7 days may be required for severe cases.

*Not FDA approved for this indication.

Syphilis

Primary chancres may involve the palate as small, firm, pink, macules or papules, which progress to form painless ulcers. Chancres heal spontaneously in 3 to 8 weeks and are highly infectious. Diagnosis is by dark-ground microscopy and serologic testing and treatment is with appropriate antibiotics.

Tumors

Benign

Benign tumors are rare in the oral cavity. Multiple neurofibromas may be seen in the oral cavity in von Recklinghausen's disease and in the multiple endocrine adenopathy syndromes (Sipple's syndrome).

Premalignant

Leukoplakia refers to white, keratotic plaquelike lesions seen in the oral cavity. The etiology is unknown. Some may be due to chronic physical (sharp edges of carious teeth) or chemical (tobacco) irritation, or chronic candidiasis. Varying degrees of dysplasia may be seen histologically. Only a small portion of leukoplakias are malignant, but all persistent lesions should be biopsied. Lesions on the tongue and floor of the mouth are more likely to become malignant. Leukokeratoses are small white plaques due to mucosal thickening caused by trauma, (cheek biting or sucking of the buccal occlusal linea alba). Single, small lesions can be treated with topical tretinoin (Retin-A).* Surgical excision, electrocautery, or vaporization by CO_2 laser may be indicated if induration or ulceration is apparent.

Erythroplasia is a red, velvety plaque involving the floor of the mouth, tongue, and the soft palate. It occurs with or without leukoplakia and diagnosis should be confirmed histologically. In 90% of cases an in situ or invasive carcinoma is demonstrable. Surgical excision is the treatment of choice. Heavy alcohol consumption and smoking may predispose to erythroplasia.

Malignant Tumor

Squamous cell carcinoma accounts for 90% of the malignant lesions of the mouth. The morphology is varied from asymptomatic red plaque with indistinct borders to white plaque or more florid ulcerations. A high index of suspicion and a willingness to obtain tissue samples promptly are necessary because 60% of oral cancers are advanced at the time of diagnosis and there is only a 30% 5-year survival rate. Extensive and mutilating surgery may be required to remove these lesions once they have developed as an aggressive, invasive state.

Vascular Lesions

Haemangioma The presence of multiple vascular tufts throughout the oral cavity suggests Rendu-Osler-Weber disease. Port-wine stain of the mucosa may appear as a part of the Sturge-Weber syndrome.

*Not FDA approved for this indication.

Treatment options include surgical excision, corticosteroid injection, and laser ablation.

Kaposi's sarcoma is a multicentric angiogenic tumor associated with HIV infection, presenting usually as red, blue, or purple patches later becoming nodular and ulcerating if traumatized, causing pain. It most commonly affects the junction of the hard and soft palate. Radiotherapy or intralesional injection with recombinant interferon (1–3 million units once a week) is the treatment of choice for isolated oral lesions. If disseminated lesions are present, chemotherapy with bleomycin (Blenoxane)* (15 mg IV twice a week up to 180-200 mg) or interferon-α-2A (3–6 million every other day) can be helpful.

Pyogenic granuloma is a pedunculated or sessile, red, painless nodule that grows rapidly and commonly affects the gingiva, lip, or tongue.

Granuloma gravidarum (pregnancy tumor) refers to an interdental pyogenic granuloma—the gingival reactions during pregnancy. Regression may take place spontaneously after delivery. Bleeding may be a problem (caused by trauma associated with eating or brushing of the teeth) and surgical removal may be necessary. Attention to oral hygiene is an important component of the management.

Pigmented Lesions

Pigmentation of the gingiva may be physiologic (in dark-skinned individual), occur during pregnancy, or while taking oral contraceptive pills. Localized pigmented lesions, such as melanotic macules, and nevi may be found on the buccal and palatal mucosa. Melanoma may occur intraorally, so a high index of suspicion is warranted with early biopsy of unstable or irregularly pigmented lesions.

GENERALIZED PIGMENTATION

Pigmentation of the oral region may be associated with the disorders listed in Table 1, the drugs listed in Table 2, amalgam tattoo (due to presence of foreign material), poor oral hygiene, carotenemia, arsenic poisoning, or scurvy.

Aphthous Ulceration

Recurrent aphthous stomatitis (RAS) is a common and difficult-to-treat ulcer of the oral cavity. Aphthous ulceration may arise in Behçet's disease, Sweet's syndrome, nutritional and mineral deficiencies, and gastrointestinal disorders. Recurrent bouts of rounded, shallow, painful oral ulcers occur at intervals of a few months to a few days. Based primarily on the size of the lesions, aphthous ulcers are classified into three types:

1. **Herpetiform ulcers** are 1 to 2 mm in size and can affect any part of the oral cavity. They often begin as grouped vesicles surrounded by a halo of erythema. These may coalesce into plaques and form ulcers that require weeks to heal. These lesions are not caused by a viral infection.
2. **Minor aphthous ulcers** are the commonest form and usually present as recurrent, multiple, small, shallow ulcerations with a yellow pseudomembranous floor on the mucolabial sulci, tongue, and nonkeratinized oral mucosa. Lesions resolve in 7 to 14 days.
3. **Major aphthous ulcers** are recurrent, large, often solitary lesions with a surrounding zone of erythema. They can occur in any area of the mouth, but particularly on the labial mucosa, tongue, or the posterior oral mucosa. Lesions begin as nodules, and subsequently form deep ulcerations, which may extend to involve underlying connective tissue and musculature. Resolution may occur with residual scar with retraction of surrounding tissue. Reduction of trauma, correction of dental defects, and meticulous oral hygiene may help to prevent RAS. Chlorhexidine (Peridex)* (0.2% W/W mouth rinse or 1% gel) can reduce the duration of the ulcers. Lidocaine gel applied three times daily can produce transient pain relief. Antihistamine solutions (Bendramine* or Chlortrimeton*) may provide sufficient topical anesthesia to allow eating. Topical tetracycline* may reduce healing times and the associated pain. Triamcinolone acetonide (Kenalog),* fluocinonide (Lidex),* and clobetasol (Temovate),* applied at 6-hour intervals are usually helpful. Sodium cromoglycate lozenges may also provide mild symptomatic relief. Oral prednisolone* 30 to 60 mg daily should be reserved for severe cases of major aphthous ulcer. Azathioprine (Imuran),* colchicines,* cyclosporine (Neoral), dapsone,* and thalidomide* have been reported to be effective but toxicity limits their clinical application.

*Not FDA approved for this indication.

TABLE 1. **Generalized Hyperpigmentation of the Oral Cavity**

Gastrointestinal polyposis—Peutz-Jeghers syndrome
Cardiomyopathy
Myxoma syndrome
Albright's syndrome
Addison's disease
Acromegaly
Cushing's disease
Nelson's disease
Hyperthyroidism
Hemochromatosis

TABLE 2. **Drugs Causing Oral Pigmentation**

Nicotine	Heroin
Busulfan	Doxorubicin
Bleomycin	Cyclophosphamide
Antimalarial	Phenothiazines
Oral contraceptives	AZT (Zidovudine)
Ketoconazole	Clofazimine
Tetracycline	Minocycline
Arsenic	Silver
Gold	Lead
Premarin	Amiodarone
Clofazimine	Nitrogen mustard

*Not FDA approved for this indication.

β-blockers (e.g., propranolol),* at low dose may have some role in reducing the frequency of recurrence of aphthous ulcers. Women with menstrual-related aphthous ulceration may benefit from an estrogen-dominant* oral contraceptive.

Chemical Burns

Salt, gum, escharotics, analgesics, or candy held in prolonged contact with the buccal mucosa and gingiva could cause chemical burn due to necrosis of tissue. These burns can be mistaken for malignant ulceration. Most of these lesions are painless.

DISORDERS OF THE TONGUE

Black Hairy Tongue

This condition is the result of hyperplasia of filiform papillae with increased pigment production by bacteria. The cause of the hyperplastic response of the papillae is not known, but it is suspected to relate to the change in microflora population. It often follows a course of antibiotic administration. Gentle cleansing twice daily with soft-bristled toothbrush and hydrogen peroxide solution is frequently satisfactory. Topical triamcinolone acetonide (Kenalog),* applied twice daily after wiping the tongue dry is also effective. A furry tongue may be seen in smokers and patients with febrile illness.

Median Rhomboid Glossitis

Median rhomboid glossitis is a dorsal midline plaquelike hypertrophy of the tongue, probably representing a form of chronic hyperplastic candidiasis.

Geographic Tongue

This is a common glossitis, which may be regarded as a variant of normal. There is cyclical atrophy and regrowth of filiform and spongiform papillae, which give the characteristic patchy lesions, surrounded by white keratotic margin. These are often multiple and typically occur on the dorsum of the tongue. Their appearance may vary within days, but the patient is often asymptomatic or experiences mild discomfort with hot, salty, or spicy foods. Geographic tongue is not related to the subsequent development of oral disease, and reassurance is usually the only therapy required with avoidance of potential irritants. The differential diagnosis of geographic tongue is listed in Table 3.

Scrotal Tongue

This is a developmental defect in which the tongue appears enlarged with multiple deep fissures or sulci. It may be seen in association with the Melkersson-Rosenthal syndrome, Sjogren's syndrome, and Down syndrome. Local hygiene is often required to remove food and debris from the fissures.

*Not FDA approved for this indication.

TABLE 3. **Differential Diagnosis of Geographic Tongue**

Lichen planus
Leukoplakia
Reiter's syndrome
Pustular psoriasis
Pityriasis rosea
Pityriasis rubra pilaris
Secondary syphilis
Miliary tuberculosis
Drug eruption

Smooth Tongue

This condition results from atrophy of the filiform papillae. The smooth tongue may be due to nutritional deficiencies or various systemic conditions (Table 4). There can be considerable discomfort, and a burning sensation may occur spontaneously, or after ingestion of sour, salty, or spicy foods.

Glossodynia

Glossodynia (paresthesia of the tongue) is a syndrome of burning or stinging sensation of the tongue with no visible lesions. Many patients with this condition suffer from psychiatric disease such as anxiety or depression. These patients should be appropriately investigated, as many will have correctable causative factors (Table 5).

Varicosity

Varicose veins on the ventral surface of the tongue are common with aging and are not of any diagnostic significance. Occasionally, a single varix may be noted as a soft purple papule that indents with firm palpation. Varices may also appear on the lateral border of the tongue or labial mucosa. No treatment is necessary once the diagnosis is established.

Lymphangioma

These lesions are usually solitary, red-yellow nodules that affect the tongue predominantly. They are

TABLE 4. **Differential Diagnosis of Smooth Tongue**

Iron deficiency anemia
Plummer-Vinson syndrome
Pernicious anemia (Hunter's glossitis)
Riboflavin deficiency
Pellagra (cardinal's tongue)
Celiac disease
Sjögren syndrome
Malnutrition
Antibiotic therapy
Cardiac failure
Amyloidosis
Syphilis

TABLE 5. **Factors Related to Glossodynia**

Pernicious anemia
Iron deficiency
Folate deficiency
Antibiotic therapy
Stomatitis medicamentosa
Xerostomia
Trigeminal neuralgia
Vascular thrombosis/spasm
Hiatus hernia
Referred pain from dental disease
Denture sore mouth

usually asymptomatic, but as they enlarge in size, pain and discomfort may be felt during speaking, chewing, and swallowing. Surgical excision is the only treatment for symptomatic patients.

SYSTEMIC DISEASES AND THE MOUTH

Hematologic Disease

Iron deficiency anemia causes a smooth tongue. In the Plummer-Vinson syndrome, koilonychiae, leukoplakia, and oral and esophageal carcinoma occur in addition to angular stomatitis. A magenta, lobulated tongue with glossodynia may be noted with pernicious anemia. Bleeding from the gingiva may be the initial manifestation of hemorrhagic diseases, whereas patients with polycythemia rubra vera may present with purple engorged gingiva. Patients with leukemia may present with gingival hyperplasia. Neutropenia can cause oral ulceration that may become extensive and necrotic.

Gastrointestinal disease: Both aphthous ulceration and nodular oral lesions, which show noncaseating granuloma, have been recorded in Crohn's disease. In ulcerative colitis, stomatitis, and pyostomatitis vegetans may be seen.

Diabetes mellitus: Gingival inflammation, periodontitis, recurrent candidiasis, and glossodynia may be seen.

Lupus erythematosus: The lower lip or the posterior buccal mucosa is most commonly involved, with erythema, superficial ulceration, or hyperkeratosis.

Amyloidosis: Macroglossia and purpuric plaques or nodules may be seen within the tongue and on other mucous membrane in primary amyloidosis.

Scleroderma: In systemic scleroderma, tissues of the mouth and lips become rigid and indurated.

Histiocytosis X: In histiocytosis X, granulomatous nodules may involve the gingiva. Mucous membrane ulceration is also observed.

DERMATOLOGIC DISEASE WITH ORAL MANIFESTATION

Pemphigus Vulgaris

A rare autoimmune skin disease, patients with pemphigus vulgaris often present with painful superficial oral erosions, which antedate skin lesions. Blisters in pemphigus are fragile and transient and the patient may be totally unaware of their existence. The most common affected sites are the palate, gingiva, and the buccal mucosa (sites of oral trauma). Diagnosis is confirmed by histology and immunofluorescence. Activity of disease is thought to be reflected in the titer of circulating antibody. It is important to exclude malignancy (e.g., lymphoma, leukemia, thymoma, and other solid tumors) because paraneoplastic pemphigus has severe mucocutaneous involvement. Early and aggressive specialist treatment is required.

Bullous Pemphigoid

This entity is more common than pemphigus. Thirty to forty percent of patients may have oral involvement, which usually develops when the disease established. Intact blisters may be seen in the oral mucosa as tense, fluid-filled blisters. Other oral lesions, such as erosion, ulcer, or desquamative gingivitis may occur. Diagnosis is confirmed by histology and immunofluorescence. A combination of tetracycline* or erythromycin* 500 mg four times daily and niacinamide* 1500 to 2000 mg/day may control this disease. Specialist referral is advised.

Cicatricial Pemphigoid

Cicatricial pemphigoid is an uncommon variant of bullous pemphigoid, which typically affects the oral and ocular mucosa. Skin lesions are uncommon. In the mouth, there are tense blisters or painful shallow erosions, typically on the gingival, buccal, or labial mucosa. Cicatricial pemphigoid is a frequent cause of desquamative gingivitis. Ocular scarring may occur, so early ophthalmologic consultation is advised.

Erythema Multiforme

Erythema multiforme is a reactive process that affects the skin and mucous membranes with an acute, self-limited course. Drugs (e.g., sulfonamides, anticonvulsants, barbiturates, and allopurinol) and infection (e.g., herpes simplex, or mycoplasma) are common precipitating factors. In the mouth, the lesions are less distinctive and the labial mucosa is typically involved, but the buccal and palatal mucosa can also be affected. Blisters, erosion, hemorrhagic crusts, or ulcerations may be manifested. Other mucosal surfaces such as conjunctiva and genitalia may be affected. Marked involvement of mucosal surfaces with severe constitutional disturbances is known as the Stevens-Johnson syndrome. Diagnosis is confirmed histologically. Swabs for viral culture may isolate herpes simplex virus, which has also been found with polymerase chain reaction (PCR) in the lesion and blood samples. Treatment is mainly supportive. Continuous oral acyclovir (Zovirax)* (400 mg twice daily) or valacyclovir (Valtrex)* (500 mg daily) are helpful to prevent recurrent herpes simplex infection. Azathioprine (Imuran)* 100 to 200 mg/day

*Not FDA approved for this indication.

can be used in patients with severe mucosal involvement. The use of systemic steroids in this condition is controversial.

Lichen Planus

Oral lichen planus affects 1% to 2% of the general adult population. Typical lesions are striations, papules, plaques, mucosal atrophy, erosions (shallow ulcers), or blisters affecting buccal mucosa, tongue, and gingiva. Lesions are usually bilateral and erosive lesions are painful and sensitive. There may be skin, genitalia, and nail involvement. Oral lichenoid lesions may be a complication of systemic medications such as nonsteroidal anti-inflammatory drugs (NSAIDs) and β-blockers. There is ongoing concern that oral lichen planus may be premalignant and biopsy is required to rule out other white or chronic ulcerative lesions, including reactive keratosis, chronic candidiasis, epithelial dysplasia, discoid lupus erythematosus, and malignancy. Treatment should include proper oral hygiene. Localized lesions may be treated with betamethasone propionate ointment* (0.05%), applied 3 to 4 times daily. Intralesional triamcinolone acetonide* (0.5 mL) can be used for persistent localized lesions. Dexamethasone* (0.025 mg) mouth rinse twice daily can be used for generalized lesions. Other topical treatments such as topical tretinoin* and cyclosporine* have also been used with limited success. Recently, topical tacrolimus (Protopic)* 0.1% ointment twice daily has been used for treatment of erosive oral lichen planus with limited local or systemic side effects. Short course of systemic steroid is used for lesions that are unresponsive to topical treatment. The combination of systemic and topical steroid therapy is often very effective. Systemic treatment with cyclosporine,* azathioprine,* retinoids,* dapsone,* and thalidomide has also been reported.

*Not FDA approved for this indication.

VENOUS ULCERS

method of
CARLOS A. CHARLES, M.D., and
ANNA F. FALABELLA, M.D.
University of Miami School of Medicine
Miami, Florida

Venous ulcers are the most common type of leg ulcer encountered in clinical practice. Up to 80% of all leg ulcers are caused by venous disease, whereas arterial disease accounts for another 10% to 25%. Less commonly, trauma, prolonged pressure, neuropathy, and malignant, inflammatory, and infectious agents are the cause of leg ulcers. Table 1 outlines the lengthy differential diagnosis of leg ulcerations. The various etiologies of leg ulcers can overlap with each other, as well as with coexisting disease, because these conditions are not mutually exclusive. Though commonly described as "venous stasis ulcers," patients with venous insufficiency actually have increased blood flow locally.

Venous blood in the lower extremities flows into a vascular system composed of three main components: the superficial, communicating, and deep veins. The long and short saphenous veins and their tributaries make up the superficial system, and these vessels are connected through smaller communicating or perforator veins to the deep system. The vessels of all three components are equipped with one-way bicuspid valves that force blood flow toward the deep system and in the cephalad direction. Blood is propelled from the legs toward the heart primarily by the pumping action of the leg muscles during ambulation; this entire system is collectively known as the calf muscle pump.

In the setting of a diseased venous system or failure of the calf muscle pump, lower extremity venous blood pressure remains elevated during ambulation. This phenomenon is known as venous hypertension. More specifically, incompetence of valves within the venous system, venous distention, deep venous outflow obstruction, calf muscle weakness, or a decrease in range of motion of the ankle all may lead to venous hypertension (Figure 1). The exact mechanism by which venous hypertension leads to ulceration is unclear, but it has been hypothesized that elevated pressure causes vascular changes that result in adherence of white blood cells to endothelial cells. This adherence may induce changes in capillary permeability and deposition of fibrin and other macromolecules around blood vessels. Extravasated macromolecules are hypothesized to bind growth factors, as well as other stimulatory and homeostatic substances, thereby rendering them physiologically "trapped" and unavailable for the healing process. Patients with venous disease may also have a systemic alteration in fibrinolysis contributing to the aforementioned processes.

EVALUATION

The diagnosis of venous ulcers is usually based solely on clinical findings and depends on a thorough history and physical examination (Figure 2). Venous ulcers are characteristically located around the medial aspect of the lower part of the leg near the ankle. Varicose veins ranging from submalleolar flare to various degrees of vessel dilation are often present. Additionally, venous ulcers are typically associated with induration, fibrosis, and pigmentation of the surrounding skin. These clinical findings are collectively known as lipodermatosclerosis. The presence of a lower leg ulcer associated with lipodermatosclerosis and/or varicose veins is highly suggestive of a venous ulcer. Other common physical findings include atrophie blanche, characterized by porcelain white scars with telangiectasia and depigmentation, and dermatitis, characterized by eczematous changes with redness, scaling, and pruritus. The shape of the leg may also provide a diagnostic clue in that the "inverted bottle shape" with associated

TABLE 1. **Differential Diagnosis of Leg Ulcers**

VASCULAR DISEASES	DRUGS–cont'd
Arterial (hypertensive atherosclerotic, vasospastic)	Drug-induced vasculitis
Venous (venous stasis ulcer)	Anticoagulant necrosis (warfarin [Coumadin], heparin)
Lymphedema	Hydroxyurea (Hydrea)
METABOLIC DISORDERS	HEMATOLOGIC ABNORMALITIES
Diabetes mellitus	Hypercoagulable states (protein C, S, antithrombin III deficiency, antigen-presenting cell resistance, prothrombin gene polymorphism)
Necrobiosis lipoidica diabeticorum	Lupus anticoagulant syndrome
Porphyria cutanea tarda	Paroxysmal nocturnal hemoglobinuria
Gout	Sickle cell anemia
Pancreatitic (pancreatitis, carcinoma)	Thalassemia
INFECTIONS	Polycythemia vera
Bacterial (especially *Staphylococcus aureus, Streptococcus*)	Leukemia
Spirochetal (syphilis)	Dysproteinemia (cryoglobulinemia, macroglobulinemia)
Fungal (deep fungal, mycetoma)	TUMORS
Opportunistic in immunocompromised hosts	Cutaneous (basal cell cancer, squamous cell cancer, sarcoma, malignant melanoma, Merkel cell)
Viral	Secondary (metastatic carcinoma, lymphoma
VASCULITIS	Kaposi's sarcoma
Hypersensitivity vasculitis	MISCELLANEOUS
Polyarteritis	Pyoderma gangrenosum
Systemic lupus erythematosus	Trauma (including factitial)
Rheumatoid vasculitis	Burns
Wegener's granulomatosis	Pressure ulcers, neuropathic ulcers
Lymphomatoid granulomatosis	Insect bites (brown recluse spider)
LYMPHEDEMA	Ulcerative lichen planus
Congenital	Bullous diseases (epidermolysis bullosa)
Postinfectious	Sweet's syndrome
Postsurgical	Idiopathic
Postirradiation	
DRUGS	
Halogens (bromide, iodide)	
Ergotism	

From Burton, CS: Leg ulcers. *In* Rakel RE, Bope ET (eds): Conn's Current Therapy 2002. Philadelphia, WB Saunders, 2002.

lipodermatosclerosis is a clinical sign of persistent venous disease (Figure 3A and B).

A definitive diagnosis of venous disease can be made by a variety of techniques, including duplex ultrasound and plethysmography. However, it is also important to exclude arterial disease because treatment with compression bandages is the mainstay of therapy, and this treatment modality should be used cautiously in patients with arterial insufficiency. A simple examination to determine arterial function is the ankle-brachial index (ABI). The ABI is obtained by dividing systolic pressure in the ankle by that in the arm, and a ratio less than 0.8 is abnormal. An ABI less than 0.7 indicates moderate arterial insufficiency. Additionally, an abnormal ABI is an independent risk factor for disease in other vascular beds such as the coronary arteries. Patients with an abnormal ABI require further evaluation. Diabetic or elderly patients may have a falsely elevated ABI as a result of calcification of the blood vessels. In these specific cases in which the ABI is overtly elevated (>1.3), further evaluation for arterial insufficiency can be accomplished by measurement of great toe arterial pressure, referred to as the toe-brachial index.

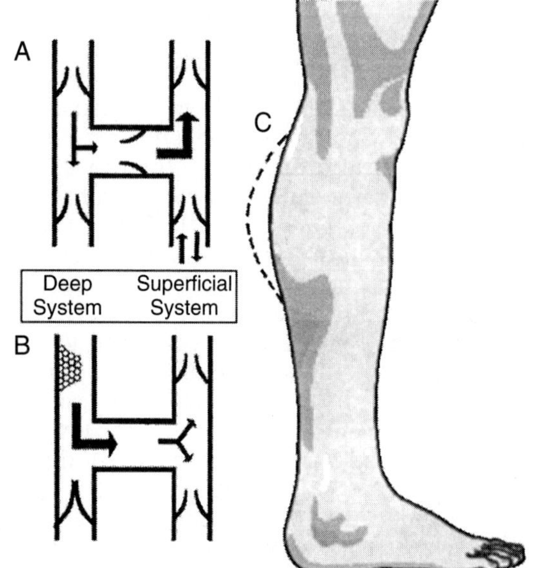

Figure 1. Mechanism of venous insufficiency. (From Valencia IC, Falabella A, Kirsner RS, Eaglstein WH: Chronic venous insufficiency and venous leg ulceration. J Am Acad Dermatol 44:401–421, 2001.)

TREATMENT

Along with healing of the venous ulcer, treatment goals include alleviation of pain, reduction of edema, and improvement of lipodermatosclerosis. Paramount to achieving these goals is reversal of the damaging effects of venous hypertension through compression

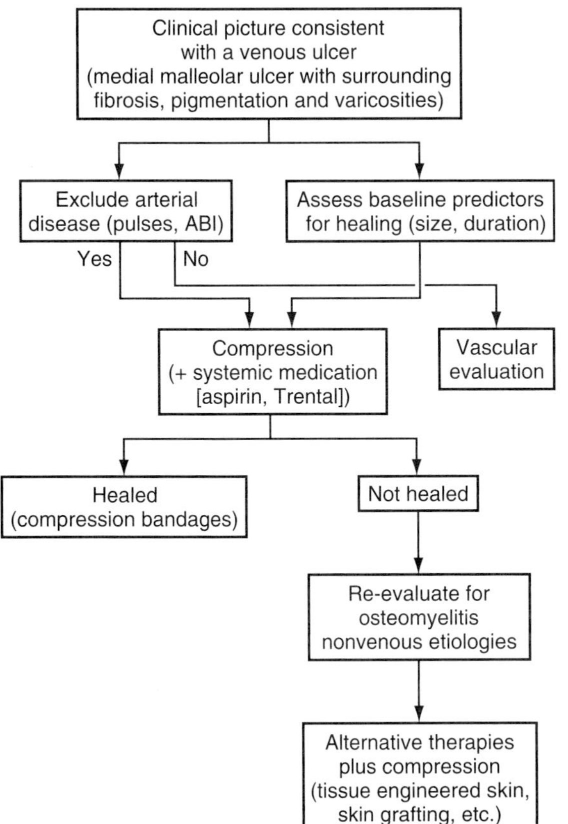

Figure 2. Simplified algorithm for the diagnosis and treatment of patients with venous ulcers.

bandages and leg elevation. The aim of compression therapy is to deliver sustained graded compression of 30 to 40 mm Hg at the ankle. The optimal method to deliver this pressure is through multilayered elastic compression bandages applied circumferentially from the toes to the knees, with the bandage covering the heel. Elastic compression bandages are superior to short stretch (inelastic) bandages in that they deliver compression both at work, when the patient is ambulating, and at rest; furthermore, they can be adjusted to provide uniform compression subsequent to a reduction in edema. Patients with associated lymphatic damage may also benefit from pneumatic compression. Systemic pharmacotherapy for the treatment of venous ulcers may be useful as an adjuvant to compression therapy. Specifically, compression bandages plus either pentoxifylline (Trental)* or aspirin* may be superior to compression bandages alone with regard to the rate of healing. Systemic antibiotics have not been shown to increase the rate of healing, and their use should be limited to ulcers with clinically proven infections such as cellulitis or osteomyelitis.

Local wound care is best achieved through the use of occlusive dressings. By providing a moist environment, occlusive dressings optimize wound healing. A wide assortment of occlusive dressings may be used, with the choice depending on several factors, including the location of the wound, the amount of exudate

*Not FDA approved for this indication.

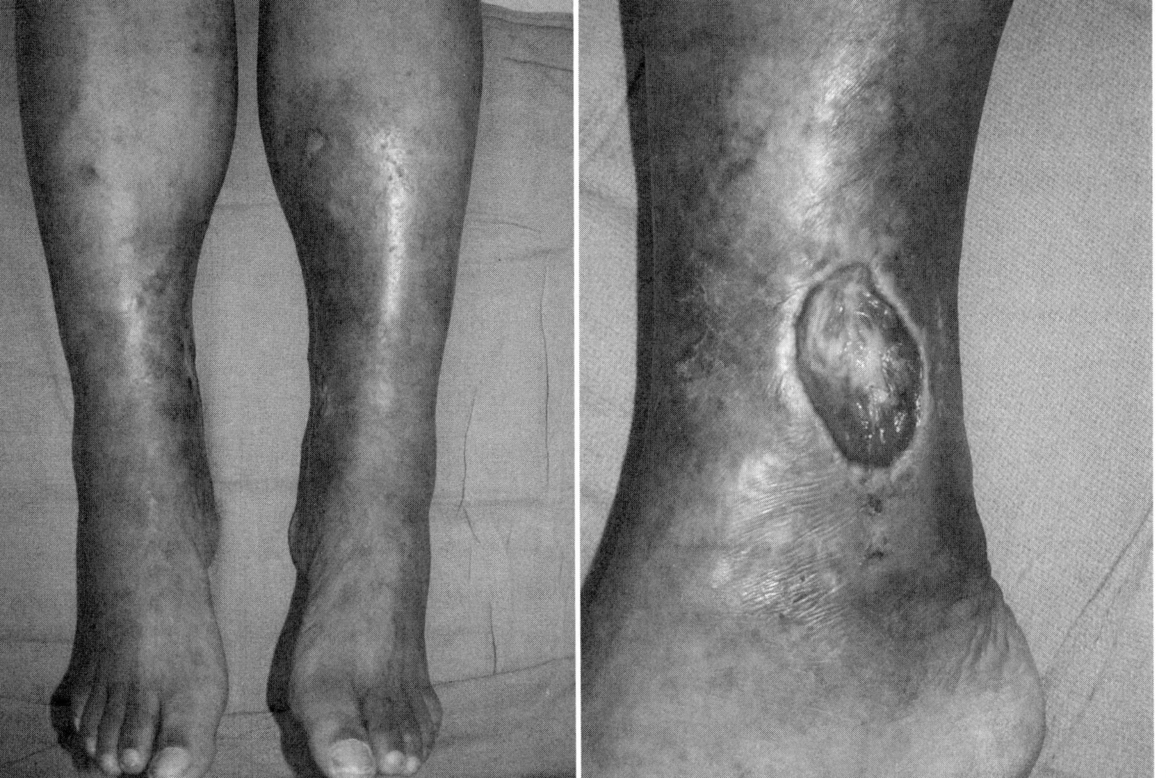

Figure 3. A, Advanced lipodermatosclerosis with the classic "inverted champagne bottle" appearance of the legs, pigmentary changes, and sclerotic, bound-down skin. **B,** Venous ulcer in a typical location, above the medial malleolus. Note the shallow wound bed with irregular borders and a base of red granulation tissue and yellow fibrinous debris.

present, and the shape and size of the wound. The fear of infection with the use of occlusive dressings is unproven. Current research has focused on the issue of wound bed preparation, or treatment of the wound bed to accelerate endogenous healing. Within this framework, the use of enzyme-containing agents such as urea and collagenase has been studied for the purpose of débridement, stimulation of granulation tissue formation and angiogenesis, and acceleration of re-epithelialization. The use of topical antiseptics and cleansing agents is controversial, and they should be applied with caution because they may prolong healing by having deleterious effects on viable cells critical to the regenerative process. However, studies on the direct effect of cadexomer iodine preparations on both human fibroblasts in culture and neonatal skin explants have shown excellent safety profiles in addition to conferring significant antimicrobial activity and stimulating the formation of granulation tissue to promote wound healing. Additionally, alternative products such as silver-impregnated dressings and topical anesthetics are commonly used agents that may be of benefit for antimicrobial activity and pain reduction, respectively, while not having any detrimental effect on wound healing.

Other clinical findings should lead the clinician to pursue different etiologies for the leg ulceration. The presence of exposed tendon or bone should prompt further workup and lead to examination for underlying osteomyelitis. Radiographs, nuclear bone scans, and biopsy for histology and culture should provide an initial assessment. Additionally, venous ulcers rarely demonstrate the presence of eschar or necrotic tissue, and these clinical findings may suggest diagnoses such as pyoderma gangrenosum, vasculitis, or other inflammatory conditions associated with cutaneous ulceration.

Studies have demonstrated that up to 40% to 50% of venous ulcers may be refractory to compression therapy alone. These refractory ulcers may be identified by baseline characteristics such as size (>5 cm^2) and duration (>6 months), as well as failure to decrease in size with 2 to 4 weeks of compression therapy. Other prognostic factors associated with failure to heal after compressive therapy include the following: a history of hip or knee replacement surgery, compromised arterial circulation (ABI <0.8), and/or the presence of fibrinous exudate on more than 50% of the wound surface. These factors should always be considered when initially evaluating a venous ulcer because they may help identify wounds that will require the attention of a wound care subspecialist or treatment with novel therapies such as tissue-engineered or autologous skin. Venous surgery or treatment with locally delivered growth factors may also be beneficial in this subset of ulcers.

Once healing occurs, patients with venous insufficiency face a significant risk of recurrence. Lifelong use of elastic compression stockings (30 to 40 mm Hg) is the mainstay of therapeutic and preventive measures; furthermore, early intervention after recurrence is critical.

PRESSURE ULCERS

method of
GERRY C. J. BENNETT, M.B.
Barts and The London Queen Mary's School of Medicine & Dentistry
London, United Kingdom

Pressure ulcers can be described as areas of dead tissue caused by pressure-induced ischemia. The relevant blood supply has been critically reduced and within a few hours a largely preventable medical injury has occurred (with significant morbidity) over bony prominences, e.g., sacrum, heels, greater trochanters, and ischial tuberosities (when sitting). This can occur however in any soft tissue subjected to sufficient internal or external pressure. The damage can also be considered a distortion injury because tissue is distorted by a bony prominence causing shear forces, which stretch and blanche the capillary beds. Friction adds to these shear stresses especially in the presence of humidity and moisture (including incontinence). The most common and important source of deep pressure is an internal bone. Pressure and tissue damage is maximal in the deep tissues and where the bones are close to the surface, e.g., in the heels, the tissue damage is full thickness from the beginning. Flaccid muscles, dehydration, and subcutaneous tissues, which are easily deformed, generate higher pressure than normal tissue.

Intrinsic factors involved in the tissue damage cascade are:

- Immobility
- Neurologic disease
- Vascular disease
- Illness
- Age
- Malnutrition

People who are unable to move (sensory loss, unconscious, ill, or restrained) are unable to respond to the pressure-ischemia pain response, which is to move, thus relieving pressure and restoring the blood supply. Patients with spinal cord injury and other neurologic disorders (multiple sclerosis) have the highest risk of pressure damage, with impaired sympathetic control probably playing a key role. People with vascular disease (including those with hypertension, smokers, and diabetics, as well as others with rheologic disorders) all have a high incidence of pressure ulcers. Prolonged pressure-induced ischemia damages endothelial cells and releases inflammatory agents with the formation of microthrombi.

Acute illness is a major precipitating factor in the development of tissue pressure injury. This can occur following a major medical challenge where microcirculatory failure can occur. Profound hypotension, secondary to peripheral vascular failure (as occurs in severe infections or trauma-induced redistribution of blood flow) may lead to multiorgan failure. However, less acute presentations of illness in older people manifest by decreased consciousness, confusion, loss of appetite, incontinence, or falls may be subsequent to an infection or dehydration. Pressure ulcers can develop rapidly with pyrexia exacerbating humidity and friction, pain inhibiting movement and increasing oxygen demand, while incontinence and diarrhea excoriate skin and increase friction. The higher prevalence of pressure ulcers in older people probably reflects the increased prevalence of illness. Body mass index is not a predictor of pressure ulcers. Not unexpectedly, malnutrition is common in patients with pressure ulcers and hypoalbuminemia is the only hematological factor shown to predict pressure injury, presumably as a marker of illness.

Extrinsic factors involved in the tissue damage cascade include:

- Time spent waiting on trolleys/stretchers
- "Nothing by mouth"
- Bed surfaces
- Repositioning
- Intensive care
- Surgery and anesthesia
- Operating tables
- Drugs
- Chair nursing
- Cushions
- Bandages and compression hosiery

Capillary closure pressures for older people and especially sick clients are not known, hence there is no *safe* pressure. Indirect measurements of damage, e.g., imaging techniques, laser Doppler flowmetry or transcutaneous gas tensions are either clinically impracticable or unavailable. It is more important to observe and document the events that precede the development of pressure damage, including medical and nursing management plans.

The majority of hospital-induced pressure ulcers occur in the first 5 days following admission and probably reflect emergency department and radiograph waits, absent pressure relief, insufficient fluids, and less-than-rapid attention to underlying illness processes. Hard hospital beds and side-to-side turning on such mattresses causes repeated high pressure damage to tissue over bony prominences. Tilting causes less tissue hypoxia though this may be more challenging in an intensive care environment. Surgery in older people, especially repair of fractured neck of femur has the highest incidence of pressure ulcer development. The medical and surgical process pre- and post-operation predisposes to tissue damage, as does the use of a standard operating table.

All drugs causing unconsciousness, drowsiness, or hypotension are potentially implicated in tissue pressure damage. Nonsteroidal anti-inflammatory drugs (NSAIDs) and high-dose steroids reduce reactive hyperemia and the healing process.

Patients who remain unwell and who cannot walk or stand unaided should spend very little time out of bed. Longer periods in a chair result in ischial tuberosity pressure ulcers. Pressure relieving cushions must be in place for high-risk patients but are not replacements for adequate bed rest and sleep. Footstools increase the pressure on the heels. Antiembolic stockings must be used cautiously and the skin reviewed regularly, especially in older people as they can cause (and hide) pressure ulcers.

TISSUE INJURY

Characteristics of superficial ulcers (grades 1 and 2):

- Nonblanchable erythema of intact skin, discoloration of skin, warmth, edema, induration, or hardness, especially in darker skin
- Partial thickness skin loss involving epidermis, dermis, or both, a superficial ulcer (abrasion or blister)

Characteristics of deep ulcers (grade 3 and 4):

- Full-thickness tissue damage is only fully apparent once the necrotic tissue has fully débrided and this can be mistaken for worsening as the wound apparently enlarges. Cellulitis can occur in the skin and deep tissues, often with an inflammatory response due to the necrotic tissue (not infection).

  Pressure ulcers are a source of bacteremia and septicemia associated with high mortality. Osteomyelitis is an increasingly recognized complication. Diagnosis may require magnetic resonance imaging, technetium bone scanning, and bone biopsy. Some superficial pressure ulcers may be unavoidable, but all relevant clinical staff are accountable if superficial ulcers worsen and form new deep ulcers.

PREVALENCE AND COST

United Kingdom prevalence studies over the last 30 years are remarkably consistent, indicating ranges between 8% to 20% with lower rates in specialist units. United States reports indicate that between 20% to 35% of elderly people have pressure ulcers at the time of admission to a nursing home. The cost to health services where a significant proportion of patients develop pressure damage is substantial. The main proportion of costs relates to prolonged stays in the hospital with studies indicating that pressure ulcers are the fourth highest cost in the Netherlands health economy and equivalent to the cost of mental health services in the United Kingdom. These figures do not include the increasing sums involved in litigations.

ASSESSMENT

Risk assessment scores describe disability rather than acute illness and none have been shown to be more effective than clinical judgment. Their most valuable use is to document the need for special care to prevent tissue injury and as a medicolegal tool. They must be used in the event of clinical deterioration. It is essential that clinicians learn to recognize patients at risk of pressure damage and that this is a multidisciplinary skill. Routine examination needs to include at-risk sites and be routine in a sick or postoperative patient. Grade 1 or 2 tissue damage indicates that the patient is at risk of irreversible pressure damage.

Prevention issues include:

- Community access to equipment
- Treatment of acute illness
- Nutrition
- Chair nursing
- Pressure relief
- Pressure relieving supports

Once recognized as at-risk of pressure damage, the pressure must be relieved immediately, in the community, as well as in nursing homes or the hospital setting. Illness must be diagnosed and treatment commenced as soon as possible. Older patients, with complex and altered presentations of disease, need rapid and expert intervention. Hydration is essential and attention to nutritional issues must be implemented as soon as is clinically practicable. In most patients, as their clinical state improves, so does their appetite. Short periods of chair nursing are appropriate, once the patient has begun to improve, and this improvement increases as mobility improves. Pressure relief needs to be available in the community, ambulance, emergency department, and on the wards. All patients assessed to be in any degree of risk should be managed on an effective support from the outset of care, which is usually the most critical period of the patient's illness. Special attention needs to be taken to prevent sheets from being used to tuck people in (via a bed cradle or use of duvets).

PRESSURE RELIEVING SUPPORTS

There are four main categories:

- Turning beds—specialist spinal injury patients only.
- Profiling beds—electrically operated, improving pressure and friction and ease of positioning.
- Constant low pressure supports, these may be either static or powered. Static soft mattresses of water, air, gel, foam, silicone beads, or fiber can show low interface pressures, but there is no evidence of their effectiveness in ill patients. Powered low pressure supports (low air and air fluidized bead beds) have been shown to be effective in relieving pressure and healing ulcers. Low-air-loss mattress overlays have also been shown to be as effective as low-air-loss beds for healing.
- Alternating pressure supports—these supports reduce pressure and reproduce the alternating high and low pressures on weight bearing areas as occurs in normal movement. Large-cell overlays and mattress replacements are effective in prevention and healing of pressure ulcers, full mattress replacement being advocated for high-risk prevention or deep ulcer management.

HEALING PRESSURE ULCERS

The factors involved include:

- Pressure relief
- Bed rest
- Pain relief
- Nutrition
- Infection

Most pressure ulcers are painful, limit mobility, and impair sleep. Effective pain relief should be started immediately and deep ulcers/damage require morphine. Regular administration will be necessary until the slough has separated and healing started (usually 2 to 4 weeks). In young people it has been calculated that twice the normal daily protein intake is required to heal a deep ulcer. Carbohydrate, vitamin C, zinc, iron, copper, magnesium, and calcium are also needed. Many nutritional factors are altered by age and illness and do not necessarily reflect intake or whole body balance. Very debilitated patients, especially with a deep ulcer present for some weeks, may benefit by an initial blood transfusion if anemic. Artificial feeding decisions should follow discussion of prognosis and client and family views.

Cellulitis, edema, pyrexia, and leukocytosis occur with new pressure injury and are a normal response to the presence of dead tissue. The discharge of foul smelling necrotic material is the first stage of healing, followed by natural débridement of necrotic fat, and so on. Routine swabbing of pressure ulcers is unnecessary and should be performed if there are signs of systemic toxicity, post-initial inflammation, or in the event of failure to heal. Methicillin-resistant *Staphylococcus aureus* (MRSA) is an increasing contamination problem. In hospitals, patients are usually isolated, although wounds usually continue to heal.

LOCAL TREATMENT

Full surgical débridement of pressure ulcers in frail older people is rarely necessary. Providing pressure is relieved, the slough separates naturally within 1 to 4 weeks. As it loosens, it should be sharply débrided with scissors or scalpel. Antiseptics, e.g., Eusol* and topical antibiotics should not be used. Proteolytic enzymes are expensive and rarely necessary. Moist wound-healing dressings decrease pain on dressing changes and the use and choice of occlusive and semiocclusive films, hydrocolloids, hydrogels, hydrofibers, and alginates should depend on the wound characteristics, e.g., amount of exudate, site, odor, and tissue base. Cavities should be loosely packed with an appropriate cavity dressing. Once the slough has separated the myofibroblasts will cause tissue contraction and a marked reduction in the size and depth of the wound.

Heel sores are usually best allowed to remain dry with attention paid to appropriate footwear. Full thickness eschars will also débride naturally. If the edges become wet and macerated, a hydrocolloid or foam will enhance further débridement and the eschar can be snipped off as it clearly separates.

The use of appropriate pressure-relieving supports are the most important issue for prevention and management. Healing agents are difficult to evaluate

*Not available in the United States.

because of the poor evidence base. Ultrasound and hyperbaric oxygen appear to confer no benefit; electrical therapy and growth factor agents indicate variable success. Cultured human skin equivalents are currently being evaluated. Some patients with deep ulcers may benefit from plastic surgery, saving many weeks to months of hospitalization.

EDUCATION

Clinical governance is a framework by which organizations and their staff are accountable for continuously improving the quality of their service. There are five components to this framework: clinical audit, clinical effectiveness, risk management, quality assurance, and the development of staff and organizations. The essential feature of pressure ulcer management is prevention, and to be successful this must form part of the emergency care of patients. Doctors need to accept responsibility for maintaining the integrity of the peripheral circulation and, hence, understand the etiology and pathology of peripheral circulatory failure. Patients at risk are found in almost every branch of medical practice. Risk management within this framework is the mechanism to identify and rectify poor quality care and lessen the physical, emotional, and financial damage associated with the process of litigation.

ATOPIC DERMATITIS

method of
ANTHONY J. MANCINI, M.D.
Northwestern University Feinberg School of Medicine
Children's Memorial Hospital
Chicago, Illinois

Atopic dermatitis (AD) is a genetically-influenced, chronically-relapsing, pruritic skin disorder. It affects 7% to 17% of school-aged children, with 60% of cases beginning within the first year of life. Three criteria are essential to making the diagnosis of AD: (1) a personal or family history of atopy (including AD, asthma and/or allergic rhinoconjunctivitis); (2) pruritus; and (3) "eczema," which is a nonspecific term for scaly, inflamed, oozing, or crusted skin. Skin findings in patients with AD include: scaly, erythematous papules and plaques, often with excoriations, crusting, and fissuring. Subacute AD and chronic AD are marked by lichenification (skin thickening with increased skin markings) and pigmentary alterations (hypo- or hyperpigmentation). Table 1 lists associated skin findings in patients with AD.

The characteristic distribution pattern varies depending on age. In infants, the face and extensor extremities predominate, with sparing of the diaper region. Toddlers and school-aged children tend to have more involvement of the antecubital and popliteal fossae, as well as facial involvement. Older children, adolescents, and adults have a similar distribution, but often with involvement of the neck, hands, and feet. Atopic dermatitis has a profound psychosocial impact on patients and families. It is a source of significant sleep disturbance (both in the patient and the parents), family discord, impaired school performance, social isolation, decreased self-esteem, and negative effects on parental work performance. There are many myths regarding its causes and therapies. Thorough education, anticipatory guidance, and psychosocial support provide the necessary framework for therapeutic success.

MANAGEMENT

The management of AD is multifactorial, and must take into account the various components of the disease. Education is paramount to any therapeutic success, and patient education materials are quite useful to this end. Patients and parents should understand that treatment of AD is supportive and not definitive, and that the natural history is one of a waxing and waning course. Identification of disease "triggers," which is often the primary goal of caretakers, is usually neither practical nor useful. The role of food allergy as an etiologic trigger is exaggerated among laypersons and some practitioners, and is probably associated in only 20% to 25% of patients with moderate-to-severe disease that is recalcitrant to therapy. The risk of blind food eliminations, especially in younger patients, should be underscored, and in patients for whom food allergy is suspected, co-management with an allergist is indicated.

DRY SKIN CARE

Adequate hydration and lubrication of the skin are important long-term principles of AD therapy. Daily, short (less than 10 minutes) baths or showers are

TABLE 1. **Associated Skin Findings in Patients With Atopic Dermatitis**

Finding	Description
Allergic shiners	Blue-gray darkening of infraorbital skin
Ichthyosis vulgaris	Polygonal scaling, mainly lower extremities
Keratosis pilaris	Hyperkeratotic follicular papules, distributed on cheeks (children), lateral arms, and dorsal thighs
Morgan-Dennie folds	Symmetric, prominent folds below margin of lower eyelids
Pityriasis alba	Hypopigmented macules and patches, most often on the face
Skin hyperlinearity	Increased markings on palms and soles
Transverse nasal crease	"Allergic salute"; secondary to nasal rubbing with allergic rhinitis
Xerosis	Dry skin, often diffuse; worse during winter months

desirable, and have many advantages, including hydration, enhanced medication penetration, bacterial débridement and bonding between parent and child. Emolliating is vital, and is most effectively achieved with thick creams or greasy ointments. Lotion-based products may be more desirable during the warmer months, especially in humid climates. Emollients should be applied at least twice daily, and as soon as possible after bathing. If anti-inflammatory agents are to be used, they should be applied to affected areas first, followed by the emollient.

TREATMENT OF INFLAMMATION

Controlling inflammation is the primary goal of AD therapy. Topical corticosteroids have long been the mainstay of therapy, and are effective and safe when used appropriately. They are usually applied twice daily, and treatment should be discontinued when the skin feels smooth (regardless of pigmentary changes). Refills should be closely monitored and regular follow-up should be arranged to assess for tachyphylaxis or side effects such as skin atrophy, telangiectases, or striae.

Ointments are usually better tolerated and more effective than creams. If topical steroid agents are used on face or fold regions (groin, axillae), they should be limited to low-strength, nonfluorinated preparations, such as hydrocortisone 1% or 2.5%, desonide 0.05% (DesOwen), or alclometasone 0.05% (Aclovate). Caution should be exercised with use of topical corticosteroids near the eyes. For affected areas on the trunk or extremities, intermediate-strength preparations are appropriate, such as triamcinolone 0.1% (Kenalog) or fluocinolone 0.025% (Synalar).* For more severely involved nonfacial, nonfold areas, more potent preparations such as fluocinonide 0.05% (Lidex), mometasone 0.1% (Elocon), or betamethasone 0.05% (Diprosone) may be indicated. These agents should be used for short, closely monitored periods of time. Scalp dermatitis can be treated with topical corticosteroid solutions, such as fluocinolone 0.01% (Synalar)* or hydrocortisone butyrate 0.1% (Locoid). Fluocinolone 0.01% in an oil base (Dermasmooth/FS)* and betamethasone 0.12% foam (Luxiq) are other options for the scalp.

*Not FDA approved for this indication.

Newer nonsteroidal topical immunomodulators (TIMs) are now available for the treatment of AD. Tacrolimus ointment (Protopic) is available in 0.03% (approved for >2 years) and 0.1% (approved for >15 years) strengths. This product is a topical preparation of the systemic immunosuppressant FK506 (Prograf), and acts via inhibition of T cell cytokine production. It is applied twice daily to affected areas. Transient stinging with application is common, and sometimes limits its use. Pimecrolimus 1% cream (Elidel) is another nonsteroidal TIM, approved in patients 2 years of age and older. It has a similar mechanism of action, and is also applied twice daily to affected areas. Application site reactions are less common, but it may be less effective in severe disease.

The newer nonsteroidal TIMs offer the advantage of being steroid free, which makes them especially ideal for periorbital therapy. Steroid-related side effects such as striae, atrophy, telangiectasia, and adrenal suppression are not an issue, and there appears to be no systemic immunosuppression when they are used as indicated. Vigilant sun protection is vital while using any topical immunomodulator, and should be stressed with use of these newer agents while long-term safety data are collected.

TREATMENT OF PRURITUS

Although topical therapies help to relieve pruritus, additional anti-itch treatment is often necessary. Patients (especially children) with AD often enter a vicious "itch-scratch" cycle, which propagates the disease and contributes to frequent secondary bacterial infection. Abrogation of pruritus is most effectively achieved with the use of oral antihistamine agents. A combination of daytime coverage with a nonsedating agent and nighttime coverage with a traditional (sedating) agent is often useful. Table 2 lists some commonly used antihistamines.

*Not FDA approved for this indication.

TABLE 2. **Antihistamines Used for Atopic Dermatitis**

Agent	Dosing	Comment
Cetirizine*	5–10 mg qd	
(Zyrtec)*	2.5–5 mg qd (2–5 yr)	Liquid: 5 mg/5 mL
Cyproheptadine	4 mg bid-tid	May increase appetite, weight gain
(Periactin)*	2 mg bid-tid (2–5 yr)	Liquid: 2 mg/5 mL
Diphenhydramine	25–50 mg tid-qid	Paradoxical hyperactivity in children
(Benadryl)*	1 mg/kg qid (children)	Liquid: 6.25 or 12.5 mg/5 mL
Doxepin*	50–100 mg qhs	
(Sinequan)	5–10 mg qhs (children)	Liquid: 10 mg/1 mL
Hydroxyzine	10–25 mg qid	Author's first choice
(Atarax, Vistaril)	0.5–1 mg/kg qid (children)	Liquid: 10 mg/5 mL
Loratadine*	10 mg qd	10 mg "Reditab" available
(Claritin)*	5 mg qd (2–5 yr)	Liquid: 5 mg/5 mL

*Not FDA approved for this indication.
Bid, twice a day; qd, every day; qid, four times daily; tid, three times daily.

TREATMENT OF INFECTION

Secondary infection with *Staphylococcus aureus* is common in patients with AD, up to 80% of whom may be carriers of this bacteria. Pustules, erosions, and crusting are the hallmarks of secondarily-infected AD. Classic "honey-yellow crusting" of impetigo is unusual. Localized infection may respond well to mupirocin 2% (Bactroban) ointment, but more extensive impetiginization often requires systemic therapy. Consideration for antimicrobial therapy must be balanced by bacterial resistance patterns, and in some instances of mild infection, withholding antibiotic therapy is a viable option. Community-acquired methicillin-resistant *S. aureus* (CA-MRSA) infections are on the increase in the United States, and are being seen in patients who lack traditional risk factors for MRSA infection (hospitalization, frequent antibiotic usage, presence of an indwelling medical device, and so on). These reports highlight the importance of the judicious use of antimicrobials and avoidance of indiscriminate therapy.

When feasible, antibiotic choice should be guided by sensitivity testing of microbial isolates. Cephalexin (Keflex) continues to be a good initial choice for most infections, with an excellent sensitivity profile and a good-tasting suspension for young children. In older individuals, dicloxacillin (Dynapen) tablets are a good initial choice. Macrolide antibiotics have variable effectiveness against *S. aureus,* dependent on regional variation. Clindamycin (Cleocin) may be indicated for resistant organisms, and most CA-MRSA isolates continue to be sensitive.

Eczema herpeticum, representing secondary superinfection of AD lesions with herpes simplex virus, presents with fever and multiple, clustered vesicles or erosions superimposed on lesions of AD. Patients can become quite ill, and therapy with systemic acyclovir (Zovirax) is indicated. Oral therapy is sufficient for mild presentations, but severe or diffuse involvement is best treated by hospitalization with intravenous acyclovir and fluids, as well as pain control.

Table 3 outlines some therapeutic vignettes for differing severities of AD.

TABLE 3. **Therapeutic Vignettes**

The following are examples of appropriate therapies for different severities of disease:

Mild Disease

Daily bathing/emolliating
Alclometasone (Aclovate) 0.05% ointment bid or desonide 0.05% ointment bid

Moderate Disease

Daily bathing/emolliation
Pimecrolimus (Elidel) 1% cream bid (face)
Fluocinolone 0.025% ointment bid (body)
Hydroxyzine (Atarax) bid and qhs as needed for pruritus

Severe Disease With Superinfection

Daily bathing/emolliating
Tacrolimus (Protopic) 0.03% ointment bid (face)
Tacrolimus 0.03% ointment or mometasone 0.1% ointment bid (body)
Cetirizine (Zyrtec)* q am
Hydroxyzine after school and qhs as needed for pruritus
Cephalexin (Keflex) tid for 7–10 days
Consider allergy testing

*Not FDA approved for this indication.
Bid, twice daily; q am, every morning; qhs, at bedtime; tid, three times a day.

SYSTEMIC THERAPY

Systemic therapies are occasionally necessary for patients with severe AD. Oral prednisone is a very effective therapy, but its use is limited by its long-term toxicities. If a brief course is necessary, it should be tapered gradually over 3 weeks to help prevent the marked rebound seen with more rapid tapers. Oral cyclosporine (2 to 4 mg/kg/day) (Neoral),* is an effective therapy for severe AD, but requires close monitoring and has many potential side effects, including hypertension, renal toxicity, gingival hyperplasia, and increased risk of infection. Its use should be limited to patients with severe, recalcitrant disease, and treatment should be discontinued as soon as feasible. Ultraviolet phototherapy (UVB, PUVA, narrow-band UVB) may be useful for some adolescents or adults with chronic refractive disease, but the risks of cumulative ultraviolet exposure make this a less-attractive option for children.

*Not FDA approved for this indication.

ERYTHEMA MULTIFORME, STEVENS-JOHNSON SYNDROME, AND TOXIC EPIDERMAL NECROLYSIS

method of
KAREN S. TARASZKA, M.D., PH.D.
Yale University School of Medicine
New Haven, Connecticut

and

JEFFREY S. DOVER, M.D.
Yale University School of Medicine
Dartmouth Medical School
Chestnut Hill, Massachusetts

Erythema multiforme (EM), Stevens-Johnson syndrome (SJS), and toxic epidermal necrolysis (TEN) encompass an overlapping spectrum of acute, self-limited exanthems. Herpes simplex virus (HSV) infection is the most common causative factor in EM, the relatively common, mild form. In contrast, adverse drug reactions are the leading cause of SJS and TEN, rare, life-threatening forms with mucocutaneous involvement. Therapeutic interventions include eliminating likely etiologic agents, as well as symptomatic and supportive care. Controlled trials are needed to validate emerging therapies for SJS and TEN.

ERYTHEMA MULTIFORME

EM is an acute, self-limited, but frequently recurrent, inflammatory dermatosis that is frequently linked to HSV infection. In 70% of patients with recurrent EM, clinical HSV lesions (oral, genital, or other) precede the exanthem by up to 10 days. Although HSV has not been cultured from keratinocytes in EM lesions, HSV proteins, DNA, and RNA can be identified. *Mycoplasma pneumoniae* infection is also associated with the spectrum of EM to SJS, but rarely TEN. Generally, *Mycoplasma* reactions involve a small percentage of body surface area, but may have more severe mucosal involvement. EM can also be due to drug hypersensitivity. Patients present with the abrupt onset of erythematous papules or plaques that are fixed in position. The lesion center becomes dusky or may blister, giving rise to the classic lesion of EM, the target lesion. The target lesion has three zones—a central dusky papule that may blister, a pale edematous middle ring, and an erythematous outer ring. The lesions are distributed symmetrically, and they usually involve the dorsal hands and feet and the extensor surfaces of the extremities. Lesions can also be present on the palms and soles and may spread centrally to involve the thighs, buttocks, and trunk. The lesions can also itch or burn. Typically, much less than 10% of the total body surface area is affected. Mucosal lesions are seen in 70% of patients and most commonly involve the oral mucosa. This benign disease typically lasts 1 to 4 weeks and is without complications. Diagnosis is made by clinical examination and skin biopsy, which reveals vacuolar degeneration of the basal layer of keratinocytes and individual necrotic keratinocytes. The differential diagnosis for EM includes acute annular urticaria, leukocytoclastic vasculitis, and bullous pemphigoid.

Therapeutic Approach

Elimination of Etiologic Factors

A careful history and review of systems should be undertaken to determine whether there is a preceding history of HSV or other viral or bacterial infection. To rule out HSV, a swab of the base of a vesicle, or ulcer, can be sent for direct fluorescence antigen (DFA) test and viral culture. In cases associated with HSV infection, once EM lesions have developed, antiviral therapy for HSV is not effective. If suspected, immunoglobulin titers for *Mycoplasma* can be sent. A detailed drug history is essential.

Supportive Care

Systemic antihistamines and analgesics may provide symptomatic relief for pruritic or painful skin lesions.

Preventive Therapy

Because the most common etiologic agent in recurrent EM is HSV infection, therapy should be targeted at controlling and preventing HSV outbreaks. Five-day oral treatment with acyclovir (Zovirax),* 200 mg five times per day, initiated at the first sign of HSV infection is beneficial in preventing recurrent EM. If treatment of recurrent HSV episodes is unsuccessful or the patient does not experience a prodrome, chronic suppression should be considered. The recommended starting dose of acyclovir is 400 mg orally twice daily. Patients with idiopathic recurrent EM have also been shown to benefit from HSV prophylaxis, suggesting that subclinical HSV episodes may trigger EM. Although their efficacy has not been specifically evaluated in EM, newer antiviral agents with enhanced bioavailability, including valacyclovir (Valtrex)* and famciclovir (Famvir)* are effective in HSV treatment and suppression and are likely to be beneficial in prevention of EM. Valacyclovir is FDA approved for treatment of herpes labialis at a dose of 2 g orally for two doses 12 hours apart at the first symptom of HSV (tingling, itching, and burning). The recommended dose for chronic suppression is valacyclovir 0.5 to 1 g orally once daily or famciclovir 250 mg orally twice daily for up to 1 year.

STEVENS-JOHNSON SYNDROME AND TOXIC EPIDERMAL NECROLYSIS

SJS and TEN are severe, acute mucocutaneous reactions. In contrast to EM, drugs are the leading etiologic agent in SJS and TEN. Based on a case-controlled study, the drugs most often associated with SJS and TEN include sulfonamides, such as trimethoprim-sulfamethoxazole and sulfasalazine, aminopenicillins, fluoroquinolones, cephalosporins, tetracyclines, imidazole antifungals, anticonvulsants (including phenytoin, valproic acid, carbamazepine, and phenobarbital), allopurinol, chlormezanone,† corticosteroids, and oxicam nonsteroidal anti-inflammatory drugs (NSAIDs). Infection (especially *Mycoplasma* in SJS), graft-versus-host disease, and vaccination are also causes of SJS and TEN. Current evidence supports a role for keratinocyte expression of Fas ligand and Fas-Fas ligand-mediated apoptosis in TEN.

SJS and TEN are often preceded by a nonspecific viral-like prodrome. An erythematous macular or maculopapular rash begins on the face, neck, and central trunk and then may spread to the extremities. Individual lesions are round to irregularly shaped macules or patches with a dusky center. Target lesions can appear at the periphery. Lesions increase in number and size and may coalesce. Large flaccid blisters form and rupture, leading to denudation and erosions. SJS refers to disease limited to less than 10% of the body surface area and TEN refers to disease involving more than 30% of the body surface area. Two or more mucosal surfaces (oral, conjunctival, urogenital, and anal—in order of frequency) are involved. Mucosal lesions can also occur throughout the pulmonary and gastrointestinal tract. Sequelae from mucosal scarring, such as blindness and esophageal or

*Not FDA approved for this indication.
†Not available in the United States.

urethral stricture, can occur. The mortality rate in TEN is approximately 30% to 40% with sepsis as the leading cause of death. Diagnosis is aided by skin biopsy or frozen section histopathologic examination of a bulla roof, which reveals extensive keratinocyte necrosis that may affect the entire epidermis. The differential diagnosis for SJS and TEN includes staphylococcal scalded-skin syndrome, toxic erythroderma, graft-versus-host disease, and generalized bullous disorders.

Therapeutic Approach

Elimination of Etiologic Factors

Suspected or potential causative drugs should be discontinued at the earliest stage. Infections, such as *Mycoplasma pneumoniae*, should be diagnosed and treated promptly.

Systemic Therapy

The use of systemic therapy in the treatment of SJS and TEN is highly controversial due to the lack of randomized, controlled trials. If systemic therapy is used, it should be implemented early in the disease, prior to extensive epidermal necrosis, and it should be stopped once disease progression is halted or if no response is noted after 2 to 4 days.

One prospective study indicates that treatment with corticosteroids increases mortality of TEN when given after extensive skin involvement and blistering has developed. Some authors have found administration of a short course of high-dose steroids (80 to 120 mg of methylprednisolone, given orally once daily and tapering over 1 week or sooner if tolerated) is useful early in the treatment of drug-induced SJS and TEN. Promising results in the treatment of TEN with early administration of intravenous immunoglobulins (IVIg [Gammagard S/D]),* (1 g/kg/d for 3 to 4 consecutive days) have been documented in several uncontrolled case series. One mechanism of IVIg may be the inhibition of Fas-Fas ligand-mediated apoptosis. Immunomodulatory treatment with cyclosporine (Neoral),* cyclophosphamide (Cytoxan),* infliximab (Remicade),* and plasmapheresis has been tried and is experimental. Thalidomide* is the only drug in the treatment of TEN that was tested in a randomized controlled trial, and the study was stopped because of excess mortality in the thalidomide group.

Supportive Care

Particular attention should be paid to early detection of infection with surveillance cultures of the skin, mucosal surfaces, blood, urine, and sputum with a low threshold for initiating antibiotic therapy. Management includes careful mucous membrane hygiene and wound care. A 1:1:1 mixture of viscous lidocaine, diphenhydramine (Benadryl)* elixir, and aluminum and magnesium hydroxide (Maalox),* used as a mouthwash, often provides relief of painful oral erosions. Depending on the severity of erosions or ulcerations, consider a petrolatum gauze dressing (Xeroform), a hydrocolloid dressing, or an absorptive dressing (Exu-Dry). When there is widespread mucocutaneous involvement, the patient should be managed in a burn unit with monitoring of fluid and electrolyte balance, thermoregulation, nutritional support, and pulmonary care (suctioning and postural drainage). The patient should be followed closely for eye involvement and, if present, ophthalmic specialist consulted. Central lines and urinary catheters should not routinely be placed, and if placed, they should be changed regularly.

Preventive Therapy

In drug-associated SJS and TEN, avoidance of the causative drug is mandatory.

*Not FDA approved for this indication.

BULLOUS DISEASES

method of
M. PETER MARINKOVICH, M.D., and
JOSEPHINE CHU, A.B.
Stanford University School of Medicine
Stanford, California

A careful clinical assessment and, as indicated, a skin biopsy with examination by routine histology, can be helpful in evaluating nonautoimmune causes of blistering, especially patients who present with blisters for the first time. Insect bites are a common cause of blistering, which often are localized to the lower extremities. Contact dermatitis can produce an abrupt onset of localized bullae. Hand and foot dermatitis, or pompholyx can produce repeated localized blistering. Lymphedema of the lower extremities or elsewhere can produce multiple bullae. When autoimmune bullous diseases are considered, they must be diagnosed with specific immunologic testing; usually this means a perilesional skin biopsy analyzed by direct immunofluorescent microscopy.

PEMPHIGUS

Pemphigus comprises a group of autoimmune blistering diseases characterized by intraepidermal skin separation. Disease pathology is caused by circulating autoantibodies that disrupt the desmogleins, important components of desmosome that function in cell-to-cell adhesion. Acantholysis, or rounding of keratinocytes in areas of intraepidermal separation, is a histologic hallmark of pemphigus, which arises as a consequence of desmosome inactivation.

PEMPHIGUS VULGARIS

Clinical and Laboratory Features

Pemphigus vulgaris, the most common pemphigus subtype, typically, but not always, presents in older individuals. Classic lesions are flaccid blisters and erosions, with or without surrounding erythema. The blisters rupture easily, so that only erosions may be observed. On physical examination, the blisters may be spread to involve neighboring areas by light digital pressure (Nikolsky's sign). The oral mucosa is the primary site of involvement in the majority of patients; however, skin of all locations is also commonly affected. Severe disease may involve other mucous membranes, such as the conjunctiva, nasal mucosa, larynx, esophagus, vulva, cervix, and rectum. Erosions may coalesce into large, painful areas of denuded skin with peripheral crusting. The lesions heal slowly, usually without scarring, and can leave areas of hypopigmentation and hyperpigmentation.

Skin biopsies demonstrate intraepidermal blisters, a mixed eosinophilic infiltrate, and characteristic acantholysis. Direct immunofluorescence performed on perilesional skin demonstrates cell surface deposits of IgG and, in 50% of patients, IgA, IgM, or C3. Indirect immunofluorescence microscopy (IDIF) demonstrates pathogenic circulating IgG autoantibodies binding with cell-to-cell junctions, which on enzyme-linked immunosorbent assay (ELISA) are shown to be directed to desmoglein 3. Many patients also have autoantibodies against desmoglein 1. It is useful to follow the titer of autoantibody detected in patient sera, either by ELISA or IDIF, because it can correlate with disease activity and patient response to therapy. Neonates born to mothers with active pemphigus vulgaris may have similar lesions; however, their disease is self-limited and requires no treatment.

PEMPHIGUS FOLIACEUS

Clinical and Laboratory Features

Pemphigus foliaceus differs from pemphigus vulgaris in that oral lesions are not seen and acantholysis takes place at a much more superficial level, in the granular cell layer. The disease course is usually chronic, lasting months to years, and is more benign than pemphigus vulgaris. It primarily affects those in the fifth or later decade of life and presents with scaly, crusted erosions on an erythematous base. Intact blisters are seldom seen. Lesions are most frequently seen on the scalp, face, and upper trunk. In severe flares, pemphigus foliaceus may also present in a generalized, cutaneous distribution. Direct immunofluorescence shows IgG and complement in the upper epidermis, localizing to the intercellular space. Indirect immunofluorescence demonstrates circulating autoantibodies that localize intercellularly to the upper epidermis. Sometimes it is difficult to distinguish pemphigus vulgaris and pemphigus foliaceus by light and immunofluorescent microscopy, and in these cases, the clinical findings are most helpful. ELISA is also helpful in distinguishing these cases because pemphigus foliaceus shows autoantibodies against desmoglein 1, but differs from pemphigus vulgaris in that it does not show antidesmoglein 3 antibodies. In Brazil, an endemic variant of pemphigus foliaceus, fogo selvagem, is thought to be transmitted by the blackfly *Simulium pruinosum*.

PEMPHIGUS ERYTHEMATOSUS

Clinical and Laboratory Features

Pemphigus erythematosus, also known as Senear-Usher syndrome, is a localized variant of pemphigus foliaceus. It often presents with a prominent, well-demarcated malar involvement similar to the malar erythema seen in patients with lupus erythematosus. The small, flaccid bullae or erosions may be thickly crusted, especially in sun-exposed areas, such as the scalp, face, and upper trunk. In most cases, the disease shows more similarities to pemphigus foliaceus than to pemphigus vulgaris. Mucous membranes are usually not involved. Photosensitivity is common in pemphigus erythematosus and approximately 30% of patients also have circulating antinuclear antibodies; however, systemic lupus erythematosus is only rarely associated with pemphigus erythematosus. Histologic analysis demonstrates acantholysis in the upper layers of the epidermis and intercellular staining with IgG and C3. Deposition of IgG at the dermal-epidermal junction is also usually seen in this disease. This disease has a better prognosis than pemphigus foliaceus, with a slow onset and progression, and a chronic course.

DRUG-INDUCED PEMPHIGUS

A careful history should be taken in patients with newly-diagnosed pemphigus to rule this out as a possible drug etiology. Thiol drugs such as D-penicillamine (Cuprimine), captopril (Capoten), and enalapril (Vasotec) cause clinical and immunologic features of pemphigus foliaceus, while nonthiol drugs such as penicillins, cephalosporins, piroxicam (Feldene), and rifampin (Rifadin) cause clinical and immunologic features similar to pemphigus vulgaris. The lesions may be extensive and may result in significant pain and burning sensations. Most patients show spontaneous recovery once the inciting agent is removed. Patients with a more chronic course may require systemic corticosteroids and/or immunosuppressive therapy.

PARANEOPLASTIC PEMPHIGUS

Paraneoplastic pemphigus is a rare autoimmune bullous disease associated with an underlying neoplasm. The most commonly associated neoplasms include non-Hodgkin's lymphoma, chronic lymphocytic leukemia, Castleman's tumor, and thymoma. The disease is always characterized by severe mucosal erosions and may also be accompanied by widespread polymorphic skin eruptions. Skin biopsies demonstrate suprabasal acantholysis and intraepithelial blister formation, and may show dyskeratotic keratinocytes throughout the layers of the epidermis as well as interface dermatitis. IgG binds to the

*Not FDA approved for this indication.

epidermis in an intercellular distribution. The disease is characterized by the presence of IgG autoantibodies against desmosomal and hemidesmosomal plakin proteins, desmogleins, and an unidentified 170-kd antigen. Diagnosis is made through a combination of direct immunofluorescent microscopy of perilesional skin biopsy, indirect immunofluorescent microscopy of patient sera on rodent epithelial tissues, and radioimmunoprecipitation of patient sera. Although paraneoplastic pemphigus is generally recalcitrant to therapy, removal of the underlying neoplasm can lead to remission. Paraneoplastic pemphigus has a high fatality rate, with deaths attributed to respiratory failure, as well as to complications associated with immunosuppressive therapy.

THERAPY OF PEMPHIGUS

Systemic corticosteroids are an important part of therapy for the pemphigus group of diseases. Most flares can be controlled with up to 1 mg/kg/d of prednisone.* As blistering activity subsides, this daily dose can be tapered gradually at a slow rate with meticulous assessment for blister recurrence. As the tapering proceeds, it is important to place patients on an alternate-day corticosteroid regimen as this will reduce systemic side effects. One should closely examine patients at frequent intervals for signs of reflaring and have them immediately report increases in blistering activity. Reflares require an increase in the dose of prednisone, sometimes back to initial levels. The long-term goal is to minimize or entirely eliminate the steroid dose, in order to reduce systemic effects. All patients receiving long-term corticosteroids should receive regular eye examinations, bone scans, and calcium supplementation, as well as appropriate treatment of osteoporosis when detected.

Immunosuppressive drugs can be useful steroid-sparing agents, especially in elderly patients at high risk for osteoporosis and other corticosteroid-induced adverse effects. A long-term complication of these treatments is the increased risk of neoplasia. Mycophenolate mofetil (CellCept),* at a dose of 2 to 3 g/d, is often effective when used in conjunction with prednisone. It is generally well tolerated, although it may cause leukopenia. Azathioprine (Imuran),* used in patients who cannot tolerate mycophenolate mofetil,* is given at a dose of 1 to 3 mg/kg/d. Hepatotoxicity, sepsis, and urinary complications are the most frequent serious complications and often occur within the first week or two of therapy. With both agents, patients should be monitored regularly with laboratory studies, including CBCs and liver function tests.

Cyclophosphamide (Cytoxan)* is generally more effective in autoimmune bullous diseases than mycophenolate mofetil* or azathioprine*; however, it has more potential systemic toxicity and patients must be carefully monitored with laboratory studies including complete blood count (CBC), chemistries, and urinalysis. Treatment usually consists of a daily dose of cyclophosphamide, 1 to 2 mg/kg/d. It is helpful for patients to take the daily dose of cyclophosphamide* by mid-day or earlier, and to push oral fluids throughout the day to flush out drug metabolites. Side effects include bone marrow suppression, urinary problems (e.g., hemorrhagic cystitis), bone marrow suppression, pulmonary fibrosis, sterility, and the increased risk of malignancies.

*Not FDA approved for this indication.

Sometimes pemphigus patients with recalcitrant disease can show significant blistering activity in the face of maximal doses of medical therapies. In these instances, plasmapheresis is a useful adjunct therapy. A typical regimen would involve six sessions of 1 volume fluid replacement given over 2 weeks. If plasma is not given as a replacement fluid, it is important to monitor fibrinogen and calcium levels during the course of therapy. To prevent rebound autoantibody production after completion of plasmapheresis, the patient should receive cyclophosphamide combined with prednisone before, during, and after therapy. Potential complications include hypotension, bleeding, electrolyte imbalances, fever, chills, pulmonary edema, and septicemia. Plasmapheresis can be administered in repeated cycles as needed to control flares of blistering.

Intravenous immunoglobulin (Gamimune N),* may be an effective adjunct therapy in patients with recalcitrant disease or flares of blisters, despite aggressive medical therapy. A loading dose of 2 g/kg can be given initially in three divided doses over 3 consecutive days. This can be followed by maintenance doses of 400 mg/kg every 3 to 4 weeks and continued until a therapeutic effect is noted.

In paraneoplastic pemphigus and drug-induced pemphigus, removal of the inciting neoplasm/drug is the treatment of choice. Systemic corticosteroids and immunosuppressive agents may also be used to decrease blistering, although paraneoplastic pemphigus is relatively resistant to such treatments.

PEMPHIGOID GROUP

Pemphigoid refers to a group of subepidermal blistering diseases characterized by tense blisters and autoantibodies directed at basement membrane zone antigens. When subepidermal bullous disease is suspected, a perilesional biopsy taken within a few millimeters of a fresh blister should be evaluated by direct immunofluorescence microscopy. Separation of biopsied skin with 1 M sodium chloride can often be performed in the diagnostic laboratory prior to direct immunofluorescent microscopy. This technique separates skin in the plane of the lamina lucida of the basement membrane and the separation helps to distinguish deeper subepidermal bullous diseases, such as epidermolysis bullosa acquisita from more superficial subepidermal bullous diseases, such as bullous pemphigoid.

*Not FDA approved for this indication.

BULLOUS PEMPHIGOID

Clinical and Laboratory Features

Bullous pemphigoid, the most common autoimmune blistering disease, is seen most often in the elderly, although younger individuals are also occasionally affected. The disease is characterized by tense nonfragile blisters, often with a preceding or concurrent urticarial plaque. The lesions almost always heal without scarring, although occasional milia can be seen. Pruritus is a common feature and can be severe. The most common sites of involvement include the trunk, proximal extremities, and flexural surfaces. Oral mucosal involvement is seen in 20% of patients. The bullae can be generalized or remain localized to one area for up to several months. Overall, the disease is chronic, with periods of exacerbation and remission, but remissions occur more frequently than with pemphigus.

A subepidermal blister with a perilesional polymorphous, eosinophil-rich, dermal infiltrate is seen on histologic examination. Direct immunofluorescence of normal-appearing, perilesional skin reveals linear staining of IgG and C3 at the epidermal basement membrane. In bullous pemphigoid, the IgG deposits localize to the epidermal side of sodium chloride-separated skin. Indirect immunofluorescence microscopy can also be used to detect circulating basement membrane zone autoantibodies in bullous pemphigoid. Immunoblot or immunoprecipitation analysis reveals circulating antibodies against one or both bullous pemphigoid antigens, BPAG1 and BPAG2.

GESTATIONAL PEMPHIGOID

Gestational pemphigoid (herpes gestationis) is a rare autoimmune bullous disease of pregnancy. The intensely pruritic lesions often develop during the second and third trimesters, but may appear at any time during pregnancy or following delivery. Patients present with periumbilical erythematous urticarial patches and plaques which progress to tense vesicles and bullae. The rash spreads peripherally, often sparing the face, palms, soles, and mucous membranes. Neonates have a slightly increased risk of premature birth and small size. They may display transient self-limited blistering. Spontaneous regression without scarring typically occurs following delivery, although in rare cases, disease may persist for years. Flares may develop with the resumption of menses, the use of oral contraceptives, and subsequent pregnancies. Histologic and immunologic findings are identical to those in bullous pemphigoid.

MUCOUS MEMBRANE PEMPHIGOID

Clinical and Laboratory Feature

Mucous membrane pemphigoid, previously termed cicatricial pemphigoid, is a group of autoimmune inflammatory, blistering diseases primarily affecting mucous membranes. It is important to identify high-risk patients, who show ocular, esophageal, laryngeal, genital, or nasopharyngeal disease from low-risk patients, whose disease is confined to the oral mucosa or oral mucosa and skin. Scarring of the mucosal surfaces is a characteristic feature. Patients with oral lesions typically present with erythematous patches, blisters, and erosions. Nasal involvement presents as erosions and crusting in the nasal vestibule. Anogenital lesions can be seen as blisters and erosions. Ocular involvement manifests as conjunctivitis, corneal epithelium keratinization, shortening of the fornices, entropion, trichiasis, symblepharon, and ankyloblepharon. Some of the most debilitating effects of mucosal scarring in mucous membrane pemphigoid include loss of vision, airway obstruction, and esophageal strictures. Cutaneous lesions consist of tense vesicles or bullae and are often found on the face, neck, and scalp. Scarring and milia formation are often present when cutaneous involvement is seen and these features differentiate this disease from bullous pemphigoid and linear IgA bullous dermatosis.

Histologic studies demonstrate subepithelial blisters which may have a significant mixed infiltrate. Immunofluorescence findings can be similar to those for bullous pemphigoid, with IgG-mediated immunoreactivity primarily at the epidermal roof of sodium chloride-separated skin, but 20% of patients with mucous membrane pemphigoid show linear deposits of IgA on direct immunofluorescence. A small subset of patients with mucous membrane pemphigoid contain autoantibodies to laminin-5, which localize to the dermal floor of split skin. It is important to identify the subset of patients with anti-laminin-5 mucous membrane pemphigoid (also termed *anti-epiligrin cicatricial pemphigoid*) because these patients appear to have an increased incidence of associated malignancies. In patients with mucous membrane pemphigoid, who show immunoreactivity to the floor of sodium chloride split skin, further studies, such as immunoblotting or ELISA can be performed in specialized centers to distinguish anti-laminin-5 mucous membrane pemphigoid from epidermolysis bullosa acquisita (described subsequently).

THERAPY OF PEMPHIGOID

Systemic corticosteroids have traditionally been the cornerstone of therapy for patients with the pemphigoid group of diseases and between 0.5 and 1 mg/kg of prednisone* can be used to halt new blister formation, followed by gradual tapering as described in pemphigus treatment (earlier). However, recent reports have shown that ultrapotent topical corticosteroids, used aggressively, appear to be as effective as systemic corticosteroids in the treatment of bullous pemphigoid patients, with a lower incidence of steroid-induced morbidity. Tetracycline* and niacinamide,* each at 2 g per day, can be effective nontoxic steroid-sparing agents in the treatment of bullous pemphigoid. Topical tacrolimus (Protopic),* may also be a useful adjunct therapy in bullous pemphigoid. In bullous

*Not FDA approved for this indication.

pemphigoid patients with more recalcitrant disease, mycophenolate mofetil (CellCept),* azathioprine (Imuran),* or cyclophosphamide (Cytoxan)* can be used as steroid-sparing agents in a manner similar to that described earlier in the treatment of pemphigus.

Therapy in mucous membrane pemphigoid varies depending on the type of disease. High-risk patients should undergo initial treatment with prednisone* (1 to 1.5 mg/kg per day) and cyclophosphamide (1 to 2 mg/kg per day) and be treated in a multidisciplinary fashion, by a team of physicians experienced in the care of the affected organ system. In patients with eye disease, cyclophosphamide can be especially effective at reducing corneal scarring, whereas prednisone is generally more effective at treating conjunctival erosions. Azathioprine (Imuran) (1 to 2 mg/kg per day) or mycophenolate mofetil (CellCept) (2 to 3 gm/day) may be substituted in patients unable to tolerate cyclophosphamide. Treatment with immunosuppressives should be maintained throughout the prednisone taper. Patients with mild disease should initially be treated with Dapsone* (50 to 200 mg per day) for 12 weeks. If the results are unsatisfactory, the patient may then be treated with prednisone and cyclophosphamide. "Low-risk" patients, with disease occurring in only oral mucosa or in oral mucosa and skin, may be treated with topical corticosteroids. Intravenous immunoglobulin (Gamimue N)* and plasmapheresis, as described, can also be effective as an adjunctive therapy in pemphigoid patients with aggressive disease, especially in high-risk mucous membrane pemphigoid patients. Steroid-sparing immunosuppressive agents are contraindicated in patients with herpes gestationis who are pregnant, and in these patients, prednisone and topical corticosteroids would need to be the main forms of therapy.

LINEAR IgA BULLOUS DERMATOSIS

Clinical and Laboratory Features

Linear IgA bullous dermatosis is an idiopathic or drug-induced autoimmune blistering disease that can affect the elderly. A variant of this disease, chronic bullous dermatosis of childhood, affects the pediatric population. Clinical manifestations consist of papulovesicles with urticarial plaques. Patients may also display an arcuate pattern with a peripheral "string of beads" grouping of blisters. Common sites of involvement for children include the lower abdomen, perineum, and anogenital areas. In adults, the trunk and limbs are typically affected. The lesions tend to be more generalized and less symmetric than those in dermatitis herpetiformis. Lesions of the oral mucosa are frequently seen, and ocular involvement may occur with scarring and even blindness. Remissions are seen more often in children, in most cases within 2 years, while diseases of adults may last from 1 to 15 years.

Histologic analysis demonstrates subepidermal blistering with a polymorphonuclear, or less commonly, an eosinophilic infiltrate. Direct immunofluorescence of perilesional as well as normal skin reveals linear deposition of IgA at the basement membrane, usually at the epidermal roof of sodium chloride-split skin, but occasionally to the dermal floor. Most, but not all, patients exhibit circulating IgA antibodies against the basement membrane zone by indirect immunofluorescent microscopy.

*Not FDA approved for this indication.

Therapy

Dapsone* is the treatment of choice in linear IgA disease at typical doses of 100 to 200 mg per day. A glucose 6 phosphate dehydrogenase (G6PD) level should be obtained prior to the beginning of therapy. A low level identifies individuals prone to extensive drug-induced hemolysis and sulfones in these patients are contraindicated. Dapsone should be started at a low dose and increased gradually, checking the CBC frequently until either a therapeutic effect is noted or undue hemolysis ensues. In the absence of preexisting anemia or other associated conditions, such as coronary artery disease, a drop in the hemoglobin of up to 1 to 2 grams in patients receiving dapsone is usually well tolerated, however care must be exercised in titrating the dose for individual patients. Sulfapyridine,† given at 1 to 2 grams per day, may be substituted in patients with normal G6PD levels who cannot tolerate dapsone. Patients taking dapsone or sulfapyridine should have CBCs checked monthly and methemoglobinemia, an occasional side effect, should also be looked for at intervals. Some patients may need additional therapy with prednisone.* Some cases show a lack of response to sulfones, and in these cases combinations of prednisone and steroid-sparing immunosuppressive agents can be used as described earlier for pemphigoid patients. Intravenous immunoglobulin* may be also be helpful as an adjuvant to combat flares of severe disease.

DERMATITIS HERPETIFORMIS

Clinical and Laboratory Features

Dermatitis herpetiformis is an autoimmune blistering disease associated with gluten-sensitive enteropathy. The age of onset is usually between the second and fourth decades of life. It is marked by pruritic, erythematous, vesicular, bullous, or papular lesions, often occurring in a herpetiform pattern. The lesions are commonly found overlying extensor surfaces, including the knees, buttocks, sacrum, back, shoulders and posterior scapula, and neck. Mucous membranes are usually not involved. Biopsy of the gastrointestinal tract reveals atrophy of the intestinal villi, but enteropathy is usually not symptomatic. Dermatitis herpetiformis is closely related to the disease celiac sprue, which causes enteropathy but no skin disease, and overlap of these diseases can be found in patients occasionally. Dermatitis herpetiformis usually follows

*Not FDA approved for this indication.
†Not available in the United States.

a lifelong course with periods of exacerbation and remission. Skin biopsy demonstrates neutrophils in the dermal papillae with neutrophil fragments, fibrin deposition, and edema. Direct immunofluorescence observation of granular IgA deposits in the dermal papillae of perilesional skin confirms the diagnosis.

Therapy

Most patients respond very well to a gluten-free diet, however this requires strict adherence. Dapsone* (100 to 200 mg/d) or, if the patient is intolerant, sulfapyridine,† is the medical therapy of choice.

EPIDERMOLYSIS BULLOSA ACQUISITA

Clinical and Laboratory Features

Epidermolysis bullosa acquisita is an acquired autoimmune blistering disease that occurs most commonly in mid-life, and is distinct from inherited epidermolysis bullosa. Patients may present with two types of skin lesions: (1) trauma-induced lesions with acral distribution that heal with scarring and milia, which is the noninflammatory presentation; and (2) generalized inflammatory vesiculobullous disease that may display a morphology similar to bullous pemphigoid. In addition, oral, anogenital, esophageal, tracheal, laryngeal, or ocular mucosa can be affected. Common mucosal pathologies caused by this disease include symblepharon, esophageal strictures, and laryngeal stenosis. Epidermolysis bullosa acquisita follows a chronic course, with periods of exacerbation and remission.

Skin biopsies display the presence of a subepidermal blister with a mixed inflammatory infiltrate. Perilesional biopsy examined by direct immunofluorescence shows a linear pattern of IgG staining, which after sodium chloride separation localizes to the dermal floor of the induced separation. Indirect immunofluorescence microscopy on salt-split human skin reveals circulating IgG antibodies. ELISA and immunoblot analysis demonstrates reactivity of autoantibodies to type VII collagen, and this is diagnostic. A subset of patients with systemic lupus erythematosus show blistering and type VII collagen autoantibodies in a manner identical to that of epidermolysis bullosa acquisita. A subset of patients with primarily mucous membrane involvement, previously diagnosed with epidermolysis bullosa acquisita, probably have mucous membrane pemphigoid, which could be differentiated by specialized immunologic tests described earlier.

Therapy

Epidermolysis bullosa acquisita shows a variable and often recalcitrant response to therapy. Oral corticosteroids with conventional steroid-sparing agents used for pemphigus is one approach that is sometimes helpful. Dapsone* and/or colchicine* (1 to 2 mg per day) may be effective for some patients and are worth a therapeutic trial because they are considerably less toxic than corticosteroids or immunosuppressive agents. Cyclosporine (Neoral),* (3 to 5 mg/kg per day) can be effective as a sole or adjunctive therapy in some patients, however renal toxicity or cytopenia can limit its use in some patients. Intravenous immunoglobulin* has been shown to be effective in epidermolysis bullosa acquisita in a number of reports. Other treatment options include combined prednisone, cyclophosphamide therapy, plasmapheresis, and photopheresis.

*Not FDA approved for this indication.
†Not available in the United States.

OTHER BULLOUS DISEASES

Porphyria Cutanea Tarda

Porphyria cutanea tarda can commonly cause bullae on the dorsal hands, head and neck, and other sun-exposed areas. Occasionally it can be associated with a scleroderma-like fibrosis. Histology shows a subepidermal separation, sometimes with dermal papillae protruding upward into the blister (festooning), and a pauci-inflammatory infiltrate. Direct immunofluorescent microscopy usually shows immunoglobulins deposited only in the dermal capillaries. Laboratory findings include elevated urinary porphyrins, which can sometimes be seen as a pink fluorescence of the urine when examined by a Wood's light. Porphyria cutanea tarda arises from deficient activity of heme-synthetic enzymes. It is often associated with hepatotoxic conditions including hepatitis, ethanol abuse, HIV infection, and hemochromatosis. Excess tissue iron appears to play an important role in this disease. The most important aspect of treatment involves sunlight avoidance because this condition is driven through phototoxic reactions. Treatment of associated liver disease and avoidance of ethanol are also important factors in therapy. Therapeutic phlebotomy is often successful in reducing excess tissue iron stores, which can decrease cutaneous blistering. Venesections are gauged at what the patient can tolerate, taking care not to induce symptoms of iatrogenic anemia, with the goal of reducing serum ferritin to the lower limit of the normal range. If phlebotomy is not possible, iron mobilization from the tissues may be facilitated through chelation with desferrioxamine. Medical therapy with antimalarials may be used alone or combined with phlebotomy in selected patients. Hydroxychloroquine (Plaquenil)* 200 to 400 mg or chloroquine (Aralen)* 125 to 250 mg twice weekly, are typical adult dosages.

Toxic Epidermal Necrolysis

Toxic epidermal necrolysis, an autoimmune disease caused by autoantibodies to Fas ligand, produces rapidly developing generalized blistering, and

*Not FDA approved for this indication.

represents a dermatologic emergency. Toxic epidermal necrolysis can be associated with graft-versus-host reaction, viral infections, measles vaccination, lymphoma, leukemia, radiotherapy, or drug reactions. Sulfonamides, sulfones, pyrazolone derivatives, antibiotics, anticonvulsants, nonsteroidal anti-inflammatory agents, allopurinol, and anti-tuberculosis drugs have all been shown to be associated with this condition. Prompt recognition of the characteristic, rapidly progressing bullous formation and skin sloughing is critically important in toxic epidermal necrolysis patients. Patients should be transferred to intensive care or burn unit to support large scale wound care and hemodynamic instability. Intravenous immunoglobulin* 2 to 3 g/kg is the only medical therapy that has proved to be effective, and its use may be lifesaving.

*Not FDA approved for this indication.

CONTACT DERMATITIS

method of
JOSEPH F. FOWLER, Jr., M.D.
University of Louisville
Louisville, Kentucky

Contact dermatitis is an inflammatory skin condition induced by direct exposure to an irritant or allergen. Although there is overlap between the categories, contact dermatitis can be either acute or chronic and can be either irritant or allergic in etiology. These four categories are important because both the clinical appearance and treatment vary with the duration and causation of the dermatitis.

ACUTE ALLERGIC CONTACT DERMATITIS

The most common cause of acute allergic contact dermatitis (ACD) in North America is poison ivy, oak, or sumac. Other common causes of ACD include exposure to nickel (especially in costume jewelry), neomycin, rubber, fragrances, and preservatives in topical products. After exposure to the allergen, specific T lymphocytes respond to antigen-presenting cells in the skin and institute the inflammatory response. This usually takes from several hours to several days. The acute inflammatory response begins with pruritus, erythema, and edema and may progress to vesicles and bullae. The severity of response depends on the degree of allergen exposure and the sensitivity of the individual.

Treatment

Symptomatic treatment starts with cool compresses or cold packs applied to the affected area. Compresses can be tap water, saline, oatmeal soaks (Aveeno and others), or Burow solution soaks (Domeboro and others). Topical corticosteroids are a mainstay of treatment of all forms of acute ACD. Because the condition is self-limited and treatment usually is needed for 7 to 10 days or less, high-potency agents applied twice daily are safe. These include clobetasol (Temovate and others), betamethasone dipropionate (Diprolene and others), and halobetasol propionate (Ultravate). Systemic corticosteroids are often needed in cases where the dermatitis is widespread or particularly uncomfortable. Prednisone may be started in doses of 40 to 60 mg daily for 5 to 7 days and is then reduced to 10 to 20 mg/day for another 5 to 7 days. Lack of adequate dosage and duration of therapy is the most common cause of relapse of the dermatitis, so prepackaged "dose packs" are not recommended. Systemic antihistamines are helpful for their sedative effects but are not very effective in relieving pruritus of ACD.

CHRONIC ALLERGIC CONTACT DERMATITIS

Chronic ACD is caused by repeated, low-level exposure to allergens. This may occur because the allergen is unrecognized or because a person is unable to avoid a known allergen, as may be the case in occupational settings. The clinical findings include erythema, scaling, thickening of the skin, and pruritus. Although history and examination are helpful, identification of specific allergens causing ACD can only be done by patch testing. In contrast to the more understood scratch or prick test, the patch test detects delayed hypersensitivity caused by T cell hypersensitivity. Small amounts of allergens are applied to specially prepared tapes (patches), which are then affixed to the back for about 48 hours. Examination of the skin after patch removal allows identification of sites where a reaction has occurred: erythema, edema, and maybe vesicles. This localized area of ACD confirms that the patient is allergic to that particular substance.

Treatment

The best treatment of chronic ACD is its prevention by protecting the skin or removing contact with the allergen (see the following section). Skin moisturizers may be helpful at controlling the scaling and cracking. Topical corticosteroids are useful, but because the process is chronic, potent agents should be avoided. Hydrocortisone derivatives such as HC butyrate (Locoid), desonide (DesOwen and others), and fluticasone propionate (Cutivate) are useful choices. Long-term use of even these lower potency agents may sometimes result in cutaneous side effects such as atrophy, and tachyphylaxis may occur. The newer "topical immunomodulators" are nonsteroidal agents that target the specific cytokines at the root of ACD. They do not have the side effects of corticosteroids and therefore may be preferable for long-term use. Whether they are as efficacious is uncertain, but they have been shown to be very useful in management of atopic dermatitis. The two products currently available in the United States are pimecrolimus cream (Elidel) and tacrolimus ointment (Protopic). Systemic corticosteroids may be used for acute exacerbations of chronic ACD, but are not recommended for chronic use because of their side effects. Ultraviolet light therapy as used for psoriasis may be very helpful in controlling chronic ACD with minimal risk. Grenz-ray, a very superficial soft x-ray treatment, is helpful for localized areas of chronic ACD, such as hand eczema. Occasionally immunosuppressive agents such as methotrexate or mycophenolate mofetil (CellSept) may be needed.

ACUTE IRRITANT CONTACT DERMATITIS

Acute irritant contact dermatitis (ICD) is essentially a chemical burn caused by the direct toxic effect of acids, alkalis, and other caustic agents. Treatment is similar to that for thermal burns.

CHRONIC IRRITANT CONTACT DERMATITIS

Chronic ICD is caused by repeated cumulative trauma to the skin. Low-level recurrent exposure to water, detergents, oils, and the like leads to depletion of the normal skin barrier. Repeated friction and other mechanical trauma may do the same. Although the inflammatory process is not primary as in ACD, after the skin barrier is broken down, inflammation occurs. The degree of irritation required to produce chronic ICD varies greatly from person to person. Those with a background of atopy or psoriasis are at especially high risk to develop ICD. The appearance of chronic ICD is similar to that of chronic ACD, although pruritus is sometimes less prominent.

Treatment

This is also similar to the treatment of chronic ACD. Special care should be taken to use good moisturizers to help rebuild the skin barrier. Certain lipids such as ceramides applied in topical agents may accelerate skin healing but much more research needs to be done to determine which ingredients are the most useful.

PREVENTION AND PROTECTION

It cannot be emphasized enough that because contact dermatitis is, by definition, caused by exposure of the skin to noxious substances, protection of the skin is critical in caring for patients with ACD or ICD. Unfortunately, we currently know very little about the best ways to protect the skin. Obviously, wearing protective gloves and other equipment is often recommended but may not always be practical. Good use of moisturizers alone may help protect the skin to some degree from water and mild chemical irritants. A variety of "barrier creams" has been promoted as skin protectants, especially in the occupational setting, but research proving their effectiveness is usually lacking. Certainly use of mild skin cleansers instead of harsh soaps should be promoted to reduce further irritation from too-frequent washing, especially in hand eczema.

The only product specifically approved by the Food and Drug Administration for prevention of ACD is a lotion containing bentoquatam (IvyBlock Lotion). This product binds urushiol, the resin that causes dermatitis from poison ivy, oak, and sumac. It may be useful in blocking other irritants and allergens but this is unproven. The lotion should be applied 30 minutes before likely exposure to the toxic plants, much as a sunscreen is applied before going outdoors.

SKIN DISEASES OF PREGNANCY

method of
LYNNE H. MORRISON, M.D.
Dermatology Department
Oregon Health & Science University
Portland, Oregon

Skin changes in pregnancy are common and may include normal cutaneous changes that occur in pregnancy, common skin diseases coincidentally developing during pregnancy, exacerbation of preexisting skin disorders, and the eruptions that are specifically associated with pregnancy. This article covers only the cutaneous diseases specifically associated with pregnancy. These can vary in severity and, to ensure an accurate diagnosis and optimize management, it is often prudent to involve the dermatologist in the care of these patients.

PRURITIC URTICARIAL PAPULES AND PLAQUES OF PREGNANCY

Pruritic urticarial papules and plaques of pregnancy (PUPPP) is a common, very pruritic eruption that typically occurs late in the third trimester of gestation and is also known as polymorphic eruption of pregnancy. It classically presents in primigravidas during the third trimester. An increased incidence of multiple pregnancies has been identified in patients with PUPPP.

The lesions of PUPPP consist of small, erythematous papules that frequently begin on the abdomen, often in the striae distensae. They may coalesce to form large, erythematous plaques. The lesions are quite pruritic, frequently interfering with the patients ability to sleep at night. The urticarial papules and plaques generally spread to involve buttocks, thighs, hips, legs, and upper inner arms, but the face is almost always spared.

Biopsies from skin lesions of PUPPP show a superficial and often mid-dermal lymphohistiocytic inflammatory infiltrate occasionally mixed with eosinophils. Epidermal changes may include mild spongiosis as well. These changes are not diagnostic in and of themselves but are consistent with the disease. There is no specific laboratory test for PUPPP, so the diagnosis rests on characteristic clinical presentation in conjunction with consistent histologic findings. It is prudent to perform biopsies for direct immunofluorescence studies if there is any suspicion of herpes gestationis.

PUPPP usually resolves soon after delivery and generally responds relatively well to treatment. It does not tend to recur in subsequent pregnancies and does not typically have a postpartum flare, as can be seen in herpes gestationis. There does not seem to be any increased incidence of fetal morbidity or mortality associated with PUPPP.

A diagnosis of PUPPP is not difficult in the classic presentation of a primigravida presenting in the late third trimester with an extremely pruritic papular eruption beginning on a woman's abdomen. In less classic cases, the differential diagnosis may include herpes gestationis, contact dermatitis, urticaria, drug eruptions, and insect bite reactions.

Frequent use of potent topical corticosteroids such as fluocinonide (Lidex) 0.05% or triamcinolone acetonide (Kenalog) 0.1% four to six times daily relieves pruritus and stops new lesion formation in most patients. As patients are improving, the therapy can be gradually tapered to less frequent treatment schedules or less potent topical steroids. Patients with very severe disease may require tapering courses of systemic corticosteroids, usually in the range of 20 to 40 mg of prednisone daily. Oral antihistamines may provide some relief but are thought to be less effective than frequent use of potent topical corticosteroids.

HERPES GESTATIONIS

Herpes gestationis is a rare antibody-mediated, autoimmune bullous disorder of pregnancy and the postpartum period which is closely related to bullous pemphigoid. Despite the name, it has no relationship to viral infection; the name refers to the characteristically grouped lesions in this disease. Its incidence has been estimated to be approximately 1 in 50,000 pregnancies, and it may present during any trimester of pregnancy, but most often occurs between the fourth and seventh month of pregnancy. Postpartum exacerbations are common, and it is important to evaluate all patients carefully at that time, including those whose disease was well controlled earlier in pregnancy. Typically the disease resolves spontaneously several weeks after delivery, but frequently flares when patients resume menses or subsequently use oral contraceptives. Herpes gestationis tends to recur in subsequent pregnancies, and when it does so, often presents earlier in gestation.

Although early reports suggested that there was an increased incidence in fetal death and premature deliveries, subsequent studies have not supported this finding, but have identified an increase in prematurity and small for gestational age infants. Most often, children born of mothers with herpes gestationis do not demonstrate skin lesions.

Herpes gestationis presents as an extremely pruritic eruption that characteristically involves the abdomen, but also may be present on palms, soles, chest, and back but rarely on the face. Typically, mucous membranes are spared. The primary lesions include erythematous papules and plaques in addition to tense blisters. Erosions may become annular to polycyclic with vesicles studded on top of urticarial plaques. Milder cases may present only with erythematous papules and plaques and limited vesicular lesions. The diseases most often confused with herpes gestationis are pruritic urticarial papules and plaques of pregnancy and erythema multiforme.

Biopsies taken from skin lesions typically show subepidermal blisters, with an eosinophil-rich infiltrate in the epidermis. Biopsies taken from urticarial lesions may show eosinophilic spongiosis only. Although these findings are typical of herpes gestationis, they are not specific for this disease and can be seen in other autoimmune, subepidermal, blistering skin diseases. It is important to perform additional biopsies of normal perilesional skin for direct immunofluorescence studies to confirm a diagnosis of herpes gestationis. Typically, these studies show continuous linear deposition of the third component of complement along epidermal basement membrane zone; approximately 30% to 40% of biopsies will also show linear deposition of IgG at the basement membrane zone. A positive direct immunofluorescence biopsy showing these findings will differentiate this disease from PUPPP and other specific dermatoses of pregnancy.

The goal of treatment in herpes gestationis is to suppress blister formation and to relieve the pruritus. Most patients require systemic steroids in doses ranging from 20 to 40 mg of prednisone* daily to accomplish this goal. Often dividing the doses of daily corticosteroids every 12 hours will allow faster improvement of symptoms in these patients. After the eruption and pruritus have been controlled, the dose of prednisone* should be tapered to the lowest dose that allows control of the disease. Patients often experience a postpartum flare of the disease, and the dose of prednisone* needs to be increased at that time or restarted if they have tapered off prednisone.* Postpartum flares of the disease may require up to 60 mg of prednisone* to gain control. The dose of steroid can be gradually tapered as the disease spontaneously regresses postpartum. If systemic steroids have been used during pregnancy, the obstetrician needs to be alerted to the possibility of adrenal insufficiency in newborns, although this does not appear to be a common problem.

Patients with very mild disease may respond adequately to frequent use of potent topical corticosteroids such as fluocinonide* .05% or triamcinolone acetonide* 0.1% used four to six times daily.

Open, wet dressings several times a day may be used to promote drying of weeping lesions. This can be followed with application of topical antibiotics and

*Not FDA approved for this indication.

nonadhesive dressings. Patients should be examined regularly for evidence of secondary bacterial infection and cultured and treated appropriately.

PRURIGO GRAVIDARUM

Prurigo gravidarum, also known as recurrent cholestasis of pregnancy, or recurrent intrahepatic cholestasis, is a hepatic condition occurring late in pregnancy, characterized by generalized pruritus and occasionally followed by jaundice. It has been estimated to occur in between 0.02% to 2.4% of pregnancies. The clinical manifestations of prurigo gravidarum consist of pruritus in the absence of primary lesions, although secondary excoriations may be seen. The pruritus may be localized at first, but subsequently tends to become generalized and the severity may vary from moderate to marked. The pruritus precedes development of clinical jaundice by about 2 to 4 weeks. Associated symptoms can include fatigue, anorexia, and occasionally nausea and vomiting. Right upper quadrant tenderness as well as light-colored stools and dark urine are also occasional associated findings. Laboratory studies may reveal elevations in hepatic transaminases and alkaline phosphatase. Generally this disease occurs in the third trimester, but has occurred as early as the first trimester. Prurigo gravidarum remits soon after delivery, but usually recurs in subsequent pregnancies or after exposure to oral contraceptives. There are reports of increased incidence of prematurity, low birth weight, and postpartum hemorrhage in patients with prurigo gravidarum. The occurrence of these events seems to be greatest in patients having both pruritus and jaundice. The cause of this disorder is not known, but is believed to be hormonally induced in susceptible individuals. The diagnosis is based on clinical and laboratory findings.

Therapy in prurigo gravidarum is aimed at symptomatic control of pruritus. Bland emollients, topical antipruritics, or topical corticosteroids often provide adequate relief of symptoms. Addition of antihistamines with or without cholestyramine may be beneficial. Because these patients have potential fat malabsorption and therefore decreased absorption of vitamin K, it has been suggested by some that administration of vitamin K before delivery could diminish the risk of postpartum hemorrhage.

IMPETIGO HERPETIFORMIS

Impetigo herpetiformis is a form of pustular psoriasis that occurs during pregnancy. It is a very rare disease but may be life-threatening. This condition often occurs in the third trimester of pregnancy but can develop also in first or second trimesters. Women with this disease do not necessarily have a personal or family history of psoriasis.

Clinically, these patients demonstrate erythematous patches and plaques with small, sterile pustules at the margins. The plaques expand peripherally with new pustules occurring at the leading edge as the old pustules centrally break down. Early lesions involve the flexural areas including groin, axillae, and anterior and posterior neck. As the lesions expand, large areas of the body can be affected including occasional involvement of mucous membranes.

Most patients have constitutional symptoms including fever, chills, nausea, vomiting, and diarrhea. Possible laboratory abnormalities include hypoalbuminemia and hypocalcemia with subsequent tetany in severe cases. Additionally, elevated white blood cell counts and sedimentation rates are commonly found in impetigo herpetiformis. Although the primary pustules in this disease are sterile, they can become secondarily infected, and, in a febrile patient, infection must be ruled out.

The disease generally resolves shortly after delivery, but can recur in subsequent pregnancies. There can be an increased risk of fetal morbidity and mortality in patients with impetigo herpetiformis. The pathologic findings are the same as that seen in pustular psoriasis. The characteristic feature is that of a collection of neutrophils in areas of spongiosis within the epidermis known as spongiform pustules of Kogoj.

The mainstay of treatment for impetigo herpetiformis consists of systemic glucocorticosteroids. Prednisone* in doses of up to 60 mg per day may be needed to control the eruption initially, but after the disease has come under control, the prednisone can be tapered. The taper should be carried out slowly to avoid flares of the disease. Patients should be evaluated for cutaneous or systemic infections and treated appropriately. Serum calcium and albumin levels should also be obtained and abnormalities corrected. The obstetrician needs to be informed if the patient has been on systemic corticosteroids during pregnancy to be alerted to the possibility of adrenal insufficiency in the newborn.

*Not FDA approved for this indication.

PRURITIS ANI AND VULVAE

method of
NEIL H. HYMAN, M.D.
Department of Surgery
University of Vermont
Burlington, Vermont

The clinical features of pruritus ani and a staggering array of suggested remedies have appeared in the literature for thousands of years. Unfortunately, relatively little progress has been made in characterizing the causative factors and in achieving consensus on what constitutes effective therapy. As such, the evaluation and treatment of an itchy perineum can be a frustrating experience for patient and physician alike.

Pruritus ani has been described in conjunction with numerous systemic illnesses (e.g., diabetes), mechanical factors (e.g., poor hygiene), food sensitivities (e.g., caffeine), dermatologic conditions (e.g., psoriasis), specific infections (e.g., pinworms), and medications (e.g., colchicine). However, in the vast majority of cases, the signs and symptoms are nonspecific and usually do not readily allow for identification of a specific causative agent. As such, treatment is often empirical and may require considerable patience.

Most cases of pruritus ani are related to dermatoses and not to definable anorectal disease. The small ulcerations and thickened, inflamed skin typically seen is usually secondary to chronic irritation and scratching rather than primarily causative. As such, patients will often mistakenly attribute their itching to anal skin tags, perianal ulcerations, or view the symptoms as a sign of "hemorrhoids."

The key to successful management is a thoughtful, systematic approach followed by a well-scripted treatment plan. Patients should be questioned about their bowel pattern, the presence of rectal bleeding or prolapse and whether they tended to emit mucus or other substances onto their perineal skin. This would help identify the occasional patient with prolapsing hemorrhoids, anal fistula, rectal prolapse, or other readily treatable cause of the itching. Inspection of the perineum may reveal a specific diagnosis such as condyloma acuminata, but most often will simply show perianal inflammation, erythema, and excoriation, or the chronic changes associated with lichenification, characterized by markedly thickened skin and accentuated cutaneous markings.

Again, most cases of pruritus ani are best thought of as related to a "skin condition." In children, many cases are caused by *Enterobius vermicularis* (pinworm) and may be readily diagnosed by microscopic examination of cellophane tape applied first thing in the morning to the perianal skin. However, in adults, a wide variety of exacerbating factors may be operative. A specific dermatosis such as eczema or psoriasis may be noted. A dietary history, with particular emphasis on caffeinated beverages, dairy products, chocolate, and tomatoes may be particularly rewarding. Many cases are associated with coffee consumption and will resolve with cessation of coffee intake. If so, coffee may be reintroduced until a threshold is defined.

Poor or more commonly excessive anal hygiene may be to blame. Many patients assume their itching must be related to inadequate cleansing and will scrub the perianal skin relentlessly and compulsively, thereby abrading and injuring the already friable epithelium. Symptoms are often exacerbated by soaps, fabrics, perfumed substances, and by reaction to various topical agents. Many patients with pruritus ani will have tried a wide array of over-the-counter topical agents; instead of being helpful, they may themselves cause a contact dermatitis, which perpetuates symptoms.

In the absence of a specific definable etiology, treatment usually starts by "de-emphasizing" the perianal skin. Excessive cleansing or wiping, particularly with harsh soaps, is discouraged, and baby wipes or a hair dryer may be used instead. Potentially causative dietary agents such as coffee are avoided, as are all perfumed toilet tissues or substances. If perianal "wetness" or moisture is a problem, an absorbent cotton ball may be applied and changed with each visit to the washroom. Because itching is often worst at night, an antihistamine (e.g., hydroxyzine hydrochloride [Vistaril]) may be prescribed at bedtime for its antipruritic and sedative effect.

Ultimately, short courses of 1% hydrocortisone ointment may be required, with higher potency steroid ointments such as triamcinolone (Kenalog) used for refractory cases. However, it must be remembered that topical steroids will cause atrophy and "rebound" inflammation, so the lowest doses and shortest effective courses should be sought.

Many of the treatment principles for pruritus ani are applicable to the management of pruritus vulvae. Vulvar itching is often causes by the layers of relatively impervious fabric in covering clothing, which traps moisture and can lead to macerated skin. However, some cases may require an analysis of vaginal secretions or fungal cultures. Recurrent vulvovaginal candidiasis may be difficult to eradicate, requiring multiple courses of topical or oral antifungals. As with the perianal skin, any suspicious lesions such as those with a scaly, plaquelike appearance should be biopsied. Bowen's disease or extramammary Paget's disease often present with chronic itching; the diagnosis is often missed, because symptoms and skin changes are often long-standing.

URTICARIA AND ANGIOEDEMA

method of
LARRY E. MILLIKAN, M.D.
Tulane University Health Sciences Center
New Orleans, Louisiana

Urticaria is a cutaneous reaction complex with obvious physical findings, and self-diagnosis is easy; the challenge is determining cause and adequate treatment. In reality it can be due to a number of conditions physical, infectious, allergic, or immune and as a secondary reaction to certain systemic diseases.

EVALUATION

Traditionally urticaria has been classified into acute and chronic. Acute is defined as less than 6 weeks' duration and chronic as more than 6 weeks' duration. Different patterns are useful in evaluation. The characteristic very superficial lesions may be very transient. With these superficial lesions one should also check for the phenomenon of dermographism. Dermographism is the appearance of hives after light trauma and its larger variant, pressure urticaria, after contact with tight belts, and tight clothing, or seat belts. Most of the physical urticaria has a very obvious pattern and one can associate them with the offending agent such as a belt, sun, cold, or heat. Dermographism is an important first step in diagnosis of any patient with urticaria. More complicated are the patients that have more lasting rather than evanescent lesions. Often these are firmer, deeper, and more erythematous and one can visualize that the perturbation is deeper in the dermis than that of the superficial dermal edema with common hives. This is the hallmark of urticarial vasculitis and the deeper involvement with larger vessels and lesions lasting for hours mandate a more aggressive workup to determine underlying systemic disease. Sometimes there is confusion between urticarial vasculitis and erythema multiforme, because both may have somewhat similar physical findings, and both urticarial vasculitis and erythema multiforme are conditions usually associated with a systemic disease. Although it is most clinician's general experience that the majority of urticaria patients go without an etiology diagnosed, one should in each case rule out serious underlining treatable etiologies such as infections, including hepatitis, and collagen vascular diseases, including lupus. In acute patients one should carefully screen agents that are ingested including foods such as certain fruits, strawberries, seafood, and medications. In my patients we initiate systemic relief (see the following section) and then as the evaluation progresses we develop a more elaborate look at underlying etiologies. In general acute urticaria patients that resolve are the most rewarding and often the ones most likely to be diagnosed related to foods or food dyes.

Chronic urticaria is the most challenging and one where diagnosis of etiology is less reliable. We generally have the patient provide a diary covering exposure or injectants. Of greatest importance in chronic urticaria are subtle ingestants including drugs and food dyes, with tartrazine being perhaps the most celebrated one. In the past, especially in Europe, challenge tests and even hospital admission with elimination diets often would result in the diagnosis of an offending food or, in some penicillin-allergic patients, minute traces of penicillin in the food chain. Usually a comprehensive history is repeated on each visit to refresh the patient's memory. The literature is replete with examples of urticaria resolving after dental surgery removing a chronic tooth abscess, chronic urinary tract infections, or sinusitis and most of this can be eliminated up front by comprehensive questionnaire and recommendations to the patient for follow-up by their dentist and other appropriate specialists. In the initial encounter it is also important to consider the role of stress. As with any other skin disease, there is a definite intensification related to personal stress. Especially in patients with dermographism, periods of high stress may result in scratching and secondary giant hives induced by the scratching. For this reason many of the most successful medications, while having some effect on the two histamine receptors (H_1, H_2), often have ataractic effects. Doxepin (Sinequan)* is useful in this area helping some with the patient's management of stress in addition to having an effect on both the histamine receptors.

*Not FDA approved for this indication.

ACUTE URTICARIA

Acute urticaria is the most potentially curable. When the etiology is obvious, the patient often does not seek medical help and may find control with topical antipruritics and diphenhydramine (Benadryl) or other over-the-counter (OTC) antihistamines. If it is widespread the symptoms may be such that patients seek medical help, for OTC preparations usually are inadequate to control their symptoms. In the emergency room parenteral intramuscular or IV diphenhydramine has always been my treatment of choice. One can see the hives disappear when diphenhydramine is given by a slow IV push (50 mg). The results are slower but usually equally effective with intramuscular diphenhydramine. This often is sufficient without the need to resort to such backup medications as the corticosteroids. If there is any suggestion of airway, lip, tongue, or throat involvement, then antihistamines are followed usually by epinephrine* and subsequently, before the patient is discharged, I usually give him or her some maintenance parenteral steroid with a prescription for oral steroid with a usual dosage equivalent of prednisone* (1 mg/kg). Usual dosage for epinephrine is 1:1000; 0.3 to 0.5 mL subcutaneously. If the patient is showing progression and signs of airway obstruction then one uses intravenous 1:10,000 epinephrine and emergency room monitoring until the patient stabilizes or admission for observation. These unstable patients may ultimately need to be hospitalized for continued IV medications and carefully observed for the possible need of airway obstruction. In many cases where the patient's symptoms are apparently progressing one should be prepared to provide airway support by intubation or tracheostomy and blood access through a patent saline drip.

CHRONIC URTICARIA

The chronic patient is one of those with long-standing "unhappy hives" and the challenge there is often to (1) relieve the symptoms and (2) determine the cause, if possible. I think it most important to carefully check each visit to make sure the urticaria is not destabilizing and note any suggestion of airway involvement. Most of these patients need chronic therapy and we now have many agents that are well tolerated and quite effective. The degree of patient symptoms determines aggressiveness of therapy. Mild chronic urticaria often responds to the H1 blocking agents of the nonsedating group. This group includes loratadine (Claritin), which I find most useful in the Redi-tab formulation, which rapidly dissolves on the tongue and useful for both adults and children. The major caveat in the use of any antihistamine in the urticaria patient is to be certain of adequate dosing. Most patients that do not get symptomatic relief from the initial treatment dosages respond with higher drug dosages. The gold standard for many years for urticaria was hydroxyzine (Vistaril).* It now has

*Not FDA approved for this indication.

essentially been replaced by its metabolite cetirizine (Zyrtec). It has a slight sedative effect, which is its only downside, but it is still the most effective agent. Additionally, fexofenadine (Allegra) shows no sedation, but a high level of effectiveness. This group of medications should be sufficient for most patients. If there still are symptoms and problems one then has to move to drugs with more side effects and greater sedation. I have found that sometimes it is necessary to use both hydroxyzine* and loratadine in those patients accepting the increased sedating side effects. Another extremely effective agent reported to have an antiserotonin effect is cyproheptadine (Periactin). When patients continue to have troublesome symptoms in spite of adequate antihistamines, the next step is H2 blockade; this can be done with such agents as cimetidine (Tagamet),* ranitidine (Zantac),* or doxepin (Sinequan).* Use these agents in the usual dosage first and then push relating to the weight of the patient. With the steps of H_1 blockade, H_2 blockade, and possible antiserotonin modification, if symptoms persist a β-active agent such as 50 mg pseudoephedrine* is added. The next step usually is corticosteroids, especially if there is any potential for airway endangerment. Initially the dosage is 1 mg/kg with quick taper down to the lowest possible maintenance therapy and the alternate-day therapy. This is then transitioned into steroid-sparing regimen with a steroid-sparing agent such as dapsone. Dapsone* used in dose of 100 mg a day overlapping with the steroids remembering that it may take 60–90 days for full dapsone effect. This then allows further reduction from daily steroids to alternate-day steroids and ultimately out. In the worst-case scenario the other drugs to be considered after very serious thought include the use of colchicine* in 0.6 mg twice a day and then the introduction of more potent agents such as azathioprine (Imuran).* In most instances the patients that require this almost heroic form of therapy are certainly candidates for consultation with regional experts in this area.

PHYSICAL URTICARIA

Pressure urticaria this with the classical manifestations of dermographism varies from a minor problem to a significant disability related to touch, pressure (seat belts, tight clothing) that can cause discomfort as well as making the patient very self-conscious. Depending on the severity, steroids, which are the gold standard for pressure urticaria, may or may not be indicated. But they remain the primary drug in these patients. The newer nonsedating antihistamines, which pass the blood-brain barrier poorly, have provided an important step in that central nervous system side effects with previously available medications created serious workplace complications. The standard treatment with loratadine 10 mg daily, desloratadine 5 mg daily, fexofenadine 60 mg twice per day or 180 mg daily, and cetirizine 10 mg daily all seem to be effective therapy. Previously the two sedating or slightly sedating drugs cyproheptadine and hydroxyzine were always the preferable agents. Start with either of these latter two as a bedtime dosage of 25 mg hydroxyzine* and 4 mg cyproheptadine, then gradually increase it to relieve symptoms or to patient's tolerance of sedating side effects. The problems with cold urticaria can be significant and even can cause airway problems with ingestion or inhalation of cold liquids or air. Therefore this mandates early workup and treatment. The patients should be evaluated for cryoproteins, cryoglobulins, or cryofibrinogen as well as cold agglutinins and the rare case of patients with syphilis mandates serologic testing in these patients. Ingestion of large amounts of cold liquids can create problems in the upper digestive tract as well as the oral pharynx and airway. Treatment to control these patients is mandatory. Follow-up testing is done using an ice cube for 5 minutes and observation for 15 minutes. Positive tests confirms the diagnosis and subsequent testing after initiating therapy will give some idea of the level of protection derived from therapy.

*Not FDA approved for this indication.

CHOLINERGIC URTICARIA

Cholinergic urticaria results from acetylcholine release during the sweating process, which gives a clinical picture of multiple small, 3- to 5-mm hives. In these patients avoid temperature extremes, minimize the sweating process, and above all else caution exposure to aspirin. Aspirin is a particular interest because the nonsteroidals may have some effect on the prostaglandin system, making these patients much more prone to reacting with urticaria after various insults. Cholinergic urticaria has, for many years, been the primary indication for the use of hydroxyzine because it began as the gold standard for the treatment of urticaria. Its derivative cetirizine should be equally effective although the amount of experience with cetirizine in this condition is still far less than that with hydroxyzine. An alternative usage of cyproheptadine (Periactin) is also an option, and in some patients one has to alternate between the agents. Cyproheptadine is of interest because it also has some apparent antiserotonin effect. A change in lifestyle to less vigorous exercise also will minimize these symptoms. It should noted that in the evaluation of a patient, presence of dermographism may significantly alter the clinical features of the urticaria, converting the small tiny papules of cholinergic urticaria into giant hives from scratching. Nonspecific treatment of pruritus also should include the use of topical forms of camphor, menthol, pramoxine, and doxepin.

AQUAGENIC URTICARIA

Aquagenic urticaria is less common and thus it has less scientific evaluation of the actual processes operative in the production of such hives. There is the possibility that the heat of the water or the sudden cooling of the skin after completion of the morning

*Not FDA approved for this indication.

shower might create aquagenic urticaria. Over the years we have found that the most significant therapeutic agent for aquagenic urticaria is the use of hydroxyzine* and the possible additional use of solar light or phototherapy. One can use the natural sun, coaching the patient and parents on the appropriate response and also educating them into the necessity and use of the various monitors that are used.

SOLAR URTICARIAS

Recommendations for solar urticaria relate to intensive evaluation to determine the spectral range of the challenging agents that produce solar urticaria, as well as serum/passive transfer. This was pioneered for many years as the primary area of evaluation and workup by the dermatologist in such cases. The association of solar challenge with appearance of hives has long been of interest, although this is a fairly uncommon condition in most physician offices. The patient continues to need protection and observation in addition to very aggressive systemic therapy including ultraviolet A and ultraviolet B and the more modern derivative, which is the use of psoralen with the ultraviolet A (PUVA) somewhat paralleling the treatment of psoriasis.

The effect of ultraviolet A from its deep penetration and PUVA has shown dramatic benefits in many skin diseases besides urticaria. The initial studies also looked at mastocytosis and the improvement in patient signs and symptoms after phototherapy and after systemic extracorporeal photopheresis. The agents used are generally the standard ultraviolet A and ultraviolet B units that are present in most dermatology departments. One always has to include hereditary angioedema or Quincke's edema in evaluation. There are two variations on this, one with the absent C1 esterase inhibitor and the other with dysfunctional C1 esterase inhibitor. Therefore workup looks at presence/absence of the proteins and at tests to measure the functional activities. Acquired urticarial syndromes need to be evaluated, for on occasion they are associated with dysproteinemia and with lymphoproliferative diseases. Similarly the entity of delayed pressure urticaria has an equally strong association with systemic disease. Testing of these patients is the same including evaluations for cold urticaria, testing for dermatographism, photo testing as appropriate, and the use of standardized weights (such as preweighted sand bags) to apply reproducible pressure to an area and evaluate the effect of the therapy to control symptoms. The traditional treatment for hereditary angioedema has been hospitalization acutely with the availability of emergency airway reconstitution with tracheostomy, and intravenous access because of the mortality that has been as high as 30%. The use of frozen plasma blood transfusions in the past were used to help replace some of the missing factors. More recently anabolic agents have been found that stimulate production of the missing enzyme and the primary agent is danazol (Danocrine* 200 mg twice daily). Alternatively, stanozolol (Winstrol* 2 mg tid) with subsequent reduction to the lowest possible dose to minimize symptoms. Treatment is important because of this significant potential for mortality.

*Not FDA approved for this indication.

ADRENERGIC URTICARIA

This rare syndrome is significant because of patients flaring when given β-adrenergic agents, usually the standard therapy. Here in the few cases reported β-blockers effectively block the urticarial response to adrenergic agents, likely affecting the prostaglandin pathway in urticariogenesis.

CONTACT URTICARIA

Contact urticaria can be sometimes easily diagnosed but can confuse. Most straightforward are the direct-contact urticaria after various contactants plants such as nettles, and animals, caterpillars, and jellyfish. In all these instances there is either an injection with histamine to the skin (in the common nettle and *Urtica* spp) or the injection of enzymes which stimulate histamine release as in the case of various caterpillar stings and jellyfish stings. Cinnamic aldehyde is another agent that can cause some of the symptoms. Of more and greater concern is the true allergic or potentially anaphylactic form of contact urticaria of which latex sensitivity has become a very prominent concern. This is especially true in health workers: more than a quarter of the people employed in Scandinavian health professions have developed a latex sensitivity. This can be due either to the latex in the gloves or small amounts of latex in the powder from the gloves. Many of these patients have associated syndromes and associated symptomatology of cross-reactions to bananas, kiwi, avocado, and chestnuts. These patients, although having significant symptoms in the skin from contact urticaria, can have potentially fatal sequelae from mucus membrane exposure to the same allergen. Testing using both contact sensitivity testing from T cell–mediated type IV reactions or the potentially fatal anaphylactic reactions (type I) with prick testing should be done to confirm or refute presumptive diagnosis. It is very important to make the diagnosis early so that syndrome does not increase in severity to become a life-threatening syndrome. Contact urticaria may respond to topical agents such as topical doxepin (Zonalon),* systemic agents such as antihistamines and antiserotonin agents, or, in the case of anaphylactic syndrome, may require systemic steroids to avert any potential fatal sequelae. In all cases of these urticarial syndromes there is an ongoing concern over cross-reactive sensitivity to nonsteroidal agents and aspirin, which this may alter testing and the patient's sensitivity because of their known effect on the prostaglandin system.

*Not FDA approved for this indication.

Because of the large number of patients whose etiology is never discerned, the physician's first duty to the patient is to control symptoms and avert life-threatening anaphylactic reactions.

PIGMENTARY DISORDERS

method of
JAMES J. NORDLUND, M.D.
Group Health Associates
Cincinnati, Ohio

The normal color of human skin can vary from white to dark black with various shades of tan and brown. Skin color is determined by a number of factors, including the amount of collagen in the papillary dermis, the presence of lipids like carotene, by the quantity of blood flow, and the type and quantity of melanin within the epidermis. Most observers consider melanin to be the primary determinant of skin color, a conclusion that is true only in those who have very dark skin.

Skin color has been divided into four (some observers use six types) types called the Fitzpatrick classification (Table 1).

This classification of skin types is based on the capacity of the individual to produce melanin. Production of melanin is inversely correlated with propensity to sunburn. Those individuals whose melanocytes produce large amounts of eumelanin tan readily and are resistant to sunburn. Those who burn easily tan poorly. It should be recognized that even those with type 4 skin color can sunburn but they do so only after prolonged exposure to intense sunlight.

There are two types of melanin: eumelanin that is black or brown, and pheomelanin that is orange in color. Eumelanin is synthesized exclusively from the amino acid tyrosine. Pheomelanin is produced from two amino acids (i.e., tyrosine and cysteine). All melanocytes and all individuals produce both types of melanin. Those individuals with type 1 skin color produce predominantly pheomelanin and a paucity of eumelanin, those with type 4 skin color mostly eumelanin.

Melanin is produced exclusively by melanocytes. The enzymatic reactions take place within lysosome-related organelles called melanosomes. The melanosomes filled with melanin are transferred into the cytoplasm of the surrounding keratinocytes. The melanocyte with surrounding keratinocytes it services has been called the epidermal melanin unit. There is another cell in the epidermis, the Langerhans cell, which is an immune macrophage. It is now clear that the three cells—the keratinocyte, Langerhans cell, and melanocyte—are the basic unit of the epidermis. This group might be called the KLM complex. The interactive functions of these three cells provides an explanation for a variety of pigmentary disorders such as postinflammatory hyper- and hypopigmentation, melasma, and pityriasis alba.

Dark skin (types 3 and 4) is characterized histologically by melanocytes and surrounding keratinocytes stuffed with large numbers of hefty melanosome replete with eumelanin. Type 1 skin color is typified by epidermal cells of the KLM complex holding fewer, smaller melanosomes containing pheomelanin and some eumelanin. Keratinocytes retain the melanin within their cytoplasm as they migrate from the basilar layer of the epidermis to the stratum corneum. It appears that melanin polymer is not degraded but is excreted from the skin by the desquamating corneocytes. Melanin production, transfer, and excretion is a complex process and at times disrupted causing various disorders of hyperpigmentation or hypopigmentation of the skin.

Abnormal skin color can be caused by many factors. Deposition of chemicals, usually medications in the epidermis or dermis, can discolor the skin. Silver, gold (for treatment of rheumatoid arthritis), cardiac medications (amiodarone), tranquilizers (Thorazine), minocycline (for treatment of acne), and numerous other medications have been observed to deposit in the skin. The discoloration can range from a lilac (chrysiasis) to blue (minocycline) or blue black (amiodarone).

Melanin itself can produce several types of hyperpigmentation. Melanocytes and melanin normally are found exclusively in the epidermis but in some disorders of hyperpigmentation they are located in the epidermis and dermis. Epidermal melanin is brown. If the excess melanin is confined to the epidermis such as observed in a café-au-lait macule, the skin will be darker brown than the surrounding skin. If the melanin or the melanocytes are located in the dermis such as occurs after many inflammatory processes, the skin takes on a gray-black or bluish-black discoloration.

Hypopigmentation is caused by two mechanisms. The first is a decrease in the amount of melanin produced by melanocytes and transferred to the surrounding keratinocytes. Mild inflammation like that which occurs in pityriasis alba is manifested as hypopigmentation. The second mechanism is partial or complete loss of melanocytes. Vitiligo is a disorder caused by the destruction of epidermal melanocytes, usually complete, resulting in depigmented skin.

TABLE 1. **Fitzpatrick Classification of Skin Types**

Skin Type	Tendency to Sunburn	Ability to Tan	Typical Ethnic Ancestry
1	Always burns	Never tans	Celts
2	Usually burns	Tans somewhat	Europeans
3	Rarely burns	Tans readily	Orientals
4	Never burns	Tans deeply	Africans and aborigines

COMMON DISORDERS OF HYPERPIGMENTATION

Melasma

Melasma is a common disorder typically affecting adult women, especially those of darker skin types. Melasma uncommonly affects men. It is confused with chloasma, a brown hyperpigmentation that occurs during pregnancy. Both conditions affected the forehead, the cheeks and malar eminences, nose, and chin—areas that are sun exposed. The dorsum of the forearms also is commonly involved. Chloasma seems to be related to high estrogen production during pregnancy. Most women with melasma have not taken hormones or been pregnant for many years before the onset of the pigmentation. The causes of melasma are unknown but might be related to photocontact allergies to common chemicals.

Melasma is divided into two basic types: epidermal and dermal. Epidermal melasma presents as brown hyperpigmentation. Dermal melasma has a blue-gray discoloration. Most individuals have a combination of both. Only the epidermal component is treatable. Dermal pigmentation is not altered by currently available medications.

The treatment of choice is hydroquinone, a molecule that inhibits the production of new melanin. It is not a bleach and has no effect on pre-existing melanin. Hydroquinone comes in many preparations such as a 3% solution (Melanex) and a 4% cream (Eldoquin Forte) that are applied twice daily. Treatment is prolonged over many months or a year. To accelerate response, applications of hydroquinone can be combined with topical steroids that also block formation of melanin. On the face nonfluorinated steroids such as desonide* 0.05% (DesOwen and Tridesilon) applied twice daily are safe for prolonged use. Applications of retinoids seem to accelerate the desquamation of pre-existing melanin. Combinations of hydroquinone, steroids, and retinoic acid (Tri-Luma) have been effectively used for treatment of melasma.

Melasma has been treated successfully with chemical peels and dermabrasion. These modalities rapidly eliminate the pre-existing melanin by removing the entire epidermis. Healing often is accompanied by postinflammatory hyperpigmentation unless the regenerating epidermis is treated with hydroquinone or other inhibitors of melanin formation.

Postinflammatory Hyperpigmentation

The melanocyte is involved in most inflammatory processes of the skin. Postinflammatory hyperpigmentation is a common sequela of such processes. It is most frequently observed in those with darker skin colors, type 3 and type 4. In dark-skinned youths, acne is accompanied by hyperpigmentation. The most important therapeutic goal is suppression of the acne. There are available several medications that suppress acne and melanin formation simultaneously. Retinoic acid* (Retin-A 0.025% or 0.05%) applied once daily can help suppress hyperpigmentation provided that it is not irritating. Azelaic acid,* a dicarboxylic acid produced by *Pityrosporum* fungi, also inhibits melanin formation. Applications of 20% azelaic acid (Azelex) once or twice daily are useful for acne and pigmentation. At times, twice-daily applications of hydroquinone 3% solution (Melanex) can be beneficial. Topical agents usually are combined with oral antibiotics such as doxycycline* 100 mg taken once or twice daily.

*Not FDA approved for this indication.

Dermatitis is defined as inflammation of the epidermis. There are many types including nummular dermatitis, atopic dermatitis, and contact dermatitis. All of these are accompanied by pigmentary changes. Epidermal (brown) and dermal (blue-gray) hyperpigmentation commonly are observed in those with dermatitis. The first therapeutic goal is suppression of the dermatitis with topical steroids applied twice daily such as triamcinolone acetonide 0.1% (Kenalog 0.1%) or fluocinonide 0.05% (Lidex 0.05%). Newer agents such as tacrolimus (Protopic 0.03% or 0.1%) or pimecrolimus (Elidel 1%) can be very useful for controlling dermatitis. Once under control, the hyperpigmentation will fade. It can be accelerated with applications of hydroquinone (3% Melanex bid or 4% Eldoquin Forte bid).

Freckles and Lentigines

Freckles are small, 2–3 mm, brown macules that form on sun-exposed skin. By histology, the only change is increased deposition of melanin in the epidermis. Typically they are seen on the face and arms but can cover the trunk as well. By definition they wax and wane with exposure to sunlight. They lighten spontaneously in winter time and are activated to appear during summer. Treatment requires minimizing sun exposure and applications of sunscreens, preferably with short- and long-wave ultraviolet protection. Applications of hydroquinone (3% Melanex solution, 4% Eldoquin Forte cream, or Tri-Luma) twice daily with rigorous sun protection will minimize freckles.

Lentigines are brown to black macules that can vary in size from 2 to 15 mm. By histology lentigines show that the epidermis is hypertrophic (called acanthosis) with increased amount of melanin. There are several types of lentigines. Some are genetic and are manifestations of syndromes like those observed in individuals with the Carney complex or the lentiginosis syndromes. Others are the result of prolonged sun exposure or blistering sunburns or follow second-degree thermal burns. These lesions are better prevented by proper sun protection than removed after the injury has occurred. Applications of lightening agents such as those for freckles will lighten but not remove these lesions. Lasers or the medication Solagé have been used successfully to remove lentigines. The Q-switched neodymium:yttrium-aluminum-garnet (at 532 nm) and the Q-switched ruby laser (694 nm) are especially effective.

*Not FDA approved for this indication.

Café-au-Lait Macules

Café-au-lait macules (CALM) are common. It has been estimated that those with type 1 or 2 skin color have an average of 0.8 CALM and those with type 3 or 4 have an average of two to three. They appear spontaneously and are brown in color with very precise borders. Most are small, less than 1 to 2 cm in longest length. Most individuals recognize them as "birthmarks." At times they can be the herald of more serious problems. Individuals with neurofibromatosis type 1 (NF-1) develop during childhood many large (>1 cm^2) CALM, by definition more than six. Most individuals with NF-1 have many more large CALM. The axillary and antecubital "freckles" are really small CALM in body folds.

CALM can be observed on the skin of individuals with many other disorders including polyostotic fibrous dysplasia, segmental neurofibromatosis, Watson's syndrome, tuberous sclerosis, the multiple lentigines syndrome, and other conditions (Table 2).

TABLE 2. **Common Disorders of Pigmentation**

Hyperpigmentation

Genetic disorders with localized hyperpigmentation

Neurofibromatosis 1–6 or more large (>1 cm^2 café-au-lait macules)
Polyostotic fibrous dysplasia—café-au-lait macules
Segmental neurofibromatosis—café-au-lait macules
Lentigo simplex—lentigines from sun exposure
Centrofacial lentiginosis—lentigines
LEOPARD syndrome, NAME and LAMB syndromes—lentigines
Carney complex—lentigines
Peutz-Jeghers syndrome—lentigines
Incontinentia pigmenti—dermal melanosis
Pigmentary demarcation lines—brown hyperpigmentation
Xeroderma pigmentosum—lentigines and freckles

Acquired disorders with diffuse or localized hyperpigmentation

Acanthosis nigricans—flexural surfaces
Atrophoderma of Pasini and Pierini—brown macules with atrophy
Becker nevus—brown hyperpigmentation with excessive hair
Café-au-lait macules—isolated
Cutaneous amyloidosis—gray brown, pruritic macules
Ephelides (freckles)
Erythema ab igne—reticulated hyperpigmentation on skin exposed to heat
Erythema dyschromicum perstans—blue macules on the trunk
Hyperpigmentation of HIV infections—diffuse brown hyperpigmentation
Morphea and scleroderma—mottled hyper- and hypopigmentation
Addison's disease—diffuse brown hyperpigmentation with adrenal insufficiency
Mycosis fungoides—diffuse hyperpigmentation associated with cutaneous lymphoma
Poikiloderma of Civatte—brown and red pigmentation on the sides of the neck
Porphyria cutanea tarda—brown hyperpigmentation associated with liver disease
Melasma—brown or gray brown hyperpigmentation on the face
Melanosis of melanoma—blue gray hyperpigmentation with metastatic melanoma
Drug pigmentation—multiple colors of drug deposition in the dermis

COMMON DISORDERS OF HYPOPIGMENTATION

Postinflammatory Hypopigmentation

At times epidermal or dermal inflammation can result in hypopigmentation. It appears that the formation of melanin is inhibited by the inflammatory process. Children and teenagers often develop poorly defined patches of hypopigmentation with a very fine scaling surface affecting the cheeks, forehead, and the upper parts of the arms or thighs. This is pityriasis (meaning scaling) alba. The histology shows a very slight infiltration of lymphocytes into the epidermis. The treatment is application of mild topical steroids such as desonide 0.05% (DesOwen or Tridesilon) twice daily for 1 to 2 months.

Seborrheic dermatitis is the most common cause of dandruff. It affects the skin of the scalp, behind the ears, the forehead, the nasolabial fold, and cheeks. The skin appears slightly flaky and often is hypopigmented. Treatment is frequent use of any of the available seborrheic shampoos and applications of hydrocortisone lotion 2.5% (Hytone lotion) once daily for several weeks and ketoconazole cream 2% (Nizoral cream) each morning for an indefinite period. The dermatitis can be suppressed for prolonged time with the ketoconazole cream and avoids the prolonged application of steroids to the face.

Vitiligo

Vitiligo is a relatively common disorder affecting about 1 per 200 individuals throughout the world. It is an acquired disorder but has a familial propensity. The disorder causes destruction of melanocytes in the epidermis that results in depigmentation of the skin. It often is first observed on the tips of the fingers and toes, on the lips, and around the mouth and eyes (acrofacial form). It can begin anywhere on the skin. It spreads to involve all parts of the body, although typically it spares the back. Occasionally individuals have total vitiligo with loss of all the melanocytes in their integument. Another type of vitiligo affects a limited part of one side of the body, called segmental vitiligo. It is not dermatomal in distribution. The causes of vitiligo of all types are not known, although some chemicals such as polyphenols used as bactericidal agents can produce depigmentation. With vitiligo, the melanocytes are gone. Repigmentation requires replacement of the melanocytes. These must come from a reservoir. The reservoir is the hair follicle. Skin such as that on the fingers, feet, lips, and genitalia has no follicles. Hair that is white has lost its complement of melanocytes and thus cannot serve as a reservoir. Thus glabrous skin and skin with white hair cannot respond to medical therapy.

There are two types of therapy. The first is topical steroids, which have been used successfully to treat skin with a reservoir. There are two approaches especially for the face. One is prolonged application of mild steroids to the affected skin such as desonide 0.05% (DesOwen)* for periods up to 3 to 4 months. The second is application of a potent steroid such as clobetasol

*Not FDA approved for this indication.

TABLE 3. **Common Disorders of Hypopigmentation**

Genetic disorders of hypo- and depigmentation
Piebaldism—mutation in c kit proto oncogene
Waardenburg syndrome—mutation in PAX 3 or MITF genes with deafness
Vitiligo vulgaris—postnatal onset of depigmentation
Albinism—defective production of melanin causing foveal atrophy and poor visual acuity
OCA 1—albinism related to mutations in tyrosinase gene
OCA 2—albinism related to p gene, possibly a transporter gene for tyrosinase
OCA 3—albinism related to mutations of TRP-1 gene
OCA 4—mutation in MATP (membrane associated transport protein)
Phenylketonuria—mutation in phenylalanine oxidase that blocks tyrosinase
Nevus depigmentosus—hypopigmented macules usually present at birth
Tuberous sclerosis—hypopigmented ash leaf spots and patches of white hair

Acquired disorders of hypo- and depigmentation
Chemical leukoderma—depigmentation from exposure to some phenols
Syphilis—necklace of Venus, hypopigmented macules associated with secondary syphilis
Leprosy—hypopigmented macules from infections by *Mycobacterium leprae*
Tinea versicolor—hypopigmented macules with fine scaling
Onchocerciasis—mottled depigmentation on the legs with inguinal adenopathy
Dermal fibrosis—deposition of collagen in the papillary dermis appears as hypopigmentation although the melanin content of the epidermis is normal
Pityriasis alba—poorly demarcated patches of hypopigmentation and scaling on the faces and extremities of young people; a form of dermatitis
Lupus erythematosus—Depigmentation in atrophic lesions
Sarcoid—hypopigmented macules overlying infiltrated plaques
Halo nevi—depigmentation surrounding a normal nevus most commonly observed in children and teenagers
Mycosis fungoides—scaly, hypopigmented patches on trunk of adults
Lichen sclerosus et atrophicus—depigmented skin associated with atrophy observed on the genitalia or other sites usually in adults
Nevus anemicus—hypopigmented macules caused by decreased blood flow

acetonide 0.05% (Temovate* cream) once daily for 1 week of the month followed by desonide for the subsequent three weeks. Both treatments are prescribed for 3 to 4 months.

Ultraviolet light also can be useful. Natural sunlight can stimulate repigmentation. The skin is exposed to summer sunlight three times a week for periods up to 30 minutes to avoid burning. Ultraviolet light can be administered in light boxes. These include narrow band ultraviolet light at 311 to 314 nm. It is administered three times each week starting at low doses (usually around 100 mJ) increasing up to tolerance. PUVA is a combination of psoralen (Oxsoralen-Ultra) and ultraviolet A. The dose of psoralen is 20 mg and the dose of UVA is started at 1 to 2 J/Rx and increased until tolerance. The administration of PUVA requires special equipment and proper training to do correctly, effectively, and safely.

*Not FDA approved for this indication.

SUNBURN

method of
BETHANY M. BERGAMO, M.D.
Assistant Professor of Dermatology
University of Alabama at Birmingham

Sunburn is the most recognized acute adverse reaction of ultraviolet radiation (UVR). Sunburn is a phototoxic reaction that is characterized by redness, warmth, pain, and swelling. This represents the inflammatory response that occurs as a result of damaging effects of UVR. UVR has been divided into three components based on differing photobiologic properties: ultraviolet C (UVC), 200–280 nm; ultraviolet B (UVB), 280–320 nm; and ultraviolet A (UVA), 320–400 nm. UVC is not present at the Earth's surface because it is absorbed by the stratospheric ozone. UVC is however present on earth in artificial sources such as hospital germicidal lamps. UVB is the component of UVR that is primarily responsible for inducing sunburn reactions. UVB and UVC do not penetrate window glass; however, UVA is completely transmitted. UVA not only augments the damaging effects of UVB, but may also induce erythema and hyperpigmentation (tanning) alone. Even though the amount of UVA required to produce erythema is 1000 times that required for UVB, its relative abundance provides a significant role in the erythema response, photoaging, and carcinogenesis. Suberythemogenic doses of both UVB and UVA may result in DNA damage in the skin.

Cutaneous vasodilation and flushing are early effects of UVR and can be measured by reflectance instruments before erythema becomes clinically apparent. Delayed effects begin a few hours after exposure and peaks about 6 to 24 hours. Blistering reactions may also occur with prolonged UVR exposure. Sunburn reactions generally begin to resolve after about a day and are often followed by clinical effects such as tanning and desquamation. The desquamation phase is often pruritic. Severe sunburn reactions can result in weakness, fever, and chills. High doses of UVR can result in rapid onset of sunburn reactions that are often more persistent. The severity of the sunburn reaction depends on several factors including the amount of UVR exposure and environmental factors. The amount of UVR exposure is determined by a variety of host and environmental factors. Host factors include the amount of inherent pigmentation, skin thickness, and antioxidant status. Individuals with fair skin and light-colored eyes generally have a higher tendency to burn. The elderly and very young often require less UVR exposure to develop a sunburn reaction. Environmental factors include the time one is exposed, environmental surroundings, and elevation. Although there is little variation in UVA, the amount of UVB varies with the time of day, elevation, clouds, and ambient humidity. Water, snow, and white sand can reflect approximately 80% of UVR and thus one can obtain enough UVR to cause sunburn even on cloudy days. There is a greater amount of

UVR exposure at higher elevations. It is estimated that UVB exposure increases by 4% for every 1000 feet above sea level.

Ultraviolet light is absorbed by proteins and DNA in the skin. The interaction of UVR with these chromophores is responsible for initiating the inflammatory response resulting in sunburn. Inflammatory mediators are released as a result of DNA damage from UVR, especially UVB and short wavelengths of UVA. UVB has its greatest effect on epidermal keratinocytes. Initially there is a decrease in keratinocyte proliferation followed by epidermal hyperplasia. Longer wavelengths in the UVA range penetrate the dermis resulting is damage to fibroblasts and endothelial cells. Mediators such as histamine, bradykinin, arachidonic acid, and prostaglandin induce a cascade of events resulting in inflammation and vasodilation. UVR induces cytokines such as interleukin (IL)-1, IL-6, IL-8, IL-10, IL-12, tumor necrosis factor-α, and others. Mutation or downregulation of the tumor suppressor gene, p53, occurs in response to UVR. Changes in cellular function occur, favoring repair of DNA. The cutaneous immune response is also inhibited by UVR. Cells that undergo sufficient cell damage undergo necrosis and cell death, or apoptosis. These cells are known as sunburn cells and are eventually lost through transepidermal elimination. Ultraviolet (UV) damage in the dermis causes disorganization and fragmentation of elastin and collagen fibers. There is also an increase in vasculature in the papillary dermis and accumulation of extracellular matrix proteins. When melanocytes are exposed to UVR, they become more dendritic, produce more melanin, and begin to proliferate.

PREVENTION AND TREATMENT

Sun exposure during peak daylight hours (10:00 AM to 4:00 PM) is perhaps the best method of prevention of sunburn. The National Meteorological Center of the National Weather Service developed the UV index. The index is a next-day forecast that estimates the amount of UVR that will reach the Earth's surface. The UV Index also considers the effects of cloud cover on anticipated UV exposure. This can be an important tool in helping to minimize overexposure to UVR.

Protective clothing and broad brimmed hats provide some sun protection. Tightly woven fabrics protect better than fabrics with a looser type of weave. Wet clothing also provides less protection because it stretches the weave, allowing UVR to penetrate more easily. Sun protective clothing lines are commercially available.

The addition of sunscreens before UVR exposure has been found to inhibit cutaneous immunosuppression, erythema, and cell death. Sun protection factor (SPF) is currently the only rating system available for comparing efficacy of commercially available sunscreens. SPF is determined by its ability to protect against UVB radiation. Protection against UVA is not taken into consideration. Because we now know that UVA plays a role in carcinogenesis and photoaging, the SPF rating system is not an optimal method for determining the efficacy of sunscreens. In theory, sunscreens with SPF 15 protect an individual by absorbing 92% of UVB radiation. The use of a sunscreen with SPF 30 will absorb an additional 5% of UVB radiation. The amount of sunscreen that was used to determine the SPF values is 2 mg/cm^2 and is about double the amount people generally apply. Sunscreens should also be reapplied every 2 hours to ensure that is providing maximal protection. The best sunscreens are ones have the broadest range of protection in the UVB and UVA range. Many sunscreens contain multiple ingredients to achieve this broad wavelength protection. Historically, sunscreens have not been very successful at blocking UVA, but there are not several agents that are effective in blocking UVA. Some of these include avobenzone and micronized titanium and zinc oxide.

The treatment of sunburn reaction depends of the severity and degree of injury. Mild erythematous reactions often require no specific treatment. Emollients are often used to help rehydrate skin. Moderate reactions can be treated with cool water compresses. Soothing baths with oatmeal, cornstarch, or baking soda may provide some relief of pain and itching. Acetaminophen can also be used for its analgesic effects, but aspirin and nonsteroidal anti-inflammatory agents such as ibuprofen are more effective in reducing the inflammatory response of sunburn. Children and teenagers should not be given aspirin or salicylate-containing medicines because of the risk for Reye's syndrome. Short courses of systemic corticosteroids such as prednisone may be used in severe sunburn reactions with or without systemic symptoms. In an average adult, prednisone 40–60 mg/day and tapered rapidly over a few days oven proves beneficial in abating the inflammatory response. Bed rest and sometimes hospitalization are sometimes required for severe sunburn reactions.

Section 14

The Nervous System

ALZHEIMER'S DISEASE

method of
ERNO S. DANIEL, M.D., PH.D.
Sansum-Santa Barbara Medical Foundation Clinic
Santa Barbara, California
University of Southern California School of Medicine
Los Angeles, California

Alzheimer's disease (AD) is a central nervous system neurodegenerative disease of older adults that causes slowly and gradually progressive dementia. Dementia is defined as an acquired abnormality in two or more cognitive functions, including memory, language, judgment, and visuospatial skills, causing overall functional decline in the presence of a clear sensorium. AD is characterized by the presence of neuritic plaques and neurofibrillary tangles in particular regions of the brain. Although the presence of plaques and tangles does not guarantee dementia of the Alzheimer type, dementia in the absence of plaques and tangles is not considered to be AD.

ETIOLOGY

The cause of AD is unknown, but the excessive deposition of beta amyloid in the form of neuritic plaques in the perineural space in characteristic regions of the central nervous system is believed to be the primary pathophysiologic mechanism. Paired helical filaments consisting of abnormally phosphorylated tau protein that forms intraneuronal neurofibrillary tangles is another significant contributory finding. There is loss of neurons, and an even more significant loss of synapses in the hippocampus, entorhinal cortex, and association areas of the neocortex, with evidence of local inflammatory response and oxidative stress. A deficiency of several neurotransmitter substances develops, primarily acetylcholine (and cholineacetyltransferase), but also norepinephrine, serotonin, dopamine, gamma-aminobutyric acid, nerve growth factor, glutamate, corticotropin releasing factor, and others.

The majority of cases are sporadic, but familial inherited forms are found in a small fraction of patients. In a few families, chromosomes 1 or 14 may have a presenilin gene mutation, or chromosome 21 may have an amyloid precursor protein gene mutation, leading to early-onset disease. Increased susceptibility is determined by chromosome 19, which carries the apolipoprotein E susceptibility gene; chromosome 12, which carries the alpha-2-macroglobulin gene; and a segment of chromosome 20, which carries the alpha-1-antichymotripsin gene. There is no evidence that AD is transmissible. Although excess aluminum is found in the brains of AD patients, this appears not to be a fundamental pathophysiologic factor. Altogether, AD may be the final result of several different pathophysiologic pathways, and its expression may depend on multiple factors leading to a similar final result. Risk factors are age, female sex, the apolipoprotein E4/E4 genotype, prior head injury, low folate and B_{12} levels, elevated homocysteine levels, and family history of dementia. Factors that appear to decrease the likelihood or delay the presentation of AD are: presence of apolipoprotein E2/E2 genotype, meticulous control of hypertension, use of statins, anti-inflammatory medicines, histamine H_2 blockers, antioxidants, moderate wine consumption, regular exercise, and the attainment of higher educational levels.

CLINICAL PRESENTATION, COURSE AND PROGNOSIS

AD generally affects older women and men, in a ratio of 1.2 to 1.5:1. The average age of onset is 75 years, with a range from 50 to 90 years, but AD is also seen rarely in younger persons. The earliest features of the disease are difficult to distinguish from the normal forgetfulness of aging, and the onset of symptomatic disease is preceded by a long preclinical phase of indeterminate duration. In older persons, the course of symptomatic disease spans an average of 8.5 years, with a range of 6 to 12 or more years, eventually ending with the death of the patient. An onset at an early age and the presence of extrapyramidal signs are associated with a more rapid decline.

For purposes of management, AD is staged as preclinical, mild, moderate, severe, and end stage. There is a great deal of heterogeneity in the progressive evolution of cognitive and behavioral signs and symptoms. The 10 warning signs of AD are noted in Table 1. Eventually, most patients develop the "five As": amnesia, anomia, aphasia, apraxia, and agnosia (visuospatial deficit), and may exhibit apathy, depression, agitation. or psychosis. Patients are generally poorly aware of their deficits. The model of the progressive cognitive and functional decline in AD as "childhood development in reverse" from the functional

TABLE 1. **Ten Warning Signs of Alzheimer's Disease***

Recent memory loss that affects job performance
Difficulty performing familiar tasks
Problems with language
Disorientation in time or place
Poor or decreased judgment
Problems with abstract thinking
Repeatedly misplacing things
Changes in mood or behavior
Changes in personality
Loss of initiative

*From the Alzheimer's Association

capacity of a 10 year old to that of an infant is easy for laypersons to understand. Patients eventually die of consequences of severe functional debilitation, most often bronchial infection and pneumonia, but the cause of death can be legally listed as AD.

DIFFERENTIAL DIAGNOSIS

Many older persons become concerned about AD when they experience forgetfulness or depression or unusual somnolence. Therefore, AD must be distinguished from age-associated memory impairment (benign senescent forgetfulness), mild cognitive impairment, and depression. Some, but not all, persons with these symptoms may eventually develop AD and therefore all should be reassessed periodically. AD must also be differentiated from delirium, which may temporarily mimic dementia, but may also occur more readily in patients with early dementia. Drugs that may impair cognition and mimic symptoms of AD include certain anticholinergics, antihypertensives, cardiac medicines, anxiolytics, hypnotics, antipsychotics, antidepressants, and anticonvulsants, as well as alcohol and some street drugs. Finally AD must be differentiated from all other causes of dementia (Table 2), primarily vascular dementia, dementia with Lewy bodies, and frontotemporal dementia. Clinical consensus criteria are available for the diagnosis of these other conditions, as well as Creutzfeldt-Jakob disease. AD is the cause of nearly two thirds of gradually progressive dementias, although it is also frequently found as mixed dementia in coexistence with vascular dementia.

DIAGNOSIS

AD is not a diagnosis of exclusion. Definitive diagnosis is established by combining clinical or historical evidence with autopsy results. The diagnosis of AD can be made with 90% or greater accuracy on clinical grounds alone. The simplest diagnostic tool is the inventory of observations of someone intimately familiar with the patient, such as a family member, friend or caregiver. Several short simple in-office or telephonic screening tests of cognition have been shown to be effective in bringing to attention mild to moderately demented patients in the primary care setting.

Diagnostic criteria for AD have been provided by several agencies. The combined National Institute of

TABLE 2. **Differential Diagnosis**

Nondementing Conditions
Age associated memory impairment (benign senescent forgetfulness)
Mild cognitive impairment
Depression
Delirium
Systemic and Brain Conditions
Gradually Progressive
Alcohol, drugs
Multi-infarct dementia
Diffuse vascular dementia
CADASIL (cerebral autosomal dominant arteriopathy with subcortical infarcts)
Binswanger's disease
Nutritional (vitamin B_{12}) deficiency
Vasculitis
Neurosyphilis
Wilson's disease
Whipple's disease
Hypothyroidism
Heavy metal poisoning
Uremic encephalopathy
Hepatic encephalopathy
Dialysis dementia
Anoxic/postanoxic dementia
Lyme disease
Amyloid angiopathy
Postcardiac bypass pump encephalopathy
Rapidly Progressive
Infection
Encephalitis
AIDS or HIV infection
Subdural hematoma/head injury
Metabolic or toxic encephalopathy
Stroke
Encephalopathy resulting from endocrine causes
Neoplasm
Paraneoplastic limbic encephalopathy
Hypoxemic injury
Hypercapnia
Progressive multifocal leukoencephalopathy
Neurodegenerative Conditions
Slowly Progressive
Alzheimer's disease
Frontotemporal dementia
Pick's disease
Normal pressure hydrocephalus
Cerebral amyloid angiopathy
Progressive subcortical gliosis
Gerstmann-Straussler
Marchiafava-Bignami
Argyrophilic grain disease
Hippocampal sclerosis
Corticobasilar degeneration
Aqueductal stenosis
Multiple sclerosis or anterior lateral sclerosis
Dementia without defined histology
With Extrapyramidal Features
Dementia with parkinsonism
Dementia with Lewy bodies
Primary progressive aphasia
Parkinson's disease
Huntington's disease
Spinocerebellar degeneration
Progressive supranuclear palsy
Rapidly Progressive
Creutzfeldt-Jakob
Spongiform encephalopathies
Inflammatory meningoencephalitis

TABLE 3. **National Institute of Neurological Disorders and Stroke—Alzheimer's Disease and Related Disorders Association Criteria for Diagnosis of Alzheimer's Disease**

Dementia established by clinical examination and documented by Mini-Mental State Examination or similar examination
Deficits in two or more areas of cognition (i.e., language, memory, perception)
Progressive worsening of memory and other cognitive functions as disease progresses, patient experiences impairment in activities of daily living and altered behavior patterns
No disturbance of consciousness
Onset between 40 and 90 years of age, but most often after age 65
Absence of other systemic disorder or brain disease that may account for deficits in memory and cognition

Neurological Disorders and Stroke-Alzheimer's Disease and Related Disorders Association criteria are listed in Table 3.

The following steps should be taken in making the diagnosis:

Establish the existence of dementia using the history as corroborated by persons who know the patient well, Mini-Mental State Examination (MMSE) and clock drawing test, or formal psychometric examination. Deficits in the ability to recall the day of the week, spell "world" backwards, and recall a list of three words are independent predictors of dementia developing within 3 years. The Mini-Cog, a three-word recall task plus a simple clock drawing test has been shown to be at least as effective as the MMSE in detecting dementia. The history is used to search for other causes of dementia, such as infections, injuries, cardiovascular problems, anoxia, alcohol use, and the use of medications and drugs.

Establish the presence and nature of progressive disease using the history from the patient and observers. Use the Hachinski scale to screen for vascular dementia.

Perform physical and neurologic examinations to confirm the absence of focal signs, presence of extrapyramidal signs, and signs of vascular disease or other conditions. Note coexisting and aggravating conditions, including impairment of vision and hearing.

Perform laboratory tests to exclude metabolic or other abnormalities. Recommended tests are a complete blood cell count, chemistry panel, thyroid test (thyroid stimulating hormone), test for cyanocobalamin (vitamin B_{12}) level, and possibly a test for syphilis. Other tests such as a human immunodeficiency virus test, measurement of arterial blood gas levels, heavy metal screening, a serologic test for Lyme disease, toxicology screening, and the erythrocyte sedimentation rate are obtained depending on clues from the history and physical examination.

Perform brain imaging generally, although this is not obligatory. Noncontrast computed tomography to rule out normal pressure hydrocephalus or a space-occupying lesion such as a chronic subdural hematoma is often sufficient. If vascular dementia or a brain tumor is suspected, magnetic resonance imaging of the brain is preferable. In questionable cases, conventional positron emission tomography (PET) of the brain showing a characteristic parietal/temporal pattern of reduced metabolic activity may be most specific, especially in early disease and sometimes even in the preclinical stage. It may help differentiate AD from conditions such as frontotemporal dementia, Pick's disease, vascular dementia, or depression. Positron emission tomography using the tracers FDDNP or PIB (Pittsburgh compound) with affinity for amyloid in the neuritic plaques may be even more specific for AD, but is used only in the research setting. Functional neuroimaging with magnetic resonance imaging and diagnostic measurement of the biomarker N-acetylaspartate by magnetic resonance spectroscopy are investigational tests.

Other testing modalities are not considered mandatory, essential, or necessary, but may be used to provide additional evidence in questionable cases.

Spinal fluid examination is not routinely performed. A diagnostic spinal tap is done in suspected cases of neurosyphilis, central nervous system acquired immune deficiency disease, or metastatic cancer. A diagnostic large-volume spinal tap may be performed in suspected cases of normal pressure hydrocephalus. Biochemical tests of the cerebrospinal fluid supporting the diagnosis of AD are available but not definitive. Decreased beta amyloid protein and increased tau protein levels in the cerebrospinal fluid are suggestive of AD but are not definitive. The appearance of a neural thread protein in the cerebrospinal fluid (upregulated in AD) may suggest and correlate with the severity of AD. Urine test for the neural thread protein is also available.

Electroencephalography (EEG) does not aid in the diagnosis of AD (EEG shows general slowing) but helps to exclude metabolic-toxic encephalopathy or a seizure disorder, to identify the characteristic encephalographic pattern of Creutzfeldt-Jakob disease and may differentiate AD from frontotemporal dementia (normal EEG). It may document seizure activity, which occurs with increased likelihood in patients with AD.

Genetic testing is not considered necessary. The apolipoprotein phenotype E4/E4 correlates with increased likelihood of AD but does not prove the diagnosis of AD, and the benefits of current treatments do not depend on genetic phenotype. Testing for chromosomal abnormalities is usually reserved for research settings.

Autopsy is the final proof of the disease and may be requested by the family or physician.

STAGING THE DISEASE AND PATIENT'S FUNCTIONAL STATE

For a comprehensive assessment of the patient with AD, several domains should be documented and assessed. These include the following.

Cognitive State

Patients should be classified as having mild cognitive impairment, or mild, moderate, severe, or terminal AD with the use of inventories such as MMSE or more extensive psychometric testing performed by someone with expertise in such examinations.

Functional State

The ability to carry out activities of daily living should be documented with the use of validated functional scales such as the Activities of Daily Living scale, Physical Self-Maintenance scale, or Functional Activities Questionnaire.

Emotional State

Concomitant mood disorders such as depression, anxiety, and behavioral problems that may require treatment should be assessed. Inventories such as the Geriatric Depression Scale (GDS), the Revised Memory and Behavior Problems Checklist, Hamilton Depression Scale, the Neuropsychiatric Inventory Q scale, or others may be used.

Coexisting Medical Problems and Overall Medical Condition

A comprehensive list of coexisting conditions that require management, with a list of prescription and nonprescription medications and supplements taken by the patient, should be compiled.

Caregiver Status

The availability of a capable caregiver is essential to the optimal care of the patient with AD. The Caregiver Burden Scale may be used as an assessment tool. On occasion an elderly caregiver may also be developing dementia, and a stressed caregiver can be the source of the patient's behavior problems.

TREATMENT

General Measures

Because AD is not curable, the focus of treatment is meticulous management of the patient at each stage to modify and slow the progress of the disease and optimize the cognitive and functional states, in the context of other medical problems the patient may have. Management of the caregiver is important in improving the outcome. To accomplish this, it is useful to see the patient and caregiver at frequent (every few months) intervals, even in the absence of significant changes in the patient's condition.

Preclinical Stage

The goal of management of susceptible individuals in the preclinical stage (e.g., those with a strong family history of early-onset disease) is to prevent and or delay the onset of AD. General measures include protection against head injury or repeated concussions. Meticulous control of vascular risk factors, including hypertension and hyperlipidemia with statins, has been shown to be important. Long-term estrogen use has been shown to reduce the likelihood of developing AD, but in combination with progestins the opposite may be true in women over 65 years of age. Studies show that nonsteroidal anti-inflammatory drugs* used for 2 years or more during a person's adult life delay the onset or reduce the likelihood of developing AD, hence both male and female patients may consider use of anti-inflammatory agents as tolerated. Taking antioxidants, particularly vitamin E,* should be considered to reduce the oxidative stresses that play a role in the evolution of AD. Use of H_2-histamine blockers* may have some preventive benefit, and it may make sense to avoid toxic exposures, such as the excessive use of aluminum-containing antacids. Overall healthy lifestyle with regular exercise, moderate calorie intake, consumption of foods rich in folate, B vitamins, and vitamin E, moderate use of alcohol, and fish in the diet should be encouraged.

Symptomatic Disease

In those with symptomatic disease, the goal is to optimize and improve the current cognitive and functional levels and slow the progression of disease. Coexisting medical conditions should be meticulously managed. For such patients, internists, family physicians, and geriatricians are generally preferred as primary physicians, with consultative help from neurologists and psychiatrists. General health maintenance measures include a healthy and nutritious diet, supplemented as needed with vitamins and minerals, avoiding excessive weight loss or weight gain, adequate dental care, control of all coexisting conditions including hidden infections (sinus, dental, prostate), regular exercise, socialization, exercising remaining mental faculties, and, possibly, deliberate memory training. The use of prescription and nonprescription medicines that impair cognition, especially anticholinergics (often prescribed for insomnia or urinary urgency), alcohol, sedatives, and hypnotics should be minimized or eliminated. Polypharmacy with unnecessary medicines including herbal products with unknown interactions, toxicities, and contaminants is to be avoided.

Disease-Modifying and Restorative Treatment

During the last decade, based on elucidation of pathophysiologic mechanisms of AD, treatment has focused on correcting documented neurochemical deficiencies and modification of degenerative central nervous system processes to improve, restore, and preserve cognitive function and slow the progressive deterioration (Table 4). At present there is no proven treatment for the pathologic deposition of amyloid, formation of neurofibrillary tangles, and deficiency of nerve growth factor. Restorative therapy is aimed primarily at correcting the deficiency of central nervous system acetylcholine. Disease-modifying treatments attempt to modify oxidative stresses, or excitotoxicity.

---

*Not FDA approved for this indication.

TABLE 4. **Current (and Future) Pharmacologic Approaches**

Current		(?Future)
Cholinesterase inhibitors		?Cholinergic
Donepezil (Aricept)	5–10 mg qd	(?Muscarinic agonists)
Galantamine (Reminyl)	4–12 mg bid	(?Nicotinic augmentation)
Rivastigmine (Exelon)	1.5–6 mg bid	(?Propentophylline)
Tacrine (Cognex)	10–40 mg qid	(?Acetyl-l-carnitine)
		?Statins
Antioxidant		
Vitamin E**	1000 IU bid	?Ampakines
		?Nerve growth factor repletion
		?Leteprinim (Neotrofin)
NMDA receptor antagonist		?Antiamyloid agents
Memantine* (Ebixa)	10 mg bid	(?Beta and gamma secretase inhibitors)
		(?Antiamyloid vaccine)
		?Clioquinol**†

*Investigational agent at this time.
**Not FDA approved for this indication.
†Available in topical form only.

Cholinergic Augmentation

Centrally acting cholinesterase inhibition is the primary available mode of treatment. Cholinesterase inhibitors (CIs) produce a temporary, modest, but measurable improvement in cognitive function, some improvement in behavioral symptoms, and some slowing of the progression of AD in patients with mild to moderately severe disease. Recently CIs have also been shown to produce similar benefits in patients with vascular dementia and dementia with Lewy bodies, but not in frontotemporal dementias. Their benefit has not been proven in severe or preterminal AD and not yet conclusively proven in mild cognitive impairment, though healthy individuals given CIs may show some improvement of scores on certain cognitive tasks. Because CIs rarely produce dramatic benefit, families and caregivers need to be informed of realistic expectations.

After a small measurable improvement in cognitive and other functions noted during the first year of treatment with CIs, the patient's cognitive function returns to pretreatment levels toward the end of the first year of continued use. Beyond that time, CIs slightly retard the rate of decline of the treated patient, possibly for 3 to 5 years, but for how long remains to be proved. There is evidence that continued use of CIs in therapeutic doses delays the need for nursing home admission in patients with AD by up to 2 years. Patients successfully treated with CIs have been shown to require reduced caregiver time. The true benefit of CIs is measured not by the rise of the patient's scores above baseline, but by the difference in scores between treated and untreated patients at various time intervals. Benefits generally are dose related, and it is desirable to try to get the patient up to the highest recommended dose. Treatment with CIs is started at the lowest recommended dose for 1 month, increasing to higher doses at monthly intervals. If the patient cannot tolerate the highest recommended dose of one CI, trial of another compound should be considered. There is no known contraindication to treating patients with AD as early in the course of the disease as possible. In fact, delay in treatment may be detrimental. Treatment should be continued as long as the probable benefit outweighs the cost and observed side effects. Sudden discontinuation of some CIs may result in rapid decline to a lower level of function. Patients not responding to one CI may respond to another. When switching from one compound to another, treatment should start at the lowest recommended dose, but may be titrated to higher doses at weekly intervals. Concurrent use of two different CIs is generally not recommended. Behavioral symptoms, such as apathy, restlessness, anxiety, delusions, depression, and irritability have been found to improve in some patients treated with CIs, leading to the use of these compounds as primary psychotropic agents in patients with dementia. In the nursing home setting, CIs may reduce the need for psychotropics.

Currently available cholinesterase inhibitors are: donepezil (Aricept), with recommended doses of 5 to 10 mg administered once per day; galantamine (Reminyl), with recommended doses of 4 to 12 mg twice a day; and rivastigmine (Exelon), with recommended doses of 1.5 to 6 mg given twice per day, with titration of dosages from lowest to highest tolerated dose at 1-month intervals. Tacrine (Cognex) though efficacious, is little used because of cumbersome dosing and need for blood tests to monitor for potential liver toxicity.

All of the cholinesterase inhibitors work by inhibiting acetylcholinesterase. Rivastigmine and tacrine also inhibit butyrylcholinesterase, the enzyme which may have increasing importance in advancing stages of AD. Galantamine additionally works as a presynaptic nicotinic receptor modulator, a mechanism that enhances presynaptic release of acetylcholine and several other neurotransmitters. Whether these additional mechanisms of action translate directly into additional clinical benefit remains to be demonstrated. Preliminary head to head study of all three agents show results similar to earlier individual studies. From individual studies, relative efficacy of CIs may be compared based on duration of benefit (i.e., how many months they keep the cognitive scores above baseline: galantamine 52 weeks, donepezil 38 to 51 weeks, rivastigmine 38 weeks), to what degree various dosage forms improve the scores relative to placebo, their efficacy in improving various behaviors, their efficacy in other dementing diseases, and their efficacy when used in combination with other medicines. The side effects of CIs are dose-related, and may include nausea (most prominent during the first few days of treatment or at the time of dosage escalation) vomiting, diarrhea, loss of appetite, weight loss, salivation, and possibly bradycardia. Taking the medication with food may reduce these side effects. Contraindications to therapy are allergy to the medicines or active peptic ulcer disease.

Other cholinergic treatments tried unsuccessfully in the past include precursor loading with lecithin* and choline,* found to be ineffective in part because of a deficiency of choline acetyltransferase in the brains of AD patients. Direct muscarinic cholinergic receptor stimulation produced more side effects and no more benefit than cholinesterase inhibition.

Cholinesterase inhibitors have also been shown to be of benefit in patients with suspected vascular dementia, dementia with Lewy bodies, Parkinson's disease with hallucinations in helping recovery from post (coronary bypass) pump encephalopathy, and some other cognitive deficiencies. The exception is frontotemporal dementia and Pick's disease, in which they have been shown to be ineffective and possibly detrimental.

Antioxidants

Alpha-tocopherol (vitamin E)* in the dose of 1000 IU twice per day was shown in a single, well-designed study of patients with moderate AD to slow deterioration in the activities of daily living, and delay progression to nursing home admission, despite no effect on the decline in cognitive measures. Treatment of symptomatic patients with mild to moderate AD with vitamin E 1000 IU twice per day is considered standard therapy. It likely provides little or no benefit in advanced cases of AD. Lower doses have potential preventive benefits in susceptible family members and healthy individuals.

Glutamate Receptor Blockade and Modulation

Excitotoxicity produced by excessive amounts of glutamate is hypothesized to contribute to neuronal cell death in AD. Memantine (Ebixa),** a moderate affinity uncompetitive N-methyl-D-aspartate antagonist that modulates glutamate levels, has been available for the treatment of dementia and Parkinson's disease in Europe for more than 10 years. A recent study in patients with moderate to severe AD showed that memantine 10 mg twice daily in combination with a stable regimen of cholinesterase therapy with donepezil significantly improved patient cognition, daily function, and global status as compared with cholinesterase treatment alone. Another study showed behavioral and functional benefits in outpatients with moderate to severe dementia on monotherapy of memantine 10 mg twice daily. An open-label extension of the same study showed that patients who switched from placebo to memantine demonstrated improvement in cognition, function, and global assessment. Memantine is reported to show significant reduction in caregiver time and significant lower rate of institutionalization. It is the first agent to show benefit in patients with moderate to severe AD (MMSE 3-14), in whom it may slow the progression of decline. It is generally well tolerated, with no clinically important differences in the incidence of side effects versus placebo. Additionally, it has pain-relieving properties. Its approval by the Food and Drug Administration is expected in the near future, and would be the first medication approved for patients with moderate to severe AD.

*Not FDA approved for this indication.
**Investigational drug in the United States.

Marginally Effective or Unproven Therapies

SELEGILINE (ELDEPRYL)*

This monoamine oxidase inhibitor has antioxidant properties and increases levels of brain catecholamines. In the same study as vitamin E, selegiline 5 mg twice per day was found to delay the progression to nursing home admission in patients with AD by a time span comparable with that of vitamin E. However, concomitant use of the two compounds produced slightly less benefit than either medication alone, and resulted in increased side effects. Given no obvious advantage over vitamin E, selegiline is seldom used in treating AD.

ESTROGENS*

Despite possible preventive benefits, double-blind studies failed to show any benefit of estrogen in patients with established AD. Estrogens may enhance benefit from cholinesterase inhibitors. The combination of estrogens and progestins may increase the likelihood of dementia in women over 65.

ANTI-INFLAMMATORIES*

Despite possible preventive benefits, anti-inflammatory agents have not shown benefit in treating established AD. A small study suggested that use of indomethacin* in patients with AD may retard progression of the disease, but not result in improvement, and was poorly tolerated due to gastrointestinal side effects. Other anti-inflammatories, including naproxen (Naprosyn),* diclofenac (Voltaren),* and the cyclooxygenase-2 inhibitor rofecoxib (Vioxx)* have shown no benefit in a 1-year study. Studies of prednisone* and hydroxychloroquine (Plaquenil)* have shown no benefit. Low-dose aspirin,* which has no significant anti-inflammatory effect, does not improve or prevent AD. However, it may allow improvement in vascular dementia.

HERBAL MEDICINES

Ginkgo biloba* is an herbal product which may produce various biochemical effects, including vasoregulatory action, antioxidant and anti-inflammatory effects, and possible neurotrophic effects. A certain extract (Egb 761) was shown in one study to produce slight improvement in cognitive scores in patients with AD, but subsequent studies failed to confirm the benefit in patients with AD or in normal elderly persons. Huperzine A,* a natural cholinesterase inhibitor, has been inadequately studied. Some herbal preparations have recently been found to be contaminated with pesticides or other agents.

*Not FDA approved for this indication.

Acetyl-L-carnitine,* which promotes acetylcholine release and is an antioxidant has not been proved to produce benefit. Nicotine* and nicotine-like compounds have been tried, but produce only transient nonsustained benefit. The antibiotic clioquinol* is being studied. It may inhibit neocortical beta amyloid accumulation.

Other medicines that do not specifically address the pathophysiologic mechanisms of the disease have been tried empirically in the past. These include ergoloid mesylates (Hydergine),* vasodilators, and chelation therapy. Trials have generally yielded marginal or unsubstantiated responses. Interactions with other agents are unknown. Therefore the use of these medicines is generally not recommended at this time.

An anti-amyloid vaccine that showed substantial promise resulted in several cases of encephalitis in human trials, and at this time the trials are on hold. The study of the possible benefit of statins* in patients with AD is currently under way.

Other interventions tried are low-flow central nervous system shunting to improve the clearance of AD associated neurotoxins, but it is not a widely accepted therapy.

Monitoring Ongoing Therapy

Disease progression may be monitored by interviews of observers, or inventories such as global impression of change, or MMSE. Continuing decline does not mean that medicine used is ineffective, because the untreated patient may have shown more rapid decline in comparison. Continued treatment is based on acceptance of published data showing that over approximately 3 years, CI-treated patients with mild to moderate AD generally remain better than untreated patients, by measures approximately equivalent to 1 to 1.5 years of disease progression.

As the disease progresses and evolves, the benefit of ongoing treatment should be periodically (e.g., every 6 months) reassessed. In the advanced stages of the disease, the medicines may no longer produce enough benefit to warrant continuation. Progression to severe or end-stage disease may warrant discontinuation of some or all medications and possibly consideration of comfort measures only.

It should be noted that there have been few formal studies of two-drug or multidrug regimens, and generally the effect of the concomitant use of multiple drugs, especially in conjunction with medicines given for other conditions is unknown. (Concurrent use of vitamin E and selegiline in patients with AD was shown to produce slightly less benefit than either agent used alone. The unexpected cardiac valve problems resulting from the concomitant use of two centrally acting appetite suppressants, fenfluramine (Pondimin)*** and phentermine (Adipex),*** also remind us to be cautious with using drug combinations). Care should be used to avoid polypharmacy and to follow the patient carefully when combinations of medicines are prescribed.

*Not FDA approved for this indication.

***Not available in the United States.

Management of Mood and Behavioral Disorders

As AD progresses, various mood and behavioral disorders may become prominent in many patients and may require intervention and treatment with medications. Some of these manifestations should lead to reconsideration of the diagnosis of AD. For example, hallucinations in the presence of evolving extrapyramidal symptoms should lead to consideration of dementia with Lewy bodies, whereas rapid development of significant personality alterations in the presence of mild dementia in a younger person should raise the question of frontotemporal dementia or Pick's disease. The most common pathologic behaviors in patients with AD are apathy (70%), agitation (60%), motor abnormalities such as pacing (40%), with delusions, disinhibited behaviors, hallucinations, and euphoria occurring less often.

Some behavior manifestations may be due to environmental factors, including impatient caregivers, and assessment and modification of these factors is advised. General considerations are optimizing the patient's sensory input with appropriate eyeglasses, hearing aids, and well-lit rooms; using structured routines, reassurance, and clear and simple communication; avoiding confrontation; and providing frequent reorientation and simple distractions. Irritability may result from the use of caffeine or alcohol or from being startled. Restlessness may be triggered by medical conditions that may cause discomfort, pain, or irritation. Sleep disturbance may be caused by excessive daytime napping, pain, nocturia, or paroxysmal nocturnal dyspnea. Pacing may be caused by urinary retention or fecal impaction. Outbursts may be caused by painful conditions or by being frightened. Urinary incontinence may result from a bladder infection or urinary retention. Patients with AD may develop myoclonic jerks and seizures, and these may be misinterpreted as behavioral problems. As a result, the management of behavioral manifestations should include a medical assessment along with environmental control measures, including education of caregivers.

Depression is often a feature of mild to moderate AD and may be improved by counseling or involvement in activities. Other mood disorders may be managed with psychosocial therapies, behavioral approaches, emotion-oriented approaches, cognition therapy, stimulation therapies, and group therapies. The simplest advice to caregivers is "the three Rs": repeat, reassure, redirect. Using lights (reduced intensity in non-sundowners and evening bright light exposure in sundowners), nature sounds, soothing music, activities, nonverbal and verbal cues, touching, and providing a pet may be tried. Suicidal ideation may present in the early stage of AD and may require special attention. A potential for violence may arise later in the illness, and firearms should be removed from the patient's access.

When these interventions have failed and there are no medical or environmental explanations for the behaviors, the use of psychotropic medications is considered. To guide the initial choice of medication, an accurate descriptive diagnosis of the patient's problem should be established. The behaviors that usually respond to treatment are depression, hallucinations, delusions, and insomnia; those that sometimes respond are apathy, anxious behaviors, episodic outbursts and aggressive behaviors, and ones that are generally refractory to treatment are wandering, repetitive questions and repetitive behaviors (Table 5).

Given the altered neurochemical state of patients with AD, the response to various psychotropic agents is idiosyncratic and unpredictable, requiring considerable individualization of treatment. The initial choice may be influenced by a history of prior benefit or untoward response to sedatives, relaxants, atypical antipsychotics, and other psychotropics taken by the patient before developing AD. Despite initial success with a medicine, as AD progresses, the patient's reaction to the medication may change. Therefore, the benefit of treatment needs periodic reassessment, and the medication may need to be changed when no longer helpful, or, in fact, counterproductive. In addition to medical considerations, the choice of medicines is governed by cost considerations, or by regulatory considerations in skilled nursing facilities.

To guide the initial choice of medication, the article by Cummings and others in *American Family Physician* (June 15, 2002, page 2525), is an excellent reference. Unconventional medicines that may be tried in refractory cases when suggested medicines fail are: mild narcotics* or barbiturates for sedation, β-blockers* for impulse control problems, and methylphenidate (Ritalin)* or ergoloid mesylates (Hydergine)* as activating agents. Note that methylphenidate may aggravate existing psychosis in AD. In cases of inappropriate sexual behavior, androgen blockers* may be tried, and trazodone (Desyrel) (which may cause priapism) discontinued. Sedatives generally cause a decline in the patient's functional state and may contribute to motor problems. In particular, benzodiazepines impair cognitive function and may contribute to falls. Antihistamines may further aggravate existing cholinergic deficit and contribute to urinary retention. Because patients with AD are more likely to have seizures than the general population, the use of medicines that lower the seizure threshold should be minimized, and medicines with antiseizure activity may be preferred in treating behavioral problems.

TABLE 5. **Choice of Medicines for Problem Behaviors**

Depression	Antidepressants (consider electroconvulsive therapy) *SSRIs in conventional doses* Citalopram (Celexa), escitalopram, (Lexapro), fluoxetine (Prozac), fluvoxamine (Luvox), paroxetine (Paxil), or sertraline (Zoloft) *Other antidepressants in conventional doses* Bupropion (Wellbutrin), mirtazapine (Remeron), nefazodone (Serzone), or venlafaxine (Effexor)
Anxiety	*Trazodone or buspirone (consider benzodiazepines or beta blocker)* Trazodone (Desyrel)* 25 mg bid to 100 bid Buspirone (BuSpar) 5 mg bid–20 mg tid Lorazepam (Ativan) 0.5 mg qd–1 mg tid Oxazepam (Serax) 5–15 mg bid Propranolol (Inderal)* 10 mg–40 mg bid
Insomnia	*Trazodone (consider hypnotics)* Trazodone (Desyrel)* 25 mg at bedtime to 150 mg at bedtime Zolpidem (Ambien) 5–10 mg at bedtime Temazepam (Restoril) 15–30 mg at bedtime
Sundowning	*Trazodone* (consider atypical antipsychotics—see psychosis)*
Delirium	*Conventional high potency antipsychotic (CHAP)* Haloperidol (Haldol)* 0.5–1 mg bid Thioridazine (Mellaril)* 10–25 mg tid
Psychosis	*Atypical antipsychotic or CHAP* Risperidone (Risperdal)* 0.25 mg qd to 0.5–1.5 mg bid Olanzapine (Zyprexa)* 2.5 mg qd–5 mg bid Quetiapine (Seroquel)* 12.5 bid–100 bid Ziprasidone (Geodon) 20–80 mg bid Aripiprazole (Abilify)** 5–15 mg Clozapine (Clozaril)* 25–50 mg qd
Aggression or anger	*Divalproex (consider typical antipsychotic, CHAP, buspirone, SSRI)* Divalproex (Depakote)* 125 mg bid—titrate to therapeutic blood level Carbamazepine (Tegretol)* 100–200 mg bid
Apathy	*Methylphenidate or ergoloid mesylate* Methylphenidate (Ritalin)* 5 mg qd–20 mg bid Ergoloid mesylate (Hydergine)* 1–4 mg tid
Inappropriate sexual behavior	*Antiandrogens (consider sedatives)* Flutamide (Eulexin)* 125 mg Leuprolide (Lupron) injectable*
Pain causing restlessness	*Acetaminophen (Tylenol), antidepressants, narcotic analgesics* (avoid propoxyphene [Darvon], meperidine [Demerol])

*Not FDA approved for this indication.
**Investigational drug in the United States.

Incontinence of Bladder and Bowel

As the disease progresses, urinary incontinence and later bowel incontinence eventually develop in most patients with AD and are often the trigger for admitting the patient to a nursing home. In the mild to moderate stage of the disease, incontinence out of proportion to cognitive deficits should lead to consideration of possible normal pressure hydrocephalus or vascular dementia. Otherwise, incontinence should receive a conventional evaluation for remediable causes such as bladder infection, overflow incontinence, urgency incontinence, bowel impaction, or prostate problems. If no remediable cause is found, accidents or bed-wetting may be reduced by regularly scheduled toileting. Bowel incontinence should trigger a search for fecal impaction or other problems such as proctitis, diverticulitis, or neoplasm. Bowel incontinence may temporarily

*Not FDA approved for this indication.

respond to the establishment of a toileting routine, with administration of a glycerin or other suppository or an enema before placing the patient on the toilet to evacuate. The use of such measures may allow the patient to be managed at home and delay admission to a nursing home.

Seizures

Ten percent or more of patients with AD may experience seizures during the course of their disease, most often in the advanced stages. If a seizure is observed, medicines that may lower the seizure threshold should be discontinued. Otherwise, conventional anticonvulsants may be used, although they sometimes result in worsening of the cognitive and functional status. Therefore, if the seizures are rare and the patient is in a safe environment, one may choose not to treat with medication. Conversely, certain anticonvulsants such as divalproex (Depakote)* are useful in the management of behavioral manifestations.

Daily Living Considerations

The role of the physician extends beyond addressing the medical and scientific issues to providing leadership in the management of the effect of the disease on the patient and family's daily living situation. The physician must encourage and guide the patient and family toward appropriate resources and therefore should be familiar with these resources. Family members should be made aware of issues that commonly arise as the disease progresses, so they can anticipate and plan for them. For patients without a family, a case manager may be needed. Referrals to the Alzheimer's Association and the Area Agencies on Aging are helpful. A partial checklist of issues to be considered follows:

Durable power of attorney for health care and financial issues should be assigned, and a primary family spokesperson designated.

Driving safety. In many states, there is a legal requirement to report a patient with cognitive impairment to the local health department or directly to the Department of Motor Vehicles. The latter is responsible for testing the patient's ability to drive. A copy of the report should be filed in the patient's medical record.

Use of hazardous appliances without supervision may necessitate the safety measure of switching off circuit breakers to such appliances when the caregiver is not present.

Living will or health care directive, including the desired intensity of care in case of illness, should be completed and may need to be updated as the disease progresses. This should include a cardiopulmonary resuscitation directive.

Conservatorship for patients without close family members or with complicated financial or legal considerations should be obtained with the help of legal counsel.

Financial planning should be instituted early to plan for health care and long-term care expenses with the help of financial consultants. In 2002 Medicare ended its practice of routinely denying claims for neurodiagnostic testing; medication management; physical, occupational, and psychologic therapy; and other treatments for patients diagnosed with AD.

Long-term care financial considerations should involve inquiring about long-term care insurance and potential Medicaid assistance.

Safe return program services are available in certain parts of the United States for patients who exhibit a tendency to wander.

Elder abuse and its legal implications are considered in case of neglect or suspected abuse by caregivers.

Liability issues may arise in the event a patient with AD injures someone.

Competency issues may arise if the patient needs to make important decisions or sign important documents such as changing a will.

Ethical issues may concern participation of the patient in research studies and whether such patients can give informed consent. Ethical issues may also arise regarding the autonomy of the patient.

Management of the Caregiver

The caregiver is pivotal to managing the patient. There is convincing evidence that a well-informed caregiver plays a significant role in improving the outcome at each stage of the illness. As such, support of the caregiver should be initiated at an early stage. Caregivers should be encouraged to attend support groups to anticipate dealing with the disease's ever-changing complexity. They should be encouraged to obtain respite or daycare help with the patient. To reinforce the importance of these suggestions, the physician should consider giving these suggestions in the form of a prescription. Caregivers should be encouraged to follow up with their own physician, with special attention to possible sleep deprivation, anxiety, depression, and alcohol use, all of which have been found with increased frequency in caregivers. Successful coping mechanisms for caregivers are a strong belief system, a flexible outlook, dependable support, and a sense of humor (Table 6).

Caregivers as well as health care professionals may keep abreast of developments through the annual report of the Alzheimer's Disease Education and

TABLE 6. **Alzheimer's Association's 10 Tips for the Caregiver**

Obtain a diagnosis as early as possible
Do legal and financial planning
Educate yourself about caregiving
Know what resources are available
Get help
Take care of yourself
Manage your stress level
Learn to let go
Be realistic
Give yourself credit, not fault

*Not FDA approved for this indication.

Referral Center of the National Institute on Aging, and through Internet Web sites such as www.alzheimer's.org. The book *The 36 Hour Day* continues to be a standard reference for caregivers. The Alzheimer's Association, Area Agencies on Aging, and help lines of pharmaceutical firms that manufacture medicines for AD are available as resources for families and patients, along with informational sources in print and on the Internet.

Nursing Home Placement

Most patients with AD eventually cannot be managed at home, and may need to be placed in a board-and-care facility and eventually in a convalescent facility or skilled nursing facility. One of the goals of patient management, and one of the measures of successful therapy, is delaying the need for placement outside the home.

Patients with dementia are often placed in nursing homes after a specific incident. This may be a fall with or without a fracture, an infection, the onset of incontinence, aggressive and agitated behavior, or wandering. Some of these may resolve, and the patient may once again be able to return home. Burnout, depression, and death of the caregiver may be other reasons.

Admission to a nursing home, because of the strange and unfamiliar surroundings, may cause increased agitation and the temporary need for increased use of psychotropics. After an adjustment period, every effort should be made to taper the administration of these extra medications.

Terminal Care

In the late stages of the disease, the patient is often reduced to the functional level of an infant. There may be an inability to feed or a risk of aspiration during feeding. At that point, the patient generally has a poor prognosis for survival, and comfort should be paramount, with life extension generally no longer a consideration. Interventions such as tube feeding in advanced AD have been shown to produce more discomfort than benefit, and informed consent for such interventions should be based on evidence of benefit versus detrimental effect shown in outcome studies, not merely on philosophic or religious considerations. Hospice services may be considered, along with discontinuation of all life-sustaining measures or medicines. Special care should be taken to prevent decubitus pressure ulcers, which may become a significant source of patient discomfort. For terminal patients with AD, there is Medicare coverage for hospice services. Medicare also provides reimbursement for physician oversight of home services when backed by proper documentation.

Expectations

AD is the focus of widespread efforts in basic research and clinical investigation. As such, management is expected to evolve significantly in the near future. Short of a cure, the goal is to retard the expression of the disease, which would substantially lower the incidence of AD. Central to the research is the elucidation of the deficits, early diagnosis with laboratory and imaging techniques, and correction of neurochemical deficits. There is also considerable effort to find memory enhancing drugs. The genetic triggers and biochemistry of deposition of long-term memory have been investigated. We may expect the development of methods or drugs to reduce beta amyloid production or aggregation with secretase inhibitors, enhance nerve cell survival with compounds that influence nerve growth factor, enhance response of neuronal receptors such as ampakines, and even possible use of neural stem cell transplants. Because of evolving changes in research and management, physicians and families are encouraged to keep abreast of new developments.

INTRACEREBRAL HEMORRHAGE

method of
GEOFFREY EUBANK, M.D.
*Neurological Associates, Inc.
Riverside Methodist Hospital
Columbus, Ohio*

Stroke is the third leading cause of death in the United States. Ischemic strokes constitute 80% of strokes, and intracranial hemorrhage (ICH) accounts for roughly 15% of strokes (with subarachnoid hemorrhage making up the last 5%). Although ICHs are less common, they carry a larger burden of mortality, with only 38% surviving beyond 1 year. Only 10% to 15% of patients have little or no disability. Approximately 50,000 ICHs occur in the United States each year, and the number is expected to increase gradually because of a number of factors. As age is a significant risk factor, the aging population will contribute to this increase. Changing racial demographics may also play a role, as the condition is 1.4 to 2.0 time more frequent in black and Asian populations.

Nomenclature can be inconsistent in dealing with this subject. In this article, the focus is on spontaneous ICH, to include all hemorrhages not related to trauma or surgery. The term hemorrhagic stroke is avoided as it can refer to a primary intracerebral hemorrhage or to a cerebral infarct with secondary hemorrhage. For the latter, the term cerebral infarct with hemorrhagic conversion is preferred.

RISK FACTORS

Hypertension is the most important risk factor for stroke, occurring in 50% to 85% depending on the study. Perhaps 50% of patients with ICH have known hypertension, with another 25% thought to have unrecognized hypertension. This risk is further increased in patients who smoke, are 55 years old or younger, and are noncompliant with their medications.

Conversely, those who have improved hypertension control have a reduced incidence of ICH, similar to what is seen in ischemic stroke.

Although alcohol in moderate amounts does not increase the risk of stroke in general, the risk for ICH does increase, especially with excessive alcohol use. Alcohol is thought to impair coagulation and perhaps affects cerebral vessel integrity. Another risk factor that is viewed differently for different stroke subtypes is serum cholesterol. Epidemiologic studies have not routinely shown an association between high serum cholesterol and stroke in general. This may be due to the fact that patients with low serum cholesterol tend to have a higher risk of bleeding, which would confound the association of increased serum cholesterol and supposed increased risk of ischemic stroke.

CLINICAL FEATURES

Stroke is defined as a sudden change in neurologic function caused by an alteration in cerebral blood flow. Certain clinical features can distinguish between the various stroke subtypes as shown in Table 1.

Although Table 1 is not inviolable, it can provide a rapid bedside assessment to direct further history and investigations. Nausea, vomiting, and meningismus are more common in ICH than ischemic infarcts. Seizures are also more common in ICH, occurring in 13% of all cases and 30% to 39% of patients with lobar hemorrhages.

Focal neurologic symptoms depend on the location of the ICH. Hemorrhages usually occur when small penetrating arteries rupture into the brain parenchyma. Table 2 summarizes the relative frequency and common signs on the basis of location.

Secondary deterioration can occur in one quarter of patients. Patients with large hematomas and intraventricular extension of hemorrhage are especially susceptible to deterioration. This can occur within the first few hours (because of rebleeding) or within the first 1 to 2 days (because of edema). Hydrocephalus may occur because of a mass effect, tissue shifts, or obstruction from intraventricular blood.

CAUSES OF INTRACRANIAL HEMORRHAGE

Hypertensive ICH, the most common type of ICH, is thought to be due to degenerative changes leading to rupture of small penetrating arteries or arterioles. The most common locations include the basal ganglia, thalamus, cerebellum, and pons. Lobar ICHs have more heterogeneous causes but are not uncommon with hypertension. Recurrence rate is approximately 2% per year, less with treatment of hypertension.

TABLE 1. **Rapid Stroke Triage Based on Presenting Symptoms**

Condition	Headache	Focal Deficit	Decreased Level of Consciousness
Ischemic infarct	–	+	–
Intracerebral hemorrhage	+	+	+
Subarachnoid hemorrhage	+	–	+

TABLE 2. **Signs and Symptoms of Intracranial Hemorrhage by Location, Listed in Order of Frequency**

Basal Ganglia (40%)
Hemiparesis
Hemisensory loss
Ipsilateral gaze deviation
Dysarthria
Aphasia (left sided)
Neglect/anosognosia (especially right)

Lobar (30%)
Variable, depending on location
Hemisensory loss, hemiparesis, hemianopsia
Neglect, aphasia, dysarthria
Seizures

Cerebellum (15%)
Ataxia, truncal or limb
Nystagmus
Nausea, vomiting

Thalamus (10%)
Hemiparesis
Hemisensory loss
Aphasia
Eye movement abnormalities
Upgaze palsy, skew deviation, and so on

Brainstem (Pons) (5%)
Coma
Quadriparesis
Pinpoint pupils
Gaze palsy, intranuclear ophthalmoplegia
Ataxia

Cerebral amyloid angiopathy is thought to be due to deposition of β-amyloid in small and medium-sized arteries in the cerebral cortex and leptomeninges, which typically leads to lobar hemorrhages. These tend to be recurrent, up to 10% per year. No specific treatment is available to decrease recurrence. It is a condition primarily of elderly persons, typically 70 years old or older.

Arteriovenous malformations involve the rupture of abnormal small vessels and can occur in various locations. Younger patients without hypertension have this as the most common cause of ICH. Risk for recurrence is up to 18%. This can be decreased with surgical excision, embolization, radiosurgery, or a combination thereof. Cavernous malformations bleed because of rupture of capillary-like vessels and have a lower rebleeding rate of 4% to 5%. Depending on location, surgery and/or radiosurgery can be used for treatment. Venous angiomas rarely bleed and when they do the recurrence is less than 0.5%. Treatment is usually not necessary.

Cerebral venous thrombosis can cause ischemic infarcts (venous infarcts), which have a relatively high risk of hemorrhagic transformation. Despite this tendency, the usual treatment is anticoagulation and, in severe cases, transvenous thrombolysis. Anticoagulation is often continued in the presence of associated hemorrhage, although large hemorrhages obviously merit more caution.

Ischemic infarct with hemorrhagic transformation is not uncommon with larger lobar infarctions. Although it is not considered to be a true primary ICH, the appearance of hemorrhage can occasionally cause clinical deterioration or changes in management. This conversion can occur spontaneously with large infarcts. In fact, autopsy studies reveal a high rate of visible hemorrhage, from frank hematoma to petechial hemorrhage. The risk of hemorrhagic conversion is higher with the use of anticoagulants for stroke, especially when boluses are given. Given the lack of proven benefit and increased risk of hemorrhage, most recent reviews on the subject of heparin* discourage the routine use of heparin for the treatment of acute cerebral infarct.

Intracranial aneurysms occasionally arise with a prominent ICH but most often with a subarachnoid hemorrhage. This is rare with other causes of ICH. Rebleeding rate is 50% in 6 months, decreasing to about 3% per year. Treatment is accomplished by surgical clipping or endovascular coiling.

Intracranial neoplasms are an uncommon cause of ICH and tend to occur with hypervascular tumors. These can be primary (glioblastoma multiforme) or metastatic (e.g., melanoma, renal cell, bronchogenic).

Coagulopathy as a cause of ICH is usually due to anticoagulant or thrombolytic therapy but rarely can be due to hereditary conditions. The risk with anticoagulation increases with age, hypertension, and prior stroke. International Normalized Ratios significantly above normal ranges can also increase the risk. Thrombolytics can cause ICH when used for myocardial infarction (0.5% to 1%) or ischemic infarcts (6% to 7%). When ICH occurs in association with thrombolysis for stroke, it typically occurs in the area of infarct. Otherwise, the ICH tends to be lobar and can be multiple. ICH with thrombolytics (and patients overly anticoagulated) often has a peculiar layered appearance on computed tomography (CT) (hyperdense on the bottom and isodense on top).

Sympathomimetic drugs, such as cocaine, amphetamines, phenylpropanolamine,** and pseudoephedrine (Sudafed), can precipitate ICH. These agents can cause an abrupt rise in blood pressure, which can overwhelm the cerebral vasculature's autoregulatory capacity. Angiography can show "beading" of vessels, although it is unclear whether this represents a vasculitic pattern versus a vasospastic pattern.

An uncommon cause of ICH is vasculitis. Ischemic infarcts may also occur. Serologic markers may or may not be present. Cerebrospinal fluid is usually abnormal (even without ICH), and angiography can show a beaded appearance. Brain biopsy is often necessary for confirmation. Treatment usually involves long-term immunosuppression.

*Not FDA approved for this indication.
**Not available in the United States.

TABLE 3. **Etiologies of Intracranial Hemorrhage by Age**

Young	Middle Aged	Elderly
Vascular malformation	Hypertension	Hypertension
Aneurysm	Vascular malformation	Amyloid angiopathy
Sympathomimetic agents	Aneurysm	Coagulopathy
		Vascular malformation
		Tumor

Age can help determine the likelihood of the cause of ICH. Table 3 illustrates the more common etiologies by age.

EVALUATION

A thorough history can help identify conditions associated with ICH (hypertension, malignancy), risk factors for coagulopathy, trauma, and so forth.

Laboratory evaluation should include a complete blood count with platelets, prothrombin time and partial thromboplastin time, erythrocyte sedimentation rate, and renal and hepatic tests. A toxicology screen should be considered, and various coagulation studies can be performed if there is concern regarding a coagulopathy.

Neuroimaging is typically done with CT scanning because of availability, speed, and ease of detection of most hemorrhages. Not only should size and location be considered, but also the presence of intraventricular blood and/or hydrocephalus should be noted. In proper hands, magnetic resonance imaging (MRI) is at least as sensitive as CT, but expertise in identifying blood or blood products at various points in time is mandatory. MRI may be able to identify vascular malformations, tumors, or evidence for old hemorrhage (which could indicate underlying amyloid angiopathy or possible previous hypertensive ICH). Cerebral angiography can help identify underlying arteriovenous malformations. In most cases of unexplained ICH (especially in those who are young and without hypertension), cerebral angiography should be performed. Also, regardless of age or hypertension history, the rare patient who has a primary intraventricular hemorrhage should undergo angiography because of the high rate of abnormalities found (>65%). Those least likely to have significant abnormalities on angiography are those who have all the following characteristics: older than 45, have hypertension, and have an ICH that is not lobar in location (e.g., basal ganglia, thalamus). The timing of angiography depends on the patient's clinical condition and timing of possible surgery.

MANAGEMENT

Initial Management in the Emergency Room or Intensive Care Unit

Initial management in the emergency room centers around initial stabilization of the patient, with attention to airway, breathing, and circulation. Although not every patient needs to be intubated, those who have a significantly decreased level of consciousness and those who have impaired protection of their airway (e.g., because of depressed reflexes) are candidates for intensive airway management. Intubation should be accomplished with short-acting agents (barbiturates, with or without lidocaine). Intubation helps to prevent secondary complications such as hypoxemia, hypercapnia, and aspiration. Ready access for hyperventilation, if needed, would be available.

Reversal of any known coagulopathies should occur as soon as possible. The offending agent (warfarin [Coumadin], heparin, antiplatelet agents, thombolytics) should be discontinued immediately upon diagnosis (or suspicion) of ICH. Depending on the condition, treatments with vitamin K, fresh frozen plasma, platelets, protamine sulfate, and cryoprecipitate may be indicated.

As the risk of deterioration is highest during the first 24 to 48 hours, patients should be monitored in a dedicated intensive care unit. Standard neurologic examination in addition to the Glasgow Coma Scale (GCS) should be performed frequently (e.g., hourly). Patients with a GCS less than 9 or with a clinical condition that is deteriorating because of increased intracranial pressure (ICP) are candidates for invasive ICP monitoring.

Management of Blood Pressure

Hemodynamic instability is unusual in the early stages of ICH. The most common hemodynamic parameter deserving of attention is severe hypertension. The development is often due to the underlying etiology (hypertension), compounded by additional contribution of physiologic stress and increased ICP (Cushing's response). Of concern is that increased blood pressure (BP) could lead to expansion of the hemorrhage. On the other hand, patients with increased ICP can have decreased cerebral perfusion pressure, and lowering the mean arterial pressure (MAP) may have a deleterious effect. BP management remains somewhat controversial, although current recommendations suggest a goal of decreasing MAP in patients with values above 130 mm Hg while maintaining cerebral perfusion pressure above 60 mm Hg. Intravenous medications such as labetalol (Normodyne) can be used, although patients who have refractory elevations in BP may require continuous nitroprusside (Nitropress).

Other Medical Management Issues

Fever should be treated aggressively as it can increase cerebral blood flow as a result of increased metabolic demands. Treatment options include acetaminophen, cooling blankets, and aggressive treatment of infection (empirical therapy for presumed source of infection, e.g., aspiration pneumonia, should be instituted as soon as suspected). Hyperglycemia should also be treated aggressively as evidence has shown that hyperglycemia can have a deleterious effect on patients with stroke. Fluid goals should be to maintain a euvolemic state. Electrolyte or acid-base status should be monitored and corrected to normal values. Agitation may lead to increases in ICP. Treatment with short-acting benzodiazepines or propofol (Diprivan) may be used. Premedicating with analgesics before painful procedures should be considered.

Pneumatic compression devices and subcutaneous heparin can decrease the risk of deep vein thrombosis and subsequent pulmonary embolism. Ulcer prophylaxis should be considered for the critically ill patient. When the patient is clinically stabilized, appropriate therapy (speech, physical, and occupational) should be instituted.

Seizure Management

Most seizures with ICH occur within the first 24 hours and are more common with lobar hemorrhages. Controversy exists in terms of prophylaxis, with some advocating prophylaxis with all ICH and others with lobar ICH. Because most seizures occur early, it is reasonable to treat with antiepileptics only if seizures occur. Phenytoin (Dilantin) (with loading doses of 20 mg/kg) is used and maintenance doses can be given to maintain adequate drug levels. Without recurrent seizures, most patients can discontinue phenytoin after 1 month. Late-onset seizures (after the first 2 weeks) often require long-term prophylaxis.

Management of Increased Intracranial Pressure

A mass effect from the hematoma, surrounding edema, and hydrocephalus can all contribute to tissue shifts and increased ICP. ICP monitoring can help direct therapies. Head position is often at 30 degrees, although this can be adjusted to optimize ICP and cerebral perfusion pressure. For patients requiring additional therapy to lower ICP, mild hyperventilation and osmotherapy can be utilized. Ventilation settings can be adjusted with a goal partial pressure of carbon dioxide (PCO_2) of 30 to 35 mm Hg. Osmotherapy is typically accomplished with mannitol. If given urgently, a dose of 1 g/kg can be given, followed by 0.25 to 0.5 g/kg every 4 to 6 hours. Serum osmolality should be monitored and mannitol held if it rises above 315 mOsm/L. Close attention needs to be paid to keeping the patient in a euvolemic state. Limited data are available for high-dose barbiturates or hypothermia at this time to provide firm recommendations.

Role of Surgical Management for Intracranial Hemorrhage

Surgical evacuation of ICH can decrease mass effect and help remove the neuropathic effects from the hematoma. This benefit can be outweighed by tissue damage caused by the surgical approach, especially for ICH involving the brainstem, thalamus, and basal ganglia. Furthermore, there is a potential for rebleeding when tissue and hematoma are removed (related to loss of local tamponade).

Surgical evacuation of cerebellar ICHs greater than 3 cm (especially those with neurologic compromise, brainstem compression, and obstructive hydrocephalus) should be strongly considered as soon as possible. Consideration for surgical evacuation should be given to younger patients with moderate to large lobar hemorrhages who deteriorate during observation. Stereotactic, endoscopic evacuation can remove hematoma with less tissue damage and holds promise to be more effective than medical therapy alone. Newer techniques, such as instilling local thrombolytics through an indwelling intracranial catheter, have shown benefit in reducing hematoma volume.

ICH remains a condition with high morbidity and mortality. Further studies need to be undertaken to see whether tissue injury can be reduced. The best approach to BP management and many other supportive medical treatments remains uncertain. Newer treatments, such as the neuroprotective drugs being studied now for ischemic stroke, if shown to be beneficial, should be evaluated. Results from trials of newer, less damaging surgical evacuation techniques and local thrombolysis or evacuation will be welcomed to see whether we can improve on the management of this devastating condition.

ISCHEMIC CEREBROVASCULAR DISEASE

method of
KEN MADDEN, M.D., PH.D.
University of Wisconsin Medical School
Marshfield Clinic
Marshfield, Wisconsin

Ischemic stroke is the third leading cause of death in the United States and is the leading cause of morbidity. Medical care of stroke patients costs many billions of dollars per year, not to mention incalculable costs in patients' quality of life and lost productivity. Traditional care for those affected by stroke has been supportive only, with primary effort directed at rehabilitation of the impaired patient. Basic science research and recent clinical trials, however, have changed the way physicians should approach the stroke patient, with regard to both acute management and prevention of subsequent cerebral infarction.

There are four primary goals for management of the patient with acute stroke. Foremost among these is the need to treat the acute arterial occlusion. Regardless of whether this can be accomplished, identification of the underlying etiology of stroke is the second goal of the patient's physician, both to serve understanding of the condition and to direct specific cerebrovascular prophylaxis. Aggressive identification and modification of the afflicted patient's vascular risk factors are a third goal. This allows physicians to minimize risk of a subsequent ischemic event involving cerebral, coronary, or systemic vasculature. Finally, physicians should direct early aggressive rehabilitation efforts in order to maximize recovery from stroke. This topic is addressed elsewhere in this text.

ACUTE INTERVENTION FOR STROKE

In 1996, recombinant tissue plasminogen activator (rt-PA, Alteplase) was approved for the intravenous treatment of acute ischemic stroke within 3 hours of the onset of ischemic symptoms. Clinical trials have also suggested that thrombolytic medication delivered by the intra-arterial route* following symptom onset may also be effective up to 6 hours in improving perfusion to the ischemic cerebral tissue bed and in improving the patient's recovery from acute stroke. Use of these treatments, however, requires a rapid coordinated effort by a team of physicians competent in the neurologic assessment of presenting patients and radiographic interpretation of their cranial imaging. Intra-arterial therapy in particular requires involvement of highly specialized physicians and is probably feasible only in tertiary medical facilities.

An important aspect of each clinical encounter is physician judgment regarding who should and who should not receive consideration for thrombolytic therapy—judgment that should be tempered by careful consideration of clinical trial data. European and Australian clinical trials have demonstrated that alternative thrombolytics such as streptokinase* are overly hazardous for use in patients with acute cerebral ischemia. A major North American trial sponsored by the National Institute of Neurological Disorders and Stroke, however, has demonstrated that use of intravenous rt-PA can result in 30% increased likelihood of nearly complete neurologic recovery from stroke, although at the risk of intracranial or major systemic hemorrhage. Physicians must understand that this and subsequent trials have served to identify a subpopulation of patients with acute stroke in which the risk-benefit consideration for this type of therapy is favorable but that treatment of patients who do not mimic characteristics of this population may well be hazardous. In this regard, use of a protocol that identifies patients appropriate for thrombolytics (Table 1) and directs appropriate medication delivery is mandatory.

The most critical aspect of clinical trial data has been time to treatment from symptom onset. Multiple attempts to establish efficacy of intravenous rt-PA beyond the 3-hour time point have been unsuccessful. Secondary analyses of trials have, in fact, suggested a linear relationship between time to treatment and expectation of benefit, with efficacy lost shortly after 3 hours. These data compel treating physicians not only to observe the 3-hour limit but also to initiate therapy as soon as possible within the treatable time frame. For institutions capable of interventional techniques, intra-arterial thrombolytic use or mechanical clot ablation techniques are justified up to 6 hours following onset of ischemic stroke symptoms, although such treatment is still considered investigational.

---

*Not FDA approved for this indication.

TABLE 1. **Protocol for Use of Recombinant Tissue Plasminogen Activator for Cerebral Ischemia**

May consider rt-PA administration:
- Ischemic stroke onset <3 h of drug administration
- Measurable deficit on NIHSS
- Computed tomography without hemorrhage or nonstroke cause of deficit
- Age >18 y

Contraindications for rt-PA:
- Symptoms minor or rapidly improving
- Seizure at onset of stroke
- Suspected aortic dissection associated with stroke
- Recent acute myocardial infarction
- Suspected subacute bacterial endocarditis or vasculitis
- Symptoms suggestive of subarachnoid hemorrhage
- Another stroke, serious head trauma, or intracranial surgery within past 3 mo
- Major surgery or serious trauma within 14 d
- Known history of intracranial hemorrhage, AVM, or aneurysm
- Gastrointestinal or urinary tract hemorrhage within 21 d
- Arterial puncture at noncompressible site within 7 d
- Lumbar puncture within 7 d
- Received heparin within 48 h and has elevated PTT
- PT >15 s or INR >1.7
- Platelet count <100,000/mm^3
- Serum glucose <50 or >400 mg/dL
- Sustained systolic blood pressure >185 mm Hg
- Sustained diastolic blood pressure >110 mm Hg
- Aggressive treatment necessary to lower blood pressure

Probable increased risk of intracranial hemorrhage:
- Very large stroke with NIHSS score >22
- Computed tomography shows evidence of large MCA territory infarction (sulcal effacement or blurring of gray-white junction in more than one third of MCA territory)

AVM, arteriovenous malformation; INR, International Normalized Ratio; MCA, middle cerebral artery; NIHSS, National Institutes of Health Stroke Scale; PT, prothrombin time; PTT, partial thromboplastin time; rt-PA, recombinant tissue plasminogen activator.

Blood pressure management has been a somewhat controversial aspect of thrombolytic protocols. Conventional wisdom in the management of stroke patients dictates that blood pressures be allowed to run well into the hypertensive range during the early phase of their medical care. Greater mean pressures are presumed to drive greater perfusion into ischemic cerebral tissue beds, which have lost autoregulatory capacity. Notably, the limits at which blood pressure elevations achieve maximal benefit before increasing risk for deleterious outcomes such as hemorrhage are unknown. This continues to be an area of clinical research in stroke. The established intravenous rt-PA protocol somewhat arbitrarily directs maximum blood pressure limits of 185/110 as exclusion criteria for treatment. Although the appropriateness of these limits remains unproved, they continue as recommended guidelines for both selection of patients and maintenance during the initial time frame following lytic therapy.

Other methods of improving cerebral perfusion to ischemic tissue beds are less proved. For patients who have not received rt-PA, liberalization of blood pressure is recommended, usually by holding antihypertensive medication during the initial phase of hospitalization. Depending on an individual's prior history of hypertension, mean arterial pressures in the range 130 to 150 torr should be allowed. Local tissue edema with associated increased intracranial pressures often accompanies cerebral ischemia and can significantly impair cerebral perfusion. Unfortunately, treatment modalities for this type of cerebral edema are largely ineffective. Hyperventilation reduces intracranial pressures by inducing cerebral vasoconstriction and decreased perfusion, not particularly a desired goal in the setting of stroke. Steroids, although quite effective for the vasogenic edema associated with neoplasm, do not lessen the cytotoxic edema associated with ischemia and may have deleterious effects through induced hyperglycemia. Hyperosmotic agents, such as mannitol, may provide short-lasting benefit but tend to accumulate eventually within the ischemic tissue bed with deleterious consequences. Some authors advocate the use of colloids such as albumin* (which may also serve as a free radical scavenger) in combination with furosemide (Lasix) to sustain longer increases in vascular oncotic pressure. Dramatic benefit cannot be expected, however. For overwhelming cerebral edema, hemicraniectomy can be considered at capable institutions.

Supplementation of thrombolytic therapy with medications that may retard neuronal injury associated with ischemia has long been a goal of physicians caring for patients with stroke. Multiple clinical trials investigating potential neuroprotective drugs have been completed. Despite compelling results from tissue culture and animal work, no such agent has demonstrated benefit in the clinical arena. This is still an area of active clinical investigation. Worsening neuronal injury related to hyperthermia or hypoxia can be minimized by close attention to medical conditions such as pneumonia and venous thrombosis as well as through the aggressive use of antipyretics.

LABORATORY INVESTIGATION OF STROKE

The standard investigation into the underlying etiology of cerebral ischemia in individual patients includes cerebral imaging, echocardiography, carotid artery imaging, and interval recording of cardiac rhythm (Table 2). Computed tomography (CT) brain imaging remains the standard initial imaging study for acute cerebral ischemia, as it is a sensitive instrument for the exclusion of hemorrhagic pathology. Magnetic resonance imaging (MRI) is substantially more sensitive for early ischemic injury within brain parenchyma and offers multiple sequences for dating onset of ischemic injury, differentiating ischemia from other pathology, and assessing vessel patency. However, MRI is often less available, less tolerated by patients, and more expensive than CT.

Ultrasonography is the most popular modality for carotid artery assessment. This procedure provides estimates of flow limitations within the common or internal carotid arteries related to atherosclerotic vessel stenosis, as well as B-mode imaging. Elevated

*Not FDA approved for this indication.

TABLE 2. **Laboratory Evaluation of Stroke**

Standard Evaluation
Cranial imaging (CT or MRI)
Carotid imaging (ultrasonography, MRA, or contrast angiography)
Transthoracic echocardiography
Cardiac monitoring (in-hospital telemetry, Holter monitoring, capture monitor)
Assessment of adequacy of control of vascular risk factors
Stroke in the Young (Additional Considerations)
Prothrombotic laboratory indicators
Transesophageal echocardiography
Toxicology screen (cocaine, amphetamines)
Vascular imaging sensitive for arterial dissection (MRA or contrast angiography)
Cerebral venous imaging (MR venography or contrast angiography)

CT, computed tomography; MRA, magnetic resonance angiography; MRI, magnetic resonance imaging.

flow velocities indicate either increased blood volumes coursing through the insonated vessel or, more commonly, increased resistance to flow as a consequence of vessel narrowing. Rough estimates of the degree of stenosis can be based on peak systolic and end-diastolic flow velocities. Unfortunately, the reliability of carotid ultrasonography varies considerably from institution to institution, secondary to variance in equipment and experience of technician and/or interpreting physician. Decision-making for carotid endarterectomy or other intervention should therefore be based on imaging from vascular laboratories that have demonstrated a high correlation between carotid ultrasonography and the gold standard conventional contrast angiography or on more reliable confirmatory studies.

Magnetic resonance angiography (MRA) provides an alternative noninvasive assessment of the carotid artery and also provides useful information on the entire cranial arterial supply. MRA, however, may also suffer from limited reliability because of tendencies toward overestimation of degree of stenosis in flow-limiting states. Thus, MRA may accurately exclude significant carotid disease but may not have the sensitivity to address particularly relevant clinical questions (such as differentiating carotid occlusion from very high grade stenosis or differentiating severity of carotid stenosis best managed by surgical revascularization from that best treated with medical prophylaxis). Such questions may require consideration of contrast angiography despite the approximate 0.5% to 2% morbidity associated with this invasive procedure. Other indications for angiography include concern about vasculitis or other vasculopathies such as arterial dissection. Transcranial Doppler sonography also enables assessment of intracranial arterial blood flow. However, it is more valuable for quantification of vessel stenosis (such as the vasospasm associated with subarachnoid hemorrhage) than documentation of arterial occlusion causing stroke. Absence of flow may be related to limitations of the bony acoustic window instead of true occlusion.

Cardiac dysrhythmias such as atrial fibrillation pose a high risk for systemic and cerebral embolization. Such rhythm disturbances are not uncommonly intermittent. An interval period of cardiac monitoring may be necessary to detect such a condition. Further investigation into possible proximal source of embolism should include transthoracic echocardiography. This noninvasive modality is particularly sensitive for assessment of left ventricular dysfunction, a common cause of local thrombosis and eventual embolization in the aging population. Emboli related to atrial pathology are more common in younger patients with stroke, an occurrence that should prompt the use of a transesophageal method of echocardiography instead.

Stroke in the young often results from mechanisms quite different from those afflicting the aging population and requires investigation into such etiologies as arterial dissection, vasculitis, and prothrombotic state. Laboratory testing for the latter include assays for antiphospholipid antibody, lupus anticoagulant, prothrombotic gene, factor V Leiden, protein C, protein S, homocysteine, and antithrombin III.

SECONDARY PREVENTION OF STROKE

Active measures to prevent recurrent cerebral thrombotic events should begin with initial contact with the patient. When hemorrhagic pathology has been excluded by imaging, antiplatelet or anticoagulant therapy can be initiated. The value of heparin in the setting of acute stroke has long been debated. Heparin has no thrombolytic activity and cannot affect the primary underlying arterial occlusion. Theoretically, its use may have value in preventing extension of the thrombotic process or preventing recurrent embolization. Clinical trials of acute anticoagulation for stroke do not support the use of heparin as a standard therapy. There may be some benefit, especially for patients with underlying pathologies such as high-grade carotid stenosis, arterial dissection, prothrombotic state, or cardiac embolization. The benefit of sustained anticoagulation, however, is countered by the accumulating incidence of hemorrhage. If heparin* is utilized, therefore, conservative degrees of anticoagulation should be targeted (i.e., activated partial thromboplastin time approximately 1.5 × control), and it should be discontinued immediately after laboratory evaluation excludes the presence of conditions that argue for long-term anticoagulation or immediate carotid endarterectomy. Systemic thrombotic events are also a concern, and pneumatic stockings or other techniques should be utilized to prevent deep venous thrombosis.

The relative merits of carotid endarterectomy have also long been debated as a means of stroke prevention. Clinical trial data have provided justification for endarterectomy by experienced surgeons with demonstrable low surgical morbidity, depending on the

*Not FDA approved for this indication.

TABLE 3. **Clinical Trials of Carotid Endarterectomy versus Medical Management**

Trial	Stenosis (%)	Stroke Incidence: Surgery (%)	Stroke Incidence: Medical (%)
Symptomatic Trial			
NASCET	70–99	9	26 (2 y)
	50–69	15.7	22.2 (5 y)
	<50	14.9	18.7 (5 y)
ECST	70–99	1.1	8.4 (3 y)
	50–69	10.1	10.5 (3 y)
	30–49	9.8	6.9 (3 y)
	<30	2.7	1.3 (3 y)
VA	>50	7.7	19.4 (1 y)
Asymptomatic Trial			
ACAS	>60	4	6.2 (2 y)
VA	>50	4.7	9.4 (4 y)

ACAS, Asymptomatic Carotid Atherosclerosis Study; ECST, European Carotid Surgery Trial; NASCET, North American Symptomatic Carotid Endarterectomy Trial; VA, Veterans Affairs Cooperative Study.

severity of stenosis and the symptomatic nature (Table 3). Major reduction in recurrent stroke risk is accomplished by endarterectomy when symptomatic patients have greater than 70% ipsilateral carotid stenosis. Modest surgical benefit can be achieved if symptomatic patients have between 50% and 70% ipsilateral stenosis or if 60% stenosis is identified in an asymptomatic patient. The safety and efficacy of carotid angioplasty with stenting are currently under investigation as an alternative to endarterectomy.

All patients who have suffered a cerebral ischemic event should be considered for a specific vascular prophylactic agent. Aspirin has traditionally been the most widely utilized drug, and its benefit has now been established for both coronary and cerebrovascular disease. Although optimal dosing has not been established, doses of 75 to 325 mg daily are most commonly recommended. Ticlopidine (Ticlid), 250 mg twice daily, is superior to aspirin for stroke prevention, although concerns about hematologic side effects have limited its use. Clopidogrel (Plavix), 75 mg daily, is similar in efficacy to aspirin for cerebrovascular disease but has greater benefit for coronary and peripheral arterial disease. Combined use of drugs with different mechanisms of platelet inhibition provides greater benefit in the prevention of subsequent vascular events. Extended-release dipyridamole-aspirin (Aggrenox), 200/25 mg twice daily, is substantially more effective in preventing recurrent stroke than aspirin alone. Aspirin combined with clopidogrel similarly improves cardiovascular prophylaxis, although its efficacy for cerebrovascular disease remains in clinical trial.

Warfarin (Coumadin) provides no more benefit than aspirin for patients without high risk factors for cardiac embolism but provides dramatically greater benefit if these risk factors are present. Most notably, the high risk of subsequent stroke in patients who have atrial fibrillation is reduced by over 60% using warfarin compared with minimal reduction by aspirin. Similar disparity of benefit may be presumed in patients with other embolism-prone cardiac pathology such as ischemic cardiomyopathy. Warfarin is also recommended for patients in whom a prothrombotic etiology of an ischemic event is suspected. Temporary anticoagulation, with conversion to antiplatelet prophylaxis at 3 to 6 months after the event, is recommended for patients who have had symptomatic arterial dissections.

The most neglected means for lowering the risk of subsequent cerebral infarction is the optimal control of medical conditions such as hypertension, diabetes mellitus, and hyperlipidemia. Aggressive use of angiotensin-converting enzyme inhibitor antihypertensives or statin-type lipid-lowering agents reduces the risk of recurrent vascular events as much as or perhaps more than the use of specific vascular prophylactic drugs. At the minimum, such drugs should be used to target normotension and acceptable lipid profiles and may be considered regardless of blood pressure or lipid status.

MANAGEMENT AND REHABILITATION OF THE STROKE SURVIVOR

method of
DAVID X. CIFU, M.D.
Virginia Commonwealth University
Richmond, Virginia

Cerebrovascular incidents are fatal in more than 150,000 individuals and cause disability in another 400,000 individuals annually, resulting in over $43 billion in direct and indirect costs. The vast majority of these individuals are aged 65 years and older, putting increasing stresses on the Medicare health insurance system (necessitating changes in Medicare reimbursement for rehabilitation known as the "prospective payment system"). By 1 year after stroke, 78% to 85% return to walking, 48% to 58% regain independence in activities of daily living, and 10% to 29% require nursing home care. Rehabilitation efforts begin as soon as individuals are admitted to the hospital and continue until they have achieved their premorbid functional status or as close to it as feasible. Early rehabilitative interventions have been clearly demonstrated to decrease mortality, morbidity, nursing home placement, and costs while increasing function and quality of life. Ongoing rehabilitation has also been shown to minimize morbidity and enhance functional independence. Services should be continued in the least restrictive setting possible until a plateau of function is achieved. Renewed rehabilitation interventions may be appropriate for a recurrence of physical impairments (e.g., painful shoulder) or for individuals who have not had access to fully integrated programs of care.

PRIMARY PREVENTION

Primary prevention of initial and subsequent strokes is one the most effective ways to decrease functional disability caused by stroke. An individual who has sustained a thrombotic stroke has a 10% likelihood of suffering a second event over the subsequent 12 months. Primary prevention should focus on addressing modifiable risk factors and the use of appropriate medications and surgery for prophylaxis. Addressing modifiable risk factors includes controlling hypertension, diabetes mellitus, hyperlipidemia, and hypercholesterolemia with education, weight loss, diet, exercise, and medications; recommending cessation of all tobacco products and moderate use of alcohol; and treating individuals with paroxysmal atrial fibrillation, cardiac valve abnormalities, and ventricular wall motion abnormalities with full anticoagulation (to prevent embolic stroke). Surgical prophylaxis with carotid endarterectomy has been shown to be appropriate for clinically asymptomatic individuals with more than 90% stenosis or symptomatic individuals (prior transient ischemic attack [TIA] or cerebrovascular accident [CVA]) with more than 70% stenosis. Anticoagulation with at least 325 mg daily of aspirin (acetylsalicylic acid [ASA]) is appropriate for all individuals older than 50 years as primary prophylaxis for (thrombotic) stroke. Individuals who have sustained a thrombotic cerebrovascular incident (TIA or CVA) while taking ASA should be given either an increased dose of ASA (up to 650 mg twice a day) or a "platelet smoother": ticlopidine (Ticlid)* or clopidogrel (Plavix).* Full anticoagulation with warfarin may be the next level of prophylaxis if these interventions are unsuccessful; however, its efficacy is not fully proved.

SECONDARY PREVENTION

Secondary prevention of medical morbidities and mortality that occur after stroke allows an increased number of individuals to participate in rehabilitation and those who participate to have fewer concomitant medical issues. Initial mortality after stroke is 30% of all strokes (highest in hemorrhagic and lowest in lacunar infarcts), 30-day mortality is 10% to 30%, and 1-year mortality is 30% to 50% of initial survivors. After 12 to 18 months, mortality is similar to that in the nonstroke population. The most common causes of early death after stroke (in declining order) are the initial stroke, a myocardial infarction (MI), pneumonia, and deep venous thrombosis (DVT) with pulmonary embolus (PE). The most common cause of late death after stroke is an MI. All individuals after stroke benefit from urgent medical management, adequate hydration and oxygenation, appropriate management of blood pressure (typically aiming for a target of 160/90), and close monitoring of electrolytes. Although acute ingestion of regular-strength (325 mg) ASA appears to enhance survivability and outcome, there is no well-established role for systemic anticoagulation (e.g., heparinization). It appears that carefully selected subpopulations of individuals after stroke may have improved mortality, morbidity, and functional outcomes with early intracranial interventions, such as tissue-type plasminogen activator. The efficacy of acute surgical evacuation of intracranial hematomas is unknown, but research suggests that it may improve outcomes in individuals who have not lost consciousness.

Deep Venous Thrombosis and Pulmonary Embolus

Thromboembolic disease is not uncommon following stroke, with DVTs occurring in approximately 40% and PEs in 15% after stroke (usually by 1 month), typically in the paretic limbs. Although poorly studied, upper extremity DVTs probably occur with nearly the same incidence as lower extremity DVTs and should be managed similarly. Rapid mobilization is a vital step in prevention, and any individual who is initially unable to return to prestroke activity (e.g., walking) must have DVT prophylaxis with low-dose unfractionated heparin (i.e., subcutaneous heparin 5000 units twice a day). Prophylaxis should begin immediately after stroke (there is no elevated bleeding risk, even in the presence of a hemorrhagic stroke or need for neurosurgical intervention) and continue until the individual is ambulating to and from the bathroom regularly or 6 weeks have passed. There is no proven indication for low-molecular-weight heparins. Intermittent compression devices may play an adjunct role to subcutaneous heparin, more often in the acute phase of recovery. Support stockings (thromboembolic disease [TED] hose) have no proven efficacy in DVT prophylaxis but may assist in controlling dependent edema. Physical examination does not provide useful information in detecting DVTs; thus, any individual who has not received appropriate prophylaxis should be screened with duplex Doppler examinations. Individuals with hemorrhagic strokes (or other sources of acute bleeding) may be fully anticoagulated by 7 days after insult, perhaps as early as 72 hours.

Aspiration Pneumonia

Aspiration pneumonia occurs in nearly 40% of individuals after stroke, usually within the first month. The incidence is highest in individuals with brainstem strokes (resulting from impairment of posterior cerebral circulation), impaired cognition or attention, a decreased level of arousal, oral motor dysfunction, and premorbid pulmonary dysfunction. The need for ventilatory support is related to both the severity of the pneumonia and the degree of hemiparesis. Radiographic findings of aspiration pneumonia may take up to 24 hours after aspiration, so aggressive antibiotic treatment (along with pulmonary toilet and ceasing all oral feeding) should be implemented on the basis of clinical parameters.

*Not FDA approved for this indication.

Predicting which individuals are likely to aspirate can be challenging. Physical examination has limited usefulness (except when performed by an experienced speech and language pathologist). Testing of cranial nerves (e.g., the gag reflex, the presence of a cough) has no significant predictive value; in fact, at least 10% of all aspirators exhibit no evidence of having just aspirated. The presence of a "wet vocal quality" may be the best prognosticator on examination. Trials of water or ice chips acutely after stroke are neither diagnostic nor recommended. A speech and language pathologist should screen all individuals with a stroke. At their recommendation, a fluoroscopic modified barium swallow examination should be performed and dietary recommendations followed. Individuals who are unable to meet their dietary or fluid requirements (i.e., require intravenous or nasogastric feeding) and are likely to need supplementation for at least 2 weeks are appropriate candidates for a percutaneous endoscopic gastric–jejunostomy (PEG-J) tube placement. Although education on appropriate techniques (e.g., small amounts of food, dry swallows between bites) and positioning (e.g., chin tuck) and monitored introduction of progressively more challenging food items are beneficial, there is no evidence that specialized interventions (e.g., thermal stimulation of the palate) work. Improvements in swallowing can continue for at least 6 months after stroke. When individuals are meeting their dietary needs orally, PEG-J tubes can be easily removed (usually in the gastroenterologist's office), but they must remain in place for at least 6 weeks after placement to decrease the likelihood of gastrocutaneous fistula formation.

Cardiac Disease

Three quarters of all stroke patients have some cardiac impairment, and 13% of stroke patients have had an acute MI. Thus, rehabilitation after stroke must also take into account elements of cardiac rehabilitation. In addition to appropriate dietary and lifestyle modifications, individuals with known cardiac disease or at elevated risk need to have appropriate pharmacologic management during rehabilitation. This can range from simple ASA prophylaxis (81 mg may be sufficient) to β-blocker use after MI. Similarly, an awareness of standard cardiac rehabilitation protocols may be necessary for some patients who have recently suffered myocardial injury. In general, even patients without acute cardiac injury need close monitoring of their initial response to rehabilitative efforts and activity. An exaggerated change in blood pressure (greater than 10 points diastolic or 20 points systolic) or pulse (greater than 20% increase) in response to basic activities of living or walking may warrant closer monitoring or cardiology consultation. Although patients' self-report scales (the Borg Self-Report Exertion Scale) have been shown to provide useful information, individuals with language or cognitive deficits as a result of their stroke typically do not provide reliable information.

Seizures

Seizures have been reported to occur in 5% to 45% of all strokes, most commonly in older adults and individuals with embolic stroke. Electroencephalography is not useful in predicting risk for seizures. There is no proven efficacy to seizure prophylaxis after stroke. If an individual undergoes a craniotomy for hematoma evacuation, 1 week of therapeutic phenytoin (Dilantin) has been shown to be effective in prophylaxis.

REHABILITATION INTERVENTIONS

Services

Longitudinal research has demonstrated that maximal neurologic recovery occurs at 11 weeks and maximal functional recovery occurs at 12.5 weeks after stroke in 95% of stroke survivors. Thus, early, comprehensive, interdisciplinary rehabilitative interventions for the first 1 to 3 months followed by more focused, often multi- or unidisciplinary services for specific persistent difficulties are most appropriate. Rapid consultation by rehabilitation services (therapist and physicians) in the first 72 hours and critical pathways embedded into acute admission orders have been demonstrated to reduce markedly urinary tract infections (e.g., remove all indwelling urinary catheters by 12 hours after stroke, catheterize for postvoid residuals > 100 mL) and aspiration pneumonias (e.g., all patients receive nothing by mouth until cleared by speech and language pathology therapists) while also reducing acute lengths of stay. Randomized, controlled trials have shown the efficacy of inpatient, interdisciplinary, comprehensive rehabilitation over the acute care medical model. Supportive data also exist for day, subacute, outpatient, and home health services for appropriate patients. Therapy services should be discontinued when an individual fails to demonstrate objective functional improvements that are maintained when the therapy is withdrawn. Typically, failure to progress for 2 weeks is justification for stopping services. If medical instability may be preventing progress, a therapy hiatus may be taken until stability is achieved.

Settings

Rehabilitation services should always be delivered in the least restrictive and least medically intensive setting that the individual can tolerate (e.g., non-inpatient settings are preferable to inpatient setting). Individuals who are medically stable enough to tolerate at least 3 hours daily of structured therapy (including physical therapy, occupational therapy, speech and language pathology, psychology, and therapeutic recreation) and who have the social supports available and the potential to regain enough functional independence to allow them to return to community dwelling are appropriate for a stay on a traditional inpatient rehabilitation unit. The interdisciplinary approach is facilitated by daily communication between team members, weekly formal meetings of all team members to discuss progress and goals, and inclusion of the patient and family members in the process. Typical lengths of stay range from 2 to 4 weeks, often followed by a 4- to 12-week period of additional services. Day rehabilitation services recreate the intensity (3 to 6 hours daily) and interdisciplinary model of inpatient care but in an outpatient setting and are appropriate for individuals who are medically stable enough to be maintained by their families at night and on weekends. Individuals who have suffered acute disability from stroke but cannot medically tolerate at least 3 hours of therapy or be maintained by their social support system at home but are felt to have potential for some (often slow) improvement are best served by lower intensity (typically 1 to 2 hours daily) subacute rehabilitation services. Subacute services are most often delivered in specialized sections of nursing homes known as skilled nursing facilities, although such specialized units are at times found on rehabilitation or acute medical units as well. Medicare (federal funding for individuals 65 years and older or those with long-term disability or end-stage renal disease), Medicaid (state funding for the medically indigent), and most commercial insurance programs provide funding for these programs as long as timely functional improvements are demonstrated.

Factors Influencing Functional Outcome

Evaluating an individual's potential for favorable recovery following stroke is an important step in determining the most appropriate setting and intensity for rehabilitation, allowing the best allocation of financial resources and social supports. Early planning for eventual discharge is vital to allow all members of the treatment to meet the patient's and family's expectations. The following factors have been associated with poorer short- and long-term functional outcomes and increased nursing home placement after stroke: age older than 65 years; prior stroke; history of acute or chronic congestive heart failure; limited social supports (including lack of a designated female caregiver); lower educational level (e.g., non–high school graduate); bladder or bowel incontinence; cognitive or perceptual deficits, visual deficits, or aphasia at 1 week; altered level of arousal initially; persistent balance deficits; need for assistance in self-grooming, feeding, or wheelchair propulsion at 1 week; and severe motor deficits (0 to 1/5 strength) initially.

COMMON MANAGEMENT ISSUES

Motor Control

The natural history of motor recovery of the limbs after stroke typically includes a progression from flaccidity (no tone and no reflexes) to hyperreflexia and hypotonia to hyperreflexia and hypertonia to synergy patterns of movement (gross motor patterns of flexion or extension elicited by noxious stimuli) to volitional control. Recovery most often begins proximally and descends distally. Unfortunately, not all individuals progress completely through these phases and thus may not achieve full motoric recovery. Flaccidity and hypotonia should be managed with appropriate positioning (e.g., elevating the distal extremity or using compressive stockings or gloves to prevent dependent edema formation), support and protection of the limb (e.g., a sling during ambulation or padded table or arm trough during sitting to maintain the integrity of the shoulder joint, gait aids or bracing to support the weakened areas of the leg), careful daily range of motion of all joints, and early introduction of therapy. A sling should be worn only if the strength of the shoulder girdle muscles is less than 2/5 and additionally only during ambulation or standing activities. Appropriate positioning and fit of the sling are important to prevent neck pain and dependent swelling in the hand. Facilitation of movement may be attempted using specific therapy techniques that include tactile stimulation (e.g., vibration, tapping), repetitive movements, use of primitive reflexes, and specific positioning of the limb. As the weakened limb regains volitional control, gradated strengthening exercises along with functional skills training are most appropriate. As noted previously, the majority of recovery occurs in the first 3 months after stroke; however, research also suggests that "forced use" of a paretic limb, which has at least enough strength to pick a washcloth off a table but has not been actively used, can result in increased strength and functional usage even years after stroke. This technique is known as constraint-induced movement therapy.

Spasticity

Hypertonia and spasticity (a type of increased tone characterized by an increase in tone linked to the rapidity of stretch) management entails all of the preceding interventions in addition to orthoses (braces) for at-risk joints (e.g., wrist, elbow, ankle) to prevent contractures and a greater frequency of joint range of motion. Although spasticity is not inherently bad (e.g., it maintains muscle bulk, decreases the incidence of DVT, and may be used as a platform for lower extremity weight bearing), when it results in the early formation of joint contractures, limits actual function (i.e., prevents an otherwise strong muscle from working), prevents appropriate hygiene (e.g., perineal care), or causes significant pain, more intensive interventions are indicated. Although infrequently utilized because of its labor intensiveness, inhibitive casting of a spastic limb can be highly effective. More commonly, systemic medications or focal neurolytic blockade is used.

When multilimb spasticity is present, a systemic approach is most beneficial. Dantrolene sodium (Dantrium), a peripherally acting muscle calcium channel blocker, is the most appropriate first-line agent and should be used in doses ranging from 25 mg daily to 100 mg four times daily. Baclofen (Lioresal), tizanidine (Zanaflex), and diazepam (Valium) are also effective but have central effects and therefore may be potentially sedating. Hepatotoxicity should be monitored with these agents. For individuals with more focal spasticity and hypertonia, the use of focal neurolytics is more practical. Phenol* (a neurodestructive alcohol derivative) may be used to reduce or block temporarily (3 to 6 months duration) individual muscle activity or all muscles innervated by a single nerve. Extremely inexpensive (i.e., $2 to $5 a limb), its usage is limited by the need for electromyographic monitoring of the placement of the phenol. Botulinum toxins A (Botox)* and B (Myobloc)* may be used to reduce or block individual muscles temporarily (2 to 4 months). Extremely expensive (e.g., >$1000 a limb), botulinum toxin does not require electromyographic monitoring. Surgical ablation of nerves or realignment of muscular attachments has no proven role in the functional management of spasticity.

Extremity Swelling and Pain

After stroke, swelling with or without pain of the paretic extremities is quite common and is typically due to dependency (lack of muscle tone and volitional contractions are unavailable to pump the venous blood back to the heart). Management should occur before the actual occurrence of the edema and includes elevation, appropriate positioning, use of compressive garments (e.g., TED hose, compressive glove), and active or passive exercises. Diuretics are not appropriate unless clearly defined cardiac dysfunction supports their usage. Naturally, the presence of DVTs must be considered, especially if appropriate prophylaxis was not used in the first 3 to 4 weeks or if the edema is recalcitrant to interventions. Other, albeit uncommon, causes that must be considered include occult fracture, heterotopic ossification (i.e., calcium deposition in the joint capsule), and cellulitis. The persistence of edema predisposes individuals to painful extremities related to the immobility it encourages (e.g., leading to adhesive capsulitis of the shoulder), an increase in muscle tone and spasticity, and the intrinsic discomfort of edema in tissues (e.g., within the metacarpophalangeal joints or across the dorsum of the foot).

Although often described, so-called reflex sympathetic dystrophy (RSD) (now known as complex regional pain syndrome) is actually a rare phenomenon, but the term is often applied to a variety of everyday painful conditions to provide a label. Because the appropriate treatment of RSD entails the same principles of management as used for any painful immobilized joint, it is preferable to leave off the negative connotation (and often overpriced and ineffective treatments) of this label and focus instead on addressing the basic issues. Far more commonly, painful shoulders are the result of prolonged immobilization with tightening of the joint capsule that responds only to progressive stretching. Intra-articular steroid or anesthetic injections of the shoulder have not been shown to be effective in placebo-controlled trials. Similarly, hand or foot pain is more commonly related to the presence of edema, abnormal perception of stimuli by the impaired brain (neuropathic pain), or tightening of joint capsules secondary to immobility. There are no shortcuts or miracle cures for these conditions other than the basic principles of pain management, gradual remobilization, desensitization techniques, edema control, tone reduction, and extensive education. Early aggressive management is highly effective but must entail education of the individuals and their families to prevent relapse.

Cognitive, Communication, and Behavioral Sequelae

Cognitive deficits occur most commonly with nondominant parietal lobe strokes and multilacunar infarction states. Parietal lobe syndromes demonstrate greater impairment of executive functioning, often with significant impulsivity and safety judgment deficits. Structured environments and schedules, family education, and frequent verbal and nonverbal cueing are the foundations of management. Pharmacologic interventions, although often utilized (i.e., antiepileptics, mood stabilizers), have limited efficacy. Multi-infarct states are a common cause of dementia and arise with more profound deficits in all areas. Management is similar; however, there may be a role for the anti-Alzheimer's disease medications (e.g., donepezil [Aricept], rivastigmine [Exelon]). Neurostimulants (e.g., methylphenidate [Ritalin]) may have a role in individuals with cognitive deficits, particularly those with attentional deficits. Communication deficits include aphasias (dominant posterior frontal and anterior temporal lobe involvement) and dysarthrias (brainstem strokes). Both are often amenable to intervention by early, intensive speech and language pathology services. These services have been clearly shown to improve aphasias for at least the first 3 months. Dysarthrias may improve for at least 6 months. Pharmacologic interventions have no proven role.

Depression may occur in up to 50% of all patients with strokes, most commonly in individuals with dominant anterior frontal lobe damage. Because symptoms may not be manifest (or be detected) for up to 12 weeks, close follow-up is recommended. Supportive counseling and antidepressant medications (most commonly selective serotonin reuptake inhibitors) have good efficacy. Medications must be used for at least 12 months in individuals with bona fide depression to prevent high rates of recurrence. Methylphenidate (Ritalin) is an appropriate intervention for medically fragile, hospitalized individuals, those with poor endurance or "motivation," or to obtain a more rapid response (usually 1 to 3 days). Switching over to a true antidepressant is recommended for long-term (minimum 1 year) care. Insomnia is not uncommon after stroke and should be managed with good sleep hygiene techniques (i.e., eliminating daytime naps, providing an appropriate environment) and, if needed, sleep medications (trazodone, zolpidem [Ambien]).

*Not FDA approved for this indication.

MANAGEMENT OF EPILEPSY IN ADOLESCENTS AND ADULTS

method of
DEAN K. NARITOKU, M.D.
Southern Illinois University School of Medicine
Springfield, Illinois

Epilepsy is one of the most common neurologic disorders and has an estimated prevalence of 0.6%. More importantly, the lifetime incidence of seizures is estimated to be approximately 10%. Thus, seizures and epilepsy are encountered in every clinical practice. Furthermore, untreated or uncontrolled epilepsy is a costly disorder that may result in severe injuries, morbidity, and death. Therefore, proper identification and management of seizures are important for all medical disciplines.

DIAGNOSIS AND CLASSIFICATION

Seizures may be defined as abnormal and uncontrolled hypersynchronous brain activity that results in a behavioral manifestation. It is a *symptom* of disordered brain regulation, and therefore it is important that underlying causes be sought. Interestingly, the ability to seize is conserved throughout nearly all animal species that possess a well-organized central nervous system and therefore must involve brain mechanisms that are present in normal individuals. In contrast, *epilepsy* is a pathologic condition in which seizures recur under relatively normal conditions, either spontaneously or after naturally occurring provocations. Thus, an increased predisposition to seizures characterizes the epileptic state. This distinction is important because symptomatic seizures, or seizures that have occurred as a result of transient conditions, usually do not warrant anticonvulsant therapy. A common example would be a seizure caused by insulin-induced hypoglycemia. The estimated recurrence rate after an unprovoked seizure is 30% to 60%, so treating patients with anticonvulsants after a first seizure would potentially subject them to unnecessary long-term therapy. Therefore, most clinicians will wait until seizures recur before starting antiepileptic drug (AED) therapy.

When approaching a patient with seizures, it is important to recognize that many conditions are mimickers of seizures, as listed in Table 1. In fact, a large percentage of patients referred to tertiary care epilepsy programs are refractory to medications, primarily because they have nonepileptic events. One of the most common differential diagnoses of seizures is syncope. Syncope can usually be distinguished clinically from seizures by its prodrome of light-headedness. However, convulsive seizures may also occur secondary to a syncopal event, thereby making the distinction less clear. Also commonly confused for seizures is panic disorder, which may cause symptoms of floating or depersonalization that are mistaken for psychic symptoms of complex partial seizures.

TABLE 1. **Common Mimickers of Seizures in Adults and Adolescents**

Syncope (with or without seizure)
Cardiogenic
Vasovagal
Panic disorder
Complex migraine
Metabolic encephalopathy
Psychogenic seizures

Because seizures are transient phenomena, the diagnosis is based initially on a history of the spells from both the patient and observers. In some valuable instances seizures occur spontaneously during an electroencephalographic (EEG) study, but unfortunately, such occurrences are rare unless continuous and prolonged recordings are performed. Interictal abnormalities (i.e., epileptiform sharp waves or spikes) may help support the diagnosis of epilepsy, but their presence or absence alone is not diagnostic. Determining whether the patient has seizures is based on careful characterization of the prodrome, the actual event, and the postdrome. A careful history will usually distinguish between the differential diagnoses of loss of consciousness.

Syncope, whether caused by cardiac or neurogenic factors, is usually preceded by light-headedness. The patient may also complain of graying out or dimming of vision. During the actual event, the patient appears pale and sweaty and, in addition, generally becomes limp. On some occasions, however, the patient may then have a tonic-clonic seizure. If no seizure occurs, the patient will generally regain consciousness quickly.

Panic disorder is a commonly confused differential diagnosis of complex partial seizures. The feelings of depersonalization and anxiety and the autonomic symptoms may resemble seizures. Vasovagal symptoms, syncope, and even secondary seizure may accompany panic attacks, thereby further confusing the diagnosis. Although complex migraine, or migraine with neurologic symptoms and loss of consciousness, is considered a disease of childhood, it may also occur in adolescents and adults.

Seizures are classified by the International Classification of Seizures (Table 2) and are broadly differentiated by whether they begin in part of the cerebral cortex (partial-onset seizures) or appear to start over the entire brain (generalized-onset seizures). Complex partial seizures are often associated

TABLE 2. **International Classification of Seizures**

Partial Onset	Generalized Onset
Simple	Absence
Complex	Primary generalized tonic-clonic
Secondary generalized tonic-clonic	Myoclonic
	Atonic
	Clonic
	Tonic
	Clonic-tonic-clonic

with an "aura," which is actually a simple partial seizure. This aura represents the start of a seizure and is perceived by the conscious brain. The symptoms of the aura reflect the area of brain onset. For example, temporal-onset seizures often start with psychic or visceral sensations or recurrent forced memories. Very often, after a complex partial seizure, patients will experience postictal confusion. During the event, patients often display automatisms, such as lip smacking and indiscriminate picking at objects. Absence seizures are generalized at onset and therefore do not have a prodrome period. Patients may also exhibit automatisms, but afterward, post-event confusion is minimal or absent. Tonic-clonic seizures consist of two phases, an initial rigid tonic phase followed by jerking of the extremities. This activity is followed by a profound postictal state. The post-event confusion and lethargy are quite distinctive; in patients with an unwitnessed episode of loss of consciousness followed by profound post-event obtundation and spontaneous recovery, a presumptive diagnosis of seizures can be made.

Complex partial seizures and absence seizures appear similar, but they differ greatly in their pathophysiology and response to specific AEDs. Complex partial seizures start with a localized onset within the cerebral cortex, whereas absence seizures are probably generated in the diencephalon. Differentiating the two seizure types may present a diagnostic difficulty. Both are characterized by staring and automatisms such as lip smacking and picking at objects. Therefore, they are easily confused, particularly in childhood, when both seizure types are commonly expressed. The presence of either an aura or a postictal state may help clinically identify the staring episode as a partial-onset seizure. A routine electroencephalogram may be helpful in classifying the seizure type; partial-onset seizures are associated with focal spikes (Figure 1), whereas primary generalized seizures are characterized by generalized high-voltage spike-and-wave discharges (Figure 2). In many cases, prolonged video and EEG recording may be necessary to diagnose the seizure type.

Myoclonic seizures are shock-like jerks. Myoclonus is commonly seen in normal individuals on falling asleep, and it is benign. However, when myoclonus occurs in the waking state, it is abnormal. It is often described by the patient as clumsiness or a twitch, especially in the morning or during drowsiness. Atonic seizures consist of sudden loss of posture and falling. They often result in injury because the loss of postural tone causes patients to strike their head.

The initial selection of medications may be made after a bona fide diagnosis of epilepsy has been made, as well as after attempts to classify the seizure type. The seizure medication is then selected according to the seizure type, as well as other considerations related to the patient. Coverage of seizure types may be considered analogous to selection of antibiotics; some of the AEDs are relatively narrow in spectrum, whereas others are broad spectrum. Selection of the wrong medication for the seizure type may lead to ineffective therapy or even worsen the seizures, especially absence or myoclonic seizures. It may be useful to select a broad-spectrum drug if an exact seizure classification cannot be made. A summary of the spectrum of coverage is presented in Table 3.

Many of the medications are recognized to be effective against different seizure types. However, the strength of the clinical evidence varies, particularly because many of the older AEDs were approved and

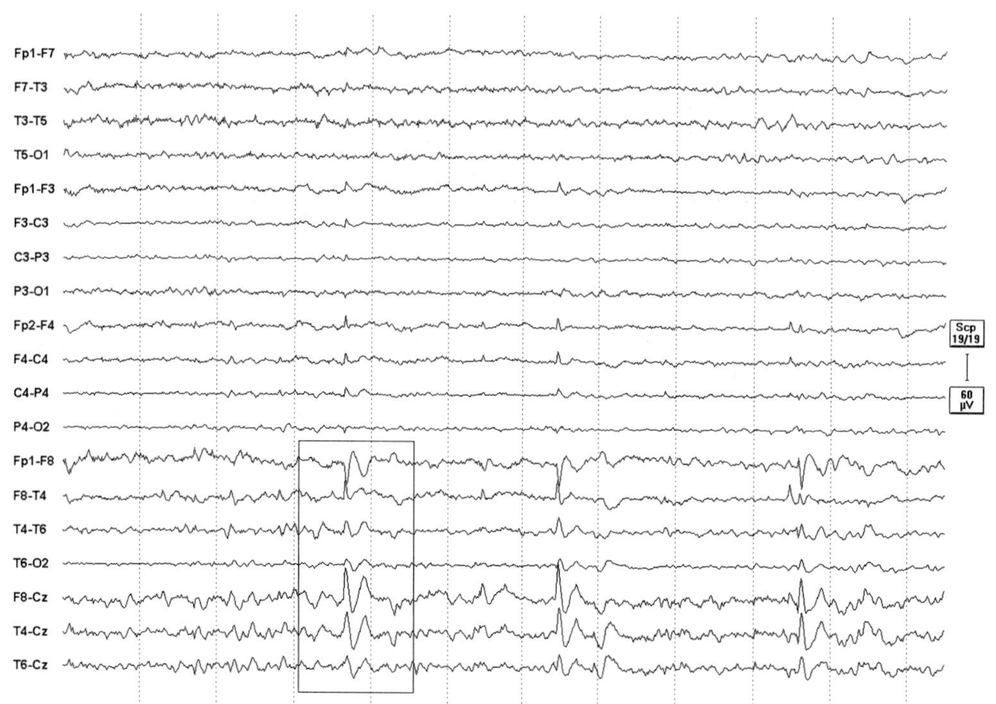

Figure 1. Focal epileptiform spikes on an electroencephalogram. This typical temporal spike is seen in a person with complex partial seizures. The abnormality is highlighted by the *box*. Localized spikes and sharp waves suggest partial-onset seizures in persons with a clinical diagnosis of epilepsy.

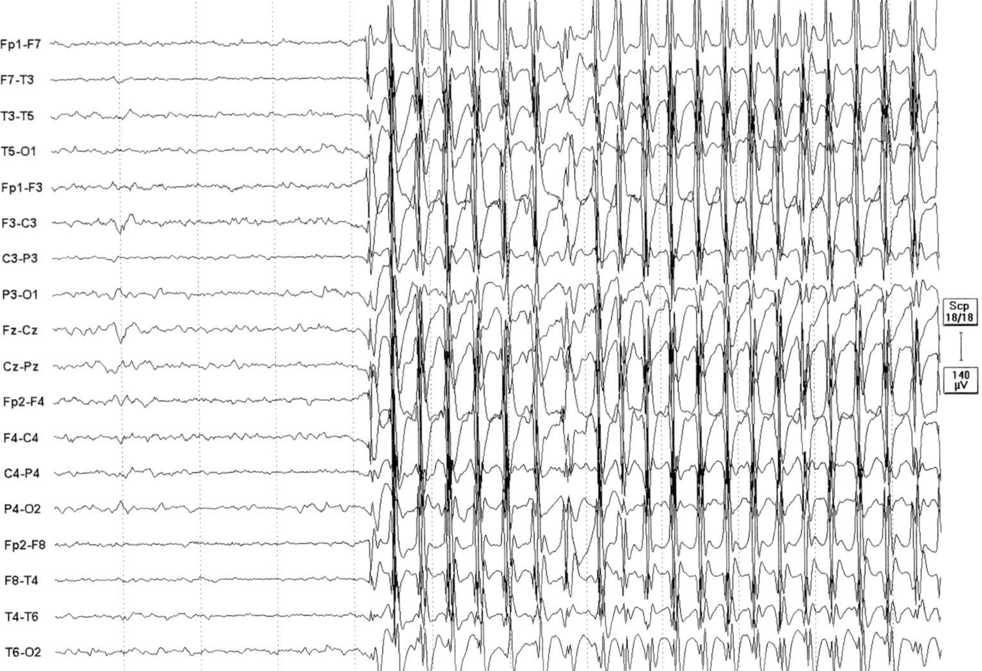

Figure 2. Generalized spike-and-wave discharge. This typical run of generalized spike-wave activity is from a person with absence seizures. Note the widespread distribution of the spike-and-wave discharges, which suggests a generalized-onset seizure.

grandfathered for their indications before the advent of rigorous clinical trials. Drugs in this category include phenytoin (Dilantin), phenobarbital, and primidone (Mysoline). Although carbamazepine (Tegretol) has not undergone registration trials for Food and Drug Administration (FDA) indications, it has been widely used as a standard comparator in recent clinical trials of new AEDs. To address the ethical considerations of clinical trials in epilepsy, most of the newer AEDs were studied and approved first as add-on therapy for patients with intractable epilepsy. Only three AEDs (valproate [Depakote], felbamate [Felbatol], and lamotrigine [Lamictal]) have gained specific FDA approval for monotherapy use, but it is reasonable to use other AEDs as single-drug therapy, depending on the individual patient response. Unfortunately, because of financial considerations, it is likely that most of the newer AEDs will not be tested or approved for FDA monotherapy indications.

TABLE 3. **Spectrum of Coverage of Antiepileptic Drugs**

		Primary Generalized-Onset Seizures			**Partial-Onset Seizures**		**Epilepsy Syndrome**
Spectrum	**Drug**	*Absence*	*Myoclonic*	*Tonic-Clonic*	*Complex Partial*	*Secondary Tonic-Clonic*	*Lennox-Gastaut*
Narrow	Ethosuximide	*N					
Limited	Carbamazepine			*	*N	*	
	Gabapentin				†A	*	
	Phenobarbital			*	*	*	
	Phenytoin			*N	*	*	
	Primidone			*	*N	*	
	Tiagabine				†A	‡	
Expanded	Lamotrigine	*		*	†A, M	†	†A
	Levetiracetam		‡	‡	†A	†	
	Felbamate		‡	‡	†A, M	†	†A
	Topiramate		‡	†A	†A	†	†A
Broad	Valproate	*A	*	*	†A, M	†	*
	Zonisamide	‡	‡	‡	†A	†	‡

*Comparative trials or extensive clinical experience.
†Randomized, double-blind placebo or active controlled trials.
‡Case series or clinical experience.
A, FDA indication for add-on therapy; M, FDA indication for monotherapy; N, FDA indication, no reference to monotherapy or add-on therapy (grandfathered).

CHARACTERISTICS OF COMMONLY USED ANTIEPILEPTIC DRUGS

Carbamazepine

Carbamazepine is one of the most widely used medications for treatment of partial-onset seizures. Its main attributes include relatively low expense and long-standing clinical experience. Although titration rates have never been formally assessed, it is clear that in at least some patients, titration should be performed slowly, with a starting dose of 200 mg twice daily (bid) titrated up to doses of 400 mg/d three times daily (tid). Carbamazepine may cause a condition similar to the syndrome of inappropriate secretion of antidiuretic hormone (SIADH), which can result in troublesome hyponatremia, especially in the elderly. Carbamazepine commonly causes a symptomatic leukopenia that should not be confused with the very rare condition fatal aplastic anemia. It is a potent inducer of the cytochrome P-450IIIA4 system, which may increase the metabolism of other medications using this pathway. Carbamazepine may autoinduce its own metabolism, thereby lowering levels a month after initial titration of therapy.

Phenytoin

Although phenytoin is one of the most commonly used medications by primary care physicians, its use has fallen out of favor with neurologists and epilepsy specialists. It is notoriously nonlinear and saturates its metabolic sites at therapeutic levels. Because of this nonlinearity, even small increases may result in large increases in its blood level (see Figure 3). As a result, phenytoin has been one of the leading causes of hospitalization for adverse drug affects. The nonlinearity of phenytoin may result in the need to draw multiple blood samples to determine levels during drug monitoring. The cost of drug monitoring may more than exceed the perceived inexpensive cost of phenytoin, and any hospitalization would nullify the savings of the medication. Phenytoin may also cause cosmetic difficulties, including gingival hyperplasia, hirsutism, and collagen abnormalities, which may result in coarsening of facial features and Dupuytren's contractures. The initial starting dose for adults is 300 mg/d, but only about a third of patients achieve levels within the "therapeutic range." When the level exceeds 10 mg/L, the dose increase should preferably be small, with no more than 30- to 60-mg increments.

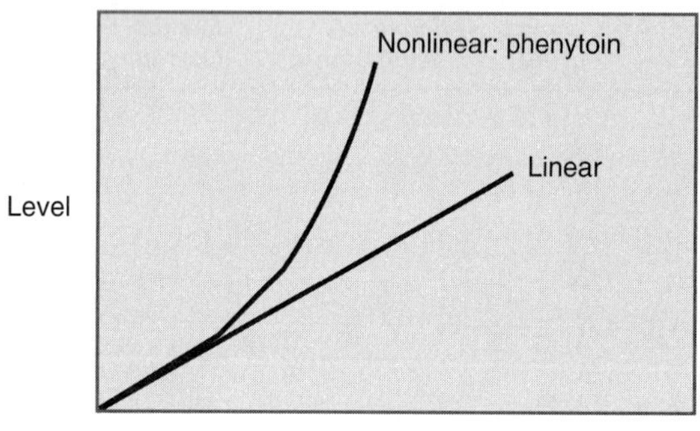

Figure 3. Nonlinear behavior of phenytoin. This figure shows hypothetical phenytoin levels as a function of dose. Note that most antiepileptic drugs follow a linear dose proportionality; that is, doubling a dose roughly doubles the resulting blood level. Phenytoin typically saturates its metabolic sites at therapeutic levels, so small increases or reductions in dose may result in large changes in levels, which may complicate therapy.

Valproate

Valproate is a broad-spectrum medication that has efficacy against all seizure types, which makes it particularly useful when the exact seizure classification is unknown or multiple seizure types exist. It is a fairly linear drug, although it exhibits reduced protein binding at high concentrations. Valproate inhibits a less commonly used subset of the P-450 system for drug metabolism and therefore tends to cause fewer interactions than the other older AEDs do. Valproate potently inhibits lamotrigine metabolism, probably by inhibiting glucuronidation, and it may raise phenobarbital levels. Overall, it is one of the most flexible drugs in that it is available in every formulation, including tablet, time-release, suspension, sprinkles, and intravenous preparations. Valproate may be loaded rapidly intravenously and is well tolerated at a rate of 3 mg/kg/min, thereby allowing the fastest initiation of any AED. At high doses it is associated with weight gain, and therefore weight monitoring and diet counseling should be provided as needed. Valproate may also increase physiologic tremor and cause temporary hair thinning. The starting daily dose of valproate is 7 to 15 mg/kg/d given either bid or tid, with an initial target dose of 15 mg/kg/d, and it may be titrated to doses up to 60 mg/kg/d.

Lamotrigine

Lamotrigine is an expanded-spectrum AED. In addition to partial and tonic-clonic seizures, it appears to be effective against absence seizures. However, it may be ineffective against myoclonic seizures and in some individuals may exacerbate or precipitate myoclonus. Lamotrigine is metabolized primarily through glucuronidation and does not inhibit or induce the P-450 system. Its metabolism, however, is strongly inhibited by valproate, and therefore special care must be exercised when adding to drug regimens with valproate. Its metabolism is also increased by inducers of the P-450 system. At the recommended rates of dose escalation, lamotrigine has an overall 0.8% risk of rash; if introduced rapidly, the rate may be as high as 10% to 15%. Because of inhibition of lamotrigine metabolism by valproate, special care must be taken to introduce lamotrigine slowly when the patient is taking valproate. The initial starting dose of lamotrigine is 25 mg/d, with increments of 25 to 50 mg weekly to reach an initial target dose of 100 mg bid., and it is titrated according to clinical response up to 150 to 250 mg bid, if needed. If valproate is used, the initial dose and rate of increase should be halved.

Topiramate

Topiramate (Topamax) is an expanded-spectrum drug that is useful against partial-onset, tonic-clonic, and myoclonic seizures. It does not appear to be effective against absence seizures. Topiramate is cleared by both the P-450 and renal systems. In general, it does not induce P-450 metabolism, but at higher doses (>200 mg/d), it may induce the metabolism of birth control medications. In some individuals, phenytoin metabolism may be inhibited by topiramate, thereby resulting in unexpectedly higher levels. When escalated too quickly, especially during AED polytherapy, it can result in significant cognitive impairment, which is generally transient. Because topiramate possesses carbonic anhydrase inhibitory properties, its use is associated with a slightly higher risk for the development of renal stones (estimated at 1.4%). The carbonic anhydrase inhibition may also result in tingling paresthesias. Topiramate is associated with weight loss, but the mechanism is unknown. The initial starting dose of topiramate is 25 to 50 mg/d, with increases of 25 to 50 mg each week to an initial target dose of 100 mg bid and titration to clinical response up to 200 to 300 mg bid.

Oxcarbazepine

Oxcarbazepine (Trileptal) is a derivative of carbamazepine that does not form an epoxide metabolite, which is believed to be more toxic than the parent compound. However, its advantages over carbamazepine for initial therapy may be more theoretic than practical, especially given the cost differential. Similar to carbamazepine, it is a limited-spectrum drug that is effective against partial-onset seizures and tonic-clonic seizures. It may also cause an SIADH-like syndrome resulting in significant hyponatremia, especially in the elderly. However, unlike carbamazepine, it does not strongly induce the P-450 system, nor does it induce asymptomatic leukopenia. The initial starting dose of oxcarbazepine is 300 mg bid, with weekly 300-mg increases to an initial target dose of 450 to 600 mg bid and titratation according to response up to 1200 mg bid.

Gabapentin

Gabapentin (Neurontin) is a limited-spectrum drug that is effective against partial-onset seizures. It is water soluble and cleared exclusively by the renal system. It has relatively low potency, and its limited absorption from the gut potentially limits its efficacy. Gabapentin has no known pharmacokinetic interactions with other medications, which may make it useful in patients with compromised hepatic function. However, caution must be taken in the elderly or other patients who may have reduced renal function, and lower doses should be used. The initial starting dose of gabapentin is 300 mg tid; in elderly and renally compromised patients, it should be reduced to 100 to 200 mg tid. The dose may be titrated upward to 1200 mg tid per clinical response.

Zonisamide

Zonisamide (Zonegran) is a broad-spectrum drug that is probably effective against all seizure types, although formal trial data are lacking for many of the primary generalized seizure types. Its main attribute is an extremely long half-life of approximately 60 hours, which allows it to be taken once daily or bid. Zonisamide is metabolized by the P-450 system, but it does not have significant interactions with other medications. It also must be titrated slowly for tolerability considerations. Zonisamide is a weak carbonic anhydrase inhibitor and is associated with an estimated 1.4% risk for kidney stones. Zonisamide is associated with weight loss, but the mechanism is unknown. The initial starting dose of 100 mg/d is clinically effective, with increases of 100 mg every 1 to 2 weeks to a daily dose of 100 to 600 mg.

Levetiracetam

Levetiracetam (Keppra) is a limited- to expanded-spectrum AED that is effective against partial-onset and tonic-clonic seizures. Early open-label data suggest that it may also be effective against some of the primary generalized seizure types, including myoclonic seizures. Levetiracetam is water soluble and predominantly cleared by the kidneys. It does not have known interactions with the P-450 system. The starting dose of levetiracetam is 500 mg bid, which is clinically effective for intractable epilepsy, and it may be titrated upward to 1500 mg bid.

Tiagabine

Tiagabine (Gabitril) is an interesting compound in that it is one of the few AEDs developed as a "rational" therapy based on its mechanism of action. It is a derivative of nipecotic acid, which blocks γ-aminobutyric acid (GABA) reuptake into neurons and glia. It is effective against partial-onset seizures. Tiagabine has a very short half-life, but clinical trials have shown no significant difference in efficacy with bid or tid dosing, and therefore the drug may be given bid. Tiagabine should be taken with food to blunt the peak effect of the medication, which may cause dizziness or drowsiness at peak doses. It is metabolized by the P-450IIIA4 system but does not induce or inhibit the metabolism of other medications. Tiagabine must be introduced slowly, with 4 mg at bedtime and 4-mg/wk increases to an initial target dose of 6 to 12 mg tid, and it may be increased further up to 56 mg/d as needed.

Barbiturates

Barbiturates, including phenobarbital and primidone, should not be routinely used in practice. Although they are inexpensive, they very frequently cause problems with sedation or cognitive impairment. They are strong inducers of the P-450 system, and phenobarbital is partially cleared by the renal system.

Barbiturates are effective against partial-onset and tonic-clonic seizures. However, given the plethora of AEDs with better tolerability profiles, this category should be considered one of the last choices for seizure therapy. The initial dose of phenobarbital is 30 mg tid with titration upward according to response.

Felbamate

Felbamate, a derivative of meprobamate, is an expanded-spectrum anticonvulsant. It has been particularly useful for childhood epilepsies, but its association with aplastic anemia and hepatotoxicity has been a source of major concern. It is a major inhibitor of the P-450 system and can cause concomitant medication levels to increase greatly, thereby resulting in toxicity. Felbamate is also associated with weight loss. Although withdrawal from the market was considered by the FDA, it continues to be available, in recognition of its value to many patients with severe epilepsy. However, it should be used only when other alternatives have failed. The initial dose of felbamate is 300 to 400 mg tid, and this dose may be titrated upward to a maximum of 1200 mg tid as needed for seizure control.

Vigabatrin*

Vigabatrin is an irreversible inhibitor of the GABA transaminase enzyme, which normally inactivates GABA. It is also the result of "rational" drug development. Vigabatrin is effective in a wide variety of seizures, including many of the severe epilepsies of infancy and early childhood. It is currently available in several countries and used on a limited basis. However, vigabatrin is associated with irreversible visual field loss, which has prevented it from being approved in the United States.

PRINCIPLES OF ANTIEPILEPTIC DRUG THERAPY

Before initiating therapy, it is important to establish whether the patient has a bona fide diagnosis of epilepsy (i.e., has episodes of recurrent seizures). Information from the history and electroencephalogram should be used to classify the seizure type to ensure appropriate drug selection. If the classification is uncertain, it may be helpful to use a broad-spectrum agent, as listed earlier. In general, most anticonvulsant drugs need to be introduced at a low dose and titrated upward slowly to the target dose. Exceptions to this guideline include fosphenytoin (Cerebyx) and valproate (Depacon), which may be loaded intravenously and are well tolerated under loading conditions. It should be noted that the suggested starting dose for some AEDs, such as levetiracetam and zonisamide, is clinically effective, although the further adjustment may be needed for optimal response. The remaining drugs require slow titration for tolerability and/or safety reasons.

*Not available in the United States.

The ultimate goal of AED therapy is freedom from seizures with no side effects. Although this goal cannot always be achieved, the clinician should continue to strive for such results. Therapy should be guided by individual patient response, as measured clinically by seizure frequency and adverse effects. A seizure diary is essential for determining the outcome of therapeutic changes. Because seizure frequency fluctuates, it is helpful to calculate a seizure index (number of seizures/duration of the interval in days from the last visit) to examine seizure trends. The patient should be questioned at each visit for signs of neurotoxicity, as outlined in the next section. AED levels are only a surrogate for clinical outcome. Although they provide feedback for rough dosing, monitoring of compliance, and evaluation of pharmacokinetic changes, they are not a substitute for the clinical endpoints of seizure frequency and side effects. In general, the lowest dose that achieves freedom from seizures will provide the most desirable results. AEDs should be titrated upward until either the best response is achieved or side effects occur.

Management of Toxicities

The most common adverse effects encountered with AED therapy are neurotoxic symptoms, including dizziness, drowsiness, blurred vision, cognitive impairment, behavioral changes, and gait unsteadiness. These effects may be related to the initial introduction of medication or be dose related. Slowing the titration rate may reduce the introduction-related toxicities, which abate as the patient builds tolerance to the adverse effects. As the dose is increased further, the patient may encounter nontransient dose-related toxicities as higher levels are achieved. It is important to remember that AED toxicity is a function of the total drug load and that the incidence of adverse effects increases with each successive anticonvulsant drug added. Recent case series have shown that the incidence of drug toxicity approaches 100% in patients taking four or more AEDs. Drug reduction should always be considered whenever the patient is receiving AED polytherapy and is having adverse effects. Similarly, reduction of concomitant medications during the introduction of a new AED improves its tolerability.

Idiosyncratic reactions are rare but often dangerous. Both aplastic anemia and fatal hepatotoxicity have been reported with all the older-generation AEDs. Although laboratory monitoring of some medications with a complete blood count and liver function studies is recommended by the FDA, it is unclear whether such studies are of value in detecting dangerous idiosyncratic reactions. Clinical vigilance is crucial to avert these rare problems. The patient and family should be instructed to contact the physician immediately should any rash, bruises, or petechiae appear, which may signal a blood dyscrasia. The hepatotoxic syndrome is a Reye-like syndrome with ataxia, drowsiness, and potential paradoxic increases in seizures. The symptoms should alert the physician to immediately reassess the condition and stop AED therapy if necessary.

Long-Term Outcome and Prognosis

Several open-label and long-term studies have looked at the prognosis of newly treated epilepsy. Interestingly, they show very similar results and suggest that about 47% of patients will respond to the initial therapy. Of the remaining patients, approximately 47% will respond to a second agent, which means that overall, approximately 30% of the population will remain resistant to two-drug trials. At this point, a patient may be considered medically intractable because only a small percentage of patients become seizure free after subsequent trials of AEDs, although many are considerably improved. Studies of patients enrolled in randomized controlled trials investigating new AEDs suggest that the rate of freedom from seizures is no higher than 5% to 7% for each successive AED. It is worthwhile noting that patients who respond to a second drug tend to be those who have failed the initial therapy as a result of adverse effects rather than efficacy. Thus, even failure to respond to the first medication predicts a poor outcome for such subsequent treatment, if the failure is due to lack of efficacy. Failure of two AEDs may earmark the patient for alternative approaches, such as epilepsy surgery. Certain pathologies are also associated with a poorer prognosis for freedom from seizures. Most notably, patients with more than one seizure focus or brain pathology are the most difficult to control.

TABLE 4. **Stages of Intravenous Pharmacologic Therapy for Status Epilepticus**

Stage	Standard (Initial Dose)	Alternative (Initial Dose)
I	Lorazepam (Ativan), 0.1 mg/kg (maximum, 4 mg)	—
II	Fosphenytoin (Cerebyx), 20 mg/kg	Valproate (Depacon), *25 mg/kg
III	Phenobarbital, *20 mg/kg	Valproate, *25 mg/kg
IV	Midazolam (Versed)*, † Pentobarbital (Nembutal)† Propofol (Diprivan)*, †	

*Not FDA approved for this indication.
†Use continuous electroencephalography to titrate to cessation of electrographic seizures.

STATUS EPILEPTICUS

Status epilepticus has traditionally been defined as either 30 minutes of continuous convulsive activity or multiple seizures without regaining consciousness. Because most seizures typically last 2 minutes or less, many centers have adopted a more rigorous definition of status epilepticus: 10 minutes of continuous seizures. This definition reflects the recognition that the prognosis for control of status epilepticus is related to how quickly therapy is instituted. Status epilepticus is a life-threatening emergency, and delay in therapy increases the risk for morbidity and mortality. The goals of therapy are to stabilize the patient and terminate the status epilepticus as quickly as possible. As with all emergencies, it is most important to

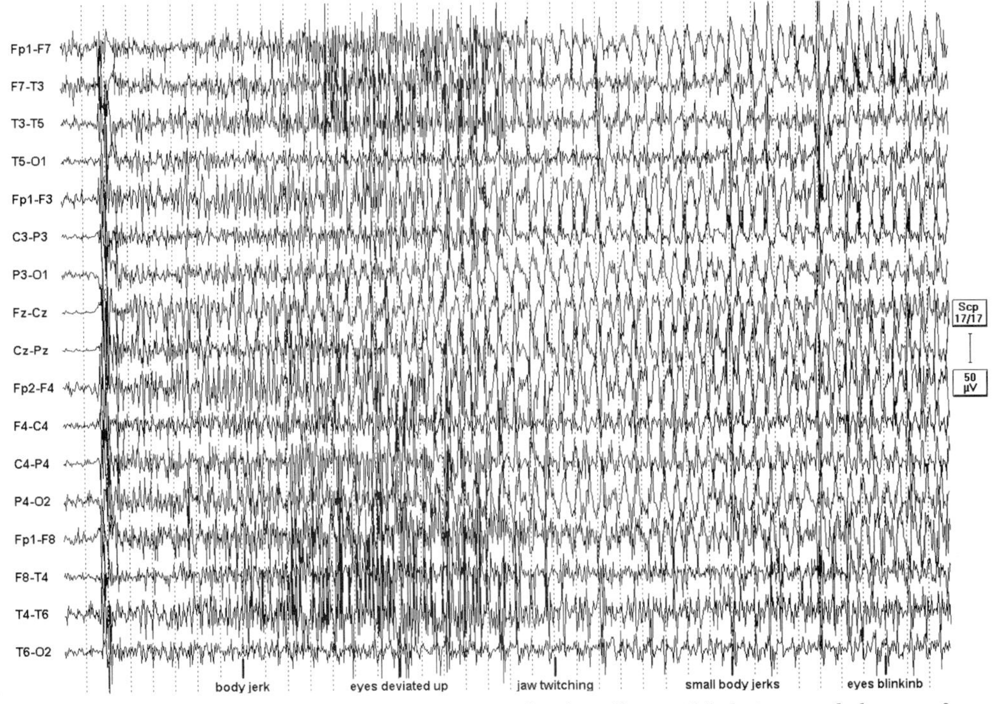

Figure 4. Electroencephalographic (EEG) monitoring during status epilepticus. Sequential electroencephalograms from a patient in convulsive status epilepticus are shown. Each line represents 1-second intervals. **A,** The EEG changes correlate with behavioral seizure episodes early in treatment.

Continued

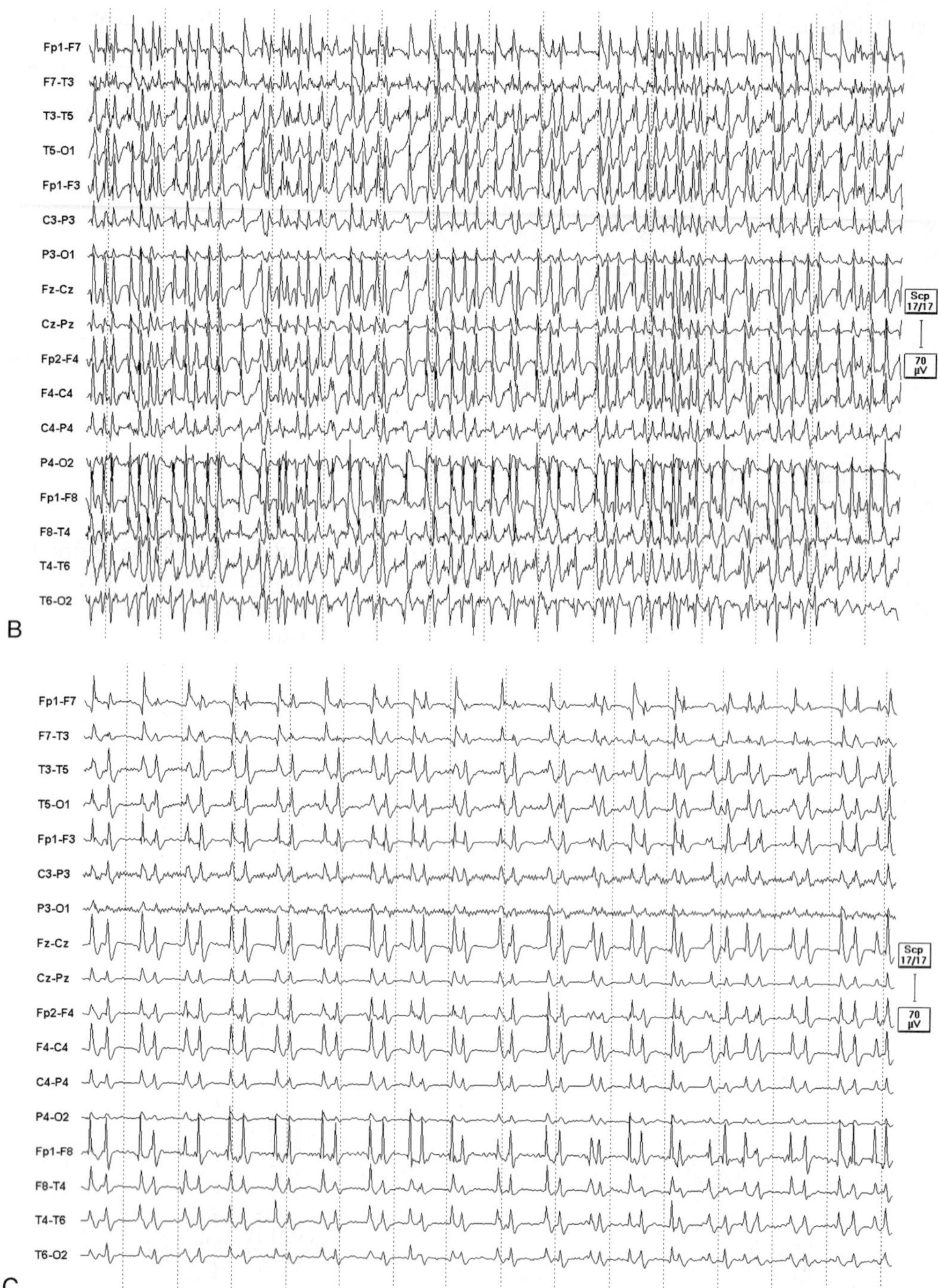

Figure 4, cont'd. **B,** The behavioral changes during seizures are minimal, but electrographic seizures persist. Without EEG monitoring, the continuation of seizure activity may not have been identified and treated properly. Later, in **C,** no behavioral seizures are observed; the electrographic seizure activity has slowed but requires further aggressive treatment. All electrographic seizure activity was eventually arrested, thus underscoring the importance of continuous EEG monitoring for proper management of status epilepticus.

first stabilize the airway, breathing, and circulation before proceeding with other therapies and studies. An intravenous line with saline is recommended in case resuscitation is necessary and for administration of anticonvulsants. When the state of the patient is in doubt, a glucose bolus and thiamine should be administered.

Pharmacologic treatment of status epilepticus may be divided into therapeutic stages as outlined in Table 4. It is crucial that *electrographic* seizures be completely eradicated because AED therapy may initially stop behavioral, but not electrographic seizures. Accordingly, the use of continuous EEG monitoring is mandated to verify the cessation of seizure activity (Figure 4). Failure to control electrographic seizures may allow the development of intractable status epilepticus and excitotoxic brain damage. In analogy to the use of electrocardiograms during cardiac emergencies, a continuous EEG monitor should now be considered the standard of care for management of status epilepticus.

Initiation of pharmacologic therapy should begin with a benzodiazepine. Lorazepam (Ativan) is currently the preferred benzodiazepine because of its long duration of action. Approximately 0.1 mg/kg (maximum of 4 mg) may be given intravenously. If this drug is unsuccessful, fosphenytoin should be given in a dose of approximately 20 mg/kg at a rate of 150 mg/min in adults. Clinical experience with intravenous valproate* suggests that it an important alternative choice for the treatment of status epilepticus because it is well tolerated and causes little hypertension. The exact place of valproate in the sequence of therapy for status epilepticus has not been determined, but it should be considered an alternative before the use of barbiturates, especially in cases of pre-existing cardiovascular instability, because of the cardiotoxicity of rapid barbiturate infusion. It may be loaded at a dose of 25 mg/kg with maintenance doses of 15 to 60 mg/kg/d in four divided doses. Valproate may be infused very rapidly at a rate of 3 mg/kg/min. Because of its short half-life, the first maintenance dose should be given approximately 1 hour after the loading dose to ensure that adequate trough levels are obtained.

If control of status epilepticus is not achieved with the aforementioned three agents, phenobarbital* therapy should be instituted with a loading dose of 20 mg/kg at a rate of 100 mg/min. Care must be taken to avoid hypotension and respiratory compromise; intubation and ventilator support are necessary. Should phenobarbital fail, anesthesia is required with either midazolam (Versed),* pentobarbital (Nembutal), or propofol (Diprivan)* under constant EEG monitoring. In the past, it was suggested that anesthesia should be titrated to a burst suppression coma pattern on the electroencephalogram. However recent case series suggest that burst suppression may increase morbidity and mortality, and it is now recommended that the dosage be titrated to cessation of electrographic seizures only. Clinical experience also suggests that midazolam may be safer than pentobarbital or propofol.

Additional studies such as brain imaging and lumbar puncture should be strongly considered. A lumbar puncture is especially necessary in patients with any suggestion of central nervous system infection or nonlocalized fever. Serum chemistry panels and infection studies may also help establish a systemic cause as a precipitant. In addition, AED levels may identify noncompliance with medications.

WHEN TO REFER

Timely referral for neurologic evaluation may be of great assistance in making an accurate diagnosis and ensuring optimal patient management. Neurologic consultation is important for a new onset of seizures because seizures are a symptom of disordered brain regulation and may be a manifestation of a latent disease process. Patients should also be referred after failure of two medications or lack of control after 6 months because such responses identify the patient as intractable. The high incidence of nonepileptic events in patients referred to tertiary care epilepsy centers underscores the importance of detailed investigation of medically intractable patients. Surgical alternatives such as lobectomy and brain stimulation may offer substantial improvement in seizure control and freedom from seizures.

In summary, seizures are commonly encountered in clinical practice. Careful and timely evaluations are crucial to achieving freedom from seizures and the best quality of life.

ACKNOWLEDGMENT

I would like to thank Judy Taylor for her assistance in preparing the manuscript.

EPILEPSY IN INFANCY AND CHILDHOOD

method of
JOHN N. GAITANIS, M.D.
Children's Hospital Boston
Boston, Massachusetts

DEFINITIONS

Seizures are self-limited clinical events resulting from abnormal and excessive firing of cortical neurons. The clinical manifestations are transient and involve motor, sensory, autonomic, or psychic changes with or without an alteration in consciousness. *Epilepsy*, on the other hand, is a condition characterized by recurrent, unprovoked epileptic seizures (Table 1).

It is important to note that epilepsy does not constitute a single entity and is instead a heterogeneous group of disorders with a multitude of etiologies and clinical manifestations. Subdivisions of epilepsy and epileptic seizures are based upon the etiology or the clinical features (Table 2). The effect of seizures on quality of life, the optimal treatment, and the prognosis

TABLE 1. **Seizure Terminology**

Seizure: A clinical event, displaying signs or symptoms, resulting from an abnormal and excessive discharge of cortical neurons.
Epilepsy: Recurrent, unprovoked seizures.
Generalized: The initial seizure discharge involves a large number of neurons throughout both hemispheres and the clinical manifestations indicate bilateral onset.
Partial: The initial seizure discharge involves a limited number of neurons in just one hemisphere.
Simple: A seizure that does not cause alteration in consciousness.
Complex: A seizure involving alteration in consciousness.
Idiopathic: Epilepsy with a genetic cause.
Cryptogenic: Nonidiopathic epilepsy without a known cause.
Symptomatic: Nonidiopathic epilepsy with a known cause (usually a brain insult or other lesion).
Tonic: Sustained posturing of a body part.
Clonic: Rhythmic jerking of a body part.
Myoclonic: Brief, irregular contractions of a body part.
Atonic: An abrupt loss of muscle tone.
Tonic-clonic: Tonic activity alternating with clonic movements.
Absence: A transient discontinuation of activity with loss of awareness.

*Not FDA approved for this indication.

TABLE 2. **Seizure Classification**

- I. Partial (Focal)
  - A. Simple
    - 1. Motor
    - 2. Sensory
    - 3. Autonomic
    - 4. Psychic
  - B. Complex
- II. Generalized
  - A. Absence
    - 1. Typical
    - 2. Atypical
  - B. Myoclonic
  - C. Clonic
  - D. Tonic
  - E. Tonic-clonic
  - F. Atonic

differ greatly between patients. It is imperative that the physician who treats epilepsy takes a careful history and explores possible etiologies in depth so that proper treatment and counseling are provided.

EPIDEMIOLOGY

Single epileptic seizures are a common clinical event, occurring in approximately 120,000 children in the United States each year. Epilepsy is diagnosed less often but is still common. Overall incidence rates of epilepsy in children vary between 73 to 134 cases per 100,000. The incidence is highest in children younger than 1 year of age.

DIAGNOSIS

The diagnosis of seizures begins with a careful history. A detailed description of the episode, focusing on its onset, progression, time course, and recovery, establishes whether seizures are a likely etiology and whether they are focal or generalized. The physical examination establishes whether neurologic dysfunction is present, indicating a symptomatic etiology. Laboratory evaluations search for things that are missed on the history and examination. Two studies are particularly valuable: electroencephalography (EEG) and magnetic resonance imaging (MRI). EEG measures the brain's electrical activity. Transient electrical disruptions (spike waves or slowing) can indicate a predisposition for seizures and help determine whether the seizures are focal or generalized. Moreover, the appearance of these disruptions can be specific for particular seizure types or epilepsy syndromes. EEG is far from a perfect test, however, and can be normal in as many as 50% of patients with known epilepsy. Similarly, patients without a history of seizures can display EEG abnormalities. Thus, the study has to be interpreted within its clinical context. MRI, on the other hand, provides a structural assessment of the brain, helping determine whether an epileptic focus is present. It is particularly useful in patients with a focal seizure onset or localized examination or EEG findings.

DIFFERENTIAL DIAGNOSIS

The first challenge in evaluating a patient with suspected seizures is to determine whether the clinical events are epileptic or nonepileptic in etiology. There are several nonepileptic events (NEEs) that resemble seizures, and the considerations change according to the patient's age.

The Neonatal Period

The diagnosis of seizures is hardest to make in neonates, in whom subtle nonspecific clinical findings, such as eye deviation, apneas, bicycling, or buccolingual movements, may be the only manifestations. Many of these subtle signs are easily misdiagnosed. Suspected seizures are actually NEEs in as many as 90% of neonates. The clinical event with the greatest specificity for epileptic seizures is focal clonic activity, which is epileptic in approximately 44% of newborns. Jitteriness, on the other hand, is nearly always a benign phenomenon. Because of the difficulty in confidently diagnosing seizures in the neonate, video EEG is often required.

Infancy

In infancy, tonic posturing is a common event and is often misdiagnosed. Without other associated signs or symptoms, tonic posturing is epileptic only 30% of the time. One common nonepileptic cause in infants is Sandifer's syndrome. This refers to abnormal tonic posturing of the neck, trunk, or limbs resulting from gastroesophageal reflux. There is often a temporal association with feeds, or there is a past history of spitting up or feeding intolerance. A gastrointestinal evaluation is needed to confirm this diagnosis.

Myoclonus is another event that is frequently misdiagnosed. Although myoclonic epilepsies can develop in infancy, there are two nonepileptic myoclonic syndromes that must be considered. These are benign neonatal sleep myoclonus and benign myoclonus of infancy. In benign neonatal sleep myoclonus, focal, multifocal, or generalized myoclonic movements occur only during sleep. Each movement is brief, lasting a second or less, but the events may cluster. They end abruptly upon awakening. The movements usually begin in the first month and subside by 6 months of age, rarely persisting into childhood. The infant is otherwise neurologically normal. Benign myoclonus of infancy, on the other hand, begins at a later age (between 3 and 15 months) and involves tonic or myoclonic movements during wakefulness. The course is self-limited and the events usually regress by age 2.

Early Childhood

Breath-holding spells are a common event in early childhood. They develop in infancy and resolve prior to school age. Although most occur in response to some upsetting incident, the preceding cause is sometimes not observed by the parent. The child displays a color change, either pallor or cyanosis. Some children have convulsive movements mimicking seizures, and many have a period of lethargy following the spell.

School Age and Adolescence

Later in childhood, most NEEs can be distinguished from seizures on the basis of a careful history or direct observation of the spells. Some include movement disorders such as motor tics, paroxysmal choreoathetosis, or focal dystonias. Narcolepsy, staring spells, complicated migraines, and syncope can also be difficult to distinguish from seizures. If all other causes have been excluded, psychogenic seizures must be considered. Many children with psychogenic seizures have epileptic seizures as well, and video EEG is often required for diagnosis.

PEDIATRIC EPILEPSY SYNDROMES

Pediatric epilepsy syndromes are defined on the basis of clinical and EEG criteria. They are important to recognize because each syndrome exhibits a characteristic treatment response and prognosis.

Febrile Seizures

Febrile seizures are the most common form of childhood seizures, affecting 2% to 4% of all children. They occur between 6 months and 5 years of age, but the peak incidence is at 18 months. Febrile seizures can be divided into simple and complex types. Simple febrile seizures are generalized, last less than 15 minutes, and do not recur within a 24-hour period. All other events are termed complex.

Overall, one third of children with a first febrile seizure experience a recurrence. Risk factors for recurrence include a family history of febrile seizures and an age of onset younger than 18 months. In children with febrile seizures, the overall risk of later epilepsy is approximately 2%. This risk is higher in the presence of neurologic or developmental abnormalities, complex febrile seizures, or a family history of epilepsy.

Most epidemiologic data indicate that febrile seizures are benign; aggressive treatment measures are not required. The simplest preventive strategy is to use analgesics during febrile illnesses. Diazepam (Valium) can also be given at the time of fever for seizure prophylaxis, but this results in only a modest reduction in recurrence. Alternatively, rectal diazepam (Diastat) can be used acutely during febrile seizures. This does not prevent the seizures from occurring, but it prevents them from becoming prolonged. Consideration can be given to using a daily antiepileptic. Phenobarbital and valproate (Depakote) are effective for this purpose, but both can cause side effects. Treatment with a daily antiepileptic agent is therefore reserved for only the most severe cases.

Infantile Spasms

Infantile spasms are an uncommon epilepsy syndrome. They typically develop during the first year, with a peak age of onset between 4 and 6 months. Brief (1 to 5 second), symmetric contractions of the trunk with extension and elevation of the arms and tonic extension of the legs characterize the typical spasm. They occur in clusters shortly after waking. During a cluster, the infant may appear irritable. The triad of infantile spasms, hypsarrhythmia (a chaotic EEG pattern), and developmental regression is termed West's syndrome. Management begins with a search for the etiology. In general, the prognosis is better in patients who do not have a discernable etiology. Two treatment options are proved to be effective: corticotropin (ACTH)* and vigabatrin (Sabril).† A course of pyridoxine* may also be considered to exclude pyridoxine-dependent seizures.

Lennox-Gastaut Syndrome

The Lennox-Gastaut syndrome develops in as many as 50% of children with infantile spasms. This syndrome, which occurs between 1 and 7 years of age, is composed of mixed seizure types, cognitive decline, and a slow spike and wave pattern on EEG (<3 Hz). The Lennox-Gastaut syndrome can be quite refractory to treatment. The outcome is poor, with mental retardation developing in 75% to 90% of affected children.

Absence Epilepsy

Typical absence seizures are manifested by a cessation of activity and unresponsiveness lasting 2 to 15 seconds, associated with 3-Hz spike and slow wave discharges on EEG. There are three epilepsy syndromes in which absence seizures are common: childhood absence epilepsy, juvenile absence epilepsy, and juvenile myoclonic epilepsy.

Childhood absence epilepsy develops between 4 and 10 years of age. Ethosuximide (Zarontin) is typically the first-line agent, but valproate (Depakote) and lamotrigine (Lamictal) are also effective. Although most children outgrow absence seizures, 15% go on to develop the lifelong syndrome of juvenile myoclonic epilepsy.

Juvenile absence epilepsy is similar but has a later age of onset (6 to 10 years). Generalized tonic-clonic seizures are more common than in childhood absence epilepsy. Valproate is the first-line treatment, with lamotrigine being an effective alternative.

Juvenile myoclonic epilepsy has an onset between 12 and 18 years. Patients can display absence, generalized tonic-clonic, and myoclonic seizures. The myoclonic jerks typically occur in the early morning hours. The EEG displays fast (3.5 to 6 Hz), generalized spike and wave or polyspike and wave activity. Unlike other absence seizure syndromes, juvenile myoclonic epilepsy is a lifelong disorder. Valproate and lamotrigine are both effective treatment options.

*Not FDA approved for this indication.
†Not available in the United States.

Benign Epilepsy with Centrotemporal Spikes

Benign epilepsy with centrotemporal spikes (BECTS) represents approximately 15% of all childhood epilepsies. As the name implies, this is a benign disorder, which, by the midteenage years, is outgrown in 100% of cases. Moreover, children with this disorder are neurologically normal and developmental regression is not seen. The most common seizure type is simple partial, involving motor or sensory symptoms of the hands or face. Generalized tonic-clonic seizures may also develop. Both seizure types commonly occur in sleep. Treatment is optional and depends largely on the presence of generalized convulsive seizures because the simple partial seizures are not harmful. Therapy is typically effective and may include carbamazepine (Tegretol) or gabapentin (Neurontin). The characteristic EEG pattern includes broad centrotemporal spikes that show an anterior-posterior dipole.

WHY TREAT SEIZURES?

When a correct diagnosis of epileptic seizures has been made, there are several reasons to treat them: (1) to lessen the risk of epilepsy-induced injury, (2) to reduce the risk of prolonged seizures (status epilepticus), (3) to prevent sudden unexplained death in epilepsy (which is fortunately a rare occurrence in children), (4) to lessen cognitive effects from frequent seizures, and (5) to improve the patient's overall quality of life. As with any medical intervention, the benefits that the patient derives from treatment need to outweigh any potential risks. The decision to treat is individualized and based on factors specific to both the seizures (type, frequency, duration) and the patient (age, compliance, level of activity).

WHEN TO TREAT?

Because epilepsy treatment is aimed at prevention, a decision to treat cannot be made without first estimating the recurrence risk. Several factors need to be considered when making this determination.

Overall, the recurrence risk following a first unprovoked seizure in childhood ranges between 44% and 64%. The recurrence risk is highest in patients with an abnormal neurologic examination, an abnormal electroencephalogram, or a remote symptomatic etiology. In patients with only a single nonsymptomatic seizure who have a normal examination and EEG, the risk of recurrent seizures is low (approximately 25%), and observation without antiepileptic medications is generally favored. Should a second seizure occur, the recurrence risk jumps to approximately 79%. Thus, treatment is often started after a second event.

HOW TO TREAT?

Once a decision has been made to treat, choosing the right antiepileptic drug (AED) becomes the next major consideration (Table 3). The optimal choice for a given patient depends on many factors, the two most important of which are efficacy and side effects. Efficacy differs depending on the seizure type. For each seizure phenotype, there is an accepted list of first-, second-, and third-line treatments (Table 4). For each class of seizures, there is often more than one

TABLE 3. **Commonly Used Antiepileptic Medications**

Agent	Pediatric Dose (mg/kg/d)	Half-Life (h)*	Dosing Schedule	Side Effects
Carbamazepine (Tegretol)	10–35	25–65 (initial) 12–17 (chronic)	bid-qid	r, hep, bd, s, n dip, hypn, ost
Clonazepam (Klonopin)	0.01–0.2	18–50	bid-tid	s, a, h, b
Ethosuximide (Zarontin)	10–15 (initial) 15–40 (maint)	30–40	qd-tid	gi, n, an, s, d, b r, bd
Gabapentin (Neurontin)	30–60	5–7	tid-qid	s, d, a, ny, wg
Lamotrigine (Lamictal)				
Off valproate:	0.6 (initial) 5–15 (maint)	7	bid	r, hep, d, a, s, n
On valproate:	0.15 (initial) 1–5 (maint)	45	qd-bid	
Levetiracetam (Keppra)†	20–60	6–8	bid	s, d, ha, b
Oxcarbazepine (Trileptal)	8–10 (initial) 20–50 (maint)	8–10	bid	r, hep, s, diz, n dip, a, ha, hyp
Topiramate (Topamax)	1–3 (initial) 5–9 (maint)	18–30	bid	s, an, ks, ps, wl
Valproic acid (Depakote)	15–60	9–20	bid-qid	hep, bd, n, s, d, wg, hl, r, gi
Zonisamide (Zonegran)†	2–4 (initial) 4–8 (maint)	50–70	qd-bid	r, bd, hep, s diz, an, n, ha wl, ks

*Half-life is based on monotherapy and assumes normal renal function.

†Not FDA approved for this indication in children.

a, ataxia; an, anorexia; b, behavioral difficulties; bd, blood dyscrasia; d, dizziness; dip, diplopia; gi, gastrointestinal distress; h, hyperactivity; ha, headache; hep, hepatotoxicity; hl, hair loss; hypn, hyponatremia; ks, kidney stones; maint, maintenance; n, nausea; ny, nystagmus; ost, osteomalacia; ps, psychomotor slowing; r, rash; s, sedation; wg, weight gain; wl, weight loss.

TABLE 4. **Which Medications for Which Seizure Types?**

Seizure Type	First-Line Therapy	Second-Line Therapy	Third-Line Therapy
Partial (all types)	CBZ, OXC	LTG, VPA, GBP, TPM, PHT	TGB, LEV, ZNS, PB
Generalized			
Tonic-clonic	VPA	LTG, TPM, PHT	PB, ZNS
Myoclonic	VPA	LTG, CZP	PB, ZNS
Tonic	VPA	LTG	CZP, TPM, ZNS
Absence (before age 10)	ESM*	VPA, LTG	ZNS, TPM
(after age 10)	VPA	LTG	ESM, TPM, ZNS
Epilepsy syndromes†			
CAE	ESM	VPA, LTG	ZNS, TPM
JAE	VPA	LTG	ESM, TPM, ZNS
JME	VPA, LTG	TPM, ZNS	CZP, PHT
Lennox-Gastaut	VPA	LTG, TPM	CZP, ZNS, FBM
Infantile spasms	ACTH, VGB	VPA, TPM, TGB, CZP	FBM, ZNS
BECTS	CBZ, GBP	VPA, PHT, CBZ	LTG, TPM

*Assuming no convulsive seizures.
†BECTS, benign epilepsy of childhood with centrotemporal spikes; CAE, childhood absence epilepsy; JAE, juvenile absence epilepsy; JME, juvenile myoclonic epilepsy.
ACTH, adrenocorticotropic hormone; CBZ, carbamazepine (Tegretol); CZP, clonazepam (Klonopin); ESM, ethosuximide (Zarontin); FBM, felbamate (Felbatol); GBP, gabapentin (Neurontin); LEV, levetiracetam (Keppra); LTG, lamotrigine (Lamictal); OXC, oxcarbazepine (Trileptal); PB, phenobarbital; PHT, phenytoin (Dilantin); TGB, tiagabine (Gabitril); VGB, vigabatrin (Sabril); ZNS, zonisamide (Zonegran).

accepted first-line therapy. Deciding which of these has the most favorable side effect profile helps narrow this choice down to a single agent. Other important considerations include the frequency of dosing, ease of administration, and cost. In children, taste and the availability of a liquid or chewable preparation can be among the most important considerations because they greatly affect compliance.

Regardless of which medication is chosen, the goal is the same—for the patient to be free of both seizures and side effects. With careful administration of the right medication, this goal can usually be achieved. In general, most AEDs are started at a low dose and increased gradually. This helps prevent side effects and allows early detection of problems if they are to develop. If side effects occur, the dose is lowered. If seizures return, the dose is raised. If neither is present, no dose change is required. Unfortunately, some patients have continued seizures and side effects, in which case a medication change is needed.

WHAT IF MEDICATION TRIALS FAIL?

Of patients who have never received an AED, approximately 47% become seizure free with the first medication given. If a second drug is needed, only 13% respond. If a third drug is used, the response rate is only 4%. A high initial seizure frequency before treatment, slowing on the EEG, and a symptomatic etiology are risk factors for developing medically intractable epilepsy.

After a patient has failed to respond to multiple AEDs, nonmedication therapies must be considered. There are three nonmedication options that are commonly used in pediatrics: the ketogenic diet, vagus nerve stimulation, and epilepsy surgery. All involve a multidisciplinary approach and require a comprehensive epilepsy center for their implementation and management.

WHEN TO DISCONTINUE THERAPY?

When seizures remain in remission during use of antiepileptic medications, the question arises of when to end treatment. Of patients who have been seizure free for over 2 years, 60% to 75% remain seizure free when medication is withdrawn. A remote symptomatic etiology and an abnormal EEG portend a higher relapse risk. Moreover, some epilepsy syndromes, such as juvenile myoclonic epilepsy, have a high relapse rate requiring a prolonged treatment course, whereas others, such as BECTS, have no chance of relapse once outgrown. The ultimate decision of withdrawing antiepileptic medications is therefore dependent on factors related to the individual patient. Yet, in most cases, 2 years of seizure freedom indicates a high likelihood of successfully weaning AEDs. If seizures are to recur, they do so within 1 year in 60% to 80% of patients. Late recurrences (more than 2 years after stopping AEDs) can develop but are rare.

ATTENTION DEFICIT HYPERACTIVITY DISORDER

method of
JUDITH A. OWENS, M.D., M.P.H., and
VICTORIA DALZELL, M.D.
Rhode Island Hospital and Brown Medical School
Providence, Rhode Island

Attention deficit hyperactivity disorder (ADHD) is among the most commonly diagnosed psychiatric conditions in childhood, affecting an estimated 4% to 12% of school-aged children in the United States. It is also a chronic and often lifelong condition, with estimated rates of persistence of symptoms into adulthood of 60% to 70% in many studies. The changes in nomenclature for this disorder over the past 50 years, from "minimal brain dysfunction (MBD)" to "hyperkinesis" to its current incarnation of ADHD, reflect an increased understanding of the neurochemical and neuropathologic basis of ADHD as well as the development of a more sophisticated and rigorous set of criteria for evaluation, diagnosis, and classification of clinical subtypes. In addition, the development and empirical testing of a variety of treatment modalities ranging from behavioral therapy to use of psychotropic agents have expanded the range of management strategies with which this disorder may be approached by the clinician in both children and adults.

Studies strongly support a neurobiologic basis for this disorder. For example, neuroimaging techniques such as positron emission tomography have demonstrated reduced cerebral glucose metabolism in individuals with ADHD in the premotor and superior prefrontal cortex, areas known to be linked to arousal-activity control. Other neural networks known to be involved in attention and in which there is evidence of altered circuitry in children with ADHD include the cerebellum and corpus callosum. Alterations in several neurotransmitters, particularly dopamine and norepinephrine, are most likely involved in producing the neurobehavioral deficits associated with ADHD. Furthermore, an increased understanding of the effects of dysfunction in specific neurotransmitters, such as the association between norepinephrine dysregulation and decreased ability to disengage and refocus attention, is beginning to lead to a more specific approach to matching target symptoms with psychopharmacologic agents.

EPIDEMIOLOGY AND RISK FACTORS

Multiple family, twin, and adoption studies have demonstrated an important genetic component in the etiology of ADHD, with an estimated hereditability in twin studies of 80%. Symptoms of ADHD are clearly more common in first-degree biologic relatives of children diagnosed with the disorder, with a two- to eightfold increased risk in parents of children with ADHD. Not all individuals with ADHD have a positive family history, but there is a suggestion that the familial type of ADHD may be more likely to persist into adulthood. A higher genetic loading may be needed to express ADHD in girls, in whom the overall prevalence of ADHD is about one half to one ninth that in boys, depending upon the sampling source. In addition, a number of other mental health disorders such as depression share common familial vulnerabilities with ADHD, and it has been postulated that bipolar disorder and conduct disorder may be a distinct familial subtype of ADHD. Several specific genes have been proposed as candidate genes for ADHD, including a number of adrenergic genes and the dopamine 4 receptor and dopamine transporter genes.

Many authors emphasize, however, that a variety of psychosocial risk factors may be as important as heredity in the pathogenesis of ADHD. These include lower socioeconomic class, marital discord and domestic violence, and sexual and physical abuse. It is likely that the cumulative effect of multiple psychosocial stressors may make the individual child more vulnerable to the expression of ADHD symptoms. Parents of children with ADHD may themselves have residual symptoms of the disorder, such as disorganization and impulsivity, which may in turn create compliance problems in carrying out behavioral treatment plans.

Certain biologic risk factors may contribute to the development of ADHD symptoms. These include prenatal alcohol and substance abuse, prematurity and birth complications, significant head trauma, central nervous system infections, iron deficiency anemia, and even relatively low levels of chronic lead exposure. More recently, an association has been demonstrated between the syndrome of general resistance to thyroid hormone and ADHD, although this familial disorder is rare. The behavioral side effects of certain medications used for chronic conditions in childhood, such as phenobarbital for seizures, may mimic symptoms of ADHD. Primary sleep disorders that result in chronic insufficient sleep or that are sleep disrupters may arise with ADHD-like symptoms of inattentiveness and hyperactivity secondary to chronic sleep deprivation and/or fragmentation; these include obstructive sleep apnea, usually related in childhood to adenotonsillar hypertrophy, and restless legs syndrome or periodic limb movement disorder.

Finally, it is important to remember that certain genetic and chromosomal disorders are associated with an increased risk of ADHD. These include fragile X syndrome (up to 80% with ADHD), Klinefelter's syndrome (primarily inattention), 47 XYY, Turner's syndrome, Angelman's syndrome, velocardiofacial syndrome (60% to 70% with ADHD), Williams' syndrome, and Smith-Magenis syndrome (severe hyperactivity). Presence of ADHD symptoms in these children should be evaluated, as appropriate treatment, including psychopharmacologic agents, may improve functional outcomes.

CLINICAL FEATURES

The hallmark of ADHD in children is the clinical constellation of *inattention*, *distractibility*, and *impulsivity*, which is frequently accompanied by physical or motor *hyperactivity*, often described as restlessness, fidgetiness, and inability to sit still. The "inattentive" component refers not only to difficulty in focusing and sustaining attention appropriately but also to a basic inability to match attention to the demands of the particular environment and to specific tasks. Children with ADHD have difficulties with selective attention and divided attention tasks, with redirecting and shifting attention, and their ability to focus is often highly motivation and interest dependent. Distractibility may manifest itself as internal preoccupation and "daydreaming" and/or inability to screen out external stimuli. Impulsivity, "acting without thinking," can be verbal or physical and often results

TABLE 1. **Diagnostic and Statistical Manual of Mental Disorders, Fourth Edition, Criteria for Attention Deficit Hyperactivity Disorder**

A. Either 1 or 2:
   1. Six (or more) of the following symptoms of *inattention* have persisted for at least 6 months to a degree that is maladaptive and inconsistent with the developmental level:
      Inattention
      a. Often fails to give close attention to details or makes careless mistakes in schoolwork, work, or other activities
      b. Often has difficulty sustaining attention in tasks or play activities
      c. Often does not seem to listen when spoken to directly
      d. Often does not follow through on instructions and fails to finish schoolwork, chores, or duties in the workplace (not because of oppositional behavior or failure to understand instructions)
      e. Often has difficulty organizing tasks and activities
      f. Often avoids, dislikes, or is reluctant to engage in tasks that require sustained mental effort (such as schoolwork or homework)
      g. Often loses things necessary for tasks or activities (e.g., toys, school assignments, pencils, books, or tools)
      h. Is often easily distracted by extraneous stimuli
      i. Is often forgetful in daily activities
   2. Six (or more) of the following symptoms of *hyperactivity-impulsivity* have persisted for at least 6 months to a degree that is maladaptive and inconsistent with the developmental level:
      Hyperactivity
      a. Often fidgets with hands or feet or squirms in seat
      b. Often leaves seat in classroom or in other situations in which remaining seated is expected
      c. Often runs about or climbs excessively in situations in which it is inappropriate (in adolescents or adults, may be limited to subjective feelings of restlessness)
      d. Often has difficulty playing or engaging in leisure activities quietly
      e. Is often "on the go" or often acts as though "driven by a motor"
      f. Often talks excessively
      Impulsivity
      g. Often blurts out answers before questions have been completed
      h. Often has difficulty awaiting turn
      i. Often interrupts or intrudes on others (e.g., butts into conversations or games)

B. Some hyperactive-impulsive or inattentive symptoms that have caused impairment were present before the age of 7 y

in a multitude of secondary behavioral concerns, such as aggressiveness with peers and disruptiveness in the classroom setting.

The *Diagnostic and Statistical Manual of Mental Disorders* IV (DSM IV) classification (Table 1) requires that six of nine inattention and/or hyperactive impulsive behaviors be present for the diagnosis. The current classification further subdivides ADHD into hyperactive/impulsive subtype, inattentive subtype, and combined subtype according to the relative prominence of more "externalizing" versus "internalizing" target symptoms. Children with predominantly inattentive ADHD usually do not have pronounced hyperactivity and, in fact, may be described as "sluggish" and "spacey." The majority of children with ADHD have the combined subtype; hyperactivity in general is more common in younger children and often subsides in adolescence.

The number and severity of symptoms of ADHD exist along a wide spectrum and can vary with age (younger children tend to be more physically active than adolescents), setting (structured versus unstructured), gender (boys are far more likely than girls to have the hyperactive/impulsive subtype of ADHD, and girls are less likely to have associated learning disabilities and co-morbid mood and disruptive disorders), and the presence or absence of co-morbid conditions. The chronicity, persistence, pervasiveness, and developmental inappropriateness of symptoms all help to distinguish the child with ADHD from the behaviorally disordered child who may be responding to an acute stress or whose behavioral problems are a reflection of inconsistent parental limit setting. By definition, with rare exceptions, the symptoms of ADHD must have been present for at least 6 months and have emerged prior to the age of 7 years, and the symptoms must be present in two or more settings to meet current diagnostic criteria.

It should be emphasized that the clinical presentation of ADHD is highly dependent upon the developmental level of the child. For example, preschoolers are more likely to present with disruptive behaviors (tantrums, aggression toward peers, destructive play), and school-aged children are more likely to present with school- and peer-related concerns (interrupting in class, academic underachievement, poor compliance with homework assignments, difficulty participating in team sports). Additional associated features of ADHD include low frustration tolerance, difficulty initiating and impersistence in completing tasks, relative resistance to rewards and punishment, and failure to "learn from one's mistakes." The failure to recognize and respond appropriately to social cues and social immaturity in addition to the impulsivity and intrusiveness can often lead to problems with peer relations. Children with ADHD are often highly inconsistent in their behavior from day to day and even hour to hour and disorganized in their approach to tasks. Understandably, these groups of symptoms eventually often lead to academic failure, especially when coupled with learning disabilities, behavior problems in school and at home, and low self-esteem.

ADHD in adolescence is characterized by a sense of inner restlessness, a disorganized approach, variability in academic performance, mental fatigue (often interpreted as "laziness" or "boredom"), difficulty working independently, excessive dependence on motivation, and difficulty in distinguishing between salient and irrelevant material ("the forest for the trees" phenomenon). Social interactions with peers are particularly problematic because of failure to attend and respond appropriately to social cues, verbal impulsivity, and difficulty in delaying gratification. Adolescents with ADHD are more likely to engage in risk-taking behavior, such as cigarette smoking, early sexual activity, and reckless driving, and the subgroup of adolescents with co-morbid conduct disorder are at especially high risk for antisocial behavior, delinquency, truancy, and substance abuse.

As noted earlier, most children with ADHD have developed symptoms, at least in retrospect, before the age of 7 years. The more severely affected youngsters, especially those with the impulsive/hyperactive subtype of ADHD, may be recognized as preschoolers. The persistence of at least some symptoms into adolescence, occurring in up to 70% of children with ADHD, and even into adulthood is now well recognized. ADHD, particularly the inattentive type, occasionally goes unrecognized until adolescence, when previously successful compensatory strategies used by the youngster become inadequate to meet the increased academic and social demands of junior and senior high school.

CO-MORBID CONDITIONS

The issue of co-morbidity in ADHD is both a complex and an important one because of the frequent coexistence of ADHD and a variety of psychiatric problems in children and adolescents, the presence of which often creates major diagnostic and management challenges and may significantly worsen functional outcomes in these children. "Pure" ADHD is now recognized to be relatively rare, even in a general population sample, and it has been estimated that almost 90% of children meeting criteria for ADHD have *at least one* co-morbid psychiatric condition and two thirds have at least two co-morbidities. Furthermore, the behavioral manifestations in childhood of ADHD and many of these psychiatric problems may overlap. For example, aggression in a preschooler may be part of the ADHD symptom constellation or may result from post-traumatic stress disorder associated with a history of sexual abuse, reflect exposure to and modeling of domestic violence in the home setting, or be a transient behavioral response to an acute stressor, such as divorce. In addition, the symptoms of the most common co-morbid conditions often show a typical developmental progression and may become evident only over time, with ADHD symptoms often developing first (in preschool age), followed by signs of oppositional defiant disorder (ages 4 to 5 years), anxiety and depression disorders (often by 5 to 7 years of age), conduct disorder (8 to 9 years of age), and finally substance abuse problems (adolescence).

Oppositional behavior, characterized by defiance, noncompliance, negativity, and difficulty in following rules, is the most common (up to 40%) co-morbid psychiatric disorder with ADHD. Conduct disorder, occurring in up to 25% of older children with ADHD, has as its central feature a basic disregard for the rights of others and is behaviorally manifested by lying, stealing, and physical aggression. Recognition and treatment of a conduct disorder are especially important because of the high risk in this group for later development of serious problems such as substance abuse and delinquency. Mood disorders are also common, including anxiety disorders such as separation anxiety and school phobia (which eventually develop in up to one third of ADHD youngsters) and depression, which occurs in up to 20% of children and adolescents with ADHD. Bipolar disorder, a serious psychiatric condition that may arise in childhood with severe ADHD-like symptoms and extreme mood lability, has been increasingly recognized to coexist with ADHD, especially in children with a family history of manic-depressive disorder.

Several other ADHD co-morbid conditions deserve comment. The prevalence of specific learning disabilities in ADHD is estimated at 10% to 35% and their presence may add significantly to the risk of academic failure. ADHD is also diagnosed in 20% to 50% of individuals with Tourette's syndrome, which is characterized by the presence of both vocal and motor tics, and is often accompanied by additional symptoms such as coprolalia (involuntary utterance of profanity) and obsessive-compulsive behavior.

Although many children presenting with ADHD in the primary care setting do not develop serious psychiatric problems, the presence of additional mental health concerns in ADHD has important implications for treatment and prognosis and should be appropriately evaluated and tracked. Referral to a child psychiatrist, psychologist, or other mental health professional may be warranted.

EVALUATION

The evaluation of children with possible ADHD may be performed by a variety of health care and mental health professionals, including child and adult psychiatrists, neurologists, and psychologists and neuropsychologists. It is most often the primary care physician, however, whom the parent or school first approaches about making the diagnosis. There is currently *no single reliable diagnostic test* for ADHD; rather, the diagnosis is based on a comprehensive clinical assessment that should include the following:

- History of the problem—including onset, type, and severity of ADHD symptoms; associated symptoms; behavior across different settings and by different observers (school, home, social situations); and current and previous attempts at behavioral management. Description of the child's typical behavior in situations that are likely to be problematic (mealtimes, chores, bedtime) may be particularly helpful.
- *Assessment* of common co-morbid conditions—including symptoms of depression or anxiety (including separation anxiety and school avoidance and school phobia), oppositional behaviors and conduct problems, and motor and vocal tics. Co-morbid psychiatric conditions such as anxiety and oppositional defiant disorder may actually be the primary diagnosis in some cases and may have a relatively greater impact on academic and social functioning than the ADHD. Therefore, successful treatment of co-morbidities may lead to significant overall improvement.
- *School history*—including previous and current academic and behavioral difficulties, history of grade retention, current educational program and setting (classroom size and child's placement in the classroom), special education services or resource help,

individualized education plan (IEP), recent report card results, academic strengths and weaknesses, homework management, peer relationships.

- *Assessment for learning disabilities*—including review of any previous educational or achievement test results and neuropsychological (e.g., IQ, language, cognitive, processing abilities) evaluation results. Because of the high prevalence of learning disabilities in ADHD (up to 35%) and the fact that some learning disabilities (such as auditory processing deficits) can mimic symptoms of ADHD, most children undergoing an ADHD evaluation should have at a minimum a screening assessment for learning problems. Any child in whom specific learning problems are suspected should have a more comprehensive neuropsychological assessment done by the school or a qualified neuropsychologist.

Although a neuropsychological evaluation cannot make the diagnosis of ADHD, certain tests, as well as trained observation of the child's testing behavior, may be helpful in substantiating the clinical impression. For example, the Freedom from Distractibility Factors subscale on the Wechsler Intelligence Scale for Children–Revised (WISC-R) IQ test, computerized attention–vigilance–reaction time tasks such as the Continuous Performance Test (CPT), and various tests that assess for errors of commission and omission may help to corroborate clinical evidence of problems with inattention and distractibility but do not in and of themselves make the diagnosis of ADHD. The description of a child who needs to be constantly "refocused," is easily frustrated, who rushes through work without checking it, fails to follow directions, and is easily distracted during a one-on-one testing session also strongly suggests the diagnosis of ADHD.

- *Family history*—including other family members with ADHD, academic problems or learning disabilities, mood or anxiety disorders, substance or alcohol abuse, thyroid disease.
- *Social history*—including educational level of parents and siblings, family constellation, marital history, history of domestic violence or sexual or physical abuse, recent or ongoing stressors in the home, family response to the child's behavior and/or academic problems.
- *Developmental history*—including major milestones, results of previous developmental evaluations.
- *Medical history*—including pregnancy and birth, significant or chronic illnesses, lead poisoning, significant head trauma, allergies, medications.
- *Physical examination*—including growth parameters, baseline vital signs, brief neurologic examination. Although ADHD may be associated with neurologic "soft signs" (e.g., clumsiness, poor fine motor coordination), their significance is unclear. In general, unless specific signs or symptoms emerge, laboratory testing, neuroimaging, or electroencephalograms (EEGs) are not indicated in the general evaluation of ADHD.
- *Sleep history*—including sleep onset difficulties, night waking, quality and duration of sleep (restless), early awakening, symptoms of obstructive sleep apnea (disruptive snoring, gasping), enuresis. Because of the high prevalence of sleep problems in children with ADHD as well as the fact that primary sleep disorders may arise with ADHD symptoms, a thorough sleep history should be part of every ADHD evaluation (see Table 2 for a simple sleep screening tool, "BEARS").
- *Child interview*—including observation of ADHD target symptoms in the office setting, oppositional or defiant behavior, general cognitive and language level, child's understanding of behavioral concerns, parent-child interactions.
- *Standard ADHD questionnaires*—including such validated instruments as the Conners' Parent and Teacher's questionnaire, which both provide information about pretreatment baseline functioning and later allow a standardized measure of treatment efficacy. The Achenbach Child Behavior Checklist (CBCL), which has parent, teacher, and self-report forms, is also an excellent screening tool for many behavioral problems, including ADHD.

The preceding assessment generally included the review of school record and previous evaluations and a 60- to 90-minute interview with the parent and child.

TREATMENT

It cannot be overemphasized that a successful treatment plan for children with ADHD involves a comprehensive approach to the behavioral, academic, social, family, and self-esteem issues that may be operative in each individual case. The primary care physician's role should be one of a case manager, coordinating medical intervention, education services, and mental health treatment components. In 2001, the American Academy of Pediatrics published clinical practice guidelines for the treatment of ADHD (Pediatrics 108:1033-1044). Emphasizing the importance of viewing ADHD as a chronic condition, the major recommendations of these practice guidelines included collaboration among clinicians, families, and educators to optimize treatment, combined behavioral and/or medication therapy for the treatment of target symptoms, and systematic monitoring of symptoms. The guidelines also stressed the clinician's role as an advocate for the child and the need to ensure the child's understanding of and cooperation with the treatment plan as an essential factor in treatment compliance.

Educational intervention by the school involves both diagnosing and addressing any specific coexisting learning disabilities and designing programs for classroom management. Parents should be strongly encouraged to become active participants in their child's educational plan. They need to be made aware of federally mandated special education services for children with ADHD-related significant academic impairment. Under the 1990 Individuals with Disabilities Education Act, children can receive services under an IEP under the "other health impaired"

TABLE 2. **BEARS Sleep Screening Algorithm***

	Examples of Developmentally Appropriate Trigger Questions		
	Toddler/Preschool (2–5 y)	*School-Aged (6–12 y)*	*Adolescent (13–18 y)*
1. **B**edtime problems	Does your child have any problems going to bed? Falling asleep?	Does your child have any problems at bedtime? (P)† Do you have any problems going to bed? (C)‡	Do you have any problems falling asleep at bedtime? (C)
2. **E**xcessive daytime sleepiness	Does your child seem overtired or sleepy a lot during the day? Does she still take naps?	Does your child have difficulty waking in the morning, seem sleepy during the day, or take naps? (P) Do you feel tired a lot? (C)	Do you feel sleepy a lot during the day? In school? While driving? (C)
3. **A**wakenings during the night	Does your child wake up a lot at night?	Does your child seem to wake up a lot at night? Any nightmares? (P) Do you wake up a lot at night? Have trouble getting back to sleep? (C)	Do you wake up a lot at night? Have trouble getting back to sleep? (C)
4. **R**egularity and duration of sleep	Does your child have a regular bedtime and wake time? What are they?	What time does your child go to bed and get up on school days? Do you think he/she is getting enough sleep? (P)	What time do you usually go to bed on school nights? Weekends? How much sleep do you usually get? (C)
5. **S**noring	Does your child snore a lot or have difficulty breathing at night?	Does your child have loud or nightly snoring or any breathing difficulties at night? (P)	Does your teenager snore loudly or nightly? (P)

*The "BEARS" instrument is divided into five major sleep domains, providing a comprehensive screen for the major sleep disorders affecting children in the 2- to 18-year-old range. Each sleep domain has a set of age-appropriate "trigger questions" for use in the clinical interview. **B**, bedtime problems; **E**, excessive daytime sleepiness; **A**, awakenings during the night; **R**, regularity and duration of sleep; **S**, snoring.

†P, parent-directed question.

‡C, child-directed question.

umbrella. The IEP, which operationalizes the stated educational goals, should be part of the patient's medical record and should be reviewed with parents periodically by the primary care physician.

An alternative route through which children with ADHD may receive classroom accommodations if the diagnosis is thought to affect classroom behavior significantly is under Section 504 of the Rehabilitation Act of 1973. Classroom accommodations generally include age- and child-specific modifications to improve attention and impulse control, enhance organizational skills and self-esteem, and increase productivity. Examples include breaking work down into smaller components, avoiding multistep directions, using a nonverbal cue (such as a pat on the shoulder) to refocus attention, seating the child in the front of the classroom, providing frequent "sit up and stretch" breaks during seated work, reinforcing orally presented material with visual aids and vice versa, establishing clear expectations and consequences for behavior and tracking these with a daily report form, allowing the child to dictate written assignments, and using a daily communication notebook to track homework assignments. Positive reinforcement and focusing on academic and extracurricular strengths are also important behavioral strategies.

Behavioral management of the child with ADHD in the home involves some of the same principles: using sticker or star charts or a token-reward system for specific target behaviors, engaging the child's attention before giving directions, anticipating and structuring problematic situations in which the child is likely to be overstimulated (e.g., holiday gatherings), and providing safe outlets for excess energy. Parents may benefit from referral to parent-training workshops or individual parent-child behavior therapy to learn these skills. Children who have particular problems with peer relationships often benefit from social skills training groups, which many schools are developing for behaviorally disordered youngsters. Individual psychotherapy referral may be necessary for children with significant self-esteem concerns and co-morbid depression, anxiety, and so forth. Family therapy can be extremely helpful to deal with problematic family relationships. The primary care physician can also provide information about adult mental health referral for identification and treatment of a parent's ADHD symptoms. Finally, parent support groups such as Children with Attention Deficit Disorder (Ch.A.D.D) are often extremely helpful in providing emotional support, practical management techniques, and information to parents.

Many parents question the role of *dietary factors*, including sugar consumption, food additives and dyes, and food allergies, in the exacerbation of ADHD symptoms. Multiple, well-controlled double-blind studies have failed to demonstrate a consistent benefit from sugar-free, allergen-free, oligoantigenic, or additive-free diets for the vast majority of children with ADHD. Most of these special diets are nutritionally adequate (although some, such as the Feingold diet, can be very restrictive and expensive). Therefore, failure to dissuade parents with scientific evidence from restricting sugar or preservatives generally does not result in harm to the child. Care should be taken, however, not to make the child feel "singled out" from siblings and peers by such dietary restrictions.

Several other proposed treatments for ADHD deserve mention; these include motor and occupational therapies, which may focus on sensory integration skills or eye movement training, and EEG biofeedback, in which children are taught to "normalize" their EEG patterns. Largely anecdotal reports of increased concentration, improved academic performance, and even increased IQ have not been empirically substantiated thus far, but these therapies do not appear to be harmful. Finally, families may choose to try other complementary and alternative medicine (CAM) such as herbal remedies and omega-3 fatty acids (Promega)* to treat ADHD. Although there are ongoing studies about the effectiveness of some of these agents, their benefit remains unclear. However, it is important for the practitioner to be aware of and to discuss any use of these therapies with families, particularly because drug interactions with conventional psychotropics may occur.

PSYCHOPHARMACOLOGY OF ATTENTION DEFICIT HYPERACTIVITY DISORDER

General Considerations

Since the first documented use of dextroamphetamine (Dexedrine) to treat hyperactivity in the late 1930s, the use of psychopharmacologic agents to treat symptoms of ADHD has risen significantly, as much as three- to sevenfold during the 1990s, depending upon the population. Psychostimulants are currently the most widely prescribed psychotropic medication in pediatrics. Despite concern about overuse, however, the rationale for the use of drug treatment in ADHD remains sound when part of a multimodal, integrated treatment plan. For many children and adolescents with ADHD, successful amelioration of symptoms by medications such as methylphenidate (Ritalin) and dextroamphetamine (Dexedrine) allows the individual to make full use of other treatment modalities, such as educational modifications, and represents the difference between academic success and failure.

In 1999 the results of a cooperative Multimodal Treatment Study of children with ADHD (MTA) were published. The study compared clinical outcomes with the following treatment modalities: carefully monitored medication management, intensive behavioral therapy, combination therapy (medication and behavior), and standard community medication management. Although improvement in symptoms was seen in all treatment groups, the results of the study suggested that the most improvement was seen in the carefully monitored medication and combination treatment arms, which were essentially equivalent in clinical outcomes. Although the results of this study underscore the importance of the role of medication in the treatment of ADHD and suggest that for many children careful medication management alone can lead to improvement in target symptoms, subsequent findings also support the existence of potential additional benefits from behavioral therapy.

Several general principles of medication management of ADHD deserve comment. First, medication should be selected on the basis of specific *target symptoms* and treatment success measured on the basis of remission of, or at least improvement in, these symptoms. Target symptoms should be well defined and measurable whenever possible (e.g., percentage of schoolwork completed, number of times out of seat) and prioritized according to the degree to which they interfere with the child's daily functioning. A standardized questionnaire such as the Conners' or daily behavioral rating charts may be especially helpful in documenting treatment success over time.

Second, age and developmental stage should be a prime consideration in drug selections. For example, pre–school-aged children tend to metabolize psychostimulants faster and may need a more frequent dosing schedule and also tend to have more unpredictable behavioral effects from these medications. Because of the risk for cardiac dysrhythmia, tricyclic antidepressants should be used with caution in prepubertal children.

Third, any medication should be started at the lower end of the dosage range and gradually titrated up at a pace commensurate with the behavioral half-life. Increased availability of longer acting preparations of both methylphenidate and dextroamphetamine (12-hour duration of action) has raised some questions regarding initiation of treatment with a short-acting versus a longer acting medication. Initial gradual titration is sometimes easier with the shorter acting preparations, but compliance may be improved with the longer acting preparations.

Fourth, medications should always be titrated to maximize the cognitive and behavioral benefits while minimizing the development of both short- and long-term side effects.

Fifth, different medications in the same class should be tried before moving on to another class of drug. Some individuals, for example, respond well to methylphenidate but not to mixed salt or dextroamphetamines and vice versa. If an individual child does not respond to several different adequate medication trials, the possibility of alternative or additional diagnoses should be strongly considered.

Sixth, medications should be initiated one at a time and effectiveness documented before combination therapy is considered in the treatment of resistant or complicated cases. Special consideration should also be given to possible drug interactions in using combination regimens. Consultation with a developmental

*Not FDA approved for this indication.

and behavioral pediatrician, child psychiatrist, or neurologist before initiating additional medication may be appropriate.

Finally, every child receiving medication for ADHD should be observed for continued medication efficacy and side effects at regular intervals (at a minimum every 3 months) when a stable dose has been reached. Some children develop tolerance to a previously effective medication or dose. A yearly trial without medication to assess continued need for drug therapy, preferably timed at a few weeks into the new school year, should be at least considered in most children. However, long-term studies have demonstrated that symptoms of ADHD often persist into adolescence and adulthood. Because these symptoms are more likely to be more subtle ones such as inattention and organizational difficulties, deterioration in functioning without medication may not be immediately apparent during a short trial without the medication.

Psychostimulants

The psychostimulants, methylphenidate (e.g., Ritalin, Ritalin LA, Concerta, Metadate) and the amphetamines (e.g., Dexedrine, Dextrostat, Desoxyn, Adderall, Adderall XR), are generally considered to be the first-line medications in the treatment of children and adolescents with ADHD (Table 3). The stimulants, at least partially through their indirect effects on the intrasynaptic availability of norepinephrine and dopamine, exert their major neurobehavioral effects by decreasing excessive variability in arousal and reactivity. Inattention, distractibility, motor hyperactivity, and behavioral intensity are all reduced by stimulants. Secondary beneficial effects include improved accuracy and speed in completing academic tasks, decreased off-task behavior, and a reduction of excessive motivation dependence. Stimulant use also often results in a decrease in oppositional, aggressive, and noncompliant behavior and an improvement in peer and family relationships.

Stimulants result in improvement or remission of ADHD symptoms in approximately 70% to 80% of individuals for whom they are appropriately prescribed. Gender does not appear to affect stimulant response. As already noted, there may be differences in individual responsiveness to the different psychostimulants. The response rate may be lower in very young children (the lower age limit for stimulant use is generally 3 years) and in adolescents and children with the inattentive type of ADHD. However, because stimulants also improve attention and reduce distractibility in non-ADHD individuals, a positive clinical response should not be taken as de facto confirmation of the diagnosis of ADHD.

Sympathomimetic agents, including pseudoephedrine (Sudafed), can potentiate the effects of stimulants and antihistamines may diminish their effectiveness. The stimulants should be used with caution in children with a seizure disorder as they may both delay absorption and increase levels of anticonvulsants. Methylphenidate can inhibit tricyclic antidepressant metabolism and result in elevated serum levels. Concern has been raised about the possible role of the combination of methylphenidate and the α_2 agonist clonidine (Catapres)* in the sudden deaths of several children receiving this combination regimen for ADHD. Although the subsequent investigation of these cases did not substantiate drug interaction as the cause of death, theoretical considerations about the possibility of hyper- or hypotensive events suggest that caution should be exercised in prescribing and monitoring dosage and timing of stimulants and clonidine together. Typically, baseline and repeated electrocardiograms (ECGs) are recommended when this combination is used.

The short-term side effects of the psychostimulants include mild headaches and abdominal discomfort (usually disappear within the first 1 to 2 weeks), irritability or depression, mild increases in blood pressure and pulse (usually clinically insignificant), appetite suppression, and sleep problems. The appetite suppression can result in significant weight loss in some children, especially initially, and may necessitate adjustment of the dosage schedule (during or after meals) and the institution of additional snack times. The relationship between psychostimulants and sleep is a complex one. Many children with ADHD are described by their parents as having significant baseline sleep difficulties, especially bedtime struggles and delayed sleep onset latency. Some children appear quite sensitive to the direct stimulant effect and may experience increased sleep difficulties while taking medication, necessitating a reduction or earlier timing of a second daily dose. Other children experience a rebound phenomenon in which behavioral symptoms of hyperactivity, impulsivity, and so forth actually increase over baseline when the noon dose wears off. If this rebound coincides with bedtime, sleep onset problems may result. These may be addressed by adding a third, smaller dose of medication late in the day to "piggyback" into bedtime. Finally, the addition of a bedtime dose of clonidine (0.025 to 0.1 mg), with its sedative effects, is becoming increasingly common in the management of ADHD-related sleep difficulties. However, any use of medication for sleep difficulties in ADHD should be combined with behavioral management strategies and instruction regarding good sleep hygiene.

Longitudinal studies showing little significant compromise in adult height suggest that concerns about significant long-term growth suppression by the psychostimulants are largely unfounded. Some clinicians continue to advocate the use of "drug holidays" on weekends and school and summer vacations to allow "catch-up" growth, but this strategy may be problematic for some children who feel particularly "out of control" without medication during these typically less structured time periods. Concerns about stimulant therapy and later substance abuse have also not been substantiated by long-term studies, although clearly ADHD itself and its co-morbid conditions

*Not FDA approved for this indication.

TABLE 3. **Attention Deficit Hyperactivity Disorder Medications***

Brand Name	Generic	Form	Strengths	Maximum Dose	Notes
Adderall	Dextroamphetamine + amphetamine (each tablet contains equal parts of dextroamphetamine saccharate, dextroamphetamine sulfate, amphetamine aspartate, and amphetamine sulfate)	Double-scored tablets	5 mg (1.25 mg of each salt)	Usually 40 mg daily in 2 or 3 divided doses	Duration of action 6–8 h Avoid giving dose with acidic foods
Adderall XR	Dextroamphetamine + amphetamine (each capsule contains equal parts dextroamphetamine saccharate, dextroamphetamine sulfate, amphetamine aspartate, and amphetamine sulfate)	Extended-release capsules	5 mg (1.25 mg of each salt) 10 mg (2.5 mg of each salt) 15 mg (3.75 mg of each salt) 20 mg (5 mg of each salt) 25 mg (6.25 mg of each salt) 30 mg (7.5 mg of each salt)	30 mg/d	Duration of action 12 h May sprinkle contents on applesauce and swallow without chewing beads
Concerta	Methylphenidate HCl	Extended-release tablets (with immediate-release outer coating)	18 mg 27 mg 36 mg 54 mg	54 mg once daily	Duration of action 12 h
Dexedrine	Dextroamphetamine sulfate	Scored tablets	5 mg	Usually 40 mg daily in 2 or 3 divided doses	Duration of action 4–6 h May switch patients to a once-daily dose of Dexedrine Spansules once titrated.
Dexedrine Spansule	Dextroamphetamine sulfate	Sustained-release capsules	5 mg 10 mg 15 mg	Usually 40 mg once daily	Duration of action 6–8 h Patients who are titrated to a maintenance dose of immediate-release dextroamphetamine may be switched to a once-daily dose of Dexedrine Spansules. Contains tartrazine
Dextrostat	Dextroamphetamine sulfate	Scored tablets Double-scored tablets	5 mg 10 mg	Usually 40 mg daily in 2 or 3 divided doses	Duration of action 4–6 h Contains tartrazine
Focalin	Dexmethylphenidate HCl	Tablets	2.5 mg 5 mg 10 mg	20 mg/d	Twice-daily dosage Single isomer methylphenidate product (use one half of racemic methylphenidate dose initially)
Metadate CD	Methylphenidate HCl	Extended-release capsules (containing immediate- and extended-release beads)	20 mg	60 mg once daily	Give one daily in the AM before breakfast May sprinkle contents on applesauce and swallow without chewing beads
Metadate ER	Methylphenidate HCl	Extended-release tablets	10 mg 20 mg	60 mg daily	Once- to twice-daily dosage
Methylin	Methylphenidate HCl	Tablets Scored tablets	5 mg 10 mg 20 mg	60 mg daily in 2 divided doses	Give before breakfast and lunch Some patients may benefit from a third dose given in the afternoon

Continued

TABLE 3. **Attention Deficit Hyperactivity Disorder Medications*—cont'd**

Brand Name	Generic	Form	Strengths	Maximum Dose	Notes
Methylin ER	Methylphenidate HCl	Extended-release tablets	10 mg 20 mg	60 mg daily in 2 divided doses	May use Methylin ER when the 8-h dose corresponds to immediate-release dose
Ritalin	Methylphenidate HCl	Tablets Scored tablets	5 mg 10 mg 20 mg	60 mg daily in 2–3 divided doses	Give before breakfast and lunch Some patients may benefit from a third dose given in the afternoon
Ritalin LA	Methylphenidate HCl	Extended-release capsules (half as immediate-release, half as delayed-release beads)	20 mg 30 mg 40 mg	60 mg once daily	Give once daily in AM May sprinkle contents on applesauce and swallow without chewing beads

*Adderall, Dexedrine, and Dextrostat are not recommended for children younger than 3 years. Adderall XR, Concerta, Cylert, Focalin, Ritalin, Methylin, and Metadate ER are not recommended for children younger than 6 years. Sustained-release and extended-release products may be swallowed whole and not crushed, chewed, or divided.

(especially conduct disorder) are risk factors for later drug and alcohol abuse. Methylphenidate, although structurally similar to cocaine, does not appear to share its addictive pharmacokinetics. However, there have been numerous anecdotal reports of recreational use of methylphenidate and amphetamines—usually "snorting" of the crushed pills by non-ADHD adolescents. In cases in which recreational use is a concern, Concerta may have an advantage over other preparations because it reportedly cannot be crushed. Clinicians should be alert, however, to the potential street value of stimulants and monitor prescription practices accordingly.

The relationship between tic disorders, including Tourette's syndrome, and psychostimulants is somewhat controversial. Currently available information suggests that tics do not generally appear de novo in a nonsusceptible individual when prescribed psychostimulants. Motor tics, when they do occur, appear to be frequently reversible after medication discontinuation. Psychostimulants are no longer contraindicated in children and adolescents with a previous history of motor or vocal tics or a family history of tics or Tourette's syndrome. Although stimulant therapy may precipitate or exacerbate tics in these individuals and symptoms should be closely monitored, the benefits of the medications often outweigh the adverse effects. Consideration can be made for addition of an α agonist if tics are thought to be disruptive or causing self-esteem or social problems.

Clinical wisdom about the duration of psychostimulant therapy for childhood ADHD has undergone some modifications in the past few years. Many adolescents and adults with ADHD continue to benefit substantially from ongoing pharmacotherapy, although target symptoms may change and the class of drug used, dose, and dosing intervals may require modification over time. Clear evidence of long-term significant improvement in academic achievement related to psychostimulant treatment, however, has been disappointingly lacking so far. Although certain academic areas (arithmetic, language and skills, likelihood of staying in school) do show long-term improvement, the most consistently identified benefits of chronic psychostimulant therapy have been in the areas of social and life skills and self-esteem.

Because of the high prevalence of co-morbid behavior problems in children with developmental disabilities, including fragile X syndrome, the use of psychostimulants to treat ADHD symptoms in mental retardation deserves special mention. Methylphenidate has been demonstrated to result in substantial clinical improvement in ADHD symptoms, especially in children with higher cognitive functioning. Although the side effects of stimulant therapy, especially social withdrawal and motor tics, tend to be more prominent and more often problematic in developmentally delayed children, the higher functioning children appear to be at lower risk. Finally, it should be noted that in this population, stimulants may sometimes worsen the child's hyperactivity and impulsivity.

Antidepressants

Antidepressants, including tricyclic antidepressants (TCAs), are generally considered to be second-line pharmacotherapy for the treatment of ADHD in children. TCAs, such as imipramine (Tofranil),* desipramine (Norpramin),* nortriptyline (Pamelor),* and amitriptyline (Elavil),* appear to exert their effect

*Not FDA approved for this indication.

by blocking presynaptic uptake of neurotransmitters, including norepinephrine and serotonin. They are used clinically in ADHD, including use in combination with other psychotropics, in a variety of situations:

- Failure to respond to adequate stimulant trial or intolerance of stimulant side effects
- High risk of stimulant abuse
- Exacerbation of tic disorder or Tourette's syndrome by psychostimulant medication (although there have been reports of tics emerging during TCA therapy as well)
- Co-morbid depression or anxiety disorder
- Strong family history of affective disorders or alcohol abuse
- Co-morbid enuresis
- Preference for continuous coverage of ADHD symptoms without rebound
- Clinician preference for availability of serum drug level monitoring (compliance issues)
- Low risk of intentional or accidental overdose by patient or family member
- Patient at low risk for cardiotoxicity (negative patient's and family's history of significant cardiac disease, sudden death)

The last two points emphasize the potential for TCAs to cause cardiac conduction abnormalities and dysrhythmias because of a quinidine-like effect. Reports of sudden death in several children younger than 12 years who were being treated with desipramine, in particular, have raised concerns about its safety. Most clinicians adhere to a conservative approach, including obtaining baseline ECGs and repeated ECGs with significant dose changes (baseline ECG limits: PR intervals no > 0.20 seconds, QRS no > 0.12 seconds; ECG with medication: QRS interval no > 30% over baseline, QTC no > 0.44–0.46); monitoring systolic (>80 mm Hg and <140 mm Hg) and diastolic blood pressures (>50 mm Hg and <85 mm Hg) and pulse (<130 bpm); and cautioning patients to avoid excessive exercise. Serum drug levels should be monitored at initiation of therapy and 5 days after significant dose changes. Although serum drug levels do not correlate well with clinical efficacy, they serve to identify the 5% to 10% of the population who are "slow metabolizers" of the TCAs.

TCAs may cause anticholinergic (dry mouth, constipation, blurred vision), antihistaminergic (sedation, weight gain), and α-adrenergic (blood pressure changes, tremor) side effects in children as well as cognitive impairment, weight loss, insomnia and nightmares, and lowering of the seizure threshold. Abrupt discontinuation of TCA administration or too infrequent dosing schedules (may need twice a day dosing to three times a day dosing in younger children) may lead to flulike withdrawal symptoms with gastrointestinal distress, agitation, and sleep disturbances.

Bupropion (Wellbutrin and Wellbutrin SR),* a relatively new antidepressant, blocks norepinephrine, dopamine, and serotonin uptake and in a few controlled clinical trials has been shown to be effective in children and adults with ADHD. It may be particularly useful in the setting of co-morbid depression, and it is thought to have relatively less potential to trigger manic symptoms in patients with co-morbid bipolar disorder. The major side effects of bupropion include irritability, insomnia, dermatitis or pruritus, edema, gastrointestinal symptoms, agitation, lowering of the seizure threshold, and possibly exacerbation of an underlying tic disorder. Venlafaxine (Effexor),* a serotonin and norepinephrine reuptake inhibitor that is an effective antidepressant and antianxiety agent in adults, is also used clinically to treat ADHD symptoms, but few data on efficacy exist. Side effects include gastrointestinal upset, irritability, and insomnia. Selective serotonin reuptake inhibitors (SSRIs) such as fluoxetine (Prozac),* paroxetine (Paxil),* sertraline (Zoloft),* and citalopram (Celexa)* have not been shown to be effective in treating the core symptoms of ADHD, although they may be helpful for treating co-morbid conditions and may be used safely in combination with psychostimulants. It should be noted that most of the antidepressants may be used in combination with stimulants, especially for co-morbid ADHD and mood-anxiety disorders, sometimes allowing a reduction in the dose of both drugs.

α_2 Agonists

Among the more recent additions to the ADHD psychopharmacologic armamentarium are the α_2 agonists, namely clonidine (Catapres)* and guanfacine (Tenex).* The α_2 agonists decrease the endogenous release of norepinephrine and bind postsynaptic receptors in the central nervous system arousal center, the locus ceruleus. They may have indirect effects on serotonin and dopamine as well.

Clonidine and guanfacine appear to be particularly effective in decreasing arousal levels in ADHD without significantly altering distractibility and attention. They are clinically most useful in the treatment of highly active, impulsive, and aggressive children with ADHD who have an early onset of symptoms and co-morbid oppositional and conduct disorders. The α_2 agonists may also be particularly helpful in treating ADHD children with a history of motor tics.

Clonidine was originally used as an antihypertensive, and thus one of its principal side effects is mild, usually clinically insignificant, hypotension and orthostatic hypotension, occasionally leading to subjective symptoms of dizziness and lightheadedness. Sedation, which may limit its effectiveness in the school setting, is the other major side effect associated with clonidine. Guanfacine, in general, appears to be both less apt to cause hypotensive symptoms and less sedating than clonidine. Other side effects of clonidine include headaches, vivid dreams and night waking, gastrointestinal symptoms, and dry mouth. Depression may occur in about 5% of patients, who usually have a

*Not FDA approved for this indication.

*Not FDA approved for this indication.

positive family history of affective disorders. Abrupt discontinuation of α_2 agonists, especially clonidine, may lead to rebound hypertension, and all patients whose medication is being discontinued should have the dosage tapered in 0.05-mg (half of a 0.1-mg tablet) increments at 1- to 3-day intervals. The patch form of clonidine may cause a local hypersensitivity reaction.

Clonidine is effective within 30 to 45 minutes and has a behavioral half-life of 3 to 6 hours, with sedation peaking at 30 to 90 minutes and the hypotensive effects at 2 to 4 hours. The usual daily dose range is 0.025- to 0.1-mg given three times to four times a day. Treatment is usually initiated with a bedtime dose and the daily dose increased every 3 days. Clinical effects may not be evident until 2 to 4 weeks into treatment, and the maximum effect may not be reached until 2 to 3 months. Clonidine is available in 0.1-, 0.2-, and 0.3-mg strengths in oral form as well as the transcutaneous patch (Catapres-TTS-1, -2, -3) form. The patch should be used only after an appropriate oral dose has been titrated. Advantages of the patch include considerable convenience (replaced every 5 to 7 days)* and less sedation. Guanfacine is usually given in 0.5- to 1-mg doses twice a day to three times a day. Tolerance may also develop, necessitating an increase in dose.

The combination regimen of methylphenidate and clonidine may be useful in treating children with both severe hyperactivity-impulsivity and significant inattentiveness, allowing up to a 40% reduction in the methylphenidate dose used. This combination may be particularly useful in reducing methylphenidate side effects, including rebound symptoms. The addition of methylphenidate may also diminish the sedative effect of clonidine. As noted earlier, clonidine has increasingly been used as a bedtime adjunct to methylphenidate in children with prolonged sleep onset delay. However, caution should be exercised in response to reports of possible severe hypo- or hypertensive episodes with this combination regimen. Clonidine should also never be used in conjunction with β-blockers. Baseline and repeated ECGs should be obtained when using α_2 agonists in combination with psychostimulants.

Atomoxetine

The selective norepinephrine reuptake inhibitor atomoxetine (Strattera) is a nonstimulant medication that has been approved for use by the Food and Drug Administration for treating ADHD in both adults and children. In double-blind, placebo-controlled studies, atomoxetine has been shown to reduce significantly core ADHD symptoms with once-daily administration. Side effects appear to be minimal and include decreased appetite, nausea or upset stomach, and fatigue; sleep-related effects appear to be less than those seen with the psychostimulants.

*Exceeds dosage recommended by the manufacturer.

TABLE 4. **Utah Criteria (Revised) for Adult Attention Deficit Hyperactivity Disorder**

Includes four symptoms of seven and at least (1) or (2)

1. Inattention persisting from childhood
2. Hyperactivity persisting from childhood
3. Inability to complete tasks
4. Impaired interpersonal relationships or inability to sustain relationships over time
5. Affective lability
6. Hot or explosive temper
7. Stress intolerance

ADULT ATTENTION DEFICIT HYPERACTIVITY DISORDER

Although much less overall is known about the clinical presentation and clinical course of adults with ADHD, both longitudinal studies and clinical experience now suggest that as many as 80% to 90% of children diagnosed with ADHD continue to have symptoms, including cognitive dysfunction, inattention, distractibility, impatience, and irritability, into adulthood. It is estimated that 10% to 20% have functional impairment significant enough to warrant a diagnosis of adult ADHD. Adults with ADHD are much more likely to manifest inattentive symptoms (90%, with about one third meeting criteria for inattentive only subtype) and to meet criteria for combined subtype (50%) than hyperactive impulsive subtype (2%). Levels of co-morbid psychiatric conditions (depressive and anxiety disorders, drug and alcohol abuse) are also high in this population. Adult ADHD, as defined by the Utah Criteria (Table 4), may result in a host of difficulties in such diverse areas as school achievement, job performance, success in intimate relationships, drug and alcohol use, legal difficulties, motor vehicle accidents, and personal satisfaction and self-esteem. It is estimated for example, that separation and divorce rates are two times higher in adults with ADHD and that these individuals are four times more likely to change jobs frequently.

Although less well studied in adults, a range of medications used in the treatment of childhood ADHD have been used successfully to treat adult ADHD, often in conjunction with behavior therapy or psychotherapy. The psychostimulant medications methylphenidate and dextroamphetamine have been the most widely studied and appear in most studies to have a statistically and clinically significant effect on reducing ADHD symptoms. Nonserotonergic antidepressants such as tricyclic antidepressants* and bupropion* have also been shown to have moderate therapeutic effects. The new nonstimulant selective norepinephrine reuptake inhibitor atomoxetine is currently the only medication specifically approved for use in adults with ADHD. Because of the high prevalence of co-morbid conditions such as depression and anxiety in adult ADHD, combination drug therapy may be necessary.

*Not FDA approved for this indication.

TREATMENT OF TOURETTE'S SYNDROME

method of
DAVID E. COMINGS, M.D.
City of Hope Medical Center
Duarte, California

Tourette's syndrome (TS) is a complex neurobehavioral disorder. Its diagnosis is based on the occurrence of motor and vocal tics almost daily for a period of at least 1 year. Coprolalia is seen in less than 10% of patients and is not required for the diagnosis. TS is a strongly genetic disorder. Like other behavioral conditions, TS is a polygenic disorder caused by the additive and epistatic effect of multiple genes interacting with the environment, each with a small effect. TS should be considered a disorder with a wide spectrum of manifestations. Thus, the feature that makes it so intriguing is the wide range of co-morbid disorders that occur in over 80% of individuals who seek medical attention. These disorders include attention deficit hyperactivity disorder (ADHD), learning disorder, obsessive-compulsive disorder (OCD) or behavior, other anxiety disorders including panic attacks and generalized anxiety disorder, mood disorders including depression and mania, sleep disorders, oppositional defiant disorder (ODD) and conduct disorder, rages, self-destructive behavior, and others. Space does not allow a discussion of the treatment of these co-morbid disorders. The focus here is on the treatment of tics.

This article is based on my personal experience over the past 25 years with the treatment of over 4000 children and adults with TS. The following are some of what I consider basic truths concerning the treatment of this complex disorder.

1. *Treatment of the whole person*. Anyone who takes on the treatment of individuals with TS should be prepared to treat the whole spectrum of co-morbid disorders because of the intimate interaction between the tics and the co-morbid behavior. Moreover, it usually works best for the patient and the physician if one person treats both disorders.
2. *Waxing and waning of tics*. The spontaneous waxing and waning of motor and vocal tics can make evaluation of the true effectiveness of medications difficult. This difficulty increases the need to use double-blind assessments when evaluating the efficacy of drugs for tics.
3. *Tics may be the least of the problems*. In most cases, the tics are often the easiest part of the spectrum to treat and are the least of the problems. Once the tics are minimized with medication, it is often the ADHD, OCD, or ODD that is the major issue in treatment.
4. *Basic pharmacology*. Many times the difference between success or failure in the treatment of TS lies less in finding exotic new treatments for difficult cases and more in understanding the best route and timing of administration of a small number of the most effective and reliable medications.
5. *Use of stimulants*. Because stimulants can make tics worse, it is often assumed that stimulants are contraindicated in the treatment of TS. In reality, the tics are often mild and easy to treat, and it is the co-morbid ADHD that causes the greatest disability. Failure to address and treat the ADHD can leave a patient significantly disabled. TS and ADHD are intimately related clinically, genetically, and pharmacologically.
6. *Exacerbation of tics by medications*. Although it is well known that stimulants can exacerbate tics in individuals with TS, it is less well appreciated that virtually every medication used in the treatment of TS and its co-morbid conditions can, in some cases, make the tics worse. Such medications include clonidine (Catapres), clonazepam (Klonopin), haloperidol (Haldol), pimozide (Orap), and risperidone (Risperdal).
7. *Polypharmacy*. The use of multiple medications used to be considered bad medical practice. However, behavioral disorders are due to the combined effect of multiple different gene variants, each affecting different neurotransmitters and other pathways and each of which may require a different medication for normalization.
8. *Drug of choice*. Clonidine,* not haloperidol or pimozide, is the drug of first choice.

Medications for the treatment of tics can be divided into two groups. Group I consists of those that are effective 60% to 80% of the time, and group II includes drugs that are less consistently effective or often ineffective.

GROUP I MEDICATIONS

In my experience, only three medications or groups of medication are included in group I. In order of preference, they are clonidine,* clonazepam,* and the typical or atypical neuroleptics (Table 1). In the following sections, the generic names are given first and the U.S. brand names are given in parentheses. They are often different in other countries.

Clonidine (Catapres)

Clonidine* is an α_2-adrenergic agonist. By stimulating presynaptic α_2-adrenergic receptors, in modest doses it results in a decrease in norepinephrine (NE) release. At higher doses it can stimulate postsynaptic α-adrenergic receptors. Clonidine is effective in the treatment of motor and vocal tics 60% to 70% of the time. However, it is a short-acting medication, and when given orally, the effects can wear off after 3 to 6 hours. Clonidine is also effective in the treatment of ADHD, and considerable evidence indicates that NE plays a significant role in ADHD. Importantly, elevated plasma levels of NE breakdown products have been associated with learning disorders in individuals with ADHD, which suggests that reducing NE levels could benefit children with learning disorders. Finally, clonidine* can be effective in the treatment of ODD, OCD, anxiety, phobias, and panic attacks. Thus,

*Not FDA approved for this indication.

TABLE 1. **Primary Groups of Drugs for the Treatment of Chronic Tics in Tourette's Syndrome**

Group	Members	Average Dose	Range
α_2-Adrenergic presynaptic receptor agonist	Clonidine patch (Catapres-TTS)*	1 TTS-1/wk	¼–4/wk
	Clonidine cream†	0.1 mg of 0.1 mg/0.1 mL/d	0.05–0.15 mL of 0.1–0.4 mg/0.1 mL 1–2×/d
	Clonidine oral (Catapres)*	0.05–0.1 mg tid	0.025–0.2 mg tid
	Guanfacine oral (Tenex)*	0.5–1 mg bid	0.25–2 mg bid–tid
Benzodiazepines	Clonazepam (Klonopin)*	0.5 mg tid	0.25–2 mg tid
	Alprazolam (Xanax)*	0.5 mg tid	0.25–2 mg tid
	Diazepam (Valium)	0.5 mg tid	0.25–5 mg tid
Typical and atypical neuroloeptics	Pimozide (Orap)	1–2 mg/d	0.25–10 mg/d
	Haloperidol (Haldol)	0.25–1 mg/d	0.25–10 mg/d
	Fluphenazine (Prolixin)*	0.5–1 mg/d	0.25–10 mg/d
	Risperidone (Risperdal)*	0.5–1 mg bid–tid	0.25–2 mg/tid
	Ziprasidone (Geodon)	20–40 mg/d	20–120 mg/d

*Not FDA approved for this indication
†Not available in the United States.

clonidine can be effective in the treatment of many of the important co-morbid conditions. It is especially relevant that clonidine is one of the very few medications that can consistently and reliably treat both tics and ADHD. This property makes it a particularly valuable alternative to the use of stimulants in the treatment of TS subjects with co-morbid ADHD. Because it is effective for such a broad range of the TS spectrum, I start treatment of most TS patients and many mild to moderately severe ADHD patients with clonidine. It covers a range of symptoms, so successful initiation of treatment with clonidine can often obviate the need to use any other medication. A number of strategies can be used to maximize the advantages of clonidine and minimize the disadvantages. With the use of these strategies, a sizable number of TS patients can be effectively treated with clonidine alone. If additional medications are needed, the dose required is often less than if a foundation of clonidine had not first been put in place.

Transdermal Clonidine (Catapres-TTS). The single major disadvantage of clonidine* is that it can be very sedating, especially when given orally. However, this side effect and the need to give frequent doses because of its short duration of action can be ameliorated by the use of transdermal clonidine, known as the Catapres Transdermal Treatment System.* It is available as TTS-1, TTS-2, and TTS-3. The latter two are equivalent to a patch two and three times the size of TTS-1. The use of a TTS-1 patch once a week is equivalent to the use of 0.1 mg of oral clonidine* per day. For children, ¼ to ½ patch per week is the usual starting dose. When the dose is right, the tics may subside within a few days. If the parents are in a hurry to get the tics under control, the dose can be increased every 1 to 2 days. If they are not so desperate, the dose is usually increased by ½ patch every week until satisfactory control of the tics or too much sedation is noted. In most cases, ½ patch has no effect, and it is thus necessary to increase to a whole patch.

*Not FDA approved for this indication.

The most common errors leading to treatment failure in treating TS subjects with the clonidine patch* are starting with a whole patch then abandoning treatment because of too much sedation or because it was ineffective. The problem with sedation can be avoided by cutting the patch and starting with less than a whole patch. The medication does not leak out of a cut patch. I have seen many cases in which a whole patch was too much, ½ patch was too little, but ¾ or ⅞ of a patch was just right. The problem with a whole patch being ineffective can often be avoided by further increasing the dose. The maximal dose is two TTS-3 patches. The average dose is one to two patches. It is common for the patch to be effective for several weeks and then lose its effectiveness. This change in effectiveness can usually be eliminated by a further increase in the dose. Only one to two such upward adjustments are typically required. Parents and patients seem to understand these changes best when told that "the dose is adjusted with a pair of scissors." It is also important to let them know that they do not need to call the doctor with every change in dose. They can be given a range to operate within, such as ½ to 2 patches.

One of the most common problems with use of the clonidine patch* is the development of a rash immediately under the patch as a result of contact dermatitis. This rash is due to an allergy to the patch material itself, not the clonidine.* It can often lead to the child complaining that the patch itches, and the patch will then be pulled off. A first line of defense against such removal is to use only the clonidine patch itself and not the large covering patch that comes in the box. In some cases, the allergy is to the covering patch rather than the clonidine patch itself. A second approach is to change the patch every 3 to 4 days instead of weekly. Because the rash sometimes occurs predominantly on days 5 to 7, earlier changing can avoid the problem. Another approach is to have the patient or parents purchase some water-based,

*Not FDA approved for this indication.

over-the-counter hydrocortisone ointment and rub it into the area where the patch is to be placed, let it dry, and then apply the patch. If all these measures fail, and they do about 20% to 30% of the time, a final very effective approach is to switch to clonidine cream.*

The patch also becomes very difficult to use in the summer when children sweat a lot or swim. Although the patch is waterproof and can resist brief showers, tub baths, and brief dips in the pool, it is not compatible with daily swims of an hour or more. These situations also call for the use of clonidine cream** or an oral form of clonidine or guanfacine (Tenex).†

Clonidine Cream.** I have had hundreds of TS patients who responded to only clonidine patches† and in whom no other medications were effective, including oral clonidine,† haloperidol, and pimozide. When only patches are effective and then a severe allergic reaction develops to the patch such that it can no longer be used, patients or parents are devastated. In the past 5 years I have found that an excellent solution to this problem is to switch to clonidine cream. It is not available at most pharmacies, but fortunately, usually at least one pharmacy in each reasonably large city does compounding and can make clonidine in cream form. If the patient had been using a TTS-1 patch, the prescription would read 0.1 mg/0.1 mL, use 0.05 to 0.15 mL on the forearm one to two times daily, with the amount being "1 month's supply." The cream is supplied in tuberculin syringes with a plastic cap. The markings allow easy dispensing of 0.1 mL. The patient, not the parent, should rub it into the forearm and make sure that no clothing comes in contact with it for 30 minutes. By this time the medication has been adsorbed into the skin and will not rub off. It will also not sweat off and will not come off in the pool. In those who swim a lot, an alternative is to use the cream after swimming each day. In some cases, morning and afternoon application of the cream is necessary to keep symptoms in check. If a compounding pharmacy is not located in your area, one might be found on the Internet. Many compounding pharmacies will fill prescriptions from any state or country.

Oral Clonidine. Oral clonidine** is the last preference for a route of administration of clonidine.** In my experience, oral clonidine is much more likely to cause an unacceptable degree of sedation than transdermal clonidine** is, probably because of the fact that blood levels rise quickly after oral administration and result in a higher blood level than what is obtained with transdermal clonidine.** Blood levels then drop and the tics return. Thus, as the parents or patients recall the day, they are either "tired or ticcing." The even blood levels obtained with transdermal clonidine** avoid this up-and-down course. Nonetheless, some patients still prefer oral clonidine. The side effects can be minimized by giving the medication in small, frequent doses such as 0.025 or 0.05 mg every 3 to 6 hours. Parents often report that they can see the medication wearing off after this time interval. They can repeat the dose as often as necessary by using a dose just under that causing tiredness. Many patients report that their physicians have previously treated their TS with oral clonidine but suggested they take it at bedtime to avoid problems with sedation. Although such administration can be effective because of the short duration of action of clonidine, it often results in less than optional control of the tics in the daytime.

Clonidine as a Sleeping Medication. In many cases, what is usually considered an undesirable side effect can become an effective therapeutic effect. Because NE is the arousal neurotransmitter, individuals with elevated central nervous system NE are often overaroused, especially children with TS and ADHD. Clonidine* can be a very effective, non–habit-forming, nonaddictive sleeping aid for such individuals. The bedtime dose usually ranges from 0.1 to 0.3 mg. Occasionally, parents complain that their TS/ADHD children wake up and roam the house in the middle of the night. Because of its short duration of action, clonidine is excellent for inducing sleep but is less effective in maintaining sleep throughout the night. A clonidine patch* can be helpful in this regard. The combination of a clonidine patch* supplemented with bedtime oral clonidine* can treat both problems of getting to sleep and staying asleep.

Although both clonidine* and guanfacine* are blood pressure medications, hypotension is rarely a troublesome side effect. Even fairly substantial doses are not associated with significant decreases in blood pressure, thus suggesting that in the absence of hypertension, only a modest decrease in blood pressure occurs. In addition, these medications have no significant effect on the QT_c interval.

Much time was devoted to the use of clonidine* because it can be so effective in the treatment of TS and its co-morbid conditions. In some children with significant motor and vocal tics, ADHD, learning problems, OCD, and ODD who are failing all their classes and are a constant visitor to the principal's office because of disruptive behavior, all these symptoms have disappeared after the use of a clonidine patch.* Equally impressive, after several months their grades may have risen to A's and B's. Some children have returned to the clinic proudly displaying plaques for "most improved student." Not all children responded this well, but many do.

Guanfacine (Tenex)

Guanfacine* is also an α_2-adrenergic agonist. It has a slightly longer duration of action than oral clonidine* does and a modestly lower incidence of sedation as a side effect. As such, it is widely used in place of oral clonidine. The usual starting dose is 0.25 to 0.5 mg three times daily (tid). Maintenance doses are usually 0.5 to 1 mg tid. Guanfacine has all the

*May be compounded by pharmacists.
**Not commercially available in the United States.
†Not FDA approved for this indication.

*Not FDA approved for this indication.

advantages of clonidine. However, as with oral clonidine, it can still be unacceptably sedating, and I prefer the clonidine patch* to both oral clonidine and oral guanfacine.*

One of the side effects of both clonidine (in any form) and guanfacine is that instead of decreasing symptoms of overarousal and hyperactivity, it can increase these symptoms. Thus, in about 5% to 10% of cases, parents report that their children are more active and more irritable and have more trouble sleeping. It has been suggested that ADHD is primarily a disorder of NE regulation and that both too little and too much NE can cause problems of inattention. Thus, if a child had a low-NE form of ADHD, clonidine* could make it worse. Alternatively, as mentioned earlier, at higher doses clonidine can have direct action on postsynaptic α-adrenergic receptors. This effect could also result in activation rather than suppression of ADHD-associated behavior.

Clonazepam (Klonopin)

Clonazepam* is one of the most frequently overlooked medications for the treatment of tics. When clonidine* is less than optimally effective, clonazepam may be the second drug of choice. The starting dose is 0.125 to 0.25 mg one to three times per day, depending on the age of the child. A common maintenance dose is 0.25 to 0.5 mg tid. As with clonidine, the major side effect is sedation. Other benzodiazepines may also be effective. Although the dependency potential of clonazepam is often a concern, it is very rare for TS individuals to request progressively higher and higher doses.

Neuroleptics

Neuroleptics such as haloperidol (Haldol), pimozide (Orap), and fluphenazine (Prolixin)* used to be the drugs of choice for treating TS. They are effective in 80% of cases. However, with the advent of the Web, parents often check out medications before using them, and the statement that permanent neurologic changes such as tardive dyskinesia can occur often frightens parents and patients so much that these neuroleptics have de facto become drugs of third choice. If clonidine* and clonazepam* have been ineffective, before neuroleptics can be used, it is often necessary to calm parents' fears of them. I have treated over 2000 TS patients with a major neuroleptic and have seen only 2 cases of mild tardive dyskinesia, both in individuals who received over 15 mg/d of haloperidol for many years. The usual doses of these medications are 0.25 to 2 mg of haloperidol, 0.5 to 4 mg of pimozide, and 0.5 to 5 mg of fluphenazine per day. Although at these low doses occasional patients may have akathisia, or extrapyramidal symptoms, I have never seen a case of tardive dyskinesia. Patients should have the QT interval monitored when taking pimozide.

*Not FDA approved for this indication.

Atypical Neuroleptics

Atypical neuroleptics have the advantage that they are much less likely to cause tardive dyskinesia, predominantly because of the fact that they cause less inhibition of dopamine D_2 receptors. However, inhibition of these receptors is the reason that neuroleptics are so effective in the treatment of tics. Of the atypical neuroleptics (risperidone [Risperdal],* olanzapine [Zyprexa],* molindone [Moban],* ziprasidone [Geodon], quetiapine [Seroquel],* clozapine [Clozaril]), risperidone* has the greatest affinity for dopamine D_2 receptors. This affinity conforms with my clinical experience that it is also the most effective atypical neuroleptic for the treatment of tics. Starting doses are usually 0.25 to 0.5 mg tid, with maintenance doses of 0.5 to 1 mg tid. Risperidone is relatively short acting. A common reason for failure of risperidone is administration of the medication only one or two times per day. If these times are in the morning and evening, recurrence of tics in the afternoon or evening may seem to be a failure of the drug. This "failure" can often be eliminated by giving a third dose at midday.

GROUP II

Group II medications are those that in my experience are effective in less than 50% of cases, are not generally available in the United States, or require special expertise. Careful attention to the use of type I medications results in control of tics in over 90% of TS cases. Group II medications and treatments, in alphabetical order, include antiandrogens, antibiotic treatment of PANDAS (pediatric autoimmune neuropsychiatric disorder associated with streptococcal infections), anticonvulsants, baclofen (Lioresal), behavioral management, β-blockers, botulinum toxin, calcium channel blockers, clomiphene citrate (Clomid), cyproterone (Androcur),† deprenyl (Eldepryl),* dronabinol (Marinol), electroencephalographic biofeedback, herbal remedies, 5-hydroxytryptophan,† lecithin, marijuana, mecamylamine (Inversine),* metoclopramide (Reglan),* naltrexone (ReVia),* nicotine patch (Habitrol),* ondansetron (Zofran),* pergolide (Permax), reserpine, selective serotonin reuptake inhibitors, tetrabenazine,‡ tramadol (Ultram), tricyclic antidepressants, and L-tryptophan. Interested readers can obtain further details from the National Library of Medicine on the Internet.

In the vast majority of cases, the motor and vocal tics of TS or the chronic motor tic disorders can be effectively treated with the use of one or more of the type I medications listed earlier. The difference between success and failure often lies less in turning to type II medications and more in paying careful attention to the pharmacologic aspects of the three type I groups of drugs.

*Not FDA approved for this indication.
†Investigational drug in the United States.
‡Not available in the United States.

HEADACHES

method of
DAWN A. MARCUS, M.D.
Multidisciplinary Headache Clinic
University of Pittsburgh Medical Center
Pittsburgh, Pennsylvania

Headache is one of the most common complaints patients bring to their doctors, affecting most adults at some time during their lives. Headache may be a symptom of systemic illness or intracranial pathologic condition or may be a primary condition, such as recurring migraine. Managing the headache patient requires establishing an appropriate diagnosis and course of treatment.

HEADACHE DIAGNOSIS

Headache diagnosis differentiates serious from benign causes of headache (Figure 1). Unfortunately, there are few headache features that identify the more severe headache. Patients with new onset, abrupt, severe headache, particularly occurring after activity, need to be screened for vascular abnormality, such as subarachnoid hemorrhage. Other causes of serious headache, such as brain tumor, often present as a mild, dull, holocranial pain, similar to tension-type headache. Often the mild headache that seems too insignificant to discuss with the doctor is the one more likely to be associated with a serious pathologic condition, as compared with the more incapacitating migraine episodes associated with vomiting and the need for bed rest.

Markers of Serious Headache

Headache should be considered as a possible marker of underlying illness when one of the following factors is present:

- New headache or change in headache pattern within the last 2 years, unrelated to change in medication
- Headache beginning after the age of 50 years
- Headache pain predominantly located in the posterior head (occiput) or neck
- Abnormalities on physical or neurologic examination

Additional evaluations are warranted when any of these factors is present. Older patients need to be screened for giant cell arteritis and intracranial lesions, such as tumors. Younger patients need to be screened for causes of increased intracranial pressure, vascular abnormalities, and systemic illness.

Testing should include laboratory screening for infection, endocrine disease, connective tissue disease, and systemic illness. Imaging studies of the head, such as magnetic resonance imaging or computed tomographic scanning, may also be needed in patients with a suspicious history or examination findings.

Benign Recurring Headache

Patients with chronic, stable headache without worrisome signs and symptoms or a negative evaluation are probably experiencing a benign recurring headache. Patients may experience a single type of headache or several distinct headache types. Patients usually have no more than two types of headache. Patients reporting more than two or three types of headache are often describing one type of headache in varying stages of severity. Patients should initially be asked whether they experience one type of headache or more than one type. Those experiencing more than one type of headache need to describe each separately to allow proper diagnosis.

Common Recurring Headaches

Common benign recurring headaches include tension-type, migraine, and post-traumatic headaches. More than 70% of adults experience tension-type headache at some time during their lives. Tension-type headache is a dull, usually bilateral, squeezing head pain that lasts for many hours to many days. Patients generally continue their daily activities during tension-type headache episodes. Although each individual headache episode is mild, experiencing frequent or daily headache is associated with significant psychological distress and reduction in quality of life.

Migraine affects about 15% of women and 5% of men. Migraine is an intermittent headache and does not occur as a chronic daily headache. Migraine may be preceded by hours to days with prodromal symptoms, including yawning, abnormal excitation or drowsiness, or cravings. About 20% of patients experience premonitory warning aura, frequently involving blind spots, sparkly or shimmering lights or lines, and, less commonly, numbness or weakness. The painful part of headache begins about 15 to 30 minutes after aura symptoms. Migraine is often a unilateral, severe, pounding pain that takes the patient to bed or significantly reduces activities. These patients often crave quiet darkness and retreat to bed with a wet washcloth placed over the forehead and eyes. Patients also report abnormal sensitivity to smells and are frequently nauseated. Each individual headache episode lasts about 6 to 12 hours, after which the patient will be headache free until the next episode. Children with migraine are more likely to experience briefer (4 to 6 hours) bilateral headache than adults. Patients typically experience no more than two migraine episodes per week. Some patients may experience the combination of migraine with tension-type headache, noticing frequent, mild tension-type headache with infrequent, incapacitating migraine.

Headache may also begin following trauma, particularly mild head injury. Headache should begin within 2 weeks of trauma, unless the patient has been hospitalized or too heavily medicated during this time to notice the headache. Typically, patients report a frank loss of consciousness or feel stunned or dazed at the time of injury. Affected patients were often unaware of impending impact and were struck when the head was

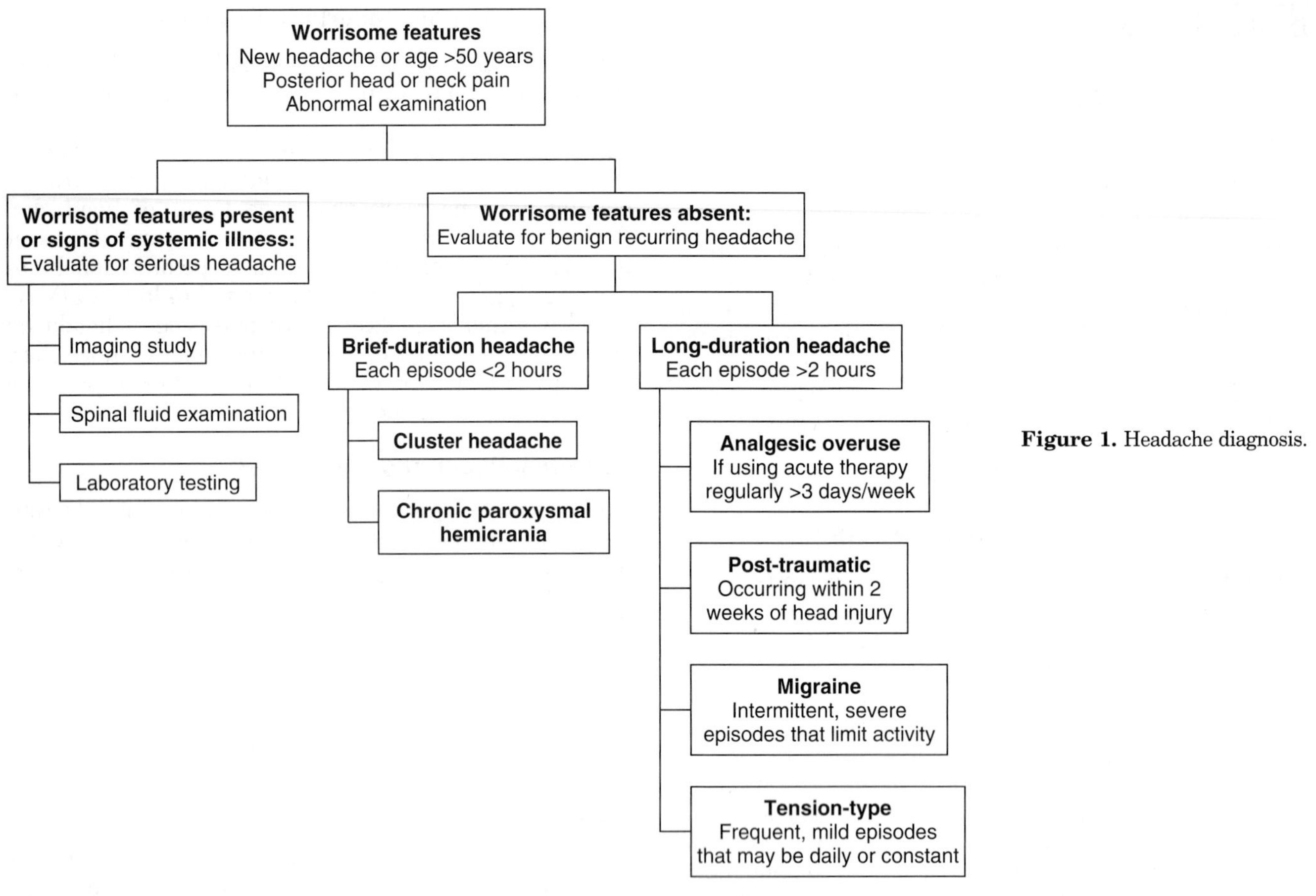

Figure 1. Headache diagnosis.

turned to the side. They may report other postconcussive symptoms in addition to headache, such as memory loss, mood disturbance, tinnitus, imbalance, or dizziness. These patients need imaging studies to rule out hemorrhage or cervical fracture. Most patients experiencing post-traumatic headache note severe, constant, incapacitating headaches for the first few weeks after head injury. Headache then becomes milder and less constant. Headache completely resolves within 6 to 12 months for most patients. One third of patients continue to experience headache 12 months after the head injury, and 15% to 20% do so after 3 years.

Patients with frequent or daily mild headache should be screened for analgesic overuse, or drug rebound, headache. Analgesic overuse headache occurs in patients with preexisting headache disorder, such as migraine or post-traumatic headache. In response to an increase in headache activity or in an effort to develop a headache prevention strategy, patients begin to use over-the-counter or prescription acute care headache medications daily or near daily. This excessive medication use results in down-regulation of headache inhibitory pathways, resulting in increased severity and frequency of headache. Patients typically respond by increasing medication consumption, which exacerbates headache. Any patient using acute care medications four or more days per week regularly for at least 6 weeks is at risk for having analgesic overuse headache. Headache symptoms will not improve until excessive medication use ceases.

Uncommon Recurring Headaches

The most common of the uncommon recurring headaches is cluster headache. Cluster headache frequently occurs at or during sleep and affects men four times as often as women. Cluster headache is experienced as brief intermittent headache. Patients report abrupt onset of excruciating, unilateral, retro-orbital pain, with each episode lasting about 30 to 60 minutes. Although each episode is brief, it is agonizingly painful and much more severe than migraine episodes. Patient behavior during cluster attacks distinguish them from migraine. Cluster headache patients are very active during attacks, showering, pacing, and sometimes literally banging their heads against the wall. Patients also can experience intense autonomic symptoms during headache episodes. Interestingly, cluster headache patients often minimize the degree of nasal congestion and profound lacrimation and rhinorrhea, whereas patients with migraine overemphasize these features. Therefore, queries about autonomic features are usually not useful diagnostically.

Episodic cluster headache occurs in groups or clusters. Patients are entirely headache free for months to years. They then awake one night after about 90 minutes of sleep with maximally intense retro-orbital pain. After 30 to 60 minutes, the pain resolves and they are asymptomatic. They return to sleep, only to wake 90 minutes later with an identical episode. Each cluster period begins with one headache nightly for the first few nights, then two nightly episodes, and finally three to four nightly episodes. After 6 weeks, the frequency of episodes reduces and the patient will again be headache free for months to years until his next cluster attack. Rarely, patients experience chronic daily cluster attacks without periods of headache remission.

Women rarely experience a similar type of excruciating, retro-orbital pain with autonomic features called chronic paroxysmal hemicrania. These episodes are brief (1 to 3 minutes) and maximally severe at onset, and they recur frequently throughout the day (about 15 episodes). These episodes resolve quickly (within several days) after treatment with indomethacin (Indocin 25 to 50 mg three times daily). Chronic paroxysmal headache, although rare, should be considered in women who present with cluster-type headache.

HEADACHE PATHOGENESIS

Serious headache occurs because of traction, inflammation, bony abnormality, or increased intracranial pressure. Benign headache occurs because of abnormalities within inhibitory pathways originating within the brainstem. In most patients, these abnormalities are believed to be genetically based. Post-traumatic headache occurs as the result of microscopic shearing forces that alter brainstem activity as the cortex moves above the relatively immobile brainstem at the time of impact. The best understood neurochemical abnormality resulting in tension-type, migraine, post-traumatic, and analgesic overuse headaches is an imbalance in serotonin.

Serotonin (5HT) is present throughout the body and is critically important for the development of headache symptoms. Plasma serotonin activates inhibitory $5HT_1$ receptors present on the dorsal raphe nucleus. Activation of $5HT_1$ receptors occurs by elevated plasma serotonin, acute analgesics, and $5HT_1$ receptor agonists (such as triptans and dihydroergotamine [Migranal]). An individual headache episode of migraine or tension-type headache begins with a drop in plasma inhibitory 5HT.

Reduction in inhibitory 5HT exposes the dorsal raphe nucleus to activation by headache trigger factors (hormones, chemicals, stress, fasting, sleep deprivation). The dorsal raphe nucleus will then release 5HT, which activates $5HT_2$ receptors. Activation of these receptors results in dilation of meningeal vessels, increased blood flow, and a pounding sensation. More importantly, these vessels stretch perivascular neurons, activating the trigeminal system, which sends pain messages to the thalamus and cortex. Headache preventive therapies, such as the antidepressants and relaxation/biofeedback, work by altering activation of the $5HT_2$ receptors (Figure 2).

Acute care medications cause an initial activation of $5HT_1$ receptors. Chronic, daily use, however, leads to down-regulation of $5HT_1$ receptors. Patients often respond with increased use of analgesics or triptans, without headache relief because the down-regulated

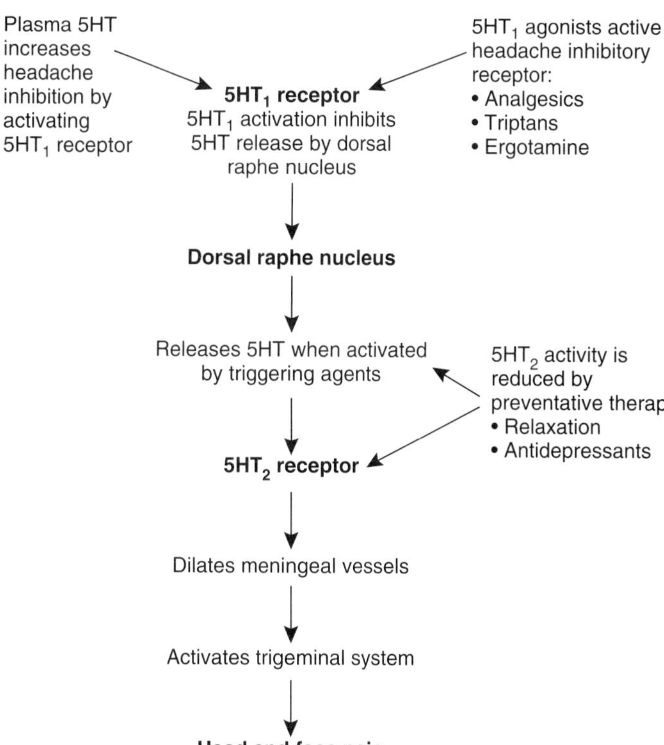

Figure 2. Headache pathogenesis. 5HT, serotonin.

$5HT_1$ receptors are unable to adequately respond to further stimulation. The delayed recovery noted after discontinuation of daily acute care medications reflects the time required to up-regulate $5HT_1$ receptors to more normal activity levels.

HEADACHE TREATMENT

The hallmark of headache treatment is education. Patients must be given a headache diagnosis and specific reassurance that the headache does not signify more ominous disease. Patients need to be informed that they can gain control over headaches through the use of both medication and nonmedication therapies. Patients who feel empowered to manage their headaches note better therapeutic response and less disability. Brief education after initial physician evaluation consisting of 30-minute education by an allied health care worker and three follow-up telephone calls to identify and address problems with therapy resulted in an incremental headache reduction by 29%, compared with standard medical therapy.

In addition to providing information about headache diagnosis, doctors must provide specific recommendations for headache treatment. Patients should be encouraged to develop effective headache coping strategies and stress management skills. Maintaining regular sleeping and eating cycles, such as avoiding fasting, often improves headache. Patients who like to sleep in on the weekends should be advised to rise at their usual time, go to the bathroom, have a small snack (juice or crackers), and then return to bed. They experience the illusion of sleeping in, with less disruption to body cycles. Avoidance of headache-provoking substances, such as caffeine (more than two cups of caffeinated beverage daily) and nicotine, should be strongly encouraged.

Patients also require specific instruction about medication use. Written instructions are ideal. Patients need to understand which medications are used for acute versus preventive therapy. Each acute care treatment should be tried for two or three headache episodes before its effectiveness is assessed. Patients should be strongly discouraged from treating only a single headache episode with a new medication, unless tolerability is poor. Most acute care medications should be initiated with the most effective dose, rather than starting with a low dose and increasing to a more effective dose with subsequent headaches. Patients will typically abandon a potentially effective therapy before achieving adequate dose with this approach.

Preventive medications, alternatively, must be taken daily. Patients should be informed that benefit will not be noticed for 2 to 3 weeks at the maximum medication dosage. Most preventive medications should be initiated at low doses, with an increasing titration schedule to improve efficacy. Traditional dogma incorrectly suggests that headache patients achieve effective pain control with very low doses of preventive medications. Antidepressants, antihypertensives, and antiepileptic medications typically must be prescribed in standard, moderate doses used for treating depression, hypertension, and epilepsy, respectively. Tizanidine (Zanaflex)* is an exception to this rule, with initiating doses of 1 mg at bedtime, titrated to 2 to 4 mg twice daily as typical effective dosages. Patients who experience benefit from preventive medication should be offered a trial of tapering their preventive agent after headaches have been well controlled for 6 months. Many patients notice continued good headache control after preventive medication discontinuation, particularly if they are also using nonmedication headache management techniques. If headaches increase during preventive medication taper, the dosage should be increased to the previously effective dose. Another tapering attempt can be done in another 6 months.

Common Recurring Headaches

Patients may experience more than one type of headache. Treatment should be designed to accommodate treatment for both infrequent headache episodes and frequent headache episodes (Figure 3). In some circumstances, patients will have only one type of headache, in other cases they may have both frequent and infrequent headaches.

Patients with frequent or daily headache must be screened for analgesic overuse headache. Headache therapies will be ineffective unless medication overuse stops. Discontinuation of analgesics results in significantly improved headache after 1 month for 30% of patients, after 2 months for 65%, and after 4 months for 82%. Analgesics may be abruptly discontinued; narcotics or butalbital should be tapered. Simultaneously, patients can be treated with daily dosing of a long-acting nonsteroidal anti-inflammatory drug (NSAID) such as nabumetone (Relafen) or etodolac (Lodine), or COX-2 drugs such as rofecoxib (Vioxx), celecoxib (Celebrex), or tramadol (Ultram) if NSAIDs are not tolerated, to prevent headache aggravation. This daily medication should continue until patients have been free of the originally offending medication for 1 month. At that point, if headache persists, standard headache preventive therapy should be started. Most patients will notice that discontinuation of daily analgesic results in loss of constant, daily headache and return of previous intermittent headaches.

Similar therapies effectively treat tension-type, migraine, and post-traumatic headaches. Specific treatment depends on headache frequency and the presence of co-morbid conditions. Infrequent headache (three or fewer headaches per week) should be treated with acute care therapy. Mild, infrequent headache often responds to analgesic combination medications. Aspirin and NSAIDs are more effective than acetaminophen, and analgesic potency is increased by combining analgesic with caffeine. Antiemetics may supplement analgesics if nausea is present. Antiemetics, such as prochlorperazine (Compazine) are more effective than metoclopramide (Reglan). Although initial treatment with antiemetics

*Not FDA approved for this indication.

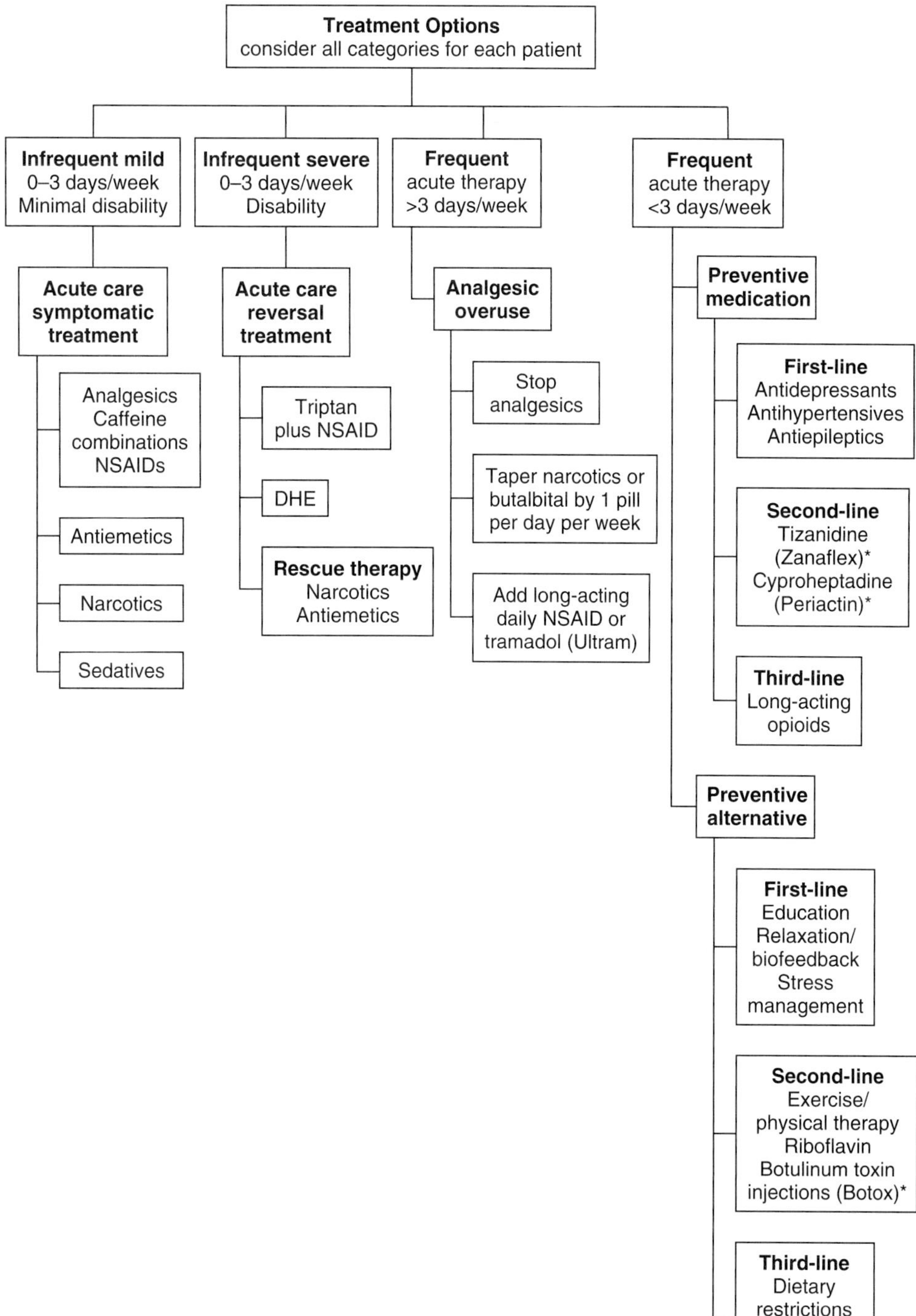

Figure 3. Headache treatment. DHE, dihydroergotamine; NSAID, nonsteroidal anti-inflammatory drug. *Not FDA approved for this indication.

alone relieves both pain and nausea of headache, symptoms will recur unless analgesic medication is also used. Therefore, antiemetics should be used as adjunctive treatment to more effective analgesic medications. Sedatives such as isometheptene combination (Midrin) may be helpful in patients for whom headache resolves after sleep and in children. Butalbital combination medications (Fiorinal, Fioricet, Esgic) are rarely helpful for headache and are readily overused. Moderate to severe headaches associated with disability (e.g., reduction in or loss of activity) are best managed with headache reversal compounds that specifically target $5HT_1$ receptors, including the triptans or dihydroergotamine (Migranal). Triptans provide rapid headache relief, whereas dihydroergotamine (Migranal) provides very long-duration relief for severe headache episodes that typically last 2 to 3 days. Neither triptans nor dihydroergotamine can be used in patients with uncontrolled hypertension or cardiovascular disease.

The most effective acute care medications include

- Analgesic with caffeine (Excedrin, ibuprofen plus coffee or cola) for mild headache
- Triptans for more severe headache
  - Fastest-acting triptans include sumatriptan (Imitrex) 6 mg subcutaneously (SC) and rizatriptan (Maxalt) 10 mg orally (PO)
  - Fast-acting triptans include sumatriptan (Imitrex) 20 mg nasal spray (NS) or 50 to 100 mg PO, zolmitriptan (Zomig) 2.5 mg PO, almotriptan (Axert) 12.5 mg PO
  - Long-duration triptans include naratriptan (Amerge) 2.5 mg and frovatriptan[†] (Frovelan) 2.5 mg PO
  - Dihydroergotamine (DHE 1 mg intramuscularly [IM] or 3 mg sublingually [SL] [specially compounded], or Migranal NS) for long-duration severe headache

Patients who fail to achieve adequate headache relief from one of these therapies should try another one. For example, only 19% of patients fail to respond to sumatriptan (Imitrex), rizatriptan (Maxalt), and zolmitriptan (Zomig). Failure to respond to one triptan does not predict failure on another triptan or failure on dihydroergotamine (Migranal). Supplementing triptan with an NSAID often speeds relief and reduces the need to redose with triptan.

Frequent headache episodes (more than three headaches weekly) should be treated with preventive therapy. The most effective therapies include:

- Antidepressants, especially tricyclics such as amitriptyline (Elavil),* imipramine (Tofranil),* or nortriptyline (Pamelor).* Bupropion (Wellbutrin)* and selective serotonin reuptake inhibitors such as paroxetine (Paxil)* and fluvoxamine (Luvox)* are moderately effective.
- Antihypertensives, especially β-blockers such as propranolol (Inderal), timolol (Blocadren), and atenolol (Tenormin).* Verapamil (Calan, Isoptin)* and lisinopril* (Prinivil, Zestril) are moderately effective.
- Gamma-amino butyric acid active antiepileptics, especially valproate (Depakote). Gabapentin (Neurontin)* is moderately effective.
- Relaxation and/or biofeedback.

Each treatment is effective for about 65% to 70% of patients. Patients failing these therapies may consider second-line therapies (see Figure 3).

Relaxation and biofeedback are effective therapies for common recurring headaches, including migraine and tension type. Patients cannot learn these techniques with self-help books; they require some instruction from a therapist. Minimal therapist contact approaches allow technique training over four sessions, with at home practice assigned in between training sessions. Efficacy of either relaxation or biofeedback matches that of standard headache preventive medications, such as antidepressants or antihypertensives. Combination of relaxation or biofeedback with preventive medication increases the effectiveness of headache reduction. Relaxation, biofeedback, and stress management are the most effective nonmedication techniques. Nicotine cessation also often improves headache because nicotine use alters endorphin activity. Dietary restriction, herbs (feverfew,* gingko biloba,* St. John's wort*), supplements (riboflavin,* calcium,* magnesium*), and exercise programs are minimally effective headache reduction therapies.

*Not FDA approved for this indication.

[†]Not available in the United States.

Patients with frequent mild, tension-type headache and infrequent migraine may require both preventive and acute care therapies. Patients using acute care medications typically use some medications for mild attacks and others for more severe episodes. Patients failing to obtain adequate relief from severe episodes with headache reversal compounds should combine an NSAID with their reversal compound. Rescue medications, such as antiemetics and narcotics, should be provided for circumstances in which acute care medications have failed, to allow home headache management.

Finally, patients with frequent or disabling headaches are at high risk for co-morbid depression and anxiety. These patients should be screened for psychological distress with self-assessment tools:

- Beck depression inventory
- Spielberger State-Trait Anxiety scales
- SCL-90 (A modified 27-item version called the SCL-27 has been validated in chronic pain patients as an effective screening tool of psychological symptoms by Hardt and Gerbershagen.)
- Online screening can be done at *http://syked.com/tests.html*.

Patients experiencing symptoms of depression and anxiety in addition to headache need to have psychological symptoms treated. Failure to treat depression and anxiety can reduce both motivation to comply with treatment recommendations and effectiveness of headache reduction therapy. Depression and anxiety will not spontaneously resolve after headache has been treated. The presence of these symptoms may provide an opportunity to choose antidepressants as preventive therapy to treat depression, anxiety, and headache.

Uncommon Recurring Headache

Cluster headache therapy focuses on headache prevention, because each individual headache episode is very severe and relatively brief. Preventive therapy should be started at the onset of the first headache within a cluster series and continued for the typical duration of the cluster, often about 6 weeks. If preventive therapy is delayed until patients have reached their peak cluster frequency, steroids must be used (e.g., prednisone 40 mg daily, tapered over 1 week). The most effective preventive medication is verapamil (Calan, Isoptin).* Alternative

*Not FDA approved for this indication.

medications can include methysergide (Sansert), valproate (Depakote),* gabapentin (Neurontin),* lithium (Eskalith),* or nightly dosing with dihydroergotamine 3 mg SL (specially compounded) or naratriptan (Amerge)* 2.5 mg PO.

Cluster headache patients should also have available fast-acting acute care medications for headaches that continue despite preventive therapy. These would include oxygen (7 L/min by face mask for 10 to 15 minutes), injectable sumatriptan (Imitrex), or butorphanol (Stadol)* nasal spray. Intranasal 4% lidocaine (Xylocaine) spray to the nostril on the painful side is occasionally helpful.

Cluster headache rarely responds to nonmedication techniques such as stress management, relaxation, or biofeedback. Most cluster headache patients are smokers, and discontinuation of nicotine products, at least during the cluster period, reduces headaches. Alcohol should also be avoided during cluster periods, as most patients have learned through personal experience of severe headache precipitated by alcohol consumption.

SUMMARY

Most chronically recurring headaches are benign headaches, such as migraine, tension-type, and posttraumatic headaches. These headaches are caused by imbalance in neurochemicals, such as serotonin. Effective therapies target activity at serotonin receptors.

New-onset headaches may be caused by a systemic illness, such as infection, or an intracranial pathologic condition. Headache needs a thorough evaluation when symptoms are new or changing, headache begins after the age of 50 years, pain is located mainly in the posterior head or neck, or the physical and neurologic examination findings are abnormal.

Headache treatment requires proper patient education about headache diagnosis and appropriate use of headache treatments. Treatments should be provided to treat both infrequent and frequent headaches. Many patients require several medications to be available so that they can effectively manage their headaches at home.

---

*Not FDA approved for this indication.

VIRAL MENINGITIS AND ENCEPHALITIS IN CHILDREN AND ADULTS

method of
JAMES F. BALE, Jr., M.D.
University of Utah School of Medicine
Primary Children's Medical Center
Salt Lake City, Utah

Many viruses cause meningitis or encephalitis in humans. In addition, several nonviral pathogens such as *Mycoplasma pneumoniae, Rickettsia rickettsiae,* and *Bartonella henselae* (the bacterium causing cat-scratch disease), as well as noninfectious conditions such as systemic lupus erythematosus and neurosarcoidosis, produce symptoms and signs that mimic viral infections of the central nervous system (CNS). These mimickers complicate the diagnostic evaluation and therapeutic management of children and adults with suspected viral meningitis or encephalitis. Table 1 lists common viral pathogens associated with meningitis or encephalitis and summarizes the microbiologic and serologic studies that can be used to detect these agents.

Before 1994, when primary encephalitis was still considered a notifiable disease in the United States, the Centers for Disease Control and Prevention received reports of 1000 to 2000 cases of viral encephalitis annually. This quantity corresponded to approximately 0.5 case per 100,000 persons living in the United States. However, the overall prevalence of viral encephalitis and meningitis in children and adults is substantially greater.

Approximately 2500 cases of herpes simplex virus type 1 (HSV-1) encephalitis, a disorder that is not considered notifiable at the national level, occur annually in the United States. Two thirds of these patients are adults, and HSV-1 thus accounts for more than 50% of the encephalitis cases in persons older than 50 years. Periodic outbreaks of viral encephalitis affect persons living in all regions of the world. In 1975, over 2500 cases of St. Louis encephalitis were reported in persons in the midwestern and eastern regions of the United States. More than 3000 human cases of West Nile virus infection, an Old World flavivirus first observed in the United States in 1999, were identified in 2002. Although only one to six cases of human rabies are detected annually in the United States, rabies causes several thousand deaths annually in developing countries.

Viral or aseptic meningitis also occurs worldwide. In most regions, the nonpolio enteroviruses (echovirus and coxsackievirus) account for most cases of viral meningitis and many cases of mild encephalitis. Nonpolio enterovirus cases cluster in the summer or fall, but because humans serve as the only reservoir for these agents, enteroviral CNS disease can be observed throughout the year. Aseptic meningitis has been linked to infections with numerous additional viruses, including the herpesviruses, the arboviruses, and lymphocytic choriomeningitis virus, a rodent-borne arenavirus, as well as to many nonviral and noninfectious conditions.

Historical information regarding a patient's residence, travel, occupational or recreational activities, and exposure to vectors provides important clues regarding the etiology of viral meningitis or encephalitis. Viruses transmitted by mosquitoes or ticks, for example, typically cause disease during the summer months in temperate climates. Many arthropod-borne viruses (collectively known as the arboviruses), such as eastern equine, western equine, St. Louis, La Crosse, Venezuelan, and Japanese encephalitis viruses, display distinctive geographic predilections, as their names imply.

TABLE 1. **Microbiologic Evaluation of Persons With Suspected Viral Encephalitis or Meningitis**

Suspected Pathogen	Diagnostic Study
HERPESVIRUSES	
Herpes simplex virus type 1 (HSV-1)	CSF PCR
Herpes simplex virus type 2 (HSV-2)	CSF PCR
Epstein-Barr virus (EBV)	CSF PCR, serum titers†
Varicella-zoster virus (VZV)	CSF PCR
Cytomegalovirus (CMV)	CSF PCR, urine/saliva culture
Human herpes virus-6 (HHV-6)	CSF PCR
Human herpes virus-7 (HHV-7)	CSF PCR
Human herpes virus-8 (HHV-8)	CSF PCR
ARTHROPOD-BORNE VIRUSES (ALPHAVIRUSES, FLAVIVIRUSES, BUNYAVIRUSES, ORBIVIRUSES)	
Western and eastern equine encephalitis viruses	Serum titers,* CSF IgM
St. Louis encephalitis virus	Serum titers
Japanese encephalitis virus	Serum titers, CSF RT-PCR, CSF IgM
West Nile virus	Serum titers, CSF RT-PCR, CSF IgM
La Crosse virus	Serum titers, CSF IgM
Tick-borne encephalitis virus group	Serum titers
Colorado tick fever	Serum titers
NONPOLIO ENTEROVIRUSES	
Echovirus and coxsackievirus	CSF RT-PCR, culture of stool and oropharyngeal secretions
EV71	Culture of stool and oropharyngeal secretions, CSF RT-PCR
OTHER	
Rabies virus	Serum titers, IFA‡, saliva RT-PCR
Measles	Serum titers, culture of oropharyngeal secretions
Lymphocytic choriomeningitis (LCM) virus	Serum titers

*Agent-specific IgM and IgG in acute and convalescent serum samples.
†Acute EBV infection can be confirmed by the presence of anti-EBV viral capsid antigen (VCA) IgG and/or IgM and the absence of anti-EBV nuclear antigen (EBNA) IgG.
‡Immunofluorescent antibody staining of skin from the nape of the neck.
CSF, cerebrospinal fluid; RT-PCR, reverse transcription polymerase chain reaction.

Certain arboviruses, such as western and eastern equine or St. Louis encephalitis viruses, occur episodically, sometimes causing massive outbreaks, whereas others, such as La Crosse and Japanese viruses, produce numerous cases of encephalitis each year. La Crosse virus, a mosquito-borne bunyavirus, causes encephalitis in children living in the Midwestern United States. Japanese encephalitis, the most common arboviral encephalitis worldwide, affects persons residing throughout Asia from Korea to India.

Cases of HSV, Epstein-Barr virus (EBV), cytomegalovirus (CMV), and varicella-zoster virus (VZV) encephalitis or meningitis also appear throughout the year and occur in persons of all ages regardless of their geographic location. Rabies virus is maintained in numerous wild animal reservoirs, including raccoons, wild canines, and bats, as well as in domestic dogs and cats in regions without compulsory vaccination. Recent human rabies cases in the United States have been imported or linked to bat rabies strains, thus emphasizing that rabies prophylaxis should be initiated after any human contact with bats.

CLINICAL FEATURES AND DIAGNOSTIC EVALUATION

The clinical manifestations of viral encephalitis in children and adults typically consist of fever, headache, vomiting, altered mental status, and seizures, either partial or generalized. Partial or focal seizures can indicate HSV-1 encephalitis, but focal seizures can also be observed with other types of viral encephalitis, including relatively benign childhood cases caused by La Crosse virus. The neurologic examination may show hyperreflexia, ataxia, cognitive disturbances, and focal deficits such as aphasia and hemiparesis.

Persons with aseptic meningitis usually have fever, headache, vomiting, and signs of meningeal irritation such as stiff neck or back pain. Other symptoms or signs, such as rash, cough, jaundice, hepatosplenomegaly, or myalgia, may be present, depending on the infectious pathogen. Children and adults with enteroviral disease commonly experience sore throat, rash, vomiting, and diarrhea. Young infants with viral CNS infections, whether encephalitis or meningitis, often have subtle, nonspecific signs such as inactivity, poor feeding, irritability, "fussy" behavior, or "high-pitched" cries.

Examination of cerebrospinal fluid (CSF) remains the most useful diagnostic procedure when evaluating patients with suspected viral CNS infection. CSF in viral meningitis or encephalitis usually shows an elevated protein content, a normal glucose content, and a lymphocytic pleocytosis. However, considerable variability can be found in the CSF findings, and in some patients the CSF can be entirely normal. Between 5% and 15% of individuals with HSV-1 encephalitis lack pleocytosis initially (with CSF cell counts $<5/\mu L$), an observation that complicates the diagnosis of HSV encephalitis, especially in young children.

Patients with CNS viral infections can have a mixed or neutrophilic pleocytosis that may resemble the CSF profile of bacterial infections. Some viruses can produce mild hypoglycorrhachia. Thus, clinicians must occasionally initiate empirical therapy consisting of antiviral agents and broad-spectrum antibiotics to cover viral and bacterial pathogens concurrently until culture and polymerase chain reaction (PCR) results become available. Erythrocytes can also be observed in the CSF, particularly in HSV encephalitis, but a hemorrhagic CSF profile generally has little diagnostic specificity.

Magnetic resonance imaging (MRI), the second essential component of the diagnostic evaluation of children and adults with suspected viral encephalitis, may show unique patterns of disease that can suggest a specific pathogen. For example, children and adults with HSV-1 encephalitis characteristically have T2 prolongation and/or gadolinium enhancement of the insular cortex, mesial temporal lobe, inferior frontal lobe, and cingulate gyrus. Patients with Japanese encephalitis display abnormalities of the thalamus, basal ganglia, and brainstem.

In other forms of viral encephalitis, MRI can be normal or demonstrate multifocal areas of T2 prolongation. Patients with the immune-mediated disorder acute disseminated encephalomyelitis (ADEM) also have multifocal areas of T2 prolongation that may involve the cerebrum, cerebellum, brainstem, and spinal cord. Approximately 15% of encephalitis cases represent ADEM. Patients with viral meningitis typically have normal MRI findings.

An electroencephalogram (EEG) should be obtained if the clinician suspects viral encephalitis, particularly when the patient has seizures. In patients older than 5 months with biopsy-proven HSV-1 encephalitis, approximately 80% have focal slowing or repetitive epileptiform discharges localized to the temporal lobes. Nearly half the children with La Crosse virus encephalitis also have focal abnormalities on the EEG, thus indicating that the diagnosis of HSV-1 encephalitis cannot rely on the EEG findings alone. Diffuse slowing of background rhythms or multifocal epileptiform discharges are commonly seen in other forms of encephalitis and in ADEM.

Children and adults with suspected viral meningitis or encephalitis require a thorough microbiologic evaluation tailored to reflect the age of the patient, the season, the geographic location, and the presence of immunocompromising conditions such as HIV infection (see Table 1). Specimens for conventional isolation of virus by culture may include urine, blood, CSF, feces, throat washings, and fluid from skin lesions, depending on the suspected virus. Serologic studies should be considered as well, but they rarely provide timely information to guide antimicrobial therapy. However, serum titers may be the only means to confirm infection with EBV, many arboviruses, and certain nonviral agents, including *M. pneumoniae*, *B. henselae*, and *Treponema pallidum*. Detection of virus-specific IgM in CSF can confirm infection with certain arboviruses, including La Crosse and St. Louis encephalitis viruses.

Examination of CSF by PCR is currently the most powerful microbiologic study for evaluating patients with suspected viral meningitis or encephalitis. PCR can be used to detect the DNA or RNA of several viruses, including HSV-1, CMV, EBV, VZV, human herpesviruses 6 and 7, and the nonpolio enteroviruses. The sensitivity of PCR, however, varies by laboratory and pathogen.

The sensitivity of CSF PCR in children and adults with HSV-1 encephalitis averages 90% to 95%, but it is only 70% to 80% in neonates with proven HSV encephalitis, in whom the encephalitis is usually due to HSV-2. By combining the results of CSF PCR and MRI, the sensitivity of detecting HSV encephalitis approaches 100% in neonates, children, and adults. Reverse transcription (RT)-PCR also has high sensitivity for the nonpolio enteroviruses. Because the sensitivity and predictive value of CSF PCR or RT-PCR for other viruses are generally lower or have not been established, clinical judgment remains the most important aspect of managing patients with suspected viral CNS infection. When doubt exists regarding the possibility of HSV-1 encephalitis, for example, full courses of acyclovir are necessary.

TREATMENT

Treatment of children and adults with viral CNS infections consists of supportive care, anticipation of potential complications, and initiation of specific antiviral chemotherapy, when available (Figure 1). Patients with clinical and CSF signs consistent with viral meningitis can often be managed as outpatients. By contrast, patients with encephalitis should be hospitalized and monitored closely for the development of increased intracranial pressure or seizures, complications that affect 15% to 50% of patients with encephalitis.

Seizures can be treated with benzodiazepines (lorazepam [Ativan] or diazepam [Valium]) at standard age- and weight-appropriate doses, such as 0.05 to 0.1 mg/kg of lorazepam administered intravenously (maximal single dose of 4 mg). Prolonged or repetitive seizures require the administration of loading doses of a maintenance anticonvulsant such as fosphenytoin (Cerebyx), 15 to 20 mg/kg of phenytoin-equivalents intravenously, or phenobarbital, 10 to 15 mg/kg intravenously in infants or toddler-aged children. Increased intracranial pressure, manifested by clinical or radiographic findings, requires mannitol, hyperventilation, or placement of an extraventricular drain.

Children with suspected HSV-1 encephalitis require treatment with acyclovir (Zovirax), 30 to 45 mg/kg/d divided every 8 hours. Doses of 1500 mg/m^2/d can be used in adolescents and adults. Neonates require higher doses, 60 mg/kg/d* divided every 8 hours, for HSV encephalitis or disseminated HSV disease. Dose reductions are necessary in patients with impaired renal function; for example, patients with creatinine clearances of 25 to 50 should receive 10 to 15 mg/kg

*Exceeds dosage recommended by the manufacturer.

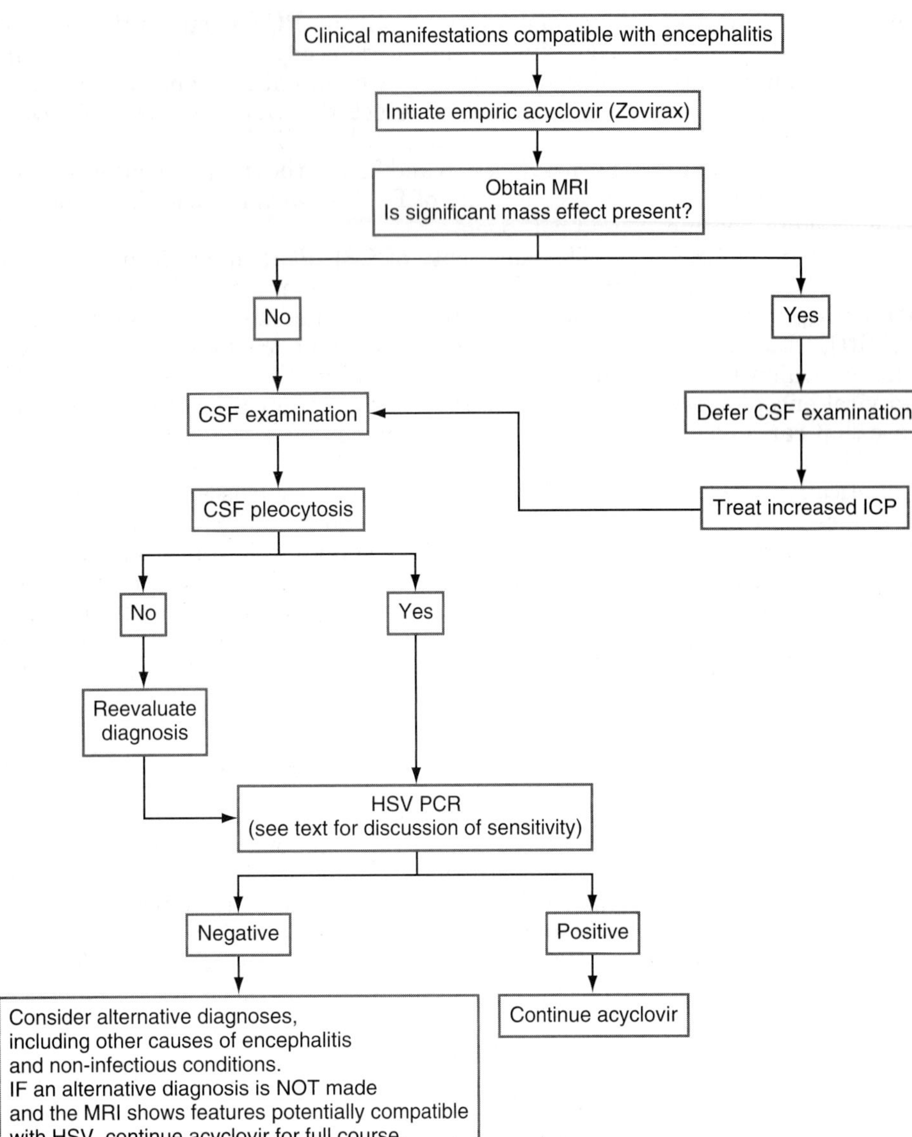

Figure 1. Approach to the initial evaluation and treatment of children and adults with suspected encephalitis. CSF, cerebrospinal fluid; HSV, herpes simplex virus; ICP, intracranial pressure; MRI, magnetic resonance imaging; PCR, polymerase chain reaction.

every 12 hours because of potential nephrotoxicity. Patients with HSV disease confirmed by PCR require therapy for 14 to 21 days.* Patients with HSV-1 or HSV-2 meningitis may also require acyclovir therapy in the regimens outlined earlier, but many such patients appear to recover spontaneously.

Patients with encephalitis caused by VZV should be treated with acyclovir,† 30 mg/kg in children younger than 1 year and 1500 mg/m^2/d in older children for 10 to 14 days. Ganciclovir (Cytovene)† at doses of 10 to 12 mg/kg/d can be considered in patients with EBV or CMV encephalitis, but the potential side effects of nephrotoxicity and myelotoxicity should be weighed cautiously against the anticipated benefits. Children and adults with severe enteroviral CNS infections, such as those caused by EV71, a particularly neurovirulent enterovirus, may receive benefit from pleconaril (Picovir),† a novel antiviral agent that possesses activity against several RNA viruses. Anecdotal information suggests that ribavirin (Virazole)† could have utility in patients with West Nile or La Crosse virus encephalitis.

Viral encephalitis has a variable prognosis that reflects several factors, including the etiologic agent, the patient's age, and the presence of underlying medical conditions. Encephalitis caused by the nonpolio enteroviruses or La Crosse virus generally has low rates of mortality and morbidity. Mortality in acyclovir-treated patients with HSV encephalitis currently averages less than 20%, but only half the survivors recover completely despite appropriate medical management. Human rabies encephalitis, rare in developed countries but common in many undeveloped regions, virtually always causes death. By contrast, patients with viral meningitis typically recover completely without specific antiviral therapy.

*Exceeds dosage recommended by the manufacturer.
†Not FDA approved for this indication.

†Not FDA approved for this indication.

MULTIPLE SCLEROSIS

method of
ROBERT P. LISAK, M.D.
Wayne State University School of Medicine
Detroit, Michigan

Multiple sclerosis (MS) is the most frequent cause of neurologic disability of young adults in the United States, Canada, and Europe other than head and spinal cord trauma. The incidence of MS varies geographically, being highest in temperate regions and in large countries such as the United States. MS is more common in the northern states than in the south. Earlier epidemiologic data indicated that the risk was related where people spent the first 15 years or so of their life, although more modern and larger studies of migration are needed to see whether this remains correct. The incidence of MS is also not evenly distributed among racial and ethnic groups, being highest in individuals of northern European origin and less common, but certainly not rare, in African Americans. It is higher in African Americans than African blacks, but whether this is related to differences in environment or interracial mixing or both is not clear. MS is rare in East Asian populations in both Japan and probably China as well as in Asian Americans. In Israel, MS is more common in Israelis of northern European origin (Ashkenazi) than in those of Mediterranean and Middle Eastern origin (Sephardim). The disease is more common in women than men, particularly the more common relapsing-remitting presentation (1.7 to 2.0:1), although in the less common later onset (older than 40 years) primary progressive form the ratio is closer to 1:1. It is estimated that there are approximately 350,000 individuals in the United States with MS. There is a suggestion that there may be an increasing incidence of MS, although it is hard to be certain that this does not simply represent better and earlier diagnosis, particularly the effect of diagnostic magnetic resonance imaging (MRI).

ETIOLOGY AND PATHOGENESIS

Despite rediscovery of the heterogeneity of the nature of the central nervous system (CNS) lesions in MS as well as the presence of axonal damage and gray matter cortical lesions, MS can still be best thought of as a disease characterized by inflammation by mononuclear cells and demyelination with *relative* sparing of axons and neurons. The etiology of MS is unknown, but immunologic and inflammatory mechanisms seem to be important in the pathogenesis of most stages of the disease. MS has been hypothesized to be the result of direct infection of the CNS with one or more infectious agents with most interest and recent investigation centering on viruses and the bacteria *Chlamydia pneumoniae*. It is fair to say that the evidence is often controversial, difficult to confirm, and sometimes indirect. Systemic infections may, however, be involved in the etiology and pathogenesis of MS through molecular mimicry in which the immune system develops antibodies and/or T cells that react with an infectious agent that shares homology in two or three dimensions with constituents of the host; in the case of MS, these constituents would be components of CNS myelin.

There is still debate about which is the critical target antigen in MS, with several candidates among those that are able to induce various types of experimental autoimmune encephalomyelitis in animals. The exact nature of the abnormalities in immunoregulation that are present in MS that allow the autoimmune and/or persistent inflammatory reactions is also incompletely understood.

As in other complex diseases, evidence continues to accumulate that there are several genes involved in MS. There is probably more than one gene that influences susceptibility to disease. In addition, there are genes that are capable of affecting severity, rate of progression, and age of onset.

CLINICAL SUBTYPES AND CLINICAL COURSE

In order to better plan clinical trials and therapy for patients on the basis of stage and subtype of disease, an international committee has suggested a classification of MS into (1) relapsing-remitting MS (RRMS), the classical presentation of dissemination in time and space in the CNS; (2) secondary progressive MS (SPMS), patients who had RRMS but now show progression (increased disability) without any clear-cut relapses (exacerbations) or have progression between relapses (stable increased residual after relapses is considered RRMS in this scheme); (3) primary progressive MS (PPMS), patients who never have clear-cut relapses but accumulate disability in one or more anatomic regions of the CNS or system (periods of relative stability or even modest improvement with physical or pharmacologic symptomatic therapy are allowed); and (4) progressive-relapsing MS (PRMS), patients who seem to have PPMS but then have a clear-cut relapse and then continue to progress. No attempt was made to define so-called benign MS because at the onset and early in the course it is usually impossible to categorize such patients. The same is true of rapidly relentlessly progressive forms of MS such as the so-called Marburg variant because these are rare. Although there are problems with this classification, it has turned out to be useful.

DIAGNOSIS

The essence of diagnosis is still basically dependent on dissemination in time and space in the CNS with the proviso that there is no better diagnosis in the judgment of a physician experienced in diagnosis of MS. With the advent of modern neuroimaging, particularly MRI, evoked potentials (EPs), and more widespread availability of sophisticated cerebrospinal fluid (CSF) analysis (oligoclonal bands, IgG index, and IgG synthesis rate) as well a serologic tests for other disorders that can imitate MS early in the course of the disease, it is now possible to make a definite diagnosis without a second clinical attack as well as PPMS. It is now also possible to predict with reasonable certainty which patients who present with what could be the first attack of MS (optic neuritis, a brainstem syndrome, myelitis, cerebellar syndrome, or a hemispheric syndrome in a young adult), a so-called clinically isolated syndrome (CIS), will develop MS on the basis of MRI and to some degree on CSF analysis.

TREATMENT

Treatment of patients with MS can be broadly divided into four categories. The first is good general health measures because MS has little effect on life expectancy. The second is symptomatic therapy designed to lessen or alleviate troubling symptoms and increase independent function. The third is treatment of relapses in order to shorten the period of disability and perhaps to lessen the disability from the relapse. Finally, there is disease-specific therapy, so-called immunomodulatory and immunosuppressive therapies.

General Health Measures

Vaccinations and Immunizations

An issue that always arises is the question of vaccinations and immunizations in patients with MS. If a patient is receiving any immunosuppressive therapy such as mitoxantrone (Novantrone), cyclophosphamide (Cytoxan), or corticosteroids, any live virus vaccines should be avoided. Killed vaccines are safe from the point of view of the immunosuppressed patient, and it can be reasonably argued the immunosuppression is a good reason to immunize such patients particularly if they might be exposed to a serious infectious agent such as pneumococcus or influenza, although their response to such immunizations might or might not be suboptimal. There is no evidence to avoid live vaccines in patients receiving immunomodulatory therapy such as glatiramer acetate (Copaxone) or interferon-β (Avonex).

For patients receiving either immunomodulatory therapy such as glatiramer acetate, interferon-β, or intravenous IgG (IGIV) or no therapy, should the patient receive attenuated live, recombinant, or killed vaccines? From the point of view of increasing relapses, there is no evidence from well-conducted prospective studies of such an effect of vaccines or immunizations. Therefore, patients who otherwise need to receive such vaccines for non–MS-related reasons or because their disability from MS is so severe as to make them likely candidates for a poor outcome if they develop influenza or pneumonia, for example, should receive the immunization. Because patients with MS often have a temporary decline in neurologic function with raised body temperature; they should have any fever resulting from vaccination, or any infection for that matter, treated with acetaminophen (Tylenol), aspirin, or a nonsteroidal anti-inflammatory agent. It has been demonstrated that viral infections are associated with subsequent relapses, not just pseudorelapses associated with fever. For that reason, some have even suggested that patients with MS be immunized against influenza even if they have no medical condition or severe MS-related disability. There are no studies that address this question, and one needs to consider the overall effectiveness of the vaccine before making such a recommendation in an otherwise healthy MS patient with little or no disability from the MS.

Symptomatic Therapy

It has been suggested that symptoms in MS can be divided into primary, secondary, and tertiary symptoms. Examples of primary symptoms are weakness, tremor, diplopia, decreased vision, ataxia, loss of sensation, paresthesias, spasticity, neurogenic bladder, fatigue, pain, and depression. Secondary symptoms, which are the result of primary symptoms, can include falls and injuries, urinary tract infections, skin breakdown, contractures, lack of sleep, and loss of intimacy. Tertiary symptoms, the outgrowth of primary and secondary symptoms, include unemployment, role changes, social isolation, divorce, loss of productivity, problems with the environment, and so on. Treatment of secondary and tertiary symptoms, although extraordinarily important, is beyond the scope of this article.

Spasticity

Spasticity is actually a neurologic sign and, if it is not interfering with the patient's function, need not necessarily be treated. With mild spasticity, simple stretching and active walking may prove to be sufficient. Physical therapy including home exercise programs is an integral part of treatment programs for MS-related spasticity of all degrees. In other patients, other treatment may be needed. I generally begin with baclofen (Lioresal) at 5 mg by mouth three times a day and after a few days generally increase to 10 mg three times a day. Depending on the patient as well as an individual patient's status and progression, larger doses are frequently required. Finding the appropriate dose, which can be as high as 50 mg four times daily,* even in partially ambulatory patients, is a matter of titrating the desired therapeutic effect of decreased symptomatic spasticity against side effects of increased weakness and sleepiness. Tizanidine (Zanaflex) is also effective but frequently causes sleepiness, particularly if it is not gradually titrated up very slowly. It may also induce hypotension, particularly postural hypotension. I start with 1 to 2 mg at bedtime for a few days before gradually increasing the dose in 1- to 2-mg increments until the patient is taking the drug three times a day. If necessary, I again increase by 1 mg per dose starting with the evening dose. For patients who have spasticity resulting in painful nighttime spasms, tizanidine with or without baclofen may prove useful and the induction of sleepiness is

*Exceeds dosage recommended by the manufacturer.

mitigated. Combinations of baclofen and tizanidine are often useful and because they have different sites of action in the CNS, modest doses of both may result in a salutary therapeutic effect without the side effects of high doses of either drug. Gabapentin (Neurontin)* may also prove helpful, particularly with paroxysmal increases in spasticity and as an adjunct to other antispasticity measures. Diazepam (Valium) (2 to 5 mg two or three times daily) may still occasionally be helpful, but higher doses are associated with considerable effect on mood and sleepiness. However, for nighttime use diazepam (5 to 10 mg at bedtime) or clonazepam (Klonopin)† may prove helpful. I have found clonazepam (0.5 to 1 mg at bedtime) also helpful in patients with MS who have periodic leg movements of sleep. Dantrolene (Dantrium) is effective in treating spasticity, but acting in the muscle it may produce increased weakness. Dantrium use is associated with hepatotoxicity, and therefore it should not be considered as a first- or second-line drug in MS. Local injection of botulinum toxin (Botox)† by a physician experienced in its use for neurologic diseases may also be helpful in selected cases. Finally, in patients in whom these medications are not effective or the dose needed to produce a satisfactory outcome is associated with unacceptable side effects, installation of a baclofen infusion pump may prove effective. Such pumps may even be used in patients who are still ambulatory with assistance.

Fatigue

Fatigue is a common and frequently disabling symptom in patients with MS, particularly those with mild to moderate disease who are still employed or active in their own activities of daily living. It is difficult to define and harder to quantitate. Although MS-related fatigue and depression are separate phenomena, patients with depression frequently describe fatigue and such fatigue should be treated with agents effective in depression such as the selective serotonin reuptake inhibitors or other agents. Another cause of fatigue is poor sleep, which in patients with MS may result from nocturia, pain, and painful spasms at night and perhaps directly from the involvement of structures within the brain. Many patients describe what can best be termed fatigability of effort. A common example is increased difficulty walking and dragging the leg the farther the patient walks. End-of-day increase in disability may also represent this phenomenon.

There is a characteristic MS-related fatigue that appears often with little effort, although heat and increased physical effort can exacerbate it. It is often overwhelming and is usually not present first thing in the morning. Resting or taking a brief nap is often effective in milder MS-related fatigue but may not always be practical. When it is more severe or when resting or napping is not an option, attempts to treat fatigue with medications may prove effective to varying degrees. Amantadine (Symmetrel)* at 100 mg daily or twice daily is often effective; the second dose should not be taken after midafternoon in order to avoid insomnia. Modafinil (Provigil),* originally developed and approved for narcolepsy and related disorders, may also be helpful in doses varying from 100 to 400 mg/d. Most patients seem to respond to and tolerate 200 mg/d. Pemoline (Cylert)* has never been shown to be particularly effective in carefully performed studies, although empirically there are patients who seem to respond. Doses vary from 18.75 mg twice or three times daily to totals of 75 mg/d. There have been reports of severe liver toxicity, and the frequent and long-term need to monitor liver function tests closely has limited its use in MS. Methylphenidate (Ritalin)* has not been shown to be effective in any large studies but there are occasional patients who seem to respond. In addition, some neurologists with considerable experience in treatment of patients with MS have observed improvement in MS-related fatigue in patients who do not otherwise seem to be depressed with fluoxetine (Prozac) (20 mg/d). Patients may have "normal" fatigue related to their own particular lifestyle, which may exacerbate MS-related fatigue. Finally, it is evident that there may be several causes of fatigue in patients with MS and attempts to sort out which ones are present increase the chances of effective therapy.

Neurogenic Bladder

Bladder dysfunction is common in patients with MS. Symptoms include urgency, frequency, hesitancy, need to double void, retention, nocturia, and incontinence. Some patients have inability to store urine; others have inability to empty. One of the most common problems is detrusor sphincter dyssynergy, a situation in which the bladder contracts but the external sphincter fails to relax and actually contracts. This not only results in difficulty in voiding but also may result in backup of pressure into the ureters. This in turn can eventually result in hydronephrosis and renal damage. Urinary retention also results in increased incidence of urinary tract infections. Mild urinary urgency and urge incontinence and dribbling can often be readily treated with oxybutynin or tolterodine. However, if the patient is retaining urine, these medications can increase urine retention. The goal is no incontinence and a postvoiding residual of less than 75 to 100 mL. Other drugs used for management of neurogenic bladder include terazosin (Hytrin),* which may increase urinary flow by relaxing the internal (bladder) sphincter, and hyoscyamine (Levsin), which blocks bladder contraction as an anticholinergic. In some patients the ideal management is frequent self-catheterization, paralyzing the bladder with oxybutynin (Ditropan) or other cholinergic drugs. This is preferable to indwelling Foley catheterization, which even with optimal care is associated with increase in urinary tract infections, bladder stones, and bladder spasms. The occasional patient

*Exceeds dosage recommended by the manufacturer.
†Not FDA approved for this indication.

*Not FDA approved for this indication.

requires a urinary bypass procedure. Urodynamic studies and involvement of a urologist are frequently necessary and helpful.

Neurogenic Bowel

Bowel complaints are common and can include urgency, fecal incontinence, constipation, and even obstipation. Secondary effects can lead to increased difficulty with hemorrhoids, rectal fissures, and related consequences of severe constipation. Mild constipation is often easily handled with appropriate diet and stool softener with or without additional fiber. A bowel training program including the use of suppositories is also helpful in constipation as well as with reducing marked episodes of fecal incontinence. Mild laxatives can be used to prevent more severe constipation, and at times stronger laxatives and enemas are required.

Sexual Dysfunction

Sexual dysfunction is another major problem for many patients and one that they frequently do not want to talk about. This is compounded by the reluctance of health workers to ask about such problems. Men may have difficulty achieving or maintaining an erection and/or ejaculation. Decreased sensation in the genital region can adversely affect sexual function in men and women, as do bladder problems. Women may have problems with lubrication and achieving orgasms. Sildenafil (Viagra) (25 to 100 mg) is often helpful in men. Counseling is helpful, and there are other techniques that can prove helpful for men and women.

Pain

Pain is not infrequent in patients with MS. The first task is to eliminate the possibility of other non-neurologic causes such as arthritis; cardiac, pulmonary, or gastrointestinal diseases; or herpes zoster. MS-related pain can be related to abnormal gait or posture standing or when seated, which can accentuate other problems such as low back pain or arthritis of the lumbar sacral or thoracic spine. A frequent cause of pain is uncontrolled spasticity including flexor or extensor spasms. This type of pain is best controlled by reducing spasticity. Neurogenic pain is also common in patients with MS and is often described as burning, tingling, paroxysmal pruritus or a diffuse deep aching. Patients with MS may have pain typical of trigeminal neuralgia and other nonspecific facial pain. Headache, usually not prominent, can accompany relapses, particularly those affecting the brainstem or rostral cervical cord.

Some patients can be successfully treated with simple analgesics or nonsteroidal anti-inflammatory drugs. In many patients other medications are needed. Several of the newer anticonvulsants (gabapentin [Neurontin],* topiramate [Topamax]*) and traditional (phenytoin [Dilantin],* carbamazepine [Tegretol]*) are often effective in reducing or even eliminating neurogenic pain. I generally start with gabapentin and gradually increase the dose to as high as 3200 mg/d in divided doses unless the patient has unacceptable side effects (sleepiness, dizziness, clouding of mentation). Gabapentin has the advantage of not being metabolized and excreted by the kidneys, is not protein bound, and does not interact with or influence the metabolism of other medications the patient may be receiving. Tricyclic antidepressants such as amitriptyline (Elavil)* (25 to 100 mg at bedtime or divided throughout the day) are also effective. In patients with facial pain, local lidocaine may be a helpful adjunct by reducing trigger points. Surgery on the trigeminal ganglion in my experience does not provide long-lasting relief as it may in idiopathic trigeminal neuralgia because the pathology is proximal to the ganglia, in the brainstem. Misoprostol (Cytotec)* 100 to 200 mg three or four times daily has been reported to be useful in trigeminal neuralgia associated with MS.

*Not FDA approved for this indication.

Tremor

Tremor is a frequent finding in patients with MS. It may range from mild to severe. It is generally related to movement and/or posture. In many patients there is also dysmetria of the limb involved, which is often the major factor in limitation of purposeful skilled use of that limb. Occupational therapy including weights on the wrist has limited effect on tremor and dysmetria. Medications including primidone (Mysoline)* (25 mg three or four times daily), diazepam (Valium)* (2 to 5 mg three times daily), and propranolol (doses ranging up to 320 mg/d), drugs useful in patients with essential tremor, have limited utility in tremor and dysmetria in MS. Reports of improvement with high doses of isoniazid (INH)* have not been confirmed; furthermore, INH can cause hepatotoxicity and if not accompanied by pyridoxine can lead to a sensory neuropathy and therefore is rarely used. Thalamotomy or thalamic stimulation may have a beneficial effect on tremor but really does not help with the equally if not more problematic dysmetria. The long-term benefit of this approach is not clear.

Paroxysmal Attacks

Patients with MS may have rapid onset of stereotype attacks such as sudden loss of strength and tone in the legs, acute dysarthria, dysphagia, and severe hemiparesis. These attacks respond well to treatment with anticonvulsants such as gabapentin (Neurontin)* and carbamazepine (Tegretol).*

Dysphagia

Dysphagia related to upper motor neuron, bulbar, and cerebellar dysfunction occurs in many patients with MS. Swallowing studies may be useful in assessing this symptom, particularly to determine whether aspiration or the potential for aspiration is present. Speech therapists or pathologists can be very helpful in assessing dysphagia and providing advice on diet and eating. In patients with severe dysphagia, a percutaneous endoscopic gastrostomy (PEG) may be necessary.

*Not FDA approved for this indication.

Disorders of Mood

Depression is common in patients with MS. In some it may be reactive, but in others it seems to be an intrinsic part of the disease symptom complex. Treatment involves pharmacologic agents, counseling, and support groups including family counseling. Patients may also exhibit inappropriate euphoria or elevated affect. Frank mania, although uncommon, does occur.

Cognitive Defects

Mild changes in cognition are common in MS and are often described as difficulty in multitasking and slowing of ability to remember things, although eventually patients say they do remember. Severe changes leading to difficulties with activities of daily living are uncommon, but the moderate defects coupled with fatigue and depression have a negative impact on employment and family activities. Depression can result in what seem to be mild cognitive defects. Treatment with cholinesterase inhibitors that are used in patients with Alzheimer's disease does not seem to have a major effect in MS, although some such as donepezil (Aricept)* (5 to 10 mg/d) that are easy to administer and with little side effects may be worth a try.

The Role of Physical and Occupational Therapy

Physical therapy can be helpful in dealing with spasticity, weakness, and gait abnormalities including imbalance. Occupational therapy can help patients deal with problems related to use of hands for fine skills and activities of daily living. Therapists are also able to help in home health evaluations to help advise on home health aids.

Pressure Sores and Decubitus Ulcers

Patients with significant disability resulting in being chair or bed bound are highly susceptible to developing pressure sores, which can then go on to decubitus ulcers. Pressure sores and decubitus ulcers are easier to prevent than to cure. Unfortunately, this requires frequent change in position, attention to seating in wheelchairs, excellent skin care, vigilance in inspection of the skin, and aggressive therapy if early pressure sores are noted.

Treatment of Relapses

There is no evidence that treatment of relapses in patients with MS has a long-term effect on disability. However, there are ample studies demonstrating that treatment of relapses with short-term corticotropin (ACTH), moderate-dose oral corticosteroids (1 mg/kg/d prednisone or equivalent), and intravenous methylprednisolone (500 to 1000 mg/d) shortens the duration of the disability associated with the relapse although not necessarily the degree of residual from the individual attack. Most studies support the concept that the very high dose intravenous (IV) corticosteroids result in more rapid improvement than ACTH or oral corticosteroids at 1 mg/kg/d. In addition, it is clear that in RRMS relapses are associated with increased disability. Therefore, treatment of relapses associated with significant increases in disability is a reasonable approach. I generally treat with 500 mg of IV methylprednisolone (Solu-Medrol) over 1½ hours every 12 hours for 10 doses for inpatients and for home treatment, because of logistics, 1 g over 1 to 1½ hours for 5 days. When appropriately studied, equivalent oral doses may well prove to be equally effective. Prophylactic treatment with a proton pump inhibitor or histamine type 2 inhibitor is generally helpful. Some patients require medication for sleep or increased anxiety during treatment. Although there are no studies demonstrating superiority of an oral taper, unless there is a relative or absolute contraindication, I recommend a taper of oral corticosteroids over a 10- to 21-day period. Intermittent IV steroids are sometimes used alone or in combination with other medications in patients with SPMS and occasionally with RRMS who are not doing well with other disease-modifying therapy, but there is no evidence for the use of chronic daily steroids.

Disease-Modifying Therapy

Relapsing-Remitting Multiple Sclerosis

The last 10 years have changed the approach to therapy of patients with RRMS with the approval of recombinant human interferon-β (IFN-β) in two different forms, three different dosing schedules, and two routes of parental administration as well as glatiramer acetate (20 mg/d given subcutaneously [SC]; previously known as copolymer 1 or Cop-1 marketed as Copaxone). These medications reduced relapses when compared with placebo and at least over the periods of the controlled "blinded" study seemed also to reduce or slow disability. There are longer term follow-up studies of glatiramer acetate (8 years) and IFN-β1a (22 or 44 μg SC three times a week, marketed as Rebif; 4 years), but there are no long, blinded or placebo-controlled prospective double-blinded studies comparing any of the IFN-β agents with glatiramer acetate. There are two studies comparing IFN-β1a (30 μg IM once a week marketed as Avonex) with IFN-β1b (250 μg SC every other day, marketed in the United States and Canada as Betaseron and in Europe as Betaferon) over 2 years using clinical (unblinded) and MRI measures (blinded) or IFN-β1a (44 μg SC three times a week) in which only the observers but not the patients were blinded for clinical outcome and the study was for only 9 months. On the other hand, in the pivotal trials of the two forms of IFN-β frequently administered SC, there was clearly a dose-response effect on clinical and MRI outcome measures. Although a study of once-weekly IM IFN-β1a showed no difference between 30 or 60 μg, unfortunately the effect of twice-weekly or three times weekly administration was not examined. Through all of this

*Not FDA approved for this indication.

one must keep in mind that these studies usually but not always have similar but not identical patients and that the outcome depends as much on how the placebo group does as how the treated group does. In addition, depending on the primary clinical outcome, one agent may be able to demonstrate an effect on disability whereas other studies were not powered for such an analysis. Differences in outcome also depend on what was looked for and when. If MRI was not examined, it does not mean that there was no effect on MRI. If gadolinium enhancement was not examined, it does not mean that the agent had no effect on gadolinium enhancement of lesions. If the first MRI time point examined was at 1 year, it does not mean that that agent has no effect on MRI until 1 year.

There have been many studies on neutralizing antibodies in patients receiving IFN-β in the different forms, doses, and routes of administration. These studies and the resulting discussions often "generate more heat than light." Different results have been reported with different antibody assays and even with the same agent in different studies. It is likely that the presence of sustained neutralizing antibodies inhibits the biologic effect, but how high a titer and what duration of the presence of these antibodies really affect short-term and more importantly long-term clinical outcome are far from clear. As of the time of this writing there are no published reports of the presence or absence of neutralizing antibodies to glatiramer acetate. In the case of both agents, assays that examine a biologic effect in in vitro studies and preferably in vivo assays examining the effect of serum IgG containing human anti–IFN-β or anti–glatiramer acetate on the animal model experimental autoimmune encephalomyelitis would be of interest because both glatiramer acetate and IFN-β inhibit this useful although admittedly not perfect model of MS.

Given these and other provisos, what do I recommend? I think that all patients who have active RRMS defined by the presence of a relapse in the last year or evidence of new or enhancing lesions should receive immunomodulatory therapy with one of these agents. Taking all of the currently available studies together, including tolerability, side effects, and adverse events, I am convinced that the patients for whom I recommend IFN therapy should be started on frequent-dose IFN (IFN-β1b 250 μg every other day or IFN-β1a 44 μg three times a week). However, if a patient is insistent on the weekly therapy, it is clearly preferable to no therapy. I am also persuaded that glatiramer acetate is as effective as the IFN therapies and perhaps more effective than the once-weekly IFN for many patients. Although glatiramer acetate currently requires daily injections, it seems to have the least side effects and significant adverse reactions. Although there are arguments about the onset of MRI versus clinical and immunologic effects, there is sufficient ambiguity about the clinical meaning of these differences in different studies that only carefully performed prospective controlled studies will answer these questions. What should be clear is that all of these drugs are imperfect in many patients, and the statement that all four agents are equivalent for groups of patients, although conceivably true, does not mean they are equally effective in individual patients. If a patient is not doing well with one agent, again a matter of judgment to define, something else needs to be considered. The issue is how long the patients should continue with treatment if they are doing well. Until an equally effective oral agent or superior parenteral or oral agent comes on the market, I suggest that my patients continue therapy indefinitely. The role of repeated MRI scans in the management of patients receiving therapy in clinical practice has not fully been defined, and in some geographic areas it is not financially practical.

Flulike reactions including fever, chills, myalgias, and headache are common with the IFN agents, particularly at the beginning of therapy. For that reason the use of acetaminophen (Tylenol) or ibuprofen (Motrin) is encouraged, as is gradually increasing the dose of the frequent-dosage forms of IFN-β. Some patients require continued use of these analgesic, antipyretic, anti-inflammatory agents as long as they are receiving IFN, although most can eventually inject IFN without the use of these drugs. Injecting at night is also helpful for most patients.

A major problem in maintaining patients with these immunomodulatory therapies is unrealistic expectations by patients, family, and unfortunately sometimes by physicians. The drugs do not treat symptoms or reverse significant disability, although some patients with minimal or modest signs (no or minimal disability) may indeed improve. Although one might argue that there could be direct or indirect (there is no evidence that these agents are present in measurable amounts in the CNS) neuroprotective or regenerative and remyelinative effects of one or more of these agents, a positive effect on reduction of new attacks and new or enlarging lesions may allow improvement through CNS plasticity at a local level (remyelination, change in sodium channels) or by activating additional neural pathways and centers, as has been shown using functional MRI.

MITOXANTRONE (NOVANTRONE)

Mitoxantrone, a chemotherapeutic agent used in T-cell leukemias and metastatic prostate cancer, has been approved for patients with SPMS but also for patients with RRMS who are showing aggressive disease (repeated relapses and/or acquiring disability). As discussed later, as a treatment for SPMS this is a potent agent with significant side effects and adverse events or reactions, and the use of this agent in most patients with RRMS should, in my opinion, not be undertaken without input from someone with extensive experience in treatment of patients with MS. The same is true for the use of cyclophosphamide (Cytoxan) in patients with RRMS doing poorly (not approved by the FDA for MS).

INTRAVENOUS IGG (GAMIMUNE N)

IGIV has been tried in different doses and dosing schedules in patients with RRMS as well as SPMS.

Some studies demonstrate reduction in relapses and MRI abnormalities. None have shown any effect on progression or progression to disability from the relapses. IGIV is expensive and is not entirely without side effects. For that reason it is best to consider IGIV experimental therapy in patients with MS. In addition, there is no evidence that IGIV reduces fixed deficits that result from prior relapses.

PLASMA EXCHANGE

There is one well-controlled small study demonstrating that patients who have a residual deficit from a relapse of demyelinating diseases of the CNS after therapy with corticosteroids improve with plasma exchange. Many of these patients did not have MS, and there was no effect on the occurrence of the next relapse. There is no evidence that plasma exchange is effective in SPMS or PPMS.

Clinically Isolated Syndrome

With the demonstration that IFN-β1a given at 22 μg SC (Rebif in the Early Treatment of Multiple Sclerosis Study Group [ETOMS] study) or 30 μg IM (Avonex in the Controlled High-Risk Subjects Avonex Multiple Sclerosis Prevention Study [CHAMPS]) once per week delays the diagnosis of MS by second defining clinical attack or new MRI lesions, the question arises of whether to treat patients with a CIS that by MRI or CSF criteria is highly likely to go on to "develop" MS (diagnosable MS; one could reasonably argue that they already have MS but it does not yet meet diagnostic criteria for definite MS) with IFN-β1a. The Food and Drug Administration has now approved Avonex for such an indication. Indeed, logic and what we know about these agents in established MS raise the issue of also using IFN-β1b or glatiramer acetate for these patients or, if choosing Rebif, using it at 22 or 44 μg three times a week because in established MS (Once Weekly Interferon for MS Study Group [OWIMS] study) 22 μg once each week SC was not better than placebo. My practice is not to prescribe therapy for patients with less than three significant MRI lesions and therefore a low chance of developing MS over the short term (2 to 5 years) but rather to observe them clinically at least every 6 months as well as repeating an MRI scan at 3 and if necessary at 6 months and then every 6 months. If a repeat MRI scan allows the patient to meet the criteria for definite MS, I then offer therapy. With patients who have a high probability of developing MS on the basis of their MRI results, I explain the issues and offer them therapy or frequent MRI and clinical follow-up as just outlined. If they have more than eight lesions, two or more large lesions, thinning of the corpus callosum, several "black holes" (hypodense lesions on T1 sequences that are not enhanced with gadolinium), or other signs of atrophy at first presentation, I suggest that they start therapy. I readily admit that this is as much art as science.

Secondary Progressive Multiple Sclerosis

The vast majority of patients with RRMS eventually experience a progressive course with or without superimposed relapses early in the progressive stage. Whether early treatment with the immunomodulatory agents would result in prevention or delay of SPMS in a large number of patients with RRMS or CIS is not yet known. We do know that some patients receiving these agents clearly develop SPMS and that patients who have a delay in diagnosis, choose not to be treated with immunomodulatory agents, are not offered therapy, or cannot afford therapy have and will continue to develop SPMS. In addition to symptomatic therapy, is there anything else to offer these individuals?

There are no studies of glatiramer acetate in patients with SPMS although there were patients whom we would now classify as having SPMS among patients with "chronic progressive MS" in a small prospective randomized study, which showed a marginal effect of treatment versus placebo.

There have been four published studies of IFN-β in SPMS. There were two with IFN-β1b. One in Europe with IFN-β1b showed a modest but statistically significant effect compared with placebo by both primary and secondary clinical outcomes as well as MRI. However, a study in North America with the same agent was negative for the primary outcome although some secondary and MRI outcomes favored active drug over placebo. A study with IFN-β1a given three times a week was negative for primary outcome, but again some secondary outcomes were statistically better in the treatment group compared with the placebo group. Finally, a study with IFN-β1a given once weekly showed superiority of active drug compared with placebo but used a different scale (multiple sclerosis functional composite, MSFC) for the primary outcome. Using the same scale as the other three studies (extended disability status scale, EDSS), there was no difference between the treated and placebo groups.

Because the other three studies did not employ the MSFC as a secondary outcome measure, the reverse comparison cannot be made. If the EDSS is the standard, there is little or no evidence of a major effect in SPMS. If the MSFC, perhaps more sensitive than the EDSS, is used, there is probably an effect of all of these agents. Given the differences in the demographics of patients in these studies and the difficulties in comparing one study with another, what do I feel is the bottom line? For patients with SPMS who are not currently receiving IFN-β and who are having superimposed relapses or enhancing lesions on MRI, I suggest high-dose frequent (three times a week or every other day) SC IFN-β, reasoning but admittedly not knowing that they should receive the highest and most frequent dosing of the agent in SPMS. If they continue to progress, particularly at the same rate, after 1 or certainly 2 years, I discontinue the treatment. One particular problem with IFN-β in SPMS or if used in PPMS (see later) is that it can increase spasticity. This increase in spasticity can generally be treated satisfactorily by initiating or increasing antispasticity therapy (see earlier), but at times the additional antispasticity therapy either is not sufficient or results in increased side effects of the antispasticity drugs. In patients who do not respond to IFN-β, do not tolerate IFN, and/or refuse to or cannot take mitoxantrone, there seems no reason not to try glatiramer acetate because it has such a high degree of tolerability and favorable side effect and adverse event-reaction profile.

MITOXANTRONE (NOVANTRONE)

Mitoxantrone has been approved for use in patients with SPMS at 12 mg/m^2 IV every 3 months. In a prospective randomized study, doses of 12 and 5 mg/m^2 every 3 months were superior to placebo in patients with progressive MS as well as RRMS not responsive to other therapy by both clinical and MRI criteria. Side effects of mitoxantrone therapy include decrease in bone marrow elements, increased susceptibility to infection, nausea and vomiting, and alopecia. Perhaps more important, mitoxantrone therapy can cause a cardiomyopathy at total lifetime doses of 100 to 140 mg/m^2. Therefore, patients who are about to undergo therapy with mitoxantrone, a drug related to doxorubicin (Adriamycin), need to have baseline assessment of cardiac function with 2D-ECHO or MUGA scans. Any patient who has abnormal baseline studies should not be treated with this agent, and patients are limited to 8 to 11 doses of the drug and need to be observed with 2D-ECHO or MUGA scans every year. Although there have been few instances of frank congestive heart failure, abnormalities in cardiac function may become manifest years later with this group of drugs. In addition, there have been a few patients treated with mitoxantrone who have developed leukemia. In patients who have rapidly progressive disease, treatment every 3 months may not be frequent enough so that patients are sometimes treated with 5, 7.5 to 8, or even 12 mg/m^2 monthly or every other month for the first several months. Patients are then given the every 3 month schedule or given the same immunomodulatory therapy or a different immunomodulatory therapy. Some continue the same immunomodulatory agent they were taking when they progressed, but I do not think this is a reasonable approach and there is no evidence to combine mitoxantrone and any immunomodulatory therapy. There are studies that suggest that combining mitoxantrone with pulse therapy with corticosteroids is superior to mitoxantrone by itself.

CYCLOPHOSPHAMIDE (CYTOXAN)*

Cyclophosphamide has a somewhat checkered history as a treatment in progressive MS. Looking at the older studies and studies in which progressive MS was subdivided using the current classification suggests that patients with rapidly progressive MS, particularly those with lesions enhanced with gadolinium or patients with RRMS who do not seem to respond to immunomodulatory therapy, seem to stabilize with cyclophosphamide. Although there are no prospective controlled randomized studies of the use of cyclophosphamide in these circumstances, it is a reasonable alternative in very rapidly progressive SPMS or unresponsive RRMS. I recommend 1 g/kg/m^2 on a monthly basis for 6 months followed by every other month for another 6 months and then giving the patient immunomodulatory therapy, probably a different therapy than the patient was receiving when rapid progression began. In addition to nausea and vomiting, there is suppression of bone marrow elements; patients may develop hemorrhage cystitis, which can generally be prevented by hydration. Again, treatment with cyclophosphamide has been reported to result in development of leukemia as well as bladder tumors, generally with total lifetime doses higher than 85 g/m^2.

*Not FDA approved for this indication.

OTHER IMMUNOSUPPRESSIVE THERAPY

There are many reports of treatment of patients with progressive MS (probably combinations of SPMS and PPMS) as well as RRMS with different cytostatic immunosuppressive agents including azathioprine (Imuran),* methotrexate (Rheumatrex),* and cladribine (Leustatin)* as well as the immunosuppressive drug cyclosporine (Sandimmune).* The overall conclusion is that there is no compelling evidence that any of these agents, particularly at doses that are safe and relatively nontoxic, are effective in MS. More recently, there have been reports of using these drugs in combination with immunomodulatory agents. As in all nonrandomized, noncontrolled studies, only safety issues can be addressed in these reports. Not only do these studies not prove that these combinations are more effective than the individual drugs, but also one can think of reasons why these combinations might be less effective than the individual agents.

COMBINATION THERAPY

Because the approved therapies are clearly only partially effective, it is natural to consider combinations of immunomodulatory agents such as a type I IFN and glatiramer acetate. In a small multicenter trial using MRI as the primary outcome, it was shown that when glatiramer acetate was added for patients treated for more than 6 months with IFN-β1a IM once per week, there was no evidence of an increase in gadolinium enhancing lesions; increased enhancement would imply that glatiramer acetate interfered with the action of IFN. It does not prove that the combination is either additive or synergistic. Therefore, I do not recommend combination therapies other than intermittent pulse corticosteroids added to immunomodulatory therapy.

INTERMITTENT PULSE THERAPY WITH CORTICOSTEROIDS

There are some studies suggesting that treating patients 1 to 3 days each month with IV methylprednisolone (1 g/d) delays progression of disability in patients with SPMS. The studies show a hint of efficacy, and it is worth considering in patients who progress with other agents, as either alternative or additive therapy.

*Not FDA approved for this indication.

Primary Progressive Multiple Sclerosis

With the discontinuation of a study of PPMS treated with glatiramer acetate because it was felt by the safety data monitoring committee that it would not be possible to demonstrate 40% superiority of glatiramer acetate over placebo, there is currently no therapy shown to be effective in slowing the progression of this type of MS. There are no positive prospective controlled randomized studies in PPMS employing IFN-β that demonstrate a positive effect of slowing of progression. Studies with various immunosuppressive agents show no or little efficacy. The observation that many of the placebo-treated patients in the study progressed at a relatively slow rate reinforces earlier natural history data from Canada showing that the rate of progression in many patients is not rapid, particularly when a patient has manifestation of clinical disease in only one functional system. Thus, at this time symptomatic therapy is the mainstay of therapy for most patients with PPMS.

Progressive-Relapsing Multiple Sclerosis

The exact relationship between PRMS, which represents approximately 4% of patients with MS, to PPMS and SPMS is unknown. I treat these patients as I do patients with SPMS.

MYASTHENIA GRAVIS

method of
VERN C. JUEL, M.D.
University of Virginia
Charlottesville, Virginia

Myasthenia gravis, the most common primary disorder of neuromuscular transmission, represents the prototypic autoimmune disorder with well characterized immunology. Four decades ago, one third of patients with myasthenia gravis died, one third had spontaneous remissions, and one third suffered progressive disease. Today, the outlook for patients with myasthenia gravis is significantly more positive, and life expectancy is nearly normal. Advances in diagnostic electrophysiology and in immunologic testing have improved diagnostic sensitivity and accuracy, and the application of immunomodulating treatments has improved prognosis.

EPIDEMIOLOGY

Myasthenia gravis has a prevalence of approximately 14 per 100,000, although the disorder is probably underdiagnosed. Myasthenia gravis has previously been characterized as a disease of younger women and older men. More accurately, myasthenia occurs at a higher rate in early adulthood in women, but in later life the incidence rates for men and women become nearly equal. The demographics of myasthenia gravis have changed somewhat with the aging of the population. The mean age of onset is now approximately 50 years, and there is a slight male predominance. Although myasthenia gravis is not inherited in a mendelian pattern, disease susceptibility is increased significantly for family members of patients with myasthenia gravis.

PATHOPHYSIOLOGY

Although rare genetic forms of myasthenia exist, most patients with myasthenia gravis have autoimmune-acquired myasthenia gravis related to immunologic attack at the postsynaptic membrane of the neuromuscular junction. Myasthenia gravis results from the production of acetylcholine receptor antibodies that bind to the postsynaptic acetylcholine receptor complex and reduce the available binding sites for acetylcholine molecules. Cross-linking of these antibodies and local complement fixation also damage the normally highly infolded postsynaptic membrane so that the membrane becomes simplified. This postsynaptic membrane damage results in a reduced concentration of acetylcholine receptors. These conformational changes reduce the probability of successful neuromuscular transmission for each quantal release of acetylcholine by the motor nerve terminal.

In myasthenia gravis and other autoimmune disorders, loss of immunologic self-tolerance occurs. The thymus is the primary organ essential for establishing self-tolerance, and thymic abnormalities have long been recognized in association with myasthenia gravis. Thymoma occurs in about 10% of patients with myasthenia gravis. Most of these thymic tumors are benign and encapsulated. About 70% of patients demonstrate thymic hyperplasia in which active germinal centers can be demonstrated. In the germinal centers, B lymphocytes interact with T helper lymphocytes to produce antibodies. Thymomas are often associated with an earlier age of onset, more fulminant disease, and higher titers of acetylcholine receptor antibodies.

CLINICAL FEATURES

Patients with myasthenia gravis present with complaints of fluctuating and fatigable weakness of specific muscle groups rather than with generalized fatigue or pain. The weakness is variable and is often worse late in the day. High body temperatures and sustained exercise may also worsen the myasthenic weakness. The majority of patients develop initial symptoms of extraocular muscle weakness. The course is frequently variable, particularly within the first year of the disease, but 75% of patients progress to weakness of oropharyngeal and limb muscles within the first 2 years. Weakness remains confined to ocular muscles in 25% of patients. Most patients reach a nadir of strength within the first year after disease onset. Initial presentations with oropharyngeal weakness and with limb weakness are more uncommon. Myasthenic symptoms and signs may worsen in a setting of thyroid disease, systemic illness, pregnancy, increased body temperature, and drugs that impair

TABLE 1. **Drugs Producing Worsening of Myasthenic Weakness**

Neuromuscular blocking agents
Antibiotics
  Aminoglycosides, particularly gentamycin
  Macrolides, particularly erythromycin and azithromycin (Zithromax)
Cardiovascular agents
  β-Blockers
  Calcium channel blockers
  Procainamide (Pronestyl)
  Quinidine
Corticosteroids
Magnesium salts
  Antacids containing magnesium
  Laxatives containing magnesium
Lithium
Iodinated contrast agents
D-Penicillamine should never be used in myasthenic patients

neuromuscular transmission (Table 1). Although such medications are not absolutely contraindicated in myasthenia gravis (with the exception of D-penicillamine), physicians should exercise caution when they must be used and recognize that myasthenic weakness may increase.

Symptoms and Physical Findings

Ocular weakness is most often manifest as fluctuating and fatigable ptosis and binocular diplopia. Many patients report difficulties with driving, reading, or watching television. Bright lights may be quite unsettling for these patients. Retrospectively, many patients report periods of blurred vision before they were able to discern dual visual images. Examination should demonstrate asymmetrical weakness of multiple extraocular muscles not attributable to a single cranial neuropathy with normal pupillary function. Ptosis is generally asymmetrical and may be associated with ipsilateral frontalis muscle contraction to help compensate for the weak levator palpebrae.

Oropharyngeal weakness may involve facial, jaw, palatal, and lingual muscles. Patients may complain of a change in voice with increased nasal quality and hoarseness. Nasal regurgitation may occur on attempts to swallow liquids, and candy or tough meats may be difficult to chew. On examination, most patients exhibit weak eye closure that can easily be overcome by the examiner. In the lower face, patients may exhibit difficulty holding air within the cheeks, and a "myasthenic snarl" may be observed with smiling attempts by the patient. The snarl follows contraction of the middle portion of the upper lip while the upper mouth corners fail to contract. Patients may assume a thoughtful resting posture by placing the thumb beneath the chin in order to hold the jaw closed in the setting of weak jaw opening muscles and neck extensors. Tongue weakness may be demonstrated with the patient's inability to protrude either cheek with the tongue. With severe tongue weakness, the tongue may not protrude beyond the lips. Neck flexor and extensor muscles are often weak in myasthenia gravis. Although the neck flexors are usually weaker, a "dropped head syndrome" related to neck extensor weakness may be observed. Weakness may involve any muscle group in the limbs, although the deltoids, triceps brachii, wrist and finger extensors, and foot dorsiflexors are often involved.

When respiration is compromised in myasthenia gravis, it is often the result of a combination of upper airway muscle weakness involving the palatal, pharyngeal, and lingual muscles along with inspiratory muscle weakness involving the diaphragm and scalenes. Myasthenic crisis, defined as respiratory failure from myasthenia gravis, is usually precipitated by infection, surgery, or rapid tapering of immune suppression. It is important to recognize the significant contribution of the upper airway muscles in patents in myasthenic crisis. Ventilatory parameters such as vital capacity and negative inspiratory flow may suggest good respiratory function while the endotracheal tube is in place. However, when the stenting effect of the endotracheal tube is eliminated after extubation, the patient may suffer respiratory compromise because of upper airway collapse.

DIAGNOSTIC TESTING

Edrophonium Chloride (Tensilon) Testing

Edrophonium testing is performed by administering up to 10 mg of intravenous edrophonium chloride (Tensilon) in the setting of suspected myasthenic weakness. The main limitation of edrophonium testing relates to choosing an objective muscle strength parameter for assessment. Accordingly, edrophonium testing is most useful in patients with significant ptosis or restricted extraocular movements which are more objectively graded. In other patterns of weakness such as limb muscle weakness, patient's volition and the muscarinic effects of edrophonium may complicate strength measurement and render the test uninterpretable.

Edrophonium testing is performed less frequently than in the past because of the availability of acetylcholine receptor antibody testing and electrophysiologic studies to support a diagnosis of myasthenia gravis. Unless significant weakness is present at the time of testing, edrophonium testing has no value. False-positive edrophonium testing has occurred in other neurologic conditions including motor neuron disease, peripheral neuropathy, and cranial neuropathy.

When edrophonium testing is performed, a needle, butterfly line, or intravenous catheter is inserted into an antecubital vein. Because of muscarinic side effects including bronchospasm and bradycardia, atropine should be readily available. An incremental dosing schedule should be utilized so that if muscle strength is clearly improved within 1 minute following any dosing increment, the test is considered positive and the procedure ended. In this way, the risk of giving excessive edrophonium and eliciting untoward muscarinic side effects is reduced. Initially, a 2-mg dose of intravenous edrophonium is given; then the patient is observed for 1 minute for improvement in the prespecified strength parameter (e.g., ptosis). If there is no improvement after 1 minute, an additional 3-mg dose of edrophonium is given. If no improvement occurs after 1 minute, the remaining 5-mg dose of edrophonium is administered.

Prior to the widespread use of immunomodulators for myasthenia gravis, edrophonium testing was routinely performed to assess whether patients were over- or underdosed with long-acting cholinesterase inhibitors such as pyridostigmine bromide (Mestinon). This practice has been largely abandoned and is potentially dangerous because cholinergic weakness may develop and result in respiratory arrest.

Electrophysiologic Testing

Repetitive nerve stimulation studies involve 2- to 3-Hz stimulation of motor or mixed nerves with measurement of the amplitude and area of the resulting compound muscle action potentials. The findings are abnormal when the amplitude of the fourth compound muscle action potential is reduced more than 10% from the baseline value. The sensitivity of this test is increased when recordings are made from clinically weak muscles. In general, proximal muscles including facial muscles, the trapezius, deltoid, and biceps brachii are more likely to exhibit abnormal findings. Overall, these studies are approximately 60% sensitive in ocular and generalized forms of myasthenia gravis. They are relatively more sensitive in generalized and relatively less sensitive in ocular myasthenia gravis.

Single-fiber electromyography is the most sensitive diagnostic test for detecting abnormal neuromuscular transmission. In single-fiber electromyography, muscle fiber action potentials generated by the same motor neuron are recorded and statistically analyzed to evaluate neuromuscular transmission. When a facial and a limb muscle are studied, single-fiber electromyography is over 97% sensitive for detecting myasthenia gravis. However, single-fiber electromyography also demonstrates abnormal neuromuscular transmission related to other motor unit disorders including motor neuropathic and myopathic processes. Thus, single-fiber electromyography must be performed and interpreted in the appropriate context. It is a time-consuming test requiring special expertise and equipment that are not available in all centers.

Antibody Testing

Acetylcholine receptor binding antibody testing in myasthenia gravis is a very specific but somewhat less sensitive diagnostic modality. Positive antibody studies confirm myasthenia gravis in a patient with appropriate symptoms and findings. In generalized myasthenia gravis, acetylcholine receptor binding antibodies are present in approximately 80% of patients, but they are present in only 55% of patients with ocular myasthenia gravis. About one half of prepubertal children with myasthenia gravis are seronegative. Acetylcholine receptor antibody titers correlate poorly with disease severity or activity, and seronegative patients do not necessarily have less severe disease. Because of this, after establishing the presence of acetylcholine receptor antibodies, we do not routinely follow antibody titers. It is reasonable to repeat antibody studies to document seroconversion in patients with initially negative antibody titers. Rare false-positive acetylcholine receptor antibodies have been observed in the setting of other autoimmune diseases such as systemic lupus erythematosus, rheumatoid arthritis, and inflammatory neuropathy. False-positive antibodies have also been reported in motor neuron disease, in patients with thymoma without myasthenia gravis, and in relatives of patients with myasthenia gravis.

Other Testing

Chest imaging studies should be performed in patients with myasthenia gravis to exclude the presence of thymoma. We obtain chest computed tomography studies, which are more sensitive than chest radiographs for delineating anterior mediastinal masses. Because myasthenia gravis often coexists with other autoimmune disorders, we perform testing for autoimmune thyroid disease, pernicious anemia, and other connective tissue diseases when clinically appropriate.

TREATMENT

As in many rare disorders, there are relatively few controlled clinical trials in myasthenia gravis. Treatment must be individualized to account for the distribution and severity of myasthenia and to consider the patient's other medical co-morbidities.

Cholinesterase Inhibitors

Cholinesterase inhibitors impair the hydrolysis of acetylcholine at the neuromuscular junction. In this way, they often provide symptomatic improvement in strength, although they do not retard the autoimmune attack on the postsynaptic membrane. Cholinesterase inhibitors are often the initial treatment in myasthenia gravis. The clinical response to cholinesterase inhibitors is often incomplete and variable between patients, in the same patient over time, and between various muscle groups within the same patient.

Pyridostigmine bromide (Mestinon) is the most commonly used cholinesterase inhibitor. Pyridostigmine is favored by most practitioners over neostigmine bromide (Prostigmin) because of fewer gastrointestinal side effects. Pyridostigmine is supplied in 60-mg scored tablets that allow smaller dosages and as a syrup (60 mg per 5 mL). The initial dosage of pyridostigmine is 30 to 60 mg every 4 to 8 hours. A timed-release pyridostigmine (Mestinon Timespan 180 mg) has been suggested for nighttime dosing in patients with significant weakness on awakening. Because of erratic absorption leading to under- or overdosing and because of the frequent tendency to overdose this medication, most practitioners disfavor its use.

The dosing schedule of pyridostigmine should be individualized in order to treat the most symptomatic muscle weakness. We typically begin with pyridostigmine 30 mg three times a day and advance slowly to a maximum dosage of about 90 mg four times a day. Patients should notice improved strength at 30 to 45 minutes after dosing, and the effects should wear off just prior to the next scheduled dose. Overdosing may cause increased weakness. If a patient becomes weaker despite increasing pyridostigmine dosages, no further increase in the dosage should be made, and an immunomodulating treatment should be considered.

Muscarinic side effects, particularly gastrointestinal symptoms of nausea, vomiting, abdominal cramping, and diarrhea, are often associated with cholinesterase inhibitor use in a dose-dependent fashion. Increased bronchial secretions and salivation may also occur. The gastrointestinal symptoms may be managed with glycopyrrolate (Robinul), diphenoxylate hydrochloride with atropine (Lomotil), and loperamide hydrochloride (Imodium).

Thymectomy

Although there is a consensus among neuromuscular specialists that myasthenic patients can benefit from thymectomy, there are differing views on the appropriate circumstances for thymectomy. Thymectomy is performed in an attempt to induce complete myasthenic remission or to reduce long-term requirements for immunosuppression. Except in very advanced age, thymectomy is recommended for all patients with thymoma. We also recommend thymectomy in all patients between puberty and age 65 years with generalized myasthenia gravis. Patients older than 65 years represent a higher surgical risk and may not respond as well to thymectomy as younger patients. Unless a thymoma is present, if the life expectancy is less than 10 years, a thymectomy should not be performed. Response to thymectomy is variable and generally occurs within the first 2 years following the procedure but may be delayed for up to 10 years. The best responses occur in young patients, in those in whom thymectomy is performed early in the course of myasthenia, and in patients without thymoma. A transsternal approach is preferred because it allows the best exposure of the mediastinum for exploration and excision of all thymic tissue. Incomplete thymic removal may reduce the benefit of thymectomy. Because transcervical and thorascopic approaches provide more limited exposure and increase the possibility of incomplete thymic removal, they are not generally favored. Although thymectomy is not generally recommended for patients with ocular myasthenia gravis, younger patients with ocular myasthenia gravis treated early may experience significant remission and not progress to generalized myasthenia.

Corticosteroids

Most myasthenic patients experience significant improvement within the first 2 months of treatment with corticosteroids. We use high-dose prednisone beginning at a dose of 1.5 to 2.0 mg/kg/d or at 60 to 80 mg/d. Improvement in strength is generally observed within 1 to 2 weeks, and peak improvement occurs at 6 to 8 weeks of treatment. At this point, the dosing may be changed to 100 to 120 mg in an alternate-day dosing schedule. Tapering to a lowest effective dose should be done slowly. In the best circumstances with rapid and complete improvement in myasthenia, the alternate-day dosage can be reduced by 20 mg/month to 60 mg every other day, then by 10 mg/month to 30 mg every other day, then by 5 mg/month to 10 to 15 mg every other day. During the taper, patients should be monitored closely for return of myasthenic weakness. In this event, the prednisone dosage may be increased and/or an adjunctive immunosuppressant medication may be initiated. Most patients require a low alternate-day dosage between 5 and 15 mg to prevent relapse of myasthenic weakness for many years or indefinitely. Although occasional patients are successfully tapered off corticosteroids without other immune suppression, most require some form of immune suppression to prevent relapse.

Corticosteroid-induced exacerbations with temporarily worsened myasthenic weakness may occur within the first 7 to 10 days of treatment with prednisone and last up to 1 week. About 25% of patients experience transient weakness after starting steroids. In most patients, the increased weakness can be monitored until it resolves and treated with cholinesterase inhibitors as necessary. In patients with oropharyngeal or respiratory weakness, however, corticosteroids may induce myasthenic crisis. Because of this, patients with oropharyngeal, respiratory, or severe generalized weakness should be hospitalized for the first week of treatment with high-dose prednisone for monitoring of vital capacity and bulbar function. Plasma exchange may be used prior to starting prednisone to prevent or to reduce the severity of steroid-induced myasthenic exacerbations and to achieve a more rapid response to prednisone. Once improvement begins after starting steroids, worsening of myasthenic weakness related to steroids is unusual.

Prednisone may also be introduced at a low dosage with slow escalation of the dose. This technique may reduce but does not eliminate the risk of steroid-related myasthenic exacerbations. In addition, a longer period of time may be required to achieve improved strength or to establish that a given patient responds to corticosteroids with this approach.

Side effects of corticosteroids are well known but are generally dose dependent. Judicious yet steady tapering to the lowest effective dosage helps to minimize these side effects. Weight gain, edema, osteoporosis, acne, insomnia, mood changes, cataracts, glucose intolerance or worsened diabetes mellitus, hyperlipidemia, and avascular necrosis of the femoral head represent the prominent adverse effects of corticosteroids. In order to help minimize these, we attempt to move the patients to alternate-day dosing as soon as feasible, encourage a diet low in sodium and fat, and prescribe supplemental calcium and vitamin D. A baseline bone density assessment is performed in postmenopausal women and is repeated every 6 to 12 months. H_2 receptor blockers are used in patients with gastritis or peptic ulcer disease.

Azathioprine (Imuran)

Azathioprine (Imuran)* inhibits T lymphocyte proliferation and is effective as a single immunomodulating treatment for myasthenia gravis or for use as a steroid-sparing agent. However, in myasthenia gravis, the effect of azathioprine is delayed for 4 to 12 months with a maximum effect at about 18 months. It may be used as an initial treatment in patients with mild symptoms controlled with cholinesterase inhibitors. For patients requiring a more rapid response, it may be used in combination with high-dose prednisone. The starting dose is 50 mg/d, and this daily dose may be increased by 50 mg each week to a target dose of 2 to 3 mg/kg/d.

A serious, idiosyncratic allergic reaction is observed in 10% to 15% of patients and necessitates stopping the medication. The reaction occurs within the first 2 weeks of treatment and is characterized by rash, fever, abdominal pain, malaise, nausea, and vomiting. The symptoms resolve within 24 hours of stopping azathioprine and recur with rechallenge. Blood monitoring for patients taking azathioprine should include blood count and transaminases weekly for the first month, then monthly for the first year, then every 3 to 6 months thereafter. Azathioprine causes myelosuppression in a dose-dependent fashion. Macrocytosis is expected and is acceptable within the therapeutic range. The dosage should be reduced if the white blood cell (WBC) count falls below 3500/mm^3, and azathioprine treatment should be interrupted for WBC counts less than 3000/mm^3. Transaminase elevations of less than twofold are permissible before dosage reductions become necessary. Pancreatitis is a rare idiosyncratic reaction with azathioprine, and evaluation with serum amylase and lipase assays should be considered for patients with persistent abdominal pain.

Cyclosporine (Sandimmune)

Cyclosporine* inhibits cell-mediated immune responses by inhibiting T helper cells and by increasing expression of T suppressor cells. Compared to azathioprine, cyclosporine produces a relatively more rapid onset of benefit at between 1 and 3 months of treatment with maximum benefit at around 6 months. The dosage is 4 to 6 mg/kg/d in two divided daily doses 12 hours apart. The target trough level is 100 to 200 ng/mL. Higher trough levels are associated with nephrotoxicity. Monthly monitoring of blood pressure, blood urea nitrogen and creatinine, and trough cyclosporine levels should be performed. The dosage should be reduced if increases in creatinine of more than 50% occur. Cyclosporine is often used in combination with alternate-day prednisone for increased effect. Side effects include nephrotoxicity, hypertension, tremor, hirsutism, and headaches. Because many medications interfere with cyclosporine metabolism, new medications should be added to a patient's regimen with caution and with monitoring of trough cyclosporine levels, blood urea nitrogen, creatinine, and blood pressure.

*Not FDA approved for this indication.

Cyclophosphamide (Cytoxan)

Cyclophosphamide* is an alkylating agent that blocks cell proliferation. It is an effective medication for myasthenia gravis, although it is not widely used because of its toxicity and the availability of safer immune suppressants. Side effects include hemorrhagic cystitis, alopecia, leukopenia, anorexia, nausea, vomiting, infections, and the potential for increased long-term risk for malignancy.

Plasma Exchange

Plasma exchange is an invasive procedure by which a patient's plasma containing antibodies is removed and replaced by albumin or fresh frozen plasma. This technique produces effective but temporary improvement in myasthenia. Plasma exchange is indicated to treat myasthenic crisis or exacerbation, to improve strength before a surgical procedure, to prevent steroid-induced exacerbation in patients with oropharyngeal or respiratory weakness, and to provide a chronic intermittent therapy in the rare patient refractory to all other treatments. The onset of improvement is variable but is usually observed within 2 to 3 days. A series of four to six exchanges is performed every other day with removal of 2 to 3 L of plasma at each session. Following a plasma exchange series, the improvement in strength is only temporary and may last several weeks at best unless an immunosuppressant is used. Repeated series of plasma exchange treatments do not produce more long-lasting improvement in myasthenia. Complications of plasma exchange are related to the need for large-bore venous access and to large fluid shifts that occur during the procedure. Venous access through temporary catheters placed in the antecubital veins significantly reduces the complications related to central venous catheters including pneumothorax, central line infections, and thrombosis.

Intravenous Immunoglobulin

High-dose intravenous immunoglobulin (IGIV)* at 2 g/kg over 2 to 5 days elicits improvement in strength in more than half of myasthenic patients in 1 week. The improvement may last for several weeks or even months. The mechanism is thought to be related to down-regulation of antibodies directed at the acetylcholine receptor and/or introduction of anti-idiotypic antibodies. IGIV is most often used as an alternative

*Not FDA approved for this indication.

to plasma exchange in patients requiring relatively rapid short-term improvement in the setting of poor venous access. IGIV is sometimes used periodically in patients who cannot tolerate or who fail other immunosuppressants. Side effects of IGIV include volume overload related to the large volumes infused because IGIV preparations are prepared as 5% to 10% solutions. The solute load is also large, and patients with preexisting renal insufficiency or diabetic nephropathy are at risk for development of acute tubular necrosis when IGIV is administered over shorter periods of time. Other side effects include headache, chills, and fever, which may be controlled by pretreatment with acetaminophen and diphenhydramine (Benadryl). Patients may experience vascular headache associated with the infusion, which often responds to triptan agents or dihydroergotamine. Some patients may experience aseptic meningitis that is self-limited. Serum immunoglobulin quantitation should be performed before IGIV infusions to exclude a selective IgA deficiency. These patients may develop anaphylaxis related to the trace amounts of IgA in the IGIV preparation and should receive other types of treatment.

Treatment Overview

Treatment of patients with ocular myasthenia gravis should begin with cholinesterase inhibitors. If symptoms are not sufficiently relieved, consider adding prednisone. In younger patients with recent onset ocular myasthenia gravis, consider thymectomy to induce remission and prevent disease progression. For patients younger than 65 years with generalized myasthenia gravis, consider thymectomy with preoperative plasma exchange if oropharyngeal or respiratory weakness is present. If weakness increases or fails to improve at 1 year after thymectomy, consider an immunosuppressant medication. For patients age 65 or older with generalized myasthenia gravis, begin treatment with cholinesterase inhibitors. If significant symptoms persist, add azathioprine if a delay in response can be tolerated. Otherwise, prednisone or cyclosporine may be used for immune suppression.

NEW THERAPIES

Mycophenolate mofetil (CellCept),* the prodrug of mycophenolate, is a selective inhibitor of inosine monophosphate dehydrogenase that selectively inhibits B and T lymphocyte proliferation. Mycophenolate mofetil is currently used to prevent transplant rejection. Preliminary studies of mycophenolate mofetil in myasthenia gravis demonstrate that it is safe and effective and that it produces significant improvement in myasthenic weakness in 4 to 8 weeks. It has a significantly faster onset of activity than azathioprine and significantly less toxicity than cyclosporine. The dosage utilized in preliminary studies has been 1000 to 1500 mg twice a day. Side effects reported in transplant studies include diarrhea and myelosuppression. A multicenter trial is currently being performed to assess the degree of improvement in myasthenic patients taking mycophenolate mofetil. The results of this trial should help to define further its role in the management of myasthenia gravis.

*Not FDA approved for this indication.

TRIGEMINAL NEURALGIA

method of
HARRY VAN LOVEREN, M.D.
University of South Florida
Tampa, Florida

Although trigeminal neuralgia (also known as tic douloureux) is a rare diagnosis that affects only 1 in 20,000 people, it is important for general practitioners and dentists to be familiar with this diagnosis. The facial pains that occur are terrible and devastating yet respond well to treatment. The myelin sheath of the trigeminal nerve is unraveling in these patients, much like an electrical wire with poor insulation. Stimulation of ordinary touch fibers causes adjacent pain fibers to fire (ephaptic transmission). To the patient, firing of the pain fibers related to ephaptic transmission is not perceptibly different from firing of the pain fibers caused by an outside stimulus such as an ice pick jammed through the face. Misdiagnosis and delayed treatment are common and lead too often to unnecessary dental extractions or nasal sinus operations in the region of pain.

DIAGNOSIS

The diagnosis of trigeminal neuralgia is rooted in the clinical history with little support from examination and no support from testing other than the exclusion of alternative or associated diagnoses. The pain of trigeminal neuralgia is *paroxysmal*, coming in sudden attacks. It has common triggers such as touching the face, washing, and brushing the teeth. Oral activities such as talking or chewing are common triggers. The character of the pain is *lancinating*, meaning sharp in quality, and is described using terms such as stabbing, jabbing, or electrical shocks. When the patient uses terms such as aching, burning, or throbbing, the clinician should become suspicious of the diagnosis. These are terms more often used to describe trigeminal neuropathies that occur after trauma to peripheral trigeminal nerve branches such as the trauma of dental extraction or surgery. Similarly, neuropathy should be suspected if the patient describes the pain as constant or chronic rather than paroxysmal. Pain is confined to the trigeminal nerve territory almost always on one side. Bilateral pain occurs in less than 1% of patients and is often associated with multiple sclerosis (MS). The three divisions of the trigeminal nerve, V1 to the eye and forehead, V2 to the nose and cheek, and V3 to the lower face, jaw, and tongue, can be affected together or individually. The most common division affected is V3 and the least common V1.

The natural history of trigeminal neuralgia is one of spontaneous remissions and exacerbations. Initial remissions are commonly as long as 6 months but remissions become progressively shorter over the years and exacerbations at least seem more severe or the patient's tolerance for the pain diminishes. The frequency of spontaneous remissions is responsible for the many pseudoremedies that have been reported.

The importance of accurate clinical diagnosis cannot be overemphasized because it represents the primary predictor of the success of treatment. Carelessly extrapolating the diagnosis to include the atypical facial pains results in unnecessary surgical procedures that leave patients with facial numbness, paresthesias, or dysesthesias in addition to their original pain complaint.

MULTIPLE SCLEROSIS

The potential association between MS and trigeminal neuralgia warrants specific attention. Approximately 5% of patients with MS can suffer from trigeminal neuralgia during the course of their illness because of a sclerotic demyelinating plaque along the trigeminal system. In 5% of these patients with MS-related tic, trigeminal neuralgia can be the first symptom of MS. Therefore, every patient with trigeminal neuralgia should be screened by a simple series of questions that can detect possible MS by highlighting other scattered episodes of neurologic dysfunction or deficit. The most common complaints involve transient unilateral visual loss or transient episodes of numbness in areas of the body outside the trigeminal distribution. The importance of detecting MS in patients with trigeminal neuralgia is related to the lower chance of success with surgical microvascular decompression because it does not address the specific cause of facial pain in this subset of patients.

EXAMINATION

The neurologic examination in trigeminal neuralgia should be normal. On rare occasion the examiner can detect a subtle sensory loss in the trigeminal sensory territory during or just after a particularly severe flurry of attacks. This is ascribed to a fatigue of the trigeminal nerve similar to a postictal Todd paralysis of brain that occurs after seizure. A severe or sustained trigeminal sensory loss should precipitate magnetic resonance imaging (MRI) to exclude the rare benign tumor or arteriovenous malformation (AVM) that can cause a secondary trigeminal neuralgia. Suspicion of a mass lesion causing secondary trigeminal neuralgia should be raised with any neurologic deficit of the cranial nerves in the patient with otherwise typical pains including facial palsy and hearing loss, which represent the two cranial nerves most likely to be affected in this location.

TESTING

It is recommended that every patient diagnosed with trigeminal neuralgia undergo MRI. This detects the rare patient who has typical pains of trigeminal neuralgia, a normal cranial nerve examination, and yet harbors a tumor or AVM as the cause. The MRI also has 98% sensitivity in detecting MS as the etiology for the pain. Radiographic evaluation specifically to determine the presence or absence of trigeminal vascular compression is neither mandatory nor routine. The proximity of arteries and veins to cranial nerves is commonplace in patients who are asymptomatic. The MRI detects the patients who are likely to have vascular compression from a tortuous dolichoectatic vertebral or basilar artery. This is useful to surgeons in counseling the preoperative patient toward reasonable expectations. Because the vertebrobasilar complex cannot be physically displaced, vascular decompression procedures are less successful and recurrence is higher. It is useful if patients understand this prior to surgery.

MEDICAL TREATMENT

Medical treatment should begin with carbamazepine (Tegretol) in divided oral doses (200 mg three times a day in young healthy patients; 100 mg three times a day in elderly patients). Dosing is titrated according to pain response, allowing 3 to 5 days for each change in dose to reach a serum steady-state level. It is not necessary to measure serum levels. The dose is escalated until either a remission is produced or signs of toxicity emerge, including nausea, lethargy, confusion, or unsteadiness. If therapeutic effect cannot be achieved before reaching toxicity, other agents should be tried. These agents include gabapentin (Neurontin), baclofen (Lioresal), and phenytoin (Dilantin). These are drugs with other primary indications, especially as antiepileptics. Their ability to decrease spontaneous firing in irritable neurons is thought to apply to suppression of ephaptic transmission in the trigeminal system of patients with trigeminal neuralgia. Narcotic analgesics are not effective in trigeminal neuralgia. Over time, nearly 75% of patients with trigeminal neuralgia fail to respond to medical treatment because of allergy, toxicity, bone marrow suppression, liver inflammation, or tolerance (tolerance refers to escalating doses with diminishing effect). During chronic medical treatment, white blood cells and liver enzymes should be evaluated biannually. When remission does occur, the patient should be instructed to taper medical treatment slowly and if possible enter a pain-free, drug-free period.

SURGICAL TREATMENT

Surgery is prescribed only when medical therapy has failed. The current best surgical treatment for trigeminal neuralgia is microvascular decompression (MVD) of the trigeminal root in the posterior fossa. Mobilizing arterial branches away from the nerve and holding them at bay with spongelike material provides a high rate of sustained relief. The actual neurophysiology behind the vascular compression theory remains poorly understood. The advantage of

MVD is the ability to stop pain without producing sensory loss. The disadvantages are related to the complications of general anesthesia and craniotomy. If the patient cannot tolerate craniotomy because of physiologic age or infirmity, a series of so-called ablative procedures can be used. These are procedures that damage the nerve in a way that produces a degree of numbness that in turn blocks pain conduction. The most commonly used is percutaneous stereotactic rhizotomy (PSR), in which an electrode is passed through the face into the trigeminal ganglion and radio frequency heat used to ablate pain fibers. Another method, percutaneous trigeminal balloon compression (PTBC), uses the pressure of a small balloon inflated in the ganglion to ablate pain fibers. Percutaneous glycerol rhizotomy (PGR) consists of injecting the chemical glycerol into the ganglion to ablate fibers. Finally, the nerve can be ablated using radiation such as in gamma knife radiosurgery (GKRS). Each of these procedures has specific indications according to the age of the patient, distribution of pain, and severity of pain. PSR is best suited to patients with pain in the V2 and V3 divisions. PTBC is best suited to patients with V1 pain because it tends to spare the corneal reflex by taking advantage of the differential sensitivity of corneal reflex fibers to pressure versus heat. GKRS has a long delay to relief, a low rate of relief compared with the other available procedures, and generally also produces facial numbness in return for relief. Therefore, GKRS should be reserved for only a few selected patients.

ACUTE FACIAL PARALYSIS (BELL'S PALSY)

method of
ANGELO FORMENTI, M.D.
Ospedale Fatebenefratelli e Oftalmico
Milan, Italy

The human face is able to express the deepest feelings, and such expression is essential to social relationships. A facial palsy will obviously therefore be a great problem, not only for patients but also for their relatives, friends, colleagues, and last but not least, their doctors.

ETIOLOGY AND DIFFERENTIAL DIAGNOSIS

The long pathway of the facial nerve from the brainstem to the facial muscles can be subdivided into two portions: intracranial and extracranial. The many relationships of the facial nerve with anatomic structures and organs often play a basic role in the etiology of facial palsy, such that Mark May could affirm: "Peripheral facial paralysis is a diagnostic challenge."

When confronted with acute facial paralysis, we have to keep in mind that Bell's palsy (BP) is a diagnosis of exclusion, and we should reserve this eponym for cases with an "unknown cause" (i.e., idiopathic palsy). The most common causes of acute peripheral paralysis are summarized in Figure 1.

On the basis of the most recent studies, we can affirm that idiopathic facial nerve paralysis (BP) is the most common mononeuritis observed in clinical practice. Nonetheless, the pathogenesis of this frequent condition, widely debated for a long time, still remains not completely clarified. The concept of BP as a mononeuritic process has been debated, and it has been suggested that BP is indeed a polyneuritis involving prominent compromise of the seventh cranial nerve. A viral or immune-related pathogenesis has been proposed, and recent evidence has lent support to the hypothesis of a pathogenetic role of herpes simplex virus (HSV), which was first suggested on the basis of serologic data in the 1970s. In particular, the HSV genome has been identified by polymerase chain reaction in the endoneural fluid of BP patients who underwent surgical decompression. Moreover, the therapeutic strategies adopted to improve the outcome of the often benign course of BP reflect the different underlying hypotheses (see later).

EVALUATION

What should be done when BP is diagnosed? First, it is necessary to quantify the degree of nerve damage and therefore the degree of paralysis. Such quantification allows us to monitor not only the functional recovery of facial muscles but also the presence of sequelae (synkinesis, contractures, hemifacial spasms). Particular attention is required because facial palsy causes a wide range of functional defects, as well as deformity of the face at rest.

An international standardized system of reporting has been difficult to create. Many authors have proposed their own scales for reporting deficits in facial function, but to date, I think that the House-Brakmann system for evaluating facial nerve deficits (1985) is the most useful. This system encompasses six levels, from I (normal) to VI (total paralysis), with a very minute description of the facial deficits for each category, at rest as well as in motion. In this way it is possible to evaluate not only the natural history of BP

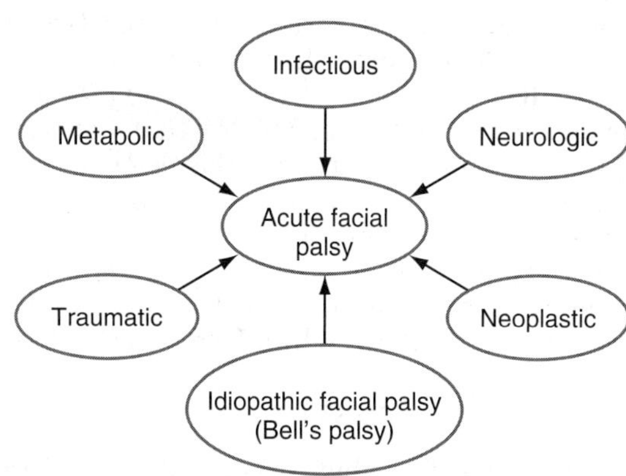

Figure 1. Most frequent causes of acute facial palsy.

but also its prognosis (it is obvious that an incomplete palsy, caused by limited injury to the nerve, will have a better outcome than a paralysis classified as type IV or V [a seriously injured nerve] in the House-Brakmann classification).

In this regard it is also very useful to perform certain electrodiagnostic tests. Electroneuromyography, also called evoked electromyography (EEMG), was introduced by Fish and Esslen (1972) to allow evoked compound muscle action potentials to be studied and recorded, with a precise quantitative assessment of the response. The amplitude of the evoked potential is expressed as a percentage of the one recorded on the normal side. If performed within 14 days after the onset of BP, EEMG has proved to be an important prognostic test. In BP, the portion of the nerve distal to the lesion continues to regularly conduct stimuli, at least for 3 days after the onset of paralysis. From the third to the fifth day, we can observe by EEMG that the amplitude of the evoked potential progressively decreases if the axons are degenerating; when the EEMG response decreases to 25% or less of the normal side, the degree of axonal degeneration will be so severe that recovery will be delayed and will very probably be incomplete. When the evoked potential is less than 10% of the normal side, only partial recovery is expected. In practice, EEMG reliably reflects the electrical changes that occur in the first 2 weeks of a facial palsy.

Fourteen days after the onset of paralysis, electromyography (EMG) becomes the test of choice because at this time, fibrillations indicate axonal degeneration. If only a few fibrillations are present, complete recovery can be expected, but when many fibrillations and few motor unit action potentials are observed, partial functional recovery and some sequelae will be expected.

In the recovery phase of facial paralysis, EEMG is not useful for monitoring and evaluating functional restoration because facial function can also return without any recordable evoked potential. In this phase EMG is the most efficient electrophysiologic test in predicting the start of recovery and the seriousness of any residual deficits. The beginning of recovery is marked by recording of polyphasic motor responses. As regeneration progresses, EMG can record abnormally large motor units (giant units), which are the result of aberrant reinnervation of some muscle fibers. This phenomenon is the basis of synkinesis, the most common sequela of facial palsy.

With the results of EEMG and a system for evaluating facial nerve deficits, it is possible to estimate the prognosis of restoration of facial function with a high degree of accuracy. On the basis of the literature and our experience, we can affirm that 90% of patients with incomplete paralysis and a response to EEMG that is greater than 10% beyond the first 2 weeks after onset of the palsy will have a satisfactory recovery; conversely, 80% of patients who in the same period have complete paralysis and an evoked potential by EEMG lower than 10% will have an unsatisfactory recovery. It is this second group of patients who require the greatest therapeutic effort to modify the natural history of the facial palsy and prevent complications from nerve degeneration.

TREATMENT

The therapeutic strategies proposed to improve the outcome of BP by accelerating recovery and decreasing the proportion of patients with permanent sequelae reflect not only the most accepted underlying etiologic hypotheses but also the doubts regarding the real nosologic entity of BP. It has repeatedly been stressed that the definition of BP covers a spectrum of clinical conditions with heterogeneous biologic and pathogenetic background. Accordingly, the inflammatory component has been addressed for many years with the use of steroids, and more recently, the infective hypothesis has been tested with antiviral drugs. In any case, while awaiting a double-blind, sufficiently extensive study with a design that can definitively demonstrate the independent and cumulative benefit of steroid-based therapy and anti-HSV treatment, it seems justified at present to propose a treatment schedule for 10 days with both drugs:

Prednisone: 1.0 mg/kg for 3 days, 0.75 mg/kg for 3 days, 0.50 mg/kg for 2 days, and 0.25 mg/kg for 2 days.
Famciclovir (Famvir)*: 500 mg three times per day.

My experience has shown that it is essential to start therapy as soon as possible, within the first 3 days and never beyond 7 days after onset of the paralysis, because the evolution of BP and the extent of recovery seem to be strictly linked to the timing of initiation of treatment.

It is important to be aware that facial paralysis can result in eye problems that could be serious if disregarded. Unsatisfactory eyelid closure can lead to corneal lesions requiring ophthalmologic treatment. In general, eye care is directed at humidification of the eye with the use of eyedrops and ointments. Particularly at night, it is very important to keep the eyelids closed with tape.

*Not FDA approved for this indication.

PARKINSONISM

method of
RONALD F. PFEIFFER, M.D.
University of Tennessee Health Science Center
Memphis, Tennessee

Parkinsonism is a general term that encompasses a variety of disease processes that display a constellation of clinical features consisting of rigidity, bradykinesia, tremor, and postural instability. These disease processes also share, at least in part, a common anatomic localization involving the basal ganglia. Parkinson's disease is the most prevalent of the parkinsonian disorders and most therapeutic modalities are based on experience in treating Parkinson's disease. Therefore, the bulk of this article focuses on the diagnosis and treatment of Parkinson's disease itself.

PARKINSON'S DISEASE

Parkinson's disease is a common neurodegenerative disorder with a prevalence rate in the general population of 100 per 100,000. In individuals older than 65 a much higher rate prevails, and it has been estimated that 1% to 2% of such persons have Parkinson's disease. The incidence of Parkinson's disease peaks between ages 70 and 79, where the incidence rate is slightly over 93 per 100,000. Although predominantly a disease of elderly persons, it is not exclusively so, and 5% to 10% of persons with Parkinson's disease experience their first symptoms prior to age 40. Men are 1.2 to 1.5 times more likely than women to have Parkinson's disease.

The etiology of Parkinson's disease is unknown, and it seems probable that there is not a single cause but that Parkinson's disease is a syndrome reflecting the clinical expression of a number of pathologic processes. Both genetic and environmental factors are probably involved in the genesis of Parkinson's disease. A number of kindreds with purely genetic parkinsonism have been identified and described, but most of these families display a variety of atypical features, including younger age of onset. A twin study has suggested that genetic factors are much more likely to be operative if an individual develops the initial clinical features prior to age 50, whereas other factors, presumably environmental, appear to be dominant in individuals who first manifest symptoms of Parkinson's disease after age 50. A number of environmental risk factors have been described in studies of Parkinson's disease, including a history of head trauma, agricultural exposure (e.g., rural living, well water consumption, farming, gardening, herbicide or pesticide exposure), and occupational exposure (e.g., steel alloy mills, wood pulp mills, welding, teaching), but the significance of these various associations is unclear and no universal risk factor has been identified. Studies have also suggested that other factors, such as smoking and caffeine consumption, may be associated with a reduced risk of developing Parkinson's disease, but the explanation for this association is also uncertain. It is likely that in most individuals both genetic factors, such as the presence of currently unidentified susceptibility genes, and environmental exposure work together to produce the clinical picture we identify as Parkinson's disease.

CLINICAL FEATURES

The clinical features of Parkinson's disease typically have an asymmetrical onset, initially appearing in one arm or leg. With time the involvement becomes bilateral, but the initially involved side often continues to be more severely affected. Tremor is the most frequent presenting feature of Parkinson's disease and is classically evident when the limb is at rest. It may be only intermittently present but is often magnified by factors such as stress and fatigue. An occasional patient may describe an internal sense of tremulousness prior to the emergence of visible tremor. Rigidity, characterized by a persistent resistance to passive joint movement, is ultimately the most common feature of Parkinson's disease. It may or may not have a cogwheeling quality and during examination can often be accentuated by reinforcement maneuvers, such as having the patient open and close the opposite hand or tap the opposite foot. Bradykinesia entails not only slowness of movement but also impaired ability to initiate and modify movement and to perform repetitive or simultaneous motor tasks. There may also be difficulty in terminating motor actions, leading to the phenomena of propulsion and festination. Patients often interpret bradykinesia as weakness even though actual weakness is not present. The fourth cardinal feature of parkinsonism, postural instability, is characterized by difficulty maintaining postural fixation and by impairment of righting reflexes, with consequent impairment of balance. It typically does not emerge until the more advanced stages of Parkinson's disease. In fact, its appearance within the first year following onset of clinical symptoms is an almost certain indication that the affected individual does not actually have Parkinson's disease but rather has one of the other parkinsonian disorders.

A rather extensive array of secondary signs also forms part of the clinical picture of Parkinson's disease, including micrographia, reduced facial expression, speech that is both soft and dysarthric, stooped posture, and the characteristic small-stepped, shuffling gait on a narrow base. Parkinson's disease is also accompanied by clinical symptoms that have little or nothing to do with motor function. These nonmotor features include derangements of autonomic function, mood, cognition, sleep, and sensation (Table 1). For some patients these nonmotor features are actually the most disabling features of the illness.

TABLE 1. **Nonmotor Features of Parkinson's Disease**

Autonomic dysfunction
Gastrointestinal
Sexual
Urinary
Cardiovascular
Thermoregulatory
Respiratory
Behavioral dysfunction
Parkinsonian personality (?)
Depression
Anxiety
Obsessive-compulsive tendencies
Dementia
Sleep-related dysfunction
Insomnia
Rapid eye movement (REM) sleep behavioral disorder
Sensory dysfunction
Visual
Olfactory
Pain
Fatigue

PATHOLOGIC FEATURES

The neuropathologic hallmark of Parkinson's disease is progressive destruction of dopaminergic neurons. Those that originate in the substantia nigra and send their axons to the caudate and putamen, forming the nigrostriatal tract, are most severely affected, but other dopaminergic pathways are also involved. The pathology of Parkinson's disease, however, is not confined to dopaminergic neuronal systems, which may explain why clinical features do not all respond equally well to drugs that enhance or mimic dopaminergic function. A characteristic microscopic pathologic feature of Parkinson's disease is the Lewy body, a cytoplasmic inclusion found in surviving dopaminergic neurons. Lewy bodies contain α-synuclein and a variety of other components and are probably the visible evidence of a cellular disturbance in Parkinson's disease involving the proteasomal system, which is responsible for degrading and disposing of damaged or unwanted proteins in neurons.

PHARMACOTHERAPY

The ideal management of any disease process is preemptive in character, either preventing disease onset or curing the disease once present. Neither is currently possible with Parkinson's disease. The next best treatment approach is to restore lost function. This is particularly important for a process such as Parkinson's disease, in which perhaps 70% of the complement of dopaminergic nigrostriatal neurons is lost before clinical symptoms ever become evident. This has led to attempts to replenish the dwindling supply of dopaminergic neurons with replacement neurons from various sources. The most widely publicized approach has been the use of fetal mesencephalic tissue, with which survival of implanted neurons has been demonstrated. However, reports of "runaway" dyskinesia (persistent involuntary movements even after stopping dopaminergic medication) have thrown this treatment approach into question. Moreover, ethical and practical concerns regarding the use and availability of fetal tissue for such procedures have prompted investigation of alternative approaches, such as the use of stem cells from various sources and employment of trophic factors and "gene therapy" techniques. All of these, however, currently remain firmly in the experimental rather than in the clinical realm.

NEUROPROTECTIVE THERAPY

Although restoring or replenishing lost neuronal function remains a goal largely for the future, the idea of protecting surviving neurons or at least slowing the progression of neuronal loss in Parkinson's disease has already been the object of several large clinical trials. Both vitamin E and riluzole (Rilutek) have been found to be ineffective as neuroprotective agents in Parkinson's disease.

The story regarding selegiline (Eldepryl), a selective inhibitor of monoamine oxidase type B (MAO-B) in doses utilized in clinical practice, is less clear. Attempts to determine whether selegiline has neuroprotective properties have been confounded by the fact that selegiline is also capable of inducing subtle improvement in clinical symptoms that may persist for a prolonged period of time after the medication is stopped. Thus, although studies have shown that selegiline can delay the need for introducing more potent symptomatic treatment such as levodopa, it has not been possible to ascertain definitively whether this is due to a neuroprotective or a symptomatic effect, even though most experts now believe the effect is primarily on symptoms.

Regardless of the mechanism involved, the employment of selegiline at a dose of 5 mg twice daily (given in the morning and at noon) is an acceptable treatment approach for the patient with newly diagnosed Parkinson's disease with minimal or no functional disability. When it is used as monotherapy, adverse effects are usually inconsequential but can include insomnia and a "wired" feeling, possibly related to metabolism of selegiline to amphetamine-related compounds. This metabolism can also produce positive urine drug screening tests in patients taking selegiline. Concerns regarding potential drug interactions have also been raised with selegiline, and life-threatening complications have been reported when selegiline and meperidine (Demerol) have been given concomitantly. If possible, it is prudent to discontinue selegiline 2 weeks before surgical or other procedures in which the use of narcotic analgesics is likely to be necessary. In emergency situations in which this is not possible, morphine should be used rather than meperidine. A "central serotonergic syndrome" has been described with concomitant use of selegiline and selective serotonin reuptake inhibitors. Use of tricyclic antidepressant medications in conjunction with selegiline has also been discouraged. However, the risk is sufficiently rare and the need to utilize some form of antidepressant treatment in Parkinson's disease patients sufficiently frequent that cautious coadministration of these drugs is felt to be acceptable by many movement disorder specialists.

Another agent currently receiving attention as a possible neuroprotective agent in Parkinson's disease is coenzyme Q10. A double-blind clinical trial in a relatively small group of patients demonstrated potential neuroprotective benefit of coenzyme Q10 at a dose of 1200 mg daily. However, the investigators in this trial view the results as only preliminary and further study with larger numbers of participants is being planned.

A considerable body of evidence has accumulated in basic laboratory studies (both cell culture and animal studies) suggesting that dopamine agonist medications (Table 2) may also have neuroprotective properties. Clinical trials of pramipexole (Mirapex), ropinirole (Requip), and pergolide (Permax), utilizing neuroimaging with either 2β-carbomethoxy-3β-(4-iodophenyl)tropane single photon emission computed tomography (β-CIT SPECT) or 18-fluorodopa positron emission tomography scanning, have also suggested a reduction in the rate of dopaminergic

TABLE 2. **Dopamine Agonist Doses**

Dopamine Agonist	Initial Dose	Maintenance Dose
Bromocriptine (Parlodel)	1.25 mg bid	5–40 mg daily
Pergolide (Permax)	0.05 mg daily	1.5–4.5 mg daily
Pramipexole (Mirapex)	0.125 mg tid	3.0–4.5 mg daily
Ropinirole (Requip)	0.25 mg tid	6–24 mg daily

neuronal loss in patients receiving dopamine agonist therapy, but the mechanism behind and clinical significance of these findings remain uncertain at this time.

SYMPTOMATIC THERAPY

During the past 35 years a growing array of medications has become available that, while not altering disease progression, is able to provide symptomatic benefit for individuals with Parkinson's disease. These medications currently represent the mainstay of the pharmacologic management of Parkinson's disease. With the exception of the anticholinergic drugs and amantadine, these agents primarily affect dopaminergic function by serving as a precursor of dopamine, by directly imitating the effect of dopamine, or by altering the metabolism of dopamine.

ANTICHOLINERGIC DRUGS

The use of anticholinergic drugs for the treatment of Parkinson's disease dates back to the 1800s, and for many years they represented the only available treatment. As newer and more effective agents have emerged, the use of these substances has diminished dramatically. The two most frequently employed anticholinergic medications in Parkinson's disease are trihexyphenidyl (Artane) and benztropine (Cogentin).

The reason for the diminishing use of these drugs is twofold. Their effectiveness is modest at best, confined primarily to tremor reduction—a 20% reduction is typical—with some possible impact on rigidity, and they have a relatively high propensity to produce adverse effects. Elderly individuals are especially sensitive to the undesirable effects of anticholinergic medications, which can include peripheral effects such as blurred vision, dry mouth, anhidrosis, constipation and urinary retention, and centrally mediated adverse effects in the form of memory impairment, confusion, and even psychosis.

A role for anticholinergic medications may still exist in the younger individual with Parkinson's disease in whom tremor is the sole or predominant clinical feature. A typical starting dose for trihexyphenidyl is 1 mg three times a day, with subsequent titration to 2 mg three times a day, and benztropine may be initiated at a dose of 0.5 mg twice daily with subsequent titration to 1 to 2 mg twice daily. It is probably prudent to avoid these medications in persons older than 60, and there is no rationale for their use in individuals without tremor.

AMANTADINE

Amantadine (Symmetrel) was initially introduced in the 1960s as an antiviral agent and subsequently noted to be effective in ameliorating symptoms of Parkinson's disease. Only relatively recently has it been recognized that a primary function of amantadine is as a glutamate antagonist.

Amantadine produces modest symptomatic improvement in tremor, rigidity, and bradykinesia in approximately two thirds of patients. There is a common perception that the benefit of amantadine often fades after several months of treatment, but investigation has not borne this out. Because of its relatively modest antiparkinson efficacy, amantadine has typically been utilized early in the course of treatment in individuals with mild Parkinson's disease. However, it can also sometimes display surprising benefit in more advanced disease when used as adjunctive therapy with traditionally more potent agents. The recognition that amantadine is a glutamate antagonist has also led to its successful employment in reducing dyskinesia in patients with levodopa-induced motor fluctuations.

Amantadine is typically prescribed at a dose of 100 mg three times a day, although a dose of 400 to 600 mg daily is sometimes used in treating dyskinesia. It is generally tolerated quite well by patients, but adverse effects certainly can occur. Some degree of pedal edema is quite common and may be prominent at times. The appearance of livedo reticularis, a purplish mottling of the skin, is a rather distinctive phenomenon in patients receiving amantadine. Cognitive dysfunction that may include confusion, nightmares, psychosis, and acute delirium may also occur; elderly individuals are especially susceptible to these psychiatric complications.

LEVODOPA AND CARBIDOPA

In the late 1950s and early 1960s a series of investigations led to recognition of the progressive nigrostriatal dopaminergic neuronal loss and consequent striatal dopamine deficiency that characterize Parkinson's disease. This recognition opened the therapeutic door, and it has now been over 35 years since levodopa, the metabolic precursor of dopamine, revolutionized Parkinson's disease treatment. It was quickly recognized that administration of levodopa by itself was inefficient because most was converted to dopamine peripherally, preventing it from reaching the brain, because dopamine itself cannot cross the blood-brain barrier. The subsequent combination of levodopa with carbidopa, a dopa decarboxylase inhibitor that does not cross the blood-brain barrier and, thus, prevents conversion of levodopa to dopamine only in the periphery, produced the combination medication, carbidopa-levodopa (Sinemet), that remains the benchmark of antiparkinson therapy today. A controlled-release carbidopa-levodopa preparation (Sinemet CR) has also been introduced to broaden the range of carbidopa-levodopa products available. In many countries outside the United States a second peripherally acting dopa decarboxylase inhibitor, benserazide, is also employed in combination with levodopa.

The initial response to carbidopa-levodopa therapy is generally quite gratifying and unmistakable. Carbidopa-levodopa is effective in alleviating the tremor, rigidity, and bradykinesia of Parkinson's disease. Individuals typically find during the early stages of carbidopa-levodopa therapy that they derive prolonged benefit from individual doses and can actually miss several doses without noticeable loss of therapeutic effect. This prolonged benefit is termed the "long-duration levodopa response" and is presumed to occur because sufficient dopaminergic nigrostriatal neurons still remain to manufacture, store, release, and reutilize the supplemental dopamine in a fashion approximating the normal state. During this early stage of treatment patients also characteristically awaken in the morning with good motor function, as if their central dopaminergic stores had been refreshed during the nighttime hours. Because of this "sleep benefit" it is usually not necessary to administer carbidopa-levodopa at bedtime during this early treatment phase. However, this often represents the quiet before the storm, and with time the tranquility of the early, smooth levodopa response gradually fades and stormier therapeutic seas arrive in the form of motor fluctuations.

Carbidopa-levodopa therapy can be initiated with either the standard or the controlled-release formulation. If the standard formulation is chosen, an initial dose schedule of one-half tablet of 25/100 carbidopa-levodopa three times a day is typically utilized; if the controlled-release formulation is employed, a dose of one tablet of 25/100 CR twice or three times daily is usual (the 25/100 CR tablet loses its controlled-release properties if it is broken in half). Nausea is the most frequently encountered adverse effect during initiation of carbidopa-levodopa therapy and is due to the peripheral conversion of levodopa to dopamine. Because it generally takes 75 to 100 mg of carbidopa daily to block this peripheral conversion adequately and the initial dosage schedules typically entail the use of less than 75 mg of carbidopa daily, additional carbidopa (Lodosyn) can be added (if available) at a dose of 25 mg with each carbidopa-levodopa tablet if nausea occurs. An alternative medication that can be used to control levodopa-induced nausea with little risk of accentuating the parkinsonism is trimethobenzamide (Tigan) in a dose of 250 to 300 mg three times a day. Conventional antinausea medications, such as prochlorperazine (Compazine) and metoclopramide (Reglan), are contraindicated in persons with Parkinson's disease because they quite predictably magnify parkinsonian symptoms.

Psychiatric toxicity in the form of hallucinations, delusions, and frank psychosis can appear at any time during carbidopa-levodopa therapy but is most likely to develop in individuals who already display some cognitive impairment as a part of their parkinsonism. If carbidopa-levodopa dosage reduction or elimination of other potential offending medications is not possible, employment of the atypical antipsychotic agent quetiapine (Seroquel) at an initial dose of 12.5 mg at bedtime with subsequent cautious titration can be initiated. Clozapine (Clozaril) is an even more effective medication in this situation, but the risk of bone marrow toxicity and the necessity for regular complete blood count measurements diminish its desirability.

Additional adverse effects from carbidopa-levodopa can include orthostatic hypotension and sleep disturbances such as excessive daytime drowsiness, insomnia, and periodic limb movements of sleep.

Long-term treatment with carbidopa-levodopa is often complicated by the emergence after a number of years of therapy of a constellation of features collectively labeled motor fluctuations. An estimated 30% of levodopa-treated patients develop motor fluctuations by 3 years, 50% by 5 years, and 80% by 10 years. Motor fluctuations can include a progressive shortening of the duration of effectiveness of a dose of carbidopa-levodopa (wearing off), the appearance of involuntary movements (dyskinesia), or ultimately the development of unpredictable and often precipitous shifts in motor performance (on-off). Treatment of levodopa-induced motor fluctuations is one of the most difficult challenges in the management of Parkinson's disease. End-of-dose wearing off can be addressed by several approaches: more frequent carbidopa-levodopa administration, switching to a carbidopa-levodopa CR preparation, adding a catechol-*O*-methyltransferase (COMT) inhibitor, adding an MAO-B inhibitor, or adding a dopamine agonist. Dealing with dyskinesia entails reducing carbidopa-levodopa dosage or adding amantadine to the treatment regimen. Because end-of-dose wearing off and peak-dose dyskinesia are often present concurrently, a combination of these treatment approaches is often necessary. For motor fluctuations that have not responded adequately to medical management, surgical treatment approaches are an option. The problems and difficulties posed by the development of motor fluctuations have prompted the investigation of treatment approaches that attempt to postpone the introduction of carbidopa-levodopa for as long as feasible. Particular focus has been directed toward the employment of dopamine agonists as first-line therapy.

DOPAMINE AGONISTS

Dopamine agonists do not rely on the function or integrity of dopaminergic neurons but rather stimulate dopamine receptors directly. Four such medications are currently available in the United States. Two are ergot derivatives: bromocriptine (Parlodel) and pergolide (Permax); two are nonergot drugs: pramipexole (Mirapex) and ropinirole (Requip). Both the benefits and adverse effect profiles of these four medications are similar.

When dopamine agonists were initially introduced they were used primarily as adjunctive therapy, added on to carbidopa-levodopa when motor fluctuations were emerging. Their longer half-lives and lower propensity to produce dyskinesia were useful in blunting the end-of-dose wearing off and involuntary movements associated with long-term carbidopa-levodopa therapy. Subsequently, multiple studies have demonstrated that dopamine agonists can also be successfully employed as initial symptomatic treatment for a significant proportion of patients with Parkinson's disease. Although many patients require supplemental carbidopa-levodopa within 1 to 2 years, it is possible to maintain a minority of individuals with dopamine agonist monotherapy for up to 4 years or longer, with a significantly reduced incidence of motor fluctuations. Even when carbidopa-levodopa supplementation is necessary the likelihood of developing motor fluctuations remains diminished, presumably because lower doses of carbidopa-levodopa are needed.

There are several potential drawbacks to the use of dopamine agonists as initial monotherapy for patients with Parkinson's disease. They are considerably more expensive than carbidopa-levodopa. As a general rule, they also need to be titrated more slowly. Although many potential adverse effects of dopamine agonists are identical to those encountered with carbidopa-levodopa, psychiatric toxicity in the form of hallucinations is more likely to occur, especially in older individuals with antecedent cognitive impairment. This has led many investigators to recommend that dopamine agonists be used with caution in individuals older than 70. There has also been some concern about the propensity of dopamine agonists to produce excessive drowsiness, and the occurrence of sudden "sleep attacks" has been described. However, the existence of such precipitous sleep episodes is controversial. It has long been known that the ergot-derived dopamine agonists (bromocriptine and pergolide) can in rare instances produce fibrotic complications such as retroperitoneal and pulmonary fibrosis. Valvular heart disease with fibroproliferative lesions has also been reported in individuals taking pergolide, although a definite cause-effect relationship has not been determined.

Although the similarities of the available dopamine agonists far outweigh their differences, there are some distinguishing features that might be important in certain situations. Pergolide has the longest half-life of the four, which might make it appealing for individuals experiencing nocturnal difficulties. Pramipexole is eliminated primarily by renal rather than hepatic routes and may, thus, be less likely to produce drug-drug interactions. It may also have antidepressant properties. Ropinirole is marketed in an extensive array of pill sizes, which makes it amenable to "gentle" titration, which might be preferable in more elderly or fragile individuals. With the introduction of the newer dopamine agonists, bromocriptine has largely been retired from the treatment scene.

CATECHOL-*O*-METHYLTRANSFERASE INHIBITORS

Although COMT is active in the metabolism of dopamine within the central nervous system, it is the metabolism of levodopa to 3-*O*-methyldopa in the periphery that is targeted by the newest class of medications to become available for the treatment of Parkinson's disease, the COMT inhibitors. Peripheral COMT inhibition results in both increased amounts of administered levodopa and reduced amounts of 3-*O*-methyldopa reaching the brain. Two such medications have been introduced, tolcapone (Tasmar) and entacapone (Comtan). Because of concerns regarding potential hepatotoxicity, however, tolcapone use has been severely limited, with monitoring of liver function studies required.

Entacapone has been shown to reduce end-of-dose wearing off when combined with carbidopa-levodopa therapy. Prolongation of the effect of a carbidopa-levodopa dose by 30 minutes is typical. Because of its short half-life, it is necessary to administer entacapone with each carbidopa-levodopa dose. The usual regimen is 200 mg with each carbidopa-levodopa dose to a maximum of 8 doses daily. Because entacapone does not have any antiparkinson activity of its own, there is no rationale for its use as monotherapy. It has been theorized that combining entacapone with carbidopa-levodopa right from the beginning of therapy might reduce the likelihood of development of motor fluctuations by providing a more constant, less pulsatile, stimulation of dopamine receptors, but this theory has yet to be fully tested.

COMT inhibitors are generally well tolerated but can accentuate levodopa-induced adverse effects. Patients who are already experiencing significant dyskinesia from carbidopa-levodopa are especially likely to experience increased dyskinesia when a COMT inhibitor is added, making a carbidopa-levodopa dosage reduction often necessary. In addition to the risk of hepatotoxicity, tolcapone can induce diarrhea in some patients, posing another deterrent to its use. Entacapone turns urine yellow, which can be a source of concern to patients if they are not forewarned.

MONOAMINE OXIDASE TYPE B INHIBITORS

The ability of selegiline (Eldepryl) to ameliorate end-of-dose wearing off of carbidopa-levodopa was first demonstrated over 25 years ago and remains its approved indication. The dosage employed and potential adverse effects of the drug in this setting are basically identical to those noted earlier, with the additional possibility that selegiline might accentuate carbidopa-levodopa–related adverse effects, much as described with entacapone.

SURGICAL THERAPY

Surgical therapy has a long history in the treatment of Parkinson's disease. The introduction of levodopa ushered in a period of relative surgical quiescence, but improvements in stereotactic surgical techniques, and especially the introduction of deep brain stimulation, have led to a resurgence of interest in surgical approaches for patients in whom medical management is no longer adequate.

Two types of surgical techniques can be employed—ablation or stimulation—and three target sites engaged: thalamus, globus pallidus, and subthalamic nucleus. Ablative procedures have the advantage of being less expensive and less complicated because no wires or other hardware are left in the patient after the procedure. They also do not require regular follow-up for adjustment of transmitter settings. However, procedures employing deep brain stimulation do not produce irreversible tissue destruction and are amenable to postoperative adjustment with improved response by changing stimulation parameters. It is also possible to perform bilateral stimulation procedures safely, which is important in the setting of Parkinson's disease because symptoms are typically bilateral. Thalamic targeting is not used extensively in Parkinson's disease because its beneficial effect is limited to tremor. Both pallidal and subthalamic targeting can produce improvement in tremor, rigidity, and bradykinesia, but perhaps the most important and useful effect is the dramatic reduction in motor fluctuations, especially dyskinesia, that is typically seen. The trend has been toward subthalamic targeting over pallidal.

It is important to emphasize that surgical treatment approaches should not be employed in individuals who have not initially responded to medical treatment. They should also not be performed in persons with significant cognitive impairment. Individuals with other forms of parkinsonism are also not candidates for surgical treatment.

TABLE 3. **Differential Diagnosis of Parkinsonism**

Neurodegenerative disorders
- Parkinsonism-plus syndromes
  - Progressive supranuclear palsy
  - Multiple system atrophy
  - Dementia with Lewy bodies
  - Corticobasal degeneration
- Alzheimer's disease

Drug-induced parkinsonism

Vascular parkinsonism

Normal pressure hydrocephalus

Repeated head trauma

Genetic disorders
- Wilson's disease
- Familial basal ganglia calcification
- Huntington's disease
- Spinocerebellar ataxias
- Dopa-responsive dystonia

Metabolic disorders
- Hypothyroidism
- Hypoparathyroidism
- Acquired hepatocerebral degeneration
- Central pontine myelinolysis

Infectious disorders
- Viral encephalitis
- AIDS
- Syphilis
- Whipple's disease
- Creutzfeldt-Jakob disease

Toxic disorders
- Manganese
- Carbon monoxide
- Cyanide
- Carbon disulfide
- *N*-Methyl-4-phenyl-1,2,3,6-tetrahydropyridine (MPTP)

NONPHARMACOLOGIC TREATMENT

Regular exercise, whether in the form of a formal physical therapy program or in a less structured setting, is an extremely important and often neglected component of the management of Parkinson's disease. Both endurance exercise (walking, swimming, running) and joint "limbering" or callisthenic-type exercises are important components of an overall program. Physical therapy evaluation can be invaluable in constructing a program that is appropriate and safe for any particular individual.

Speech therapy, occupational therapy, and music therapy are additional disciplines that have much to offer for certain individuals with Parkinson's disease. Participation in local Parkinson's disease support groups can be an important educational and social resource for patients and family members. Caregiver groups that often exist within the structure of such support organizations can also be tremendously beneficial for spouses struggling to deal with the stress and hardships of caring for individuals with Parkinson's disease.

OTHER PARKINSONIAN SYNDROMES

Treatment of the other parkinsonian syndromes is generally disappointing. Although individuals with multiple system atrophy may initially respond to carbidopa-levodopa, the response is generally suboptimal and wanes relatively rapidly. Employment of medications such as fludrocortisone (Florinef) and midodrine (ProAmatine) may reduce orthostatic hypotension and improve life quality. Individuals with progressive supranuclear palsy and corticobasal degeneration generally show no significant response to any of the antiparkinson agents. The parkinsonian features of persons with dementia with Lewy bodies (diffuse Lewy body disease) may sometimes respond to carbidopa-levodopa, but these individuals can be exquisitely prone to psychiatric toxicity, even at very low carbidopa-levodopa doses.

Day-to-day management of Parkinson's disease demands the type of close patient-physician relationship that is becoming increasingly difficult to maintain in today's medical environment. Treatment choices can be most effectively made when the physician is familiar with not only the increasing array of medications but also the nuances of disease symptoms in individual patients. Regular communication with patients and caregivers is vital. Although we cannot currently cure Parkinson's disease or with certainty even slow its progression, it is possible with judicious use of medication and other treatment modalities, along with meticulous attention to detail, to provide most individuals with Parkinson's disease a quality of life that, although far from ideal, is both meaningful and manageable.

The differential diagnosis of parkinsonism is outlined in Table 3.

PERIPHERAL NEUROPATHIES

method of
COLIN CHALK, M.D., C.M.
McGill University
Montreal, Canada

Disorders of the peripheral nervous system are among the most common neurologic problems in general medical practice. These disorders can be broadly divided into those affecting single nerves or nerve roots (mononeuropathies or radiculopathies) and those affecting several nerves or the entire peripheral nervous system (polyneuropathies). Some therapies for peripheral nerve disorders are specific to the disorder, but there are also therapies that are broadly applicable to many of these conditions. Accordingly, this article is divided into one main section in which diagnosis-dependent treatments are considered, followed by a second section in which generally applicable (diagnosis-independent) measures are described.

DIAGNOSIS-DEPENDENT THERAPIES

Dividing peripheral nerve disorders into the mononeuropathies and the polyneuropathies is convenient, but more importantly, the division reflects different etiologies. Most mononeuropathies are the result of mechanical trauma or compression of the nerve (e.g., compression of the median nerve in the carpal tunnel), whereas polyneuropathies have a large array of potential causes.

Mononeuropathies

Mononeuropathies affect patients of all ages who are otherwise healthy and usually cause troublesome symptoms rather than major disability. The most common cause of mononeuropathy is nerve compression, so surgical treatment to relieve nerve compression is often under consideration for these patients. Treatment of the four most common mononeuropathies is considered in the following paragraphs.

Median Neuropathy at the Wrist (Carpal Tunnel Syndrome). The main symptom of carpal tunnel syndrome is numbness in the hand. The numbness is initially intermittent, occurring especially at night, but may gradually become continuous. Some patients clearly describe numbness in the thumb, index finger, and middle finger, corresponding to the median nerve distribution, but often the numbness seems to involve the entire hand. Shaking the hand to gain relief is highly suggestive of carpal tunnel syndrome. More advanced median nerve injury also results in weakness of thenar muscles, affecting functions that require a good pincer grasp.

Patients with intermittent, mild symptoms may need nothing other than reassurance; the condition tends to worsen with time, but this is quite variable. A light-weight splint, worn on the flexor surface of the wrist and designed to prevent wrist flexion (which increases median nerve compression in the carpal tunnel), is often effective in patients with predominantly nocturnal symptoms. The splint is usually worn only at night, as it is cumbersome during the day. If symptoms are still troublesome despite a wrist splint, one option is local corticosteroid injection of the carpal ligament (e.g., methylprednisolone [Depo-Medrol] 40 mg). This can provide relief for up to several months. Finally, surgical decompression of the median nerve by sectioning the carpal ligament may be needed. In the hands of an experienced surgeon, this is a simple outpatient procedure with a very high rate of success in relieving carpal tunnel syndrome symptoms. If prolonged, severe median nerve compression has occurred, resulting in significant axonal loss, symptom relief may be incomplete.

Ulnar Neuropathy at the Elbow (Cubital Tunnel Syndrome). Patients with ulnar neuropathy at the elbow present with numbness of the medial hand and two fingers and weakness of the interosseous muscles. Some patients with this syndrome have a clear antecedent history of elbow trauma, but in most the ulnar neuropathy develops insidiously, and it is assumed to be due to many episodes of minor trauma. The common habit of leaning on one's elbow when reading, driving, and so forth may lead to ulnar neuropathy in people whose nerves are superficially located.

Education of the patient about the anatomy of the ulnar nerve at the elbow and correction of a habit of leaning on the elbow leads to improvement in many patients. Sometimes a hockey or skateboarding elbow pad worn at night is helpful. If symptoms and signs worsen despite these measures, ulnar nerve surgery can be considered. Unlike carpal tunnel surgery, however, the results of surgery are less certain, as reflected by the existence of several different surgical procedures.

Peroneal Neuropathy at the Fibular Head. Here the main symptoms are foot drop and numbness on the dorsum of the foot. Like ulnar neuropathy at the elbow, in peroneal neuropathy at the fibular head, there may be a clear antecedent history of trauma to the knee, but often this mononeuropathy is ascribed to repeated minor trauma, particularly related to sitting with the legs crossed. Generally speaking, the natural history of peroneal neuropathy at the fibular head is favorable, especially if leg crossing can be stopped. Surgical exploration is reserved for patients whose condition worsens during follow-up.

Facial Neuropathy (Bell's Palsy). Bell's palsy is an inflammatory process, unlike the compressive mononeuropathies. The cause is unknown, although some indirect evidence implicates herpes simplex virus. Occasionally, acute facial neuropathy is not Bell's palsy but is a manifestation of herpes zoster reactivation, Lyme disease, or sarcoidosis. The natural history of Bell's palsy for most patients is complete recovery within several weeks, but in about 15%, some facial weakness remains. Corticosteroids are widely prescribed for Bell's palsy, an entirely rational practice, although the evidence that this actually improves the condition's natural history is debatable. For most patients, it is reasonable to use a short course of oral corticosteroids (e.g., prednisone 60 mg daily, decreasing by 10 mg steps every 2 days until 0); there is probably little or no benefit if steroids are started more than 14 days after onset of facial weakness. Because of the possibility that herpes simplex virus may be involved in Bell's palsy, some physicians advocate treatment with an antiviral (e.g., acyclovir [Zovirax] 800 mg orally five times daily for 7 days) in addition to prednisone. Based on one controlled trial, there may be a marginal advantage to this approach.

Other cranial nerves besides the facial, particularly the sixth and third nerves, are sometimes affected by what is presumed to be an acute inflammatory process. As with Bell's palsy, these cranial mononeuropathies generally have a self-limited natural history. Whether corticosteroids are beneficial is unknown.

Polyneuropathies

Diagnosis of a specific cause of a patient's polyneuropathy can be difficult, as the list of possible causes is long, and the clinical features are often nonspecific. For example, almost all of the 100 or so causes of polyneuropathy can produce the classic glove-and-stocking pattern of distal sensorimotor symptoms and signs. Although it is beyond the scope of this article to provide a comprehensive account of the clinical features and investigation of the many varieties of polyneuropathy, the differential diagnosis can often be simplified by asking three key questions in every patient.

1. *Do the patient's symptoms and signs fit into a pattern other than a chronic, symmetrical, distal sensorimotor polyneuropathy?* If so, the list of possible causes is likely to be much shorter. Examples of such distinctive patterns include the syndrome of multiple mononeuropathies, acute-onset polyneuropathy, or predominantly sensory ataxic polyneuropathy.
2. *Do the nerve conduction studies suggest that the polyneuropathy is demyelinating?* Nerve conduction studies are an essential part of the investigation of any patient with polyneuropathy. Relatively few types of polyneuropathy are demyelinating, and the associated clinical features usually allow one to easily narrow the differential diagnosis to a few diagnoses.
3. *Could the patient have an inherited neuropathy?* Inherited neuropathy is common and often unrecognized, often because the possibility is not considered. As inherited neuropathies are generally benign, with very slow progression over decades, patients often present for evaluation for the first time in middle or even advanced age. A "negative" family history does not exclude the possibility, as the patient may have a recessive disorder, paternity may be unclear, or, most often, the neuropathy is present but unrecognized in the family.

There are a number of ways to classify the polyneuropathies. One approach is to separate inherited from acquired polyneuropathies and to then subdivide the acquired causes into four main categories: metabolic disorders, toxins and deficiency states, infections, and immune-inflammatory processes. The discussion that follows uses this broad classification scheme, highlighting those polyneuropathies for which there are specific treatments or therapeutic issues. For essentially all of these conditions, one or more of the generally applicable, diagnosis-independent treatments discussed at the conclusion of this article can also be considered.

Inherited Polyneuropathies

There have been significant advances in knowledge about the genetics of the inherited neuropathies in the last 15 years, and genes for several of these disorders are now known. A precise understanding of why altered function of the known genes produces neuropathy is an active area of scientific investigation. Gene dosage appears to be important in the diseases caused by altered expression of the gene for the peripheral myelin protein PMP-22. Patients with the most common form of hereditary motor and sensory neuropathy type 1 (Charcot-Marie-Tooth disease type 1A) have three copies of the PMP-22 gene, whereas patients with a deletion of this gene (i.e., only one copy) have a quite different syndrome, hereditary susceptibility to pressure palsies. As with many genetic diseases, the severity of the phenotype produced by the same genetic defect can be highly variable, and the factors that contribute to this variability are not understood.

The advances made in the genetics of inherited neuropathies have not yet been translated into specific therapies. In the near future, the inherited neuropathies seem unlikely candidates for gene replacement or manipulation, when one balances the likely risks of such therapies against the relatively benign natural history of most of these disorders. Nevertheless, establishing that a patient has an inherited neuropathy, whether or not genotyping is available, is important for several reasons: a clear diagnosis relieves patient worry and prevents further unnecessary investigation; there may be implications for family planning; and one can generally be reassuring about the benign long-term prognosis.

Acquired Polyneuropathies

Metabolic Disorders

Diabetic Polyneuropathy. Diabetic polyneuropathy is a common complication of diabetes. In the population-based Rochester Diabetic Neuropathy Study, the prevalence of polyneuropathy in diabetic patients was about 50%, although only about one third of these patients were symptomatic. In other studies, estimates of prevalence range from 10% to 75%, depending on the population studied, how the condition is defined, and what techniques are used to detect it. Diabetic polyneuropathy begins insidiously and progresses slowly, the main clinical features being distal, symmetrical sensory loss (often painful) plus mild distal weakness. Compressive mononeuropathies (e.g., ulnar neuropathy at the elbow, median neuropathy at the wrist) are frequently superimposed. In some diabetic patients, other less common peripheral nerve syndromes (see later discussion) may dominate the clinical picture, but usually against a background of diabetic polyneuropathy.

Despite intensive study, the pathogenesis of diabetic polyneuropathy remains incompletely understood. The two main hypotheses have been that (1) diabetic polyneuropathy is an ischemic disorder, caused by a vasculopathy affecting nerve microvascular supply, analogous to diabetic retinopathy; or that (2) hyperglycemia and related biochemical changes in the nerve microenvironment are responsible for nerve malfunction and injury. These hypotheses are not mutually exclusive. Although there is evidence from human and animal studies to support both mechanisms, at present the case for an ischemic basis for diabetic polyneuropathy is stronger.

Ideally, treatment of diabetic neuropathy would be preventative. The Diabetes Control and Complications Trial found that tight glucose control with multiple insulin injections or insulin pumps seemed to decrease the proportion of persons with type I diabetes who eventually developed polyneuropathy. In persons with type II diabetes, on the other hand, controlled evidence for a preventative effect of tight glucose control is lacking. In patients with established diabetic polyneuropathy, good glucose control is routinely advised. While it is hard to find fault with this advice, it must be admitted that diabetic polyneuropathy persists and progresses even in most patients with meticulous control. There is some evidence that polyneuropathy may improve in the long term in diabetic patients treated with pancreas transplantation.

There have been numerous clinical trials of drugs targeting one of the putative mechanisms in the pathogenesis of diabetic polyneuropathy. Many of these studies had important methodologic flaws, such as imprecise or unreliable measures of peripheral nerve function, or insufficient length of follow-up. There have been more than a dozen trials of aldose reductase inhibitors,* which prevent metabolism of glucose to polyol sugars hypothesized to be deleterious to nerve. In human trials, a small improvement in motor nerve conduction velocity was found, but the clinical significance of this is unclear, and no consistent improvement in clinical symptoms or signs has been demonstrated. Other recent large negative trials have included acylcarnitine* and recombinant human nerve growth factor.* A promising agent is alpha-lipoic acid,* an antioxidant, for which clinical trials are currently underway.

The main focus in treatment of diabetic polyneuropathy remains symptom management, particularly the treatment of neuropathic pain. The general measures for neuropathic pain are all applicable to painful diabetic polyneuropathy. Meticulous care of the feet to prevent complications such as plantar ulcers or osteomyelitis are important in any patient with sensory loss from a polyneuropathy, but in patients with diabetic polyneuropathy, foot care is even more important, as concomitant peripheral vascular disease is almost universal.

Many diabetic patients have abnormal autonomic nervous system function in addition to polyneuropathy. Autonomic neuropathy is not unique to diabetes, but diabetes is by far the most common cause. Dysautonomia can have various manifestations, including orthostatic hypotension, erectile impotence and disturbance of ejaculation in men (or less well-studied sexual dysfunction in women), postgustatory sweating, intestinal dysmotility, and altered cardiac function (especially loss of sinus arrhythmia). The severity of diabetic autonomic neuropathy does not appear to correlate with the severity of diabetic polyneuropathy.

Orthostatic hypotension may be the most disabling symptom of autonomic neuropathy. Management includes patient education and strategies to increase circulating blood volume, such as added dietary salt, sleeping with the head of the bed elevated to 30 degrees, or wearing support hose. If these measures are inadequate, fludrocortisone acetate (Florinef),† 0.1 to 0.2 mg daily, can be added. The vasopressor midodrine (ProAmatine), 2.5 to 10 mg three times daily, is reserved for more refractory patients.

Several less common peripheral nerve syndromes can occur in diabetic patients, including lumbosacral plexopathy (or diabetic amyotrophy), truncal neuropathy, and oculomotor neuropathy. These are usually superimposed on a background of diabetic polyneuropathy but sometimes develop relatively soon after the onset of diabetes. These syndromes generally have a self-limited course lasting months. Their pathogenesis has long been assumed to be ischemic, but there is now increasing evidence, at least for lumbosacral plexopathy, of an inflammatory cause. It is usually necessary to exclude other possibilities before diagnosing these syndromes (e.g., ruling out a posterior communicating artery aneurysm in a diabetic patient with an oculomotor palsy). Pain management is often a major therapeutic issue. Because of the evidence pointing to an inflammatory process, there is an increasing trend to treat diabetic lumbosacral plexopathy with corticosteroids (e.g., prednisone 60 mg daily for 2 to 3 months, then tapering by 10 mg per month). Given the self-limited natural history of lumbosacral plexopathy, it can be difficult to know whether improvement is in fact due to prednisone; a controlled trial of corticosteroids in this setting is underway.

Polyneuropathies due to Other Metabolic Disorders. Polyneuropathy in the setting of chronic renal failure has become uncommon since the widespread availability of dialysis and renal transplantation. Uremic neuropathy is a distal, symmetrical, axonal neuropathy in which sensory symptoms and signs are prominent and motor weakness is mild. The biochemical basis of uremic neuropathy is unclear.

*Investigational drug in the United States.

†Not FDA approved for this indication.

In general, dialysis will stabilize or slow the progression of uremic neuropathy, while transplantation can be expected to improve symptoms and signs slowly.

Failure of other organ systems (e.g., cardiopulmonary, hepatic, hematopoietic) and electrolyte derangements are generally not associated with development of polyneuropathy. However, an axonal sensorimotor polyneuropathy, sometimes severe, can occur in critically ill patients with sepsis and multiorgan failure (critical illness polyneuropathy). There is no specific treatment for critical illness polyneuropathy, although if sepsis is successfully treated and organ failure is reversed, gradual recovery of peripheral nerve function seems to be the rule. A mild polyneuropathy can occur in patients with hypothyroidism and in those with acromegaly; correction of the hormonal disturbances probably improves these polyneuropathies, although this has not been well studied.

Toxins or Deficiency States

The most common type of toxic neuropathy encountered in current practice is iatrogenic, that is, neuropathy as a side effect of therapeutic drugs. Numerous drugs can produce peripheral neuropathy as a side effect, so a careful drug history is important in all patients with polyneuropathy. Drugs for which there is reasonable evidence of peripheral nerve toxicity are listed in Table 1; note that the propensity to cause neuropathy is quite different from one drug to another. The clinical picture of a toxic neuropathy is nonspecific, usually being distal, sensorimotor, and symmetrical. Nerve conduction studies show axon loss. Clearly one must establish that exposure to the putative neurotoxin began before the onset of the neuropathy. The exposure duration and dose needed to result in neuropathy are variable and depend on the particular medication and on individual susceptibility.

The essential therapeutic maneuver in the treatment of drug-induced neuropathy is obviously to stop exposure to the offending agent or agents. Slow improvement over months can be expected, although residual symptoms and signs are frequent. General measures for treatment of neuropathic pain (see later) are often needed. In some patients, the neuropathy will continue to worsen initially after they stop taking the neurotoxin (so-called coasting), before the expected slow improvement begins.

The mechanistic details of how a given drug produces neuropathy are mostly unknown. For some antineoplastic drugs, the propensity to cause neuropathy can be the dose-limiting factor, and there is some hope that pretreatment with neuroprotective agents such as neurotrophins might prevent the neuropathy and allow higher doses to be used. A neuroprotective approach has been used with some success in animals (e.g., the neurotrophin NT-3 can prevent cisplatin-induced neuropathy in mice), but is not yet available in humans.

Ethanol is often considered to be a cause of neuropathy. While there is little doubt that a distal, symmetrical, often painful neuropathy occurs in some alcoholic people, it is unclear whether the culprit is the ethanol, the associated malnutrition, or other factors. Animals chronically fed large quantities of ethanol but who are otherwise well nourished do not develop neuropathy. On the other hand, alcoholic neuropathy still occurs in countries where beer and spirits are supplemented with B vitamins. Treatment of alcoholic neuropathy is the treatment of alcoholism and includes cessation of alcohol consumption, proper nutrition, and treatment of related psychological issues.

Poisoning by salts and organic compounds containing arsenic, lead, or thallium can cause axonal neuropathies. Most cases evolve over months, but more acute presentations can be seen if large doses of the poison are ingested. Patients usually have systemic features such as diarrhea, abdominal pain, myelosuppression, or cutaneous signs in addition to the neuropathy, which is often painful. Diagnosis depends on demonstrating increased levels of the suspected element in hair or nails. The main therapeutic maneuver is to stop exposure; it is not unusual to discover that the patient is being deliberately poisoned. Chelating agents such as British anti-Lewisite (Bal in oil), EDTA, or penicillamine (Cuprimine)* can be used to promote excretion of the toxic element, but there is no consensus about which is the most effective.

Vitamin deficiency, particularly of thiamine (B_1), is a well-established cause of neuropathy in the setting of severe malnutrition. Vitamin B_{12} deficiency also produces a mild axonal neuropathy, but the major neurologic findings in B_{12} deficiency are those of a myelopathy. There is no physiologic basis for the routine prescription of multivitamins for patients who are not malnourished. In large doses, in fact, pyridoxine (vitamin B_6) is neurotoxic, producing a severe ataxic sensory neuropathy.

Infectious Diseases

HIV Infection. Peripheral nerve syndromes are frequent in patients with HIV. Most common is a distal, symmetrical, mostly sensory polyneuropathy, which can be a direct or indirect effect of HIV infection, as

*Not FDA approved for this indication.

TABLE 1. **Drugs That May Produce Polyneuropathy**

Antineoplastics	**Drugs for Rheumatologic Diseases**
Cisplatin (Platinol)	Chloroquine (Aralen)
Suramin (Metaret)	Colchicine
Taxoids (docetaxel [Taxotere], paclitaxel [Taxol])	Gold (sodium thiomalate) [Aurolate]
Vinca alkaloids (vincristine [Oncovin], vinblastine [Velban])	Thalidomide (Thalomid)
Antimicrobials	**Miscellaneous**
Chloramphenicol (Chloromycetin)	Amiodarone (Cordarone)
Dapsone	Disulfiram (Antabuse)
Didanosine (ddI) (Videx)	Perhexilene*
Isoniazid (Nydrazid)	Phenytoin (Dilantin)
Metronidazole (Flagyl)	Pyridoxine (vitamin B_6; in megadose quantities)
Nitrofurantoin (Macrodantin)	Simvastatin (Zocor)
Stavudine (d4T) (Zerit)	
Zalcitabine (ddc) (Hivid)	

*Not available in the United States.

well as an adverse effect of several antiretroviral drugs (see Table 1). As with antineoplastic drugs, neuropathy is frequently the dose-limiting side effect with these antiretroviral agents. In patients whose polyneuropathy is thought to be due to HIV rather than antiretroviral drugs, HIV treatment may stabilize or improve the neuropathy. A recent phase II trial of recombinant human nerve growth factor in HIV-associated sensory polyneuropathy showed improvement in pain and in sensory signs.

Several less common immune-inflammatory peripheral nervous system syndromes occur in HIV patients. Acute and chronic inflammatory demyelinating polyneuropathies, similar to those in the non-HIV population (see later), appear to respond well to plasma exchange or intravenous gamma globulin (BayGam). Direct infection of nerve and nerve roots by cytomegalovirus can occur in advanced HIV disease, producing an acute lumbosacral polyradiculopathy with paraplegia and incontinence. Cytomegalovirus is also intimately involved in the pathogenesis of a vasculitic syndrome of multiple mononeuropathies. These cytomegalovirus-related syndromes are usually treated with drugs such as ganciclovir (Cytovene) 5 mg/kg IV twice daily for 14 to 21 days. In some patients improvement occurs, although this may be limited by the general debility of the patient with advanced HIV.

Herpes Zoster. Reactivation of latent herpes zoster virus in trigeminal or spinal ganglia produces a characteristic dermatomal vesicular skin eruption and pain. Sometimes there is motor weakness in the corresponding myotome. Herpes zoster is normally self-limited, with resolution of the skin eruption and pain within several weeks. Some patients, however, develop postherpetic neuralgia, usually defined as persistence of pain for more than 8 weeks after onset of the skin lesions. This is particularly likely in the elderly (up to 45% of patients older than 65 years develop postherpetic neuralgia). Postherpetic neuralgia is managed with the usual drugs for neuropathic pain (see later), although success is often limited. Topical local anesthetic preparations (e.g., EMLA cream,* an oil-water emulsion of lidocaine and prilocaine) provide at least temporary relief but are inconvenient for many patients. Topical capsaicin (Zostrix) is helpful for some patients. It should be applied four times daily to the painful area and usually will cause worsening of the burning discomfort for the first few applications. Capsaicin ointment cannot be used on the face. There is good evidence from controlled trials that treatment of acute herpes zoster with antiviral drugs (famciclovir [Famvir] 500 mg PO three times daily for 7 days, or acyclovir [Zovirax] 800 mg PO five times daily for 7 days) substantially lowers the fraction of patients who develop postherpetic neuralgia. Addition of corticosteroids to these antivirals in the treatment of acute zoster confers no additional benefit.

Lyme Disease. Infection by the spirochete *Borrelia burgdorferi* causes arthralgia, skin rash, heart block, and peripheral nerve dysfunction. Acutely, *B. burgdorferi* infection manifests as facial neuropathy, often bilateral, which resolves spontaneously. In endemic areas, Lyme disease rivals Bell's palsy in frequency as the cause of facial palsy. If untreated, Lyme disease may evolve into a generalized sensorimotor axonal polyradiculoneuropathy. Diagnosis is dependent on serologic proof of *B. burgdorferi* infection, cerebrospinal fluid pleocytosis (especially in early stages), and a positive response to appropriate antimicrobials. Early stages of Lyme disease, including facial palsy, are treated with oral antibiotics (doxycycline 100 mg twice daily for 10 to 30 days, or amoxicillin 500 mg three times daily for 10 to 30 days); late Lyme disease, with cerebrospinal fluid pleocytosis or polyradiculopathy, requires intravenous antibiotics (ceftriaxone [Rocephin] 2 g daily for 14 to 21 days).

*Not FDA approved for this indication.

Leprosy. Infection of peripheral nerve by *Mycobacterium leprae* is among the leading causes of peripheral neuropathy worldwide. Although leprosy is now rare in North America and Western Europe, newly diagnosed leprosy is seen from time to time in patients who have emigrated from endemic areas such as the Indian subcontinent. Leprosy characteristically affects cutaneous sensory nerves in the coolest parts of the body, producing a patchy distribution of dense sensory loss unlike any other type of neuropathy. Biopsy of skin or nerve is needed for diagnosis. Leprosy can be cured with appropriate antibiotics, although treatment must be continued for 6 to 9 months. A multiple-drug regimen, typically rifampin (Rifadin)* plus dapsone and sometimes clofazimine (Lamprene), is usually employed, and should be supervised by a physician experienced with the management of leprosy. Education of the patient and family members is also important, because of the stigma associated with the diagnosis. It is of particular importance to emphasize that the disease is not highly contagious, as fears of infection can lead to patients becoming socially isolated.

Immune-Inflammatory Processes

Guillain-Barré Syndrome. Guillain-Barré syndrome (GBS) is the most common nontraumatic cause of acute quadriparesis in the Western world. The central pathophysiologic process is an immunologically mediated attack on peripheral nerve myelin; in most cases, it is presumed that an antecedent infection triggers the patient's immune response, which is subsequently misdirected at peripheral nerve. A number of bacterial and viral infections have been implicated, of which *Campylobacter jejuni* enteritis is the most common.

The clinical course of GBS is characterized by the acute onset of motor and sensory symptoms, most often distally in the limbs. There is progressive worsening over several days, a plateau period lasting days to weeks, and then slow spontaneous improvement. Variations on this classic pattern of "ascending paralysis" are common and can cause diagnostic confusion,

*Not FDA approved for this indication.

particularly in patients with predominant cranial nerve involvement. One year after onset, about 85% of patients will have recovered fully or have only minor symptoms and signs. A small number are left with permanent major disability.

The most important treatment for GBS is meticulous medical and nursing care to prevent complications arising in patients who are bed-bound and paralyzed, for example, urinary and pulmonary infections, venous thromboembolism, and cutaneous pressure sores. The main advance in GBS therapeutics in the last 50 years has been assisted ventilation, which has reduced the mortality rate from about 30% to less than 5%. The possibility of ventilatory failure must always be borne in mind in patients with GBS, particularly when the patient's deficits are still progressing. It is important to monitor such patients closely, preferably in a setting where intubation and ventilation are available around the clock.

In addition to these important supportive measures, therapies that aim to abrogate the immune process in GBS have been evaluated in several large clinical trials over the past 20 years. Both plasma exchange and intravenous immunoglobulin (IGIV; Gamimune N)* were found to have similar advantages over supportive treatment of GBS, reducing the duration of assisted ventilation by 2 weeks and hastening the recovery to a state of independent ambulation by about 30 days. Both treatments must be given early in the course of the illness, preferably within 14 days of onset of symptoms. The dose of IGIV is 0.4 g/kg daily for 5 consecutive days. With plasma exchange, one aims to remove about 10 L of plasma, usually in five consecutive daily sessions. Because IGIV is technically much easier to administer than plasma exchange, and the benefits of the two treatments are similar, IGIV is now generally preferred. Combined treatment (plasma exchange followed by IGIV infusions) appears to offer no advantage over either treatment alone. Corticosteroids are beneficial in animal models of GBS, but in human trials, no benefit could be shown. Therefore, the use of corticosteroids in GBS is not recommended.

Chronic Inflammatory Demyelinating Polyradiculoneuropathy (CIDP). CIDP shares some features with GBS, as it is an immune-mediated disease in which attack on peripheral nerve myelin results in weakness and sensory loss. Unlike GBS, however, CIDP begins insidiously and progresses over weeks to months. Some patients follow a relapsing-remitting course, but in most the neurologic deficits slowly worsen with time. Cranial nerve and respiratory involvement, which are common in patients with GBS, are rare in patients with CIDP.

Several of the treatments used in GBS are also effective in CIDP, but the approach to treatment is different. CIDP, like many non-neurologic autoimmune diseases, usually must be treated for many months, as the disease does not spontaneously remit, and none of the treatments currently available are able to terminate the abnormal immune process giving rise to the disease. Plasma exchange and IGIV (Gamimune)* can each bring about substantial improvement in most patients with CIDP, but the benefit of a single treatment is short-lived, and repeated treatments are needed. Because IGIV is easier to administer, it is probably the treatment of choice. A typical regimen might involve 0.4 g/kg per treatment, given twice per week for 3 weeks, then once a week for 9 more weeks. The frequency of subsequent treatments would be determined by the patient's clinical response, with most patients requiring a treatment every 2 to 4 weeks.

Corticosteroids are also effective in treating CIDP, but the response is slower than that with IGIV or plasma exchange, and the complications of chronic corticosteroid use often arise. Sometimes a judicious combination of corticosteroids (e.g., prednisone 60 mg daily, tapering after 2 to 3 months by monthly steps of 5 mg to as low a dose as possible) and periodic IGIV treatments provides the best balance between benefits, side effects, and patient convenience. Other immunosuppressive drugs (azathioprine [Imuran],* cyclosporin [Neoral, Sandimmune],* and mycophenolate [CellCept]*) are also sometimes used in treating CIDP, but controlled evidence for their efficacy is lacking.

Vasculitic Neuropathy. Peripheral neuropathy is a frequent and often prominent feature of systemic vasculitides, particularly polyarteritis nodosa, as well as Churg-Strauss syndrome, Wegener's granulomatosis, and rheumatoid vasculitis. Classically, vasculitis affects individual nerves in different limbs in a stepwise fashion (the syndrome of multiple mononeuropathies), although up to one third of patients with vasculitic neuropathy have a symmetrical, distal pattern. Diagnosis hinges on showing inflammatory cell infiltration and blood vessel wall necrosis in a nerve biopsy. Signs of an associated systemic illness (e.g., fever, weight loss, glomerular disease, rash, arthralgias) are often present.

Peripheral nerve involvement in systemic vasculitis can cause significant disability, but it is not life threatening, and the disease's non-neurologic features are usually the primary focus of treatment. Immunosuppressive drugs are the mainstay, usually prednisone (1 to 1.5 mg/kg PO daily), often combined with cyclophosphamide (Cytoxan)* (50 to 100 mg PO daily). Some practitioners advocate using intravenous infusions of either agent at 1- to 4-week intervals (e.g., methylprednisolone [Solu-Medrol]* 500 mg IV once a month; cyclophosphamide (Cytoxan) 10 mg/kg IV every 7 to 10 days). Although there is general consensus that immunosuppression is effective in systemic vasculitis, the relative merits of the regimens described have not been evaluated in controlled trials. Vasculitis produces ischemic nerve injury and axonal degeneration. Successful control of the pathologic inflammatory response by immunosuppressants results in stability of the peripheral nerve deficits and no signs of new nerve involvement. Recovery of peripheral nerve function can be expected, but it is slow (many months) and often incomplete.

---

*Not FDA approved for this indication.

*Not FDA approved for this indication.

Polyneuropathy Associated with Other Connective Tissue Diseases. In addition to the vasculitides, polyneuropathy can be a feature of several other connective tissue diseases. Nerve biopsies from patients with polyneuropathy and Sjögren's syndrome generally show evidence of perivascular inflammation and sometimes frank vasculitis, but the benefits of immunosuppression (e.g., corticosteroids) are less convincing in this setting than in systemic vasculitis. A mild polyneuropathy can develop in some patients with systemic lupus erythematosus, mixed connective tissue disease, or scleroderma. Based on limited pathologic data, these neuropathies are also assumed to be immune mediated, but the details are not known. Whether treatment of the connective tissue disease benefits the neuropathy is difficult to assess.

Some unusual peripheral nerve syndromes can occur in patients with connective tissue diseases, including trigeminal sensory neuropathy (Sjögren's syndrome, scleroderma, mixed connective tissue disease) and dorsal root ganglionopathy (Sjögren's syndrome). The latter results from lymphocytic infiltration of ganglia, but a benefit from immune therapy has not been clearly shown.

Monoclonal Protein–Associated Neuropathy. A monoclonal gammopathy in a patient without an identifiable hematologic or lymphoproliferative disease is known as a *monoclonal gammopathy of undetermined significance* (MGUS), because a substantial minority of such patients do eventually develop a lymphoproliferative disease. About 10% of patients with MGUS have a polyneuropathy, and in these patients, it is assumed that the monoclonal protein plays a role in the neuropathy's pathogenesis, a notion that is supported by epidemiologic and some experimental evidence. Most patients with MGUS neuropathy have a distal, sensorimotor process, often asymmetrical, with axonal electrophysiology. Less often, MGUS neuropathy can resemble CIDP, with demyelinating nerve conduction studies. As a general rule, IgM MGUS neuropathy tends to feature more nerve conduction slowing and more impairment of proprioception than when the MGUS neuropathy is IgG or IgA mediated. A controlled trial of plasma exchange (twice weekly for 3 weeks) showed benefit for IgG and IgA MGUS neuropathy, but not for IgM patients. IVIG is also used to treat MGUS neuropathy (e.g., 0.4 g/kg weekly for 6 to 12 weeks); this may have efficacy comparable with plasma exchange, but controlled data are lacking. Treatments that target the clone of plasma cells producing the monoclonal protein (chlorambucil [Leukeran],* prednisone,* α-interferon*) are advocated by some neurologists, but evidence of effectiveness has not been convincing.

Patients whose monoclonal gammopathy is associated with a hematologic disease most often have multiple myeloma, a plasma cell malignancy characterized by osteolytic bone lesions, hypercalcemia, and renal failure. Patients with typical multiple myeloma occasionally have a mild neuropathy, but in an uncommon variety of myeloma, osteosclerotic myeloma, a demyelinating polyneuropathy resembling CIDP is frequent. Patients with osteosclerotic myeloma often have localized disease amenable to radiation therapy, and in some patients the associated polyneuropathy also improves.

Amyloid Polyneuropathy. There are two main types of amyloid polyneuropathy: familial amyloid polyneuropathy, caused by point mutations in the gene for transthyretin, and polyneuropathy secondary to systemic amyloidosis, in which the amyloid is composed of immunoglobulin light chains. Both types of amyloid neuropathy commonly produce significant autonomic dysfunction in addition to sensory and motor deficits. Diagnosis is by nerve biopsy, with characterization of the amyloid type by immunohistochemical methods. A successful method to remove amyloid from nerve and other tissues has not yet been devised. Liver transplantation has been employed with some success in familial amyloid polyneuropathy. Systemic amyloidosis is often treated with prednisone and alkylating agents such as chlorambucil (Leukeran),* but the impact on the disease is uncertain, and most patients die because of cardiac or renal involvement.

Polyneuropathy Associated with Other Hematologic Diseases. Occasionally neuropathy will develop in patients with hematologic diseases, particularly lymphoma. Some of these patients have a monoclonal gammopathy, which presumably is a variant of MGUS neuropathy. Other patients with lymphoma and polyneuropathy prove to have lymphomatous invasion of peripheral nerve, usually involving nerve roots or cranial nerves. Still other patients have neither a monoclonal gammopathy nor malignant invasion of nerve; it is assumed that these neuropathies are also immune mediated, but the mechanisms are not known. In all these situations, treatment of the underlying disorder is the main focus, although adding plasma exchange or IGIV* in the treatment of patients with a monoclonal gammopathy can be considered. The response of the neuropathy to successful treatment of the hematologic disease is unpredictable, although major neurologic improvement can sometimes occur in a patient with lymphomatous invasion of nerve.

Paraneoplastic Neuropathy. Several uncommon neurologic syndromes can arise in patients with malignancies, particularly ovarian and small cell lung cancers. Neurologic derangement in the paraneoplastic syndromes is not due to invasion of the nervous system by the cancer, nor is it a result of cancer treatment. Instead, these syndromes arise as a byproduct of the immune system's attempts to contain the neoplasm, presumably owing to immunologic cross-reactivity between the tumor and nervous tissue. The best-known peripheral nervous system paraneoplastic syndrome is paraneoplastic sensory neuronopathy, in which dorsal root ganglia neurons are destroyed by a T lymphocyte–mediated process, resulting in an ataxic

*Not FDA approved for this indication.

*Not FDA approved for this indication.

sensory neuropathy. Dysautonomia and central nervous system dysfunction (limbic encephalitis) often coexist with the sensory neuronopathy. Most patients with this syndrome have an underlying small cell lung cancer, sometimes at a localized and potentially curable stage. Treatment of the small cell cancer may prevent worsening of the neuropathy, but improvement does not occur. Immunomodulatory treatments (corticosteroids, IGIV,* plasma exchange) appear to have no benefit. From time to time, a neoplasm is found in a patient with an unexplained progressive sensorimotor neuropathy; some of these cases may be true paraneoplastic syndromes, but this can be difficult to prove.

GENERALLY APPLICABLE (DIAGNOSIS-INDEPENDENT) THERAPIES

In this concluding section, therapies that are useful in many types of neuropathy, regardless of diagnosis, are described. The principal focus is on treatment of neuropathic pain, a challenging and common problem. Strategies to compensate for motor weakness are also considered.

Neuropathic Pain

Pain is a common symptom in many types of neuropathy. It is often pain, rather than motor, sensory, or autonomic deficits, that is the patient's main concern, so a strategy to manage neuropathic pain is important. It is easy for both patient and physician to become demoralized by chronic neuropathic pain, but it is possible to have some meaningful impact on pain in most patients.

Patient education is an important aspect of management. Many patients interpret the presence of pain as a sign of severe disease and assume that they face inexorable, progressive loss of function, culminating in a state of helpless dependency. In fact, most painful neuropathies are noteworthy for the relative *lack* of significant neurologic deficit: weakness tends to be minimal and very distal, and demonstrable sensory loss is often rather minor, involving only the distal parts of the feet. In general, these deficits do not worsen, or they do so only very slowly (over decades), such that one can reassure the patient that ambulation is likely to be preserved, and that important loss of limb function is not expected. Reassurance about the prognosis may have more therapeutic benefit in some patients than any other intervention.

Nonpharmacologic measures can provide some relief to many patients. Shoes with a spacious fit or open-toed sandals may decrease neuropathic foot pain, whereas tight shoes tend to aggravate the symptoms. Prolonged weight bearing often worsens neuropathic pain, and modifications at work (e.g., frequent sitting breaks for jobs requiring standing) can be explored. Soaking the feet in cold tap water for 20 to 30 minutes before bed may temporarily diminish symptoms and allow the patient to get to sleep. Less often, warm or hot water soaks are helpful, and some patients find cold alternating with hot tap water ("contrast soaks") to be more effective. None of these maneuvers are likely to completely abolish neuropathic pain, but they are cheap and harmless, and patients should be encouraged to try them.

*Not FDA approved for this indication.

Several classes of medicines can be tried for neuropathic pain. Patients should be counseled that complete abolition of pain by medication is unlikely; rather, one hopes to reduce pain to the point where it is tolerable or nonintrusive. Tricyclic agents* such as amitriptyline (Elavil) or nortriptyline (Aventyl) can be considered benchmarks against which other agents are compared. The doses generally effective for pain (10 to 30 mg at bedtime) are considerably less than the usual antidepressant doses, which may minimize side effects. The main side effects are dry mouth and somnolence; the latter is often beneficial in patients whose pain is compounded by poor sleep. An adequate trial of a tricyclic requires a 2- to 3-month period.

Some anticonvulsants can be helpful, particularly when lancinating pain is a prominent complaint. Sustained-release carbamazepine (Tegretol-XR)* may be effective as a single bedtime dose (200 to 400 mg). Gabapentin (Neurontin)* is probably of similar efficacy to amitriptyline and may be better tolerated. The effective dose range is wide, with some experiencing benefit with as little as 100 mg three times daily, and others having increasing benefit without side effects in doses up to 1200 mg four times daily. Another new anticonvulsant, topiramate (Topamax),* 100 to 200 mg twice daily, shows some promise, although experience is limited. Third-line agents for neuropathic pain include baclofen (Lioresal),* 10 to 20 mg four times daily, and mexiletine (Mexitil)* 100 to 400 mg four times daily. Simple analgesics (e.g., aspirin or acetaminophen 300 mg two to four times daily) offer additional relief to some patients and can be combined with any of the above-mentioned drugs. An occasional patient is helped by topical capsaicin ointment (Zostrix), but most find it to be ineffective or too troublesome for regular use.

Treatments for Muscle Weakness

The ankle-foot orthosis (AFO) is perhaps the most underprescribed but effective therapy in neurology. AFOs should be considered in every patient with weakness of ankle dorsiflexion. There are several types of AFO. The most commonly used device is made of rigid but lightweight plastic; it slides into the patient's shoe and is fastened to the back of the calf with straps, and it holds the ankle joint fixed at 90 degrees. The obvious benefit of an AFO is preventing the toes or foot from catching on the ground during the swing phase of gait. The patient with a foot drop compensates by lifting the knee higher than normal (the classic "steppage gait"); an AFO

*Not FDA approved for this indication.

minimizes the patient's need to alter the gait pattern, making walking more efficient and easier. Patients with bilateral ankle weakness (the usual situation in polyneuropathy) often experience a sense of instability or imbalance when walking, in addition to the expected symptoms of foot drop. Bilateral AFOs often improve the patient's sense of stability when standing or walking.

Ensuring that an AFO is properly fitted is essential. This is generally best done by an experienced orthotist. Some patients are concerned about the stigma of wearing a brace, although an AFO is essentially invisible when the person is wearing long pants. Patients who worry that wearing the AFO will weaken their muscles can be reassured that, if anything, the improved ease of walking will ensure that the weak muscles will in fact be used more than without an AFO. If there is only mild dorsiflexion weakness, AFOs may produce more inconvenience than benefit.

Somewhat analogous orthoses for wrist drop are also available, although polyneuropathies sufficiently severe to produce significant weakness of wrist extension are uncommon outside of specialized neuromuscular clinics. Unfortunately, wrist drop orthoses are generally less helpful than AFOs, as the main functional problem in such patients is usually due to the concurrent intrinsic hand muscle weakness, which a wrist drop orthosis helps only indirectly.

In selected situations, especially when there is patchy weakness in the upper limbs, surgical tendon transfers can be worthwhile. For example, severe weakness of thumb opposition results in an important functional loss for the hand. If finger flexor strength is relatively preserved, transfer of a finger flexor tendon to the thumb will allow some thumb opposition, albeit imperfect. The net effect can be a significant gain in hand function. Clearly the uses of the tendon transfer approach are limited, but consultation with an experienced hand surgeon is a therapeutic option that is probably underutilized.

Patients often ask about the benefit of exercise for muscle weakness. There is no evidence that exercise per se reverses or reduces the muscle weakness or atrophy produced by denervation, and there is evidence that intense exercise to the point of exhaustion is actually harmful. Nevertheless, regular medium aerobic and stretching exercises do help to optimize function in minimally or unaffected muscles, as well as having cardiovascular and psychological benefits. A reasonable guideline is two or three 30-minute exercise sessions per week. A physiotherapist, occupational therapist, or physiatrist may help patients tailor their exercise to their specific needs.

ACUTE TRAUMATIC BRAIN INJURY IN ADULTS

method of
ROGER HARTL, M.D., and
JAMSHID GHAJAR, M.D., PH.D.
Weill Medical College of Cornell University
New York Presbyterian Hospital
New York, New York

The terms *head injury* and *traumatic brain injury* (TBI) have been used synonymously, with the latter term used now commonly as a better descriptor. Traumatic brain injury is graded as mild, moderate, or severe based on the level of consciousness or the Glasgow Coma Scale (GCS) score after resuscitation (Table 1). Mild TBI is characterized by GCS scores between 13 and 15. In most cases it represents a concussion, and there is full neurologic recovery, although many patients reveal short-term memory and concentration difficulties. Patients with moderate TBI are typically stuporous and lethargic with a GCS score between 9 and 13. A comatose patient unable to open his or her eyes or follow commands, with a GCS score of less than 9, by definition has a severe TBI.

Over the past two decades, it has become increasingly clear that patients with TBI are susceptible to post-traumatic arterial hypotension, hypoxia, and brain swelling. All major advances in the care of these patients have been achieved by reducing the severity of these secondary insults on the injured central nervous system. Rapid resuscitation of trauma patients in the field and direct transport to a major trauma center and improved critical care management in the hospital with intracranial pressure monitoring seem to have cut down the rate of mortality from up to 50% in the 1970s and 1980s to between 15% and 25% in most recent series. The development of scientifically based management protocols for the treatment of patients with TBI holds considerable promise for further improvement in outcome.

The goal of this article is to familiarize the reader with the basic principles of TBI management. In this article we refer to four recently published, evidence-based documents containing guidelines for the prehospital and in-hospital surgical and medical management of patients with severe TBI. These documents can be accessed via the Internet at www.braintrauma.org.

EPIDEMIOLOGY

About 1.6 million people sustain a TBI each year in the United States, and 270,000 require hospitalization. With about 52,000 deaths per year, TBI is the most common cause of death and disability in young people and accounts for about one third of all trauma deaths. The costs of TBI to society are immense; neurotrauma is a serious public health problem requiring continuing improvement in the care of injured patients. Motor vehicle accidents are the major cause

TABLE 1. **Glasgow Coma Scale**

Score	Eyes Open	Best Verbal Response	Best Motor Response
6	—	—	Obeys commands
5	—	Oriented & converses	Localizes painful stimuli
4	Spontaneously	Disoriented & converses	Flexion withdrawal
3	To verbal command	Inappropriate words	Flexion abnormal
2	To painful stimuli	Incomprehensible sounds	Extension
1	No response	No response	No response

of TBI, particularly in young people. Falls are the leading cause of death and disability from TBI in people older than 65 years.

PATHOPHYSIOLOGY: SECONDARY BRAIN DAMAGE

Neurologic injury not only occurs during the impact (primary injury) but also evolves over the following hours and days (secondary brain injury). Within the first days and weeks after TBI, the brain is extremely vulnerable to decreases in blood pressure and oxygenation that are well-tolerated by the noninjured central nervous system. Secondary brain damage is the most dominant cause of TBI in-hospital death. The most important insults that may lead to secondary brain damage and poor outcome are listed in Table 2. Many of these insults are preventable. In the prehospital phase, hypoxia and arterial hypotension have been shown to be the most significant secondary insults. Studies have reported that between 27% and 55% of patients were hypoxemic (arterial oxygen concentration < 90%) at the scene, in the ambulance, or on arrival in the emergency room. Arterial hypotension is defined as a single systolic blood pressure reading of less than 90 mm Hg. Hypotensive episodes were observed in 16% and 32% of patients with severe TBI at the time of hospital arrival and during surgical procedures, respectively. A single hypotensive episode has been shown to be associated with increased morbidity rate and a doubling of the mortality rate.

Recommendation: The mean arterial blood pressure in patients with severe TBI should always be maintained above 90 mm Hg to keep the cerebral perfusion pressure at approximately 70 mm Hg.

Soon after the primary injury, brain swelling occurs. Brain swelling can be due to vascular engorgement or to an increase in brain water content, called *brain edema*. Depending on the underlying mechanism, it is possible to distinguish several types of brain swelling:

- Swelling caused by hyperemia or venous congestion, or both
- Vasogenic brain edema
- Cytotoxic brain edema
- Interstitial brain edema

Disruption of the blood-brain barrier within minutes after TBI leads to accumulation of fluid in the extravascular compartment and vasogenic edema. Vasogenic edema can also develop later around areas of contused brain tissue and hemorrhage. Despite the effectiveness of steroids to treat vasogenic edema in patients with brain tumors, they have not proven to be of benefit in patients with TBI. The main type of brain swelling after TBI is probably due to cytotoxic edema. This type of edema is characterized by a failure of sodium/potassium pumps to maintain intracellular hemostasis. This leads to influx of ions and water into cells and initiates a self-destructive cascade culminating in progressive ischemia and intracranial hypertension. Several pharmacologic agents that interfere with this cascade, such as calcium antagonists, free-radical scavengers, and *N*-methyl-D-aspartate antagonists have been tested, but none have been proven effective.

Recommendation: The lack of pharmacologic agents that are available to treat patients with TBI reinforces the importance of optimal critical care management and monitoring and treatment of brain pressure, blood pressure, and oxygenation to maintain and improve cerebral perfusion.

TABLE 2. **Secondary Insults After Traumatic Brain Injury (TBI)**

Secondary Insult	Critical Values in TBI	Main Cause
Arterial hypotension	Systolic blood pressure < 90 mm Hg	Blood loss, sepsis, cardiac failure, spinal cord injury, brainstem injury
Hypoxemia	Arterial O_2 saturation < 90%, $Pa{O_2}$ <60 mm Hg, apnea, cyanosis	Hypoventilation, thoracic injury, aspiration
Hypocapnia	Sustained $Pa{CO_2}$ <25 mm Hg	Induced or spontaneous hyperventilation
Intracranial hypertension	ICP > 20–25 mm Hg	Mass lesion or cerebral swelling

Abbreviation: ICP, intracranial pressure.

MANAGEMENT

Assessment of the Patient with Traumatic Brain Injury

A short summary of a typical neurotrauma evaluation with possible critical findings is summarized in Table 3. The goal of the immediate management is to:

- Determine the severity of the primary TBI
- Identify patients at risk for deterioration
- Prevent secondary brain damage
- Identify associated injuries

Emergency room patients with mild or moderate TBI or suspected TBI need to be followed very closely for neurologic deterioration, ideally with neurochecks every 15 minutes. A complete trauma workup should be initiated if there is any suspicion of associated injuries. Nausea or vomiting, progressive headaches, restlessness, pupillary asymmetry, seizures, and increasing lethargy should be interpreted as signs of neurodeterioration, and a head computed tomography (CT) scan should be obtained immediately. It is important to remember that with expanding intracranial mass lesions, pupillary changes can precede a significant change in mental status. Blood alcohol levels and urine toxicology screen should be considered in all patients presenting with TBI. Routine blood tests, including coagulation parameters, should be obtained in patients with moderate and severe TBI and in patients with associated injuries. Tetanus toxoid must be administered if there are any associated open wounds. Immobilization of the cervical spine using a hard collar is mandatory in all patients with head injury. All patients with severe TBI need radiographic evaluation of the craniocervical junction down to T1. Any complaint of neck pain in patients with mild or moderate TBI should also lead to a radiographic assessment of the cervical spine.

Patients with Mild Traumatic Brain Injury

The majority of patients seen in the emergency department with a history of head injury have a mild or moderate TBI. The category of mild TBI includes patients who are awake with GCS scores between 13 and 15 without an intracranial pathologic lesion, a focal neurologic deficit, and other intracranial complications such as seizures. They may be amnesic for the event. Studies have shown that only 3% to 13% of patients in this category will have an abnormality on their head CT scan that can be attributed to the trauma. The management algorithm for patients with mild TBI is depicted in Figure 1.

Patients lacking a history of loss of consciousness, with a GCS score of 15 and normal clinical examination findings, who do not show any of the findings listed in Table 4 can be sent home with a head injury instruction sheet provided a "responsible individual" will remain with the patient for the first 24 hours (Table 5). The discharge instructions should be carefully reviewed with the patient and his or her companions. Patients who present with a GCS score of 13 or 14 who do not improve to a GCS score of 15 within 6 hours after TBI should be admitted for observation.

With a history of loss of consciousness, up to 18% of patients show CT abnormalities and 5% require surgical evacuation of the lesion. Any patient presenting with a history of loss of consciousness or any of the moderate or high risk findings listed in Table 4 will undergo CT of the head. Skull radiographs are not recommended for the routine evaluation of TBI patients. Cervical spine radiographic studies are performed in patients with neck pain or extremity weakness. Patients with a normal head CT scan and a GCS score of 15 can be sent home, provided a responsible individual is available who will observe the patient, as outlined in Table 6.

At our institution, every patient admitted for observation with a contusion or an extra-axial collection such as an epidural hematoma or subdural hematoma is admitted to the intensive care unit. A repeat head CT scan is obtained approximately 6 to 12 hours after admission. Patients with a small traumatic subarachnoid hemorrhage located over the hemispheres with normal examination findings do not always need a repeat CT scan. Patients with abnormal head CT

TABLE 3. **Immediate Assessment and Treatment of Patients with Traumatic Brain Injury**

Parameter	Critical Findings	Immediate Intervention
1. Resuscitation		
Oxygenation/ventilation	Apnea,cyanosis, oxygen saturation <90%	Intubation if hypoxemic despite supplemental O_2, no hyperventilation
Blood pressure	SBP <90 mm Hg	Fluid resuscitation
2. Primary Survey/Postresuscitation		
Spinal stability	Pain, step-off, external signs of trauma to neck, mechanism	Immobilization, radiographs
Postresuscitation GCS score	<9	Intubation, normoventilation, head CT
Motor examination, pupillary diameter, light reflex, direct orbital trauma	Suspect cerebral herniation: flaccidity or motor posturing and asymmetrical or fixed and dilated pupils	Short-term hyperventilation +/– mannitol, if herniation suspected
3. Placement of lines, urinary and gastric catheters, and cervical spine, chest, and pelvis radiographs		
4. Secondary survey/detailed neurologic examination		

Abbreviations: CT, computed tomography; GCS, Glasgow Coma Scale; SBP, systolic blood pressure.

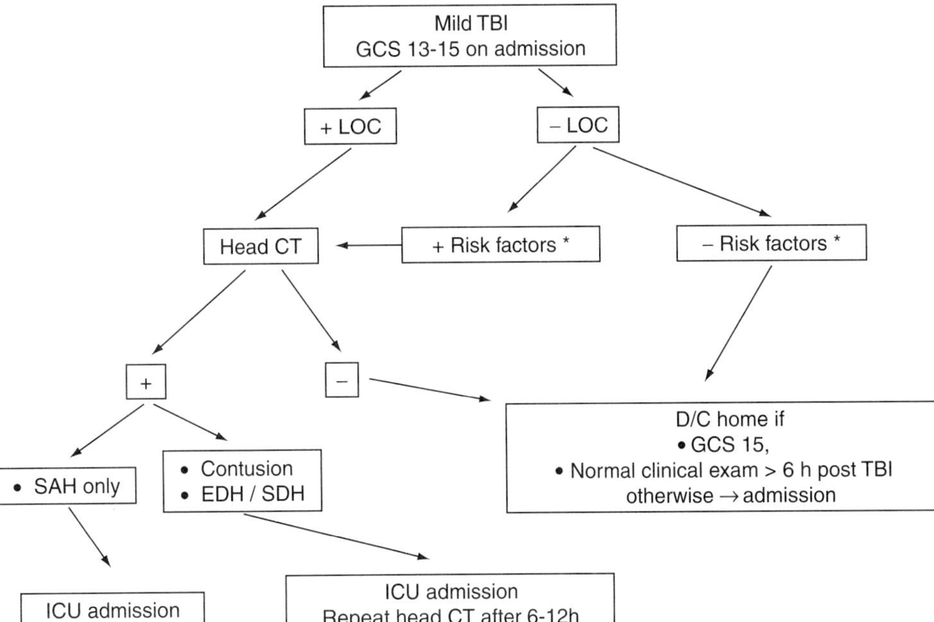

Figure 1. Treatment algorithm for the management of patients with mild traumatic brain injury (TBI). *Risk factors are listed in Table 4. CT, computed tomography; D/C, discharge (home); EDH, epidural hematoma; GCS, Glasgow Coma Scale; ICU, intensive care unit; LOC, loss of consciousness; SAH, subarachnoid hemorrhage; SDH, subdural hematoma.

findings with disease-related or pharmacologically induced coagulopathy undergo neurologic observation in the hospital for at least 2 days.

Patients with Moderate Traumatic Brain Injury

Approximately 10% of patients with TBI will fall into the category of moderate TBI with a GCS score between 9 and 12. These patients all undergo CT scanning of their head and are admitted to the intensive care unit. Approximately 40% of patients with moderate TBI will have abnormal head CT findings, and 8% will require surgical treatment. Up to 20% of patients with moderate TBI will deteriorate and become comatose. Follow-up CT scans are obtained in all patients with moderate TBI when there is neurologic deterioration or before the patient is discharged.

TABLE 4. **Findings Associated with Risks for Poor Outcome After Traumatic Brain Injury**

Low Risk	Moderate Risk	High Risk
GCS score 15	GCS score 9–14	GCS score 3–8
Mild headache/ dizziness	Progressive headache	Focal neurologic deficit
Scalp injuries	Alcohol, drug intoxication	Abnormal CT scan
	Seizure	Pupillary abnormality
	Vomiting	SBP < 90 mm Hg
	Age <2 years	Sao_2 < 90%
	Multitrauma	
	Coagulopathy	
	Facial fractures	

Abbreviation: CT, computed tomography; GCS, Glasgow Coma Scale; SBP, systolic blood pressure.

Rakel and Bope: Conn's Current Therapy 2004. Copyright 2004 by Elsevier Inc.

Patients with Severe Traumatic Brain Injury

Prehospital Management

The prehospital management of patients with severe TBI is outlined in Figure 2. Rapid and physiologic resuscitation is the first priority in these patients. Following stabilization of airway, breathing, and circulation, the GCS score should be determined by direct verbal or physical interaction with the patient. If the patient does not respond to verbal commands, the physician or paramedic should apply blunt

TABLE 5. **Head Injury Instructions**

Although no evidence of any serious head injury is present at this time, careful attention for the next 24–48 hours is advised, as evidence of head injury may appear several hours following an injury. Of particular importance are the following:

1. A responsible individual should remain with the patient for the first 24 hours
2. No alcohol should be taken for the next 48 hours
3. No sedatives or pain medicines other than Tylenol unless prescribed by the doctor should be taken for the next 48 hours
4. Awaken the patient every 2 hours through the first 8 hours and ask his/her name, where he/she is, and the date. This should be rechecked every 6 hours for the next 24 hours

The patient should return to the emergency room immediately for re-evaluation if any of the following symptoms occur:

1. Drowsiness or mental confusion
2. Difficulty in arousing the patient
3. Recurrent vomiting
4. Blurred vision or double vision
5. Increasingly severe headache
6. Drainage of blood or fluid from the nose or ears
7. Weakness of arms or legs
8. Convulsions
9. Pupils of the eyes become unequal in size
10. Loss of balance
11. Fever with or without a stiff neck

TABLE 6. **Treatment Algorithm for Patients with Intracranial Hypertension**

In all Patients with GCS Score < 9	Add if ICP > 20 mm Hg	Add if ICP > 25 mm Hg	Add for Persistent ICP > 25 mm Hg	Add for Persistent ICP > 25 mm Hg and/or Pupillary Abnormalities
ICP monitoring				
Elevate head of bed 30 degrees	Ventricular CSF drainage	Neuromuscular blockade: vecuronium (Norcuron), atracurium (Tracrium)	Moderate hypothermia, core temperature 34–36°C	High-dose propofol (Diprivan) infusion
Maintain euvolemia and hemodynamic stability, keep CVP 5–10 mm Hg	Sedation: midazolam (Versed) *or* lorazepam (Ativan)	Mannitol 0.25–1 gm/kg IV over 5–10 minutes q4–6 h PRN. Serum osmolarity 300–320 mOsm/L; serum sodium 150–155 mEq/L	Hyperventilation to Pa_{CO_2} 30–35 mm Hg	Hyperventilation to Pa_{CO_2} 25–30 mm Hg
Pa_{O_2} >90 mm Hg	Analgesia: fentanyl (Sublimaze) *or* morphine			Consider hypertonic saline bolus infusion Consider decompressive craniectomy
Pa_{CO_2} 35–40 mm Hg				
Systolic blood pressure > 90 mm Hg	"CPP management": Inotropic and pressor support to maintain CPP (dopamine [Intropin] 5–20 μg/kg/min, norepinephrine [Levophed] 0.05–0.5 μg/kg/min			
CPP approximately 70 mm Hg	Repeat head CT to exclude operable mass lesion			

Abbreviations: CPP, cerebral perfusion pressure; CSF, cerebrospinal fluid; CT, computed tomography; CVP, central venous pressure; ICP, intracranial pressure; GCS, Glasgow Coma Scale.

pressure to the nail bed or pinch the anterior axillary skin to elicit eye opening. Patients with a GCS score between 9 and 13 should be transported to a trauma center, and patients with a GCS score of less than 9 should be brought to a trauma center with the following TBI capabilities:

- 24-hour CT scanning capability
- 24-hour available operating room and prompt neurosurgical care
- The ability to monitor intracranial pressure and treat intracranial hypertension

Comatose patients with a GCS score less than 9 should be intubated. Adult patients who respond to nail bed pressure or axillary pinch with abnormal extension, or are flaccid, or have asymmetric or dilated pupils should be hyperventilated at a rate of 20 breaths per minute. All patients should have their oxygenation and blood pressure assessed at least every 5 minutes. Their oxygen saturation should be maintained above 90% and systolic blood pressure should be kept above 90 mm Hg (see Table 3).

In-Hospital Management

Initial Management in the Emergency Department

Maintaining brain perfusion or, put bluntly, "squeezing oxygenated blood through swollen brain" is the guiding principle in managing comatose patients with severe TBI.

The cornerstones of the resuscitation of the severely head injured patient are:

- Resuscitation (airway, breathing, circulation)
- Primary survey with cervical spine control and brief neurologic assessment
- Secondary survey with complete neurologic examination and determination of the GCS score (see Table 3)

General principles of the TBI workup are:

- Normocapnia should be maintained. Unless there are signs of cerebral herniation (pupillary asymmetry, dilated/fixed pupils, and/or extensor posturing or flaccidity to noxious stimuli) patients should not be hyperventilated and the arterial P_{CO_2} should be maintained around 35 mm Hg.
- Isotonic fluids should be used for resuscitation to avoid free water overload.
- CT is the imaging study of choice to detect skull fractures and intracranial injury with hemorrhage and to assess the necessity of surgical evacuation of a mass lesion. A head CT scan can also demonstrate findings that are closely associated with intracranial hypertension, such as obliterated basal cisterns, compressed cerebral ventricles, and midline shift (Figure 3).
- All comatose patients with an abnormal CT scan and a GCS score of 8 or less should undergo intracranial pressure (ICP) monitoring.

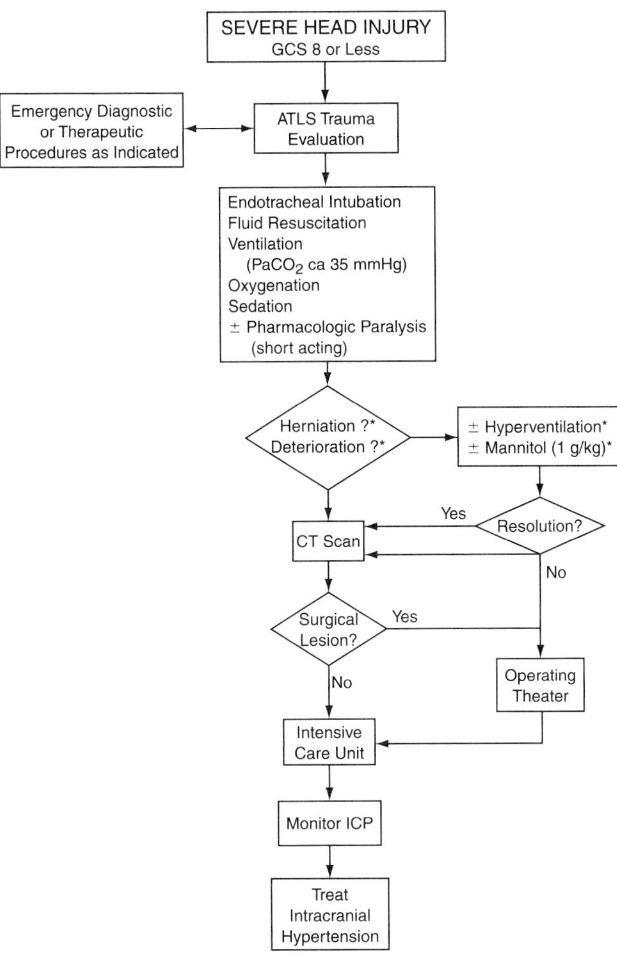

Figure 2. Initial resuscitation of patients with severe traumatic brain injury. *Only in the presence of signs of herniation or progressive neurologic deterioration not attributable to extracranial factors. ATLS, Advanced Trauma Life Support—American College of Surgeons; CT, computed tomography; GCS, Glasgow Coma Scale; ICP, intracranial pressure.

- Plain radiographs of the cervical spine should be obtained as soon as possible, and a CT scan of suspicious areas should be obtained.
- Once the patient has been stabilized, a careful physical examination should be conducted.

Computed Tomography Scan Assessment

After resuscitation, all stable patients with severe TBI should get a CT scan of the head as soon as possible to identify:

- A life-threatening mass lesion that requires surgical evacuation
- Evidence of raised ICP
- The degree of intracranial injury, to determine prognostic indicators of outcome

Approximately 10% of initial head CT scans in patients with severe TBI will not show any abnormalities. The absence of abnormalities on CT scan at admission does not preclude increased ICP. Significant new lesions and increased ICP may develop in 40% of patients with initially normal head CT scan. In addition, patients with normal CT findings, systolic blood pressure lower than 90 mm Hg, age greater than 40 years, or motor posturing are at the same risk for intracranial hypertension as those with abnormal head CT findings.

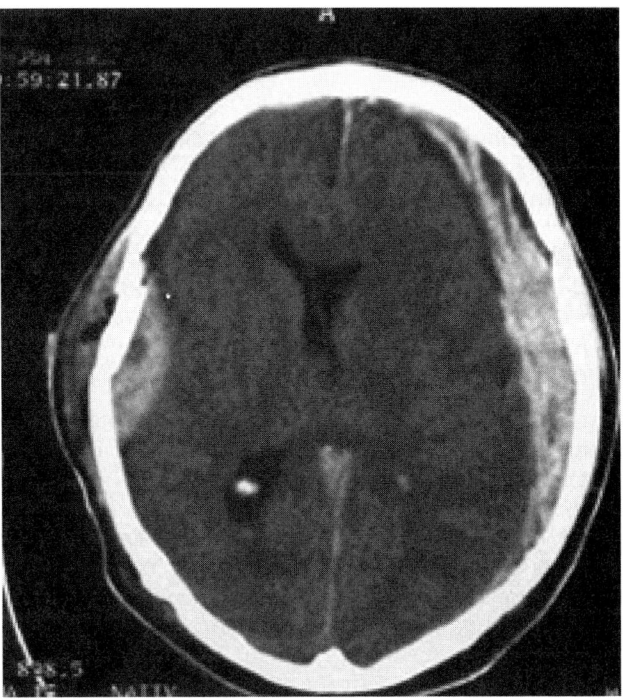

Figure 3. Head computed tomography scan of a patient with severe traumatic brain injury demonstrating right-sided acute epidural hematoma (left side of picture) with skull fracture and left-sided acute subdural hematoma. There is significant midline shift.

Intracranial Pressure Monitoring and Treatment of Elevated Intracranial Pressure

Comatose head injury patients (GCS score 3 to 8) with abnormal CT scans should undergo ICP monitoring for the following reasons:

- Helps in the earlier detection of intracranial mass lesions
- Can limit the indiscriminate use of therapies to control ICP, which themselves can be potentially harmful
- Can reduce ICP by cerebrospinal fluid drainage and thus improve cerebral perfusion
- Helps in determining prognosis
- May improve outcome

Elevated ICP is present in the majority of severely head-injured patients. Cerebral perfusion pressure is defined as the mean arterial blood pressure minus ICP. This physiologic variable defines the pressure gradient driving cerebral blood flow and metabolite delivery and is therefore closely related to cerebral ischemia. A threshold for cerebral perfusion pressure of approximately 60 mm Hg for adults is currently recommended.

Recommendation: ICP monitoring is appropriate in severe head injury patients (GCS score

3 to 8) with an abnormal CT scan, or a normal CT scan if two or more of the following are noted upon admission:

- Systolic blood pressure less than 90 mm Hg
- Age greater than 40 years
- Unilateral or bilateral motor posturing

Intracranial pressure treatment should be initiated at an upper threshold of 20 or 25 mm Hg. Cerebral perfusion pressure (mean arterial pressure minus ICP) should be maintained at approximately 60 mm Hg.

Increased ICP should be treated vigorously. The management of the typical TBI patient with ICP monitoring at our institution is outlined in Table 7. Hyperventilation should not be used routinely in these patients because of the risk of further compromising cerebral perfusion. We do use hyperventilation only for brief periods when there is acute neurologic deterioration or if intracranial hypertension is refractory to other treatment interventions. Under these circumstances, we use intraparenchymal brain tissue oxygen monitoring to titrate the degree of hyperventilation and to avoid cerebral ischemia (see Table 7).

Recommendation: In the absence of increased ICP, chronic prolonged hyperventilation therapy ($Paco_2 \leq 25$ mm Hg) should be avoided. The use of prophylactic hyperventilation ($Paco_2 \leq 35$ mm Hg) therapy during the first 24 hours after severe TBI should be avoided because it can compromise cerebral perfusion.

Glucocorticoids have not been shown to improve outcome after severe TBI.

Recommendation: The use of glucocorticoids is not recommended for improving outcome or reducing intracranial pressure in patients with severe TBI.

Intracranial Pressure Monitoring Technology. The ICP monitoring devices can be ranked based on their accuracy, stability, and ability to drain cerebrospinal fluid. With the current state of technology, the ventricular catheter connected to an external strain gauge is the most accurate, low-cost, and reliable method of monitoring ICP. It also allows therapeutic cerebrospinal fluid drainage. ICP transduction via fiberoptic or strain gauge devices placed in ventricular catheters provide similar benefits, but at a higher cost. Parenchymal ICP monitors are generally accurate and are easily placed. Subdural, subarachnoid, and epidural devices are less accurate.

Barbiturate Coma. High-dose barbiturate therapy may be considered in hemodynamically stable, salvageable, severe TBI patients with intracranial hypertension refractory to maximal medical and surgical ICP-lowering therapy. Barbiturates appear to exert their cerebral protective and ICP-lowering effects through several distinct mechanisms: alterations in vascular tone, suppression of metabolism,

TABLE 7. **Typical Orders for Patients with Severe Traumatic Brain Injury (TBI)**

Admit to Neuro/Trauma intensive care unit

Monitoring and notifications

- Check vital signs and neurostratus q1h, call HO for neurochange
- Check temperature q4h, call for T > 38.3°C. If T >38.3°C, remove sheets, use cooling blankets, fan and/or ice packings
- Monitor end tidal CO_2. Call for $Paco_2$ < 30 mm Hg
- Notify for SBP > 180 or SBP < 90
- Specify ventriculostomy settings
- Monitor CPP, call for CPP < 70 mm Hg
- Monitor CVP, call for CVP < 5 or CVP > 10 mm Hg
- If Swan Ganz catheter in place, measure cardiac parameters q4 hours, call for wedge pressure < 8 and > 15 mm Hg
- Strict I's and O's, call for UO > 200 mL/hr × 2 hours

Activity

- Bedrest with HOB 30 degrees
- Log roll, spine precautions
- Cervical collar

Nursing

- Foley catheter
- Knee high stockings and/or pneumatic compression devices
- Daily weights
- 2–4 L O_2 per nasal cannula
- Orogastric tube, nasogastric tube if no basilar skull fracture

Diet

- Start tube feedings within 24–36 h after TBI

Maintenance IV fluids

- D5 Normal saline +/− 20 mEq/L KCl at 1–2 mL/h, typically 80–120 mL

Medication

- Stool softener
- Docusate sodium (Colace) 200 mg PO bid

Antiemetic

- Trimethobenzamide (Tigan) 200 mg IM q8h prn
- Prochlorperazine (Compazine) 5–10 mg IM q6h prn

Analgesia

- Codeine 30–60 mg IM/PO q3h prn
- Morphine 1–6 mg IV/IM q4–6h prn or IV drip up to 5–10 mg/h
- Fentanyl (Sublimaze) 50–150 μg bolus, then 30–100 μg/h maintenance

Antipyretics

- Acetaminophen (Tylenol) 600–1000 mg PO/PR q6h prn if T >38.3°C
- Ibuprofen 400 mg NG/PR q8h prn if T >38.3°C

Sedation

- Midazolam (Versed) drip 1–2 mg/h
- Lorazepam (Ativan) 1 mg PO bid–tid
- Diazepam (Valium) 2–10 mg PO bid

GI prophylaxis (a recent review recommended sucralfate > continuous cimetidine > intermittent H_2 blockers)

- Sucralfate (Carafate) 1 g PO qid
- Cimetidine (Tagamet) continuous infusion 37.5–100 mg/h IV
- Famotidine (Pepcid) 20 mg PO/IV bid

Seizure prophylaxis

- Phenytoin (Dilantin) 300 mg PO qd

Arterial hypertension

- Labetalol (Trandate) 10 mg IV q15 min for SBP > 180 mm Hg prn, hold for HR < 60 beats/min
- Hydralazine (Apresoline) 10 mg IV q15 min for SBP > 180 prn, hold for HR > 90 beats/min; may increase ICP and CBF

Others

- Lidocaine protocol for suctioning

Labs

- CBC, Coags, T&C, SMA-10, Tox screen, ETOH level

Ventilator settings

and inhibition of free radical–mediated lipid peroxidation. The most important effect may relate to coupling of cerebral blood flow to regional metabolic demands, such that the lower the metabolic requirements, the less the cerebral blood flow and related cerebral blood volume with subsequent beneficial effects on ICP and global cerebral perfusion.

There is a poor correlation between serum level, therapeutic benefit, and systemic complications. The risk of arterial hypotension induced by peripheral vasodilation is high. A reliable form of monitoring is the electroencephalographic pattern of burst suppression. Near-maximal reductions in cerebral metabolism and cerebral blood flow occur when burst suppression is induced. To conduct a reliable brain death examination, pentobarbital (Nembutal) levels should be 1 mg/dL or less or 10 μg/mL or less.

High-Dose Propofol. In recent years, propofol (Diprivan) has gained popularity as an alternative to barbiturates in patients with intracranial hypertension refractory to maximal medical and surgical ICP-lowering therapy. The main advantages of propofol is that it is short acting. Like other anesthetics, it can cause hypotension, and, even though ICP decreases, overall cerebral perfusion pressure may drop. Prolonged use of propofol can cause pancreatitis. Hepatic and pancreatic enzymes should be monitored. Propofol should not be used in pediatric patients.

Mannitol. Mannitol is effective for control of raised ICP after severe TBI. Limited data suggest that intermittent boluses may be more effective than continuous infusion. Effective doses range from 0.25 to 1 g/kg body weight. Hypovolemia should be avoided by fluid replacement. Serum osmolarity should be kept below 320 mOsm to avoid renal failure. Euvolemia should be maintained by adequate fluid replacement. A Foley catheter has to be placed in these patients. ICP reduction reaches a maximum approximately 30 to 60 minutes after bolus infusion and persists between 90 minutes and 6 hours, or longer. Mannitol together with furosemide (Lasix) may cause rapid diuresis and depletion of intravascular volume and electrolytes and is therefore not recommended.

> *Recommendation: The indications for the use of mannitol prior to ICP monitoring are signs of transtentorial herniation or progressive neurologic deterioration not attributable to a systemic pathologic condition. Euvolemia should be maintained by adequate fluid replacement. Intermittent bolus doses may be more effective for raised ICP than continuous infusions. Effective doses range from 0.25 to 1 g/kg body weight.*

Hypertonic Saline. Hypertonic saline has found its place as a second-tier therapy in the treatment of intracranial hypertension resistant to conventional treatment maneuvers. Hypertonic saline has been used both as bolus infusion for treatment of acutely elevated ICP and as continuous infusion of 1.8 to 3% saline to increase serum osmolarity. Hypertonic saline decreases ICP by reducing brain water content. Clinical data demonstrate that bolus infusion reliably decreases ICP in patients in whom mannitol has lost its efficacy. A hyperosmolar state with serum osmolarities well above 320 mOsm/L may develop but seems to be tolerated well as long as euvolemia and arterial normotension are maintained. We do currently use bolus infusions of up to 250 mL of 5% or 7.5% saline over 5 to 10 minutes every 6 hours in patients who do not respond to mannitol or in patients who are hemodynamically unstable.

Nutritional Support

Studies have shown that not feeding severely head-injured patients by the first week increases mortality. It is our practice to initiate tube feedings within the first 2 days after TBI.

> *Recommendation: Replace 140% of resting metabolism expenditure in nonparalyzed patients and 100% of resting metabolism expenditure in paralyzed patients using enteral or parenteral formulas containing at least 15% of calories as protein by the seventh day after injury. Jejunal feeding by gastrojejunostomy is preferable because of ease of use and avoidance of gastric intolerance.*

Treatment of Seizures

Post-traumatic seizures (PTS) are divided into early (<7 days after trauma) and late seizures (>7 days after trauma). In recent TBI studies that followed high-risk patients up to 36 months, the incidence of early PTS varied between 4% and 25%, and the incidence of late PTS varied between 9% to 42% in untreated patients. Prophylactic use of phenytoin (Dilantin), carbamazepine (Tegretol), or phenobarbital is not recommended for preventing late PTS. Anticonvulsants may be used to prevent *early* PTS in patients at high risk for seizures following head injury. Phenytoin and carbamazepine have been demonstrated to be effective in this setting. However, the available evidence does not indicate that prevention of early PTS improves outcome following head injury. Routine seizure prophylaxis later than 1 week following head injury is therefore not recommended. If late PTS occurs, patients should be managed in accordance with standard approaches to patients with new-onset seizures. We do not use routine seizure prophylaxis after TBI, mainly out of concern of potential side effects such as drug fever and anaphylaxis. Fever may develop 1 to 8 weeks after exposure to phenytoin, phenobarbital, or carbamazepine.

> *Recommendation: Prophylactic use of phenytoin (Dilantin), carbamazepine (Tegretol), or phenobarbital is not recommended for preventing late PTS. Anticonvulsants such as phenytoin and carbamazepine can be used to prevent early PTS in patients at high risk for seizures following TBI.*

Cervical Spine Assessment

Immobilization of the cervical spine using a hard collar is mandatory in all patients with TBI. In fully conscious patients who are not intoxicated and

- Do not complain of neck pain
- Do not reveal bony cervical tenderness
- Do not have peripheral sensory or motor abnormalities on examination
- Have a pain-free full range of neck movements, the cervical spine is cleared clinically without any further studies.

Six percent of primary head injuries are associated with cervical spine injury. All seriously head-injured patients should be treated as if a concomitant cervical spine injury is present until proven otherwise. A wooden or metal backboard is used to immobilize the thoracic and lumbar spine, since 25% to 30% of spine injuries are located in that region. Patients should be taken off the backboard once they have been evaluated in the emergency department. It is important to remember that 15% of patients with an identified spine injury will have a second injury at some other site. Therefore, any abnormality detected in the cervical spine requires a complete set of spine radiographs.

All patients complaining of neck pain or tenderness and all comatose patients with TBI should have the following set of cervical spine radiographs:

- Lateral view revealing the base of the occiput to the upper border of T1
- Anteroposterior view from C2 to T1
- Open-mouth odontoid view revealing the lateral masses of C1 and the complete odontoid process

In the conscious and cooperative patient with neck pain who is neurologically intact, these films should be followed by flexion and extension views.

A thin-cut axial CT scan with sagittal reconstruction should be obtained through suspicious areas or for poor visualization on plain radiographs. This combination of studies can provide a false-negative rate of only 0.1%. In comatose patients, the craniocervical junction should be scanned. It is our practice to remove the hard collar in comatose patients if all radiologic studies are negative. If we expect the patient to be fully awake within a few days, we leave the cervical collar on and wait until we can perform a reliable examination.

Surgical Management of Acute Traumatic Brain Injury

The decision as to whether an intracranial lesion requires surgical evacuation can be difficult and is based on the patient's GCS score, pupillary examination findings, co-morbidities, CT findings, age, and, in delayed decisions, ICP. Neurologic deterioration over time is also an important factor influencing the decision to operate. Trauma patients presenting to the emergency department with altered mental status, pupillary asymmetry, and abnormal flexion or extension are at high risk for an intracranial mass lesion, and it is our practice to notify the operating room even before obtaining a CT scan that an emergency craniotomy will most likely be necessary.

This discussion of the surgical management has been organized according to the traditional literature-based classification of post-traumatic mass lesions: namely, epidural hematoma (EDH), acute subdural hematoma (SDH), intraparenchymal lesions (contusion, intracerebral hematoma), acute posterior fossa mass lesions, and depressed fractures of the skull. In many patients with severe or moderate TBI, more than one of these acute post-traumatic mass lesions may coexist at the same time. For these reasons, each patient requires individual management, and, even more than in other areas of TBI management, neurosurgical judgment is required to formulate an optimal treatment plan for each patient.

Epidural Hematoma

The incidence of surgical and nonsurgical EDH among TBI patients is around 3%. Among patients in coma, up to 9% harbored an EDH requiring craniotomy. The peak incidence of EDH is in the second decade and the mean age of patients with EDH is between 20 and 30 years of age. Traffic-related accidents, falls, and assaults account for the majority of all cases of EDH. EDH usually results from injury to the middle meningeal artery but can also be due to bleeding from the middle meningeal vein, the diploic veins, or the venous sinuses. In patients with EDH, one third to one half are comatose on admission or immediately before surgery. The classically described "lucid interval," which describes a patient who is initially unconscious, then wakes up and secondarily deteriorates, is seen in approximately one half of patients undergoing surgery for EDH.

Clot thickness, hematoma volume, and midline shift (MLS) on the preoperative CT scan are related to outcome. Noncomatose patients without focal neurologic deficits and with an acute EDH with a thickness of less than 15 mm, an MLS less than 5 mm, and a hematoma volume less than 30 mL can be managed nonsurgically with serial CT scanning and close neurologic evaluation in a neurosurgical center. The first follow-up CT scan in nonsurgical patients should be obtained within 6 to 8 hours after TBI. Temporal location of an EDH is associated with failure of nonsurgical management and should lower the threshold for surgery. Patients with a GCS score less than 9 and an EDH larger than 30 mL should undergo immediate surgical evacuation of the lesion. All patients, regardless of GCS score, should be considered for surgery if the volume of their EDH exceeds 30 mL. Patients with an EDH volume less than 30 mL should be considered for surgery but may be managed successfully without surgery in selected cases. Time from neurologic deterioration to surgery correlates with outcome. In these patients, surgical evacuation should be done as soon as possible, since every hour of delay in surgery is associated with progressively worse outcome.

Acute Subdural Hematoma

Subdural hematomas are diagnosed on a CT scan as extracerebral, hyperdense, crescentic collections between the dura and the brain parenchyma. They can be divided into acute and chronic lesions. The incidence of acute SDH is between 12% and 29% in patients admitted with severe TBI. The mean age is between 31 and 47 years, with the vast majority of patients being male. Most SDHs are caused by motor vehicle-related accidents, falls, and assaults. Falls have been identified as the main cause of traumatic SDH in patients older than 75 years. Between 37% and 80% of patients with acute SDH present with initial GCS scores of 8 or lower. Clot thickness or volume and MLS on the preoperative CT scan correlate with outcome. Patients with SDH presenting with a clot thickness of greater than 10 mm or MLS greater than 5 mm should undergo surgical evacuation, regardless of their GCS. Patients who present in a coma (GCS score < 9) but with a SDH with a thickness of less than 10 mm and MLS less than 5 mm can be treated nonsurgically, providing that they undergo ICP monitoring, they are neurologically stable since injury, they have no pupillary abnormalities, and they have no intracranial hypertension (ICP > 20 mm Hg).

Traumatic Parenchymal Lesions

Traumatic parenchymal mass lesions occur in up to 10% of all patients with TBI and 13% to 35% of patients with severe TBI. Most small parenchymal lesions do not require surgical evacuation. However, the development of mass effect from larger lesions may result in secondary brain injury, placing the patient at risk of further neurologic deterioration, herniation, and death. Parenchymal lesions tend to evolve, and the timing of the surgery affects the outcome. Patients with parenchymal mass lesions and signs of progressive neurologic deterioration referable to the lesion, medically refractory intracranial hypertension, or signs of mass effect on CT scan should be treated operatively. Comatose patients with frontal or temporal contusions greater than 20 mL in volume and with MLS of 5 mm or cisternal compression on CT scan, or both, and patients with any lesion greater than 50 mL in volume should be treated surgically. Patients with parenchymal mass lesions who do not show evidence for neurologic compromise, have controlled ICP, and have no significant signs of mass effect on CT scan can be managed nonsurgically.

Posterior Fossa Mass Lesions

Less than 3% of patients with TBI present with posterior fossa lesions. The vast majority of these are posterior fossa epidural hematomas. It is important to recognize these lesions early on, because patients can undergo rapid clinical deterioration due to the limited size of the posterior fossa and the propensity for these lesions to produce brainstem compression. Patients with fourth ventricular mass effect on CT scan or with neurologic dysfunction or deterioration referable to the lesion should undergo a suboccipital craniectomy as soon as possible. Patients without significant mass effect on CT scan and without signs of neurologic dysfunction can be managed by close observation and serial imaging.

Depressed Skull Fractures

Depressed skull fractures complicate up to 6% of head injuries, and the presence of skull fracture is associated with a higher incidence of intracranial lesions, neurologic deficit, and poorer outcome. Patients with open skull fractures depressed greater than the thickness of the skull should undergo surgical intervention to prevent infection. Patients with open depressed fractures should be covered with antibiotic prophylaxis.

Decompressive Craniectomy for Control of Intracranial Hypertension

Decompressive procedures, such as subtemporal decompression, temporal lobectomy, and hemispheric decompressive craniectomy, are surgical procedures that have been used to treat patients with refractory intracranial hypertension and diffuse parenchymal injury. Decompressive craniectomy may be very effective if it is done early after TBI in young patients who are expected to develop postoperative brain swelling and intracranial hypertension.

Early Prognostic Indicators

Outcome from TBI is frequently described using the Glasgow Outcome Scale at 6 months following TBI (Table 8). This is a widely accepted and standardized scale that is of value for the clinical description of patients and also for medicolegal documentation and research purposes. The Glasgow Outcome Scale is poor for assessing patients with mild TBI. In these patients, more refined outcome measures are used that describe functional status based on neuropsychological testing, cognitive function, return-to-work data, and productivity.

Patients with mild TBI frequently perform poorly on complicated tasks requiring prolonged attention and rapid response times, but this difficulty usually

TABLE 8. **Glasgow Outcome Scale**

Score	Rating	Definition
5	Good Recovery	Resumption of normal life despite minor deficits.
4	Moderate Disability	Disabled but independent. Can work in sheltered setting.
3	Severe Disability	Conscious but severely disabled. Dependent for daily support.
2	Persistent Vegetative	No conscious behavior.
1	Death	

resolves within 1 month after injury. Postconcussive symptoms such as headache, dizziness, and memory problems occur in 50% of patients after mild TBI and persist at 3 months in about 33% of patients. Taken together, these data indicate that outcome from mild brain injury may not be as favorable as previously thought. A link has been proposed between post-concussional symptoms and psychiatric sequelae of TBI such as depression and physical manifestations of anxiety.

The most important early presenting factors influencing outcome from severe TBI are:

- Age
- GCS score
- Pupillary examination findings
- The presence of arterial hypotension
- CT scan findings

Studies show that the probability of poor outcome increases with decreasing admission GCS score in a continuous, stepwise manner below a GCS score of 9. Patients with very low GCS scores have a mortality rate between 70% and 90%, but up to 10% may survive with Glasgow Outcome Scale scores of 4 or 5. Increasing age is a strong independent factor in prognosis from severe TBI, with a significant increase in poor outcome in patients older than 60 years of age. This is not explained by the increased frequency of systemic complications in older patients. Several studies confirm that among comatose patients with acute SDH, no patient over the age of 75 who preoperatively showed signs of tentorial herniation made a good recovery.

The pupillary diameter and the pupilloconstrictor light reflex can prognosticate outcome from severe TBI. Bilaterally unreactive pupils following resuscitation on admission are associated with a greater than 90% chance of poor outcome.

A systolic blood pressure less than 90 mm Hg measured after severe TBI on the way to the hospital or in-hospital has been associated with an almost 70% likelihood of poor outcome. Combined with hypoxia, this likelihood increases to 79%. A single recording of arterial hypotension doubles the rate of mortality from severe TBI.

Among these early prognostic indicators of outcome, arterial hypotension is the only factor that can be significantly affected by therapeutic intervention.

The CT scan findings associated with poor outcome from severe TBI are

- Compressed or absent basal cisterns
- Traumatic subarachnoid hemorrhage
- MLS greater than 5 mm

Following admission, ICP greater than 20 mm Hg is a poor prognostic indicator. The rate of mortality from epidural hematoma requiring surgery is around 10% (range 7% to 12.5%). The rate of mortality from acute SDH is between 40% and 60%. The mortality rate among patients with acute SDH presenting to the hospital in coma with subsequent surgical evacuation is between 57% and 68%.

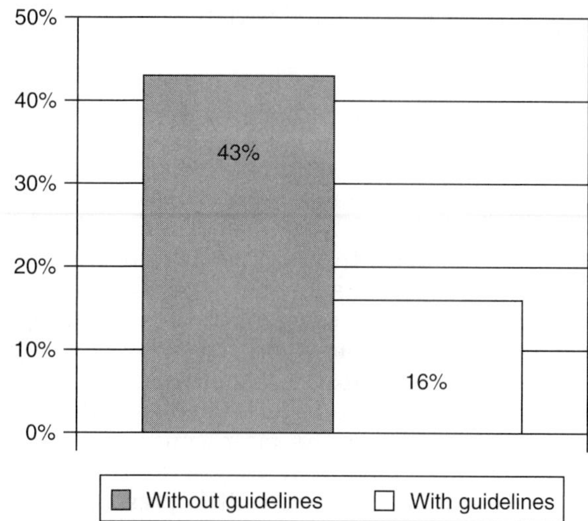

Figure 4. Mortality rate at 6 months following severe traumatic brain injury in 37 patients treated before (left, *gray column*) and 56 patients treated after (right, *white column*) introduction of management guidelines. Scientific evidence–based medical care reduced deaths by more than 50%. (From Palmer S, Bader M, Qureshi A, et al: The impact on outcomes in a community hospital setting of using the AANS traumatic brain injury guidelines. J Trauma 50:657–664, 2001.)

Overall, the mortality rate from severe TBI has been reduced from up to 50% in the 1970s and 1980s to between 15% and 25% in most recent series. In the absence of any pharmacological breakthrough, this improvement is attributed to more effective resuscitation in the field, rapid transport of TBI patients to trauma hospitals, more widely accepted ICP monitoring, and improvements in critical care management. In a recent study of 93 patients with severe TBI, the 6-month mortality rate was reduced 50% by the introduction of protocol guidelines for the management of severe TBI (Figure 4). The treatment guidelines supported ICP monitoring, adequate volume resuscitation, aggressive treatment of low blood pressure and oxygenation, avoidance of extreme hyperventilation, and early nutritional intervention. Multidisciplinary, comprehensive clinical pathways based on scientifically based treatment guidelines for TBI streamline patient care, standardize critical care management, and hold the potential for significantly improving patient outcome and reducing hospital costs.

Improvement in outcome from TBI is a result of advances in critical care management, imaging, and the reorganization of trauma systems. Early recognition and treatment of cerebral hypoperfusion and intracranial hypertension are key to managing these patients. Medical personnel in the prehospital and in-hospital setting should be aware of and trained in these principles of TBI care. The next advance will arrive with the further development and implementation of evidence-based management guidelines, which serve as the basis for standardizing acute care. This will then allow the conduction of prospective randomized clinical trials that can provide further evidence to develop and strengthen guideline recommendations.

ACUTE HEAD INJURIES IN CHILDREN

method of
RASHID M. JANJUA, M.D., and
THOMAS M. MORIARTY, M.D., PH.D.
University of Louisville
Louisville, Kentucky

Traumatic brain injury (TBI) remains an important cause of morbidity and mortality in pediatric patients. According to the Centers for Disease Control and Prevention, an estimated 3000 children and youth die of TBI; 29,000 are hospitalized and 400,000 are treated in hospital emergency departments. Currently, no population-based studies of the outcomes of TBI in children and youth are available to provide national estimates of TBI-related disability and document the need for services. In comparison, TBI leads to more than 6 times the number of deaths related to HIV/AIDS, 20 times the number of deaths from asthma, and 38 times the number of deaths from cystic fibrosis. TBI is the most common cause of acquired disability in pediatric patients, with a peak incidence in children younger than 5 years and those in mid to late adolescence, and it occurs most frequently in the 14- to 24-year-old age range. The leading cause of TBI in infants is falls, in contrast to adolescents, in whom participation in traffic (bicycle) and outdoor activities leads to transportation being the principal cause (Figure 1). Although several aspects in the management of pediatric TBI are identical to those in adults, the differences may be challenging.

DEFINITIONS

TBI can be classified into three categories based on the severity of the injury and the subsequent clinical condition of the patient.

Mild TBI is defined as head trauma with a clinical examination score on the Glasgow Coma Scale (GCS) of 13 to 15. A score of 9 to 12 on the GCS defines *moderate* TBI, whereas 8 or less is regarded as *severe* TBI. This latter group usually has more significant trauma and may have more extensive injury on their radiologic workup. In children younger than 3 years, the eye-opening and motor response subscales are identical to the GCS, but the verbal response subscale rates behavior/affect in these preverbal populations (Tables 1 and 2).

The most common structural abnormalities that cause these clinical conditions are *diffuse axonal injury,* which occurs as a result of a lagging brain as the skull moves; the lagging brain causes brain structures to tear, particularly at the gray and white matter junction, and the cell bodies become disconnected from their axons. A *contusion* can be the result of a direct impact to the head and is essentially a bruised part of the brain. Occasionally, contusions may require surgical evacuation. A *penetrating injury* to the brain occurs from the impact of a bullet, knife, or other sharp object that forces hair, skin, bone, and fragments from the object into the brain, with firearms being the single largest cause. All these mechanisms may not only cause damage to brain tissue but can also lead to extra-axial hemorrhage, such as *subdural* and *epidural hematomas,* which in turn may prove to be mass lesions endangering the brain and thus requiring evacuation. *Skull fractures* are commonly seen in pediatric patients. Only 0.1% of the fractures do not heal and are considered "growing skull fractures," which require surgical repair.

These mechanisms are identical to those seen in the adults. However, in infants, the developing brain is more susceptible because of the following reasons:

- Infants' heads are large and heavy and account for about 25% of their total body weight. Their neck muscles are too weak to support such a disproportionately large head.
- Infants' skulls are relatively thin and absorb less energy when traumatized, and they may convey more energy to the underlying brain.
- Infants' brains are immature and more easily injured.
- Infants' blood vessels around the brain are more susceptible to tearing than those of older children and adults.

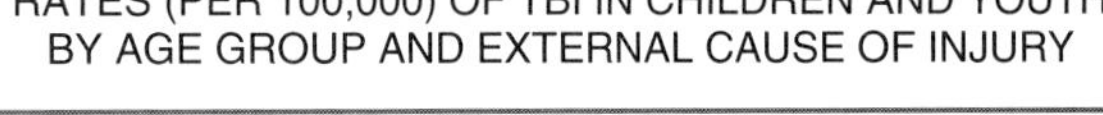

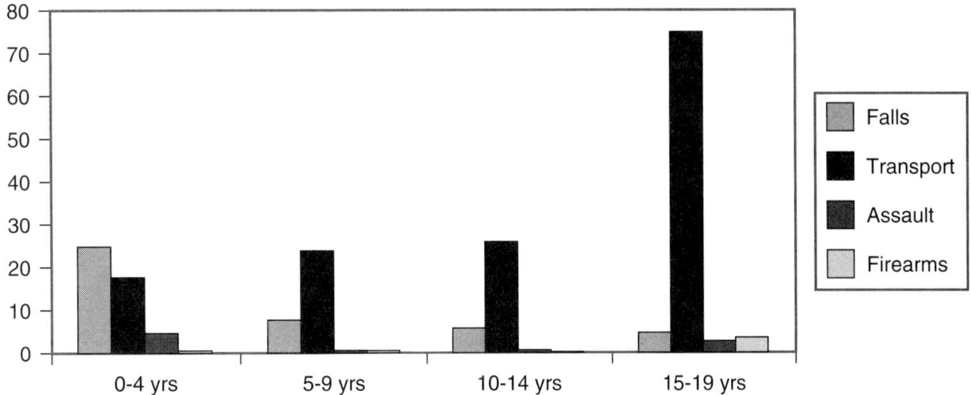

Figure 1. Rates (per 100,000) of traumatic brain injury in children and youth by age group and external cause of injury.

TABLE 1. **Glasgow Coma Scale for Children**

Score	Eyes Open	Best Verbal Response in Adults	Best Verbal Response in Children <36 mo	Best Verbal Response in Infants and Preschoolers	Best Motor Response
6	—	—	—	—	Obeys commands
5	—	Oriented and converses	Smiles, interacts	Babbles/gestures	Localizes painful stimuli
4	Spontaneously	Disoriented and converses	Cries, interacts	Cries for needs	Flexion withdrawal
3	To verbal command	Inappropriate words	Consolable, moans	Cries, nonspecific	Flexion abnormal
2	To painful stimuli	Incomprehensible sounds	Irritable, restless	Sounds	Extension
1	No response	No response	No response	No response	No response

MANAGEMENT

Treatment of TBI encompasses intensive care unit admission and management of possibly raised intracranial pressure. Treatment is individualized to the specific injuries of each patient. In general, the following guidelines are used:

Mild TBI. Patients with mild TBI usually fare well and require an overnight stay in the hospital. If any intracranial hemorrhage (intraparenchymal, subarachnoid, subdural or a contusion) is present on initial head computed tomography (CT), seizure prophylaxis is initiated with a loading dose of phenytoin (Dilantin), 20 mg/kg, followed by 2 mg/kg three times daily for the duration of 1 week, and CT is repeated the following day.

Moderate TBI. Alongside measures that are taken for children with mild TBI, this category of patients needs more intense surveillance and treatment. Most patients have a more severe injury and can deteriorate despite aggressive management; brain swelling (with or without the presence of contusions) can lead to deterioration of the neurologic condition (see "Severe TBI") and thus the necessity for intubation.

The following measures aimed at avoiding excess rises in intracranial pressure need to be taken to ensure optimal care:

- The head of the bed should be raised up to 30 degrees to facilitate venous outflow from the cranium.
- Plasma phenytoin levels between 15 and 20 μg/mL should be ensured because generalized seizures can lead to vascular engorgement and a rise in intracranial pressure.
- Aggressive monitoring and correction of electrolyte disturbances should be instituted.
- Low blood oxygen saturation and blood pressure drops should be avoided. The latter can lead to reflex vasodilation in the brain with a subsequent rise in cerebral blood volume and thus intracranial blood pressure.
- Patient agitation needs to be treated with low-dose, short-acting sedatives (propofol [Diprivan]) or opioids (fentanyl).
- The use of hypotonic intravenous solutions and hypervolemia should be avoided.
- Empirical intravenous mannitol is an optional, though controversial treatment.

In younger children, a fair initial condition may be misleading because children, unlike adults, may not show a slow decline in their condition but, instead, may deteriorate very rapidly.

Severe TBI. Recommendations for the treatment of severe TBI have been outlined in guidelines for the management of severe traumatic brain injury by the Joint Section on Neurotrauma and Critical Care of the American Association of Neurological Surgery for adults. Comparative guidelines for children are pending. For now, the adult parameters are followed with minor variations.

Aside from the aforementioned measures, these patients usually require ventilatory assistance and are therefore intubated and sedated. As a neurologic examination cannot be performed, monitoring of the condition of the injured brain is achieved by invasive monitoring of intracranial pressure. Such monitoring is performed by inserting a catheter into the cerebrospinal fluid–filled lateral ventricles with simultaneous measurement of intracranial pressure. This treatment principle is based on upholding satisfactory perfusion of brain tissue, or maintenance of cerebral perfusion pressure.

TABLE 2. **Glasgow Coma Scale in Adolescents and Adults**

Score	Best Motor Response	Best Verbal Response	Best Eye-Opening Response
6	Obeys commands	—	—
5	Localizes stimulus	Oriented	—
4	Withdraws from stimulus	Conversant but confused	Open spontaneously
3	Flexes arm	States recognizable words or phases	Open to voice
2		Makes unintelligible sounds	Open to painful stimulus
1	No response	No response	Remain closed

Serious consideration needs to be given to evacuating any subdural, epidural, or intraparenchymal hemorrhage in these patients. The initial condition of the child at arrival may be such that emergency evacuation may be warranted.

If no single mass lesion is present but generalized brain swelling with focal contusions is noted, decompressive craniotomy may be an option. In this procedure, the part of the osseous cranium overlying the most aggravated brain tissue is removed to allow the nervous tissue to swell without compromising its blood supply.

Treatment with intravenous boluses of mannitol is warranted at a dosage of 1 g/kg every 4 to 6 hours. Care should be given to rising serum osmolarity because values higher than 320 are associated with renal failure. This treatment regimen is upheld until the intracranial pressure has dropped to a satisfactory level and the patient can be extubated.

Prevention. A recent poll commissioned by the Brain Injury Association has revealed that the American public greatly underestimates the magnitude and importance of TBI. Great effort is being made by institutions such as the Think First Foundation and the Centers for Disease Control and Prevention to educate individuals, community leaders, and creators of public policy.

More information can be found at *www.thinkfirst.org*.

Post-Traumatic Seizure Prophylaxis. The incidence of early (less than 7 days after trauma) post-traumatic seizures is high, and some evidence supports the potential benefits of preventing seizures following head injury. Ample evidence in the literature supports the benefit of phenytoin and carbamazepine (Tegretol) for *early* post-traumatic seizures but is lacking for *late* seizures. Children with any traumatic intracranial pathology are treated for 1 week with phenytoin. If the seizure activity continues, changes are made in the regimen and anti-seizure medication is continued for approximately 3 months. Thereafter, an electroencephalogram is obtained to assess the epileptic activity of the brain.

Post-Hospitalization Recommendations. Most patients with TBI eventually require short or longer term inpatient rehabilitation. After this phase, patients should at all costs attempt to avoid any circumstances that may lead to a recurrent brain injury because the prognosis after such injuries is much poorer in patients who have suffered TBI in the past 6 months. Patients with decompressive craniotomies are fitted with cushioning helmets.

Social Aspects. Children with various degrees of cognitive and physical disabilities and their parents are confronted with challenges from their environment that can lead to distress and social isolation with subsequent developmental decline. Many organizations are available as sources for information and guidance. The role of the family physician and pediatrician is pivotal in this care. Some of these organizations can be found on www.biausa.org and www.braintrauma.org.

BRAIN TUMORS

method of
ARNOLD C. PAULINO, M.D.
Emory University
and
Children's Healthcare of Atlanta
Atlanta, Georgia

INCIDENCE

Brain tumors can be divided into two general categories. Primary brain tumors originate in the brain, with an incidence of 11.3 cases per 100,000 person-years. It is estimated that 35,500 new cases are diagnosed in the United States each year. The most common tumors are meningioma (27%), glioblastoma multiforme (22%), other malignant astrocytomas (17%), pituitary gland neoplasms (10%), and nerve sheath tumors (7%). In children, the incidence of primary brain tumors is 3.7 cases per 100,000 person-years, with an estimated 2900 new cases annually. Primary brain tumors comprise the second most common group of neoplasms in children. The most common tumors in children are astrocytoma (38%), medulloblastoma (20%), brainstem glioma (10%), ependymoma (9%), anaplastic astrocytoma and glioblastoma multiforme (6%) and craniopharyngioma (6%).

The second category of brain tumors is brain metastases. In adults, brain metastases are the most common cause of brain tumors, being 5 to 10 times more frequent than primary brain tumors. These tumors develop from cells originating in an organ outside the central nervous system and spread to the brain through hematogenous metastasis. The most common primary tumors that spread to the brain, originate from the lung (48%), breast (15%), melanoma (9%), and colon/rectum (5%). Approximately 10% of brain metastases are without a known primary lesion at initial patient presentation. Brain metastases in children are rare and occur in approximately 5% of neuroblastomas and sarcomas.

ETIOLOGY

A number of brain tumors are associated with a recognized neurocutaneous or genetic syndrome at patient presentation (Table 1). Exposure to vinyl chloride and previous radiation therapy to the scalp for tinea capitis have also been found to increase the likelihood of certain types of brain tumors. Transplant patients and those with acquired immunodeficiency syndrome (AIDS) have increased risks for primary central nervous system lymphoma.

CLINICAL PRESENTATION

Patients with seizures are a presenting symptom in approximately 20% of patients with supratentorial tumors, especially in low-grade tumors and those arising from the temporal lobe. Patients with headaches are a common presenting symptom and typically occur

TABLE 1. **Neurocutaneous and Genetic Syndromes Associated with Brain Tumors**

Syndrome	Types of Tumor
Neurofibromatosis, type 1	Optic pathway glioma, low grade gliomas of the thalamus, cerebral hemisphere and cerebellum
Neurofibromatosis, type 2	Acoustic neuroma, ependymoma, astrocytoma
Tuberous sclerosis	Subependymal giant cell astrocytoma
Li-Fraumeni syndrome	Malignant glioma and sarcoma, breast cancer, leukemia
Turcot syndrome	Medulloblastoma, malignant glioma, astrocytoma, and colorectal adenocarcinoma
Gorlin syndrome	Medulloblastoma and basal cell carcinoma

in early morning. Frontal and temporal lobe tumors tend to cause headaches in the frontal, retro-orbital or temporal regions, whereas patients with infratentorial tumors have headaches located in the occipital and retroauricular regions. Gastrointestinal symptoms such as nausea, loss of appetite, and queasiness can occur. Projectile vomiting may be seen in children. Headaches associated with vomiting may be a manifestation of increased intracranial pressure, secondary to obstruction of cerebrospinal fluid pathways.

Focal symptoms and signs can occur and depend on the location of the tumor. Patients with tumors of the frontal lobe can present with hemiplegia and personality changes. Tumors of the parietal lobe can alter sensory and perceptual functions, whereas those located in the occipital lobe can cause visual aberrations. Tumors located in the temporal lobe can impair spatial judgment, recent memory, and aggressive behavior. Tumors of the posterior fossa may disrupt cranial nerve and cerebellar function.

IMAGING AND WORK-UP

Magnetic resonance imaging (MRI) is the imaging modality of choice for diagnosis and follow-up of brain tumors. The administration of gadolinium diethylene pentaacetic acid (Gd-DPTA) increases the sensitivity of MRI. Meningiomas usually demonstrate T_1 isointensity to hypointensity and proton density and T_2 isointensity to hyperintensity with prominent gadolinium enhancement. Patients with glioblastomas often present with tumors showing irregular nodular ring enhancement, a necrotic center, and surrounding vasogenic edema. Pilocytic astrocytomas are well defined and circumscribed with T_2 hyperintensity. Imaging characteristics of astrocytomas, which may indicate a higher grade, include: density or intensity heterogeneity, irregular shape, poor margination, mass effect, edema, hemorrhage, and ringlike enhancement. Patients with primary central nervous system (CNS) lymphoma may present with multifocal periventricular lesions with T_2 isointensity and surrounding hyperintensity.

The workup of certain types of tumors may include imaging and cytology to assess leptomeningeal dissemination. MRI of the spine and cerebrospinal fluid (CSF) cytology from a lumbar tap are part of the routine studies done for medulloblastomas and other primitive neuroectodermal tumors, ependymomas, and germ cell tumors. Serum and CSF markers such as beta-human chorionic gonadotropin (bhCG) and α-fetoprotein may be helpful in determining the type of germ cell tumor. Pure germinomas do not have elevated α-fetoprotein levels but occasionally may have slightly elevated bhCG markers. On the other hand an elevated α-fetoprotein means that a non-germinomatous germ cell component is present, such as an endodermal sinus or yolk sac tumor.

PATHOLOGY

There are many different histologic types of tumors that occur in the brain. Table 2 summarizes the most common histologic types. In some neoplasms, mixed histologies can occur such as an oligoastrocytoma or a mixed germ cell tumor. Pineoblastomas, which are a type of pineal parenchymal tumor, are actually primitive neuroectodermal tumors (PNET).

TABLE 2. **Types of Brain Tumor**

Astrocytomas
Pilocytic astrocytoma
Diffuse astrocytoma
Anaplastic astrocytoma
Glioblastoma multiforme
Oligodendroglial Tumors
Oligodendroglioma
Anaplastic oligodendroglioma
Ependymal Tumors
Ependymoma
Anaplastic ependymoma
Myxopapillary ependymoma
Choroid Plexus Tumors
Choroid plexus papilloma
Choroid plexus carcinoma
Pineal Parenchymal Tumors
Pineocytoma
Embryonal Tumors
Medulloblastoma
Supratentorial primitive neuroectodermal tumor (PNET)
Atypical teratoid/rhabdoid tumor
Meningeal Tumors
Meningioma
Hemangiopericytoma
Sellar Tumors
Craniopharyngioma
Pituitary adenoma
Tumors of the Cranial and Peripheral Nerves
Schwannoma
Neurofibroma
Germ Cell Tumors
Germinoma
Non-germinomatous germ cell tumors
Metastatic Tumors to the Brain

Ependymoblastoma, likewise, belongs to the family of PNET and is not an ependymal tumor.

TREATMENT

Steroids

Corticosteroids are indicated in patients with symptomatic peritumoral edema. Corticosteroids reduce edema via two mechanisms. First, they reduce the permeability of tumor capillaries, limiting the leakage of water, sodium, and protein into the peritumoral extracellular space. Second, steroids facilitate the transport of fluid into the ventricular system. The drug of choice is dexamethasone (Decadron) because of its long half-life. Most symptomatic patients are started at a dose of 16 mg/d in four divided doses with improvement within 24 to 72 hours after initiation of dexamethasone. Dexamethasone may have an oncolytic effect in patients with CNS lymphoma. Prolonged steroid use should be avoided if possible in the brain tumor patient because of potential complications, such as myopathy and peptic ulceration.

Observation

When the patient is not symptomatic and the tumor is benign, such as a small convexity meningioma, observation with serial MRI scans may be a reasonable option as long as the tumor is not enlarging and not producing symptoms. Close observation is a reasonable approach for very young children with neurofibromatosis and low-grade gliomas, provided the child is not symptomatic and the tumor is not increasing in size on serial MRI scans. Observation is particularly attractive in this setting because it may delay initiation of radiation therapy, which may impair the child's neurocognitive and neuroendocrine state. Sometimes, tumors can be observed with serial MRI examination after supportive care, such as in the case of a focal tectal plate glioma after CSF diversion to alleviate symptoms.

Surgery

The surgical team plays an important role in the management of brain tumors. First, surgery may be needed to establish patency of CSF pathways; second, surgery is diagnostic and may be paramount in cytoreduction of disease. Patients who have hydrocephalus may need diversion of CSF in the form of a ventriculoperitoneal (VP) shunt; other shunts that are available include ventriculocisternal, ventriculoatrial, and ventriculopleural shunts. For many brain tumors, maximal surgical resection is desirable with the exception of radioresponsive tumors such as germinomas and CNS lymphomas or tumors, which are not amenable to resection because of morbidity such as a diffuse pontine glioma. After complete resection, no adjuvant therapy is usually needed for pilocytic astrocytoma, meningioma, low-grade gliomas, and craniopharyngioma. Patients with high-grade glioma, ependymoma, or PNET need adjuvant radiation therapy (RT), with or without chemotherapy, even after complete resection. For patients with a solitary brain metastasis and no other site of disease, surgical resection followed by postoperative conventional external beam RT has been shown to improve survival when compared with conventional external beam RT alone. Patients who undergo a subtotal resection for low-grade gliomas may be observed or given RT. The advent of stereotactic neurosurgical techniques has made it possible for better resections, allowing the ability to safely remove tumors without much neurologic morbidity.

Radiation Therapy

Radiation therapy (RT) is an important modality in the treatment of brain tumors. Teletherapy or external beam radiation therapy is the most common form of treatment; photons from a linear accelerator are usually employed. Stereotactic radiosurgery and fractionated stereotactic RT are forms of teletherapy. In Loma Linda and Boston, proton therapy is available. Protons have a Bragg peak, unlike photons, which means less radiation dose beyond the target volume; this reduction of high-dose volume may be critical in the brain and in young children. The other form of RT is brachytherapy, which utilizes a radioisotope next to the target; radioactive seeds may be implanted in the tumor bed. In some instances, radioactive liquid such as phosphorus-32 may be instilled in a cyst, such as a craniopharyngioma. Radiation acts directly to destroy tumor cell DNA or indirectly by creating free radicals that destroy DNA. Free radical formation is most effective in the presence of oxygen. Hypoxic regions in the tumor may be more radioresistant because of this phenomenon.

External beam radiation therapy is usually given 5 days a week. The total dose to be delivered is divided into smaller doses so that the normal surrounding tissues would be able to tolerate the treatment. The fraction size or the daily dose is the main determinant of late effects of RT. Table 3 shows some common dose fractionation schemes in radiotherapy. Stereotactic radiosurgery using a modified linear accelerator or a gamma knife (201 cobalt-60 sources) is given in one treatment to a very focused target, usually less than 4 cm in maximal diameter. Intensity-modulated radiation therapy (IMRT) is a newer method of conformal RT that utilizes an inverse planning algorithm.

Patients who have completely resected high-grade gliomas, medulloblastoma, and ependymoma require postoperative RT. For subtotally resected meningioma and craniopharyngioma, postoperative RT increases the probability of local control. For subtotally resected low-grade glioma, postoperative RT can delay local recurrence but probably does not have an impact on survival.

Chemotherapy

In many childhood brain tumors, chemotherapy has been used to either improve outcome or decrease amount and/or volume of radiotherapy. For standard-risk medulloblastoma, for example, a lower craniospinal

TABLE 3. **Common Radiotherapy Fractionation Schemes**

Type of Tumor	Dose; Fractionation
Low-grade gliomas	45–54 Gy; 25–30 fractions over 5 to 6 wks
High-grade gliomas	60 Gy; 30 fractions over 6 wks
Meningioma	54 Gy; 30 fractions over 6 wks
Medulloblastoma	54–55.8 Gy; 30–31 fractions over 6–6.2 wks
Ependymoma	54 Gy; 30 fractions over 6 wks
Pituitary adenoma	45–50.4 Gy; 25–28 fractions over 5–5.6 wks
Brainstem glioma	54 Gy; 30 fractions over 6 wks
Brain metastases	30 Gy; 10 fractions over 2 wks

dose can be delivered with the use of chemotherapy compared with a higher dose using RT alone. Neoadjuvant cisplatin-based chemotherapy, followed by localized RT can be used instead of craniospinal RT for pure germinomas with similar cure rates. Chemotherapy can also be used in infants with brain tumors to delay initiation of RT. For patients with optic pathway gliomas, for example, carboplatin (Paraplatin),* chemotherapy has been shown to reduce tumor burden and delay initiation of RT.

*Not FDA approved for this indication.

For adult brain tumors, chemotherapy has produced modest benefit in high-grade gliomas. Both carmustine (BCNU) and a regimen of procarbazine (Matulane),* lomustine (CCNU), and vincristine (Oncovin)* (PCV) have been employed with about an equal survival outcome but with more toxicity with PCV. Current protocols are investigating the use of temozolomide (Temodar). In anaplastic oligodendroglioma, PCV chemotherapy has been found to be of some benefit. For CNS lymphoma, high-dose methotrexate-based regimens with RT have been reported to have better median survival outcome when compared with historical series of RT alone. There are some studies that show tamoxifen (Nolvadex),* mifepristone (Mifeprex),* and hydroxyurea (Hydrea)* may have efficacy in meningiomas. In order for chemotherapy to be more effective in the treatment of most brain tumors, two problems must be overcome: drug effectiveness and drug delivery. For these reasons, novel agents and methods of drug delivery are needed. Currently trials that involve gene therapy, differentiation agents, immunomodulators, and monoclonal antibody-delivered radioisotopes are in progress.

*Not FDA approved for this indication.

Section 15

The Locomotor System

RHEUMATOID ARTHRITIS

method of
THEODORE PINCUS, M.D.
Vanderbilt University Medical Center
Nashville, Tennessee

and

TUULIKKI SOKKA, M.D., PH.D.
Jyväskylä Central Hospital
Jyväskylä, Finland

Rheumatoid arthritis (RA) is a chronic disease in which dysregulation of immune function is associated with a chronic systemic inflammatory response, affecting joints and other organs. If untreated, chronic inflammation results in damage to joints and other organs, with a natural history of severe long-term outcomes of functional declines, work disability, and premature death in most patients. Since the 1980s, a traditional view that RA could be controlled in most patients with aspirin or other nonsteroidal anti-inflammatory drugs (NSAIDS), so that disease-modifying antirheumatic drugs (DMARDs) traditionally were not used until after 2 to 5 years of disease, has been replaced by an approach involving "tight control" of inflammatory activity with methotrexate and new DMARDs. This approach aims to reduce, and possibly prevent, damage to joints and other organs in most patients, analogous to the modern approach to hypertension and diabetes, in which control of elevated blood pressure or blood glucose (which are consequences of a dysregulation) reduces mortality rates and vascular damage. Lifelong therapy is required, because the etiology of the dysregulation remains unknown and persistent, as in hypertension and diabetes, but the outlook for patients at this time is much better than in previous decades.

The traditional, conservative approach to RA until the mid-1980s was based, in part, on evidence that many patients with inflammatory arthritis have a self-limited process rather than progressive disease, as well as on recognition that traditional DMARDs, such as injectable gold salts and penicillamine, had low rates of long-term effectiveness and high rates of toxicity. During the mid-1980s, it became apparent that most patients with symptoms for longer than 3 to 6 months rarely experienced spontaneous remission, and short-term drug efficacy of available DMARDs did not provide long-term effectiveness to prevent joint damage and poor outcomes.

The contemporary approach to patients is based on methotrexate as the anchor drug, a far more effective and less toxic drug than earlier DMARDs. New DMARDs have been introduced, including cyclosporine (Neoral) and leflunomide (Arava), and the biological agents etanercept (Enbrel), infliximab (Remicade), anakinra (Kineret), and adalimumab (Humira). Perhaps as important, a new approach to RA has emphasized *early* use of available therapies, often in combinations, to control inflammation as completely as possible to prevent long-term damage. In addition, joint replacement surgery has been an important advance for patients with severely damaged joints, although the need for surgery in RA appears to be declining with improved medical therapy. The outlook for patients with RA is considerably brighter than it was 15 years ago.

EARLY DIAGNOSIS—THE FIRST STEP TO EARLY CONTROL

Although the primary purpose of this article is to summarize current therapy, a few points regarding diagnosis of RA appear critical to understand the contemporary approach to treatment:

1. The most important information to make a diagnosis of RA is derived from a history and physical examination, in contrast to most diseases, in which a definitive diagnosis is based on data from high-technology sources, such as blood pressure, a laboratory test, and/or imaging data. The seven American College of Rheumatology (ACR) classification criteria for RA, in which a patient meeting four of the criteria would be classified as having RA, are (1) morning stiffness ≥1 hour, (2) symmetric joint swelling for 6 weeks, (3) hand joint swelling, (4) swelling in three or more joint areas lasting for 6 weeks or more, (5) rheumatoid nodules, (6) positive rheumatoid factor, and (7) radiographic erosions. Five of these criteria are clinical measures, one a laboratory test, and one imaging data. Therefore, a patient may meet four of the seven criteria to be classified as having RA without any laboratory or radiographic abnormalities. Conversely, a diagnosis of RA cannot be made without clinical evidence of disease. Further, the ACR criteria may not be sensitive for a diagnosis of early RA, and at least two in five patients have normal erythrocyte sedimentation rate (ESR) or C-reactive protein (CRP) at presentation.

2. In population studies, most people who have acutely swollen joints, including more than half of people who meet criteria for RA, have a self-limited condition, with no evidence of disease seen 3 to 5 years later. Therefore, most people with swollen joints may have a postviral or reactive arthritis that does *not* develop into progressive inflammatory disease, and many never see a physician about this problem. By contrast, most people who have sustained symptoms for 3 to 6 months or more are likely to have a progressive disease.

3. Most people who present to a general physician with joint discomfort do not have RA. A general physician may see only one to five new cases of RA per year versus dozens of patients with conditions not associated with generalized inflammation, such as fibromyalgia and soft tissue conditions such as bursitis, tendonitis, trauma, or osteoarthritis. If a patient reports pain in a "squeezing" test of hands (metacarpophalangeal and proximal interphalangeal joints) or feet (metatarsophalangeal joints), the patient should be seen by a specialist. In fact, the most effective diagnostic measure for a person with possible early RA may not be a radiograph or laboratory test but rather an evaluation by a specialist or generalist with extensive experience with the disease.

4. Any evidence of joint swelling should lead to consideration of possible early RA after infection, reactive arthritis, and other bases for joint swelling are excluded. By the time joint deformity and/or radiographic evidence of erosion are seen, there is already irreversible joint damage. Treatment before joint damage appears optimal.

5. Poor long-term outcomes, including work disability and premature mortality, are predicted more effectively by severe functional disability assessed on a patient questionnaire than by laboratory or radiographic abnormalities, although poor status according to these measures also indicates a poor long-term prognosis.

NONPHARMACOLOGIC THERAPY

Although emphasis of this article and all medical practice in the treatment of RA involves drugs, it is important at the outset to emphasize that nondrug therapy is a valuable component of management in RA (and all chronic diseases). Sympathetic support of an understanding physician and his or her staff, including appropriate encouragement that it is possible to lead a near-normal life with appropriate adjustments of activities and behaviors, is of value to all patients. Further interaction with other health care professionals, including a physical therapist, occupational therapist, social worker, and nurse educator, may prove very helpful for some patients.

Specific therapies have included occupational therapy for individuals with problems of the upper extremity in joint preservation, ergonomic considerations, and use of assistive devices. Patients with family issues and disability may benefit from consultation with social workers. Pharmacists can help teach patients to understand the risks and benefits of drugs. Nurse educators can help patients with understanding of drugs, disease processes, and prognoses. Patients with vocational problems may benefit from interactions with vocational rehabilitation counselors.

Traditional physical therapy included heat and cold therapy, splints, range of motion exercises, and other exercise programs. Aerobic exercise with muscle strength training has been found to be associated not only with improved cardiovascular fitness but also with better RA status. Patient self-management through physical exercises should be implemented as part of patient care. Earlier directives to avoid or limit exercise are incorrect for most RA patients. In postoperative situations, physical therapy is necessary for rehabilitation. However, many health care professionals have little or no training in the management of arthritis, so it is desirable to identify a therapist with experience in dealing with RA patients to provide optimal benefit to the patient.

GENERAL PRINCIPLES OF DRUG THERAPY

Several general principles, as follows, characterize the contemporary approach to patients with RA:

1. Therapy to control inflammation should be directed to tight control, with a goal of "prevention" of joint damage. Improvement at a 20% level (ACR 20) versus placebo is sufficient for approval of marketing through the Food and Drug Administration (FDA), but this level of control usually is not sufficient to prevent long-term damage, which requires more extensive control of inflammation in most patients. The goal of total remission is desirable, although "near-remission" status may be acceptable for many patients.

2. The treatment of RA differs from the treatment of neoplastic disease, in that 80% control may lead to excellent clinical control in RA, whereas 90% to 99% of disease must be eradicated in neoplasia. Hence lower doses of methotrexate and other drugs with less toxicity are possible in the treatment of RA.

3. Once damage is present in a joint, drug therapy may prevent further damage but cannot reverse loss of cartilage and subluxation due to damage of soft tissue structures. When damage is extensive, joint surgery may be the best therapy for that specific joint, although continued medical therapy usually is needed to control generalized inflammation.

4. The "anchor drug" is methotrexate, the most effective DMARD, as well as, ironically, among DMARDs with the lowest level of toxicities, particularly with use of concomitant folic acid. Traditional DMARDs such as gold salts, penicillamine, and azathioprine are less likely than methotrexate to be efficacious and considerably more likely to induce toxicities. Hydroxychloroquine, sulfasalazine, and minocycline may have somewhat less toxicity, but they also have less efficacy. In general, it is desirable for all patients with RA to take as high a dose of weekly methotrexate as needed or tolerated.

5. Availability of new DMARDs such as cyclosporine and leflunomide, as well as biological anti–tumor

necrosis factor-alpha (TNF-α) agents, etanercept, infliximab, adalimumab, and the interleukin-1 (IL-1) receptor antagonist anakinra, has greatly added to the armamentarium for RA, although each of these drugs is not necessarily effective in all patients. A large percentage of patients are controlled with methotrexate and do not appear to require biological agents.

6. Long-term high-dose corticosteroid therapy (>10 mg for more than a few weeks) should be avoided in treatment of RA. By contrast, benefits of low-dose corticosteroid therapy, in doses of 5 mg or less, are often greater than possible harm and may be continued over many years, particularly with therapy for osteopenia. However, long-term low-dose use of corticosteroid therapy remains controversial.

7. Therapy must be individualized for each patient. Results of randomized, controlled clinical trials and clinical observational studies are presented for *groups* of patients, and the response of *individual* patients to different agents varies considerably.

8. Therapy to control inflammation must be continued indefinitely in most patients, as is the case with other dysregulatory diseases such as hypertension and diabetes. This includes maintenance of drugs through intercurrent illnesses, as well as elective and nonelective surgery. When patients appear to be in remission, withdrawal of therapy can be tried very cautiously (e.g., prednisone 1 mg every 3 months or methotrexate 2.5 mg every 3 months); at some point, most patients will relapse as therapy is withdrawn.

9. A "preventive" effort to reduce or avoid damage through control of inflammation is begun as soon as there is evidence of joint swelling and causes other than RA, such as infection and reactive arthritis, have been excluded. Some patients may be treated unnecessarily using a preventive approach. However, risks from the "side effects" of RA are substantially greater than those from the side effects of contemporary DMARDs, and substantial benefits may be seen in many patients who were to develop RA.

10. Monitoring of patient status over time is important. Quantitative monitoring may include joint counts for swelling, tenderness, and deformity; radiographs of hands and feet every 1 to 5 years; laboratory tests for inflammation such as ESR or CRP; and patient self-report questionnaires to assess functional capacity, pain, global status, and morning stiffness. A useful assessment tool in clinical practice is a health assessment questionnaire or a multidimensional version designed to provide simplified scoring in routine clinical settings.

DISEASE-MODIFYING ANTIRHEUMATIC DRUGS (DMARDs)

Traditional discussions of RA therapy begin with NSAIDs. However, as current philosophy of treatment generally emphasizes early and aggressive use of DMARDs, we begin with DMARDs, which may be classified into the following five categories:

1. Methotrexate
2. Agents used in mild disease or in combination with methotrexate
   a. Hydroxychloroquine (Plaquenil)
   b. Sulfasalazine (Azulfidine)
   c. Minocycline (Minocin)
3. Traditional DMARDs—limited general use at this time
   a. Gold salts (Myochrysine, Solganal, Auranofin)
   b. Penicillamine (Cuprimine, Depen)
   c. Azathioprine (Imuran)
4. New small-molecule DMARDs, often used in combination with methotrexate
   a. Cyclosporine (Neoral)
   b. Leflunomide (Arava)
   c. Other transplantation drugs—tacrolimus (FK506, Prograf), mycophenolate mofetil (CellCept)
5. Biological agents—usually used in combination with methotrexate
   a. Anti-TNF agents
      i. Etanercept (Enbrel)
      ii. Infliximab (Remicade)
      iii. Adalimumab (Humira)
   b. IL-1 receptor antagonist—anakinra (Kineret)

Methotrexate

Methotrexate, an antimetabolite discovered more than 40 years ago, is generally the first-line DMARD in most patients with RA at this time. The usual starting dose is 7.5 to 10 mg PO weekly orally in two or three doses given every 12 hours and may be increased to as high as 30 mg weekly. At least 80% of patients have some improvement with methotrexate. Parenteral therapy may be effective to reduce gastrointestinal complications and usually enhances efficacy. Furthermore, parenteral methotrexate is usually less expensive than tablets. All patients treated with methotrexate are also treated with folic acid (1 to 3 mg/d).

Methotrexate is used in the management of neoplastic diseases, including breast cancer and leukemia, and therefore may appear to health professionals and patients to be a "drastic" therapy. The primary mechanism of action of weekly methotrexate in RA appears to involve anti-inflammatory rather than antimetabolite actions, and evidence of actual immunosuppression in doses used to treat RA is unusual. Methotrexate is a minimally toxic drug at doses used in RA for most patients, safer than many NSAIDs. Any patient who can take methotrexate should be given a dose to control inflammation as completely as possible, or the maximum dose tolerated, up to 30 mg, if complete control is not seen.

The common toxicities of methotrexate include gastrointestinal distress, oral ulcers, and hair loss. These problems limit dosage of methotrexate but can usually be controlled by reduction of the methotrexate dose. In patients who have significant gastrointestinal distress, parenteral methotrexate, up to 30 mg per week, is usually better tolerated and also less expensive. Nonetheless, about 20% to 30% of patients do not tolerate more than 7.5 mg of weekly methotrexate and are maintained at lower doses.

The more potentially severe life-threatening complications include cytopenias; liver toxicity, particularly in patients who have excessive use of alcohol; methotrexate pneumonia; and the hypothetical possibility of increased malignancies. In practice, these complications are rare, particularly with the use of folic acid. Cytopenias are most unusual with small doses of weekly methotrexate. It appears likely that any increase in malignancies associated with methotrexate is at most marginal and may not be present at all.

Methotrexate pneumonitis is a toxic reaction that may occur in up to 1% of patients, generally within the first year of treatment. Symptoms include dyspnea, tachypnea, fever, and dry cough. A diffuse interstitial pattern in a chest radiograph distinguishes methotrexate pneumonitis from bacterial pneumonia. Methotrexate pneumonitis is a potentially fatal condition with mortality of 10% to 20%. All patients who are treated with methotrexate should be informed of the risk of pneumonitis, the most common severe side effect of methotrexate. This complication has been seen less frequently in recent years, perhaps secondary to use of folic acid and treatment of patients who had systemic disease.

Liver toxicity is unusual, even in patients who consume one or two alcoholic drinks per day. If liver enzyme levels are elevated to less than twice normal, they usually return to normal levels without adjustment of dose. If elevated to more than three times normal values, the dose is reduced and these generally revert to normal. Liver biopsies are rarely needed. The guidelines recommend monitoring rheumatologic status and liver function every 4 to 8 weeks, but in practice, blood tests are often obtained only every 3 to 4 months.

In the authors' clinical practice, more than 70% of patients have continued with long-term methotrexate for at least 5 years. Discontinuation may result from limited efficacy or toxicities of intractable oral ulcers, unacceptable hair loss, or development of nodulosis, which in some patients responds to discontinuation of methotrexate.

Agents Used in Mild Cases or in Combination with Methotrexate

Hydroxychloroquine

Hydroxychloroquine (Plaquenil) is an antirheumatic drug derived from chloroquine. Its efficacy in RA was initially identified by travelers who took the drug as prophylaxis for malaria. Hydroxychloroquine is well tolerated, although it is generally insufficient to provide adequate benefit as a single DMARD. The usual dose is 200 mg twice daily or 400 mg once daily. In general, hydroxychloroquine is used in combination with methotrexate. A formal clinical trial indicated that the combination of methotrexate, hydroxychloroquine, and sulfasalazine resulted in clinical improvement that was similar to the level seen with biological agents, although direct comparisons are not available.

Side effects of hydroxychloroquine may include rash, gastrointestinal discomfort, headaches, neuromyopathy, and retinopathy, though most of these are unusual. It has been traditionally recommended that patients have routine ophthalmologic slit-lamp examination every 6 to 12 months to monitor visual fields, but that is no longer recommended in certain countries because retinopathy is quite rare and patients who experience this complication may recognize a diminution in their visual field clinically.

Sulfasalazine

Sulfasalazine (Azulfidine) is a conjugate of 5-aminosalicylic acid and sulfapyridine, which has disease-modifying activity. It had been the mainstay of RA treatment in Europe until recent years but is now supplanted by methotrexate in many settings because methotrexate appears to be more effective and better tolerated. As noted earlier, the combination of sulfasalazine, hydroxychloroquine, and methotrexate has been shown to have efficacy similar to biological agents (although not compared directly).

Treatment is generally begun at 1000 mg/d and increased to 2000 to 3000 mg/d in two or three doses. Gastrointestinal intolerance, headache, and rash are the primary limiting toxicities. Gastrointestinal distress is common at doses higher than 2000 mg/d, even with enteric-coated tablets and limits the use of higher doses in many patients. Sulfasalazine should not be administered to patients with sulfa allergy. It may add to efficacy of methotrexate when used in combination.

Minocycline

Minocycline has been found to have efficacy in patients with RA compared to placebo, although the level of benefit is relatively limited except in early disease. The mechanism of action appears to involve interference with metalloproteinase enzymes involved in destruction rather than antibiotic actions. Minocycline is used primarily in patients with early RA and may be used in combination with methotrexate.

Traditional DMARDs

Gold Salts

Parenteral gold salts were introduced for the treatment of RA in the 1930s, initially based on a rationale of anti–tubercle bacilli effects because RA was thought to be a mycobacterial infectious disease. In some sense, gold injections are the only true "remission-inducing" therapy, leaving a patient free of symptoms without any further therapy. However, remissions were seen in only 10% to 20% of patients and generally were sustained in fewer than 5%. After 2 years of treatment, 80% to 90% of patients treated with parenteral gold were no longer taking this drug because of loss of efficacy or toxicity. Gold thiomalate (Myochrysine) is generally administered as a test dose of 10 mg the first week, 25 mg the second week, and 50 mg/week thereafter. The traditional practice was to discontinue injections when the total dose reached 1000 mg (20 weeks). In recent years, the practice has been to continue doses of 25 or 50 mg every 2 to 4 weeks.

Parenteral gold salts lead to clinical improvement without actual remission in about 50% of patients, no response at all in about 30% to 40%, and remission in 10% to 20%, as noted earlier. At this time, most rheumatologists in the United States have fewer than 5% of patients taking parenteral gold therapy.

Parenteral gold is associated with serious toxicities in 20% to 30% of patients, including rash, mucositis, proteinuria, pneumonitis, and life-threatening cytopenias in some patients, which were sometimes fatal. Acute "nitritoid" reactions seen with gold thiomalate were less common with aurothioglucose, which is no longer available.

Auranofin, or oral gold was introduced in the late 1970s. In clinical trials, auranofin appeared to have efficacy similar to parenteral gold salts but was seen primarily in patients with new-onset RA, who were overrepresented in clinical trials, and again it was short-lived. Auranofin is administered in 3-mg tablets, one to three per day in single or divided doses. Gastrointestinal intolerance with diarrhea was commonly seen with auranofin, which is hardly used at this time.

Penicillamine

Penicillamine was introduced for treatment of RA in the 1970s because it uncoupled sulfhydryl groups seen in rheumatoid factor and thereby reduced autoantibody activity. Penicillamine is traditionally administered in a "go low, go slow" approach, beginning at 250 mg a day and increasing the dose every 4 weeks up to 750 mg and, occasionally, up to 1000 mg/d. Penicillamine is effective in about 20% of patients, with 40% experiencing mild benefit and about 40% discontinuing because of toxicities. Toxicities of penicillamine include gastrointestinal intolerance, nephritis, and cytopenias. Penicillamine is rarely used for RA at this time because it is less effective and considerably more likely to induce toxic side effects than is methotrexate.

Azathioprine

Azathioprine, the first antimetabolite introduced for widespread use in RA, is a purine analogue that is converted to 6-mercaptopurine in vivo and is thought to have efficacy in RA due to its antimetabolite properties. Generally azathioprine is initiated at 50 mg/d and increased every 2 weeks by 50 mg, to a maximum of 200 mg/d. Weekly methotrexate appears far superior to daily azathioprine in most patients, although there is not a molecular explanation for this phenomenon. The toxicities include gastrointestinal intolerance, cytopenias, and possible predisposition to malignancy.

At this time, azathioprine is used primarily in patients who do not tolerate methotrexate. Its use may lead to substantial long-term benefit in some patients, and it may be used in combination with methotrexate.

New Small-Molecule Immunosuppressive DMARDs

Cyclosporine

Cyclosporine is an immunosuppressive drug widely used in clinical organ transplantation. Cyclosporine has efficacy as a single drug in RA, and it was the first shown to have efficacy in combination with methotrexate in patients who had incomplete responses to methotrexate. It is administered as the newer microemulsion preparation, Neoral, rather than the older preparation, Sandimmune. The starting dose is 2.5 mg/kg per day, in two divided doses, with a maximum of 5 mg/kg per day.

The primary toxicities of cyclosporine are renal, with increased blood pressure and decreased creatinine clearance. The dose is reduced by protocol whenever there is a 30% increase in creatinine or sustained increase in blood pressure. However, even with this precaution most patients who take cyclosporine develop hypertension and reduction in creatinine clearance after 24 months and are forced to discontinue cyclosporine, which limits its use in RA. It may be used as "bridge therapy" during disease flares, generally in combination with methotrexate.

Leflunomide

Leflunomide (Arava) is an immunomodulatory drug that interferes via a metabolite with a pyrimidine synthesis pathway, affecting T cells more than B cells. The usual dose is 20 mg/d; an initial "loading dose" of 100 mg for 3 days is generally no longer used. Leflunomide has efficacy comparable to methotrexate in clinical trials but has a higher likelihood of toxicities, including diarrhea, alopecia, liver toxicity, and hypertension.

Leflunomide is very helpful in the 10% to 20% of patients with RA who do not tolerate methotrexate. It may be used in combination with biological agents. The addition of leflunomide to methotrexate in partial responders increases efficacy in combination, with no substantial increase in toxicity compared to leflunomide monotherapy, even hepatic toxicity, although vigilance is required.

Other Transplantation Drugs

There are reports of efficacy in patients with RA for other drugs used in organ transplantation, including tacrolimus (FK506, Prograf) and mycophenolate mofetil (CellCept), which have immunosuppressive activity. These drugs may generally be used in combination with methotrexate in patients who appear refractory to other therapies. Further studies of these drugs for use in RA have been largely supplanted by targeted therapy with anti-TNF biological agents, but they may have a place in management of some patients with RA.

Biological Agents

An important recent development in rheumatology has been the synthesis of biological agents that provide targeted therapies for different components of the inflammatory cascade. The two cytokines for which biological agents have been found to have greatest efficacy are TNF-α and IL-1-β. Three biological agents are directed to TNF-α—etanercept, infliximab, and adalimumab—and one to IL-1-β—anakinra.

Etanercept

Etanercept is a soluble 75-kD TNF-α receptor fused to the Fc portion of an IgG1 that neutralizes lymphotoxin-α and TNF-α. Etanercept has been documented in clinical trials to have substantial efficacy used as a single DMARD and in combination with methotrexate in patients who had experienced partial responses to methotrexate. In early RA, etanercept is somewhat more efficacious than methotrexate. It is administered as a subcutaneous injection, 25 mg per injection, twice a week. Generally patients self-administer the injection, although some may receive their injections from a family member, friend, or health professional.

Some patients have very dramatic, almost "miraculous" responses to etanercept, particularly if there is very little organ damage. However, at least 20% to 40% of patients do not appear to respond, and there is no method at present to predict whether a patient will respond or not. If patients have not reached a state of near remission after 2 or 3 months of two DMARDs, generally including methotrexate and hydroxychloroquine, it is recommended that they be given an anti-TNF agent or leflunomide. Etanercept is generally well tolerated. A few patients experience injection site reactions.

The use of etanercept is limited in part by its substantial cost of more than $1200 per month. Many insurance payers require that patients "fail" at least two DMARDs prior to authorizing the use of etanercept. This practice may involve delays of up to 1 year, which may be deleterious in a number of patients, with evidence that delays of even 3 months result in greater damage 3 to 5 years later.

The primary toxicity of etanercept is based on its anti-TNF action to compromise the capacity of a patient to fight infections, particularly granulomatous types. There has been a slight increase in cases of tuberculosis with the use of etanercept as well as infliximab and adalimumab. The anti-TNF activity appears to interfere with granuloma formation, and patients are also at risk for fungal infections, including histoplasmosis and coccidioidomycosis, as well as *Listeria*. Because of concern about reactivation of tuberculosis, many rheumatologists recommend use of skin tests and/or chest radiographs at baseline. Patients may also develop antinuclear antibodies, although clinical lupus beyond serositis is generally not seen. There are reports of optic neuritis and other demyelination occurring with the use of anti-TNF agents, and it is recommended that these agents be discontinued if patients develop demyelinating conditions. In addition, aggravation of congestive heart failure has been reported with anti-TNF agents.

Infliximab

Infliximab is a chimeric IgG1-kappa monoclonal antibody that specifically neutralizes TNF-α. It is administered as an intravenous infusion at baseline, 2 and 6 weeks later, and every 8 weeks thereafter. It is recommended that infliximab be administered in combination with methotrexate.

Clinical trials did not indicate statistically significant differences whether infusions were administered every 4 or 8 weeks or whether the dose of infliximab was 3 or 10 mg/kg. Therefore, the recommended dosage is 3 mg/kg every 8 weeks. However, many patients appear to benefit from doses higher than 3 mg/kg administered more frequently than every 8 weeks—up to every 4 weeks. Escalation of both the dose and frequency is common in practice.

As is the case with etanercept, some patients respond to infliximab with dramatic benefits, and some patients do not show any significant benefit. Again, a most important consideration is the high cost. At this time, Medicare reimburses treatment with infliximab but not with etanercept, and this is an important consideration in elderly patients, most of whom cannot afford to pay for these treatments out of pocket.

The toxicities of infliximab are also based in large part on their anti-TNF activity. Higher than expected prevalence of tuberculosis and other chronic granulomatous diseases has been reported, and vigilant monitoring for infection is indicated, with a pretreatment chest radiograph and/or tuberculosis skin test, as with infliximab. There are also reports of autoantibodies, optic neuritis, and congestive heart failure, as with other anti-TNF agents. Rare anaphylactic reactions have been reported during infusion with infliximab. Infliximab has been approved for use only with methotrexate (in part as a strategy to prevent development of antibodies over time, although it has efficacy by itself, as well as with methotrexate) or leflunomide if a patient cannot tolerate methotrexate.

Adalimumab

Adalimumab is a newly approved monoclonal anti-TNF antibody that is distinguished by being a fully human monoclonal antibody. It has also been documented to have efficacy in clinical trials as a single agent and in combination with methotrexate. It is administered as a subcutaneous injection, 40 mg per injection, every other week.

Although adalimumab is a fully human antibody, patients who receive adalimumab may develop autoantibodies, but a clinical new-onset autoimmune disease during adalimumab treatment is rare. At this time, long-term experience with the use of adalimumab is limited. Increased susceptibility to infection, particularly granulomatous infection, as well as development of autoantibodies, optic neuritis, and congestive heart failure, as seen with other anti-TNF agents, remain a concern.

Anakinra

Anakinra is an IL-1β receptor antagonist that interferes with the action of IL-1. It has efficacy in clinical trials compared to placebo, both as a single agent and with methotrexate in combination.

Nonetheless, many patients do not respond to IL-1 receptor antagonist treatment, and fewer "dramatic" responses are seen compared to treatment with anti-TNF agents, suggesting that anti-TNF may be a proximal cytokine in the inflammatory cascade in a larger proportion of patients than is IL-1.

There exist animal models of inflammatory arthritis that respond more effectively to IL-1 blockade than to anti-TNF blockade, as well as models in which the combination of anti-IL-1 and anti-TNF activity has substantially greater efficacy than blockade of either cytokine alone. However, human studies suggest that combination anti-TNF and anti-IL-1 therapy is associated with increased toxicity and no greater benefit than single agents.

The toxicities of anakinra include local skin reactions and increased susceptibility to infection, as with the anti-TNF agents.

GLUCOCORTICOSTEROIDS

Treatment of RA with corticosteroids has evoked controversy for half a century. Initial clinical results in 1948 indicated spectacular clinical improvement, and the Nobel Prize in Medicine was awarded to Hench and Kendall shortly thereafter. Clinical trials in the 1950s indicated that corticosteroids had disease-modifying properties in RA by retarding progression of radiographic damage. However, it was soon recognized that toxicities associated with long-term use of corticosteroids in pharmacologic doses of prednisone of 20 to 40 mg, commonly used at the time, almost invariably outweighed any benefits. By the late 1950s, clinicians were taught that corticosteroids had no place in long-term management of most patients with RA.

A reassessment of corticosteroids in RA has occurred over the last 2 decades. Long-term therapy with high doses of corticosteroids is clearly undesirable for all patients with RA. However, many patients appear to benefit from therapy with very low doses, in the range of 5 mg/d or less, which may be described as "physiologic" rather than "pharmacologic" doses. The usual starting dose used by the authors for most patients is 3 mg, given in 1-mg pills (not available in many countries other than the United States), which appears quite satisfactory for a large percentage of patients. If the patient has very severe disease, 5 mg or even rarely 10 mg may be given, but 10 mg is regarded as a "high dose" unless there is life-threatening extra-articular disease or vasculitis. Although many authorities regard corticosteroids as a temporary bridge rather than a long-term therapy in RA, long-term, low-dose corticosteroids are used in many patients over long periods, since the basic dysregulation remains uncontrolled.

Some studies suggest that people with RA do not make normal glucocorticoid responses to stress, which may indicate why "physiologic" doses of corticosteroids are of benefit to many patients with RA. Low-dose corticosteroids appear to be well tolerated and to be associated with no additional prevalence of hypertension, diabetes, or cataracts over more than a decade, compared to RA patients not treated with corticosteroids. There remains concern about osteoporosis, and therapy for osteopenia should be considered in all patients taking corticosteroids over long periods. A "trade-off" of joint preservation for mild bone loss may be justified for many patients. The adverse effects of corticosteroids in low doses include skin thinning and bruising, which many patients again accept as justified in terms of disease modification but may become intolerable for some patients. Long-term use of low-dose corticosteroids may be appropriate for many patients with RA, although this remains controversial.

Intra-articular corticosteroid injections may be helpful to provide symptomatic relief when one joint is disproportionately affected compared to other joints. There are reports that intra-articular corticosteroid injection may be useful in early undifferentiated monoarthritis to distinguish self-limited disease from persistent inflammatory arthritis.

INTRA-ARTICULAR THERAPY WITH ALKYLATING AGENTS AND RADIOISOTOPES

Intra-articular therapy with alkylating agents such as thiotepa and radioisotopes such as yttrium and dysprosium have been used in selected centers. However, intra-articular therapy appears to have become less common as more effective DMARDs have become available.

NONSTEROIDAL ANTI-INFLAMMATORY DRUGS (NSAIDs)

As recently as 1985, aspirin and NSAIDs were recommended for several years before turning to DMARDs. It is now recognized that NSAIDs do not control the disease process, or they control only a limited level of inflammation, and are useful primarily only to relieve symptoms. Only about two thirds of patients under the care of rheumatologists take NSAIDs, many on an as-needed rather than regular basis.

NSAIDs reduce inflammation by inhibiting cyclooxygenase (COX) enzymes required for synthesis of prostaglandins, which are major mediators of inflammation stimulated by cytokines such as TNF and IL-1. Prostaglandins also have beneficial effects, such as protecting the lining of the stomach from acid and ulceration, enhancing fluid excretion by the kidney, and maintaining balance in the central nervous system. Traditional NSAIDs inhibit both COX-1 and COX-2 enzymes and may result in side effects such as gastrointestinal bleeding, hypertension, generalized edema, and headache by the same mechanisms that led to beneficial effects. Because of the widespread use of NSAIDs, the magnitude of adverse gastrointestinal events associated with NSAIDs is substantial, said to result in as many deaths as from acquired immunodeficiency syndrome or Hodgkin's disease in the United States.

The problem of gastrointestinal adverse events associated with NSAIDs was addressed initially by (1) the use of salicylate salts, such as sodium salicylate (Disalcid, Trilisate), that did not block prostaglandins; (2) the addition of misoprostol (Cytotec), a prostaglandin analogue, which protected the lining of the stomach; (3) the addition of proton pump inhibitors, which appeared to block the adverse events caused by NSAIDs; and (4) a recommendation that acetaminophen (Tylenol) be used in lieu of NSAIDs when possible.

An important advance resulted from recognition that there were at least two types of cyclooxygenases: COX-1, a primary constitutive enzyme that protects the lining of the stomach, and COX-2, the primary enzyme leading to inflammation. COX-2–selective drugs that inhibit COX-2, the primary basis of inflammation, but spare COX-1, have been developed, including celecoxib (Celebrex), rofecoxib (Vioxx), and valdecoxib (Bextra). Inhibition of COX-2 is associated with reduction of inflammation and lower risk of gastrointestinal events, but nonetheless with potential adverse events, as it now appears that COX-2 is expressed constitutively in certain organs, including the kidney, reproductive organs, and central nervous system. One major concern has been a higher incidence of cardiovascular events associated with high doses of rofecoxib (Vioxx).

In general, the most effective pain relief for RA is control of inflammation with DMARDs, such as methotrexate and low-dose prednisone. Patients with chronic arthritis pain generally find NSAIDs to be superior to analgesics and opiates for pain relief.

OVERALL STRATEGY IN MANAGEMENT OF RHEUMATOID ARTHRITIS

The management of a typical patient may vary somewhat according to severity of disease. In general, it is desirable to introduce one drug at a time so that if there is toxicity, it is obvious which drug may be causing it. In patients with very severe disease, this caution is overridden by a desire to give the patient optimal therapy to gain rapid control of the inflammatory process.

The authors have a practice that has been termed *rapid step-up therapy for rheumatoid arthritis*. The principle is to begin a drug and generally, if there is poor response or no response after 2 to 3 months, to add or change the drug every 2 to 3 months. The initial drug may be methotrexate 7.5 to 10 mg/week or low-dose prednisone 3 mg/d. If prednisone is begun and is effective, methotrexate is added at the next visit. In patients with moderately severe disease, prednisone 5 to 10 mg and methotrexate in doses of 10 mg or more are begun. Visits are arranged every 2 to 3 months, and new therapies are added, including leflunomide or anti-TNF therapy, if control of inflammation is not adequate. By the third visit patients are taking low-dose corticosteroids, methotrexate, and leflunomide or anti-TNF therapy. This approach may not be optimal in the sense that anti-TNF therapy may be indicated even in patients with apparently mild early disease, but this has not been studied extensively, and the costs and potential long-term toxicities may limit such a practice.

With evidence from both clinical trials and long-term clinical studies that DMARD therapy will retard radiographic progression and apparent mortality associated with RA, it is now the practice to recommend early DMARD therapy in all patients. This practice appears to have greatly improved the outlook and outcomes for patients with RA.

JUVENILE RHEUMATOID ARTHRITIS

method of
C. EGLA RABINOVICH, M.D., M.P.H.
Duke University Medical Center
Durham, North Carolina

CLASSIFICATION AND DIAGNOSIS

Juvenile rheumatoid arthritis (JRA) has been called juvenile chronic arthritis in countries outside of the United States, with recently proposed reclassification to Juvenile Idiopathic Arthritis (JIA). The American College of Rheumatology still recognizes the terminology JRA, the nomenclature used in this article. Estimates of prevalence run between 30 and 220 per 100,000. JRA can be divided into three different subtypes (Table 1). The diagnosis of JRA is made when a child younger than 16 years of age has arthritis (swelling in a joint or pain, erythema, and heat in a joint associated with loss of motion) for at least 6 consecutive weeks and other etiologies for arthritis (e.g., malignancy, trauma, or infection) are excluded. Pediatric spondyloarthropathies, including psoriatic arthritis and HLA-B27-related arthritis, affect large weight-bearing joints and fingers in a "sausage-like" manner, and are associated with tendonitis and are not discussed further here.

Pauciarticular JRA is arthritis occurring in up to four joints within the first 6 months after presentation. This disease has an excellent prognosis. When children with pauciarticular JRA develop arthritis in more than four joints, it is called "extended pauciarticular" arthritis and, in general, it has a less positive prognosis. Polyarticular JRA is defined as arthritis occurring in at least five joints within the first 6 months after disease presentation. The prognosis in this subtype is variable; rheumatoid factor positivity is associated with the poorest prognosis. Systemic JRA is characterized by daily or twice-daily high-spiking fevers; a salmon-colored evanescent rash accompanying the fever; high peripheral white blood cell counts, platelet counts, and sedimentation rates; and arthritis in at least one joint. The prognosis of systemic JRA is extremely variable with children appearing ill and with fevers. Macrophage activation syndrome (MAS) is a rare, but potentially lethal, complication of systemic JRA. MAS is characterized by persistent, unremitting fever, mental status changes, elevated

TABLE 1. **Subtypes of JRA**

Subtype	% of JRA	F:M	Peak Age of Onset (yrs)	Number of Joints Affected	Serologic Markers	Extra-Articular Manifestations
Pauciarticular	60	5:1	1-3	1-4	ANA (50-70%)	Chronic uveitis (20%)
Polyarticular	30	3:1	1-3, 8-10	$\geq$5	ANA (40-50%) RF (<10%)	Chronic uveitis (5%), fevers, pleuritis, pericarditis
Systemic	10	1:1	No peak	Any	High WBCs, ↑ESR, plts	High fevers, rash, polyserositis, hepatosplenomegaly, lymphadenopathy

ANA, antinuclear antibody; RF, rheumatoid factor; WBC, white blood cells; ESR, erythrocyte sedimentation rate; plts, platelets.

liver enzymes (along with a fall in sedimentation rate), leukopenia, thrombocytopenia, and disseminated intravascular coagulation syndrome.

GENERAL TREATMENT GUIDELINES

Treatment of JRA is individually tailored, but in general depends on the subtype and the individual course, along with the presence of risk factors for adverse outcome (Table 2). There is a paucity of controlled clinical trials for the treatment of JRA, with treatment based on individual and collective experience. Etiology of JRA is unknown; it is believed to occur in genetically susceptible children after a trigger, such as trauma or infection. Treatment is aimed at controlling inflammation, decreasing disability, and preventing or stabilizing contractures and erosive joint disease, with attention paid to the psychological impact of JRA on the child and family. Management of JRA is best handled in a multidisciplinary clinic with a team that includes a physical therapist, occupational therapist, social worker and/or psychologist, nurse specialist, and pediatric rheumatologist. In addition, a knowledgeable orthopedic surgeon for consultation is necessary. Careful attention must be paid to regular ophthalmologic examinations, as the uveitis associated with JRA is asymptomatic until scarring has occurred. The frequency of screening ophthalmologic visits for children with JRA without known uveitis is outlined in Table 3, and children with uveitis are followed more closely as determined by the ophthalmologist.

In addition to pharmacologic therapy, physical and occupational therapy are important adjunctive interventions for increasing range, strength, and function of affected joints. In a child with a knee or wrist contracture, extension resting splints are made by the therapist and worn while sleeping. Dynamic splinting is generally to be avoided because it may cause joint subluxation. Occasionally, serial casting is needed for resistant joint contractures not due to irreversible damage. The cast should be changed frequently, with close monitoring and an accompanying aggressive physical therapy or occupational therapy program. A leg-length discrepancy is seen in a growing child having asymmetrical knee arthritis with the affected leg growing faster. Inserting a shoe lift in the shorter leg prevents compensatory scoliosis. The leg length discrepancy often diminishes over time, as long as the arthritis is quiescent. Cognitive-behavioral therapy may be useful in treating pain associated with arthritis.

TABLE 2. **Prognostic Factors for Poorer Outcomes in Juvenile Rheumatoid Arthritis**

Positive rheumatoid factor
Persistence of systemic symptoms >6 months
Platelet counts >600,000/mm^3 at 6 months for systemic disease
Subcutaneous nodules
Early erosions
Long duration of active disease
Polyarticular presentation in an older child

The ultimate treatment goal is to achieve remission in children utilizing the right combination of medications. There is no "cookbook recipe" for the treatment of JRA. Therapy needs to be tailored to the individual child and his or her family with discussion of benefits, along with potential side effects of the medications. It is important that the family be in agreement with the therapy because it increases compliance. Too often remission cannot be achieved, despite aggressive therapy. Recent studies suggest that 30% of children with JRA continue with active arthritis as adults. The practitioner needs to balance potential medication side effects in the growing child with the potential morbidity of arthritis.

PAUCIARTICULAR JUVENILE RHEUMATOID ARTHRITIS

Children with this subtype have the best joint prognosis. First-line therapy is a nonsteroidal anti-inflammatory drug (NSAID). The NSAID should be continued until there has been no sign of active arthritis for at least 3 months. Intra-articular (IA) joint injection with a long-acting corticosteroid (usually under anesthesia, especially in a younger child) should be considered if a contracture is present or if there are contraindications to NSAID use; intra-articular injection is used by some specialists as first-line therapy. If a joint flares, if it is partially responsive to the NSAID, or if the child develops significant side effects to the NSAID, IA joint injection is a good option; consideration

TABLE 3. **Frequency of Screening Ophthalmologic Visits in JRA**

	Age of Onset	
	≤7 years	**>7 years**
+ANA	q 3 mo × 4 yrs, then q 6 mo × 3 yr, then yearly	q 6 mo × 4 yrs, then yearly
–ANA	q 6 mo × 7 yrs, then yearly	q 6 mo × 4 yrs, then yearly
Systemic JRA	Yearly	Yearly

ANA, antinuclear antibody; JRA, juvenile rheumatoid arthritis; mo, months; q, every; yrs, years.

may be given to reinjection two to three times per year. For persistent disease that is unresponsive to NSAIDs and IA injections, a second-line agent may be added. Milder second-line agents that may be effective in pauciarticular JRA include sulfasalazine (Azulfidine) and hydroxychloroquine (Plaquenil).* These are slow-acting agents that may take 2 to 3 months to see full effect. In the child who does not respond fully to any of the above therapies, methotrexate (MTX) (Rheumatrex) may be considered, with or without IA injection. Once a clinical remission is obtained, the child needs to stay on the drugs for at least 6 months with a slow taper over 3 to 12 months. Methotrexate is also useful in recalcitrant cases of uveitis, even in those without active joint disease.

POLYARTICULAR JUVENILE RHEUMATOID ARTHRITIS

Children with polyarticular JRA are generally treated more aggressively with earlier initiation of a second-line agent. This is true especially if risk factors indicating a poorer outcome are present. An NSAID remains initial therapy with consideration of adding methotrexate for those presenting with a delay in diagnosis and/or extensive involvement and disability. Alternative second-line agents include sulfasalazine and hydroxychloroquine; these medications are often used in combination with either each other or MTX. IA steroid injections are considered either for a few troublesome joints or as palliative therapy while waiting for full effect of a second-line agent. Etanercept (Enbrel) is an acceptable alternative second-line agent; limitations to its use include cost and availability. Etanercept and MTX can be used together; usually etanercept is added to MTX for partial or nonresponders. For severe polyarticular JRA that is unresponsive to this regimen, other aggressive drug therapies may be used, including cyclosporine (Neoral),* infliximab (Remicade),* leflunomide (Arava),* azathioprine (Imuran),* and, rarely, cyclophosphamide (Cytoxan).* No controlled studies of these drugs in JRA exist at this time. Daily corticosteroid administration is best avoided in JRA. Weekly intravenous pulses of methylprednisolone may produce fewer side effects than daily oral administration and is used to maintain mobility in the most severely affected children.

*Not FDA approved for this indication.

SYSTEMIC JUVENILE RHEUMATOID ARTHRITIS

Systemic JRA differs in that the constitutional symptoms of fever and malaise can be an overwhelming aspect of the disease. It has an unpredictable course, ranging from weeks to years. The disease may be monocyclic, polycyclic, or unremitting. The degree of arthritis varies from mild arthritis present only during systemic flares to a progressive, destructive polyarthritis. Children may be quite ill and unable to go to school without extensive support services.

NSAIDs continue to be first-line therapy, with the caveat that aspirin is characteristically hepatotoxic in these patients. Systemic corticosteroids, given as intravenous pulses, help with fever and systemic symptoms. Malignancy and infection as the causes of fevers must be carefully ruled out before initiation of corticosteroids. Daily administration of corticosteroids is best avoided unless a pericardial effusion is present. Pulse steroids are initiated daily for 3 days, and then administered weekly. Following white blood cell counts and sedimentation rates may be useful in monitoring disease activity and guiding steroid taper. MTX is generally started at the initiation of steroids. For children not responding to the above regimen, etanercept is added promptly. For those who don't respond to etanercept or who lose response over time, infliximab* infusions may be useful. In the child with severe systemic JRA, cyclophosphamide pulses may be given either every month or every 3 months in combination with methylprednisolone pulses. Other medications to consider include cyclosporine,* thalidomide,* and leflunomide.* Sulfasalazine is associated with a higher incidence of rashes and intolerance in children with systemic JRA. A child with signs of MAS should be treated aggressively with systemic steroids and cyclosporine.

DRUG COMPLICATIONS AND MONITORING

NSAIDs

Nonsteroidal anti-inflammatory drugs are the mainstay of therapy for JRA (Table 4). It helps compliance to prescribe an NSAID that is given once or twice a day; taste is also an important factor for children. FDA-approved choices are limited to ibuprofen

*Not FDA approved for this indication.

TABLE 4. **Selected Commonly Used NSAIDs for JRA**

Drug	Dose (mg/kg)	Frequency	Maximum Dose	Preparation (mg)
Naproxen (Naprosyn, Aleve)	15-20	bid	500 mg bid	125/5 mL, 220, 250, 375, 500
Ibuprofen (Advil, Motrin)	40	tid	800 mg tid	100/5 mL, 50, 100, 200, 400, 600, 800
Tolmetin (Tolectin)	30-40	tid	600 mg tid	200, 400, 600
Indomethacin (Indocin)	2	bid	75 mg bid	25/5 mL, 25, 50
Indomethacin (Indocin SR)	2-3	qd or bid	75 mg bid	75
Aspirin	80-100	tid	1800 mg tid	81, 325, 500, 650, 975
Diclofenac (Voltaren)	2-3	bid	150 mg bid	25, 50, 75
Nabumetone (Relafen)	25	qd or bid	1000 mg bid	500, 750
Celecoxib (Celebrex)	?	bid	200 mg bid	100, 200
Rofecoxib (Vioxx)	?	qd	25 mg qd	12.5/5 mL, 25/5 mL, 12.5, 25

bid, twice daily; qd, every day; tid, three times daily.

(Motrin, Advil), naproxen (Naprosyn, Aleve), aspirin, and tolmetin (Tolectin). However, clinicians often prescribe other NSAIDs available on the market, especially in older children. The association of aspirin with Reye syndrome has frightened many parents and clinicians away from the drug; varicella and influenza vaccinations should be given before initiation of aspirin therapy. Indomethacin (Indocin) is useful in treating recalcitrant fevers and pericarditis in systemic JRA.

NSAIDs work by inhibiting both cyclooxygenase (COX)-1 and COX-2 pathways. Newer, selective NSAIDs have their main effect on inhibition of COX-2, decreasing gastrointestinal side effects. Pediatric trials have not been performed to establish dosage. Celecoxib (Celebrex)* and rofecoxib (Vioxx)* are both COX-2–specific drugs that may be used in older children.

NSAIDs should always be administered with food to protect against gastritis, the most common side effect. To treat NSAID-induced gastritis, an H_2 blocker, proton pump inhibitor, misoprostol (Cytotec), or sulfacrate (Carafate) may be used in conjunction with the NSAID. In fair-skinned, blue-eyed children pseudoporphyria (fragility of the skin in sun-exposed areas associated with depressed scars during healing) is seen with the propionic acid NSAIDs, especially naproxen (Naprosyn) and, to a lesser extent, nabumetone (Relafen). Central nervous system side effects seen with all NSAIDs include excessive sleepiness, difficulty concentrating, and other behavior changes. Less common adverse effects of NSAIDs include hepatotoxicity, nephrotoxicity, and, rarely, leukopenia. A blood count, liver panel, and a urinalysis should be monitored twice a year in children chronically taking NSAIDs.

Sulfasalazine

Sulfasalazine (Azulfidine) contains both a sulfa and an aspirin component. It is administered twice daily at a dose of 40 to 50 mg/kg per day. It is available in a 500-mg pill and can be formulated as a liquid. It has been associated with rash, usually not severe, but can cause Stevens-Johnson syndrome. Other toxicities include bone marrow suppression, hepatotoxicity, photosensitivity, and abdominal distress. Starting dose of sulfasalazine is generally 20 mg/kg/d; if after 2 to 4 weeks a check of blood count and liver transaminases is normal, the dose is increased to 40 mg/kg/d. Monthly blood counts and liver transaminases should be monitored until the child has been on the drug for 3 months, then every 3 months thereafter.

*Not FDA approved for this indication.

Hydroxychloroquine

Hydroxychloroquine (Plaquenil)* is given at doses of 5 to 6 mg/kg/d (maximum dose is 400 mg/d) as a single dose. It is available only in pill form; pharmacists can compound it into a liquid. Side effects include abdominal pain and headaches. Retinal toxicity has been described, patients first presenting with color discrimination problems. Yearly eye examination should be performed by an ophthalmologist.

Methotrexate

Methotrexate (Rheumatrex), an inhibitor of folate metabolism, is given once a week either orally, via subcutaneously, or intravenously. Starting dose is generally 10 mg/m^2 and may be increased to 1 mg/kg. It has been an effective, relatively safe drug in the therapy of JRA. Common side effects include elevation of liver transaminases, leukopenia, stomatitis, nausea and vomiting, malaise, fatigue, chills, fever, dizziness, photosensitivity, and rash. Folic acid, 1 mg by mouth (PO) daily, should be given along with MTX because it decreases the frequency and severity of side effects. Leucovorin (Wellcovorin) (5 mg PO) may be given 12 to 24 hours after MTX in children having immediate side effects. Premedication with antiemetics, such as ondansetron (Zofran), is necessary in a few patients. Serious side effects include hepatotoxicity, pancytopenia, nephrotoxicity, immunosuppression with increased infections, pneumonitis, pulmonary fibrosis, Stevens-Johnson syndrome, toxic epidermal necrolysis, and erythema multiforme. There have been reports of methotrexate-associated lymphoma, which responds to withdrawal of the drug.

Children starting methotrexate need to have monthly monitoring of their serum transaminases and

*Not FDA approved for this indication.

complete blood counts. One should wait 4 to 5 days after administration of methotrexate to have blood studies drawn, as MTX may cause mild, clinically insignificant, transient elevations of the transaminases. For children on chronic, stable doses, the frequency of toxicity screening may be decreased to every 6 to 8 weeks. The family should be warned about increased hepatotoxicity with alcohol intake and girls of reproductive age should be counseled about reliable contraception. Drugs containing sulfonamides should be avoided because they may potentiate MTX toxicity.

Glucocorticoids

Corticosteroids promote osteoporosis, decrease linear growth, and increase the risk of obesity, hypertension, cataract formation, avascular necrosis, glaucoma, and striae. However, steroids do not prevent joint damage; it is best to avoid corticosteroids in children with JRA. When needed, pulse intravenous doses may be more effective, with fewer side effects than daily oral administration. Doses of 30 mg/kg, maximum 1 gram of methylprednisolone, are administered intravenously over 1 hour with monitoring of blood pressure every 15 minutes until 30 minutes after the infusion is complete. Besides hypertension, facial flushing, diffuse erythema, myalgias, mood swings, and fatigue may be seen for 24 hours. Low-dose daily prednisone is sometimes needed in children with polyarticular or systemic JRA. It is best decreased slowly with tapering to every-other-day dosing before discontinuation. Linear growth, bone density assessment, and ophthalmologic examinations should be monitored every 6 months in children on chronic corticosteroids.

Triamcinolone hexacetonide (Aristospan) is the steroid of choice for intra-articular injection. Doses range from 5 to 40 mg† depending on the size of the child and the joint(s) affected. It must never be used in a joint suspected of being septic. Adverse effects include skin atrophy at the injection site, introduction of infection, and bruising. Rarely, a chemical synovitis may be precipitated by the injection, which resolves within days.

Biologics

Etanercept (Enbrel) is an antitumor necrosis factor-alpha (anti TNF-α) biologic approved for use in polyarticular JRA. It is given biweekly via subcutaneous injection at a dose of 0.4 mg/kg, maximum dose of 25 mg, often used in combination with MTX. Common reactions include injection site pain and erythema, rash, abdominal pain, and vomiting. More serious reactions include reactivation of tuberculosis, sepsis, and other serious infections, including opportunistic infections. A purified protein derivative test should be done before initiation of therapy. Etanercept is stopped temporarily with any serious infections requiring hospitalization or intravenous antibiotics. Infliximab (Remicade)* is another anti-TNF-α agent used with MTX or other second-line agents in severe polyarticular or systemic JRA that is not responding to conventional therapy. It is given intravenously in doses ranging from 3 mg/kg/dose to 10 mg/kg/dose. It is initially given 2 weeks apart, then every 4 to 8 weeks. It has side effects similar to etanercept in terms of infection; in addition, it may cause a lupus-like syndrome and a hypersensitivity reaction, along with fever, chills, nausea and vomiting, back pain, myalgias, dizziness, hypotension, hypertension, and elevated liver transaminases. Use of doses up to 20 mg/kg have been reported in systemic JRA, but should be used with caution.

†Exceeds dosage recommended by the manufacturer.

Cyclosporine

Cyclosporine (Neoral)* is a T-cell modulator used in severe, nonresponsive, polyarticular and systemic JRA and in MAS. It is given twice daily at doses from 2 mg/kg to 7 mg/kg.† In children less than 5 years it may be harder to obtain therapeutic levels without administering the drug three times daily at doses up to 7 mg/kg/d. Cyclosporine should be started at the lowest dose and titrated up. Trough serum levels are monitored periodically. Common side effects include hirsutism, gum hyperplasia, acne, abdominal pain, and hypertension. More serious side effects include nephrotoxicity, hepatotoxicity, anaphylaxis, malignancy, immunosuppression, and cytopenias. Blood counts, electrolyte levels (including BUN and creatinine), liver transaminases, urinalysis, and blood pressure should be monitored at regular intervals.

Leflunomide

Leflunomide (Arava)* is a pyrimidine synthesis modulator. It has not been studied in pediatric populations but is used in older children. It is given at a dose of 10 to 20 mg daily in adults. It has a very long half-life and is potentially teratogenic. Common side effects include diarrhea, elevated liver transaminases, alopecia, and rash.

Cyclophosphamide

Cyclophosphamide (Cytoxan)* use has been reported in systemic JRA and polyarticular JRA. It is an option for those children who have failed all conventional therapies. It is given in monthly intravenous pulses in doses from 500 mg to 1000 mg/m^2. Hemorrhagic cystitis, nausea and vomiting, infertility, and leukopenia are all potential side effects. Care must be taken to hydrate the child well with an adequate antiemetic regimen after infusion. A blood count must be checked 10 days after therapy to evaluate the degree of leukopenia induced by the drug.

*Not FDA approved for this indication.
†Exceeds dosage recommended by the manufacturer.

ANKYLOSING SPONDYLITIS

method of
ANDREW KEAT, M.D.
Northwick Park Hospital
Middlesex, United Kingdom

Results of treating ankylosing spondylitis (AS) are often far from satisfactory. Early diagnosis is essential if a patient is to have a reasonable chance of maintaining mobility, posture, and lifestyle. The prospect exists, however, of enabling a young patient with early disease to anticipate a life not far removed from that of healthy peers. But for a patient with established disease, treatment is at best palliative. Thus, in a disease with slow and often subtle deterioration, management involves the whole gamut of the physician's art, including motivation, long-term record keeping, personal support, and occupational advice in addition to soundly based treatment ranging from physical therapy through conventional drug therapy to biologic therapy.

THE SPONDYLOARTHROPATHIES

AS is the central member of the spondyloarthropathy family. This cluster of disorders shares key clinical and pathologic features, notably capacity to involve the sacroiliac joints and spine, enthesitis, characteristic lower limb oligoarthritis, episodic ocular inflammation, clinical and subclinical bowel inflammation, and psoriasiform skin and mucus membrane lesions (Table 1). Familial clustering occurs and predisposition to all members of the family is associated with the HLA-B27 gene. The spondyloarthropathy family constitutes the second most common form of inflammatory arthritis.

TABLE 1. **Amor Criteria for Classification of Spondyloarthritides***

Past or current clinical manifestations	Points
Back pain at night and/or back stiffness in the morning	1
Asymmetric oligoarthritis	2
Gluteal pain without other features, or	1
Alternating gluteal pain	2
Sausage-like finger or toe	2
Heel pain or other enthesopathy	2
Iritis	2
Nongonococcal urethritis or cervicitis within 1 month before onset of arthritis	1
Diarrhea within 1 month before onset of arthritis	1
Past or current psoriasis and/or balanitis and/or inflammatory bowel disease	2
Roentgenographic changes	
Sacroiliitis (stage 2 or more if bilateral, stage 3 or more if unilateral)	2
Predisposing genetic factors	
Presence of the HLA-B27 antigen and/or positive family history of ankylosing spondylitis, Reiter's syndrome, psoriasis, uveitis, or chronic bowel disease	2
Response to treatment	
Improvement within 48 hours after initiation of a nonsteroidal anti-inflammatory drug	2

*A score of 6 points or more merits a diagnosis of spondyloarthropathy.

According to the prominence of spinal involvement, psoriasis, overt inflammatory bowel disease, or a predisposing gastrointestinal or genitourinary infection, the principal forms of spondyloarthropathy are designated: ankylosing spondylitis, psoriatic arthritis, enteropathic arthritis, or reactive arthritis/Reiter's syndrome. Typical forms of spondyloarthropathy may occur in children, although in both adults and children undifferentiated forms of spondyloarthropathy occur. In contrast to rheumatoid disease, patients characteristically lack IgM rheumatoid factor.

For practical purposes, treatment of patients with this group of conditions is dependent on the dominant lesions present because no single approach is appropriate for all aspects of the disease or for all patients. Critical analysis of the clinical problems, therefore, guides the selection of treatment.

KEY LESIONS

Sacroiliitis

This is a *sine qua non* for the diagnosis of AS. It occurs in a minority of patients with other spondyloarthropathies. Patients with sacroiliitis usually present in the late teens or twenties, with buttock pain that may be aggravated by standing or activity and may awaken the patient from sleep. Characteristic radiographic appearances may take several years to develop, although MRI scanning may show earlier changes.

Spondylitis

Spinal features of AS seldom appear before the age of 18 years and onset after age 40 years is rare. Inflammatory back pain is characterized by insidious onset, persistence, exacerbation with inactivity, and improvement with exercise. Spinal stiffness and restriction typically ascend the spine and may include costovertebral joints and referred pain around the chest. Vertebral osteoporosis occurs early in disease, and severe disease leads to spinal rigidity with increased risk of vertebral fracture.

As with sacroiliac joints, radiographic diagnostic features are slow to appear but evidence of osteitis associated with spinal enthesitis may be demonstrated earlier in the disease by magnetic resonance imaging (MRI).

Synovitis

Peripheral synovitis is characterized by the distribution of joints affected rather than by histologic changes. Oligoarticular, asymmetrical, and sometimes episodic involvement of hips, knees, ankles, and metatarsophalangeal joints is characteristic, although histologically the lesions are indistinguishable from typical rheumatoid disease. Upper limb joints are affected only when psoriasis is present. Dactylitis in one or more toes or fingers may last for many months and cause severe symptoms.

Enthesitis

Inflammation at sites of attachment between tendons or ligaments and bones is a dominant feature of AS. It accounts for much of the pain, stiffness, and restriction both at sacroiliac and spinal joints and at peripheral sites, such as the heel. Radiographically, such lesions lead initially to a small area of local osteopenia, which is subsequently replaced by a bony spur within the enthesis. In joints such as the knee, it is important to differentiate pain due to patellar enthesitis from that of synovitis.

Systemic Features

Fatigue, sleep deprivation, and depression are common. So, too, is impairment of family and working life, with failure of career progression, part-time working, and early retirement. Osteoporosis occurs early in disease and, uncommonly, amyloidosis may develop later, especially in those with persistent active axial and peripheral disease. Subclinical bowel inflammation occurs in the majority of individuals with AS but does not require treatment. Overt ulcerative colitis or Crohn's disease may require specific treatment, as may psoriasis and inflammatory eye lesions. Subtle carditis may be an incidental finding, although aortic valve disease, occurring in approximately 1% of people with AS, may require specialist cardiologic assessment and treatment.

DIAGNOSIS AND DIFFERENTIAL DIAGNOSIS

Clinical features may suggest a spondyloarthropathy, which may be diagnosed according to the Amor criteria (see Table 1). Strictly, the diagnosis of AS depends on the New York criteria. However, probable or early disease may be diagnosed on the basis of the presence of inflammatory back or buttock pain that is relieved by exercise or nonsteroidal anti-inflammatory drugs, with restricted spinal movements. A history of iritis, psoriasis, inflammatory bowel disease, or a family history of spondyloarthropathy, increases the confidence of the diagnosis. Early evidence of bilateral sacroiliitis is best achieved by MRI or computed tomography scanning because classic radiographic changes may take years to become apparent.

When the clinical suspicion of AS is high, the presence of the HLA-B27 antigen enhances the likelihood of this diagnosis. In patients with ill-defined back pain, testing for the HLA-B27 antigen may be misleading and should be avoided.

TREATMENT

In some patients, specific treatment is unnecessary. In all, however, a careful explanation of the diagnosis, encouragement to adopt a physically active lifestyle, and long-term monitoring to detect subtle spinal restriction and deformity are essential. Specific approaches to treatment are dependent upon the particular features present in the individual. Thus, a careful assessment of the objectives of treatment is vital in planning the management of patients with spondyloarthropathy.

Active Sacroiliitis or Spondylitis

Physical activity delays ankylosis and imparts a sense of well-being. However, regular exercises are difficult and unattractive for young, busy adults and motivation by both physician and physical therapist is, therefore, a key aspect of treatment. Membership in local self-help groups is useful for some patients. A daily routine of stretches helps to maintain flexibility and patients should be encouraged to pursue some regular sporting activity, such as swimming. Assessment and instruction by a physical therapist help to identify particular problems which may require specific home exercise or therapy.

Nonsteroidal anti-inflammatory drugs (NSAIDs) are usually effective at reducing pain and stiffness. Because there is considerable variability of effect, it is worth prescribing brief trial periods of perhaps 1 week of several NSAIDs to assess efficacy and tolerability. Pain and stiffness during the night and first thing in the morning may be helped by an NSAID with a long half-life such as piroxicam (Feldene)* or celecoxib (Celebrex)* or in a sustained-relief preparation such as diclofenac (Voltaren),* ibuprofen (Motrin),* or indomethacin (Indocin) taken after the evening meal. Once-daily dosage may be sufficient, though for many individuals, twice-daily dosage with agents such as diclofenac, 75 mg SR twice daily, or indomethacin, 75 mg twice daily provides better symptom control. Phenylbutazone is now of limited availability, although may still be effective at 100 mg three times daily when other agents are not. Treatment with phenylbutazone,‡ however, necessitates blood monitoring of full blood count at least every three months.

Gastroprotection is desirable in the elderly and for those with dyspepsia, past history of upper gastrointestinal bleeding, and peptic ulceration or perforation. This may be achieved by using a combined preparation of a nonsteroidal, e.g., diclofenac with misoprostol (Arthrotec), by the addition of a proton pump inhibitor or H_2 receptor antagonist with a nonselective cyclooxygenase inhibitor, or by prescribing a selective COX-2 inhibitor, such as celecoxib or rofecoxib (Vioxx).* Although having fewer gastrointestinal side effects, the remaining toxicity profile of COX-2 inhibitors is similar to that of older NSAIDs, and these agents may be more costly than older drugs used on their own.

When control of symptoms and disease progression is still inadequate in spite of maximal NSAID therapy, second-line treatment should be instituted. Oral steroid therapy may be valuable, although it should be restricted to short courses of less than 6 weeks. Alternatively, steroid may be administered

*Not FDA approved for this indication.
‡Not available in the United States.

by intramuscular injections of depot steroid preparations such as depot prednisolone (Depo-Medrol), 80 to 120 mg, or by single intravenous pulses of 250 to 500 mg methylprednisolone (Solu-Medrol). Such pulses of treatment may help to reverse progressive disruptive symptoms or enable grossly restricted patients to benefit more fully from intensive physical therapy programs and may be used as a temporary adjunct when starting a second-line agent. In fact, no drug has been shown to truly modify the course of AS, although sulfasalazine (Azulfidine)* has a demonstrable effect on symptom control. This agent should be introduced incrementally up to a full dose of 3 g daily† with monitoring of full blood count and liver function tests every 4 to 6 weeks. Methotrexate (Rheumatrex)* has no demonstrable benefit for spinal disease and there are no grounds for using other antirheumatoid drugs, such as gold and hydroxychloroquine (Plaquenil),* for spinal disease, although these agents may be useful in the treatment of peripheral arthritis.

Progressive, poorly responsive spinal disease may respond well to TNF blockade treatment with infliximab (Remicade) or etanercept (Enbrel). However, there are no agreed-on criteria nor protocols, and licensing for use in spondyloarthropathies may vary from country to country.

Recent studies have demonstrated some therapeutic efficacy of pamidronate (Aredia)* given as 60 mg infusions every 3 months and thalidomide (Thalomid)* at a dose of 100 mg to 200 mg orally daily. In the latter case, of course, women of childbearing potential must be excluded absolutely and regular monitoring for neurotoxicity should be carried out.

Rarely, intractable pain at one or both sacroiliac joints may be helped by intra-articular injection of steroid under imaging control.

Established Long-Standing Disease

Symptoms in those with long-standing disease may be due to spinal rigidity, flexed posture, or fracture. Acute exacerbation of back pain in such individuals should be attributed to fracture until proved otherwise.

Even in the presence of complete spinal ankylosis, vigorous exercise regimens may still maintain general mobility and a sense of well-being. Severe flexion deformity, at any level of the spine, may have profound effects on activities of daily living, pain, and self-esteem. Provided that assessment and surgery can be carried out by an experienced spinal team, corrective surgery can produce remarkable results with acceptable morbidity and mortality rates and should be considered for those with severe spinal deformities. Spinal fracture may occasionally provide the opportunity for surgical fixation of the spine in a more extended position without the need for osteotomy. Where flexed posture is exacerbated or caused by flexion deformities at the hips, useful postural improvement may be achieved by bilateral total hip replacement.

*Not FDA approved for this indication.
†Exceeds dosage recommended by the manufacturer.

Peripheral Arthritis

NSAIDs are usually helpful. Where a single joint (such as the knee) is symptomatic, a local steroid injection, with or without NSAIDs, may suffice. Persistent monoarthritis may be helped by medical synovectomy, using either osmic acid or yttrium instillation, although improvement tends to be short-lived, as with arthroscopic surgical synovectomy. Persistent mono- or oligoarthritis, in spite of maximal NSAID therapy, may respond to weekly oral or parenteral methotrexate,* 7.5 to 25 mg weekly, or to oral sulfasalazine* 2 to 3 g daily. As an alternative, azathioprine (Imuran),* 1 to 3 mg/kg, may be helpful. In these instances, regular blood monitoring is essential. There is little clear evidence that antibiotic therapy is of benefit.

Oligo- or polyarticular disease that is progressive, in spite of use of two conventional DMARDs in maximum tolerated doses, may respond to TNF blockade. As with spinal disease, there are no agreed-on criteria or protocols and licensing for use in spondyloarthropathies may vary from country to country. Current evidence indicates, however, that a satisfactory anti-inflammatory effect is likely to be achieved in 75% to 80% of recipients. As in rheumatoid arthritis, careful case selection, screening, and monitoring are essential.

Profoundly destructive changes at peripheral joints with a substantial effect on mobility and pain may be treated successfully with surgery.

Enthesitis and Dactylitis

Troublesome peripheral enthesitis at the calcaneal insertion of the plantar fascia and at the patella may respond to local steroid injections. At the Achilles tendon insertion, carefully placed steroid injection may also be effective, although here and at the patella tendon, great care should be taken to avoid injecting *into* the tendon because this may predispose tendon to rupture.

Dactylitis may improve with a short course (less than 6 weeks) of oral steroid.

PREGNANCY

AS tends not to remit during pregnancy. When possible, pregnancy should be planned in light of continuing symptoms and need for treatment and the prospect of a prolonged drug-free period should be tested prior to conception. The avoidance of all medication during pregnancy must be regarded as the gold standard. For many, however, continued use of nonsteroidals is essential. The potential risk of oligohydramnios and premature closure of the ductus arteriosus should be recognized. Sulfasalazine and other agents, including TNF blockers, should be withdrawn 6 months prior to conception. Oral steroids may provide the best option for the control of symptoms if NSAIDs are insufficient. Every effort should be made to maintain daily stretching and a regular physical exercise routine throughout pregnancy.

*Not FDA approved for this indication.

Osteoporosis

Because osteoporosis is a recognized complication of AS in both men and women, all patients should undergo assessment of risk factors and a measurement of bone density at the spine and hip on at least one occasion. Treatment should be the same as for postmenopausal osteoporosis. Thus, those patients with bone mineral density (BMD) T scores of less than –1 or greater than –2.5 should receive calcium and vitamin D supplements, whereas those with T scores of less than –2.5 should receive a bisphosphonate or hormone replacement treatment. Advanced bony changes may cause spinal BMD measurements to be spuriously high, so that results at an uninvolved hip may provide a more reliable guide to treatment.

Fatigue, Depression, and Quality of Life

Disturbed sleep is common among people with AS and may be compounded by anxiety, depression, or frustration. Tricyclic antidepressants such as amitriptyline (Elavil), 10 mg to 25 mg, at night may improve fatigue, sleep, and a feeling of well-being. Supportive psychotherapy, group membership, and intensive treatment programs may bolster morale and motivation. The reduced capacity of sufferers to secure and hold a job, to work full-time, and to secure promotion should be recognized and appropriate support provided. However, maintaining the patient's motivation to exercise regularly remains one of the most demanding prospects for all concerned.

TEMPOROMANDIBULAR DISORDERS

method of
JEFFREY P. OKESON, D.M.D.
University of Kentucky College of Dentistry
Lexington, Kentucky

Temporomandibular disorder (TMD) is a collective term that includes a number of clinical complaints involving the muscles of mastication, the temporomandibular joints (TMJ), and/or associated orofacial structures. Other commonly used terms are *Costen's syndrome, TMJ dysfunction*, and *craniomandibular disorders*. Temporomandibular disorders are a major cause of nondental pain in the orofacial region and are considered to be a subclassification of musculoskeletal disorders. In many TMD patients, the most common complaint is not the temporomandibular joints but rather the muscles of mastication. Therefore, the terms TMJ dysfunction or TMJ disorder are actually inappropriate for many of these complaints. It is for this reason that the American Dental Association has adopted the term *temporomandibular disorder*.

Signs and symptoms associated with temporomandibular disorders are a common source of pain complaints in the head and orofacial structures. These complaints can be associated with general joint problems and somatization. Approximately 50% of patients suffering from TMDs do not first consult with a dentist, but seek advice for the problem from a physician. The family physician should be able to appropriately diagnose many TM disorders. In many instances, the physician can provide valuable information and simple therapies that will reduce the patient's TMD symptoms. In other instances, it is appropriate to refer the patient to a dentist for additional evaluation and treatment.

EPIDEMIOLOGIC FINDINGS FOR TEMPOROMANDIBULAR DISORDERS

Cross-sectional population-based studies reveal that 40% to 75% of adult populations having at least one sign of temporomandibular joint dysfunction (jaw movement abnormalities, joint noise, tenderness on palpation, and so on) and approximately 33% have at least one symptom (face pain, joint pain, and so on). Many of these signs and symptoms are not troublesome for the individual, with only 3% to 7% of the population seeking any advise or care. Although in the general population women seem to have only a slightly greater incidence of TMD symptoms, women seek care for TMD more often than men at a ratio ranging from 3:1 to 9:1. For many patients, temporomandibular disorders are self-limited, or are associated with symptoms that fluctuate over time without evidence of progression. Although many of these disorders are self-limiting, the health care provider can provide conservative therapies that will minimize the patient's painful experience.

SIGNS AND SYMPTOMS OF TEMPOROMANDIBULAR DISORDERS

The primary signs and symptoms associated with TMD originate from the masticatory structures and are associated with jaw function (Table 1). Pain during opening of the mouth or when chewing is common. Some individuals will even report difficulty speaking or singing. Patients often report pain in the preauricular areas, face, and/or temples. TMJ sounds are frequently described as clicking, popping, grating, or crepitus, and locking of the jaw during opening or closing can be demonstrated. Patients frequently report painful jaw muscles and, on occasion, may even

TABLE 1. **Symptoms Associated with Temporomandibular Disorders**

Primary Symptoms
Facial muscle pain
Preauricular (TMJ) pain
TMJ sounds; jaw clicking, popping, catching, or locking
Limited mouth opening
Increased pain associated with chewing
Secondary Symptoms
Earache
Headache
Neck ache

TMJ, temporomandibular joint.

report a sudden change in their bite, coincidental with the onset of the painful condition.

It is important to appreciate that pain associated with most TM disorders is increased with jaw function. Because this is a condition of the musculoskeletal structures, function of these structures generally increases the pain. When a patient's pain complaint is not influenced by jaw function, other sources of orofacial pain should be suspected.

The spectrum of TMD often includes commonly associated complaints such as headache, neck ache, or earache. These associated complaints are often referred pains and must be differentiated from primary pains. As a general rule, referred pains associated with TM disorders are increased with any activity that provokes the TM disorder pain. Therefore, if the patient reports that the headache is aggravated by jaw function, it may very well represent a secondary pain related to the TM disorder. Likewise, if the secondary symptom is unaffected by jaw use, one should question its relationship to the TM disorder and be suspicious of two separate pain conditions. Pain or dysfunction due to nonmusculoskeletal causes such as otolaryngologic, neurologic, vascular, neoplastic, or infectious disease in the orofacial region is not considered a primary temporomandibular disorder even though musculoskeletal pain may be present. It should be remembered, however, that TM disorders often coexist with other craniofacial and orofacial pain disorders.

ANATOMY AND PATHOPHYSIOLOGY OF TEMPOROMANDIBULAR DISORDERS

The temporomandibular joint is formed by the mandibular condyle fitting into the mandibular fossa of the temporal bone. The movement of this joint is quite complex because it allows hinging movement in one plane and, at the same time, allows gliding movements in another plane.

Separating these two bones from direct articulation is the articular disk. The articular disk is composed of dense, fibrous connective tissue devoid of any blood vessels or nerve fibers. The articular disk is attached posteriorly to a region of loose connective tissue that is highly vascularized and well innervated, known as the *retrodiskal tissue*. The anterior region of the disk is attached to the superior lateral pterygoid muscle.

The movement of the mandible is accomplished by four pairs of muscles termed the *muscles of mastication*: the masseter, temporalis, medial pterygoid, and lateral pterygoid. Although not considered to be muscles of mastication, the digastric muscles also play an important role in mandibular function. The masseter, temporalis, and medial pterygoid muscles elevate the mandible and, therefore, provide the major forces used for chewing and other jaw functions. The inferior lateral pterygoid muscles provide protrusive movement of the mandible and the digastric muscles serve to depress the mandible (open the mouth).

When discussing the pathophysiology of TMD one needs to consider two main categories: joint pathophysiology and muscle pathophysiology. Because etiologic considerations and treatment strategies are different for these conditions, they will be presented separately.

Pathophysiology of Intracapsular Temporomandibular Joint Pain Disorders

Several common arthritic conditions, such as rheumatoid arthritis, traumatic arthritis, hyperuricemia, and psoriatic arthritis, can affect the temporomandibular joint. These conditions, however, are not nearly as common as local osteoarthritis. As with most other joints, osteoarthritis results from overloading the articular surface of the joint, thus breaking down the dense fibrous articular surface and ultimately affecting the subarticular bone. In the TMJ, this overloading commonly occurs as a result of an alteration in the morphology and position of the articular disk. In the healthy TMJ, the disk maintains its position on the condyle during movement because of its morphology (i.e., the thicker anterior and posterior borders) and interarticular pressure maintained by the elevator muscles. If, however, the morphology of the disk is altered and the diskal ligaments become elongated, the disk can be displaced from its normal position between the condyle and fossa. If the disk is displaced, normal opening and closing of the mouth can result in an unusual transitory movement between the condyle and the disk that is felt as a click or a pop. Disk displacements that result in joint sounds may or may not be painful. When pain is present, it is thought to be related to either loading forces applied to the highly vascularized retrodiscal tissues or a general inflammatory response of the surrounding soft tissues (capsulitis or synovitis).

Pathophysiology of Masticatory Muscle Pain Disorders

The muscles of mastication are a very common source of TMD pain. Understanding the pathophysiology of muscle pain, however, is very complex and still not well understood. The simple explanation of muscle spasm does not account for most TMD muscle pain complaints. It appears that a better explanation would include a central nervous system (CNS) effect on the muscle that results in an increase in peripheral nociceptive activity originating from the muscle tissue itself. This explanation more accurately accounts for the high levels of emotional stress that are commonly associated with TMD muscle pain complaints. In other words, an increase in emotional stress activates the autonomic nervous system, which, in turn, seems to be associated with changes in muscle nociception.

These masticatory muscle pain conditions are further complicated when one considers the unique masticatory muscle activity known as bruxism. Bruxism is the subconscious, often rhythmic, grinding or gnashing of the teeth. This type of muscle activity is considered to be parafunctional and may also occur as a simple static loading of the teeth known as clenching. This activity commonly occurs while sleeping but may also be present during the day. These parafunctional activities alone can represent a significant source of masticatory muscle pain, and certainly bruxism in the presence of CNS-induced muscle pain can further accentuate the patient's muscle pain complaints.

ETIOLOGIC CONSIDERATIONS OF TEMPOROMANDIBULAR DISORDERS

Because TMD represents a group of disorders, there are multiple etiologies that may be associated. Problems arising from intracapsular conditions (e.g., clicking, popping, catching, or locking) may be associated with various types of trauma. Gross trauma, such as a blow to the chin, can immediately alter ligamentous structures of the joint, leading to joint sounds. Trauma may also be associated with more subtle injury, such as stretching, twisting, or compressing forces during eating, yawning, yelling, or prolonged mouth opening.

When the patient's chief complaint is muscle pain, etiologic factors other than trauma should be considered. Masticatory muscle pain disorders have etiologic considerations similar to other muscle pain disorders of the neck and back. Emotional stress seems to play a significant role for many patients. This may explain why patients often report that their painful symptoms fluctuate greatly over time. Although most TMD patients do not have a major psychiatric disorder, psychological factors can certainly enhance the pain condition. The clinician needs to consider such factors as anxiety, depression, secondary gain, somatization, and hypochondriasis. Psychosocial factors may predispose certain individuals to TMD and may also perpetuate TMD once symptoms have become established. A careful consideration of psychosocial factors is, therefore, important in the evaluation and treatment of every TMD patient.

Temporomandibular disorders have a few unique etiologic factors that distinguish them from other musculoskeletal disorders. One such factor is the occlusal relationship of the teeth. Traditionally, it was felt that malocclusion was the primary etiologic factor responsible for TMD. Recent investigations do not support this concept, however. Still, there are certain instances when occlusal instability of the teeth can contribute to a TM disorder. This may be true in patients both with and without teeth. Poorly fitting dental prostheses can also contribute to occlusal instability. The occlusal condition should be suspected, especially if the pain problem began with a change in the patient's occlusion (e.g., a dental appointment).

HISTORY AND EXAMINATION FOR TEMPOROMANDIBULAR DISORDERS

All patients reporting pain in the orofacial structures should be screened for TMD. This can be accomplished with a brief history and physical examination. The screening questions and examination are performed to rule in or out the possibility of a TM disorder. If a positive response is found, a more extensive history and examination are indicated. Table 2 lists questions that should be asked during a screening assessment for TMD. Any positive response should be followed by additional clarifying questions.

Patients experiencing orofacial pain should also be briefly examined for any clinical signs associated with TMD. The clinician can easily palpate a few sites to assess tenderness or pain, as well as assess for jaw mobility. The masseter muscles can be palpated bilaterally while asking the patient to report any pain or tenderness. The same assessment should be made for the temporal regions, as well as the preauricular (TMJ) areas. While the hands are over the preauricular areas, the patient should be asked to repeatedly open and close the mouth. The presence of joint sounds should be noted and it should be determined whether these sounds are associated with joint pain.

A simple measurement of mouth opening should then be made. This can be accomplished by placing a millimeter ruler on the lower anterior teeth and asking the patient to open as wide as possible. The distance should be measured between the maxillary and mandibular anterior teeth. It is generally accepted that less than 40 mm is considered a restricted mouth opening.

It is also helpful to inspect the teeth for significant wear, mobility, or decay that may be related to the pain condition. The clinician should examine the buccal mucosa for ridging and the lateral aspect of the tongue for scalloping. These are often signs of clenching and bruxism. A general inspection for symmetry and alignment of the face, jaws, and dental arches may also be helpful. A summary of this screening examination is found in Table 3.

MANAGEMENT CONSIDERATIONS FOR TEMPOROMANDIBULAR DISORDERS

Most recent studies suggest that TM disorders are generally self-limiting and symptoms often fluctuate over time. Understanding this natural course does not

TABLE 2. **Recommended Screening Questionnaire for Temporomandibular Disorders***

1. Do you have difficulty, pain, or both when opening your mouth, for instance when yawning?
2. Does your jaw "get stuck," "locked," or "go out"?
3. Do you have difficulty, pain, or both when chewing, talking, or using your jaws?
4. Are you aware of noises in the jaw joints?
5. Do your jaws regularly feel stiff, tight, or tired?
6. Do you have pain in or about the ears, temples, or cheeks?
7. Do you have frequent headaches, neck aches, or toothaches?
8. Have you had a recent injury to your head, neck, or jaw?
9. Have you been aware of any recent changes in your bite?
10. Have you been previously treated for unexplained facial pain or a jaw joint problem?

*All patients reporting pain in the orofacial region should be screened for temporomandibular disorder with a questionnaire that includes these questions. The decision to complete a comprehensive history and clinical examination depends on the number of positive responses and the apparent seriousness of the problem for the patient. It should be noted that a positive response to any question may be sufficient to warrant a comprehensive examination, if it is of concern to the patient, or if it is viewed as clinically significant by the physician.

TABLE 3. **Recommended Screening Examination Procedures for TM Disorders***

1. Palpate for tenderness in the masseter and temporalis muscles.
2. Palpate for preauricular (TMJ) tenderness.
3. Measure range of mouth opening. (Note any incoordination in the movements.)
4. Auscultate and palpate for TMJ sounds (i.e., clicking or crepitus).
5. Note excessive occlusal wear, excessive tooth mobility, buccal mucosal ridging, or lateral tongue scalloping.
6. Inspect symmetry and alignment of the face, jaws, and dental arches.

*All patients with face pain should be briefly screened for temporomandibular disorder using this or a similar cursory clinical examination. The need for a comprehensive history and clinical examination depends on the number of positive findings and the clinical significance of each finding.

TMJ, temporomandibular joint.

mean these conditions should be ignored. TMD can be a very painful condition leading to a significant decrease in the patient's quality of life. Understanding the natural course of TMD does suggest, however, that therapy may not need to be very aggressive. In general, initial therapy should begin very conservatively and escalate only when therapy fails to relieve the symptoms.

When the physician identifies a patient with a TM disorder, he or she has two options. The physician can elect to treat the patient or refer the patient to a dentist who specializes in TMD for further evaluation and treatment. The decision to refer the patient should be based on whether the patient needs any unique care provided only in a dental office. The following are some indications for referral to a dentist:

1. History of trauma to the face related to the onset of the pain condition
2. The presence of significant temporomandibular joint sounds during function
3. A feeling of jaw catching or locking during mouth opening
4. The report of a sudden change in the occlusal contacts of the teeth
5. The presence of significant occlusal instability
6. Significant findings related to the teeth (i.e., tooth mobility, tooth sensitivity, tooth decay, and tooth wear)
7. Significant pain in the jaws/masticatory muscles upon awakening.
8. The presence of an orofacial pain condition that is aggravated by jaw function and has been present for more than several months.

The specific therapy for a temporomandibular disorder varies according to the precise type of disorder identified. In other words, masticatory muscle pain is managed somewhat differently than intracapsular pain. Generally, however, the initial therapy for any type of TMD should be directed toward the relief of pain and the improvement of function. This initial, conservative therapy can be divided into three general types: patient education, pharmacologic therapy, and physical therapy.

Patient Education

It is very important that patients have an appreciation for the factors that may be associated with their disorder, as well as the natural course of the disorder. Patients should be reassured and, if necessary, convinced by appropriate tests that they are not suffering from a malignancy. Properly educated patients can contribute greatly to their own treatment. For example, knowing that emotional stress is an influencing factor in many TM disorders can help the patient understand the reason for daily fluctuations of pain intensity. Attention should be directed toward changing their response to stress or, when possible, reducing their exposure to stressful conditions. Patients with pain during chewing should be told to begin a softer diet, to chew slower, and to eat smaller bites. As a general rule, the patient should be told "if it hurts, don't do it." Continued pain can contribute to the cycling of pain and should always be avoided. The patient should be instructed to let the jaw muscles relax, maintaining the teeth apart. This will discourage bruxing activities and minimize loading of the teeth and joints.

When pain is associated with a clicking TM joint, the patient should be informed of the biomechanics of the joint. This information often allows the patient to select functional activities that are less traumatic to the joint structures. For example, some patients may report that the pain and clicking are less when they chew on a particular side of the mouth. When this occurs, they should be encouraged to continue this type of chewing.

Pharmacologic Therapy

Pharmacologic therapy can be an effective adjunct in managing symptoms associated with TM disorders. Patients should be aware that medication alone will not likely solve or cure the problem. Medication, however, in conjunction with appropriate physical therapy and definitive treatment does offer the most complete approach to many TMD problems. Mild analgesics are often helpful for many TM disorders. Control of pain is not only appreciated by the patient but also reduces the likelihood of other complicating pain disorders such as muscle co-contraction, referred pain, and central sensitization.

Nonsteroidal anti-inflammatory drugs (NSAIDs) are very helpful with many TM disorders. Included in this category are aspirin,* acetaminophen,* and ibuprofen.* Ibuprofen (i.e., Motrin, Advil, and Nuprin) is often very effective in reducing musculoskeletal pain. A dosage of 600 to 800 mg three times a day for 3 to 5 days commonly reduces pain and stops the cyclic effects of the deep pain input. The newer COX-2 inhibitors (i.e., celecoxib [Celebrex],* rofecoxib [Vioxx],* and valdecoxib [Bextra]*) can also be useful.

Physical Therapy

Many patients with TMD receive symptom relief with very simple physical therapy methods. Simple instructions for the use of moist heat and/or cold can

*Not FDA approved for this indication.

be very helpful. Surface heat can be applied by laying a hot, moist towel over the symptomatic area. A hot water bottle wrap inside the towel will help maintain the heat. This combination should remain in place for 10 to 15 minutes, not to exceed 30 minutes. An electric heating pad may be used, but care should be taken not to leave it on the face too long. Patients should be discouraged from using the heating pad while sleeping because prolonged use is likely to cause burns.

Like thermotherapy, coolant therapy can provide a simple and often effective method of reducing pain. Ice should be applied directly to the symptomatic joint and/or muscles and moved in a circular motion without pressure to the tissues. The patient will initially experience an uncomfortable feeling that will quickly turn into a burning sensation. Continued icing will result in a mild aching and then numbness. When numbness begins the ice should be removed. The ice should not be left on the tissues for longer than 5 minutes. After a period of warming, a second cold application may be desirable.

The physician should be aware that many TM disorders respond to the use of orthopedic appliances (i.e., occlusal appliances, bite guards, splints). These appliances are made by the dentist and are custom fabricated for each patient. There are several types of appliances available. Each is specific for the type of TM disorder present. The dentist should be consulted for this type of therapy.

Other Therapeutic Considerations

Sometimes TM disorders can become chronic and, as with other chronic pain conditions, may then be best managed by a multidisciplinary approach. If the patient reports a long history of TMD complaints, the physician should consider referring the patient to a dentist associated with a team of therapists, such as a psychologist, physical therapist, and even a chronic pain physician. Generally, chronic TMD patients are not managed well by the simple initial therapies discussed in this article. Often other factors, such as mechanical conditions within the TM joints or psychological factors, need to be addressed. The physician who attempts to manage these conditions in the private practice setting may become very frustrated with the results. It is, therefore, recommended that if the patient's history suggests chronicity or if initial therapy fails to reduce the patient's symptoms, referral is indicated.

BURSITIS, TENDONITIS, MYOFASCIAL PAIN, AND FIBROMYALGIA

method of
ROBERT T. SCHOEN, M.D.
Yale University School of Medicine
New Haven, Connecticut

Musculoskeletal pain is common. Whereas some patients have degenerative, inflammatory, or infectious arthritis as the cause of pain, many others have the conditions grouped together by the term *soft tissue rheumatism*. These disorders may be local (bursitis and tendonitis), regional (myofascial pain), or generalized (fibromyalgia). Because they cause pain and occur frequently, these conditions are an important source of anxiety and disability. There is a spectrum of diagnostic complexity ranging from straight- forward (e.g., pain over the lateral epicondyle of the elbow) to complex (e.g., intractable neck pain). The challenge of diagnosis is increased by limited diagnostic laboratory tests. But success in the diagnosis and treatment of soft tissue rheumatic syndromes can be gratifying. For some patients, rest and reassurance will be associated with a self-limited syndrome. For others, prompt and appropriate intervention will reduce pain, anxiety, and morbidity.

Bursitis and Tendonitis

A bursa is a closed sac or envelope lined with synovial membrane and containing fluid, usually found in areas subject to friction. Bursae are often found where a tendon passes over a bone. A tendon is a fibrous cord or band that connects a muscle to a bone or other structure. It consists of fascicles of very densely arranged, almost parallel, collagen fibers, tendon cells, and ground substance. Because of the proximity of tendons and bursa, tendonitis and bursitis often coexist. For example, *rotator cuff tendonitis* can lead to *subacromial bursitis*.

Bursitis and tendonitis are usually suspected because of local tenderness at sites where these structures are present. Swelling is noted when bursitis and tendonitis occur close to the body surface (e.g., *prepatellar bursitis*), but swelling is not appreciated for deeper structures (e.g., *trochanteric bursitis*). For bursitis and tendonitis, there is often preserved passive range of motion but reduced active range of motion. In contrast, a decrease in both active and passive range of motion is more typical for structural joint abnormalities. As part of the history and physical examination, it is important to determine whether bursitis and tendonitis arise as an isolated finding in a previously healthy patient or whether this problem is associated with systemic diseases such as gout or rheumatoid arthritis.

Whenever possible, bursal fluid should be obtained for synovial analysis, including culture, Gram stain, glucose, white blood cell count, and crystal evaluation. As in septic arthritis, a bursal fluid white blood cell count of greater than 50,000/mm^3 provides strong preliminary evidence of infection, but infected bursae may also have significantly lower white blood cell counts. In patients with tendonitis and bursitis, plain radiographs often demonstrate calcium deposition or associated degenerative joint disease. Diagnostic laboratory evaluation should also be used to assess coexistent systemic disease (e.g., diabetes, alcoholism, or rheumatoid arthritis) which may predispose to bursitis and tendonitis.

There are hundreds of bursae and tendons but the approach to bursitis and tendonitis emphasizes specific clinical syndromes in a small number, the most common of which occur in the shoulder, the elbow, the hip, the knee, and the ankle and foot.

Shoulder

Rotator cuff tendonitis is the most common cause of shoulder pain. This syndrome may be acute or chronic. There is pain on active abduction. Calcific deposits in the supraspinatus tendon are seen in some patients, particularly with acute symptom onset. In older patients or as a result of repetitive strain, rotator cuff tendonitis may become chronic. Patients complain of continuous pain, although this is usually increased by abduction and internal rotation. Rotator cuff tendonitis is associated with *acromial bursitis* when inflammation spreads from the supraspinatus tendon to the subacromial bursa. *Rotator cuff tears* may occur acutely as the result of trauma, but at least one half of patients with a rotator cuff tear have no antecedent history of trauma. Typically, age-associated degeneration of the rotator cuff is responsible. A diagnosis of a ruptured rotator cuff can be established by an abnormal arthrogram that shows a communication between the glenohumeral joint and the subacromial bursa. Diagnostic ultrasonography and magnetic resonance imaging can also help identify rotator cuff tears.

Adhesive capsulitis, also known as "frozen shoulder," refers to a syndrome of generalized pain, loss of active and passive range of motion, and muscle atrophy. Adhesive capsulitis is often associated with inflammatory arthritis, diabetes, immobility, and depression. *Bicipital tendonitis* is a tenosynovitis of the long head of the biceps in which the tendon is frayed and fibrotic. There is anterior shoulder pain and local tenderness over the bicipital groove. A snap over the tendon may be noted in the shoulder when the arm is passively abducted to 90 degrees. Rupture of the long head of the biceps tendon is a common complication and produces a bulbous enlargement of the lateral half of the muscle.

Elbow

The olecranon bursa at the point of the elbow is a frequent location for bursitis. Because of its superficial location, the bursa characteristically develops swelling, erythema, and tenderness. *Olecranon bursitis* may be idiopathic or post-traumatic, but rheumatoid arthritis, gout, and sepsis should be considered. Infection of the bursa can follow an abrasion or the introduction of a foreign body or occur in association with cellulitis. Whereas most patients with olecranon bursitis have acute syndromes, chronic or recurrent olecranon bursitis is seen with repetitive trauma or rheumatoid arthritis. *Lateral epicondylitis* results from degeneration of the common extensor tendons, particularly the extensor carpi radialis brevis tendon. This form of "tennis elbow" results from activities of daily living (shaking hands, lifting a suitcase, gardening, and so on). *Medial epicondylitis*, which involves the flexor carpi radialis tendon ("golfer's elbow"), is less common.

Wrist and Hand

A *ganglion* can develop from cystic swelling of a tendon sheath or joint over the dorsum of the wrist. *De Quervain's tenosynovitis* is tenosynovitis of the abductor pollicis longus and extensor pollicis brevis tendons. It typically results from repetitive overuse and may be associated with pregnancy, trauma, and systemic diseases, such as rheumatoid arthritis. Pain is noted over the radial side of the wrist during pinching or thumb and wrist movement. Tenosynovitis occurs in other flexor and extensor tendons of the wrists. The findings vary depending on which tendons are involved.

Hip

In the hip, the trochanteric bursa lies deep between the tendon of the gluteus maximus and the posterior lateral prominence of the greater trochanter. Although common, *trochanteric bursitis* often goes undiagnosed. The main symptom is aching over the lateral thigh and hip and is usually associated with point tenderness on palpation. Pain may be increased with abduction and external rotation of the hip. Trochanteric bursitis often affects middle-aged and elderly patients and may be associated with stress, osteoarthritis of the lumbar spine or hip, leg length discrepancy, and scoliosis. *Ischiogluteal bursitis* ("weaver's bottom") is caused by trauma or prolonged sitting on hard surfaces, resulting in pain in the bursa over the ischial prominence. Point tenderness over the bursa is found.

Knee

Prepatellar bursitis ("housemaid's knee") is usually an acute swelling of the prepatellar bursa located between the patella and the overlying skin. It usually results from irritating trauma but, like the olecranon bursa, the prepatellar bursa is an important location for septic bursitis and crystal-induced diseases such as gout. In a small percentage of patients, prepatellar bursitis becomes chronic with erythema and induration of the overlying skin. *Anserine bursitis* affects a superficial bursa at the base of the medial tibial plateau. Anserine bursitis is usually found in patients with coexistent osteoarthritis of the knees, obesity, and an abnormal gait. Although often not recognized, anserine bursitis, rather than associated osteoarthritis, may be the principal cause of knee pain in obese patients with osteoarthritis. A *popliteal cyst* ("Baker's cyst") is a cystic swelling of the popliteal fossa best appreciated by having the patient stand and examining this area from behind. Any knee condition having a synovial effusion can be complicated by a popliteal cyst because of a natural communication between the knee joint and the semimembranosus-gastrocnemius bursa found in many individuals.

Ankle and Feet

Achilles' tendonitis usually results from trauma, sports activities, or improperly fitting shoes. There may be associated inflammatory arthritis in some patients. Pain, swelling, and tenderness occur over the Achilles' tendon at its attachments and proximally. Dorsiflexion of the ankle increases the pain. Rupture of the Achilles' tendon can occur. Often there is an audible snap followed by difficulty in walking and standing on the toes. Swelling and edema develop. Ultrasound can be used to differentiate full from partial thickness tears.

TREATMENT

In many instances, bursitis and tendonitis improve with removal of aggravating factors and joint protection. Patient education in body mechanics is therefore important. Explanation of the likely duration of symptoms is also helpful. If co-morbid systemic illnesses are present, these must be recognized and treated. The inflammation and pain of bursitis and tendonitis can be treated with nonsteroidal anti-inflammatory drugs including ibuprofen (Motrin)* and naproxen (Naprosyn) and the newer COX-2 selective agents rofecoxib (Vioxx)* and celecoxib (Celebrex).* In patients with acute bursitis and tendonitis, local injection with lidocaine,* corticosteroids, or both can provide benefit. Corticosteroid injection should be avoided in tendonitis where tendon rupture is a risk (such as bicipital tendonitis and Achilles' tendonitis). Physical therapy is often helpful to teach joint protection and to improve flexibility, strength, and endurance with repetitive exercise.

Septic bursitis is treated just as septic arthritis with identification of the causative organism and appropriate antibiotic therapy. Most cases of septic arthritis are caused by *Staphylococcus aureus* and other gram-positive organisms, but gram-negative infection, particularly in immunocompromised or diabetic patients, is also seen. As in septic arthritis, it is important to adequately drain a septic bursa. Repeated aspiration is often necessary. In some patients open surgical drainage or bursectomy may be necessary. The decision whether to treat patients with oral or parenteral antibiotics is based on the severity of infection, the presence of any systemic symptoms, and the virulence of the causative organism.

*Not FDA approved for this indication.

Myofascial Pain and Fibromyalgia

Myofascial pain syndrome and fibromyalgia are soft tissue pain disorders that cause musculoskeletal pain. These conditions are common and controversial. Patients look well and have no obvious abnormalities on physical examination or laboratory or diagnostic testing. The etiology of pain is unknown and many of these patients suffer from depression. Many physicians believe that these conditions are psychogenic in nature.

Myofascial Pain Syndrome

Myofascial pain syndrome may be a regional form of fibromyalgia. Myofascial pain syndrome is said to be characterized by localized areas of deep muscle tenderness—"trigger points"—that can be aggravated by palpation on physical examination. Myofascial pain syndrome may differ from fibromyalgia in that therapies that successfully ameliorate trigger point pain routinely alleviate the syndrome, whereas in fibromyalgia it is not usually possible to successfully treat specific areas of local tenderness. But many believe that the evaluation and management of myofascial pain cannot be separated from fibromyalgia. Both myofascial pain and fibromyalgia are syndromes, not specific disease entities. For example, tension headaches, idiopathic low back pain, neck pain, and temporomandibular joint disease may be examples of myofascial pain. In this review, the treatment of myofascial pain syndrome and fibromyalgia will be considered together.

Fibromyalgia

Fibromyalgia is a chronic musculoskeletal syndrome characterized by diffuse pain and tender points. There is no evidence of synovitis or myositis. Physical examination, laboratory analysis, and radiographic abnormalities are unrevealing. Eighty to 90 percent of fibromyalgia patients are women, typically between the ages of 30 and 50. Fibromyalgia is characterized by chronic, widespread musculoskeletal pain. Although the pain is chronic, it may vary in intensity. Patients have difficulty distinguishing between muscle and joint pain and may report symptoms of joint swelling, although such swelling is not apparent on examination.

Fibromyalgia patients are said to have a specific finding on physical examination—"tender points" which are areas of diffuse tenderness at discrete anatomic sites. It is said that patients with fibromyalgia are more tender than healthy controls at these anatomic sites. In 1990, the American College of Rheumatology published diagnostic criteria for fibromyalgia in which widespread musculoskeletal pain and excess tenderness in at least 11 of 18 predefined anatomic sites were reported to be highly specific and sensitive in differentiating fibromyalgia patients from controls. It should be noted that although these criteria have become widely used in clinical practice, they were validated only for use in research. In some clinical situations (e.g., patients involved in litigation or seeking disability), using criteria that rely on self-assessed reporting of subjective pain is probably not valid. Many fibromyalgia patients have associated symptoms such as fatigue, sleep disorder, headaches, irritable bowel syndrome, anxiety, and depression. Neurologic symptoms such as paresthesias, subjective weakness, and headaches are also common.

Fibromyalgia is often a diagnosis of exclusion. It is a clinical challenge not only to distinguish diseases such as rheumatoid arthritis, polymyalgia rheumatica, hypothyroidism, and neuropathy from fibromyalgia but also to recognize the presence of fibromyalgia in other patients and avoid never-ending diagnostic testing. As described above, myofascial pain syndrome may be a regional form of fibromyalgia. Chronic fatigue syndrome also shares considerable overlap with fibromyalgia.

TREATMENT

There is a spectrum of opinion among physicians about the diagnosis and treatment of myofascial pain syndrome and fibromyalgia. Some physicians believe that these disorders are rigorously defined diseases with an organic, if incompletely understood, pathogenesis. Others consider fibromyalgia to be aches and pains in people who cannot cope. For still others, the diagnosis of fibromyalgia is an example of mass hysteria. Given this diagnostic ambivalence, recommendations about management will be subjective. What follows is a highly personal approach to the management of fibromyalgia in the form of ten suggestions (Table 1).

Fibromyalgia: Ten Management Suggestions

1. Accept fibromyalgia as a syndrome diagnosed by exclusion. Many patients present to physicians with widespread musculoskeletal pain, fatigue, difficulty with sleep, and depressive symptoms. The recognition and acceptance of fibromyalgia by physicians allow labeling that can be informative and reassuring. If fibromyalgia does not exist, it needs to be invented. Many other diseases can cause some of the same symptoms, but experienced clinicians acquire skill in separating fibromyalgia from diseases with similar symptoms.

2. Define ownership of the problem and patient goals. The treatment of fibromyalgia has analogies to counseling for obesity or smoking cessation. While the physician can provide education and some relief with medication, fibromyalgia is a chronic, subjective pain syndrome for which patients bear the greatest responsibility for their own improvement. Not all patients accept the diagnosis of fibromyalgia as real and the success of treatment varies from patient to patient. By the time fibromyalgia is diagnosed, most of the patients' symptoms have become chronic. It is helpful for the physician to explain that symptomatic improvement can often be achieved, but that the improvement will not occur overnight and that patience, on the part of both the patient and the physician, is necessary.

3. Emphasize benignity and reassurance. The diagnosis of fibromyalgia should be reassuring. This diagnosis rules out more serious diseases such as rheumatoid arthritis or multiple sclerosis. Patients can be helped with treatment. The physician should recognize and empathize with the patient's pain, but many patients are unnecessarily frightened by the concept that fibromyalgia is an incurable, intractable source of unremitting pain.

4. Assess patterns of sleep. Most patients with fibromyalgia have problems with the quantity and quality of sleep. Improving sleep through regular habits, stress avoidance, medication, and exercise provides significant symptomatic improvement.

5. Exclude infection and avoid antibiotics. Chronic fatigue syndrome and chronic Lyme disease are two current examples in which nonspecific symptoms of fatigue, musculoskeletal pain, and vague neurologic symptoms are ascribed to infectious agents without scientific evidence. If a physician suspects that a patient has a specific infection, diagnostic testing should be done to evaluate this possibility. If not, avoid therapeutic misadventure and refrain from treating infections that do not exist.

6. Avoid disability and litigation. Patients with fibromyalgia should be reassured. Efforts should be made to reduce their pain. In my opinion, fibromyalgia is not disabling. Occasional patients benefit from short-term, self-limited disability from work or other responsibilities to allow them to gain greater endurance. Beyond this, however, physicians should lead their patients away from the dependency and limitations of long-term disability. A related problem is the destructive concept of post-traumatic fibromyalgia, a diagnosis which has no pathogenic validation but has become an epidemic problem for our civil justice system.

7. Recognize mental illness. Many patients with fibromyalgia have some degree of depression. The clinician treating fibromyalgia can have a positive impact on depression. Sometimes, however, fibromyalgia is diagnosed in individuals who have serious psychiatric disease. This is a mistake. The physician who is an expert in managing musculoskeletal pain should typically refer patients with serious mental illness to mental health professionals.

8. Avoid narcotics. While fibromyalgia is a "pain" syndrome, fibromyalgia patients do not benefit from "pain" pills. The use of narcotic analgesics has the risk

TABLE 1. **Fibromyalgia: Ten Management Suggestions**

Accept fibromyalgia as a syndrome diagnosed by exclusion
Define ownership of the problem and patient goals
Emphasize benignity and reassurance
Assess patterns of sleep
Exclude infection and avoid antibiotics
Avoid disability and litigation
Recognize mental illness
Avoid narcotics
Emphasize physical conditioning
Consider low-dose amitriptyline*

*Not FDA approved for this indication.

of becoming open ended and will probably aggravate pre-existing depression. Narcotics should be avoided. Nonsteroidal anti-inflammatory drugs (NSAIDs) are also usually not effective.

9. Emphasize physical conditioning. Several prospective, well controlled studies demonstrate that low-impact physical conditioning reduces pain and improves function in fibromyalgia. It is important to assess each patient's aptitude and interests and to find physical activities for which there can be a regular, sustained commitment. Physical activity relieves stress, improves sleep, and reduces deconditioning. It approaches fibromyalgia as a symptom complex rather than a disease and has virtually no side effects.

10. Consider low-dose amitriptyline. Unlike NSAIDs and narcotics, low-dose antidepressant medication relieves pain in fibromyalgia patients. Often there is improved sleep, more energy, and less pain. Amitriptyline (Elavil) and other tricyclic antidepressants are the best studied and probably most effective antidepressants for fibromyalgia patients.

OSTEOARTHRITIS

method of
SHARI MIURA LING, M.D., and
JOAN M. BATHON, M.D.
Johns Hopkins University School of Medicine
Baltimore, Maryland

Osteoarthritis is the most common form of arthritis in the United States and the most common cause of surgical knee and hip replacements. The prevalence of osteoarthritis increases with age. Given the prolonged life expectancy in the United States and the aging of the "baby boom" cohort, the prevalence of osteoarthritis is expected to increase. By the year 2020, it is projected that 59 million Americans will suffer from osteoarthritis. Treatment options for osteoarthritis are targeted primarily to reduction of pain and preservation of function. Because there are few proven interventions that will slow the progress of osteoarthritis, many affected patients will require knee or hip replacement surgery. Treatment of osteoarthritis thus constitutes a huge economic burden to society. This review will highlight the efficacy and safety of current treatments for osteoarthritis (OA), and will focus primarily on peripheral (rather than spinal) osteoarthritis.

CLINICAL PRESENTATION AND DIFFERENTIAL DIAGNOSIS

Before age 50, men have a higher prevalence and incidence of osteoarthritis than do women. After age 50, the prevalence and incidence are higher in women. In general, risk factors for the development of osteoarthritis of the peripheral joints include age, weight, family history of osteoarthritis in a first-degree relative, prior injury to the knee, and occupational trauma.

Osteoarthritis commonly affects the knee, hip, first carpometacarpal joint, first metatarsal-phalangeal joint, distal and proximal interphalangeal joints, and cervical and lumbar spine. The most common initial symptoms of osteoarthritis are morning stiffness, and stiffness following prolonged inactivity (known as the "gel" phenomenon), of the affected joint(s). Stiffness or "gelling" rarely persists for more than 30 minutes. As osteoarthritis progresses in severity, patients report pain with movement of the joint and resolution of pain upon resting the joint. In advanced disease, patients often report pain at rest and pain that awakens them from sleep. Symptoms of "giving way" or locking may also be reported and usually signal internal derangement of the joint, such as a meniscal tear in the knee.

Physical examination of a joint with early osteoarthritis may not reveal any abnormalities. Alternatively, a small, cool effusion may be present. As the disease progresses, joint line tenderness, crepitus, and bony prominence will usually be evident. Valgus or varus deformity and decreased range of motion of the affected joint will indicate severe end-stage disease.

Radiographic characteristics of osteoarthritis include osteophytes at the joint margin, joint space narrowing, subchondral sclerosis, and cysts. The osteophyte is the most specific radiographic marker of osteoarthritis, although it is considered a rather late manifestation of the disease process. Radiographic narrowing of the joint space in an osteoarthritic joint is usually asymmetric; for example, medial, but not lateral, compartmental narrowing is frequently seen in osteoarthritis of the knee. The American College of Rheumatology has set forth classification criteria that integrate the clinical and radiographic characteristics of the disease to aid in the identification of patients with symptomatic osteoarthritis. These criteria are summarized in Table 1.

Radiographic evidence of osteoarthritis is very common in older populations and is frequently asymptomatic. Other conditions, such as tendonitis or bursitis, that cause articular or periarticular pain may coexist in patients with osteoarthritis and should be carefully excluded. Arthritis of the metacarpal-phalangeal, wrist, elbow, ankle, or glenohumeral joint is rarely due to osteoarthritis, and other causes, such as rheumatoid arthritis, should be investigated. Morning stiffness lasting more than 1 hour and constitutional symptoms, such as weight loss, fatigue, fever and loss of appetite may be a harbinger of systemic inflammatory conditions such as rheumatoid arthritis, polymyalgia rheumatica, or lupus. A joint effusion that is accompanied by warmth and erythema should prompt an evaluation for inflammatory types of arthritis including rheumatoid arthritis, gout, pseudogout, psoriatic arthritis, or infection. Aspiration of the joint will aid in distinguishing osteoarthritis from these conditions. Generally, the total white blood cell count in an osteoarthritic joint will not exceed 200 to 300/mm^3, while an inflammatory arthritis will exhibit counts of greater than 2000/mm^3.

TABLE 1. **Criteria for the Diagnosis of Osteoarthritis of the Hand, Knee, and Hip**

Hand	Knee	Hip
Hand pain, aching or stiffness	Knee pain	Hip pain
AND	AND	AND
Hard tissue enlargement of two or more joints	Radiographic osteophytes	Two or more of the following:
AND	AND	ESR <10 mm/h
Fewer than three swollen MCP joints	One or more of the following:	Radiographic femoral or acetabular osteophytes
AND	Age ≥50 yrs	Radiographic joint space narrowing
Two or more DIP joints with hard tissue enlargement	Morning stiffness <30 minutes	
OR	Crepitus on motion	
Deformity in two or more *select joints		

*Select joints: DIP, distal interphalangeal; PIP, proximal interphalangeal; and CMC, first carpometacarpal.
ESR, erythrocyte sedimentation rate; MCP, metacarpophalangeal.

Early Diagnosis of Osteoarthritis: Radiographic and Laboratory Tools

Conventional radiography remains the definitive procedure for the diagnosis of osteoarthritis, but it is limited by relative insensitivity. Magnetic resonance imaging (MRI) offers promise for earlier detection of osteoarthritis because focal defects in cartilage can be identified and changes in cartilage volume over time can be quantified. Furthermore, MRI has contributed to our understanding of bone edema as a cause of pain in osteoarthritis. Standardized methods for assessing and interpreting cartilage and bone abnormalities at baseline and over time are still lacking, however. There is also considerable interest in identifying an inexpensive and accurate biologic marker that would facilitate the early identification of osteoarthritis and/or the identification of individuals at risk for rapid progression of the disease. Considerable work is ongoing in this regard but, to date, no single biomarker for serum, urine, or synovial fluid has distinguished itself alone, or in combination with other biomarkers, as both a highly sensitive and highly specific marker for osteoarthritis.

MANAGEMENT OF OSTEOARTHRITIS

The goals of the management of osteoarthritis are to reduce pain and to maintain or improve function. A combination of nonpharmacologic and pharmacologic approaches is usually recommended. Education of patients about the disease process, and self-management courses offered by the Arthritis Foundation, can be powerful adjunctive strategies.

Nonpharmacologic Interventions

PHYSICAL AND OCCUPATIONAL THERAPY

Physical therapy is a useful adjunctive strategy for managing arthritis symptoms and maximizing function. Manual therapy and other modalities such as local heat or ice and ultrasound to an affected joint may be useful in relieving pain and increasing range of motion. Physical and occupational therapists will also counsel the patient on techniques to safely improve and maintain function by increasing muscle strength and range of motion of the joint. The physical therapist focuses on lower extremity function and will also evaluate the patient's need for devices to overcome mobility limitations, such as a raised toilet seat, shower and bathtub bars, and walking devices such as canes. An occupational therapist should be consulted for advice regarding upper extremity limitations and can recommend devices such as jar openers and "hand extenders."

WEIGHT MANAGEMENT

Several population-based studies have identified obesity as a risk factor for the development and progression of knee, hip, and even hand osteoarthritis. It is estimated that persons in the highest quintile of body weight have up to ten times the risk of knee osteoarthritis than those in the lowest quintile. From 1960 to 1999 in the United States, the percentage of adults who are overweight (body mass index [BMI] of 25 to 30 kg/m^2) increased from 44% to 61%, and the percentage who are obese (BMI >30 kg/m^2) increased from 13% to 27%. Furthermore, the onset of obesity is occurring at an earlier age. These trends are likely to increase the numbers, and lower the age, of individuals at risk of developing osteoarthritis of the weight-bearing joints.

Weight loss in obese individuals with osteoarthritis of the knee has been associated in epidemiologic studies with improvement in pain and slowing of disease progression. Consequently, weight reduction is recommended for all overweight patients with osteoarthritis of the weight-bearing joints. Unfortunately, this can be difficult to achieve because patients with chronic knee or hip pain tend to be sedentary and consequently may gain, rather than lose, weight. A combined program of diet and exercise is usually necessary. A 10% reduction in weight is a reasonable objective and should be achieved at a rate not to exceed 1 to 2 pounds per week. In many cases, a structured weight management program with counseling may be necessary to achieve weight loss.

EXERCISE

Light or moderate physical activity in patients with osteoarthritis has not been associated with worsening symptoms or with joint injury in short-term clinical trials, and may have significant health benefits. Consequently, exercise is currently recommended for all patients with osteoarthritis of the lower extremities.

For example, in a controlled, randomized study of community-residing adults with symptomatic knee osteoarthritis, those randomized to aerobic or resistive exercise training for 3 months experienced greater reduction in pain and self-reported disability and greater improvements in aerobic performance, mobility, and mood than those randomized to educational classes without exercise. Other studies have demonstrated that resistive muscle strengthening improves gait, strength, and overall function. On the other hand, a recent report derived from the Framingham data set, in which very heavy physical activity was associated with a higher risk for radiographic knee osteoarthritis, suggested that physical exertion may be detrimental. Interestingly, the risk was the highest for individuals in the upper third of body mass index.

Low-impact activities, such as water-resistive exercises and bicycle training, also promote muscle tone and strength, neuromuscular function, and cardiovascular endurance without injury to the joints. Moreover, exercise need not be conducted in a single, prolonged high-intensity session but can be accrued in a series of short moderate-intensity bouts throughout the day. For example, three vigorous 10-minute walks per day can achieve health benefits equivalent to one 30-minute walk per day. Other strategies of moderate-intensity activity have also been shown to lessen pain, reduce disability, improve fitness, and enhance psychological well-being. The Surgeon General currently recommends that people of all ages strive to accumulate 30 minutes of moderate-intensity lifestyle activity throughout the day on most days of the week. This new approach to exercise, often termed "lifestyle activity," can include all leisure, occupational, and household activities that are at least moderate to vigorous in intensity. Examples include brisk walking, raking leaves, and gardening.

COMPLEMENTARY AND ALTERNATIVE APPROACHES

As many as 66% of patients with rheumatic diseases were reported in a recent study to utilize complementary and alternative treatments, including acupuncture, magnets, mind-body exercises, and nutritional supplements. Except for glucosamine* and chondroitin sulfate* (discussed subsequently), the efficacy of most therapies in the management of osteoarthritis is unstudied or unproven, and therefore are not standard recommendations for the management of osteoarthritis. However, to the extent that they are likely to cause few adverse events and provide a means for patients to self-manage and cope with their disease, they should not be discounted.

Pharmacologic Therapy

The goals of pharmacologic management in osteoarthritis are to relieve pain and to slow progression of disease. There are multiple strategies for analgesia in osteoarthritis; however, glucosamine is the only therapeutic agent demonstrated to potentially slow disease progression.

*Not FDA approved for this indication.

ACETAMINOPHEN, NSAIDS, AND COX-2 INHIBITORS

The guidelines of the American College of Rheumatology recognize acetaminophen* (up to 4000 mg/d) as the analgesic of choice for symptomatic osteoarthritis. This recommendation is based on studies demonstrating the superiority of acetaminophen to placebo, and its equivalence to nonsteroidal anti-inflammatory agents (NSAIDs) for reducing osteoarthritis-related pain, as well as the superior gastrointestinal safety profile of acetaminophen compared to NSAIDs. In patients with moderate to severe disease, however, acetaminophen may be inadequate for pain control, and NSAIDs, or the more recently developed inhibitors of cyclooxygenase-2 (coxibs), may be more beneficial.

Pain and inflammation in the osteoarthritic joint are believed to be mediated, at least in part, by overproduction of prostanoids. In addition to their inflammatory actions, however, prostanoids also serve important physiologic roles in intestinal and renal homeostasis and platelet aggregation. Consequently, reduction of prostanoid levels in nonarticular organs can result in the well-recognized side effects of NSAIDs—that is, gastrointestinal ulceration, renal impairment, and prolonged bleeding time. Older adults are at a significantly higher risk for these NSAID-associated side effects by virtue of multiple co-morbid illnesses, concurrent pharmacologic therapies, and diminished physiologic reserve.

Prostanoids involved in maintaining the gastric lining and in platelet aggregation are produced by cyclooxygenase-1 (COX-1), whereas COX-2 is the isoenzyme primarily upregulated in inflammatory states. Conventional NSAIDs inhibit prostanoid synthesis via inactivation of both COX-1 and COX-2, whereas the newer class of NSAIDs, the coxibs, specifically inhibit COX-2. Coxibs (celecoxib [Celebrex], rofecoxib [Vioxx], and valdecoxib [Bextra]) were developed, therefore, as a novel anti-inflammatory strategy that would minimize GI side effects. Indeed, in controlled clinical trials, treatment with celecoxib or rofecoxib was associated with significantly fewer endoscopically proven and clinically symptomatic gastric ulcers when compared with NSAIDs. Relative efficacies in reducing osteoarthritis-related pain were equivalent in coxib and NSAID-treated groups. In the CLASS study (celecoxib [Celebrex] versus ibuprofen [Advil] or diclofenac [Voltaren] in osteoarthritis and rheumatoid arthritis), symptomatic ulcers occurred in 1.4%, and complicated ulcers in 0.44%, of celecoxib-treated participants who did not use concomitant aspirin, whereas these rates in NSAID-treated participants were 2.91% and 1.27%, respectively. However, in participants taking concomitant low-dose aspirin for cardioprotection, the GI protective effect of celecoxib was lost. In the Vioxx Gastrointestinal Outcomes Research (VIGOR) study (rofecoxib versus naproxen in rheumatoid arthritis), concomitant aspirin treatment was not allowed, and

*Not FDA approved for this indication.

the incidence of symptomatic and complicated gastric ulcers was significantly lower in the rofecoxib-treated group.

Importantly, however, in the VIGOR trial, a higher incidence of myocardial infarctions was observed in the rofecoxib-treated group (0.4% versus 0.1%, respectively). In fact, 35% of these infarctions occurred in the 4% of trial participants who would have been candidates for low-dose aspirin for cardioprotection. Whether the difference in rates of myocardial infarction was due to a hypercoagulable effect of rofecoxib or a cardioprotective effect of naproxen remains a matter of debate, although several recent reports suggest the latter. In any case, a potential conundrum exists in the treatment of arthritis in which a trade-off between cardiovascular and gastrointestinal morbidities must be considered.

It is currently recommended that, for arthritis patients with, or at high risk for, coronary artery disease who are treated with coxibs, low-dose aspirin (81 mg/d) should be added. However, because low-dose aspirin will likely reduce or negate the gastrointestinal protection afforded by the coxib, selective COX-2 inhibition appears to offer no advantage over conventional NSAIDs in this type of patient. Conventional NSAIDs offer less cardioprotection than aspirin, and co-treatment with low-dose aspirin is still recommended in cardiac patients taking these drugs. The addition of aspirin to conventional NSAIDs may further enhance the risk for gastrointestinal ulcers and bleeds, however. An important risk factor identified in epidemiologic studies for NSAID-associated bleeding gastric ulcers is co-morbid cardiac disease. Therefore, in patients with co-morbid heart disease and osteoarthritis who are co-treated with low-dose aspirin and a conventional NSAID, the addition of a gastroprotective agent is strongly recommended. Options for gastrointestinal prophylaxis include misoprostol (Cytotec), proton pump inhibitors (e.g., omeprazole [Prilosec]* and lansoprazole [Prevacid]*), and histamine H_2 receptor blockers (e.g., ranitidine [Zantac]* and famotidine [Pepsid]*). All three classes of drugs have been demonstrated to provide effective antiulcer prophylaxis. Misoprostol, at the recommended dose of 200 µg four times daily, may be poorly tolerated due to diarrhea, and the cost of the proton pump inhibitors may be prohibitive.

For osteoarthritis patients at low risk for cardiac disease, but at high risk for NSAID-associated gastrointestinal ulcers, a selective COX-2 inhibitor offers a clear advantage over conventional NSAIDs. Risk factors for NSAID-associated gastrointestinal side effects include age over 65, a prior history of gastrointestinal ulceration or bleeding, and concomitant treatment with corticosteroids. Alternatively, the addition of a gastroprotective agent to a conventional NSAID may afford a level of gastroprotection equivalent to coxibs. A recent study was conducted in arthritis patients with prior ulcer bleeds to assess the relative incidence of recurrent bleeds over 6 months associated with celecoxib 200 mg twice daily compared with diclofenac 75 mg twice daily plus omeprazole 20 mg daily. Celecoxib proved to be as effective as diclofenac plus omeprazole in preventing recurrence of ulcer bleeding. However, the annualized incidence of rebleed in both groups was disturbingly high at 10%. Thus, careful vigilance for GI bleeds in high-risk patients is warranted regardless of the class of COX inhibitor.

*Not FDA approved for this indication.

Renal side effects including exacerbation of hypertension, peripheral edema, and renal failure are well recognized risks of NSAID use, particularly in individuals with advanced age, pre-existing renal insufficiency, and hypovolemic states, such as congestive heart failure. Both COX-1 and COX-2 are expressed in the kidney and appear to be important in regulating water and salt homeostasis. Thus, selective inhibition of COX-2 would not be expected to afford any advantage over nonselective COX inhibitors with regard to maintenance of renal function. Indeed, a number of studies have demonstrated comparable rates of edema, hypertension, and decline in renal function with celecoxib or rofecoxib compared with nonselective NSAIDs. Thus, both NSAIDs and coxibs should be used cautiously in patients at risk for renal side effects. Acetaminophen is the preferred analgesic for these patients, although a recent study implicated acetaminophen as a dose-dependent risk factor for chronic renal failure. Individuals taking acetaminophen 1.4 g daily or more had a five times greater odds of renal failure than nonusers. The relationship was most profound for those with diabetes mellitus or other underlying pre-existing renal disease. Widespread acceptance of these findings will require confirmation from additional independent clinical studies.

Glucosamine and chondroitin sulfate:* Glucosamine is an amino-monosaccharide component of articular cartilage. Glucosamine stimulates proteoglycan synthesis by chondrocytes in vitro and, in animal models of arthritis, has mild anti-inflammatory effects. Short-term clinical trials consistently demonstrate superiority of glucosamine over placebo in alleviating osteoarthritis-related joint pain. Two randomized, placebo-controlled clinical trials in early knee osteoarthritis have now demonstrated a reduction in the rate of joint space narrowing over 2 to 3 years in the glucosamine-treated participants compared with placebo controls. Although the methodology for assessing joint space width in these studies has been questioned, these studies suggest that glucosamine may alter the natural history of osteoarthritis by slowing cartilage degradation. It seems reasonable to recommend glucosamine (500 mg three times daily) for patients with symptomatic knee osteoarthritis, particularly in view of its excellent safety profile.

Frequently sold in combination with glucosamine, chondroitin sulfate* is a proteoglycan component of articular cartilage. Chondroitin sulfate has also been shown in a number of short-term clinical trials to be superior to placebo, and equivalent to NSAIDs, in

*Not FDA approved for this indication.

relieving joint pain associated with osteoarthritis. Interestingly, and in contrast to NSAIDs, the analgesic effect of chondroitin sulfate may persist for several months after the neutraceutical is discontinued. No long-term studies examining the effect of chondroitin sulfate on radiographic progression are available. The usual dose is 1200 mg daily.

Because glucosamine and chondroitin sulfate are sold in the United States as over-the-counter neutraceuticals, manufacture of these supplements is not as tightly regulated as prescription drugs, and cost is not generally reimbursable by third-party prescription plans. The cost of the two agents combined can be prohibitive for many patients.

INTRA-ARTICULAR THERAPIES

Judicious use of intra-articular glucocorticoid injections is appropriate for osteoarthritis patients who are not candidates for, or who have inadequate responses to, oral analgesics or anti-inflammatory agents. Intra-articular corticosteroids may be particularly useful in patients who have joint effusion and local signs of inflammation. Another potentially useful compound that is administered by intra-articular injection is hyaluronic acid, and several formulations are currently available. A series of three to five weekly injections can provide a degree of pain relief comparable to NSAIDs for up to 6 months in some patients with mild to moderate knee osteoarthritis. Post-injection inflammation and infection are potential, albeit rare, complications.

NARCOTIC ANALGESICS

Slow-release formulations of narcotics administered in low doses, such as oxycodone SR* 10 mg, have been shown in several short-term studies to be relatively safe and efficacious for patients with moderate to severe osteoarthritis of the knee, in whom pain is inadequately controlled by acetaminophen or NSAIDs alone. Improvements in pain and quality of sleep were comparable for short-versus long-acting narcotic preparations, but the incidence of GI side effects, such as constipation, was lower with the latter. These agents may be particularly useful for chronic management of patients with severe knee or hip osteoarthritis who are not surgical candidates due to co-morbid cardiac or pulmonary illness.

SURGICAL MANAGEMENT

Surgical intervention should be considered for patients with limited function and persistent pain. Irrigation and débridement have been argued by some as an effective means of pain management for osteoarthritis of the knee, but these procedures have recently come under scrutiny. Tidal irrigation of the knee (performed at the bedside rather than surgically) was no more effective in relieving pain or improving function than sham irrigation. In a recent surgical study, patients with knee osteoarthritis were randomized to undergo arthroscopic lavage, arthroscopic débridement, or sham surgery. No significant differences were observed in reduction of pain or improvement in self-reported disability or function among the treatment groups. Although patients with suspected meniscal tears (based on reports of locking and give-way weakness) may still warrant arthroscopic evaluation and treatment, arthroscopic treatment is no longer justified as a general strategy for pain management in osteoarthritis.

Tibial osteotomy is frequently recommended for patients with knee osteoarthritis who have isolated disease of the medial compartment and a relatively small varus angulation (less than 10 degrees) and stable ligamentous structures. Knee arthroplasty (joint replacement) is recommended for patients with more extensive disease, more severe varus or any valgus deformity, or ligamentous instability, and for those in whom tibial osteotomy has provided inadequate relief of pain. Hip arthroplasty is recommended for patients with advanced osteoarthritis of the hip. Older patients who have not yet developed appreciable muscle weakness or cardiovascular deconditioning and who can medically withstand the stress of surgery are ideal surgical candidates. Knee and hip prostheses have a life span of approximately 10 to 15 years. Revision surgery will be required in most patients who live past this time frame. Transplantation of autologous chondrocytes has been used successfully to repair discrete defects in articular cartilage, such as those resulting from twisting injuries. However, because the area of cartilage loss in osteoarthritis can be quite extensive and because older chondrocytes are less metabolically active than younger chondrocytes, it remains doubtful that transplantation will be practical in the treatment of osteoarthritis.

NEW TARGETS

A number of molecules have been implicated in the pathogenesis of OA by virtue of their abilities to promote degradation, or suppress repair, of cartilage. These include proinflammatory cytokines, matrix metalloproteinases, growth factors, and some oncogenes. Molecular strategies that will promote the synthesis of cartilage matrix components such as type II collagen and proteoglycans, inhibit apoptosis of chondrocytes, and suppress the production or activity of matrix-degrading enzymes are sorely needed in this disease. Active efforts to identify novel therapies such as these are currently under way.

CONCLUSIONS

Osteoarthritis remains the most prevalent articular disease of older adults. Recommended treatments include safe and adequate pain relief using systemic and local therapies, and medical and rehabilitative interventions to compensate for functional deficits. Biologic markers that will detect early disease and enable early intervention with pharmacologic agents that modify, or halt, disease progression are much needed.

*Not FDA approved for this indication.

POLYMYALGIA RHEUMATICA AND GIANT CELL ARTERITIS

method of
THOMAS G. WIMMER, M.D., and
S. LOUIS BRIDGES, Jr., M.D., Ph.D.
University of Alabama at Birmingham
Birmingham, Alabama

Polymyalgia rheumatica (PMR) is a syndrome of proximal muscle aching and stiffness in individuals older than 50 years of age. Giant cell arteritis (GCA) is a panarteritis mostly affecting large-sized arteries that also typically affects people older than 50 years of age. Symptoms include new-onset headache, jaw claudication, temporal artery tenderness, and visual changes. About 10% to 15% of PMR patients develop GCA, and up to one half of patients with GCA have concomitant PMR. Both conditions are more common in whites than African-Americans. PMR may be difficult to distinguish from seronegative rheumatoid arthritis.

DIAGNOSIS

Patients with PMR characteristically present with progressive, symmetrical, dull aching in muscle of the proximal hip or shoulder girdle, torso, or neck, and it is worse after inactivity. Other symptoms include low-grade fever, fatigue, weight loss, and synovitis. Weakness is not a feature, but muscle strength may seem diminished secondary to pain. There may be tenderness over affected regions. Laboratory findings include elevated erythrocyte sedimentation rate (ESR) and C-reactive protein (CRP), normocytic anemia, and thrombocytosis. Selected diagnostic criteria for PMR are shown in Table 1; the differential diagnosis is shown in Table 2.

Common features of GCA include fatigue, weight loss, fever, new-onset headaches, tender temporal or occipital arteries, jaw claudication, diplopia, blurred vision, and visual loss. Permanent visual loss is present in up to 20% of cases. Other manifestations may include tongue or throat pain, claudication, chronic cough, tenosynovitis, thoracic aortic aneurysms, and transient ischemic attacks or stroke. Tender or thickened temporal or occipital arteries, bruits over the aortic arch branches, and mild synovitis may be noted. Laboratory findings include elevated Westergren ESR (frequently above 100 mm/h) and CRP. Normal ESR has been reported in approximately 5% of patients with GCA. Other common laboratory findings include normochromic anemia and thrombocytosis. The differential diagnosis of GCA is shown in Table 2.

ACR classification criteria for GCA (Table 3) were designed to distinguish it from other forms of systemic vasculitis, but may be useful in diagnosing individual patients. Temporal artery biopsy is highly recommended in all suspected cases. If possible, 2 to 3 cm should be obtained and multiple sections examined, because the disease may be segmental. The contralateral artery may be biopsied if the first biopsy is negative. Histopathology typically shows transmural infiltration of lymphocytes and macrophages and fragmentation of the internal elastic lamina. Multinucleated giant cells are often present, but are not necessary for diagnosis.

Table 1. **Simple Diagnostic Criteria for Polymyalgia Rheumatica**

- Age at onset ≥50 years
- Symmetric ache/pain for at least 1 month found in two of three muscle groups below, with associated morning stiffness lasting >30 minutes:
  - Neck or torso
  - Shoulders or proximal arms
  - Hips or proximal thighs
- ESR > 40 mm/hour (Westergren)
- Prompt, dramatic response to glucocorticoids (equivalent to prednisone 20 mg once a day or less)

ESR, erythrocyte sedimentation rate.

Table 2. **Conditions in the Differential Diagnosis of Polymyalgia Rheumatica and Giant Cell Arteritis**

Polymyalgia Rheumatica	Giant Cell Arteritis
Seronegative rheumatoid arthritis	Polyarteritis nodosa
Polymyositis	Wegener's granulomatosis
Hypothyroidism	Takayasu's arteritis
Endocarditis	Hypersensitivity vasculitis
Paraneoplastic syndromes	Amyloidosis
Multiple myeloma	Lyme disease
Bursitis/tendonitis	
Remitting seronegative symmetrical synovitis with pitting edema (RS_3PE) syndrome	
Amyloidosis	
Fibromyalgia	

TREATMENT

PMR responds almost immediately to glucocorticoids. Oral prednisone* should be started at 15 to 20 mg every morning. Lack of rapid response should

Table 3. **Classification Criteria for Giant Cell Arteritis**

Age >50 years at disease onset	Development of symptoms or findings beginning at age 50 or older
New headache	New onset or new type of localized pain in the head
Temporal artery abnormality	Temporal artery tenderness to palpation or decreased pulsation unrelated to arteriosclerosis of cervical arteries
Elevated ESR	ESR > 50 mm/hour (Westergren)
Abnormal artery biopsy	Biopsy specimen with artery showing vasculitis characterized by a predominance of mononuclear cell infiltration or granulomatous inflammation, usually with multinucleated giant cells

For classification purposes, a patient with vasculitis shall be said to have GCA if at least three of these five criteria are present. The presence of any three or more criteria yields a sensitivity of 93.5% and a specificity of 91.2%. From Arthritis Rheum 33:1122-1128, 1990.

ESR, erythrocyte sedimentation rate; GCA, giant cell arteritis.

*Not FDA approved for this indication.

prompt reconsideration of the diagnosis. Once symptoms are controlled for 2 to 4 weeks, the dose is reduced by 10% every 2 to 4 weeks. Once 10 mg daily is reached, the dose can be tapered by 1 mg/d monthly. As many as 25% to 50% of patients relapse; some evidence suggests that relapse is more prevalent in fast tapers. ESR should begin to normalize within 1 week of therapy. Continued elevation of ESR without symptoms does not justify continuation of glucocorticoids, but vigilance for recurrence of symptoms is necessary.

Once the diagnosis of GCA is suspected, prednisone,* 40 to 60 mg daily should be started immediately in order to prevent visual loss. Consultation with an ophthalmologist should be initiated emergently, but treatment should not be delayed while awaiting biopsy, because it can be performed up to 1 week after initiating therapy without decreasing its diagnostic usefulness. If visual loss is apparent or suspected, 1 gram methylprednisolone (Solu-Medrol)* intravenously daily for 3 days should be considered. Once symptoms disappear and ESR begins to normalize, the prednisone dose should be tapered by 10 mg/d every 14 days to an initial goal of 40 mg/d. Once at 40 mg daily, a decrease of approximately 10% every 1 to 2 weeks should be attempted. Alternate-day dosing should be avoided.

If clinical findings indicate recurrent inflammation, the dose may be increased. Although treatment is usually given for 1 to 2 years, some patients require long-term use of 10 mg/d of prednisone. Some patients may relapse (20% to 50%), usually within the first year of therapy.

TOXICITY

Calcium (1000 to 1500 mg/d) and vitamin D (400 to 800 IU/d) should be instituted at the start of glucocorticoid therapy to minimize risk of osteoporosis. If there are risk factors for osteoporosis, baseline bone mineral density should be measured. Antiresorptive therapy is recommended for all patients receiving more than 5 mg/d of prednisone for greater than 3 months. Other side effects of glucocorticoids include: glucose intolerance, infections, hypertension, weight gain, cataract formation, and mental status changes. The efficacy of disease-modifying drugs, such as methotrexate for refractory disease or as glucocorticoid-sparing agents, is unclear and remains controversial.

*Not FDA approved for this indication.

OSTEOMYELITIS

method of
ED SEPTIMUS, M.D.
Infectious Diseases, Memorial Hermann Healthcare System
Baylor College of Medicine
Houston, Texas

Despite recent advances in antimicrobial therapy and surgical techniques, osteomyelitis continues to pose a challenge to clinicians. The condition may at times be difficult to diagnose, yet if undiagnosed, it may progress to a chronic stage, with serious short- and long-term consequences to the patient. Osteomyelitis is usually caused by microorganisms that reach the bone by one of three routes: hematogenous, contiguous focus of infection, or direct inoculation secondary to trauma or surgery.

Osteomyelitis can be classified as acute or chronic depending on the presentation and clinical findings. If the initial acute episode of osteomyelitis is diagnosed early and appropriate antimicrobial therapy administered, the infection usually can be eradicated with minimal residual sequelae. However, if treatment is delayed, bone necrosis can occur, making eradication of the infection much more difficult and leading to the chronic phase of osteomyelitis, which is characterized by draining sinuses and recurrent episodes. Many investigators resist the word cure in osteomyelitis, because infection can recur years after apparently successful treatment.

An alternative classification system has been proposed by Cierny and Mader (Table 1). This classification system takes into account the anatomic extent of disease and the status of the host. There are four anatomic types combined with three physiologic host stages.

Stage 1 is termed medullary osteomyelitis associated with early hematogenous osteomyelitis. Most of these cases can be treated with antibiotics alone. In stage 2, or superficial osteomyelitis, the infection usually results from a contiguous soft-tissue infection. Necrosis is limited to exposed surfaces at the base of the wound. Stage 2 osteomyelitis generally requires superficial débridement, appropriate antimicrobial therapy, and coverage with a local or microvascular flap. Stage 3, or localized osteomyelitis, is defined by full-thickness cortical necrosis. This usually results from trauma, but can also result from evolving stage 1 and 2 disease. Stage 3 osteomyelitis requires débridement and appropriate antimicrobial therapy. Surgery does not usually result in instability of the infected bone. Stage 4, or diffuse osteomyelitis, represents necrosis through and through with loss of bone stability. Stage 4 requires débridement, dead space obliteration with bone stabilization, and appropriate antimicrobial therapy.

In the alternative classification system, patients are classified as A, B, or C hosts. A hosts are those patients with no underlying metabolic or immunologic disorders. B hosts are patients with localized or systemic diseases.

TABLE 1. **Cierny-Mader Classification System**

Anatomic type
Stage 1, medullary osteomyelitis
Stage 2, superficial osteomyelitis
Stage 3, localized osteomyelitis
Stage 4, diffuse osteomyelitis
Physiologic class
A host: normal host
B host
Systemic compromise (Bs)
Local compromise (Bl)
C host: treatment worse than the disease
Systemic (Bs)
Malnutrition
Renal, liver failure
Diabetes mellitus
Chronic hypoxemia
Immune deficiency
Malignancy
Extremes of age
Immunosuppression
Tobacco use
Intravenous drug use
Local compromise (Bl)
Chronic lymphedema
Venous stasis
Major vessel compromise
Arteritis
Extensive scarring
Radiation fibrosis
Small-vessel disease
Complete loss of local sensation

It is important to improve factors and diseases to make a B host more like an A host. The last category, C hosts, represents patients for whom the treatment of the bone infection is worse than the disease itself.

ACUTE HEMATOGENOUS OSTEOMYELITIS

More than 80% of cases of acute hematogenous osteomyelitis occur in the long bones of people younger then age 20, with a second smaller peak in persons more than 50 years of age in whom the primary focus is the axial skeleton. In children, the site of involvement is characteristically the metaphysis of rapidly growing long bones. Several factors appear to contribute to this predilection: high blood flow in the metaphyseal region, sluggish blood flow in the postcapillary venous sinusoids, and reduced active phagocytic cells lining the capillary loops. Trauma also may cause local hemorrhage and further impair bacterial clearance. Most children present with fever, pain on motion, and local tenderness. A history of prior trauma to the affected limb is present in approximately one third of patients. *Staphylococcus aureus, Streptococcus pyogenes,* and *Haemophilus influenzae* are the most common organisms isolated (Table 2). However, the incidence of *Haemophilus influenzae* is decreasing because of the new *H. influenzae* vaccine now given to children.

Neonatal osteomyelitis presents with few systemic symptoms. Fever is often absent. Local findings may include some swelling and failure to move the affected extremity. Joint involvement is present in 60% to 70% of cases because of the absence of epiphyseal plates in this age group. Group B streptococcus, *S. aureus*, and *Escherichia coli* are the most frequently reported organisms.

TABLE 2. **Microbiology**

Group or condition	Organism(s)
Neonates*	*Escherichia coli, Staphylococcus aureus, Streptococcus agalactiae*
Children*	*S. aureus,* streptococci
Adults*	*S. aureus,* Enterobacteriaceae
Sickle cell*	*Salmonella* spp., *S. aureus*
Intravenous drug abuse*	*S. aureus, Pseudomonas aeruginosa* Enterobacteriaceae, fungi
Open fracture	*S. aureus,* Enterobacteriaceae
Puncture of foot	*P. aeruginosa*
Animal or human bite	*Pasteurella multocida* *Eikenella corrodens*
Rheumatoid arthritis	*S. aureus*
Foreign body	Coagulase-negative staph, propionibacterium
Vascular insufficiency	Mixed aerobic/anaerobic bacteria
Diabetic foot lesion	Mixed aerobic/anaerobic bacteria
Decubitus ulcers	Mixed aerobic/anaerobic bacteria
Immunocompromised	Fungi, Group G strep, Enterobacteriaceae

*Hematogenous.

Acute hematogenous osteomyelitis in adults is different from that in children in that it usually affects the vertebral spine and infrequently the long bones. The prevalence of vertebral osteomyelitis in adults is attributed to the fact that organisms can reach the vertebral spine directly from segmental arteries supplying the vertebrae, which bifurcate to supply two adjacent vertebral bodies. Therefore, the disease frequently involves the intravertebral disc and the two adjacent vertebral bodies. The lumbar vertebrae are most commonly involved, followed by the thoracic and cervical vertebrae. The disease usually begins insidiously with progressive, dull, continuous back pain. Less commonly, the back pain may be of rapid onset, occasionally accompanied by neurologic symptoms. On physical exam, localized pain and tenderness of the involved site are present in more than 90% of patients. Some patients may also have severe muscle spasm over the affected area. Fever and elevated white blood cell count are documented in a minority of patients. If the infection extends posteriorly, compression of the cord may develop, necessitating emergency surgical decompression. In the normal host, *S. aureus* is the most commonly documented organism (see Table 2). In intravenous drug abusers, *Pseudomonas aeruginosa* and *S. aureus* are the most common, and in patients with urinary tract infections, *Enterobacteriaceae* spp. are the most common organisms.

CONTIGUOUS OSTEOMYELITIS

Contiguous osteomyelitis is caused by secondary extension of a soft-tissue infection into adjacent bone.

The majority of patients in this category have diabetes mellitus or peripheral vascular disease. Most patients are generally older than 40 years of age. Patients usually present with local erythema and swelling in the affected area of variable duration. Unlike hematogenous osteomyelitis, in which a single organism is usually identified, osteomyelitis secondary to a contiguous focus often is associated with multiple pathogens. *S. aureus* is still the most common organism, but aerobic gram-negative bacilli and anaerobes also may be cultured (see Table 2). Other examples of contiguous osteomyelitis include decubitus ulcers with osteomyelitis of the sacrum and heels and mandibular osteomyelitis secondary to odontogenic infections.

DIRECT INOCULATION

Osteomyelitis secondary to direct inoculation can result from open fractures, puncture wounds, and orthopedic surgery. Open fractures pose a particular challenge. By definition, the wound is contaminated, which increases the risk for infection. The bacteriology in this setting can be very diverse and polymicrobial. Puncture injuries of the foot, especially by stepping on a nail, have been associated with osteomyelitis because of *Pseudomonas aeruginosa*. Animal bites, especially from cats, can result in osteomyelitis because of *Pasteurella multocida,* and osteomyelitis secondary to human bites, especially from closed-fist injuries, is associated with osteomyelitis because of *Eikenella corrodens* (see Table 2).

DIAGNOSIS

To manage patients with any form of osteomyelitis, the need for accurate microbiology cannot be overemphasized. In acute hematogenous osteomyelitis, blood cultures may be positive in up to 50% of patients. If a joint effusion is present, an arthrocentesis should be performed to obtain fluid for analysis, including culture. If blood cultures are negative, a needle aspirate of the affected area may yield the pathogen; however, if this is negative, a percutaneous or open biopsy may be necessary to determine the pathogen. This is especially important in vertebral osteomyelitis, where a broad range of organisms may be involved. Other laboratory data may be of limited value. Leukocytosis may be present and the sedimentation rate and C-reactive protein are usually elevated, but these tests are not specific for the diagnosis of osteomyelitis.

In patients with contiguous osteomyelitis, surface cultures of decubitus ulcers and diabetic/vascular ulcers may be misleading, making biopsies or aspirates imperative. Sinus tract cultures are reliable for *S. aureus* but not for predicting gram-negative organisms causing osteomyelitis. For patients with osteomyelitis resulting from direct inoculation, deep cultures by aspiration, biopsy, or intraoperative samples are preferred (Table 3).

TABLE 3. **Methods for Confirming Diagnosis of Osteomyelitis**

Procedure	Sensitivity (%)	Specificity (%)
Blood culture	50	>95
Arthrocentesis	75	>95
Needle aspiration	60	>95
Surgical bone biopsy	90	>95
Wound or sinus tract	100	25-90

IMAGING STUDIES

One of the problems in making an early diagnosis of osteomyelitis by plain radiographs is that radiographic findings are normal in the early stages of disease. At least 50% of the bone must be destroyed before radiographs show typical lytic changes. Radiographic improvement can lag behind clinical response as well. In contiguous osteomyelitis and chronic osteomyelitis, the radiographic changes may be very subtle. Comparison with prior radiographs can be very useful.

The use of ^{99m}technetium scans (bone scans) has provided clinicians with a sensitive study for demonstrating early inflammatory disease. Bone scans may be positive as early as 24 hours after the onset of symptoms. A positive bone scan is not pathognomonic for osteomyelitis because a positive bone scan can be seen with fractures, tumors, infarcts, and trauma. It is less specific in settings of complicated disease (i.e., overlying cellulitis, trauma, diabetic feet). Gallium scans show increased uptake in areas of neutrophils, macrophages, and tumors. Gallium does not distinguish bone inflammation from cellulitis well. Indium-labeled white cell scans also have decreased sensitivity and specificity compared with bone scans in uncomplicated cases. Patients with chronic osteomyelitis often have negative indium scans. Computed tomography (CT) can play a role in the diagnosis of osteomyelitis. CT can show medullary destruction and necrotic bone, but image distortion can occur because of artifacts caused by bony fragments or metal. Magnetic resonance imaging (MRI) has become the imaging study of choice in difficult cases. MRI can differentiate bone and soft-tissue infection, often a problem with other radionuclide studies. The typical appearance of osteomyelitis is an area of abnormal marrow with decreased T_1-weighted images and increased T_2-weighted images (Table 4).

TABLE 4. **Imaging Studies for Osteomyelitis**

	Sensitivity (%)	Specificity (%)
Bone scan		
Uncomplicated	94	95
Complicated	95	33
Gallium scan	81	50-70
Indium scan	88	80
MRI	95	88

TREATMENT

In acute hematogenous osteomyelitis in children and vertebral osteomyelitis, treatment is primarily medical. In acute hematogenous osteomyelitis in children, surgical intervention is indicated if the patient does not respond within 2 to 3 days to appropriate antimicrobial therapy. In vertebral osteomyelitis, open surgical intervention is usually not necessary unless there is an extension of the infection, such as a paravertebral or epidural abscess, especially with any neurologic symptoms. After the organism has been identified, appropriate susceptibility studies should be performed to determine the most suitable antibiotic (see the following section). The patient should be treated for 4 to 6 weeks with intravenous therapy or 4 to 6 weeks after the last major surgical intervention. Oral antibiotics have been used successfully in treating hematogenous osteomyelitis in children; however, this should be conducted under carefully controlled situations. It is still recommended that the patient receive 1 to 2 weeks of intravenous therapy before changing to an oral drug.

In contiguous and chronic osteomyelitis, the major problem is infected necrotic bone with poor blood supply. Control of infection is difficult until adequate débridement and drainage has been accomplished and infected hardware removed if present. Management of dead space to replace dead tissue and fibrosis with well-vascularized tissue is critical to long-term success. Muscle flaps may be used to fill in dead space and provide adequate wound closure. The patient should be treated with 4 to 6 weeks of antibiotic therapy after the last major débridement.

Antibiotic-impregnated beads have been used to deliver a high concentration of antibiotics to the affected site and temporarily fill in dead space. The beads are usually removed within 2 to 4 weeks. Hyperbaric oxygen therapy may have a role where marginal or low oxygen tensions are present.

As discussed previously, establishment of the microbiologic diagnosis cannot be overemphasized (Table 5). The most common organism is *S. aureus*. For oxacillin (methicillin)-sensitive strains, treatment with nafcillin (Unipen),* cefazolin (Ancef), or clindamycin (Cleocin) is preferred. For osteomyelitis resulting from oxacillin-resistant *S. aureus*, treatment is more problematic. Vancomycin (Vancocin) remains the drug of choice with or without rifampin (Rifadin). Trimethoprim-sulfamethoxazole TMP-SMX (Bactrim)* plus rifampin,* clindamycin (if susceptible), or linezolid (Zyvox)* offer alternatives. Ciprofloxacin (Cipro) plus rifampin for staphylococcal infections related to orthopedic implants given for 3 to 6 months has been very effective. Penicillin or clindamycin remain the drugs of choice for the beta-hemolytic *Streptococcus*.

For osteomyelitis resulting from gram-negative organisms, therapy should be based on the sensitivities of the infecting organism. For polymicrobial infections with anaerobic and aerobic pathogens, an effective anaerobic drug should be part of the antimicrobial regimen, such as metronidazole (Flagyl), clindamycin, imipenem (Primaxin), or a beta-lactam beta-lactamase inhibitor (e.g., ampicillin/sulbactam [Unasyn], piperacillin/tazobactam [Zosyn]).*

Quinolones have been used with increasing frequency in the treatment of osteomyelitis. The published success for osteomyelitis resulting from quinolone-susceptible Enterobacteriaceae is more than 90%; however, the success for *Pseudomonas aeruginosa* and *S. aureus* is less than 80%. Furthermore, the development of resistance to quinolones on therapy has been observed with both *P. aeruginosa* and *S. aureus*.

PREVENTION

Antimicrobial prophylaxis with an antistaphylococcal agent given preoperatively (within 1 hour before the surgical incision) for patients undergoing either joint replacement or open reduction and internal fixation for closed fractures has been shown to reduce the incidence of postoperative surgical site infections. Antimicrobial prophylaxis has also decreased infection rates in patients with compound or open fractures.

Patients with diabetes mellitus can reduce the risk for osteomyelitis with tight glycemic control and meticulous foot care.

*Not FDA approved for this indication.

TABLE 5. **Initial Antimicrobial Choice for Osteomyelitis (Adult Dose)**

Organism	Antibiotic of Choice	Alternative(s)
Staphylococcus aureus, oxacillin sensitive	Nafcillin* (Unipen) 2 g q4–6h	Cefazolin (Ancef)
S. aureus, oxacillin resistant	Vancomycin (Vancocin) 1 g q 12 h	TMP-SMX (Bactrim) + rifampin (Rifadin) or linezolid (Zyvox)
Enterococcus spp.	Ampicillin* 2 g q 6 h	Vancomycin or linezolid*
Beta-hemolytic Streptococcus	Penicillin* 2 MU q 4–6 h or clindamycin (Cleocin) 600–900 mg q 8 h	Cefazolin
Enterobacteriaceae	Ceftriaxone (Rocephin) 1–2 g daily	Quinolone
Pseudomonas spp.	Ceftazidime (Fortaz) 2 g q 8 h or piperacillin/tazobactam* (Zosyn) 4.5 g q 6 h	Ciprofloxacin (Cipro) or imipenem (Primaxin) and cilastatin
Anaerobes	Metronidazole (Flagyl) 500–750 mg q 8 h	Clindamycin or imipenem and cilastatin or ampicillin/sulbactam (Unasyn)

*Not FDA approved for this indication.

COMMON SPORTS INJURIES

method of
CHRIS G. KOUTURES, M.D.
Pediatrics and Sports Medicine, Gladstien and Koutures
Team Physician, California State University, Fullerton
Anaheim Hills, California

Active individuals frequently express concern over both acute sporting injuries and chronic conditions that impair sports participation. This review discusses appropriate history and physical examination techniques, along with pertinent evaluation tools and rehabilitation goals to enable safe and appropriate return to activity. Certain age-related conditions will also be discussed to help direct the practitioner toward a diagnosis and management plan.

REVIEWING THE INJURY

With most sporting injuries, a diagnosis can be made after a focused physical examination, which often serves to confirm what was learned from a complete patient history.

In the case of acute trauma, it is important to identify the precise mechanism of injury because characteristic biomechanical events can readily lead to the proper diagnosis. Inquire about the disposition of the patient immediately after the injury—the presence and character of the pain, deformity, or swelling—and whether the athlete was able to return to activity. An inability to return to play or, with lower extremity injuries, an inability to bear weight often suggests a more serious injury. Inquire about any modalities (ice, heat, wraps, elevation) used immediately afterward because they may affect the results of physical examination. Finally, review any previous history of injury to the same region because improperly rehabilitated past injuries may predispose the athlete to subsequent disability.

With a more chronic condition, the practitioner must gain an understanding of the training and technical demands placed on the patient. Focus on the period leading up to the injury, with an emphasis on recent changes in the duration, frequency, and intensity of activity. Poor sporting technique combined with training errors (too much, too fast, too soon) leads to fatigue and stress of an overused region—proper diagnosis and rehabilitation require an appreciation of all the factors that contribute to injury. Appropriate quantification of pain by using numerical (1 to 10) pain scales or the presence of pain relative to activity can help in both assessing the initial disability and measuring progress throughout the rehabilitation process.

PRINCIPLES OF TREATMENT AND REHABILITATION

Management of any sporting injury is a stepwise process that attempts to not only correct the acute disability but also modify longer-standing factors that predisposed the individual to injury. The following

R Relative Rest (below level of pain, may use other body parts or alternate activities that do not stress injured region)
I Ice (repeat 20 minutes on, 40 minutes off)
Immobilization (bracing or splinting, if needed)
C Compression (ace wrap +/− foam pad to reduce swelling)
Crutches (if needed for lower extremity injuries, maximum 2–3 days unless longer interval is indicated)
E Elevation (above the level of the heart)

Figure 1. RICE mnemonic for care of acute injuries.

nonoperative rehabilitation principles can be used in the great majority of sporting injuries—even in those initially managed with surgical repair.

The RICE mnemonic (Figure 1) can be used to reduce the initial pain and swelling. Nonsteroidal anti-inflammatory drugs (NSAIDs) can also reduce pain and inflammation, although no substantial data favor a particular agent, nor does any evidence support scheduled NSAID administration versus as-needed dosing. Longer-term use of these agents may have associated side effects, namely, gastrointestinal and hepatic damage, that may require monitoring. Ultrasound, massage, and iontophoresis are other anti-inflammatory modalities used by physical therapists and athletic trainers in the initial stages of an injury.

Subsequent stages of rehabilitation focus on range of motion, strength, flexibility, and proprioceptive/neuromuscular conditioning. It is important to adhere to the criteria for advancement in each stage and start slowly at each stage, especially when returning to a sport-specific activity. Often, eager athletes (and those around them) desire a quick return to the sport, but a hasty return can lead to chronic disability or further injury from incomplete and improper rehabilitation.

DISCUSSION OF COMMON INJURIES BY REGION

Head Injuries

Any direct blow to the head or whiplash injury from violent neck or torso motion may result in a concussion (aka: mild traumatic brain injury). Symptoms range from frank loss of consciousness or diminished sensorium to more subtle signs such as poor concentration, emotional lability, dizziness, headache, altered balance, and nausea.

Any individual with possible concussion symptoms must be immediately removed from activity. Initial or sideline evaluation should test general orientation, the ability to remember new information, and recall of recent events, along with physical evaluation of strength, balance, and rapidly alternating movements. In the office setting, a complete neurologic examination should be performed, with brain computed tomography or magnetic resonance imaging (MRI) indicated for significant deficits, although the results of such studies are unremarkable in most cases of mild traumatic brain injury.

Most head injury symptoms resolve within days of the traumatic event, but some individuals will suffer prolonged post-concussive syndromes consisting of headaches, vertigo, concentration issues, poor sleep, and mood/personality changes. Neurologic or psychiatric consultation may help in these cases, and formal neuropsychologic evaluation is being used more frequently to identify postinjury deficits, especially in situations in which pre-injury baseline testing can be used as a comparison.

Given the risk of serious morbidity and even mortality from subsequent concussions without adequate healing of a primary concussion, no athlete should be returned to play until all symptoms and deficits have completely cleared. After an appropriate symptom-free waiting period has passed, gradual return is indicated, starting with light, noncontact activity and progressing to more strenuous contact activity if the symptoms do not return.

Shoulder Injuries

Common traumatic injuries to the shoulder region include acromioclavicular joint disruptions (aka: separated shoulder) and glenohumeral joint dislocation (aka: shoulder dislocation). Acromioclavicular joint injuries are often due to a direct blow to the lateral aspect of the shoulder and involve disruption of the joint capsule and possibly the supporting ligaments. Patients will have localized acromioclavicular pain with an inability to raise the shoulder above 90 degrees in either flexion or abduction. A visible prominence is noted with more severe joint disruptions, and focused acromioclavicular joint radiographs can rule out associated clavicular fracture. The patient must regain full, pain-free shoulder range of motion before return to play (usually 2 to 6 weeks), with additional padding of the affected joint indicated for contact sports.

An anterior position of the humeral head relative to the glenoid fossa is the most common type of sport-related shoulder dislocation, and it is usually due to a posterior blow to the abducted, externally rotated upper part of the arm. Immediate on-field reduction is indicated in a skeletally mature (>18 year old) athlete with no open skin lesions or gross neurologic compromise—a delay in attempting reduction often mandates the use of muscle relaxants and narcotics in an emergency room setting. Radiographs can confirm the position of the humeral head and evaluate for associated fractures of the humeral head or the glenoid rim. Post-dislocation management is somewhat controversial. Because some studies report a 90% redislocation rate in patients younger than 25 years, many authorities recommend surgical stabilization of first-time shoulder dislocations in this active age group. Older or less active patients may fare better with nonoperative management consisting of rotator cuff strengthening and avoidance of at-risk activities.

Overuse of the shoulder in overhead motions such as throwing, overhand tennis volley/serve, and freestyle swimming may lead to the triad of rotator cuff weakness, subacromial impingement, and glenohumeral multidirectional instability. Weakness of the rotator cuff muscles allows superior motion of the humeral head toward the acromial process, thereby contributing to impingement of the supraspinatus tendon. This weakness also allows increased motion of the humeral head relative to the glenoid fossa, especially in extremes of internal or external shoulder rotation.

Examination of the shoulder begins with an evaluation of range of motion, followed by strength testing of the four rotator cuff muscles. Further stress testing is described in Table 1.

Management of shoulder injuries begins with reduction or cessation of the offending activity and strengthening of both the rotator cuff muscles and scapular stabilizing muscles. On return to activity, attention to proper sport technique is required. Subacromial corticosteroid injections may help with impingement. Surgical evaluation is suggested in patients with a frank rotator cuff tear or those with poor progression of symptoms after 3 to 4 months of physical therapy.

Elbow Epicondylitis

Pain at the medial epicondylar origin of the forearm flexors is commonly seen in school-aged and adolescent throwers as a result of the valgus stress placed on the elbow with overhead throwing. Similar pain may

TABLE 1. **Shoulder Evaluation**

Suspected Injury	Test Name	Technique	Finding
Anterior glenohumeral laxity	Apprehension	Patient sitting either upright or supine and 90 degrees of shoulder abduction and elbow flexion with the fist pointing upward. Place posterior force on the elbow	Patient discomfort or excessive anterior motion of the humerus relative to the glenoid suggests anterior laxity
Rotator cuff impingement	Neer	Patient upright, shoulder at 90 degrees abduction and 30 degrees forward flexion. Fist pointing downward and the humerus rotated into extreme internal rotation.	Pain or crepitus suggests supraspinatus impingement under the acromial process
	Hawkins	Patient upright, arm extended against the side of the body. Place in extreme internal rotation, then passively bring the arm into full overhead flexion.	Pain or crepitus suggests supraspinatus impingement under the acromial process

also be seen in the trail elbow of golfers. Examination reveals focal tenderness at the medial epicondyle that is worsened with resisted wrist flexion and pronation. One must distinguish this injury from a tear of the medial collateral ligament, in which the injured elbow has increased valgus laxity of the elbow in comparison to the noninjured arm (Table 2). Evaluate the ipsilateral shoulder for rotator cuff weakness that can contribute to poor throwing technique and additional stress on the elbow. Obtain radiographs in skeletally immature athletes to rule out apophyseal or epiphyseal injuries to the developing elbow.

The lateral epicondyle is stressed in sports involving forearm and wrist extension, such as tennis backhand strokes. Pain is usually noted a few centimeters above the tip of the lateral epicondyle and may be worsened with resisted extension of the wrist and third digit.

Rehabilitation of epicondylar injuries includes flexor and extensor strengthening and stretching, anti-inflammatory modalities, and particular attention to proper sporting technique. Counterforce braces applied below the elbow may help in both conditions, whereas the value of serial corticosteroid injections for lateral epicondylitis is somewhat controversial.

Spondylolysis

Excessive hyperextension or torso rotation may predispose a young athlete to spondylolysis–stress fracture of the pars interarticularis, most commonly seen at L4 or L5. Localized pain without radiation, initially with activity before progressing to constant pain, is the usual manifestation. Hyperlordotic lumbar curves, tight hamstrings, and pain on single-leg stance with lumbar hyperextension and flexion of the opposite knee (stork test) are common physical findings. Plain radiographs may be normal even in advanced cases, and many authorities recommend single photon emission computed tomography (SPECT) of bone to make the diagnosis. Activity restriction, hamstring stretching, and rigid braces that prevent lumbar hyperextension or excessive lordosis are often used in the several-month treatment phase. Pain-free range of motion at rest is required before any return to sporting activity.

Acute Knee Pain and Swelling

Anterior Cruciate Ligament Tear

Complete tear of the anterior cruciate ligament (ACL) is the most common cause of a rapid-onset suprapatellar knee effusion within 1 to 2 hours after either landing and twisting on an extended knee or planting and cutting on the knee followed by an audible pop and immediate discomfort. Younger female athletes are statistically more prone to ACL tears than their sport- and age-matched male counterparts, although the reason for this discrepancy is not completely understood.

TABLE 2. **Grading of Ligament Sprains**

Grade	Focal Tenderness	Laxity
1	Present	None
2	Present	Increased with firm endpoint
3	Variable	Increased with no endpoint

The diagnosis of an incompetent ACL can be made by the Lachman test (Table 3). Often, meniscal tears or sprains of the collateral ligaments accompany ACL injury.

In athletes who wish to return to sports that require jumping, twisting, or cutting skills, surgical reconstruction of the ACL is the favored treatment. Nonoperative rehabilitation and bracing leave a high risk of subsequent instability and further meniscal and articular cartilage injury.

Meniscal Tears

A meniscal tear often results from axial loads placed on a flexed knee with sudden turning or twisting; the medial meniscus is torn more frequently than the lateral. In adults older than 40 years, degenerative meniscal tears can occur without any precise injury or trauma. Focal knee swelling and pain at the femoral-tibial joint line with a sensation of loose bodies catching in that area are common initial concerns. The McMurray, squat, and Apley tests (Table 3) are used to clinically diagnose meniscal tears, but given the relatively low sensitivity of these tests, MRI is often used to further identify the injury.

Nonoperative rehabilitation may allow full recovery from some tears, but larger or unstable tears often require surgical repair. Thus, many advocate orthopedic consultation in cases of suspected or documented meniscal injuries.

Collateral Ligament Injuries

A direct blow to the lateral aspect of the knee can cause a valgus stress that injures the medial collateral ligament (MCL). The patient will report difficulty walking and focal tenderness at the most medial aspect of the femoral-tibial joint line. Apply stress to the MCL as discussed in Table 3, with grading as discussed in Table 2. Virtually all isolated MCL sprains can be treated nonoperatively, with full recovery taking from 2 weeks (grade 1 sprain) to 2 months (grade 3 sprain).

Chronic Anterior Knee Pain

Osgood-Schlatter disease, or focal pain in the area where the patellar tendon inserts into the tibial tubercle, is frequently seen in skeletally immature athletes, usually during periods of a growth spurt or intense physical activity. The remainder of the physical examination may reveal a prominent tibial tubercle, quadriceps weakness (especially the vastus medialis oblique [VMO]), and hamstring tightness. Radiographs are unnecessary in uncomplicated cases. Ice, hamstring stretches, quadriceps strengthening, and counterforce bracing can help reduce the immediate pain, and this disorder remits after full ossification of the tibial tuberosity at the end of puberty.

TABLE 3. **Examination of the Knee**

Structure Tested	Test Name	Technique	Finding
Anterior cruciate ligament	Lachman	Stabilize the underside of the femur with one hand; the lower hand pulls the tibia forward relative to the femur	Lack of a firm endpoint implies an incompetent ACL
Meniscus	McMurray	Start with the knee in full flexion, then extend while placing pressure on the joint line	Focal pain and crepitus at the joint line indicate a possibly torn meniscus
	Squat	Patient squats into bilateral full knee flexion	Pain at the joint line with flexion
	Apley	Patient in the prone position, flex the knee to 90 degrees, then place an axial load compressing the tibia toward the femur	Pain or crepitus at the joint line, sensation of a foreign body at the joint line
Medial collateral ligament	Valgus at 30 degrees knee flexion	Bend knee to 30 degrees, apply valgus stress	Pain and laxity suggest isolated MCL sprain
	Valgus at full knee extension	Valgus stress to the fully extended knee	Pain and laxity suggest MCL sprain plus injury to other significant supporting structures

Athletes of all ages may suffer from patellofemoral pain syndrome, a constellation of vague, peripatellar pain worsened with running uphill/upstairs or after prolonged sitting with knee flexion. Focal swelling about the patella is common, and the physical examination may again show hamstring tightness or weak quadriceps/VMO. Treatment includes hamstring stretching, quadriceps/VMO strengthening, and correction of other predisposing biomechanical issues—such as taping/bracing for patellar hypermobility and arch supports for midfoot hyperpronation.

Ankle and Hindfoot Pain

Acute Ankle Sprain

Inversion ankle injuries with resultant sprains of the lateral anterior talofibular ligament and/or the calcaneofibular ligament are among the most common sports injuries. Injuries to the deltoid ligament on the medial aspect of the ankle are far less common. The history and physical examination should focus on the ability to bear weight—the ability to take four or more steps after an ankle injury is strongly correlated with the absence of a fracture—and the precise location of the pain. Pain in the posterior portion of the lateral malleolus in a non–weight-bearing patient is more suggestive of a possible fracture.

Stress testing of the ankle is described in Table 4, with grading of ligament sprains reviewed in Table 2.

TABLE 4. **Ankle Stress Testing**

Test Position	Structure Tested
Varus ankle stress with the foot in plantar flexion	Anterior talofibular ligament laxity
Varus ankle stress with the foot in dorsiflexion	Calcaneofibular ligament laxity
With the foot in neutral position, pull the calcaneus forward relative to the tibia (anterior drawer test)	Laxity of the anterior talofibular ligament and calcaneofibular ligament
Varus ankle stress, foot in neutral position	Medial deltoid ligament stability

Immediate application of ice, compression with an elastic bandage and a horseshoe foam splint, and elevation can reduce the swelling and discomfort considerably. Active rehabilitation of ankle sprains is discussed in Figure 2.

Achilles Tendonitis and Sever's Syndrome

Sever's syndrome consists of focal pain and inflammation at the Achilles tendon insertion to the immature apophysis of the posterior calcaneus. Symptoms tend to occur in the preadolescent and early teen years and worsen with prolonged running or jumping. These patients are likely to have tightness in the gastrocnemius-soleus muscle, so Achilles tendon and calf stretches are indicated for longer pain relief. Direct application of ice along with the use of heel cups or heel wedges in athletic shoes can help reduce pain, as can semirigid arch supports in patients with increased pronation (flatfoot). Radiographs are rarely needed, and the syndrome remits on reaching skeletal maturity.

Pain along with inflammation in the midsubstance of the Achilles tendon is more common in mature athletes, especially runners and jumpers, and is often

INITIAL EXERCISES

ALPHABET (use big toe to draw all the letters of the alphabet)
ALPHABET WITH RESISTANCE (use inner tube, elastic band, or large towel to provide resistance to drawing letters with big toe)
ACHILLES TENDON STRETCHING
BALANCE ON INJURED ANKLE (stand only on injured ankle for 15–30 seconds)

MORE ADVANCED EXERCISES

CONTINUE ACHILLES TENDON STRETCHING
HEEL RAISE (hold on to chair, rise up on toes of injured ankle, slowly lower heel back to the floor. For more challenge, do without support of chair.)
SINGLE LEG HOP (hop on injured ankle without pain)
SHUTTLE HOP (place box or ball on floor, hop side-to-side over object for 10–30 repetitions)
BALANCE AND CATCH (while balancing on injured ankle, have someone toss ball to patient)

Figure 2. Ankle rehabilitation exercises.

due to overuse or a rapid increase in sports activity. The pain is insidious in onset—a rapid onset of sharp pain should suggest complete Achilles tendon rupture versus Achilles tendonitis. Examination begins with placing the patient in a prone position and squeezing the calf muscle belly; the absence of ankle plantar flexion indicates Achilles rupture (Thompson test). Local swelling and crepitus along with focal pain are the hallmarks of Achilles tendonitis, and treatment consists of ice and anti-inflammatory drugs plus stretching of the calf-Achilles region. Cessation of the offending activities, often for several months, may be needed to reduce the symptoms, with gradual return to activity thereafter.

Section 16

Obstetrics and Gynecology

ANTEPARTUM CARE

method of
PAUL J. WENDEL, M.D.,
NANCY ANDREWS COLLINS, M.D., and
KATRINA R. DAVIS, M.D.
University of Arkansas for Medical Sciences
Little Rock, Arkansas

Prenatal care is designed to maximize the probability that every pregnancy produces a healthy baby without compromising the health of the mother. To achieve this goal, prenatal care should be thought of as encompassing evaluations and interventions prior to conception (preconceptual care) and after pregnancy has been diagnosed. In 1991 the U.S. Department of Health and Human Services released the recommendations of their expert panel convened to review the content of prenatal care in the United States. The panel concluded that a significant portion of maternal conditions (i.e., medical and behavioral) that can potentially lead to poor pregnancy outcomes could be identified and altered before conception.

PRECONCEPTUAL CARE

Significant anatomic, physiologic, and psychosocial changes occur throughout the course of pregnancy. As a consequence, various underlying maternal conditions may be affected both positively and negatively by the pregnancy. Thus, addressing these issues and conditions prior to conception allows the greatest potential for a favorable outcome. The key components of preconceptual care as defined by the American College of Obstetricians and Gynecologists (ACOG) are listed in Table 1.

TERMINOLOGY

The mean duration of a normal pregnancy is calculated from the first day of the last normal menstrual period. A normal pregnancy lasts approximately 280 days or 40 weeks from the first day of the last menstrual period. An estimate of the expected date of delivery is arrived at by adding 7 days to the date of the first day of the last normal menstrual period and counting back 3 months (Nägele's rule). It has become customary to divide pregnancy into three equal trimesters of approximately three calendar months each. All subsequent prenatal care is based on the precise knowledge of the age of the fetus; therefore, for ideal obstetric management, it is imperative to know the gestational age at any given time during pregnancy. Thus, early prenatal care makes it possible to assign gestational age through an accurate history of the last menstrual period and physical assessment of uterine size.

THE INITIAL PRENATAL VISIT

The initial prenatal visit is perhaps the most important visit of this care sequence. At this time, the relationship between the patient and the health care provider is established. It is the time to establish the goals of assessing the health of both the mother and the fetus, establishing the gestational age of the fetus, and initiating a plan for continuing obstetric care. To do this, a comprehensive medical and obstetric history must be obtained. The medical history should inquire about any prior hospitalizations, surgical procedures, underlying medical conditions, or current diseases that are being followed by a medical caregiver. Any family history of birth defects, mental retardation, or developmental delays should be obtained. The obstetric history should document the number, duration, and outcomes of all prior pregnancies, including infant weights, delivery methods, and pregnancy complications. Any prior abdominal surgeries should be investigated, and the uterine scar type of any prior cesarean section should be documented to determine whether the patient is a candidate for a subsequent vaginal birth.

A complete physical examination of the patient should be performed at the first prenatal visit. Any examination should include a routine evaluation of all the major organ systems, with special attention paid to the genital tract. A pelvic examination should include assessment of the vulva and any associated physical findings, evaluations of the vagina and cervix, as well as a Papanicolaou (Pap) smear. Ideally, any early examination should include a bimanual examination to determine the patency, length, and consistency of the external cervix as well as the uterine size. This examination also helps to confirm the gestational age of the pregnancy. In addition to the Pap smear, a gonorrhea culture should be obtained. Any findings suggestive of other sexually transmitted diseases may prompt culturing for *Chlamydia* or *Trichomonas*.

TABLE 1. **Components of Preconceptional Care**

Systematic identification of preconceptional risks through assessment of reproductive, family and medical histories; nutritional status; drug exposures; and social concerns of all fertile women
Provision of education based on risks
Discussion of possible effects of pregnancy on existing medical conditions for both the prospective mother and the fetus and introduction of interventions, if appropriate and desired
Discussion of genetic concerns and referral, if appropriate and desired
Determination of immunity to rubella and immunization, if indicated
Determination of hepatitis status and immunization, if desired
Laboratory tests as indicated
Nutritional counseling on appropriate weight for height, sources of folic acid, and avoidance of vitamin oversupplementation; referral for in-depth counseling, if appropriate and desired
Discussion of social, financial, and psychological issues in preparation for pregnancy
Discussion regarding desired birth spacing and real and perceived barriers to achieving desires, including problems with contraceptive use
Emphasis on importance of early and continuous prenatal care and discussion of how care may be structured on the basis of the woman's risks and concerns
Recommendation for women to keep menstrual calendar

From Cunningham FG, MacDonald PC, Gant NF, et al: Williams Obstetrics, 20th ed. Norwalk, CT, Appleton & Lange, 1997, p 228.

The first prenatal visit is an ideal time to obtain a host of laboratory tests, which include a hemoglobin and hematocrit with platelets; a urinalysis, including a microscopic examination and culture; blood group and D typing; indirect Coombs; syphilis serology; hepatitis B serology; and voluntary HIV testing. Selective populations should undergo testing for sickle cell anemia, diabetes, hemoglobinopathies, and tuberculosis.

Knowledge gathered from a history and physical examination allows the caregiver to provide a risk assessment program for each patient. Typically, pregnancies that include underlying preexisting medical illness or previous poor pregnancy performance may be categorized as high risk and may be referred on for consultation.

SUBSEQUENT PRENATAL CARE

Traditionally, women with pregnancies at low risk for adverse outcomes have been seen on a monthly basis until 28 weeks, then every 2 weeks until 35 weeks and weekly thereafter. If prenatal care is initiated early, this typically results in 13 to 15 visits. One of the recommendations of the expert panel on prenatal care was to modify this schedule. It was their belief that a woman should be seen early in pregnancy to be screened for underlying conditions. She should return at 10 to 12 weeks to be offered chorionic villus sampling and electronic identification of fetal heart tones. The next visit should occur in the interval from 16 to 20 weeks, when maternal serum screening and ultrasonography may be performed. The next important visit is at 26 to 28 weeks, during which time the diabetes screen, complete blood count, and Rh screen could be repeated, along with Rh_0(D) immune globulin (RhoGAM) administration, if necessary. Finally, visits in the third trimester can be performed every 2 weeks to monitor fundal height growth, fetal activity, and blood pressure. The clinician should remain flexible in the assigning of subsequent visits depending on the performance of the pregnancy and underlying conditions or complications that may arise.

PRENATAL SURVEILLANCE

Follow-up visits are designed to determine the well-being of both the mother and the fetus. Therefore, information that it is especially important to obtain from the fetal aspect comprises heart rate, size of the fetus (actual and rate of change), amount of amniotic fluid, presenting part and station (late in pregnancy), and fetal activity. From the maternal standpoint, the following information should be obtained: blood pressure, weight, general well-being, and distance to the uterine fundus from the symphysis pubis. Late in pregnancy, a pelvic examination provides potentially important information regarding confirmation of the presenting part, station of the presenting part, clinical assessment of the pelvis in relation to the fetus, and the consistency, effacement, and dilatation of the cervix.

GENERAL GUIDELINES DURING PREGNANCY

In addition to the physical examination and medical history obtained at the first prenatal visit, information should be provided to the patient regarding a host of topics in order to optimize the potential for a successful pregnancy performance.

Nutrition

In general, a well-balanced diet in pregnancy provides the majority of the Food and Drug Administration recommended daily allowances of dietary requirements. The Institute of Medicine concluded that iron was the only nutrient whose dietary requirement during pregnancy could not be met by diet alone. It is recommended that 30 to 60 mg of elemental iron be supplied on a daily basis. In the preconceptional period, the Centers for Disease Control and Prevention recommends dietary supplementation of 400 mcg of folic acid for approximately 4 weeks before and 3 months after conception for all women in an effort to prevent neural tube defects; for women who previously conceived a fetus with a neural tube defect, this should be increased to 4.0 mg. Additional nutritional supplements are unnecessary and indeed could be harmful; certain minerals and vitamins (including zinc; selenium; and vitamins A, B_6, C, and D) may produce toxic effects in excess amounts.

Weight Gain

In 1990, a committee of the National Academy of Sciences published its recommendations for weight gain during pregnancy. It recommended weight gains of 28 to 40 pounds for underweight women, 25 to 35 pounds for normal-weight women, and 15 to 25 pounds for overweight women. These categories were based on body mass index (weight [kg] divided by height [m^2]), defined by prepregnancy weight. Underweight women had an index less than 19.8 kg/m^2, and overweight women exceeded 26 kg/m^2.

Exercise

As a rule, it is not necessary for the pregnant woman to limit exercise provided that she does not become excessively fatigued or risk injury to herself or her fetus. The ACOG recommends that women who are accustomed to aerobic exercise before pregnancy should be allowed to continue this during pregnancy; however, caution should be taken against starting new exercise programs or intensifying training efforts during pregnancy. Women should avoid exercises that are performed in the supine position.

Employment

As with exercise, pregnant women should be encouraged to work throughout their pregnancy up until the time of delivery. Care should be taken to provide a healthy working environment, free from excessive physical exertion, prolonged standing, and exposure to occupational hazards. Limitations on employment and hours worked should be individualized to the patient, depending on the health of the mother.

Travel

In low-risk pregnancies, there is no reason to limit travel for a pregnant woman as long as she has access to medical care. There is essentially no risk to the fetus in a pressurized cabin of an airplane. Whether traveling by car, train, or airplane, women should be encouraged to walk at least every 2 hours. Travel in a car should be the same as in the nonpregnant state; passengers should be restrained with three-point seat belts. The lap belt portion of the restraining belt should be placed under the abdomen and across the upper thighs; the upper shoulder belt should be snugly applied between the breasts. International travel should be limited only by access to medical care and exposure to areas with endemic diseases. Patients requiring vaccines for international travel should consult their physician regarding the nature of the vaccine because of the potential for harmful effects from live attenuated virus vaccines.

Sexual Activity

Whenever a threatened abortion or preterm labor is present, any erotic stimulation should be avoided because it may produce uterine contractions. Otherwise, it has generally been accepted that in healthy, pregnant women, sexual activity usually does no harm. Although uterine activity may transiently increase following erotic stimulation, this is usually self-limited. In pregnancies complicated by placenta previa and threatened preterm delivery, coitus should be avoided.

Smoking

In general, smoking leads to decreased birth weight by an average of 200 g; consequently, smoking should be discouraged for all pregnant patients. Nicotine replacement therapies, such as patches and chewing gums, have been reported to be effective in achieving smoking cessation in pregnancy.

Alcohol

Because alcohol use during pregnancy may be harmful to the fetus, the Surgeon General recommends that women who are pregnant or considering pregnancy abstain from using any alcoholic beverages.

Caffeine

The Fourth International Caffeine Workshop concluded that there was no evidence that caffeine increases teratogenic or reproductive risk. Most studies on human pregnancy report no association between caffeine consumption and early pregnancy wastage, birth defects, or low birth weight. Patients should be encouraged to take a commonsense approach in their daily intake of caffeine in pregnancy.

COMMON COMPLAINTS IN PREGNANCY

Nausea and Vomiting

Nausea and vomiting are common in the first half of pregnancy. Typically, they have a self-limited course and begin to subside after the 14th to 16th week of pregnancy. The etiology continues to be unclear. Supportive therapy with oral and rectal antiemetics usually proves beneficial. Promethazine (Phenergan), 25 to 50 mg orally or rectally every 6 to 8 hours, proves helpful in most cases. The restriction to clear liquids and the addition of metoclopramide (Reglan) orally may be of benefit in some recalcitrant cases. Intravenous feeding and hospitalization may be necessary in unusual cases.

Back Pain

Low back pain is common, especially as pregnancy progresses. Significant movement of the skeleton and softening of the fibroelastic cartilages are hormonally mediated. Women should be instructed on proper body mechanics when lifting, rising, and lying down. Occasionally, supportive braces and physical therapy may be of some benefit.

Constipation

Constipation is a result of delayed gastric emptying and increased intestinal transit time, which are both hormonally and mechanically mediated. Both processes result in greater resorption of water from the gastrointestinal tract, resulting in hard stools and constipation. Typically, constipation responds well to increasing fluid intake and eating smaller, more frequent meals. The addition of bulk to the diet, through either high-fiber foods or supplements, usually proves helpful. Stool softeners may be beneficial.

Hemorrhoids

Hemorrhoids are varicosities of the rectal veins; they may appear for the first time during pregnancy. Their development or exacerbation is undoubtedly related to the increased pressure in the rectal veins caused by the obstruction of the venous return by the enlarging uterus. Constipation typically promotes their development or makes them more symptomatic. Pain and swelling are usually relieved by topically applied anesthetics, warm soaks, and stool softeners. Occasionally, thrombosis of the rectal vein may require excision under topical anesthesia.

Heartburn

Heartburn is probably the most common complaint in pregnant women. It is caused by reflux of gastric contents into the lower esophagus, made worse by the upward displacement of the stomach and compression of the uterus against the lower esophageal sphincter. Antacid preparations of aluminum hydroxide and magnesium hydroxide (Mylanta) usually provide considerable relief. H_2 blockers should be reserved for mothers who do not respond to oral antacids.

PRENATAL DIAGNOSIS

Approximately 3% to 5% of all newborns are delivered with some form of birth defect, whether it is major or minor. Only about 25 years ago, a fetal anomaly was first diagnosed in utero. With the development of increasingly sophisticated imaging technology, especially ultrasonography, fetal anomalies are diagnosed regularly. At present, however, no authoritative body recommends the use of routine ultrasonographic examination for population-based screening for congenital anomalies. As maternal age increases, there is an increasing risk of delivering a baby with an autosomal trisomy such as Down syndrome. The current standard of care is to offer amniocentesis for fetal karyotype to all women who will be 35 years of age or older at the time of delivery. All women who are older than 35 should be offered an amniocentesis. Maternal serum screening programs have been developed in attempts to identify fetuses at risk for neural tube defects, trisomies, and abdominal wall defects. Neural tube defects are usually seen in 1 to 2 of 1000 infants in the United States and 1 to 2 of 100 in Great Britain. An elevated maternal serum α-fetoprotein (MS-AFP), that is, greater than 2.5 multiples of the median (MOM), identifies patients at risk for delivering an infant with neural tube defects or abdominal wall defect.

Shortly after the initiation of MS-AFP screening in the United States, it was noted that low MS-AFP values (i.e., <0.5 MOM) may identify as many as 30% of mothers at risk for delivering a fetus with an autosomal trisomy. The addition of human chorionic gonadotropin and unconjugated estriol to the MS-AFP has made it possible to identify up to 60% to 70% of fetuses with chromosomal abnormalities. This program has proved extremely beneficial to the roughly 80% of women in the United States who deliver chromosomally abnormal babies without known risk factors. Unfortunately, the positive predictive value of these serum screens is low; as a result, only 1 in 60 to 70 abnormal screens results in identification of a trisomic fetus. Universal application of maternal screening for fetal anomalies and trisomies would result in 5% to 10% of all pregnant women undergoing amniocentesis.

The advent of genetic testing has now increased the number of diseases that can be potentially identified through prenatal testing. Currently there are over 500 genetic diseases that can be identified, either through direct gene mapping or through linkage testing. Consultation with a geneticist is important, as the list of potentially identifiable genetic diseases continues to increase rapidly.

ULTRASONOGRAPHY

Ultrasonography is perhaps the most revolutionary development in prenatal care during this century. The advantages of routine ultrasonographic screening include less frequent labor inductions for post-term pregnancy, earlier detection of fetal growth restriction, and identification of malformed fetuses. No clear-cut guidelines exist that define which women should receive an ultrasound examination or how many should be performed during a pregnancy. However, Table 2 lists the components of a basic ultrasound examination according to the trimester of the pregnancy in which it is performed. Regardless of the controversy, in general, the earlier the ultrasound examination is performed, the greater the accuracy in determining gestational age. Information obtained

TABLE 2. **Components of Basic Ultrasound Examination According to Trimester of Pregnancy**

First Trimester	Second and Third Trimesters
1. Gestational sac location	1. Fetal number
2. Embryo identification	2. Presentation
3. Crown-rump length	3. Fetal heart motion
4. Fetal heart motion	4. Placental location
5. Fetal number	5. Amnionic fluid volume
6. Uterus and adnexal evaluation	6. Gestational age
	7. Survey of fetal anatomy
	8. Evaluation for maternal pelvic masses

Modified from Cunningham FG, MacDonald PC, Gant NF, et al: Williams Obstetrics, 20th ed. Norwalk, CT, Appleton & Lange, 1997, p 1024.

at less than 18 weeks' gestational age typically has a margin of error less than 10 days. Studies performed in the third trimester may have a margin of error of roughly 3.5 weeks.

VAGINAL BLEEDING IN PREGNANCY

The significance of vaginal bleeding depends on the trimester in which the bleeding occurs. First-trimester vaginal bleeding can be from a variety of sources, including eversion of the endocervical canal, threatened abortion, and fetal death. Infectious etiologies, such as gonorrhea or chlamydial infections, may cause inflammatory cervicitis, which produces bleeding. Second-trimester vaginal bleeding may be a sign of continued threatened abortion or missed abortion. Other causes that require investigation include preterm cervical dilatation and cervical incompetence as well as preterm labor producing cervical change. A placenta previa may also be a cause of midtrimester vaginal bleeding. It is usually described as painless vaginal bleeding that may or may not be associated with uterine activity. An ultrasound examination should be performed in order to identify the location of the placenta before performing a pelvic examination. Again, careful speculum examination identifies signs of cervical infections, trauma, or neoplasms. Third-trimester vaginal bleeding is a common event. Placenta previa needs to be excluded and other causes sought. Cervical dilatation and labor should be ruled out as a sign of any bleeding. Finally, bright red bleeding associated with increased uterine tone and pain may be a sign of placental abruption. Placental abruption is usually associated with hypertensive diseases, trauma, and use of illicit drugs, especially cocaine.

TERATOGENS AND RADIATION EXPOSURE

A teratogen is any agent or factor that produces a permanent alteration in form or function of an organism when exposure to the agent or factor occurs in the embryonic or fetal period. Pregnancy is divided into the ovum period (from fertilization to implantation), the embryotic period (from the second through the eighth week) and the fetal period (from 8 weeks until term). Typically, agents that affect the ovum produce an all-or-nothing phenomenon. The major impact of teratogens occurs during the embryotic period. The factors that affect whether a drug has teratogenic effects depend on whether the fetus is exposed to quantities sufficient to cause it developmental anomalies. Many factors play a role in the accumulation of the drug or its metabolites to potentially toxic levels in the fetal compartment. These include the degrees of maternal absorption and metabolism, protein binding and storage, molecular size, electrical charge, and lipid solubility, all which affect the degree of placental transfer. Any drug given to pregnant women should be thoroughly researched by the caregiver before exposing the woman and her fetus to it. As with all medications in pregnancy, the potential benefit to be gained from maternal exposure should be weighed against the potential side effects to the fetus. Medications with known fetal effects should be used only after consultation with medical specialists and with clear indications.

Unfortunately, radiologic procedures are performed during early pregnancy before the pregnancy is diagnosed. As with medications, radiologic procedures may have defined specific risks based on the fetal dose of radiation. When calculating the dose of ionizing radiation from x-rays, it is important to consider the type of study, the type and age of the equipment, the distance of the organ in question from the source of radiation, the thickness of the body part penetrated, and the method or technique employed in the study. Current evidence suggests that there is no increased risk to the fetus with regard to congenital malformation, growth restriction, or abortion from ionizing radiation at a dose less than 5 rads to the fetus. A standard chest radiograph involves a dose exposure of less than 0.05 rads. Currently, no single diagnostic procedure results in a radiation dose significant to threaten the well-being or development of an embryo or fetus.

INFECTIONS IN PREGNANCY

Varicella Virus

Varicella infection in adults tends to be more severe than in children. There is evidence that the infection may be especially severe in pregnancy. Serious sequelae, such as the development of pneumonitis in the mother, may occur. Maternal chickenpox may infect the fetus by transplacental infection. In early pregnancy, infection may result in severe congenital malformations, including chorioretinitis, cerebral cortical atrophy, and limb defects. Administration of varicella zoster immune globulin (VZIG) may prevent or attenuate the varicella infection in mothers if given within 96 hours of exposure. The dose is 125 units per 10 kg given intramuscularly. The maximum dose is 625 units intramuscularly. If practical, maternal varicella IgG titers should be assessed prior to VZIG administration.

Parvovirus

Human B19 parvovirus causes erythema infectiosum or fifth disease. The maternal infection is usually associated with a rash, accompanying arthralgias, and many nonspecific symptoms. However, maternal infection may also be associated with adverse pregnancy outcomes, including abortion and fetal death. Diagnosis is confirmed by serologically demonstrating the presence of IgM parvovirus-specific antibodies. If fetal hydrops develops, fetal transfusion may be considered. Currently, there is no known maternal treatment for the disease.

Cytomegalovirus

Cytomegalovirus (CMV) is the most common cause of perinatal infection and may be found in as many as 2% of all neonates. Maternal CMV infection is characterized by fever, pharyngitis, lymphadenopathy, and polyarthritis. The risk of seroconversion among susceptible women during pregnancy is roughly 1% to 4%. Immunity from prior infection can be demonstrated in as many as 85% of pregnant women. Congenital CMV infection causes a syndrome that includes low birth weight, microcephaly, intracranial calcifications, chorioretinitis, and mental retardation. This syndrome is seen more commonly in mothers with primary infection in pregnancy and may be present in up to 20% of infants whose mother demonstrates primary infection during pregnancy. Recurrent infection in the mother is rarely associated with clinical sequelae. No effective therapy for maternal infection is known. Primary infection is diagnosed by a fourfold increase in IgG titers in paired acute and convalescent serum or by the identification of IgM CMV antibody in maternal serum. Recurrent infection is usually not accompanied by IgM antibody production.

Toxoplasmosis

Toxoplasmosis gondii infection is transmitted by eating infected raw or undercooked meat or through contact with infected cat feces. Maternal immunity is usually protective against intrauterine infection. Maternal infection is characterized by fatigue, muscle pain, and lymphadenopathy, although subclinical infection may be present. At birth, affected infants usually have evidence of generalized disease with low birth weight, hepatosplenomegaly, and various neurologic complications. The presence of *Toxoplasma* IgG antibody confers immunity for the mother. The most accurate method of diagnosis currently is a polymerase chain reaction (PCR). There is some evidence that maternal treatment with spiramycin* may be effective in preventing fetal infection and/or modifying its severity. Treatment has also been demonstrated to be effective with pyrimethamine (Daraprim) plus sulfadiazine.

Syphilis

Syphilis is a treponemal infection that can produce profound effects on the pregnancy by causing an endarteritis that results in preterm labor, fetal death, and neonatal infection by a transplacental or perinatal route. Fortunately, syphilis is highly preventable and susceptible to therapy. Diagnosis is made by serologic screening with such tests as the Venereal Disease Research Laboratory or the rapid plasma reagin, usually at the first prenatal visit. This screen is required by law in most areas. Positive findings should be confirmed by fluorescent treponemal antibody absorption or a microhemagglutination assay–*Treponema pallidum* preparation. Penicillin remains the treatment of choice. Intramuscular penicillin G cures early maternal infection and prevents neonatal syphilis in 98% of cases. Primary and secondary syphilis should be treated with 2.4 million units of benzathine penicillin G (Bicillin L-A) intramuscularly for 1 to 2 weeks. Syphilis of more than 1 year's duration should be treated with three sequential doses. Women with penicillin allergies should be referred for therapy.

*Not available in the United States.

Gonorrhea

In most cases of new gonococcal infection in pregnancy, the infection is limited to the lower genital tract. Acute salpingitis rarely develops because of obliteration of the uterine cavity after 8 weeks' gestational age. However, there is some evidence that pregnancy may place the patient at an increased risk for systemic infection. There is an association between gonococcal infection, septic abortion, preterm delivery, premature rupture of membranes, chorioamnionitis, and postpartum infection. Treatment of uncomplicated gonococcal infection includes ceftriaxone (Rocephin) 125 mg intramuscularly or cefixime (Suprax) 400 mg orally in a single dose. Patients with a positive gonorrhea culture should be screened for other sexually transmitted diseases.

Chlamydial Infections

Genital infection with *Chlamydia trachomatis* is the most common sexually transmitted bacterial disease in women of reproductive age. Cultures are positive in as many as a quarter of pregnant women. PCR testing of cervical secretions is now the detection method of choice. The role of routine screening for *C. trachomatis* during pregnancy remains unclear. However, there appears to be some evidence that it is linked to preterm delivery, premature rupture of membranes, and chorioamnionitis. Current treatment guidelines include erythromycin base (E-Mycin) 500 mg orally four times per day for 7 days or the new macrolide antibiotic azithromycin (Zithromax), 1 g orally as a single dose.

Herpes Simplex Virus

The management of herpes simplex virus (HSV) infection in pregnancy continues to evolve. The distinction between type 1 and type 2 herpetic infections has become blurred. Both virus types may produce maternal genital and neonatal infection. Most serious sequelae result from primary or first-episode infection in pregnancy. Primary infection is typically associated with more significant maternal symptoms along with a greater potential for vertical transmission to the fetus. A primary herpetic outbreak in pregnancy may be associated with a 25% to 40% rate of transmission to the infant if delivered over an active lesion, whereas recurrent lesions typically produce neonatal infection in only 3% to 5% of cases. Current management schemes continue to advocate cesarean delivery if herpetic vesicles or ulcers, whether primary or recurrent, are present at the time of rupture of membranes or labor. In the absence of a clinical lesion or prodromal symptoms, vaginal delivery is usually allowed. Diagnosis of a herpetic lesion should be confirmed by a tissue culture. The development of PCR assay for herpes simplex virus shows promise.

The ACOG Practice Bulletin in October 1999 recommended that women with primary HSV during pregnancy be treated with antiviral therapy. Furthermore, women at or beyond 36 weeks of gestation who are at risk for recurrent HSV may benefit from antiviral therapy as well. Numerous agents are available for the treatment of genital herpes, but none have received approval for use in pregnancy by the U.S. Food and Drug Administration. However, valacyclovir (Valtrex) and famciclovir (Famvir) (class B medications) and acyclovir (class C medication) have been approved for the treatment of primary genital herpes, the treatment of episodes of recurrent disease, and daily treatment for suppression of outbreaks of recurrent genital herpes.

Human Immunodeficiency Virus

HIV infection rates among young women of reproductive age are increasing more than in any other subgroup of the population because of transmission through heterosexual contact. As a consequence, all pregnant women should be counseled regarding HIV infection and offered screening. A positive enzyme-linked immunosorbent assay test should be repeated and, if positive a second time, confirmed with a Western blot analysis. A confirmatory finding on the Western blot indicates current infection. Protocols for the treatment of HIV-positive women in pregnancy have demonstrated decreased vertical transmission from the mother to the infant by greater than 68%. More recently, emphasis has shifted to include not only fetal well-being but also the most efficacious therapy for the pregnant woman. Research has shown that triple chemotherapy improves short-term survival rates and decreases morbidity in asymptomatic HIV-infected patients.

Current recommendations according to the Perinatal HIV Guidelines Working Group (2000, 2001) are that combination therapy with two nucleoside analogue reverse transcriptase inhibitors—zidovudine (AZT), zalcitabine (ddC), didanosine (ddI), stavudine (Zerit), lamivudine (3TC), abacavir (Ziagen)—plus either a non-nucleoside analogue—nevirapine (Viramune), delavirdine (Rescriptor), efavirenz (Sustiva)—or a protease inhibitor—indinavir (Norvir), ritonavir (Invirase), saquinavir, nelfinavir (Viracept), amprenavir (Agenerase)—be offered to pregnant women. During the intrapartum period, women who have had combination therapy should continue to receive zidovudine, 2 mg/kg intravenously, followed by continuous infusion of 1 mg/kg/hour until delivery. Those who have not had antepartum therapy should be considered for alternative therapies to include a regimen for the infant. Studies have also shown a reduced vertical HIV transmission rate when cesarean delivery was compared with other delivery methods. As a result, in 2000 the ACOG concluded that scheduled cesarean section should be discussed and recommended for HIV-infected women with an HIV-1 RNA load greater than 1000 copies/mL. Scheduled delivery may be offered as early as 38 weeks to lessen the likelihood of membrane rupture and/or labor. Neonatal care depends upon the antepartum and intrapartum drug received by the mother and should be supervised by a pediatrician. Postpartum mothers should be referred to a specialist for consideration of possible multiple-drug regimens and follow-up.

GESTATIONAL DIABETES

Gestational diabetes is defined as carbohydrate intolerance of variable severity with onset or first recognition during pregnancy. Undoubtedly, some women with gestational diabetes have previously unrecognized overt diabetes. There is neither agreement about the most appropriate diagnostic criteria for gestational diabetes nor consensus regarding the most appropriate women to be screened for this disorder. Whether universal screening or screening based on maternal risk factors is employed, any program should be instituted between the 24th and 28th weeks of gestational age. Screening programs involving risk factors should include age older than 30, family history of diabetes, prior macrosomic fetus, infant malformed or stillborn, obesity, hypertension, or glycosuria. The patients undergoing screening should be given a 50-g oral glucose tolerance test between the 24th and 28th weeks without regard to the time of day or last meal. A plasma value at 1 hour exceeding 140 mg/dL is used as the cutoff for a positive test. The diagnosis of gestational diabetes is made using a 100-g, 3-hour oral glucose tolerance test. Women with a previous history of gestational diabetes may benefit from earlier screening. If screening is performed early in pregnancy and yields a normal value, subsequent screening should still be performed at 24 to 28 weeks. If a 100-g, 3-hour oral glucose tolerance test is performed, it should be done after an overnight fast. Typically, the cutoff values for a positive 3-hour glucose tolerance test are plasma values (mg/dL): fasting 95, 1 hour 180, 2 hour 155, 3 hour 140. A positive test is defined as two or more values that are abnormal. Because women with gestational diabetes may not have fasting hyperglycemia during the time of organogenesis, the fetus may not be at any increased risk for fetal anomalies as are fetuses of women with overt diabetes. Similarly, whereas pregnant women with overt diabetes are at a greater risk for fetal death, this danger does not appear to be apparent in women with postprandial hyperglycemia only (gestational diabetes class A1).

Current management strategies for the treatment of gestational diabetes are aimed primarily at preventing macrosomia and the associated risks for birth trauma related to shoulder dystocia. Fetuses of diabetic mothers are anthropometrically different from other large-for-gestational-age infants. Typically, the infants of diabetic mothers have excess fat deposition on the shoulders and trunk, predisposing the fetuses to shoulder dystocia. These processes are consequences of maternal hyperglycemia resulting in fetal hyperinsulinemia, which in turn stimulates excessive somatic growth. Women who have fasting plasma glucose levels over 105 mg/dL or a 2-hour postprandial value over 120 mg/dL may benefit from dietary counseling and the addition of insulin. Women with a diagnosis of gestational diabetes should initially be started on the American Diabetes Association diet of 30 to 35 kcal/day as determined by the patient's ideal body weight. Any decision to add insulin should be undertaken after the initiation of this diet and monitoring of fasting values and 2-hour postprandial values. New evidence shows possible promise in the use of oral hypoglycemic agents, such as metformin (Glucophage), in the treatment of gestational diabetes under certain circumstances. More studies are needed before definitive recommendations can be given.

The decision on whether to perform antenatal fetal testing to prevent fetal losses should be individualized according to the patient. There is no evidence that antenatal fetal testing is required in gestational diabetics who are diet controlled. Expert opinion is divided on whether fetuses born to mothers who require insulin require fetal testing in the third trimester. It is currently our practice not to include fetal testing as a part of their management if glucose levels are well controlled and there is no suspicion of fetal macrosomia. In addition, there is no evidence to support the fact that fetuses born to mothers with gestational diabetes have delayed lung maturity. As a result, amniotic fluid testing for lung maturity is not required in gestational diabetics prior to delivery. Management in labor should include control of maternal blood sugar using intravenous insulin if needed to decrease the risk of fetal hypoglycemia in the neonatal period.

The effect of gestational diabetes on future outcome is important. It has been estimated that 50% of women with gestational diabetes experience overt diabetes within 20 years of delivery. As a result, women should be evaluated with a 75-g oral glucose tolerance test within 3 months of delivery. In addition, the recurrence of gestational diabetes in subsequent pregnancies has been documented to be as high as 20% to 30%.

HYPERTENSIVE DISORDERS IN PREGNANCY

Hypertensive disorders complicating pregnancy are common and form one of the deadly triad that includes hemorrhage and infection, which are responsible for the majority of maternal deaths. Because of the potentially severe sequelae of this diagnosis, the development of hypertension in a previously normotensive pregnant woman should and must be considered potentially dangerous to both the mother and the fetus. Pregnancy-induced hypertension (PIH) is divided into three categories: hypertension alone, preeclampsia, and eclampsia. The diagnosis of PIH is made when the blood pressure is 140/90 mm Hg or greater. The diagnosis of preeclampsia has traditionally required the identification of PIH plus proteinuria or generalized edema. However, because generalized edema is such a common finding, its presence should not validate, nor should its absence exclude, the diagnosis of preeclampsia.

Proteinuria is defined as more than 300 mg of protein in a 24-hour period or 100 mg/dL in two random urine specimens collected 6 hours apart. The degree of proteinuria may fluctuate widely over 24 hours; thus, a single random sample may fail to demonstrate significant proteinuria. Chronic hypertension in pregnancy is defined as the presence of hypertension (>140/90 mm Hg) either preceding pregnancy or detected before 20 weeks of pregnancy. The presence or absence of other associated symptoms and/or the identification of abnormalities in specified laboratory tests is used to assess the severity of PIH or preeclampsia. The key indicators that differentiate mild from severe preeclampsia are listed in Table 3. Management of PIH should be individualized on a patient-by-patient basis. Management of preeclampsia should take into account the severity of the disorder as assessed by the presence or absence of other conditions, identified in Table 3, the duration of the gestation, and the condition of the cervix. When the diagnosis of severe preeclampsia is made, hospitalization and prompt delivery should be undertaken in almost all cases. Unless the pregnancy is at the extreme limits of prematurity or the disease has not met severe criteria, expectant management and careful surveillance of the mother may prove beneficial in order to obtain greater fetal maturity.

Unfortunately, drug therapy for early mild preeclampsia and/or severe preeclampsia has been disappointing. Almost universally, the addition of antihypertensive agents fails to treat the underlying cause of the PIH and has failed to yield improvements in mean pregnancy prolongation, gestational age at delivery, or birth weight. It is important to keep in

TABLE 3. **Pregnancy-Induced Hypertension: Indications of Severity**

Abnormality	Mild	Severe
Diastolic blood pressure	<100 mg Hg	110 mm Hg or higher
Proteinuria	Trace to 1+	Persistent 2+ or more
Headache	Absent	Present
Visual disturbances	Absent	Present
Upper abdominal pain	Absent	Present
Oliguria	Absent	Present
Convulsions	Absent	Present (eclampsia)
Serum creatinine	Normal	Elevated
Thrombocytopenia	Absent	Present
Hyperbilirubinemia	Absent	Present
Liver enzyme elevation	Minimal	Marked
Fetal growth restriction	Absent	Obvious
Pulmonary edema	Absent	Present

Modified from Cunningham FG, MacDonald PC, Gant NF, et al: Williams Obstetrics, 20th ed. Norwalk, CT, Appleton & Lange, 1997, p 695.

mind that preeclampsia is a multisystem disorder that includes hypertension; it is not, strictly speaking, merely a hypertensive disorder with accompanying edema and/or proteinuria. Consequently, enthusiasm for the treatment of preeclampsia through pharmacologic agents has not been great. As part of any treatment algorithm for patients with PIH, intramuscular glucocorticoids to enhance fetal lung maturity and prevent intracranial hemorrhage should be used. These glucocorticoids do not seem to affect the cause of maternal hypertension.

During labor, women with PIH or preeclampsia should be given intravenous magnesium sulfate to prevent seizure activity. The usual dose is 4 g intravenously as a loading dose over 20 minutes, followed by a continuous intravenous maintenance dose of 2 g per hour. As long as urinary output is adequate (i.e., >30 mL per hour with a serum creatinine of <1.2), serum magnesium levels need not be measured. Preeclamptic patients managed expectantly should have their blood pressure, proteinuria, creatinine, liver functions, and platelet counts monitored closely. In addition, some form of fetal surveillance should be performed on a regular basis to avoid potential perinatal morbidity or mortality. In women who are between 32 and 34 weeks of gestational age, testing for fetal lung maturity may be appropriate as an indication of whether to deliver. After 34 weeks' gestational age, PIH with complications is usually best remedied by delivery. In the postpartum period, magnesium sulfate therapy should be continued for 24 hours. Intravenous hydralazine (Apresoline) may be given intermittently as needed for diastolic blood pressures over 110 mm Hg or systolic values over 170 mm Hg. Patients may be discharged when there is evidence that severe hypertension is showing a downward trend or laboratory values begin to normalize. Follow-up should be individualized according to the severity of the disease.

PRETERM DELIVERY

Premature birth in the United States is defined as any delivery prior to 37 weeks and low birth weight is defined as any birth less than 2500 g. The great majority of mortality and serious morbidity from preterm birth occurs prior to 34 weeks. Approximately 8% to 10% of all live births in the United States are characterized by low birth weight. The underlying etiology of preterm labor and preterm birth is poorly understood; consequently, interventions to prevent it have been disappointing. Associated maternal conditions, such as low socioeconomic status, nonwhite race, poor nutrition, multiple gestation, maternal smoking and alcohol use, as well as poor prenatal care attendance, have been linked to preterm labor and birth. It is now thought that ascending genital tract infections may be an etiologic factor in some cases of preterm labor. Current interventional strategies are being aimed at the early midtrimester. It is during this time that patients are being offered screenings for vaginal infections. It is theorized that intravaginal infections, such as chlamydia, bacterial vaginosis, gonorrhea, and mycoplasma, may be responsible for ascending infections that tip off a biochemical cascade that produces uterine activity. Whether these strategies can prevent preterm delivery will be answered with time. Clinical interventions to treat these infections are beginning to show promise but should be considered investigational at this time.

Programs designed to identify patients at risk for preterm delivery generally use scoring systems that identify predisposing factors. Although they may be useful for identification purposes, interventions to prevent preterm delivery based on these have been disappointing. Also, programs designed to identify early uterine activity through either self-palpation or electronic monitors have been disappointing. Although these are good at identifying uterine activity, there are still few interventions that can prevent this uterine activity from resulting in a preterm delivery.

When uterine activity has begun, efforts must be made to determine the underlying cause. In as many as 50% of cases, no significant underlying etiology is identified. Strategies to determine an infectious etiology include vaginal cultures as well as amniocentesis. Debate continues on whether treatment of intrauterine amniotic infection can prevent preterm delivery. However, if intrauterine infection is identified, intravenous antibiotics should be considered. Typically, women are initially started on intravenous fluids and given intravenous sedation as necessary. If this therapy proves ineffective, the decision of whether to include an intravenous tocolytic agent should be undertaken. Currently, the tocolytic agents include β-sympathomimetics (i.e., ritodrine [Yutopar] and terbutaline [Brethine]*), nonsteroidal anti-inflammatory agents (i.e., indomethacin [Indocin]*), calcium channel blockers (i.e., nifedipine [Procardia]*), and magnesium sulfate. Although data have failed to prove conclusively that tocolytic therapy arrests labor for more than 48 to 72 hours, it should not be misconstrued as a reason not to treat the patient. This 48- to 72-hour delay makes it possible to institute intramuscular corticosteroid treatment, thus decreasing the risk of death, respiratory distress syndrome, and intraventricular hemorrhage in preterm infants. Current recommendations as issued by the National Institutes of Health Consensus Development Conference (2000) are that a single course of antenatal steroids (i.e., two doses of 12 mg of betamethasone [Celestone Soluspan]* intramuscularly 24 hours apart or four doses of 6 mg of dexamethasone intramuscularly 12 hours apart) be given to all pregnant women between 24 and 34 weeks of gestation who are at risk of preterm delivery within 7 days.

New strategies that show promise in the prediction of preterm delivery include the identification of fetal fibronectin in the cervix and vagina and measurement of cervical length by vaginal ultrasonography. As with identification and treatment of infections in the genital tract, these methods are not yet proved to

*Not FDA approved for this indication.

decrease the rate of preterm birth and should therefore continue to be considered investigational.

ECTOPIC PREGNANCY

method of
ELIZABETH KENNARD, M.D.
The Ohio State University
Columbus, Ohio

Ectopic pregnancy is the leading cause of pregnancy-related deaths in the first trimester. Despite advances and great success in treatment, the condition is still misdiagnosed and undiagnosed. Early diagnosis and prompt treatment are essential.

RISK FACTORS AND EPIDEMIOLOGY

Risk factors include prior tubal surgery, prior ectopic pregnancy, prior salpingitis, and known pelvic adhesions. Patients with infertility and assisted reproduction are also at increased risk. Nonwhite women as well as women older than 35 have an increased risk for ectopic pregnancy. If a patient has an intrauterine device, a positive pregnancy test is more likely to signal an ectopic than intrauterine pregnancy. Most patients with an ectopic pregnancy do not have any known risk factors.

EARLY DIAGNOSIS

It is imperative to recognize a potential ectopic pregnancy and monitor patients closely. Most women who have an ectopic pregnancy do *not* have vaginal bleeding and do not experience the classical triad of pain, bleeding, and adnexal mass. The standard way to diagnose this problem is through a combination of serial β-human chorionic gonadotropin (β-hCG) levels and vaginal ultrasonography.

The rate of β-hCG rise during the first 4 weeks after ovulation is well established and approximately doubles every 48 hours. The lower limit of normal rise is approximately 67% every 48 hours. Most of the time, a normal rise in levels indicates a normal pregnancy, although there may be a 13% chance of an ectopic pregnancy when levels rise normally.

Because it is possible to have an ectopic pregnancy with normally rising β-hCG levels, vaginal ultrasonography must be combined with serial β-hCG levels to improve the detection of ectopic pregnancy. At a level of 1500 IU/L, there should be a visible gestational sac. With accurate gestational age, this can be very helpful. If a patient is certain of her date of menses or of conception, she should have a gestational sac 24 days after conception, and if none is visible the pregnancy is usually ectopic. Vaginal ultrasonography may also identify an adnexal mass, although it is possible to confuse a corpus luteum of the ovary with an ectopic pregnancy. Should the adnexal mass be larger than 4 cm or contain an embryo with cardiac activity, treatment is usually surgical.

TREATMENT

Ectopic pregnancies are usually treated either surgically or medically. Expectant management is reserved for patients who are carefully informed about their risks. They should have falling β-hCG titers, no evidence of rupture, and no evidence of bleeding. Most patients should have medical or surgical treatment when their ectopic pregnancy is diagnosed.

Medical treatment using methotrexate* was reported over 20 years ago, and numerous clinical trials have demonstrated success in approximately 90% of ectopic pregnancies that are ≤3 cm in size, unruptured, with β-hCG levels lower than 5000 mIU/mL. Common guidelines for using methotrexate are listed in Tables 1 and 2. Methotrexate is usually administered as a single dose of 50 mg/m^2 given intramuscularly. Serum β-hCG levels are determined on day 4 and day 7 and weekly thereafter until negative. There should be a decline of at least 15% by day 7 or a second dose may be given.

Methotrexate may rarely result in bone marrow suppression. Stomatitis, nausea, gastrointestinal upset, and transient increase in liver function tests may also occur. However, the most common complication of methotrexate treatment of ectopic pregnancy is failure to resolve the ectopic pregnancy and possible rupture.

Surgical treatment involves either salpingostomy or salpingectomy through laparoscopy or laparotomy. The success of the procedure depends on the location in the tube and ease of removal. Ampullary ectopic pregnancies are usually outside the lumen of the tube and are easier to remove than isthmic ectopic pregnancies. Laparotomy and laparoscopy achieve comparable results in resolution of ectopic pregnancies and in achievement of future intrauterine pregnancies. A salpingectomy should be performed if childbearing is not desired or in the case of uncontrolled bleeding or a severely damaged tube. If a patient has a second ectopic pregnancy in the same tube, a salpingectomy is usually recommended.

Surgery for ectopic pregnancy should never be delayed in cases of hemodynamic instability or for a

*Not FDA approved for this indication.

TABLE 1. **Selection of Patients for Methotrexate* Treatment**

Hemodynamically stable with no evidence of tubal rupture
Reliable patient who is able to reach health care facilities promptly
Patient should desire maintenance of fertility or avoidance of surgery
Ectopic mass does not exceed 4 cm, β-human chorionic gonadotropin level <10,000 mIU/mL, no cardiac activity in the mass
No evidence of an intrauterine pregnancy

*Not FDA approved for this indication.

TABLE 2. **Management of Methotrexate*-Treated Pregnancy**

Baseline liver and renal function tests, complete blood count, and platelets
Advise patient to cease folic acid–containing vitamins and avoid alcohol
Administer RhoGAM if indicated
Plan for d 4 and d 7 β-hCG levels, retreat if levels do not decline by 15% by d 7
Follow β-hCG levels until they return to negative

*Not FDA approved for this indication.
β-hCG, β-human chorionic gonadotropin; RhoGAM, $Rh_0(D)$ immune globulin.

patient who desires prompt resolution of her diagnosed ectopic pregnancy.

PERSISTENT ECTOPIC PREGNANCY

With medical or conservative surgical treatment of ectopic pregnancy there is a risk of persistent trophoblast tissue. Any patient who does not undergo a salpingectomy should have her β-hCG levels monitored until they decline to zero. Up to 15% of patients may require further treatment. If the patient is hemodynamically stable with no evidence of ruptured ectopic pregnancy, she may be treated with a dose of methotrexate.

FUTURE PROSPECTS

After one ectopic pregnancy, a patient has a 10% chance of a second ectopic pregnancy. Should she have a second ectopic pregnancy, her risk of a third is at least 30% to 40% and she has a significant risk of experiencing difficulty conceiving. A salpingectomy should be considered along with a recommendation for in vitro fertilization in the future.

VAGINAL BLEEDING IN LATE PREGNANCY

method of
STEPHEN T. VERMILLION, M.D.
Medical University of South Carolina
Charleston, South Carolina

Hemorrhage occurring in the third trimester of pregnancy complicates approximately 6% of all pregnancies. Possible etiologies include placenta previa, placental abruption, minor cervical trauma attributed to labor-induced changes, genital lesions, and rarely vasa previa. Understanding the physiologic changes that affect the cardiovascular system during the third trimester is essential in developing a plan of management. During pregnancy, the uterus receives about 25% of the cardiac output or approximately 500 mL of blood per minute. Consequently, an obstetric hemorrhage in the third trimester can have disastrous results for the mother as well as the fetus. The physician must be able to implement support for the maternal cardiovascular system quickly, develop a differential diagnosis to ascertain the source of bleeding, and then provide the best treatment for the mother and fetus.

The first issue is basic life support for the mother. Most patients with a third-trimester hemorrhage do not have any airway or breathing difficulties, but administering oxygen (6 to 8 L by face mask) may temporize the onset of maternal tissue hypoxia and increase the oxygen delivery to the fetus. Maintaining adequate intravascular volume is more problematic. Intravenous access should be established immediately with two large-gauge intravenous catheters to facilitate transfusion of blood products if necessary.

The average pregnant female can tolerate a 15% volume loss (1000 mL) without any hemodynamic alteration. With a 20% to 25% volume loss (1200 to 1500 mL), the pregnant patient demonstrates mild tachycardia, slightly increased respiratory rate, and orthostatic hypotension. However, the only change in the patient's blood pressure may be a more narrow pulse pressure. With 30% to 35% volume loss (2000 mL), the patient becomes overtly hypotensive and markedly tachycardic (120 to 160 bpm). When the volume deficit exceeds 40% (2500 mL), the patient may have no palpable blood pressure or pulse in the extremities. Unless volume therapy is quickly initiated, circulatory collapse and cardiac arrest soon follow. Monitoring urine output with a Foley catheter can provide important clinical information. As renal perfusion declines, urine output often decreases before changes in the patient's hemodynamic parameters are noted. In addition, the physician must be mindful of other underlying medical conditions, such as preeclampsia, anemia, or cardiovascular disease, which could alter the response to hemorrhage.

To assess quickly the potential complication of disseminated intravascular coagulopathy, a sample should be drawn in a red-top tube. If the blood firmly clots within 7 minutes, the patient is not yet coagulopathic. In addition, a type and crossmatch, a complete blood count (CBC), platelet count, prothrombin time (PT), and partial thromboplastin time (PTT) should be obtained. In Rh-negative patients, a Kleihauer-Betke test should be ordered and Rh immunoglobin administered accordingly. An arterial blood gas can be also useful as the oxygen tension is usually normal but the pH, carbon dioxide, and bicarbonate usually reflect some degree of metabolic acidosis. A base deficit of −6 to −8 indicates shock and the need for aggressive fluid and blood replacement. Base excesses greater than −8 usually signify impending cardiovascular collapse.

The clinician should initially estimate the amount of blood loss the patient has experienced and develop a plan for volume replacement. Volume replacement can be initiated with crystalloid solutions such as lactated Ringer's or 0.9% normal saline. In general, 3 mL of a crystalloid solution replaces the volume of 1 mL of whole blood. One milliliter of colloid solutions, such as hetastarch or albumin, replaces the volume of 1 mL of whole blood. Although both crystalloids and colloids may be used for volume expansion and improved circulation, neither is a substitute for the oxygen-carrying capacity of maternal red blood cells. Consequently, the physician may consider a blood transfusion earlier in the pregnant patient to maintain adequate oxygen delivery to the placenta and fetus.

Ideally, whole blood is the most physiologic therapy for an antepartum hemorrhage, but today blood component therapy is normally the only option. One unit of packed red blood cells is expected to increase the maternal hemoglobin by 1 g/dL. If a transfusion is needed urgently, type-specific blood can be safely administered to a patient with a known negative antibody screen with minimal transfusion risk. Platelets and fresh frozen plasma should be administered for clinical evidence of disseminated intravascular coagulopathy. Prophylactic transfusion with fresh frozen plasma and platelets is no longer recommended.

Only after the mother has been stabilized should the physician focus attention on fetal well-being. Most cases of apparent fetal distress resolve with maternal stabilization and subsequent in utero resuscitation of the fetus. Unfortunately, many care providers deliver the fetus prior to maternal stabilization, thus increasing the frequency of delivering a fetus unnecessarily by cesarean. This may further jeopardize the maternal stabilization effort because of the additional stress and blood loss from emergent surgery.

After maternal stabilization, the final step in managing third-trimester bleeding should be determining the etiology. An ultrasound examination should be performed to determine placental location. If the relationship between the placental edge and the internal os is not well visualized, a transvaginal or translabial approach may be carefully employed. A skilled sonographer should be able to detect readily a placenta previa. Conversely, visualization of an abruptio placentae is a much more difficult task and unreliable. A large retroplacental clot must be present before an abruption is detectable by ultrasonography. Most cases of significant placental abruption manifest with clinical symptoms prior to ultrasonographic evidence, making the utility of ultrasonography somewhat limited.

A placenta previa is usually associated with painless vaginal bleeding and occurs in 1 in 250 live births. When the diagnosis of placenta previa is made, management options depend on the gestational age, the amount of bleeding, fetal condition, and fetal presentation. At term, a major hemorrhage (≥750 mL) or nonreassuring fetal status after adequate maternal volume resuscitation should prompt the physician to consider an urgent cesarean delivery. Management decisions are more difficult in the preterm patient. With a stable mother and fetus, the obstetrician may consider an amniocentesis for fetal lung maturation between 34 and 37 weeks of gestation before proceeding to delivery. With immaturity or gestational age less than 34 weeks, expectant management is reasonable. In the presence of uterine activity and prematurity, tocolytics with either magnesium sulfate or indomethacin (Indocin P.O.) may be considered. Although β-mimetics have been used, the associated tachycardia complicates maternal evaluation. Corticosteroid administration to enhance fetal lung development is warranted for patients at less than 34 weeks. Maternal blood transfusion to maintain the hematocrit greater than 30% provides a margin of safety in expectantly managed patients.

Historically, a double setup has been advocated to determine the possibility of a vaginal delivery; however, this is rarely indicated because of current high-resolution sonography. However, a double setup may be useful for patients with a marginal previa or a very low-lying placenta. Otherwise, a cesarean delivery should be the choice of delivery. The type of uterine incision depends on the fetal lie and the position of the previa. For a fetal back-down transverse lie or anterior complete previa, a low vertical uterine incision is usually preferable to limit the blood loss and aid with delivery of a malpresenting fetus. For a posterior previa and all other presentations, we prefer a low transverse uterine incision.

The obstetrician should be aware that a placenta previa is associated with a higher incidence of placenta accreta, especially if the patient has an anterior previa and one or more prior cesarean sections. Ideally, the patient can be evaluated antenatally by ultrasonography or magnetic resonance imaging to determine whether the placenta invades the myometrium. If either modality suggests an accreta, the positive predictive value is high. However, the sensitivity as well as the depth of invasion is underestimated using these radiographic techniques. If an accreta is diagnosed prior to surgery, blood loss can be reduced if the placenta is left in situ while performing the cesarean hysterectomy.

Management of a placental abruption depends upon the degree of placental separation. Grade 1 abruption is associated with minimal uterine bleeding and uterine activity, no signs of hypovolemia, and reassuring fetal status. As with the previa, management of the patient is dependent of gestational age and maternal and fetal status. In a term patient, we would consider oxytocin (Pitocin) augmentation and delivery because of concern that the abruption may further separate the placenta and limit the maternal-fetal perfusion. In the preterm patient with uterine activity, tocolysis may be considered. We would follow the same guidelines for tocolysis that we discussed in the management of a previa. Grade 2 abruption is associated with mild to moderate uterine bleeding, frequent uterine contractions or tetanic uterine contractions, 20% to 25% volume loss, and occasionally evidence of early disseminated intravascular coagulopathy. The fetal heart rate pattern is usually nonreassuring. If vaginal delivery is imminent, it is the preferred mode of delivery. However, a cesarean delivery must often be performed because of nonreassuring fetal status remote from delivery. In a patient with early disseminated intravascular coagulopathy, the surgeon should consider a vertical skin incision, as this incision is more hemostatic than a Pfannenstiel incision. Grade 3 abruption is associated with moderate to severe uterine bleeding, maternal hypotension, and fetal death in utero. As with all classifications of abruption, the bleeding may be concealed and thus estimation of blood loss on the basis of vaginal bleeding is unreliable.

A rare cause of vaginal bleeding is a vasa praevia. This condition occurs when the placenta has a velamentous cord insertion and the vessels cross the internal cervical os. The vessels can rupture with either spontaneous or artificial rupture of membranes. Because all of the blood is fetal in origin, abrupt changes in the fetal heart rate tracing occur. The obstetrician must have a high index of suspicion to diagnosis this cause of vaginal bleeding. Immediate delivery by cesarean is warranted, and the pediatric team must be ready for volume resuscitation of the infant after birth. Under the best circumstances, perinatal morbidity and mortality are high.

Although abruptio placentae and placenta previa account for the majority of significant vaginal bleeding in the third trimester, other causes should be considered. The patient may have lower genital tract trauma, cervical cancer, or leiomyoma. In such cases, the same principles of maternal and fetal evaluation should be observed. However, treatment needs to be individualized on the basis of the source of vaginal bleeding.

HYPERTENSIVE DISORDERS OF PREGNANCY

method of
PHILLIP J. SHUBERT, M.D., and
DAVID N. HACKNEY, M.D.
The Ohio State University
Columbus, Ohio

The word eclampsia is from the Greek for "lightning." The appropriateness of this metaphor is evident to anyone who has ever witnessed the devastating and sometimes rapid effect that severe preeclampsia-eclampsia can have on a previously healthy mother and fetus. Despite an incidence in pregnancy of nearly 10%, preeclampsia remains one of medicine's most resilient and frustrating enigmas. Not only is the etiology unknown, but the proper management strategy remains unclear as well.

Preeclampsia can affect virtually every organ system in the human body, and the list of potential severe complications is long (Table 1). Thus, the practitioner of obstetrics must be familiar with the fundamental aspects of this disorder and have a low threshold for performing further evaluations of patients with minimal signs and symptoms (Table 2). Aggressive surveillance, however, does not necessarily translate into aggressive management and intervention.

TABLE 1. **Severe Criteria**

Blood pressure >160/110 mm Hg on two occasions 6 h apart
5 gm of protein in a 24-h collection
Oliguria (<500 mL urine per 24 h)
Cerebral or visual disturbances, eclampsia
Pulmonary edema
Persistent epigastric or right upper quadrant pain
Impaired liver function, syndrome of hemolysis, elevated liver enzymes, and low platelets (HELLP)
Thrombocytopenia
Intrauterine growth restriction, nonreassuring fetal well-being

This is especially true in regard to the fact that no proven prevention strategies exist and, unfortunately, the only cure remains delivery of the fetus and placenta. This article reviews the preeclamptic differential diagnosis and diagnostic criteria as well as management of patients with hypertensive disorders, eclampsia, and other emergencies.

PREECLAMPTIC RISK FACTORS AND THEORIES OF ETIOLOGY

Despite decades of research, the etiology of preeclampsia remains unsolved. Although the disease usually manifests itself in the third trimester, the underlying pathologic process probably begins at a much earlier state of placental development. Studies have consistently demonstrated a failed placental invasion of the maternal spiral arteries and deciduas. Preeclamptic patients often have otherwise unexplained elevations in maternal serum α-fetoprotein, perhaps secondary to abnormal placentation. Later in the pregnancy, multiorgan endothelial dysfunction occurs producing thrombus formation, vasospasm, and increased vascular permeability. This process accounts for the clinical manifestations of preeclampsia, such as renal dysfunction and seizures. Both the impaired placental development and the endothelial dysfunction, however, are probably manifestations themselves of a more fundamental and mysterious process.

Insight into the etiology of preeclampsia can be obtained through its risk factors, and many of these point to an immunologic basis for the disease. Preeclamptic patients tend to be nulliparas or pregnant with the child of a new father, implying an association with paternal antigen exposure. Multifetal pregnancy, molar gestations, and the occurrence of preeclampsia in a previous pregnancy also pose an increased risk. Conversely, immunosuppressed and untreated HIV-positive patients tend to have a lower incidence of the disease. Other risk factors, however,

TABLE 2. **Symptoms of Preeclampsia**

Headache
Visual disturbances
Subjective increase in upper extremity or facial edema
Nausea, emesis
Right upper quadrant or epigastric pain

lack an obvious immunologic association. These include obesity, chronic hypertension, chronic renal disease, diabetes, and thrombophilias.

CLASSIFICATION AND CRITERIA

Hypertension in pregnancy is generally divided into four categories: chronic hypertension, preeclampsia, gestational hypertension, and preeclampsia superimposed upon chronic hypertension, as outlined in Table 3. Pregnancy-induced hypertension, an ill-defined phrase traditionally encompassing both gestational hypertension and preeclampsia, is considered outdated and should be avoided.

The diagnosis of chronic hypertension (CHTN) would ideally be made prior to conception. Unfortunately, the first obstetric visit is often the first time that women, being generally young and healthy, have seen a physician in years. CHTN in pregnancy is thus defined as hypertension (blood pressure [BP] >140/90 mm Hg) diagnosed before pregnancy, developing before 20 weeks' gestation, or persisting more than 6 weeks post partum. The diagnosis technically cannot be made in a patient who presents with newly elevated BP and late prenatal care (>20 weeks). Likewise, a woman who presents de novo at 16 to 20 weeks with BP in the 130s/80s mm Hg would also not achieve the CHTN diagnosis. Such a patient, however, may actually have preconceptual hypertension and is experiencing the physiologic nadir, and caution will be warranted in the third trimester.

Gestational hypertension (GHTN) is new hypertension first diagnosed after 20 weeks of pregnancy without proteinuria (<300 mg per 24 hours) or other signs of preeclampsia and which resolves post partum. It is a diagnosis of exclusion that can truly be made only after delivery of the fetus and placenta. In the absence of other complications or very high BPs, GHTN alone does not confer an increased risk to the mother or fetus.

Preeclampsia was traditionally diagnosed by its classical triad: hypertension, proteinuria, and edema. Edema, however, is too prevalent and nonspecific in the third trimester and is no longer incorporated into diagnostic criteria. The accepted definition is new hypertension (BP >140/90 mm Hg) after 20 weeks' gestation with greater than 300 mg of protein in a 24-hour urine collection or greater than 2+ on urine dip (preferably free from contaminant and infection). A relative increase in BP that does not actually exceed 140/90 mm Hg no longer qualifies as hypertension. These definitions presume that preeclampsia will not develop before 20 weeks' gestation, which is generally true with the exception of molar pregnancies.

After the initial diagnosis, preeclampsia is then further divided into mild and severe cases. The diagnostic criterion for severe preeclampsia is listed in Table 1 and is worthy of memorization by anyone who practices obstetrics. The laboratory studies used to differentiate mild from severe preeclampsia usually include 24-hour urine protein quantification, platelets, liver function tests (LFTs), lactate dehydrogenase, blood urea nitrogen (BUN), creatinine (Cr), and uric acid. In the absence of thrombocytopenia, coagulation studies (prothrombin time, partial thromboplastin time, International Normalized Ratio) are typically not needed. It is imperative that patients diagnosed with preeclampsia undergo fetal evaluations. Preeclampsia with associated intrauterine growth restriction (IUGR) generally warrants delivery regardless of gestational age.

The diagnosis of preeclampsia superimposed upon CHTN is often fraught with clinical uncertainty. The usual definitions involve new-onset proteinuria in a CHTN patient with a previously normal 24-hour collection or new nephrotic range proteinuria in a patient with previous renal disease, as well as worsening BP control or other "severe" preeclampsia criteria. If the patient's CHTN is itself secondary to an underlying disorder, such as lupus or a glomerulonephropathy, the differentiation between new preeclampsia and a worsening chronic disease can be extremely difficult. Because a diagnosis of severe preeclampsia superimposed upon CHTN may necessitate delivery of the fetus, consultation with high-risk obstetrics, nephrology, or other specialties is warranted in these situations.

Tonic-clonic seizures or a significant alteration in mental status in a woman with preeclampsia and without other causes of seizure (i.e., drug withdrawal) defines eclampsia. HELLP syndrome is a syndrome of hemolysis, elevated liver enzymes, and low platelets. Neither eclampsia nor HELLP syndrome is a disease genuinely separate from preeclampsia; instead, they represent extreme manifestations in different organ systems.

TABLE 3. **Categories and Definitions of Hypertension**

Chronic hypertension (HTN): HTN (>140/90 mm Hg) diagnosed before pregnancy or HTN before 20 wk gestation or persisting more than 6 wk post partum
Preeclampsia: HTN after 20 wk gestation with >300 mg protein in 24-h urine collection
Gestational HTN: HTN after 20 wk gestation and resolving within 6 wk post partum without proteinuria or other signs of preeclampsia
HELLP syndrome: Preeclampsia plus (aspartate transaminase [AST] > 72 or bilirubin > 1.2 or lactate dehydrogenase > 600) and platelets [PLT] < 150,000. Note: Some practitioners use PLT < 100,000 and standard deviation cutoffs of AST.
Eclampsia: New-onset tonic-clonic seizures in a preeclamptic patient not attributable to another source.

DIFFERENTIAL DIAGNOSIS OF PREECLAMPSIA

Because many different organ systems are involved, many different diseases can mimic preeclampsia and vice versa. Extreme pain, in general, transiently increases a patient's BP and may produce nausea as well. Both migraine attacks and gallbladder disease can mimic preeclampsia by arising with headache and right upper quadrant pain, respectively, along with nausea and hypertension. The elevated BPs in these situations should become normal with pain control and this, along with the history and lack of proteinuria, allows one to rule out preeclampsia.

Pyelonephritis and nephrolithiasis may cause proteinuria, as well as pain-associated hypertension and abdominal pain. In addition to the normalization of BP with pain control, the fever that accompanies pyelonephritis and the hematuria seen in nephrolithiasis do not occur with preeclampsia.

Differentiating preeclampsia from worsening primary renal disease can be very difficult. Preeclampsia, fortunately, is rarely associated with renal casts or an "active" urinary sediment, which may help distinguish it from a primary glomerulonephropathy. Complement levels and double-stranded DNA (dsDNA) can help differentiate a lupus flare.

The differential diagnosis of thrombocytopenia includes gestational thrombocytopenia (GTP), idiopathic thrombocytopenia (ITP), transient thrombocytopenia with purpura (TTP), and hemolytic-uremic syndrome (HUS) in addition to preeclampsia and HELLP syndrome. GTP is an idiopathic although generally benign disorder that involves decreased platelet counts throughout gestation, including the first trimester. It is thus important to check first-trimester platelet levels before ascribing thrombocytopenia to severe preeclampsia. TTP and HUS, although rare, are potentially life threatening. Whereas patients with HELLP may have very low platelets, they usually lack purpural skin lesions, mental status changes, and fever. In cases of TTP-HUS, plasma transfusions and exchanges can be lifesaving.

Acute fatty liver of pregnancy (AFL) is another rare but potentially fatal disorder that must be recognized promptly. Patients usually present in the third trimester with nausea, emesis, right upper quadrant pain, and occasionally hypertension. LFTs are predictably elevated and coagulation disorders may exist as well, thus causing confusion with HELLP syndrome. As AFL progresses, however, the patient becomes profoundly hypoglycemic and jaundiced, neither of which is characteristic of preeclampsia. The liver damage of AFL progresses relentlessly until the delivery of the fetus and placenta and then sometimes continues afterward. Once it is diagnosed, delivery must be performed without delay and regardless of gestational age in order to prevent permanent liver failure and potential maternal death.

THE OBSTETRIC PATIENT WITH CHRONIC HYPERTENSION

There are several important decisions that must be made when first encountering a pregnant patient with CHTN: What baseline laboratory studies are in order? What changes should be made in the patient's antihypertensive medications? Is a referral or transfer of care to a high-risk obstetric specialist needed?

Many pregnant patients with CHTN have been previously diagnosed and evaluated, but for some women the diagnosis may be new. Although most cases are "essential hypertension," a standard evaluation, including a detailed physical examination and laboratory studies, is still required. Substance abuse, especially cocaine, is unfortunately not uncommon and may also cause BP elevations. For patients with known lupus, measurements of baseline complement levels (C3, C4) and dsDNA are important, especially if one needs to differentiate new-onset preeclampsia from a lupus flare later in pregnancy.

Renal function should be evaluated in any new CHTN patient through BUN and Cr measurements, 24-hour urine protein quantification, and Cr clearance. Kidney biopsies, although not contraindicated, have a higher complication rate in pregnancy secondary to increased renal blood flow and are generally deferred until the postpartum period.

The initiation or discontinuation of antihypertensive medications in the pregnant patient with CHTN is a matter of controversy. Control of mild CHTN during pregnancy is of maternal benefit only and has never been demonstrated to improve obstetric outcomes. For this reason, initiation of antihypertensives in the newly diagnosed gravid female with CHTN requires BPs that are higher than those of a nonpregnant patient for the maternal benefits to outweigh the potential fetal risks. The exact BP required is controversial, although almost every obstetrician would treat first-trimester BPs of 160s/110s and/or labile pressures. Likewise, the CHTN patient with mild disease who has been well controlled may be a candidate for a trial of medication discontinuation in the first trimester.

Table 4 lists the antihypertensives commonly used in pregnancy. Methyldopa (Aldomet) enjoys the most extensive data with regard to fetal safety and is often used. β-Blockers, especially labetalol, are also generally considered safe. Angiotensin-converting enzyme inhibitors, on the other hand, are teratogenic and absolutely contraindicated in pregnancy.

A general plan for the pregnancy can be formulated after baseline evaluations and medication changes have been performed. The majority of patients with otherwise uncomplicated CHTN enjoy a benign pregnancy, although they are at increased risk for the development of preeclampsia (see Table 2). In addition, they should have frequent determinations of BP and urine protein. Any new symptoms, increased proteinuria, or BP elevations should prompt an evaluation for superimposed preeclampsia, as outlined in

TABLE 4. **Commonly Used Antihypertensives**

1. Antiadrenergics: Methyldopa (Aldomet)
   Initial dose: 250 mg bid
   Comments: Best safety profile
2. β-Blockers: Labetalol (Trandate)
   Initial dose: 100 mg PO bid, 20–40 mg IV q10min for emergent HTN
   Comments: Atenolol (Tenormin) should not be used
3. Calcium channel blockers: Nifedipine (Procardia)
   Initial dose: 20 mg qd of Procardia XL or 10 mg tid
   Comments: Cannot be used concurrently with a magnesium infusion
4. Vasodilators: Hydralazine (Apresoline)
   Initial dose: 5–10 mg IV q10–20min
   Comments: Used for emergent HTN

the preceding section. In the absence of preeclampsia or worsening BP control, delivery is initiated at term in the presence of a favorable cervix or after 40 weeks.

Optimal antepartum fetal monitoring in the otherwise uncomplicated CHTN patient is currently unclear. Patients should, at a minimum, be instructed in daily fetal kick counts and undergo nonstress tests (NSTs) if there is any concern about fetal well-being. Serial ultrasound studies for growth and amniotic fluid as well as weekly or twice-weekly NSTs are absolutely indicated in a patient with worsening HTN, proteinuria, or superimposed preeclampsia.

PREECLAMPTIC ANTENATAL MANAGEMENT

Once the diagnosis of preeclampsia or preeclampsia superimposed upon CTHN has been made (see earlier), one must decide whether or not to deliver the fetus. Despite decades of scientific research, preeclampsia remains a disease with no cure other than ending the pregnancy.

Three general principles should guide one's decision making. (1) Any patient with preeclampsia who is at term (>37 weeks) or has had fetal lung maturity documented by amniocentesis should be delivered; (2) conservative management should be abandoned if there is evidence that the fetus is not benefiting from the uterus, that is, the development of IUGR or nonreassuring fetal well-being (NRFWB); and (3) the pregnancy should be ended if the mother's life becomes acutely endangered by preeclampsia. Table 5 lists situations in which conservative management is contraindicated and the fetus should be delivered regardless of gestational age.

In the absence of severe criteria or fetal indications, mild preeclampsia can safely be continued until term (>37 weeks). Betamethasone (Celestone) should be given to enhance fetal maturity when preeclampsia is diagnosed at less then 34 weeks' gestational age. Amniocentesis can be performed if desired prior to 37 weeks to document fetal pulmonary maturation and allow earlier delivery. Patients with mild preeclampsia need to be placed on bed rest and undergo continual surveillance for severe disease. Indicated testing includes serial nonstress tests and ultrasonography for fetal weight and amnionic fluid analysis. A 24-hour urine protein quantification and preeclampsia laboratory tests (see earlier) should be performed at least twice weekly.

TABLE 5. **Situations in Which Conservative Management Is Contraindicated**

Associated prolonged premature rupture of membranes, preterm labor
Intrauterine growth restriction, nonreassuring fetal well-being
Eclampsia
Syndrome of hemolysis, elevated liver enzymes, and low platelets (HELLP)
Pulmonary edema
Disseminated intravascular coagulation
Renal failure

When preeclampsia becomes severe, delivery is uniformly recommended when the patient is past 34 weeks' gestation, has documented fetal pulmonary maturity, or a live-threatening maternal condition exists (see Table 5). The conservative management of patients with severe disease at less than 34 weeks' gestation is highly controversial within obstetrics. The benefits of prolonged fetal maturation must be weighed against the potential fetal and maternal risks and vary depending upon the actual severe criteria met as well as the estimated fetal weight and gestational age.

Antihypertensives may be initiated for patients who are remote from term and are severe by BP criteria only. When the decision has been made to deliver the fetus, one can still often wait for 48 hours to obtain the maximum fetal benefits from antenatal betamethasone (Celestone). Intravenous magnesium should be given during this interval. If a prolonged labor induction is anticipated, steps such as cervical prostaglandin administration may be started prior to 48 hours.

LABOR AND DELIVERY MANAGEMENT OF PREECLAMPSIA

Blinded, randomized trials have proved that intravenous magnesium sulfate infusions provide the most effective seizure prophylaxis in women with preeclampsia. In the absence of contraindications, such as myasthenia gravis, magnesium sulfate should be administered to every preeclamptic woman in labor or undergoing cesarean section and be continued for 24 hours post partum. Four grams are given as a loading dose followed by an infusion of 2 g/hour.

The greatest risk of magnesium infusion is the development of hypermagnesemia from decreased renal secretion. Thus, all women receiving an infusion need to have hourly recordings of their urine output and an indwelling catheter. Deep tendon reflexes (DTRs) and pulmonary examinations should be performed regularly. Loss of DTRs precedes more serious effects such as respiratory depression. A serum magnesium level should be checked if the urine output falls or if the patient has clinical signs of overdose. Therapeutic and toxic serum levels of magnesium are listed in Table 6. If life-threatening magnesium toxicity is encountered, calcium gluconate can be given as an antidote. Most cases, however, can be managed by decreasing the infusion rate or temporarily holding the infusion.

All methods of labor induction, including cervical prostaglandins and oxytocin (Pitocin) infusions, are safe in preeclamptic patients. Although magnesium

TABLE 6. **Magnesium Levels**

5–10 mg/dL	therapeutic
8–12 mg/dL	loss of deep tendon reflexes
10–12 mg/dL	mental status changes
15–17 mg/dL	respiratory impairment
30–35 mg/dL	cardiac arrest

infusions have uterine relaxation effects and are also used clinically to stop preterm labor, this can be overcome through an adequate oxytocin infusion. Magnesium should never be withheld for fear of prolonging labor. Even in the presence of severe disease or actual eclamptic seizures, cesarean sections should be reserved for the standard obstetric indications. An exception would be the patient for whom labor induction could take hours if not days (i.e., a primigravida with an unfavorable cervix) and who is developing increasingly severe disease.

In the absence of significant thrombocytopenia or coagulation disorders, epidural anesthesia is safe in preeclamptic patients. Because normal platelet counts can fall during the course of a labor induction, consideration should be given to early epidural placement.

Magnesium crosses the placenta and sedates the fetus. Decreased fetal heart rate (FHR) variability and loss of reactivity are not uncommon. Decelerations of FHR, especially late decelerations, can never be attributed to magnesium infusions and require further evaluations.

The risk of eclamptic seizures continues post partum, and thus magnesium infusions are generally continued for 24 hours after delivery. In the presence of eclampsia, HELLP syndrome, or other especially severe situations, the length of infusion may be extended to 48 hours or longer. During this time, regular assessment of urine output, DTRs, and pulmonary edema is needed. The BP should eventually become normal after delivery in patients with preeclampsia, and thus antihypertensives are usually not needed.

ECLAMPSIA AND HYPERTENSIVE EMERGENCIES

With improved treatments for obstetric hemorrhage and infections, hypertensive disorders have become one of the most common causes of maternal mortality in developed countries. Eclamptic seizures are tonic-clonic in nature and without focal deficits or localizing symptoms and usually last 1 to 2 minutes. The etiology of these seizures is uncertain and contentious. The development of coma or other significant mental status changes, including blindness, also meets the definition of eclampsia. When the diagnosis is established, delivery of the fetus is indicated regardless of gestational age.

Management of the seizing pregnant patient is not unlike that of the nongravid woman. Oxygen should be administered, the airway should be secured, if possible, and the patient should be situated in a manner that minimizes self-harm and on the left-hand side. Fetal distress during and immediately after an eclamptic seizure is more often a rule than an exception. FHT tracings usually improve after conclusion of the seizure, and one should resist the temptation to intervene for the fetus during an active convulsion because maternal morbidity would be very high.

Intravenous magnesium not only is the agent of choice for seizure prophylaxis but also is used for seizure treatment. Six grams are given as a loading dose, followed by an infusion of 2 g/hour. For patients who seize while already receiving a prophylactic infusion, an additional 2-g load of magnesium should be given followed by a determination of serum magnesium levels. Additional antiepileptics are not usually necessary except in the rare events of repetitive seizures despite adequate magnesium therapy or life-threatening status epilepticus.

Plans for delivery should be made when the mother has been stabilized. Consideration should be given to transferring the patient to a tertiary care center, especially if the fetus is remote from delivery. Vaginal delivery is associated with less maternal morbidity and should be attempted when feasible. Most eclamptic patients stabilize after initiation of magnesium therapy and can safely undergo labor induction. Cesarean section should be entertained when the patient has an unfavorable cervix, is not responding to initial induction efforts, or is suffering recurrent seizures.

HELLP syndrome is another manifestation of severe preeclampsia and is also generally considered an absolute indication for delivery. Unlike the situation in eclampsia, however, labor induction does not necessarily have to be immediate and, if the mother is otherwise stable, one can attempt to obtain the 48 hours of maximum fetal benefit from betamethasone (Celestone). Serial laboratory analysis is needed if conservative management is attempted, and delivery should be performed if progressively severe thrombocytopenia is encountered. A transient "steroid effect" is often seen after betamethasone (Celestone) administration with increasing platelet levels.

As with eclampsia, vaginal delivery is the preferred route of delivery, and cervical ripening can be performed while one is awaiting the maximum steroid effect. Platelet transfusions are avoided if possible because they are rapidly consumed by the underlying disease process and there is a risk of formation of antiplatelet antibodies. If a cesarean section is planned, however, platelets should ideally be at least 50,000, and preoperative transfusion may be necessary. Epidural anesthesia is generally contraindicated with severe thrombocytopenia. Consideration should be given to the placement of an early epidural when the diagnosis of HELLP syndrome is made in the event of further decreases of platelets. After delivery, the platelets may continue to fall for another 24 to 28 hours but always eventually return to normal.

Subcapsular hematoma, rupture of Glisson's capsule, and complete hepatic rupture are the most feared consequences of HELLP syndrome. They usually arise with acute worsening right upper quadrant pain or new shoulder pain with deteriorating vital signs or shock. Emergent laparotomy and general surgery consultation are needed. Of note, although right upper quadrant tenderness is important in screening patients for severe preeclampsia, when the diagnosis of HELLP syndrome is made, palpation of the right upper quadrant should be avoided.

BPs that are consistently greater than 160/110 mm Hg pose a danger to the patient and need to be corrected. Antihypertensive therapy is covered more completely earlier and in Table 4. For emergent treatments, intravenous labetalol (Normodyne) and hydralazine (Apresoline) are most often used. One should be careful in overcorrecting severe hypertension. The fetal placental perfusion often acclimates itself to higher pressures and fetal distress may be encountered in these situations if pressures fall below 140/90 mm Hg.

CONCLUSION

Hypertension disorders of pregnancy encompass a wide range of diagnostic and therapeutic dilemmas. A high index of suspicion and subsequent diligence are required for timely diagnosis and appropriate management.

POSTPARTUM CARE

method of
CHARLES E. DRISCOLL, M.D.
Centra Health, Inc. and University of Virginia
Lynchburg, Virginia

The usual postpartum period requires careful follow-up care beginning immediately after delivery of the placenta and continuing until 6 to 8 weeks following the birth. The length of this period is defined by the *puerperium*, which is the time needed for the anatomic and physiologic changes of pregnancy to revert to the normal state. Some postpartum problems, however, can be delayed in appearance for months beyond this time (e.g., anemia, sexual readjustment, thyroiditis, and depression). Care is usually managed in the hospital (48 to 72 hours), home, and medical office (4 to 6 weeks after birth) with mapping of tasks for routine medical care, care of complications, psychological care, education, and family and social support. Some medical urgencies may require a visit in the emergency department. This method of care describes the tasks pertinent to each clinical setting. Table 1 provides an overview.

HOSPITAL CARE

The first few hours after delivery are a critical time in which to monitor the patient for *hypotension, hemorrhage (overt* or *concealed), dyspnea, fever, preeclampsia,* and *urinary retention.* Pulse, blood pressure, respiratory rate, temperature, lochia, urination, and pain status are monitored every 15 minutes until the patient stabilizes and then every 4 to 6 hours; the physician is alerted immediately if unexpected findings appear. Particular attention is required when conduction or regional anesthesia has been used, as the patient may not be aware of her own condition, and also when the patient complains of more severe pain than anticipated. The following should be investigated:

- *Hypotension* may be secondary to vagal response, hypovolemia, or an anesthetic reaction. The first ambulation after delivery should be observed and assisted. Treatment of hypotension includes placing the patient in Trendelenburg's position and giving a 500-mL bolus of intravenous (IV) crystalloid with normal saline or lactated Ringer's solution. The caregiver should exercise caution and observe for pulmonary edema with a history of prolonged oxytocin (Pitocin), terbutaline (Brethine), or magnesium sulfate usage. If hypotension is due to blood loss, it is managed according to the hemorrhage protocol.
- *Hemorrhage* occurs in approximately 4% of deliveries and is defined as more than 500 mL of blood loss or a change of more than 10% from the pre- to postpartum hematocrit values. Hemorrhage may be secondary to uterine atony (most common), laceration, hematoma, and rarely bleeding diatheses. Risk factors include prolonged labor, overdistended uterus, multiparity, amnionitis, retained placental fragments, instrumentation, history of prior postpartum hemorrhage, and use of uterine relaxants (e.g., magnesium sulfate). Anticipatory management is the best course of action with placement of an IV catheter for access *before* delivery has occurred. The labia, vagina, and uterus should be explored in all bleeding patients to identify and stem the source of bleeding; a concealed hemorrhage of up to 3 units is possible. Crystalloid solution IV should be delivered to restore blood volume, and oxytocics (Table 2) are

TABLE 1. **Components of Postpartum Care**

Location of Care	Duration	Goals
Hospital care	24–48 h for routine vaginal delivery 72 h for cesarean section	Minimize risks of infection, hemorrhage, and pain Bowel-bladder function and lactation established Begin education of family
Home care	Following discharge from hospital	Establish self-sufficiency, renew contraception, and educate concerning urgencies requiring a physician visit
Office care	At 4–6 wk from delivery	Examine for healing, check for adjustment to new baby, contraception, lactation
Emergency department	When needed	Management of bleeding and other urgencies

TABLE 2. **Oxytocics Used for Control of Uterine Atony**

Drug	Dose	Maintenance	Contraindications
Oxytocin (Pitocin)	10 U IM or infuse 10 to 40 U in 1 L of IV fluid	IV infusion maintained 1–4 h	None
Methylergonovine (Methergine)	0.2 mg IM	Repeat q2–4h	Hypertension, toxemia
Prostaglandin $F_{2\alpha}$ (carboprost; Hemabate)	0.25 mg IM	Repeat q15–90min	Cardiac or pulmonary disease
Prostaglandin E_2 (Prostin E2)	20-mg suppository inserted into rectum	Repeat q2–4h	Hypotension (use $PGF_{2\alpha}$ instead)

used and blood product replacement (red cells, platelets, or fresh frozen plasma) arranged if hemoglobin falls to less than 7 g/dL or a coagulopathy is suspected.

- *Dyspnea* may mean embolization of amniotic fluid (AFE), a thrombotic pulmonary embolus, or exacerbation of reactive airway disease. Embolization is suspected in the presence of respiratory distress, apprehension, chest pressure, a history of prior deep venous thrombosis (DVT), and the signs of cardiovascular collapse. AFE is a rare but catastrophic event with 80% mortality. If suspected, 100% O_2 should be administered, endotracheal intubation with ventilator support arranged, hypotension treated with crystalloid, and the disseminated intravascular coagulation that invariably accompanies this condition managed. Embolization of thrombus requires antithrombolytic or anticoagulation therapy. Acute asthma is manageable with nebulized albuterol (Proventil).
- A temperature in the range of 99° F to 100° F can be normal within the first 24 hours after delivery, but *fever* (temperature >100° F) requires diagnosis and management. Infection rates are approximately 5.5% after vaginal delivery (in descending frequency, mastitis, urinary tract infection [UTI], episiotomy site infection, endometritis) and 7.5% after cesarean birth (surgical site infection, mastitis, UTI, endometritis). A search for DVT (legs and pelvic veins) should be included in the diagnostic workup. Between 10% to 20% of all postpartum infections appear during the hospitalization; the rest manifest after discharge. One common hospital scenario is febrile chorioamnionitis during labor leading to endometritis and parametritis. Broad-spectrum IV antibiotic regimens (e.g., ampicillin-sulbactam [Unasyn] 2 g every 6 hours *or* ticarcillin-clavulanate [Timentin] 3.1 g every 6 hours *or* clindamycin [Cleocin] 900 mg plus gentamicin [Garamycin] 1 mg/kg every 8 hours) are given until the patient has been afebrile for 48 hours. Mastitis is treated with antibiotics that cover *Staphylococcus* (e.g., cefazolin [Ancef], or dicloxacillin [Dycill]).
- *Postpartum preeclampsia or eclampsia* accounts for 25% of cases and occurs within 1 week of delivery. Blood pressures higher than 140/90 mm Hg, edema of the face and hands, hyperreflexia, and albuminuria alert the physician to begin treatment. Magnesium sulfate remains the mainstay of therapy, giving 4 g slowly IV over 15 to 30 minutes until hyperreflexia resolves and following with an IV infusion of 1 to 3 g per hour keeping serum magnesium levels between 4 and 7 mEq/L. Calcium gluconate (1 g IV push) is kept at the bedside to counteract overtreatment with magnesium sulfate. If blood pressure does not respond to the magnesium sulfate, IV hydralazine (Apresoline) (40 mg/L) is infused to titrate the blood pressure to about 130/80 mm Hg. Ringer's solution IV fluid is given to maintain urinary outputs of higher than 50 mL/hour.
- *Urinary retention* is not uncommon after the trauma of delivery or as a result of anesthetics used. If the patient does not void within 6 hours of delivery, in-and-out single catheterizations are preferable to Foley retention catheters to minimize risk for UTI.
- *Other considerations* for hospital care prior to discharge are noted in Table 3.

HOME CARE

The agenda for home care is established with discharge planning and education or by follow-up phone consultation. The best management is to provide anticipatory guidance regarding the concerns most women express post partum. Nurse visitation at home is particularly important for patients with early hospital discharge (<36 hours), those with language or cultural needs not met in the hospital environment, and those at risk for developing problems (e.g., the mother with a history of a prior postpartum depression). The following topics are recommended for education:

1. Gentle reentry into sexuality after healing.
2. Avoid putting anything in vagina until lochia changes from bloody to serous.
3. "Dry vagina" occurs with lactation and requires use of sexual lubricant.
4. Call the physician in the event of chills; fever (temperature >100° F); mastitis; heavy uterine bleeding; signs of infection in incision; calf warmth, redness, tenderness, or swelling; inordinate pain; dysuria; obstipation; significant depression or adjustment problems; abdominal pain; and purulent lochia.
5. Return of ovulation schedule and contraception appropriate to nursing status.
6. Bowel regularity and laxative recommendations.
7. Incontinence occurs in 20% to 30% of new mothers; teach pelvic floor exercises.

TABLE 3. **Other Considerations for Hospital Care**

Topic	Recommendations
Pain control (perineum, breast)	Ice to the perineum initially, then hot sitz baths, ibuprofen (Motrin) 600–800 mg q6-8h, tight breast binder applied.
Sleeplessness	Quiet, dark environment and relaxation with soft music; if medication required, use short-acting zolpidem (Ambien) 5–10 mg at bedtime.
Rh-negative mother giving birth to Rh-positive infant	Administer $Rh_0(D)$ immune globulin (RhoGAM) 300 μg within 72 h of delivery.
Rubella status nonimmune or unknown	Administer 1 dose of rubella vaccine.
Hemorrhoids and bowel movements	Use stool softeners, adequate liquid intake, laxative, and encourage ambulation. Hemorrhoid creams or witch hazel pads may help. Excise thrombosed external hemorrhoid.
Anemia	Continue prenatal vitamins and add ferrous sulfate 325 mg 1–3 daily with orange juice.
Postpartum "blues"	Explain as a normal occurrence; role model to family how to be supportive.
Lactation	Use lactation consultant for first-time breast-feeders; feed on demand; lanolin moisturizing ointment or wet tea bags for sore nipples; supportive nursing bra; increased fluid intake; teach breast milk expression techniques.

8. Stress and anger management.
9. Exercise and reconditioning.
10. Available local services, support groups, and Internet resources (Table 4).

OFFICE CARE

The first scheduled office visit can be at 4 to 6 weeks post partum. Provision of care for maternal concerns probably outweighs the disadvantages associated with a 4-week visit. The 4-week visit has the advantages of early intervention for stress management, encouragement for continuation of breast-feeding, reinforcement of education agenda, and examination of the progress of healing in the puerperium. If healing of the perineum permits, reassurance can be given for earlier return to sexual intimacy when desired. The disadvantage of a 4-week interval is that diaphragm fitting requires a second visit in 4 to 6 more weeks and sometimes lochia is still too heavy in nonlactating women to do Pap testing. Physical examination should include blood pressure, weight, palpation of the thyroid for evidence of thyroiditis, breast examination, auscultation of the heart for appearance of new murmurs, examination of legs for swelling and tenderness, and examination of the abdomen for muscle tone and healing if a cesarean delivery was done. Preventive health issues (e.g., weight control, smoking) should be addressed and urine and blood count checked if indicated.

TABLE 4. **Community and Internet Resources**

Your hospital nursery and lactation consultant phone numbers
La Leche League 847-519-7730 or http://www.lalecheleague.org
Women's Health Information http://www.4women.gov/pregnancy/index.htm
Patient Information http://www.familydoctor.org
Women, Infants and Children 703-305-2746 or http://www.fns.usda.gov/wic/menu/contacts/coor/coor.htm
International Lactation Consultants http://www.ilca.org
Postpartum Support International http://www.postpartum.net
Postpartum Education for Parents, especially the links to other groups http://www.sbpep.org

RESUSCITATION OF THE NEONATE

method of
COLONEL STEPHEN M. GOLDEN, M.D., USAF, MC
Department of Pediatrics
David Grant Air Force Medical Center
Travis AFB, California

The views expressed in this manuscript are those of the author and do not reflect the official policy of the U.S. Government, the Department of Defense, or the Department of the Air Force.

The purpose of neonatal resuscitation is to support and restore normal cellular function during the transition from uterine to extrauterine existence. Neonatal resuscitation is a set of sequential psychomotor skills. Familiarity with physiologic changes that occur around the time of birth enables members of the resuscitation team to better understand the reasons for the sequence of resuscitative actions. This knowledge is of practical value when making therapeutic decisions in caring for infants who do not respond to initial resuscitative efforts. Additionally, difficult resuscitations require a coordinated team effort with each team member interacting in a constructive manner. Therefore, successful resuscitation is the culmination of several components: familiarity with fetal/neonatal physiology, practiced manual skills, presence of proper equipment, preparation, leadership, and teamwork.

PHYSIOLOGY

In utero, oxygenated blood (with a pO_2 only in the low 30 torr range) is carried to fetus from the placenta via the umbilical vein. The umbilical venous blood passes through the liver, through the ductus venosus

TABLE 1. **Risk Factors for Neonatal Resuscitation**

Maternal Factors	Antepartum Factors	Perinatal Factors
Insulin-dependent diabetes	Multiple gestation	Preterm labor
Fever/infection	Fetal malformations	Fetal distress
Hypertension	Oligo/polyhydramnios	Prolapsed cord
Vaginal bleeding	Prolonged rupture of membranes	Abruptio placentae
Drug abuse	Fetal size: small/large for gestational age	Meconium stained amniotic fluid
No or late prenatal care	Abnormal fetal presentation	Emergent operative delivery
Severe systemic diseases	Abnormal stress test	
Isoimmunization		

and enters the inferior vena cava; much of this relatively oxygenated blood then passes through the right atrium and foramen ovale into the left atrium and finally flows into the left ventricle and out through the aorta. This pathway results in delivery of the most oxygenated blood to the fetal brain. Because aortic blood flow has continuity with the low-pressure placenta via the umbilical arteries, the systemic circuit is the low pressure circuit, in utero. Conversely, because of the relatively low fetal blood pH and pO_2, the pulmonary vascular bed is constricted and offers high resistance to flow. Because of this high pulmonary vascular resistance, approximately 10% of the right ventricular output (largely received from the superior vena cava) flows into the fetal lungs. The remainder passes through the ductus arteriosus (DA) and enters the proximal descending aorta, where it mixes with the more oxygenated aortic blood. At birth, clamping of the umbilical cord immediately transforms the systemic circulation into a high-resistance circuit. The newborn then enters a phase of transitional circulation in which the ductus arteriosus gradually closes and the pulmonary vascular resistance (PVR) rapidly decreases, enabling increased pulmonary blood flow and oxygenation. Decreased PVR and closure of the DA are dependent upon two factors: normalization of both oxygenation and pH. The relevance of these physiologic processes to resuscitation steps is clear: initiation of effective ventilation is necessary for oxygenation and exhalation of carbon dioxide (which, in excess, will cause respiratory acidosis and continued constriction of the pulmonary vascular bed). Pulmonary fluid must also be absorbed from the alveolar spaces. Ventilation decreases hydrostatic pressure in the pulmonary circuit and improvement of pulmonary blood flow improves alveolar fluid absorption. Further measures such as volume expansion and medications may be required to correct severe metabolic acidosis and to support cardiac output.

ASPHYXIA AND APNEA

Fetal and neonatal asphyxia occur when there is inadequate cellular perfusion and oxygenation; it is biochemically characterized by hypoxia, hypercarbia, and metabolic acidosis. Both the fetus and newborn may initially be capable of compensating for the hypoxia with tachycardia and vasoconstriction—reflexes that maintain perfusion of vital organs. Without resolution, metabolic acidosis worsens and both the heart rate and blood pressure begin to fall. Intrauterine asphyxia is clinically characterized by alterations in fetal heart rate, passing meconium (in term or near-term gestations), gasping respirations, and, finally, apnea. This first apneic episode is termed primary apnea. If the asphyxic insult does not resolve, the fetal heart rate may fall, there may be a series of spontaneous deep gasps followed by a second apneic period: secondary apnea. In the delivery room, apneic newborns are in a state of primary or secondary apnea. Infants with primary apnea have not suffered from physiologic decompensation and although they may be cyanotic or bradycardic, spontaneous respirations can be induced by vigorous drying or a brief

TABLE 2. **Equipment Used During Delivery Room Neonatal Resuscitation**

Precheck: Presence, Functionality, Cleanliness
Thermal environment
Warm room temperature
Overhead radiant warmer or heat lamps
Towels, warmed blankets, stocking caps
Clear airway
Suction apparatus (bulb syringe, suction devices)
Meconium aspirator attachment
Suction catheters (use largest practical for infant's size: 6, 8, 10 Fr)
Breathing (ventilation)
Self-inflating bag or anesthesia bag with manometer (preferred)
Oxygen
Neonatal face masks—newborn and premature sizes
Laryngoscope
Straight blades, sizes 00, 0, and 1
Endotracheal tubes; sizes 2.5, 3.0, 3.5, and 4.0
Stethoscope
Circulation
Umbilical catheterization set
Intravenous solutions (and associated lines, needles, syringes)
50% dextrose in water, 10% dextrose in water, normal saline
Drugs (see Table 3)
Miscellaneous equipment
Sterile gloves
Stylets (for endotracheal tubes)
Tape, scissors, alcohol swabs, skin prep
Light source
Oximeter

period of positive pressure ventilation. In contrast, infants born with secondary apnea have suffered from more severe and prolonged axphyxic insults. These infants are often more profoundly bradycardic, have markedly diminished muscle tone, moderate to severe acidosis, and will not initiate spontaneous ventilation after stimulation or initial bagging. Depending upon the severity of the asphyxia, the PVR may remain elevated, lung fluid clearance delayed, and additional fluid may leak into the lungs because of capillary damage. These infants often require prolonged bagging or intubation, increased initial inspiratory pressures, correction of hypovolemia and resuscitative drugs. Fortunately, the vast majority of infants will respond to stimulation, suctioning and a few inspiratory breaths. However, the resuscitation team must have all equipment and medications readily available or accessible to effectively manage the unexpected, asphyxiated infant birth (Tables 1 to 3).

APGAR SCORE

The Apgar score (Table 4) provides an objective, quantitative measure of an infant's condition in the first minutes after birth. Resuscitation should not be interrupted to determine an Apgar score. The score is most useful in assessing an infant's response to resuscitative interventions. A rising score—especially heart rate, muscle tone and respiratory effort—are important indicators of infant improvement. A decreasing score is extremely serious and requires immediate reassessment of interventions.

ABCs OF RESUSCITATION

The essential initial efforts of resuscitation are geared toward:

1. Lung expansion and initiation of ventilation and oxygenation: the "primacy of ventilation"
2. Maintaining adequate cardiac output and tissue perfusion
3. Concurrent with items 1 and 2, avoiding hyper- or hypothermia and avoiding hypoglycemia

The sequence of resuscitation actions follows the "ABCs" (airway, breathing, and circulation); however, assessments of an infant's physiologic status (e.g., respirations, heart rate, tone, color) are done concurrently and continuously throughout the resuscitation process. An initial rapid wiping of the newborn's face and chest will provide a dry stable platform for bagging and for performing external cardiac massage. Quickly drying will also decrease evaporative heat loss. If possible, resuscitation should be performed under a pre-heated, radiant warmer.

Drying must not delay airway management and ventilation in the apneic and/or bradycardic infant.

A: Airway

Rapidly and immediately clear the airway of fluid by bulb suction or catheter. Use the largest catheter size practical (e.g., size 10 Fr). Small-lumen catheters are inefficient, and prolonged suctioning can stimulate

TABLE 3. **Drugs for Resuscitation/Stabilization**

Medication	Concentration	Dosage/Route	Indications	Comment
Epinephrine	1:10,000	Endotracheal umbilical venous catheter/0.1–0.3 mL/kg/dose	Asystole Bradycardia inunresponsive to inventilation	Effective via endotracheal tube; Dilute dose with 1–3 mL of normal saline for endotracheal use Do not wait for intravenous access Do not wait for accurate weight: preterm/SGA, give 0.5 mL; term/LGA, give 1.0 mL May repeat dosage every 3–5 minutes
Volume expanders Normal saline Ringer's lactate Whole blood		Umbilical venous catheter or UAC/10 mL/kg		Use for hypovolemia or shock Acute blood loss requires acute blood replacement May repeat dosage
Glucose	10%	Intravenous; 2 mL/kg 5% or 10% dextrose in saline in maintenance fluids	Hypoglycemia	Documented hypoglycemia Post-resuscitation fluids; Early maintenance fluids in LGA/SGA neonates
Sodium bicarbonate	0.5 mEq/mL	Intravenous; 2 mL/kg	Documented metabolic acidosis Severe asphyxia Prolonged resuscitation	Must have effective ventilation; Hypertonic: Administer slowly ~2 mL/min
Surfactant (Survanta)	No dilution	Endotracheal; 4 mL/kg: 2 mL/kg in each mainstem bronchus Or, 4 mL in one dose in extreme situations	Documented or suspected respiratory distress syndrome	May be administered in delivery room; may be useful in respiratory distress resulting from meconium aspiration

LGA, large for gestational age; SGA, small for gestational age.

TABLE 4. **Apgar Score**

Sign	0	1	2
Heart rate	Absent	<100 beats/minute	>100 beats/minute
Respiratory effort	Absent	Slow or irregular	Cry
Muscle tone	Flaccid	Some flexion	Active; good tone
Reflex irritability (using suction catheter or bulb syringe)	No response	Grimace	Cough or sneeze
Color	Pale or cyanotic	Pink body; blue extremities	Totally pink

reflexes that result in bradycardia and hypotension. Place the infant's head in a neutral or slightly extended position (the "sniffing" position). A small towel roll beneath the shoulders may assist in getting the infant in a sniffing position, but is usually unnecessary and can waste precious time if not prepositioned.

B: Breathing (Positive Pressure Ventilation—PPV)

Indications for PPV include: apnea, gasping respirations, or bradycardia (<100 beats/minute). An infant with primary apnea may start spontaneous respirations with the stimulation provided by rubbing or drying—or after a few effective PPV breaths. Infants with secondary apnea will need prolonged face mask PPV or eventual endotracheal intubation and ventilation. Both neonatal-sized self-inflating and anesthesia PPV bags are effective. Advantages and disadvantages of each type are shown in Table 5. When preparing anesthesia bags, an oxygen source flow rate of 8–10 L/min with a the bag's release valve set for a resultant continuous positive airway pressure (CPAP) of 8–10 cm H_2O provides adequate initial flows for bagging or allowing an infant to breathe against CPAP (Figure 1). An effective technique of securing the face mask and providing jaw-thrust when performing bag-mask PPV is shown in Figure 2.

Inspiratory pressures are variable and are related to the infant's size, lung compliance, and opening pressures needed for initial lung expansion. Initial opening pressures of 60–80 cm H_2O (or more) may be needed for an asphyxiated, term infant whose lungs are filled with fluid. The mean initial inspiratory pressure for a term, apneic infant is around 40 cm H_2O. Spontaneously breathing infants can often be ventilated with initial pressures of 25–30 cm H_2O. After the lung's opening pressure is reached, subsequent breaths require less pressure. An inline manometer is an invaluable tool in assessing the pressure being delivered and in adjusting it. As a general clinical guide, pressures must be sufficient to create visible chest wall movement (not excessive); pressures are usually adequate if one can auscultate breath sounds. An increasing heart rate is the best indicator of effective ventilation.

Pressures needed to ventilate premature infants are not well-defined and range from 14 to 30 cm H_2O. If a premature infant has spontaneous ventilations after a few PPV breaths and a good heart rate (>100/min), one can try delivering CPAP via an anesthesia bag; at times intubation can be avoided with this technique.

Forty to 60 breaths/min is the generally accepted initial rate of ventilation. The rate can be slowed as the infant's heart rate increases and spontaneous respirations begin.

Intubation

Intubation is the only way to ensure airway control. Indications for intubation include: anticipated need for positive pressure mechanical ventilation, administration of surfactant, intratracheal meconium aspiration, ineffective manual bag ventilation, upper airway obstruction, and need for chest compression during resuscitation. A guide for endotracheal tube size and

TABLE 5. **Positive Pressure Ventilation**

Anesthesia Bags	Self-inflating Bags
Advantages:	*Advantages:*
Can deliver 100% oxygen	Ease of use
Control over inspiratory pressures and time	Self-inflation (not dependent upon external source of air or oxygen)
Inline manometer	
Can deliver continuous positive airway pressure (CPAP)	
Disadvantages:	*Disadvantages:*
Requires practice	Need oxygen reservoir attachment
Requires external compressed oxygen source	Poor feel of lung compliance
Small changes in flow-control valve can lead to underinflation or excessively high pressures	Poor control of inspiratory pressures
	Difficult to retrofit with inline manometer or CPAP devices

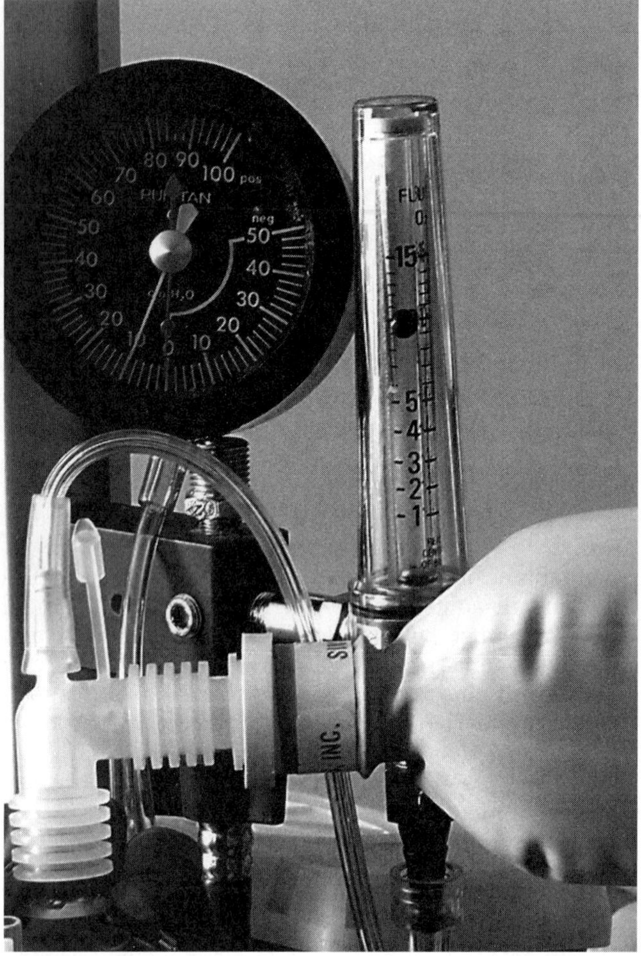

Figure 1. Anesthesia bag preparation. Setting the initial flow rate to 8–10 liters/minute and the end-respiratory pressure to 8–10 cm/H_2O allows for effective bag filling while providing positive pressure ventilation.

depth of insertion are shown in Table 6. The endotracheal tube's position should be evaluated at the bedside by auscultation: breath sounds must be equal on each side. After breath sounds are determined to be equal, the tube's position must be compulsively "guarded" until the tube is taped into position (Figure 3). The tube's position should be confirmed by chest radiograph; but this does not have to be

TABLE 6. **Endotracheal Tube Guide Approximate Internal Diameter and Depth of Insertion**

Birth Weight (grams)	Depth of Insertion (cm from lip)	Gestational Age (weeks)	Tube Size (mm internal diameter)
500	6–6.5	<25	2.5
<1000	**6**–7 cm	**25**	**2.5**
>**1000**	**7** cm	**30**	**3.0**
>**2000**	**8** cm	**35**	3.0–**3.5**
>**3000**	**9** cm	**40**	3.5–**4.0**
>**4000**	**10** cm	>40	4.0

Numbers in **bold** type highlight the numerical sequence to aid in memorization.

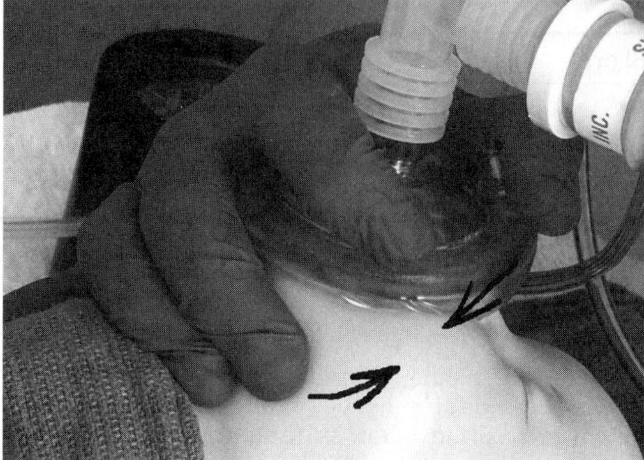

Figure 2. Proper placement and seal of face mask. The thumb and third finger (which is on the mandible or ramus of the mandible) are being squeezed towards each other. These combined force vectors create a tight seal without any net downward force on the mouth or jaw. The resuscitator maintains an upward force on his/her forearm. The net result of tensing the forearm towards the resuscitator is an effective "jaw thrust" vector which tends to keep the posterior tongue from obstructing the airway.

performed in the delivery room if the infant's condition is improving.

Oxygen

One hundred percent oxygen (or the maximum oxygen concentration available) is used for resuscitation. Resuscitations have been successful using room air; therefore, ventilation should not be delayed if an oxygen source is not available. Oxygen concentration may be gradually decreased in infants successfully resuscitated to the percentage needed to maintain normoxia.

Interference

A distended stomach can hinder diaphragmatic movement; rapid placement of a nasogastric (NG) or orogastric (OG) tube will suffice for decompression. However, placement of an OG or NG tube must be timed so as not to interfere with the process of intubation or performance of manual bag-mask-ventilation (BMV). Likewise, drying the infant's torso and extremities must not interfere with these essential processes. The resuscitator providing ventilation must control the sequence and timing of these actions (see Resuscitation Team Management).

C: Circulation

External Cardiac Massage

After 30 seconds of effective PPV, external cardiac massage is begun if the heart rate is less than 60 beats/minute. The two techniques of external cardiac massage—two thumb-chest encircling and the two finger technique—are shown in Figures 4 and 5. The thumbs or fingers are placed on the infant's sternum below the nipple line and above the xiphoid process; the chest is compressed one third of its diameter.

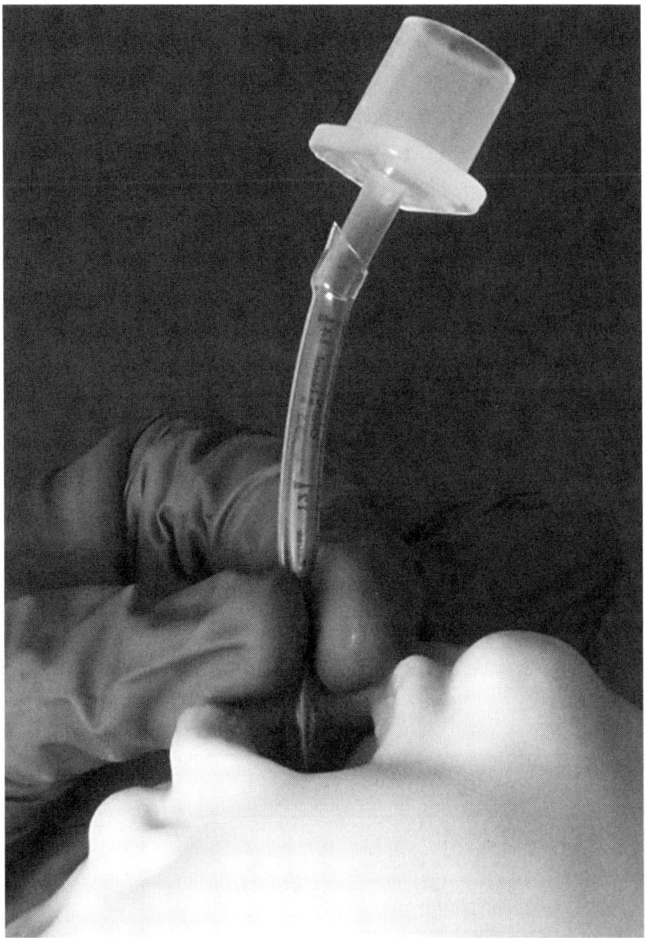

Figure 3. "Guarding" the endotracheal tube. Until the E-T tube is securely taped in place, it must be prevented from slipping during bagging.

Chest compressions are coordinated with ventilation with a breath:compression ratio of 3:1 This sequence is rapidly performed with three compressions and one inhalation breath performed in two seconds—this will result in 30 breaths/min and 90 compressions/minute. The two-thumb technique is felt to provide better

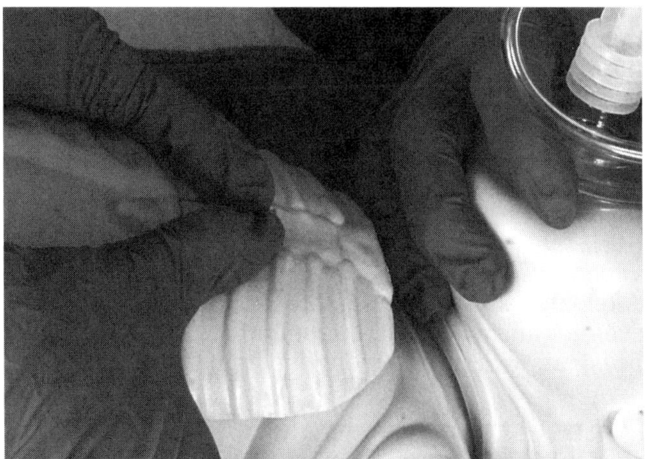

Figure 4. Two-thumb chest-encircling external cardiac massage. This is the preferred technique. Note that the thumbs are above the xyphoid process and are in the mid-sternum region.

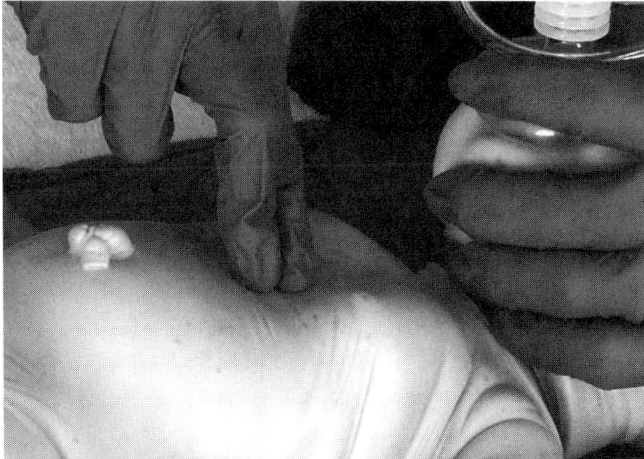

Figure 5. Two-finger external cardiac massage. Fingers are above xyphoid process; approximately one finger width beneath the nipple line. This technique is useful when an umbilical catheter is being inserted.

cardiac output and a more controlled depth of compression. However, if an umbilical line is being inserted during cardiac compression, the two-finger technique is more practical as it allows the compressor to stand aside and provides physical access to the infant's abdominal area. If the heart rate does not begin to increase after 30 seconds of external cardiac massage and ventilation, 1:10,000 epinephrine is administered either via the endotracheal (ET) tube or umbilical vein (see Drugs, Table 3).

Volume Expansion

Indications for volume expansion are: pallor, poor capillary filling, tachycardia or bradycardia, known or suspected blood loss/hemorrhage, or hypotension. Do not wait for hypotension to be proven before giving fluids. Acute blood loss should be replaced as soon as possible with red blood cells. If fetal blood loss is suspected and time permits, O-negative blood (cross-matched against the mother) can be made available for immediate administration.

The umbilical vein provides the most rapid vascular access. The umbilical vein is usually easily accessed and a saline filled, air-free umbilical venous catheter (UVC), or sterile feeding tube if a UVC is not available, can be gently and quickly inserted into the umbilical vein (Figure 6). Ideally, the UVC should be advanced until there is a free-flow of blood upon aspiration; however, with the exception of sodium bicarbonate, which is very hypertonic, isotonic fluids, blood, and epinephrine can be administered without documentation of catheter position so long as there seems to be no resistance to the fluid push. Intraosseous needle insertion is not routinely performed, but is an acceptable method of access if UVC is unsuccessful.

D: Drugs

Epinephrine is the primary drug of resuscitation. It is rapidly administered via ET tube or UVC if an

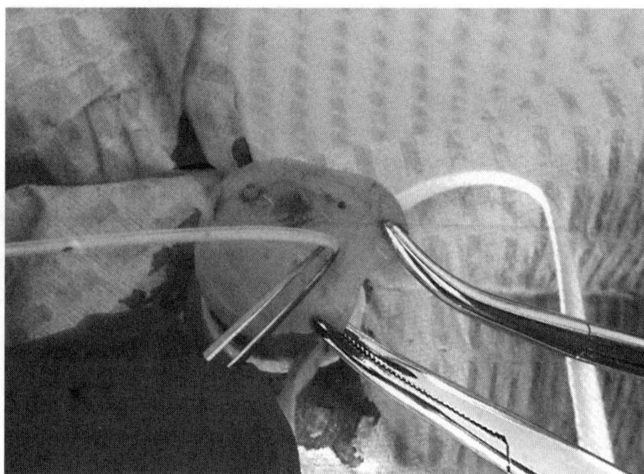

Figure 6. Umbilical vein catheterization. The umbilical vein is the preferred route for immediate venous access for drug medication and volume administraion.

infant remains bradycardic after effective BVM or ET tube bagging. Only 1:10,000 epinephrine is recommended for neonates. Use the higher dose, 0.3 mL/kg, when administering via ET route folowed by 1–2 mL normal saline flush. In the sequence of resuscitative steps, an infant receiving epinephrine will already be receiving manual ventilation and external cardiac massage. Volume-expanding fluids will either have been administered or will be in the process of being drawn up for administration.

Naloxone (Narcan) is rarely needed; it is only given to otherwise stable infants whose apnea appears to be solely related to recent maternal narcotic administration. Do not give Narcan to infants born to women with known or suspected drug abuse or women on methadone maintenance therapy because it may precipitate seizures.

Surfactant (Survanta) may be given in the delivery room to premature infants with respiratory distress. All infants who require resuscitation should be monitored for hypoglycemia. Intravenous glucose should be started on those who needed volume expansion or drugs for resuscitation.

E: Evaluation/Evacuation

Resuscitation is a sequence of continual assessments, therapeutic interventions, and reassessments of the responses to the actions taken (Figure 7). When an infant in not improving, one must look for "errors" or complications. First, visually walk from the wall oxygen outlet to the infant: Is the oxygen flowing? Are the manometer line and all air/oxygen lines attached? The mnemonic "DOPE" helps evaluate common complications:

D: Is the endotracheal tube **D**islodged? Is it in the right or left mainstem bronchus?

O: Is the endotracheal tube **O**bstructed?

P: Is there a **P**neumothorax? If a tension pneumothorax is diagnosed, it must be **E**vacuated.

E: Is the **E**sophagus intubated?

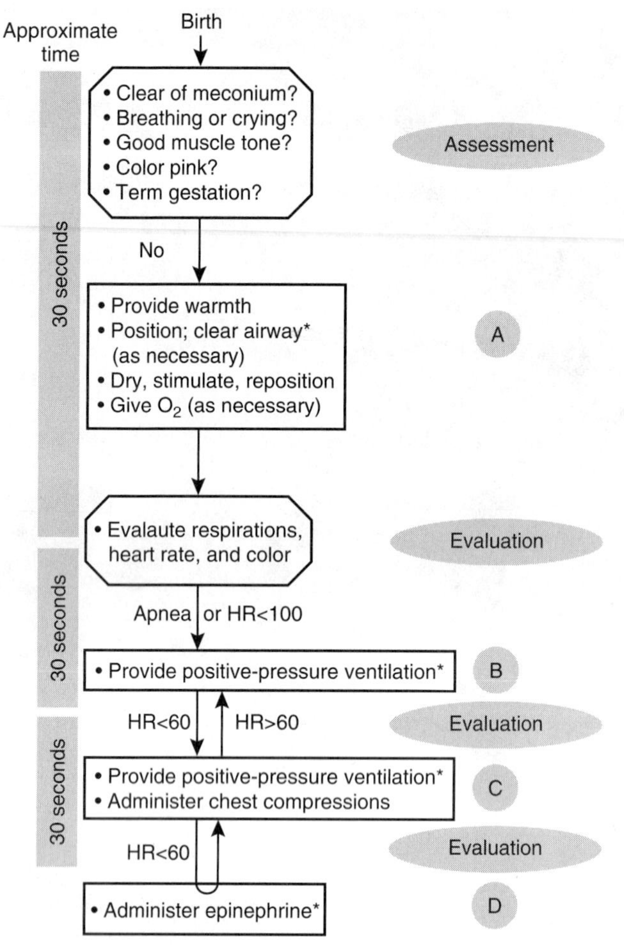

Figure 7. Resuscitation sequence. From Textbook of Neonatal Resuscitation, 4th Edition. American Academy of Pediatrics.

MECONIUM

An infant can aspirate meconium in utero or upon its first breath. Rapid suctioning of the oropharynx upon delivery of the head may prevent or minimize meconium aspiration. A vigorous, crying infant does not require laryngeal intubation and suctioning. However, a limp, bradycardic, or apneic infant should be immediately intubated and suction then applied to the ET tube. If thick meconium enters the tube, continue suctioning until the meconium flow stops. Remove the tube and immediately reintubate with a fresh tube. This process must be repeated until thick, viscous, obstructive meconium is no longer obtained. After the tube remains patent during suctioning—even if scanty flecks of meconium are seen—PPV can be begun without removing the final tube.

RESUSCITATION TEAM MANAGEMENT

All deliveries should be attended by an individual skilled in initiating resuscitation and whose primary responsibility is assessment of the neonate immediately

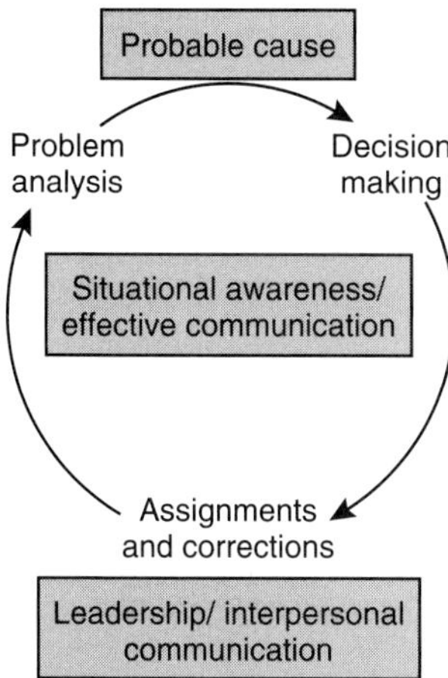

Figure 8. Resuscitation Team Management.

after birth. The most senior or experienced resuscitator customarily stands at the infant's head and is in charge of the airway and directs the resuscitative interventions. Resuscitation of the critically ill infant is a team effort. The team must coordinate activities, interact effectively, and communicate with one another. Wide variation in team members' experience, education, professional responsibilities, and technical skills must not be allowed to hinder the team's function. Degradation of team function—or behavioral problems—can be grouped into categories of: interpersonal communication, situational awareness and leadership. Barriers to interpersonal communication can be caused by status differential (differences in professional background) or personality conflicts. Team members must not involve personalities in communicating relevant clinical data. The team leader must listen to comments and data presented and give feedback to the sender—either verbally or by gesture. Lack of acknowledgment of a message may cause the sender to be hesitant in relaying further observations or suggestions. Situational awareness is an understanding of what events are occurring at the moment and the relationship of immediate events to what has happened in the past and what may happen in the future. Situational awareness is based upon one's past experiences and involvement in the current event—and will affect the decision process. Boredom, complacency, and uncertainty can degrade situational awareness; the team leader should support new team members and clarify issues to give them a holistic perspective of the care being given and planned. Teams are lead by a designated leader—the most senior or experienced person present. However, leader-follower roles are interchangeable. A functional leader is the person who has the most information about the current situation and can modify the decision process by their influence. A functional follower temporarily defers to the person with the most information or immediate skill set. All team members must be concerned about "what" is right, not "who" is right. Recommendations by team members are not to be considered as a challenge to the designated leader. These interactions are shown in Figure 8.

CARE OF THE HIGH-RISK NEONATE

method of
TOMMY LEONARD, Jr., M.D.
Baylor College of Medicine
Houston, Texas

More than 400,000 infants in the United States are born with conditions that classify them as high-risk neonates. High-risk neonates are infants requiring complex medical and surgical treatment. Ideally, their care should be provided in a hospital commensurate with their medical and surgical needs and managed by a neonatologist. Unavoidably, infants are delivered in situations that are not optimal for successful management, thus the potential for high morbidity and mortality. Current guidelines for regional perinatal services (Table 1) may assist the primary care provider in making an appropriate and timely referral.

A carefully taken maternal history may with some degree of accuracy predict which infants will require a higher level of care. Many circumstances, both maternal and neonatal, will alert the provider to conditions that require strong consideration for transferring the mother before delivery (Table 2). The most experienced provider should assess the mother for imminence of delivery and risk of transport. Factors to consider before transporting the mother are gravida status, parity, dilation and effacement, well-being of the mother and infant, and the time required for transport. If it is not possible to transport the mother before delivery, it is the provider's responsibility to plan for, receive, stabilize, and coordinate transport of the critically ill neonate.

Time is precious and becomes one of the early constraints during the planning phase. One way to maximize the time available is to have a pre-existing plan for such an event. Once delivery has occurred, the focus must be on management of the airway, breathing, and circulation (ABCs) of the infant.

It is imperative to have a health care provider who is technically competent and to have the appropriate equipment available to execute the pre-existing resuscitation and transport plan. Technical competence comes from having the necessary training and ongoing updates in specific areas of concern. Managing critically ill neonates is well addressed in the Neonatal Resuscitation Program (NRP) sponsored by the American Heart Association and the American Academy of Pediatrics. If an institution is involved in obstetric care, regardless of the level, it is highly recommended that the staff be certified as NRP providers and receive the necessary updates. Another necessity for a successful outcome is the availability of appropriate-sized equipment. As a minimum, the equipment listed in Table 3 is recommended.

The prenatal history is also vital in the planning phase. Many disorders that exist during pregnancy can give clues to potential abnormalities in the newborn. Premature labor with delivery of an infant less than 37 weeks' gestation has an increased risk of hyaline membrane disease that is inversely proportional

TABLE 1. **Levels of Inpatient Perinatal Care**

Basic Perinatal Center	Specialty Perinatal Center	Subspecialty Perinatal Center
Function Includes:	*Function Includes:*	*Function Includes:*
Management of newborns with uncomplicated conditions and those requiring emergency resuscitation and/or stabilization for transport	Management of newborns with selected complications and conditions Expanded capabilities could include: Moderately ill newborns with problems expected to resolve rapidly	Management of normal newborns, moderately ill newborns, and extremely ill newborns
Risk assessment to identify need for consultation/referral	Extremely ill newborns requiring stabilization before transfer Recovering infants who can be transferred from a perinatal center	Neonatal intensive care unit staffed and equipped to treat critically ill neonates with a sufficient intermediate care area for convalescing and moderately ill neonates
Capability to resuscitate and stabilize infants in the delivery room and/or nursery with formal education in resuscitation such as the NRP	Consultation and/or referral to a subspecialty center for infants requiring ventilation for >6 h Risk assessment with consultation and referral based on guidelines	Provision of continuing education relative to neonatal care and stabilization
Continuing education consistent with the patient population served	Continuing education consistent with the population served	

Additional guidelines apply to obstetric services and the support services. This table addresses only inpatient neonatal services.

Abbreviation: NRP, Neonatal Resuscitation Program.

Adapted from Toward improving the outcome of pregnancy: The 90's and beyond. March of Dimes Birth Defects Foundation, 1993. From Khan A, Denson S: Care of the high-risk neonate. In Rakel RE (ed): Conn's Current Therapy 1999. Philadelphia, WB Saunders, 1999.

TABLE 2. **Perinatal Risk Factors for Subspecialty Intensive Care**

	Maternal	Fetal/Neonatal
Antepartum	Previous abnormal pregnancies	Congenital anomalies
	Diabetes, thyroid disease	Multiple gestation
	Hypertension/toxemia	Fetal growth restriction
	Immune thrombocytopenia	Polyhydramnios
	Collagen vascular, autoimmune disease	Oligohydramnios
	Substance abuse/smoking	
	Rh isoimmunization	
	Cardiovascular disease	
	Myasthenia gravis, myotonic dystrophy	
	Epilepsy	
	Pulmonary disease with hypoxemia or hypercapnia	
	Renal or other chronic disease while taking medications	
	Vaginal colonization with *Chlamydia*, *Ureaplasma*, or group B hemolytic streptococci	
	Infection: bacterial (gonorrhea, syphilis, tuberculosis), viral (rubella, cytomegalovirus, varicella), parasitic (toxoplasmosis)	
Intrapartum	Fever/chorioamnionitis	Fetal distress
	Bleeding from placental abruption or previa	Meconium-stained amniotic fluid
	Prolonged or premature rupture of membranes	Pulmonary immaturity
	Premature labor	Perinatal depression
	Herpes genitalis	Breech/malpresentation
	Hypotension/shock	Prolapsed umbilical cord
	Operative delivery (forceps, vacuum, cesarean section)	Fetal blood loss
Postnatal		Birth asphyxia
		Hypotension/shock
		Metabolic acidosis, hypoglycemia, hypothermia
		Respiratory distress
		Cyanosis
		Congenital anomalies
		Prematurity/postmaturity
		Large or small for gestational age
		Infection/sepsis
		Anemia/polycythemia
		Nonimmune hydrops
		Seizures

TABLE 3. **Neonatal Resuscitation Supplies and Equipment**

Suction equipment: bulb syringe, mechanical suction and tubing, suction catheters (5 or 6, 8, and 10 or 12 F), 8-F feeding tube and 10-mL syringe, meconium aspirator device
Bag-and-mask equipment: neonatal resuscitation bag with a pressure-release valve or pressure manometer (the bag must be capable of delivering 90% to 100% oxygen), face masks (newborn and premature sizes; masks with cushioned rim preferred), oxygen with flowmeter (flow rate up to 10 L/min) and tubing (including portable oxygen cylinders)
Intubation equipment: laryngoscope with straight blades (no. 0 for preterm and no. 1 for term), extra bulbs and batteries for laryngoscope, tracheal tubes (2.5, 3.0, 3.5, and 4.0 mm ID), stylet (optional), scissors, tape or securing device for tracheal tube, alcohol sponges, CO_2 detector (optional), laryngeal mask airway (optional)
Medications: epinephrine 1:10,000; isotonic crystalloid (normal saline or Ringer's lactate); sodium bicarbonate 4.2%; nalaxone hydrochloride; normal saline; dextrose 10%; normal saline "fish" or "bullet" (optional); 5-F feeding tube (optional)
Umbilical vessel catheterization supplies: sterile gloves, scalped or scissors, providone-iodine solution, umbilical tape, umbilical catheters (3.5 and 5 F), three-way stopcock, syringes (1, 3, 5, 10, 20, and 50 mL), needles (25, 21, and 18 G) or puncture device for needleless system
Miscellaneous: gloves and appropriate personal protection; radiant warmer or other heat source; firm, padded resuscitation surface; clock (timer optional); warmed linens; stethoscope; tape (1/2 or 3/4 in); cardiac monitor and electrodes and/or pulse oximeter with probe (optional for delivery room); oropharyngeal airways

Data from Pediatrics 2000;106(3):29.

to gestational age. The infant of a diabetic mother has a risk not only of premature lung disease but also macrosomia and an increased risk of dystocia, asphyxia, hypoglycemia, cyanotic congenital heart disease, and caudal regression.

Receiving a critical neonate requires focus on the ABCs. Within the first 30 seconds, the adequacy of the airway should be assessed. An infant less than 28 weeks' gestation usually requires assisted bag-and-mask ventilation, followed by tracheal intubation. The infant initially establishes a reasonable breathing effort, but because of surfactant deficiency, respiratory failure ensues. The distress is indicated by chest retractions, nasal flaring, grunting, and central cyanosis without supplemental oxygen. In this situation, it is necessary to provide oxygen at 100% and proceed with interventions to minimize the stress of heat loss and increased oxygen consumption. Ongoing assessment of the adequacy of breathing is essential. If increased work of breathing or apnea is observed, the infant must be intubated without delay. Although in some instances providing continuous distending airway pressure may support some infants and avoid the need for early tracheal intubation, the usual treatment of apnea is intubation.

The adequacy of circulation is determined first by checking the heart rate. If the heart rate is less than 60 beats per minute, chest compressions are indicated. Any infant with a sustained heart rate less than 100 should receive positive-pressure ventilation, which can be provided by bag and mask for a short period until endotracheal intubation can be accomplished. If the heart rate is 60 beats per minute or less in spite of chest compressions and positive-pressure ventilation, epinephrine (1:10,000), 0.1 to 0.3 mL/kg, is indicated. Initially, it can be administered through the endotracheal tube. Dosing can be repeated every 3 to 5 minutes until the heart rate is 100 beats per minute or more. Seldom is this amount of intervention required in the delivery suite. Usually, with oxygenation and positive-pressure ventilation, the infant responds readily with improved color and an increased heart rate. If hypovolemia is suspected, venous access for the administration of a volume expander is immediately required. The most accessible access route would be the umbilical vein. Once access is accomplished, the infant must be given a volume expander, 10 to 20 mL/kg of normal saline infused slowly over a period of 5 to 10 minutes. This dose may be repeated after clinical assessment and observation for a response. If ongoing blood loss is documented, the infant should be reassessed and volume replacement administered. The umbilical vein catheter is secured with tape and/or suture. A quick reference for all the interventions just described can be obtained in Figure 1.

FLUID AND ELECTROLYTES

Once the infant has been successfully stabilized, attention turns to fluid and electrolyte balance. The initial focus is on the water needs of the infant. Physicians are well aware of the accepted weight loss of 5% to 10% in the first week of life in a full-term infant; however, premature infants can lose up to 20% of their birth weight in the first week. Inadequate caloric intake plays some role in this loss of weight, but the major factor is contraction of the extracellular fluid space (ECF). Insensible water loss (IWL) plays a significant role in this contraction of the ECF space. The starting rate for maintenance fluids is 5% to 10% dextrose in water at 80 to 100 mL/kg/d. This rate of fluid administration should provide 4 to 8 mg of glucose per kilogram per minute. It should also be remembered that IWL is inversely related to gestational age. It is crucial to track the infant's weight to appreciate the dramatic fluid loss, particularly in premature infants. By also monitoring urine output, weight loss, and serum sodium, IWL can be better compensated. Certain factors may exaggerate IWL, including lack of humidity and the use of phototherapy. Acute management of a critically ill infant is confined to such a short period before transport that a detailed endeavor into the fine-tuning of fluids and electrolytes is beyond the scope of this writing. If the infant remains in your care for longer than 24 hours, it is recommended that sodium, potassium, and calcium be added to the administered fluids. The recommendation for sodium is 1 to 3 mEq/kg/d; potassium, 1 to 2 mEq/kg/d; and calcium, 200 mg/kg/d of 10% calcium gluconate. These additives need to be included in the dextrose solution that will be administered over a 24-hour period.

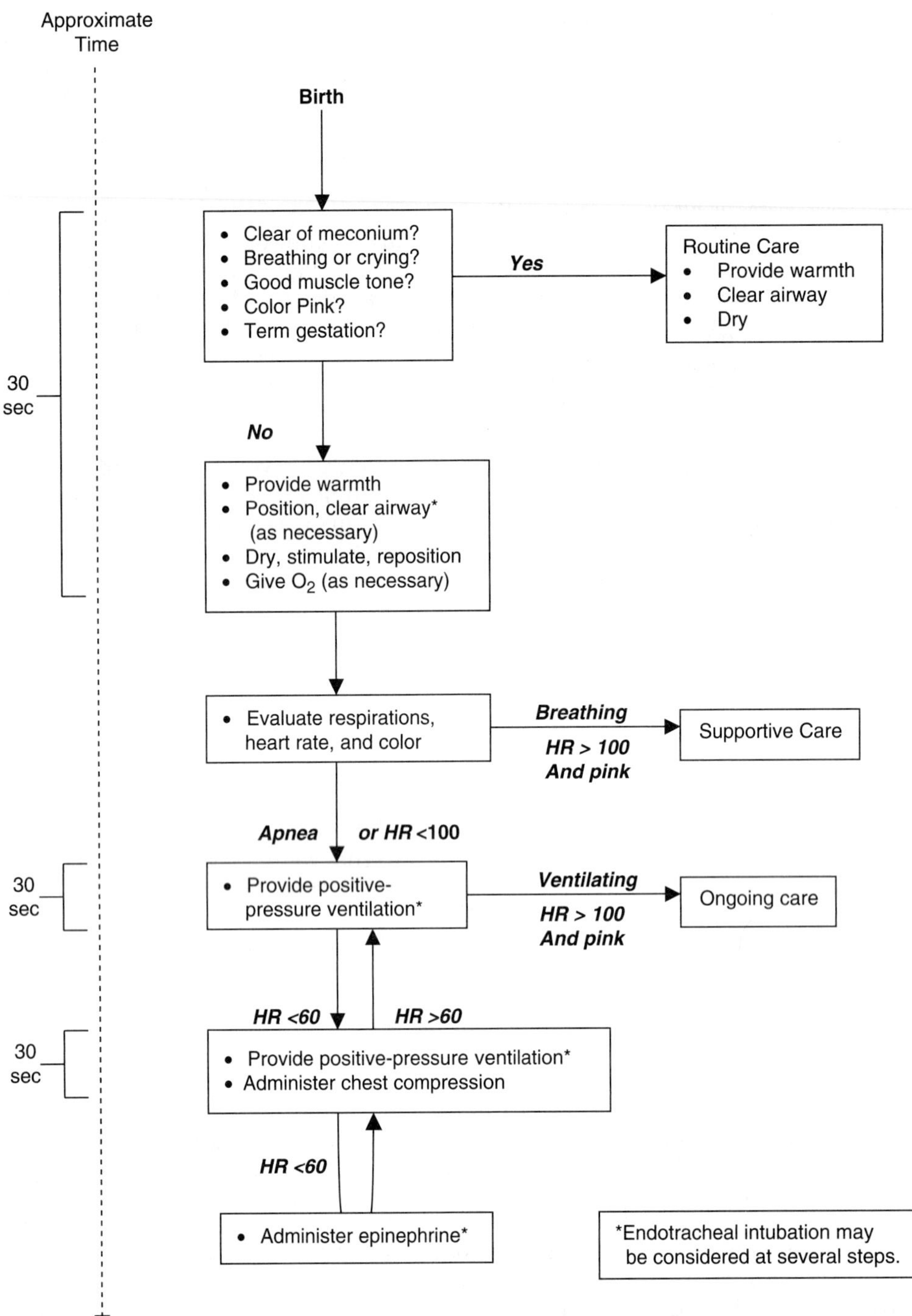

Figure 1. Algorithm for resuscitation of a newly born infant. Abbreviation: HR = heart rate. (Modified from Kattwinkel I (ed): Textbook of Neonatal Resuscitation, 4th ed. Chicago, American Heart Association and American Academy of Pediatrics, 2000.)

CYANOTIC NEWBORN

Cyanosis is classically defined as a bluish discoloration of the skin and mucous membranes resulting from the presence of at least 3 to 5 g/dL of reduced hemoglobin in the systemic capillaries. It is important to distinguish cyanosis as central or peripheral. Peripheral cyanosis is often associated with a response to a cool environment; however, it can also be associated with slow capillary blood flow and a reduction in oxyhemoglobin at a local level. Central cyanosis can be related to a number of conditions, and it would be prudent to be aware of these entities (Table 4).

If cyanosis is suspected, the best approach is to consider infection first as an etiology. Assuming that the ABCs of managing an acutely ill newborn have been accomplished, a more in-depth evaluation should follow. Because sepsis can have many signs and symptoms, trying to sort them out may be difficult, and the time wasted is not beneficial. This in-depth evaluation needs to include a sepsis workup; complete blood count; blood, urine, and spinal fluid cultures; and administration of antibiotics. Occasionally, an infant's condition will not withstand the positioning for a lumbar puncture, so in these situations, institution of antibiotics should proceed without delay after the blood culture. The antibiotics of choice are ampicillin and an aminoglycoside. Depending on the maternal history, age at evaluation, and other clinical signs such as skin rash, bleeding diathesis, and seizures, herpesvirus must be considered and appropriate cultures from the conjunctiva, oropharynx, and rectum obtained. In addition, acyclovir (Zovirax) must be initiated at a dosage of 20 mg/kg every 8 hours.

After the initiation of antibiotics, the hyperoxia test is performed. Placing the patient in an ambient oxygen environment of 100% oxygen under an oxygen hood for 5 minutes and obtaining an arterial blood gas measurement can accomplish the hyperoxia test. If the initial arterial blood gas has a PaO_2 greater than 150 mm Hg, the presence of cyanotic congenital heart disease is unlikely. If it is less than 150 mm Hg, the ability to exclude a right-to-left shunt based on the hyperoxia is limited. Initiating nasal continuous positive airway pressure at 6 cm H_2O for 15 minutes and repeating the arterial blood gas determination may be helpful. In the absence of cyanotic congenital heart disease, a significant increase in PaO_2 may be observed. If PCO_2 is greater than 60 mm Hg, intubate and proceed with the hyperoxia test. It must be remembered that hypercapnia and acidemia, metabolic acidosis, hypoxia, and hypothermia are potent stimulants to pulmonary vasoconstriction. The resulting condition of persistent pulmonary hypertension of the newborn can easily be mistaken for cyanotic congenital heart disease. Regardless, the appropriate intervention is to transport this infant to a neonatal intensive care unit for further evaluation and care. Care for such an infant at the community hospital level is not recommended.

MECONIUM ASPIRATION

Passage of meconium before delivery occurs in 10% to 15% of newborns and may lead to significant morbidity and mortality. Although passage of meconium may represent fetal hypoxia and fetal distress, most delivered infants have no discernible problems. The task for the provider is to act timely and appropriately for infants requiring direct tracheal suctioning.

Management of these infants is controversial; however, consensus has been reached regarding the principle of suctioning the nose and oropharynx. It is not required or of benefit for the obstetrician to try to distinguish between watery and particulate meconium. All infants with meconium-stained amniotic fluid should have their nose and oropharynx thoroughly suctioned with a 10 French or larger suction catheter. A growing body of evidence suggests that for a vigorous infant, the need for direct tracheal suctioning is uncertain. As a matter of fact, this once vigorous infant is more likely to become depressed. For a depressed infant with thick or particulate meconium, clearing the tracheobronchial tree by direct tracheal suctioning may avoid significant morbidity and potential mortality. Tracheal intubation requires an experienced and skilled provider at the delivery. Prevalent in these infants initially is the mechanical effect caused by meconium. This particulate matter in the airway results in occlusion of the distal airways with subsequent air trapping, ventilation-perfusion inequalities, overdistention of compliant alveoli, and ultimately, air leaks. All these events add to the instability of such a patient and the potential for acute worsening of the clinical course. Ventilation-perfusion inequalities result in hypoxia and a dramatic increase in pulmonary vascular resistance, decreased pulmonary blood flow, and persistent pulmonary hypertension of the newborn. Interventions such as inhaled nitric oxide and extracorporeal membrane oxygenation are available at some centers and may avert the dismal outcome in such a scenario.

HYPOGLYCEMIA

A newborn's preparation for extrauterine life requires many adaptations, but glucose homeostasis is critical. Inadequate adaptation results in markedly and potentially prolonged hypoglycemic episodes leading to difficulty maintaining body temperature, respiration, muscular activity, and plasma glucose concentrations, as well as potentially devastating central nervous system injury. In utero, the fetus is dependent on the supply of glucose obtained by glucose transport across the placenta. Normally, the amount of glucose through transplacental transport meets the necessary requirements. By the 12th week of fetal life, the enzymatic capacity for gluconeogenesis and glycogenolysis is present. The absolute levels of gluconeogenesis enzymes are far lower than the adult levels and therefore produce very little glucose under normal circumstances.

From a clinical standpoint, defining hypoglycemia is critical. During the first 6 hours of life, glucose values fall to 50 to 60 mg/dL. Values less than 50 mg/dL should be interpreted as hypoglycemia. Remember that whole blood glucose is 10% to 15% lower than the plasma level. Because red blood cells use glucose, delay in assessing the specimen may result in a falsely low reported value. Once hypoglycemia is identified, appropriate management includes a maintenance infusion of glucose at a rate of 6 to 8 mg/kg/min, with the infusion increased until the serum glucose is stable at a value greater than 50 mg/dL. In a symptomatic infant, administration of 2 mL/kg of 10% dextrose in water intravenously as a minibolus followed by continuous infusion of glucose at a rate of 6 to 8 mg/kg/min is recommended. Serum glucose levels continued to be monitored and the infusion of glucose is increased as required to maintain levels greater than 50 mg/dL. For most infants, 6 to 12 mg/kg/min of glucose administered as a continuous infusion is sufficient to reach a steady state. Infants with congenital hyperinsulinism or Beckwith-Wiedemann syndrome (islet cell hyperplasia and secondary hyperinsulinism), infants of diabetic mothers, and small-for-gestational-age infants may require glucose infusions greater than 12 mg/kg/min. If the hypoglycemia is refractory to the increased infusion of glucose, it is essential to draw

TABLE 4. **Causes of Neonatal Cyanosis**

Category	Examples	Signs	Responses to Hyperoxia Test	Chest Radiograph	Arterial Blood Gases
Heart disease with right-to-left shunt; *decreased* pulmonary blood flow	Tetralogy of Fallot Pulmonary atresia Tricuspid insufficiency	Hyperpnea Heart murmur Soft S_2	Minimal to nil	Variable heart size Diminished PVMs	pH normal or high P_{CO_2} normal or high
Heart disease with right-to-left shunt; *increased* pulmonary blood flow	*d*-Transposition Anomalous pulmonary venous return	Tachypnea Loud S_2 Variable heart murmur	Minimal	Large heart (unless obstructed with TAPVD) Increased PVMs	pH normal or low P_{CO_2} normal or high
Heart disease with heart failure; ventilation-perfusion mismatch	Coarctation syndrome Large left-to-right shunt Supraventicular tachycardia	Tachypnea Shock Heart murmur	Good response (Pa_{O_2}>150)	Large heart Rule out pneumonia Pulmonary edema	pH low P_{CO_2} high
Primary pulmonary disease	RDS Group B streptococci Meconium aspiration Pneumothorax	Tachypnea Retractions Grunting, etc.	Good response (may need CPAP to prove)	Diagnostic appearance	pH low P_{CO_2} high
Metabolic disease	Hypoglycemia Methemoglobinemia	Variable: Tachypnea Flaccidity Jitteriness, etc.	Minimal	Normal or large heart	pH normal or low P_{CO_2} normal
Polycythemia	Twin-twin transfusion Intrauterine growth retardation	Plethora Signs of congestive heart failure	Minimal	Large heart Normal PVMs	pH normal or low P_{CO_2} normal
Infection	Sepsis Myocarditis	Shock Marked peripheral cyanosis	Good	Large heart (unless hypoadrenal) Pulmonary edema	pH low P_{CO_2} high
Persistent pulmonary hypertension	Meconium aspiration LGA baby Maternal salicylates	Hyperpnea Differential cyanosis	Variable—transiently good (with CPAP)	Normal heart size Decreased PVMs	pH low P_{CO_2} may be elevated
Neurologic disease	Intracranial bleeding Seizure disorder	Tachypnea Focal signs Apnea	Good	Normal	pH low P_{CO_2} elevated

Abbreviations: CPAP, continuous positive airway pressure; LGA, large for gestational age; PVMs, pulmonary vascular markings; RDS, respiratory syndrome; TAPVD, total anomalous pulmonary venous drainage.

From Burg F, Polin R, Yoder M: Workbook in Practical Neonatology 2001. Philadelphia, WB Saunders, 2001. Modified from Lees MH: Cyanosis of the newborn infant. J Pediatr 77:484, 1970.

blood for an insulin level while the infant is hypoglycemic, which may provide a significant clue regarding why a steady state cannot be achieved.

SEPSIS

Infections cause a significant amount of morbidity and mortality in the neonatal period. When dealing with neonates, it is important to not ignore any cultured pathogen without weighing the risk of no intervention. It should be borne in mind that the infant is assuming the greatest risk.

Primarily invasive bacterial infections occur in the bloodstream, but 25% of these bacteremic infants can also have associated meningitis. The occurrence rate of bacterial sepsis is about 2 to 3 per 1000 live births. The incidence appears low; however, because of the incredible risk to the infant, the provider must consider infection early, perform the necessary evaluation, and provide prophylactic antibiotics.

The potential list of bacteria causing sepsis is numerous. Most causative bacteria, 60% to 70%, are group B β-hemolytic streptococci (GBS) and *Escherichia coli* (K1 strain). Other causative agents are *Staphylococcus epidermidis* and *Staphylococcus aureus*. An appreciation for the etiologies provides a better understanding of the recommendations for empirical antibiotic coverage.

Risk factors for sepsis can be maternal and/or neonatal in origin. Maternal risks factors include prolonged rupture of fetal membranes, colonization with GBS, and chorioamnionitis. Prolonged rupture of membranes is associated with a 1% incidence of sepsis. The longer the membranes are ruptured, the greater the risk for sepsis. Chorioamnionitis is suspected with a purulent or foul-smelling amniotic fluid, fetal tachycardia, uterine tenderness, and/or a maternal temperature greater than 100.4° F. Epidural anesthesia is commonly associated with a 15-fold increase in intrapartum and postpartum fever. Although this association is strong, it is not exact, and by no means should it be used to defer intervention.

GBS has demanded a significant amount of attention in the newborn period. This attention is reserved for GBS because of its significant mortality of 5% to 15%. Attempts at reducing the adverse impact of GBS include identification of colonized mothers at 35 to 37 weeks' gestation by cervical culture and the use of intrapartum penicillin. This strategy, endorsed by the American College of Obstetrics and Gynecology and the Centers for Disease Control and Prevention, is effective, but 25% of cases in colonized mothers may not be identified. GBS can also cause pneumonia with or without bacteremia or meningitis and can have a sudden onset and a fulminant course.

Unfortunately, every infant requiring resuscitation cannot be identified. Therefore, it is critical to take the time, when not faced with a critically ill neonate, to plan for such an event. This planning phase must address equipment and personnel issues. It is also imperative to evaluate performance during an actual resuscitation and identify weak areas for future planning and training cycles. This process is continuous; it is aimed at improving the performance of the team and results in improved outcomes for the newborn.

NORMAL INFANT FEEDING

method of
NEAL S. LELEIKO, M.D., PH.D., and
CHRISTINE M. HARDY, M.S., R.D., L.D.N.
The Hasbro Children's Hospital/Rhode Island Hospital and The Brown Medical School
Providence, Rhode Island

BREASTFEEDING

Breast milk is the ideal form of nutrition for the newborn. Commercial formula manufacturers invariably compare their products with breast milk. Breast milk maintains a considerable level of nutritional superiority above its commercially prepared counterparts. Seventy percent of new mothers are reportedly nursing their newborns at discharge from the hospital. The number declines to approximately 30% at 6 months of age.

During the first few days after birth, the mothers' breasts produce colostrum. Colostrum is physiologically appropriate for the newborn and, although generally of low volume, contains many constituents that are advantageous to the newborn. Colostrum is produced for approximately 3 days. It is gradually followed by transitional milk. Transitional milk, which is higher in protein than mature milk, is soon followed by mature human milk. The nutrient composition of mature milk varies with time as well as from the beginning of a feeding to the end. Milk delivered early in a feeding (fore milk) contains more protein, and milk taken at the end of a feeding contains more fat (hind milk). This is one of the reasons why it is important for a mother to empty at least one breast of its milk before starting her infant on her other breast. (This approach also stimulates the production of additional milk.) The protein composition of breast milk differs considerably from that of cow milk and is of a much higher quality. The protein in many infant formulas is "humanized" to make it more closely resemble human milk protein. The principal carbohydrate in breast milk is lactose, which is present in greater quantity than in cow milk formula. Lactose (which contains galactose) may enhance calcium absorption. Total fat content is similar in breast milk and formula, but the fat contained in breast milk tends to reflect maternal dietary fat composition. Caloric density of common commercial formulas is adjusted to be similar to that of breast milk, about 20 kcal/ounce or 0.67 cal/mL.

Added benefits of breast-feeding include its nominal cost, ease of preparation, and regulation of satiety. A few proponents have focused on a study suggesting a very small but perhaps significant advantage in neurodevelopment.

Breast-feeding usually does not require special preparation or sterilization compared with commercial formulas, although breast milk may be expressed and refrigerated or frozen for later use. Breast-feeding ad libitum permits the infant to regulate its caloric intake on the basis of hunger and satiety, not on the need to finish a specific volume of formula in a bottle.

The successful initiation and continuation of breast-feeding require both prenatal and postpartum strategies. Prenatal education and support should begin early, especially for first-time mothers. These efforts are the responsibility of the obstetrician, nurse midwife, or family practitioner. Breast examination during an early prenatal examination should allow the prospective mother to voice her concerns and questions regarding her ability to breast-feed. Breast-feeding should be strongly encouraged and negative feelings explored. For the mother who, for whatever reason, chooses to use infant formula, reassurance about the safety and adequacy of the formula is appropriate. There is no reason to make a mother feel inadequate if she is unable to nurse or chooses not to breast-feed.

Breast-feeding should be attempted shortly after delivery, preferably within the first 30 minutes. Frequent nursing, every 2 to 3 hours, helps establish the mother's milk supply as well as her level of confidence, improving the likelihood of success after discharge from the hospital. No supplements such as sugar water, sterile water, or formula should be given for the first few days following birth. This helps the infant to develop an effective suckling ability, which is quite different from the sucking that occurs when an infant uses a bottle. Early, in-hospital, lactation support is important to help the new mother become comfortable with breast-feeding as well as prepare her for potential difficulties she may encounter at home. Continuing lactation support at home is also extremely important for overcoming any problems encountered that might result in discontinuation in the early postpartum period. The American Academy of Pediatrics currently recommends that breast-feeding continue exclusively for the first 6 months, followed by supplementation with age-appropriate solid foods until 12 months of age whenever possible.

Contraindications to breast milk feeding are few. These are listed in Table 1.

TABLE 1. **Contraindications to Breast-Feeding**

1. Infant medical diagnosis:
   Inborn errors of metabolism (i.e., galactosemia)
2. Maternal medical diagnosis
   HIV, AIDS
   Untreated tuberculosis
3. Maternal medications
   Antineoplastics: cisplatin, cyclophosphamide
   Benzodiazepines
   Ergot alkaloids: ergotamine, ergonovine
   Illegal drugs: amphetamines, cocaine, heroin, methadone, marijuana, phencyclidine
   Alcohol

TABLE 2. **Infant Formulas (Examples)**

1. Formulas for healthy premature infants
   (Generally contain increased protein, vitamin D, calcium, and phosphorus, slightly more calories)
   Enfamil EnfaCare
   Enfamil Premature
   Similac Neosure
2. Cow milk formulas
   (Same quantities of water and energy as breast milk, but whey/casein ratio may differ.)
   America's Store brand (formerly SMA)
   Carnation Good Start
   Enfamil LIPIL
   Enfamil LactoFree
   Gerber Baby formula
   Similac
   Similac Lactosefree
   Similac PM 60/40
3. Soy protein formulas
   (Soy offers an alternative protein but little other advantage.)
   America's Store brand
   Carnation Alsoy
   Gerber Soy Formula
   Isomil
   ProSobee
4. Casein hydrolysate formulas
   (These are specialty formulas that should be used only for specific indications)
   Alimentum
   Nutramigen
   Pregestimil
5. Free amino acid formulas
   (Like the hydrolysates, these are highly specialized formulas that are appropriate only for special situations. Their use requires careful monitoring of growth and development by a pediatric specialist.)
   Elecare
   Neocate

FORMULA FEEDING

Nutritional adequacy of competing commercially prepared infant formulas is generally assured because of federal rules. Because all formulas must comply with known standards for nutritional adequacy, marketing strategies must emphasize differences in formula that are not established or universally agreed upon. Standards for nutritional adequacy utilize mature breast milk as the control solution. Infant formulas are designed to meet all of an infant's nutrient requirements during the first year of life. The variety of infant formulas has grown rapidly over the past several years. Formulas may vary by the type and amount of protein, carbohydrate, or fat they contain in addition to variation in certain electrolytes, vitamins, or minerals. Infants who are formula fed should receive only iron-fortified formula.

The different formula classifications are listed in Table 2.

SOLID FEEDINGS

The age at introduction of solid foods is determined according to fading of the extrusion reflex. The fading of this reflex may vary considerably from infant to infant. Successful introduction of solids is unlikely before this reflex disappears. Extrusion of solids introduced too soon is likely to be misinterpreted as a sign that an infant dislikes a particular food. This may have the unfortunate consequence of causing caretakers to abandon nutritious foods without good reason. There are no absolute rules for feeding in the first year of life, and only guidelines can be offered. The importance of developing good eating habits for all of childhood and adult life should be emphasized. Iron-fortified infant cereal is often the first food offered as it is easily prepared, and because its texture is readily adjusted it is well accepted. By the time most infants begin solids they benefit from added iron as stores deposited in utero become depleted, especially in infants who are exclusively breast-fed. The cereal can be offered at appropriate mealtimes (i.e., breakfast or lunch). It is best to avoid combinations of foods or introducing too many new foods too fast. Commercially prepared baby foods are totally unnecessary but are convenience foods that a parent may elect to use.

The use of fruit juice is not indicated during the first year of life. It is best considered as "sugar" water with fruit flavoring (perhaps with some additional vitamin C) and treated as such.

VITAMIN AND MINERAL SUPPLEMENTS

Healthy premature infants have increased nutrient requirements that often cannot be met by breast milk. Breast milk fortifiers have been developed that can be added to expressed breast milk to provide more protein, calcium, and vitamin D to meet the increased needs of these infants.

Term infants who consume adequate breast milk or formula for normal growth also receive adequate vitamins and minerals to meet their requirements in this volume. As mentioned earlier, iron stores become depleted by approximately 6 months of age, necessitating the introduction of iron-fortified solids. It is unnecessary to provide an iron supplement if iron-fortified cereal is consumed in adequate amounts. Some infants may benefit from supplemental vitamin D. After 6 months, infants who are fed infant formula prepared with nonfluoridated water require supplemental fluoride.

DISEASES OF THE BREAST

method of
RACHE SIMMONS, M.D., and
MICHAEL OSBORNE, M.D.
The New York–Presbyterian Hospital and The Weill Medical College of Cornell University
New York, New York

BENIGN BREAST CHANGES

A great variety of benign breast conditions are grouped together into the catchall term "fibrocystic disease" and are detected in most normal women at some point during their reproductive years. An appreciation of the spectrum of benign disorders and any associated risk of breast cancer is necessary so that patients can be given appropriate treatment and counseling.

Breast Cysts

Cysts within the breast are a common finding in premenopausal women. Benign cysts are often tender and fluctuate with the menstrual cycle. Cysts may be detected either on physical examination as a palpable, smooth, mobile nodule or by breast ultrasound. They may appear as a solitary nodule or in a cluster. Confirmation of the diagnosis of a cyst should be made by needle aspiration of the cystic fluid or by noting the characteristic sonographic appearance. A cyst does not need further intervention if it does not have internal echoes on ultrasound or if nonbloody fluid is aspirated and the palpable mass resolves.

Fibroadenoma

Fibroadenomas are benign tumors commonly found in young women. They are characteristically detected on physical examination as a well-circumscribed, mobile, palpable mass. They pose no increased risk of breast cancer and do not mandate surgical removal unless desired by the patient.

Epithelial Hyperplasia, Lobular Carcinoma In Situ, Radial Scar

Epithelial hyperplasia, with or without atypia, and lobular carcinoma in situ (LCIS, lobular neoplasia) typically do not produce a palpable mass or mammographic abnormality, and they are diagnosed incidentally after biopsy of another lesion. Radial scars are usually mammographically manifested as a stellate mass and can thus mimic a malignancy.

Epithelial hyperplasia with and without atypia, LCIS, and radial scars are associated with an increased risk for the future development of breast cancer. Women with epithelial hyperplasia but without atypical hyperplasia (AH) have an increased relative risk of 1.3, whereas those with AH have a 4.3 relative risk of breast cancer and those with AH and a family history of breast cancer have a relative risk of 11 when compared with women without proliferative disease. In women in whom LCIS is diagnosed, subsequent invasive carcinoma will develop in approximately 30% within 20 years, and the risk is equal in the ipsilateral and the contralateral breast.

For epithelial hyperplasia with atypia, radial scars, and LCIS, a policy of close observation is the most commonly recommended management. In such a program, women should be trained to carry out breast self-examination (BSE) and have appropriate annual mammographic screening and regular examinations every 6 months by their physician.

The results of the National Surgical Breast and Bowel Project (NSABP) Breast Cancer Prevention

Trial P-1 showed that women at increased risk for breast cancer could decrease their risk by taking tamoxifen (Nolvadex). In this double-blind randomized trial, women taking tamoxifen had an approximately 50% reduction in the subsequent risk of breast cancer. The use of tamoxifen may be appropriate in selected patients with AH, LCIS, or radial scar to decrease their subsequent risk. Clinical assessment of the potential risks and benefits is necessary when recommending tamoxifen as a preventive agent.

RISK FACTORS FOR BREAST CANCER

It is estimated that 80% of women in whom breast cancer develops have no documented risk factors. However, women who have a personal or strong familial history of breast cancer are at increased risk. Women known to have the *BRCA1* or *BRCA2* genetic mutation have an 85% lifetime risk of breast cancer, as well as an increased risk of ovarian cancer. Women with a previous breast biopsy revealing a diagnosis of epithelial hyperplasia, LCIS, or radial scars have a higher risk of subsequent breast cancer. Reproductive factors such as menarche before 12 years of age, menopause after the age of 55, nulliparity, and first pregnancy after the age of 30 are associated with a minimal elevation in breast cancer risk. Radiation exposure such as previous radiation therapy for lymphoma, especially during adolescence, has been shown to elevate a woman's risk of subsequent breast cancer.

Screening Techniques for Detection of Breast Cancer

Screening for breast cancer includes imaging techniques such as mammography and ultrasound, BSE, and physical examination by a physician. The use of screening mammography has been shown in large clinical trials such as the Health Insurance Plan of the New York Breast Screening Project to reduce mortality. However, it is estimated that 10% to 15% of breast cancer cases are not detectable on screening mammography, thus emphasizing the importance of physical breast examination by a physician and BSE.

Physical examination by a physician and BSE by the patient should include both visual inspection and manual examination of the breast. On inspection, signs of breast malignancy include skin/nipple retraction or discoloration, nipple discharge/crusting, or peau d'orange edema of the breast. On palpation, any asymmetric mass of the breast or axilla should be regarded as a potential malignancy that deserves further evaluation.

Current recommendations are for a woman to perform BSE and physical examination at 18 years of age and to initiate annual mammography at the age of 40. If a woman has a first-degree relative with a diagnosis of breast cancer at an early age, screening mammography at a younger age may be appropriate.

BIOPSY TECHNIQUES FOR A BREAST LESION

Any suspicious mammographic, sonographic, or palpable lesion should have a tissue diagnosis performed to rule out breast cancer. Breast cancer can also be manifested as a serous or bloody nipple discharge without any palpable or image-detectable lesion, and such women should undergo surgical evaluation. A diagnostic biopsy can be performed by several methods.

For nonpalpable lesions, an image-guided needle biopsy can be performed with the assistance of breast ultrasound or mammographic stereotactic techniques. The biopsy technique can be either fine-needle aspiration (FNA) or core biopsy to sample the lesion. If the lesion is palpable, FNA or core biopsy can also be performed without the assistance of breast imaging.

Because of the limited sensitivity of FNA in comparison to core biopsy and its inability to distinguish invasive and noninvasive disease, many surgeons prefer a core biopsy to establish a diagnosis. A core biopsy without evidence of invasion does not exclude the diagnosis because of the technique's limited sampling. Core biopsy samples provide additional information about the histologic grade of the tumor and the status of estrogen and progesterone receptors.

Breast lesions can also be diagnosed by excisional biopsy, which can be facilitated by ultrasound or mammographic localization of wire placement in nonpalpable lesions.

BREAST CANCER

Incidence

It is estimated that breast cancer will develop in one in nine women living in the United States if they live to be 90 years old. The average age at diagnosis of breast cancer is 64 years, and it is more commonly diagnosed with increasing age. Breast cancer is more frequently found in women with a family history of premenopausal breast cancer in a first-degree relative, in those with a known high-risk genetic mutations such as *BRCA1/BRCA2*, or in women with previously diagnosed high-risk pathology.

Breast cancer is designated as stage 0, I, II, III, or IV by the American Joint Committee on Cancer TMN system. This system categorizes breast cancer by its invasive or noninvasive character, tumor size, axillary lymph node status, and the presence of metastatic disease (Table 1). Overall survival with breast cancer is related to stage.

Histology

Ductal Carcinoma In Situ

Ductal carcinoma in situ (DCIS, intraductal carcinoma) is noninvasive breast cancer and is designated stage 0. Historically, DCIS represented only about 5% of breast cancer cases, whereas today it represents 20% to 30%. This rise is predominately due to the increasing use of screening mammography because

DCIS is most often detected as mammographic microcalcifications.

Invasive Breast Cancer

The most common type of infiltrating carcinoma is ductal—not otherwise specified (IFDC-NOS), which represents 85% of all invasive breast cancer. Infiltrating lobular carcinoma originates from the lobular structures of the breast and accounts for 15% of all invasive breast cancer. Other less common subtypes represent less than 10% and include tubular, medullary, mucinous, and papillary carcinoma. Additional rare subtypes of breast cancer include inflammatory carcinoma, malignant phylloides tumor, sarcoma, lymphoma, and Paget's disease.

SURGICAL TREATMENT OF THE BREAST

A significant paradigm shift in the treatment of breast cancer has occurred over the past several decades. The Halsted paradigm, popularized at the beginning of the 20th century, hypothesized that breast cancer spreads in a contiguous fashion from the breast to the axillary lymph nodes and then to distant sites elsewhere in the body. This theory has been modified by the Fisher paradigm, which views breast cancer as systemic from very early in the course of the disease; the axillary lymph nodes act not as a barrier but as indicators of disease aggressiveness. The Halsted paradigm promotes more intensive local treatment to eradicate the cancer, whereas the Fisher

TABLE 1. **TNM Staging System for Breast Cancer**

Primary Tumor (T)	
TX	Primary tumor cannot be assessed
T0	No evidence of primary tumor
Tis	Carcinoma in situ
Tis (DCIS)	Ductal carcinoma in situ
Tis (LCIS)	Lobular carcinoma in situ
TIS (Paget)	Paget's disease of the nipple with no tumor *Note:* Paget's disease associated with a tumor is classified according to the size of the tumor
T1	Tumor 2 cm or less in greatest dimension
T1mic	Microinvasion 0.1 cm or less in greatest dimension
T1a	Tumor more than 0.1 cm but not more than 0.5 cm in greatest dimension
T1b	Tumor more than 0.5 cm but not more than 1 cm in greatest dimension
T1c	Tumor more than 1 cm but not more than 2 cm in greatest dimension
T2	Tumor more than 2 cm but not more than 5 cm in greatest dimension
T3	Tumor more than 5 cm in greatest dimension
T4	Tumor of any size with direct extension to chest wall or skin, only as described below
T4a	Extension to chest wall, not including pectoralis muscle
T4b	Edema (including peau d'orange) or ulceration of the skin of the breast, or satellite skin nodules confined to the same breast
T4c	Both T4a and T4b
T4d	Inflammatory carcinoma
Regional Lymph Nodes (N)	
NX	Regional lymph nodes cannot be assessed (e.g., previously removed)
N0	No regional lymph node metastasis
N1	Metastasis in movable ipsilateral axillary lymph node(s)
N2	Metastases in ipsilateral axillary lymph nodes fixed or matted or in clinically apparent* ipsilateral internal mammary nodes in the absence of clinically evident axillary lymph node metastasis
N2a	Metastasis in ipsilateral axillary lymph nodes fixed to one another (matted) or to other structures
N2b	Metastasis only in clinically apparent* ipsilateral internal mammary nodes in the absence of clinically evident axillary lymph node metastasis
N3	Metastasis in ipsilateral infraclavicular lymph node(s), or in clinically apparent* ipsilateral internal mammary lymph node(s) and in the presence of clinically evident axillary lymph node metastasis; or metastasis in ipsilateral supraclavicular lymph node(s) with or without axillary or internal mammary lymph node involvement
Regional Lymph Nodes (pN0)[†]	
pNX	Regional lymph nodes cannot be assessed (e.g., previously removed or not removed for pathologic study)
pN0	No regional lymph node metastasis histologically, no additional examination for isolated tumor cell (ITC)[‡]
pN0(i−)	No regional lymph node metastasis histologically, negative IHC
pN0(i+)	No regional lymph node metastasis histologically, positive IHC, no IHC cluster greater than 0.2 mm
pN0(mol−)	No regional lymph node metastasis histologically, negative molecular findings (RT-PCR)[§]
pN0(mol+)	No regional lymph node metastasis histologically, positive molecular findings (RT-PCR)[§]
pN1mi	Micrometastasis (greater than 0.2 mm, none greater than 2.0 mm)
pN1	Metastasis in 1 to 3 axillary lymph nodes, and/or in internal mammary nodes with microscopic disease detected by sentinel lymph node dissection but not clinically apparent[‖]
pN1a	Metastases in 1 to 3 axillary lymph nodes
pN1b	Metastases in internal mammary nodes with microscopic disease detected by sentinel lymph node dissection but not clinically apparent[‖]
pN1c	Metastasis in 1 to 3 axillary lymph nodes and in internal mammary lymph nodes with microscopic disease detected by sentinel lymph node dissection but not clinically apparent[‖,¶]
pN2	Metastasis in 4 to 9 axillary lymph nodes, or in clinically apparent* internal mammary lymph nodes in the absence of axillary lymph node metastasis
pN2a	Metastasis in 4 to 9 axillary lymph nodes (at least 1 tumor deposit greater than 2.0 mm)

Continued

TABLE 1. **TNM Staging System for Breast Cancer—cont'd**

pN2b	Metastasis in clinically apparent* internal mammary lymph nodes in the absence of axillary lymph node metastasis
pN3	Metastasis in 10 or more axillary lymph nodes, or in infraclavicular lymph nodes, or in clinically apparent* ipsilateral internal mammary lymph nodes in the presence of 1 or more positive axillary lymph nodes; or in more than 3 axillary lymph nodes with clinically negative microscopic metastasis in internal mammary lymph nodes; or in ipsilateral supraclavicular lymph nodes
pN3a	Metastasis in 10 or more axillary lymph nodes (at least 1 tumor deposit greater than 2.0 mm), or metastasis to the infraclavicular lymph nodes
pN3b	Metastasis in clinically apparent* ipsilateral internal mammary lymph nodes or in the presence of 1 or more positive axillary lymph nodes; or in more than 3 axillary lymph nodes and in internal mammary lymph nodes with microscopic disease detected by sentinel lymph node dissection but not clinically apparent
pN3c	Metastasis in ipsilateral supraclavicular lymph nodes

Distant Metastasis (M)

MX	Distant metastasis cannot be assessed
M0	No distant metastasis
M1	Distant metastasis

Stage Grouping

0	Tis	N0	M0
I	T1**	N0	M0
II A	T0	N1	M0
	T1**	N1	M0
	T2	N0	M0
II B	T2	N1	M0
	T3	N0	M0
IIIA	T0	N2	M0
	T1**	N2	M0
	T2	N2	M0
	T3	N1	M0
	T3	N2	M0
IIIB	T4	N0	M0
	T4	N1	M0
	T4	N2	M0
IIIC	Any T	N3	M0
IV	Any T	Any N	M1

*Clinically apparent is defined as detected by imaging studies (excluding lymphoscintigraphy) or by clinical examination.
†Classification is based on axillary lymph node dissection with or without sentinel lymph node dissection. Classification based solely on sentinel lymph node dissection without subsequent axillary lymph node dissection is designated (sn) for sentinel node. For example, pN0(I+)(sn).
‡Isolated tumor cells (ITC) are defined as single cell clusters not greater than 0.2 mm, usually detected only by immunohistochemical (IHC) or molecular methods, but which may be verified on hematoxylin and eosin stains. ITCs do not usually show evidence of metastatic activity (e.g., proliferation or stromal reaction).
§RT-PCR = reverse transcriptase–polymerase chain reaction.
||Not clinically apparent is defined as not detected by imaging studies (excluding lymphoscintigraphy) or by clinical examination.
¶If associated with greater than 3 positive axillary lymph nodes, the internal mammary nodes are classified as pN3b to reflect increased tumor burden.
**T1 includes T1mic
From Greene FL, et at (eds): AJCC Cancer Staging Manual, 6th ed. New York, Springer-Verlag, 2002.

paradigm promotes less aggressive local treatment with the addition of systemic treatment in most women even with relatively early disease. Because of this philosophy change and the detection of earlier disease through diligent screening techniques, surgical treatment of breast cancer has progressed toward less radical surgery and more adjuvant therapy, with equal or better outcomes.

Breast Conservation

Most small noninvasive and invasive breast cancers are treated by breast conservation, which consists of wide local excision with negative surgical margins and irradiation of the breast. Studies to date, including the NSABP B-06 and B-17 trials and the Milan Institute Quadrantectomy versus Radical Mastectomy Trial, as well as other clinical trials, show no statistically significant difference in patient survival with mastectomy or breast conservation.

Because of the multicentricity of breast cancer, the addition of radiation treatment to wide local excision in patients with noninvasive and invasive carcinoma is currently the standard of treatment. The NSABP B-06 and B-17 trials evaluated local recurrence of small noninvasive and invasive tumors with and without irradiation after lumpectomy and found that patients who did not undergo radiation therapy had a significantly higher rate of local recurrence. Limited data support excision alone in small, well-differentiated DCIS with surgical margins of at least 1 cm.

Mastectomy

Some breast cancer patients have contraindications to breast conservation, and the recommendation for treatment would be mastectomy with or without immediate reconstruction. Some of these contraindications include previous radiation treatment to the breast area, pregnancy, extensive microcalcifications, an inability to achieve tumor-free margins, and multicentricity, defined as the presence of two or more separate tumors in different quadrants of the breast. A relative contraindication to radiotherapy in breast conservation includes connective tissue disorders because of a higher incidence of tissue damage. Another factor favoring mastectomy can be patient preference.

Total mastectomy surgically removes the breast parenchyma, pectoral fascia, nipple, and the areola complex. A modified radical mastectomy includes axillary dissection. A radical mastectomy, which is rarely used currently, includes removal of the pectoralis major and minor muscles and axillary dissection.

Breast Reconstruction

Any patient recommended to have a mastectomy should be offered the option of immediate or delayed reconstruction and referred to a plastic and reconstructive surgeon to discuss which techniques would be appropriate on an individual basis. One commonly used method of breast reconstruction is a tissue expander/breast implant. In this procedure, a tissue expander is placed beneath the pectoralis muscles, and expansions are performed over a period of several weeks to months to stretch the subpectoral pocket to accommodate the permanent implant. The permanent saline or silicone implant is then inserted as a secondary procedure.

Another method of breast reconstruction is the transverse rectus abdominis myocutaneous (TRAM) flap, which involves the transfer of skin, fat, and muscle from the lower part of the abdomen to create a reconstructed breast. This procedure can be performed as a free flap with the arterial and venous supply anastomosed to vessels in the axilla or as a pedicle flap with the arterial and venous supply from the superior epigastric vessels. Other types of flap reconstructions include latissimus dorsi or gluteal flaps. Reconstruction of the nipple and areola is often performed as a later procedure.

Surgical Treatment of the Axilla

The status of the axilla should be assessed for metastases in any patient with invasive breast cancer for several reasons. The status of the axillary lymph nodes is important in determining the patient's stage of disease. The presence or absence of axillary lymph node metastases is predictive of the prognosis and facilitates decisions by the medical oncology team regarding adjuvant therapy. Surgical removal of metastatic nodes in the axilla significantly decreases the possibility of axillary recurrence. Axillary dissection may improve overall survival, but this issue is debated in the medical literature.

Sentinel Lymph Node Biopsy

Traditionally, axillary dissection has been performed on all patients with invasive breast cancer as an important predictor of prognosis. Sentinel lymphadenectomy or "sentinel lymph node biopsy" (SLNB) identifies the first, or "sentinel," lymph node or nodes in the axillary chain to receive drainage from the breast cancer and thus the most likely to contain metastases. The technique of SLNB is performed by the injection of isosulfan or methylene blue dye and/or radioactive isotope to localize the sentinel lymph node.

SLNB has been shown by multiple studies to accurately predict the presence of axillary metastases in T1-2 breast cancer. SLNB offers a less invasive method to assess the status of the axilla and is associated with fewer complications than axillary node dissection is.

Axillary Dissection

It is typically recommended that patients who have metastatic cells on SLNB undergo complete axillary lymph node dissection (ALND). Alternatively, if a patient is not a candidate for SLNB, ALND should be performed. Contraindications to SLNB include T3 breast cancer, palpable suspicious axillary lymph nodes, and previous axillary surgery because of axillary scar tissue and potential inaccuracy of the technique. SLNB is also contraindicated in pregnancy because of a lack of data regarding fetal safety.

Axillary dissection involves the removal of 10 to 30 lymph nodes from the axilla. The potential risk of axillary dissection includes the accumulation of a seroma, ipsilateral arm lymphedema, and numbness around the area of the intercostal brachial innervation if the nerve is sacrificed at the time of surgery. Because of the lifetime increased chance of arm lymphedema and possible infection, it is recommended that patients avoid any trauma or procedures such as venipuncture or blood pressure measurements on the ipsilateral arm.

Bone Marrow Aspiration

Axillary lymph node metastases have historically been the most important indicator of prognosis in breast cancer patients. Bone marrow micrometastases obtained by bone marrow aspiration have also been shown to predict distant recurrence and prognosis.

Bone marrow sampling is performed under sedation and local or general anesthesia at the time of breast cancer surgery. A small skin incision is made on each of the patient's anterior iliac crests to introduce the aspiration needle. The needle (Illinois 14 gauge) is advanced within the iliac crest and aspiration is performed. An ideal yield for evaluation is 6 mL from each side. Cytospins of these cells are prepared from this aspirate and stained with monoclonal antibodies against cytokeratin for analysis by immunohistochemistry.

Several studies have shown the combination of bone marrow micrometastases and axillary lymph node status to predict distant relapse and survival. This information can be used in conjunction with axillary lymph node status to assess risk and offer systemic therapeutic options to breast cancer patients.

ADJUVANT THERAPY

Adjuvant therapy is used to treat patients with a substantial likelihood for the development of metastatic disease. Most medical oncologists consider this risk sufficient in node-negative patients with a tumor diameter of 1 cm or larger and in those with nodal metastases to justify adjuvant chemotherapy or hormonal therapy.

Hormonal therapy such as tamoxifen is commonly used as adjuvant treatment in early breast cancer patients with estrogen receptor–positive tumors. The recommended length of treatment for node-negative patients is 5 years. Additionally, it can be used as a chemopreventive agent to decrease the chance of an additional ipsilateral tumor developing in patients undergoing breast conservation or to decrease the possibility of contralateral breast cancer.

Recommendations regarding tamoxifen, chemotherapy alone, or a combination of both are dependent on the clinical judgment of the treating medical oncologist. Consideration should be given to the likelihood of systemic recurrence based on nodal status, tumor size, and tumor grade. Estrogen receptor positivity of the tumor is predictive of a response to hormonal therapy, and Her-2/Neu may determine the type of appropriate chemotherapy. Another factor is the patient's age and any co-morbid diseases that would decrease the patient's tolerance to a course of chemotherapy.

SURVEILLANCE AFTER A DIAGNOSIS OF BREAST CANCER

Surveillance should continue after diagnosis and treatment of breast cancer to detect local recurrence or a new primary breast cancer in either the ipsilateral or contralateral breast. The National Comprehensive Cancer Network guidelines recommend that patients continue diligent monthly self-examinations and that a physician perform a physical examination at 4- to 6-month intervals to assess for evidence of local recurrence and symptoms of metastatic disease. The ipsilateral arm should be evaluated to detect early signs of lymphedema and initiate appropriate management. Mammography should be performed every 6 months on the ipsilateral conserved breast for 2 years and on the contralateral breast annually. Bone and computed tomographic scans and other tumor markers should be performed only on patients with symptomatic systemic disease because of the lack of evidence of improved survival with early detection of distant metastases.

SPECIAL TOPICS IN BREAST DISEASE

Gynecomastia

Gynecomastia is the unilateral or bilateral benign enlargement of male breast tissue. The etiology of gynecomastia is often related to various substances, including exogenous hormones, alcohol, and marijuana use, or it may be idiopathic. The main concern is to rule out the diagnosis of male breast cancer. Once breast cancer has been excluded, no treatment is indicated for gynecomastia. If medication and lifestyle etiologies have been eliminated without remission of the gynecomastia, the excess breast tissue may be surgically removed for cosmetic considerations if desirable.

Male Breast Cancer

Carcinoma of the male breast represents 1% of all breast cancers. Because men are not routinely screened for breast cancer as women are, the diagnosis is often delayed. The most common manifestation of male breast cancer is a painless, firm, subareolar breast mass. The differential diagnosis is gynecomastia. Breast imaging with mammography and/or ultrasound may be helpful in rendering a diagnosis inasmuch as the appearance of male breast cancer is a stellate, irregular solid mass. Any suspicious breast mass in a male patient should undergo diagnostic biopsy as with a female patient. If a malignancy is diagnosed, standard treatment is mastectomy with assessment of the axillary nodes by SLNB or axillary dissection. Most cases of male breast cancer are estrogen receptor positive, and recommendations for adjuvant chemotherapy or hormonal therapy should be based on criteria similar to those for breast cancer in female patients.

Breast Cancer in Pregnancy

Pregnancy-associated breast cancer represents 2% of all breast cancer diagnoses. Frequently, the breast cancer is diagnosed at a late stage because of the difficulty of examination of the breast in pregnant women and avoidance of mammography during pregnancy. Any suspicious lesion noted during pregnancy should be subjected to biopsy in the same fashion as in a nongravid woman. Radiation therapy should not be administered during pregnancy, so breast conservation is generally contraindicated unless the diagnosis is made within a few weeks of delivery. Surgical treatment with mastectomy and axillary dissection is the standard treatment of breast cancer during pregnancy. Adjuvant chemotherapy can be delivered with selective agents during the second and third trimesters. The prognosis is similar to that of nongravid women in whom breast cancer is diagnosed at a comparable stage.

Inflammatory Breast Cancer

The classic manifestation of inflammatory breast cancer is erythema, edema, peau d'orange, and calor of the breast resembling an infectious process. Malignant cells within the dermal lymphatic vessels of the breast confirm the diagnosis. The usual pathology of the associated carcinoma is IFDC-NOS. Inflammatory carcinoma is a very aggressive type of breast cancer, with over 90% of patients having positive axillary lymph nodes at diagnosis. The recommended treatment is multimodality therapy, with chemotherapy preceding surgery. Surgical treatment is mastectomy and is followed by radiation therapy and often additional chemotherapy.

Locally Advanced Breast Cancer

Patients with N2 or N3 nodal status or those with four or more positive axillary nodes, T3 or T4 tumors, or involvement of the pectoralis fascia are said to have locally advanced breast cancer (LABC). The recommended treatment for patients with LABC is neoadjuvant chemotherapy, which is administered before surgical treatment. The NSABP B-18 trial demonstrated that in LABC patients randomized to neoadjuvant or postoperative chemotherapy, neoadjuvant chemotherapy decreased the size of the tumor in 80% of patients, with 36% having complete clinical disappearance of their tumor. Multiple studies, including the B-18 trial, have shown that neoadjuvant chemotherapy increases the possibility of breast conservation in women with large tumors. Neoadjuvant therapy has no impact on overall survival in patients with LABC.

ENDOMETRIOSIS

method of
JULIA V. JOHNSON, M.D.
Reproductive Endocrinology
Department of Obstetrics and Gynecology
University of Vermont College of Medicine
Burlington, Vermont

Endometriosis is defined as ectopic endometrial tissue, including glands and stroma, located outside the uterine cavity. Although the frequency of endometriosis in the general population is not certain, it is estimated to occur in 30% to 50% of women with unexplained infertility and is found at laparoscopy in up to 70% of women with undiagnosed pelvic pain.

Although endometriosis is a common disorder in women, the understanding of its pathophysiology, methods for diagnosis, and treatment options are limited. It is also a heterogeneous disease, with the symptoms matching poorly with the severity of the disease. The lesions are most commonly found as implants on the pelvic peritoneum and implants or cysts on the ovaries, although also found on the bowel and bladder serosa, appendix, upper abdominal cavity, lymph nodes, and extrapelvic sites. Despite the variations in presentation and the effectiveness of treatment, active research is ongoing to understand of the etiology of endometriosis.

PATHOGENESIS

The initial explanation for the pathogenesis of endometriosis was postulated by J. Sampson in 1927 with his article: *Peritoneal Endometriosis due to Menstrual Dissemination of Endometrial Tissue into the Peritoneal Cavity*. He theorized that endometrial tissue, passing through the fallopian tubes, could implant onto the pelvic peritoneum. It is now known that retrograde menstruation, as described by Sampson, actually occurs in at least 90% of women. This raises the question of why more women do not develop endometriosis in the peritoneal cavity. Several theories have been proposed to explain the ability of endometrial tissue to attach in the abdominal cavity. In some women, an excessive amount of retrograde menstruation resulting from a mullerian anomaly or obstructed menstrual outflow, explains the placement of endometrial cells in the pelvic cavity. It is also known that endometriosis can occur in surgical wounds, such as laparotomy scars and vaginal or vulvar incisions, after uterine surgery. This confirms that endometrial cells can implant in tissues outside the uterus. The presence of endometriosis in women with normal anatomy, however, cannot be explained by retrograde implantation alone.

Endometrium can also reach the pelvic cavity by direct extension or through lymphatic and vascular channels. Adenomyosis, endometrial tissue within the uterine myometrium, demonstrates that endometrium can spread to adjacent tissue. It is also known that endometrial cells can be found in the lymph glands in 7% of women. The presence of endometrium in blood vessels and the lymphatic system may explain the rare cases of endometriosis outside the abdominal cavity. The presence of endometrium outside the uterus has also been explained as the metaplasia of peritoneal tissue to endometrial tissue, thus explaining endometriosis in areas throughout the abdominal cavity. It has also been postulated that cell rests of mullerian origin can transformed into endometrial cells explaining the very rare finding of endometriosis in males.

These interesting theories of pathogenesis do not explain the common occurrence of this disease in women. Genetic factors may explain the frequency of endometriosis in family groups. Linkage analysis and global gene profiling studies are ongoing, and a Web site is being developed for the genetic epidemiology of endometriosis. Another component in the development of endometriosis may be an alteration in the immune system in women with this disease. Studies have identified alterations in peritoneal fluid lymphocytes and macrophages, growth factors, natural killer cells, cytokines, and interleukins in women with endometriosis. These changes may partially explain the etiology for the disease and the symptoms associated with endometriosis. Changes within the endometrial cells, such as increased production of matrix metalloproteinases, may allow the cells to implant in the pelvis. These exciting areas of research promise to define the pathogenesis and potentially optimize treatment choices for endometriosis.

CLINICAL PRESENTATION

Endometriosis is classically defined by the volume of implants, the presence and size of endometriomas (ovarian cysts), and the extent of adhesions. The Revised Classification of Endometriosis from the American Society of Reproductive Medicine (ARSM; formally the American Fertility Society or AFS) describes the definition of minimal (stage I), mild (stage II), moderate (stage III), and severe disease (stage IV). The ASRM classification is illustrated in Figures 1 and 2. The scoring system at the time of surgery based on the size of lesions, the depth of the implants, the size of ovarian lesions, the extent of ovarian and tubal adhesions, and the degree of cul-de-sac obliteration. Lesions have a varied appearance being red, red-pink, clear, white, yellow-black, black, and blue. Lesions can be superficial or have deep penetration into the adjacent tissue. Most women have multiple types of endometriosis implants.

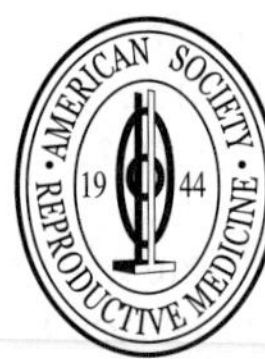

AMERICAN SOCIETY FOR REPRODUCTIVE MEDICINE
REVISED CLASSIFICATION OF ENDOMETRIOSIS

Patients' Name ____________________ Date ____________________

Stage I (Minimal) - 1–5
Stage II (Mild) - 6–15
Stage III (Moderate) - 16–40
Stage IV (Severe) - > 40

Laparoscopy ______ Laparotomy ______ Photography ______

Recommended treatment ____________________

Total ____________ Prognosis ____________

	ENDOMETRIOSIS	< 1cm	1–3cm	<3cm
Peritoneum	Superficial	1	2	4
	Deep	2	4	6
Ovary	R Superficial	1	2	4
	Deep	4	16	20
	L Superficial	1	2	4
	Deep	4	16	20
	POSTERIOR CULDESAC OBLITERATION	Partial		Complete
		4		40
	ADHESIONS	$< \frac{1}{3}$ Enclosure	$\frac{1}{3}$–$\frac{2}{3}$ Enclosure	$> \frac{2}{3}$ Enclosure
Ovary	R Filmy	1	2	4
	Dense	4	8	16
	L Filmy	1	2	4
	Dense	4	8	16
Tube	R Filmy	1	2	4
	Dense	4*	8*	16
	L Filmy	1	2	4
	Dense	4*	8*	16

*If the fimbriated end of the fallopian tube is completely closed, change the point assignment to 16.

Denote appearance of superficial implant types as red [(R), red, red-pink, flamelike, vesicular blobs, clear vesicles], white [(W), opacifications, peritoneal defects, yellow-brown], or black [(B) black, hemosiderin deposits, blue]. Denote percent of total described as R__%, W__% and B__%. Total should equal 100%.

Denote appearance of of superficial implant types as red [(R), red, red-pink, flamelike, vesicular blobs, clear vesic

Additional Endometriosis: ____________________

Associated pathology: ____________________

L To be used with normal tubes and ovaries R

L To be used with abnormal tubes and/or ovaries R

Figure 1. American Society for Reproductive Medicine revised classification of endometriosis.

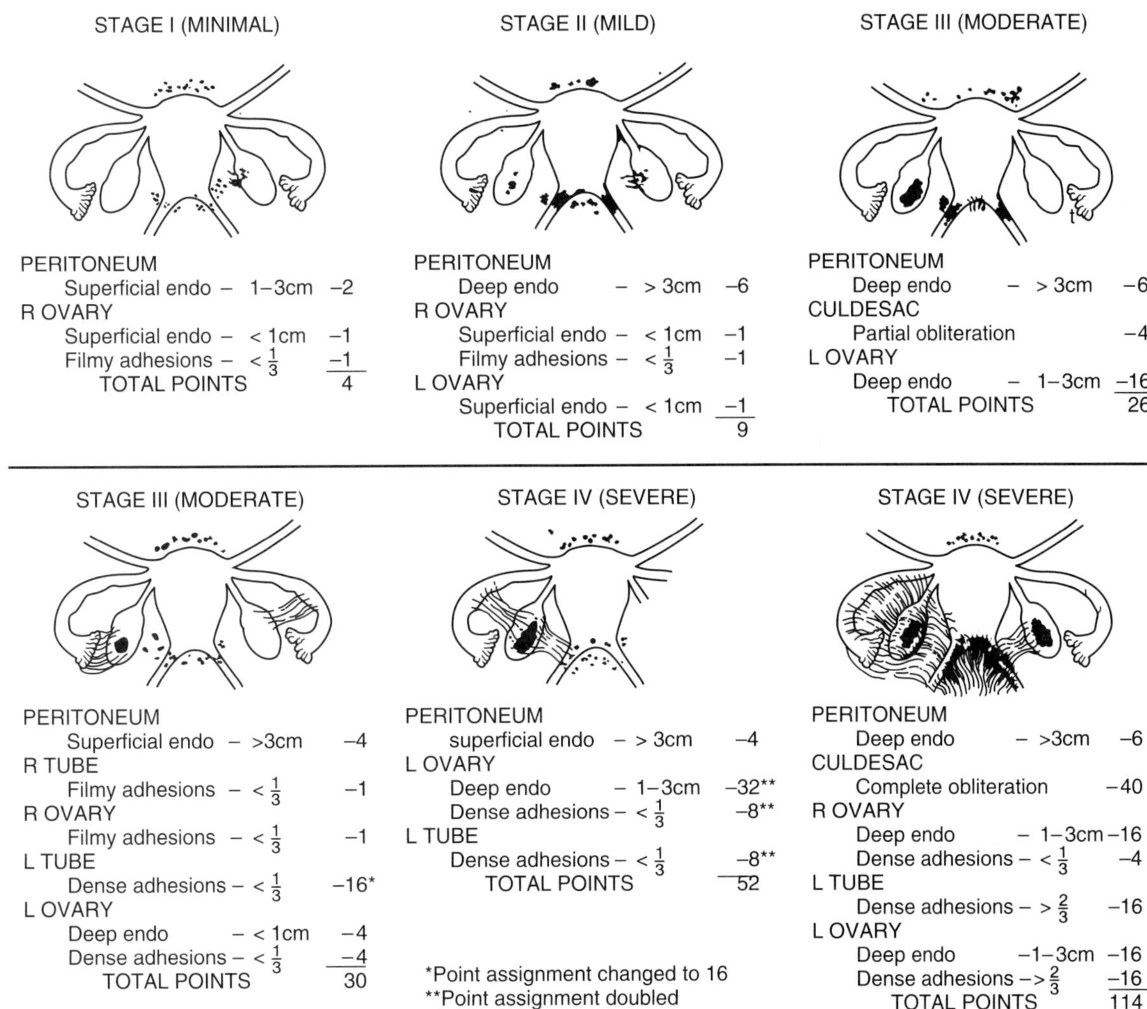

Figure 2. American Society for Reproductive Medicine scoring system.

Symptoms are not consistent with the scoring system. Although women with stage III and IV are more likely to have severe dysmenorrhea, pain can be severe for women with stage I and II disease. Infertility is associated with all stages of endometriosis, although severe adhesions associated with stage IV (score >70) rarely results in spontaneous pregnancy. The classification is not ideal for determining the best mode of treatment, but allows appropriate communication between providers on the extent of the disease.

DIAGNOSIS

Although endometriosis can only be diagnosed with certainty at surgery or biopsy of lesions, signs and symptoms can suggest the disease. Women with symptoms suggesting endometriosis can be treated without surgical confirmation. The classic history includes worsening dysmenorrhea and dyspareunia that advances to pain throughout the menstrual cycle. Pain can vary to include lower back pain, upper thigh pain, dysuria, dyschezia, and mid-abdominal pain. For all women presenting with chronic pelvic pain, it is critical to rule out pregnancy, urinary tract, gastrointestinal, and musculoskeletal causes. Chronic pelvic pain is more common in women with a history of sexual abuse, so it is important to obtain this history from all women presenting with pain. The pelvic exam may demonstrate pain or nodular lesions in the cul-de-sac, an ovarian mass, or fixation of the pelvic organs. Ultrasound can be used to confirm the presence of a possible endometrioma, but cannot identify endometrial implants.

CA 125 levels have been used for the diagnosis and follow-up for women with endometriosis. Commonly, the CA 125 level is mildly elevated in women with any peritoneal lesion. The CA 125 level has primarily been used to demonstrate the efficacy of therapy and the presence of recurrence. Another glycoprotein, CA 19-9, has been shown to be a potential marker for endometriosis.

Endometriosis is not consistently associated with pelvic pain or dysmenorrhea, and it should be considered in women with unexplained infertility. Although endometriosis is found in 30% to 50% of women with unexplained infertility, it is unclear if all stages of endometriosis are associated with infertility. Extensive adhesions, associated with stage IV disease, can affect tubal patency and the release of the oocyte at ovulation. Lysis of adhesions increases the chance of pregnancy after surgery, confirming the effect of severe disease on fertility. A recent multicenter trial also demonstrated increased pregnancy rates in women with stage I and II disease after laparoscopic removal of implants. This suggests that even minimal and mild endometriosis can adversely affect fertility. Although surgical treatment may not be the most effective therapy to optimize fertility, women with unexplained infertility may be considered for surgical diagnosis and treatment.

MEDICAL THERAPY

The medical treatments for endometriosis are moderately effective, as listed in Table 1. Unfortunately all of these therapies affect ovarian function and therefore delay pregnancy. For women not desiring pregnancy, or willing to delay conception, medical therapy is an option. There is considerable discussion regarding the use of medications for the treatment of endometriosis without surgically confirming the disease. Certainly it is reasonable to use oral contraceptives or progestins to treat pelvic pain before confirming the presence of endometriosis. Often nonsteroidal anti-inflammatories are added to hormonal suppression as a treatment for undiagnosed pelvic pain. Oral contraceptives are effective in up to 80% of women. Oral contraceptives are often given as a pseudopregnancy regimen, as a continuous medication, with no placebo week of pills.

Progestins, including norethindrone acetate (NEA) (Aygestin) and medroxyprogesterone acetate (MPA) (Provera),* are also effective for the treatment of pain resulting from endometriosis. Approximately 90% of women have an improvement in pain with 5 to 15 milligrams of NEA daily. MPA, as an oral preparation or a 150 mg depot injection given every 90 days, is effective in 90% of women. Desogestrel and cyproterone acetate, progestins that are not available in the United States, have also been shown to be effective treatments for pelvic pain. Although the other medical therapies are recommended for only 6 months, oral contraceptives and progestins can be used for extended periods. Studies are limited, but these medications are often used after surgical therapy to less the risk of endometriosis recurrence for women not desiring pregnancy. Side effects, including breast tenderness, bloating, weight gain, mood changes, headache, and decreased libido, can occur these medications.

*Not FDA approved for this indication.

Danazol (Danocrine),* a synthetic androgen, suppressives gonadotropin release, prevents ovulation, and inhibits ovarian steroid production. The typical dose is 600 to 800 mg daily for 6 months. Pain relief has been documented in various studies between 70% and 100%. Surgical studies have demonstrated a decrease in endometriosis implants after therapy. Side effects, as expected with an androgenic agent, can include weight gain, oily skin, acne, hirsutism, and breast atrophy. Rarely, deepening of the voice can occur.

Gonadotropin releasing hormone agonists (GnRHa) effectively stop the release of gonadotropins and cause "temporary menopause." These agents, available by injection or intranasal spray, act to downregulate the pituitary production of follicle-stimulating hormone and luteinizing hormone. Studies suggest up to 95% of women have improvement in pain with this medication. Recent studies suggest increased pregnancy rates in women using this medication for 3 months before in vitro fertilization (IVF). This medication is limited because of a decrease in bone density with extended use, limiting the usage to 6 months. The hypoestrogenic side effects include hot flushes, sleep disturbance, mood changes, and vaginal dryness. Add-back therapy with estrogen and progestin therapy have been added to prevent bone loss and to minimize side effects.

Medical therapy has been combined with surgical therapy to attempt to improve pain relief and improve subsequent fertility. Limited studies do suggest that medical therapy with GnRH agonists may improve long-term pain relief after surgery, but the combination of surgery and medical therapy appear less likely to improve the chance for pregnancy than surgery alone.

TABLE 1. **Medical Treatment of Endometriosis**

Nonsteroidal anti-inflammatories	Oral
Oral contraceptives	Cyclic or continuous
Progestins	Oral or injectable
Norethindrone acetate (Aygestin)	
Medroxyprogesterone acetate (Provera)*	
Androgens	Oral
Danazol (Danocrine)	
Gonadotropin-releasing hormone agonist	Injectable or intranasal
Leuprolide acetate (Lupron)	
Buserelin	

*Not FDA approved for this indication.

SURGICAL THERAPY

As well as diagnosing endometriosis, surgery allows treatment of the disease. Removal of implants, either by cautery or laser ablation, improved pain in 85% of women. Unlike medical therapy, surgical therapy allows the removal of endometriomas and lysis of adhesions. Studies have demonstrated that laparoscopic surgery is equivalent to a laparotomy for the treatment of pelvic pain for women with stage IV disease. This suggests that outpatient surgery by laparoscopy is the first choice for surgical ablation of endometriosis.

Women with recurrent endometriosis, who do not desire fertility, may elect to undergo definitive therapy by hysterectomy and bilateral oophorectomy. Ninety percent of women have resolution of pain after the removal of the uterus and ovaries. The effectiveness is less successful if the ovaries are not removed, with 30% to 40% of women having recurrent pain.

*Not FDA approved for this indication.

Recurrence of pain after hysterectomy alone may require an additional procedure to remove the ovaries.

MANAGEMENT OF INFERTILITY

There is considerable discussion regarding the association between infertility and endometriosis. Studies have shown that, after the diagnosis of endometriosis, up to 70% of women with primary infertility and 80% with secondary infertility will conceive in 5 years. Although many women will eventually conceive, there is a decrease in per cycle fecundity in women with endometriosis, as compared with the general population, prolonging the time required to achieve pregnancy. This is especially concerning for women with decreased fertility based on advancing maternal age. Although women with endometriosis can elect to have no therapy, infertility treatment is often recommended.

Despite the possible increase in fertility after surgery for endometriosis per cycle fecundity is still reduced. After laparoscopic ablation of endometriosis, only 31% of women conceived within 36 months. Women may elect to attempt pregnancy for a period of time after surgery, but other infertility therapy may shorten the time to conception.

Infertility treatment for women with endometriosis is similar to the treatment options for unexplained infertility, as listed in Table 2. Studies demonstrate that the chance for pregnancy without therapy is 3% per month, with clomiphene citrate (Clomid) and intrauterine inseminations 6% to 9% per month, and with injectable gonadotropins 9% to 14% per month. The highest pregnancy rate per cycle of treatment occurs with assisted reproductive technologies. Both gamete intrafallopian transfer (GIFT) and IVF are effective treatments for endometriosis. The most recent data demonstrate greater than 25% per cycle fecundity for GIFT and IVF therapy. Studies have examined the effectiveness of medical and surgical therapy before GIFT or IVF and offer limited support to the use of GnRHa prior to infertility therapy.

CONCLUSION

Endometriosis is a common gynecologic disorder that can cause pelvic pain and infertility. Although the pathogenesis of endometriosis is not yet known, recent studies suggest a genetic link and an association with changes in the immune system. A thorough history and physical can strongly suggest endometriosis, allowing treatment with oral contraceptives or progestins before surgical diagnosis. Women with ongoing pain or recurrent endometriosis are effectively treated with medical therapy including danazol, an oral androgen, and gonadotropin-releasing hormone agonist. Women who have completed childbearing may elect to have definitive surgery with hysterectomy and oophorectomy. For women with infertility, endometriosis can be diagnosed and treated by laparoscopic surgery. To shorten the time to conception, women may elect to undergo infertility treatment after the diagnosis of endometriosis. The most effective infertility therapies for women with endometriosis are the assisted reproductive technologies.

TABLE 2. **Treatment of Infertility for Women with Endometriosis**

No therapy
Laparoscopy
Cautery or laser ablation of implants
Lysis of adhesions
Medical therapy
Clomiphene (Clomid)/intrauterine insemination
Injectable gonadotropins
Assisted reproductive technologies
In vitro fertilization
Gamete intrafallopian transfer

DYSFUNCTIONAL UTERINE BLEEDING

method of
CHAD I. FRIEDMAN, M.D.
The Ohio State University
Columbus, Ohio

CLASSIFICATION

This article deals exclusively with abnormal uterine bleeding in the reproductive-age female. Various terminology exists to describe abnormal bleeding: menorrhagia (heavy or prolonged bleeding), metrorrhagia (bleeding in between periods), polymenorrhea (frequent bleeding), and so forth. Although descriptive, these terms provide little insight for diagnosis, etiology, or treatment. For this discussion I categorize abnormal bleeding into (1) anovulatory bleeding, (2) ovulatory bleeding that is excessive (quantity or duration), and (3) abnormally timed bleeding associated with ovulatory cyclicity. Other causes of bleeding (pregnancy-related bleeding, postmenopausal bleeding, and pharmacologic-contraceptive bleeding) are dealt with in other articles and are not the focus of this discussion.

Most complaints of abnormal uterine bleeding are not emergencies and allow time for determination of whether the woman is ovulatory or anovulatory. Ovulatory function can be assessed by numerous methods. The least expensive include a history of prolonged oligomenorrhea in the absence of pregnancy preceding the bleeding episode (suggestive of anovulation), basal body temperature charting (high specificity, low sensitivity), and self-evaluation of cervical mucus. More reliable tests of ovulatory function include serum or salivary progesterone, urinary pregnanediol levels, or, the most commonly used one in this situation, endometrial biopsy. These later studies, to be reliable, must be performed during the luteal phase, ideally between 4 to 10 days after ovulation or before the next bleeding episode. Basal body temperature charts, luteinizing hormone (LH) predictor kits, or premenstrual symptom charting may be helpful in timing the diagnostic tests. The importance of laboratory confirmation of ovulatory function is highlighted by studies showing that 25% of presumed anovulatory bleeders have secretory endometrial biopsies and that 20% of hirsute women with regular cyclic bleeding may be anovulatory.

ANOVULATORY BLEEDING

The most common cause of anovulatory bleeding is polycystic ovary disease. Other causes include mild hyperprolactinemia, thyroid disorders, granulosa cell tumors, bulimia, and exogenous estrogen treatment. Hypoestrogenic states such as ovarian failure, anorexia nervosa, prolactinomas, and hypopituitarism commonly arise as amenorrhea rather than abnormal bleeding. The evaluation of anovulatory states is detailed elsewhere. Treatment of anovulatory bleeding should focus on correcting the cause of anovulation as well as treatment of the symptomatic bleeding.

Women with anovulatory bleeding represent a situation of unopposed estrogen with an increased risk of endometrial hyperplasia or endometrial cancer. Women younger than 25 years with a history of less than 1 year of anovulatory status are at extremely low risk of endometrial carcinoma or atypical hyperplasia. An endometrial biopsy to exclude endometrial neoplastic changes is suggested for most anovulatory women older than 25 with abnormal bleeding.

Progestins are the mainstay of symptomatic treatment as well as avoidance of endometrial carcinoma. Hormonal contraceptives are perhaps the easiest means for establishing controlled regular cyclic bleeding. For those in whom hormonal contraceptives (oral, patch, or ring) are contraindicated or not well tolerated, cyclic progestins administered for 14 days every 4 to 6 weeks can be utilized: medroxyprogesterone (Provera) 5 to 10 mg/d, norethindrone (Aygestin) 5 mg/d, or micronized progesterone (Prometrium) 400 mg at bedtime. When bleeding is very heavy during the initial presentation, conjugated estrogen (Premarin) (2.5 to 5 mg for 5 days) may be utilized beginning 2 days before the progestin or oral contraceptive to control the bleeding. In the absence of a treatment plan capable of restoring ovulatory cyclicity, exogenous progestins (hormonal contraceptives or progestin only) need to be administered throughout the reproductive life span of anovulatory women.

EXCESSIVE OVULATORY BLEEDING

The differential diagnosis of excessive ovulatory bleeding focuses on anatomic abnormalities (fibroids, adenomyosis), coagulopathies, infections, and hypothyroidism. As in all cases of abnormal bleeding, pregnancy must be ruled out. A major problem in the evaluation of excessive ovulatory bleeding (>80 mL of blood) is documenting the complaint. Estimates of the amount of bleeding by both the patient and physician are notoriously unreliable except in the extreme. Anemia is strongly supportive of excessive bleeding but has many causes. Iron and folic acid supplementation, although integral in the treatment of heavy menstrual bleeding, may also prevent documentation of the patient's complaint.

Routine pelvic examination is helpful for determining the presence of fibroids or the suggestion of adenomyosis. Imaging procedures (transvaginal ultrasonography or magnetic resonance imaging) are, however, often necessary to evaluate for smaller submucosal fibroid and the elusive adenomyosis. Coagulatory function should be assessed by complete blood count (CBC), prothrombin time, activated partial thromboplastin time, and a von Willebrand panel. This is extremely important in adolescents. Hematologic consultation may be considered if other signs or symptoms of a coagulation defect exist. Endometrial biopsy can be used to confirm ovulatory function while evaluating for neoplastic processes and infection. A thyroid-stimulating hormone test can be obtained to complete the initial assessment. For a majority of women complaining of excessive menstrual bleeding, no cause is found clinically. Studies support an imbalance in prostaglandins, metalloproteinase inhibitors, or angiogenic factors contributing to excessive uterine bleeding.

Nonsurgical treatment options for excessive menstruation rely on hormonal therapy, antiprostaglandins, and procoagulants. Oral contraceptives typically decrease the amount of bleeding compared with ovulatory cycles. By extending the duration of active medication (i.e., from 21 to 42 days) the number of bleeding episodes can be decreased. Introduction of progestin-releasing intrauterine devices (Progestasert)* provides another highly effective hormonal means for reducing menstrual blood loss with the potential for rapid reversibility when removed. Depo Provera (medroxyprogesterone)* may be used to create an amenorrheic state in up to 60% of women. However, the prolonged action of Depo Provera makes future treatment difficult if this treatment option is unsuccessful in alleviating the patient's global symptoms. Gonadotropin-releasing hormone agonists may also be used to control excessive menstrual bleeding, but the high cost makes them unacceptable for long-term therapy. It is noteworthy that luteal progestin supplementation in ovulatory women has inconsistently been shown to be of any benefit in limiting menstrual bleeding.

Antiprostaglandins (i.e., mefenamic acid [Ponstel]* 500 mg three times a day, ibuprofen [Motrin]* 1200 mg/d) have been shown to reduce blood loss mildly (20%) in women with menorrhagia. Although the effect is limited, the associated reduction in dysmenorrhea may significantly reduce the overall menstrual complaints. The oral antifibrinolytic tranexamic acid (Cyklokapron)* (1 g/day for 3 days) is an agent commonly used in Europe for excessive menstrual bleeding with high efficacy. Regrettably, it is not easily obtainable in the United States. For women with von Willebrand's deficiency, administration of

*Not FDA approved for this indication.

DDAVP (desmopressin) around the time of menses is of some benefit.

For many women, medical treatment is inadequate, inconvenient, or associated with excessive side effects. Endometrial ablation, uterine artery embolization, myomectomy, and hysterectomy are reasonable alternatives for these women when childbearing is completed.

ABNORMALLY TIMED BLEEDING ASSOCIATED WITH OVULATORY CYCLICITY

Bleeding in between endogenous progesterone-induced withdrawal bleeding may be caused by several readily recognizable entities: cervical polyps, endometrial polyps, cervical carcinoma, submucosal fibroids, functioning ovarian cysts, cervicitis, and endometriosis. Premenstrual spotting not infrequently is associated with endometriosis, reflecting the numerous biochemical abnormalities described with eutopic endometrium from subjects with endometriosis. Preovulatory bleeding induced by the fall of estrogen prior to the LH surge may also be suspected on the basis of timing and its typically light character.

Evaluation consists of exclusion of pregnancy (i.e., intrauterine, ectopic, choriocarcinoma) and then visualization of the lower genital tract and cervix with cytologic evaluation (i.e., Pap smear) and sexually transmitted disease (STD) specimens, bimanual examination, and, in the absence of a readily identified cause, uterine cavity evaluation (hydrosonogram or hysteroscopy) with an endometrial biopsy. Laparoscopic evaluation and treatment of endometriosis are performed when dysmenorrhea, dyspareunia, or cul-de-sac nodularity is present.

Treatment is often surgical involving removal of polyps or fibroids at hysteroscopy, occasional antibiotic treatment, and, in the case of preovulatory bleeding, supplementation with estrogen (micronized estradiol [Estrace] 2 mg for 3 days) commencing the day before the usual onset of bleeding. When a benign-appearing cyst is present, observation with reevaluation in a month is appropriate.

PROFUSE UTERINE HEMORRHAGE

Rarely we are faced with profuse uterine hemorrhage in the nonpregnant female, which mandates immediate intervention. In this situation, after a rapid history and physical examination, intravenous access for fluid resuscitation and laboratory studies is achieved. Initial laboratory studies include a CBC, platelets, human chorionic gonadotropin, prothrombin time, partial thromboplastin time, von Willebrand panel, type and crossmatch, liver function test, and creatinine. Pelvic examination should exclude any gross lesions (laceration, gestational trophoblast tumor, pedunculated fibroid, cervical cancer, large fibroid) as well as the extent of bleeding. A Foley catheter appropriate for the uterine size can be placed in an intracavitary fashion and inflated with saline to compress the endometrium provided pregnancy is excluded. If uterine artery embolization is not feasible within the institution, vasopressin (Pitressin)* 3 mL (10 units in 20 mL of 1% lidocaine) may be injected at 2, 4, 8, and 10 o'clock paracervically to reduce the hemorrhage and reduce the discomfort of uterine distention. When uterine artery embolization is feasible, vasopressin should be avoided as it compromises the procedure. Conjugate estrogen (Premarin) (25 mg) intravenous every 6 hours has been suggested as an additional means to reduce uterine bleeding and should be initiated. Blood and coagulation factor for replacement may also be infused on the basis of clinical status and laboratory studies. Ultrasonography should now be performed to assess for anatomic abnormalities in addition to establishing proper placement of the Foley catheter within the fundus if placed. Failure to control the bleeding significantly at this point requires surgical (hysteroscopy, uterine artery ligation, dilation and curettage, or hysterectomy) or radiologic (embolization) intervention. Endometrial biopsy or hysteroscopy with sampling is required but can be performed at 12 to 24 hours following stabilization when the catheter is removed.

*Not FDA approved for this indication.

AMENORRHEA

method of
DEAN MOUTOS, M.D.
University of Arkansas for Medical Sciences
Little Rock, Arkansas

Amenorrhea occurs in approximately 5% of reproductive-aged women and is defined as (1) absent menses for 6 months, (2) absent menses for 3 months in a woman previously having regular menses, or (3) no menstrual period by 16 years of age. Primary amenorrhea refers to women who have never experienced menses, whereas secondary amenorrhea refers to the cessation of menses in a previously menstruating woman. Although this classification implies distinct etiologies for each category, the two have considerable overlap. The diagnostic workup for amenorrhea is similar regardless of whether it is primary or secondary. Remember that pregnancy is the most common cause of amenorrhea, and a pregnancy test should be performed in all reproductive-aged women with amenorrhea.

NORMAL MENSTRUAL CYCLE

Regular cyclical menstruation is the result of a complex series of endocrine events orchestrated to prepare the endometrium for implantation of an embryo. Control of the cycle originates in the hypothalamus. The arcuate nucleus secretes gonadotropin-releasing hormone (GnRH) in a pulsatile fashion every 60 to 90 minutes. Pulsatile release is critical; an increase or decrease in pulse frequency may result in amenorrhea. The hypothalamus is subject to neurohormonal input from higher brain centers and to external environmental factors that have the potential to disrupt the pulsatile release of GnRH. GnRH stimulates the secretion of follicle-stimulating hormone (FSH) and luteinizing hormone (LH) by the pituitary. FSH stimulates follicular development and selection of the dominant follicle, which secretes estradiol, thereby leading to endometrial proliferation. The midcycle rise in estradiol triggers a surge of pituitary LH resulting in ovulation. The corpus luteum secretes progesterone, which induces the secretory changes in the endometrium necessary for implantation of an embryo. In the absence of pregnancy, steroid secretion by the corpus luteum declines 14 days after ovulation, with subsequent breakdown of the endometrium and menstrual bleeding. As the new cycle ensues and the dominant follicle begins secreting estradiol, the endometrium is regenerated, menses stop, and the process repeats itself.

The physical manifestation of amenorrhea may represent a problem with the uterus, the gonads, the pituitary, or the hypothalamus. The goal of the workup outlined in the next section is to accurately and cost-effectively identify which component of the reproductive axis is malfunctioning.

ETIOLOGY OF AMENORRHEA

Thyroid and Prolactin. Thyroid dysfunction (usually hypothyroid) can cause menstrual abnormalities, including amenorrhea. Hyperprolactinemia inhibits the pulsatile release of GnRH, which results in menstrual abnormalities ranging from luteal phase deficiency to amenorrhea. The higher the prolactin level, the more profound the menstrual derangement. Not all patients with elevated prolactin will have galactorrhea, so prolactin should be measured in all women with amenorrhea. Thyrotropin-releasing hormone (TRH) is a potent stimulator of both thyroid-stimulating hormone (TSH) and prolactin. Patients with primary hypothyroidism may have moderate elevations in prolactin as a result of an increase in TRH. If prolactin is elevated, TSH should be measured.

Hypothalamus. Amenorrhea secondary to hypothalamic dysfunction is characterized by normal prolactin, low or low-normal FSH and LH, and low estrogen levels. A disturbance in the pulsatile release of GnRH caused by physical or psychological stress is a common cause of hypothalamic amenorrhea. Elevated corticotropin-releasing hormone (CRH) is thought to inhibit GnRH pulsatility during times of stress. Amenorrhea usually resolves when the stress is relieved. Exercise-induced amenorrhea, another form of hypothalamic dysfunction, is usually evident from the patient's history. The amount and intensity of exercise directly correlate with the degree of menstrual dysfunction, which can range from luteal phase insufficiency to amenorrhea. The mechanism of this disorder appears to be related to a combination of restricted caloric intake, a low percentage of body fat, and large energy expenditure. Exercise-induced amenorrhea is a hypoestrogenic state that can result in osteoporosis and bone fractures. Menstrual function usually improves with a decrease in exercise intensity, even with no change in body weight.

Eating disorders are frequently associated with menstrual disturbances. The most severe eating disorder, anorexia nervosa, is usually accompanied by amenorrhea, which may precede, coincide with, or follow the actual weight loss. Hormonal characteristics include low FSH, LH, estradiol, and triiodothyronine (T_3); normal prolactin, TSH, and thyroxine (T_4); and high reverse T_3 and cortisol. Resolution of the anorexia usually results in return of normal menstrual function, although 30% of patients remain amenorrheic even after weight gain.

Isolated gonadotropin deficiency is probably due to GnRH deficiency in the hypothalamus, which results in an absence of pituitary FSH and LH secretion. Patients have primary amenorrhea and deficient breast development because of a lack of estrogen production. If anosmia is present, the condition is called Kallmann's syndrome. Pseudocyesis (false pregnancy) is a rare cause of amenorrhea, presumably hypothalamic in origin. Patients have many of the physical signs of pregnancy, including amenorrhea and abdominal distention, but they are not pregnant. The hormone profile in these patients is variable. With appropriate psychological counseling, the condition is reversible.

Pituitary. Pituitary adenomas, usually prolactin secreting, may cause amenorrhea. Other pituitary tumors, including growth hormone- and adrenocorticotropic hormone (ACTH)-secreting, may also be associated with amenorrhea. Radiologic imaging of the pituitary is indicated if prolactin levels are elevated. Empty sella syndrome is due to a congenital defect in the sellar diaphragm that results in herniation of the subarachnoid space into the pituitary fossa. Radiologic studies reveal an enlarged sella turcica with the pituitary gland flattened against the pituitary fossa. Most patients with empty sella syndrome have normal endocrine function, although hyperprolactinemia may be seen. Sheehan's syndrome is infarction of the pituitary gland after hypovolemic shock in the postpartum period. Patients will not lactate and will have persistent postpartum amenorrhea. Other anterior pituitary hormones, including TSH and ACTH, may also be deficient in Sheehan's syndrome.

Ovary. The most frequent ovarian disorder associated with amenorrhea is polycystic ovarian (PCO) syndrome. Hyperandrogenism and chronic anovulation are the hallmarks of PCO syndrome. Although most PCO patients have oligomenorrhea, some may have amenorrhea. Symptoms of PCO syndrome usually begin during the teenage years and may become more prominent with age. PCO patients have chronic estrogen stimulation of the endometrium without the balancing effect of progesterone. They may have prolonged episodes of amenorrhea punctuated with episodes of hypermenorrhea.

Abnormalities of the X chromosome will result in ovarian failure with FSH and LH levels in the menopausal range. Patients with pure Turner's syndrome (45,XO) will have primary amenorrhea and sexual infantilism. Turner mosaics (46,XX/45,XO) may have secondary amenorrhea and normal sexual development, and fertility may be possible. Deletions of the short or long arm of the X chromosome may also lead to ovarian failure. Patients with pure gonadal dysgenesis will have fibrous bands of tissue (streak gonads) replacing the ovaries. These patients will have primary amenorrhea and sexual infantilism. Their karyotype may be either 46,XX or 46,XY, but the external phenotype will be infantile female.

A karyotype should be obtained in all patients with primary amenorrhea and elevated gonadotropin levels. Approximately 50% will have a chromosomal abnormality. It is important to determine whether a Y chromosome cell line is present because the risk of gonadal tumors is increased. Removal of the gonads is indicated in such patients. It is arguable whether older patients with secondary amenorrhea and elevated gonadotropins should have a karyotype performed. Chromosome abnormalities will occasionally be found, but most such cases of premature ovarian failure are idiopathic. Patients who have received therapeutic doses of irradiation or chemotherapy may experience premature ovarian failure. The amount of irradiation or chemotherapy that the ovaries will tolerate is both dose and age dependent. Younger women tolerate larger doses without undergoing ovarian failure.

Androgen-secreting ovarian (and less commonly adrenal) tumors may result in amenorrhea. Signs of androgen excess such as hirsutism, acne, and oily skin are usually present. Signs of virilization, including clitoromegaly, temporal balding, deepening of the voice, and decreased breast size, may be seen. An important clue to the presence of a tumor is the rapidity of development of the androgenic manifestations. Symptoms in patients with androgen-secreting tumors usually develop over the course of several months, whereas those in patients with PCO syndrome develop slowly over many years. Total testosterone and dehydroepiandrosterone sulfate (DHEAS) levels should be measured in patients suspected of having androgen-secreting tumors. A total testosterone level greater than 200 ng/dL, a DHEAS level greater than 700 μg/dL, or rapidly developing symptoms should prompt radiologic evaluation of the ovaries and adrenals.

Uterus and Outflow Tract. Congenital malformations of the müllerian ducts (uterus, cervix, upper part of the vagina) will usually be associated with amenorrhea. Complete absence of the müllerian ducts is known as Rokitansky's syndrome. These patients have a short blind vaginal pouch without a uterus or cervix. Other obstructive malformations such as cervical atresia, a transverse vaginal septum, and an imperforate hymen will be manifested as amenorrhea, often in conjunction with pelvic pain caused by obstructed menstrual flow. A key feature is the development of normal secondary sexual characteristics because of the presence of normally functioning ovaries. Cervical stenosis obstructing the outflow of menstrual blood may be an acquired condition in patients with a history of cone biopsy or cryotherapy of the cervix. The diagnosis is confirmed by an inability to pass a uterine sound past the cervical canal.

Intrauterine adhesions obliterating the uterine cavity (Asherman's syndrome) may result in hypomenorrhea or amenorrhea. A history of dilation and curettage in conjunction with a recent pregnancy is usually noted. Abdominal myomectomy may rarely lead to obliteration of the uterine cavity. If extension of uterine fibroids into the uterine cavity is not recognized during the course of performing a myomectomy, the endometrial cavity can be inadvertently resected or sutured and amenorrhea will result.

Patients with complete androgen insensitivity (also known as testicular feminization) have primary amenorrhea and a seemingly normal female phenotype. On closer inspection, they will have a short blind-ending vagina, absent müllerian structures, scant pubic and axillary hair, and pale areolae. Male gonads can be found in either the abdomen or the inguinal canal in these 46,XY patients. Gonadotropin levels will be normal, and testosterone will be in the normal male range. A mutation in the androgen receptor renders testosterone biologically inactive. These patients will feminize at puberty as a result of peripheral conversion of androgens to estrogens. The gonads should be removed after puberty to prevent the development of gonadal tumors.

Enzyme Deficiencies. Various adrenal enzyme deficiencies may be associated with amenorrhea and abnormal sexual development, including 21-hydroxylase, 11β-hydroxylase, 17-ketosteroid reductase, 17α-hydroxylase, and 17,20-desmolase. The karyotype may be 46,XX or 46,XY.

DIAGNOSTIC EVALUATION

A careful history and physical examination will suggest the diagnosis in most cases. The patient's general physical appearance, including height, weight, and body mass index, should be noted. Careful attention should be paid to the presence of breast tissue. The breasts are very sensitive to estrogen, so the presence of breast tissue indicates at least previous exposure to estrogen. Signs of androgen excess such as hirsutism, acne, clitoromegaly, and temporal balding should be sought. The presence of galactorrhea suggests a prolactin disorder. A pelvic examination should allow confirmation of an intact uterus, cervix, and vagina. Cervical stenosis can be ruled out by gently passing a uterine sound through the cervical canal. If the presence of normal müllerian structures is in doubt, pelvic ultrasound will usually clarify the anatomy. After pregnancy has been ruled out, the following guidelines should allow the correct diagnosis to be made.

Step 1

TSH and prolactin should be measured. If the TSH level is elevated, replacement with levothyroxine (Synthroid) at a dose of 1.5 μg/kg/d is indicated. TSH testing should be repeated 6 weeks after the start of therapy. If prolactin is elevated, a careful medication history should be obtained because numerous drugs can cause elevations in prolactin. If a repeat morning fasting prolactin level is still elevated, either computed tomography (CT) or magnetic resonance imaging (MRI) of the pituitary should be performed to look for a pituitary adenoma.

Step 2

If TSH and prolactin are normal, proceed with a progestin challenge. Medroxyprogesterone acetate (Provera) is given orally at a dose of 10 mg/d for 7 days. Menstrual bleeding should occur within 2 to 7 days after stopping use of the drug. Any amount of bleeding is considered a positive response that indicates an intact uterine outflow tract and the presence of endometrium that is estrogen primed. As an alternative to medroxyprogesterone, a single intramuscular injection of 200 mg of progesterone in oil can be given. A positive progestin challenge indicates anovulation as the etiology of the amenorrhea. If the patient does not desire pregnancy, periodic exposure of the endometrium to progestins is necessary to prevent endometrial hyperplasia and cancer. Medroxyprogesterone acetate is given orally at a dose of 5 to 10 mg/d for 12 days each month. Oral micronized progesterone (Prometrium), 200 mg/d for 12 days, may also be used to induce cyclical withdrawal bleeding. Neither of these drugs provides contraception. Patients with chronic anovulation may ovulate sporadically, and fertility is possible. If a patient fails to have withdrawal bleeding after she has been taking cyclical progestins, pregnancy should be ruled out. If contraception is necessary, combination oral contraceptive pills (OCPs) should be given. If fertility is desired, clomiphene citrate (Serophene, Clomid) is given at a dose of 50 mg/d for 5 days to induce ovulation. The dose may be increased by 50 mg each cycle up to a maximum of 200 mg/d for 5 days to induce ovulation. Approximately 80% of patients will ovulate with clomiphene. Exogenous gonadotropin therapy is required for patients who do not ovulate with clomiphene.

Step 3

A negative progestin challenge indicates either an anatomic problem with the uterus or an endometrium that is not estrogen primed. Sequential estrogen and progestin should be given next. Conjugated estrogens (Premarin)* are administered at a dose of 2.5 mg/d orally for 21 days in conjunction with medroxyprogesterone acetate, 10 mg/d orally for the last 5 days. Combination OCPs should be avoided because they do not provide sequential exposure of the endometrium to estrogen followed by progestin. Failure to have withdrawal bleeding indicates a uterine problem. The most likely cause in someone who was previously menstruating is Asherman's syndrome. Hysteroscopy or hysterosalpingography will confirm the diagnosis. Treatment is surgical excision of the adhesions with a hysteroscope.

Step 4

Positive bleeding with sequential estrogen/progestin indicates a functioning endometrium that was not estrogen primed. FSH and LH should be measured. Elevated gonadotropin levels with FSH higher than LH indicate ovarian failure. Depending on the patient's age and clinical history, a karyotype may be considered. Ovarian failure is irreversible, and standard menopausal hormone replacement therapy should be started to prevent osteoporosis and alleviate other symptoms of estrogen deficiency. If fertility is desired, in vitro fertilization with the use of donor oocytes is the only option.

Low or low-normal gonadotropin levels indicate a pituitary or hypothalamic problem. Risks factors for hypothalamic dysfunction such as stress, weight loss, eating disorders, and others should be sought. In the absence of an identifiable cause, CT or MRI of the brain should be performed to rule out a mass lesion. These patients are hypoestrogenic and are at risk for the usual consequences of estrogen deficiency. Interestingly, they do not usually have hot flashes despite menopausal estrogen levels. Estrogen, usually in the form of OCPs, is given if fertility is not desired. If fertility is desired, induction of ovulation is indicated. Clomiphene citrate may be tried, but these patients usually require exogenous gonadotropins to induce ovulation. It should be emphasized that if the factor precipitating hypothalamic amenorrhea is stress, the amenorrhea will resolve when the stress is relieved. If weight loss or high-intensity exercise is the cause, lifestyle modifications should be emphasized before attempts at medical induction of ovulation.

DYSMENORRHEA

method of
THAIS BROWN TONORE, M.D.
University of Mississippi School of Medicine
Jackson, Mississippi

Dysmenorrhea refers to pain during the menstrual cycle. This is characterized by crampy suprapubic lower abdominal pain. It is described as spasmodic and sharp pain that may radiate to the lower back or thigh areas. It occurs at the start of menstruation and usually lasts 1 to 2 days. Nausea, vomiting, diarrhea, fatigue, headaches, and lightheadedness may accompany it. Dysmenorrhea usually starts within 3 years of menarche when regular ovulatory cycles are established.

The prevalence of dysmenorrhea ranges from 50% to 90%. From 5% to 15% of women find their daily activities limited because of the pain and symptoms they experience with their monthly menses. These numbers may be low because of the over-the-counter availability of non-steroidal anti-inflammatory drugs (NSAIDs). Access to these medications allows patients the option of self-treatment, and the condition may not be brought to the physician's attention if the patient is experiencing relief of her symptoms.

The pain with menstruation is caused by release of prostaglandins from the sloughing cells of the endometrium. Estrogen and then progesterone stimulation of the endometrial cells during an ovulatory cycle result in increased stores of arachidonic acid, which is a precursor to prostaglandin production. Prostaglandin $F_{2\alpha}$ ($PGF_{2\alpha}$) and prostaglandin E_2 (PGE_2) are made by the endometrial cells and upon release stimulate uterine contractions that decrease the blood supply in the muscles and result in muscle ischemia and pain. The severity of the dysmenorrhea correlates with the levels of prostaglandins. The symptoms are more severe in the first 2 days of the cycle when the prostaglandin levels are highest. The bronchial, bowel, and vascular smooth muscles can also be affected by the prostaglandins and cause symptoms of bronchoconstriction, nausea, vomiting, diarrhea, and hypertension.

In diagnosing dysmenorrhea, a careful history should include the characteristics of the pain and its relationship to the beginning of the menstrual cycle. Other problems need to be excluded, such as infections and pains during other parts of the cycle. In primary dysmenorrhea, the physical examination and pelvic examination should be normal. There are no diagnostic tests for confirmation. If pelvic pathology is identified by the history or physical examination, the pain is termed secondary dysmenorrhea.

Beginning therapy with education and reassurance helps with understanding the process that is occurring and with compliance. Placebo has been effective in treating dysmenorrhea, but the effects fade with each successive cycle. Improvement went from 84% in the first cycle to 29%, 16%, and 10% in each of the following cycles.

Because prostaglandins play a role in the genesis of the pain, a trial of NSAIDs should give partial, if not complete, relief. Success rates vary from 64% to 100%. Most studies show that 80% to 86% of the patients maintained relief of pain with use of NSAIDs. Response to NSAIDs can be helpful in confirming the diagnosis of primary dysmenorrhea. The NSAIDs are usually started at the onset of menses and continued for 1 to 2 days into the cycle. Many women report better symptom control if the medications are started 1 to 2 days prior to menses.

TABLE 1. **Nonsteroidal Anti-Inflammatory Drugs Used to Treat Dysmenorrhea**

Class of Nonsteroidals	Dosages
Phenylpropionic Acid Derivatives	
Ibuprofen (Advil, Ibuprin, Motrin)	400–800 mg q4–8h
Naproxen (Naprosyn)	500 mg, then 250 mg q6–8h
Naproxen sodium (Anaprox, Naprelan, Aleve)	275–550 mg q8–12h
Fenamates	
Mefenamic acid (Ponstel)	500 mg, then 250 mg q6h
Cyclooxygenase (COX-2) Inhibitors	
Celecoxib (Celebrex)	400 mg, then 200 mg q12h
Rofecoxib (Vioxx)	25–50 mg qd
Valdecoxib (Bextra)	20 mg q12h

Three classes of NSAIDs have proved effective: fenamates, phenylpropionic acid derivatives, and cyclooxygenase (COX-2) inhibitors. The fenamates (mefenamic acid [Ponstel]) and the phenylpropionic acid derivatives (ibuprofen [Advil], naproxen [Naprosyn], and naproxen sodium [Anaprox]) both inhibit prostaglandin synthesis. The fenamates also block prostaglandin action. A reasonable approach is to try the phenylpropionic acid derivatives first and, if relief is not complete, to try one of the fenamates. Patients who have been using over-the-counter medications and have not achieved relief may not have been taking high enough doses. The cyclooxygenase inhibitors (valdecoxib [Bextra], rofecoxib [Vioxx], and celecoxib [Celebrex]) have also been approved for use in treating dysmenorrhea. Table 1 gives choices and dosages of these medications. Contraindications to these medicines include allergy to the drugs, pregnancy, ulcers, and asthma.

If NSAIDs do not provide complete relief of pain, oral contraceptives can be considered. When contraception is also needed, oral contraceptives may be the first choice of treatment. Birth control pills inhibit ovulation, decrease the thickness of the uterine lining, and decrease the amount of prostaglandins present.

TABLE 2. **Alternative Treatments for Dysmenorrhea**

Modality/Supplement	No. in Study	Dosage	Effects
TENS unit	126		42%–60% moderate relief, decreased NSAID dosage
Laparoscopic-presacral neuronectomy	88		33%–88% decreased pain
Acupuncture	43		91% improved, 41% decreased analgesics
Omega-3 fatty acids*	181 dietary, 42 supplements	No dosage specified	Decrease in pain with supplements
Transdermal nitroglycerin (Nitro-Dur)*	65	0.1 to 0.2 mg/h	90% effective 20% with headache
Thiamine (B1)*	556	100 mg/d × 90 d	87% cured 2 mo later (India)
Magnesium supplements*	30	No dosage specified	84% decreased symptoms
Vitamin E*	100	500 units/d	Decreased pain severity
Low-fat vegetarian diet	33		Decreased menstrual pain and duration

*Not FDA approved for this indication.
TENS, transcutaneous electrical nerve stimulation.

It may take two or three cycles to achieve maximum results. NSAIDs can be used with contraceptive pills for added benefits.

Lack of response to NSAIDs and oral contraceptives is an indication to look for other pathology. Ten percent of women still have primary dysmenorrhea despite adequate doses of these medications. To determine whether secondary dysmenorrhea is present, sonography or laparoscopic surgery may be necessary. Secondary dysmenorrhea usually occurs after a woman has had normal periods for some time. The pain is caused by an abnormality in the uterus, tubes, or ovaries. Causes of secondary dysmenorrhea are endometriosis, adenomyosis, chronic pelvic inflammatory disease, leiomyomata, and cervical stenosis. The management plan should address the pathology associated with the pain. (See discussion of clinical condition in appropriate chapters in this book.)

Patients are becoming more involved in their own treatments and are using alternative methods and supplements. There have been numerous small trials of alternative medications and modalities for the treatment of dysmenorrhea. Table 2 shows supplements and modalities that have been shown to be more effective than placebo in relieving dysmenorrhea. Physicians should ask patients about their use of alternative therapies.

Dysmenorrhea is a common gynecologic complaint. Treatment of the disorder is usually successful. Taking a good history, recognizing the disorder, and prescribing adequate medications improves outcome and patients' satisfaction.

PREMENSTRUAL DYSPHORIA

method of
URIEL HALBREICH, M.D.
State University of New York at Buffalo
Buffalo, New York

Premenstrual syndromes (PMSs) are clusters of symptoms and signs that appear during the late luteal phase of the menstrual cycle. More than 80% of women of reproductive age report some changes premenstrually. In about 10% of women the symptoms are severe and distressful to a point that treatment is sought and necessary. Mood and behavior changes are most prominent; in 3% to 8% of women they reach the level of a disorder that is currently defined in the psychiatric nomenclature as premenstrual dysphoric disorder (PMDD). PMDD may be conceived of as a severe subtype of PMS. Strict diagnostic criteria for PMDD were developed by the American Psychiatric Association (APA) as part of its *Diagnostic and Statistical Manual of Mental Disorders* (DSM) IV system. Criteria for PMS were published by the American College of Obstetrics and Gynecology (ACOG). PMS may first be reported during adolescence and be present until menopause. It does not appear before menarche, during pregnancy, during periods of amenorrhea, or following menopause.

During the last two decades there has been substantial progress in awareness, understanding, and management of PMS and PMDD that has resulted in treatment modalities that in clinical trials were shown to be efficacious in about 60% of women who met strict research criteria for PMS-PMDD. In day-to-day clinical practice, the rate of response is presumably higher if adequate diagnosis and proper treatment are provided.

DIAGNOSTIC DEFINITION OF PREMENSTRUAL SYNDROME AND PREMENSTRUAL DYSPHORIC DISORDER

The ACOG diagnostic criteria for PMS require that the patient reports at least 1 of 10 mood (depression, angry outbursts, irritability, anxiety, confusion, and social withdrawal) and somatic symptoms (breast tenderness, abdominal bloating, headache, and swelling of extremities) during the 5 days before menses, in each of three prior menstrual cycles. The symptoms should be relieved within 4 days of menses onset, without recurrence until at least cycle day 13; they should occur reproducibly during two cycles of prospective recording; and dysfunction in social or economic performance should be identified. Symptoms should be present in the absence of any pharmacologic therapy, hormone ingestion, or drug or alcohol abuse.

The DSM IV diagnostic criteria of PMDD follow a similar principle with an emphasis on mood and behavior. They require 1 year duration of symptoms that are present for the majority of cycles. At least 5 of 11 symptoms must occur during the week before menses and remit within days of menses. At least one of these symptoms should be depressed mood or hopelessness, irritability, tension or anxiety, or affective lability. Symptoms should interfere seriously with work, social activities, or relationships and not be an exacerbation of another disorder. They should be confirmed by prospective daily ratings during at least two consecutive symptomatic cycles.

For clinical practice, the diagnostic definition of PMS is:

Any symptom or cluster of symptoms that:

1. Appear cyclically, repeatedly, and consistently during the luteal phase of the menstrual cycle.
2. Are relieved shortly following the beginning of menses.
3. Do not exist for at least a week that includes the midfollicular phase.
4. Cause emotional or physical distress, suffering, or impairment of daily functioning.
5. Luteal phase occurrence and cyclicity are confirmed by prospective daily monitoring.

It should be noted that the duration of the symptomatic period may vary from 1 day prior to menses to the entire length of the luteal phase and the beginning of the next follicular phase. Therefore, for clinical practice no strict cutoff criteria should be exercised as long as the symptoms are consistently premenstrual. Even a woman who usually reports very severe PMS may have some cycles with no or mild symptoms.

ETIOLOGY AND PATHOPHYSIOLOGY

The exact etiology and underlying processes leading to PMS have not yet been definitively determined. It is plausible that multifaceted, multidimensional interactive processes are involved. Genetics plays an important role in the propensity to develop PMS and its specific phenotypes. Vulnerability is dynamically evolving; it might be increased by early life experiences (high prevalence of reported sexual and physical abuse during childhood, as well as other past traumas, was suggested) as well as accumulation of other stressful occurrences. Gonadal hormones and their menstrually related fluctuations play a major role in triggering PMS. The general pattern of gonadal hormone secretion in women with PMS is within normal limits. However, vulnerable women may demonstrate altered sensitivity to changes in gonadal hormones and related systems that do not affect most women. Relatively high levels of progesterone or some progesterone anxiogenic metabolites were suggested, as well as a premenstrual decrease in anxiolytic progestogens. Altered rate of fluctuation of gonadal hormones as well as their pulsatility has been suggested.

Estrogens and progestins influence and interact with various brain neurotransmitter systems as well as other central and peripheral processes. Activity of these system may fluctuate along with the fluctuations in activity of gonadal hormones. Clinically relevant changes have been demonstrated in the serotonergic and γ-aminobutyric acid systems and to some degree also in the dopaminergic, cholinergic, noradrenergic, and renin-angiotensin systems as well as in neuronal excitability. Women with PMS probably have a trait of amended cognition and coping style. Environmental inputs—stressful as well as pleasant—may influence the appearance or severity of PMS in a given cycle.

CLINICAL PRESENTATION

Over 300 diverse symptoms and signs have been reported as appearing premenstrually. To my knowledge, none of these symptoms is unique to the premenstrual period. PMS is defined by the *timing* of symptoms and not by their nature.

The most prevalent premenstrual psychological symptoms are irritability, anxiety, depression, and impulsivity. The most prominent physical symptoms are breast tenderness, sense of bloatedness, and headache. However, any symptom or cluster of symptoms to which a woman is vulnerable may appear premenstrually, including increased or decreased sleep and energy, increased or decreased appetite, depression, and hypomania or mania. The nature of symptoms and their clusters are usually consistent within each woman.

The individual vulnerability to specific phenotypes is underscored by reports of episodes of numerous physical disorders that in some women may appear only or mostly premenstrually. They include epilepsy, asthma, migraine headache, and others. Episodes of these so-called catamenial disorders or molimina may also appear during other periods of a woman's life, especially during stress. Their relation with PMS is still debatable although they may share similar triggers. There is also controversy regarding mental syndromes that are not exclusive to the premenstrual period but also appear with no connection to the menstrual cycle phase. It has been reported that the prevalence of several depressions and anxiety disorders is higher in women with PMS or PMDD and vice versa. Many women with chronic or repeated mental disorders have few or less severe episodes not premenstrually with exacerbations or increased severity premenstrually. These observations may point to shared vulnerability and the same triggers for the disordered state. Currently, most clinical investigators clearly differentiate between them and "pure" PMDD, a distinction that has clinical implications.

DIAGNOSTIC PROCEDURES

The diagnostic process for PMS is unique in the emphasis on timing and cyclicity and not on the nature of phenomena—symptoms and signs. There are also no specific pathognomonic laboratory tests yet. The two formalized diagnostic criteria systems (the DSM IV and ACOG's) call for prospective monitoring of symptoms for at least two cycles. There are a number of daily rating forms (DRFs) that have been published mostly for research purposes but are also useful for clinical diagnosis. All are based on subjective self-report by the patient. An applicable DRF should at least include the ACOG symptoms. It is important that the patient adds the specific symptoms that are her most severe individual complaints as well as impairment in home, social, and work activities and distress. All symptoms of the DRF should be noted every day before bedtime, preferably with a measure of severity (e.g., 0, not at all; 1, mild; 2, severe; 3, most severe). Days of bleeding should be noted.

In order to shorten the period until the final diagnosis, it is preferable to mail the DRF to the patient at the time of scheduling the first appointment, with instructions.

A first office visit should preferably be scheduled for the expected midfollicular phase in order to obtain a physician's observation of a nonsymptomatic period and exclude a chronic noncyclic disorder.

During this initial visit, physical and mental histories are taken and physical examination is performed—mostly to rule out other diagnoses. See Table 1. Obstetric and gynecologic history should also include inquiries about any symptoms during pregnancy and postpartum periods and adverse effects of hormonal contraceptives—all may be associated with vulnerability to PMS.

TABLE 1. **Differential Diagnosis of Premenstrual Syndrome**

General Medical Conditions
Dysmenorrhea
Endometriosis
Polycystic ovaries
Some oral contraceptives
Hypothyroidism
Hyperglycemia
Anemia
Exacerbation of chronic disorders (e.g., autoimmune diseases such as systemic lupus erythematosus)
Mental Disorders with Premenstrual Exacerbations
Dysthymic disorder
Bipolar disorder
Anxiety disorders
Somatoform disorder
Personality disorders
Major depressive disorder
Substance abuse

Blood and urine tests to rule out the disorders in Table 1 should also be performed at the first visit. For women who first seek treatment in their 40s, serum levels of follicle-stimulating hormone should be determined to evaluate a possible contribution of perimenopausal status.

No pharmacologic treatment should be initiated at that visit. However, education and information on PMS are of utmost importance. General measures for enhancement of well-being and changes in lifestyle may be initiated. Because they are effective for women who have mild to moderate PMS, these procedures might also serve as a diagnostic aid. They are addressed in the section on management.

A second office visit should be scheduled for the expected late luteal–symptomatic phase of the next menstrual cycle. This allows two cycles of prospective daily monitoring of symptoms as well as the physician's observation in a reported symptomatic period as compared with the first visit in a nonsymptomatic period. During this second visit the DRFs are reviewed with the patient and the cyclic pattern is confirmed.

In addition to confirmation of cyclicity, severity of impairment and/or distress is determined for treatment decision.

If the patient has severe symptoms during both office visits, PMS is not confirmed and a chronic disease exists unless the patient reports a stressful situation during the midfollicular visit that might influence symptom severity. In that case, daily monitoring of symptoms should continue for a third cycle. Similarly, if no severe symptoms are observed during the two office visits, the diagnosis of PMS is not confirmed unless the patient had a delightful vacation or other happy occasion during the late luteal phase—an external influence that can reduce the severity of symptoms in some women. When PMS is confirmed, effective treatment is available and should be recommended.

MANAGEMENT OF PREMENSTRUAL SYNDROME

Three main treatment modalities may be applied for treatment of PMS-PMDD: (1) nonpharmacologic, general enhancement of well-being and lifestyle; (2) symptomatic pharmacologic treatment; and (3) hormonal interventions, mostly for suppression of ovulation, which is presumably the trigger of symptoms. The recommended treatments are presented in Table 2.

General measures may already be initiated at the first visit. If they are effective, no other pharmacologic treatment is necessary, which is the case in women with mild to moderate PMS. They include education (which may be performed with brochures from ACOG as well as other organizations). Regular exercise, improved stress management, and relaxation are helpful. Multivitamins and calcium carbonate 1200 mg/d may be recommended. Dietary modifications such as restricted salt intake, decreased caffeine and alcohol, as well as frequent smaller meals instead of heavy meals have not been confirmed as specific treatment for PMS but should be considered to be beneficial for any person. Family members should preferably be involved in the treatment for enhancement of social support. Environment and coping skills may be discussed with attempts for improvement. If available and affordable, cognitive-behavioral treatment has been claimed to be effective.

Women with confirmed severe PMS need pharmacologic interventions. For women with mostly mood and behavioral symptoms, selective serotonergic reuptake inhibitors (SSRIs) are currently the first line of treatment. There is some claim that the SSRIs are also efficacious for alleviation of physical premenstrual symptoms; however, it is still unclear whether this is not a carryover of improvement in mood symptoms. The treatment of PMDD with SSRIs is different from the use of these medications for treatment of depression and anxiety in three main ways: (1) for PMDD intermittent treatment limited to the luteal phase of the menstrual cycle is as efficacious as continuous treatment, (2) doses are in the lower range, and (3) improvement may be noticed in the first treatment cycle, within a few days.

Fluoxetine (Prozac,* Sarafem) 20 mg/d and sertraline (Zoloft for PMDD) 50 to 100 mg/d have been approved by the Food and Drug Administration (FDA) for treatment of PMDD and are the first choice. However, paroxetine (Paxil)* (20 mg/d), citalopram (Celexa)* (20 mg/d), and the combined serotonin-norepinephrine reuptake inhibitor venlafaxine (Effexor)* (50 to 150 mg/d) are probably equally efficacious, as is the serotonergic tricyclic antidepressant clomipramine (Anafranil).* Once-weekly fluoxetine (90 mg enteric coated*) has been shown to be effective when given twice, 14 and 7 days before expected menses, but not when given only once, 7 days before menses.

*Not FDA approved for this indication.

TABLE 2. **Management of Premenstrual Syndrome**

For predominately mood symptoms	
Fluoxetine (Prozac,* Sarafem)	20 mg/d for 14 last days of each cycle
Sertraline (Zoloft for PMDD)	50–100 mg/d for 14 last days of each cycle
Fluoxetine once weekly*	90 mg at days 14 and 7 prior to next menses.
Also	
Paroxetine (Paxil)*	20 mg/d
Citalopram (Celexa)*	20 mg/d
Venlafaxine (Effexor)*	50–150 mg/d
Alprazolam (Xanax)*	0.25–1.0 mg q.i.d. for 1 wk before menses
For bloatedness, edema	
Spironolactone (Aldactone)*	100 mg/d
For mastalgia	
Bromocriptine (Parlodel)*	1.25 mg–7.5 mg/d, luteal
General	
Gonadotropin-releasing hormone agonists:	
Leuprolide acetate (Lupron Depot)*	3.75 mg IM at d 2 of cycle and every 30 d
General enhancement of well-being and lifestyle	
Education of patient	
Regular exercise	
Stress management and relaxation	
Dietary modification	
Multivitamins and calcium carbonate (1200 mg/d)	
Improved social support and environment	
Nonpharmacologic treatment	
Improved coping skills	
Cognitive-behavioral therapy	

*Not FDA approved for this indication.

In clinical trials, the efficacy of SSRIs has been shown to be about 60%. It is probably higher in daily practice. In long-term continuous treatment decreased libido was reported as the most disturbing adverse effect (45% of patients). Other common adverse effects are headache, insomnia, fatigue, and decreased concentration.

For women who do not respond to an SSRI, the benzodiazepine alprazolam (Xanax)* may be prescribed. For PMDD, alprazolam should be prescribed only during the late luteal phase at a dosage of 0.25 to 1.0 mg four times daily and discontinued following the beginning of the next menses. No dependence or withdrawal effects were reported with this regimen. Noradrenergic or dopaminergic antidepressants, such as desipramine (Norpramin),* maprotiline (Ludiomil),* and bupropion (Wellbutrin SR),* have not been shown to be effective as treatment of PMDD. When mastalgia is the main complaint, the dopaminergic agonist bromocriptine (Parlodel)* (1.25 to 7.5 mg twice a day) may be effective. Spironolactone (Aldactone)* (100 mg/d) may be tried for bloatedness and reported edema. However, for treatment of mood and most physical symptoms its efficacy is at best controversial.

HORMONAL INTERVENTION

If symptomatic treatment is not effective, ovulation suppressants are indicted. When PMS is very severe, suppression of ovulation may be initiated as a first line of treatment.

*Not FDA approved for this indication.

Gonadotropin-releasing hormone (GnRH) agonists, such as leuprolide acetate (Lupron Depot),* 3.75 mg intramuscularly at day 2 of the menstrual cycle and then every 30 days; are highly effective. However, they are costly and, most important, they cause medical menopause. The iatrogenic hypoestrogenic state causes menopause-like symptoms such as hot flashes, vaginal dryness, and some headache and decreased well-being. Long-term treatment causes a decrease in bone mineral density and eventually osteoporosis and possibly an increased risk of cardiovascular disorders. An add-back treatment similar to hormonal replacement therapy or tibolone[†] may be effective for the adverse effects. But whether or not it affects the GnRH therapeutic efficacy is still undecided. Ovariectomy has been reported to be highly effective in eliminating PMS, but castration is unjustified when reversible medical interventions are equally effective.

The androgenic compound danazol (Danocrine)* in dosages of 200 to 600 mg was reported to be an effective treatment when anovulatory status was achieved, but its adverse effects (mood changes, weight gain, fluid retention, acne, virilization) render it undesirable. (Its use in the luteal phase at a low dose is ineffective.) Other hormonal interventions that were shown to be ineffective were progesterone* (despite its popular use) and thyroid hormones.

Oral contraceptives* are widely used for ovulation suppression. Some monophasic preparations are effective, depending on the progestin used. Sequential

*Not FDA approved for this indication.
[†]Investigational drug in the United States.

preparations are probably ineffective. At the time of preparation of this article, several contraceptive preparations are being studied in clinical trials. Results are still unknown.

MENOPAUSE

method of
R. DON GAMBRELL, JR., M.D., FACOG
Medical College of Georgia
Augusta, Georgia

After the menopause, which is defined as 1 year of amenorrhea in midlife, the average woman still has one third of her life span ahead. However, women's experience of the menopause and its effects on their remaining years vary widely. The declining ovarian function can be rapid for some and slower for others. Surgical menopause, caused by bilateral oophorectomy during the reproductive years, usually results in a rapid onset of severe symptoms. Some women may produce sufficient endogenous estrogens to remain asymptomatic, but others experience a variety of disturbances during the climacteric, a term in current use for the premenopausal, menopausal, and postmenopausal period.

These symptoms may include:

- Hot flushes (or flashes)
- Insomnia
- Night sweats
- Depression
- Vaginal irritation or dryness
- Irritability

After increasing numbers of estrogen replacements in observational studies during the 1980s and 1990s, indicating the many benefits of treatment of menopause with estrogens, early in the 21st century questions and controversies arose again. The first critics stated that decreased risk of heart disease and stroke was due not to estrogen replacement but to the healthy user effect. Women who seek hormone replacement take better care of themselves, watch their weight, avoid cholesterol, exercise, do not smoke, and use alcohol moderately, if at all. Reports such as those of the Heart and Estrogen/Progestin Replacement Study (HERS) and the Women's Health Initiative (WHI) indicate adverse effects such as increased cardiovascular disease and breast cancer instead of decreased risk of myocardial infarction and stroke. This has led to a disturbing trend across the country: "The lowest effective dosage for the shortest period of time." This thinking arises because it is thought that treating menopausal symptoms until a woman "gets through" the menopause is the only use of estrogen. After 45 years of clinical research and practice, I am convinced that when the proper regimens and dosages are used, there are many benefits from estrogen other than alleviating symptoms such as preventing:

- Genital atrophy
- Osteoporosis
- Cardiovascular disease
- Alzheimer's disease
- Psychogenic manifestations
- Colorectal cancer
- Macular degeneration of retina
- Cataracts

ADVERSE EFFECTS

Until the report of the WHI being discontinued in July 2002, it was estimated that 15 million women in the United States were using estrogen. Over the next few months, up to 50% of these 15 million stopped their hormones, many without consulting their physicians. If they did consult their physicians, many doctors did not know what to tell their patients and some even recommended the discontinuation of hormones. The intended 8½ year WHI study was stopped after 5.2 years because of a perceived increased hazard ratio (HR) of 1.26 (95% confidence interval [CI], 1.00 to 1.59) of breast cancer and an HR of 1.29 (95% CI, 1.02 to 1.63) for cardiovascular disease. When these confidence intervals were adjusted for other variables, they lost all significance, 0.83 to 1.92 for breast cancer and 0.85 to 1.97 for coronary heart disease. The mean of 5.2 years of follow-up is too short an interval to show anything about estrogens increasing the risk of breast cancer. The longest any subject had used Prempro was 6½ years, and many were diagnosed after only 2 to 3 years of hormone replacement therapy (HRT) (Table 1). On the basis of doubling times of 7 to 8 years for carcinoma of the breast, the majority of the 290 cases of breast cancer, out of 16,000 women, most likely had malignant cells in their mammary tissues at the onset of the study. Although it might be argued that the estrogen-progestogen hormones could accelerate the growth of already malignant cells, there are no data to support this concept. In August 2002 we published a study of 69 patients with breast cancer in our practice who were treated with estrogens for up to 32 years. They had three recurrences and three deaths. Compare these with the 32 patients whom we could observe for 11 years, whose physicians had convinced them not to take estrogen because of their breast cancer. There were six recurrences and six deaths in this nonhormone group. A review of 54 studies of HRT and breast cancer by Trudy Bush, a

TABLE 1. **Invasive Breast Cancer**

	Number of Patients (Annualized Percentage)	
Year	***Hormone Replacement Therapy***	***Placebo***
1	11 (0.13)	17 (0.21)
2	26 (0.31)	30 (0.38)
3	28 (0.34)	23 (0.29)
4	40 (0.50)	22 (0.29)
5	34 (0.57)	12 (0.22)
6+	27 (0.53)	20 (0.43)

Table 2. **Coronary Heart Disease**

Year	Number of Patients (Annualized Percentage)	
	Hormone Replacement Therapy	*Placebo*
1	43 (0.51)	23 (0.29)
2	36 (0.43)	30 (0.38)
3	20 (0.24)	18 (0.23)
4	25 (0.32)	24 (0.32)
5	23 (0.39)	9 (0.16)
6+	17 (0.33)	18 (0.42)

well-known and respected epidemiologist at Johns Hopkins University, observed in 2001 that estrogen use up to 15 years or more does not increase the risk of breast cancer. She also confirmed that when breast cancer was diagnosed in hormone users, the prognosis was greatly improved, with no studies to the contrary.

The increased risk of cardiovascular disease observed in both the HERS and WHI studies was probably due to the hormones used. In both studies, continuous combined HRT (CCHRT) (Table 2) was used with conjugated estrogens 0.625 mg and medroxyprogesterone acetate 2.5 mg in every tablet (Prempro). Unopposed estrogen has direct beneficial effects upon coronary arteries in addition to improvement in lipids and lipoproteins: decreased total cholesterol and low-density lipoprotein cholesterol with increase in high-density lipoprotein (HDL) cholesterol. Estrogens:

- Improve vascular blood flow
- Increase velocity of blood flow
- Dilate coronary arteries
- Increase cardiac output
- Increase endothelium-derived relaxing factor
- Inhibit atherosclerosis progression
- Decrease platelet adhesion
- Reduce vascular resistance
- Inhibit coronary thrombosis

Studies from Wake Forest in monkeys indicated that progestogens may block many of these effects in addition to producing down-regulation of estrogen receptors when the progestogen is given continuously as in CCHRT.

The primary reason why progestogens were added to estrogen replacement was to prevent estrogen-induced endometrial cancer. The sequential methods (Table 3) are very endometrial-protective and may even reduce the risk of breast cancer. However, 97% of woman given sequential HRT have withdrawal menstrual periods until age 60, after which withdrawal bleeding occurs in only 60% after age 65. Because women do not want to resume or continue menstrual periods, the continuous combined regimen (CCHRT) was devised. For the first 6 months women in their early 50s usually have breakthrough bleeding with this regimen, but by 6 months 60% to 65% become amenorrheic. Unfortunately, after a year or two of amenorrhea, some women using CCHRT start bleeding again. After appropriate evaluation by endometrial biopsy and/or ultrasonography, these women usually

Table 3. **Methods of Hormone Administration**

Method	Estrogen	Progestogen
Cyclic sequential	1st–25th month	13th–25th month
Continuous sequential	Every day	1st–14th month
Continuous combined	Every day	Every day
Cyclic combined	1st–25th month	1st–25th month
Continuous interrupted	Every day	3 days out of 6 or 7

have to use one of the sequential regimens. CCHRT is not fully endometrial-protective because more than 110 cases of endometrial cancer have been reported. Prempro, which is representative of this regimen, was the hormone combination used in the Postmenopausal Estrogen/Progestin Interventions (PEPI) study, HERS, and the WHI. It was alleged that Prempro increased breast cancer risk (see Table 1), which is most likely not true because of the premature termination of this part of the WHI study after 5.2 years. Prempro probably did increase the risk of cardiovascular disease (see Table 2) because of down-regulation of estrogen receptors in the coronary arteries from the continuous use of progestogen. The medroxyprogesterone acetate (Provera) also had a partial blockage of the estrogen-induced cardiovascular benefits.

Cyclic combined HRT, in which the progestogen with or without the estrogen is discontinued after the 25th of the month, is clinically superior to CCHRT because 75% of women become amenorrheic in 4 months, compared with 65% of the CCHRT users at 6 months. In the 25% of cyclic combined users who do not stop withdrawal bleeding; it is usually only a light flow on the 26th and 27th of the month. This regimen is the most popular one in France with approximately 400,000 users and maintains amenorrhea in 85% to 95% of patients after the sixth month of treatment. The cyclic combined regimen should be more endometrial-protective because it allows shedding of any buildup of the endometrium, allows up-regulation of progestogen receptors after suppression with continuous progestogen, and reduces angiogenesis in the endometrium. An innovative new regimen is continuous estrogen with interrupted or pulsed progestogens. Continuous progestogens can produce continuous down-regulation of progesterone receptors as well as estrogen receptors and therefore may not be fully endometrial-protective. Interrupting the progestogen for 3 out of 6 days allows up-regulation of progesterone receptors to occur intermittently. An oral preparation of 17β–estradiol 1 mg used alone for 3 days and combined with norgestimate 0.09 mg for 3 days (Ortho-Prefest) was effective in producing amenorrhea. Bleeding control improved over time with 69% of women free of bleeding (irrespective of spotting) the first month, 69% free of bleeding by 6 months, and 80% with no bleeding after 12 months.

NONORAL ESTROGENS

Estrogen vaginal cream is the longest available and probably the most useful of the nonoral estrogens.

With creams, estrogens are well absorbed through the vaginal mucosa so that good systemic levels are obtained as well as local beneficial effects. Vaginal creams probably provide the quickest response and subsequent relief of symptoms of atrophic vaginitis, such as:

- Vaginal irritation
- Vaginal dryness
- Pruritus
- Dyspareunia

Rarely is estrogen vaginal cream used for primary therapy, although it could be used in that way; it is mostly used secondary to oral estrogens where vaginal symptoms persist.

The transdermal system of estrogen replacement therapy is another form of nonoral administration. There are now many different systems and multiple dosages. Change is twice weekly for most; however, weekly patches are available. The dosages range from 0.025 to 0.1 mg. The lower dosages may be used for estrogen supplementation in the perimenopausal years; however, for replacement to prevent osteoporosis and provide a sense of well-being, the 0.1-mg patch is preferred. Although there are few or no undesirable effects with transdermal systems, endometrial proliferation is normal and an oral progestogen must be given for 10 to 13 days each month. Transdermal estradiol takes longer to produce a rise in HDL-cholesterol than do oral estrogens; however, over the long term, patches should be just as protective from atherosclerotic heart disease, especially with the 0.1-mg estradiol dosage. There is a combination patch of estradiol-norethindrone acetate (CombiPatch) used as CCHRT, which may not be fully endometrial-protective, just like the CCHRT pills. It is preferred to use it as a cyclic combined therapy by prescribing in seven out of the eight 3½-day changes. The last 3½ days of the 28-day cycle can be substituted with an estradiol-only 0.05- or 0.1-mg patch. As with the oral CCHRT pills, using the combined patch in this way provides a greater percentage of amenorrhea with less breakthrough bleeding, usually only spotting on the 26th or 27th day of the month.

MANAGEMENT OF HORMONE REPLACEMENT SIDE EFFECTS

In addition to resumption of bleeding, side effects of hormone replacement are a major reason for discontinuation of therapy. These include breast tenderness, edema or bloating, premenstrual syndrome–like symptoms, headaches, cramping, abdominal pressure, irritability, depression, and lethargy. Many of these are related to fluid retention, and 50% of patients respond to a mild diuretic such as 25 to 50 mg of either spironolactone (Aldactone)* or hydrochorthiazide* for 7 to 10 days before menses. Should this not be effective, the dosage of progestogen can be lowered when norethindrone acetate (Aygestin)* is being used, from

*Not FDA approved for this indication.

TABLE 4. **Available Progestogens**

Progestogen	Available Strength (mg)	Minimum Effective Dosage
Medroxyprogesterone acetate (Provera)	2.5, 5, 10	10 mg daily
Norethindrone acetate (Aygestin)	5	2.5 mg daily
Megestrol acetate (Megace)	20, 40	40 mg daily
Norgestrel (Ovrette)	0.075	0.150 mg daily
Norethindrone (Micronor)	0.35	1.05 mg daily
Progesterone vaginal suppositories*	25, 50	25 mg bid
Oral micronized progesterone (Prometrium)	100, 200	300 mg in divided doses
Vaginal micronized progesterone gel 8% (Crinone)	90	90 mg daily

*May be compounded by pharmacists.

5 to 2.5 mg, or even 1.0 mg* of norethindrone. However, the lowest dosage of medroxyprogesterone acetate (Provera)† that fully protects the endometrium in the sequential regimens is 10 mg for 12 to 14 days. Other progestogens can be used or the route of administration can be changed (Table 4). Progestogen-only oral contraceptive pills can be used to provide the lowest dosage of progestogen. A side effect–free progestogen can be found for almost every estrogen user, but sometimes it may be necessary to use the progestogen-only oral contraceptives (two or three daily for the 12 to 14 days).

USE OF ANDROGENS

Estrogens give relief of most menopausal symptoms; however, it sometimes becomes necessary to add androgens to estrogen therapy. Up to 75% of estrogen production is lost after menopause, but up to 50% of androgen production can also be lost when ovaries cease to function or are surgically removed. If symptoms persist, it is best to add a low dose of androgen rather than continue increasing the estrogen dosage beyond 1.25 mg of conjugated estrogens (Premarin). Potential benefits of androgens include alleviation of:

- Hot flashes
- Lethargy
- Endogenous depression
- Nocturia and incontinence
- Kraurosis vulvae (with use of 1% to 2% testosterone cream)
- Headaches (migrainoid)
- Fibrocystic disease of the breast

Although estrogens alleviate both hot flashes and genital atrophy, the addition of an androgen helps overcome fatigue. When estrogens are thought to be contraindicated, as in patients with breast cancer (although this is rapidly changing), androgens alone

*Not available in this dosage.
†Not FDA approved for this indication.

may be helpful to relieve vasomotor symptoms and improve the psyche. However, they are of little value in treatment of genital atrophy and probably do not prevent osteoporosis in the dosages that can be used.

Some postmenopausal women complain of hirsutism before any hormone replacement. This is probably due to a relative imbalance of endogenous estrogens and androgens such that estrogen levels decrease more than androgen levels. Typically manifested by an increase in upper lip hair or small moustache, this usually lessens with estrogen replacement. Androgen therapy can exacerbate preexisting hirsutism, acne, and oiliness of the skin. If there are good results from the androgen but worsening of hirsutism or acne, reducing the androgen dosage and/or increasing the estrogen dosage may help. Spironolactone (Aldactone)* 50 mg twice daily may also be added to the estrogen-androgen combination so that the benefits of the androgen can be continued. A new cream with eflornithine HCl (Vaniqa) is also quite effective in treating facial hair. Oral preparations of esterified estrogens, 1.25 mg methyltestosterone, 2.5 mg (Estratest) and esterified estrogens, 0.625 mg–methyl testosterone, 1.25 mg (Estratest H.S.) are balanced preparations with minimal side effects. Fluoxymesterone (Halotestin)* 2 mg can be added to conjugated estrogens (Premarin) 0.625 mg or other oral estrogens. Injectable estrogen-androgen preparations are also available, but they are more irregular in the duration of symptom relief than the oral preparations.

*Not FDA approved for this indication.

VULVOVAGINITIS

method of
DAVID A. BAKER, M.D.
State University of New York at Stony Brook
Stony Brook, New York

Vulvovaginitis brings large numbers of women to see their health care provider. Over the last several decades with the availability of numerous over-the-counter preparations, most patients medicate themselves to treat their symptoms. However, it is clear that the majority of patients make the wrong diagnosis. They use the wrong medications and delay bringing their symptoms and complaints to the attention of the clinician; as a result, many women will experience complications from their vaginal infection. Therefore, the clinician needs to take this condition (vulvovaginitis) seriously and view the patient as one with a significant medical, physiologic, and social problem that may lead not only to significant medical conditions and complications but also to significant interpersonal problems.

An accurate diagnosis is required to provide proper and correct treatment of this condition. Symptoms presented to the health care provider by phone can be very nonspecific and may lead to an improper diagnosis and treatment. The three major categories of vaginitis in the United States (Figure 1) are those caused predominately by candidiasis, trichomoniasis, and bacterial vaginosis (BV). Of these three abnormal symptomatic manifestations, BV is the most common in the United States. Many patients mistake BV for *Candida* infections and take over-the-counter antifungal preparations, which are costly and ineffective. Patients do not appreciate the significance of this most common condition: BV may lead to important medical complications not only during pregnancy but also when the patient is not pregnant. Of the three conditions, the only one that is considered a sexually transmitted disease (STD) is trichomoniasis. BV is associated with other STDs.

The goal of therapy is to not only treat or control the organism that is abnormally colonizing or growing in the vagina but also return the vagina to normal vaginal colonization. This objective may be difficult, and one of the major problems of recurrent vaginal infection is our inability to colonize the lower genital tract with healthy bacteria. The normal vagina has an acidic pH that is produced by a combination of normal host flora and the species *Lactobacillus,* which produces lactic acid. The importance of *Lactobacillus* strains that produce not only lactic acid but also hydrogen peroxide cannot be overemphasized; they maintain the lower genital tract flora and act as a protective barrier to the acquisition of certain STDs, including HIV. It is therefore the goal of the treating clinician to eradicate the patient's symptoms, control the abnormal vaginal colonization, and try to propagate normal lower genital tract flora. Women with normal lower genital tract flora containing lactobacilli producing lactic acid and hydrogen peroxide were less likely to contract chlamydiosis, trichomoniasis, and symptomatic candidiasis. In addition, the prevalence of gonorrhea, chlamydiosis, and trichomoniasis was significantly lower in women who had normal vaginal *Lactobacillus* flora during pregnancy.

BACTERIAL VAGINOSIS

The term given to abnormal colonization of the lower genital tract with anaerobic bacteria is *bacterial vaginosis*. However, a more meaningful definition of BV may be one that includes an inflammatory component of this anaerobic bacterial overgrowth. Currently, approximately 50% of women in the United States who visit a clinician for treatment of vaginitis have BV. It is a polymicrobial infection involving an increase in anaerobic bacteria, loss of the normal *Lactobacillus* flora, and consequently, an imbalance in the vaginal ecosystem. The absence or a decreased number of lactobacilli facilitates the overgrowth of pathogenic organism, which are predominately anaerobic bacteria.

The exact factors that trigger the overgrowth of anaerobic bacteria are still not fully understood. Douching can lead to a disturbance in the delicate balance of lower genital tract organisms. Other risk factors for BV include trichomoniasis, other STDs,

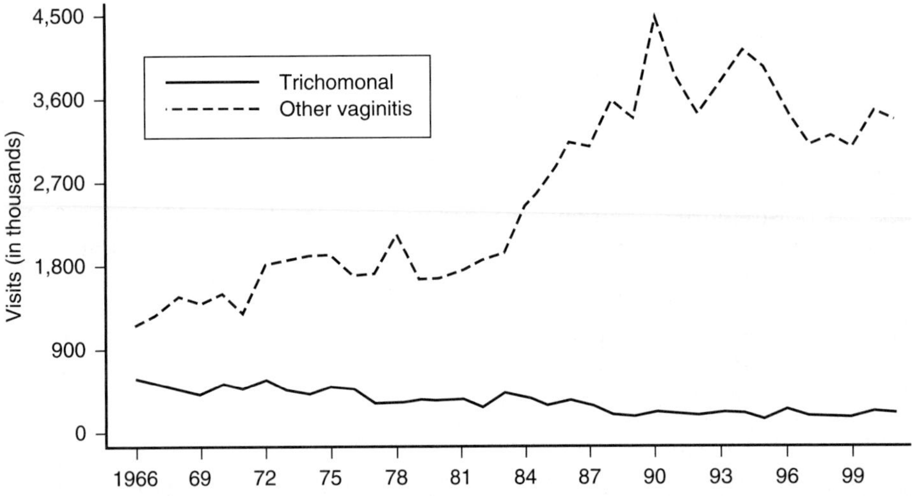

Figure 1.

early sexual experience, multiple sexual partners, and the use of an intrauterine contraceptive device.

Diagnosis

Proper diagnosis is important for the treatment and eradication of BV. The diagnosis can be made during vaginal examination and does not require expensive and elaborate techniques. The current 2002 Centers for Disease Control and Prevention (CDC) STD treatment guidelines require three of the following symptoms or signs for diagnosis: a homogeneous, white, noninflammatory discharge that coats the vaginal walls smoothly; the presence of clue cells on microscopic examination; a pH of vaginal secretions of less than 4.5; and a fishy odor of the vaginal discharge before or after the addition of 10% KOH (the whiff test). Gram stain is an acceptable laboratory method for diagnosing BV. However, culture is not recommended as a diagnostic tool. In addition, cervical Papanicolaou tests have limited clinical utility for the diagnosis of BV because of low sensitivity. Other commercially available tests add to the cost and rarely aid the clinician in diagnosing this vaginal infection.

Treatment

The goal of therapy is to not only control this anaerobic infection but also relieve vaginal symptoms, lessen the risk of infectious complications after procedures, and reduce the risk of development of other infectious complications, HIV, and other STDs. All women who have symptomatic disease require treatment. Because of the increased risk of postoperative infectious complications associated with BV, it is suggested that before surgical procedures are performed on women, they be screened and treated for BV, in addition to undergoing other routine prophylactic measures.

BV during pregnancy has been associated with adverse pregnancy outcomes, including preterm labor, premature rupture of membranes, and postpartum infections. Therapy during pregnancy has the potential of reducing these potential risks, as well as reducing the risk of acquiring STDs and HIV during pregnancy. The CDC has given recommendations for the treatment of nonpregnant and pregnant women with BV (Table 1). Patients need to be informed that clindamycin (Cleocin) cream and ovules are oil-based preparations that may interfere with the efficiency of latex condoms and diaphragms. In addition, oral and topical metronidazole (Flagyl) regimens are equally efficacious. Studies of vaginal clindamycin cream appear to demonstrate that it is less efficacious than metronidazole regimens. Short-course therapy for BV in the form of metronidazole, 2 g orally in a single dose, has been proposed. The clinician must recognize that metronidazole, 2 g in a single dose, is an alternative regimen because of its lower efficacy in the treatment of BV. Unfortunately, at the current time, no

TABLE 1. **Bacterial Vaginosis: Treatment Regimens**

RECOMMENDED REGIMENS, NONPREGNANT
Metronidazole (Flagyl), 500 mg orally twice a day for 7 d
or
Metronidazole (Metro-Gel), 0.75% gel, 1 full applicator (5 g) intravaginally once a day for 5 d
or
Clindamycin (Cleocin), 2% cream, 1 full applicator (5 g) intravaginally at bedtime for 7 d
ALTERNATIVE REGIMENS, NONPREGNANT
Metronidazole, 2 g orally in a single dose
or
Clindamycin, 300 mg orally twice a day for 7 d
or
Clindamycin ovules, 100 g intravaginally once at bedtime for 3 d
RECOMMENDED REGIMENS, PREGNANT
Metronidazole, 250 mg orally three times a day for 7 d
or
Clindamycin, 300 mg orally twice a day for 7 d

Note: Patients should be advised to avoid consuming alcohol during treatment with metronidazole and for 24 hours thereafter. Clindamycin cream and ovules are oil based and might weaken latex condoms and diaphragms: Refer to condom product labeling for additional information.

From Centers for Disease Control and Prevention: Sexually transmitted diseases treatment guidelines 2002. MMWR Morb Mortal Wkly Rep 51:42–48, 2002.

preparation, either intravaginal or oral, is able to induce reversion to the normal lower genital tract vaginal flora.

BV is not considered an STD, and therefore routine treatment of sex partners is not currently recommended. When using clindamycin and metronidazole, one must differentiate between side effects and allergic reactions. Metronidazole gel (MetroGel) may be appropriate for patients who have side effects with oral metronidazole, but it should not be used in a patient allergic to metronidazole.

Oral regimens are recommended (Table 1) for pregnant women. Topical clindamycin (Cleocin vaginal cream) is contraindicated in pregnancy because of the potential overgrowth of gram-negative aerobic bacteria *(Escherichia coli)* in the vagina. Patients who have BV should be offered testing for HIV and other STDs. Patients with HIV should be screened and treated for BV with the same regimens as those who are HIV negative.

TRICHOMONIASIS

The incidence of trichomoniasis has slowly declined in the United States since the mid 1960s and has remained at a low level over the past decade. Trichomoniasis is caused by the protozoan *Trichomonas vaginalis*. Women who are infected usually have a vaginal discharge and specific symptoms, in contrast to men, who are generally asymptomatic. *T. vaginalis* is a pear-shaped flagellated protozoon that is usually identified in wet mounts by a rapid swaying motion and the presence of polymorphonuclear leukocytes. Growth is typically enhanced by anaerobic conditions and an elevated pH. The incubation period ranges from 4 to 28 days. The clinician needs to recognize that infection with this organism occurs not only in the vagina but also in the urethra, Skene's glands, and the bladder. In men, the urethra is the most common site. However, the prostrate and epididymis may also be infected, and the organism may be detected in semen and urine. Trichomoniasis is an STD transmitted through sexual contact, with infection documented in 85% of female partners of infected men. Risk factors for trichomoniasis are the presence of other STDS, an increased number of sexual partners, the presence of BV, smoking, and a vaginal pH over 4.5.

Diagnosis

The patient usually has a discharge, odor, and vulvar itching with or without dysuria. The discharge is yellow-green with a frothy appearance. Further evaluation of the patient reveals that the pH of the vagina is over 4.5, the amine test may be positive, and on wet preparations, the organism and an increase in the white blood cell count (greater than 10 per high-power field) are usually found. Wet preparations and Pap smears have an approximately 50% to 60% sensitivity and greater than 90% specificity. Other techniques are in development that should better enable the clinician to diagnose this infection. Trichomoniasis in pregnant women has been associated with adverse pregnancy outcomes, specifically, preterm rupture of membranes, preterm labor, and preterm delivery. In addition, studies have shown that the presence of trichomoniasis is associated with an increased risk of acquiring HIV, so patients in whom trichomoniasis has been diagnosed should be screened for other STDs, and HIV testing should be encouraged.

TABLE 2. **Trichomoniasis: Treatment Regimens**

RECOMMENDED REGIMEN
Metronidazole (Flagyl), 2 g orally in a single dose
ALTERNATIVE REGIMEN
Metronidazole, 500 mg twice a day for 7 d

From Centers for Disease Control and Prevention: Sexually transmitted diseases treatment guidelines 2002. MMWR Morb Mortal Wkly Rep 51:42–48, 2002.

Treatment

Current CDC treatment guidelines are presented in Table 2 The metronidazole regimen recommended has resulted in cure rates of approximately 90% to 95%. Because trichomoniasis is an STD, treatment of sexual partners is mandatory. Metronidazole gel has an efficacy of approximately 50% for the treatment of trichomoniasis. Because the organism may be found in locations other than the vagina, such treatment is less efficacious and not recommended. Women who fail oral therapy may repeat a 7-day course of therapy with topical metronidazole. Because metronidazole is currently the only approved therapy in the United States, patients with allergic reactions to metronidazole may be managed by desensitization. Newer medications and therapies for this condition are in development and may be of assistance in patients with allergic reactions or the emerging problem of metronidazole-resistant trichomoniasis.

CANDIDIASIS

Most patients think that their symptoms are associated with a yeast infection, but in reality, studies show that 75% of patients with chronic candidiasis have another etiologic agent for their problems. However, candidiasis is still one of the most common vaginal infections and is usually treated initially with over-the-counter or alternative regimens. Patients who cannot control the infection or experience recurrent symptoms generally seek medical assistance. The CDC has classified vulvovaginal candidiasis (VVC) as uncomplicated VVC or complicated VVC (Table 3). This classification is based on clinical findings, microbiology, host factors, and response to therapy. Approximately 10% to 20% of women will have complicated VVC.

Diagnosis and Treatment

Pruritus and an inflammatory reaction suggest the diagnosis of candidal vaginitis. A white cheesy

TABLE 3. **Classification of Vulvovaginal Candidiasis (VVC)**

Uncomplicated	Complicated
Sporadic or infrequent VVC	Recurrent VVC
or	*or*
Mild-to-moderate VVC	Severe VVC
or	*or*
Likely to be *Candida albicans*	Non-*albicans* candidiasis
or	*or*
Non-immunocompromised women	Women with uncontrolled diabetes, debilitation, or immunosuppression or those who are pregnant

From Centers for Disease Control and Prevention: Sexually transmitted diseases treatment guidelines 2002. MMWR Morb Mortal Wkly Rep 51:42–48, 2002.

TABLE 4. **Vulvovaginal Candidiasis: Recommended Treatment Regimens**

INTRAVAGINAL AGENTS

Butoconazole (Mycelex), 2 % cream, 5 g intravaginally for 3 d*
or
Butoconazole 2% cream, 5 g (butoconazole—sustained release), single intravaginal application,
or
Clotrimazole (Gyne-Lotrimin), 1% cream, 5 g intravaginally for 7–14 d*
or
Clotrimazole, 100-mg vaginal tablet for 7 d
or
Clotrimazole, 100-mg vaginal tablet, 2 tablets for 3 d
or
Clotrimazole, 500-mg vaginal tablet, 1 tablet in a single application
or
Miconazole (Monistat), 2% cream, 5 g intravaginally for 7 d*
or
Miconazole, 100-mg vaginal suppository, 1 suppository for 7 d*
or
Miconazole, 200-mg vaginal suppository, 1 suppository for 3 d*
or
Nystatin, 100,000-U vaginal tablet, 1 tablet for 14 d
or
Tioconazole (Vagistat), 6.5% ointment, 5 g intravaginally in a single application*
or
Terconazole (Terazol), 0.4% cream, 5 g intravaginally for 7 d
or
Terconazole, 0.8% cream, 5 g intravginally for 3 d
or
Terconazole, 80-mg vaginal suppository, 1 suppository for 3 d

ORAL AGENT

Fluconazole (Diflucan), 150-mg oral tablet, 1 tablet in single dose

Note: The creams and suppositories in these regimens are oil based and may weaken latex condoms and diaphragms. Refer to condom product labeling for further information.

*Preparations for intravaginal administration of butoconazole, clotrimazole, miconazole, and tioconazole are available over the counter (OTC). Self-medication with OTC preparations should be advised only for women in whom VVC has previously been diagnosed and who have a recurrence of the same symptoms. Any woman whose symptoms persist after using an OTC preparation or who has a recurrence of symptoms within 2 months should seek medical care. Unnecessary or inappropriate use of OTC preparations is common and can lead to a delay in treatment of other etiologies of vulvovaginitis that could result in adverse clinical outcomes.

From Centers for Disease Control and Prevention. Sexually transmitted disease treatment guidelines 2002. MMWR Morb Mortal Wkly Rep 51:42–48, 2002.

discharge is usually what drives the patient to buy an over-the-counter antifungal preparation. The clinician needs to use additional modalities for diagnosis, including a wet preparation with 10% KOH, Gram stain or culture, and determination of vaginal pH (less than 4.5). Because a significant number of women are colonized with *Candida,* culture in the absence of symptoms is not clinically relevant. Most patients with uncomplicated VVC have no precipitating factor; however, VVC commonly develops after antibiotic use. The CDC has recommended numerous regimens (Table 4) for the treatment of uncomplicated VVC, including 14 topical regimens and 1 single-dose oral regimen. VVC is not acquired through sexual activity, and therefore treatment of the partner is not usually recommended.

Complicated VVC is usually defined as four or more episodes of symptomatic VVC each year and should occur in only a small percentage of women. Most patients with recurrent VVC have no apparent predisposing or underlying conditions. Culture may be important in determining the appropriate treatment and management of these patients. Non-*albicans* species of *Candida* are found in only 10% to 20% of patients with recurrent VVC. Different therapeutic regimens for a longer duration may be of benefit in treating recurrent VVC. The use of antifungals for maintenance therapy or in specific daily or weekly recommended regimens can be considered for up to 6 months. However, side effects and the toxicity of oral medications need to be taken into account. Once maintenance therapy is discontinued, VVC will recur in upward of 40% of women.

Non-fluconazole azole drugs are recommended as first-line therapy for non-*albicans* VVC. In this specific clinical situation, 600 mg of boric acid* by capsule intravaginally once daily for 2 weeks may be beneficial.

Specific investigation to evaluate for pregnancy, HIV infection, and systemic immunocompromising conditions such as diabetes is important in managing vulvovaginitis.

*Not available in the United States. May be compounded by pharmacists.

CHLAMYDIA TRACHOMATIS

method of
STEPHANIE N. TAYLOR, M.D.
Louisiana State University School of Medicine
New Orleans, Louisiana

Chlamydia trachomatis is a sexually transmitted and obligate intracellular organism that is the most common reportable infectious disease in the United States. In 2001, 783,242 cases were reported to the Centers for Disease Control and Prevention (CDC). The reported rate of chlamydial infections also increased from 78.5 per 100,000 to 435.2 per 100,000 from 1987 to 2001. The reasons for this increase are multifactorial and include increased use of more sensitive nucleic acid amplification tests, increased chlamydia screening, improved reporting, and continued high disease burden. Many cases remain undetected as a result of asymptomatic and unreported disease, and it is estimated that there are about 4 million cases per year in the United States. It is critical that these chlamydial infections be detected and treated because of the serious complications such as pelvic inflammatory disease (PID), ectopic pregnancy, tubal infertility, and enhanced HIV transmission.

SCREENING RECOMMENDATIONS

Asymptomatic chlamydial infection is common in both men and women. Some estimate that in women 70% or more of endocervical infections may be asymptomatic, and there are similar estimates of asymptomatic infections in men. Because chlamydial infections occur frequently among adolescents and young adults, they represent a priority population with regard to routine screening. In addition, because noninvasive, urine-based diagnostic tests that do not require examination are now available, screening should be offered in nontraditional settings such as high schools, emergency rooms, community centers, malls, and mobile units. In essence, chlamydial screening should be brought to difficult-to-reach adolescent and young adult populations who are commonly asymptomatic and do not present for medical attention. Screening for asymptomatic chlamydial infection has also been shown to be cost effective and decreases PID. In addition, reduction in the prevalence of chlamydial infection has been demonstrated with the implementation of extensive screening programs in the Pacific Northwest and elsewhere.

The CDC recommendations for chlamydial screening and rescreening are presented in Table 1. In addition to screening and treatment of patients with clinical manifestations of chlamydia and their partners, annual screening is recommended for all sexually active adolescent women, sexually active 20- to 25-year-old women, and older women with risk factors such as new or multiple sex partners. The American Academy of Pediatrics expands this annual sexually transmitted disease screening to include all sexually active adolescents.

Another issue that has attracted attention is the high prevalence of chlamydial infection in patients who have been recently treated for chlamydia. Recurrent infection has been noted in up to 20% to 30% of women within 6 months of their initial infection. Most of these infections are the result of reinfection secondary to contact with untreated partners or sexual activity in networks with a high prevalence of disease. These repeated infections have been shown to increase the risk of PID and other complications. For these reasons, the CDC now recommends that health care providers consider advising all women treated for chlamydial infection to be rescreened 3 to 4 months after treatment.

TABLE 1. **Chlamydia Screening Recommendations**

Routine Screening
Patients with mucopurulent cervicitis or urethritis
Partners of patients with cervicitis or urethritis
Sexually active asymptomatic adolescent women (annual)
Sexually active 20- to 25-y-old women (annual)
Older women with risk factors (new sex partner or multiple sex partners)
CDC Rescreening Recommendations
Consideration should be given to advising all women with chlamydial infection to be rescreened 3–4 mo after treatment (especially high priority for adolescents)
Providers strongly encouraged to rescreen all women treated for chlamydial infection whenever they next present for care within the following 12 mo

CDC, Centers for Disease Control and Prevention.

Adapted from the 2002 CDC Sexually Transmitted Diseases Treatment Guidelines. MMWR Morb Mortal Wkly Rep 51:RR-6, 2002.

CLINICAL MANIFESTATIONS

The clinical manifestations of *C. trachomatis* genital tract infections are similar in presentation to those of *Neisseria gonorrhoeae* except that chlamydial infections tend to be characterized by milder symptoms, less abrupt onset, and are often asymptomatic. Both organisms prefer infecting columnar or transitional epithelial cells of the cervix and urethra with extension to the endometrium, fallopian tubes, epididymis, peritoneum, and rectum. Both organisms also cause conjunctivitis and, rarely, systemic manifestations such as perihepatitis and reactive arthritis. Table 2 outlines the clinical manifestation of chlamydial infections in men and women. Infections of the genital tract are primarily caused by serovars D through K, and serovars L1, L2, and L3 are associated with lymphogranuloma venereum.

Mucopurulent cervicitis is the most common clinical manifestation of chlamydial infection in women. Most of these cases are asymptomatic, but it has been demonstrated that a least one third of women have local signs of infection. These signs are characterized

TABLE 2. **Clinical Manifestations of *Chlamydia trachomatis* Infection**

Men
Urethritis (nongonococcal urethritis [NGU])
Epididymitis
Conjunctivitis
Proctitis
Reiter's syndrome (urethritis, conjunctivitis, arthritis, characteristic skin lesions)
Lymphogranuloma venereum (lymphotrophic serovars L1, L2, and L3)
Women
Cervicitis
Pelvic inflammatory disease (salpingitis, endometritis)
Acute urethral syndrome (urethritis)
Conjunctivitis
Bartholinitis
Perihepatitis
Reactive arthritis
Lymphogranuloma venereum (lymphotrophic serovars L1, L2, and L3)

by mucopurulent cervical discharge, abnormal vaginal discharge and/or bleeding (e.g., postcoital bleeding), and hypertrophic ectopy of the cervical os that results in edema, congestion, friability, and easy cervical bleeding upon examination. Cervical ectopy, or the extension of columnar epithelium beyond the os, may predispose to women to chlamydial infection by exposing susceptible cells to the organism. Conversely, chlamydial infection may indeed cause cervical ectopy.

Ascension of infection into the upper genital tract occurs in 20% to 40% of women and causes PID. Extensive tubal inflammation and scarring have also been demonstrated in the absence of symptoms. Chlamydial PID is therefore often "silent" and occurs three times as often as symptomatic PID. Unfortunately, the complications of silent PID, ectopic pregnancy and infertility, remain the same as those of its symptomatic counterpart and provide the impetus for screening and treatment of asymptomatic chlamydial infection. For more on information on this topic, please see the following article on PID.

Chlamydial urethritis occurs in both men and women and is responsible for 15% to 55% of cases of nongonococcal urethritis. Symptoms usually begin within 7 to 10 days after exposure to an infected partner. Although commonly asymptomatic in men, the infection is characterized by dysuria, a thin, clear urethral discharge that can sometimes be purulent or minimally cloudy, a Gram stain of a urethral swab with more than 5 white blood cells (WBCs) per oil immersion field in the absence of intracellular diplococci, and a positive leukocyte esterase test or microscopic examination of first-void urine with more than 10 WBCs per high-power field. Chlamydia also causes urethritis in women that usually asymptomatic but can occur as the acute urethral syndrome. This syndrome mimics a urinary tract infection or acute cystitis with dysuria, frequency, or hesitancy, but the urine culture reveals less than 10^5 organisms/mL.

Another infection caused by chlamydia is epididymitis, and it occurs in about 1% of men who develop this upper genital tract infection. This infection is considered the equivalent of PID and arises with unilateral scrotal pain, swelling, and fever in young men who often have an associated urethritis. In addition, chlamydia causes conjunctivitis, proctitis, and Reiter's syndrome in men; lymphogranuloma venereum (a nondescript genital ulcer followed by extensive inguinal adenopathy); and reactive arthritis and perihepatitis in women.

DIAGNOSIS

Automated methods for the detection and amplification of chlamydia DNA or RNA represent exciting developments in the arena of chlamydial diagnostic testing. These methods can be used on cervical, urethral, and urine specimens from both men and women. Although the organism can be detected by other means such as culture, enzyme-linked immunoassay, and direct immunofluorescence, amplification methods have surpassed them all as the screening test of choice with increased sensitivities and high specificities. In addition, they have changed the approach to chlamydial screening and prevention by allowing the examination of self-collected vaginal swabs or tampons and noninvasive specimens such as urine in nontraditional settings such as high schools and community centers.

TABLE 3. **Treatment Regimens for Uncomplicated Chlamydial Infections**

Urethritis or Cervicitis
Recommended regimens:
Azithromycin (Zithromax) 1 g orally in a single dose or doxycycline (Vibramycin) 100 mg orally bid for 7 d
Alternative regimens:
Erythromycin base (Ery-Tab) 500 mg orally qid for 7 d
or
Erythromycin ethylsuccinate (E.E.S.) 800 mg orally qid for 7 d
or
Ofloxacin (Floxin) 300 mg bid for 7 d or levofloxacin 500 mg qd for 7 d
Chlamydial Infections in Pregnancy
Recommended:
Erythromycin base 500 mg orally qid for 7 d
or
Amoxicillin 500 mg orally tid for 7 d
Alternative regimens:
Erythromycin base 250 mg orally qid for 14 d
or
Erythromycin ethylsuccinate 800 mg orally qid for 7 days or 400 mg qid for 14 d
or
Azithromycin 1 g orally, single dose

*Adapted from the 2002 CDC Sexually Transmitted Diseases Treatment Guidelines. MMWR Morb Mortal Wkly Rep 51:RR-6, 2002.

TREATMENT

The 2002 CDC Sexually Transmitted Diseases Treatment Guidelines for uncomplicated chlamydial infection are summarized in Table 3. The mainstay of therapy remains azithromycin (Zithromax), 1 g orally once or doxycycline (Vibramycin) 100 mg twice a day orally for 7 days. Azithromycin offers the distinct advantage of being a single dose and allows directly observed therapy. This is particularly attractive for adolescents, less compliant patients, and those who are asymptomatic. Patients should abstain from sexual intercourse for 7 days after receiving single-dose therapy. Erythromycin (Ery-Tab), ofloxacin (Floxin), and levofloxacin (Levaquin)* are alternative treatment options.

The recommended regimens for treatment in pregnancy are erythromycin or amoxicillin. Azithromycin is widely used, and clinical practice and preliminary data suggest that it is safe and effective. Doxycycline and the quinolones are contraindicated in pregnancy. Erythromycin is poorly tolerated and amoxicillin is a static drug against chlamydia. For these reasons, it is recommended that all pregnant women undergo repeated testing 3 weeks after completion of treatment.

*Not FDA approved for this indication.

PELVIC INFLAMMATORY DISEASE

method of
OSCAR D. ALMEIDA, Jr., M.D.
University of South Alabama College of Medicine
Mobile, Alabama

Pelvic inflammatory disease (PID) is among the most menacing infections of the female reproductive tract. Overall, the incidence of acute PID is about 1% to 2% in sexually active women, highest in the midteens through 20s. There is a decline in the number of cases of PID with advancing age, a stable monogamous relationship, in women who use oral contraceptives, when the male sexual partner uses condoms, and with use of other barrier methods such as diaphragms and spermicides.

The ascending pelvic infection is not limited to salpingitis and endometritis but can encompass tubo-ovarian abscess, pelvic peritonitis, and perihepatitis (Fitz-Hugh-Curtis syndrome). Acute PID is accompanied by moderate to severe pelvic and abdominal pain, painful and frequent urination, vaginal discharge, nausea, and fever. With chronic PID the patient may experience mild intermittent low abdomen pain, irregular menses, dyspareunia, back pain, vaginal discharge, and infertility.

Endometriosis, a common cause of acute and chronic pelvic pain, may mimic the symptoms of PID. Acute PID is the most common complication of sexually transmitted diseases (STDs). Although most cases have a polymicrobial origin, sexually transmitted organisms, most commonly *Chlamydia trachomatis* and *Neisseria gonorrhoeae*, are often suspected as the catalysts for the development of this disease. Risk factors for PID include age at first coitus, number of sex partners or sexual encounters, marital status, and previous history of PID.

As a result of the acute and chronic symptoms, PID is responsible for over 2 million doctor visits and thousands of surgical procedures annually. A primary concern in the reproductive-age patient with PID is that the disease may cause tubal infertility. Other sequelae include ectopic pregnancy and chronic pelvic pain. Although mortality ascribed to PID is rare today because of the available pharmacologic armamentarium, such tragic complications may occur secondary to the development of acute respiratory distress syndrome.

ETIOLOGY

Approximately 85% of PID occurs naturally in sexually active women. Although most cases have a polymicrobial origin, the slower growing *C. trachomatis* and faster growing *N. gonorrhoeae* are frequently isolated. Other causative organisms implicated include endogenous aerobic and anaerobic bacteria and genital *Mycoplasma* species. Although pelvic tuberculosis is a rare etiology of PID in the United States today, it should be considered when treating individuals from developing countries or in those who have recently traveled to these places and present with these signs and symptoms.

The remaining15% of PID arises following minor surgical procedures that inflict a break in the cervical mucus barrier allowing the vaginal flora to colonize in the upper genital tract. This has been noted following endometrial biopsy, dilation and curettage, placement of an intrauterine device, hysteroscopy, and hysterosalpingography. Increased douching has been implicated.

DIAGNOSIS

The diagnosis of acute PID is usually made on the basis of clinical history and physical examination. Although laparoscopy is the most accurate technique for visualizing the pelvis and thus confirming the diagnosis of PID, it has some limitations during the early part of the disease process. For example, endometritis cannot be diagnosed through the laparoscope. However, it is extremely helpful in ruling out other disease entities and surgical emergencies such as appendicitis. The perplexity of diagnosing PID is due to the large spectrum of signs and symptoms presented by these patients. The diagnosis of PID should be entertained in women who present with pelvic pain and inflammation of the lower reproductive tract when no other clear etiology can be discerned. Pelvic pain and abdominal pain are the most common symptoms observed in acute PID. The differential diagnosis of acute PID can involve other common gynecologic disorders (Table 1). The Centers for Disease Control and Prevention (CDC) have established minimum criteria for the initiation of empirical treatment of PID in sexually active women and those at increased risk for STDs (Table 2).

Acute PID begins suddenly and tends to be more severe, whereas chronic PID is a low-grade infection that may cause only mild pain and sometimes backache. Fitz-Hugh-Curtis syndrome consists of inflammation and adhesions around the liver. Patients with this complication of PID experience pain in the right upper quadrant and pleuritic pain. Acute cholecystitis or pneumonia can produce signs and symptoms similar to those of perihepatitis.

TREATMENT

The objective in the treatment of PID is to resolve the acute infection and prevent or limit its sequelae. Depending on the severity of the disease, treatment requires a medical and at times a surgical approach.

Table 1. **Differential Diagnosis of Acute Pelvic Inflammatory Disease**

Endometriosis
Acute appendicitis
Ectopic pregnancy
Ruptured ovarian cyst
Adnexal torsion
Crohn's disease

TABLE 2. **Centers for Disease Control and Prevention Criteria for Empirical Treatment of Pelvic Inflammatory Disease**

Minimum Criteria

Cervical motion tenderness
Uterine tenderness
Adnexal tenderness

Additional Criteria

Documentation of cervical infection with *C. trachomatis* or *N. gonorrhoeae*
Oral temperature > 101°F (>38.3°C)
Cervical or vaginal mucopurulent discharge
Elevated erythrocyte sedimentation rate
Elevated C-reactive protein
Presence of white blood cells on saline wet preparation

Specific Criteria

Laparoscopic evidence of PID
Endometrial biopsy confirmed endometritis
Transvaginal ultrasonography or magnetic resonance imaging
Findings suggestive of PID

PID, pelvic inflammatory disease.

Empirical treatment should commence as soon as the minimum criterion threshold has been met, even before laboratory documentation of the causative organism or organisms is available. A diagnosis of PID underscores the urgency to treat the sex partner or partners as well. All treatment regimens must provide broad-spectrum coverage of likely organisms including *C. trachomatis* and *N. gonorrhoeae*, anaerobes, gram-negative facultative bacteria, and streptococci. The CDC has developed criteria for hospitalization of patients with PID (Table 3). Because a negative bacteriologic screen does not rule out upper genital tract infection, parenteral and oral regimens must be efficacious against *C. trachomatis* and *N. gonorrhoeae*. The CDC guidelines contain several parenteral regimens for the treatment of PID (Table 4). Doxycycline should be administered orally whenever possible because of pain associated with parenteral infusion. Parenteral therapy may be discontinued 24 hours following clinical improvement. Outpatient oral therapy can be used in most cases of PID. The CDC guidelines include several regimens for oral treatment (Table 5). The complete course of oral therapy should consist of 14 days. Patients who do not show a clinical response to oral treatment within 72 hours should be administered parenteral therapy and reevaluated to confirm the diagnosis of PID.

TABLE 3. **Criteria for Hospitalization of Patients with Pelvic Inflammatory Disease**

Severe illness
Nausea, vomiting
High fever
Presence of tubo-ovarian abscess
Noncompliance
Inability to tolerate outpatient therapy
Pregnancy
Immunosuppression
Failure of oral antimicrobial therapy
Cannot rule out surgical emergency

TABLE 4. **Parenteral Therapy Regimens for Pelvic Inflammatory Disease**

Regimen A

Cefotetan (Cefotan) 2 g IV every 12 h
or
Cefoxitin (Mefoxin) 2 g IV every 6 h
plus
Doxycycline (Vibramycin) 100 mg or IV every 12 h

Regimen B

Clindamycin (Cleocin) 900 mg IV every 8 h
plus
Gentamicin loading dose IV or IM (2 mg/kg body weight) followed by a maintenance dose (1.5 mg/kg) every 8 h. Single daily dosing may be substituted.

Alternative Regimens

a. Ofloxacin (Floxin) 400 mg IV every 12 h
or
Levofloxacin (Levaquin) 500 mg IV once daily
with or without
Metronidazole (Flagyl) 500 mg IV every 8 h
b. Ampicillin/sulbactam (Unasyn) 3 g IV every 6 h
plus
Doxycycline 100 mg orally or IV every 12 h

Severe cases of PID and those that are unresponsive to medical therapy may require surgical intervention. Table 6 highlights these surgical options. Laparoscopy is generally utilized to establish or clarify the diagnosis. Laparotomy is frequently used to manage a ruptured tubo-ovarian abscess.

In cases in which vaginal drainage of a pelvic abscess is desirable, posterior colpotomy may be the procedure of choice. However, there are established criteria for selecting surgical candidates for this procedure. These include the following: (1) the abscess must be localized in the midline, (2) the abscess must be adjacent to the cul-de-sac and should dissect in such a manner that pus does not flow transperitoneally, and (3) the abscess should be cystic in order to obtain satisfactory drainage. Patients requiring definitive treatment after failed medical therapy may require a unilateral or bilateral salpingo-oophorectomy and at times an abdominal hysterectomy.

COUNSELING

Appropriate counseling of the patient with PID is critical in order to prevent similar episodes from occurring in the future. She should be provided literature containing an explanation of the disease process, risks, prevention, and treatments. Patients diagnosed with PID should be advised to avoid unprotected

TABLE 5. **Oral Therapy Regimens for Pelvic Inflammatory Disease**

Ofloxacin (Floxin) 400 mg orally twice daily for 14 d
or
Levofloxacin (Levaquin) 500 mg orally once daily for 14 d
with or without
Metronidazole (Flagyl) 500 mg orally twice daily for 14 d

Table 6. **Surgical Options for Pelvic Inflammatory Disease**

Laparoscopy
Laparotomy
Posterior colpotomy
Salpingo-oophorectomy
Total abdominal hysterectomy, bilateral salpingo-oophorectomy

sexual intercourse until they and their sexual partner or partners have completed treatment and follow-up. In addition, these patients should be counseled and offered screening for other STDs including HIV, hepatitis C, and syphilis. Whenever possible, the sexual partners should also be counseled and encouraged to see their personal physician.

LEIOMYOMAS

method of
BRUCE R. CARR, M.D., and
DEREK A. HAAS, M.D.
University of Texas Southwestern Medical Center at Dallas
Dallas, Texas

EPIDEMIOLOGY

Uterine leiomyomas remain one of the most common conditions affecting women of reproductive age. Their frequency ranges from 20% to 40% in women older than 30. Pathologic examination of surgical specimens reveals the prevalence to be as high as 77%. In the United States, 30% of women have had a hysterectomy by the age of 60 years with the majority performed to treat fibroids. Black women have over a threefold greater frequency of myomas compared with white women. Obesity is strongly associated with leiomyomas, with the risk being three times greater in women weighing more than 70 kg.

CLINICAL MANIFESTATIONS

The majority of leiomyomas do not cause significant morbidity. Symptoms are divided into three categories: abnormal uterine bleeding, pelvic pressure and pain, and reproductive dysfunction. The bleeding pattern most characteristic of myomas is menorrhagia. Intermenstrual bleeding is not as common and should be investigated to rule out endometrial disease. Symptoms are more often related to the location than the size of the leiomyoma. The location is usually defined in relation to the uterine wall: subserosal, intramural, or submucosal. Generally, these tumors do not cause pain but can lead to pressure sensations. As a myoma enlarges, it may impinge on surrounding organs and lead to problems such as urinary frequency (bladder), constipation (rectum), or hydronephrosis (ureter). Acute pain can occur in the rare case of myoma degeneration or when there is torsion of a pedunculated fibroid. If the endometrial cavity is distorted by submucous myomas, the risk of infertility is increased.

PATHOPHYSIOLOGY

The histology of leiomyomas is characterized by well-differentiated smooth muscle cells arranged in interlacing bundles with uniform, cigar-shaped nuclei showing little or no mitotic activity (0 to 4 mitotic figures per 10 high-power fields) and no cytologic atypia. Collagenous extracellular matrix tends to be more prominent in myomas. The karyotypic discordance between myomas and leiomyosarcomas suggest that the two tumors arise from distinct pathogenetic pathways. A malignant leiomyosarcoma is hypercellular and less fascicular and contains atypical smooth muscle cells with hyperchromatic, enlarged nuclei.

The pathogenesis of leiomyomas includes two processes: transformation of normal myocytes into abnormal myocytes and their subsequent growth by clonal expansion. The mechanisms controlling growth are unclear but probably involve a genetic predisposition, steroid hormones (estrogen and progesterone), peptide growth factors, and the availability of an adequate blood supply. These are tumors largely confined to women of reproductive age. Myomas have not been described in prepubertal girls. They enlarge after exposure to estrogens or during pregnancy. In addition, they regress during menopause and after gonadotropin-releasing hormone (GnRH) agonist treatment. Progesterone as well as estradiol up-regulates the cell proliferating activity in leiomyoma cell cultures with the mitotic activity highest during the luteal phase.

Specific chromosomal regions have nonrandom abnormalities in up to 40% of tumors, most commonly chromosomes 6, 7, 12, and 14. Leiomyomas represent independent monoclonal lesions; multiple tumors from the same uterus often have different chromosomal abnormalities. Rearrangements occur in already existing tumors and are secondary events in tumor progression. A primary genetic change may be responsible for tumor growth in genetically susceptible cells; however, this susceptibility gene or genes remain to be identified. Growth-promoting effects of the steroid hormones are mediated through the local production of specific growth factors (Table 1).

DIAGNOSIS

The myomatous uterus can often be appreciated on pelvic examination to be large or irregularly shaped. Radiographic imaging to confirm the diagnosis is an option. For the asymptomatic, mildly enlarged uterus that does not obscure palpation of the ovaries, expectant management is acceptable. Transvaginal sonography and transvaginal sonohystography (especially good for submucosal fibroids and polyps) are good initial methods. Transabdominal ultrasonography may be better for uteri greater than 12 weeks in size.

TABLE 1. **Growth Factors and Gene Products Linked to Leiomyoma Formation or Growth**

Factor or Product	Action
EGF	Mitogenic activity in reproductive tissues Increased amounts during secretory phase Decreased levels after GnRH-a treatment
TGF-β	Stimulates expression of fibronectin, collagen Increased amounts in luteal phase leiomyoma samples Decreased amounts after GnRH-a treatment
bFGF	Stimulates mitogenesis, differentiation of fibroblasts and smooth muscle cells Higher amounts in leiomyoma versus matched myometrium
Bcl-2	Apoptosis-inhibiting gene product Overexpressed in leiomyoma relative to normal myometrium Up-regulated by progesterone
PPARs	Increased expression in leiomyoma cells Can be activated in target tissues by estrogen
HMGI-C	High-mobility-group protein type I-C encodes a protein acting as an architectural transcription factor Rearranged in a variety of benign or locally aggressive mesenchymal tumors Critical gene involved in chromosomal 12 translocations
Wnt7a	Gene that guides development of female reproductive tract Critical role in uterine smooth muscle patterning 67% of human leiomyoma showed decreased messenger RNA levels
DNA methylation changes	Two genomic fragments identified that frequently undergo methylation changes in leiomyoma
MMPs, TIMPs	TGF-β1 increases TIMP-1 and decrease MMP-1,3 Favored an antidegradation state of ECM (fibronectin-promoting role)

Abbreviation: bFGF, basic fibroblast growth factor; ECM, extracellular membrane; EGF, epidermal growth factor; GnRH-a, gonadotropin-releasing hormone agonist; HMG, high-mobility-group proteins; MMP, matrix metalloproteinase; PPAR, peroxisome proliferator-activted receptor; TGF, transforming growth factor; TIMP, tissue inhibitor of metalloproteinase.

MANAGEMENT

The myomatous uterus is managed expectantly unless symptoms arise. Size and location of the myoma, presenting symptoms, and age and reproductive desires of the patient all determine treatment. The three main approaches to symptomatic fibroids are medical, surgical, and through interventional radiology. Medical therapy is generally tried first.

GnRH agonists (i.e., leuprolide acetate [Lupron Depot], 3.75 mg every month by intramuscular injection for 2 to 6 months) have been the mainstay of medical therapy, resulting in significant reduction in uterine size (35% to 65%) as well as inducing amenorrhea in most women. A measurable response is seen by 1 to 2 months with maximal effect by 3 to 4 months. The most common side effects have been those of hypoestrogenism (i.e., hot flushes, vaginal dryness). In addition, GnRH agonist treatment for 6 months can cause a 6% loss in trabecular bone, not all of which is reversible on discontinuation. To counteract this, hormone replacement therapy can be added back to alleviate these long-term side effects. Most authors recommend using GnRH agonists first to attain uterine shrinkage (12 weeks) and then adding back estrogen and progestin (low doses equivalent to menopausal hormone replacement therapy). After cessation of GnRH agonist therapy, the uterus rapidly returns to pretreatment volume. For this reason, GnRH agonist therapy has been recommended as a preoperative therapy to improve the hemoglobin level, decrease the estimated blood loss at surgery, decrease the need for a vertical incision, and convert a hysterectomy from an abdominal to a vaginal approach.

Surgical therapy for the treatment of leiomyoma has focused on either myomectomy for women wishing to retain their uterus or hysterectomy. Hysterectomy eliminates both the symptoms and the chance of recurrence. Myomectomy can be approached abdominally, laparoscopically, or hysteroscopically, depending on the location and size. The goal of myomectomy is to remove as many myomas as possible through the least number of incisions. The rate of recurrence of myomas by ultrasonography after abdominal myomectomy is high (about 50% at 5 years), and postoperative adhesions are common. Laparoscopic myomectomy should be reserved for cases with a small number of subserosal or intramural fibroids no bigger than 6 to 8 cm in diameter with a total uterine size of 16 weeks or less. Submucosal myomas are ideally approached hysteroscopically. More than one hysteroscopic procedure may be necessary if the myoma is large or extends deep into the myometrium.

The third avenue of treatment for leiomyoma involves uterine artery embolization performed by interventional radiology. Uterine fibroids appear to be particularly sensitive to the effects of the acute ischemia produced by embolization and undergo necrosis. The response of fibroids is variable (mean decrease of 30% to 50%) and it appears to persist. There has been a significant incidence of morbidity and mortality following the procedure. Complications include fibroid expulsion through the cervix, fibroid necrosis, postprocedure pain requiring hospital admission, uterine abscess formation, and fever.

There have not been studies with sufficient long-term follow-up to know the recurrence rate. Pregnancies have been reported following the procedure. However, because of the risk of premature menopause, it is reserved for women not desiring future fertility.

ENDOMETRIAL CANCER

method of
JAMES J. BURKE, II, M.D., and
DONALD G. GALLUP, M.D.
Mercer School of Medicine (Savannah)
Memorial Health University Medical Center
Savannah, Georgia

Endometrial cancer is the most common gynecologic cancer in the United States, with an estimated 40,100 new cases reported each year. Although approximately 80% of these cases are diagnosed as stage I disease, 6800 women will succumb of their disease annually.

Endometrial cancer is subdivided into two histologically and clinically separate groups. Type I endometrial cancer is directly related to an increased estrogenous state. This type of endometrial cancer is the most common and is usually found at an earlier stage, and treatment results in a more favorable outcome. Type II endometrial carcinoma is a more virulent type of carcinoma characterized by early metastasis, and it typically has a worse prognosis.

EPIDEMIOLOGY, CLINICAL FEATURES, AND DIAGNOSIS

Type I Endometrial Carcinoma

Endometrial carcinoma is a heterogeneous mix of several histologic types with various clinical outcomes. This more common type of endometrial carcinoma represents approximately 90% of all endometrial cancers and is associated with a hyperestrogenic state. Table 1 lists risk factors associated with type I endometrial carcinoma. In the 1970s it was found that giving estrogen preparations without progestin for hormone replacement therapy led to at least a six times greater chance of endometrial carcinoma developing. Similarly, women who are obese have an increased risk of endometrial carcinoma as a result of peripheral conversion of androstenedione to estrone in peripheral adipose tissue by 5α-reductase enzyme activity. Finally, women who have untreated atypical endometrial hyperplasia, a well-known precursor to type I endometrial carcinoma, have a 29 times greater chance of endometrial carcinoma developing. Hence, intervention when this precursor is found can prevent endometrial cancer.

TABLE 1. **Risk Factors for the Development of Endometrial Carcinoma**

Risk Factors	RR
Overweight (age 50–59)	
By 20–50 lb	3
By >50 lb	10
Nulliparity vs. multiparity	5
Menopause after age 52	2
Diabetes	3
Unopposed estrogen replacement	6
Combination OCP	0.5

OCP, oral contraceptive preparation; RR, relative risk.

Although 90% of women with this type of carcinoma initially have painless, postmenopausal vaginal bleeding or some form of vaginal discharge, most postmenopausal vaginal bleeding is related to conditions other than malignancy. Nonetheless, all postmenopausal bleeding needs further evaluation. The gold standard is endometrial biopsy, usually carried out in the office with minimal patient discomfort. However, should the results of this type of in-office biopsy still be equivocal or performance of the biopsy not be possible because of cervical stenosis, formal fractional dilation and curettage should be performed. Another modality used for assessment of postmenopausal bleeding is transvaginal ultrasound to measure the thickness of the endometrium. Endometrial stripes found to be thicker than 5 mm require endometrial sampling because of the higher likelihood of malignancy.

Type II Endometrial Carcinoma

Unlike type I endometrial carcinoma, type II is not related to an increased estrogenic state and encompasses several histologic variants that are quite aggressive. These carcinomas tend to have either serous, papillary serous, or clear cell histology and typically occur in women older than 70 years. Fortunately, carcinomas of these types account for less than 10% of all endometrial cancers, but unfortunately, they contribute the majority of deaths from endometrial cancer. Because of the aggressive nature of these cancers, most have metastasized before initial evaluation and diagnosis and spread in a fashion similar to ovarian carcinoma.

As with type I endometrial carcinoma, type II carcinomas are commonly manifested as painless, postmenopausal vaginal bleeding or vaginal discharge. However, patients may have no bleeding at all but instead have nonspecific gastrointestinal symptoms such as nausea and vomiting, constipation, early satiety, abdominal bloating, and abdominal pain. All these symptoms point to intra-abdominal metastasis, common with this type of endometrial carcinoma. In these patients, early computed tomography (CT) can aid in the diagnosis. Even when these carcinomas have not spread and are limited to the endometrium or endometrial polyps, the risk of recurrence is high.

STAGING AND TREATMENT

Staging

Recognizing that clinical staging did not take into account pathologic or surgical prognostic information, the Gynecologic Oncology Group (GOG) conducted two large prospective surgical staging trials in the 1980s. In 1988, the Fédération Internationale de Gynécologie et d'Obstétrique (FIGO) adopted the surgical staging of endometrial cancer (Table 2). Surgical staging involves obtaining pelvic washings, extrafascial hysterectomy, bilateral salpingo-oophorectomy,

TABLE 2. **FIGO Surgical Staging Classification for Endometrial Carcinoma**

Stage IA	Tumor limited to the endometrium
Stage IB	Invasion to less than half the myometrium
Stage IC	Invasion equal to or more than half the myometrium
Stage IIA	Endocervical glandular involvement only
Stage IIB	Cervical stromal invasion
Stage IIIA	Tumor invading the serosa of the corpus uteri and/or adnexa and/or positive cytologic findings
Stage IIIB	Vaginal metastases
Stage IIIC	Metastases to the pelvic and/or paraortic lymph nodes
Stage IVA	Tumor invasion of the bladder and/or bowel mucosa
Stage IVB	Distant metastases, including intra-abdominal metastasis and/or metastasis to the inguinal lymph nodes

FIGO, Federation Internationale de Gynécologie et d'Obstétrique.

TABLE 3. **Distribution of Endometrial Cancer by Stage**

Stage I	72.8%
Stage II	10.9%
Stage III	13.1%
Stage IV	3.2%

and lymph node sampling from the pelvic and para-aortic regions. In addition, if high-risk histology or gross spread of disease is present at the time of surgery (common with type II endometrial cancers), removal of the omentum is recommended. Table 3 shows the typical stage distribution for endometrial carcinoma.

Adjuvant Therapy

Radiotherapy is currently the mainstay of adjuvant therapy for early-stage endometrial carcinoma at risk for recurrence. Several trials have examined hormonal therapy or chemotherapy in an adjuvant setting for early-stage disease, but none has shown any benefit in reducing recurrences.

Although 75% of endometrial carcinomas are found to be confined to the uterus after surgical staging, some of these patients will be at risk for recurrence and failure with surgical treatment only (Figure 1). Patients found to be at high risk for recurrence are treated with whole-pelvic radiotherapy after surgery, whereas patients who are at "intermediate" risk usually do not need radiotherapy, provided that they have been surgically staged. However, any adjuvant therapy for this group of patients remains controversial.

Advanced-Stage or Recurrent Disease

A study conducted by the GOG showed that 36% of patients who were found to have metastasis to the para-aortic lymph nodes (stage IIIC) and were treated with radiotherapy were tumor free at 5 years. Similarly, if only pelvic lymph node metastasis (stage IIIC) was found and treated with radiotherapy, 72% would be alive at 5 years.

For serous or clear cell carcinomas found to have extrauterine spread at the time of surgery, "debulking" the metastasis and treating with chemotherapeutic regimens used for ovarian cancer have been shown to increase progression-free survival in several case series. Patients with gross intra-abdominal spread of endometrioid carcinoma generally have a grim prognosis and have not been shown to have prolonged survival with radiotherapy or chemotherapy. Therefore, these patients should be offered participation in clinical trials.

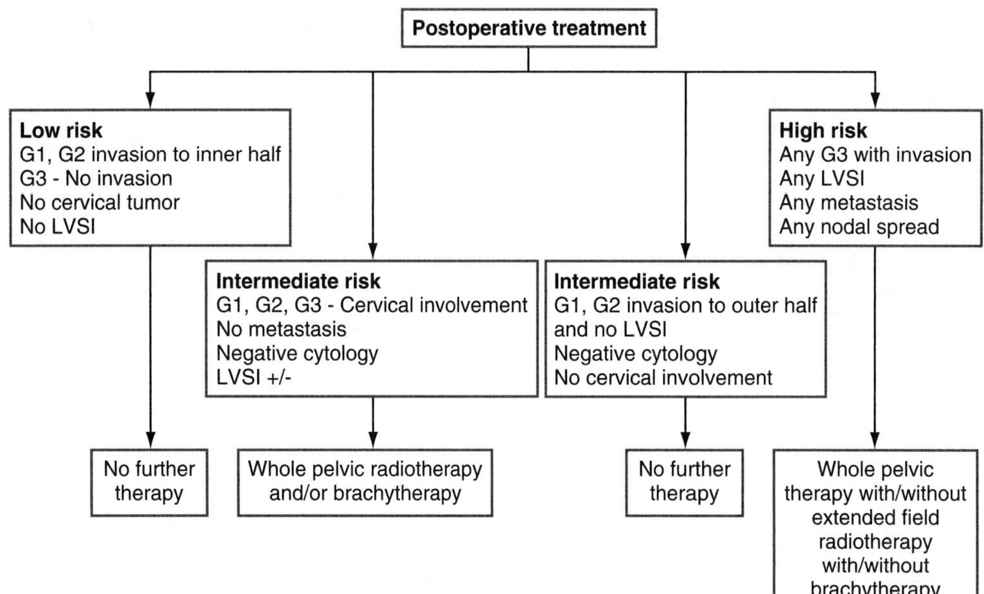

Figure 1. Postoperative treatment scheme at Memorial Health University Medical Center for surgical stage I endometrial carcinoma. G, grade; LVSI, lymphovascular space involvement.

In most patients in whom cancer recurs, it will do so within 3 years of initial treatment. Unfortunately, if the recurrence is any place other than the pelvis (vaginal apex), the likelihood of long-term cure is poor. Depending on the location of the recurrence, radiotherapy, surgery, hormonal therapy, or chemotherapy can be used. Progestins have been studied for the treatment of recurrent disease but have demonstrated modest responses of limited duration.

Follow-Up

Of the endometrial carcinomas that recur, most will do so within the first 3 years after treatment. Typically, the site of recurrence is in the pelvis, with the vaginal apex being the most common location. Unfortunately, a number of patients will have recurrence at distant sites, and the chest and upper part of the abdomen are the most common areas. Thus, patients treated for endometrial carcinoma are usually monitored closely for 5 years. At Memorial Health University Medical Center, we use an assessment program in which patients are seen every 3 months for the first year, every 4 months for the second year, and every 6 months until 5 years has elapsed since completion of treatment. In addition, a Pap smear is performed at every visit, and chest radiographs are obtained annually for the first 2 years. Furthermore, annual mammography as well as counseling for screening colonoscopy is carried out. CT scanning is not generally used for surveillance in follow-up because of its high cost and low yield of detection. However, patients with abdominal symptoms may be assessed with CT because the likelihood of finding pathology is greater. For patients with advanced disease or high-risk histologic features, serum measurement of CA 125 may be considered. Table 4 shows 5-year survival rates of patients with endometrial carcinoma by stage.

Tamoxifen (Nolvadex)

The National Surgical Adjuvant Breast and Bowel Project (NSABP) conducted a prevention trial with tamoxifen known as the P-1 trial. In this randomized, double-blind prospective trial, women with high-risk family histories were treated with tamoxifen or placebo for 5 years. The trial demonstrated a 49% reduced risk for breast cancer, but a 2.5 times greater risk for endometrial carcinoma. Most of the endometrial carcinomas detected were stage I carcinomas, were of endometrioid histology (type I endometrial carcinoma), and were successfully treated with surgery. Additionally, other nonmalignant endometrial abnormalities were detected.

TABLE 4. **Endometrial Cancer: Five-Year Survival Rate by Stage**

Stage	5-Year Survival Rate
Stage IA	91%
Stage IB	88%
Stage 1C	81%
Stage II	72%
Stage III	51%
Stage IV	9%

In addition to the use of tamoxifen for prevention of breast cancer, many women who have receptor-positive breast carcinomas are using tamoxifen for adjuvant treatment.

The question arises of how one monitors patients taking tamoxifen? The consensus has been to not perform transvaginal ultrasonography or endometrial sampling in women who are asymptomatic. However, women who are taking tamoxifen and experience vaginal bleeding need to have an immediate evaluation by endometrial sampling to rule out endometrial carcinoma.

Although endometrial carcinoma remains the most common gynecologic malignancy in the United States, it is also the most curable because of its low stage at diagnosis. Surgery remains the primary treatment modality for this type of carcinoma, with adjuvant radiotherapy reserved for patients at high risk for recurrent disease after surgery. Chemotherapeutic and hormonal agents have been used to palliate advanced-stage or recurrent disease, but durable, long-term survival has not been demonstrated. Finally, women who are taking tamoxifen for prophylaxis or adjuvant treatment of breast carcinoma need no special surveillance for the development of endometrial carcinoma. However, should any postmenopausal or abnormal vaginal bleeding occur in this group of women, immediate evaluation by endometrial sampling is required.

CANCER OF THE UTERINE CERVIX

method of
JEFFREY G. BELL, M.D.
Riverside Methodist Hospital and Ohio State University Columbus, Ohio

EPIDEMIOLOGY

Although invasive cancer of the cervix remains a leading cause of death in many countries, both the incidence of the disease and the mortality from this cancer have declined over several decades in the United States as a result of successful screening programs. In the year 2000 the incidence of cervical cancer was 10 per 100,000 in the standard population, and the mortality from cervical cancer was 3.3 per 100,000. The approximate absolute numbers are 13,000 new cases of cervical cancer per year and 4100 deaths per year. Both the incidence of the disease and the mortality rate are higher for blacks and Hispanics than for white Americans. The probability of a woman developing invasive cervical cancer over her lifetime is 1 in 117, but this probability is age dependent, with the greatest risk between ages 40 and 49 (1 in 288).

The etiology of cervical cancer is closely associated with the human papillomavirus (HPV) that is sexually transmitted. Over 90% of squamous carcinomas of the cervix have HPV DNA within the cells. Invasive cancer is preceded by a phase of cellular dysplasia that may exist for years before the transition into invasive disease. Tissue samples from the dysplastic areas on the cervix, termed squamous intraepithelial lesions (SILs), also contain cellular HPV DNA. Almost all factors that increase a person's risk of cervical cancer are associated with increased exposure to HPV: multiple sexual partners, early age of coitus, contraceptive use, socioeconomic status, other venereal diseases, cigarette smoking. The latter, cigarette smoking, may be related to cervical cancer not only because of the indirect association with increased sexual activity but also because of carcinogenic cofactors found in the tobacco or possible mitigation of cervical mucosal immunologic factors that protect against HPV.

PATHOPHYSIOLOGY

The HPV family consists of more than 50 subtypes classified as either low risk or high risk on the basis of their association with dysplasia and cancer. High-grade SILs and cancers contain high-risk HPV DNA more frequently than low-risk subtypes. HPV DNA produces oncogenic proteins, most notably E6 and E7, that interfere with normal cells' tumor suppressor genes, *p53* and *Rb* (retinoblastoma gene). This interaction results in dysplastic cellular growth producing an SIL. Cervical cells most susceptible to HPV damage are located in the transformation zone where columnar cells are undergoing metaplasia to become squamous cells. Dysplastic cells or SILs are confined to the epithelium, during which time they may regress spontaneously or be successfully eradicated by a variety of local treatments. For reasons not thoroughly understood at this time but presumably related to carcinogenic cofactors, some dysplastic cells attain the potential to invade the basement membrane of the epithelium. From this point the cancer cells can invade the stroma of the cervix, causing a local mass or ulcer, or invade the lymphovascular spaces, through which they can metastasize to the pelvic lymph nodes. Hematogenous spread is much less likely but can result in metastasis to liver, lung, bone, and brain.

CLINICAL FEATURES

Surprisingly, despite the widespread use of Pap smears in our screening programs, only 20% of patients who present with invasive cervical cancer are asymptomatic. The most common symptom is vaginal bleeding. Other symptoms include irregular menses, postcoital bleeding, vaginal discharge, and pain. Vaginal discharge may be watery, pink, purulent, or mucoid and sometimes malodorous. Pelvic pain associated with cervical cancer is a late symptom related to advanced disease involving adjacent organs or pelvic nerves.

Physical findings are usually confined to the pelvic examination, although advanced disease may be associated with adenopathy in either the supraclavicular or groin area. The size and shape of the cervix may vary greatly. Obviously, microinvasive or minimally invasive cancers do not distort the overall cervix. Cancers arising within the endocervical canal may produce bulky firm cervices that have normal-appearing ectocervical epithelium, so palpation of the cervix is an important part of the examination. These cancers are the so-called barrel-shaped tumors. Gross lesions of the cervix may arise as ulcerations, flat lesions, or exophytic tumors. A watery, bloody, or purulent discharge is often present with gross tumors.

The diagnosis of cervical cancer requires a tissue specimen by biopsy. Although a Pap smear may demonstrate "carcinoma" cells, only a tissue specimen can verify invasive cancer. Errors in diagnosing carcinoma often arise from ignoring persistent symptoms such as vaginal discharge or irregular bleeding, especially postcoital bleeding. A good endocervical Pap and/or endocervical curettage is necessary to evaluate postcoital bleeding in a patient with a normal-appearing cervix. On the other hand, a biopsy is mandator for any cervical gross lesion. "Erosion" or cervicitis should be a diagnosis of exclusion only if a biopsy confirms the absence of cancer. Reliance on a Pap smear for diagnosis when a lesion is present is a common clinical error. If a biopsy of a grossly visible lesion diagnoses invasive cancer, the patient should *not* have a cone biopsy; this is another frequent clinical error. A Pap smear showing dysplastic or SIL cells is an indication for colposcopy to look for invasive cancer. If a colposcopically directed biopsy of a grossly normal-appearing cervix diagnoses or suggests invasive cancer, the patient should undergo conization to determine the depth of invasion.

HISTOLOGY

The most frequent histologic type of cervical cancer is squamous, accounting for 80% to 85% of all cases. Adenocarcinomas constitute 10% to 15% of cancers, and the remaining few percent consist of rare types such as adenosquamous, sarcoma, lymphoma, and neuroendocrine (carcinoid and small cell). Rarely, the cervix is the site of metastasis from another primary cancer. Although somewhat controversial, most authorities believe that the prognosis for squamous carcinomas and that for adenocarcinomas are similar after stratifying for stage and tumor size. On the other hand, adenosquamous carcinomas tend to be more aggressive cancers associated with poorer survival. Small cell carcinomas of the cervix carry the worst prognosis, 0% to 15% survival even for stage I cancer.

PRETREATMENT STAGING AND EVALUATION

The stage of disease is the most important prognostic factor, generally because the stage is related to the risk of the cancer metastasizing to the pelvic or aortic lymph nodes; lymph node status is the most important histologic prognostic indicator. Because the majority of patients with cervical cancer receive radiation therapy, pretreatment staging uses only clinical parameters rather than surgical findings. Acceptable clinical staging procedures include pelvic examination, intravenous pyelogram, chest radiograph, cystoscopy, and sigmoidoscopy. Sophisticated imaging such as computed tomography (CT), magnetic resonance imaging, bone scans, and lymphangiograms are not used for staging diagnosis for two main reasons; they are not internationally available, and they are not uniformly accurate in diagnosis. CT scans are common pretreatment evaluations in patients with stage II to IV cancers. Their sensitivity in detecting lymph node metastasis is approximately 65%. Evaluation of suspicious lymph nodes may involve CT-guided percutaneous biopsy or retroperitoneal selective lymph node dissection. This information may alter or define treatment, but it does not change the clinical stage based on the accepted procedures.

Gynecologic oncologists employ FIGO (International Federation of Obstetricians and Gynecologists) staging for treatment planning (Table 1). The stage is based on the natural route of cancer progression and the risk of lymph node metastasis. Besides the stage of disease, the lymph node status is the most important prognostic factor. The incidence of lymph node metastases relates directly to the depth of stromal invasion and to the stage (Table 2). Some institutions employ retroperitoneal surgical exploration to assess the nodal status more accurately than is possible with imaging. Those institutions believe that the advantages of surgical staging are (1) the ability to tailor the radiotherapy fields to areas of documented nodal disease and (2) the ability to remove grossly enlarged nodes, which may be incurable with radiotherapy alone. Nonrandomized trials indicate a survival benefit for patients with documented aortic node metastases who receive extended field radiotherapy compared with those receiving only pelvic radiotherapy.

TABLE 1. **FIGO Staging for Carcinoma of the Cervix (1995)**

Stage 0	Carcinoma in situ, intraepithelial carcinoma
Stage I	Cancer confined to the cervix
Ia1	Microscopic invasion of stroma measuring 3 mm or less in depth and 7 mm or less in width
Ia2	Microscopic invasion of stroma measuring >3 mm in depth but not greater than 5 mm in depth nor greater than 7 mm in width
Ib1	Lesions greater than in Ia2 but not greater than 4 cm in size
Ib2	Lesions greater than 4 cm in size
Stage II	Cancer extends beyond the cervix
IIa	Cancer involves the upper two thirds of the vagina
IIb	Obvious parametrial extension
Stage III	Extension of cancer to pelvic wall or lower vagina
IIIa	Cancer involves lower one third of vagina
IIIb	Cancer extends to pelvic wall or hydronephrosis or nonfunctioning kidney
Stage IV	
IVa	Cancer involves the bladder or rectal mucosa
IVb	Cancer metastasis to distant organs

FIGO, Federation Internationale de Gynécologie et d'Obstétrique.

TABLE 2. **Relationship between Stromal Invasion or Stage and the Incidence of Lymph Node Metastasis**

Invasion or Stage	Pelvic Nodes (% positive)	Aortic Nodes (% positive)
Less than 3 mm	0–1	
3–5 mm	2.5–5	
6–10 mm	4–8	
11–15 mm	10–25	
Ib1	15–25	5–10
Ib2	30–50	15–20
IIa	15–25	5–10
IIb	30–45	20
III	50	30

TREATMENT

All three basic treatment modalities, surgery, radiotherapy, and chemotherapy, play important roles in the management of cervical cancer. Selection of therapy is based upon stage of disease, patient's age, and patient's medical condition.

Most patients with minimally invasive disease, termed "microinvasion," are young and often wish to maintain fertility. In 1995, FIGO redefined stage Ia cancers to identify a set of patients with risk of extracervical disease low enough to allow treatment by conservative surgery. Thus, because the risk of nodal metastasis in stage Ia1 lesions is less than 1%, surgical treatment may be cone biopsy for patients desiring preservation of the uterus and standard hysterectomy for those who do not wish to maintain fertility. Microinvasive adenocarcinoma, in contrast to squamous carcinoma, is a difficult diagnosis for most pathologists, and the acceptance of conservative treatment by conization has been controversial. Patients so treated by conization require extremely close surveillance, and the chance of recurrent cancer is higher than for squamous cancers.

Generally, either radical surgery or radiotherapy is an appropriate selection for patients with stage Ia2, Ib1, Ib2, and IIa. Once again, the patient's age and medical status are important factors for the decision. Surgical treatment has the clear advantage of preserving ovarian function. Radical hysterectomy involves removing some portion of the parametrium and vagina with the uterus. Pelvic lymphadenectomy is an integral part of the radical surgery for these stages. For stage Ia2, which is a microscopic cancer, most gyn/oncologists modify the radical hysterectomy by removing less parametrium and vagina than necessary for macroscopic cancers. Stage Ib2 cancers are a special consideration because of the size (greater than 4 cm), which makes surgical resection often technically difficult. For this reason, some institutions elect to treat these larger cancers with combination chemotherapy and radiotherapy, termed chemoradiotherapy, to reduce the tumor mass, followed by standard hysterectomy. The addition of weekly cisplatin

(Platinol) chemotherapy to pelvic radiotherapy reduces the risk of both recurrence and death by 50% compared with radiotherapy alone.

Following radical hysterectomy, some patients may require adjuvant pelvic radiotherapy. Although the ultimate goal of radical surgical treatment is to effect cure while avoiding multimodality therapy, several pathologic factors indicate a need for additional adjuvant radiotherapy; these factors are positive lymph nodes, positive surgical margins, large size of the cervical cancer, deep invasion into the cervix, and presence of cervical stromal lymphovascular space invasion. Even when the lymph nodes are normal, patients with large cancers deeply invading the cervix and/or invading the lymphovascular spaces have a significantly increased risk of cancer recurrence. Patients with combinations of these pathologic risk factors should receive postoperative pelvic radiotherapy that has proved to reduce the risk of recurrence by 50%.

The standard therapy for advanced disease, stages IIb to IV, has become chemoradiotherapy. Patients receive concurrent weekly cisplatin (Platinol)* or cisplatin with 5-fluorouracil (Adrucil)* while undergoing pelvic radiotherapy. The radiation therapy typically consists of 45 to 50 Gy administered over 25 days, followed by one or two intracavitary tandem treatments over 24 to 48 hours that deliver an additional 30 to 35 Gy to point A (a point 2 cm lateral to the internal cervical os).

SURVIVAL

Survival is related to stage and lymph node status. General 5-year survival rates are shown in Table 3. These numbers come from literature on radical surgery and radiotherapy without concurrent chemotherapy. Most oncologists believe that the prognosis for early-stage cancer treated by surgery is similar to that for radiotherapy. The survival for stage I cancer treated by radical hysterectomy and pelvic lymphadenectomy depends upon the lymph node status and the other pathologic factors mentioned in the preceding treatment section. The 5-year survival for patients with normal lymph nodes and low-risk cervical factors is approximately 90%. Patients with normal lymph nodes but high-risk cervical factors experience a 2-year disease-free survival of 88% when treated by postoperative pelvic radiation. In contrast, the prognosis for patients with positive nodes falls to approximately 65%. Because postoperative pelvic radiotherapy has not convincingly improved that survival, researchers are investigating postoperative chemoradiotherapy for these patients with positive pelvic nodes.

Reports on chemoradiotherapy for advanced disease indicate that the addition of chemotherapy to standard radiation reduces the risk of death by 45%. The approximate 4-year survival for locally advanced disease (stages IIb to IVa) treated by chemoradiation is 60%.

*Not FDA approved for this indication.

TABLE 3. **Five-Year Survival Rates for Cervical Cancer by Stage**

Stage	Survival (%)
Ia1	99–100
Ia2	95
Ib1	85–90
Ib2	65–75
IIa	75–80
IIb	65
IIIa	45
IIIb	35
IV	15

SURVEILLANCE

After primary treatment by either surgery or radiotherapy or chemoradiotherapy to standard radiation, patients return every 3 to 4 months for 2 years, then semiannually for an additional 3 years. Physical examination and Pap smear are routine at each visit, annual chest radiography is typical, and other imaging studies such as CT and intravenous pyelograms are discretionary, based upon symptoms and physical findings.

RECURRENT CANCER

Three fourths of recurrent cancers are diagnosed within the first 18 months after therapy and 90% within 3 years. Sites of recurrence in descending order of incidence are the pelvis, liver, lung, bone, abdominal cavity, lymph nodes, and brain.

The treatment for localized recurrent cancer in the central pelvis following primary radiation or chemoradiation is pelvic exenteration; this is the surgical removal of the uterus, vagina, bladder, and rectum, or some combination of those organs. Preoperative and intraoperative assessment for metastatic disease excludes nearly three fourths of candidate patients from the operation. Patients who do undergo exenteration experience a 40% to 60% 5-year survival.

Pelvic recurrence following primary surgical treatment usually involves the pelvic wall. These patients are candidates for radiation, either by teletherapy or interstitial technique, possibly combined with chemotherapy. Again, other sites of metastatic disease may alter the plan for pelvic treatment. Ten percent to 15% of patients may survive 5 years.

Treatment of distant metastatic cancer is problematic because the chance of cure is essentially nonexistent; therapy is usually palliative. Radiation therapy to bone or brain often relieves pain and neurologic symptoms. Chemotherapy, either cisplatin (Platinol) alone or cisplatin with paclitaxel (Taxol), may palliate or temporarily control recurrent cancer in other metastatic sites or the pelvis previously radiated. The expected response rate is 10% to 30%, with duration of response lasting only 4 to 6 months.

NEOPLASMS OF THE VULVA

method of
DAVID E. COHN, M.D., and
LARRY J. COPELAND, M.D.
The Ohio State University College of Medicine and Public Health
Columbus, Ohio

Overall, vulvar neoplasms are rare. These disorders can be benign or malignant and are derived from various histologic sites. Standard management for most vulvar neoplasms is surgical removal, with the radicality of the excision determined by the behavior of the tumor. High rates of wound breakdown, disfiguring cosmetic changes, and chronic lymphedema of the lower extremities have led to modifications in the approach to these lesions in an effort to maximize cure while minimizing adverse outcomes. Because both benign and malignant vulvar neoplasms can vary in their appearance, any vulvar abnormality should have a biopsy initially to minimize the risk of conservative treatment of a lesion that should be managed surgically.

BENIGN TUMORS OF THE VULVA

Cystic Neoplasms

A cyst of Bartholin's duct is the most common large cystic neoplasm of the vulva. They occur in approximately 2% of women as an asymptomatic mass in the lateral inferior aspects of the labia minora and vagina. Therapy for these benign cysts is generally reserved for women who become symptomatic (because of obstruction and infection of the gland) and when there is a suspicion of adenocarcinoma (which is rare in women younger than 40 years). Symptoms consistent with a Bartholin's gland abscess include acute vulvar pain and tenderness, especially while walking. Signs include a mass in the region of Bartholin's gland that is erythematous and tender, often with fluctuence. Treatment for these situations is aimed at establishing a route of drainage from the gland to the vaginal vestibule, accomplished either by everting the edges of the duct and suturing them to the vagina (marsupialization) or by inserting a drainage catheter (Word catheter) into the abscess.

The most common small cystic vulvar neoplasm is an epidermal inclusion cyst that appears on the labia majora as pale nodules that contain desquamated cyst lining. Therapy is reserved for women in whom these cysts become symptomatic and require excision. Other less common cysts include remnants of the mesonephric ducts (Gartner's duct cyst) that occur in the vaginal vestibule. Inclusion cysts occur after trauma or a procedure to the vulva, most commonly after an episiotomy.

Solid Neoplasms

Fibromas and lipomas are the most common solid tumors of the vulva and are most commonly found on the labia majora. These tumors can be observed when they are small but are usually excised when they are large. Hidradenomas are rare vulvar tumors arising from the apocrine sweat glands, in contrast to syringomas, which arise from the eccrine glands. These tumors are benign and managed with excisional biopsy for histologic diagnosis and therapy. Endometriosis can rarely occur in the vulva and appear as small firm nodules that vary in color. Most commonly, implants occur at the site of previous obstetric trauma, mainly in the episiotomy scar. Symptoms of vulvar endometriosis are similar to those experienced with endometriosis in other locations; cyclic pain, tenderness, and enlargement of the vulvar mass are common.

Lichen Sclerosus

Lichen sclerosus is a common benign condition of the vulva that tends to be multifocal and to have multiple recurrences. Clinically, the vulva appears white. Treatment is generally with topical fluorinated corticosteroids (0.025% triamcinolone acetonide [Aristocort]* twice daily for 1 to 2 weeks) to remedy the inflammatory and pruritic symptoms, followed by topical testosterone* (2% testosterone propionate in petrolatum,† used twice daily).

Paget's Disease

Extramammary Paget's disease of the vulva occurs most frequently in the sixth and seventh decades of life. During its early phase, the patient is often asymptomatic; when pruritus begins, lesions occur often over much of the vulva. The typical appearance is that of a velvety red epithelium interspersed with patches. Although Paget's disease is an intraepithelial disorder, approximately 20% of patients have an adenocarcinoma of the underlying apocrine glands. Thus, simple vulvar excision in which the superficial subcutaneous tissues (1 to 1.5 cm) are removed in addition to the epithelium is the procedure of choice for Paget's disease. Some recommend evaluation of the surgical margins with frozen section at the time of surgery with an attempt at attaining negative pathologic margins, although many have abandoned this technique because recurrences occur frequently, even with negative margins. Along with the risk of synchronous adenocarcinoma, a concomitant carcinoma of the breast, rectum, colon, or cervix can be present in up to 25% of cases. Therefore, exclusion of these lesions is imperative in women diagnosed with Paget's disease.

Condylomata

Vulvar condylomata (genital warts) are a common problem faced by medical professionals. They are characteristically raised, fleshy lesions that can cover

*Not FDA approved for this indication.
†May be compounded by pharmacists.

the entire vulva. They are spread by sexual contact and are highly contagious. The underlying pathogenesis is related to infection with low-risk human papillomavirus (HPV) strains, typically types 6 and 11. In the immunocompetent host, infection with HPV is often asymptomatic, but in women with HIV, pregnancy, diabetes, or taking immunosuppressive medications, condylomata often become apparent. Treatment of condylomata is aimed at the destruction of the lesions. Ablative therapies include the use of trichloracetic acid (Tri-Chlor), cryotherapy, laser ablation, ultrasonic surgical aspirator, or podophyllin (Podocon-25). Simple vulvectomy has also been used in the treatment of condyloma, although significant scarring often results from the extensive resection needed to treat multifocal disease. Immune modifiers such as 5% imiquimod (Aldara) for 16 weeks have been used in the treatment of genital warts with up to 75% complete resolution and in general excellent satisfaction on the part of the patient. Topical 5-fluorouracil (1%) (Fluoroplex)* in a vaginal hydrophilic gel† can also be applied to eradicate vulvar warts effectively. Biopsy should always be considered to eliminate the possibility of malignancy.

PREINVASIVE LESIONS

Vulvar Intraepithelial Neoplasia

Squamous intraepithelial neoplasia of the vulva is becoming a more commonly identified condition, especially in younger women. Vulvar intraepithelial neoplasia (VIN) III is commonly associated with high-risk HPV strains, typically types 16 and 18. Although sometimes asymptomatic, most women experience pruritus, pain, or irritation with VIN. Clinically, lesions appear flat, white, pigmented, or reddened on gross inspection. With the application of 4% acetic acid, dysplastic epithelium is highlighted. On the basis of the degree of replacement of normal epithelium with dysplasia, VIN is classified as VIN I (inner one third thickness dysplastic epithelium), VIN II (middle one third) and VIN III (carcinoma in situ, Bowen's disease, outer one third or entire epithelium replaced by dysplasia). Because of the "field effect" in which all genital tract tissues are at risk for the development of dysplasia, careful evaluation of the cervix and vagina is necessary prior to the treatment of vulvar dysplasia.

The treatment of VIN is based on ablation of the abnormal epithelium. Small lesions are most simply treated by local excision, but resection of larger or multifocal lesions may lead to significant cosmetic and functional problems. Hence, laser vaporization is a popular treatment for women with larger or multifocal lesions. This treatment method produces excellent cosmetic results and is particularly advantageous for lesions of the clitoris or periclitoral skin. Regardless of the efficacy of the initial treatment, it is the nature of the disease for de novo lesions to develop subsequently. Because laser vaporization, in contrast to excision, does not provide tissue for confirmation of diagnosis, it is important that the physician be confident the disease process is preinvasive as up to 20% of women presenting for therapy for VIN III have histologic evidence of invasive cancer. For this reason, it is prudent to obtain multiple biopsy specimens prior to vaporization. Topical chemotherapy has also been advocated as a treatment of multifocal or large lesions. Topical 5-fluorouracil (5%, Efudex)* is applied twice daily until it causes an inflammatory response (experienced as symptoms similar to those of a sunburn), usually within 7 days. Over the next 4 to 6 days, the skin reaction worsens and then culminates in an exfoliative end stage. Following treatment, recurrent disease is more likely in women who smoke, and smoking cessation should be recommended prior to initiation of therapy. Reliable follow-up is imperative after treatment to detect foci of persistent disease and to identify new lesions.

*Not FDA approved for this indication.
†May be compounded by pharmacists.

MALIGNANT LESIONS

Invasive Squamous Cell Carcinoma

Vulvar cancer is a rare disease, accounting for less than 5% of all gynecologic malignancies. Over 90% of these cancers are squamous in histology, and most occur in older women. Risk factors for the disease include smoking, VIN, HPV, immunosuppression, and lichen sclerosus. Symptoms often include pruritus, pain, dysuria, and bloody vaginal discharge. Physical examination often reveals a nodule or raised ulceration; however, because benign conditions can simulate cancer, histologic confirmation is mandatory. Vulvar cancer may be relatively slow growing and spread by both direct infiltration of adjacent tissue and through the lymphatics in an orderly fashion from the inguinal to femoral to pelvic nodes. The incidence of regional lymph nodes varies with depth of tumor invasion (Table 1), diameter of the lesion (Table 2), and FIGO (International Federation of Gynecology and Obstetrics) stage (Table 3). The surgicopathologic factors that predict nodal spread are important as it is related to the surgical management of vulvar cancer. Vulvar cancer is staged surgically, and classified using the tumor, nodes, and metastasis (TNM) system (Table 4) as proposed by the International Union Against Cancer and the FIGO system (Table 5), and therefore includes information regarding the primary tumor as a well as the regional lymph nodes.

*Not FDA approved for this indication.

TABLE 1. **Incidence of Regional Node Metastases by Depth of Tumor Invasion**

Depth of Invasion (mm)	% Positive Inguinal Nodes
<1	1–5
1–3	10–15
3–5	15–30
5–10	30–45
>10	>40

TABLE 2. **Incidence of Regional Node Metastases by Tumor Diameter**

Tumor Diameter (cm)	% Positive Inguinal Nodes
<1	0–15
1–2	5–20
2–3	25–35
3–5	35–50
>5	>50

TABLE 3. **Incidence of Regional Node Metastases by FIGO Stage**

FIGO Stage	% Positive Inguinal Nodes
I	5–10
II	20–30
III	55–70
IV	40–100

FIGO, International Federation of Gynecology and Obstetrics.

TABLE 4. **TNM Classification of Vulvar Carcinoma**

T PRIMARY TUMOR	
Tis	Carcinoma in situ
T1	Confined to vulva, diameter ≤2 cm
T2	Confined to vulva, diameter >2 cm
T3	Adjacent spread to urethra, vagina, perineum, or anus (any size)
T4	Infiltration of upper urethral mucosa, bladder, rectum, or bone
N REGIONAL LYMPH NODES	
N0	No lymph node metastasis
N1	Unilateral regional lymph node metastasis
N2	Bilateral regional lymph node metastasis
M DISTANT METASTASES	
M0	No clinical metastases
M1	Distant metastasis (including pelvic lymph node metastasis)

TNM, tumor, nodes, and metastasis.

After histologic confirmation of malignancy, surgical management of vulvar cancer is generally undertaken. Significant modifications of the treatment of vulvar cancer have been developed over the last 50 years, with the en bloc resection of primary tumor and lymph nodes being abandoned in favor of the management of these sites through separate incisions and also with less radical excisions of the primary vulvar tumor, with resultant decreased morbidity without sacrificing survival. Current investigations include the technique of lymphatic mapping with sentinel lymph node dissection, in which the first lymph node encountered draining the vulva serves as a surrogate for the entire groin; if this node is pathologically negative, there is in theory no need for complete lymphadenectomy and the attendant morbidity of the procedure. For patients with a small primary tumor that invades less than 1 mm, the risk of nodal metastasis is too low to justify lymphadenectomy. Postoperative treatment is assigned on the basis of the pathologic status of the lymph nodes and

TABLE 5. **FIGO Classification (with Corresponding TNM Classification) for Vulvar Carcinoma**

Stage I (T1N0M0)	Tumor confined to vulva and/or perineum, 2 cm or less in greatest dimension, nodes are negative
Stage IA	Stromal invasion no greater than 1 mm
Stage IB	Stromal invasion greater than 1 mm
Stage II (T2N0M0)	Tumor confined to the vulva and/or perineum, more than 2 cm in greatest dimension, nodes are negative
Stage III	
T3N0M0	Tumor of any size with adjacent spread to the lower urethra and/or the vagina, or the anus
T3N1M0	Unilateral regional lymph node metastasis
T2N1M0	
Stage IVA	
T1N2M0	Tumor invades any of the following:
T2N2M0	Upper urethra, bladder mucosa, rectal mucosa, pelvic bone, and/or bilateral regional node metastasis
T3N2M0	
T4 any N M0	
Stage IVB	
Any T any N M1	Any distant metastasis including pelvic lymph nodes

FIGO, International Federation of Gynecology and Obstetrics; TNM, tumor, nodes, and metastasis.

margins of the primary resection. Disease in these sites requires postoperative radiation therapy to the pelvic nodes, groin nodes, and possibly perineum. For large primary tumors, preoperative radiation therapy can lead to a decrease in size that allows a less morbid resection. Survival is based on stage at diagnosis (Table 6).

Invasive Adenocarcinoma

Vulvar adenocarcinoma is a rare disease, accounting for less than 1% of vulvar cancers. These malignancies arise from Bartholin's gland most commonly and occur in women older than 40 years. Exclusion of other sites of primary or metastatic adenocarcinoma is necessary given the rarity of vulvar adenocarcinoma. Therapy is similar to that outlined for squamous cell cancer of the vulva.

Malignant Melanoma

Malignant melanoma is the second most common histologic type of vulvar cancer and accounts for

TABLE 6. **Survival Rate by FIGO Stage for Patients with Invasive Squamous Cell Vulvar Cancer**

FIGO Stage	% Surviving 5 years
I	70–90
II	50–80
III	30–50
IV	10–15

FIGO, International Federation of Gynecology and Obstetrics.

approximately 5% of vulvar malignancies. The melanomas are usually pigmented, raised, and may ulcerate. The prognosis is related to the histologic type of the lesion, lesion size, and depth of invasion. Treatment includes surgical excision, by either radical excision or radical vulvectomy. When the depth of invasion exceeds 0.75 mm, the risk of lymphatic spread increases, justifying lymphadenectomy. Clinical trials investigating the role of adjuvant therapy are under way.

Basal Cell Carcinoma

This tumor exhibits local growth only and is best treated by wide local excision. The lesion should be carefully examined pathologically because the presence of squamous elements changes the diagnosis, prognosis, and therapy, as they should be managed similarly to squamous cell cancers.

Sarcoma

Sarcomas of the vulvar are rare, accounting for only 1% to 2% of vulvar malignancies. The majority are leiomyosarcomas, which do not metastasize early; however, following excision they are prone to local recurrences. Alveolar rhabdomyosarcomas occur in adolescents and can be confused with Bartholin's gland abnormalities. Because of their rapid spread, the best hope for cure is early diagnosis.

CONTRACEPTION

method of
E. J. CHANEY, M.D.
University of Kansas School of Medicine
Wichita, Kansas

The history of contraception can be traced to ancient writings. The Kahun Papyrus describes a pessary made of crocodile dung and fermented dough. These writings, dating from 1850 BC, also referred to vaginal plugs of honey, gum, and acacia bark. The use of Queen Ann's lace, or wild carrots, as an oral contraceptive was mentioned over 2000 years ago by Hippocrates. In the Book of Genesis (38:9) is a reference to coitus interruptus. In addition, the use of charms and amulets was not uncommon. Many plants and other substances have been used as oral contraceptives, and some have been toxic and resulted in death to the user (Figure 1).

BEHAVIORAL METHODS

Abstinence

Absence of sexual intercourse is the only perfect contraceptive technique, and although it is used by 200 million women worldwide, it is not an option for sexually active individuals.

Coitus Interruptus (Withdrawal)

Use of this method cannot be considered a reliable contraceptive technique. Typical failure rates have been estimated at 17% to 19%, but other reports indicate failure rates as high as 25%. This method requires cooperation, discipline, dedication, and thorough patient education.

Family Planning

Avoidance of intercourse during the female "fertile period," the time during which an ovum is available for fertilization, has been used by couples for many years. This method assumes that the period of possible fertilization can be determined by various observations such as cervical mucus, basal body temperature, and menstrual rhythm. If sexual intercourse is avoided during that fertile period, conception will be prevented. Meticulous observations and strict avoidance of sexual activity may be required during that period. The typical-use failure rate averages 22%.

Lactation

For a period after birth while a women is lactating, ovulation is retarded. However, that time is unpredictable, and it is not useful as a reliable contraceptive technique.

BARRIER METHODS

Male Condoms

Early condoms were made of animal membranes and were used to protect against disease. Gabriello Fallopius in 1564 recommended the use of linen sheaths as protection against syphilis. If the story about a "Dr. Condom," who is said to have developed a cloth sheath for King Charles II to prevent illegitimate offspring, is true, it would be the first known use of a condom for contraception.

A variety of materials have been used for condoms, including cloth, linen, animal membranes, and, more recently, latex. Latex condoms are available and affordable.

The use of condoms has increased in the past few years, and the number manufactured annually probably exceeds 20 billion. The use of condoms as a contraceptive has increased in the last 20 years. Condoms may be somewhat effective in the prevention of sexually transmitted diseases (STDs), and this factor has probably added to the increase in use.

Because of increasing latex allergies, a polyurethane condom has been developed. A recent study found that the "typical-use" failure rate for both types of condoms was not statistically significantly different (4.8% for polyurethane and 6.3% for latex). The polyurethane condom had a higher clinical failure rate and more breakage and slippage in first-time users. The study concluded that latex condoms appeared to be superior but, for couples with latex sensitivity, polyurethane condoms are an effective alternative.

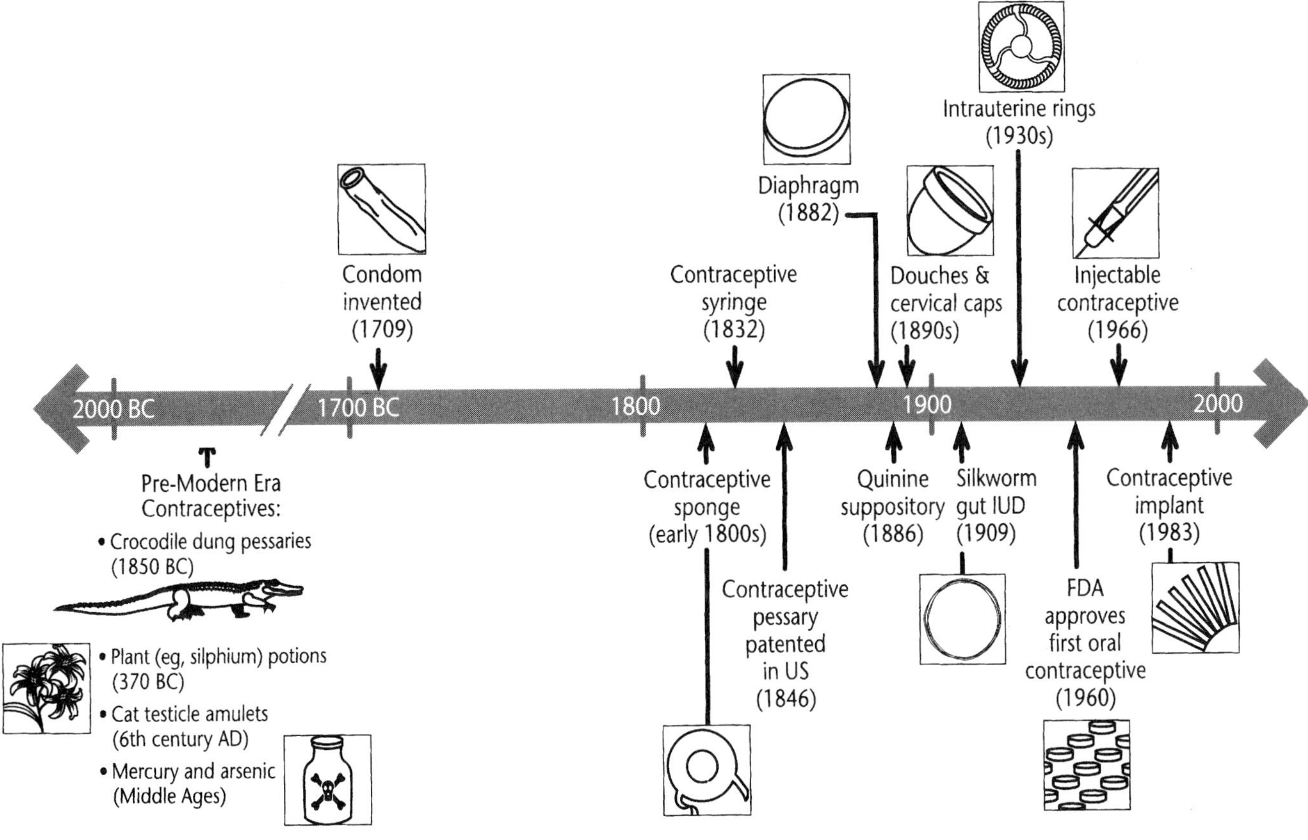

Figure 1. Contraceptive development through the ages.

Female Condoms

In January 1992, the Ob-Gyn Devices Panel of Experts of the Food and Drug Administration (FDA) recommended approval of a new method of female contraception. The FDA gave approval in May 1993 for the female condom. This rapid approval was given under new guidelines to more quickly introduce devices that have the potential of decreasing the spread of STDs.

In August 1994, female condoms were available over the counter to the public. They offer the same benefits as male condoms, but are the first condom that allowed complete control by the woman. It has contraceptive value and value in preventing STDs. Females may be more susceptible than males to the heterosexual transmission of HIV, and this device is targeted at women who want to protect themselves against HIV infection when their partner refuses to use a condom. The device consist of a thin polyurethane sheath with flexible rings at both ends. The closed end is inserted into the vagina much the same as a diaphragm. The sheath then covers the cervix, vaginal wall, and the labia, with the other ring lying outside the vagina (Figure 2). Several studies are investigating the efficacy of female condoms in the prevention of pregnancy and STDs, as well as comparing them against the male condom.

The devise does not require a prescription or a visit to a health care provider and has a failure rate of about the same as a diaphragm, vaginal sponge, or cervical cap. The FDA labeling indicates a typical-use failure rate of 21% and a perfect-use failure rate of 5%.

Other Female Barrier Methods

Women have used a variety of barrier methods over the centuries. Contraceptive sponges, pessaries, cervical caps, and diaphragms have all been used. In the

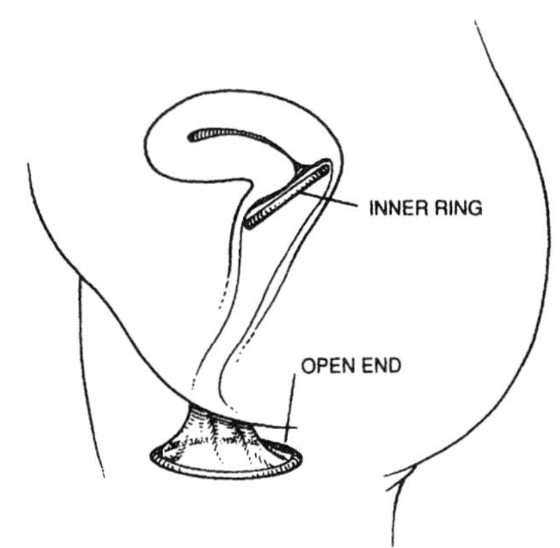

Figure 2. Position of properly inserted female condom.

1880s, the "Mensinga Diaphragm" was described and used as originally designed for many decades. By 1940, a third of all married couples in America were using diaphragms.

With the introduction of oral contraceptives (OCs) and intrauterine contraceptive devices (IUDs) and the increasing use of condoms, the use of diaphragms has decreased to less than 2% today. The typical-use failure rate averages 16%. Diaphragms require fitting by a professional and should be used along with a spermicidal gel.

VAGINAL SPERMICIDAL AGENTS

Today, only 1% of married couples use spermicidal agents alone. At one time, more than 90 spermicidal products were available, but only 3 are on the market now.

Nonoxynol 9, octoxynol 9, and menfegol* are available. These products are mainly recommended to be used along with a diaphragm or cervical cap. Their effectiveness when used alone is 24% to 26% in 6 months. The development of more reliable and acceptable methods of contraception has reduced the use of these agents.

INTRAUTERINE CONTRACEPTIVE DEVICES

The use of a device inserted into the uterine cavity for the purpose of preventing pregnancy is a 20th century development. In the early 1900s the first true IUD, made of two coarse strands of silkworm gut wound into a ring and capped with celluloid, was described. Little progress was made in this type of contraceptive until after World War II. In 1962, the "Lippes Loop" was made available and became the most widely prescribed IUD in the United States.

The value of copper in increasing an IUD's effectiveness in preventing pregnancy was recognized, and Dr. Howard Tatum proposed a T-shaped IUD with the addition of copper to decrease the risk of pregnancy. The inclusion of slow-releasing progesterone in the IUD helped reduce the amount of cramping and blood loss. In the early 1970s, around 7% of U.S. couples were using IUDs. In 1999 that percentage fell to less than 1%. Current worldwide use is approaching 100 million. The 90% decrease in U.S. use is related to medical liability issues regarding this form of contraception. The multifilament tail of the Dalkon shield was accused of causing an increase in pelvic inflammatory disease (PID), which seems less likely now than originally thought, and modern IUDs use monofilament tails. New evidence indicates that the risk of PID is associated not so much with the string on the device but rather with the process of insertion. A 1992 study by the World Health Organization suggested that a higher risk of PID occurs during the first 20 days after insertion and that the risk is low and uniform during all other times after insertion. Some recommended the use of prophylactic antibiotics, but recent studies have not shown such measures to be of significant value.

The complication of uterine perforation occurs in about 1 to 3 per 1000 insertions and is related to operator training and experience. Use of this method is also complicated by a decrease in training of IUD insertion techniques in both obstetric-gynecologic and family practice residents.

Increase use of this method is further hampered because many companies discontinued the production of IUDs as a result of legal liability issues. In the summer of 2001, the progesterone-releasing IUD (Progestasert) was discontinued, with the last units expiring on September 1, 2001. It had a typical-use failure rate of 2% to 3% each year and required replacement annually.

A levonorgestrel-releasing IUD (Mirena) with 5 years between insertions was approved in late 2000 in the United States. The typical-use failure rate is 0.14% the first year with a cumulative 0.71% rate for 5 years. The third-generation copper IUD ParaGard T380A is one of the most effective IUD ever used in the United States, with a first-year failure rate of 0.5%, and the duration of effectiveness was extended from the original 4 years of use to 10 years in 1994. The package insert for T380A is not required to list a history of previous ectopic pregnancy as a contraindication to its use.

The manner in which an IUD prevents pregnancy has been investigated but is not completely understood. Recent evidence indicates that the device interferes with reproductive activity before fertilization.

As with any method of use, complications can develop, including uterine perforation, which usually occurs at time of insertion and is related to the skill of the operator. Spontaneous expulsion occurs mainly within 3 months of insertion, with 3.3 to 7.1 expulsions per 100 woman-years of use of the copper T380A.

Many of the complication can be reduced by careful attention to proper selection of patients who wish to use this form of contraception. Absolute contraindications are listed in Table 1. Relative contraindications such as multiple sexual partners and exposure to STDs must be a consideration in patient selection. With careful screening, counseling before insertion, and insertion by qualified person using sterile technique, the consensus of a recent international conference on intrauterine contraceptives was that when used within the guidelines, the IUD is a safe, highly efficacious, and cost-effective method of contraception. Several new IUDs are being investigated, including a copper device that has no solid frame. This device is expected to cause less pain and bleeding.

TABLE 1. **Absolute Contraindications to Use of an Intrauterine Device**

Malignancy of the uterus or cervix
Suspected or known pregnancy
Active pelvic inflammatory disease
Vaginal bleeding of unknown etiology

*Not available in the United States.

IMPLANTS AND INJECTABLE HORMONAL METHODS

Subdermal Implants

Research into the safety and efficacy of subdermal implants was conducted in the late 1960s. Silastic tubing was chosen because it had been observed to allow for prolonged release of hydrophilic drugs.

Levonorgestrel (Norplant) was selected as the progestational drug because it had been widely used in OCs and extensive data on its safety were available. In December 1990, the FDA gave approval for hormonal implants. Contraceptive protection occurs within 24 hours if the insertion is performed in the first 7 days of the menstrual cycle. Protection lasts for 5 years, and the failure rate is reported as 0.2% for the first and second years of use, 0.9% in the third year, 0.5% for the forth year, and 1.2% for the fifth year.

The current implants have had some difficulties that have been greatly exaggerated by litigation. Although menstrual irregularities are common, they are seldom of any great significance. Infections at the implant site are very infrequent and occur about 0.7% of the time. Other side effects such as weight gain, headache, nausea, and depression have been reported, but the most publicized problem has involved removal of the implants. Although removal is usually a short, simple, and atraumatic office procedure, it can be difficult and may require a longer time. It is the highly visible litigation issue that has resulted in a decrease in both acceptance and availability of these devices.

In 1995 the FDA conducted an extensive evaluation of implant safety. The findings indicated that when the implants were used as directed, they were safe and effective.

Future implants are being evaluated that will reduce the number of capsules and make them more ridged. Investigators are evaluating both one and two rod implants. The two-rod system (Norplant II) contains levonorgestrel and can be used for 5 years, with pregnancy rates and side effects comparable to those of the old six-rod system.

Other investigators are studying biodegradable compounds. All these new methods may be delayed in production because of lawsuits.

INJECTABLE HORMONAL CONTRACEPTIVES

Medroxyprogesterone acetate (Depo-Provera) was granted FDA approval in 1992. This long-acting injectable drug is a highly effective and safe contraceptive with a failure rate of less than 1% per year. The usual dosage is 150 mg every 3 months. Contraceptive levels persist for up to 14 weeks after injection. A combination of 25 mg medroxyprogesterone acetate and 5 mg estradiol cypionate (Lunelle) is given every 28 days and has a first-year failure rate of less than 0.01%.

As with any drug, side effects do occur, and irregular bleeding is very common with this method. These irregular episodes decrease with continued use of the drug. Other side effects are similar to those seen with implants and OCs containing progestational agents. These side effects account for a third of patients discontinuing the injections at the end of 1 year and half discontinuing by the end of the second year.

The most troublesome potential side effect is the potential loss of bone density in younger users. The relative hypoestrogenic state that occurs with this drug has been questioned with regard to its possible contribution to bone density loss. Several studies have been reported, but with greatly different conclusions. The amount and significance of the bone density loss remain unclear at this time. New injectable agents are being investigated such as combined estrogen and progestin, as well as longer acting progestin-only methods. A 200-mg injection of norethindrone enanthate (Noristerat)* was effective for 2 months with a pregnancy rate of 0.4% at 12 and 24 months of use. Other compounds being studied are even longer acting and suppress ovulation for over 8 months. The use of microspheres or microcapsules that contain one or more hormones is also under investigation.

ORAL CONTRACEPTIVE PILLS

The development of OCs has been a slow and sometimes painful process. In the 1920s it was shown by an Austrian scientist that if ovarian extracts were given to animals, ovulation would be inhibited. The death of the original investigator, the Nazi occupation of Austria, and the lack of a practicable source of hormones all helped delay further development of this science. Advancements in steroid chemistry allowed progesterone to be produced from plants. Before that discovery, the ovaries of over 2000 pregnant pigs were required to produce 1 mg of progesterone. In 1944, a Mexican-based company (Syntex) was founded and produced 3 mg of progesterone from 5 gallons of syrup made from Mexican yams.

In 1951, the oral active progestational agent norethindrone was patented, and in 1953, a company (G.D. Searle) applied for a patent for norethynodrel, another progestational agent. Dr. Gregory Pincus and Dr. John Rock began a large-scale clinical trial in Puerto Rico to evaluate the effectiveness and safety of these new contraceptive agents. At that time in the United States, contraceptive research was hindered by very strong political, religious, and legal opposition.

The original supply of progestin in that trial was contaminated by a small amount of mestranol equal to 150 mg of estrogen. When the contamination was removed, women began to have breakthrough bleeding, so the estrogen was retained to correct that problem. Thus began the use of combined OCs.

The first FDA approval of norethynodrel (Enovid)* and norethindrone (Norlutin),* both with mestranol, was for the regulation of "gynecologic disorders." Two years later, the FDA granted approval to Searle for the indication of contraception, and the age of OCs

*Not available in the United States.

commenced. Within a year after approval, OCs were used by over 400,000 U.S. women.

By 1968, 3.8 million U.S. women were using "the pill." In that year over 99% of all OC prescriptions in the United States contained 50 mg of estrogen. In 1998, only 1.4% of OC prescriptions were for pills containing 50 mg or more of estrogen.

OCs are safe, highly effective, and easy to use and have added health benefits. Of all the methods that require regular action by the user, OCs have the lowest failure rates. Typical-use failure rates are 4% at 6 months and 7% after 12 months of use.

Some of the health benefits are well documented, such as protection against benign breast disease, iron loss anemia, ovarian and endometrial cancer, and ectopic pregnancy. Evidence is growing that OCs also offer protection against osteoporosis and possibly against the development of colorectal cancer, uterine fibroids, and premenopausal rheumatoid arthritis. Most women and many health care providers do not realize that for many women the risk of pregnancy generally outweighs the risk of taking OCs.

However, it is the continuing controversy about the relationship between estrogen and breast cancer that concerns both patients and physicians. Despite increasing evidence that the risk of cancer of the breast with OCs is negligible, this possibility continues to be a factor in acceptance and use of this method.

A multitude of OC preparations are available, and it behooves the health care provider to carefully review the patient's needs and match the requirements of the patient with the appropriate medication. Such selection demands careful attention to obtaining a complete family history, sexual history, and future childbearing desires, as well as a complete physical examination and appropriated follow-up.

NONREVERSIBLE METHODS

Sterilization by surgery on either the vas deferens or fallopian tubes is a very common form of contraception in the United States. Although patients should consider these procedures to be nonreversible and permanent, neither is absolutely true, particularly with tubal surgery. Data indicate that the overall 10-year failure rate for tubal ligation is about 19 per 1000 procedures and, in young women, about 50+ per 1000 operations.

Vasectomies are also common, with a study in 1995 reporting that almost one in five white men who were married to a woman of childbearing age had had a vasectomy. Although at one time some concern existed about the possible connection of vasectomies with cardiovascular disease, the recent Physicians Health Study found no evidence that such an association exists.

Because the fields of reproductive physiology and steroid chemistry are rapidly advancing, primary care physicians must keep abreast of these advances. They are the first line of contact to a great many woman and families during the reproductive years and must not only be knowledgeable and aware of new development and methods but also be prepared to evaluate each patient's physical and emotional contraceptive needs, as well as educating their patients.

Section 17
Psychiatric Disorders

ALCOHOLISM

method of
KATHERINE A. McQUEEN, M.D.
Baylor College of Medicine
Houston, Texas

The use and misuse of alcohol are common in our society. Half of all Americans drink alcohol, and at least 6% of the population currently meet the criteria for alcohol abuse or dependence (Figure 1). Alcohol consumption in the United States was lowest in 1934, at the peak of the Depression and the end of Prohibition, and highest in 1980, after a period when many states lowered the legal drinking age to 18. The economic cost of alcohol abuse and dependence is high, estimated at over $165 billion a year. Although the health benefits of light to moderate consumption are clear—a decrease in both cardiovascular and all-cause mortality—misuse of alcohol is responsible for 100,000 deaths each year.

Alcoholism, as defined by the American Society of Addiction Medicine, is "a primary, chronic disease with genetic, psychosocial, and environmental factors influencing its development and manifestations. The disease is often progressive and fatal. It is characterized by continuous or periodic impaired control over drinking, preoccupation with the drug alcohol, use of alcohol despite adverse consequences, and distortions in thinking, most notably denial." The term *alcoholism* is most often applied to the diagnosis of alcohol dependence, but alcohol problems occur on a spectrum from use through dependence. It is important to understand this entire spectrum to properly diagnose, prevent the progression of, and treat an individual patient's alcohol problem.

PHARMACOLOGY AND MEDICAL COMPLICATIONS

Alcohol is a central nervous system depressant that acts on at least six separate neurotransmitter systems. Acute administration leads to increased levels of dopamine, serotonin, and norepinephrine; increased activity in the inhibitory transmitter system involving γ-aminobutyric acid (GABA); and inhibition of the *N*-methyl-D-aspartate (NMDA) receptor. Chronic use can lead to depletion of these neurotransmitters and down-regulation of GABA and NMDA receptors. Metabolism, blood levels, and impairment from alcohol are related to gender, body mass, consumption with food, and tolerance. Acute effects range from impaired coordination to memory lapses, coma, and death (Table 1).

As consumption of alcohol exceeds two drinks a day, damage to various organ systems may be detectable. A standard drink is one 12-oz beer, one 5-oz glass of wine, or 1½ oz of distilled spirits. Chronic alcohol use is associated with increased gastrointestinal, cardiovascular, psychiatric, and neurologic problems, as well as a marked increase in the incidence of accidents, suicides, and homicides. The most common problems encountered in primary care are listed in Table 2.

ETIOLOGY AND NATURAL HISTORY OF ALCOHOL DEPENDENCE

The etiology of alcohol dependence is multifactorial. Genetics, environment, and sociocultural factors all play a role in the development and prognosis of this disease. This disorder has been shown to run strongly within families, with a threefold to fourfold higher risk of alcoholism in the adopted-away children of parents with alcoholism in comparison to controls. Several candidate genes have been identified. It is likely that a combination of genes places an individual at markedly increased risk and that these genetic factors interact with the environment to give a final level of risk.

Environmental and sociocultural factors consistently correlated with alcohol abuse and dependence include peer and parental values, religion, availability, poverty, depression, and high levels of job stress. Alcohol dependence is a chronic medical illness characterized by periods of abstinence and excess. Drinking often begins in the teenage years, and alcohol-related medical, psychiatric, and social problems appear in the second and third decades. The first treatment episode frequently takes place early in the fourth decade, and individuals with alcohol dependence have a 15-year reduction in life expectancy. Not all individuals who experience problems with alcohol will become alcohol dependent, however, and therefore a thorough understanding of diagnostic criteria and effective screening approaches is vital.

DIAGNOSIS

Alcohol problems occur on a spectrum and may be classified into a number of categories, including at-risk or hazardous drinking, harmful drinking, alcohol

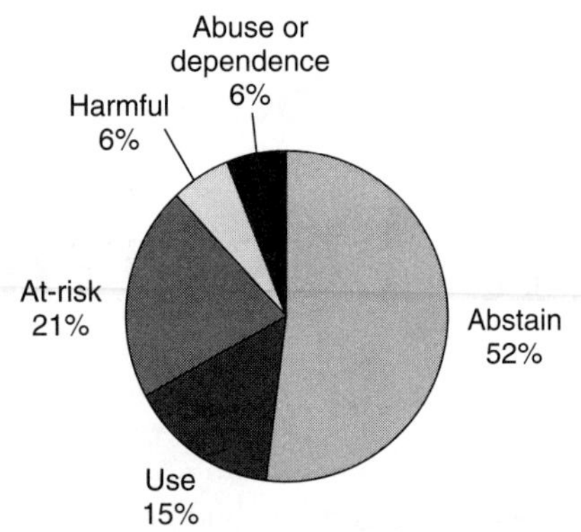

Figure 1. U.S. patterns of alcohol consumption. (Data from 2001 National Household Survey on Drug Abuse.)

abuse, and alcohol dependence (Table 3). The hallmark of alcohol abuse is a pattern of recurrent use despite the consequences and, for alcohol dependence, a total loss of control. In primary care settings, the incidence of at-risk drinking is estimated at 9%; harmful drinking, 8%; and alcohol abuse or dependence, 5%.

Alcohol use disorders are easier to identify in patients with problems such as pancreatitis or cirrhosis. However, most health, family, and social problems related to alcohol use occur in nondependent drinkers. These patients benefit significantly from early detection and intervention, as do their families and society. The role of the general practitioner is outlined in Figure 2.

A number of groups, including the National Institute on Alcohol Abuse and Alcoholism (NIAAA), the U.S. Preventative Services Task Force, and the American Academy of Family Physicians, reviewed the issue of screening and have recommended screening of all adolescent and adult patients for problematic use of alcohol.

The most effective screening method for detecting alcohol problems is to elicit an alcohol history by asking quantity and frequency questions and using a standardized screening instrument. Questions should be asked in a directed, nonjudgmental manner and are most acceptable in the context of other screening questions about smoking, diet, and exercise. Formal screening instruments, such as the CAGE questionnaire (Have you ever felt that you should **C**ut down on your drinking? Have people **A**nnoyed you by criticizing your drinking? Have you ever felt bad or **G**uilty about your drinking? and Have you ever taken a drink the first thing in the morning [**E**ye-opener] to steady your nerves or get rid of a hangover?—one yes suggests a need for further assessment), the Alcohol Use Disorders Identification Test (AUDIT), and the CRAFFT focus on the social and behavioral aspects of alcohol problems and provide greater accuracy than do quantity and frequency questions alone, laboratory tests, or clinical detection. The AUDIT (Table 4) seems to perform better in a variety of primary care settings because of increased sensitivity for both hazardous drinking and alcohol problems among adolescents, women, and some minorities. The CRAFFT (Have you ever ridden in a **C**ar driven by someone [including

TABLE 1. **Impairment by Blood-Alcohol Level**

Blood Alcohol Level (mg/100 mL Blood)	Effect
20-99	Impaired coordination
100-199	Ataxia, impaired judgment
200-299	Slurred speech, difficulty ambulating, labile mood, nausea and vomiting
300-399	Blackouts, decreased level of consciousness
>400	Coma and death

TABLE 2. **Signs and Symptoms of an Alcohol Problem**

System	Signs and Symptoms
Cardiovascular	Hypertension, atrial fibrillation, cardiomyopathy
Endocrine	Hypertriglyceridemia, erectile dysfunction, hyperuricemia
Gastrointestinal	Nausea, vomiting, pain, hepatitis, cirrhosis, portal hypertension, peptic ulcer disease, pancreatitis
Gynecologic	Spontaneous abortion, fetal alcohol syndrome
Hematologic	Macrocytic anemia, thrombocytopenia
Neurologic	Headache, withdrawal, Wernicke's encephalopathy, Korsakoff's psychosis, dementia, myopathy, peripheral neuropathy
Oncologic	Neoplasms of the head and neck, esophagus, stomach, pancreas, liver
Psychiatric	Depression, anxiety, abuse of other substances, antisocial personality disorder
Social/family	Loss of job, family conflict, social isolation, children with learning disorders, school and peer problems

TABLE 3. **Spectrum of Alcohol Problems**

Diagnosis	Criteria
At-risk (NIAAA)	Men >14/wk or >4/occasion Women >7/wk or >3/occasion Elders >7/wk or >1/occasion
Harmful (WHO)	Drinking at levels causing physical or psychologic harm
Alcohol abuse (DSM-IV)	Recurrent pattern of use leading to ≥1: Failure to fulfill major role obligations Use in hazardous situations Legal problems Use despite social problems
Alcohol dependence (DSM-IV)	Maladaptive pattern of use leading to ≥3 over a 12-mo period: Tolerance Withdrawal Great deal of time spent obtaining, using, and recovering Drinking more and longer than intended Important activities given up because of alcohol Desire and/or attempts to cut down Use despite knowledge of physical or psychologic harm

DSM-IV, *Diagnostic and Statistical Manual of Mental Disorders:* NIAAA, National Institute on Alcohol Abuse and Alcoholism; WHO, World Health Organization.

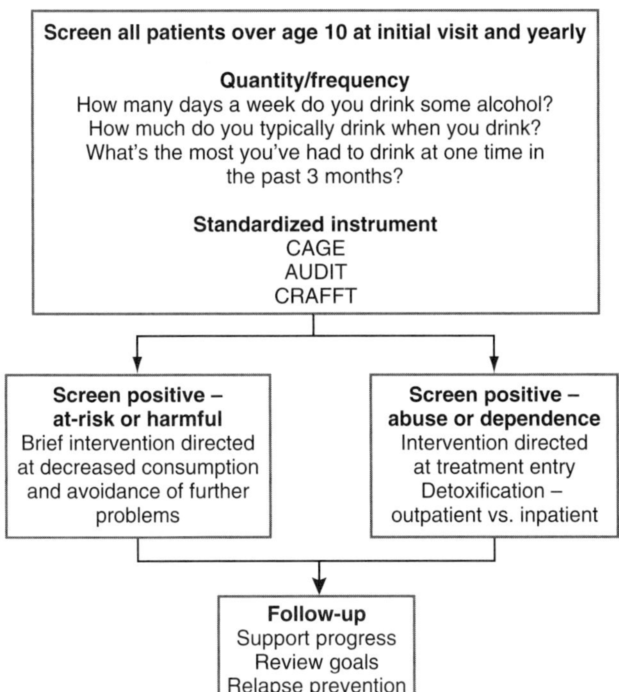

Screen all patients over age 10 at initial visit and yearly
Quantity/frequency
How many days a week do you drink some alcohol?
How much do you typically drink when you drink?
What's the most you've had to drink at one time in the past 3 months?
Standardized instrument
CAGE
AUDIT
CRAFFT
Screen positive – at-risk or harmful
Brief intervention directed at decreased consumption and avoidance of further problems
Screen positive – abuse or dependence
Intervention directed at treatment entry
Detoxification – outpatient vs. inpatient
Follow-up
Support progress
Review goals
Relapse prevention

Figure 2. Role of the general practitioner. AUDIT, Alcohol Use Disorders Identification Test; CAGE, see text; CRAFFT, see text.

yourself] who was "high" or had been using alcohol or drugs? Do you ever use alcohol or drugs to **R**elax, feel better about yourself, or fit in? Do you ever use alcohol or drugs while you are by yourself, **A**lone? Do you ever **F**orget things you did while using alcohol or drugs? Do your family or **F**riends ever tell you that you should cut down on your drinking or drug use? and Have you gotten into **T**rouble while you were using alcohol or drugs?—two or more yes answers suggest a serious problem) was designed specifically for use in adolescents.

Laboratory tests such as γ-glutamyltransferase, liver transaminases, and mean corpuscular volume may be used. Limitations include cost and low sensitivity in nondependent individuals. These tests are most useful after a positive screen to help document the scope and course of a problem. Physical examination provides little evidence to suggest an alcohol problem in the early stages.

BRIEF INTERVENTION

A brief intervention is a time-limited, patient-centered counseling strategy that focuses on changing behavior. It is not unique to the treatment of alcohol problems, but recent meta-analyses have confirmed that brief interventions are effective at reducing alcohol consumption and alcohol-related problems. For example, the World Health Organization studied 1490 at-risk drinkers in 10 nations and demonstrated that screening with 5 minutes of brief advice decreased consumption by 21%. Fleming and colleagues demonstrated that not only did brief advice decrease consumption among at-risk drinkers but that it also produced a net benefit per patient of $947. Although many different frameworks may be used for brief interventions, most share common elements, including feedback about the negative effects of alcohol, expressions of empathy and optimism, options to change, advice about cutting down or abstaining from alcohol, a discussion of the patient's reaction to feedback, and a follow-up plan. Written materials and referral to local support groups are very helpful. For more detailed information, a free copy of The Physician's Guide to Helping Patients with Alcohol Problems is available at www.niaaa.nih.gov/publications/physicn.htm.

Brief intervention for alcohol-related problems is particularly useful in three different clinical situations: to reduce consumption in at-risk and harmful drinkers, to support abstinence for those in a rehabilitation program, and to facilitate referral of dependent drinkers to a specialist or treatment program.

DETOXIFICATION AND WITHDRAWAL

Detoxification is an important step in the treatment of patients with alcohol dependence. Outpatient detoxification has been demonstrated to be as efficacious as inpatient detoxification, but with decreased cost. Patients with a history of severe withdrawal, alcoholic liver disease, severe medical or psychiatric co-morbidity, and little social support require inpatient detoxification. For all other patients, the regimen to be outlined will assist the clinician in appropriately triaging and managing detoxification and withdrawal.

Alcohol withdrawal is a well-described syndrome that occurs in more than half the patients entering detoxification. Criteria for alcohol withdrawal in the fourth edition of the *Diagnostic and Statistical Manual of Mental Disorders* (DSM-IV) include two main components: a history of cessation or reduction of alcohol consumption and a complex of symptoms that include autonomic hyperactivity, tremor, nausea and vomiting, and possibly hallucinations and seizures. The severity of withdrawal is a dose-related phenomenon, and previous episodes of severe withdrawal are predictive of future severe withdrawal. Mild withdrawal is characterized by weakness, nausea, and tremor. The most severe form of withdrawal, delirium tremens, occurs in less than 5% of patients managed with benzodiazepines, but in more than 15% of patients who receive no pharmacotherapy. Benzodiazepines reduce withdrawal severity, as well as the incidence of delirium and seizures. Three main strategies are used for dosing of benzodiazepines: fixed-schedule dosing, front loading, and symptom-triggered dosing (Table 5). Several studies have demonstrated the effectiveness of these strategies, but a symptom-triggered approach results in less medication and a significantly shorter duration of treatment. Few differences are found between the results of medium- and long-acting benzodiazepines, and chlordiazepoxide (Librium), lorazepam (Ativan),*

*Not FDA approved for this indication.

TABLE 4. **Alcohol Use Disorders Identification Test—AUDIT**

Please circle the answer that is correct for you

1. How often do you have a drink containing alcohol?

Never	Monthly or less	2-4 times/mo	2-3 times/wk	≥4 times/wk

2. How many drinks containing alcohol do you have on a typical day when you are drinking?

1 or 2	3 or 4	5 or 6	7-9	≥10

3. How often do you have ≥6 drinks on one occasion?

Never	Less than monthly	Monthly	2-3 times/wk	≥4 times/wk

4. How often during the last year have you found that you were not able to stop drinking once you had started?

Never	Less than monthly	Monthly	2-3 times/wk	≥4 times/wk

5. How often during the last year have you failed to do what was normally expected of you because of drinking?

Never	Less than monthly	Monthly	2-3 times/wk	≥4 times/wk

6. How often during the last year have you needed a first drink in the morning to get yourself going after a heavy drinking session?

Never	Less than monthly	Monthly	2-3 times/wk	≥4 times/wk

7. How often during the last year have you had a feeling of guilt or remorse after drinking?

Never	Less than monthly	Monthly	2-3 times/wk	≥4 times/wk

8. How often during the last year have you been unable to remember what happened the night before because you had been drinking?

Never	Less than monthly	Monthly	2-3 times/wk	≥4 times/wk

9. Have you or someone else been injured as a result of your drinking?

No	Yes, but not in the last year	Yes, during the last year

10. Has a relative or friend, doctor, or other health care worker been concerned about your drinking or suggested that you cut down?

No	Yes, but not in the last year	Yes, during the last year

Scoring AUDIT: Questions 1-8 are scored 0, 1, 2, 3, or 4. Questions 9 and 10 are scored 0, 2, or 4 only.

	0	1	2	3	4
Question 1	Never	Monthly or less	2-4 times/mo	2-3 times/wk	≥4 times/wk
Question 2	1 or 2	3 or 4	5 or 6	7-9	≥10
Questions 3-8	Never	Less than monthly	Monthly	Weekly	Daily or almost daily
Questions 9-10	No		Yes, but not in the last year		Yes, during the last year

A score of 8 or more indicates a strong likelihood of an alcohol problem.

Data from Babor TF, de la Fuente JR, Saunders J, Grant M: The Alcohol Use Disorders Identification Test: Guidelines for Use in Primary Health Care. Geneva, World Health Organization, 1992.

and diazepam (Valium) are all effective. Symptom-triggered therapy is directed by the severity of withdrawal as measured by a standardized instrument such as the revised Clinical Institute Withdrawal Assessment—Alcohol (CIWA-Ar). Patients with scores under 8 to 10 can be managed as outpatients with supportive nonpharmacologic therapy and continued monitoring. A score of 10 to 15 suggests the need for benzodiazepines, and scores over 15 occur in patients with a significant risk for severe withdrawal, including delirium tremens.

Supportive care should include monitoring of electrolyte and fluid status, nutritional support, and motivation to achieve long-term abstinence. Though uncommon, Wernicke's encephalopathy (ataxia, delirium, and ophthalmoplegia) and Korsakoff's syndrome are severe complications. Both can be prevented, and severity decreased, by the administration of an initial parenteral dose of thiamine before glucose and then daily oral thiamine.

TABLE 5. **Treatment Strategies for Alcohol Withdrawal**

Method	Medication and Dosage
Fixed schedule	Chlordiazepoxide (Librium), 50-100 mg qid × 1 d, then 25-50 mg qid × 2 d
Front loading	Lorazepam (Ativan),* 2 mg q20min until symptoms resolve
Symptom triggered	Chlordiazepoxide, 25-100 mg q1-3h when CIWA-Ar ≥8
Severe withdrawal/ delirium tremens	Lorazepam,* 2 mg IV, then 1-2 mg IV q10min until calm, *or* diazepam (Valium), 10 mg IV, then 5 mg IV q10min (ICU care recommended)

*Not FDA approved for this indication.

CIWA-Ar, revised Clinical Institute Withdrawal Assessment—Alcohol; ICU, intensive care unit.

REHABILITATION

Most patients with alcohol dependence will require a more intensive counseling approach than can be delivered in the primary care setting. Of the estimated 18 million people who need treatment of an alcohol-related problem, less than a fourth get help. The cost offsets and benefits of treatment are important to consider. When compared with patients treated for alcohol dependence, an untreated patient incurs health care costs at least 100% higher. Clinicians should be familiar with the type of programs available and the need for continued follow-up and a program of relapse prevention.

Three common psychotherapeutic approaches are 12-step facilitation, motivational enhancement therapy, and cognitive behavioral therapy. Twelve-step facilitation therapy is based on the principles of Alcoholics Anonymous (AA), and key components include peer support, admission of loss of control, and commitment to abstinence. Motivational enhancement therapy bolsters a commitment to change by exploring the pros and cons of drinking alcohol and developing discrepancy between the behavior of drinking alcohol and the patient's goals. Cognitive behavioral therapy assists patients in identifying risk factors for drinking and developing tools to prevent relapse.

These therapies were evaluated in Project Matching Alcoholism Treatment to Client Heterogeneity (MATCH), and the results demonstrated considerable improvement with all three therapies, but no significant differences between treatments. Referral should be based on available resources and patient preference. Rehabilitation can be performed on an inpatient or outpatient basis. Matching of patients to the most appropriate program is based on the severity of addiction, medical and psychiatric co-morbidity, and the availability of resources. Distinction should be made between treatment and participation in a self-help group. Self-help groups are complementary to both intensive psychotherapeutic and pharmacologic interventions. AA is readily available and has been of unquestionable value to many people suffering from an addictive disorder. Becoming familiar with the 12 steps of AA by attending an open meeting can assist clinicians in understanding more about the disease of alcohol dependence and in referring patients to 12-step programs. Having literature available, providing a list of meetings, and following up after a referral can support patients in initiating and maintaining sobriety.

Many medications have been evaluated for use in alcohol dependence, and they have a role as part of a comprehensive rehabilitation program. Optimal benefit from any medication occurs in the context of supportive psychotherapy. The two main Food and Drug Administration–approved pharmacologic agents used to decrease craving and relapse are disulfiram (Antabuse) and naltrexone (ReVia). Disulfiram is an aversive agent that inhibits the metabolism of alcohol. The usual dose of disulfiram is 250 mg once a day. Drinking while taking disulfiram produces flushing, palpitations, nausea, and vomiting. Disulfiram should not be prescribed for patients with cirrhosis or other chronic medical conditions such as heart disease. Naltrexone is an opiate antagonist that theoretically blocks some of the euphoria of drinking, thereby leading to fewer relapses and fewer drinks per relapse. The usual dose of naltrexone is 50 mg once a day. A third agent, acamprosate,* is awaiting approval.

*Not available in the United States.

Acamprosate works through the GABA neurotransmitter system and has been extensively tested in Europe. A number of other medications such as antidepressants and anticonvulsants have also been studied, but the results are conflicting, and currently, no data support the widespread use of these medications for alcohol dependence without co-morbid depression.

Primary care providers are in a unique position to provide ongoing support for patients in recovery. Skills that help in preventing relapses include maintaining a nonjudgmental and empathetic approach, reinforcing success, and identifying "triggers" (reasons) for relapse and methods to decrease or remove triggers. Two very important triggers for relapse are psychiatric illness and smoking.

Patients with alcohol dependence should be screened for co-morbid depression, anxiety, and post-traumatic stress disorder. Psychiatric problems may be either primary or secondary to alcohol. The distinction is difficult during periods of heavy drinking, and treatment ideally should be guided by a mental health professional with experience in both addiction and general psychiatry.

Studies by Hughes and associates have found that 80% of alcoholics smoke. Smoking more than one pack per day should prompt further investigation into alcohol consumption, and all drinkers should be queried about tobacco use. Alcohol and tobacco in combination increase the risk associated with cancer and cardiovascular and infectious diseases. In fact, data show that smoking actually kills more alcoholics than alcohol does. Recent research supports the efficacy of stopping both smoking and drinking together.

In summary, excessive alcohol use has medical, social, and legal consequences. The information in this chapter is intended to aid in the diagnosis, intervention, treatment, and referral of a spectrum of alcohol-related problems. Caring for patients and families adversely affected by alcohol is an excellent opportunity for the generalist physician because of the prevalence of the problem and the tremendous potential for successful intervention by a primary care provider.

DRUG ABUSE

method of
MIKHAIL V. NICKITA, M.D., and
FRANCES R. LEVIN, M.D.
College of Physicians and Surgeons of Columbia University
New York State Psychiatric Institute
New York, New York

Substance abuse and alcohol disorders are major problems in the United States, with costs in excess of $300 billion annually. In the United States, 18% of the population experiences a substance-related or alcohol disorder at some point in their lives. Furthermore, an average of 20% of patients in general medical facilities present with alcohol or substance use disorders.

The knowledge of how to identify, diagnose, treat, and prevent drug-related problems may give health care providers the necessary confidence to deal successfully with substance use disorders.

IDENTIFICATION AND DIAGNOSIS

Health care providers may encounter patients with substance use disorders in the following situations: (1) medical complications of drug use, such as thrombosis or hypertension; (2) drug-seeking behavior including requests for opioids or benzodiazepines or vague complaints of insomnia or pain; (3) accidents secondary to drug use (e.g., falls, driving while impaired); and (4) emergency room settings (e.g., overdoses). The identification of a drug problem is the first step in helping patients. This can be an especially difficult problem for the middle-class substance abuser. An important approach is to take the time to gather a substance use history for every patient, particularly those with complaints of pain. If the problematic use of drugs is suspected, gathering additional information from a collateral source such as a spouse can be crucial. Another significant indicator of an increased risk of a drug problem is a history of antisocial problems beginning at an early age. In a patient in whom drug misuse is suspected, the clinician should look for physical signs of misuse (e.g., needle marks, perforated septum, miosis). Useful tools in identifying drugs of abuse are blood, urine, and hair screenings as objective measures of a drug's presence. Blood, the most invasive, gives readings of current drug levels and is most useful in emergency room settings; urine can stay positive for 2 to 3 days (cocaine, heroin) or for days to weeks (marijuana). Hair testing is of no use for current impairment because it takes approximately 5 days for drugs to show up in a person's hair, but once they appear, they will continue to be detectable in new hair growth for approximately 90 days.

The diagnosis of a substance use disorder is based on clinical criteria provided by the fourth edition of the *Diagnostic and Statistical Manual of Mental Disorders* (DSM-IV), which identifies two groups of disorders: abuse and dependence (Tables 1 and 2).

OPIOIDS

The semisynthetic drug *heroin* is the most commonly abused illicit opiate. Reports indicate increased use, largely because of increased purity, which makes non-injectable routes such as snorting and smoking more readily available. If used regularly, this drug rapidly produces tolerance and dependence. Heroin may lead to a significant reduction in pain perception, sedation, and significant euphoria, particularly when it is used intravenously. Other common effects of heroin are constipation, drowsiness, decreased appetite and libido, and respiratory depression. Heroin can be lethal in an

TABLE 1. **DSM-IV Diagnostic Criteria for Substance Dependence**

A maladaptive pattern of substance use, leading to clinically significant impairment or distress, as manifested by three (or more) of the following, occurring at any time in the same 12-month period:

1. Tolerance, as defined by either of the following:
   a. A need for markedly increased amounts of the substance to achieve intoxication or desired effect
   b. Markedly diminished effect with continued use of the same amount of the substance
2. Withdrawal, as manifested by either of the following:
   a. The characteristic withdrawal syndrome for the substance
   b. The same (or closely related) substance is taken to relieve or avoid withdrawal symptoms
3. The substance is often taken in larger amounts or over a longer period than was intended.
4. There is a persistent desire or unsuccessful efforts to cut down or control substance use.
5. A great deal of time is spent in activities necessary to obtain the substance (e.g., visiting multiple doctors or driving long distances), use the substance (e.g., chain-smoking), or recover from its effects.
6. Important social, occupational, or recreational activities are given up or reduced because of substance use.
7. The substance use is continued despite knowledge of having a persistent or recurrent physical or psychological problem that is likely to have been caused or exacerbated by the substance (e.g., current cocaine use despite recognition of cocaine-induced depression or continued drinking despite recognition that ulcer was made worse by alcohol consumption).

Specify if:
With physiological dependence: evidence of tolerance or withdrawal (i.e., either item 1 or 2 is present)
Without physiological dependence: no evidence of tolerance or withdrawal (i.e., neither item 1 nor 2 is present)

Course specifiers:
Early full remission
Early partial remission
Sustained full remission
Sustained partial remission
On agonist therapy
In a controlled environment

TABLE 2. **DSM-IV Diagnostic Criteria for Substance Abuse**

A. A maladaptive pattern of substance use leading to clinically significant impairment or distress, as manifested by one (or more) of the following occurring within a 12-month period:

1. Recurrent substance use resulting in a failure to fulfill major role obligations at work, school, or home (e.g., repeated absences or poor work performance related to substance use; substance-related absences, suspensions, or expulsions from school; neglect of children or household)
2. Recurrent substance use in situations in which it is physically hazardous (e.g., driving an automobile or operating a machine when impaired by substance use)
3. Recurrent substance-related legal problems (e.g., arrests for substance-related disorderly conduct)
4. Continued substance use despite having persistent or recurrent social or interpersonal problems caused or exacerbated by the effects of the substance (e.g., arguments with spouse about consequences of intoxication, physical fights)

B. The symptoms have never met the criteria for substance dependence for this class of substance.

Reprinted with permission from the Diagnostic and Statistical Manual of Mental Disorders, 4th ed. Copyright 2000, American Psychiatric Association.

overdose. The characteristic signs of overdose include shallow respirations, pupillary miosis, bradycardia, a decrease in body temperature, and varying degrees of clouded consciousness up to a complete absence of responsiveness to external stimulation.

The first step in treatment of opiate overdose should be establishing basic life support with a respirator and other emergency procedures. The definitive treatment for opiate overdose is the narcotic antagonist naloxone, given in an initial dose of 0.4 mg (1 mL) or 0.01 mg/kg intravenously or intramuscularly if the intravenous route is not available; this dose can be repeated every 2 to 3 minutes, as indicated by clinical symptoms. The effects of naloxone last 2 to 3 hours. It is important to monitor the patient for at least 24 hours after a heroin overdose and 72 hours after an overdose of long-acting opioids such as methadone because of the possible recurrence of opioid toxicity.

Although opioid withdrawal symptoms are not life-threatening, they are associated with pronounced craving for heroin and rapid relapse. The symptoms can include dysphoria, nausea, vomiting, sweating, "goose flesh," musculoskeletal pains, spasms, severe abdominal cramps, dilated pupils, yawning, and agitation. These symptoms peak at 36 to 72 hours and begin to subside over about 5 to 7 days. Before treatment of the withdrawal syndrome is initiated, patients must receive a thorough physical examination with specific attention to liver and neurologic functions and identification of local and systemic infections. The severity and chronicity of the heroin dependence should be evaluated. There are several different approaches to treating heroin withdrawal, depending on the assessment. These approaches may include:

1. Readministration of sufficient opiate medication on day 1 of treatment with gradual taper of the drug over the next 5 to 10 days. Because of cross-tolerance, any opiate will work, but many physicians prefer to use long-acting drugs such as methadone. Most patients require between 20 and 40 mg of methadone orally given on day 1. After a few days of a stabilized drug dose, the opiate is then reduced by 20% to 25% daily.

2. The use of the α_2-adrenergic agonist clonidine. Doses of approximately 5 μg/kg (usual range, 0.3 to 1.2 mg/d in three to four divided doses) decrease many of the autonomic components of the opioid withdrawal syndrome. However, clonidine is less effective in reducing muscle pain, lethargy, and insomnia.

3. Buprenorphine, a partial opioid receptor agonist/antagonist, was approved by the U.S. Food and Drug Administration (FDA) for office-based management of opioid withdrawal or maintenance in sublingual tablets of 2 and 8 mg. The medication should not be started until the patient is at least in mild withdrawal (usually 12 hours after the last heroin dose or 24 to 36 hours after the last methadone dose of no higher than 30 to 40 mg/d). The initial dose, usually 4 or 8 mg of buprenorphine, can be increased up to a total of 16 mg on day 1, depending on the patient. Patients treated with this medication experience little or no withdrawal, and cravings are significantly diminished. In contrast to clonidine, buprenorphine does not seriously affect blood pressure and reduces subjective and physiologic withdrawal symptoms as much as or more than clonidine. There are certain restrictions regarding availability and training for prescription providers accessible elsewhere. Because it is only a partial agonist, too rapid an increase in the dose on day 1 or 2 can worsen rather than alleviate withdrawal.

After initial treatment of withdrawal symptoms, several approaches are used to help maintain abstinence from heroin. The choice depends on the motivation of the patient and the chronicity of the opioid addiction. Patients with sufficient motivation and a relatively short period of using an opioid may be tried on naltrexone, approved by the FDA in 1984 for the treatment of narcotic addiction. Before beginning naltrexone, to avoid precipitating withdrawal, the patient must not have taken short-acting agonists such as heroin for at least 5 days and methadone for 10 to 14 days. Two common dosing regimens are 50 mg/d or 100 mg on Monday and Wednesday and 150 mg on Friday. Compliance with naltrexone can be an issue, which can be handled by supervised intake such as by a significant other. For patients with less external motivation and an extended period of opioid dependence, maintenance on methadone or buprenorphine may be preferred. A restricted therapeutic community can be of significant help to patients, but it usually requires external motivating factors to enter treatment. An alternative to methadone is LAAM (*l*-acetyl-α-methadol), a synthetic opioid agonist, approved for maintenance treatment in 1993. LAAM has a half-life of about 2.5 days, and this allows for administration less frequently than methadone and a reduction in clinic visits. However, because LAAM has a potential for cardiotoxicity with prolongation of the QT interval and induction of arrhythmia, newer FDA guidelines require regular electrocardiographic monitoring and state that LAAM should not be considered a first-line treatment. Buprenorphine, especially the combination form that contains naloxone, is permitted to be prescribed in office-based or clinic-based settings with physician training. Up to a 30-day prescription is permitted for appropriate patients. In any case, it is important to establish a therapeutic, nonjudgmental relationship with the patient as a basis for carrying out successful recovery. Medications need to be supplemented with psychosocial interventions when appropriate.

BENZODIAZEPINES AND OTHER SEDATIVE-HYPNOTICS AND ANXIOLYTICS

This is a clinically diverse group of frequently prescribed medications used for treatment of various medical conditions. When indicated, many patients can be maintained on *benzodiazepines* without either abuse or escalation of doses. However, in some patients, especially those with a prior history of alcoholism or other substance abuse, use of these drugs can be problematic. In these patients, the medications are more likely to be abused. These agents can produce physical dependence when they are taken in higher than usual doses or for prolonged periods. Additionally, benzodiazepines may be used by addicted patients as an adjunct to their primary drugs of choice, for instance, to mitigate the adverse effects of cocaine or to produce a drunken state with methadone. The intoxication syndromes induced by the sedative-hypnotics are quite similar and include sluggishness, slurred speech, unsteady gait, impairment in attention, memory, and reaction time, and sometimes disinhibition. The best way to confirm the diagnosis of intoxication is to obtain a blood sample for substance screening. In case of overdose, basic life support measures should be started. Since its introduction in the early 1990s, the effective treatment of overdose includes the benzodiazepine antagonist flumazenil, 0.2 mg (2 mL) intravenously over 15 seconds, with repeated doses up to 3 mg.

Some patients who have taken a benzodiazepine in therapeutic doses for a long period can abruptly discontinue it without developing withdrawal symptoms. However, for others, cessation or marked reduction of the benzodiazepine may produce a withdrawal syndrome, which is qualitatively similar for all sedative-hypnotics and can include anxiety, tremors, insomnia, anorexia, nausea, vomiting, orthostasis, seizures, delirium, hyperpyrexia, and even death. The risk of withdrawal symptoms increases with length and amount of use. Symptoms typically begin 12 to 40 hours after the last dose, depending on the half-life of a substance, and they peak in intensity with short-acting benzodiazepines between 24 and 72 hours and with long-acting agents on the fifth to eighth days. The withdrawal effects are rapidly reversed with the administration of benzodiazepines. There are four strategies for treating dependence on sedative-hypnotics. The first is the gradual withdrawal technique. For patients treated with benzodiazepines for longer than 2 to 3 months, the dose should be decreased no faster than 10% per week, until these drugs are at 10% to 20% of their peak level. At this point, further reduction in the benzodiazepine dose should be slower. The second approach is to substitute another longer-acting benzodiazepine. With this strategy, clonazepam has gained popularity. This medication is introduced on day 1 of the treatment, with the appropriate dose equivalent to the dose of the sedative-hypnotic, and then it is gradually withdrawn. The third method is to substitute an anticonvulsant such as carbamazepine or valproate. The fourth method is using phenobarbital or another long-acting barbiturate as a substitute for the abused agent and then gradually withdrawing it. Treatment with sedative-hypnotics and anxiolytics should include an advance discussion with patients of the possibility of withdrawal symptoms when these agents are discontinued.

CANNABIS

Cannabis is the most commonly used illicit substance in the world. Epidemiologic studies suggest that cannabis dependence occurs in 9% of persons who try marijuana. Cannabis is usually the first illicit drug of experimentation for adolescents in the United States, and its use is usually preceded by alcohol and cigarettes (also illegal for adolescents). The prevalence of cannabis use increased throughout the 1990s, although from 2000 to 2002 it reached a plateau.

Symptoms of cannabis intoxication include euphoria, anxiety, a sensation of slowed time, and impaired judgment, as well as increased appetite, tachycardia, dry mouth, and conjunctival injection. Acute adverse effects of marijuana use include paranoid ideations, impaired short-term memory, hallucinations, and generalized anxiety with panic attacks or agitation. Cannabis intoxication is a self-limiting condition. Symptoms of intoxication, even when complicated by psychotic or anxiety disorders, usually remit as cannabis is metabolized and is eliminated from the body.

If a state of cannabis intoxication comes to clinical attention, no treatment is usually necessary other than observation, reality testing by friends and family, and reassurance that symptoms are caused by the drug and will stop. Anxiolytic agents occasionally are needed. If symptoms persist for more than 24 to 48 hours after acute cannabis intoxication, the possibility of another psychiatric diagnosis must be considered. Cannabis has been shown to cause relapse in patients with stabilized schizophrenia.

There is no proven targeted pharmacologic treatment of long-term cannabis use. Pure marijuana abuse or dependence rarely requires inpatient treatment and detoxification. However, inpatient laboratory studies suggest that heavy long-term marijuana users who cease using cannabis experience increased irritability, anxiety, insomnia, and decreased food intake, symptoms that may promote continued cannabis use. Outpatient treatment interventions have included self-help 12-step groups, family therapy, individual therapy, and periodic urine testing to monitor abstinence. The cannabinoid agonist dronabinol (a schedule III controlled substance) may help with craving and withdrawal during early abstinence, or it may be used in an off-label capacity for prolonged maintenance.

STIMULANTS

Cocaine and *methamphetamine* are the most commonly abused illicit stimulants in the United States. Although epidemiologic data suggest that overall use of cocaine is declining, the drug still produces the greatest number of illicit drug-related admissions to the emergency room. Further, among arrestees, cocaine is the most common illicit substance found in urine toxicology testing. Cocaine, methamphetamine, and other stimulants produce quite similar physiologic and behavioral effects. All stimulants produce dose-related elevation of mood and dose-related increase in cardiac rate and blood pressure, although the risk of having a stimulant-induced myocardial infarction is not related to dose. High doses of stimulants can produce lethal hypertension and hyperpyrexia. Common psychiatric symptoms of intoxication include euphoria or affective blunting, changes in sociability, hypervigilance, interpersonal sensitivity, anxiety, tension and anger, and impaired judgment. Physiologic changes are usually tachycardia, pupillary dilatation, elevated blood pressure, perspiration or chills, nausea or vomiting, muscular weakness, respiratory depression, chest pain or cardiac arrhythmias, confusion, seizures, dystonia, or coma.

Treatment of acute intoxication is symptomatic, with close monitoring of patients with a tendency for developing cardiac and respiratory complications. Treatment of stimulant overdose can be a medical emergency, which may require treatment in an intensive care unit. The choice of treatment depends on the clinical signs and symptoms. Hyperthermia requires ambient cooling procedures or dantrolene. Intravenous propranolol, up to 1.0 mg, and calcium channel blockers have been shown to be effective for control of cardiovascular complications. For agitation, anxiety, and paranoia, which typically last for 3 to 5 days, benzodiazepines are the preferred choice. Use of neuroleptics or other medications with a tendency to lower the seizure threshold can complicate more than help the clinical picture. In case of seizures, diazepam, 10 mg intravenously, has been effective in acute management. Symptoms of stimulant withdrawal do not usually present a medical danger. After a binge, patients characteristically experience extreme exhaustion with depression, agitation, and anxiety, followed by a desire for sleep. Clinically, the symptoms resemble those of a major depressive episode, except for the comparatively brief duration. If a patient is brought to clinical attention, management during this phase consists of observation, especially because of the possibility of suicidal ideation. After providing an opportunity for sleep, the clinician should ensure that neurovegetative symptoms and suicidal ideations are no longer present. In most cases, this is usually done in an emergency room. The principles of stimulant rehabilitation are similar to the principles used with other varieties of drug dependence and require combined efforts by family, physicians, psychiatrists, and other healthcare providers. Not all stimulant users require extensive rehabilitative efforts; some patients who are not severely dependent may respond to external pressures.

No pharmacologic agent has shown adequate effectiveness in the treatment of stimulant dependence, although many different medications have been tried. Different pharmacologic approaches have included: (1) treating withdrawal symptoms, (2) targeting psychiatric co-morbidity, and (3) decreasing craving. Different cognitive-behavioral approaches and contingency contracting have been successfully used to manage stimulant abuse. Individual and group psychotherapy, family, and self-help group assistance programs are often useful to promote remission from stimulant use.

CLUB DRUGS

Club drugs are primarily synthetic substances that continue to gain popularity among young adults at nightclubs, bars, and raves (all-night dance parties). These substances often include, but are not limited to, 3,4-methylenedioxymethamphetamine (MDMA), γ-hydroxybutyrate (GHB), phencyclidine (PCP), ketamine, lysergic acid diethylamide (LSD), and flunitrazepam (Rohypnol). The nation's top monitoring mechanisms report that use of these drugs is on the rise, with a dramatic increase in emergency room admissions. Contrary to common belief, no club drug is benign. Club drugs can cause serious physical and psychological problems and even death. The following is a short overview of selected preparations.

MDMA, with street names such as "ecstasy," "XTC," "X," "Eve" or "lover's speed," has both stimulant and psychedelic effects. MDMA is taken orally, usually in tablets or capsules, although it can be injected. It can cause euphoria, feelings of well-being, and enhanced mental and emotional clarity. In high doses, MDMA can cause a marked increase in body temperature, muscle tension, involuntary teeth clenching, nausea, vomiting, increased heart rate and blood pressure, blurred vision, faintness, tremors, convulsions, and chills or sweating. Psychological difficulties can include irrational or violent behavior, depression, depersonalization, hallucinations, confusion, severe anxiety, and paranoia. An MDMA high can last 6 to 24 hours, although the average duration is usually around 3 to 4 hours. Several episodes of death from MDMA use were reported after users developed malignant hyperthermia with rhabdomyolysis and kidney failure.

PCP is an easily synthesized anesthetic with hallucinogenic properties. A localized increase in its use has been observed. It is taken orally, by smoking, or by intravenous injection. The most common street preparation, "angel dust," is a white granular powder. The effects of low-dose PCP administration last 4 to 6 hours and include agitation, excitement, impaired motor coordination, dysarthria, and analgesia. Examination of a user may reveal horizontal or vertical nystagmus, blushing, diaphoresis, and hyperacusis. Behavioral changes frequently include distortions of body image, disorganization of thinking, and a feeling of estrangement. Abusers often use PCP in higher or repeated doses, which can lead to hypersalivation, vomiting, myoclonus, fever, stupor, or coma. Overdose can also cause convulsions, opisthotonos, and decerebrate posturing, which may be followed by prolonged coma. Confirmation of PCP use is possible by determination of PCP levels in serum or urine. Death from PCP overdose may occur as a consequence of some combination of pharyngeal hypersecretion, hyperthermia, respiratory depression, severe hypertension, seizures, hypertensive encephalopathy, and intracerebral hemorrhage. Rhabdomyolysis may take place and may cause renal failure as a result of myoglobinemia.

LSD is a potent hallucinogen commonly referred to as "acid." It can be sold as tablets, capsules, liquid, and thin squares of gelatin, or it can be absorbed on colorful paper to be licked. Effects of LSD, a "high" or "trip," can last anywhere from 3 to 12 hours. Users may have tachycardia, hypertension, papillary dilation, tremor, and hyperpyrexia within minutes of LSD ingestion. Psychological effects are varying, but they often consist of bizarre perceptual and mood changes, including visual illusions, synesthesias, and extreme lability of mood. "Flashbacks," both perceptual and affective, can occur for months after the last use. The emergency room mentions of LSD use are most frequently associated with developing panic episodes, which can persist up to 24 hours. There are no clinical reports of death caused by the direct effect of LSD.

GHB, with street names "G," "Georgia home boy," "Gook," "liquid ecstasy," "easy lay," and "grievous bodily harm," is a central nervous system depressant. GHB is usually sold as a slightly salty, clear liquid; however, it can be obtained in capsule form or as grainy, white to sandy-colored powder. Once GHB is ingested, its effects last 1 to 3 hours. GHB produces disinhibition, euphoria, and sedation. When it is taken at higher doses, hypothermia, bradycardia, amnesia, coma, seizures, nausea, and respiratory depression can occur. GHB has been involved in poisonings, overdoses, date rapes, and death. Because of rapid metabolism, GHB leaves no traces in the urine after about 4 to 5 hours.

Ketamine is another drug that is used in rave or party settings. It is a legally sold anesthetic intended for veterinary use. This drug can be injected or snorted. Its slang terms include "special K," "vitamin K," and "super K." Users experience dreamlike states, visual distortions, and hallucinations, which can last anywhere from 30 minutes to 2 hours. At larger doses, ketamine can produce delirium, amnesia, impaired motor functioning, high blood pressure, depression, and potentially fatal respiratory problems.

Rohypnol (flunitrazepam), a benzodiazepine, is not legally available in the United States, but it is currently licensed in numerous other countries. It has been connected with drug-facilitated sexual assaults, rape, and robbery. It is known as "rophies," "roofies," "Roche," and "forget-me-pill." Rohypnol is tasteless and odorless, and it is dissolved easily in beverages. A dose of the drug as small as 1 mg can impair a victim for 8 to 12 hours. Users of Rohypnol first may feel intoxicated, then sleepy. Rohypnol can cause slurred speech, impaired judgment, and difficulty with walking. Especially when this agent is mixed with other drugs such as alcohol, deep sedation, decreased blood pressure, respiratory distress, amnesia, and death can occur.

The principles of treatment of other drug overdoses are also applied to a club drug emergency to a large extent. Any club drug overdose requires prompt life support measures including treatment of coma, respiratory depression, seizures, severe hypertension, and malignant hyperthermia in a hospital intensive care unit. If the drugs were taken orally, gastric lavage can be done. Acidification of urine increases the excretion rate of PCP. For Rohypnol overdose, there is an antidote, flumazenil. Acute psychosis and severe behavioral reactions with a club drug use should be considered a psychiatric emergency. These conditions should be treated in a protective, nonstimulating environment with use of reassurance and support. If needed, a benzodiazepine, such as lorazepam, can be given. Most patients who have mild to moderate symptoms of acute intoxication will improve rapidly. Intoxicated patients should be observed until their mental status has remained normal for several hours. Some persons who use club drugs will develop abuse and dependence and may be helped with standard psychotherapeutic approaches. However, at present, there are few empirical studies to guide treatment. Although no targeted treatment has been developed, club drug abuse and dependence, like all other chemical dependence problems, may require long-term interventions.

SUMMARY

Health care providers face two main dilemmas when they encounter substance-related conditions in their patients: to identify accurately those patients who need treatment and to provide the best treatment option possible. To resolve these dilemmas successfully is not always easy because of the complexity of the substance-related disorders, the high level of co-morbidity, and the presence of several barriers to detection and treatment. This chapter has offered a brief, pragmatic outline to help health care providers to expand their diagnostic and treatment repertoire. Continuing efforts to develop and improve the diagnostic and treatment options for health care providers and for patients suffering from substance-related conditions are likely to result in major improvements.

ACKNOWLEDGMENT

We are most thankful to our divisional director, Herbert D. Kleber, M.D., for his helpful review of the manuscript.

ANXIETY DISORDERS

method of
NEIL R. LIEBOWITZ, M.D.
Connecticut Anxiety and Depression Treatment Center
University of Connecticut
Farmington, Connecticut

Anxiety is one of the most common psychiatric symptoms reported in patients. Accurate patient assessment is important for making the best treatment decisions because patients often mislabel their symptoms and use the terms *anxiety* and *depression* interchangeably. Even when labeled correctly, anxiety may be a symptom of obsessive-compulsive disorder (OCD), panic attacks, unipolar or bipolar depression, or psychosis. The significance of misdiagnosis becomes gravely evident when a patient with panic attacks becomes acutely manic after being given an antidepressant.

This article is a brief guide to understanding anxiety-related symptoms, as they help predict response to treatment. It is a compilation of clinical experience learned from many psychiatrists and supported by the author's own work with patients. It focuses on assessment of symptoms that should complement the reader's knowledge of *Diagnostic and Statistical Manual of Mental Disorders* (DSM-IV) criteria.

ASSESSMENT OF THE PATIENT

The initial assessment should include past psychiatric treatment, medical history, family history, social/occupational history, and symptom profile. The psychiatric history should include past medication trials with details of dosage, duration, and response. Previously successful treatment is the best predictor of future response to the same treatment. Careful attention to the effect of any medication trial may help guide the clinician in selecting another medication with a more beneficial mechanism of action. Questions regarding previous hospitalization, substance abuse, suicide attempts, and physical, emotional, and/or sexual abuse can be brief and directed.

The medical history may identify conditions that contribute to psychiatric symptoms, such as neurologic or endocrine abnormalities. A complete query into the use of medications and supplements may reveal anxiogenic agents such as β-adrenergic asthma medications, steroids, or supplements with ephedra,* caffeine, or ma huang.* Some may have drug interactions with pharmacotherapeutic agents. Extensive medical complaints may reflect somatization disorder or a history of physical or sexual abuse.

The family history is best taken with a genogram to keep track of biologic family relationships. The genogram may suggest hereditary psychiatric or substance abuse conditions that may have typical or atypical manifestations. A positive response to medication by a first-degree relative is the second best predictor of response behind previous medication response in an identified patient.

The social/occupational history serves many purposes. It provides a quick assessment of past functional ability and current level of disability. Questions regarding social support, religious involvement, and hobbies help guide the clinician in recommending activities to support the patient's recovery and highlight loss of motivation and interests. Information about the level of exercise, nutrition, and drug and alcohol use may point to reasons for treatment failure. Any amount of drug use and alcohol consumption in excess of two drinks for a woman or four for a man per 24-hour period are reliable predictors of treatment failure. Vitamin deficiency (usually B vitamins) as a result of chronically poor nutrition may pose another reason for lack of response to treatment.

SYMPTOM ASSESSMENT

Most of the history needs to be taken with directive questions to obtain a complete description of the symptoms, including the onset, duration, exacerbating and ameliorating factors, and level of dysfunction. The following paragraphs contain descriptions of specific symptoms that are commonly confused when interviewing an anxious patient. Proper identification of these symptoms will affect the choice of treatment.

Panic Attacks. Panic attacks are discrete episodes of severe anxiety that often appear out of the blue or in previously feared situations. The anxiety symptoms reach peak intensity in 10 minutes or less and fade over the course of 1 hour. A single panic attack never lasts all day. However, a patient may have multiple panic attacks within a day and suffer enduring anticipatory anxiety. No other medical symptom has this exact pattern. Angina is the closest differential diagnosis, but this condition usually has an exertional precipitant and less rapid rise in symptoms. Have the patient graph the intensity over time if the pattern of anxiety is at all in doubt. Symptoms of panic can be divided into physical (increased heart rate, shortness of breath, numbness and tingling, blurred vision, or gastrointestinal discomfort with urgency) and cognitive (fear, sense of doom, feeling unreal or detached, anger or aggression, or the urge to flee).

Obsessions and Compulsions. Compulsions are repetitive behaviors that the patient feels driven to do, usually to prevent some feared harm. An example is repetitive checking of door locks or the stove beyond one or two times. Obsessions are repetitive thoughts or images that are intrusive and distressing to the patient. They are usually the same thoughts repeated over and over again, such as repeating a prayer over and over if another thought interrupts. Patients are generally embarrassed by these thoughts and behaviors and will not volunteer these symptoms without direct questioning. It is helpful to ask: "Do you do any behavior repetitively or have any intrusive, obsessive thoughts that distress you? If so, how much time do you waste per day because of this symptom?" Consider

*Not FDA approved for this indication.

treatment of any distressing thoughts (e.g., intrusive, violent thoughts) or symptoms that waste over 20 minutes per day. Obsessions differ from delusions in the patient's awareness of their senseless nature (i.e., ego-dystonic). Delusions are strongly held false beliefs that persist despite lack of supporting evidence (i.e., ego-syntonic).

Simple Paranoia Versus True Paranoia. Patients with panic attacks will often say that they get "paranoid" when going to crowded places. Usually they are describing "simple paranoia," which reflects one's sense of being extremely self-conscious that others are able to tell that they are nervous. Such behavior is not a psychotic symptom, and unless accompanied by agitation, it is not an indication for any antipsychotic medication. True paranoia is the delusional belief that there is a conspiracy against the patient, who often has inconsistent circumstantial evidence to support the belief. Simple paranoia is a nonpsychotic fear that the patient realizes is irrational, like an obsession.

Agitation Versus Anxiety. Anxiety is a cognitive symptom involving fear, worry, distress, or apprehension. It is usually felt in relationship to a stressful situation or conflict. Agitation is a physical symptom that involves restlessness or an inability to sit still or relax. Agitation is easy to observe. Anxiety is usually present in the context of agitation, but the reverse is not true. Agitation is often a symptom of a psychotic process, and its presence should lead to a more thorough exploration of psychotic symptoms such as paranoia, hallucinations, and delusions.

Trauma Symptoms. Nightmares and flashback-reliving phenomena are characteristic of recent or past trauma. In addition, patients startle easily and may have panic-like symptoms. After acute trauma, patients may have agitation and paranoia. These psychotic symptoms are usually of brief duration and of a fluctuating nature. It is important to elicit a history of trauma because medications alone are going to be of limited benefit for post-traumatic stress disorder (PTSD) and dosages are often different than for treatment of other disorders with similar anxiety and psychotic symptoms.

Social Anxiety Versus Agoraphobia. Social anxiety disorder can be viewed as a type of OCD in which patients obsess about what other people are thinking of them. They realize that such thinking is unrealistic (i.e., not a delusion) but are unable to resist the self-conscious thoughts. Agoraphobia is a learned avoidance because of fear of having a panic attack in the feared situation. Patients with agoraphobia avoid going to social situations for fear that they would not be able to leave easily if they have a panic attack. Patients with social anxiety avoid social situations because of fear that others would have a negative opinion of them.

Anxiety Versus Depression. These symptoms usually coexist, but it is useful to identify the primary affect or the sequence of symptoms. Patients will often state that the anxiety occurs first, followed by despair over their inability to cope with the anxiety. Anxiety is characterized by nervousness, worry, and fear. It is a high-energy state that often leads to fatigue. Anxiety is usually worse in the afternoon as life stressors progress and more often has associated initial insomnia (i.e., difficulty falling asleep). Depression is a low-energy state with loss of drive and motivation and has associated terminal insomnia (i.e., early-morning awakening). Depression is usually worse in the AM, and patients frequently complain of nonspecific pain symptoms. (Treatment of depression is not covered in this article.)

Bipolar Disorder Screening. In any assessment of anxiety, it is important to look for clues for the elusive bipolar disorder. Some patients with bipolar disorder experience their "highs" as dysphoric mania, with the major complaint being severe anxiety. Bipolar disorder may have been diagnosed or suspected in family members. Other clues include a history of cyclical symptoms, most typically anxiety with high energy in the spring and lows in the winter; severe postpartum symptoms; migraines, especially in a cyclical pattern; and a history of agitation triggered by antidepressants that persists beyond 2 weeks. (Patients with panic disorder will have worse panic for up to 2 weeks after starting antidepressant medications, but in bipolar patients, the panic persists beyond 2 weeks.) The response to antidepressants is often erratic in bipolar disorder, with medications losing effectiveness after several weeks to months of a good response or patients not responding at all to medication that previously worked. (Treatment of suspected bipolar disorder is not covered in this article.)

Attention-Deficit/Hyperactivity Disorder. Occasionally, a clinician encounters an adult patient who complains of mind racing, insomnia, poor concentration, and anxiety and reports getting very tired when taking selective serotonin reuptake inhibitors (SSRIs). The hyperactivity and impulsivity may look like bipolar disorder, but the symptoms are not cyclical and can be traced to childhood. These patients report anxiety relief from tobacco. Attention-deficit/hyperactivity disorder is one condition in which stimulant medication or bupropion (Wellbutrin)* may dramatically relieve the anxiety and irritability, as well as help focus attention.

Performance Anxiety. Patients who report anxiety only in situations in which they have to give a presentation or performance usually have considerable anticipatory anxiety with noradrenergic symptoms of a rapid heart rate, sweating, and obvious tremors. The symptoms of performance anxiety resemble panic attacks but are sustained as long as the individual is in the spotlight. The use of propranolol (Inderal),* 20 to 40 mg 1 hour before the situation, helps prevent these symptoms without the cognitive dulling or sedation that may occur with benzodiazepines.

PSYCHOTHERAPY PARADIGMS

Anxiety is a normal part of life and serves as a motivational signal. If an individual loses a job or is in a bad relationship that demands unrealistic

*Not FDA approved for this indication.

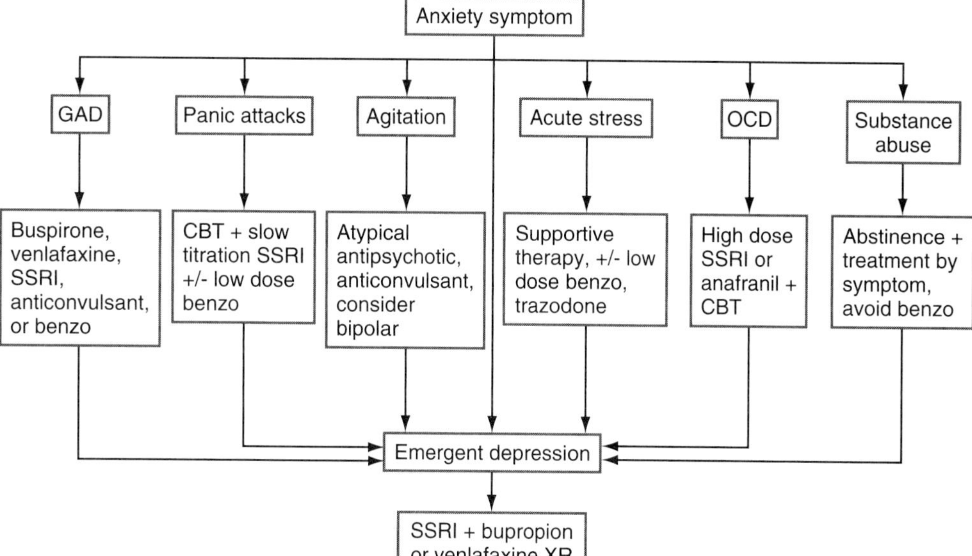

Figure 1. Treatment algorithm for anxiety disorders. CBT = cognitive-behavioral therapy; GAD = generalized anxiety disorder; OCD = obsessive-compulsive disorder; SSRI = selective serotonin reuptake inhibitor; benzo = benzodiazepine.

expectations, anxiety signals the need to make decisions about resolving these problems. Supportive counseling may help a patient better understand the nature of the conflict and appreciate alternative solutions. In these situations, therapy is the main treatment, and any pharmacotherapy should be limited and brief, such as low-dose benzodiazepine or a sleeping medication.

Panic attacks require specific cognitive-behavioral therapy (CBT). This approach is educational and embodies the concept that the panic symptoms are the body's natural alarm system going off falsely. In genetically vulnerable individuals, excess stress causes this alarm to reset more sensitively. Medication can help reset the alarm, but therapy is needed to prevent and reverse avoidance and reduce the perceived danger from situations. Explaining that a panic attack is a real condition that lasts under 1 hour and causes no harm can help reduce the fear that may trigger another attack. Avoidance is the major source of the disability, not the actual brief panic attack. To prevent the development of conditioned avoidance, patients should be encouraged to remain in situations until the attacks pass. Once panic attacks are controlled by medication, gradual exposure to feared situations is essential to recovery. Overmedication must be avoided because it interferes with this cognitive reframing and motivation. Relaxation techniques help reduce the anticipatory anxiety but do little for the actual panic attack. (Panic disorder is covered in more detail in another article.)

CBT is also the treatment of choice for OCD and social anxiety. The book *Brain Lock* by Jeffrey Schwartz (1997) provides a self-help manual to apply CBT for OCD. Exposure to feared situations is essential in the treatment of OCD. PTSD requires a more complicated psychotherapy process involving traumatic stress debriefing acutely and a combination of supportive, insight-oriented, and CBT techniques over an extended period. Medications are targeted at the most severe symptoms but should not overly sedate the patient, which interferes with the therapeutic process (Figure 1).

PHARMACOTHERAPY STRATEGIES

SSRIs are the main treatment of anxiety. No evidence has shown one SSRI to be superior to another; however, SSRIs have significant differences in side effects and drug interactions. Escitalopram (Lexapro)* and citalopram (Celexa)* are associated with the least inhibition of cytochrome P-450 and the least protein binding, in addition to having a favorable side effect profile. Sertraline (Zoloft)* is a good alternative. Paroxetine (Paxil)* and fluoxetine (Prozac)* are associated with very significant inhibition of P-450IID6, which makes polypharmacy more complicated. Many psychiatrists believe that paroxetine may cause more weight gain and sexual inhibition than the other drugs do. The author has seen several severe drug interactions with both paroxetine and fluoxetine and suggests avoiding these medications in the elderly and patients taking multiple medications.

Patients with a history of past or present *panic attacks* have a high likelihood of having the panic worsen in the first 2 weeks of treatment until receptor down-regulation occurs. It is important to give these patients realistic expectations about the course of the response to therapy and begin clonazepam (Klonopin), 0.25 mg twice daily (bid), on the day before initiation of the SSRI. Having realistic expectations encourages an adequate medication trial and prevents jumping from medication to medication. Clonazepam may be tapered after 1 month if a good response is obtained from the SSRI. Although SSRIs are well tolerated, care should be taken to not overmedicate patients because over-medication results in a flattening of affect, low motivation, worsening of sexual side effects, cognitive dulling, and weight gain.

In *OCD, PTSD,* and *social anxiety* (not complicated by panic attacks), the starting dose of SSRIs can be

*Not FDA approved for this indication.

TABLE 1. **Selective Medications for Treatment of Anxiety Disorders**

Medication	Starting Dose	Target Dose (Indication)	Comment
SSRIs			
Escitalopram (Lexapro)	5 mg	10–20 mg (panic, GAD) 20 mg (OCD, PTSD)*	Most selective SSRI, least drug interaction
Citalopram (Celexa)	10 mg	20–60 mg (high end for OCD)*	More sedation than with Lexapro
Sertraline (Zoloft)	25 mg	50–200 mg (high end for OCD)	Diarrhea
Dual reuptake inhibitor			
Venlafaxine (Effexor XR)	37.5 mg	75–150 mg (anxiety) 225–375 mg (depression)	More energizing than SSRI Useful for associated pain, migraine, fibromyalgia, IBS
Benzodiazepine			
Clonazepam (Klonopin)	0.25 mg bid	0.5–1.5 mg	Lower doses more effective for panic; tolerance at any dose for GAD* if used regularly; 20-h half-life allows bid dosing
Buspirone (BuSpar)	7.5 mg bid	Up to 30 mg bid (higher dose for alcoholics)	Take with food to reduce dizziness
Anticonvulsant			
Valproic acid (Depakote)*	250 mg bid or 500 mg extended release	500–1500 mg	Levels may be less than "therapeutic" for anxiety, agitation, OCD augmentation
Propranolol (Inderal)*	20 mg	20–80 mg	For performance anxiety, use prn 1 h before event
Atypical antipsychotic			
Risperidone (Risperdal)*	0.25–0.5 mg	0.25–1.5 mg	For OCD augmentation, agitation, and racing thoughts
Quetiapine (Seroquel)	25 mg	25–100 mg	A safer thioridazine (Mellaril) for agitation

*Not FDA approved for this indication.
GAD = generalized anxiety disorder; IBS = irritable bowel syndrome; OCD = obsessive-compulsive disorder; PTSD = post-traumatic stress disorder; SSRI = selective serotonin reuptake inhibitor.

higher. Doses at or above the upper limits are often needed for remission of symptoms. Clonazepam* can be given to patients without a history of substance abuse as needed, not to exceed 1.5 mg/d in divided doses. If this dose is not adequate or the patient has a history of substance abuse, alternative medications may be used such as buspirone (BuSpar),* valproic acid (Depakote),* and gabapentin (Neurontin*—keep the dose below 1800 mg because some dependence may be evident above this dose). Agitation or other psychotic symptoms are treated with low dosages of an atypical antipsychotic medication (e.g., risperidone [Risperdal], olanzapine [Zyprexa], quetiapine [Seroquel]).

Several medications are useful augmenters of SSRIs. Trazodone (Desyrel),* 25 to 150 mg, makes a safe, nonaddicting sleeping pill that also has anxiolytic effects. Studies in Italy have shown trazodone, 25 mg three times daily (tid), to be equivalent to diazepam (Valium), 5 mg tid, for treatment of anxiety. Buspirone, 15 to 30 mg bid, is particularly helpful in alcoholic patients and as an add-on with SSRIs for residual *generalized anxiety.* Start with 7.5 mg bid taken with food to reduce the major side effect of dizziness. Quetiapine (Seroquel), 25 to 100 mg, can help with *agitation* and severe anxiety when clonazepam is not adequate. In *OCD,* severe obsessing, racing thoughts often benefit from low-dose risperidone, 0.5 to 1 mg at bedtime.

Generalized anxiety disorder occurs in two major forms. The first has an obsessional quality and is associated with panic-like symptoms. This form is best treated with an SSRI augmented, if needed, by one of the aforementioned medications. The second form has an agitated and depressive quality. The worrying takes the form of elaborate negative dwelling as opposed to repetitive obsessing. These patients are generally more dysfunctional. This more severe generalized anxiety disorder is best treated with a dual reuptake inhibitor such as venlafaxine (Effexor XR, 75 to 225 mg in the AM) or a tricyclic antidepressant (e.g., nortriptyline [Aventyl],* 50 to 150 mg). These agents are good for treating migraines, fibromyalgia, chronic pain, and the irritable bowel–associated diarrhea that often accompanies anxiety disorders.

Emergent *depressive symptoms* are common in patients with anxiety. Some patients will return after several months of successful treatment and report that the medication has stopped working. Careful evaluation usually finds that the anxiety symptoms are in good control but the patient is suffering from low motivation, low energy, and other depressive symptoms. These symptoms can be treated with the addition of a

*Not FDA approved for this indication.

*Not FDA approved for this indication.

norepinephrine agent such as bupropion (Wellbutrin SR, 150 to 300 mg) or Effexor XR. If given alone, these medications have a high likelihood of worsening the anxiety, but their energizing norepinephrine effect is balanced by combination with an anxiety-reducing serotonergic agent. When starting Wellbutrin SR, 150 mg, the dose of SSRI can be reduced by half. If the anxiety worsens, the SSRI is returned to the original dose. If the depression has not remitted, Wellbutrin SR is raised to 150 mg bid or Effexor XR is tried with a target dose of 225 mg/d. An adequate trial of Effexor XR requires a dose of at least 225 mg to obtain enough norepinephrine effect to treat the depression. Some patients get too anxious with this higher dose of Effexor and may benefit from a combination of low-dose Effexor with an SSRI (Table 1).

CONCLUSION

Anxiety can be a symptom of many different conditions ranging from situational conflicts to psychotic disorders. Careful assessment is needed at the initial evaluation, as well as at each follow-up visit. Serotonin appears to be the primary neurotransmitter regulating the anxiety level, panic, and OCD. Norepinephrine and dopamine are involved in motivation, drive, and agitation. Effective treatment involves finding the right balance of neurotransmitter effect and attention to symptom shifts during treatment. Most anxious patients require a combination of medications and psychotherapy for the best outcome.

BULIMIA NERVOSA

method of
JOEL YAGER, M.D.
University of New Mexico School of Medicine
Albuquerque, New Mexico

Although *bulimia nervosa* as now conceptualized was first described in the 1950s, interest in the disorder has grown considerably as its prevalence has increased greatly. In recent years, many female celebrities suffering from bulimia nervosa have been highly publicized, so virtually every girl and woman in the United States is aware of these disorders and their dangers.

EPIDEMIOLOGY

The lifetime prevalence among women ranges from 1.1% to 4.2%. Subclinical cases are much more prevalent; individual symptoms such as binge eating, restrictive dieting, purging, laxative and diuretic abuse, and compulsive exercise are seen in 20% to 30% of some female subgroups such as members of select college sororities or gymnasts. In clinical settings, 90% to 95% of cases are in girls and women, but in some community samples, the percentage of male patients may reach 20% to 30%.

DIAGNOSIS AND CLINICAL FEATURES

Diagnosis requires: (1) recurrent episodes of binge eating, consisting of consuming much more food than most people would eat during a similar discrete period of time (e.g., 2 hours) and under similar circumstances; (2) sensing that during the episode one's eating is out of control, with an inability to stop or control what or how much one is eating; (3) recurrent inappropriate compensatory behavior to prevent weight gain, such as self-induced vomiting; misuse of laxatives, diuretics, enemas, or other medications; fasting; or excessive exercise; and (4) personal self-evaluation unduly influenced by body shape and weight. Furthermore, eating binges and inappropriate compensatory behaviors must both occur, on average, at least twice a week for 3 months. The *purging type* of bulimia nervosa requires self-induced vomiting or the misuse of laxatives, diuretics, or enemas. The *nonpurging type* requires the use of other inappropriate compensatory behaviors, such as fasting or excessive exercise, but it lacks the purging behaviors mentioned earlier. If the disturbances occur exclusively during episodes of anorexia nervosa, the diagnosis is more appropriately *anorexia nervosa, binge-eating/purging type.*

Binge eating disorder, a syndrome essentially meeting criteria for binge eating without compensatory behaviors and closely corresponding to *compulsive overeating*, is currently diagnosed as an "Eating Disorder Not Otherwise Specified."

Bulimia nervosa typically starts in the teens and early adulthood, but later onsets occur. This disorder now appears to be evenly distributed across socioeconomic groups and is seen commonly in different racial groups.

Although bulimia nervosa and anorexia nervosa are separate disorders, they often appear in a continuum of self-starvation and binge-purge cycles: up to 50% of patients with anorexia nervosa have binge eating and purging symptoms, and many patients with bulimia nervosa previously experienced at least subclinical forms of anorexia nervosa. Weight preoccupation and body dissatisfaction are common to both disorders. However, many patients with bulimia nervosa never have anorexia nervosa but, in contrast, were previously overweight.

Eating binges often entail at least 2000 kcal of high-calorie foods per binge, some as high as 10,000 kcal. Aside from eating binges, most patients eat restricted diets containing fewer calories than are required for energy and weight maintenance. Self-induced vomiting occurs in about 80%, and about 30% to 40% misuse laxatives or diuretics (notoriously ineffective for losing calories, but effective at causing fluid and electrolyte depletion, thereby reducing weight quickly). Some patients exercise compulsively for hours daily. Although criteria require binge-purge episodes at least twice per week for 3 consecutive months, many patients seeking care binge and purge daily or multiple times per day, often for years. Patients are typically ashamed and secretive about these problems. When untreated, the disorder is often chronic, lasting years to decades, but some degree of spontaneous improvement may occur. Outcomes related to treatment are discussed later.

ASSOCIATED MEDICAL FINDINGS

Patients may develop significant medical complications, especially if they are undernourished, most notably gastrointestinal, metabolic, and cardiac abnormalities. Serum amylase elevations of 10% to 40% (largely of salivary gland origin) may serve as crude indicators of vomiting activity. Dehydration with hypokalemic, hypochloremic alkalosis may result from vomiting and laxative use, and it may require rehydration and electrolyte replacement. Long-term ipecac use to induce vomiting may result in toxic myopathies, cardiomyopathy, and death. Esophageal and gastric irritation and bleeding may occur; rarely, death has resulted from esophageal or gastric rupture. Laxative abuse may damage haustral muscles in the large intestine and may result in pseudo-Hirschsprung's bowel dysfunction. Long-term anthraquinone-containing laxative misuse may cause melanosis coli and possibly increased rates of colon cancer. When chronic, severe laxative and/or diuretic use is terminated abruptly, patients may develop significant bloating and edema, with rapid gains of 10 to 15 lb. Hypomagnesemia and hypophosphatemia, especially in laxative abusers, may contribute to neuropathic or central nervous system symptoms. Menstrual irregularities and amenorrhea are frequently seen, even in patients of normal weight.

Common physical findings include: (1) chubby facial appearance ("squirrel facies"), resulting from edematous benign hyperplasia of overstimulated parotid and sublingual glands; (2) caries, most notably of the front teeth, resulting from enamel erosion by vomitus-associated gastric acid; and (3) scarred dorsal surfaces of the hands near the knuckles, resulting from dental abrasions associated with repeated self-induced vomiting.

CONCURRENT PSYCHIATRIC CONDITIONS

Patients seen at treatment centers frequently have multiple psychiatric co-morbidities. Co-morbid major depressions and/or dysthymias occur in 50% to 75%, anxiety disorders in 30% to 43%, chemical dependency in 30% to 37%, and personality disorders or notable personality trait disturbances in 42% to 75%. Sexual abuse has been reported in 20% to 50%. Up to 15% of patients, described as "multi-impulsive," suffer from low frustration tolerance and impulsivity involving money, sex, anger, and self-mutilation.

Dysfunctional families are common. Substance abuse and mood disorders occur in more than 30% of first-degree relatives, and obesity and obsessive-compulsive disorders occur frequently in these families. Female relatives are at a 4 to 12 times increased risk of eating disorders.

ETIOLOGY AND PATHOGENESIS

Theories explaining bulimia nervosa have implicated biologic, psychological, and social causes.

Biologic Theories

Higher concordance in monozygotic (more than 50%) than dizygotic (14% to 27%) twins suggests genetic factors, although the nature of inherited vulnerabilities is obscure. Eating disorders are transmitted in families, but familial transmission alone may reflect environmental as well as genetic influences. Abnormalities concerning serotonin, opioid peptides, and various stress hormones have been proposed. However, studies involving patients who have fully recovered in terms of weight and behavior virtually always show these parameters returning to normal.

Because of frequent co-occurrence, bulimia nervosa has been proposed as a "variant" of mood disorders or obsessive-compulsive disorders. Prior tendencies toward obesity may contribute. Aside from these theories, the major biologic stimulus leading to binge eating involves self-imposed hunger resulting from restrictive eating.

Psychological Theories

Numerous factors have been suggested. Vulnerability may be related to temperamental and constitutional factors including proneness toward shyness, timidity, anxiety, and perfectionism. Further difficulties may be fostered by problematic parenting including various degrees of neglect as well as psychological, physical, and sexual abuse. Some families communicate destructively, in which vulnerable family members are strongly criticized and are blamed for all family difficulties, including their disorders.

Because many families use food for stress reduction, some children learn to reduce tension and frustration by eating excessively, maladaptive responses involving classical or operant conditioning. The anxieties generated by eating binges are, in turn, relieved by purging. Patients may also learn to seek associated sensations including heightened arousal with binge-eating, abdominal distention after a binge, and feelings of emptying or emptiness with purging.

Poor self-esteem, low self-worth, and pervasive shame have been associated with teasing about appearance in childhood (by parents, other relatives, peers), and may be associated with distorted self-perceptions (e.g., tendency to misperceive oneself as much fatter than in reality), which bring on ruminative negative thoughts leading to disparaged physical appearance and destructive eating patterns. Examples include such thoughts as: "If I gain 1 lb, everyone will notice how fat and ugly I am," and "I overate a little, so now it doesn't matter and I'll let myself go whole hog." Patients may also show distorted interocepts (e.g., difficulty in realistically identifying sensations involving hunger and satiety) and difficulties in accurately identifying and acknowledging some emotional states (e.g., anger).

Adolescents less competent to deal with age-related tasks involving identity development, life direction, separating from family, and sexual pressures may feel overwhelmed and may resort to the immature coping of bulimic behaviors.

Social and Cultural Factors

These disorders have increased dramatically in recent decades, paralleling society's increased valuing of thinner fashion models and female celebrities. Although no single factor accounts for all findings, many find support in clinical observations, and each has informed interventions.

ASSESSMENT AND MANAGEMENT: THE ROLE OF THE PRIMARY PHYSICIAN

Primary care physicians play major roles in prevention, detection, and management:

1. Given the high prevalence of subclinical as well as full-syndrome bulimia nervosa, primary physicians should remain alert to excessive concerns about dieting and appearance in young female patients; physicians should routinely question them about their desired weights, dieting and exercise practices, and use of laxatives; and they should educate these patients about healthy nutrition and the dangers of unrealistic dieting. Young women with mood disorders, anxiety, substance abuse, and other psychological problems are at particular risk for eating disorders.
2. Danger signs include compulsive eating, menstrual irregularities, desire to lose 10 to 15 lb more than reasonable, overconcern with weight or physical appearance, misuse of laxatives or diuretics, psychological disturbances, and any of the characteristic physical findings described earlier.
3. Once bulimia nervosa is suspected, patients merit a physical examination and laboratory tests including electrolytes, blood count, thyroid, calcium, magnesium, and amylase and, for thin patients, an electrocardiogram. Occult laxative abuse may be detected by stool examination for phenolphthalein.
4. Psychiatric consultation and referral: Most patients with serious eating disorders warrant consultation with a psychiatrist or psychologist knowledgeable about eating disorders to guide the patient, family, and physicians about the nature, severity, and prognosis of the disorder, treatment options; and recommendations for psychosocial and medical management. Consultation is mandatory when patients fail to respond to competent attempts at outpatient management, when psychological and/or physical status deteriorates, and when severe depression, suicidal ideation, and/or significant family problems are present.
5. General treatment strategies: Primary care physicians work conjointly with mental health professionals and dietitians knowledgeable about eating disorders to develop comprehensive outpatient programs. With motivated patients, such team approaches are quite successful. The primary care physician's role is to educate, counsel, refer, and monitor physical status and laboratory tests and, in the absence of psychiatric involvement, to prescribe and monitor antidepressant medications if indicated. Primary care physicians vary considerably in willingness and ability to assume more intense involvement with psychological and family issues.

TREATMENT OPTIONS

Treatment planning starts with comprehensive assessment, and the strategies employed in a given patient should be targeted to nutrition and physical status, eating behaviors, emotions and thoughts, and related psychiatric and family problems. Treatment usually includes education, dietary counseling, cognitive-behavioral therapy (CBT) and other psychotherapies, and often medications. The best outcomes have been associated with combinations of CBT and medications. If they are not used concurrently from the start and a patient shows little response to CBT alone in a month or so, medications should be strongly considered. Many clinicians start with medication as well as therapy, particularly if a patient is depressed or anxious or has a family history of depression. The best programs combine these elements pragmatically. The following discussion is organized around the management of problems related to specific eating disorders.

Nutritional and Physical Status

Dietary interventions and behavior change usually deal with these problems satisfactorily. Weight optimization should be a central, early goal in treating underweight patients; management includes frank discussions of the patient's motivations and of healthy and desirable weight ranges. Patients with clear biologic and familial tendencies to be overweight may need to gain some weight, usually 5 to 10 lb, if their food obsessions, binge episodes, and moodiness are to subside; this weight is usually far less than patients fear, but more than they desire.

Bingeing, Purging, and Overexercise Behaviors

Nutritional counseling, CBT, and psychopharmacologic interventions are frequently combined. Some excellent "guided self-help" books based on CBT principles are readily available, and up to 20% of patients make significant improvement through working with these programs independently. Patients do better working at these programs with a trained clinician as a guide. More intensive outpatient programs for bulimia nervosa are also employed in which patients attend various highly structured group programs several hours each day for several weeks.

Typical CBT programs require 12 to 20 weekly or biweekly sessions, followed by half a year to a year of monthly sessions, to bolster relapse prevention during times that patients are most likely to have a relapse. Patients are actively educated about weight regulation, dieting, and the adverse consequences of bulimia, and they develop and practice specified eating plans. Treatment starts by establishing the patient's control over eating using such techniques as *self-monitoring* (keeping detailed symptom-relevant diaries), *exposure plus response prevention* (eating until satiated without being allowed to purge), *prescribing patterns of regular eating*, and *stimulus* (or *"cue"*) *control measures* (avoiding situations likely to stimulate binges). These interventions often alleviate many symptoms, partly by reducing the hunger that stimulates binges.

Distorted and Maladaptive Thoughts and Emotions

CBT treatments next attempt to restructure patients' unrealistic and distorted thoughts (e.g., assumptions and expectations) and to instill more effective modes of coping. Other psychological techniques including interpersonal psychotherapies have proven effectiveness, and some psychodynamic therapies may be useful. Interpersonal psychotherapy (IPT) is a brief, evidence-based therapy focusing on clarifying and resolving interpersonal disputes, actual and imagined losses, grief, and complicated bereavement, role transitions such as moving away to college, and interpersonal deficits, essentially personality quirks that interfere with fulfilling relationships. Although short-term results with CBT offer greater symptom improvement, IPT also yields good results over the long run. In practice, most clinicians combine elements of both CBT and IPT. Furthermore, most CBT and IPT programs use important psychodynamic psychotherapy principles, acknowledging and attending to psychological resistances, conflicts, and distortions. After initial nutritional, behavioral, and cognitive-emotional problems are resolved, further treatment emphasizes maintaining gains and preventing relapse through prescriptive relapse prevention techniques.

The overall success rate of these methods varies considerably. For those completing the programs, about 50% to 90% experience about 70% reduction in bingeing and purging frequency. About one third become fully symptom-free. In long-term follow-up, 70% to 75% of those treated maintain recovery, although some recidivism is seen, particularly at times of severe stress.

Associated Psychiatric Problems

These problems are also assessed and managed with psychotherapies and medications as indicated.

Psychopharmacologic Approaches

The largest controlled studies have shown selective serotonin reuptake inhibitors to be effective in treating bulimia nervosa by achieving reductions of 50% to 75% in rates of bingeing and vomiting; complete abstinence occurs only in about 30% of patients treated with medication alone. Furthermore, higher doses, such as 60 mg/d of fluoxetine (Prozac), are more effective than doses of 20 mg/d, the usual antidepressant dose. Many older controlled studies showed that tricyclic antidepressants (particularly imipramine [Tofranil]* and desipramine [Norpramin]* in doses of 200 to 300 mg/d), monoamine oxidase inhibitors (particularly phenelzine [Nardil]* at 60 to 90 mg/d and isocarboxizid [Marplan]* at 60 mg/d), and trazodone (Desyrel),* at 200 to 400 mg/d, were also useful in bulimia nervosa, but they are less commonly prescribed because of their adverse effects. Common problems include medication noncompliance and maintenance of adequate serum levels in the presence of persistent vomiting. The antidepressant bupropion is associated with an increased seizure risk and is contraindicated in actively purging patients.

Hospitalization

Hospitalization is rarely necessary for patients with uncomplicated bulimia nervosa. Indications to hospitalize patients include failure to respond to adequate outpatient treatment trials, other worrisome medical complications not manageable in outpatient settings, and other psychiatric indications such as suicidal ideation.

SUGGESTED READINGS

American Psychiatric Association: Practice guideline for the treatment of patients with eating disorders (revision). Am J Psychiatry 157(Suppl):1-39, 2000 (http://www.psych.org/clin_res/guide.bk.cfm).

Hay P, Bacaltchuk J: Bulimia nervosa. Clin Evid 7:834-845, 2002.

*Not FDA approved for this indication.

DELIRIUM

method of
JAMES A. BOURGEOIS, O.D., M.D., and
ROBERT E. HALES, M.D.
University of California, Davis, Medical Center
Sacramento, California

DEFINITION

Delirium is classified in the current psychiatric nomenclature system in the *Diagnostic and Statistical Manual of Mental Disorders* (DSM-IV-TR) as a cognitive disorder. Unlike most dementia syndromes (with which it is frequently co-morbid), delirium is usually an episodic illness with an acute to subacute onset. The symptoms of delirium often have a fluctuating course and typically resolve once the associated precipitating systemic disturbance is corrected. Because of the systemic context of its clinical features, delirium is best conceptualized as "neuropsychiatric expression of systemic illness" with symptoms that call for aggressive evaluation and management strategies.

EPIDEMIOLOGY

The risk of delirium developing increases with age, complexity of the medical and/or surgical illness, and the use of medications. In addition, the risk is increased by central nervous system abnormalities such as dementia, Parkinson's disease, and traumatic brain injury. Other high-risk states for delirium include post-cardiotomy status, severe burns, and prolonged stay in the intensive care unit.

ETIOLOGY

Delirium may be conceptualized as a disturbance in the "body-brain circuit" (Figure 1). As such, any "local" disturbance in cardiac, respiratory, renal, hepatic, vascular, or cerebral function and/or any "systemic" disturbance such as anemia, infection, shock, poisoning, medications, or drug intoxication/withdrawal may lead to delirium. Less dramatic and thus often less obvious to the clinician are the "psychophysiologic" contributors to delirium, including factors such as sleep deprivation, sensory deprivation, social isolation, and rapid, discontinuous changes in the patient's environment.

PATHOPHYSIOLOGY

Functionally, delirium can be descriptively understood as a syndrome of acetylcholine deficiency combined with dopamine excess. This model accounts for the derangement in cognitive function (functional acetylcholine deficit) plus the intrusion of actively psychotic symptoms such as hallucinations and delusions (functional dopamine excess). Delirium following exposure to anticholinergic agents and the treatment of delirium with antipsychotic agents support this acetylcholine deficiency–dopamine excess model. However, this model fails to fully account for the variable manifestations of delirium, as well as the role of pharmacologic agents not acting through dopamine or acetylcholine mechanisms (e.g., benzodiazepines) to be useful treatments of delirium.

CLINICAL SIGNS AND SYMPTOMS

According to DSM-IV-TR, clinical features required for a diagnosis of delirium include the following:

1. Disturbance in consciousness with a reduced ability to focus, sustain, or shift attention

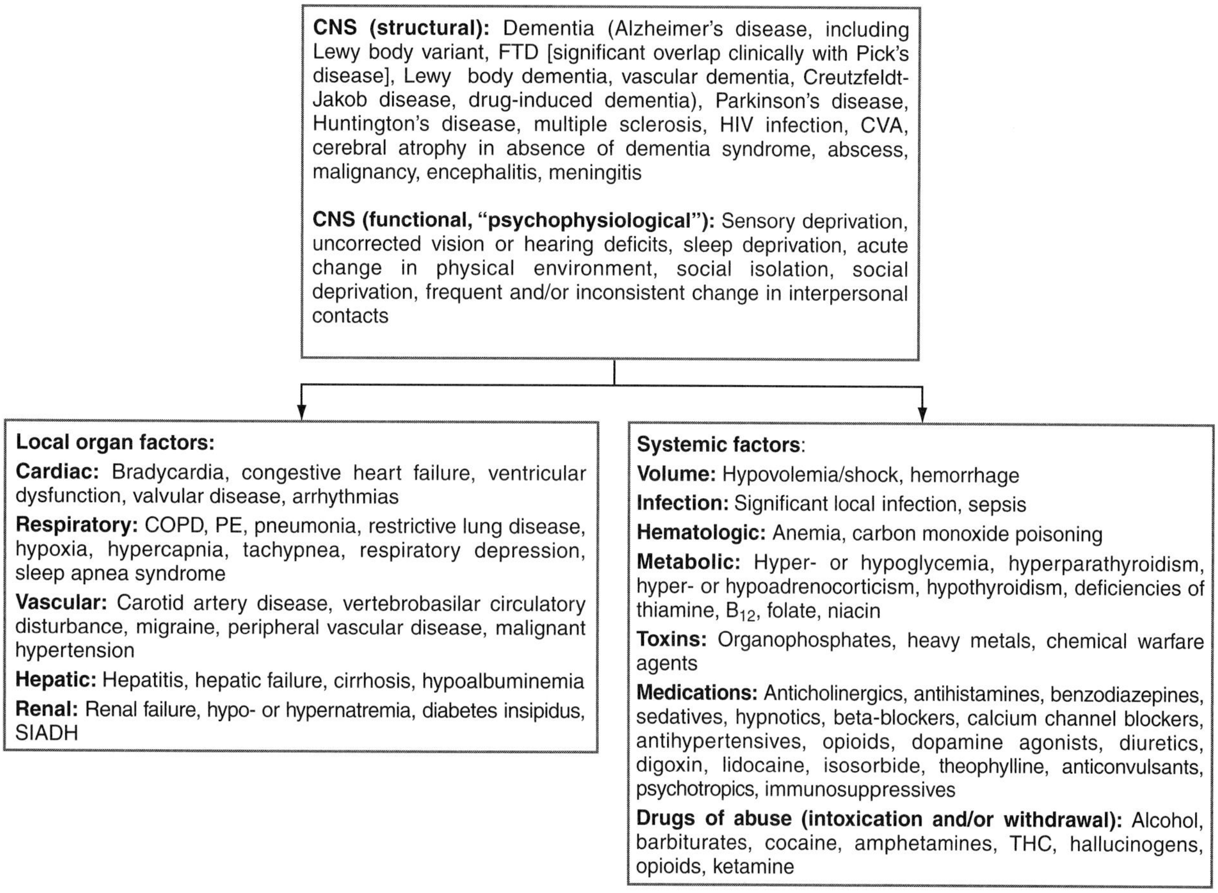

CNS (structural): Dementia (Alzheimer's disease, including Lewy body variant, FTD [significant overlap clinically with Pick's disease], Lewy body dementia, vascular dementia, Creutzfeldt-Jakob disease, drug-induced dementia), Parkinson's disease, Huntington's disease, multiple sclerosis, HIV infection, CVA, cerebral atrophy in absence of dementia syndrome, abscess, malignancy, encephalitis, meningitis

CNS (functional, "psychophysiological"): Sensory deprivation, uncorrected vision or hearing deficits, sleep deprivation, acute change in physical environment, social isolation, social deprivation, frequent and/or inconsistent change in interpersonal contacts

Local organ factors:

Cardiac: Bradycardia, congestive heart failure, ventricular dysfunction, valvular disease, arrhythmias

Respiratory: COPD, PE, pneumonia, restrictive lung disease, hypoxia, hypercapnia, tachypnea, respiratory depression, sleep apnea syndrome

Vascular: Carotid artery disease, vertebrobasilar circulatory disturbance, migraine, peripheral vascular disease, malignant hypertension

Hepatic: Hepatitis, hepatic failure, cirrhosis, hypoalbuminemia

Renal: Renal failure, hypo- or hypernatremia, diabetes insipidus, SIADH

Systemic factors:

Volume: Hypovolemia/shock, hemorrhage

Infection: Significant local infection, sepsis

Hematologic: Anemia, carbon monoxide poisoning

Metabolic: Hyper- or hypoglycemia, hyperparathyroidism, hyper- or hypoadrenocorticism, hypothyroidism, deficiencies of thiamine, B_{12}, folate, niacin

Toxins: Organophosphates, heavy metals, chemical warfare agents

Medications: Anticholinergics, antihistamines, benzodiazepines, sedatives, hypnotics, beta-blockers, calcium channel blockers, antihypertensives, opioids, dopamine agonists, diuretics, digoxin, lidocaine, isosorbide, theophylline, anticonvulsants, psychotropics, immunosuppressives

Drugs of abuse (intoxication and/or withdrawal): Alcohol, barbiturates, cocaine, amphetamines, THC, hallucinogens, opioids, ketamine

Figure 1. Central nervous system, local organ, and systemic factors in delirium. CNS, central nervous system; COPD, chronic obstructive pulmonary disease; CVA, cerebrovascular accident; FTD, frontotemporal dementia; HIV, human immunodeficiency virus; PE, pulmonary embolism; SIADH, syndrome of inappropriate antidiuretic hormone secretion; THC, tetrohydrocannabinol.

2. Change in cognition or development of a perceptual disturbance not better accounted for by dementia
3. Symptoms developing over a short period and fluctuating during the course of a day
4. Symptoms that are a direct physiologic consequence of a general medical condition

Specific subtypes of delirium described in DSM-IV-TR include (1) delirium caused by substance intoxication, (2) delirium resulting from substance withdrawal, (3) delirium caused by multiple etiologies, and (4) delirium not otherwise specified. Though not included in DSM-IV-TR, patients with delirium can manifest symptoms in either a hyperactive or hypoactive state. "Hyperactive" delirium is characterized by psychomotor agitation, restlessness, decreased sleep, more dramatic hallucinations, and acting-out behavior. "Hypoactive" delirium symptoms include excessive sleep, decreased psychomotor activity, and relatively greater cognitive impairment. The hyperactive type is more likely to come to clinical attention early in a hospitalization because of the patient's more disruptive behavior. The hypoactive type may initially escape detection unless physicians and nurses incorporate cognitive screening examinations into routine practice.

TABLE 1. **Clinical Workup of Delirium**

History of present illness
History of medication/drug exposure
Description of psychiatric symptoms
Mental status examination: Appearance/behavior, speech/language, thought process and content, mood and affect, quantitative assessment of cognitive status with a standardized instrument (e.g., MMSE), judgment/insight
Correction/reversal of metabolic/structural/infectious/functional etiology
Avoidance/minimization of "delirogenic" medications, e.g., anticholinergics, antihistamines, opioids, β-blockers, calcium channel blockers, dopamine agonists
Laboratory tests: Electrolytes, BUN/Cr, liver function tests, albumin, PT/PTT, TSH, vitamin B_{12}, folate, UA, toxicology, NH_4, GGTP, CBC/differential, ABG, pulse oximetry, CSF analysis; drug levels of TCAs, digoxin, theophylline, anticonvulsants, acetaminophen, and ASA; blood, urine cultures; CSF analysis/culture in selected cases
Radiology: CT of the head (unenhanced is generally adequate), MRI of the head, CXR; cardiac and carotid ultrasound in selected cases
Other assessments: ECG and CXR, with EEG considered in ambiguous cases; the role of functional neuroimaging (SPECT, PET scanning) awaits definition and is not universally available

ABG, arterial blood gases; ASA, acetylsalicylic acid; BUN, blood urea nitrogen; CBC, complete blood count; Cr, creatinine; CSF, cerebrospinal fluid; CT, computed tomography; CXR, chest x-ray; ECG, electrocardiography; EEG, electroencephalography; GGTP, γ-glutamyl transpeptidase; MMSE, Mini-Mental State Examination; PET, positron emission tomography; PT, prothrombin time; PTT, partial thromboplastin time; SPECT, single photon emission computed tomography; TCA, tricyclic antidepressant; TSH, thyroid-stimulating hormone; UA, urinalysis.

EVALUATION AND MANAGEMENT

Evaluation and management of delirium are approached differently from other psychiatric illnesses for two reasons. First, evaluation of delirium is intimately commingled with assessment of the associated systemic condition. As such, the physician should take a thorough and systems-based approach, as described in Table 1. Second, evaluation of delirium is inextricably linked with clinical management, and a patient's response to treatment interventions should guide further evaluation.

The clinical history should focus on the sequences of clinical events (e.g., new-onset illnesses, medication changes, environmental alterations) temporally connected with the emergence of delirium symptoms. A history of cognitive impairment and/or previous episodes of delirium are especially important variables that may indicate a pattern of vulnerability to delirium.

With regard to laboratory and radiologic testing, it is better to obtain a number of "screening" laboratory studies of blood and urine, pulse oximetry/arterial blood gases, chest radiography, and electrocardiography (Table 1). Neuroimaging need not be obtained early in every case, but it should be readily performed if the delirium does not resolve when a clear precipitant is corrected. Delirium occurring in a patient at risk for dementia should increase the urgency to obtain a neuroimaging assessment even more. Usually, nonenhanced computed tomography of the head will be adequate. Other studies of supplemental value in certain more ambiguous cases of delirium include an electroencephalogram, cerebrospinal fluid studies, and when available, functional neuroimaging.

Management principles are outlined in Table 2 and include both behavioral and psychopharmacologic therapies. Behavioral management generally consists of provision of a safe and nonthreatening environment, external reality testing by staff, provision of external cueing to assist in reorientation, and simulation of a normal light-dark (hence sleep-wake) cycle. Psychopharmacologic interventions can be considered either symptom specific (e.g., antipsychotic* agents for psychotic symptoms) or nonspecific (e.g., combinations of antipsychotic* agents and benzodiazepines* for most routine cases of delirium). Doses of medications should be ordered on both a scheduled and an as-needed basis. It is generally best to treat delirium symptoms aggressively and to then wean medications to the lowest effective dose. Once delirium has resolved, medications should be maintained for several days and then discontinued for a period of medication-free observation.

For delirium caused by withdrawal from alcohol, benzodiazepines, or sedative/hypnotics, benzodiazepine* monotherapy in doses adequate to control the hyperadrenergic "rebound state" is often adequate. If psychotic symptoms are noted, antipsychotic agents should be added. In patients with delirium caused by a different etiology or by multiple etiologies, an antipsychotic* agent plus adjunctive use of a benzodiazepine* is preferred. When needed, combination therapy has a synergistic effect, and the total medication burden may be much less than if a single agent were used. Some patients are at risk for QT_c prolongation as a result of antipsychotic therapy, so electrocardiographic

*Not FDA approved for this indication.

TABLE 2. **Management of Delirium**

Behavioral: Constant observation, consideration of restraints for safety, vital signs and behavioral/mental status assessment every 4 h, reorientation of patient on every encounter, judicious use of radio/TV/other electronic media, placement near window, alteration of ambient light levels to simulate light/dark cycle, placement of familiar objects in room, regular visitation by family and friends

Psychopharmacologic: Lower doses may be needed for elderly patients, those with neurologic illnesses, and "hypoactive" symptoms.

Benzodiazepines for sedative/hypnotic, alcohol, or benzodiazepine withdrawal: Short–half-life agent, e.g., lorazepam (Ativan),* 1-4 mg IV/IM/PO q6h on schedule plus the same dose q4h prn for continued withdrawal symptoms. Titrate to effect; increase the dose for agitation, and decrease the dose for sedation.

Antipsychotics with consideration of adjunctive use of benzodiazepines for most cases of delirium: High-potency antipsychotic, e.g., haloperidol (Haldol),* 5 mg IV/IM/PO q6h on schedule plus q4h prn for continued symptoms; titrate dose to effect. Cases of "hypoactive" delirium and delirium in elderly/demented patients may respond to a lower starting dose of haloperidol,* e.g., 1 mg q12h. If antipsychotic monotherapy fails to control delirium symptoms, combination therapy consisting of haloperidol, 5 mg, plus lorazepam,* 1 mg IV/IM/PO q6h, on schedule plus q4h prn for continued symptoms. Titrate to effect, increase dose(s) for continued symptoms, and decrease dose(s) for excess sedation. Monitor electrocardiogram for increased QT_c. An evolving approach is atypical antipsychotic(s) in lieu of haloperidol because of a lower risk of extrapyramidal side effects and generally greater tolerability. Risperidone (Risperdal),* 2 mg; olanzapine (Zyprexa),* 5 mg; and quetiapine (Seroquel),* 25 mg, have an effect approximately equivalent to that of haloperidol, 5 mg. These agents are available only in PO form, although risperidone is available in an elixir and olanzapine in a rapidly dissolving tablet (Zyprexa Zydis). Ziprasidone (Geodon),* 10 mg PO q6h, is available both PO and IM and may be an atypical parenteral choice for NPO patients.

Alternative medications for specific circumstances: These uses are considered anecdotal. (1) Valproate (Depacon),* 10-15 mg/kg/24 h IV in bid dosing for delirium in cases in which benzodiazepines are excessively sedating and/or antipsychotics are associated with cardiac conduction defects. (2) Donepezil (Aricept),* 5-10 mg/d PO for cases of anticholinergic toxicity and/or pre-existing dementia. (3) Chloral hydrate (generic only),* 500-1000 mg PO qhs for persistent nighttime insomnia and agitation refractory to conventional management.

Post-recovery psychiatric workup: Thorough examination for predisposing psychiatric illness, specifically, dementia, psychotic disorders, amnestic disorders, and substance-induced illness.

*Not FDA approved for this indication.

monitoring is needed. Because of persistent systemic illness (e.g., chronic liver failure and disseminated malignancy), certain patients may be at risk for chronic delirium, and they may be candidates for continued psychopharmacologic treatment. In such cases, antipsychotics should be continued and benzodiazepines discontinued.

The post-delirium period is a critical one. The cognitive examination should be repeated, and any persistent cognitive deficits should lead to a workup for dementia and consideration of psychopharmacologic interventions. The recovered patient should also be examined for residual psychotic symptoms. If present, the diagnosis of a psychotic disorder should be assumed and the patient given an extended course of treatment with an atypical antipsychotic agent.

MOOD DISORDERS

method of
JAMES M. MARTINEZ, M.D., and
LAUREN B. MARANGELL, M.D.
Baylor College of Medicine
Houston, Texas

MAJOR DEPRESSIVE DISORDER

Major depressive disorder is a common, brain-based disorder that is distinct from normal sadness. By definition, major depressive episodes last 2 weeks or more, although most last months to years. Symptoms include persistent feelings of sadness or loss of interest in and pleasure from usual activities, with disruptions in sleep, energy level, concentration, appetite, and motor activity. Symptom severity is sufficient to cause subjective distress or functional impairment. Associated features include feelings of helplessness, hopelessness, worthlessness, excessive guilt or self-blame, anxiety, and suicidal thoughts. In severe depression, psychotic symptoms may be present, such as auditory hallucinations or delusional beliefs.

Major depressive disorder affects up to 12% of boys and men and 20% to 25% of girls and women at some point during their lives. The disorder often begins in early adulthood and follows a chronic, recurrent course. As such, it is a major cause of disability worldwide and is associated with significant individual, familial, and societal costs. Common co-morbid psychiatric illnesses include anxiety disorders and substance abuse. The prevalence of major depressive disorder increases as medical co-morbidity increases. Data suggest that co-morbid major depressive disorder worsens the morbidity and mortality of nonpsychiatric illnesses, such as cardiovascular disease. This article provides an overview of treatments for major depressive disorder.

Pharmacologic Treatments

All available antidepressants facilitate monoamine neurotransmission, although the mechanisms by which these changes lead to an antidepressant response are unknown and likely involve changes in second-messenger systems and gene transcription. Antidepressants are categorized according to their specific actions on monoamine receptors, reuptake pumps, or catabolic enzymes, typically for serotonin and/or norepinephrine. The major classes of antidepressants and their available formulations are shown in Table 1.

Selective Serotonin Reuptake Inhibitors

The *selective serotonin reuptake inhibitors* (SSRIs) have been available in the United States since the 1980s. These agents are considered first-line antidepressants by many clinicians because of their once-daily dosing schedule (except fluvoxamine*), the minimal need for dose titration, relative safety in overdose, improved

*Not FDA approved for this indication.

TABLE 1. **Available Formulations of Selected Antidepressant Medications**

Medication (Trade Name)	Dosage Formulations
Selective Serotonin Reuptake Inhibitors	
Fluoxetine	
Immediate-release (Prozac, Sarafem)	10-, 20-, 40-mg capsules; 20 mg/5 mL liquid
Delayed-release (Prozac Weekly)	90-mg capsules
Sertraline (Zoloft)	25-, 50-, 100-mg tablets; 20 mg/mL liquid
Citalopram (Celexa)	10-, 20-, 40-mg tablets; 2 mg/mL liquid
Escitalopram (Lexapro)	5-, 10-, 20-mg tablets
Paroxetine	
Immediate-release (Paxil)	10-, 20-, 30-, 40-mg tablets; 10 mg/5 mL liquid
Controlled-release (Paxil CR)	12.5-, 25-, 37.5-mg tablets
Fluvoxamine (Luvox)	25-, 50-, 100-mg tablets
Newer Antidepressants	
Mirtazapine (Remeron, Remeron SolTab)	15-, 30-, 45-mg tablets
Bupropion	
Immediate-release (Wellbutrin)	75-, 100-mg tablets
Sustained-release (Wellbutrin SR)	100-, 150-, 200-mg tablets
Venlafaxine	
Immediate-release (Effexor)	25-, 37.5-, 50-, 75-, 100-mg tablets
Extended-release (Effexor XR)	37.5-, 75-, 150-mg capsules
Nefazodone (Serzone)	50-, 100-, 150-, 200-, 250-mg tablets
Trazodone (Desyrel)	50-, 100-, 150-, 300-mg tablets
Tricyclic Antidepressants	
Amitriptyline (Elavil, Endep)*	10-, 25-, 50-, 75-, 100-, 150-mg tablets
Clomipramine (Anafranil)	25-, 50-, 75-mg tablets
Desipramine (Norpramin)	10-, 25-, 50-, 75-, 100-, 150-mg tablets
Imipramine (Tofranil)	10-, 25-, 50-, 75-, 100-, 125-, 150-mg tablets
Nortriptyline (Aventyl, Pamelor)	10-, 25-, 50-, 75-mg capsules
Monoamine Oxidase Inhibitors	
Phenelzine (Nardil)	15-mg tablets
Tranylcypromine (Parnate)	10-mg tablets

*Not available in the United States.

tolerability compared with tricyclic antidepressants (TCAs) and monoamine oxidase inhibitors (MAOIs), and broad spectrum of efficacy in treating other disorders, including many major anxiety disorders.

The SSRIs potently and selectively block the presynaptic reuptake of serotonin without significant antihistaminic, anti–α-adrenergic, and antimuscarinic effects. Most side effects are transient and include nausea, vomiting, diarrhea or constipation, headaches, insomnia or somnolence, sweating, anxiety, and vivid dreams. Dose-related sexual side effects, such as decreased libido or delayed ejaculation in men and anorgasmia in women, are also common and typically do not resolve without intervention. Management strategies for treatment-related sexual dysfunction, although not well-studied, include SSRI dose reduction and the addition of (or switch to) antidepressants not associated with sexual dysfunction, such as bupropion (Wellbutrin, Wellbutrin SR), nefazodone (Serzone), or mirtazapine (Remeron). Other management strategies include the addition of a psychostimulant,* sildenafil* (Viagra) or buspirone (Buspar).*

An uncomfortable, although not life-threatening, discontinuation syndrome of flulike symptoms, including nausea, irritability, anxiety, paresthesias, and muscle aches, can occur after the abrupt cessation of SSRIs with short half-lives (e.g., paroxetine). This syndrome can be minimized by gradually tapering the dose when discontinuing an SSRI.

An apathy syndrome with symptoms of decreased initiative and a sense of emotional blunting or "flatness" has been described with the long-term use of SSRIs. This syndrome can be distinguished from a recurrence of depression based on the absence of sadness and neurovegetative signs and symptoms of depression. The underlying mechanism of this syndrome is unknown, but it may involve serotonergic modulation of frontal lobe dopamine activity. Management strategies include SSRI dose reduction or the addition of a stimulant* or olanzapine (Zyprexa).* This syndrome should be distinguished from a recurrence or exacerbation of depressive symptoms, which would warrant an SSRI dose increase or another intervention aimed at targeting depression.

Although SSRIs share serotonin reuptake inhibition properties, a broad spectrum of efficacy, and some common side effects, the individual agents are structurally unrelated and have important differences in pharmacokinetic and pharmacodynamic properties, including the potential for drug-drug interactions (Table 2). Additionally, some persons may preferentially respond to one SSRI and not to another.

The SSRIs can be initiated at potentially effective dosages (see Table 3). Thus, the clinician should wait at least 4 weeks after initiating treatment to determine the degree of response before considering a dose escalation. If no response is seen within 4 weeks, an upward dose titration is indicated (increase by 10-mg increments for paroxetine and escitalopram, 10- to 20-mg increments for fluoxetine, 12.5-mg increments for paroxetine CR, 20-mg increments for citalopram, and 25- to 50-mg increments for sertraline). If a partial response is noted, the clinician should continue the SSRI at the given dose for an additional 2 to 3 weeks to see whether further improvement occurs and to avoid the risk of additional side effects. Patients taking fluoxetine 20 mg daily who wish to take the delayed-release formulation (Prozac Weekly) can be started on the 90-mg capsule approximately 7 days after the last dose of 20 mg.

Venlafaxine (Effexor, Effexor XR)

Venlafaxine inhibits presynaptic serotonin reuptake and, at higher therapeutic doses, norepinephrine reuptake. Advantages of venlafaxine include low protein binding and minimal hepatic cytochrome P-450

*Not FDA approved for this indication.

TABLE 2. **Pharmacokinetic and Pharmacodynamic Differences Among Selective Serotonin Reuptake Inhibitors**

Medication	Half-life* (h)	Protein Binding (%)	Cytochrome P-450 Enzyme Inhibition
Fluoxetine (Prozac)	4-16 d	>90%	2C9/10, 2C19, 2D6
Sertraline (Zoloft)	26-66 h	>90%	2D6
Citalopram (Celexa)	35 h	80%	None
Escitalopram (Lexapro)	27-32 h	56%	None
Paroxetine (Paxil)	21 h	>90%	2D6
Fluvoxamine (Luvox)	15 h	80%	1A2, 2C9/10, 2C19, 3A4

*Half-lives listed include active metabolites where applicable.

isoenzyme inhibition. Side effects are similar to those of the SSRIs, including sexual dysfunction, serious drug-drug interactions with MAOIs, and a discontinuation syndrome on abrupt cessation of the drug. Additionally, there is a dose-dependent risk of hypertension, particularly at daily doses of 300 mg or greater.

Venlafaxine is available in immediate- and extended-release formulations. The extended-release formulation is preferred because of once-daily dosing and improved tolerability. Unlike most SSRIs, venlafaxine appears to have a linear dose-response curve. Venlafaxine XR can be started at 75 mg once daily (37.5 mg/d if prominent anxiety is present) and increased in 75-mg increments on a weekly basis based on tolerability and response. The recommended dose range is 75 to 225 mg/d (see Table 3), although clinicians often titrate beyond this range, particularly if a partial response occurs within the recommended range.

Bupropion (Wellbutrin, Wellbutrin SR, Zyban)

Bupropion facilitates dopaminergic and noradrenergic neurotransmission without significant antihistaminic, antimuscarinic, and anti–α-adrenergic effects. Because of its lack of direct serotonergic activity, bupropion differs from the SSRIs in its spectrum of efficacy and side effect profile. Bupropion is generally well tolerated and does not cause sexual dysfunction or significant weight gain. Common side effects include agitation, headaches, insomnia, gastrointestinal upset, and dizziness. Bupropion is also associated with a risk of generalized seizures at high doses, a risk that can be minimized by following the recommended titration schedule and avoiding bupropion use in patients with an uncontrolled seizure disorder, a history of severe head trauma, and an active eating disorder or in combination with medications or substances of abuse that lower the seizure threshold. Bupropion is moderately protein bound and inhibits the hepatic cytochrome P-450 isoenzyme 2D6.

Bupropion is available in immediate- and sustained-release formulations. The sustained-release formulation (which allows for twice-daily dosing) can be initiated at 150 mg every morning and increased to 150 mg twice daily (with doses separated by at least 8 hours) no sooner than 4 days after starting treatment. The maximum daily dose of Wellbutrin SR is 200 mg twice daily, and no single dose should exceed 200 mg. Unlike the SSRIs, bupropion is not effective in treating co-morbid anxiety disorders. Bupropion should also be avoided in psychotic depression, because the facilitation of dopaminergic activity can worsen psychosis.

Mirtazapine (Remeron, Remeron SolTabs)

Mirtazapine facilitates noradrenergic and serotonergic neurotransmission by antagonizing presynaptic α_2-receptors. In addition, mirtazapine blocks postsynaptic serotonergic 5-HT-2 and 5-HT-3 receptors. Side effects may include prominent sedation and weight gain, dizziness, dry mouth, and constipation. There is also a rare risk of agranulocytosis. Mirtazapine lacks sexual side effects and significant cytochrome P-450 isoenzyme inhibition.

Mirtazapine can be initiated at 15 mg/night and titrated upward in 15-mg increments to a maximum dose of 45 mg/night. Patients should be informed of the potential for significant sedation and weight gain.

Nefazodone (Serzone)

Nefazodone blocks presynaptic serotonin and norepinephrine reuptake and antagonizes postsynaptic serotonergic 5-HT-2 receptors. Like bupropion and mirtazapine, nefazodone does not cause sexual dysfunction. Common side effects include sedation, dizziness, dry mouth, and nausea. Nefazodone also blocks α_1-adrenergic receptors and may cause orthostatic hypotension. Significant hepatic transaminase elevations warrant treatment discontinuation, because case reports of liver failure have been associated with nefazodone. Nefazodone may be associated with drug-drug interactions because of its high protein binding and inhibition of the hepatic cytochrome P-450 isoenzyme 3A3/4. Additionally, nefazodone (like SSRIs) should not be administered in combination with MAOIs.

Nefazodone has a short half-life and requires twice-daily dosing. Unlike SSRIs, nefazodone must be started at a subtherapeutic dose of 50 mg twice daily and titrated upward in 50-mg twice-daily increments on a weekly basis to a target dose range of 150 to 300 mg twice daily.

Trazodone (Desyrel)

Trazodone modulates serotonergic activity, but it is chemically distinct from TCAs and SSRIs. Side effects include prominent sedation, blurred vision, hypotension, dry mouth, dizziness, fatigue, and nausea. Trazodone has also been associated with priapism and arrhythmias. Trazodone is not considered a first-line medication for depression at this time. However, it is often prescribed at low doses (25 to 100 mg) for the short-term treatment of insomnia.*

Tricyclic Antidepressants

TCAs were among the earliest antidepressants available, but they fell out of favor as first-line antidepressants when antidepressants with improved tolerability, safety, and dosing regimens became available. However, TCAs are thought to be as effective as newer antidepressants and may be reasonable options for patients who have responded favorably to them in the past or who have failed to adequately respond to newer antidepressants. TCAs are also commonly used in the treatment of neuropathic pain.

Most of the side effects of TCAs are related to their antagonism of histaminic, muscarinic, and α_1-adrenergic receptors. These side effects include sedation, weight gain, constipation, dry mouth, urinary retention, tachycardia, blurred vision, dizziness, and orthostatic hypotension. TCAs are also associated with conduction delays and quinidine-like antiarrhythmic effects and should not be used in patients with significant cardiovascular disease or bundle branch blocks. TCAs should also be avoided in patients with narrow-angle glaucoma and prostate hypertrophy. Drug-drug interactions may occur when TCAs are administered concomitantly with cytochrome P-450 2D6 inhibitors (the primary metabolic route for TCAs), leading to increased TCA levels.

Overdose with TCAs can lead to anticholinergic delirium, ventricular arrhythmias, significant hypotension, seizures, and death. A TCA overdose constitutes a medical emergency and requires close clinical and cardiac monitoring. Patients with a prolonged QRS interval may be at increased risk for ventricular arrhythmias.

Baseline evaluation before initiating a TCA regimen includes a medical evaluation to rule out significant cardiovascular disease, prostate hypertrophy, and narrow-angle glaucoma. An electrocardiogram should be done in patients 40 years of age or older to exclude the presence of bundle branch blocks. All TCAs listed in Table 3 can be started at 25 mg/d, followed by weekly titration through their respective dose ranges based on tolerability and response (use divided dosing). Daily doses should not exceed 250 mg for clomipramine* (owing to a dose-related risk of seizures) and 150 mg for nortriptyline. Therapeutic blood levels exist for nortriptyline (50 to 150 ng/mL) and imipramine (combined imipramine plus desipramine level greater than 200 ng/mL).

Monoamine Oxidase Inhibitors

The MAOIs available for the treatment of major depression in the United States include phenelzine (Nardil) and tranylcypromine (Parnate). These agents nonselectively and irreversibly inhibit MAO-A and MAO-B enzymes. MAOIs have numerous side effects, including orthostatic hypotension, dry mouth, insomnia, headache, peripheral edema, weight gain, and sexual dysfunction. These agents are currently only rarely used, but they are important because of the propensity for serious adverse reactions that may present in primary care settings. Table 3 gives dose recommendations for MAOIs and other antidepressants.

Potentially serious complications with MAOIs are the *serotonin syndrome,* a life-threatening reaction that can occur when serotonergic agents are combined, particularly SSRI-MAOI or meperidine-MAOI combinations, and the *hypertensive crisis*. Signs and symptoms of the serotonin syndrome include altered mental status, agitation, diaphoresis, hyperthermia, flushing, hypertonicity, and myoclonus. Treatment involves the immediate discontinuation of serotonergic agents and supportive measures. A hypertensive crisis may occur when patients taking an MAOI consume foods high in tyramine, such as aged cheeses and meats, sauerkraut, soy sauce, and fava beans. This reaction occurs because nonselective inhibition of both MAO-A and MAO-B inhibits the metabolism of tyramine, which may then displace norepinephrine in presynaptic stores and lead to marked noradrenergic neurotransmission. This reaction may also occur when patients concomitantly take MAOIs and sympathomimetic agents. Symptoms of a hypertensive crisis include severe headache, sweating, and elevated blood pressure. If the reaction is severe enough, cerebral hemorrhage can occur.

Nonpharmacologic Treatments

Psychotherapy

Numerous individual and group psychotherapeutic interventions may be helpful in the treatment of patients with major depression, including interpersonal psychotherapy, behavioral and cognitive-behavioral psychotherapy, psychodynamic psychotherapy, and marital therapy (a thorough discussion of the various psychotherapeutic approaches is beyond the scope of this section). These interventions may be helpful alone or in combination with antidepressant medications. In patients with severe depression, the combination of psychotherapy and antidepressant medication may be more effective than either intervention alone. Clinicians should consider psychotherapy as a treatment option for their patients with major depression and should make appropriate referrals as indicated.

Electroconvulsive Therapy

Electroconvulsive therapy is a relatively safe and effective treatment for many patients. The most common significant side effects are cognitive impairment, including postictal confusion and retrograde or anterograde amnesia, as well as those side effects and risks associated with general anesthesia. Despite its efficacy, electroconvulsive therapy is often reserved for patients who have failed to respond to other treatment interventions, for severely depressed patients

*Not FDA approved for this indication.

TABLE 3. **Starting Dose and Dose Ranges for Selected Antidepressant Medications**

Medication (Trade Name)	Typical Daily Antidepressant Dose (mg) Starting Dose	Dose Range
Selective Serotonin Reuptake Inhibitors		
Fluoxetine		
Immediate-release (Prozac, Sarafem)	10-20	20-80
Delayed-release (Prozac Weekly)	90*	
Sertraline (Zoloft)	25-50	50-200
Citalopram (Celexa)	20	20-60
Escitalopram (Lexapro)	10	10-20
Paroxetine		
Immediate-release (Paxil)	10	10-50
Controlled-release (Paxil CR)	12.5	12.5-62.5
Newer Antidepressants		
Mirtazapine (Remeron; Remeron SolTab)	15	15-45
Bupropion		
Immediate-release (Wellbutrin)	100 bid	100-150 tid
Sustained-release (Wellbutrin SR)	150	150-200 bid
Venlafaxine		
Immediate-release (Effexor)	37.5 bid	75 bid-tid
Extended-release (Effexor XR)	37.5-75	75-225
Nefazodone (Serzone)	50 bid	150-300 bid
Trazodone (Desyrel)	50	150-200 bid
Tricyclic Antidepressnts		
Amitriptyline (Elavil)	25	100-300†
Clomipramine (Anafranil)	25	100-250
Desipramine (Norpramin)	25	100-300
Imipramine (Tofranil)	25	100-300†
Nortriptyline (Pamelor, Aventyl)	25	50-150
Monoamine Oxidase Inhibitors		
Phenelzine (Nardil)	15	15-60
Tranylcypromine (Parnate)	10	30-60

*Prozac Weekly 90-mg capsules are administered once weekly.
†Exceeds dosage recommended by the manufacturer.
bid, twice-daily dosing; tid, three times per day dosing.

with psychotic or catatonic features, for patients with significant suicidality, for elderly patients, and for pregnant patients who do not want to take antidepressant medications.

Treatment Approaches for Patients With Major Depression

Antidepressants have generally been considered to be similarly effective in treating major depression, although some evidence suggests differences among antidepressants in remission rates and preferential responses to certain types of depression (e.g., depression with atypical features). Likewise, clinical experience has demonstrated that individual responses to antidepressants vary, even to antidepressants with similar mechanisms of action. Nevertheless, clinicians often choose an antidepressant based on other factors, including safety, tolerability, dosing schedule, potential for drug-drug interactions, history of prior antidepressant response in an individual patient or close family member, and the presence of co-morbid illnesses that may respond (positively or negatively) to particular antidepressant medications. The goals of treatment are to achieve complete remission of acute depressive episodes (with symptom resolution and functional recovery) and to prevent relapses or recurrences.

Acute Major Depressive Episode

Treatment options should be discussed with the patient before initiating treatment, and patients who choose psychotherapy (either alone or in combination with medication management) should be referred to clinicians who are trained in depression-specific psychotherapies, such as cognitive-behavioral or interpersonal modalities. Pharmacologic treatment can be initiated with any of the available antidepressants, although an SSRI or one of the other newer agents is preferred. The antidepressant response is often delayed for 4 to 6 weeks, although 4 weeks is a reasonable period to evaluate the response. If there is no response after 4 weeks of treatment, the clinician should titrate the dose upward and then evaluate the patient's response through the antidepressant's dose range. If a partial response is seen after 4 weeks of treatment, the clinician should continue treatment at the present dose for an additional 2 weeks to see whether further improvement occurs.

If a partial, but inadequate, response is achieved despite titrating throughout the antidepressant's dose range, many clinicians attempt to augment the antidepressant with a second medication. Both lithium (Eskalith)* and triiodothyronine (Cytomel; thyroid hormone supplementation)* have controlled data supporting their use as augmenting agents. Lithium should be started at low doses (600 mg/d) and evaluated for at least 2 weeks before further upward dose titration. Triiodothyronine should be used in low doses as well (up to 25 μg/d). The goal of thyroid supplementation is to augment the antidepressant but not iatrogenically induce a hyperthyroid state. Less well studied augmentation strategies include stimulants and buspirone. Antidepressant combinations are also used, although most combinations are not well studied.

If an antidepressant is ineffective throughout its dose range, the clinician should switch to a different antidepressant. Switching from one SSRI to a second SSRI is reasonable, although a second SSRI trial failure suggests a switch to a different antidepressant class. If several antidepressants have been ineffective, the clinician should consider referring the patient for electroconvulsive therapy. Patients with psychotic depressions typically require an antipsychotic medication in combination with the antidepressant.

Dysthymia

The term *dysthymia* is used to describe a chronic, mild to moderate state of depression lasting 2 years or longer that does not fully meet criteria for major depression but can still be quite distressing and impairing. Antidepressants, alone or in combination with psychotherapy, may be effective in treating these states as well.

Continuation and Maintenance Treatment

Once an acute major depressive episode is in complete remission, treatment should be continued for at least 6 to 12 months at the doses that were effective for the acute episode. The length of treatment beyond this time depends largely on the patient's history of illness. Patients with a single depressive episode in their lifetime have a 50% chance of having another episode at some point. A trial period without antidepressants may be reasonable if such patients desire it. Patients with three or more lifetime depressive episodes, or those with a history of a severe, treatment-resistant depressive episode, should consider indefinite maintenance treatment to prevent recurrence, especially if there is a positive family history of major depression.

BIPOLAR DISORDER

Bipolar disorder is a chronic, recurrent illness characterized by the presence of both *depressive episodes* and manic or hypomanic episodes. *Manic episodes* last a week or longer and are characterized by a markedly elevated or irritable mood, increased energy level, decreased need for sleep, mood lability, distractibility, impulsivity, talkativeness, racing thoughts, psychomotor agitation, and increased goal-directed activity. Manic persons often engage in pleasurable, but potentially destructive activities, such as increased sexual activity and spending sprees. Psychotic symptoms, such as delusions of grandeur, can also be present. Patients with severe episodes often require hospitalization. Manic episodes with significant depressive symptoms are called *mixed episodes*. Mild episodes with manic symptoms that do not significantly impair someone's functioning or require hospitalization are called *hypomanic episodes*.

Bipolar disorder often begins at an early age and follows a chronic, recurrent course. It is equally common in male and female patients and is found in all socioeconomic and cultural backgrounds. Medications with mood-stabilizing properties are currently the standard of care in the treatment of bipolar disorder. Antidepressants should not be used unless a mood stabilizer with antimanic properties is used simultaneously.

Pharmacologic Treatments

Lithium (Lithium Carbonate, Lithobid, Eskalith, Eskalith CR)

Lithium has been a standard treatment option for bipolar disorder for several decades. It is effective in the treatment of acute mania and bipolar depression and, in the maintenance phase, to prevent recurrence of mood episodes. Because lithium is a salt that is excreted unchanged in the urine, it is a reasonable first-line choice for patients with significant hepatic impairment. Side effects include weight gain, nausea, diarrhea, fine tremor, polyuria and polydipsia, nephrogenic diabetes insipidus (from inhibition of vasopressin), mild cognitive impairment, acne, alopecia, and exacerbation of psoriasis. Long-term use of lithium can lead to hypothyroidism, which is typically reversible. Severe side effects may include arrhythmias, sinus node dysfunction, and pseudotumor cerebri. Possible laboratory abnormalities include low triiodothyronine and thyroxine levels, elevated thyroid-stimulating hormone levels, proteinuria, and benign T-wave flattening or inversion on the electrocardiogram. Renal morphologic changes can also occur, but therapeutic doses of lithium are not thought to cause renal failure. Contraindications include severe cardiovascular disease, unstable renal disease, dehydration, and sodium depletion.

Lithium toxicity is associated with high serum lithium levels. Mild toxicity (approximately 1.5 mEq/L or greater) includes sedation, vomiting, hyperreflexia, gait instability, tremors, and muscle weakness. More severe toxicity may involve ataxia, dysarthria, and myoclonus. Treatment of mild lithium toxicity in patients with normal renal functioning involves the brief cessation of lithium for 24 to 48 hours and close observation with evaluation of vital signs, neurologic status, serum electrolytes and renal function tests, serum lithium level, and an electrocardiogram.

*Not FDA approved for this indication.

Intravenous hydration with normal saline solution may be necessary to help remove lithium. Resumption of lithium treatment after mild toxicity should begin at low doses and under close monitoring. Severe toxicity with serum lithium levels higher than 3.0 mEq/L is life-threatening and may require hemodialysis to remove lithium.

Teratogenicity with lithium includes the risk of Ebstein's anomaly, a cardiac defect involving the tricuspid valve. The risk-benefit ratio should be discussed with women planning pregnancy, and the plan for treatment during pregnancy should be individualized based on the patient's history of illness. Lithium is also excreted in breast milk and should not be used by nursing mothers.

Lithium may be associated with numerous drug-drug interactions. Many commonly used medications can increase serum lithium levels, including thiazide diuretics, angiotensin-converting enzyme inhibitors, nonsteroidal anti-inflammatory drugs, and cyclooxygenase-2 inhibitors.

Baseline evaluation before starting lithium should include a complete blood cell count, renal function tests (blood urea nitrogen and creatinine), serum thyroid-stimulating hormone level, and an electrocardiogram for patients with a history of cardiovascular disease or those 40 years of age and older. Lithium is administered at a dose to target a therapeutic serum blood level between 0.6 and 1.2 mEq/L. Patients can be started on lithium carbonate at 300 mg twice daily or 600 mg at bedtime. Lithium levels should be checked 5 days after a dose increase and drawn approximately 12 hours after a dose. Titration should proceed in increments of 300 mg/d approximately weekly until clinical response is achieved and a therapeutic serum level is reached. Available lithium formulations recommend twice-daily (Lithobid, Eskalith CR) or thrice-daily dosing (lithium carbonate), although clinicians often switch to a once-daily dosing schedule (typically at bedtime) once the patient is clinically stable and no further dose titration is required. Controlled-release preparations may be better tolerated as a result of less fluctuation in serum lithium levels.

Valproate (Valproic Acid, Depakene, Depakote, Depakote ER)

Valproate is an anticonvulsant that is approved for use in the treatment of acute mania, although it is also used as maintenance treatment to prevent mood episodes. Valproate, like lithium, is considered a first-line medication for the treatment of bipolar disorder. It is often preferred as an initial treatment option in manic patients with marked irritability, patients in a rapid-cycling state (four or more discrete mood episodes in the preceding 12 months), patients with renal impairment, and patients with a history of numerous prior mood episodes.

Side effects associated with valproate include nausea, sedation, dizziness, vomiting, abdominal pain, anorexia, weight gain, sedation, tremor, diplopia, blurred vision, and alopecia. Rare cases of hepatotoxicity and acute pancreatitis have also been reported. Hematologic adverse events may include thrombocytopenia and coagulation problems. Pregnant women should avoid valproate in the first trimester because of an increased risk of neural tube defects.

Several potential drug-drug interactions are associated with valproate. Valproate is hepatically metabolized, and inducers of enzymes involved in the glucuronidation of valproate, such as carbamazepine (Tegretol) and phenytoin (Dilantin), can increase valproate clearance. Valproate can inhibit the metabolism of other anticonvulsants, including phenytoin, phenobarbital, and ethosuximide, and it can increase levels of carbamazepine's 10,11-epoxide metabolite. Additionally, valproate can more than double the half-life of lamotrigine (Lamictal), thus increasing the potential for rash. Valproate is also highly protein bound and can displace other protein-bound drugs, including warfarin (Coumadin) and tolbutamide (Orinase).

Baseline evaluation before initiating valproate therapy should include a complete blood count with differential, liver function tests, and, in women of childbearing potential, a pregnancy test. Valproate can be initiated at 250 mg three times daily or 500 mg at bedtime and titrated upward in increments of 250 to 500 mg/d on a weekly basis according to tolerability, response, and a target therapeutic serum valproate level of 50 to 120 μg/mL.

Olanzapine (Zyprexa)

Olanzapine is an atypical antipsychotic medication that is approved for use in the treatment of acute mania, though emerging data suggest a role for olanzapine in the treatment of bipolar depression as well. Response in mania is independent of psychosis.

Like other antipsychotic medications with dopamine D_2 receptor-blocking properties, olanzapine carries a risk of dystonic reactions, extrapyramidal side effects, neuroleptic malignant syndrome, and tardive dyskinesia. However, the risks of extrapyramidal side effects and tardive dyskinesia appear to be much lower with olanzapine and other atypical antipsychotics compared with conventional antipsychotics, such as haloperidol (Haldol). Other potential side effects include sedation, dry mouth, constipation, dizziness, weight gain, and orthostatic hypotension. There have also been reports of new-onset hyperglycemia and diabetic ketoacidosis with olanzapine (and with other atypical antipsychotics), as well as hyperlipidemia. There are no clear monitoring guidelines, although clinicians may consider evaluating serum glucose and lipid indices at baseline and throughout treatment.

Olanzapine is unlikely to cause clinically significant cytochrome P-450–mediated drug interactions. However, carbamazepine may increase the clearance of olanzapine as a result of cytochrome P-450 1A2 and 3A3/4 isoenzyme induction. In addition, the sedative effects of olanzapine may be potentiated by the concomitant use of other sedating medications or substances of abuse.

For outpatients, olanzapine treatment should be initiated at 5 mg every night for 1 week and increased in increments of 5 mg/d, based on tolerability and response to a target dose range of 15 to 20 mg/d.

Carbamazepine (Tegretol)

Carbamazepine* is an anticonvulsant that is often used as a second-line alternative to lithium, valproate, and olanzapine in the treatment of acute mania and as maintenance treatment in bipolar disorder. Side effects include nausea, vomiting, sedation, dizziness, and rash. Potentially serious hematologic abnormalities may include leukopenia, thrombocytopenia, and (rarely) aplastic anemia or agranulocytosis. Other serious adverse events include hepatotoxicity and teratogenicity, including neural tube and craniofacial defects. Thus, carbamazepine is contraindicated in patients with significant hepatic disease; patients at risk of hematologic abnormalities, including patients taking medications that may cause bone marrow suppression; and patients who are pregnant, especially during the first trimester.

Carbamazepine is associated with the potential for numerous drug-drug interactions. It is metabolized primarily by the cytochrome P-450 3A3/4 isoenzyme, and drugs that inhibit this enzyme may increase carbamazepine levels. Carbamazepine is an inducer of hepatic cytochrome P-450 isoenzymes, and it can lead to the increased metabolism of other medications, including numerous anticonvulsants and oral contraceptives. Carbamazepine can also induce its own metabolism, leading to declining blood levels and the need for dosage adjustment approximately 10 to 14 days after the initiation of treatment.

Carbamazepine should be initiated at 200 mg twice daily and titrated in increments of 200 mg/d on a weekly basis, based on clinical response and tolerability (maximum recommended daily dose: 1200 mg) after baseline blood cell count indices and serum hepatic transaminase levels have been assessed and a diagnosis of pregnancy has been excluded. Serum blood levels do not correlate with response, but monitoring them may be useful in avoiding toxicity and in monitoring for autoinduction.

Oxcarbazepine (Trileptal) is a derivative of carbamazepine that has less cytochrome P-450 isoenzyme induction, no autoinduction, and improved tolerability. Side effects may include sedation, dizziness, blurred vision, rash, and hyponatremia. Available data support its use in acute mania, but its effectiveness as maintenance therapy in bipolar disorder is unclear. The dose conversion from carbamazepine to oxcarbazepine is approximately 1:1.5. Oxcarbazepine* is typically initiated at 150 mg twice daily and is titrated in increments of 300 mg/d at weekly intervals, based on response and tolerability to a target dose range of 900 to 2400 mg/d (divided twice daily).

*Not FDA approved for this indication.

Lamotrigine (Lamictal)

Lamotrigine* is an anticonvulsant with data supporting its use in the treatment of bipolar depression and possibly in rapid cycling states, particularly in bipolar II disorder. Lamotrigine is generally well tolerated. Side effects may include dizziness, blurred vision, and headaches. Additionally, approximately 10% of patients taking lamotrigine may experience a rash. Although most rashes are benign, there is a small risk of the potentially life-threatening Stevens-Johnson syndrome. Factors that may be associated with the risk for developing a rash include high lamotrigine starting doses, rapid dose titration, and concomitant valproate use.

Other Anticonvulsants and Atypical Antipsychotic Medications

Several other anticonvulsants (including gabapentin,* topiramate,* zonisamide,* and tiagabine*) and atypical antipsychotic medications (including riseridone,* quetiapine,* ziprasidone,* and clozaril*) have received interest as potential treatments for mood disorders, although none have compelling controlled data suggesting efficacy as monotherapy in the treatment of bipolar disorder to date. However, clinicians often use these agents in combination with first-line medications in patients with a chronic and severe, treatment-resistant course of illness.

Approach to Treatment of the Patient With Bipolar Disorder

As with the treatment of major depression, the goals of treatment in bipolar disorder are to achieve complete symptom remission and functional recovery from acute mood episodes and to prevent mood episode relapses or recurrences.

Acute Manic or Mixed Episodes

Acute manic or mixed episodes should be treated initially with lithium, valproate, or olanzapine.* Hospitalization may be required in severe cases. Patients who fail to respond to monotherapy should be treated with the combination of two first-line agents. Antidepressant medications should be discontinued because they may worsen mania or exacerbate mood cycling.

Rapid-Cycling States

Patients with four or more mood episodes in a 12-month period are said to be in a rapid-cycling state. This state occurs in approximately 10% to 15% of patients with bipolar disorder and is often difficult to treat. Rapid-cycling states may be exacerbated by uncontrolled hypothyroidism and antidepressant medications, and these possibilities should be considered during treatment. Valproate and olanzapine are often preferred over lithium,* although combination treatment may be necessary.

*Not FDA approved for this indication.

Acute Depressive Episodes

Acute depressive episodes in patients with bipolar disorder pose an interesting treatment challenge: traditional antidepressants, if used alone, may accelerate mood cycling or may cause an affective switch into (hypo)mania. Thus, the initial treatment of bipolar depression involves the initiation (or optimization) of a first-line mood-stabilizing agent, such as lithium,* valproate,* and olanzapine,* or the use of lamotrigine.* For patients who fail to respond to this strategy, the addition of an SSRI or other non-TCA antidepressant may be indicated.

Continuation and Maintenance Treatment

Lithium* and valproate* are generally considered the standard treatment options for maintenance therapy in bipolar disorder. However, clinicians often continue the medications that were effective in the most recent mood episode as a maintenance regimen. Discontinuation of medications that were used to treat certain target symptoms may be attempted during the maintenance phase. Additionally, the need for ongoing antidepressant therapy during the maintenance phase of treatment should be evaluated for each patient based on the individual history of illness. Attention to psychosocial factors and psychoeducation is critically important for the optimal long-term management of bipolar disorder.

*Not FDA approved for this indication.

SCHIZOPHRENIA

method of
MICHAEL B. KNABLE, D.O.
Stanley Medical Research Institute
Bethesda, Maryland

Schizophrenia is a common neuropsychiatric disorder affecting approximately 1% of the population. In the United States, medical care for people with schizophrenia costs about $65 billion annually, and about 100,000 people with schizophrenia are hospitalized at any given time. The origin of schizophrenia, like that of many "complex diseases," is incompletely understood. However, an inherited predisposition to the disorder appears to be mediated by several genes that individually convey a small degree of risk. In addition, environmental factors such as fetal hypoxia, viral infection, and malnutrition may contribute to disease risk.

SECOND-GENERATION ANTIPSYCHOTIC DRUGS

The positive symptoms of psychosis (hallucinations and delusions) are probably related to hyperactivity of dopamine in subcortical brain regions, because drugs that antagonize dopamine in these regions readily ameliorate symptoms in most patients. All antipsychotic drugs with proven efficacy in schizophrenia are antagonists of dopamine D_2 receptors.

The second-generation or atypical antipsychotic drugs are generally selected as first treatments for schizophrenia. These drugs are considered atypical because of their reduced propensity for extrapyramidal side effects when compared with older drugs. Atypical drugs may also be associated with a broader spectrum of efficacy, better compliance, fewer relapses, and fewer hospitalizations.

Risperidone (Risperdal)

Risperidone is a high-affinity antagonist at dopamine D_2 receptors and at serotonin 5-HT-2_A receptors. This pharmacologic profile has been proposed as a defining feature of atypical antipsychotic drugs. In a meta-analysis of controlled trials comparing risperidone with typical antipsychotic drugs (usually haloperidol [Haldol]), risperidone demonstrated superior efficacy for positive, negative, cognitive, and mood symptoms in patients with chronic schizophrenia. However, if one controls for the high doses of typical antipsychotics used as comparators in these trials, the superiority of risperidone is more difficult to demonstrate. Risperidone was also superior to haloperidol in preventing symptomatic relapse in a long-term prospective study. Although limited data are available, risperidone does not appear to have superior efficacy when compared with other second-generation drugs or in patients with treatment-refractory schizophrenia.

Risperidone is better tolerated than first-generation antipsychotic drugs. However, extrapyramidal side effects are more common with risperidone than with other atypical drugs. This feature may limit its use in patients with a prior history of extrapyramidal side effects, in patients with underlying primary movement disorders, and in the elderly. Risperidone is more likely than other atypical antipsychotics to produce hyperprolactinemia, amenorrhea, and galactorrhea. Weight gain, sedation, and cardiac conduction abnormalities are less common with risperidone than with other second-generation drugs.

Olanzapine (Zyprexa)

Olanzapine is an antagonist at D_2 and 5-HT-2_A receptors, but it also has high affinity at histamine and muscarinic acetylcholine receptors. This pharmacologic profile is similar to that of clozapine (Clozaril), the prototype of atypical antipsychotics. Some studies have suggested that olanzapine has superior efficacy compared with first-generation drugs, especially for negative symptoms, but systematic reviews and meta-analyses have not reliably supported this contention. Olanzapine has been shown to be superior to haloperidol for the prevention of relapse during long-term maintenance treatment. Olanzapine has not shown superior efficacy when compared with other second-generation antipsychotics or for treatment-refractory patients.

The incidence of extrapyramidal and cardiac side effects is very low with olanzapine. Weight gain, however, is a significant disadvantage. Weight gain tends to become maximal after 9 to 12 months and may reach a total of 25 to 30 pounds. Weight gain is associated with an increased risk of diabetes mellitus, diabetic ketoacidosis, hypertension, hyperlipidemia, and coronary artery disease. Patients with pre-existing obesity, diabetes, and hyperlipidemia are therefore not ideal candidates for olanzapine treatment, and careful monitoring for these adverse events should be undertaken in all patients.

Quetiapine (Seroquel)

In addition to 5-HT-2_A and D_2 receptor antagonism, quetiapine has substantial affinity at histamine receptors and lacks affinity at muscarinic receptors. The efficacy of quetiapine is equivalent to that of first-generation antipsychotics and risperidone. It has not been compared directly with other second-generation drugs, nor has it been evaluated in long-term, controlled studies of relapse prevention. Quetiapine was superior to haloperidol in one study of patients with an incomplete response to first-generation antipsychotics.

Quetiapine is unlikely to cause extrapyramidal side effects, prolactin elevation, or cardiac conduction abnormalities. Weight gain has not been systematically evaluated, but it appears to be less common with quetiapine than with olanzapine or clozapine. The sedative properties of quetiapine can be an advantage for patients with agitation, but these effects are experienced as unpleasant by others. In patients who are very sensitive to extrapyramidal side effects or who have had neuroleptic malignant syndrome, quetiapine may be a good choice because it has the lowest D_2 receptor affinity of the second-generation drugs. Lens opacities were observed in animal studies with quetiapine, so ophthalmologic examination should be obtained periodically in patients receiving long-term treatment with this agent.

Ziprasidone (Geodon)

Ziprasidone blocks 5-HT-2_A and D_2 receptors and uniquely inhibits serotonin and norepinephrine reuptake, as antidepressants do. Ziprasidone is superior to placebo, but it has not been evaluated systematically in comparison with first-generation or other second-generation drugs. In one published comparison with haloperidol, ziprasidone had greater efficacy for negative symptoms. Ziprasidone has not been evaluated in long-term, controlled studies of relapse prevention or in treatment-refractory patients. Ziprasidone is the only second-generation antipsychotic for which a parenteral formulation has been marketed.

Ziprasidone is unlikely to cause extrapyramidal side effects, prolactin elevation, or weight gain. Ziprasidone is often experienced as an activating or alerting drug, which can be advantageous for patients who are abulic or depressed. Ziprasidone is associated with a greater prolongation of the QT_c interval compared with risperidone, olanzapine, quetiapine, and haloperidol. Fewer than 1% of patients enrolled in clinical trials of ziprasidone developed a QT_c interval greater than 500 milliseconds. However, because a prolonged QT_c interval is associated with an elevated risk of torsades de pointes and other arrhythmias, ziprasidone should be used with caution in patients with cardiac conduction abnormalities; a pre-existing, prolonged QT_c interval; hypokalemia; or hypomagnesemia.

Aripiprazole (Abilify)

Aripiprazole is the latest addition to the list of second-generation antipsychotic drugs. It may be considered a third-generation drug because it possesses a novel pharmacologic property not present in the other drugs. Aripiprazole is thought to act as a dopamine stabilizer because it is a partial agonist at D_2 receptors. Aripiprazole is also a partial agonist at 5-HT-1a receptors and an antagonist at 5-HT-2 receptors.

Only one published study of aripiprazole has demonstrated superior efficacy compared with placebo, but not with haloperidol. Aripiprazole treatment was associated with very low rates of extrapyramidal side effects, weight gain, sedation, hyperprolactinemia, and electrocardiographic abnormalities.

Clozapine (Clozaril)

Clozapine is the prototypical second-generation antipsychotic. It has the usual profile of greater 5-HT-2_A than D_2 antagonism. It is also an antagonist at various other dopamine, acetylcholine, histamine, and adrenergic receptors. In systematic meta-analyses, clozapine demonstrated efficacy superior to that of first-generation drugs in both short-term and long-term studies. Superior efficacy compared with other second-generation drugs has not been conclusively demonstrated. Clozapine is the only antipsychotic drug for which superior efficacy in treatment-resistant patients has been demonstrated.

Clozapine treatment is usually reserved for severely ill or treatment-refractory patients, because of its tendency to induce neutropenia or agranulocytosis. This side effect, which occurs in fewer than 1% of patients receiving the drug, requires weekly monitoring of the white blood cell count through a national registry program. Clozapine treatment is also commonly associated with seizures, sedation, anticholinergic side effects, and weight gain. Clozapine is the only second-generation antipsychotic for which a correlation has been established between clinical efficacy and serum concentration of the drug.

FIRST-GENERATION ANTIPSYCHOTIC DRUGS

First-generation antipsychotics are infrequently prescribed for patients with newly diagnosed schizophrenia, but these drugs are still used commonly in other settings. Some patients respond well to first-generation drugs, but not to second-generation drugs, and a history of prior response to a particular antipsychotic is a compelling reason to use the drug again. Several first-generation drugs (e.g., haloperidol, chlorpromazine, fluphenazine) are available in parenteral formulations and are commonly used in agitated patients. Haloperidol and fluphenazine are also available in long-acting depot intramuscular formulations that can be administered biweekly or monthly in patients who are unable to comply with daily oral therapy.

ADJUNCTIVE STRATEGIES

Many patients treated with antipsychotic drugs have residual symptoms or co-morbid symptoms of anxiety, depression, or cognitive difficulties. Therefore, it is very common for patients to have prescriptions for several agents. Generally, this practice has evolved naturally and is not governed by systematic studies. Common augmentation strategies with commercially available drugs are summarized in the following sections. Augmentation of antipsychotic drugs with other drugs acting on cortical dopamine systems, the nicotinic acetylcholine system, and certain aspects of glutamate neurotransmission are under active pursuit in research settings.

Antipsychotic Drug Combinations

It is reasonable to hypothesize that the efficacy of second-generation antipsychotics may be due to factors other than D_2 antagonism; therefore, the addition of a more potent D_2 antagonist may improve efficacy in treatment-resistant patients. Controlled trials have supported this hypothesis when sulpiride[†] (a selective D_2 blocker not available in the United States) or chlorpromazine was added to clozapine. Improvement in psychotic symptoms has also been reported in uncontrolled trials that combined risperidone, pimozide,* or loxapine with clozapine. There are no controlled trials examining the combination of multiple second-generation antipsychotics.

Antidepressants

Antidepressants are commonly added to antipsychotic drugs in the treatment of schizophrenia, but the literature supporting this practice is generally of poor quality. The addition of a tricyclic antidepressant (e.g., desipramine [Norpramin] or imipramine [Tofranil]) to a first-generation antipsychotic for the treatment of depressive symptoms in schizophrenia is supported by several controlled studies. Selective serotonin reuptake inhibitors have been combined with antipsychotics in several controlled trials designed to improve residual negative symptoms. Fluoxetine (Prozac) and fluvoxamine (Luvox)* have demonstrated modest improvements in negative symptoms, but sertraline (Zoloft) and citalopram (Celexa) have not. Novel antidepressants such as mirtazapine (Remeron) and bupropion (Wellbutrin) have improved negative symptoms in some preliminary studies.

*Not FDA approved for this indication.
†Not available in the United States.

Lithium, Anticonvulsants, and Benzodiazepines

Early studies reported that lithium augmentation of antipsychotics was associated with improvement in psychotic, mood, and anxiety symptoms. More recent controlled studies have not replicated these results. Adjunctive lithium treatment is a reasonable approach in patients with prominent affective symptoms or impulsivity. Likewise, valproic acid (Depakene) and carbamazepine (Tegretol) may be prescribed to such patients or to patients who have concomitant structural brain disease or seizures. Valproic acid treatment was beneficial in one study of acutely ill schizophrenic patients, but the drug did not demonstrate beneficial effects in controlled studies with chronically ill patients. One controlled trial reported beneficial effects of carbamazepine in schizophrenic patients with electroencephalographic abnormalities. Some case reports have indicated that topiramate (Topamax)* and lamotrigine (Lamictal)* augmentation may benefit some patients, but controlled data are lacking. Benzodiazepines are frequently prescribed to reduce agitation in acute psychosis. However, the long-term use of adjunctive benzodiazepines for control of antipsychotic drugs is not supported by consistent findings in the literature.

*Not FDA approved for this indication.

PANIC DISORDER

method of
MANUEL E. TANCER, M.D., and
SHAHID HUSSAIN, M.D.
Wayne State University School of Medicine
Detroit, Michigan

Anxiety disorders are among the most common psychiatric illnesses seen by primary care practitioners. Patients with panic attacks often present initially to primary care physicians or emergency departments because of sudden physical symptoms. *Panic attacks* are paroxysmal episodes of marked anxiety with at least four somatic or psychosensory symptoms that reach a peak within 10 minutes and then dissipate (Table 1).

DIAGNOSIS

Panic attacks can be a symptom of medical conditions (e.g., hypothyroidism or hyperthyroidism, hypoxia, hypoglycemia), side effect of medications or intoxication

TABLE 1. **Diagnostic Criteria for Panic Attack**

A discrete period of intense fear or discomfort, starting abruptly, reaching a crescendo within 10 minutes, and associated with at least four of the following signs and symptoms:

1. Palpitations, pounding heart, or accelerated heart rate
2. Sweating
3. Trembling or shaking
4. Sensations of shortness of breath or smothering
5. Feeling of choking
6. Chest pain or discomfort
7. Nausea or abdominal distress
8. Feeling dizzy, unsteady, lightheaded, or faint
9. Derealization (feelings of unreality) or depersonalization (being detached from oneself)
10. Fear of losing control or going crazy
11. Fear of dying
12. Paresthesias (numbness or tingling sensations)
13. Chills or hot flashes

Adapted from the Diagnostic and Statistical Manual, 4th edition (DSM-IV).

from substances (Table 2), or the result of withdrawal from medications and substances of abuse (Table 3). It is essential that the symptoms of anxiety be evaluated by a detailed history, physical examination, and appropriate laboratory evaluation. Panic disorder must be included in the differential diagnosis of chest pain, dizziness, shortness of breath, and "fainting spells."

In the patient's medical history, attention should be paid to the use of medications (prescription and over the counter), ethanol and drug use (amounts and patterns), and caffeine use. Changes in medications or medication doses may result in panic attacks. The same is also true for use of illicit drugs such as cocaine. Reduction or elimination of caffeine can be an effective therapeutic intervention for many people. It is also important to ask about the patient's use of herbal compounds (Tables 4 and 5).

The physical examination should focus on ruling out "organic" causes for the presenting symptoms. Particular attention should be paid to the cardiac examination. Targeted laboratory studies should be done to exclude any suspected medical conditions, and an electroencephalogram may be necessary in some patients.

Panic disorder is a syndrome characterized by recurrent, initially unexpected, panic attacks. At first, the panic attacks are unexpected, but over time they may become situationally cued or predisposed. Panic attacks may also occur at night (*nocturnal panic*). *Agoraphobia,* defined as the avoidance of situations and/or places associated with panic attacks, is a common complication of panic disorder and contributes significantly to its morbidity. The diagnostic criteria for panic disorder given in the fourth edition of the American Psychiatric Association's *Diagnostic and Statistical Manual of Mental Disorders* (DSM-IV) are listed in Table 6.

Panic disorder has a lifetime prevalence of 3.5% of the population. The peak age at onset is between 18 and 35 years, although it can begin earlier. There is a 2:1 or 3:1 female-male ratio in the prevalence of panic disorder, and this illness tends to show some genetic concordance.

Panic disorder has a highly variable course of illness: some patients experience episodic symptoms, and others experience chronic, unremitting symptoms. As a group, these patients make frequent use of health care resources. Patients with panic disorder are at increased risk of being depressed; most studies report that 50% to 75% of these patients have histories of major depression. This co-morbidity has been blamed in large part for the significantly elevated rate of suicide in panic disorder, and suicidal ideation must be inquired about openly in these patients. There is also an increased risk of substance abuse in panic disorder, specifically alcohol abuse or dependence in up to 30% of patients.

The presence of panic attacks in a patient should alert the clinician to look carefully for symptoms of depression and of drug and/or ethanol abuse or dependence. The presence of co-morbid conditions worsens the prognosis and often influences treatment choices. Patients with atypical features, especially attacks occurring at a young age (less than 20 years) with a particularly fearful component, also need to be evaluated for psychosis, bipolar illness (significantly

TABLE 2. **Medications and Drugs Associated with Anxiety Symptoms**

Corticosteroids	Nonsteroidal anti-inflammatory agents
Antihypertensives	Birth control pills
Lidocaine	Selective serotonin reuptake inhibitors
Caffeine	Analgesics containing caffeine
Cocaine	Stimulants
Marijuana	Catecholamines

TABLE 3. **Withdrawal from Medications and Substances Associated with Anxiety Symptoms**

Corticosteroids
β-Blockers
Opiates
Cocaine
Alcohol
Benzodiazepines
Barbiturates
Selective serotonin reuptake inhibitors

TABLE 4. **Herbal Compounds Used for the Treatment of Anxiety Disorders**

Compound	Adverse Effects
Kava kava*	Sedation, extrapyramidal symptoms, ataxia, paralysis (toxicity)
St. John's wort*	Photosensitivity, serotonin syndrome when combined with serotonergic agents
Valerian*	Sedation, withdrawal syndrome (similar to that from benzodiazepines)

*Not FDA approved for this indication.

TABLE 5. **Herbal Compounds in Common Use That Are Known to Cause Anxiety**

Compound	Active Ingredient	Use
Yohimbe	Yohimbine	Aphrodisiac
Ephedra	Ephedrine	Weight loss and energy boost
Guarana	Caffeine	Energy boost

more common than in the general population), obsessive-compulsive disorder, and post-traumatic stress disorder.

TREATMENT

Panic disorder can be treated either with medication or with nonpharmacologic therapies. Of the nonmedication treatments, cognitive-behavioral therapy has been shown to be the most effective. There is no way of determining beforehand who will respond better to which treatment, and the patient's choices need to be taken into account in this matter. It is unclear whether combined treatment offers any added benefit. If a patient with panic disorder is not showing any clinical improvement after 6 to 8 weeks with one treatment modality, a reassessment of the patient and a shift in treatment modalities are probably warranted. Patients with exclusively nocturnal panic attacks should be prescribed pharmacotherapy.

Pharmacotherapy

Pharmacotherapy can be quite effective in the treatment of panic disorder, particularly in blocking unexpected panic attacks. It is, however, less successful in the treatment of agoraphobia. Antidepressant medications and high-potency benzodiazepines have been the most widely studied and used agents (Table 7). The selective serotonin reuptake inhibitors (SSRIs) are the first-line agents for the treatment of panic disorder. Both paroxetine (Paxil) and sertraline (Zoloft) have been approved by the U.S. Food and Drug Administration (FDA) for the treatment of panic disorder. Other SSRIs are known to have similar effects. Antidepressants take 4 to 6 weeks for full effects to be seen. Some patients treated with SSRIs experience excessive arousal, so starting with a low dose—one fourth to one half the typical starting dose—is recommended. Evening dosing may help people who experience excessive arousal. Patients must be warned about the possibility of sexual dysfunction and monitored for the emergence of treatment-related hypomania/mania (decreased sleep with increased energy, excessive talkativeness, irritability or euphoria, spending, grandiosity). The SSRI discontinuation syndrome is well documented and necessitates close monitoring when patients stop taking these medications.

The high-potency benzodiazepines alprazolam (Xanax) and clonazepam (Klonopin) are also FDA approved for the treatment of panic disorder. The benzodiazepines work rapidly (within 1 week) and may be valuable for patients with rapidly progressing symptoms or in patients unable to tolerate antidepressant medications. Benzodiazepines should be used cautiously in patients with a history of alcohol abuse. These drugs should not be used as monotherapy in patients with co-morbid major depressive disorder. It is important that patients take benzodiazepines on a regular basis to prevent attacks from occurring rather than giving these drugs on an as-needed basis, because patients often tend to wait until it is too late to abort the attack.

Some patients with panic disorder with rapidly escalating or severe symptoms require combination pharmacotherapy, usually an SSRI combined with a benzodiazepine. After 6 to 8 weeks, the antidepressant should be fully effective, and gradual benzodiazepine tapering can begin.

It is becoming clear that panic disorder is a chronic condition, but data remain insufficient to make predictions about recurrence risks. As such, a 9- to 12-month treatment period after remission, or longer if clinically suitable, is recommended. Discontinuing medication is ideally done in a planned, phased fashion, with patient education and family involvement, when possible.

TABLE 6. **Diagnostic Requirements for Panic Disorder**

1. Recurrent, unexpected panic attacks
2. One of the panic attacks is followed by 1 month of:
   a. Worry about subsequent attacks
   b. Worry about the implications of the attack (e.g., having a heart attack or losing control)
   c. Significant change in behavior related to the attacks
3. The absence of an organic (direct physiologic effect of a drug or medication or a general medical condition) basis for the attacks
4. Symptoms not better accounted for by another mental disorder
5. Panic disorder can be further characterized by the presence or absence of agoraphobia.

Adapted from the Diagnostic and Statistical Manual, 4th edition (DSM-IV).

Cognitive-Behavioral Therapy

Cognitive-behavioral therapy can be conducted individually or in groups and is equally effective in either format. The cognitive part of cognitive-behavioral therapy involves identifying misinterpreted thoughts (racing heartbeat = heart attack) and helping the patient to adopt a more realistic understanding of the symptoms. The behavioral view of panic disorder is that the extreme symptoms of the panic attack are responsible for the escape or avoidance behaviors. Treatment involves graduated, real-life exposure to the fearful situations until habituation or tolerance develops. Cognitive-behavioral therapy thus involves a commitment from patients to place themselves in uncomfortable situations. This approach requires support from an empathic and trained clinician.

TABLE 7. **Medications for the Treatment of Panic Disorder**

Drug Class	Drug	Dose Range	FDA-Indicated
TCA	Desipramine (Norpramin)*	50-300 mg/d	No
TCA	Imipramine (Tofranil)*	50-300 mg/d	No
SSRI	Fluoxetine (Prozac)*	5-40 mg/d	No
SSRI	Fluvoxamine (Luvox)*	25-150 mg/d	No
SSRI	Paroxetine (Paxil)	10-40 mg/d	Yes
SSRI	Sertraline (Zoloft)	25-150 mg/d	Yes
SSRI	Citalopram (Celexa)*	10-40 mg/d	No
MAOI	Phenelzine (Nardil)*	30-90 mg/d	No
Benzodiazepine	Alprazolam (Xanax)	1.5-6 mg/d	Yes
Benzodiazepine	Clonazepam (Klonopin)*	1.5-6 mg/d	Yes
Benzodiazepine	Diazepam (Valium)*	15-60 mg/d	No

*Not FDA approved for this indication.

MAOI, monoamine oxidase inhibitor; SSRI, selective serotonin reuptake inhibitor; TCA, tricyclic antidepressant.

Patient Education

Patient education is an essential part of the treatment of patients with panic disorder. Patients *should* be given a definitive diagnosis and should *not* be told that there is "nothing wrong with them." Patients should be told that antidepressants may take 4 to 6 weeks to act. In many patients, the learned avoidance behavior may persist long after the panic attacks have ceased. For these patients, it is important to recommend gradual exposure at their own pace. There are also various self-help books available about panic disorder.

Section 18
Physical and Chemical Injuries

BURNS

method of
NICHOLAS A. MEYER, M.D., F.A.C.S.
University of Wisconsin Hospital and Clinics
Madison, Wisconsin

Despite the preventive efforts of educators, lawmakers, and health care providers, burn injuries continue to be a significant source of morbidity and mortality. Annually, 1.5 million burn injuries are reported in the United States, approximately 3000 of which result in death. Worldwide, 282,000 deaths occurred in 1999 from burn injury, thus making burns the second leading cause of death after trauma in children and young adults. Although these statistics are sobering, improvements in both short-term and long-term care of patients with burns has resulted in dramatically increased survival rates as well as improved quality of life for survivors. In the early 1970s, an 80% total body surface area burn was associated with 100% mortality. Today, patients with an 80% total body surface area burn have greater than a 50% chance of survival. In addition to decreased mortality, survivors of large and less severe burns benefit from today's better understanding of wound healing and from the improved medical treatment and reconstructive techniques that have resulted from this knowledge.

PREVENTION

Although most burn injuries continue to result from avoidable accidents, significant progress has been made in burn prevention since the early 1970s. Proven examples of effective intervention in private homes include the widespread installation of smoke detectors and the government regulation of hot water heat temperature settings. In public buildings, laws requiring sprinkler systems and smoke detectors have led to a decrease in the prevalence and severity of fires. All these interventions have resulted in a decreased incidence of burn-related injuries, including those involving scald burns and smoke inhalation.

Locally, educational programs teaching the "stop, drop, and roll" technique and fire safety in schools are thought to lessen burn severity and incidence. Much more needs to be done, however. Education in electrical safety and safe handling of flammable substances is sadly lacking, especially in developing countries.

The role of the primary care physician is to reinforce the need for smoke detectors and the need for child safety protective devices where appropriate, including, but not limited to, electrical outlet covers, safety covers for hot water spigots, and protective fencing around fireplaces and wood-burning stoves. Parents need to be warned and educated to place flammable and corrosive agents (e.g., gasoline, mineral spirits, acids, matches, cigarette lighters) out of reach of children and to educate children about the dangers of playing with such materials. High-risk groups include young children (less than 5 years old), who have a disproportionately higher rate of contact and scald injuries than adults. Teenage boys tend to have a high incidence of flame burns caused by activities such as igniting aerosol cans, jumping over burning leaves, and playing with fire. Electrical and chemical burns occur mostly in the setting of employment and in very young children, whereas house fires tend to affect all age groups similarly.

WOUND ASSESSMENT

The severity of a burn is defined by both the depth and the extent of injury (Table 1). *First-degree burns*, typified by the common sunburn, damage the outer layers of the epithelium but preserve the barrier function of the skin. They can be painful but do not require wound care other than soothing moisturizers. *Second-degree* or *partial-thickness burns* produce complete epithelial separation and may involve partial damage to the underlying dermis. Blisters under which the dermis is moist, pink, and very tender are clinical characteristics of second-degree burns. *Third-degree burns* destroy the entire thickness of epidermis and dermis and leave no skin elements from which the skin can regenerate. These deep burns are characteristically dry, pale, and insensate or can even appear black and charred on presentation after a flame injury.

By destroying the barrier function of the skin, both second-degree and third degree burns create an open wound prone to microbial invasion, fluid loss, inflammation, and pain. The extent of the wound is quantified

TABLE 1. **Clinical Assessment of Burn Depth**

Burn Depth	Appearance	Pain	Time to Epithelialize	Tissue Destruction
First-degree	Red, dry, blanches to pressure	Moderate	—	Partial epidermis
Second-degree (partial-thickness)	Blisters, pink, moist, blanches to pressure	Severe	<2 to 3 wk	Total epidermis, partial dermis
Third-degree (full-thickness)	Red, white, or black, dry, does not blanch to pressure	Minimal	>3 wk to never	Total epidermis, total dermis

as a percentage of the total body surface area. The *rule of nines* is a quick and easily remembered method to assess burn size by measuring the relative involvement of discrete parts of the body (Table 2). In this model, each body part comprises a percentage of total body surface area equal to a multiple of nine. Determining the total body surface area of a burn is imperative because it is directly related to the morbidity and mortality of the patient.

OUTPATIENT TREATMENT OF SMALL BURNS

Small burns are defined as those involving less than 10% total body surface area, superficial in depth, and not fitting the criteria identified in Table 3 as appropriate for transfer to a burn center. The wounds of second- and third-degree burns are open and are prone to infection, pain, contracture, and scar formation. Treatment is primarily directed at wound hygiene, analgesia, maintaining mobility, and, once healed, the use of topical pressure. Burn wounds inevitably become colonized with bacteria, which, if allowed to propagate to large colonies, can slow wound healing and can predispose to infection. Initial wound débridement and washing twice daily with a dilute antiseptic such as 1% chlorhexidine* will keep bacterial numbers to a minimum by mechanical removal of both bacteria and nonviable substrate. Tetanus immunization status should be ascertained, and a booster should be given according to the recommendations of the American College of Surgeons. Prophylactic use of systemic antibiotics is not indicated; however, empirical antibiotic use is justified for burn cellulitis evidenced by erythema progressing beyond 1 to 2 cm from the burn edge.

*May be compounded by pharmacists or diluted 1:1, 2% chlorhexidine:saline.

Wound Treatments

A moist wound heals faster and is less painful than a dry wound. Topical antibacterial ointments and creams (e.g., bacitracin zinc ointment, silver sulfadiazine [Silvadene]) can be applied twice daily after wound cleansing to keep the wound moist and bacterial counts low. Alternative dressings include biologic dressings, which are produced from human or animal tissue (e.g., human allograft skin, porcine xenograft skin, compound membranes [Biobrane and TransCyte]) and adhere through protein-protein bonds. Biologic dressings succeed only when they are applied to a clean, sterile wound base. The advantages of biologic dressings are immediate wound closure, less pain, and no need for dressing changes. The disadvantages include high cost and infection or failure if the dressings are applied to a contaminated or nonviable base.

Analgesia

Pain is typically severe after second-degree burns. Frequent (every 5 to 10 minutes) small doses of intravenous narcotics (e.g., up to 0.1 mg/kg morphine) may be necessary to titrate analgesia for initial wound débridement. Subsequent wound care can usually be managed with short-acting oral narcotics such as oxycodone (Roxicodone) and hydrocodone and acetaminophen (Vicodin) 30 minutes before dressing changes. Long-acting narcotics (OxyContin, MS Contin)

TABLE 2. **Clinical Assessment of Burn Extent (Rule of Nines)**

Body Part	Percentage of Total Body Surface Area (%)
Head	9
Torso, anterior	18
Torso, posterior	18
Arm, right	9
Arm, left	9
Leg, right	18
Leg, left	18
Genitals	1
Total	100

TABLE 3. **American Burn Association Criteria for Transfer to a Burn Center**

- Second-degree burns over more than 10% of total body surface area
- Third-degree burns
- Burns to face, hands, feet, genitalia, perineum, or major joints
- Electric injury (lightning included)
- Chemical burns
- Inhalation injuries
- Burns accompanied by pre-existing medical conditions
- Burns accompanied by trauma, in which burn injury poses the greatest risk of morbidity or mortality
- Burns in children in hospitals without pediatric services
- Burns in patients with special social, emotional, or rehabilitative needs

Adapted from the American Burn Association Guidelines for Operation of Burn Units. Please see http://www.ameriburn.org/pub/guidelinesops.pdf (first page).

work well to maintain a steady level of analgesia between wound care procedures.

Mobilization

Open wounds begin to contract after the first week and can produce contractures, especially when burns are located over or near joints. Active and passive stretching as well as routine use of the burned extremity function to minimize this phenomenon. If a burn wound takes longer than 2 to 3 weeks to re-epithelialize, operative intervention will usually produce a better outcome. Once the wound has healed, scar maturation can take up to a year and should be managed as described later.

Most burn injuries can be treated successfully with simple wound care. More complicated burn injuries such as large burns, nonthermal burns, and deep burns are best treated in burn centers to take advantage of appropriate expertise and the multidisciplinary approach available at these institutions. The American Burn Association has identified a list of criteria that warrant transfer to a burn center (see Table 3).

TREATMENT OF LARGE BURNS

Large burns are defined as a total burn extent greater than 10% to 20% of the total body surface area. This is the threshold at which the induced inflammatory response becomes systemic and causes massive fluid shifts as capillaries become leaky in response to inflammatory signals. Therefore, replacement of the displaced intravascular volume is paramount to survival of the patient with a large burn. Intravascular access must be secured early, and isotonic fluid resuscitation is begun with lactated Ringer's solution, which has an electrolyte makeup most consistent with that of serum. Attempts to resuscitate with normal saline are complicated by progressive hyperchloremic metabolic acidosis. An estimation of the first 24-hour fluid needs is provided by the following formula:

$$4 \times (\text{weight in kilograms}) \times (\text{percentage of total body surface area burned})$$

Half of this volume is needed in the first 8 hours after the burn, with the remaining half delivered over the next 16 hours. This formula provides a guideline from which active fluid resuscitation should be titrated to maintain adequate organ perfusion. A urine output between 0.5 and 1.0 mL/kg (1.0 to 1.5 mL/kg in children) usually reflects an appropriate resuscitation rate during the first 24 hours after the burn injury. Additional parameters that can indicate inadequate fluid resuscitation include tachycardia and hypotension, lactic acidosis, and hemoconcentration.

Progressive edema formation can eventually compromise the airway, especially when burns are larger than 50% of total body surface area and involve the head and neck. Appropriate fluid resuscitation should not be withheld to minimize this effect. Instead, the airway should be controlled with endotracheal intubation if facial and upper airway swelling is imminent but before the act of intubation is compromised. Signs of a threatened airway include stridor, hoarseness, and depressed mental status and should prompt immediate intubation.

Hypothermia is a common, significant problem that develops insidiously during transport and evaluation of victims of burns. Many factors contribute to this effect, including high evaporative losses, vasodilatation at the wound base, routine exposure of the patient for wound assessment, and the use of cold, wet dressings. Every effort should be made to keep the patient warm. The evaluation room should be kept at 90°F, and the patient should be exposed briefly only when necessary. Removal of wet clothing and replacement with warm, dry sheets and blankets are appropriate during evaluation and before transport. Application of antibiotic ointment is best delayed until evaluation at a burn center. Prophylactic intravenous antibiotics are also not indicated.

Circumferentially burned extremities are at risk of developing compartment syndrome secondary to continued edema formation within a nonelastic eschar (the leathery skin denatured from the burn). Once signs of impaired circulation develop (pain with passive movement, distal numbness, and loss of distal capillary refill and pulses) or an internal tissue pressure breaches 30 to 35 mm Hg, escharotomy is indicated to relieve the pressure. Escharotomies are best oriented longitudinally along the extremities crossing the joints laterally and medially. Because it takes time for edema to develop, escharotomy is rarely necessary within the first 12 hours after a burn. If tissue pressures are not high, this procedure should be delayed until the patient has arrived at the burn center.

All burns are painful, even if they are mostly third-degree burns. Attention to adequate analgesia should begin once vital signs are confirmed. Morphine has a rapid onset and relatively long action and for many years has been the mainstay of analgesia in patients with burns. Large amounts of narcotics are often necessary, but they should be tempered by depressed mental status, hypotension, and respiratory depression in these patients. Concern for narcotic addiction at this time is irrelevant. Best results are achieved by administering frequent (every 5 to 10 minutes) small, intravenous doses (0.05 to 0.1 mg/kg morphine) while continuously reassessing for the drug's effect. Intravenous drug delivery is the most reliable route in the setting of burn shock.

SPECIAL TOPICS

Inhalation Injury

No single factor has more influence on mortality of burn victims than inhalation injury. Most thermal energy is effectively dissipated in the upper airways before reaching the lower airways. The toxins in smoke, however, can cause significant damage to the respiratory epithelium. History of the injury is highly predictive of inhalation injury when the victim was trapped in a closed, smoky space or if found unconscious from anoxia.

Signs and laboratory values that suggest inhalation injury include carbonaceous sputum, a hoarse voice, soot in the pharynx, and an arterial carboxyhemoglobin value greater than 10%. Confirmatory diagnostic tests include flexible bronchoscopy and xenon perfusion scan, the necessity of which is controversial because treatment is essentially supportive.

Treatment of inhalation injury involves supplemental oxygen, aggressive pulmonary suctioning, and mobilization of secretions. Bronchospasm precipitated by smoke may respond to inhaled bronchodilators. Although not necessary for all patients, endotracheal intubation is indicated for patients with any sign of airway or breathing compromise such as poor oxygenation, depressed mental status, or stridor. Percussive modes of ventilation have been shown to be more beneficial than standard ventilatory modes. Patients with high levels of carboxyhemoglobin (greater than 20%) are treated with endotracheal intubation and 100% oxygen until levels return to normal. Hyperbaric treatment of carbon monoxide poisoning (200% oxygen) is controversial and is thought to be unsafe for patients with large burns because of the complexity of their care and the limited access to patients who are in the hyperbaric chamber.

Chemical Burns

Most chemical burns are either from acid or from alkali; the latter tends to produce deeper injury. The onset can be insidious because many patients have contact with the chemical for hours before they experience symptoms. Initial treatment for these injuries should be aimed at preventing further burning by removing the patient's contaminated clothing and brushing off any dry chemical, followed by copious saline irrigation for at least 1 hour. Once the wound pH is neutral, as confirmed by litmus paper applied to the moist surface, the burn wound should be washed and dressed as described previously. Hydrofluoric acid burns, however, require special wound care. Hydrofluoric acid is an agent used for cleaning metal in industrial, farm, and car detailing applications. This acid has considerable penetration through the skin and can be neutralized only by calcium; therefore, treatment is aimed at increasing the calcium concentration of the tissues. For mild injuries, topical calcium gluconate gel (Calgonate) application changed every couple of hours is effective and when the injury is isolated to the hands; the gel can be held in place under a rubber glove. For more severe injuries, intra-arterial delivery of calcium gluconate* with management in an intensive care unit may be necessary. Treatment should continue until symptoms of pain resolve, which is thought to correlate with cessation of active tissue destruction.

Tar Burns

A common occupational hazard in the roofing and paving industry is a hot tar burn. Injury is minimized by immediate immersion in cool water for a few minutes to cool the adherent tar. Removal of the tar with a petroleum-based, surface active solvent (De-Solv-It) is nonirritating to the wound and is very effective. Care of the open wound is as described previously.

Electrical Burns

Electrical injury occurs in two forms: flash and current. Flash burns are generally less severe and result from the intense flash of heat and light that emanate from an electrical arc. The temperature is very high, although the duration is brief. Burns to exposed skin are usually second-degree burns, except when clothing is ignited, continues to burn, and thus causes deeper injury.

Electrical current burns are classified into low-voltage and high-voltage injuries. Low voltage (less than 1000 volts) rarely causes significant tissue damage, but it can precipitate cardiac arrhythmias, transient peripheral nerve symptoms, and shallow cutaneous burns. Electrocardiography, neurologic examination, and local wound care are the basic medical interventions. Twenty-four-hour cardiac monitoring is suggested when a history of syncope accompanies the injury or when changes are noted on the electrocardiogram.

High voltage (greater than 1000 volts) can produce extensive tissue damage. Characteristics of high-voltage injuries are entrance and exit sites consisting of focal third-degree burns with evidence of tissue vaporization sometimes extending into the deep tissues. Occult destruction can follow the haphazard path of the current from one focal wound to another, inciting complications including: (1) deep muscle necrosis leading to myoglobinemia and compartment syndrome, (2) peripheral nerve damage, (3) bone injury, (4) cardiac arrhythmias, (5) bowel perforation, and (6) lumbar spinal fractures. The possibility of extensive internal injuries beyond the extent of the cutaneous burns should prompt cautious treatment decisions. To minimize myoglobin toxicity to the kidneys, a high urine output should be maintained (1.5 to 2 mL/kg/hour) by increasing the rate of resuscitative fluid delivery when the urine is a dark burgundy or cola color characteristic of myoglobinuria. Electrocardiography and continuous cardiac monitoring are useful to screen for arrhythmias. Roentgenography of the lumbar spine can screen for lumbar fractures. Full neurologic assessment should be performed to evaluate for nerve injuries. Findings of distal numbness and paresthesias, pain with passive movement, and/or decreased capillary refill indicate compartment syndrome, at which time compartment pressures should be measured and fasciotomy performed in patients with tissue pressures greater than 35 mm Hg.

Gunpowder Burns

Close-range gunpowder explosions often produce burns accompanied by implantation of carbon particles in viable dermis. If not removed within 12 to 24 hours, these dermal implants will produce a

*Not FDA-approved for this indication.

permanent tattoo. Effective cleansing of the wound often requires vigorous scrubbing that patients can tolerate only when they are under general anesthesia in the operating room. Therefore, prompt consultation with a surgeon is mandatory for optimal cosmetic outcome.

SCAR MANAGEMENT

Healed burn wounds can produce scars often accompanied by discomfort, dysfunction, and disfigurement. Therapy to minimize scarring is indicated if, by 6 weeks, a raised, erythematous scar is evident (hypertrophic scar). Current scar therapies include massage, use of topical silicone, and pressure. Massage should be performed as often as possible, but at least four times per day for 10 to 15 minutes per session, and is facilitated by the use of moisturizer. For stubborn scars, topical silicone sheets have some effect if they are left in contact for extended periods. More extensive scars are best treated with constant-pressure therapy (20 to 25 mm Hg) by means of a custom-made elastic garment or plastic mold. When the scar extends over or close to a joint, full range of motion must be maintained by actively stretching out any tightness two to four times per day. Because contraction begins early in the healing process, stretching exercises are begun immediately after injury. Formal physical or occupational therapy should be enlisted when necessary. Most scar therapy should be delivered continuously until hyperemia of the scar resolves, usually 1 year after injury.

PSYCHOLOGICAL AND SOCIAL ISSUES

Understandably, psychological distress is common in patients with burns. Not only are burn injuries very painful, but also they are frequently accompanied by anxious concerns of permanent functional disability and disfigurement. Patients often relive the injury over and over again, a form of post-traumatic stress disorder. Psychological stress is aggravated when injuries physically preclude the patient from returning to previous employment, when the patient's home has been destroyed, or when loved ones have also been burned. For these and other reasons, both psychological counseling and social work assistance can be invaluable.

In many burn injuries, especially those involving children and the elderly, burns are sustained in an abusive or neglectful situation. It is estimated that 10% to 20% of all childhood burn injuries are secondary to abuse or neglect. Health care practitioners must maintain a high level of suspicion when they evaluate patients with burn injuries in these at-risk populations. A common form of child abuse is a dip injury in which the child is forcibly held under hot water for a significant amount of time; this injury creates second- or third-degree burns in well-demarcated, circumscribed patterns. Contact burns can also be associated with abuse and classically present as multiple small burns and/or burn scars in various stages of healing consistent with ongoing, repeated injury, usually from hot metal or cigarettes. Abuse must also be suspected when a delay in seeking medical assistance occurs or when repeated statements describing the incident are inconsistent. Engagement of experienced psychologists and/or social workers in cases in which abuse is suspected is invaluable, to protect both the patient from further injury and the family members and caregivers from false accusations. Clearly, great sensitivity is needed in such situations.

RECONSTRUCTION

Excessive scarring and contracture formation after deep burn injuries and skin grafting are often corrected by further reconstructive operations, sometimes years after the initial injury. Children are especially prone to contracture development, because bone growth under unyielding burn scars can produce tightness across joints and can limit movement. For these reasons, patients with burns require follow-up in burn centers for many years.

Small, shallow burns make up most burn injuries. Simple wound care to keep the wound clean and moist and the use of analgesics are frequently all that are needed to treat small burns. Large burns, nonthermal burns, and burns in critical locations require more complicated, multidisciplinary care. Such patients should be transferred to burn centers that are equipped to handle these complicated needs.

HIGH-ALTITUDE ILLNESS

method of
PETER H. HACKETT, M.D.
University of Colorado Health Sciences Center
Denver, Colorado

The term *high-altitude illness* encompasses clinical syndromes that occur on ascent to high altitude, generally higher than 2500 m. These syndromes reflect derangements of physiology resulting from the decreased partial pressure of oxygen in the thinner air. The syndromes include those affecting the brain (acute mountain sickness [AMS] and high-altitude cerebral edema [HACE]) and those affecting the lung (high-altitude pulmonary edema [HAPE] and high-altitude pulmonary hypertension [HAPH]). Chronic mountain polycythemia (CMP) is a condition affecting only long-term residents.

ACUTE MOUNTAIN SICKNESS AND HIGH-ALTITUDE CEREBRAL EDEMA

AMS is the most common high-altitude illness, striking as many as 25% of those who sleep at 2750 m, 40% of those sleeping at 3000 m, and 70% of those who make a rapid ascent from low altitude to 4000 m. Day trips to high altitude are much less likely to induce AMS. Risk factors for AMS include residence at altitudes lower than 1000 m, abrupt ascent (low altitude to more than 2500 m in 1 day), physical exertion, and a past history of AMS. Gender and age have little effect, although persons more than 50 years old are slightly less susceptible. Physical fitness is not protective. The elderly, persons with cardiovascular and respiratory diseases, patients with diabetes, and pregnant women, among others with common medical conditions, are not particularly predisposed to develop AMS. Altitude exposure within the previous week, especially for more than 2 days, will aid acclimatization and helps to prevent AMS.

The diagnosis of AMS is based on the setting of a recent gain in altitude and on typical symptoms (Table 1). No physical findings confirm AMS. Because the symptoms are nonspecific, other diagnoses must always be considered, especially when duration at a given altitude exceeds 3 to 4 days, by which time the patient should be relatively acclimatized. Symptoms do not correlate well with pulse oximetry; although low oxygen saturation is more often associated with symptoms, many patients who are ill have normal pulse oximetry values for the altitude. The usual course of AMS is resolution over 12 to 48 hours as acclimatization proceeds, as long as no further ascent takes place while the patient is symptomatic.

HACE is defined as progressive neurologic deterioration in someone with AMS (or HAPE) and is characterized by a change in consciousness and by the presence of truncal ataxia (see Table 1). HACE typically develops over 2 to 3 days and is often associated with pulmonary edema. The onset of coma from initial ataxia and confusion may be as rapid as 8 to 12 hours. Death results from brain herniation.

TABLE 1. **Diagnostic Criteria for High-Altitude Illness**

Acute Mountain Sickness

Recent gain in altitude in an unacclimatized person
Headache plus at least one of the following: anorexia, nausea, or vomiting; insomnia; dizziness; or fatigue

High-Altitude Cerebral Edema

Progression of neurologic symptoms and signs in a person with acute mountain sickness or high-altitude pulmonary edema, characterized by a change in consciousness and ataxia

High-Altitude Pulmonary Edema

Recent gain in altitude in an unacclimatized person
Two or more of the following symptoms: dyspnea at rest, cough, weakness, decreased exercise performance, chest tightness, or congestion
Two or more of the following signs: rales or wheezing in one or more lung fields, central cyanosis, tachypnea, tachycardia, or pulse oximetry oxygen saturation more than 10 points below normal for the altitude

High-Altitude Pulmonary Hypertension

Asymptomatic: a high-altitude resident with elevated pulmonary arterial pressure but without symptoms; possible right axis deviation or right ventricular hypertrophy on electrocardiogram
Symptomatic: a high altitude resident (infant, child, or adult) with elevated pulmonary arterial pressure and symptoms, either mild (dyspnea on exertion and chest tightness) or severe (cor pulmonale and right heart failure)

Chronic Mountain Polycythemia (Chronic Mountain Sickness)

A high-altitude resident with a hemoglobin concentration >20 g/dL and headaches, dizziness, fatigue, poor exercise performance, and impaired cerebral function

Exactly what causes AMS and HACE is unknown. Clinically, they seem to represent ends of a continuous spectrum. However, magnetic resonance imaging has documented reversible white matter edema in patients with HACE and severe AMS, but not in persons with mild to moderate AMS. Whether this finding reflects a limitation of these techniques to demonstrate very early edema or whether the pathophysiology of early AMS is different from that of HACE is still unknown. AMS is associated with a poor ventilatory response to hypoxia, elevated antidiuretic hormone and aldosterone, and fluid retention.

Management of AMS is based on three principles: (1) stop ascent when symptoms develop, (2) descend to a lower altitude if symptoms progress despite rest or treatment, and (3) descend immediately if the patient shows any sign of HACE. Descent is the definitive treatment but is not always necessary or possible. Supplemental oxygen and various medications will also help to resolve AMS and, to some extent, HACE (Tables 2 and 3). AMS can be treated effectively by using portable hyperbaric bags, which simulate descent to a lower altitude. Persons who have recovered from AMS can often ascend successfully afterward, especially with acetazolamide (Diamox) prophylaxis. Persons with HACE who do not rapidly and completely recover on descent, or those with focal neurologic deficits, should be hospitalized for a complete evaluation including magnetic resonance imaging.

The most effective preventive measure for AMS is slow, staged ascent, to allow time for acclimatization. Experts recommend not going directly from low altitude to more than 2750 m sleeping altitude in 1 day. They also recommend moving the sleeping altitude upward no more than 700 m per day once above 3000 m, with an extra day taken for acclimatization every 1000 m or so. These general guidelines are too slow for some persons and too fast for those with the genetic disposition to poor acclimatization and AMS. Currently, only past experience at altitude identifies these susceptible persons. Agents useful for chemical prophylaxis are listed in Table 3. Indications for prophylaxis include a past history of AMS or HACE or unavoidable abrupt ascent. Acetazolamide, the agent of choice for prevention of AMS, is also useful for treatment when it is given early in the illness and thus offers an alternative to prophylaxis.

HIGH-ALTITUDE PULMONARY EDEMA

HAPE accounts for most deaths from high-altitude illness. HAPE is noncardiogenic, hydrostatic edema caused by hypoxia-induced changes in the pulmonary circulation. Current thinking is that pulmonary hypertension caused by uneven pulmonary arteriolar vasoconstriction, combined with pulmonary venous constriction, leads to capillary hypertension and a reversible leak in the fragile capillaries. HAPE is preceded or accompanied by AMS 50% of the time;

TABLE 2. **Management of Acute High-Altitude Illness**

Clinical Presentation	Management
Mild Acute Mountain Sickness Mild to moderate headache with nausea, dizziness, or fatigue within first 24 h of ascent to high altitude (>2500 m)	Stop ascent, rest, and acclimatize, or descend 500 m or more Speed acclimatization with acetazolamide (Diamox), 125-250 mg PO bid Treat symptoms with mild analgesics and antiemetics Or use combination of these approaches
Moderate Acute Mountain Sickness Moderate to severe headache with marked nausea or vomiting, weakness, dizziness, lassitude, and peripheral edema 12-24 h after rapid ascent to high altitude	Stop ascent, rest, treat medically, or descend 500 m or more Give acetazolamide (Diamox), 250 mg PO bid, or dexamethasone (Decadron),* 4 mg PO or IM q6h, or both Administer low-flow oxygen (1-2 L/min) or use portable hyperbaric chamber Treat symptoms Or use combination of these approaches
High-Altitude Cerebral Edema Confusion, lassitude, and ataxia 48 h after ascent to high altitude; had acute mountain sickness first 2 d	Start immediate descent or evacuation If descent delayed or impossible, use portable hyperbaric chamber and/or administer oxygen (2-4 L/min) Administer dexamethasone (Decadron), 8 mg IM, IV, or PO initially, then 4 mg q6h
High-Altitude Pulmonary Edema Cough, weakness, dyspnea, chest congestion 60 h after arrival at 2750 m	Administer oxygen (2-4 L/min, to keep arterial oxygen saturation >90%) Start immediate descent, minimizing exertion and cold stress If descent delayed or impossible, or if oxygen unavailable, use portable hyperbaric chamber If descent or oxygen unavailable, administer nifedipine (Procardia, Adalat),* 10 mg PO initially, then 30 mg extended-release formulation q12h Albuterol (Proventil)* inhaler, four to six puffs q4h

*Not FDA-approved for this indication.

TABLE 3. **Medications for Acute High-Altitude Illness**

Agent	Indication	Dose	Adverse Effects	Comments
Acetazolamide (Diamox)	Prevention of AMS	125-250 mg PO bid a day beginning 24 h before ascent until 48 h at altitude	Common: paresthesias, polyuria, altered taste of carbonated beverages Precautions: sulfonamide reactions possible; avoided in breast-feeding; can decrease therapeutic levels of lithium	Can be taken episodically for symptoms; no rebound effect; pregnancy category C
	Treatment of AMS	250 mg PO q8-12h		
	Treatment of pediatric AMS	2.5 mg/kg body weight PO q12h		
	Treatment of periodic breathing	125 mg PO 1 h before bed		
Dexamethasone (Decadron)*	Treatment of AMS	4 mg q6h PO, IM, or IV	Mood changes; hyperglycemia; dyspepsia	Rapidly improves AMS symptoms; can be lifesaving in HACE; may improve HACE enough to facilitate descent; no value in HAPE; pregnancy category C
	Treatment of HACE	8 mg initially, then 4 mg q6h PO, IM, or IV		
	Treatment of pediatric HACE	1-2 mg/kg body weight initially, then 0.25-0.5 mg/kg q6h PO, IM, or IV, not to exceed 16 mg/d		
Ginkgo biloba[†]	Prevention of AMS	80-120 mg PO bid starting 5 d before ascent and continuing to highest altitude	Occasional headache; rare reports of bleeding	Requires further study; preparations vary
Nifedipine (Procardia, Adalat)*	Prevention of HAPE	20-30 mg extended-release PO q12h	Reflex tachycardia; hypotension (uncommon)	No value in AMS or HACE; not necessary if supplemental oxygen available; pregnancy category C
	Treatment of HAPE	10 mg PO initially, then 20-30 mg extended-release PO q12h		
Promethazine (Phenergan)	Symptomatic treatment of nausea and vomiting	25-50 mg PO, IM, IV, or rectally q6h	Causes sedation; extrapyramidal reactions may occur with high doses	Pregnancy category C
Zolpidem (Ambien)	Treatment of insomnia	10 mg PO	Rare, short-acting	Does not depress ventilation at high altitude; pregnancy category B

*Not FDA-approved for this indication.
[†]Available as a dietary supplement and not yet approved for this indication.
AMS, acute mountain sickness; HACE, high-altitude cerebral edema; HAPE, high-altitude pulmonary edema.

10% to 20% of patients with HAPE develop cerebral edema. Risk factors for HAPE include abrupt ascent, overexertion, and a past history of HAPE. Girls and women have lower incidence of HAPE than do boys and men. HAPE-susceptible persons demonstrate increased pulmonary vasoreactivity to hypoxia at low and high altitude, greater pulmonary hypertension, and lower ventilation on ascent to high altitude. Scientists have demonstrated an association between certain genotypes and HAPE susceptibility.

The diagnosis of HAPE while still early in its course and most easily treated requires a high index of suspicion. A decrease in exercise performance coupled with a dry cough is sufficient to raise consideration of HAPE. Crackles may be present at this time, most often in the right middle lobe of the lung. As the illness progresses, dyspnea at rest becomes noticeable, as well as tachycardia, tachypnea, and, in late stages, pink, frothy sputum. Drowsiness is usually the first neurologic symptom, followed by confusion and then ataxia if HACE develops. The differential diagnosis includes respiratory infections, asthma, mucus plugging, pulmonary embolus, acute myocardial infarction, and heart failure. The mortality from HAPE is high, generally because the victim is in a remote and inaccessible region and is without oxygen. In contrast, HAPE in ski resorts is rarely fatal because of the proximity of medical care and supplemental oxygen.

Improving oxygenation is the highest priority for treating HAPE (see Table 2). Breathing supplemental oxygen quickly reduces pulmonary artery pressure, raises arterial oxygenation, protects the brain, and is lifesaving. In fact, in Colorado ski resorts, the usual care for mild to moderate HAPE is to keep the patient at high altitude and to administer oxygen by concentrator or compressed gas in the patient's hotel room. This approach requires 2 to 3 days, but it allows the patient to remain with the family and not completely spoil the vacation. For severe HAPE, defined as an oxygen requirement of greater than 4 to 5 L/minute to maintain normal oxygen saturation, or the presence of HACE, patients are transferred to hospital at lower altitude. If oxygen is not available, immediate descent with minimal exertion by the victim is the best strategy, with or without medication. Hyperbaric bags are also useful. Drugs that reduce pulmonary artery pressure are adjunctive treatment for HAPE; none are nearly as effective as oxygen or descent. These include nifedipine (Adalat),* nitric oxide (INOmax),* and epoprostenol (Flolan),* with sildenafil (Viagra)* currently under investigation because it blocks hypoxic pulmonary hypertension. Salmeterol (Serevent)* has been found effective for prevention of HAPE, presumably because β-agonists up-regulate transport of alveolar fluid back to the interstitial space. Given this mechanism, it seems likely that β-agonist drugs will help to improve clinical HAPE. Because these agents are safe and easy to use, I recommend them for the treatment of HAPE (see Tables 2 and 3). Positive airway pressure devices help to improve gas exchange in HAPE and are useful when oxygen supplementation and descent are not available. Once HAPE has resolved, patients sometimes resume skiing or climbing, even reaching summits. An episode of HAPE demonstrates one's susceptibility to the condition, and although it is not a contraindication to a subsequent ascent, caution is warranted. Persons with repeated episodes should consider prophylaxis with nifedipine and perhaps with salmeterol as well.

*Not FDA-approved for this indication.

HIGH-ALTITUDE PULMONARY HYPERTENSION

Unlike the altitude illnesses already discussed, HAPH is a problem of longer-term high-altitude visitors or residents. Certain genotypes are associated with exaggerated pulmonary hypertension during exposure to hypoxia, and pulmonary hypertension persists in these persons even with long-term exposure. Although persons with mild HAPH are asymptomatic, some go on to develop severe clinical problems. *Subacute infantile mountain sickness* was a term used to describe Chinese infants who, when brought to the altitude of the Tibetan plateau, developed cor pulmonale and right heart failure, with a high mortality. The same syndrome, resulting from severe pulmonary hypertension, develops in Indian soldiers on transfer to high altitude, generally within the first 6 to 12 months. The only effective treatment to date is relocation to lower altitude, whereas oxygen and diuretics may offer temporizing measures. Less severe HAPH can result in dyspnea on exertion and chest tightness, and it can occur in tourists as well as residents.

CHRONIC MOUNTAIN POLYCYTHEMIA

CMP is defined as excessive polycythemia in a high-altitude resident. Whereas hemoglobin concentration is elevated in all high-altitude residents, those with CMP have values greater than 20 g/dL. Symptoms include headache, insomnia, dizziness, fatigue, and impaired cerebral function, all of which resolve with relocation to lower altitude or phlebotomy to reduce hematocrit. Greater hypoxemia and pulmonary hypertension are also present. Symptoms are attributed to increased blood viscosity. What causes the condition is unclear. Many cases of CMP are secondary, and the excessive polycythemia is the result of lung disease, sleep-disordered breathing, or other primary problems. Patients with primary CMP, also called chronic mountain sickness, may have idiopathic hypoventilation causing greater hypoxemia or a disorder of erythropoietin regulation. The World Health Organization has recognized CMP as a public health problem of high-altitude regions of the world.

DISTURBANCES DUE TO COLD

method of
GORDON G. GIESBRECHT, PH.D.
University of Manitoba
Winnipeg, Manitoba, Canada

For many clinicians, the book on disturbances due to cold has been closed for some time. Many preeminent scientists and physicians wrote extensively about accidental hypothermia and frostbite from the Second World War until the 1980s. With the scientific emphasis shifting to cellular and molecular biology, less work has been done on whole-body human research in the past 20 years. Thus, many present-day physicians base clinical decisions on older literature, and, sometimes, on isolated anecdotes. In many cases, dogma has emerged that is difficult to amend, even in the face of recent research and evidence-based medicine. This update addresses prehospital and emergency department care for cold disturbances.

ACCIDENTAL HYPOTHERMIA

Etiology

The decrease in body core temperature (T_{co}) during accidental hypothermia can result from cold water immersion (head above water), cold water submersion (head below water; cold water near-drowning), and exposure to cold environments. Hypothermia onset depends mainly on the imbalance between increased heat loss and decreased heat production. Heat loss can be increased by environmental factors (especially the combination of cold, wet, and wind), inadequacy of clothing insulation (which is attenuated if wet), lean body composition, or some skin diseases. Heat production can be deleteriously affected by age, malnutrition, sleep deprivation, medical illness, trauma, and several pharmacologic agents.

Because of their higher body surface-to-mass ratio, children cool faster than adults. During complete submersion in cold water, this factor is advantageous, as children will cool faster and thus benefit more from cold-induced protection from hypoxic brain damage. On the other hand, adults have the advantage during cold water head-out immersion or exposure to cold air, as they will become hypothermic at a slower rate.

When long-term cold exposure induces a reduction in shivering rate or ability to exercise, overall heat production decreases and the rate of core cooling increases.

Pathophysiology

The primary effect of body core cooling is a decrease in tissue metabolism and gradual inhibition of neural transmission and control. However, in the intact conscious condition, the secondary responses to skin cooling predominate initially. Therefore, sudden cooling of the skin initiates shivering thermogenesis, with increased metabolism ($\dot{V}O_2$), minute ventilation ($\dot{V}_E$), heart rate (f_c), cardiac output, and mean arterial pressure. The primary effects of cooling can be seen during anesthesia or at lower core temperatures (i.e., TC_o <30°C [86°F]) when shivering ceases and $\dot{V}O_2$, $\dot{V}_E$, f_c, mean arterial pressure, and cardiac output decrease with the fall in core temperature, and total peripheral resistance increases. During cooling, there can be a considerable loss of intravenous volume due to extravascular fluid shifts and renal diuresis, thus increasing hematocrit and blood viscosity and decreasing systemic perfusion.

Other effects include coagulopathies caused by depressed enzymatic function of clotting factors and weakened clot strength due to platelet malfunction. Thus, trauma with significant bleeding carries an increased risk of shock in the hypothermic victim. Although hypothermia may provide some protection for brain trauma or ischemia (i.e., following stroke or cardiac arrest), it is not protective after severe truncal trauma.

Classification

The following classification system for hypothermia is helpful because it is based on physiologic thresholds and is related to treatment protocols. Temperature, however, should not be the sole criterion for a clinical classification (see later). In mild hypothermia (T_{co} 35 to 32°C [95 to 90°F]) thermoregulatory mechanisms (i.e., shivering) operate fully, with development of ataxia, dysarthria, and apathy. In moderate hypothermia (T_{co} 32 to 28°C [90 to 82°F]), the effectiveness of the thermoregulatory system diminishes until it fails, the primary effect of body cooling becomes evident, there is a progressive decrease in level of consciousness, and atrial fibrillation and other cardiac dysrhythmias occur. In severe hypothermia (T_{co} <28°C [82°F]), consciousness is generally lost, shivering is absent, acid-base disturbances develop, and the heart is susceptible to ventricular fibrillation (either spontaneous or caused by mechanical stimuli) or asystole. Death from hypothermia is generally from cardiorespiratory failure.

Treatment

Prehospital Paramedical Care

One complicating factor in paramedical care is that of an unconscious patient at a possible crime scene. There may be a tendency to assume the victim is dead and to preserve the scene for analysis. However, it is more important to assume the victim is resuscitatable, to begin treatment, and to transport the patient to advanced medical care immediately.

The paramedical personnel should apply electrocardiographic leads and keep the patient horizontal to prevent episodes of perirescue collapse. They should start an intravenous infusion with 250 to 500 mL of 5% dextrose in warmed normal saline solution. Lactated Ringer's solution should be avoided because a cold liver cannot metabolize lactate. Inhalation of warmed humidified air/oxygen could be initiated if available. Although inhalation warming will not significantly warm the body core, cardiorespiratory and thermoregulatory control may improve because of direct warming of upper airway and brainstem structures. Ventilatory support is also provided.

If a patient is severely hypothermic, endogenous heat production will be minimal and external heat is required to reverse the fall in T_{co}. The attending personnel should remove all wet clothes gently, preferably by cutting them off, and wrap the patient in effective insulation. The decision to actively heat the patient depends on the expected elapsed time until arrival at an advanced medical care facility. If transport will take more than about 30 minutes and circulation is intact, active warming should be initiated. If power is available in rescue/transport vehicles (e.g., helicopter, airplane, ambulance) the use of forced-air warming and resistive heating devices could be used to apply heat to the torso only.

Some practitioners believe that such warming may be dangerous, and the advice to prevent "uncontrolled superficial warming" is common. First, if shivering is absent, the patient's T_{co} will continue to decrease substantially and remain low for several hours even if the patient is dry and insulated. Second, with the limited amounts of heat available during prehospital transport, there is no danger of warming too rapidly or inducing cardiovascular collapse due to vasodilation.

At low T_{co}, the heart may beat slowly and weakly, making it difficult to obtain a pulse. If heart activity is not apparent in a hypothermic victim, one must not start cardiopulmonary resuscitation unless it is clear that the heart is not beating. Premature initiation of chest compressions may induce ventricular fibrillation. One should feel for a carotid pulse for at least 1 minute or, preferably, use an electrocardiographic monitor to determine whether there is a viable cardiac rhythm.

Respiration is evidence of an active heart (Figure 1). In the absence of respiration, 1 to 2 minutes of ventilation may improve cardiac status to the point that heart beats may be detected. If signs of respiration and heart activity are still not seen, the attending personnel should start cardiopulmonary resuscitation. Once it is determined that cardiopulmonary resuscitation is necessary, chest compressions should follow the standard recommended frequency. Care must be taken not to hyperventilate the patient, as resulting hypocapnia may increase the tendency for ventricular fibrillation. One can avoid hyperventilation either by using mouth-to-mouth breathing at normothermic rates or by ventilating with air or 100% oxygen at about half of the normothermic rate.

Rarely, intubation has triggered ventricular fibrillation, but never following preoxygenation of the patient. If conditions warrant, intubation should proceed.

It should be standard practice to measure core temperature in cold victims. Esophageal temperature is the best noninvasive measure (see later) and can be easily obtained by standard portable telethermometers. An accurate core temperature is valuable for determining whether unconsciousness is due to hypothermia or other causes.

It is very important to provide the advanced medical facility with medical information during prehospital transport. If coordinated properly, the emergency department personnel can be ready to commence aggressive therapy immediately on patient admission.

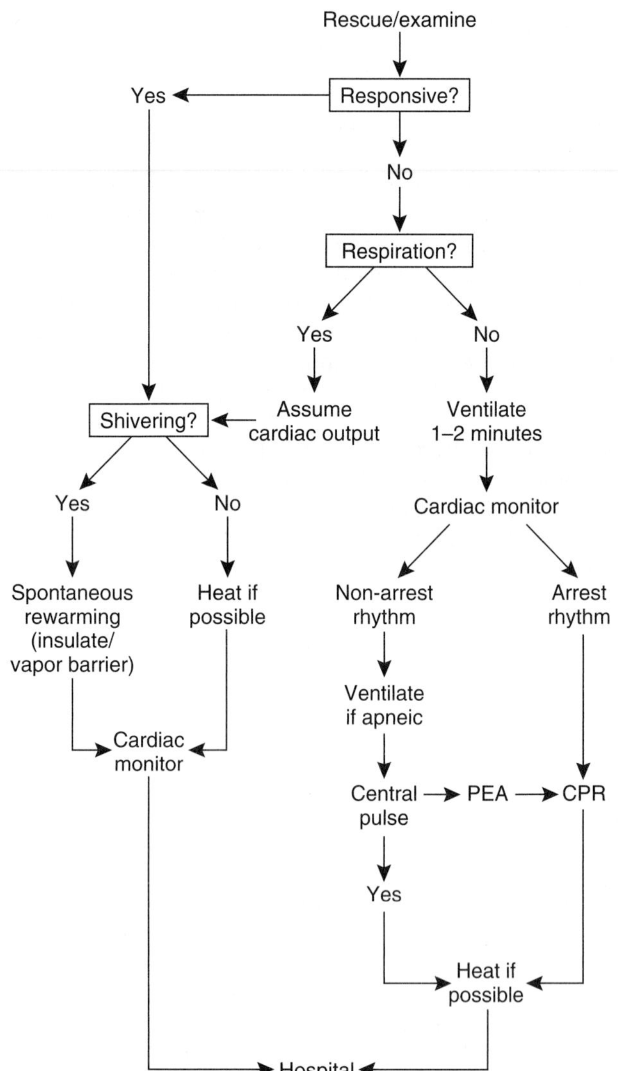

Figure 1. Emergency Medical Service (EMS) algorithm for hypothermia treatment. CPR, cardiopulmonary resuscitation; PEA, pulseless electrical activity.

Emergency Department Care

The main priorities for treatment are to arrest the fall in core temperature and to establish a steady, safe rewarming rate while maintaining the stability of the cardiovascular system and providing sufficient physiologic support (i.e., oxygenation, correction of metabolic and electrolyte imbalances, and intravenous volume replenishment).

Hypothermia should not be classified on the basis of temperature alone. Patients should be primarily classified by level of consciousness and cardiovascular stability, with core temperature used as an adjunctive diagnostic tool. A more important factor regarding core temperature may not be its present value but, rather, the direction in which it is going. Core temperature varies depending on where it is measured. Rectal temperature (T_{re}) is most commonly used in clinical settings, but T_{re} lags behind esophageal temperature (T_{es}) during non–steady state conditions, with T_{re} being higher than T_{es} during cooling but lower during warming, sometimes by several degrees. The greatest inaccuracy occurs during the transition from cooling to warming (the period when treatment decisions are often made in the emergency department). Heart and esophageal temperature may be rising but T_{re} will continue to decrease for up to 1 hour. Basing treatment on T_{re} values may result in too early use of invasive methods that could be avoided by waiting or measuring T_{es}.

A cardiac monitor (preferably 12-lead) should be attached and intravenous catheters inserted as required. Arterial blood gases are taken without correcting for temperature. The most important laboratory measures are blood sugar and electrolytes. Other, less important measures include urea, complete blood cell count, creatinine, serum calcium, serum magnesium, serum amylase, prothrombin and partial thromboplastin times, platelet count, and fibrinogen levels. Nasogastric tube insertion is indicated in cases of moderate or severe hypothermia, and indwelling bladder catheters with urine meters are necessary to monitor urine output. In cases of mild to moderate hypothermia, noninvasive heat sources may be sufficient. In severe cases in which cardiorespiratory activity is present, invasive measures such as arteriovenous fistula (otherwise known as continuous arteriovenous rewarming) and body cavity lavage are warranted. In the case of cardiac arrest, cardiopulmonary bypass is preferred for rewarming and cardiorespiratory support.

The pharmacologic effects of various drugs are decreased at lower temperatures because of increased protein binding. In addition, clearance is also diminished to such a degree that drugs will be less effective at low temperatures and may reach toxic levels following rewarming. It is generally accepted that the most effective agent during hypothermia for treating ventricular fibrillation is bretylium tosylate because of its direct effects on the myocardium. Although data are sparse, bretylium infusion of 10 g/kg has resulted in chemical ventricular defibrillation in hypothermic patients.

Defibrillation is usually ineffective for myocardial temperatures below 30°C (86°F). Furthermore, repeated defibrillatory shocks may damage the myocardium. Defibrillation should be limited to three shocks at 200 joules (J), 300 J, and 360 J, consecutively, in patients colder than 30°C (86°F). If this is not successful, one should assume that the victim must be rewarmed before further attempts are made.

In all cases, once treatment has been initiated, resuscitation efforts should not be discontinued until core temperature has been raised to at least 32°C (90°F).

FROSTBITE

Etiology

Frostbite describes the freezing of peripheral tissue. There are many risk factors for frostbite. External factors include low ambient temperature, wind chill, duration of exposure, clothing (either low insulation value or a tight fit that restricts blood supply), immobilization, direct contact with metal, or wetness. Physiologic factors include dehydration, race, illness, drug or ethanol ingestion, circulatory deficits, extreme fatigue, and previous episodes of frostbite. Frostbite may be unavoidable in some emergency situations, such as being stranded on a mountainside in a storm. Many cases could be avoided, however, such as those caused by drug- or alcohol-induced unconsciousness or merely neglecting to care for cold extremities.

Pathology

Tissue damage relates to the tissue destroyed during freezing itself and to post-thaw problems with circulatory insufficiency and release of inflammatory mediators consistent with a reperfusion injury. The process of ice crystal formation depends on rate of freezing. During rapid freezing (i.e., within minutes) ice crystals form predominantly intracellularly, which can cause direct physical destruction of the cells. Slower freezing (over hours to days) results in larger ice crystal formation in the interstitium. If this condition persists, cellular water can be drawn into the interstitium, leading to intracellular dehydration, toxic concentrations of electrolytes, membrane collapse, and cell destruction.

Following thawing, circulation to the affected area may be compromised because of physical destruction of microvasculature during freezing, deposition of capillary microthrombi, or damage to the vascular endothelium. Reversal of the direct freezing injury is dependent on blood-borne oxygen and nutrients. Thawing may lead to a condition similar to reperfusion injury, with formation of arachidonic acid metabolites and oxygen free radicals. For instance, prostaglandin $F_{2\alpha}$ and thromboxane A_2 lead to vasoconstriction, platelet aggregation, and vessel thrombosis, which potentiates cellular hypoxia and death.

Classification, Signs, and Symptoms

Although frostbite is often described by clinical presentation, these classifications do not guarantee prediction of final outcome. First-degree frostbite involves numbness, erythema, and often edema. Second-degree injury is usually confined to the epidermal layers of skin and produces clear blisters (usually extending to the end of the digits), surrounded by erythema and edema. Third-degree frostbite usually extends beneath the dermal vascular plexus and results in purple, blood-containing blisters (which often do not extend to the end of the digits). Fourth-degree injury extends below the dermal layer to muscle and bone and leads to mummification.

In the field, differentiation between superficial and deep frostbite is important, as a person can remain in the field once superficial frostbite is reversed. Evacuation is advised for all cases of deep (second- to fourth-degree) frostbite. Skin color will generally progress from pink to red to pale white to yellow. Sensation changes from cold, to prickly pain, to more severe pain, to numbness, to total anesthesia. At this point, the skin is in jeopardy of freezing. Skin texture changes from soft and pliable to stiff and hard. Joints will progressively become fixed and immobile.

In the hospital, the part may be frozen and be cold, stiff, anesthetic, immobile, and pale yellow. If thawing has already occurred, the part may be swollen, painful, partially immobile, pale, dusky, and cyanotic, and blebs may have already developed.

Treatment

In the field, care should be taken to guarantee the prevention of refreezing before thawing is attempted. It would be better to let the part remain frozen, even for days, rather than risk refreezing, as the ultimate tissue damage will be much worse.

Regardless of the location, rapid warming in 40 to 42°C (104 to 108°F) water is indicated, provided refreezing can be avoided. This process can be extremely painful. If pain is a problem, the water temperature can be safely reduced to 32 to 38°C (90 to 100°F) with little or no effect on subsequent prognosis. A whirlpool bath is preferred and the water should contain an antiseptic soap such as Hibiclens. The affected part should be warmed until vascular flushing reaches the tips of the digits (usually within 30 minutes) or a line of pale demarcation persists between warmed and unwarmed tissue (inability to rewarm a part is a very poor prognostic sign). Pain may be significant during rewarming, and morphine or meperidine (Demerol) can be given intravenously or intramuscularly as indicated.

After rewarming, one should dry the area carefully and leave the limb exposed on clean sheets and protected with appropriate bed cradles. Pledgets can be placed between the digits to prevent maceration unless the swelling could cause compression.

One must take extreme care to maintain the affected area under very clean or aseptic conditions. All blebs should be left intact in the hope that the fluid will be absorbed. Blood-filled blisters indicate severe underlying injury and should be left intact to prevent infection. Ruptured blebs should be débrided and treated with topical aloe vera (Dermaide aloe) or a specific thromboxane inhibitor. Penicillin (500,000 U) is administered every 6 hours for the first 72 hours, and subsequently if signs of infection ensue.

Following rewarming, the clinician should elevate the injured extremities above the level of the patient's heart to minimize edema and avoid any further trauma to the area. Ibuprofen (Motrin) 400 mg should be given every 6 hours for several days. This drug inhibits the arachidonic acid cascade, promotes fibrinolysis, and provides some analgesia. Intravenous low molecular weight dextran (1 L) can be given within the first 24 hours to prevent or reverse erythrocyte clumping and increased blood viscosity. Antitetanus prophylaxis is also indicted.

Hydrotherapy should be conducted in a whirlpool bath at about 40°C (104°F) for 30 to 45 minutes, twice a day. This will assist physiologic separation of necrotic tissues from newly formed epithelium below. Daily physiotherapy should be started immediately to promote joint motion.

Tissue edema appears within 3 hours of rewarming and may last 5 or more days. Bullae may appear 6 to 24 hours after rewarming. After 9 to 15 days, frostbitten skin becomes black and hard, and a dry eschar forms. Mummification occurs and a line of demarcation forms within 22 to 45 days.

One should delay surgical involvement, beyond minor débridement, as long as possible. The old maxim "frozen in January, amputate in June" may not be temporally correct but is the principle to be followed so as not to destroy salvageable tissue. Technetium-99m scans of the affected extremity done shortly after the patient arrives, after 2 to 3 days, and after 2 to 3 weeks may provide good prognostic information and help in the decision about whether or when to amputate. If an eschar becomes constrictive, it should be incised with lateral or dorsal slits to permit joint movement. Severe edema may increase intracompartmental pressure (P_{IC}) to the point of preventing cellular perfusion and causing a risk of amputation of nonfrostbitten tissue. If the P_{IC} increases above 35 mm Hg, extensive fasciotomy opening of all major compartments may save a limb that would otherwise require amputation.

The decision to amputate should be based on the presence of gangrene with a clear demarcation line and with a viable tissue proximal to the line of demarcation. Frequently, the area of healthy tissue is separated from the gangrenous area by a narrow line of pink granulation tissue. Amputation should be delayed until the tissue is dry and not edematous. It is important that amputation be done through viable, nondraining, uninfected tissue. If gangrene is "wet," it is because of infection, and the patient must receive massive doses of antibiotics and have a guillotine amputation with revision later.

The level of amputation is functionally important, and salvage of a few centimeters is very important, especially in the hands. Attempts at early amputation may lead to the unnecessary removal of viable and perhaps functionally valuable tissue. Amputations may have to be revised and plastic surgery may be necessary to reconstruct digits and stumps to increase the functional efficiency of the limbs.

DISTURBANCES DUE TO HEAT

method of
MICHAEL P. WAINSCOTT, M.D.
University of Texas Southwestern Medical Center
Dallas, Texas

The spectrum of heat illness encompasses a broad range from heat cramps to life-threatening heat stroke. The summer of 1995 brought a record heat wave that generated an estimated 750 deaths in Chicago. *Hyperthermia* is a temperature in excess of the normal range of 36°C (96.8°F) to 37.5°C (99.5°F). Temperatures higher than 41°C (105°F) may be life-threatening.

THERMOREGULATION

Control of thermoregulation resides within the hypothalamus, which stimulates cutaneous vasodilation and sweating through the autonomic nervous system in response to elevation of blood temperature. Blood flow to the skin may increase 20-fold. Cooling normally occurs by transfer of heat from the skin by radiation, convection, and evaporation. As the ambient temperature exceeds the body's temperature, a rise in body temperature may occur in response to radiation and convection of heat from the environment. When the humidity rises, the body's ability to cool through evaporation is diminished.

PREDISPOSING FACTORS

Many factors predispose to heat illness, often by impairing thermoregulation. Heat production within the body increases as a result of exercise, drugs such as sympathomimetics, fever, exertional states such as drug-induced agitation, and muscular rigidity states such as malignant hyperthermia and neuroleptic malignant syndrome. The muscular rigidity states cause hyperthermia without high ambient temperature and are not included in this discussion. Table 1 is a list of predisposing factors to heat illness.

HEAT EXHAUSTION

Heat exhaustion is a relatively common disorder in patients exposed to high ambient temperature who do not adequately replace fluid and electrolyte losses. Classic descriptions of heat exhaustion suggest two types: water depletion and salt depletion. It is more practical to view patients with heat exhaustion as suffering from volume depletion, with electrolyte disturbances based on fluid and electrolyte intake versus losses.

Clinically, the patient has systemic symptoms including fatigue, headache, dizziness, weakness, nausea, vomiting, muscle cramps, lightheadedness, and possibly syncope. Evaluation may reveal diaphoresis, orthostatic hypotension, and tachycardia. The patient's temperature may be normal or elevated up to 40°C (104°F). Mental status is normal. If mental status changes are present, the patient must be treated for heat stroke.

In addition to rest and removal of the patient to a cool environment, treatment is directed at volume replacement, usually with intravenous saline solutions. Laboratory studies direct the electrolyte management. Elevated blood urea nitrogen and hemoconcentration are common. Although uncommon, severe hypernatremia associated with extremely limited fluid intake may be seen and must be treated slowly, to avoid cerebral edema.

Patients with heat exhaustion are monitored by vital signs, symptom relief, and urine output. Hospitalization is usually not necessary unless there are complicating medical conditions, such as impaired renal or cardiac function, significant electrolyte disturbances, underlying illness, injuries, or extremes of age.

TABLE 1. **Factors Predisposing to Heat-Related Illness**

Increased heat production
Hot, humid, windless environment
Lack of acclimatization or physical conditioning
Dehydration
Cardiovascular disease
Extremes of age
Obesity
Inappropriate clothing or external equipment
Skin diseases
Medications or drugs of abuse

HEAT STROKE WITH HIGH AMBIENT TEMPERATURE

Heat stroke includes a temperature higher than 41°C (105.8°F), and mental status changes. The literature suggests that (regardless of cause) it is a form of hyperthermia associated with a systemic inflammatory response leading to a syndrome of multiorgan dysfunction in which encephalopathy predominates. As organ temperatures reach 42°C (107.6°F), enzyme denaturation, protein coagulation, cell dysfunction, lipid liquefaction, and tissue damage begin to occur. Cell injury depends on the maximum temperature reached and the duration of exposure.

Two epidemiologically distinct types of heat stroke associated with high ambient temperatures are described: exertional and nonexertional. Patients with *exertional heat stroke* are typically young people who exerted themselves intensely in a hot, humid environment. Predisposing factors are mentioned previously. Sweating is common. Major metabolic disturbances can occur, including the following: lactic acidosis, respiratory alkalosis (from hyperventilation), hypoglycemia, hypocalcemia, hypokalemia (from aldosterone effect) or hyperkalemia (from muscle cell damage and renal failure), and hypophosphatemia (from renal injury). Other findings can include highly elevated creatinine kinase, aspartate aminotransferase, and lactate dehydrogenase levels, rhabdomyolysis with associated myoglobinuric renal failure, hepatic necrosis, and disseminated intravascular coagulation.

Patients with *nonexertional heat stroke* are usually elderly or chronically ill and sedentary. Elderly patients have diminished cardiac output, decreased ability to sweat, and decreased ability to vasoregulate. They may have impaired awareness of their surroundings and of the development of heat illness. Medications may predispose them to heat illness because of negative effects on cardiac output (β-blockers) or on sweating (anticholinergics) or because of volume depletion (diuretics). Nonexertional heat stroke may be indolent in its onset and may be associated with significant volume depletion. Acute renal failure is less common with nonexertional heat stroke, but it remains no less life-threatening.

In both types of heat stroke, by definition, central nervous system dysfunction is present. Patients may present with confusion, bizarre behavior, combativeness, hallucinations, delirium, stupor, seizures, and coma. Ataxia may be a manifestation of acute cerebellar injury. The duration of coma is a predictor of mortality.

Regardless of the type or cause of heat stroke, treatment is the same. Interventions are made for problems with the airway, breathing, or circulation. Oxygen therapy is initiated. Cardiac and pulse oximetry monitors are placed. Intravenous access is obtained, and isotonic solutions such as normal saline are started. Body temperature is recorded using thermometers capable of measuring temperatures higher than 41°C (105.8°F), usually rectally. Because cooling may be started by prehospital personnel, the first recorded temperature may be lower than 41°C (105.8°F). A Foley catheter is inserted into the bladder to monitor urine output.

It is critical that patients with heat stroke are quickly recognized and cooled. The patient's clothing should be removed, and the patient should be rapidly cooled to 39°C (102.2°F). Ice water immersion is the classic method used to cool these patients. The patient's trunk and extremities are immersed or partially immersed while the head remains above water. An open body bag may be used for this purpose. Cooling should be stopped when the patient's core temperature reaches 39°C (102.2°F) because the patient will continue to cool even after removal from the ice water.

Another cooling method is evaporative cooling, using fans and tepid water continuously applied by spray bottles or sponged onto the skin. This approach is better tolerated than ice water immersion by the conscious patient. The literature on the effectiveness of this technique is more limited than for ice water immersion, and there are no controlled studies comparing the effects of the various cooling techniques on cooling times and outcomes. Ice may also be placed in strategic locations such as the groin and axilla to assist in the cooling process if immersion or near immersion is not desired. Cold gastric lavage, cold colonic lavage, and cold peritoneal lavage are also described but are rarely used.

Illnesses or injuries that potentially contributed to the development of heat stroke should be sought and treated. Complications of heat stroke should be anticipated. Renal function is monitored. Rhabdomyolysis is classically treated with fluids, alkalinization of the urine, and mannitol. Patients with heat stroke should be admitted to an intensive care setting. Patients who are no longer hyperthermic on arrival to the hospital should be admitted for observation and monitored for complications.

Future studies on the treatment of heat stoke will include the potential role and suppression of inflammatory cytokines and antipyretics, as well as investigations of the mechanisms of coagulation disorders and endothelial cell injury. Stress-response proteins are another area of investigation.

PREVENTION

Prevention of heat illness is focused on high-risk groups and situations, including the following: identification of high-risk environments; education of elderly patients and their caretakers; limits on activity on hot, humid days; education of parents on dangers of heat and small children; and evaluation of other predisposing factors to heat illness.

SPIDER BITES AND SCORPION STINGS

method of
LUCINDA S. BUESCHER, M.D.
Southern Illinois University School of Medicine
Springfield, Illinois

SPIDER BITES

More than 30,000 species of spiders exist; most are venomous, but few are considered a hazard to human beings. When someone encounters a spider with chelicerae (jaws) long enough to penetrate the skin, the envenomation may be painful but is rarely dangerous. The site of the bite is usually erythematous, edematous, and tender. Minor spider bites are sufficiently treated with gentle wound cleansing, resting and elevating the affected body part, applying cold compresses, using nonsteroidal anti-inflammatory agents for pain and swelling, administering tetanus prophylaxis (if indicated), and prescribing antibiotics if secondary infection is suspected. It is crucial for the patient to bring in the spider for identification whenever possible because significant morbidity can result from bites by species of *Loxosceles* (fiddleback or violin spiders) and *Latrodectus* (widow spiders).

Loxosceles Envenomation

Although the brown recluse spider, *Loxosceles reclusa*, is the most notable and widespread of this genus, at least four other species in the United States are known to cause cutaneous necrosis (necrotic arachnidism). These spiders are most prevalent in the south-central United States but have been reported in most states. They prefer a warm, dry habitat outdoors in a protected niche, but as they migrate north, they move indoors. These spiders spin inconspicuous matted webs. As its name implies, the spider is reclusive and is a nocturnal feeder. Encounters with human beings are rare, and bites usually result when the spider is trapped against the skin (often after occupying clothing left on the floor overnight).

Loxosceles spiders are tan or gray and have a distinctive dark brown, violin-shaped marking on the dorsal cephalothorax (*L. unicolor* has a very subtle marking). Another distinguishing feature is the presence of six eyes, rather than the usual eight found in most arachnids. The body measures 10 to

15 mm in length, and its leg span may be greater than 25 mm.

The actual *Loxosceles* bite usually goes unnoticed and often occurs on the lower abdomen, thigh, or axilla. Six to 12 hours after the bite, local signs and symptoms appear, including pruritus, pain, edema, erythema, and induration. A pustule or vesicle may appear at the bite site. When necrotic arachnidism is imminent, the center of the lesion becomes mottled dark blue or purple, surrounded by a white halo and finally a large area of reactive erythema, which is somewhat irregular in configuration because of gravitational effects. Over the ensuing 2 or 3 days, the darkened skin progresses to frank cutaneous necrosis, with stellate ulceration and eschar formation, often requiring months to heal.

Systemic signs and symptoms such as headache, malaise, arthralgias, myalgias, fever, and a generalized, faintly papular eruption may accompany many bites, but viscerocutaneous loxoscelism is rare. This syndrome affects primarily children, who may present with massive hemolysis. This can eventuate in renal failure, which may not appear until 2 to 3 days after the bite. Other findings include leukocytosis, leukopenia, thrombocytopenia, disseminated intravascular coagulation, convulsions, and coma.

Venom isolated from *L. reclusa* contains numerous enzymes, but that responsible for cutaneous necrosis and hemolysis is sphingomyelinase D. This enzyme binds to target cell membranes and causes structural alterations that presumably initiate an inflammatory reaction. Neutrophil activation is essential for the development of cutaneous inflammation and necrosis after envenomation; complement, arachidonic acid metabolites, and lymphokines are also likely participants.

Treatment

Because most *Loxosceles* bites are trivial, the same initial care noted earlier will suffice (i.e., cleansing, rest, elevation, cool compresses), and this approach should be employed until the lesion resolves. These measures should greatly diminish pain, but analgesics are often required. Administration of tetanus toxoid may be indicated, and antibiotics are necessary if wound infection is suspected.

Perhaps the most important management aspect in cases of cutaneous necrosis is careful consideration of the differential diagnosis. The definitive diagnosis of an arachnid bite is made only when there is identification of a captured spider. Other causes include trauma, infection (e.g., with herpesviruses or bacteria), and pyoderma gangrenosum.

Surgical excision and grafting are rarely necessary and are contraindicated in the early stages of necrosis, when graft failure is likely. Surgical intervention should be reserved for late eschars that fail to heal by secondary intention.

Patients with suspected systemic loxoscelism may have hemolysis and renal compromise. Treatment is supportive. Serial laboratory evaluations should include complete blood cell counts and urinalysis. Hydration is essential to maintain adequate renal perfusion. Systemic steroids may minimize hemolysis (especially in children) and may protect renal function. Treatments for viscerocutaneous loxoscelism such as dapsone,* hyperbaric oxygen, and antivenin are occasionally reported to be useful, but none of these have proven beneficial in controlled clinical trials.

Latrodectus Envenomation

Five widow spiders inhabit the United States. *Latrodectus mactans* is the most common species and can be found throughout the country, especially in the southern states. *Latrodectus variolus* is the northern black widow, and *Latrodectus hesperus* is the western black widow. These three species are all similar in appearance. The brown widow (*Latrodectus geometricus*) may be found in Florida and California, whereas the red widow (*Latrodectus bishopi*) is limited to Florida. These spiders establish webs in dark, protected spaces indoors and out.

Female black widow spiders are shiny, with the characteristic, but variable, red or orange hourglass marking on the abdomen. Mature arachnids have a 3- to 4-cm leg span. Males are approximately half this size; thus, their bites rarely result in significant symptoms.

The actual bite by a mature female widow is mild. A blue or red macule surrounded by a white halo and a faint urticarial eruption may ensue. Other local signs include piloerection, focal perspiration, and lymphangitis.

Neurotoxic signs and symptoms may begin within an hour, peak by 6 hours, and usually remit after 24 hours. Severe cramps and muscle contractions gradually spread from the inoculation site; that is, patients with an upper extremity bite will suffer from pleuritic pain and respiratory difficulty, whereas those with lower extremity bites may have abdominal rigidity mimicking an acute abdomen, but distention and severe tenderness will be lacking. Some authorities suggest that burning of the volar feet is a characteristic symptom of latrodectism. Additional findings are headache, anxiety, dizziness, diaphoresis, nausea, vomiting, salivation, lacrimation, respiratory distress, fever, priapism, hyperactive deep tendon reflexes, urinary retention, tachycardia, tremors, hypertension, paresthesias, and coma. Death is rare, occurring in less than 1% of patients bitten.

Á-Latrotoxin, a neurotoxin, is the venom released by black widow spiders. It induces a massive, calcium-dependent release of acetylcholine and catecholamines from synaptic terminals and blocks transmitter reuptake as well.

Treatment

Early application of ice packs to the bite site may slow the absorption of venom. Tetanus immunization status should be assessed, and the patient should be monitored for signs of shock. Pain relief is the focus of management, and patients require oral or, occasionally,

*Not FDA-approved for this indication.

intravenous analgesics (e.g., morphine or fentanyl). Sedatives (e.g., benzodiazepines) may also be beneficial. Some pain may persist for several weeks and may necessitate appropriate outpatient management. Suspected cellulitis at the bite site requires systemic antibiotics.

Antivenin (produced in horses) is available and is not species-specific. Because antivenin can cause anaphylaxis and serum sickness, it is reserved for those patients with potential for severe complications (e.g., infants, young children, pregnant women, the elderly, and patients with hypertensive heart disease or respiratory distress). Those patients at risk of complications should be hospitalized and monitored for renal failure, convulsions, cardiac and respiratory failure, cerebral hemorrhage, and local cellulitis.

SCORPION STINGS

Scorpions have a crablike appearance, with pincers on the front appendages, a segmented body and tail with a bulbous terminal segment, and a distal curved stinger. They vary in size from 2 to 10 cm. *Centruroides exilicauda (Centruroides sculpturatus)* is the only deadly species in the United States. It is yellowish brown and less than 6 cm in length. This arthropod resides in southern Arizona, western New Mexico, and Mexico. The common striped scorpion *Centruroides vittatus* is the most commonly encountered scorpion in southwestern states and has an extremely painful, nonfatal sting.

Scorpions are known to burrow into small crevices only to emerge at night to feed on insects and spiders. They may enter homes, especially attics that provide cool, dark niches. They may appear around sinks, bathtubs, and toilets in their quest for water.

Most scorpion stings cause immediate sharp pain and local edema and erythema, but unless the patient has an allergy to the venom, stings are rarely of medical importance. Regional lymph node enlargement, local itching, paresthesias, fever, nausea, and vomiting may follow. The more deadly species inject venom with greater neurotoxic and hemolytic activity. Systemic effects may not appear until 2 to 20 hours after envenomation. The patient may experience drowsiness, partial paralysis, muscle twitching, sialorrhea, perspiration, hypertension, tachycardia, and convulsions. Death may result from respiratory paralysis, peripheral vascular failure, or myocarditis.

Treatment

To minimize the absorption of venom, patients should remain calm and should apply ice and pressure to the sting site. Antivenin (produced at Arizona State University by inoculation of goats with *C. sculpturatus* venom) is species-specific and can be administered in cases of severe envenomation and in young children, but it is not FDA-approved. There is a high incidence of allergic hypersensitivity and serum sickness to the antivenin. Midazolam (Versed) bolus followed by continuous infusion (to induce a light sleep state) can suppress involuntary movements. This approach requires prior assurance of adequate airway, breathing, and circulation and then continuous cardiopulmonary monitoring.

Supportive measures and careful monitoring for relapse and deterioration are mandatory. Oxygen and positive-pressure breathing may be necessary for patients with impending respiratory failure. Tachycardia and severe hypertension may require temporary treatment with β-blockers and α-blockers, respectively. Antiepileptic drugs are indicated to control seizures. Opiates and other narcotics are contraindicated because they have a synergistic effect with the venom.

SNAKE VENOM POISONING

method of
TERENCE M. DAVIDSON, M.D.
University of California, San Diego
VA San Diego Health Care System
San Diego, California

There are approximately 45,000 snakebites annually in the United States. Approximately 10,000 involve venomous snakes. Approximately 10 deaths are reported on an annual basis. The majority of snakes habitating the United States are ecologically important for maintaining a balance in the rodent population, are of little to no harm to humans, and are an important part of the balance of nature. Many harmless snakes are needlessly destroyed by those who believe that all snakes are bad or by those who mistake them for venomous serpents. Education and discouragement of this practice are encouraged.

The vast majority of venomous snakes belong to two families. These are the vipers, such as the Northern American rattlesnake, family Viperidae, and the elapids, family Elapidae, such as the cobra and the Australian tiger snake. Although there are 250 to 300 species of venomous snakes belonging to these two families, the vast majority of venomous snakes and venomous snakebites in the United States involve the rattlesnakes and their close relatives, the cottonmouth and the water moccasin.

Coral snakes, belonging to the family Elapidae, are present in both the Western and the Eastern United States. Only the eastern coral snake is large enough to inflict a venomous bite. One hundred or so coral snake bites are reported annually.

There are an increasing number of exotic snakes in the United States; many are kept illegally in private collections. Exotic snakebites are being increasingly reported throughout the United States. It is recommended that the U.S. physician know two resources: The U.S. Poison Control Centers maintain expertise and important networking capabilities for the evaluation and management of snakebite. Where expertise is lacking and where questions arise, this is an important resource. I have written protocols for the evaluation and management of snakebite around the world. This resource can be accessed on the Internet. Go to http://www.drdavidson.org and click on Snakebite Protocols or go to http://www-surgery.ucsd.edu/ent/DAVIDSON/Snake/Index.htm.

As rattlesnake bite is the most common venomous snake bite in the United States, the majority of what follows focuses on the evaluation and management for rattlesnakes, copperheads, and water moccasins. Rattlesnakes are cold-blooded animals. They hibernate in the winter, emerging in the spring and returning in the fall. Rattlesnakes are distributed throughout the Southern half of the United States, but in some regions they inhabit areas up to the Canadian border.

The majority of snake bite victims fall into three categories: (1) Young adult males who own these animals as pets. The typical scenario is that following alcohol consumption, the owner attempts to handle the snake or play the game of "who is faster." These individuals present bitten on the hand and intoxicated. (2) Children, typically male, who are bitten while attempting to catch or handle a snake. These bites are typically located on the upper extremity. (3) Hikers, outdoor workers, and others moving around in snake-inhabited country. These bites can be seen on the lower extremity or occasionally on the upper extremity, as occurs when one is reaching to pick up rocks, logs, brush, or other objects.

Death from snake bite is extremely uncommon, but significant tissue destruction with substantial morbidity in the untreated cases is extremely common. Therefore, proper evaluation and management are important.

First aid and field management involve the following rules:

1. Do not panic.
2. Remove the bitten victim from the area of the snake to avoid a second bite.
3. Remove constricting jewelry such as rings and watches.
4. Apply lymphatic retardant.
5. Transport to a medical facility.

Getting away from the snake and remaining calm are important. It is of no value to kill the snake. It is of no value to bring the snake to the emergency department. Both scenarios can lead to being bitten a second time by the same or another snake. The area of the bite will swell, and if jewelry is not removed immediately, it may cause problems and will have to be cut off at a later time. There is enormous discussion about the value of constricting bands or lymphatic retardants. Those who believe in lymphatic retardants believe in them strongly. Those who oppose lymphatic retardants oppose them equally strongly. Definitive, scientific investigation does not exist for U.S. rattlesnakes.

For the Elapidae bites, it is widely accepted that wrap and immobilization delays systemic onset of symptoms in areas such as Asia, Africa, and Australia, where mortality is common in the untreated bite victim, especially for those bites occurring in areas far away from definitive medical care. In the United States, rattlesnake bite mortality is uncommon. A band applied as a tourniquet or as a constricting band, which then tightens with swelling and becomes a tourniquet, will potentially cause serious consequences. However, a lymphatic retardant or constricting band such as a 1-inch Penrose drain, as used in vena puncture, will slow down venom absorption and, if properly applied, is an important adjunct to first aid.

Morbidity and mortality do not occur for hours or even days. Therefore, transportation to a medical facility for definitive treatment is important but does not need to be conducted in a crisis fashion. Helicopters and dangerous transportation are not generally required. Particularly with a lymphatic retardant in place, a 12- to 24-hour delay before the institution of medical treatment is acceptable. The victim should be transported expeditiously, but there is no need to incur added danger by hurried evacuation.

There are many myths regarding the management of snakebite. Cryotherapy is contraindicated because it enhances tissue destruction. Electric shock therapy is contraindicated. Once reported by *The Lancet* to be of value, this type of therapy makes no physiologic sense. Electric shock treatment has failed to provide any significant improvement and has resulted in reported deaths. Incision and suction is contraindicated. The Sawyer pump extractor, developed in Europe for bee sting extraction, was touted as a first-aid treatment. The pump is of little value, but it also poses little harm. Some question the value of carrying antivenin in the field. This is generally discouraged unless 10 to 20 vials are carried and the medical kit contains all of the necessary equipment for cardiopulmonary resuscitation.

Evaluation in a medical facility begins with a history confirming that snake bite occurred. Hysterical people are often mistaken about what bit them. The signs and symptoms of rattlesnake bite are listed in Table 1.

The initial signs and symptoms of snake bite include pain with typical onset in 5 to 10 minutes and swelling, also with typical onset within 5 to 10 minutes. As the venom is absorbed, additional proteolytic activity is

TABLE 1. **Signs and Symptoms of Rattlesnake Bite**

Fang marks
Swelling and edema
Pain
Numbness or tingling of lips or affected part
Ecchymosis
Decreased blood platelets
Decreased fibrinogen
Increased fibrin split products
Fasciculations
Vesiculations/blebs
Increased blood clotting time
Proteinuria
Hematuria
Necrosis
Unconsciousness
Convulsions

seen with bleb formation and extension of the edema up the bitten extremity. The majority of venoms are hemotoxic. They lyse fibrinogen and consume platelets. Subcutaneous hemorrhage is noted as a bluish discoloration. Blebs can be filled with serosanguineous fluid. Systemic effects of venom include third spacing of fluid with hemoconcentration, decreased serum potassium, and increased serum calcium and circumoral tingling, probably as a result of the electrolyte changes. If a severe bite is allowed to progress, hypotension, cardiovascular collapse, coma, and death are seen.

Neurotoxic symptoms are rarely seen except in the most severe case of rattlesnake bite. Systemic effects of anticoagulation include bleeding from the gums, hemoptysis, hematuria, and bleeding from needle puncture sites.

Approximately 20% of rattlesnake bites inflict no envenomation. These are often termed *dry bites*. In such cases, no local or systemic symptoms will be noted. If any symptoms are noted, laboratory evaluation is instituted. This includes a complete blood cell count, electrolytes, calcium, some measure of hepatic and renal function, and a coagulation profile. The most important monitor of coagulation difficulties is the quantitative platelet count. However, fibrinogen and fibrin split products are often useful monitors of the progression of envenomation. Intrinsic and extrinsic bleeding measures such as prothrombin time, partial thromboplastin time, and International Normalized Ratio (INR) are rarely abnormal unless coagulopathy is advanced. Laboratory data should be collected periodically and are sometimes useful in monitoring the progression of envenomation and the therapy.

Mild bites are those in which signs and symptoms are restricted to the bite site, typically the distal extremity. Moderate bites are those with symptoms extending up the extremity either as swelling blebs or fasciculations. More advanced or severe bites are those with systemic manifestations, typically coagulopathy, hypotension, and generalized muscular fasciculation. Mild bites can be observed. This is not uncommon with water moccasin and cottonmouth bites. However, once symptoms advance to involve the proximal extremity, more aggressive therapy is recommended.

The mainstay of medical therapy is the intravenous infusion of antivenin. In the majority of the world, skin testing is not used. However, skin testing is typically practiced in the United States. Assuming horse serum sensitivity is not identified, the most commonly available antivenin is the Wyeth Crotalidae Antivenin. This is effective against all North American pit vipers. The Wyeth Antivenin is an immune serum obtained from horses. It is infused intravenously, and the amount required is determined by monitoring the signs and symptoms of envenomation.

The antivenin is seemingly weak. It is recommended that antivenin treatment employ 5-vial aliquots. In the case of the mildest of bites, the initial treatment may begin with 5 vials, but in the case of more advanced bites, treatment should begin with 10 vials. The average rattlesnake treatment in the United States employs 20 vials. If a therapeutic mistake is made, it is giving too little too slowly. Five vials of antivenin are diluted in 50 mL of diluent or normal saline. The antivenin is typically infused at a rate of 1 vial every 7 to 10 minutes. The signs and symptoms of envenomation are then monitored. The antivenin will typically halt progression without reversing many of the signs and symptoms. Once the antivenin infusion is completed, one must monitor the patient for progression of the symptoms. Pain is a very sensitive symptom. Edema is an insensitive sign. Progression of edema is a sensitive sign. Muscular fasciculation is typically not sensitive. Circumoral tingling is an insensitive symptom. Quantitative platelets are a sensitive laboratory sign, as is bleeding from the gums or at the bite site or blood in the urine. Antivenin infusion is continued in 5-vial aliquots. As much as 5 to 10 vials of antivenin can be delivered per hour. Once the patient is stabilized and the progression of symptoms halted, the patient is monitored in an intensive care setting. The following morning, laboratory values are repeated, the patient is evaluated, and, if all is well on both accounts, the patient may be discharged to home.

Immediate allergic reactions are uncommon. Some patients respond negatively to a rapid infusion of antivenin. In these cases, simply stopping the infusion and restarting 10 to 15 minutes later at a slower rate is beneficial. Acute anaphylaxis is sometimes seen. These cases can often be extremely difficult to manage and can be fatal. In these cases, the antivenin infusion must be stopped. Steroids, vasopressors, antihistamines, and fluids should all be available and administered appropriately. Delayed cutaneous allergic reactions are common, occurring in 20% to 30% of treated patients. Patients typically present with pruritus and urticaria 7 to 20 days following treatment. Antihistamines are theoretically the first line of treatment. A short course of systemic steroids is the most effective treatment.

A number of special circumstances and conditions can arise. If the patient is skin-test positive, the inexperienced snake bite physician is strongly encouraged to: (1) call the local poison control center and (2) request assistance from a colleague with experience in snake bite. In these cases, antivenin can very often be administered, but it must be delivered in a diluted concentration, such as 1 vial in 100 mL of lactated Ringer's solution and must be administered extremely slowly, such as 1 mL per minute for 5 minutes, wait 10 minutes, then 1 mL per minute for the first vial. Many individuals with positive skin reactions will not demonstrate systemic reactions. However, those that do will have extremely serious reactions, which can be fatal.

In cases of moderate and advanced bites, extremity edema can progress to a point where arterial pulses are not palpable and may even be difficult to hear by Doppler. There is always concern that a compartment syndrome has evolved and that surgical intervention is indicated.

Invariably, capillary perfusion persists. This is best checked at the fingernail beds. Most likely, wick measurements will show that the subcutaneous pressures are elevated, but the compartment pressures are not raised above 30 mm. Fasciotomy is virtually never indicated, with the possible exception of the extremely uncommon bite in which venom is delivered into the muscle compartment. This is extremely uncommon in North American pit viper bites.

Excision of the bite site was once recommended as a surgical therapy. Certainly if one conducts a wide excision soon after envenomation, the need for systemic antivenin might be obviated. The resultant scar is not a reasonable trade off. I would rather have 20 vials of antivenin than cut off my finger or all my skin on my dorsal hand or foot. Surgical excision is therefore not indicated.

The 10 or so deaths per year from snake bite occur predominantly in two circumstances. In the first, an intravenous bite is inflicted and the patient succumbs within 15 to 20 minutes. In the second, a large snake inflicts a large bite with a lethal venom infusion and the patient either fails to report for medical therapy or is so far removed from medical therapy that medical therapy is not provided in a timely fashion.

The intravenous infusions can be managed by early recognition and treatment with 1 gm of methylprednisolone (Solu-Medrol) intravenously followed by 20 vials of antivenin administered by intravenous push over 5 to 10 minutes.

Treatment of coral and exotic snake bites follows identical principles. Assuming one knows the inflicting snake, one need only know the signs and symptoms and then administer the specific antivenin in appropriate quantities. As exotic antivenins are not typically available in the United States, this can be problematic. Poison control centers are the best resources for these cases. Effective antivenin is available for the management of the Eastern coral snake.

A new crotalid antivenin, marketed under the name of CroFab, is currently commercially available. CroFab is a highly purified immunoglobulin derived from sheep. Treatment principles are the same as those of the Wyeth Antivenin. However, the antivenin appears to be cleared more rapidly; therefore, as venom is absorbed, signs and symptoms may reappear and a repeat treatment may be required the following day. CroFab costs more per vial, and, if retreatment is necessary, treatment becomes substantially more expensive. Nonetheless, this is hopefully the treatment paradigm of the future and is already used in many facilities.

As in many fields of medicine, prevention is always wise. Individuals in areas infested by snakes should be encouraged to remain sober, dress sensibly, and watch where they are reaching and stepping. Proper clothing for snake-infested areas includes long pants and, for most situations, ankle high boots. In heavily infested areas in which the individual may be required to travel through brush, a mid-calf boot theoretically offers greater protection.

HAZARDOUS MARINE CREATURES

method of
GABRIELLE HAWDON, M.B., B.S., B.MED.SC., M.P.H.
University of Melbourne
Victoria, Australia

JELLYFISH

Chirodropoids (Box Jellyfish and *Chiropsalmus* Species)

Box Jellyfish or Sea Wasp (Chironex fleckeri)

The box jellyfish *(Chironex fleckeri)* is the most dangerous jellyfish and arguably the most dangerous venomous creature in the world. Its sting may cause death from cardiorespiratory arrest within minutes. It is found during the summer months (October to May) in the coastal waters of northern Australia, but not on the Great Barrier Reef. The true range of the box jellyfish is unknown but may extend to Papua New Guinea, the Philippines, and Penang, where it may have caused several deaths. It is a large cubozoan jellyfish weighing up to 6 kg and measuring about 20 to 30 cm across the bell. It has four bundles of tentacles that may number 60, and the tentacles may stretch to 2 m. Each tentacle contains many millions of nematocysts, or stinging cells, that discharge venom on contact. Nematocysts are used by jellyfish to deliver toxin into their prey (small fish or prawns). The stinging apparatus consists of a "harpoon" on a thread coiled inside the stinging cell attached to a reservoir containing venom. On contact with the victim, the stinging cell discharges its harpoon into the skin and injects venom. Contact with a large amount of tentacular material over a wide surface area can result in massive envenomation.

The mechanisms of toxicity are poorly understood, but death is thought to be due to respiratory failure, possibly central in origin, or to direct cardiotoxicity leading to atrioventricular conduction disturbances or to paralysis of the cardiac muscle in systole. Patients may become unconscious before they can leave the water or run out of the water and collapse on the beach. In addition to cardiotoxic and neurotoxic properties, the venom contains dermatonecrotic and hemolytic components.

Most stings occur in the summer months in shallow water near the beach and are particularly common in children. (In two series in the 1970s, the average age of box jellyfish sting victims was 14 years, with a median age of 11 years.) More than 60 fatalities have been recorded in Australia, the most recent occurring in January 2000, when a 5-year-old child experienced massive envenomation and died on a beach near Cairns. The diagnosis is usually straightforward but may be assisted (including postmortem cases) by the identification of nematocysts obtained by the application of adhesive tape to affected areas of skin.

Contact with tentacles of the box jellyfish results in severe localized pain, often associated with vigorous attempts by the patient to remove the tentacles, which may make the envenomation worse by inducing the discharge of additional nematocysts. Pain increases over about a 15-minute period, even after removal of the tentacles.

Wide (0.5 to 1 cm) erythematous lines with associated wheals are visible where the tentacles have been in contact with the skin. The total area of skin involvement may provide an indication of the severity of the envenomation. Most stings are minor and result in only pain and skin changes. When the initial skin vesiculation and wheals subside, full-thickness dermal necrosis often results in scarring and pigmentation changes. Ice packs are useful for pain relief after inactivation of the nematocysts. In more severe envenomation, confusion, agitation, unconsciousness, and collapse with respiratory failure and/or cardiac arrest may be seen. Death can occur within 5 minutes after massive envenomation.

Because of the rapidity of onset of symptoms, immediate first aid is vital, and cardiopulmonary resuscitation may be required. Any remaining undischarged nematocysts should be inactivated with large quantities of dilute (3% to 5%) acetic acid (i.e., household vinegar) for at least 30 seconds once the patient has been safely removed from the water. Alcohol should never be used because it induces further nematocyst discharge. After inactivation, tentacular material may be removed, preferably with gloves. If antivenom is not available immediately, pressure-immobilization first aid may be used after the nematocysts have been inactivated, although the often wide area of tentacular contact may render this method less effective.

Antivenom may be administered by lifesaving or other paramedical personnel at the scene by the intramuscular route, although intravenous administration is preferable if appropriately skilled personnel are available. The antivenom (produced by CSL Ltd, Australia) has been available since 1970 and consists of purified sheep immunoglobulin. No adverse reactions have been reported after its use in more than 100 cases. Its efficacy has been established experimentally by in vitro neutralization and subsequent protection of experimental animals. Indications for box jellyfish antivenom include cardiorespiratory arrest or cardiac arrhythmias; difficulty with breathing, speech, or swallowing; severe pain; extensive skin lesions; or skin lesions in cosmetically important areas such as the face, neck, hands, and forearms. Early administration of antivenom may result in reduced pain and decreased scarring from the dermatonecrosis. Silver sulfadiazine (Silvadene) cream is recommended for the treatment of skin lesions.

In the hospital, intravenous antivenom should be administered promptly if it has not already been given or if the patient remains symptomatic. Assisted ventilation and narcotic analgesia may be required.

The use of ancillary agents such as verapamil (Calan)* is controversial. Research, including prophylaxis and rescue experiments in animals, has provided contradictory results, and verapamil is not currently recommended. Clinical experience with verapamil is lacking. Animal experimental results do not support the use of antihistamines or corticosteroids to reduce dermatonecrotic activity.

Stings may be prevented by avoiding swimming during the box jellyfish season (approximately October to May), particularly at unpatrolled or unnetted beaches. Specially designed stinger suits or pantyhose provide protection for those who must enter the water (e.g., lifeguards).

*Not FDA-approved for this indication.

Chiropsalmus Species

Similar to the box jellyfish, members of this genus are chirodropoids (box-shaped jellyfish with multiple tentacles at each corner). They are smaller and less dangerous, though still capable of causing severe injuries and death. *Chiropsalmus quadrigatus* is the most common species. The bell may measure 7 cm, and the number of tentacles on each of the pedalia (fleshy arms) seldom exceeds nine. The tentacles are shorter and finer than those of *C. fleckeri.* Its venom contains lethal, dermatonecrotic, and hemolytic properties in approximately the same proportions as *Chironex* venom, but the venom output of *Chiropsalmus* is much less (Barnes estimated in 1966 that the stinging potential of *C. quadrigatus* was approximately 10% that of *C. fleckeri*), and the toxicity of the venom in mice (as tested by Freeman and Turner in 1972) was approximately one sixth the toxicity of *Chironex* venom. Stinging results in severe pain and shock, but the illness is less severe than that caused by the box jellyfish. Residual scarring is usually minimal. No deaths from the sting of members of this genus have been reported in Australia, although deaths have been reported in the Philippines and Japan, and a child died in Mexico within 40 minutes of being stung by a jellyfish believed to have been *C. quadrumanus.* Box jellyfish antivenom has been experimentally shown to neutralize *Chiropsalmus* venom, but clinical experience is lacking.

Carybdeids (Irukandji, Jimble, Morbakka)

Carybdeids are box jellyfish (cubozoans) that are differentiated from chirodropoids by the presence of a single tentacle at each corner of the bell. Carybdeids of medical importance include the Irukandji *(Carukia barnesi)*, the Jimble *(Carybdea rastoni)*, and the Morbakka (*Tamoya* species).

Irukandji (Carukia barnesi)

C. barnesi (called the Irukandji) is a small carybdeid jellyfish responsible for an unusual and dramatic syndrome observed in individuals after they were stung in northern Australia, especially north Queensland. The bell may measure 2 cm and the tentacles 35 cm. Nematocysts are present on the bell as well as the tentacles. In contrast to *C. fleckeri*, Irukandji have been found mostly in the deeper waters of the reef, although they may be swept inshore by prevailing currents. Little is known of the biology and lifestyle of this jellyfish or its venom.

Many people have been affected by the Irukandji syndrome, including several hundred in north

Queensland in the summer of 1991 and the summer of 1992. Every summer, more than 60 people with this potentially fatal syndrome are hospitalized. The sting itself is only moderately painful, with little associated tissue damage. Rather than linear wheals or vesiculation, an area of erythema about 5 cm in diameter may be visible at the site. Approximately 30 minutes later, a complex of systemic symptoms develop, including severe back and abdominal pain, limb or joint pain, nausea and vomiting, profuse sweating, and agitation. Victims may also experience numbness or paresthesia. Hypertension and tachycardia are observed frequently and are thought to be related to catecholamine release.

A second phase may be observed in severe cases 6 to 18 hours after the sting. This phase consists of cardiac failure and acute pulmonary edema. Victims may require hospitalization for analgesia and sometimes intravenous antihypertensive therapy; α-blocking agents such as phentolamine (Regitine) have been used for this purpose. Supraventricular tachycardia and transient dilated cardiomyopathy have been reported after Irukandji stings, and it has been suggested that serial echocardiography be performed to monitor the progress of severely affected patients.

First aid consists of analgesia and reassurance. The role of vinegar in deactivating undischarged nematocysts remains uncertain, with initial work proving inconclusive. Vinegar is currently recommended because it may reduce further discharge of nematocysts. Analgesia is usually required and may need to be given intravenously when the pain is severe. No definitive treatment is currently available for the Irukandji syndrome. Box jellyfish antivenom appears to be ineffective. Recovery typically occurs after 1 to 2 days, and no fatalities have been recorded. A similar syndrome has been described elsewhere in the Pacific, although the causative organisms are unknown.

Jimble (Carybdea rastoni)

C. rastoni is a small chirodropoid jellyfish (approximately 2 cm across) with four tentacles measuring up to 30 cm. These jellyfish are distributed throughout the warmer waters of the Pacific, from Japan to Hawaii. A similar species, *Carybdea marsupialis*, is found in the Atlantic. They are often observed in groups and are seen most commonly at the surface at dawn and dusk.

The venom has been shown to cause the release of endogenous catecholamines and the influx of calcium ions into smooth muscle. Stings cause moderate pain for 2 hours, with associated swelling and redness. Skin changes may take several weeks to resolve, and pigmentation may remain for even longer. No deaths have been recorded, although an Irukandji-like syndrome has been described anecdotally after stings from this species. Treatment consists of the application of vinegar to inactivate the nematocysts and the use of local anesthetic ointment for extensive lesions.

Morbakka (Tamoya Species)

Also called the fire jelly, *Tamoya* species are carybdeids found in northern Australian waters. The bell measures up to 12 cm across and the tentacles 60 cm. Stings result in severe burning pain and a wheal and red flare resembling a burn. Respiratory distress and back pain have been reported. Vesiculation, pruritus, and dermal necrosis may ensue. Treatment consists of the application of vinegar and local analgesic agents such as ice packs or topical anesthetic creams.

Portuguese Man-of-War or Bluebottle (*Physalia* Species)

The Portuguese man-of-war, or bluebottle, is well known throughout the Pacific and Atlantic oceans for causing painful stings. It is not a true jellyfish, but a colony of individual organisms. The float measures 2 to 15 cm and keeps the animal on the surface. The main or fishing tentacle may be 10 m long and is responsible for most of the stings. There are probably two species, the smaller *Physalia utriculus*, with a single fishing tentacle, and a larger species, *Physalia physalis*, with multiple tentacles. The venom contains lethal and hemolytic components and has been shown to produce nerve conduction disturbances, flaccid paralysis, and smooth muscle contraction in experimental animals.

Swimmers may be stung when bluebottles are blown inshore, sometimes in large numbers. Stings are also possible from specimens washed up on beaches, even after a few days. In human envenomation, pain is the most prominent feature, along with localized skin lesions with a *string of beads* appearance: discrete wheals surrounded by erythema. Pain may involve the entire limb or trunk and may last for several hours. Systemic symptoms are uncommon but may include headache, nausea and vomiting, abdominal pain, and (occasionally) collapse. First aid consists of removal of the tentacles, preferably with forceps. Vinegar is not recommended because it may cause some discharge of nematocysts. Analgesia may be required, although most stings respond to ice packs and/or topical anesthetic agents. No fatalities have been confirmed in the Pacific, but several deaths, occurring within minutes of stings, have been attributed to the larger Atlantic *P. physalis* on the southeast coast of the United States.

Other Jellyfish

Widely distributed throughout the world in tropical and temperate waters, the mauve blubber or mauve stinger *(Pelagia noctiluca)* is a multicolored jellyfish that usually measures approximately 12 cm across the bell. Little is known about the venom. Contact with the tentacles or bell causes local pain, wheals, and urticaria. Recurrent skin eruptions have been reported, but no deaths or serious illnesses. An epidemic of stings by this species occurred in 1978 along the coast of Yugoslavia, when an estimated 250,000 people were stung. No serious injuries were reported. Recommended treatment includes the use of ice packs (not vinegar) and simple analgesia.

The sea blubber or hairy stinger, lion's mane, and sea nettle (*Cyanea* species) are widely distributed in coastal waters throughout the world. They have a flattened or platelike bell and multiple delicate, hairy tentacles. The bell may be 30 cm across in Australian jellyfish and significantly larger in the cold-water Antarctic or Atlantic jellyfish. Stinging results in severe pain that may last an hour. Nausea and abdominal pain sometimes occur, as do sweating, muscle cramps, and breathing difficulties. No deaths have been attributed to this creature. Ice packs, analgesia, and supportive care are the recommended treatment.

Many jellyfish inhabit the tropical and temperate waters of the world. Commonly encountered jellyfish include *Catostylus mosaicus, Pseudorhiza haeckeli, Olindias singularis, Chrysaora* species, *Aurelia* species, and *Cassiopeia* species. Most stings by these jellyfish result in only local pain, skin welts, and erythema; however, nausea, vomiting, and headaches may sometimes occur. First aid consists of the local application of ice packs or iced water and supportive care, such as analgesia, as required.

The purpose of applying vinegar to jellyfish stings is to prevent the firing of undischarged nematocysts (stinging cells) and the injection of more venom into the victim. Vinegar does not decrease the pain or diminish the effects of the venom; it only helps prevent the injection of additional venom.

STONEFISH AND OTHER STINGING FISH

Stonefish (*Synanceja* Species)

Stonefish are found in warm coastal waters throughout the Indo-Pacific region and may be described as the world's most dangerous stinging fish. Ambush predators, they are extremely well camouflaged and look like rocks or coral. They dig themselves into the surrounding sand or mud, which makes them almost impossible to see. They average around 20 cm in length.

Stonefish venom is purely for defense and plays no role in feeding activities. Thirteen dorsal spines project from venom glands along the back, and when the fish is disturbed, the spines become erect. When the spines are pressed, venom is involuntarily expelled, along with integumentary material. Stonefish venom has been shown to cause depression of the cardiovascular and neuromuscular systems, as well as hemolysis and increased vascular permeability. It also has a direct effect on muscle and contains a variety of enzymes, including hyaluronidase. The main feature of stonefish envenomation, however, is pain.

Stonefish envenomation is relatively common in tropical waters in the Pacific. Men tend to be overrepresented among victims, probably because of occupational or recreational fishing activities, and almost all stings are sustained on the limbs. The sting is immediately extremely painful, and swelling develops rapidly. The severity of the symptoms is related to the depth of penetration of the spines and the number of spines involved. Systemic effects of the venom may include muscle weakness, paralysis, and shock. Fatalities have been recorded in the Indo-Pacific region.

First aid consisting of bathing or immersing the stung area in hot water may be effective, but hospitalization for intravenous narcotic analgesia, local anesthetic infiltration (without adrenaline), or regional nerve blockade may be required. All stonefish stings should receive medical attention. Definitive management is administration of stonefish antivenom (produced by CSL, Ltd, Australia, from the venom of *Syanceja trachynis*), which is usually given intramuscularly.

Indications for antivenom include severe pain, systemic symptoms, or signs of envenomation (weakness, paralysis) or multiple punctures indicating the discharge of several spines and injection of a larger amount of venom. Recommended doses are 2000 U (1 ampule) for one to two spine punctures, 4000 U for three to four punctures, and 6000 U for five to six punctures. Premedication with subcutaneous epinephrine is recommended. The antivenom may be given by the intravenous route if the pain is severe or the patient is in shock. Antivenom is not universally available outside Australia, and supportive care plus analgesia may be all that is possible.

GENERAL MANAGEMENT OF WOUNDS INFLICTED BY MARINE ORGANISMS (INCLUDING STONEFISH, STINGING FISH, CORAL, AND ECHINODERMS)

Tetanus prophylaxis should be initiated if the patient's immunization status is not current. Severe stings may produce an area of tissue necrosis, particularly if medical treatment or antivenom administration is delayed. This necrosis may require surgical débridement or skin grafting. Consideration should be given to the presence of a foreign body (i.e., broken spines or integument) within the wound, which should be determined by viewing radiographs if possible. Infection is relatively common after skin trauma from marine creatures. Deep wounds or those more than 6 hours old when initially seen should be regarded as potentially contaminated. In addition to *Staphylococcus* and *Streptococcus* species, marine microorganisms, including *Vibrio, Aeromonas, Plesiomonas*, and other gram-negative bacilli, should be considered when ordering wound cultures (special saline culture media may be required) or prescribing antibiotics. Suitable antibiotics include tetracyclines, ciprofloxacin (Cipro), trimethoprim-sulfamethoxazole combinations (Bactrim; check for allergies, particularly to sulfonamides), broad-spectrum (third-generation) cephalosporins, aminoglycosides, chloramphenicol, and carbapenems. Clostridial infection should also be considered when necrotic tissue is present.

STINGING FISH

Numerous stinging fish are distributed throughout the tropical and temperate waters of the world. Similar to the stonefish, most possess spines associated with venom glands or sacs for defensive purposes. Little is known about the venom of most of these fish, and no specific antivenom exists for any but the stonefish. Deaths have been reported in connection with weaver fish, zebra fish, catfish, and stonefish.

The major clinical feature of these fish stings is immediate severe pain, which may be prolonged and difficult to manage, even with narcotic analgesia. The pain usually subsides within 24 hours, but swelling may persist for several days to weeks.

Pain from most fish stings is reduced by bathing the stung area in hot (not scalding) water. (The temperature of the water should be tested with the other limb first.) The mechanism by which pain is reduced is unclear, but no attempt should be made to restrict the movement of venom because such restriction may worsen pain and necrosis at the site. Pain relief from severe fish stings may require infiltration with a local anesthetic (without epinephrine) or a regional nerve block. All but the most trivial fish stings require medical attention. Foreign material and bacteria may be deposited in the wound, sometimes quite deeply. As with stonefish stings, tetanus prophylaxis should be updated if required, and the wound should be examined for signs of infection or retained foreign material in the form of broken spines. Radiographs should be obtained if possible. Envenomation by the spines of a fish is possible several days after the fish has been killed, even after it has been refrigerated. Spines that have been removed from the fish along with the venom apparatus are also capable of envenomation.

Common stinging fish include the following:

- *Notesthes robusta* (bullrout or kroki, also known as scorpion fish, wasp fish, rock cod)
- *Scorpaena cardinalis* (red rock cod)
- *Pterois volitans* (butterfly cod, lionfish, zebra fish)
- *Hydrolagus lemures* (rat fish or bight ghostshark)
- *Siganus lineatus* (rabbit fish)
- *Centropogon* species (fortescues)
- *Glyptauchen* species (goblinfish)
- Acanthuridae family (surgeonfish)
- Catfish (multiple species, including *Plotosus lineatus, Paraplotosus, Cnidoglanis macrocephalus, Tachysurus, Euristhmus, Tandanus, Neosilurus*)
- *Enoplosus armatus* (zebra fish, old wife)
- *Gymnapistes marmoratus* (scorpion fish, soldier fish)
- *Batrachomeus dubius*, *Halophryne diemensis* (frogfish or toadfish)
- Platycephalidae family (flatheads)
- *Inimicus species* (ghouls)
- *Neosebastes pandus* (gurnard perch, gurnard scorpion fish)
- *Trachinus* species (weaver fish)
- *Scorpaena guttata* (Californian scorpion fish)
- *Heterodontus portjacksoni* (Port Jackson shark)

STINGRAYS (MULTIPLE SPECIES)

Stingrays are found throughout the world and are named for the venomous barbs present on the dorsum of their tails. Although they are venomous, the major clinical problem is often related to mechanical trauma from the sting itself, which may produce deep-penetrating injuries, severe lacerations, and/or subsequent infection, including tetanus. Fatalities from penetrating chest or abdominal wounds by stingray barbs have been recorded. Envenomation may result in increasing local pain (which may spread to involve the entire limb), swelling, and a characteristic bluish white appearance of the wound. Systemic symptoms are rare but may include nausea and vomiting, salivation, diarrhea, sweating, muscle cramps, syncope, cardiac arrhythmias, and convulsions. Immersion of the stung area in hot water, as for stinging fish, may provide temporary pain relief. Treatment consists of analgesia, tetanus prophylaxis, radiographs, and surgical exploration and débridement if necessary. (All penetrating chest and abdominal wounds should be explored.) Contaminated wounds may become infected with poorly characterized marine bacteria requiring special culture media. Consideration should therefore be given to antibiotic prophylaxis in contaminated wounds, particularly if medical treatment has been delayed. No antivenom is available for stingray envenomation.

SEA SNAKES (FAMILY HYDROPHIIDAE)

Sea snakes are common in the western Pacific and Indian oceans, particularly in warmer waters; they are not found in the Atlantic. Around 60 species have been identified. The most common sea snake worldwide is the yellow-bellied sea snake *Pelamis platurus*, which is found in warmer waters throughout the Pacific. It is unusual among sea snakes in that it is found far out to sea, whereas most other species prefer shallower coastal waters.

Sea snakes are readily identified by their flattened tails and valvular, upward-facing nostrils. Many are brightly colored. They are excellent swimmers and divers (100 m) and feed on fish and eels or crustaceans. Sea snakes may absorb 22% of their oxygen requirement through their skin, which they shed much more frequently than land snakes do, sometimes every 2 weeks. The young are born alive at sea except for those of the banded sea krait *(Laticauda colubrina)*, which comes ashore to lay its eggs. All sea snakes are venomous, although the venom output of many species is quite low. Species dangerous to human beings include *Enhydrina schistosa* (considered the most dangerous), *Aipysurus laevis, Astrotia stokesii, Lapemis curtus*, and *P. platurus.*

Human envenomation is relatively uncommon except in those using traditional techniques such as net fishing by hand. The number of cases worldwide is unknown. As is the case with terrestrial snake bites, sea snake bites often do not result in clinically significant envenomation. The bite itself is not usually particularly painful and may go unnoticed, thus distinguishing it from envenomation by stinging fish or jellyfish, both of which generally cause immediate and often excruciating pain. The bite site is inconspicuous, with minimal swelling or tissue reaction, although the fangs are fragile and may sometimes break off in the wound. If sufficient venom has been injected to produce clinical illness, it is usually apparent within

2 hours of the bite. Rhabdomyolysis is a major feature of sea snake envenomation and results in muscle pain, tenderness, and sometimes spasm, typically within 30 to 60 minutes. Pain on passive movement of the limb or other muscles follows, and myoglobinuria develops after 3 to 6 hours, as does elevation of plasma creatine kinase and serum potassium. Neurologic impairment mediated by postsynaptic neurotoxins and manifested as ptosis, diplopia, dysarthria, and weakness may also occur, as well as headache, sweating, nausea, and vomiting.

Pressure-immobilization first aid should be used and left in situ until the patient reaches medical care. Incision and suction have no place in the treatment of sea snake bites or any other envenomation. Envenomation may be treated by the intravenous infusion of diluted sea snake antivenom (based on the venom of the beaked sea snake *E. schistosa*) or tiger snake antivenom (both produced by CSL Ltd, Australia). In the case of the latter, 2 ampules should be given initially. Prophylaxis against allergic reactions to the venom (composed of equine immune globulin) should be considered. Subcutaneous epinephrine (0.3 to 0.5 mL of a 1:1000 solution for an adult, 0.005 mg/kg for a child) is recommended, particularly in those with previous exposure or allergy to equine serum. Supportive measures such as intubation and ventilation for respiratory failure or the treatment of hyperkalemia may be required.

OCTOPUSES (CLASS CEPHALOPODA)

More than 600 species of cephalopods are found throughout the world, including octopuses, squid, cuttlefish, and nautiluses. With the exception of the blue-ringed octopus (genus *Hapalochlaena*, discussed subsequently), cephalopods pose little threat to human beings. Bites by nonvenomous octopuses are reported rarely. (Nine cases were found in a world literature review in 1971.) Effects range from local pain to swelling and numbness of the entire bitten limb. The saliva contains a variety of substances, including octopamine, serotonin, and hyaluronidase, and the ink produced by octopuses may cause irritation of the skin. Suckers on the limbs may cause injury, particularly to the eyes or sensitive skin. Octopuses are strong, and it is possible that divers might be injured or drowned if unable to escape the grip of a large octopus, although no deaths in this manner have been reliably reported.

Blue-Ringed Octopuses (*Hapalochlaena* Species)

Blue-ringed octopuses are small (20 cm) brown octopuses on which brilliant blue ring-shaped markings develop when disturbed. The genus is found throughout Australia's coastal waters and north at least as far as the equator. At least six species of *Hapalochlaena* have been described; *H. maculosa, H. lunulata*, and *H. fasciata* have been studied in some depth, but little is known about the other three as yet unnamed species.

The blue-ringed octopus is found in tidal rock pools and is attractive, especially to children and tourists, who are at risk of envenomation when they pick up the octopus. Bites may also occur if the creature is trodden on by waders.

The blue-ringed octopus' salivary glands contain tetrodotoxin, which causes motor paralysis because of neuronal sodium channel blockade. (See the section on tetrodotoxin poisoning under Poisoning by Ingestion of Marine Creatures for a more complete description of the toxin and its effects.) Other toxins may also be present in the saliva. The toxin, which is normally used by the octopus to subdue its prey of crabs, is injected when a human victim is bitten, typically while handling the octopus. The initial bite is not painful and may be unnoticed. Within about 10 minutes, symptoms of poisoning begin to develop, including weakness and numbness around the face, accompanied by nausea and vomiting. Cerebellar signs were reported in one case. Severe envenomation may progress rapidly to generalized flaccid paralysis and respiratory failure. Death may occur in 30 minutes. The patient may be paralyzed completely, sometimes with fixed dilated pupils, but the sensorium remains intact until hypoxia or hypercapnia supervenes, and care should be taken to avoid negative remarks that may distress an alert but paralyzed patient. First aid using the pressure-immobilization technique is recommended for blue-ringed octopus envenomation. Prolonged artificial respiration may be required before medical aid can be reached. Respiratory failure and any risk of pulmonary aspiration are indications for endotracheal intubation and mechanical ventilation until the effects of the venom wear off, usually within several hours to days. No antivenom is available for clinical use, although an experimental antibody has been produced in Hawaii. Envenomation is uncommon (one series from Australia reported 11 cases up to 1983, including 2 fatalities).

CONE SHELLS (*CONUS* SPECIES)

Cone shells or, more correctly, cone snails are predatory gastropods (Conidae family) that live mainly in shallow tropical and subtropical reef waters of the Indo-Pacific. More than 600 varieties have been identified. They are distinguished by a characteristically marked cone-shaped shell, which ranges from a few centimeters to 23 cm in length. They are attractive shells and may be picked up by children or visitors to the reef who are unaware of the danger. Some of the more dangerous *Conus* species include the following:

C. geographus
C. stercusmuscarium
C. magus
C. textile
C. omaria
C. tulipa
C. striatus
C. marmoreus

Cone snails usually hunt nocturnally and kill their prey of worms, fish, octopus, and other gastropods with venom that they inject by radula teeth (resembling small harpoons) held in their proboscis. The venom apparatus consists of a muscular venom bulb that forces venom down a long duct or gland toward the radula sac, which contains 20 developing radular teeth. The chitinous tooth, shaped and barbed like a harpoon, is soaked in venom and gripped at the tip of the proboscis, which drives it into the prey. Venom is pushed along the hollow tooth to emerge at the tip.

The venom consists of numerous small (12 to 30 amino acids) neurotoxic peptides called *conotoxins.* They are classified into α, γ, δ, κ, μ, σ, υ, ω, conopressin, and conantokin based on their structure and mode of action. The actions of some of the conotoxins are summarized in Table 1. Different species' venom contains different combinations of conotoxins, probably related to their different prey. The major actions of cone snail venom are to block neuronal and neuromuscular transmission, thereby resulting in paralysis of the prey.

Stings in humans are uncommon. In 1963, one author reported 37 cases worldwide, including 7 deaths. Another author cites more than 70 cases reported worldwide, with 26 deaths. *C. geographus* and *C. textile* are implicated most commonly in human fatalities. Stings are usually associated with handling of the attractive cone shells. A sharp pain is felt initially, and the stung area may become swollen and pale or cyanotic. Numbness may follow the initial pain. Symptoms and signs of neurologic impairment, including weakness, lack of coordination, and disturbances in vision, speech, and hearing, may progress rapidly. Less common systemic symptoms include nausea and generalized pruritus. Severe envenomation may result in death within hours secondary to respiratory paralysis. Survivors may experience weakness and numbness for several days to weeks.

In the event of a cone snail sting, pressure-immobilization first aid should be applied and left in place until resuscitation facilities are available because assisted ventilation may be required. Several patients have recovered after a period of mechanical ventilation.

TABLE 1. **Classification of Conotoxins**

Class	Action
α Conotoxins	Competitively block muscle and vertebrate neuronal nicotinic acetylcholine receptors
γ Conotoxins	Activate pacemaker cationic channel
δ Conotoxins	Activate predominantly mollusc sodium channels
κ Conotoxins	Block potassium channels
μ Conotoxins	Block vertebrate muscle/nerve sodium channels
σ Conotoxins	Inhibit 5-HT_3 channel
υ Conotoxins	Noncompetitively block muscle acetylcholine receptors
ω Conotoxins	Block N-type or P/Q-type vertebrate calcium channels
Conopressin	Vasopressin agonist
Conatokin	Inhibit vertebrate NMDA-glutamate channels

Abbreviation: NMDA = *N*-Methyl-D-Aspartate.

After Sutherland SK, Tibballs J: Australian Animal Toxins. Oxford, Oxford University Press, 2001.

No antivenom or other specific treatment is available for cone snail stings. The wound should be regarded as potentially contaminated, and tetanus prophylaxis should be updated if required. Infection may occur, and foreign bodies and marine microorganisms should be considered.

Conotoxins have been the subject of intense interest for the development of scientific probes and drugs. Trials are currently under way to investigate the use of conotoxins and their derivatives in the treatment of pain and stroke.

VENOMOUS CREATURES

Echinoderms

Echinoderms are marine invertebrates with radial symmetry and spines. They include starfish and sea urchins.

Crown of Thorns Starfish (Acanthaster planci)

The only significantly venomous starfish known, the large (40-cm) crown of thorns starfish inhabits coral reefs of the Indo-Pacific. It has 13 to 17 arms and is covered with sharp spines. The integument surrounding the spines contains glandular cells filled with venom, about which little is known. Spines penetrating the skin may break off and become embedded. Local pain may be severe and may last for several hours. Vomiting is a major feature of envenomation and may be protracted. Treatment is similar to that recommended for fish stings. Wounds commonly become infected.

Sea Urchins (Family Diadematidae)

Sea urchins are round-bodied creatures with mobile spines that project from the body. They are found all over the world, but the species considered medically significant are all tropical or subtropical. An important genus is *Diadema*, whose long (30-cm) fragile spines snap off easily and become embedded in the skin. Venom glands have not been identified, but immediate burning pain follows a sting, along with erythema and swelling. Systemic effects such as nausea and weakness may occur, and infection is common. Pain and tenderness may persist for days to weeks. The leather urchins (multiple species) have venom glands associated with their short spines. Treatment is similar to that recommended for stinging fish injuries, including immersion in hot water for first aid.

Considered the most dangerous of the sea urchins, the flower sea urchin *(Toxopneustes pileolus)* is found throughout the Indo-Pacific, including Japan. Although the spines are not venomous, the pedicellariae *(seizing organs)*, which form the "flowers" between the spines, are poisonous on ingestion or contact. Severe, radiating pain and systemic effects, including collapse, paralysis, and respiratory distress, have been described. It is said to have caused death. Management is supportive.

Coral (Order Scleractinia)

Although they possess nematocysts, the stinging apparatus of coral is too small to be considered dangerous to human beings. However, contact with some coral may cause wheals, erythema, pain, and swelling. The application of vinegar is recommended for these minor injuries. Cuts sustained on coral also represent a hazard because they are slow to heal and are particularly prone to infection. Cuts should be cleaned thoroughly as soon as possible and antiseptic applied. Tetanus immune status should be checked, and prophylactic antibiotics with activity against marine microorganisms should be considered.

Sea Anemones (Order Actinaria)

Many anemones can cause painful stings, rash, and itching on contact. Stings from *Actindendron plumosum*, the stinging anemone of the Great Barrier Reef, may be painful for a week. Nausea and shock have been reported in association with Australian sea anemones. Some anemone proteins interact with the sodium channels of excitable tissue. A Mediterranean species reportedly causes skin necrosis, as does a species from Japan. Ingestion of one (uncooked) Pacific species proved fatal.

Sea Bathers' Eruption (Sea Lice)

Sea bathers' eruption, or sea lice, refers to a condition of contact dermatitis observed on covered areas of the body after swimming in the ocean. It is thought to be related to exposure to the larval forms of some sea anemones or jellyfish.

Family Milleporidae (Fire Coral or False Coral)

Fire coral or false coral is a hydrozoan that grows in plantlike colonies in shallow tropical waters and causes pain, swelling, and erythema on contact. Nausea, vomiting, and collapse have been reported. Treatment consists of the application of vinegar and topical analgesia.

Stinging Seaweed *(Aglaophenia cupressina)* and Fire Weed *(Lytocarpus philippinus)*

Stinging seaweed and fire weed are fernlike colonies of hydrozoans that are common in tropical waters and produce pain, erythema, and blistering on contact. Fever, malaise, and gastrointestinal symptoms may occur. Topical anesthetic creams and steroid creams are recommended, but vinegar is not.

Glaucus *(Glaucus atlanticus)*

The glaucus is a small (about 3-cm) nudibranch found in oceans worldwide. It ingests nematocysts from other creatures such as *Physalia* and passes them to its appendages, where they are used to sting prey. *Glaucilla marginata*, a similar creature found in the Pacific, also uses recycled nematocysts in this way. Human envenomation results in similar, but usually less severe, symptoms as those seen in stings by the creature from which the nematocysts originated. The usual linear pattern of wheals or erythema is not seen. Vinegar is recommended for first aid treatment.

Stinging Sponges (Class Demospongiae)

Contact with many species of sponges may produce irritation of the skin. This irritation occurs as a result of penetration of the skin by siliceous spicules coated with toxin. *Neofibularia mordens* is considered to be the most dangerous Australian sponge. Initial contact is unremarkable, but after approximately 1 hour, a prickling sensation develops, followed by severe contact dermatitis. Resolution may take a week or more, and desquamation may occur. *Lissodendoryx* and *Haliclona* species have also been associated with severe contact dermatitis. No specific treatment exists. Antibiotics or topical steroids have not been shown to alter the course of the illness. Severe cases may require analgesia and immobilization.

Marine Worms (Class Polychaeta)

Many species of marine worms are covered with setae (stinging bristles) that readily detach and may lodge in the skin and produce irritation. Blistering, rash, and swelling may occur. Some bristles may be removed by the application of adhesive tape to the affected area. Alcohol or alkaline solutions are said to produce relief. Marine worms also bite, and in the case of the larger species (1.5 m), the bites may be severe.

OTHER DANGEROUS BUT NONVENOMOUS MARINE CREATURES

Many marine creatures, though not venomous, pose danger to human beings. Extensive trauma and death are well known in relation to sharks, and deaths from shark attacks are probably under-recognized. Many other marine creatures are also capable of inflicting severe trauma, including barracuda, moray eels, needlefish, stingrays (see earlier), electric rays and eels, and many other large carnivorous fish. Estuarine crocodiles *(Crocodylus porosus)* have been known to attack and kill humans on beaches in northern Australia, Papua New Guinea, and Southeast Asia. Treatment issues revolve around management of the blood loss and hypovolemic shock and infection of contaminated wounds, often with tissue deficit or necrosis. Near-drowning and, in the case of scuba divers, decompression illness may complicate the management of trauma or illness caused by marine animals.

POISONING BY INGESTION OF MARINE CREATURES

Tetrodotoxin Poisoning

Tetrodotoxin is a highly toxic compound found in the flesh and organs of hundreds of species of marine creatures throughout most of the world. It is also the toxin responsible for paralysis related to bites by the blue-ringed octopus and is found in the skin glands of the Californian newt (*Taricha* species) and in the skin of some Central American frogs (*Atelopus* species), as well as in the Pacific goby and other marine creatures, including starfish, crabs, and flatworms. Many tetrodotoxic fish inflate their bodies with water or air in response to a threat, thus resulting in common names such as puffer fish, globe fish, toadfish, or balloon fish. Some are covered with spikes and are called porcupine fish. Large eyes and the apparent absence of scales are characteristic of this group of fish, as is fusion of the teeth into four large beaklike teeth at the front of the mouth, hence the order classification tetraodontiforms (*tetra* = four; *odont* = teeth). In these fish, tetrodotoxin is present in highest concentration in the liver, intestines, ovaries, and skin, but the flesh may be contaminated when the fish is caught or handled.

The major effect of tetrodotoxin is to block sodium channels in motor nerves, which leads to motor paralysis and, ultimately, respiratory failure. Sensory conduction and autonomic nerve conduction are also affected. The onset of symptoms usually occurs within 10 to 45 minutes of ingestion and may progress from numbness or tingling around the mouth through numbness of the face and other areas and early motor paralysis and incoordination to widespread paralysis with associated hypotension and respiratory failure. Death has been reported 17 minutes after the ingestion of puffer fish, but the typical course of the illness is slower, with progression over a period of several hours or longer.

The most well-known instances of tetrodotoxin poisoning occur in Japan, where some toadfish, fugu, are considered a delicacy. The tingling or numbness around the mouth resulting from the ingestion of small amounts of tetrodotoxin is said to add to the culinary experience. Despite the requirement of a special license to prepare these fish, death from respiratory failure secondary to tetrodotoxin poisoning still occurs. Between 1955 and 1975, 3000 cases of tetrodotoxin poisoning were reported in Japan, with a case-fatality rate of 51%. With the advent of improved supportive care and mechanical ventilation, the death rate has declined markedly.

The diagnosis is usually obvious, particularly if several people are involved. A history of recent ingestion of tetrodotoxic fish and the characteristic syndrome of numbness and paralysis are the main features at initial evaluation. Tetrodotoxin poisoning may be distinguished from ciguatera by the type of fish ingested and by the characteristic reversal of temperature perception (cold perceived as hot) common in ciguatera patients. Tetrodotoxin may be detected in fish or in gastrointestinal contents by high-performance liquid chromatography, which is sometimes used in postmortem investigations.

No specific antivenom for tetrodotoxin is commercially available (although experimental monoclonal antibodies* have been used in animals), and treatment is supportive. Treatment may include evacuation of stomach contents, either by the induction of emesis (only in fully conscious patients with neurologic function adequate to protect the airway) or by gastric lavage, with the airway secured by endotracheal intubation if required. Intubation may be necessary if the patient is unable to swallow and is at risk for aspiration of saliva. Mechanical ventilation is required for patients with evidence of ventilatory failure (increasing hypercapnia or hypoxia). Because the problem is predominantly motor paralysis, the patient's conscious state is likely to be preserved until quite late in the illness. Care should be taken to ensure adequate sedation for intubation and ventilation and to avoid careless remarks in the presence of the paralyzed patient. Hypotension secondary to vasodilation may necessitate the administration of intravenous plasma volume expanders. As with any paralyzed patient, scrupulous pressure care and eye care are mandatory. Anticholinesterases† have on occasion been administered for the treatment of tetrodotoxin poisoning, but with little clinical or theoretical basis for their use.

Ciguatera

Ciguatera is an illness that occurs after the consumption of fish whose flesh contains a toxin called ciguatoxin, which is produced by the dinoflagellate *Gambierdiscus toxicus* and converted from a precursor in the muscle of the fish. Ciguatoxin is concentrated up the food chain from plankton-feeding organisms to larger fish that feed on them. It may be present in high concentrations in the bodies of large predatory fish. The toxin is not destroyed by cooking and is undetectable by taste.

Hundreds of species of tropical marine fish have been implicated in ciguatera outbreaks. Reef fish such as coral trout (*Plectropomus* species), mackerel (*Scomberomorus* species), and barracuda (*Sphyraena jello*) are commonly involved. Although the illness typically occurs within 30 degrees north or south of the equator, the transport of fish to destinations outside these latitudes means that ciguatera may also be present beyond this range. The diagnosis may be delayed in these cases because of lack of familiarity with the illness.

Ciguatoxins are a group of lipophilic polycyclic ethers produced in precursor form (gambiertoxins) by some strains of *G. toxicus* and metabolized to the more potent ciguatoxins by fish. Their mechanism of action is related to membrane depolarization resulting from increased sodium permeability.

Ciguatera is a variable illness in which gastrointestinal and/or neurologic effects usually predominate. Neurologic symptoms may include paresthesia, arthralgia, myalgia, weakness, vertigo, and ataxia. A characteristic sensory disturbance or dysesthesia,

*Investigational drug in the United States.
†Not FDA approved for this indication.

with an inability to discriminate temperatures or altered temperature perception such that cold feels like hot, occurs frequently, and a proportion of patients describe painful or loose-feeling teeth. Gastrointestinal disturbance with nausea, vomiting, and diarrhea is common. Cardiovascular effects may include hypotension and bradycardia, and rash, itch, and desquamation also occur, as well as a variety of constitutional symptoms. Symptoms typically develop within 12 hours of ingestion of contaminated fish and resolve over a period of several days to weeks. Weakness and paresthesia, in particular, may be slower to resolve. In severe cases, death from respiratory failure may occur. Mortality rates of 12% have been reported, but with improvement in health care, death is now uncommon.

Treatment of ciguatera is mainly supportive. If the patient is conscious and able to protect the airway, vomiting should be induced. Intravenous fluid replacement is necessary for patients with severe gastrointestinal disturbance, and mechanical ventilation is sometimes required in those with severe neurologic impairment. In mildly affected patients, very cold or hot fluids should be avoided because of the patient's inability to discriminate temperature.

Several drugs, including corticosteroids, antihistamines, calcium gluconate, and atropine, have been used in the treatment of ciguatera, although none have been the subject of controlled trials. The most widely used treatment has been intravenous infusion of mannitol. Several case reports have suggested neurologic improvement after the infusion of mannitol, although recurrences are sometimes reported. The mechanism of action is unknown. No simple test can be used for detection of ciguatoxin. Bioassays, chromatography, and spectroscopy have been used in the laboratory. A simple enzyme immunoassay has been developed for the testing of fish, but it is of limited usefulness in practice.

Ciguatera is a significant public health problem in the Pacific, where fish form an important part of the diet. It also interferes with the fishing industry. The incidence is variable geographically as well as seasonally, and increases may be related to disturbances in tropical reefs by storms or by human activity such as construction of jetties and possibly nuclear testing in the south Pacific. Reported rates vary from 5 cases per 10,000 in Miami to around 100 per 10,000 on some Pacific atolls. Similar to tetrodotoxin poisoning, it may be unrecognized outside endemic areas. Rapid transport of reef fish to markets outside the tropics has resulted in cases of ciguatera in temperate areas such as Melbourne, Australia, and England.

Shellfish Poisoning

Marine intoxication accounted for 13.8% of all foodborne outbreaks of disease in the United States from 1972 through 1982. Of these cases, 7.4% were due to shellfish poisoning. The true incidence of shellfish poisoning worldwide is unknown, although in 1974 it was estimated that approximately 1600 cases and 300 deaths occur per annum. Case-fatality rates of 8.5% to 23.2% have been reported in the past. More recent series (1968 to 1990) provide an aggregate case-fatality rate of 5.9%. Mortality is possibly higher in children. It is likely that deaths have decreased with improvements in medical care (particularly intensive care) since this estimate was made. The incidence of shellfish poisoning in Western countries is also thought to have decreased because of the institution of safety measures such as inspections and quarantines and because of increased awareness. Most cases in the West are not related to commercial fishing but to the ingestion of shellfish collected by amateurs.

The toxins involved in shellfish poisoning are produced by dinoflagellates (unicellular phytoplankton). Around 20 of the more than 1200 known species of dinoflagellates produce toxins that may cause significant illness in human beings. They are heat stable (and not destroyed by cooking) and accumulate in filter-feeding shellfish, usually bivalved mollusks such as clams, mussels, oysters, scallops, and cockles. Outbreaks are generally seasonal and occur most commonly in the warmer months. Illness usually follows the ingestion of contaminated shellfish within 30 minutes to 3 hours. Four major syndromes have been associated with shellfish poisoning.

Paralytic Shellfish Poisoning

The dinoflagellate species most commonly associated with paralytic shellfish poisoning (PSP) are *Alexandrium catenella, Alexandrium tamerense, Pyrodinium bahamense, Pyrodinium bahamense* (var. *compressum*), and occasionally, *Gymnodinium catenatum* and *Cochlodinium catenatum.* The toxins are heat-stable, water-soluble, tetrahydropurine compounds, the principal toxin of which is saxitoxin (named after the butter clam *Saxidomus gigantea*). Many derivatives of these toxins exist and are called gonyautoxins (named after the genus *Gonyaulax*, now *Alexandrium*). The toxins block the propagation of nerve and muscle action potentials by interfering with membrane sodium ion channels, thereby causing reduced conduction velocity and reduced amplitude of motor and sensory impulses in peripheral nerves.

The clinical manifestation of PSP is similar to that of ciguatera and tetrodotoxin poisoning, with neurologic, cardiovascular, and respiratory problems. Fatalities have occurred secondary to respiratory failure. In the United States in 1971 through 1977, 32% of patients with PSP required hospitalization, and 6% required mechanical ventilation. No specific treatment is available, although animal experiments point to the possible usefulness of antibodies or other saxitoxin-binding proteins and the drug 4-aminopyridine, which facilitates neurotransmitter release at synapses.

Neurotoxic Shellfish Poisoning

The dinoflagellate organism *Gymnodinium breve* (or *Ptychodiscus brevis*) produces toxins that cause neurotoxic shellfish poisoning (NSP). The principal toxins responsible for NSP are at least two heat-stable brevetoxins different from saxitoxin in structure and clinical effect. They are similar in structure to ciguatoxin; are heat stable, lipid soluble, acid stable, and base labile; and activate sodium channels in parasympathetic nerves (and possibly adrenergic nerve fibers) by keeping "h" gates open.

The syndrome has been described mostly from the west coast of Florida. It is a milder form of shellfish poisoning than PSP. Brevetoxins are also unusual in that they can cause bronchospasm in response to inhaled toxin. No specific treatment is currently available, although a polyclonal antiserum has been used successfully in animal studies.

Diarrheic Shellfish Poisoning

Diarrheic shellfish poisoning is a variant of shellfish poisoning that occurs mostly in Japan but also in Europe and Mexico in association with *Diniphysis* species and *Prorocentrum* species in mussels. It is caused by a group of fat-soluble toxins that are derivatives of okadaic acid but distinct from saxitoxins and brevetoxins. The diarrhea is thought to be due to the release of sodium from intestinal cells. Gastrointestinal disturbance with nausea, vomiting, diarrhea, and fever begins within about 30 minutes and lasts for 8 hours or more. No specific treatment is known.

Amnestic (Encephalopathic) Shellfish Poisoning

Amnestic shellfish poisoning is a relatively recently (1987) described syndrome associated with mussels containing domoic acid produced by the diatom *Nitzschia pungens (F. multiseries)* from Prince Edward Island, Canada. Domoic acid has structural similarities to glutamic acid and may act as an excitatory neurotransmitter. It is also a potent depolarizing agent of spinal cord ventral root neurons.

In patients who were observed, gastrointestinal symptoms, headache, and memory loss were characteristic. In severe cases, hemiparesis, seizures, ophthalmoplegia, and altered consciousness develop, and four fatalities have been reported. Survivors were left with severe anterograde memory deficits. Severe neuronal necrosis was seen in the hippocampus and amygdaloid nucleus and in the dorsal medial nucleus of the thalamus in poisoned patients.

Scombrotoxism

Scombrotoxism is a form of poisoning that occurs when histamine is produced enzymatically from histidine in fish muscle as a result of contamination of the muscle with enteric bacteria during processing. Scombroid fish (family Scombridae) include mackerel, tuna, and bonito. Other fish, including anchovies and sardines (Engraulidae) and bluefish (Pomatomidae), have also been linked to outbreaks of scombrotoxism. It is reportedly the most significant cause of illness associated with seafood in the United States and Canada.

Symptoms and signs related to histamine intoxication include headache, dizziness, nausea and vomiting, diarrhea, erythema, flushing and sweating, urticaria, pruritus, bronchospasm, respiratory distress, palpitations, shock, and death (although death is rare). The illness typically begins within about 30 minutes of ingestion and usually lasts 8 to 12 hours. Scombroid poisoning may be difficult to differentiate from seafood allergy. Careful note of any history of ingestion and clinical manifestations should be taken. Treatment consists of the administration of antihistamines, intravenous fluids, and supportive care. Bronchospasm or hypotension may require epinephrine and bronchodilators. No deaths have been reported.

Other Fish Poisonings

Many other marine creatures have been associated with poisoning. Most of these illnesses do not have any specific antidote, and treatment consists of emesis and supportive care.

Clupeiotoxism

Clupeiotoxism, associated with herrings and anchovies (family Clupeidae), may cause nausea and vomiting, diarrhea, abdominal pain, dilated pupils, paresthesia, muscle cramps, paralysis, coma, and death. The toxin is unknown, possibly planktonic in origin. Clupeiotoxism has been described in the Indo-Pacific and the Caribbean Sea.

Gempylotoxic Fish (Family Gempylidae)

The oil contained in the flesh of these pelagic mackerel may cause diarrhea.

Ichthyotoxism

Nausea, vomiting, diarrhea, abdominal pain, cramps, hypotension, and cyanosis have been described after ingestion of the roe or gonads of some freshwater fish (including sturgeon, pike, gar, and carp) and some marine fish (blenny, sculpin).

Ichthyohemotoxism

Behavioral changes, nausea, vomiting, and diarrhea have been described after drinking eel's blood. The cause or toxin is unknown.

Toxic Crabs

Several marine toxins, including saxitoxin, gonyautoxin, and tetrodotoxin, may accumulate or be produced in crabs. Ingestion of toxic crabs may result in neurologic or gastrointestinal disturbances as described earlier. Various tropical Indo-Pacific species have been implicated.

Toxic Snails

Saxitoxin, gonyautoxin, and tetrodotoxin have been isolated from some species of marine snails. The species *Babylonia japonica* produces surugatoxins (glycosides) that cause atropine-like effects.

Turtle Poisoning

Ingestion of the flesh, blood, or organs of several species of sea turtles (order Chelonia) has been associated with poisoning characterized by a ciguatera-like illness, including nausea, vomiting, dysphagia, and acute stomatitis. The toxin has been named chelonitoxin, but little is known about it. Sporadic outbreaks, mostly from remote locations, have resulted in mortality rates of 7% to 28%. No specific treatment is available.

Elasmobranch Poisoning

A ciguatera-like illness with a predominance of neurologic symptoms has been described after ingestion of the liver of large sharks and rays (elasmobranchs). Mass poisonings in Madagascar resulted in dozens of deaths. Two liposoluble toxins distinct from ciguatoxin were isolated.

Hypervitaminosis A

High levels of vitamin A accumulated in the livers of many marine mammals, including seals, whales, and dolphins, as well as in polar bears, arctic foxes, huskies, and sharks, if ingested by human beings, may cause illness resulting in headache, vomiting, diarrhea, and drowsiness. Extensive desquamation is characteristic. Death may occur in severe cases.

MEDICAL TOXICOLOGY: INGESTIONS, INHALATIONS, AND DERMAL AND OCULAR ABSORPTIONS

method of
HOWARD C. MOFENSON, M.D., D.A.B.M.T.,
THOMAS R. CARACCIO, PHARM. D., D.A.B.A.T.,
MICHAEL McGUIGAN, M.D., D.A.B.M.T., and
JOSEPH GREENSHER, M.D.
Long Island Regional Poison and Drug Information Center
Mineola, New York

INTRODUCTION AND EPIDEMIOLOGY

According to the national Toxic Exposure Surveillance System (TESS), almost 2.2 million potentially toxic exposures were reported last year to Poison Control Centers throughout the United States. Poisonings were responsible for almost 920 deaths and more than 475,000 hospitalizations. Poisoning accounts for 2% to 5% of pediatric hospital admissions, 10% of adult admissions, 5% of hospital admissions in the elderly (>65 years of age), and 5% of ambulance calls. In one urban hospital, drug-related emergencies accounted for 38% of the emergency department visits. An evaluation of a medical intensive care unit and step-down unit over a 3-month period indicated that poisonings accounted for 19.7% of admissions.

The largest number of fatalities resulting from poisoning reported to the TESS are caused by analgesics. The other principal toxicologic causes of fatalities are antidepressants, sedative hypnotics/antipsychotics, stimulants/street drugs, cardiovascular agents, and alcohols. Less than 1% of overdose cases reaching the hospitals result in fatality. However, patients presenting in deep coma to medical care facilities have a fatality rate of 13% to 35%. The largest single cause of coma of inapparent etiology is drug poisoning.

Pharmaceutical preparations are involved in 40% of poisonings. The number one pharmaceutical agent involved in exposures is acetaminophen. The severity of the manifestations of acute poisoning exposures varies greatly depending on whether the poisoning was intentional or unintentional. Unintentional exposures make up 85% to 90% of all poisoning exposures. The majority of cases are acute, occurring in children younger than 5 years of age, in the home, and resulting in no or minor toxicity. Many are actually ingestions of relatively nontoxic substances that require minimal medical care. Intentional poisonings, such as suicides, constitute 10% to 15% of exposures and may require the highest standards of medical and nursing care and the use of sophisticated equipment for recovery. Intentional ingestions are often of multiple substances and frequently include ethanol, acetaminophen, and aspirin. Suicides make up 52% of the reported fatalities. About 25% of suicides are attempted with drugs. Sixty percent of patients who take a drug overdose use their own medication and 15% use drugs prescribed for close relatives. The majority of the drug-related suicide attempts involve a central nervous system (CNS) depressant, and coma management is vital to the treatment.

ASSESSMENT AND MAINTENANCE OF THE VITAL FUNCTIONS

The initial assessment of all patients in medical emergencies follows the principles of basic and advanced cardiac life support. The adequacy of the patient's airway, degree of ventilation, and circulatory status should be determined. The vital functions should be established and maintained. Vital signs should be measured frequently and should include body core temperature. The assessment of vital functions should include the rate numbers (e.g., respiratory rate) and indications of effectiveness (e.g., depth of respirations and degree of gas exchange). Table 1 gives important measurements and vital signs.

Level of consciousness should be assessed by immediate AVPU (Alert, responds to Verbal stimuli, responds to Painful stimuli, and Unconscious). If the patient is unconscious, one must assess the severity of the unconsciousness by the Glasgow Coma Scale (Table 2).

If the patient is comatose, management requires administering 100% oxygen, establishing vascular access, and obtaining blood for pertinent laboratory studies. The administration of glucose, thiamine, and naloxone as well as intubation to protect the airway should be considered. Pertinent laboratory studies include arterial blood gases (ABG), electrocardiography

TABLE 1. **Important Measurements and Vital Signs**

Age	Body Surface Area (m²)	Weight (kg)	Height (cm)	Pulse (bpm) resting	Blood Pressure: *Hypotension*	Blood Pressure: Hypertension *Significant*	Blood Pressure: Hypertension *Severe*	*Respiratory rate (rpm)*
Newborn	0.19	3.5	50	70–190	<40/60	>96	>106	30–60
1 mo–6 mo	0.30	4–7	50–65	80–160	<45/70	>104	>110	30–50
6 mo–l y	0.38	7–10	65–75	80–160	<45/70	>104	>110	20–40
1–2 y	0.50–0.55	10–12	75–85	80–140	<47/74	>74/112	>82/118	20–40
3–5 y	0.54–0.68	15–20	90–108	80–120	<52/80	>76/116	>84/124	20–40
6–9 y	0.68–0.85	20–28	122–133	75–115	<60/90	>82/122	>86/130	16–25
10–12 y	1.00–1.07	30–40	138–147	70–110	<60/90	>82/126	>90/134	16–25
13–15 y	1.07–1.22	42–50	152–160	60–100	<60/90	>86/136	>92/144	16–20
16–18 y	1.30–1.60	53–60	160–170	60–100	<60/90	>92/142	>98/150	12–16
Adult	1.40–1.70	60–70	160–170	60–100	<60/90	>90/140	>120/210	10–16

Data from Nadas A: Pediatric Cardiology, 3rd ed. Philadephia, WB Saunders, 1976; Blumer JL (ed): A Practice Guide to Pediatric Intensive Care. St Louis, Mosby, 1990; AAP and ACEP: Respiratory Distress in APLS Pediatric Emergency Medicine Course, 1993; Second Task Force: Blood pressure control in children–1987, Pediatr 79:1, 1987; Linakis JG: Hypertension. In Fliesher GR, Ludwig S (eds); Textbook of Pediatric Emergency Medicine, 3rd ed. Baltimore, Williams & Wilkins 1993.

(ECG), determination of blood glucose level, electrolytes, renal and liver tests, and acetaminophen plasma concentration in all cases of intentional ingestions. Radiography of the chest and abdomen may be useful. The severity of a stimulant's effects can also be assessed and should be documented to follow the trend.

The examiner should completely expose the patient by removing clothes and other items that interfere with a full evaluation. One should look for clues to etiology in the clothes and include the hat and shoes.

PREVENTION OF ABSORPTION AND REDUCTION OF LOCAL DAMAGE

Exposure

Poisoning exposure routes include ingestion (70%), dermal (8%), ophthalmologic (5%), inhalation (6%), insect bites and stings (4%), and parenteral injections (0.4%). The effect of the toxin may be local, systemic, or both.

Local effects (skin, eyes, mucosa of respiratory or gastrointestinal tract) occur where contact is made with the poisonous substance. Local effects are nonspecific chemical reactions that depend on the chemical properties (e.g., pH), concentration, contact time, and type of exposed surface.

Systemic effects occur when the poison is absorbed into the body and depends on the dose, the distribution, and the functional reserve of the organ systems. Shock and hypoxia are part of systemic toxicity.

Delayed Toxic Action

Therapeutic doses of most pharmaceuticals are absorbed within 90 minutes. However, the patient with exposure to a potential toxin may be asymptomatic at

TABLE 2. **Glasgow Coma Scale**

Scale	Adult Response	Score	Pediatric, 0–1 Years
Eye opening	Spontaneous	4	Spontaneous
	To verbal command	3	To shout
	To pain	2	To pain
	None	1	No response
Motor response			
To verbal command	Obeys	6	
To painful stimuli	Localized pain	5	Localized pain
	Flexion withdrawal	4	Flexion withdrawal
	Decorticate flexion	3	Decorticate flexion
	Decerebrate extension	2	Decerebrate flexion
	None	1	None
Verbal response: adult	Oriented and converses	5	Cries, smiles, coos
	Disoriented but converses	4	Cries or screams
	Inappropriate words	3	Inappropriate sounds
	Incomprehensible sounds	2	Grunts
	None	1	Gives no response
Verbal response: child	Oriented	5	
	Words or babbles	4	
	Vocal sounds	3	
	Cries or moans to stimuli	2	
	None	1	

Data from Teasdale G, Jennett B: Assessment of coma impaired consciousness. Lancet 2:83, 1974; Simpson D, Reilly P: Pediatric coma scale. Lancet 2:450, 1982; Seidel J: Preparing for pediatric emergencies. Pediatr Rev 16:470, 1995.

this time because a sufficient amount has not yet been absorbed or metabolized to produce toxicity at the time the patient presents for care.

Absorption can be significantly delayed under the following circumstances:

1. Drugs with anticholinergic properties (e.g., antihistamines, belladonna alkaloids, diphenoxylate with atropine [Lomotil], phenothiazines, and tricyclic antidepressants).
2. Modified release preparations such as sustained-release, enteric-coated, and controlled-release formulations have delayed and prolonged absorption.
3. Concretions may form (e.g., salicylates, iron, glutethimide, and meprobamate [Equanil]) that can delay absorption and prolong the toxic effects. Large quantities of drugs tend to be absorbed more slowly than small quantities.

Some substances must be metabolized into a toxic metabolite (acetaminophen, acetonitrile, ethylene glycol, methanol, methylene chloride, parathion, and paraquat). In some cases, time is required to produce a toxic effect on organ systems (*Amanita phalloides* mushrooms, carbon tetrachloride, colchicine, digoxin [Lanoxin], heavy metals, monoamine oxidase inhibitors, and oral hypoglycemic agents).

Initial Management

1. Stabilization of airway, breathing, and circulation and protection of same.
2. Identification of specific toxin or toxic syndrome.
3. Initial treatment: $D_{50}W$, consider thiamine, naloxone (Narcan), oxygen, and antidotes if needed.
4. Physical assessment.
5. Decontamination: Gastrointestinal tract, skin, eyes.

Decontamination

In the asymptomatic patient who has been exposed to a toxic substance, decontamination procedures should be considered if the patient has been exposed to potentially toxic substances in toxic amounts.

Ocular exposure should be immediately treated with water irrigation for 15 to 20 minutes with the eyelids fully retracted. One should not use neutralizing chemicals. All caustic and corrosive injuries should be evaluated with fluorescein dye and by an ophthalmologist.

Dermal exposure is treated immediately with copious water irrigation for 30 minutes, not a forceful flushing. Shampooing the hair, cleansing the fingernails, navel, and perineum, and irrigating the eyes are necessary in the case of an extensive exposure. The clothes should be specially bagged and may have to be discarded. Leather goods can become irreversibly contaminated and must be abandoned. Caustic (alkali) exposures can require hours of irrigation. Dermal absorption can occur with pesticides, hydrocarbons, and cyanide.

Injection exposures (e.g., snake envenomation) can be treated with venom extracts. Venom extractors can be used within minutes of envenomation, and proximal lymphatic constricting bands or elastic wraps can be used to delay lymphatic flow and immobilize the extremity. Cold packs and tourniquets should not be used and incision is generally not recommended. Substances of abuse may be injected intravenously or subcutaneously. In these cases, little decontamination can be done.

Inhalation exposure to toxic substances is managed by immediate removal of the victim from the contaminated environment by protected rescuers.

Gastrointestinal exposure is the most common route of poisoning. Gastrointestinal decontamination historically has been be done by gastric emptying: induction of emesis, gastric lavage, administration of activated charcoal, and the use of cathartics or whole bowel irrigation. No procedure is routine; it should be individualized for each case. If no attempt is made to decontaminate the patient, the reason should be clearly documented on the medical record (e.g., time elapsed, past peak of action, ineffectiveness, or risk of procedure).

Gastric Emptying Procedures

The gastric emptying procedure used is influenced by the age of the patient, the effectiveness of the procedure, the time of ingestion (gastric emptying is usually ineffective after 1 hour postingestion), the patient's clinical status (time of peak effect has passed or the patient's condition is too unstable), formulation of the substance ingested (regular release versus modified release), the amount ingested, and the rapidity of onset of CNS depression or stimulation (convulsions). Most studies show that only 30% (range, 19% to 62%) of the ingested toxin is removed by gastric emptying under optimal conditions. It has not been demonstrated that the choice of procedure improved the outcome.

A mnemonic for gathering information is STATS:

S—substance
T—type of formulation
A—amount and age
T—time of ingestion
S—signs and symptoms

The examiner should attempt to obtain AMPLE information about the patient:

A—age and allergies
M—available medications
P—past medical history including pregnancy, psychiatric illnesses, substance abuse, or intentional ingestions
L—time of last meal, which may influence absorption and the onset and peak action
E—events leading to present condition

The intent of the patient should also be determined.

The Regional Poison Center should be consulted for the exact ingredients of the ingested substance and the latest management. The treatment information on the labels of products and in the Physician's Desk Reference are notoriously inaccurate.

Ipecac Syrup

Syrup of ipecac–induced emesis has virtually no use in the emergency department. Although at one time it was considered most useful in young children with a recent witnessed ingestion, it is advised only within 1 hour of ingestion of known agents only when a toxic amount is involved. Current guidelines from the American Association of Poison Control Centers has significantly limited the indications for inducing emesis because the risk most often exceeds the benefit derived from this procedure. The Poison Control Center should be called before one induces emesis.

Contraindications or situations in which induction of emesis are inappropriate include the following:

- Ingestion of caustic substance
- Loss of airway protective reflexes because of ingestion of substances that can produce rapid onset of CNS depression (e.g., short-acting benzodiazepines, barbiturates, nonbarbiturate sedative-hypnotics, opioids, tricyclic antidepressants) or convulsions (e.g., camphor [Ponstel], chloroquine [Aralen], codeine, isoniazid [Nydrazid], mefenamic acid, nicotine, propoxyphene [Darvon], organophosphate insecticides, strychnine, and tricyclic antidepressants)
- Ingestion of low-viscosity petroleum distillates (e.g., gasoline, lighter fluid, kerosene)
- Significant vomiting prior to presentation or hematemesis
- Age under 6 months (no established dose, safety, or efficacy data)
- Ingestion of foreign bodies (emesis is ineffective and may lead to aspiration)
- Clinical conditions including neurologic impairment, hemodynamic instability, increased intracranial pressure, and hypertension
- Delay in presentation (more than 1 hour postingestion)

The dose of syrup of ipecac in the 6- to 9-month-old infant is 5 mL; in the 9- to 12-month-old, 10 mL; and in the 1- to 12-year-old, 15 mL. In children older than 12 years and in adults, the dose is 30 mL. The dose can be repeated once if the child does not vomit in 15 to 20 minutes. The vomitus should be inspected for remnants of pills or toxic substances, and the appearance and odor should be documented. When not available, 30 mL of mild dishwashing soap (not dishwasher detergent) can be used, although it is less effective.

Complications are very rare but include aspiration, protracted vomiting, rarely cardiac toxicity with long-term abuse, pneumothorax, gastric rupture, diaphragmatic hernia, intracranial hemorrhage, and Mallory-Weiss tears.

Gastric Lavage

Gastric lavage should be considered only when life-threatening amounts of substances were involved, when the benefits outweigh the risks, when it can be performed within 1 hour of the ingestion, and when no contraindications exist.

The contraindications are similar to those for ipecac-induced emesis. However, gastric lavage can be accomplished after the insertion of an endotracheal tube in cases of CNS depression or controlled convulsions. The patient should be placed with the head lower than the hips in a left-lateral decubitus position. The location of the tube should be confirmed by radiography, if necessary, and suctioning equipment should be available.

Contraindications to gastric lavage include the following:

- Ingestion of caustic substances (risk of esophageal perforation)
- Uncontrolled convulsions, because of the danger of aspiration and injury during the procedure
- Ingestion of low-viscosity petroleum distillate products
- CNS depression or absent protective airway reflexes, without endotracheal protection
- Significant cardiac dysrhythmias
- Significant emesis or hematemesis prior to presentation
- Delay in presentation (more than 1 hour postingestion)

SIZE OF TUBE

The best results with gastric lavage are obtained with the largest possible orogastric tube that can be reasonably passed (nasogastric tubes are not large enough to remove solid material). In adults, a large-bore orogastric Lavacuator hose or a No. 42 French Ewald tube should be used; in young children, orogastric tubes are generally too small to remove solid material and gastric lavage is not recommended.

The amount of fluid used varies with the patient's age and size. In general, aliquots of 50 to 100 mL per lavage are used in adults. Larger amounts of fluid may force the toxin past the pylorus. Lavage fluid is 0.9% saline.

Complications are rare and may include respiratory depression, aspiration pneumonitis, cardiac dysrhythmias due to increased vagal tone, esophageal-gastric tears and perforation, laryngospasm, and mediastinitis.

Activated Charcoal

Oral activated charcoal adsorbs the toxin onto its surface before absorption. According to recent guidelines set forth by the American Academy of Clinical Toxicology, activated charcoal should not be used routinely. Its use is indicated only if a toxic amount of substance has been ingested and is optimally effective within 1 hour of the ingestion. Because of the slow absorption of large quantities of toxin, activated charcoal may be beneficial after 1 hour postingestion.

Activated charcoal does not effectively adsorb small molecules or molecules lacking carbon (Table 3). Activated charcoal adsorption may be diminished by milk, cocoa powder, and ice cream.

There are a few relative contraindications to the use of activated charcoal:

1. Ingestion of caustics and corrosives, which may produce vomiting or cling to the mucosa and falsely appear as a burn on endoscopy.

TABLE 3. **Substances Poorly Adsorbed by Activated Charcoal**

C	**Caustics and corrosives**
H	**Heavy metals** (arsenic, iron, lead, mercury)
A	**Alcohols** (ethanol, methanol, isopropanol) and glycols (ethylene glycols)
R	**Rapid onset of absorption** (cyanide and strychnine)
C	**Chlorine and iodine**
O	**Others insoluble in water** (substances in tablet form)
A	**Aliphatic hydrocarbons** (petroleum distillates)
L	**Laxatives** (sodium, magnesium, potassium, and lithium)

2. Comatose patient, in whom the airway must be secured prior to activated charcoal administration.
3. Patient without presence of bowel sounds.

Note: Activated charcoal was shown not to interfere with effectiveness of *N*-acetylcysteine in cases of acetaminophen overdose, so it is no longer contraindicated as was thought in the past.

The usual initial adult dose is 60 to 100 g and the dose for children is 15 to 30 g. It is administered orally as a slurry mixed with water or by nasogastric or orogastric tube. Caution: Be sure the tube is in the stomach. Cathartics are not necessary.

Although repeated dosing with activated charcoal may decrease the half-life and increases the clearance of phenobarbital, dapsone, quinidine, theophylline, and carbamazepine (Tegretol), recent guidelines indicate there is insufficient evidence to support the use of multiple-dose activated charcoal unless a life-threatening amount of one of the substances mentioned is involved. At present there are no controlled studies that demonstrate that multiple-dose activated charcoal or cathartics alter the clinical course of an intoxication. The dose varies from 0.25 to 0.50 g/kg every 1 to 4 hours, and continuous nasogastric tube infusion of 0.25 to 0.5 g/kg/hr has been used to decrease vomiting.

Gastrointestinal dialysis is the diffusion of the toxin from the higher concentration in the serum of the mesenteric vessels to the lower levels in the gastrointestinal tract mucosal cell and subsequently into the gastrointestinal lumen, where the concentration has been lowered by intraluminal adsorption of activated charcoal.

Complications of treatment with activated charcoal include vomiting in 50% of cases, desorption (especially with weak acids in intestine), and aspiration (at least a dozen cases of aspiration have been reported). There are many cases of unreported pulmonary aspirations and "charcoal lungs," intestinal obstruction or pseudoobstruction (three cases reports with multiple dosing, none with a single dose), empyema following esophageal perforation, and hypermagnesemia and hypernatremia, which have been associated with repeated concurrent doses of activated charcoal and saline cathartics. Catharsis was used to hasten the elimination of any remaining toxin in the gastrointestinal tract. There are no studies to demonstrate the effectiveness of cathartics, and they are no longer recommended as a form of gastrointestinal decontamination.

Whole-Bowel Irrigation

With whole bowel irrigation, solutions of polyethylene glycol (PEG) with balanced electrolytes are used to cleanse the bowel without causing shifts in fluids and electrolytes. The procedure is not approved by the U.S. Food and Drug Administration for this purpose.

INDICATIONS

The procedure has been studied and used successfully in cases of iron overdose when abdominal radiographs reveal incomplete emptying of excess iron. There are additional indications for other types of ingestions, such as with body-packing of illicit drugs (e.g., cocaine, heroin).

The procedure is to administer the solution (GoLYTELY or Colyte), orally or by nasogastric tube, in a dose of 0.5 L per hour in children younger than 5 years of age and 2 L per hour in adolescents and adults for 5 hours. The end point is reached when the rectal effluent is clear or radiopaque materials can no longer be seen in the gastrointestinal tract on abdominal radiographs.

CONTRAINDICATIONS

These measures should not be used if there is extensive hematemesis, ileus, or signs of bowel obstruction, perforation, or peritonitis. Animal experiments in which PEG was added to activated charcoal indicated that activated charcoal–salicylates and activated charcoal–theophylline combinations resulted in decreased adsorption and desorption of salicylate and theophylline and no therapeutic benefit over activated charcoal alone. Polyethylene solutions are bound by activated charcoal in vitro, decreasing the efficacy of activated charcoal.

Dilutional treatment is indicated for the immediate management of caustic and corrosive poisonings but is otherwise not useful. The administration of diluting fluid above 30 mL in children and 250 mL in adults may produce vomiting, reexposing the vital tissues to the effects of local damage and possible aspiration.

Neutralization has not been proved to be safe or effective.

Endoscopy and surgery have been required in the case of body-packer obstruction, intestinal ischemia produced by cocaine ingestion, and iron local caustic action.

DIFFERENTIAL DIAGNOSIS OF POISONS ON THE BASIS OF CENTRAL NERVOUS SYSTEM MANIFESTATIONS

Neurologic parameters help to classify and assess the need for supportive treatment as well as provide diagnostic clues to the etiology. Table 4 lists the effects of CNS depressants, CNS stimulants, hallucinogens, and autonomic nervous system anticholinergics and cholinergics.

Central nervous system depressants are cholinergics, opioids, sedative-hypnotics, and sympatholytic agents. The hallmarks are lethargy, sedation, stupor,

TABLE 4. **Agents with Central Nervous System (CNS) Effects**

Agents	General Manifestations	Agents	General Manifestations
CNS Depressants		*Hallucinogens*	
Alcohols and glycols (S-H)	Bradycardia	Amphetamines‡	Tachycardia and dysrhythmias
Anticonvulsants (S-H)	Bradypnea	Anticholinergics	Tachypnea
Antidysrhythmics (S-H)	Shallow respirations	Cardiac glycosides	Hypertension
Antihypertensives (S-H)	Hypotension	Cocaine	Hallucinations, usually visual
Barbiturates (S-H)	Hypothermia	Ethanol withdrawal	Disorientation
Benzodiazepines (S-H)	Flaccid coma	Hydrocarbon inhalation (abuse)	Panic reaction
Butyrophenones (Syly)	Miosis	Mescaline (peyote)	Toxic psychosis
β-Adrenergic blockers (Syly)	Hypoactive bowel sounds	Mushrooms (psilocybin)	Moist skin
Calcium channel blockers (Syly)		Phencyclidine	Mydriasis (reactive)
Digitalis (Syly)			Hyperthermia
Opioids			Flashbacks
Lithium (mixed)		*Anticholinergics*	
Muscle relaxants			
Phenothiazines (Syly)		Antihistamines	Tachycardia, dysrhythmias rare
Nonbarbiturate/benzodiazepine sedative-hypnotics (chloral hydrate, glutethimide, methaqualone, methyprylon, ethchlorvynol, bromide)		Antispasmodic gastrointestinal preparations	Tachypnea
		Antiparkinsonian preparations	Hypertension (mild)
		Atropine	Hyperthermia
Tricyclic antidepressants (late Syly)		Cyclobenzaprine (Flexeril)	Hallucinations ("mad as a hatter")
CNS Stimulants		Mydriatic ophthalmologic agents	Mydriasis (unreactive) ("blind as a bat")
Amphetamines (Sy)	Tachycardia		
Anticholinergics*	Tachypnea and dysrhythmias	Over-the-counter sleep agents	Flushed skin ("red as a beet")
		Plants (*Datura* spp)/mushrooms	Dry skin and mouth ("dry as a bone")
Cocaine (Sy)	Hypertension		
Camphor (mixed)	Convulsions	Phenothiazines (early)	Hypoactive bowel sounds
Ergot alkaloids (Sy)	Toxic psychosis	Scopolamine	Urinary retention
Isoniazid (mixed)	Mydriasis (reactive)	Tricyclic/cyclic antidepressants (early)	Lilliputian hallucinations ("little people")
Lithium (mixed)	Agitation and restlessness		
Lysergic acid diethylamide (H)	Moist skin	*Cholinergics*	
Hallucinogens (H)	Tremors	Bethanechol (Urecholine)	Bradycardia (muscarinic)
Mescaline and synthetic analogs		Carbamate insecticides (Carbaryl)	Tachycardia (nicotinic effect)
Metals (arsenic, lead, mercury)			
Methylphenidate (Ritalin) (Sy)		Edrophonium	Miosis (muscarinic)
Monoamine oxidase inhibitors (Sy)		Organophosphate insecticides (Malathion, parathion)	Diarrhea (muscarinic)
Pemoline (Cylert) (Sy)			
Phencyclidine (H)†		Parasympathetic agents (physostigmine, pyridostigmine)	Hypertension (variable)
Salicylates (mixed)			
Strychnine (mixed)			
Sympathomimetics (Sy) (phenylpropanolamine, theophylline, caffeine, thyroid)		Toxic mushrooms (*Clitocybe* spp.)	Hyperactive bowel sounds
Withdrawal from ethanol, beta-adrenergic blockers, clonidine, opioids, sedative-hypnotics (W)			Excess urination (muscarinic)
			Excess salivation (muscarinic)
			Lacrimation (muscarinic)
			Bronchospasm (muscarinic)
			Muscle fasciculations (nicotinic)
			Paralysis (nicotinic)

H = hallucinogen; S-H = sedative-hyprotic; Sy = sympathomemetic; Syly = Sympatholytic; W = withdrawal.
*Anticholinergics produce dry skin and mucosa and decreased bowel sounds.
†Phencyclidine may produce miosis.
‡The amphetamine hybrids are methylene dioxymethamphetamine (MDMA, ecstasy, "ADAM") and methylene dioxyamphetamine (MDA, "Eve"), which have been recently associated with deaths.

and coma. In exception to the manifestations listed in Table 4, (1) barbiturates may produce an initial tachycardia; (2) convulsions are produced by codeine, propoxyphene (Darvon), meperidine (Demerol), glutethimide, phenothiazines, methaqualone, and tricyclic and cyclic antidepressants; (3) benzodiazepines rarely produce coma that will interfere with cardiorespiratory functions; and (4) pulmonary edema is common with opioids and sedative-hypnotics.

The CNS stimulants are anticholinergic, hallucinogenic, sympathomimetic, and withdrawal agents. The hallmarks of CNS stimulants are convulsions and hyperactivity.

There is considerable overlapping of effects among the various hallucinogens, but the major hallmark manifestation is hallucinations.

GUIDELINES FOR IN-HOSPITAL DISPOSITION

Classification of patients as high risk depends on clinical judgment. Any patient who needs cardiorespiratory support or has a persistently altered mental status for 3 hours or more should be considered for intensive care.

Guidelines for admitting patients older than 14 years of age to an intensive care unit, after 2 to 3 hours in emergency department, include the following:

1. Need for intubation
2. Seizures
3. Unresponsiveness to verbal stimuli
4. Arterial carbon dioxide pressure greater than 45 mm Hg
5. Cardiac conduction or rhythm disturbances (any rhythm except sinus arrhythmia)
6. Close monitoring of vital signs during antidotal therapy or elimination procedures
7. The need for continuous monitoring
8. QRS interval greater than 0.10 second, in cases of tricyclic antidepressant poisoning
9. Systolic blood pressure less than 80 mm Hg
10. Hypoxia, hypercarbia, acid-base imbalance, or metabolic abnormalities
11. Extremes of temperature
12. Progressive deterioration or significant underlying medical disorders

USE OF ANTIDOTES

Antidotes are available for only a relatively small number of poisons. An antidote is not a substitute for good supportive care. Table 5 summarizes the commonly used antidotes, their indications, and their methods of administration. The Regional Poison Control Center can give further information on these antidotes.

ENHANCEMENT OF ELIMINATION

The acceptable methods for elimination of absorbed toxic substances are dialysis, hemoperfusion, exchange transfusion, plasmapheresis, enzyme induction, and inhibition. Methods of increasing urinary excretion of toxic chemicals and drugs have been studied extensively, but the other modalities have not been well evaluated.

In general, these methods are needed in only a minority of cases and should be reserved for life-threatening circumstances when a definite benefit is anticipated.

Dialysis

Dialysis is the extrarenal means of removing certain substances from the body, and it can substitute for the kidney when renal failure occurs. Dialysis is not the first measure instituted; however, it may be lifesaving later in the course of a severe intoxication. It is needed in only a minority of intoxicated patients.

Peritoneal dialysis utilizes the peritoneum as the membrane for dialysis. It is only 1/20 as effective as hemodialysis. It is easier to use and less hazardous to the patient but also less effective in removing the toxin; thus, it is rarely used except in small infants.

Hemodialysis is the most effective dialysis method but requires experience with sophisticated equipment. Blood is circulated past a semipermeable extracorporeal membrane. Substances are removed by diffusion down a concentration gradient. Anticoagulation with heparin is necessary. Flow rates of 300 to 500 mL/min can be achieved, and clearance rates may reach 200 or 300 mL/min.

Dialyzable substances easily diffuse across the dialysis membrane and have the following characteristics: (1) a molecular weight less than 500 daltons and preferably less than 350; (2) a volume of distribution less than 1 L/kg; (3) protein binding less than 50%; (4) high water solubility (low lipid solubility); and (5) high plasma concentration and a toxicity that correlates reasonably with the plasma concentration. Considerations for hemodialysis and hemoperfusion are cases of serious ingestions (the nephrologist should be notified immediately), and cases involving a compound that is ingested in a potentially lethal dose and the rapid removal of which may improve the prognosis. Examples of the latter are ethylene glycol 1.4 mL/kg 100% solution or equivalent and methanol 6 mL/kg 100% solution or equivalent. Common dialyzable substances include alcohol, bromides, lithium, and salicylates.

The patient-related criteria for dialysis are (1) anticipated prolonged coma and the likelihood of complications, (2) renal compromise (toxin excreted or metabolized by kidneys and dialyzable chelating agents in heavy metal poisoning), (3) laboratory confirmation of lethal blood concentration, (4) lethal dose poisoning with an agent with delayed toxicity or known to be metabolized into a more toxic metabolite (e.g., ethylene glycol, methanol), (5) hepatic impairment when the agent is metabolized by the liver, and clinical deterioration despite optimal supportive medical management. Table 6 gives plasma concentrations above which removal by extracorporeal measures should be considered.

The contraindications to hemodialysis include the following: (1) substances are not dialyzable, (2) effective antidotes are available, (3) patient is hemodynamically unstable (e.g., shock), (4) presence of coagulopathy because heparinization is required.

Hemodialysis also has a role in correcting disturbances that are not amenable to appropriate medical management. These are easily remembered by the "vowel" mnemonic:

A—refractory acid-base disturbances
E—refractory electrolyte disturbances
I—intoxication with dialyzable substances (e.g., ethanol, ethylene glycol, isopropyl alcohol, methanol, lithium, and salicylates)
O—overhydration
U—uremia

Complications of dialysis include hemorrhage, thrombosis, air embolism, hypotension, infections, electrolyte imbalance, thrombocytopenia, and removal of therapeutic medications.

Hemoperfusion

Hemoperfusion is the parenteral form of oral activated charcoal. Heparinization is necessary. The patient's blood is routed extracorporeally through an

TABLE 5. **Initial Doses of Antidotes for Common Poisonings**

Antidote	Use	Dose	Route	Adverse Reactions/Comments
***N*-Acetyl cysteine (NAC, Mucomyst):** Stock level to treat 70 kg adult for 24 h: 25 vials, 20%, 30 mL	Acetaminophen, carbon tetrachloride (experimental)	140/mg/kg loading, followed by 70 mg/kg every 4 h for 17 doses	PO	Nausea, vomiting Dilute to 5% with sweet juice or flat cola.
Atropine: Stock level to treat 70 kg adult for 24 h: 1 g (1 mg/mL in 1, 10 mL)	Organophosphate and carbamate pesticides; bradydysrthythmics, β-adrenergics, calcium channel blockers	*Child:* 0.02–0.05 mg/kg repeated q5–10 min to max of 2 mg as necessary until cessation of secretions. *Adult:* 1–2 mg q5–10 min as necessary. Dilute in 1–2 mL of 0.9% saline for ET instillation. *IV infusion dose:* Place 8 mg of atropine in 100 mL D_5W or saline. Conc. = 0.08 mg/mL; dose range = 0.02–0.08 mg/kg/h or 0.25–1 mL/kg/h. Severe poisoning may require supplemental doses of IV atropine intermittently in doses of 1–5 mg until drying of secretions occurs	IV/ET	Tachycardia, dry mouth, blurred vision, and urinary retention Ensure adequate ventilation before administration.
Calcium chloride (10%): Stock level to treat 70 kg adult for 24 h:10 vials 1 g (1.35 mEq/mL)	Hypocalcemia, fluoride, calcium channel blockers, β-blockers, oxalates, ethylene glycol, hypermagnesemia	0.1–0.2 mL/kg (10–20 mg/kg) slow push every 10 min up to max 10 mL (1 g). Since calcium response lasts 15 minutes, some may require continuous infusion 0.2 mL/kg/h up to maximum of 10 mL/hr while monitoring for dysrhythmias and hypotension.	IV	Administer slowly with BP and ECG monitoring and have magnesium available to reverse calcium effects Tissue irritation, hypotension, dysrhythmias from rapid injection Contraindications: digitalis glycoside intoxication
Calcium gluconate (10%) Stock level to treat 70 kg adult for 24 h: 20 vials 1 g (0.45 mEq/mL)	Hypocalcemia, fluoride, calcium channel blockers, hydrofluoric acid; black widow envenomation	0.3–0.4 mL/kg (30–40 mg/kg) slow push; repeat as needed up to max dose 10–20 m (1–2 g)	1V	Same comments as calcium chloride
Infiltration of calcium gluconate	Hydrofluoric acid skin exposure	Dose: Infiltrate each square cm of affected dermis/ subcutaneous tissue with about 0.5 ml, of 10% calcium gluconate using a 30-gauge needle. Repeat as needed to control pain.	Infiltrate	
Intra-arterial calcium gluconate	Hydrofluoric acid skin exposure	Infuse 20 mL of 10% calcium gluconate (not chloride) diluted in 250 mL D_5W via the radial or brachial artery proximal to the injury over 3–4 hours.		Alternatively, dilute 10 mL of 10% calcium gluconate with 40–50 mL of D_5W.
Calcium gluconate gel Stock level: 3.5 g	Hydrofluoric acid skin exposure	2.5 g USP powder added to 100 mL water-soluble lubricating jelly, e.g., K-Y Jelly or Lubifax (or 3.5 mg into 150 mL). Some use 6 g of calcium carbonate in 100 g of lubricant. Place injured hand in surgical glove filled with gel. Apply q4h. If pain persists, calcium gluconate injection may be needed (above).	Dermal	Powder is available from Spectrum Pharmaceutical. Co. in California: 800-772-8786. Commercial preparation of Ca gluconate gel is available from Pharmascience in Montreal, Quebec: 514-340-1114.
Cyanide antidote kit: Stock level to treat	Cyanide Hydrogen sulfide (nitrites are given only)	Amyl nitrite: 1 crushable ampule for 30 secs of every min. Use new amp q3min.	Inhalation	If methemoglobinemia occurs, do not use methylene blue to correct this because it releases cyanide.

Continued

TABLE 5. **Initial Doses of Antidotes for Common Poisonings—cont'd**

Antidote	Use	Dose	Route	Adverse Reactions/Comments
70 kg adult for 24 h: 2 Lilly Cyanide Antidote kits	Do not use sodium thiosulfate for hydrogen sulfide Individual portions of the kit can be used in certain circumstances (consult PCC)	May omit step if venous access is established.		
	Cyanide Hydrogen sulfide (nitrites are given only) Do not use sodium thiosulfate for hydrogen sulfide Individual portions of the kit can be used in certain circumstances (consult PCC)	Sodium nitrite: *Child:* 0.33 mL/kg of 3% solution if hemoglobin level is not known, otherwise based on tables with product. *Adult:* up to 300 mg (10 mL). Dilute nitrite in 100 mL 0.9% saline, administer slowly at 5 mL/min. Slow infusion if fall in BP.	IV	If methemoglobinemia occurs, do not use methylene blue to correct this because it releases cyanide.
	Do not use sodium thiosulfate for hydrogen sulfide Individual portions of the Kit can be used in certain circumstances (consult PCC)	Sodium thiosulfate: *Child:* 1.6 mL/kg of 25% solution, may be repeated every 30–60 min to a maximum of 12.5 g or 50 mL in adult. Administer over 20 min.	IV	Nausea, dizziness, headache. Tachycardia, muscle rigidity, and bronchospasm (rapid administration).
Dantrolene sodium (Dantrium): Stock level to treat 70 kg adult for 24 h: 700 mg, 35 vials (20 mg/vial)	Malignant hyperthermia	2–3 mg/kg IV rapidly. Repeat loading dose every 10 minutes, if necessary up to a maximum total dose of 10 mg/kg. When temperature and heart rate decrease, slow the infusion of 1–2 mg/kg every 6 hours for 24–48 h until all evidence of malignant hyperthermia syndrome has subsided. Follow with oral doses 1–2 mg/kg four times a day for 24 h as necessary.	IV/PO	Hepatotoxicity occurs with cumulative dose of 10 mg/kg Thrombophlebitis (best given in central line) Available as 20 mg lyophilized dantrolene powder for reconstitution, which contains 3 g mannitol and sodium hydroxide in 70 mL vial. Mix with 60 mL sterile distilled water without a bacteriostatic agent and protect from light. Use within 6 hours after reconstituted.
Deferoxamine (Desferal): Stock level to treat 70 kg adult for 24 h: 17 vials (500 mg/amp).	Iron	IV infusion of 15 mg/kg/h (3 mL/kg/hr: 500 mg in 100 mL D_5W) max 6 g/day. Rates of >45 mg/kg/h if conc >1000 μg/dL	Preferred IV; avoid therapy >24 hr	Hypotension (minimized by avoiding rapid infusion rates) DFO challenge test 50 mg/kg is unreliable if negative.
Diazepam (Valium): Stock level to treat 70 kg adult for 24 h: 200 mg, 5 mg/mL; 2, 10 mL	Any intoxication that provokes seizures when specific therapy is not available, e.g., amphetamines, PCP, barbiturate and alcohol withdrawal. Chloroquine poisoning.	Adult, 5–10 mg IV (max 20 mg) at a rate of 5 mg/min until seizure is controlled. May be repeated 2 or 3 times. Child, 0.1–0.3 mg/kg up to 10 mg IV slowly over 2 min.	IV	Confusion, somnolence, coma, hypotension. Intramuscular absorption is erratic. Establish airway and administer 100% oxygen and glucose.
Digoxin-specific Fab antibodies (Digibind): Stock level to treat 70 kg adult for 24 h: 20 vials.	Digoxin, digitoxin, oleander tea with the following: (1) Imminent cardiac arrest or shock, (2) hyperkalemia >5.0 mEq/L, (3) serum digoxin >5 ng/mL (child) at 8–12 h post-ingestion in adults, (4) digitalis delirium, (5) ingestion over 10 mg in adults or 4 mg in child, (6) bradycardia or second- or	(1) If amount ingested is known total dose × bioavailability (0.8) = body burden. The body burden ÷ 0.6 (0.5 mg of digoxin is bound by 1 vial of 38 mg of FAB) = # vials needed. (2) If amount is unknown but the steady state serum concentration is known in ng/mL: Digoxin: ng/ml: (5.6 L/kg Vd) × (wt kg) = μg body burden Body burden ÷ 100 = mg body burden/0.5 = # vials needed.	IV	Allergic reactions (rare), return of condition being treated with digitalis glycoside. Administer by infusion over 30 minutes through a 0.22 μm filter. If cardiac arrest imminent, may administer by bolus. Consult PCC for more details.

TABLE 5. **Initial Doses of Antidotes for Common Poisonings—cont'd**

Antidote	Use	Dose	Route	Adverse Reactions/Comments
	third-degree heart block unresponsive to atropine, (7) life-threatening digitoxin or oleander poisoning.	Digitoxin body burden = ng/mL × (0.56 L/kg Vd) × (wt kg) Body burden ÷ 1000 = mg body burden/0.5 = # vials needed. (3) If the amount is not known, it is administered in life-threatening situations as 10 vials (400 mg) IV in saline over 30 minutes in adults. If cardiac arrest is imminent, administer 20 vials (adult) as a bolus.		
Dimercaprol (BAL in peanut oil): Stock level to treat 70 kg adult for 24 h: 1200 mg (4 amps - 100 mg/mL 10% in oil in 3 mL amp)	Chelating agent for arsenic, mercury, and lead.	3–5 mg/kg q4h usually for 5–10 d	Deep IM	Local infection site pain and sterile abscess, nausea, vomiting, fever, salivation, hypertension, and nephrotoxicity (alkalinize urine)
2,3 Dimercapto-succinic acid (DMSA succimer): 100 mg/capsule; 20 capsules	Used as a chelating agent for lead, especially blood lead levels >45 μg/dL. May also be used for symptomatic mercury exposure	10 mg/kg 3× daily for 5 days followed by 10 mg/kg 2× daily for 14 days.	PO	Precautions: monitor AST/ALT; use with caution in G6PD-deficient patients. Avoid concurrent iron therapy. Relatively safe antidote, rarely severe, uncommon minor skin rashes may occur.
Diphenhydramine (Benadryl) Antiparkinsonian action. Stock level to treat a 70 kg adult for 24 h: 5 vials (10 mg/mL, 10 mL each)	Used to treat extrapyramidal symptoms and dystonia induced by phenothiazines, phencyclidine, and related drugs.	Children: 1–2 mg/kg IV slowly over 5 minutes up to maximum 50 mg followed by 5 mg/kg/24h orally divided every 6 hours up to 300 mg/24h *Adults:* 50 mg IV followed by 50 mg orally four times daily for 5–7 days. Note: Symptoms abate within 2–5 minutes after IV.	IV	Fatal dose, 20–40 mg/kg. Dry mouth, drowsiness.
Ethanol (ethyl alcohol): Stock level to treat 70 kg adult for 24 h:3 bottles 10% (1 L each)	Methanol, ethylene glycol	10 mL/kg loading dose concurrently with 1.4 mL/kg (average) infusion of 10% ethanol (consult PCC for more details)	IV	Nausea, vomiting, sedation Use 0.22 μm filter if preparing from bulk 100% ethanol
Flumazenil (Romazicon): Stock level to treat 70 kg adult for 24 h: 4 vials (0.1 mg/mL, 10 mL)	Benzodiazepines (may also be beneficial in the treatment of hepatic encephalopathy)	Administer 0.2 mg (2 mL) IV over 30 sec (pediatric dose not established 0.01 mg/kg), then wait 3 min for a response, then if desired consciousness is not achieved, administer 0.3 mg (3 mL) over 30 sec, then wait 3 min for response, then if desired consciousness is not achieved, administer 0.5 mg (5 mL) over 30 sec at 60-sec intervals up to a maximum cumulative dose of 3 mg (30 mL) (1 mg in children). Because effects last only 1–5 hours, if patient responds monitor carefully over next 6 hours for resedation. If multiple repeated doses, consider a continuous infusion of 0.2–1 mg/h.	IV	Nausea, vomiting, facial flushing, agitation, headache, dizziness, seizures, and death. It is not recommended to improve ventilation. Its role in CNS depression needs to be clarified. It should not be used routinely in comatose patients. It is **contraindicated** in cyclic antidepressant intoxications, stimulant overdose, long-term benzodiazepine use (may precipitate life-threatening withdrawal), if benzodiazepines are used to control seizures, in head trauma.
Folic acid (Folvite):	Methanol/ ethylene	1 mg/kg up to 50 mg q4h for 6 doses.	IV	Uncommon

Continued

TABLE 5. **Initial Doses of Antidotes for Common Poisonings—cont'd**

Antidote	Use	Dose	Route	Adverse Reactions/Comments
Stock level to treat 70 kg adult for 24 h: 4 100-mg vials	glycol (investigational)			
Fomepizole (4-MP, Antizol): Stock level to treat 70 kg adult: 4 1.5-mL vials (1 gm/mL)	Ethylene glycol Methanol	Loading dose: 15 mg/kg (0.015 mL/kg) IV followed by maintanence dose of 10 mg/kg (0.01 mL/kg every 12 hours for 4 doses, then 15 mg/kg every 12 hours until ethylene glycol levels are <20 mg/dL. Fomipazole can be given to patients undergoing hemodialysis (dose q4hr).	IV	Suggested: co-administer folate 50 mg IV (child 1 mg/kg), thiamine 100 mg/d (child 50 mg), and pyridoxine 50 mg IV/IM q6h until intoxication is resolved. Monitor for urinary oxalate crystals. Adverse reactions include headache, nausea, and dizziness. Antizole should be diluted in 100 mL 0.9% saline or D_5W and mixed well. Antizole should not be given undiluted.
Glucagon: Stock level to treat 70 kg adult for 24 h: (10 vials, 10 units)	β-Blocker, calcium channel blocker	3–10 mg in adult, then infuse 2–5 mg/h (0.05–0.1 mg/kg child, then infuse 0.07 mg/kg/h) Large doses up to 100 mg/24h used	IV	Use D_5W, not 0.9% saline, to reconstitute the glucagon (rather than diluent of Eli Lilly, which contains phenol). Vomiting precautions.
Magnesium sulfate: Stock level to treat 70 kg adult for 24 h: approx 25 g (50 mL of 50% or 200 mL of 12.5%)	Torsades de pointes	*Adult:* 2 g (20 mL of 20%) over 20 min. If no response in 10 min, repeat and follow by continuous infusion 1 g/h. *Children:* 25–50 mg/kg initially and maintenance is 30–60 mg/kg/24h) (0.25–0.5 mEq/kg/24h) up to 1000 mg/24h. (Dose not studied in controlled fashion)	IV	Use with caution if renal impairment is present.
Methylene blue: Stock level to treat 70 kg adult for 24 h: 5 amps (10 mg/10 mL)	Methemoglobinemia	0.1–0.2 mL/kg of 1% solution, slow infusion, may be repeated every 30–60 min	IV	Nausea, vomiting, headache, dizziness
Naloxone (Narcan): Stock level to treat 70 kg adult for 24 h: 3 vials (1 mg/mL, 10 mL)	Comatose patient; decreased respirations <12; opioids	In postoperative opioid depression reversal, IV 0.1–0.5 μg/kg every 2 minutes as needed and may repeat up to a total dose of 1 μg/kg In **suspected overdose,** administer IV 0.1 mg/kg in a child under 5 years of age up to 2 mg, in older children and adults administer 2 mg every 2 min up to a total of 10–20 mg. Can also be administered into the endotracheal tube. If no response by 10 mg, a pure opioid intoxication is unlikely. **If opioid abuse** is suspected, **restraints** should be in place before administration; **initial dose** 0.1 mg to avoid withdrawal and violent behavior. The initial dose is then doubled every minute progressively to a total of 10 mg. **A continuous infusion** has been advocated because many opioids outlast the short half-life of naloxone (30–60 minutes). The **naloxone infusion hourly rate** to produce a response is equal to the effective dose required (improvement in ventilation and arousal). An additional dose may be required in 15–30 minutes as a bolus.	IV, ET	**Larger doses** of naloxone may be required for more poorly antagonized synthetic opioid drugs: buprenorphine (Buprenex), codeine, dextromethorphan, fentanyl, pentazocine (Talwin), propoxyphene (Darvon), diphenoxylate, nalbuphine (Nubain), new potent "designer" drugs or long-acting opioids such as methadone (Dolophine) **Complications.** Although naloxone is safe and effective, there are rare reports of complications (<1%) of pulmonary edema, seizures, hypertension, cardiac arrest, and sudden death. The infusions are titrated to avoid respiratory depression and opioid withdrawal manifestations. Tapering of infusions can be attempted after 12 hours and when the patient's condition has been stabilized.

TABLE 5. **Initial Doses of Antidotes for Common Poisonings—cont'd**

Antidote	Use	Dose	Route	Adverse Reactions/Comments
Physostigmine (Antilirium): Stock level to treat 70 kg adult for 24 hrs: 2–4 mg (2 mL each)	Anticholinergic agents (not routinely used, only indicated if life-threatening complications)	*Child:* 0.02 mg/kg slow push to max 2 mg q30–60min; *Adult:* 1–2 mg q5min to max 6 mg	IV	Bradycardia, asystole, seizures, bronchospasm, vomiting, headaches. Do not use for cyclic antidepressants.
Pralidoxime (2PAM, Protopan): Stock level to treat 70 kg adult for 24 h: 12 vials (1 gm per 20 mL)	Organophosphates	Child <- 12 yr, 25–50 mg/kg max (4 mg/min); > 12 yr, 1–2 g/ dose in 250 mL of 0.9% saline over 5–10 min. Max 200 mg/min. Repeat q6–12h for 24–48 h. Max adult 6 g/day. Alternative: Maintenance infusion 1 g in 100 ml, of 0.9% saline at 5–20 mg/kg/h (0.5–12 mL/kg/hr) up to max 500 mg/h or 50 mL/h. Titrate to desired response. End point is absence of fasciculations and return of muscle strength.	IV	Nausea, dizziness, headache; tachycardia, muscle rigidity, bronchospasm (rapid administration).
Pyridoxine (vitamin B_6): Stock level to treat 70 kg adult for 24 h: 100 mg/mL 10% solution. For a 70 kg patient, 10 g = 10 vials	Seizures from isoniazid or *Gyromitra* mushrooms; ethylene glycol	*Isoniazid: Unknown amt ingested:* 5 g (70 mg/kg) in 50 mL D_5W over 5 min + diazepam 0.3 mg/kg IV at rate of 1 mg/min in child or 10 mg dose at rate up to 5 mg/min in adults. Use different site (synergism). May repeat q5–20min until seizure controlled. Up to 375 mg/kg have been given (52 g). *Known amount:* 1 g for each gram isoniazid ingested over 5 min with diazepam (dose above) *Gyromitra mushroom:* Child 25 mg/kg or 2–5 g, adults IV over 15–30 min to max 20 g. *Ethylene glycol:* 100 mg IV daily	IV	After seizure is controlled, administer remainder of pyridoxine 1g/1g isoniazid total 5 g as infusion over 60 min. Adverse reactions uncommon; do not administer in same bottle as sodium bicarbonate. For *Gyromitra* mushrooms, some use PO 25 mg/kg/day early when mushroom ingestion is suspected.
Sodium bicarbonate ($NaHCO_3$): Stock level to treat 70 kg adult for 24 h: 10 ampules or syringes (500 mEq)	Tricyclic antidepressant cardiotoxicity (QRS> 0.12 sec; ventricular tachycardia, severe conduction disturbances); metabolic acidosis; phenothiazine toxicity	1–2 mEq/kg undiluted as a bolus. If no effect on cardiotoxicity, repeat twice a few minutes apart.	IV	Monitor sodium, potassium, and blood pH because fatal alkalemia and hyponatremia have been reported.
	Salicylate: to keep blood pH 7.5–7.55 (not >7.55) and urine pH 7.5–8.0. Alkalinization recommended if salicylate conc. >40 mg/dL in acute poisoning and at lower levels if symptomatic in chronic intoxication. 2 mEq/kg will raise blood pH 0.1 unit.	*Adult* with clear physical signs and laboratory findings of acute moderate or severe salicylism: Bolus 1–2 mEq/kg followed by infusion of 100–150 mEq $NaHCO_3$ added to 1 liter of 5% dextrose at rate of 200–300 mL/h *Child:* Bolus same as adult followed by 1–2 mEq/kg in infusion of 20 mL/kg/h 5% dextrose in 0.45% saline. Add potassium when patient voids. Rate and amount of the initial infusion, if patient		Monitor **both** urine and blood pH. Do not use the urine pH alone to assess the need for alkalinization because of the paradoxical aciduria that may occur. Adjust the urine pH to 7.5–8 by $NaHCO_3$ infusion. After urine output established, add potassium 40 mEq/L.

Continued

TABLE 5. **Initial Doses of Antidotes for Common Poisonings—cont'd**

Antidote	Use	Dose	Route	Adverse Reactions/Comments
		is volume depleted: 1 h to acheive urine output of 2 mL/kg/h and urine pH 7–8. In mild cases without acidosis and urine pH >6 administer 5% dextrose in 0.9% saline with 50 mEq/L or 1 mEq/kg $NaHCO_3$ as maintanence to replace on going renal loses. If **acidemia** is present and pH <7.2, add 2 mEq/kg as loading dose followed by 2 mEq/kg q3 to 4h to keep pH at 7.5–7.55. If acidemia is present, recommend isotonic $NaHCO_3$, 3 Ampules to 1 liter of D_5W @10–15 mL/kg/h or sufficient to produce normal urine flow and a urine pH of 7.5 or higher.		
	Long-acting barbiturates: Phenobarbital and primidone (Mysoline) Note: Alkalinization is not effective for the short or intermediate-acting barbiturates	$NaHCO_3$: 2 mEq/kg during the first hour or 100 mEq in 1 L of D_5W with 40 mEq/L potassium at rate of 100 mL/hr in adults. Adequate potassium is necessary to accomplish alkalinization	IV	Additional sodium bicarbonate and potassium chloride may be needed. Adjust the urine pH to 7.5–8 by $NaHCO_3$ infusion
Thiamine 100 mg/mL, 2 vials	Thiamine deficiency, ethylene glycol poisoning, alcoholism	100 mg IV followed with 100 mg IW/IM for 5–7 days in an alcoholic and followed by 100 mg a day orally.	IV/IM	
Vitamin K_1 (AquaMephyton) 10 mg/1–5 mL; 5 mg tablets	Warfarin anticoagulant or rodenticide toxicity	Oral 0.4 mg/kg/dose child, 10–25 mg adults. If evidence of bleeding, administer vitamin K_1 SC, IV 0.6 mg/kg/dose child and up to 25–50 mg adults for 6 hours depending on severity	PO/SC, IV	Give vitamin K daily until PT/INR are normal. Examine stools and urine for evidence of bleeding.

ALT = alanine aminotransferase; amp = ampule; AST = aspartate aminotransferase; BAL = British antilewisite; BP = blood pressure; Conc. = concentration; ECG = electrocardiogram; ET = endotracheal; G6PD = glucose-6-phosphate dehydrogenase; IM = intramuscular; IV = intravenous; PCC = poison control center; PO = oral; PT = Prothrombin time; SC = subcutaneous.

outflow arterial catheter through a filter-adsorbing cartridge (charcoal or resin) and returned through a venous catheter. Cartridges must be changed every 4 hours. The blood glucose, electrolytes, calcium, and albumin levels; complete blood cell count; platelets; and serum and urine osmolarity must be carefully monitored. This procedure has extended extracorporeal removal to a large range of substances that were formerly either poorly dialyzable or nondialyzable. It is not limited by molecular weight, water solubility, or protein binding, but it is limited by a volume distribution greater than 400 L, plasma concentration, and rate of flow through the filter. Activated charcoal cartridges are the primary type of hemoperfusion that is currently available in the United States.

The patient-related criteria for hemoperfusion are (1) anticipated prolonged coma and the likelihood of complications, (2) laboratory confirmation of lethal blood concentrations, (3) hepatic impairment when an agent is metabolized by the liver, and (4) clinical deterioration despite optimally supportive medical management.

The contraindications are similar to those for hemodialysis.

Limited data are available as to which toxins are best treated with hemoperfusion. Hemoperfusion has proved useful in treating glutethimide intoxication, phenobarbital overdose, and carbamazepine, phenytoin, and theophylline intoxication.

Complications include hemorrhage, thrombocytopenia, hypotension, infection, leukopenia, depressed phagocytic activity of granulocytes, decreased immunoglobulin levels, hypoglycemia, hypothermia, hypocalcemia, pulmonary edema, and air and charcoal embolism.

TABLE 6. **Plasma Concentrations Above Which Removal by Extracorporeal Measures Should Be Considered**

Drug	**Plasma Concentration**	**Protein Binding (%)**	**Volume Distribution (L/kg)**	**Method of Choice**
Amanitin	NA	25	1.0	**HP**
Ethanol	500–700 mg/dL	0	0.3	HD
Ethchlorvynol	150 μg/mL	35–50	3–4	**HP**
Ethylene glycol	25–50 μg/mL	0	0.6	HD
Glutethimide	100 μg/mL	50	2.7	**HP**
Isopropyl alcohol	400 mg/dL	0	0.7	HD
Lithium	4 mEq/L	0	0.7	HD
Meprobamate (Equanil)	100 μg/mL	0	NA	**HP**
Methanol	50 mg/dL	0	0.7	HD
Methaqualone	40 μg/dL	20–60	6.0	**HP**
Other barbiturates	50 μg/dL	50	0–1	**HP**
Paraquat	0.1 mg/dL	poor	2.8	**HP** > HD
Phenobarbital	100 μg/dL	50	0.9	**HP** > HD
Salicylates	80–100 mg/dL	90	0.2	HD > **HP**
Theophylline		0	0.5	
Chronic	40–60 μg/mL			**HP**
Acute	80–100 μg/mL			**HP**
Trichlorethanol	250 μg/mL	70	0.6	**HP**

HD = hemodialysis; **HP** = hemoperfusion; **HP** > HD hemoperfusion preferred over hemodialysis

Note: Cartridges for charcoal hemoperfusion are not readily available anymore in most locations, so hemodialysis may be substituted in these situations. In mixed or chronic drug overdoses, extracorporeal measures may be considered at lower drug concentrations.

Data from Winchester JF: Active methods for detoxification. In Haddad LM; Winchester JF (eds). Clinical Management of Poisoning and Drug Overdose; 2nd ed. Philadelphia, W B. Saunders, 1990; Balsam L, Cortitsidis GN, Fienfeld DA: Role of hemodialysis and hemoperfusion in the treatment of intoxications. Contem Manag Crit Care 1:61, 1991.

Hemofiltration

Continuous arteriovenous or venovenous hemodiafiltration (CAVHD or CVVHD, respectively) has been suggested as an alternative to conventional hemodialysis when the need for rapid removal of the drug is less urgent. These procedures, like peritoneal dialysis, are minimally invasive, have no significant impact on hemodynamics, and can be carried out continuously for many hours. Their role in the management of acute poisoning remains uncertain, however.

Plasmapheresis

Plasmapheresis consists of removal of a volume of blood. All the extracted components are returned to the blood except the plasma, which is replaced with a colloid protein solution. There are limited clinical data on guidelines and efficacy in toxicology. Centrifugal and membrane separators of cellular elements are used. It can be as effective as hemodialysis or hemoperfusion for removing toxins that have high protein binding, and it may be useful for toxins not filtered by hemodialysis and hemoperfusion.

Plasmapheresis has been anecdotally used in treating intoxications with the following agents: paraquat (removed 10%), propranolol (removed 30%), quinine (removed 10%), L-thyroxine (removed 30%), and salicylate (removed 10%). It has been shown to remove less than 10% of digoxin, phenobarbital, prednisolone, and tobramycin. Complications include infection, allergic reactions including anaphylaxis, hemorrhagic disorders, thrombocytopenia, embolus and thrombus, hypervolemia and hypovolemia, dysrhythmias, syncope, tetany, paresthesia, pneumothorax, adult respiratory distress syndrome, and seizures.

SUPPORTIVE CARE, OBSERVATION, AND THERAPY FOR COMPLICATIONS

Altered Mental Status

If airway protective reflexes are absent, endotracheal intubation is indicated for a comatose patient or a patient with altered mental status. If respirations are ineffective, ventilation should be instituted, and if hypoxemia persists, supplemental oxygen is indicated. If a cyanotic patient fails to respond to oxygen, the practitioner should consider methemoglobinemia.

Hypoglycemia

Hypoglycemia accompanies many poisonings, including with ethanol (especially in children), clonidine (Catapres), insulin, organophosphates, salicylates, sulfonylureas, and the unripe fruit or seed of a Jamaican plant called ackee. If hypoglycemia is present or suspected, glucose should be administered immediately as a intravenous bolus. Doses are as follows: in a neonate, 10% glucose (5 mL/kg); in a child, 25% glucose 0.25 g/kg (2 mL/kg); and in an adults, 50% glucose 0.5 g/kg (1 mL/kg).

A bedside capillary test for blood glucose is performed to detect hypoglycemia, and the sample is sent to the laboratory for confirmation. If the glucose reagent strip visually reads less than 150 mg/dL, one administers glucose. Venous blood should be used rather than capillary blood for the bedside test if the patient is in shock or is hypotensive. Large amounts of glucose given rapidly to nondiabetic patients may cause a transient reactive hypoglycemia and hyperkalemia and may accentuate damage in ischemic cerebrovascular and cardiac tissue. If focal neurologic signs are present, it may be prudent to withhold glucose, since hypoglycemia causes focal signs in less than 10% of cases.

Thiamine Deficiency Encephalopathy

Thiamine is administered to avoid precipitating thiamine deficiency encephalopathy (Wernicke-Korsakoff syndrome) in alcohol abusers and in malnourished patients. The overall incidence of thiamine deficiency in ethanol abusers is 12%. Thiamine 100 mg intravenously should be administered around the time of the glucose administration but not necessarily before the glucose. The clinician should be prepared to manage the anaphylaxis that sometimes is caused by thiamine, although it is extremely rare.

Opioid Reactions

Naloxone (Narcan) reverses CNS and respiratory depression, miosis, bradycardia, and decreased gastrointestinal peristalsis caused by opioids acting through μ, κ, and δ receptors. It also affects endogenous opioid peptides (endorphins and enkephalins), which accounts for the variable responses reported in patients with intoxications from ethanol, benzodiazepines, clonidine (Catapres), captopril (Capoten), and valproic acid (Depakote) and in patients with spinal cord injuries. There is a high sensitivity for predicting a response if pinpoint pupils and circumstantial evidence of opioid abuse (e.g., track marks) are present.

In cases of suspected overdose, naloxone 0.1 mg/kg is administered intravenously initially in a child younger than 5 years of age. The dose can be repeated in 2 minutes, if necessary up to a total dose of 2 mg. In older children and adults, the dose is 2 mg every 2 minutes for five doses up to a total of 10 mg. Naloxone can also be administered into an endotracheal tube if intravenous access is unavailable. If there is no response after 10 mg, a pure opioid intoxication is unlikely. If opioid abuse is suspected, restraints should be in place before the administration of naloxone, and it is recommended that the initial dose be 0.1 to 0.2 mg to avoid withdrawal and violent behavior. The initial dose is then doubled every minute progressively to a total of 10 mg. Naloxone may unmask concomitant sympathomimetic intoxication as well as withdrawal.

Larger doses of naloxone may be required for more poorly antagonized synthetic opioid drugs: buprenorphine (Buprenex), codeine, dextromethorphan, fentanyl and its derivates, pentazocine (Talwin), propoxyphene (Darvon), diphenoxylate, nalbuphine (Nubain), and long-acting opioids such as methadone (Dolophine).

Indications for a continuous infusion include a second dose for recurrent respiratory depression, exposure to poorly antagonized opioids, a large overdose, and decreased opioid metabolism, as with impaired liver function. A continuous infusion has been advocated because many opioids outlast the short half-life of naloxone (30 to 60 minutes). The hourly rate of naloxone infusion is equal to the effective dose required to produce a response (improvement in ventilation and arousal). An additional dose may be required in 15 to 30 minutes as a bolus. The infusions are titrated to avoid respiratory depression and opioid withdrawal manifestations. Tapering of infusions can be attempted after 12 hours and when the patient's condition has been stabilized.

Although naloxone is safe and effective, there are rare reports of complications (less than 1%) of pulmonary edema, seizures, hypertension, cardiac arrest, and sudden death.

Agents Whose Roles Are Not Clarified

Nalmefene (Revex), a long-acting parenteral opioid antagonist that the Food and Drug Administration has approved, is undergoing investigation, but its role in the treatment of comatose patients and patients with opioid overdose is not clear. It is 16 times more potent than naloxone, and its duration of action is up to 8 hours (half-life 10.8 hours, versus naloxone 1 hour).

Flumazenil (Romazicon) is a pure competitive benzodiazepine antagonist. It has been demonstrated to be safe and effective for reversing benzodiazepine-induced sedation. It is not recommended to improve ventilation. Its role in cases of CNS depression needs to be clarified. It should not be used routinely in comatose patients and is not an essential ingredient of the coma therapeutic regimen. It is contraindicated in cases of co-ingestion of cyclic antidepressant intoxication, stimulant overdose, and long-term benzodiazepine use (may precipitate life-threatening withdrawal) if benzodiazepines are used to control seizures. There is a concern about the potential for seizures and cardiac dysrhythmias that may occur in these settings.

LABORATORY AND RADIOGRAPHIC STUDIES

An electrocardiogram (ECG) should be obtained to identify dysrhythmias or conduction delays from cardiotoxic medications. If aspiration pneumonia (history of loss of consciousness, unarousable state, vomiting) or noncardiac pulmonary edema is suspected, a chest radiograph is needed. Electrolyte and glucose concentrations in the blood, the anion gap, acid-base balance, the arterial blood gas (ABG) profile (if patient has respiratory distress or altered mental status), and serum osmolality should be measured if a toxic alcohol ingestion is suspected. Table 7 lists appropriate testing on the basis of clinical toxicologic presentation. All laboratory specimens should be carefully labeled, including time and date. For potential legal cases, a "chain of custody" must be established. Assessment of the laboratory studies may provide a clue to the etiologic agent.

TABLE 7. **Patient Condition/Systemic Toxin and Appropriate Tests**

Condition	Tests
Comatose	Toxicologic tests (acetaminophen, sedative-hypnotic, ethanol, opioids, benzodiazepine), glucose.
Respiratory toxicity	Spirometry, FEV_1, arterial blood gases, chest radiograph, monitor O_2 saturation
Cardiac toxicity	ECG 12-lead and monitoring, echocardiogram, serial cardiac enzymes (if evidence or suspicion of a myocardial infarction), hemodynamic monitoring
Hepatic toxicity	Enzymes (AST, ALT, GGT), ammonia, albumin, bilirubin, glucose, PT, PTT, amylase
Nephrotoxicity	BUN, creatinine, electrolytes (Na, F, Mg, Ca, PO_4), serum and urine osmolarity, 24-hour urine for heavy metals if suspected, creatine kinase, serum and urine myoglobin, urinalysis and urinary sodium
Bleeding	Platelets, PT, PTT, bleeding time, fibrin split products, fibrinogen, type and match

ALT = alanine aminotransaminase; AST = aspartate aminotransaminase; BUN = blood urea nitrogen; GGT = γ-glutamyltransferase; PT = prothrombin time; PTT = partial thromboplastin time.

Electrolyte, Acid-Base, and Osmolality Disturbances

Electrolyte and acid-base disturbances should be evaluated and corrected. Metabolic acidosis (usually low or normal pH with a low or normal/high $Pa{CO_2}$ and low HCO_3) with an increased anion gap is seen with many agents in cases of overdose.

The anion gap is an estimate of those anions other than chloride and HCO_3 necessary to counterbalance the positive charge of sodium. It serves as clue to causes, compensations, and complications. The anion gap (AG) is calculated from the standard serum electrolytes by subtracting the total CO_2 (which reflects the actual measured bicarbonate) and chloride from the sodium: $(Na - [Cl + HCO_3]) = AG$. The potassium is usually not used in the calculation because it may be hemolyzed and is an intracellular cation. The lack of anion gap does not exclude a toxic etiology.

The normal gap is usually 7 to 11 mEq/L by flame photometer. However, there has been a "lowering" of the normal anion gap to 7 ± 4 mEq/L by the newer techniques (e.g., ion selective electrodes or colorimetric titration). Some studies have found anion gaps to be relatively insensitive for determining the presence of toxins.

It is important to recognize anion gap toxins, such as salicylates, methanol, and ethylene glycol, because they have specific antidotes, and hemodialysis is effective in management of cases of overdose with these agents.

Table 8 lists the reasons for increased anion gap, decreased anion gap, or no gap. The most common cause of a decreased anion gap is laboratory error. Lactic acidosis produces the largest anion gap and can result from any poisoning that results in hypoxia, hypoglycemia, or convulsions.

Other blood chemistry derangements that suggest certain intoxications are listed in Table 9.

Serum osmolality is a measure of the number of molecules of solute per kilogram of solvent, or mOsm/kg water. The osmolarity is molecules of solute per liter of solution, or mOsm/L water at a specified temperature. Osmolarity is usually the calculated value and osmolality is usually a measured value. They are considered interchangeable where 1 L equals 1 kg. The normal serum osmolality is 280 to 290 mOsm/kg. The freezing point serum osmolarity measurement specimen and the serum electrolytes specimens for calculation should be drawn simultaneously.

The serum osmolal gap is defined as the difference between the measured osmolality determined by the freezing point method and the calculated osmolarity. It is determined by the following formula:

$$(\text{Sodium} \times 2) + (\text{BUN}/3) + (\text{Glucose}/20),$$

(where BUN is blood urea nitrogen).

This gap estimate is normally within 10 mOsm of the simultaneously measured serum osmolality. Ethanol, if present, may be included in the equation to

TABLE 8. **Etiologies of Metabolic Acidosis**

Normal Anion Gap Hyperchloremic	Increased-Anion Gap Normochloremic	Decreased-Anion Gap
Acidifying agents	Methanol	Laboratory error†
Adrenal insufficiency	Uremia*	Intoxication—bromine, lithium
Anhydrase inhibitors	Diabetic ketoacidosis*	Protein abnormal
Fistula	Paraldehyde,* phenformin	Sodium low
Osteotomies	Isoniazid	
Obstructive uropathies	Iron	
Renal tubular acidosis	Lactic acidosis†	
Diarrhea, uncomplicated*	Ethanol,* ethylene glycol*	
Dilutional	Salicylates, starvation solvents	
Sulfamylon		

*Indicates hyperosmolar situation. Recent studies have found the anion gap may be relatively insensitive for determining the presence of toxins.

†Lactic acidosis can be produced by intoxications of the following: carbon monoxide, cyanide, hydrogen sulfide, hypoxia, ibuprofen, iron, isoniazid, phenformin, salicylates, seizures, theophylline.

Table 9. **Blood Chemistry Derangements in Toxicology**

Derangement	Toxin
Acetonemia without acidosis	Acetone or isopropyl alcohol
Hypomagnesemia	Ethanol, digitalis
Hypocalcemia	Ethylene glycol, oxalate, fluoride
Hyperkalemia	β-blockers, acute digitalis, renal failure
Hypokalemia	Diuretics, salicylism, sympathomimetics, theophylline, corticosteroids, chronic digitalis
Hyperglycemia	Diazoxide, glucagon, iron, isoniazid, organophosphate insecticides, phenylurea insecticides, phenytoin (Dilantin), salicylates, sympathomimetic agents, thyroid, vasopressors
Hypoglycemia	β-blockers, ethanol, insulin, isoniazid, oral hypoglycemic agents, salicylates
Rhabdomyolysis	Amphetamines, ethanol, cocaine, or phencyclidine, elevated creatine phosphokinase

eliminate its influence on the osmolal gap (the ethanol concentration divided by 4.6; Table 10).

The osmolal gap is not valid in cases of shock and postmortem state. Metabolic disorders such as hyperglycemia, uremia, and dehydration increase the osmolarity but usually do not cause gaps greater than 10 mOsm/kg. A gap greater than 10 mOsm/mL suggests that unidentified osmolal-acting substances are present: acetone, ethanol, ethylene glycol, glycerin, isopropyl alcohol, isoniazid, ethanol, mannitol, methanol, and trichloroethane. Alcohols and glycols should be sought when the degree of obtundation exceeds that expected from the blood ethanol concentration or when other clinical conditions exist: visual loss (methanol), metabolic acidosis (methanol and ethylene glycol), or renal failure (ethylene glycol).

A falsely elevated osmolal gap can be produced by other low molecular weight un-ionized substances (dextran, diuretics, sorbitol, ketones), hyperlipidemia, and unmeasured electrolytes (e.g., magnesium).

Note: A normal osmolal gap may be reported in the presence of toxic alcohol or glycol poisoning, if the parent compound is already metabolized. This situation can occur when the osmolal gap is measured after a significant time has elapsed since the ingestion. In cases of alcohol and glycol intoxication, an early osmolar gap is due to the relatively nontoxic parent drug and delayed metabolic acidosis, and an anion gap is due to the more toxic metabolites.

Table 10. **Conversion Factors for Alcohols and Glycols**

Alcohol/ Glycol	1 mg/dL in blood raises osmolality mOsm/L	Molecular Weight	Conversion Factor
Ethanol	0.228	40	4.6
Methanol	0.327	32	3.2
Ethylene glycol	0.190	62	6.2
Isopropanol	0.176	60	6.0
Acetone	0.182	58	5.8
Propylene glycol	not available	72	7.2

Example: Methanol osmolality. Subtract the calculated osmolality from the measured serum osmolarity (freezing point method) = osmolar gap × 3.2 (1/10th molecular weight) = estimated serum methanol concentration. Note: This equation is often not considered very reliable in predicting the actual measured blood concentration of these alcohols or glycols.

The serum concentration is calculated as mg/dL = mOsm gap × MW of substance divided by 10.

Radiographic Studies

Chest and neck radiographs are useful for suspected pathologic conditions such as aspiration pneumonia, pulmonary edema, and foreign bodies and to determine the location of the endotracheal tube. Abdominal radiographs can be used to detect radiopaque substances.

The mnemonic for radiopaque substances seen on abdominal radiographs is CHIPES:

C: chlorides and chloral hydrate
H: heavy metals (arsenic, barium, iron, lead, mercury, zinc)
I: iodides
P: PlayDoh, Pepto-Bismol, phenothiazine (inconsistent)
E: enteric-coated tablets
S: sodium, potassium, and other elements in tablet form (bismuth, calcium, potassium) and solvents containing chlorides (e.g., carbon tetrachloride)

Toxicologic Studies

Routine blood and urine screening is of little practical value in the initial care of the poisoned patient. Specific toxicologic analyses and quantitative levels of certain drugs may be extremely helpful. One should always ask oneself the following questions: (1) How will the result of the test alter the management? and (2) Can the result of the test be returned in time to have a positive effect on therapy?

Owing to long turnaround time, lack of availability, factors contributing to unreliability, and the risk of serious morbidity without supportive clinical management, toxicology screening is estimated to affect management in less than 15% of cases of drug overdoses or poisonings. Toxicology screening may look specifically for only 40 to 50 drugs out of more than 10,000 possible drugs or toxins and more than several million chemicals. To detect many different drugs, toxic screens usually include methods with broad specificity, and sensitivity may be poor for some drugs, resulting in false-negative or false-positive findings. On the other hand, some drugs present in therapeutic amounts may be detected on the screen, even though they are causing no clinical symptoms. Because many agents are not sought or detected during a toxicologic screening, a negative result does not always rule out poisonings. The specificity of toxicologic tests is dependent on the method and the laboratory. The presence of other drugs, drug metabolites, disease states, or incorrect sampling may cause erroneous results.

For the average toxicologic laboratory, false negative results occur at a rate of 10% to 30% and false-positives at a rate of 0% to 10%. The positive screen predictive value is about 90%. A negative toxicology screen does not exclude a poisoning. The negative predictive value of toxicologic screening is about 70%. For example, the following benzodiazepines may not be detected by some routine immunoassay benzodiazepine screening tests: alprazolam (Xanax), clonazepam (Klonopin), temazepam (Restoril), and triazolam (Halcion).

The "toxic urine screen" is generally a qualitative urine test for several common drugs, usually substances of abuse (cocaine and metabolites, opioids, amphetamines, benzodiazepines, barbiturates, and phencyclidine). Results of these tests are usually available within 2 to 6 hours. Since these tests may vary with each hospital and community, the physician should determine exactly which substances are included in the toxic urine screen of his or her laboratory. Tests for ethylene glycol, red blood cell cholinesterase, and serum cyanide are not readily available.

For cases of ingestion of certain substances, quantitative blood levels should be obtained at specific times after the ingestion to avoid spurious low values in the distribution phase, which result from incomplete absorption. The detection time for drugs is influenced by many variables, such as type of substance, formulation, amount, time since ingestion, duration of exposure, and half-life. For many drugs, the detection time is measured in days after the exposure.

COMMON POISONS

Acetaminophen (Paracetamol, *N*-acetyl-paraaminophenol)

Toxic Mechanism

At therapeutic doses of acetaminophen, less than 5% is metabolized by P450-2E1 to a toxic reactive oxidizing metabolite, *N*-acetyl-p-benzoquinoneimine (NAPQI). In a case of overdose, there is not sufficient glutathione available to reduce the excess NAPQI into nontoxic conjugate, and so it forms covalent bonds with hepatic intracellular proteins to produce centrilobular necrosis. Renal damage is caused by a similar mechanism.

Toxic Dose

The therapeutic dose of acetaminophen is 10 to 15 mg/kg, maximum five doses in 24 hours for a maximum total daily dose of 4 g. An acute single toxic dose is greater than 140 mg/kg, possibly greater than 200 mg/kg in a child younger than 5 years. Factors affecting the P450 enzymes include enzyme inducers such as barbiturates and phenytoin (Dilantin), ingestion of isoniazid, and alcoholism. Factors that decrease glutathione stores (alcoholism, malnutrition, and HIV infection) contribute to the toxicity of acetaminophen. Alcoholics ingesting 3 to 4 g/day of acetaminophen for a few days can have depleted glutathione stores and require *N*-acetylcysteine therapy at 50% below hepatotoxic blood acetaminophen levels on the nomogram.

Kinetics

Peak plasma concentration is usually reached 2 to 4 hours after an overdose. Volume distribution is 0.9 L/kg, and protein binding is less than 50% (albumin).

Route of elimination is by hepatic metabolism to an inactive nontoxic glucuronide conjugate and inactive nontoxic sulfate metabolite by two saturable pathways; less than 5% is metabolized into reactive metabolite NAPQI. In patients younger than 6 years of age, metabolic elimination occurs to a greater degree by conjugation via the sulfate pathway.

The half-life of acetaminophen is 1 to 3 hours.

Manifestations

The four phases of the intoxication's clinical course may overlap, and the absence of a phase does not exclude toxicity.

- Phase I occurs within 0.5 to 24 hours after ingestion and may consist of a few hours of malaise, diaphoresis, nausea, and vomiting or produce no symptoms. CNS depression or coma is not a feature.
- Phase II occurs 24 to 48 hours after ingestion and is a period of diminished symptoms. The liver enzymes, serum aspartate aminotransferase (AST) (earliest), and serum alanine aminotransferase (ALT) may increase as early as 4 hours or as late as 36 hours after ingestion.
- Phase III occurs at 48 to 96 hours with peak liver function abnormalities at 72 to 96 hours. The degree of elevation of the hepatic enzymes generally correlates with outcome, but not always. Recovery starts at about 4 days unless hepatic failure develops. Less than 1% of patients with a history of overdose develop fulminant hepatotoxicity.
- Phase IV occurs at 4 to 14 days, with hepatic enzyme abnormalities resolving. If extensive liver damage has occurred, sepsis and disseminated intravascular coagulation may ensue.

Transient renal failure may develop at 5 to 7 days with or without evidence of hepatic damage. Rare cases of myocarditis and pancreatitis have been reported. Death can occur at 7 to 14 days.

Laboratory Investigations

The therapeutic reference range is 10 to 20 μg/mL. For toxic levels, see the nomogram presented in Figure 1.

Appropriate and reliable methods for analysis are radioimmunoassay, high-pressure liquid chromatography, and gas chromatography. Spectroscopic assays often give falsely elevated values: bilirubin, salicylate, salicylamide, diflunisal (Dolobid), phenols, and methyldopa (Aldomet) increase the acetaminophen level. Each 1 mg/dL increase in creatinine increases the acetaminophen plasma level 30 μg/mL.

If a toxic acetaminophen level is reached, liver profile (including AST, ALT, bilirubin, and prothrombin time), serum amylase, and blood glucose must be monitored. A complete blood cell count (CBC); platelet

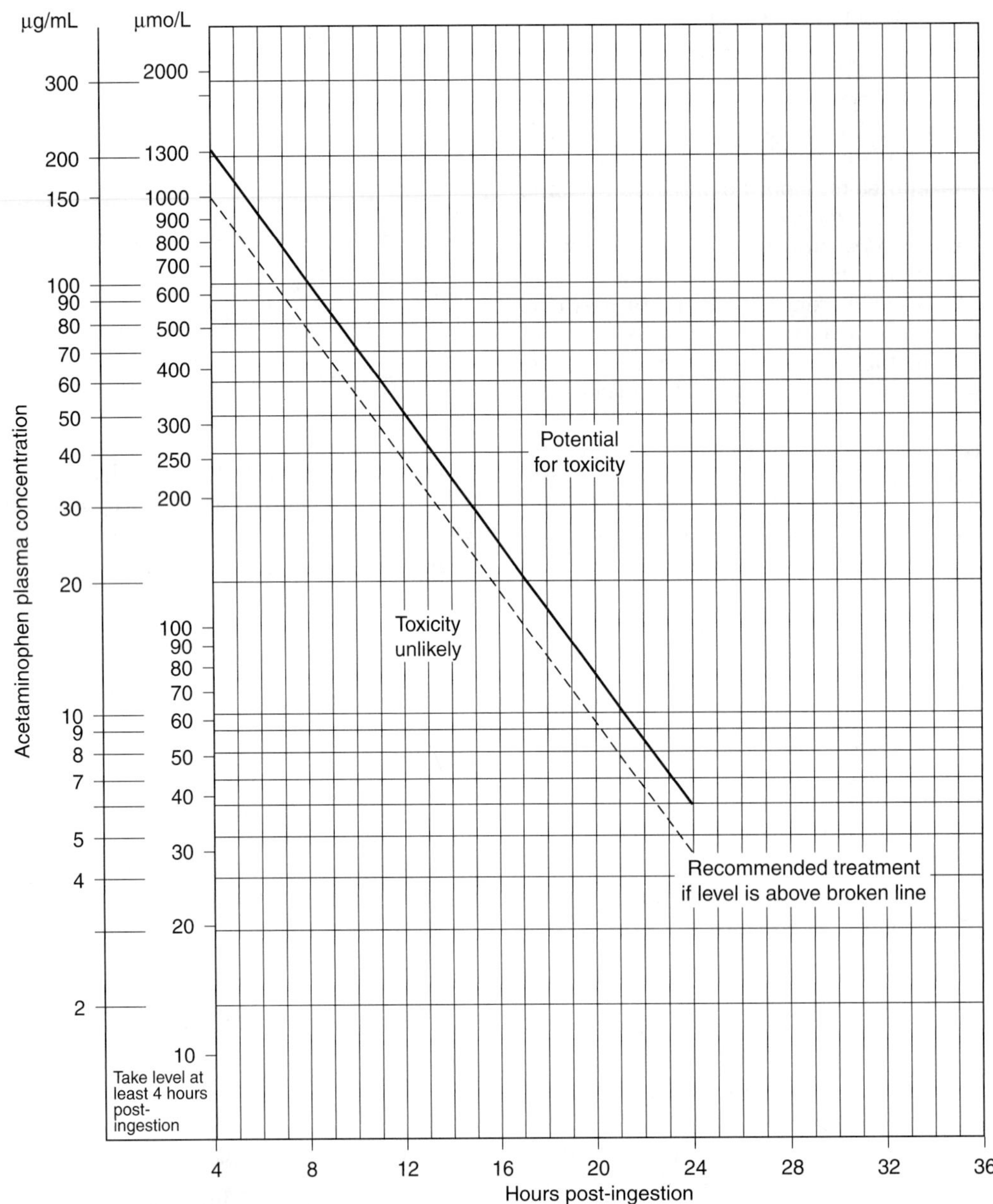

Figure 1. Nomogram for acetaminophen intoxication. *N*-acetylcysteine therapy is started if levels and time coordinates are above the lower line on the nomogram. Continue and complete therapy even if subsequent values fall below the toxic zone. The nomogram is useful only in cases of acute single ingestion. Levels in serum drawn before 4 hours may not represent peak levels. (From Rumack BH, Matthew H: Acetaminophen poisoning and toxicity. Pediatrics 55:871, 1975.)

count; phosphate, electrolytes, and bicarbonate level measurements; ECG; and urinalysis are indicated.

Management

Gastrointestinal Decontamination. Although ipecac-induced emesis may be useful within 30 minutes of ingestion of the toxic substance, we do not advise it because it could result in vomiting of the activated charcoal. Gastric lavage is not necessary. Studies have indicated that activated charcoal is useful within 1 hour after ingestion. Activated charcoal does adsorb *N*-acetylcysteine (NAC) if given together, but this is not clinically important. However, if activated charcoal needs to be given along with NAC separate the administration of activated charcoal from the administration of NAC by 1 to 2 hours to avoid vomiting.

***N*-acetylcysteine (Mucomyst)** (Table 11). NAC, a derivative of the amino acid cysteine, acts as a sulfhydryl donor for glutathione synthesis, as surrogate glutathione, and may increase the nontoxic sulfation pathway resulting in conjugation of NAPQI. Oral NAC should be administered within the first 8 hours after a toxic amount of acetaminophen has been ingested. NAC can be started while one awaits the results of the blood test for acetaminophen plasma concentration, but there is no advantage to giving it before 8 hours. If the acetaminophen concentration result after 4 hours following ingestion is above the upper line on the modified Rumack-Matthew nomogram

TABLE 11. **Protocol for *N*-Acetylcysteine Administration**

Route	Loading Dose	Maintenance Dose	Course	FDA Approval
Oral	140 mg/kg	70 mg/kg every 4 h	72 hr	Yes
Intravenous* (England, Canada)	150 mg/kg over 15 min	50 mg/kg over 4 h followed by 100 mg/kg over 16 h	20 hr	No
Intravenous* (Investigative in US)	140 mg/kg	70 mg/kg every 4 h	48 hr	No

*Not FDA approved for this indication.

(see Figure 1), one should continue with a maintenance course. Repeat blood specimens should be obtained 4 hours after the initial level is measured if it is greater than 20 mg/mL, which is below the therapy line, because of unexpected delays in the peak by food and co-ingestants. Intravenous NAC (see Table 11) has been used in Europe and Canada for about 30 years but is not approved in the United States. There have been a few cases of anaphylactoid reaction and death by the intravenous route.

Variations in Therapy

In patients with chronic alcoholism, it is recommended that NAC treatment be administered at 50% below the upper toxic line on the nomogram.

If emesis occurs within 1 hour after NAC administration, the dose should be repeated. To avoid emesis, the proper dilution from 20% to 5% NAC must be used, and it should be served in a palatable vehicle, in a covered container through a straw. If this administration is unsuccessful, a slow drip over 30 to 60 minutes through a nasogastric tube or a fluoroscopically placed nasoduodenal tube can be used. Antiemetics can be used if necessary: metoclopramide (Reglan) 10 mg per dose intravenously one half-hour before administration of NAC (in children, 0.1 mg/kg; maximum, 0.5 mg/kg/day) or ondansetron (Zofran) 32 mg (0.15 mg/kg) by infusion over 15 minutes and repeated for three doses if necessary. The side effects of these antiemetics include anaphylaxis and increases in liver enzymes.

Some investigators recommend variable durations of NAC therapy, stopping the therapy if serial acetaminophen blood concentrations become nondetectable and the liver enzyme levels (ALT and AST) remain normal after 24 to 36 hours.

There is a loss of efficacy if NAC is initiated 8 or 10 hours postingestion, but the loss is not complete, and NAC may be initiated 36 hours or more after ingestion. Late treatment (after 24 hours) has been shown to decrease the rates of morbidity and mortality in patients with fulminant liver failure due to acetaminophen and other agents.

Extended Relief formulations ("ER" embossed on caplet) contain 325 mg of acetaminophen for immediate release and 325 mg for delayed release. A single 4-hour postingestion serum acetaminophen concentration can underestimate the level because ER formulations can have secondary delayed peaks. In cases of overdose of the ER formulation, it is recommended that additional acetaminophen levels be obtained at 4-hour intervals after the initial level is measured. If any level is in the toxic zone, therapy should be initiated.

It is recommended that pregnant patients with toxic plasma concentrations of acetaminophen be treated with NAC to prevent hepatotoxicity in both fetus and mother. The available data suggest no teratogenicity to NAC or acetaminophen.

Indications for NAC therapy in cases of chronic intoxication are a history of ingestion of 3 to 4 g for several days with elevated liver enzyme levels (AST and ALT). The acetaminophen blood concentration is often low in these cases because of the extended time lapse since ingestion and should not be plotted on the Rumack-Matthew nomogram. Patients with a history of chronic alcoholism or those on chronic enzyme inducers may also present with elevated liver enzyme levels and should be considered for NAC therapy if they have a history of taking acetaminophen on a chronic basis, since they are considered to be at a greater risk for hepatotoxicity despite a low acetaminophen blood concentration.

Specific support care may be needed to treat liver failure, pancreatitis, transient renal failure, and myocarditis.

Liver transplantation has a definite but limited role in patients with acute acetaminophen overdose. A retrospective analysis determined that a continuing rise in the prothrombin time (4-day peak, 180 seconds), a pH of less than 7.3 2 days after the overdose, a serum creatinine level of greater than 3.3 mg/dL, severe hepatic encephalopathy, and disturbed coagulation factor VII/V ratio greater than 30 suggest a poor prognosis and may be indicators for hepatology consultation for consideration of liver transplantation.

Extracorporeal measures are not expected to be of benefit.

Disposition

Adults who have ingested more than 140 mg/kg and children younger than 6 years of age who have ingested more than 200 mg/kg should receive therapy within 8 hours postingestion or until the results of the 4-hour postingestion acetaminophen plasma concentration is known.

Amphetamines

The amphetamines include illicit methamphetamine ("Ice"), diet pills, and formulations under various trade names. Analogues include MDMA (3,4 methylenedioxymethamphetamine, known as "ectasy," "XTC," "Adam") and MDA (3,4-methylenedioxy-amphetamine, known as "Eve"). MDA is a common hallucinogen and euphoriant "club drug" used at "raves," which are all-night dances. Use of methamphetamine and designer analogues is on the rise, especially among young people, between the ages of 12 and 25 years. Other similar stimulants are phenylpropanolamine and cocaine.

Toxic Mechanism

Amphetamines have a direct CNS stimulant effect and a sympathetic nervous system effect by releasing catecholamines from alpha (α) and beta (β) adrenergic nerve terminals but inhibiting their reuptake.

Hallucinogenic MDMA has an additional hazard of serotonin effect (refer to serotonin syndrome in the SSRI section). MDMA also affects the dopamine system in the brain. Because of its effects on 5-hydroxytryptamine, dopamine, and norepinephrine, MDMA can lead to serotonin syndrome associated with malignant hyperthermia and rhabdomyolysis, which contributes to the potentially life-threatening hyperthermia observed in several patients who have used MDMA.

Phenylpropanolamine stimulates only the β-adrenergic receptors.

Toxic Dose

In children, the toxic dose of dextroamphetamine is 1 mg/kg; In adults, the toxic dose is 5 mg/kg. The potentially fatal dose of dextroamphetamine is 12 mg/kg.

Kinetics

Amphetamine is a weak base with pKa of 8 to 10. Onset of action is 30 to 60 minutes, and peak effects are 2 to 4 hours. The volume distribution is 2 to 3 L/kg.

Through hepatic metabolism, 60% of the substance is metabolized into a hydroxylated metabolite that may be responsible for psychotic effects.

The half-life of amphetamines is pH dependent—8 to 10 hours in acid urine (pH <6.0) and 16 to 31 hours in alkaline urine (pH >7.5). Excretion is by the kidney—30% to 40% at alkaline urine pH and 50% to 70% at acid urine pH.

Manifestations

Effects are seen within 30 to 60 minutes following ingestion.

Neurologic manifestations include restlessness, irritation and agitation, tremors and hyperreflexia, and auditory and visual hallucinations. Hyperpyrexia may precede seizures, convulsions, paranoia, violence, intracranial hemorrhage, psychosis, and self-destructive behavior. Paranoid psychosis and cerebral vasculitis occur with chronic abuse.

MDMA is often adulterated with cocaine, heroin, or ketamine, or a combination of these, to create a variety of mood alterations. This possibility must be taken into consideration when one manages patients with MDMA ingestions, as the symptom complex may reflect both CNS stimulation and CNS depression.

Other manifestations include dilated but reactive pupils, cardiac dysrhythmias (supraventricular and ventricular), tachycardia, and hypertension, rhabdomyolysis, and myoglobinuria.

Laboratory Investigations

The clinician should monitor ECG and cardiac readings, ABG and oxygen saturation, electrolytes, blood glucose, BUN, creatinine, creatine kinase, cardiac fraction if there is chest pain, and liver profile. Also, one should evaluate for rhabdomyolysis and check urine for myoglobin, cocaine and metabolites, and other substances of abuse. The peak plasma concentration of amphetamines is 10 to 50 ng/mL 1 to 2 hours after ingestion of 10 to 25 mg. The toxic plasma concentration is 200 ng/mL. When the rapid immunoassays are used, cross-reactions can occur with amphetamine derivatives (e.g., MDA, "ecstasy"), brompheniramine (Dimetane), chlorpromazine (Thorazine), ephedrine, phenylpropanolamine, phentermine (Adipex-P), phenmetrazine, ranitidine (Zantac), and Vicks Inhaler (L-desoxyephedrine). False-positive results may occur.

Management

Management is similar to management for cocaine intoxication. Supportive care includes blood pressure and temperature control, cardiac monitoring, and seizure precautions. Diazepam (Valium) can be administered. Gastrointestinal decontamination can be undertaken with activated charcoal administered up to 1 hour after ingestion.

Anxiety, agitation, and convulsions are treated with diazepam. If diazepam fails to control seizures, neuromuscular blockers can be used and the electroencephalogram (EEG) monitored for nonmotor seizures. One should avoid neuroleptic phenothiazines and butyrophenone, which can lower the seizure threshold.

Hypertension and tachycardia are usually transient and can be managed by titration of diazepam. Nitroprusside can be used for hypertensive crisis at a maximum infusion rate of 10 μg/kg/minute for 10 minutes followed with a lower infusion rate of 0.3 to 2 mg/kg/minute. Myocardial ischemia is managed by oxygen, vascular access, benzodiazepines, and nitroglycerin. Aspirin and thrombolytics are not routinely recommended because of the danger of intracranial hemorrhage. It is important to distinguish between angina and true ischemia. Delayed hypotension can be treated with fluids and vasopressors if needed. Life-threatening tachydysrhythmias may respond to an α-blocker such as phentolamine (Regitine) 5 mg IV for adults or 0.1 mg/kg IV for children and a short-acting β-blocker such as esmolol (Brevibloc) 500 μg/kg IV over 1 minute for adults or 300 to 500 μg/kg over 1 minute for children. Ventricular dysrhythmias may respond to lidocaine or, in a severely hemodynamically compromised patient, immediate synchronized electrical cardioversion.

Rhabdomyolysis and myoglobinuria are treated with fluids, alkaline diuresis, and diuretics. Hyperthermia is treated with external cooling and cool 100% humidified oxygen. More extensive therapy may be needed in severe cases. If focal neurologic symptoms are present, the possibility of a cerebrovascular accident should be considered and a CT scan of the head should be obtained.

Paranoid ideation and threatening behavior should be treated with rapid tranquilization using a benzodiazepine. One should observe for suicidal depression that may follow intoxication and may require suicide precautions.

Extracorporeal measures are of no benefit.

Disposition

Symptomatic patients should be observed on a monitored unit until the symptoms resolve and then observed for a short time after resolution for relapse.

Anticholinergic Agents

Drugs with anticholinergic properties include antihistamines (H_1 blockers), neuroleptics (phenothiazines), tricyclic antidepressants, antiparkinsonism drugs (trihexyphenidyl [Artane], benztropine [Cogentin]), ophthalmic products (atropine), and a number of common plants.

The antihistamines are divided into the sedating anticholinergic types, and the nonsedating single daily dose types. The sedating types include ethanolamines (e.g., diphenhydramine [Benadryl], dimenhydrinate [Dramamine], and clemastine [Tavist]), ethylenediamines (e.g., tripelennamine [Pyribenzamine]), alkylamines (e.g., chlorpheniramine [Chlor-Trimeton], brompheniramine [Dimetane]), piperazines (e.g., cyclizine [Marezine], hydroxyzine [Atarax], and meclizine [Antivert]), and phenothiazine (e.g., Phenergan). The nonsedating types include astemizole (Hismanal), terfenadine (Seldane), loratadine (Claritin), fexofenadine (Allegra), and cetirizine (Zyrtec).

The anticholinergic plants include jimsonweed (*Datura stramonium*), deadly nightshade (*Atropa belladonna*), henbane (*Hyoscyamus niger*), and antispasmodic agents for the bowel (atropine derivatives).

Toxic Mechanism

By competitive inhibition, anticholinergics block the action of acetylcholine on postsynaptic cholinergic receptor sites. The toxic mechanism primarily involves the peripheral and CNS muscarinic receptors. H_1 sedating-type agents also depress or stimulate the CNS, and in large overdoses some have cardiac membrane–depressant effects (e.g., diphenhydramine [Benadryl]) and α-adrenergic receptor blockade effects (e.g., promethazine [Phenergan]). Nonsedating agents produce peripheral H_1 blockade but do not possess anticholinergic or sedating actions. The original agents terfenadine (Seldane) and astemizole (Hismanal) were recently removed from the market because of the severe cardiac dysrhythmias associated with their use, especially when used in combination with macrolide antibiotics and certain antifungal agents such as ketoconazole (Nizoral), which inhibit hepatic metabolism or excretion. The newer nonsedating agents, including loratadine (Claritin), fexofenadine (Allegra), and cetirizine (Zyrtec), have not been reported to cause the severe drug interactions associated with terfenadine and astemizole.

Toxic Dose

The estimated toxic oral dose of atropine is 0.05 mg/kg in children and more than 2 mg in adults. The minimal estimated lethal dose of atropine is more than 10 mg in adults and more than 2 mg in children. Other synthetic anticholinergic agents are less toxic, and the fatal dose varies from 10 to 100 mg.

The estimated toxic oral dose of diphenhydramine (Benadryl) in a child is 15 mg/kg, and the potential lethal amount is 25 mg/kg. In an adult, the potential lethal amount is 2.8 g. Ingestion of five times the single dose of an antihistamine is toxic.

For the nonsedating agents, an overdose of 3360 mg of terfenadine was reported in an adult who developed ventricular tachycardia and fibrillation that responded to lidocaine and defibrillation. A 1500 mg overdose produced hypotension. Cases of delayed serious dysrhythmias (torsades de pointes) have been reported with doses of more than 200 mg of astemizole. The toxic doses of fexofenadine (Allegra), cetirizine, and loratadine (Claritin) need to be established.

Kinetics

The onset of absorption of intravenous atropine is in 2 to 4 minutes. Peak effects on salivation after intravenous or intramuscular administration is at 30 to 60 minutes.

Onset of absorption after oral ingestion is 30 to 60 minutes, peak action is 1 to 3 hours, and duration of action is 4 to 6 hours, but symptoms are prolonged in cases of overdose or with sustained-release preparations.

The onset of absorption of diphenhydramine is in 15 minutes to 1 hour, with a peak of action in 1 to 4 hours. Volume distribution is 3.3 to 6.8 L/kg, and protein binding is 75% to 80%. Ninety-eight percent of diphenhydramine is metabolized via the liver by *N*-demethylation. Interactions with erythromycin, ketoconazole (Nizoral), and derivatives produce excessive blood levels of the antihistamine and ventricular dysrhythmias.

The half-life of diphenhydramine is 3 to 10 hours.

The chemical structure of nonsedating agents prevents their entry into the CNS. Absorption begins in 1 hour, with peak effects in 4 in 6 hours. The duration of action is greater than 24 hours.

These agents are metabolized in the gastrointestinal tract and liver. Protein binding is greater than 90%. The plasma half-life 3.5 hours. Only 1% is excreted unchanged; 60% of that is excreted in the feces and 40% in the urine.

Manifestations

Anticholinergic signs are hyperpyrexia ("hot as a hare"), mydriasis ("blind as a bat"), flushing of skin ("red as a beet"), dry mucosa and skin ("dry as a bone"), "Lilliputian type" hallucinations and delirium ("mad as a hatter"), coma, dysphagia, tachycardia, moderate hypertension, and rarely convulsions and urinary retention. Other effects include jaundice (cyproheptadine [Periactin]), dystonia (diphenhydramine [Benadryl]), rhabdomyolysis (doxylamine), and, in large doses, cardiotoxic effects (diphenhydramine).

Overdose with nonsedating agents produces headache and confusion, nausea, and dysrhythmias (e.g., torsades de pointes).

Laboratory Investigations

Monitoring of ABG (in cases of respiratory depression), electrolytes, glucose, and the ECG should be undertaken. Anticholinergic drugs and plants are not routinely included on screens for substances of abuse.

Management

For patients in respiratory failure, intubation and assisted ventilation should be instituted. Gastrointestinal decontamination can be instituted. Caution must be taken with emesis in cases of diphenhydramine (Benadryl) overdose because of the drug's rapid onset of action and risk of seizures. If bowel sounds are present for up to 1 hour after ingestion, activated charcoal can be given. Seizures can be controlled with benzodiazepines (diazepam [Valium] or lorazepam [Ativan]).

The administration of physostigmine (Antilirium) is not routine and is reserved for life-threatening anticholinergic effects that are refractory to conventional treatments. It should be administered with adequate monitoring and resuscitative equipment available. The use of physostigmine should be avoided if a tricyclic antidepressant is present because of increased toxicity. Urinary retention should be relieved by catheterization to avoid reabsorption of the drug and additional toxicity.

Supraventricular tachycardia should be treated only if the patient is hemodynamically unstable. Ventricular dysrhythmias can be controlled with lidocaine or cardioversion. Sodium bicarbonate 1 to 2 mEq/kg IV may be useful for myocardial depression and QRS prolongation. Torsades de pointes, especially when associated with terfenadine and astemizole ingestion, has been treated with magnesium sulfate 4 g or 40 mL 10% solution intravenously over 10 to 20 minutes and countershock if the patient fails to respond.

Hyperpyrexia is controlled by external cooling. Hemodialysis and hemoperfusion are not effective.

Disposition

Antihistamine H_1 Antagonists. Symptomatic patients should be observed on a monitored unit until the symptoms resolve, then observed for a short time (3 to 4 hours) after resolution for relapse.

Nonsedating Agents. All asymptomatic children who acutely ingest more than the maximal adult dose and all symptomatic children should be referred to a health care facility for a minimum of 6 hours' observation as well as cardiac monitoring. Asymptomatic adults who acutely ingest more than twice the maximal adult daily dose should be monitored for a minimum of 6 hours. All symptomatic patients should be monitored for as long as there are symptoms present.

Barbiturates

Barbiturates have been used as sedatives, anesthetic agents, and anticonvulsants, but their use is declining as safer, more effective drugs become available.

Toxic Mechanism

Barbiturates are γ-amino butyric acid (GABA) agonists (increasing the chloride flow and inhibiting depolarization). They enhance the CNS depressant effect of GABA and depress the cardiovascular system.

Toxic Dose

The shorter acting barbiturates (including the intermediate acting agents) and their hypnotic doses are as follows: amobarbital (Amytal), 100 to 200 mg; aprobarbital (Alurate), 50 to 100 mg; butabarbital (Butisol), 50 to 100 mg; butalbital, 100 to 200 mg; pentobarbital (Nembutal), 100 to 200 mg; secobarbital (Seconal), 100 to 200 mg. They cause toxicity at lower doses than long-acting barbiturates and have a minimum toxic dose of 6 mg/kg; the fatal adult dose is 3 to 6 g.

The long-acting barbiturates and their doses include mephobarbital (Mebaral), 50 to 100 mg, and phenobarbital, 100 to 200 mg. Their minimum toxic dose is greater than 10 mg/kg, and the fatal adult dose is 6 to 10 g. A general rule is that an amount five times the hypnotic dose is toxic and an amount 10 times the hypnotic dose is potentially fatal. Methohexital and thiopental are ultrashort-acting parenteral preparations and are not discussed.

Kinetics

The barbiturates are enzyme inducers. Short-acting barbiturates are highly lipid-soluble, penetrate the brain readily, and have shorter elimination times. Onset of action is in 10 to 30 minutes, with a peak at 1 to 2 hours. Duration of action is 3 to 8 hours. The volume distribution of short-acting barbiturate is 0.8 to 1.5 L/kg; pKa is about 8. Mean half-life varies from 8 to 48 hours.

Long-acting agents have longer elimination times and can be used as anticonvulsants. Onset of action is in 20 to 60 minutes, with a peak at 1 to 6 hours. In cases of overdose, the peak can be at 10 hours. Usual duration of action is 8 to 12 hours. Volume distribution is 0.8 L/kg, and half-life is 11 to 120 hours. The pKa of phenobarbital is 7.2. Alkalinization of urine promotes its excretion.

Manifestations

Mild intoxication resembles alcohol intoxication and includes ataxia, slurred speech, and depressed cognition. Severe intoxication causes slow respirations, coma, and loss of reflexes (except pupillary light reflex).

Other manifestations include hypotension (vasodilation), hypothermia, hypoglycemia, and death by respiratory arrest.

Laboratory Investigations

Most barbiturates are detected on routine drug screens and can be measured in most hospital laboratories. Investigation should include barbiturate level; ABG; toxicology screen, including acetaminophen; glucose, electrolyte, BUN, creatinine, and creatine kinase levels; and urine pH. The minimum toxic plasma levels are greater than 10 μg/mL for short-acting barbiturates and greater than 40 μg/dL for long-acting agents. Fatal levels are 30 μg/mL for short-acting barbiturates and 80 to 150 μg/mL for long-acting agents. Both short-acting and long-acting agents can be detected in urine 24 to 72 hours after ingestion, and long-acting agents can be detected up to 7 days.

Management

Vital functions must be established and maintained. Intensive supportive care including intubation and assisted ventilation should dominate the management. All stuporous and comatose patients should have glucose (for hypoglycemia), thiamine (if chronically alcoholic), and naloxone (Narcan) (in case of an opioid ingestion) intravenously and should be admitted to the intensive care unit. Emesis should be avoided especially in cases of ingestion of the shorter-acting barbiturates. Activated charcoal followed by MDAC (0.5 g/kg) every 2 to 4 hours has been shown to reduce the serum half-life of phenobarbital by 50%, but its effect on clinical course is undetermined.

Fluids should be administered to correct dehydration and hypotension. Vasopressors may be necessary to correct severe hypotension, and hemodynamic monitoring may be needed. The patient must be observed carefully for fluid overload. Alkalinization (ion trapping) is used only for phenobarbital (pKa 7.2) but not for short-acting barbiturates. Sodium bicarbonate, 1 to 2 mEq/kg IV in 500 mL of 5% dextrose in adults or 10 to 15 mL/kg in children during the first hour, followed by sufficient bicarbonate to keep the urinary pH at 7.5 to 8.0, enhances excretion of phenobarbital and shortens the half-life by 50%. Diuresis is not advocated because of the danger of cerebral or pulmonary edema.

Hemodialysis shortens the half-life to 8 to 14 hours, and charcoal hemoperfusion shortens the half-life to 6 to 8 hours for long-acting barbiturates such as phenobarbital. Both procedures may be effective in patients with both long-acting and short-acting barbiturate ingestion. If the patient does not respond to supportive measures or if the phenobarbital plasma concentration is greater than 150 μg/mL, both procedures may be tried to shorten the half-life.

Bullae are treated as a local second-degree skin burn. Hypothermia should be treated.

Disposition

All comatose patients should be admitted to the intensive care unit. Awake and oriented patients with an overdose of short-acting agents should be observed for at least 6 asymptomatic hours; overdose of long-acting agents warrants observation for at least 12 asymptomatic hours because of the potential for delayed absorption. In the case of an intentional overdose, psychiatric clearance is needed before the patient can be discharged. Chronic use can lead to tolerance, physical dependency, and withdrawal and necessitates follow-up.

Benzodiazepines

Benzodiazepines are used as anxiolytics, sedatives, and relaxants.

Toxic Mechanism

The GABA agonists produce CNS depression and increase chloride flow, inhibiting depolarization.

Flunitrazepam (Rohypnol; street name "roofies") is a long-acting benzodiazepine agonist sold by prescription in more than 60 countries worldwide, but it is not legally available in the United States.

Toxic Dose

The long-acting benzodiazepines (half-life >24 hours) and their maximum therapeutic doses are as follows: chlordiazepoxide (Librium), 50 mg; chlorazepate (Tranxene), 30 mg; clonazepam (Klonopin), 20 mg; diazepam (Valium), 10 mg in adults or 0.2 mg/kg in children; flurazepam (Dalmane), 30 mg; and prazepam, 20 mg.

The short-acting benzodiazepines (half-life 10 to 24 hours) and their doses include the following: alprazolam (Xanax), 0.5 mg, and lorazepam (Ativan), 4 mg in adults or 0.05 mg/kg in children, which act similar to the long-acting benzodiazepines.

The ultrashort-acting benzodiazepines (half-life <10 hours) are more toxic and include temazepam (Restoril), 30 mg; triazolam (Halcion), 0.5 mg; midazolam (Versed), 0.2 mg/kg; and oxazepam (Serax), 30 mg.

In cases of overdose of short- and long-acting agents, 10 to 20 times the therapeutic dose (>1500 mg diazepam or 2000 mg chlordiazepoxide) have been ingested with resulting mild coma but without respiratory depression. Fatalities are rare, and most patients recover within 24 to 36 hours after overdose. Asymptomatic nonintentional overdoses of less than five times the therapeutic dose can be seen. Ultrashort-acting agents have produced respiratory arrest and coma within 1 hour after ingestion of 5 mg of triazolam (Halcion) and death with ingestion of as little as 10 mg. Midazolam (Versed) and diazepam (Valium) by rapid intravenous injection have produced respiratory arrest.

Kinetics

Onset of CNS depression is usually in 30 to 120 minutes; peak action usually occurs within 1 to 3 hours when ingestion is by the oral route. The volume distribution varies from 0.26 to 6 L/kg (LA, 1.1 L/kg); protein binding is 70% to 99%. For flunitrazepam, the onset of action is in 0.5 to 2 hours, oral peak is in 2 hours, and duration 8 hours or more. The half-life of flunitrazepam is 20 to 30 hours, volume distribution is 3.3 to 5.5 L/kg, and 80% is protein bound. Flunitrazepam can be identified in urine 4 to 30 days after ingestion.

Manifestations

Neurologic manifestations include ataxia, slurred speech, and CNS depression. Deep coma leading to respiratory depression suggests the presence of short-acting benzodiazepines or other CNS depressants. In elderly persons, the therapeutic doses can produce toxicity and can have an additive effect with other CNS depressants. Chronic use can lead to tolerance, physical dependency, and withdrawal.

Laboratory Investigations

Most benzodiazepines can be detected in urine drug screens. Quantitative blood levels are not useful. Some of the immunoassay urinary screens cannot detect all of the new benzodiazepines currently available. A consultation with the laboratory analyst is warranted if a specific case occurs in which the test result is negative but benzodiazepine use is suspected by the patient's history. Situations in which benzodiazepines may not be detected include ingestion of a low dose (e.g., <10 mg), rapid elimination, and a different or no metabolite. Some immunoassay methods can produce a false-positive finding for the benzodiazepines when nonsteroidal anti-inflammatory drugs (tolmetin [Tolectin], naproxen [Aleve], etodolac [Lodine], and fenoprofen [Nalfon]) are used. If this is a concern, the laboratory analyst should be consulted.

In cases in which "date rape" drugs such as flunitrazepam are suspected, a police crime or reference laboratory should be consulted for testing.

Management

Emesis and gastric lavage should be avoided. Activated charcoal can be useful only if given early before the peak time of absorption occurs. Supportive treatment should be instituted but rarely requires intubation or assisted ventilation.

Flumazenil (Romazicon) is a specific benzodiazepine receptor antagonist that blocks the chloride flow and inhibitor of GABA neurotransmitters. It reverses the sedative effects of benzodiazepines, zolpidem (Ambien), and endogenous benzodiazepines associated with hepatic encephalopathy. It is not recommended to reverse benzodiazepine-induced hypoventilation. The manufacturer advises that flumazenil be used with caution in cases of overdose with possible benzodiazepine dependency (because it can precipitate life-threatening withdrawal), if cyclic antidepressant use is suspected, or if a patient has a known seizure disorder.

Disposition

If the patient is comatose, he or she must be admitted to the intensive care unit. If the overdose was intentional, psychiatric clearance is needed before the patient can be discharged.

β-Adrenergic Blockers (β-Blocker)

β-Blockers are used in the treatment of hypertension and of a number of systemic and ophthalmologic disorders. Properties of β-blockers include the factors listed in Table 12.

Lipid-soluble drugs have CNS effects, active metabolites, longer duration of action, and interactions (e.g., propranolol). Cardioselectivity is lost in overdose. Intrinsic partial agonist agents (e.g., pindolol) may initially produce tachycardia and hypertension. Cardiac membrane depressive effect (quinidine-like) occurs in cases of overdose but not at therapeutic doses (e.g., with metoprolol or sotalol). α-Blocking effect is weak (e.g., with labetalol or acebutolol).

Toxic Mechanism

β-Blockers compete with the catecholamines for receptor sites and block receptor action in the bronchi, the vascular smooth muscle, and the myocardium.

Toxic Dose

Ingestions of greater than twice the maximum recommended daily therapeutic dose are considered toxic (see Table 12). Ingestion of 1 mg/kg propranolol in a child may produce hypoglycemia. Fatalities have been reported in adults with 7.5 g of metoprolol. The most toxic agent is sotalol, and the least toxic is atenolol.

Kinetics

Regular-release formulations usually cause symptoms within 2 hours. Propranolol's onset of action is 20 to 30 minutes and peak is at 1 to 4 hours, but it may be delayed by co-ingestants. The onset of action with sustained-release preparations may be delayed to 6 hours and the peak to 12 to 16 hours. Volume distribution is 1 to 5.6 L/kg. Protein binding is variable, from 5% to 93%.

Metabolism

Atenolol (Tenormin), nadolol (Corgard), and santalol (Betapace) have enterohepatic recirculation. The duration of action for regular-acting agents is 4 to 6 hours, but in cases of overdose it may be 24 to 48 hours. The duration of action for sustained-release agents is 24 to 48 hours.

The regular preparation with the longest half-life is nadolol, at 12 to 24 hours and the one with the shortest half-life is esmolol, at 5 to 10 minutes.

Manifestations

See Toxic Properties and Table 12.

Highly lipid-soluble agents produce coma and seizures. Bradycardia and hypotension are the major cardiac symptoms and may lead to cardiogenic shock. Intrinsic partial agonists initially may give tachycardia and hypertension. ECG changes include atrioventricular conduction delay or asystole. Membrane-depressant effects produce prolonged QRS and QT interval, which may result in torsades de pointes. Sotalol produces a very prolonged QT interval. Bronchospasm may occur in patients with reactive airway disease with any β-blocker because the selectivity is lost in overdose. Other manifestations include hypoglycemia (because β-blockers block catecholamine counter-regulatory mechanisms) and hyperkalemia.

Laboratory Investigations

Measurements of blood levels are not readily available or useful. ECG and cardiac monitoring should be maintained, and blood glucose and electrolytes, BUN,

TABLE 12. **Pharmacologic and Toxic Properties of β-Blockers**

Blocker	Maximum Solubility	Therapeutic Plasma Level	Lipid Solubility	Intrinsic Sympathomimetic Activity (Partial Agonist)	Membrane Stabilizing Effect β-Selective		Cardiac Selectivity
					β_1	β_2	α-Selective
Acebutolol (Sectral)	800 mg	200–2000 ng/mL	Moderate	+	+	+	+
Alprenolol*	800 mg	50–200 ng/mL	Moderate	2+	+	–	–
Atenolol (Tenormin)	100 mg	200–500 ng/mL	Low	–	–	2+	–
Betaxolol (Kerlone)	20 mg	NA	Low	+	–	+	–
Carteolol (Cartrol)	10 mg	NA	No	+	–	–	–
Esmolol (Brevibloc) (Class II antidysrhythmic, IV only)			Low	–	–	+	–
Labetalol (Trandate)	800 mg	50–500 ng/mL	Low	+	+/–	–	+
Levobunolol (AKBeta eyedrop) (Eye drops 0.25% and 0.5%)	20 mg	NA	No	–	–	–	–
Metoprolol (Lopressor)			Moderate	–	–	2+	–
Nadolol (Corgard)	320 mg	20–40 ng/mL	Low	–	–	–	–
Oxyprenolol*	480 mg	80–100 ng/mL	Moderate	2+	+	–	–
Pindolol (Visken)	60 mg	50–150 ng/mL	Moderate	3+	+/–	–	–
Propranolol (Inderal) (Class II antidysrhythmic)	360 mg	50–100 ng/mL	High	–	2+	–	–
Sotalol (Betapace) (Class II antidysrhythmic)	480 mg	500–4000 ng/mL	Low	–	–	–	–
Timolol (Blocadren)	60 mg	5–10 ng/mL	Low	–	+/–	–	–

*Not available in the United States.

and creatinine levels should be monitored, as well as ABG if there are respiratory symptoms.

Management

Vital functions must be established and maintained. Vascular access, baseline ECG, and continuous cardiac and blood pressure monitoring should be established. A pacemaker must be available. Gastrointestinal decontamination can be undertaken initially with activated charcoal up to 1 hour after ingestion. MDAC is no longer recommended, based on the latest guidelines. Whole-bowel irrigation can be considered in cases of large overdoses with sustained-release preparations, but there are no studies evaluating the efficacy of intervention.

If there are cardiovascular disturbances, a cardiac consultation should be obtained. Class IA antidysrhythmic agents (procainamide, quinidine) and III (bretylium) are not recommended. Hypotension is treated with fluids initially, although it usually does not respond. Frequently, glucagon and cardiac pacing are needed. Bradycardia in asymptomatic, hemodynamically stable patients requires no therapy. It is not predictive of the future course of the disease. If the patient is unstable (has hypotension or a high-degree atrioventricular block), atropine 0.02 mg/kg (up to 2 mg) in adults, glucagon, and a pacemaker can be used. In case of ventricular tachycardia, overdrive pacing can be used. A wide QRS interval may respond to sodium bicarbonate. Torsades de pointes (associated with sotalol) may respond to magnesium sulfate and overdrive pacing. Prophylactic magnesium for prolonged QT interval has been suggested, but there are no data. Epinephrine must not be used because an unopposed α effect may occur.

Hypotension and myocardial depression are managed by correction of dysrhythmias, Trendelenburg position, fluids, glucagon, or amrinone (Inocor), or a combination of these. Hemodynamic monitoring with a Swan-Ganz catheter or arterial line may be necessary to manage fluid therapy.

Glucagon is the initial drug of choice. It works through adenyl cyclase and bypasses catecholamine receptors; therefore, it is not affected by β-blockers. Glucagon increases cardiac contractility and heart rate. It is given as an intravenous bolus of 5 to 10 mg* over 1 minute and followed by a continuous infusion of 1 to 5 mg/h (in children, 0.15 mg/kg followed by 0.05 to 0.1 mg/kg/h). In large doses and in infusion therapy D5W, sterile water, or saline should be used as a dilutant to reconstitute glucagon in place of the 0.2% phenol diluent provided with some drugs. Effects are seen within minutes. It can be used with other agents such as amrinone.

Amrinone (Inocor) inhibits phosphodiesterase enzyme, which metabolizes cyclic AMP. It is administered as a bolus of 0.15 to 2 mg/kg (0.15 to 0.4 mL/kg) intravenously, followed by infusion of 5 to 10 μg/kg/min.

Hypoglycemia should be treated with intravenous glucose. Life-threatening hyperkalemia is treated with calcium (avoid if digoxin is present), bicarbonate, and glucose or insulin. Convulsions can be controlled with diazepam or phenobarbital. If bronchospasm is present, β_2 nebulized bronchodilators are given.

Extraordinary measures such as intra-aortic balloon pump support can be instituted. Extracorporeal measures can be undertaken. Hemodialysis for cases of atenolol, acebutolol, nadolol, and sotalol (low volume

*Exceeds dosage recommended by the manufacturer.

distribution, low protein binding) ingestion may be helpful, particularly when there is evidence of renal failure. Hemodialysis is not effective for propranolol, metoprolol and timolol.

Prenalterol† has successfully reversed both bradycardia and hypotension but is not currently available in the United States.

Disposition

Asymptomatic patients with history of overdose require baseline ECG and continuous cardiac monitoring for at least 6 hours with regular-release preparations and for 24 hours with sustained-release preparations. Symptomatic patients should be observed with cardiac monitoring for 24 hours. If seizures or abnormal rhythm or vital signs are present, the patient should be admitted to the intensive care unit.

Calcium Channel Blockers

Calcium channel blockers are used in the treatment of effort angina, supraventricular tachycardia, and hypertension.

Toxic Mechanism

Calcium channel blockers reduce influx of calcium through the slow channels in membranes of the myocardium, the atrioventricular nodes, and the vascular smooth muscles and result in peripheral, systemic, and coronary vasodilation, impaired cardiac conduction, and depression of cardiac contractility. All calcium channel blockers have vasodilatory action, but only bepridil, diltiazem, and verapamil depress myocardial contractility and cause atrioventricular block.

Toxic Dose

Any ingested amount greater than the maximum daily dose has the potential of severe toxicity. The maximum oral daily doses in adults and toxic doses in children of each are as follows: amlodipine (Norvasc), 10 mg for adults and more than 0.25 mg/kg for children; bepridil (Vascor), 400 mg for adults and more than 5.7 mg/kg for children; diltiazem (Cardizem), 360 mg for adults (toxic dose > 2 g) and more than 6 mg/kg for children; felodipine (Plendil), 40 mg for adults and more than 0.56 mg/kg for children; isradipine (DynaCirc), 40 mg for adults and more than 0.4 mg/kg for children; nicardipine (Cardene), 120 mg for adults and more than 0.85 mg/kg for children; nifedipine (Procardia), 120 mg for adults and more than 2 mg/kg for children; nimodipine (Nimotop), 360 mg for adults and more than 0.85 mg/kg for children; nitrendipine (Bayress),† 80 mg for adults and more than 1.14 mg/kg for children; and verapamil (Calan), 480 mg for adults and 15 mg/kg for children.

Kinetics

Onset of action of regular-release preparations varies: for verapamil it is 60 to 120 minutes, for nifedipine 20 minutes, and for diltiazem 15 minutes after ingestion. Peak effect for verapamil is 2 to 4 hours, for nifedipine 60 to 90 minutes, and for diltiazem 30 to 60 minutes, but the peak action may be delayed for 6 to 8 hours. Duration of action is up to 36 hours. The onset of action for sustained-release preparations is usually 4 hours but may be delayed, and peak effect is at 12 to 24 hours. In cases of massive overdose, concretions and prolonged toxicity can develop.

Volume distribution varies from 3 to 7 L/kg. Hepatic elimination half-life varies from 3 to 7 hours. Patients receiving digitalis and calcium channel blockers run the risk of digitalis toxicity, since calcium channel blockers increase digitalis levels.

Manifestations

Cardiac manifestations include hypotension, bradycardia, and conduction disturbances occurring 30 minutes to 5 hours after ingestion. A prolonged PR interval is an early finding and may occur at therapeutic doses. Torsades de pointes has been reported. All degrees of blocks may occur and may be delayed up to 16 hours. Lactic acidosis may be present. Calcium channel blockers do not affect intraventricular conduction, so the QRS interval is usually not affected.

Hypocalcemia is rarely present. Hyperglycemia may be present because of interference in calcium-dependent insulin release. Mental status changes, headaches, seizures, hemiparesis, and CNS depression may occur.

Laboratory Investigations

Specific drug levels are not readily available and are not useful. Monitor blood sugar, electrolytes, calcium, ABG, pulse oximetry, creatinine, and BUN, and also use hemodynamic monitoring, ECG and cardiac monitoring.

Management

Vital functions must be established and maintained. Baseline ECG readings should be obtained and continuous cardiac and blood pressure monitoring maintained. A pacemaker should be available. Cardiology consultation should be sought.

Gastrointestinal decontamination with activated charcoal is recommended. If a large dose of a sustained-release preparation was ingested, whole-bowel irrigation can be considered, but its effectiveness has not been investigated.

If the patient is symptomatic, *immediate* cardiology consult must be obtained, because a pacemaker and hemodynamic monitoring may be needed. In the case of heart block, atropine is rarely effective and isoproterenol (Isuprel) may produce vasodilation. The use of a pacemaker should be considered early.

Hypotension and bradycardia can be treated with positioning, fluids, and calcium gluconate or chloride, glucagon, amrinone (Inocor), and ventricular pacing. Calcium salts must be avoided if digoxin is present. Calcium usually reverses depressed myocardial contractility but may not reverse nodal depression or peripheral vasodilation. Calcium chloride can be given in a 10% solution, 0.1 to 0.2 mL/kg up to 10 mL in an

†Not available in the United States.

adult, or calcium gluconate in a 10% solution 0.3 to 0.4 mL/kg up to 20 mL in an adult. Administration is intravenous, over 5 to 10 minutes. One should monitor for dysrhythmias, hypotension, and the serum ionized calcium. The aim is to increase calcium 4 mg/dL to a maximum of 13 mg/dL. The calcium response lasts 15 minutes and may require repeated doses or a continuous calcium gluconate infusion 0.2 mL/kg/h up to maximum of 10 mL/h.

If calcium fails, glucagon can be tried for its positive inotropic and chronotropic effect, or both. Amrinone (Inocor), an inotropic agent, may reverse the effects of calcium channel blockers. An effective dose is 0.15 mg to 2 mg/kg (0.15 to 0.4 mL/kg) by intravenous bolus followed by infusion of 5 to 10 μg/kg/min.

In case of hypotension, fluids, norepinephrine (Levophed), and epinephrine may be required. Amrinone and glucagon have been tried alone and in combination. Dobutamine and dopamine are often ineffective.

Extracorporeal measures (e.g., hemodialysis and charcoal hemoperfusion) are not useful, but extraordinary measures such as intra-aortic balloon pump and cardiopulmonary bypass have been used successfully.

For cases of calcium channel blocker toxicity that fail to respond to aggressive management, recent studies demonstrate that insulin and glucose have therapeutic value. The suggested dose range for insulin is to infuse regular insulin at 0.5 IU/kg/h with a simultaneous infusion of glucose 1 g/kg/h, with glucose monitoring every 30 minutes for at least the first 4 hours of administration and subsequent glucose adjustment to maintain euglycemia (70 to 100 mg/dL). Potassium levels should be monitored regularly, as they may shift in response to the insulin.

Disposition

Patients who have ingested regular-release preparations should be monitored for at least 6 hours and those who have ingested sustained-release preparations should be monitored for 24 hours after the ingestion. Intentional overdose necessitates psychiatric clearance. Symptomatic patients should be admitted to the intensive care unit.

Carbon Monoxide

Carbon monoxide is an odorless, colorless gas produced from incomplete combustion; it is also an in vivo metabolic breakdown product of methylene chloride used in paint removers.

Toxic Mechanism

Carbon monoxide's affinity for hemoglobin is 240 times greater than that of oxygen. It shifts the oxygen dissociation curve to the left, which impairs hemoglobin release of oxygen to tissues and inhibits the cytochrome oxidase enzymes.

Toxic Dose and Manifestations

Table 13 describes the manifestations of carbon monoxide toxicity. Exposure to 0.5% for a few minutes is lethal. Sequelae correlate with the patient's level of consciousness at presentation. ECG abnormalities may be noted. Creatine kinase is often elevated, and rhabdomyolysis and myoglobinuria may occur.

The carboxyhemoglobin (COHb) expresses in percentage the extent to which carbon monoxide has bound with the total hemoglobin. This may be misleadingly low in the anemic patient with less hemoglobin than normal. The patient's presentation is a more reliable indicator of severity than the COHb level. The manifestations listed in Table 13 for each level are in addition to those listed at the level above. The COHb may not correlate reliably with the severity of the intoxication, and linking symptoms to specific levels of COHb frequently leads to inaccurate conclusions. A level of carbon monoxide greater than 40% is usually associated with obvious intoxication.

Kinetics

The natural metabolism of the body produces small amounts of COHb, less than 2% for nonsmokers and 5% to 9% for smokers.

Carbon monoxide is rapidly absorbed through the lungs. The rate of absorption is directly related to alveolar ventilation. Elimination also occurs through the lungs. The half-life of COHb in room air (21% oxygen) is 5 to 6 hours; in 100% oxygen, it is 90 minutes; in hyperbaric pressure at 3 atmospheres oxygen, it is 20 to 30 minutes.

Laboratory Investigations

An ABG reading may show metabolic acidosis and normal oxygen tension. In cases of significant poisoning, the ABG, electrolytes, blood glucose, serum creatine kinase and cardiac enzymes, renal function tests, and liver function tests should be monitored. A urinalysis and test for myoglobinuria should be obtained. Chest radiograph can be useful in cases of smoke inhalation or if the patient is being considered for hyperbaric chamber. ECG monitoring should be maintained, especially if the patient is older than

TABLE 13. **Carbon Monoxide Exposure and Possible Manifestations**

COHb Saturation (%)	Manifestations
3.5	None
5	Slight headache, decreased exercise tolerance
10	Slight headache, dyspnea on vigorous exertion, may impair driving skills
10–20	Moderate dyspnea on exertion, throbbing, temporal headache
20–30	Severe headache, syncope, dizziness, visual changes, weakness, nausea, vomiting, altered judgement
30–40	Vertigo, ataxia, blurred vision, confusion, loss of consciousness
40–50	Confusion, tachycardia, tachypnea, coma, convulsions
50–60	Cheyne-Stokes, coma, convulsions, shock, apnea
60–70	Coma, convulsions, respiratory and heart failure, death

40 years, has a history of cardiac disease, or has moderate to severe symptoms. Which toxicology studies are used is based on symptoms and circumstances. COHb should be monitored during and at the end of therapy. The pulse oximeter has two wavelengths and overestimates oxyhemoglobin saturation in carbon monoxide poisoning. The true oxygen saturation is determined by blood gas analysis, which measures the oxygen bound to hemoglobin. The co-oximeter measures four wavelengths and separates out COHb and the other hemoglobin binding agents from oxyhemoglobin. Fetal hemoglobin has a greater affinity for carbon monoxide than adult hemoglobin and may falsely elevate the COHb as much as 4% in young infants.

Management

The first step is to adequately protect the rescuer. The patient must be removed from the contaminated area, and his or her vital functions must be established.

The mainstay of treatment is 100% oxygen via a nonrebreathing mask with an oxygen reservoir or endotracheal tube. All patients receive 100% oxygen until the COHb level is 5% or less. Assisted ventilation may be necessary. ABG and COHb should be monitored and the present COHb level determined. Note: A near-normal COHb level does not exclude significant carbon monoxide poisoning, especially if the measurement is taken several hours after termination of exposure or if oxygen has been administered prior to obtaining the sample.

The exposed pregnant woman should be kept on 100% oxygen for several hours after the COHb level is almost 0, because carbon monoxide concentrates in the fetus and oxygen is needed longer to ensure elimination of the carbon monoxide from fetal circulation. The fetus must be monitored, because carbon monoxide and hypoxia are potentially teratogenic.

Metabolic acidosis should be treated with sodium bicarbonate only if the pH is below 7.2 after correction of hypoxia and adequate ventilation. Acidosis shifts the oxygen dissociation curve to the right and facilitates oxygen delivery to the tissues.

The decision to use the hyperbaric oxygen chamber must be made on the basis of the ability to handle other acute emergencies that may coexist in the patient and of the severity of the poisoning. The standard of care for persons exposed to carbon monoxide has yet to be determined, but most authorities recommend using the hyperbaric oxygen chamber under any of the following conditions:

- If the patient is in a coma or has a history of loss of consciousness or seizures
- If there is cardiovascular dysfunction (clinical ischemic chest pain or ECG evidence of ischemia)
- If the patient has metabolic acidosis
- If symptoms persist despite 100% oxygen therapy
- In a child, if the initial COHb is greater than 15%
- In symptomatic patients with preexisting ischemia
- If there are signs of maternal or fetal distress regardless of COHb level (infants and fetus are a special problem because fetal hemoglobin has greater affinity for carbon monoxide)

Although controversial, a neurologic-cognitive examination has been used to help determine which patients with low carbon monoxide levels should receive more aggressive therapy. Testing should include the following: general orientation memory testing, involving address, phone number, date of birth, and present date; and cognitive testing, involving counting by 7s, digit span, and forward and backward spelling of three-letter and four-letter words. Patients with delayed neurologic sequelae or recurrent symptoms up to 3 weeks may benefit from hyperbaric oxygen chamber treatment.

Seizures and cerebral edema must be treated.

Disposition

Patients with no or mild symptoms who become asymptomatic after a few hours of oxygen therapy and have a carbon monoxide level less than 10%, and normal physical and neurologic-cognitive examination findings can be discharged, but they should be instructed to return if any signs of neurologic dysfunction appear. Patients with carbon monoxide poisoning requiring treatment need follow-up neuropsychiatric examinations.

Caustics and Corrosives

The terms *caustic* and *corrosive* are used interchangeably and can be divided into acids and alkalis. The US Consumer Product Safety Commission Labeling Recommendations on containers for acids and alkalis indicate the potential for producing serious damage, as follows:

- Caution—weak irritant
- Warning—strong irritant
- Danger—corrosive

Some common acids with corrosive potential include acetic acid, formic acid, glycolic acid, hydrochloric acid, mercuric chloride, nitric acid, oxalic acid, phosphoric acid, sulfuric acid (battery acid), zinc chloride, and zinc sulfate. Some common alkalis with corrosive potential include ammonia, calcium carbide, calcium hydroxide (dry), calcium oxide, potassium hydroxide (lye), and sodium hydroxide (lye).

Toxic Mechanism

Acids produce mucosal coagulation necrosis and may be absorbed systemically; they do not penetrate deeply. Injury to the gastric mucosa is more likely, although specific sites of injury for acids and alkalis are not clearly defined.

Alkalis produce liquefaction necrosis and saponification and penetrate deeply. The esophageal mucosa is likely to be damaged. Oropharyngeal and esophageal damage is more frequently caused by solids than by liquids. Liquids produce superficial, circumferential burns and gastric damage.

Toxic Dose

The toxicity is determined by concentration, contact time, and pH. Significant injury is more likely with a substance that has a pH of less than 2 or greater than 12, with a prolonged contact time, and with large volumes.

Manifestations

The absence of oral burns does not exclude the possibility of esophageal or gastric damage. General clinical findings are stridor; dysphagia; drooling; oropharyngeal, retrosternal, and epigastric pain; and ocular and oral burns. Alkali burns are yellow, soapy, frothy lesions. Acid burns are gray-white and later form an eschar. Abdominal tenderness and guarding may be present if perforation has happened.

Laboratory Investigations

If acid ingestion has taken place, the patient's acid-base balance and electrolyte status should be determined. If pulmonary symptoms are present, a chest radiograph, ABG measurement, and pulse oximetry are called for.

Management

It is recommended that the container be brought to the examination, as the substance must be identified and the pH of the substance, vomitus, tears, or saliva tested.

If the acid or alkali has been ingested, all gastrointestinal decontamination procedures are contraindicated except for immediate rinse, removal of substance from the mouth, and dilution with small amounts (sips) of milk or water. The examiner should check for ocular and dermal involvement. Contraindications to oral dilution are dysphagias, respiratory distress, obtundation, or shock. If there is ocular involvement one should immediately irrigate the eye with tepid water for at least 30 minutes, perform fluorescein stain of eye, and consult an ophthalmologist. If there is dermal involvement, one should immediately remove contaminated clothes and irrigate the skin with tepid water for at least 15 minutes. Consultation with a burn specialist is called for.

In cases of acid ingestion, some authorities advocate a small flexible nasogastric tube and aspiration within 30 minutes after ingestion.

Patients should receive only intravenous fluids following dilution until endoscopic consultation is obtained. Endoscopy is valuable to predict damage and risk of stricture. The indications are controversial, with some authorities recommending it in all cases of caustic ingestions regardless of symptoms, and others selectively using clinical features such as vomiting, stridor, drooling, and oral or facial lesions as criteria. We recommend endoscopy for all symptomatic patients or patients with intentional ingestions. Endoscopy may be performed immediately if the patient is symptomatic, but it is usually done 12 to 48 hours postingestion.

The use of corticosteroids is considered controversial. Some feel they may be useful for patients with second-degree circumferential burns. They recommend starting with hydrocortisone sodium succinate (Solu-Cortef) intravenously 10 to 20 mg/kg/d within 48 hours and changing to oral prednisolone 2 mg/kg/d for 3 weeks before tapering the dose. We do not usually recommend using corticosteroids because they have not been shown to be effective.

Tetanus prophylaxis should be provided if the patient requires it for wound care. Antibiotics are not useful prophylactically. Contrast studies are not useful in the first few days and may interfere with endoscopic evaluation; later, they can be used to assess the severity of damage.

Emergency medical therapy includes agents to inhibit collagen formation and intraluminal stents. Esophageal and gastric outlet dilation may be needed if there is evidence of stricture. Bougienage of the esophagus, however, has been associated with brain abscess. Interposition of the colon may be necessary if dilation fails to provide an adequate-sized passage.

Management of inhalation cases requires immediate removal from the environment, administration of humid supplemental oxygen, and observation for airway obstruction and noncardiac pulmonary edema. Radiographic and ABG evaluation should be obtained when appropriate. Intubation and respiratory support may be required.

Certain caustics produce systemic disturbances. Formaldehyde causes metabolic acidosis, hydrofluoric acid causes hypocalcemia and renal damage, oxalic acid causes hypocalcemia, phenol causes hepatic and renal damage, and picric acid causes renal injury.

Disposition

Infants and small children should be medically evaluated and observed. All symptomatic patients should be admitted. If they have severe symptoms or danger of airway compromise, they should be admitted to the intensive care unit. After endoscopy, if no damage is detected, the patient may be discharged when he or she can tolerate oral feedings. Intentional exposures require psychiatric evaluation before the patient can be discharged.

Cocaine (Benzoylmethylecgonine)

Cocaine is derived from the leaves of *Erythroxylon coca* and *Truxillo coca*. "Body packing" refers to the placement of many small packages of contraband cocaine for concealment in the gastrointestinal tract or other areas for illicit transport. "Body stuffing" refers to spontaneous ingestion of substances for the purpose of hiding evidence.

Toxic Mechanism

Cocaine directly stimulates the CNS presynaptic sympathetic neurons to release catecholamines and acetylcholine, while it blocks the presynaptic reuptake of the catecholamines; it blocks the sodium channels along neuronal membranes; and it increases platelet aggregation. Long-term use depletes the CNS of dopamine.

Toxic Dose

The maximum mucosal local anesthetic therapeutic dose of cocaine is 200 mg or 2 mL of a 10% solution. Although CNS effects can occur at relatively low local anesthetic doses (50 to 95 mg), they are more common with doses greater than 1 mg/kg; cardiac effects can occur with doses greater than 1 mg/kg. The potential fatal dose is 1200 mg intranasally, but death has occurred with 20 mg parenterally.

Kinetics

Cocaine is well absorbed by all routes, including nasal insufflation, and oral, dermal, and inhalation routes (Table 14). Protein binding is 8.7%, and volume distribution is 1.5 L/kg.

Cocaine is metabolized by plasma and liver cholinesterase to the inactive metabolites ecgonine methyl ester and benzoylecgonine. Plasma pseudocholinesterase is congenitally deficient in 3% of the population and decreased in fetuses, young infants, the elderly, pregnant people, and people with liver disease. These enzyme-deficient individuals are at increased risk for life-threatening cocaine toxicity.

Ten percent of cocaine is excreted unchanged. Cocaine and ethanol undergo liver synthesis to form cocaethylene, a metabolite with a half-life three times longer than that of cocaine. It may account for some of cocaine's cardiotoxicity and appears to be more lethal than cocaine or ethanol alone.

Manifestations

The CNS manifestation of cocaine ingestion are euphoria, hyperactivity, agitation, convulsions, and intracranial hemorrhage. Mydriasis and septal perforation can occur, as well as cardiac dysrhythmias, hypertension, and hypotension (with severe overdose). Chest pain is frequent, but only 5.8% of patients have true myocardial ischemia and infarction. Other manifestations include vasoconstriction, hyperthermia (because of increased metabolic rate), ischemic bowel perforation if the substance is ingested, rhabdomyolysis, myoglobinuria, and renal failure. In pregnant users, premature labor and abruptio placentae can occur.

Body cavity packing should be suspected in cases of prolonged toxicity.

Mortality can result from cerebrovascular accidents, coronary artery spasm, myocardial injury, or lethal dysrhythmias.

Laboratory Investigations

Monitoring of the ECG and cardiac rhythms, ABG, oxygen saturation, electrolytes, blood glucose, BUN, creatinine, and creatine kinase levels should be maintained. One should monitor cardiac fraction if the patient has chest pain, as well as the liver profile, and the urine for myoglobin. Intravenous drug users should have HIV and hepatitis virus testing.

Urine should be tested for cocaine and metabolites and other substances of abuse, and abdominal radiographs or ultrasonogram should be ordered for body packers. If the urine sample was collected more than 12 hours after cocaine intake, it will contain little or no cocaine. If cocaine is present, cocaine has been used within the past 12 hours. Cocaine's metabolite benzoylecgonine may be detected within 4 hours after a single nasal insufflation and up to 48 to 114 hours. Cross-reactions with some herbal teas, lidocaine, and droperidol (Inapsine) may give false-positive results by some immunoassay methods.

Management

Supportive care includes blood pressure, cardiac, and thermal monitoring and seizure precautions. Diazepam (Valium) is the drug of choice for treatment of cocaine toxicity agitation, seizures, dysrhythmias; doses are 10 to 30 mg intravenously at 2.5 mg/minute for adults and 0.2 to 0.5 mg/kg at 1 mg/minute up to 10 mg for a child.

Gastrointestinal decontamination should be instituted, if the cocaine was ingested, by administration of activated charcoal. MDAC may adsorb cocaine leakage in body stuffers or body packers. Whole-bowel irrigation with polyethylene glycol solution (PEG) has been used in body packers and stuffers if the contraband is in a firm container. If the packages are not visible on plain radiographs of the abdomen, a contrast study or CT scan can help to confirm successful passage. Cocaine in the nasal passage can be removed with an applicator dipped in a non–water-soluble product (lubricating jelly) if this is done within a few minutes after application.

In body packers and stuffers, venous access must be secured, and drugs must be readily available for treating life-threatening manifestations until the contraband is passed in the stool. Surgical removal may be indicated if the packet does not pass the pylorus, in an asymptomatic body packer, or in the case of intestinal obstruction.

Hypertension and tachycardia are usually transient and can be managed by careful titration of diazepam. Nitroprusside may be used for severe hypertension. Myocardial ischemia is managed by oxygen, vascular access, benzodiazepines, and nitroglycerin. Aspirin and thrombolysis are not routinely recommended because of the danger of intracranial hemorrhage.

Dysrhythmias are usually supraventricular (SVT) and do not require specific management. Adenosine is ineffective. Life-threatening tachydysrhythmias may respond to phentolamine (Regitine) 5 mg IV bolus in

TABLE 14. **The Different Routes and Kinetics of Cocaine**

Type	Route	Onset	Peak (min)	Half-life (min)	Duration (min)
Cocaine leaf	Oral, chewing	20–30 min	45–90	NA	240–360
Hydrochloride	Insufflation	1–3 min	5–10	78	60–90
	Ingestion	20–30 min	50–90	54	sustained
	Intravenous	30–120 sec	5–11	36	60–90
Free base/crack	Smoking	5–10 sec	5–11	—	up to 20
Coca paste	Smoking	Unknown	—	—	—

adults or 0.1 mg/kg in children at 5- to 10-minute intervals. Phentolamine also relieves coronary artery spasm and myocardial ischemia. Electrical synchronized cardioversion should be considered for patients with hemodynamically unstable dysrhythmias. Lidocaine is not recommended initially but may be used after 3 hours for ventricular tachycardia. Wide complex QRS ventricular tachycardia may be treated with sodium bicarbonate 2 mEq/kg as a bolus. β-Adrenergic blockers are not recommended.

Anxiety, agitation, and convulsions can be treated with diazepam. If diazepam fails to control seizures, neuromuscular blockers can be used. The EEG should be monitored for nonmotor seizure activity. For hyperthermia, external cooling and cool humidified 100% oxygen should be administered. Neuromuscular paralysis to control seizures will reduce temperature. Dantrolene and antipyretics are not recommended. Rhabdomyolysis and myoglobinuria are treated with fluids, alkaline diuresis, and diuretics.

If the patient is pregnant, the fetus must be monitored and the patient observed for spontaneous abortion.

Paranoid ideation and threatening behavior should be treated with rapid tranquilization. The patient should be observed for suicidal depression that may follow intoxication and may require suicide precautions. If focal neurologic manifestations are present, one should consider the possibility of a cerebrovascular accident and obtain a CT scan.

Extracorporeal clearance techniques are of no benefit.

Disposition

Patients with mild intoxication or a brief seizure that does not require treatment who become asymptomatic may be discharged after 6 hours with appropriate psychosocial follow-up. If cardiac or cerebral ischemic manifestations are present, the patient should be monitored in the intensive care unit. Body packers and stuffers require care in the intensive care unit until passage of the contraband.

Cyanide

Hydrogen cyanide is a byproduct of burning plastic and wools in residential fires. Hydrocyanic acid is the liquefied form of hydrogen cyanide. Cyanide salts can be found in ore extraction. Nitriles, such as acetonitrile (artificial nail removers) are metabolized in the body to produce cyanide. Cyanogenic glycosides are present in some fruit stones (such as amygdalin in apricots, peaches, and apples). Sodium nitroprusside, the antihypertensive vasodilator, contains five cyanide groups.

Toxic Mechanism

Cyanide blocks the cellular electron transport mechanism and cellular respiration by inhibiting the mitochondrial ferricytochrome oxidase system and other enzymes. This results in cellular hypoxia and lactic acidosis. Note: Citrus fruit seeds form cyanide in the presence of intestinal β-glucosidase (the seeds are harmful only if the capsule is broken).

Toxic Dose

The ingestion of 1 mg/kg or 50 mg of hydrogen cyanide can produce death within 15 minutes. The lethal dose of potassium cyanide is 200 mg. Five to 10 mL of 84% acetonitrile is lethal. Infusions of sodium nitroprusside in rates above 2 μg/kg/minute may cause cyanide to accumulate to toxic concentrations in critically ill patients.

Kinetics

Cyanide is rapidly absorbed by all routes. In the stomach, it forms hydrocyanic acid. Volume distribution is 1.5 L/kg. Protein binding is 60%. Cyanide is detoxified by metabolism in the liver via the mitochondrial thiosulfate-rhodanese pathway, which catalyzes the transfer of sulfur donor to cyanide, forming the less toxic irreversible thiocyanate that is excreted in the urine. Cyanide is also detoxified by reacting with hydroxocobalamin (vitamin B_{12a}) to form cyanocobalamin (vitamin B_{12}).

The cyanide elimination half-life from the blood is 1.2 hours. The elimination route is through the lungs.

Manifestations

Hydrogen cyanide has the distinctive odor of bitter almonds or silver polish. Manifestations of cyanide intoxication include hypertension, cardiac dysrhythmias, various ECG abnormalities, headache, hyperpnea, seizures, stupor, pulmonary edema, and flushing. Cyanosis is absent or appears late.

Laboratory Investigations

The examiner should obtain and monitor ABGs, oxygen saturation, blood lactate, hemoglobin, blood glucose, and electrolytes. Lactic acidemia, a decrease in the arterial-venous oxygen difference, and bright red venous blood occurs. If smoke inhalation is the possible source of cyanide exposure, COHb and methemoglobin (MetHb) concentrations should be measured.

Cyanide levels in whole blood, red blood cells, or serum are not useful in the acute management because the determinations are not readily available. Specific cyanide blood levels are as follows: smokers have less than 0.5 μg/mL; a patient with flushing and tachycardia has 0.5 to 1.0 μg/mL, one with obtundation has 1.0 to 2.5 μg/mL, and one in coma and who has died has more than 2.5 μg/mL.

Management

If the cyanide was inhaled, the patient must be removed from the contaminated atmosphere. Attendants should not administer mouth-to-mouth resuscitation. Rescuers and attendants must be protected. Immediate administration of 100% oxygen is called for and oxygen should be continued during and after the administration of the antidote. The clinician must decide whether to use any or all components of the cyanide antidote kit.

The mechanism of action of the antidote kit is twofold: to produce methemoglobinemia and to provide a sulfur substrate for the detoxification of cyanide. The nitrites make methemoglobin, which has a greater affinity for cyanide than does the cytochrome oxidase enzymes. The combination of methemoglobin and cyanide forms cyanomethemoglobin. Sodium thiosulfate provides a sulfur substrate for the rhodanese enzyme, which converts cyanide into the relatively nontoxic sodium thiocyanate, which is excreted by the kidney.

The procedure for using the antidote kit is as follows:

Step 1: Amyl nitrite inhalant perles is only a temporizing measure (forms only 2% to 5% methemoglobin) and it can be omitted if venous access is established. Alternate 100% oxygen and the inhalant for 30 seconds each minute. Use a new perle every 3 minutes.

Step 2: Sodium nitrite ampule is indicated for cyanide exposures, except for cases of residential fires, smoke inhalation, and nitroprusside or acetonitrile poisonings. It is administered intravenously to produce methemoglobin of 20% to 30% at 35 to 70 minutes after administration. A dose of 10 mL of 3% solution of sodium nitrite for adults and 0.33 mL/kg of 3% solution for children is diluted to 100 mL 0.9% saline and administered slowly intravenously at 5 mL/min. If hypotension develops, the infusion should be slowed.

Step 3: Sodium thiosulfate is useful alone in cases of smoke inhalation, nitroprusside toxicity, and acetonitrile toxicity and should not be used at all in cases of hydrogen sulfide poisoning. The administration dose is 12.5 g of sodium thiosulfate or 50 mL of 25% solution for adults and 1.65 mL/kg of 25% solution for children intravenously over 10 to 20 minutes.

If cyanide symptoms recur, further treatment with nitrites or the perles is controversial. Some authorities suggest repeating the antidotes in 30 minutes at half of the initial dose, but others do not advise this for lack of efficacy. The child dosage regimen on the package insert must be carefully followed.

One hour after antidotes are administered, the methemoglobin level should be obtained and should not exceed 20%. Methylene blue should not be used to reverse excessive methemoglobin.

Gastrointestinal decontamination of oral ingestion by activated charcoal is recommended but is not very effective because of the rapidity of absorption. Seizures are treated with intravenous diazepam. Acidosis should be treated with sodium bicarbonate if it does not rapidly resolve with therapy. There is no role for hyperbaric oxygen or hemodialysis or hemoperfusion.

Other antidotes include hydroxocobalamin (vitamin B_{12a}) (Cyanokit), which has proven effective when given immediately after exposure in large doses of 4 g (50 mg/kg) or 50 times the amount of cyanide exposure with 8 g of sodium thiosulfate. Hydroxocobalamin has FDA orphan drug approval.

Disposition

Asymptomatic patients should be observed for a minimum of 3 hours. Patients who ingest nitrile compounds must be observed for 24 hours. Patients requiring antidote administration should be admitted to the intensive care unit.

Digitalis

Cardiac glycosides are found in cardiac medications, common plants, and the skin of the Bufo toad.

Toxic Mechanism

Cardiac glycosides inhibit the enzyme sodium/potassium–adenosine triphosphase (ATPase), leading to intracellular potassium loss and increased intracellular sodium and producing phase 4 depolarization, increased automaticity, and ectopy. There is increased intracellular calcium and potentiation of contractility. Pacemaker cells are inhibited, and the refractory period is prolonged, leading to atrioventricular blocks. There is increased vagal tone.

Toxic Dose

Digoxin total digitalizing dose, the dose required to achieve therapeutic blood levels of 0.6 to 2.0 ng/mL, is 0.75 to 1.25 mg or 10 to 15 μg/kg for patients older than 10 years of age; 40 to 50 μg/kg for patients younger than 2 years of age; and 30 to 40 μg/kg for patients 2 to 10 years of age.

The acute single toxic dose is greater than 0.07 mg/kg or greater than 2 or 3 mg in an adult, but 2 mg in a child or 4 mg in an adult usually produces only mild toxicity. One to 3 mg or more may be found in a few leaves of oleander or foxglove. Serious and fatal overdoses are more than 4 mg in a child and more than 10 mg in an adult.

Acute digitoxin ingestion of 10 to 35 mg has produced severe toxicity and death. Digitoxin therapeutic steady state is 15 to 25 ng/mL. In cases of chronic or acute-on-chronic ingestions in patients with cardiac disease, more than 2 mg may produce toxicity; however, toxicity can develop within therapeutic range on chronic therapy.

Patients at greatest risk of overdose include those with cardiac disease, those with electrolyte abnormalities (low potassium, low magnesium, low T_4, high calcium), those with renal impairment, and those on amiodarone (Cordarone), quinidine, erythromycin, tetracycline, calcium channel blockers, and β-blockers.

Kinetics

Digoxin is a metabolite of digitoxin. In cases of oral overdose, the typical onset is 30 minutes, with peak effects in 3 to 12 hours. Duration is 3 to 4 days. Intravenous onset is in 5 to 30 minutes; peak level is immediate, and peak effect is at 1.5 to 3 hours.

Volume distribution is 5 to 6 L/kg. The cardiac-to-plasma ratio is 30:1. After an acute ingestion overdose, the serum concentration is not reflective of tissue concentration for at least 6 hours or more, and steady state is 12 to 16 hours after last dose.

Sixty percent to 80% of the parent compound is excreted unchanged in the urine. The elimination half-life is 30 to 50 hours.

Manifestations

Onset of manifestations is usually within 2 hours but may be delayed up to 12 hours.

Gastrointestinal effects of nausea and vomiting are frequently present in cases of acute ingestion but may also occur in cases of chronic ingestion. The "digitalis effect" on ECG is scooped ST segments and PR prolongation; in cases of overdose, any dysrhythmia or block is possible but none are characteristic. Bradycardia occurs in patients with acute overdose with healthy hearts; supraventricular tachycardia occurs in patients with existing heart disease or chronic overdose. Ventricular tachycardia is seen only in cases of severe poisoning.

The CNS effects include headaches, visual disturbances, and colored halo vision. Hyperkalemia occurs following acute overdose and correlates with digoxin level and outcome. Among patients with serum potassium levels of less than 5.0 mEq/L, all survive. If the level is 5 to 5.5, 50% survive, and if the level is greater than 5.5, all die. Hypokalemia is commonly seen with chronic intoxication. Patients with normal digitalis levels may have toxicity in the presence of hypokalemia.

Chronic intoxications are more likely to produce scotoma, color perception disturbances, yellow vision, halos, delirium, hallucinations or psychosis, tachycardia, and hypokalemia.

Laboratory Investigations

Continuous monitoring of ECG, pulse, and blood pressure is called for. Blood glucose, electrolytes, calcium, magnesium, BUN, and creatinine levels should also be monitored. An initial digoxin level should be measured on patient presentation and repeated thereafter. Levels should be measured more than 6 hours postingestion because earlier values do not reflect tissue distribution. Digoxin clinical toxicity is usually associated with serum digoxin levels of greater than 3.5 ng/mL in adults.

An endogenous digoxin-like substance cross-reacts in most common immunoassays (not with high-pressure liquid chromatography) and values as high as 4.1 ng/mL have been reported in newborns, patients with chronic renal failure, patients with abnormal immunoglobulins, and women in the third trimester of pregnancy.

Management

A cardiology consult should be obtained and a pacemaker should be readily available.

In undertaking gastrointestinal decontamination, excessive vagal stimulation should be avoided (e.g., emesis and gastric lavage). Activated charcoal should be administered, and if a nasogastric tube is required for the activated charcoal, pretreatment with atropine (0.02 mg/kg in children and 0.5 mg in adults) should be considered.

Digoxin-specific antibody fragments (Fab, Digibind) 38 mg binds 0.5 mg digoxin and then is excreted through the kidneys. The onset of action is within 30 minutes. Problems associated with Fab therapy are mainly from withdrawal of digoxin and worsening heart failure, hypokalemia, decrease in glucose (if the patient has low glycogen stores), and allergic reactions (very rare). Digitalis administered after Fab therapy is bound and may be inactivated for 5 to 7 days.

Absolute indications for Fab therapy include the following:

- Life-threatening malignant (hemodynamically unstable) dysrhythmias
- Ventricular dysrhythmias, unstable severe bradycardia, or second- or third-degree blocks unresponsive to atropine or rapid deterioration in clinical status
- Life-threatening digitoxin and oleander poisonings

Relative indications for Fab therapy include the following:

- Ingestions greater than 4 mg in a child and 10 mg in an adult
- Serum potassium level greater than 5.0 mEq/L
- Serum digoxin level greater than 10 ng/mL in adults or greater than 5 ng/mL in children 6 hours after an acute ingestion
- Digitalis delirium and thrombocytopenia response

Digoxin-specific Fab fragments therapy can be administered as a bolus through a 22-μm filter if the case is a critical emergency. If the case is less urgent, then it can be administered over 30 minutes. An empiric dose is 10 vials in adults and 5 vials in a child for an unknown amount ingested in a symptomatic patient with history of a digoxin overdose.

To calculate the dose in the case of a known ingestion, the following equation is used:

$$\text{Amount (total mg)} \times (0.8) = \text{body burden}$$

If liquid capsules were taken or the substance was given intravenously the 80% bioavailability figure is not used. Instead, the body burden divided by 0.5 (0.5 mg digoxin is bound by 1 vial of 38 mg of Fab) equals the number of vials needed.

If the amount unknown but the steady state serum concentration is known, the following equations are used:

For Digoxin

$$\text{Digoxin ng/mL} \times (5.6\ \text{L/kg Vd}) \times (\text{wt kg}) = \text{mg body burden}$$
$$\text{Body burden} \div 1000 = \text{mg body burden}$$
$$\text{Body burden}/0.5 = \text{number of vials needed}$$

For Digitoxin

$$\text{Digitoxin ng/mL} \times (0.56\ \text{L/kg Vd}) \times (\text{wt kg}) = \text{mg body burden}$$
$$\text{Body burden} \div 1000 = \text{mg body burden}$$
$$\text{Body burden}/0.5 = \text{number of vials needed}$$

Antidysrhythmic agents or a pacemaker should be used only if Fab therapy fails. For ventricular tachydysrhythmias, electrolyte disturbances should be corrected by the administration of lidocaine or phenytoin.

For torsades de pointes, magnesium sulfate 20 mL 20% IV can be given slowly over 20 minutes (or 25 to 50 mg/kg in a child), titrated to control the dysrhythmia. Magnesium should be discontinued if hypotension, heart block, or decreased deep tendon reflexes are present. Magnesium is used with caution if the patient has renal impairment.

Unstable bradycardia and second-degree and third-degree atrioventricular block should be treated by Fab first. A pacemaker should be available if necessary. Isoproterenol should be avoided because it causes dysrhythmias. Cardioversion is used with caution, starting at a setting of 5 to 10 joules. The patient should be pretreated with lidocaine, if possible, because cardioversion may precipitate ventricular fibrillation or asystole.

Potassium disturbances are due to a shift, not a change, in total body potassium. Hyperkalemia (>5.0 mEq/L) is treated with Fab only. Calcium must never be used, and insulin/glucose and sodium bicarbonate should not be used concomitantly with Fab because they may produce severe life-threatening hypokalemia. Sodium polystyrene sulfonate (Kayexalate) should not be used. Hypokalemia must be treated with caution because it may be cardioprotective. Treatment can be administered if the patient has ventricular dysrhythmias or a serum potassium level less than 3.0 mEq/L and atrioventricular block.

Extracorporeal procedures are ineffective. Hemodialysis is used for severe or refractory hyperkalemia.

One must never use antidysrhythmic types Ia (procainamide, quinidine, disopyramide [Norpace], amiodarone [Cordarone]), Ic (propafenone [Rythmol], flecainide [Tambocor]), II (β-blockers), or IV (calcium channel blockers). Class Ib drugs (lidocaine, phenytoin [Dilantin], mexiletine [Mexitil], and tocainide [Tonocard]) can be used.

Disposition

Consult with a poison control center and a cardiologist experienced with digoxin-specific Fab fragments is warranted. All patients with significant dysrhythmias, symptoms, elevated serum digoxin concentration, or elevated serum potassium level should be admitted to the intensive care unit.

Ethanol

Table 15 lists the features of alcohols and glycols.

Toxic Mechanism

Ethanol has CNS depressant and anesthetic effects. Ethanol stimulates the gamma aminobutyric acid (GABA) system. It promotes cutaneous vasodilation (contributes to hypothermia), stimulates secretion of gastric juice (gastritis), inhibits the secretion of the antidiuretic hormone, inhibits gluconeogenesis (hypoglycemia), and influences fat metabolism (lipidemia).

Toxic Dose

A dose of 1 mL/kg of absolute ethanol (100% ethanol, or 200 proof) gives a blood ethanol concentration of 100 mg/dL. A potentially fatal dose is 3 g/kg for children or 6 g/kg for adults. Children are more prone to developing hypoglycemia than adults.

Kinetics

Onset of action is 30 to 60 minutes after ingestion; peak action is 90 minutes on empty stomach. Volume distribution is 0.6 L/kg. The major route of elimination (>90%) is by hepatic oxidative metabolism. The first step is by the enzyme alcohol dehydrogenase, which converts ethanol to acetaldehyde. Alcohol dehydrogenase metabolizes ethanol at a constant rate of 12 to 20 mg/dL/hour (12 to 15 mg/dL/hour in nondrinkers, 15 to 30 mg/d/hour in social drinkers, 30 to 50 mg/dL/hour in heavy drinkers, and 25 to 30 mg/dL/hour in children). At very low blood ethanol concentration (<30 mg/dL), the metabolism is by first-order kinetics. In the second step, acetaldehyde is metabolized by acetaldehyde dehydrogenase to acetic acid, which is metabolized by the Krebs cycle to carbon dioxide and water. The enzyme steps are nicotinamide adenine dinucleotide–dependent, which interferes with gluconeogenesis. Less than 10% of ethanol is excreted unchanged by the kidneys.

TABLE 15. **Summary of Alcohol and Glycol Features**

	Methanol	Isopropanol	Ethanol	Ethylene glycol
Principal Uses	Gas line antifreeze, Sterno, windshield de-icer	Solvent jewelry cleaner, rubbing alcohol	Beverage, solvent	Radiator antifreeze, windshield de-icer
Specific Gravity	0.719	0.785	0.789	1.12
Fatal Dose	1 mL/kg 100%	3 mL/kg 100%	5 mL/kg 100%	1.4 mL/kg
Inebriation	+/–	2+	2+	1+
Metabolic Change		Hyperglycemia	Hypoglycemia	Hypocalcemia
Metabolic Acidosis	4+	0	1+	2+
Anion Gap	4+	+/–	2+	4+
Ketosis	Ketobutyric	Acetone	Hydroxybutyric	None
Gastrointestinal Tract	Pancreatitis	Hemorrhagic gastritis	Gastritis	
Osmolality*	0.337	0.176	0.228	0.190

*1 mL/dL of substances raises freezing point osmolarity of serum. The validity of the correlation of osmolality with blood concentrations has been questioned.

The relationship between blood ethanol concentration (BEC) and dose (amount ingested) can be calculated as follows:

BEC (mg/dL) = amt ingested (mL) × % ethanol product × SG (0.79) / Vd (0.6 L/kg) × body wt (kg)

Dose (amt ingested) = BEC (mg/dL) × Vd (0.6) × body wt (kg) / % ethanol × specific gravity (0.79)

Manifestations

Clinical signs of acute ethanol intoxication are given in Table 16.

Chronic alcoholic patients tolerate higher blood ethanol concentration, and correlation with manifestations is not valid. Rapid interview for alcoholism is the *CAGE questions:*

- C—Have you felt the need to *C*ut down?
- A—Have others *A*nnoyed you by criticism of you drinking?
- G—Have you felt *G*uilty about your drinking?
- E—Have you ever had morning *E*ye-opening drink to steady your nerves or get rid of a hangover?

Two affirmative answers indicate probable alcoholism.

Laboratory Investigations

The blood ethanol concentration should be specifically requested and followed. Gas chromatography or a breathalyzer test gives rapid reliable results if no belching or vomiting is present. Enzymatic methods do not differentiate between the alcohols. ABG, electrolytes, and glucose should be measured, the anion and osmolar gap determined (measure by freezing point depression, not vapor pressure), and a check for ketosis made.

Management

The examiner should inquire about trauma and disulfiram use. The patient must be protected from aspiration and hypoxia. Vital functions must be established and maintained. The patient may require intubation and assisted ventilation.

Gastrointestinal decontamination plays no role in the management of ethanol intoxication.

If the patient is comatose, glucose should be administered intravenously, 1 mL/kg 50% glucose in adults and 2 mL/kg 25% glucose in children. Thiamine, 100 mg intravenously, is administered if the patient has a history of chronic alcoholism, malnutrition, or suspected eating disorders to prevent Wernicke-Korsakoff syndrome. Naloxone (Narcan) has produced a partial inconsistent response but is not recommended for known alcoholics.

General supportive care includes administration of fluids to correct hydration and hypotension and correction of electrolyte abnormalities and acid-base imbalance. Vasopressors and plasma expanders may be necessary to correct severe hypotension. Hypomagnesemia is frequent in chronic alcoholics. In case of hypomagnesemia, a loading dose of 2 g magnesium sulfate 10% is administered by intravenous solution over 5 minutes in the intensive care unit with blood pressure and cardiac monitoring and calcium chloride 10% on hand in case of overdose. This is followed with constant infusion of 6 g of 10% solution over 3 to 4 hours. Caution must be taken with the use of magnesium if renal failure is present.

Hypothermic patients should be warmed. See the section on the general treatment of poisoning.

Hemodialysis can be used in severe cases when conventional therapy is ineffective (rarely needed).

Repeated or prolonged seizures should be treated with diazepam (Valium). The brief "rum fits" do not need long-term anticonvulsant therapy. Repeated seizures or focal neurologic findings may warrant skull radiographs, lumbar puncture, and CT scan of the head, depending on the clinical findings. Withdrawal is treated with hydration and large doses of chlordiazepoxide (Librium) 50 to 100 mg or diazepam (Valium) 2 to 10 mg intravenously; these doses may be repeated in 2 to 4 hours. Very large doses of benzodiazepines may be required for delirium tremors. Withdrawal can occur in presence of elevated blood ethanol concentration and can be fatal if left untreated.

Chest radiograph is warranted to determine whether aspiration pneumonia is present. Renal and liver function tests and bilirubin level measurement should be made.

TABLE 16. **Clinical Signs in the Nontolerant Ethanol Drinker**

Ethanol Blood Conc. (mg/dL)*	Manifestations
>25	Euphoria
>47	***Mild incoordination,*** sensory and motor impairment
>50	Increased risk of motor vehicle accidents
>100	Ataxia (legal toxic level in many localities)
>150	***Moderate incoordination,*** slow reaction time
>200	Drowsiness and confusion
>300	Severe incoordination, stupor, blurred vision
>500	***Flaccid coma,*** respiratory failure, hypotension; may be fatal

*Ethanol concentrations sometimes reported in %.

Note: mg/% is not equivalent to mg/dL because ethanol weighs less than water (specific gravity 0.79). A 1% ethanol concentration is 790 mg/d and 0.1% is 79 mg/d. There is great variation in individual behavior at different blood ethanol levels. Behavior is dependent on tolerance and other factors.

Disposition

Clinical severity (e.g., intubation, assisted ventilation, aspiration pneumonia) should determine the level of hospital care needed. Young children with significant unintentional exposure to ethanol (calculated to reach a blood ethanol concentration of 50 mg/dL) should have blood ethanol concentration obtained and blood glucose levels monitored for hypoglycemia frequently for 4 hours after ingestion. Patients with acute ethanol intoxication seldom require admission unless a complication is present. However, intoxicated patients should not be discharged until they are fully functional (can walk, talk, and think independently), have suicide potential evaluated, have proper disposition environment, and have a sober escort.

Ethylene Glycol

Ethylene glycol is found in solvents, de-icers, radiator antifreeze (95%), and air-conditioning units. Ethylene glycol is a sweet-tasting, colorless, water-soluble liquid with a sweet aromatic aroma.

Toxic Mechanism

Ethylene glycol is oxidized by alcohol dehydrogenase to glycolaldehyde, which is metabolized to glycolic acid and glyoxylic acid. Glyoxylic acid is metabolized to oxalic acid via a pyridoxine-dependent pathway to glycine and by thiamine and magnesium-dependent pathways to α-hydroxy-ketoadipic acid. The metabolites of ethylene glycol produce a profound metabolic acidosis, increased anion gap, hypocalcemia, and oxalate crystals, which deposit in tissues (particularly the kidney).

Toxic Dose

The ingestion of 0.1 mL/kg 100% ethylene glycol can result in a toxic serum ethylene glycol concentration of 20 mg/dL, Ingestion of 3.0 mL (less than 1 teaspoonful or swallow) of a 100% solution in a 10 kg child or 30 mL of 100% ethylene glycol in an adult produces a serum ethylene glycol concentration of 50 mg/dL, a concentration that requires hemodialysis. The fatal amount is 1.4 mL/kg of 100% solution.

Kinetics

Absorption is via dermal, inhalation, and ingestion routes. Ethylene glycol is rapidly absorbed from the gastrointestinal tract. Onset is usually in 30 minutes but may be delayed by co-ingestion of food and ethanol. The usual peak level is at 2 hours. Volume distribution is 0.65 to 0.8 L/kg.

For metabolism, see Toxic Mechanism.

The half-life of ethylene glycol without ethanol is 3 to 8 hours; with ethanol, it is 17 hours, and with hemodialysis it is 2.5 hours. Renal clearance is 3.2 mL/kg/minute. About 20% to 50% is excreted unchanged in the urine. The relationship between serum ethylene glycol concentration (SEGC) and dose (amount ingested) can be calculated as follows:

0.12 mL/kg of 100% = SEGC 10 mg/dL

Manifestations

Phase I. The onset of manifestations is 30 minutes to several hours longer after ingestion with concomitant ethanol ingestion. The patient may be inebriated. Hypocalcemia, tetany, and calcium oxalate and hippuric acid crystals in urine can be seen within 4 to 8 hours but are not always present. Early, before metabolism of ethylene glycol, an osmolal gap may be present (see Laboratory Investigations). Later, the metabolites of ethylene glycol produce changes starting 4 to 12 hours following ingestion, including an anion gap, metabolic acidosis, coma, convulsions, cardiac disturbances, and pulmonary and cerebral edema. Since fluorescein is added to some antifreeze, the presence of fluorescence may be a clue to ethylene glycol exposure. Recently, however, it has been shown that fluorescent urine is not a reliable indicator of ethylene glycol ingestion and should not be used as a screen.

Phase II. After 12 to 36 hours, cardiopulmonary deterioration occurs, with pulmonary edema and congestive heart failure.

Phase III. Phase III occurs 36 to 72 hours after ingestion, with pulmonary edema and oliguric renal failure from oxalate crystal deposition and tubular necrosis predominating.

Phase IV. Neurologic sequelae may occur rarely, especially in patients who fail to receive early antidotal therapy. The onset ranges from 6 to 10 days after ingestion. Findings include facial diplegia, hearing loss, bilateral visual disturbances, elevated cerebrospinal fluid pressure with or without elevated protein levels and pleocytosis, vomiting, hyperreflexia, dysphagia, and ataxia.

Laboratory Investigations

Blood glucose and electrolytes should be monitored. Urinalysis should look for oxalate ("envelope") and monohydrate ("hemp seed") crystals. Urine fluorescence is not reliable as a screen. ABG, ethylene glycol, and ethanol levels, plasma osmolarity (using freezing point depression method), calcium, BUN, and creatinine should be measured. A serum ethylene glycol concentration of 20 mg/dL is toxic (ethylene glycol levels are very difficult to obtain). If possible, a glycolate level should be obtained. Cross-reactions with propylene glycol, a vehicle in many liquids and intravenous medications (phenytoin [Dilantin], diazepam [Valium]), other glycols, and triglycerides may produce spurious ethylene glycol levels. False-positive ethylene glycol values may occur with colorimetric or gas chromatography using an OV-17 column in the presence of propylene glycol.

The following equations can be used to calculate the osmolality, osmolal gap, and ethylene glycol level:

2 (Na+ mEq/L) + (Blood glucose mg/dL)/20 + (BUN mg/dL)/3 = Total calculated osmolality (mOsmL/L)

Osmolar Gap = measured osmolality (by freezing point depression method) − calculated osmolality

A gap greater than 10 is abnormal. Note: if ethanol is involved, add ethanol level/4.6 to the calculated equation.

An increased osmolal gap is produced by the following common substances: acetone, dextran, dimethyl sulfoxide, diuretics, ethanol, ethyl ether, ethylene glycol, isopropanol, paraldehyde, mannitol, methanol, sorbitol, and trichloroethane. Table 10 gives the conversion factors for these substances.

Although a specific blood level of ethylene glycol in milligrams per deciliter can be estimated using the equation below, this is not considered to be a reliable method and should not take the place of obtaining a measured ethylene glycol blood concentration.

$$\text{osmolar gap} \times \text{conversion factor} = \text{serum concentration}$$

Caution: The accuracy of the ethylene glycol estimated decreases as the ethylene glycol levels decrease. The toxic metabolites are not osmotically active, and patients presenting late may show signs of severe toxicity without an elevated osmolar gap.

The anion gap can be calculated using the following equation:

$$Na - (Cl + HCO_3) = \text{anion gap}$$

The normal gap is 8 to 12. Potassium is not used because it is a small amount and may be hemolyzed. Table 8 lists factors that may account for an increased or a decreased anion gap.

Management

Vital functions should be established and maintained. The airway must be protected, and assisted ventilation can be used, if necessary. Gastrointestinal decontamination has limited role. Only gastric aspiration can be used within 60 minutes after ingestion. Activated charcoal is not effective.

Baseline measurements of serum electrolytes and calcium, glucose, ABGs, ethanol, serum ethylene glycol concentration (may be difficult to obtain readily in some institutions), and methanol concentrations should be obtained. In the first few hours, the measured serum osmolality should be determined and compared to calculated osmolality (see osmolality equation, earlier). If seizures occur, one should measure serum calcium (preferably ionized calcium) and treat with intravenous diazepam. If the patient has hypocalcemic seizures, he or she should also be treated with 10 to 20 mL 10% calcium gluconate (0.2 to 0.3 mL/kg in children) slowly intravenously, with the dose repeated as needed. Metabolic acidosis should be corrected with intravenous sodium bicarbonate.

Ethanol therapy should be initiated immediately if fomepizole (Antizol) is unavailable (see next paragraph). Alcohol dehydrogenase has a greater affinity for ethanol than ethylene glycol. Therefore, ethanol blocks the metabolism of ethylene glycol. Ethanol therapy is called for if there is a history of ingestion of 0.1 mL/kg of 100% ethylene glycol, serum ethylene glycol concentration is greater than 20 mg/dL, there is an osmolar gap not accounted for by other alcohols or factors (e.g., hyperlipidemia), metabolic acidosis is present with an increased anion gap, or there are oxalate crystals in the urine. Ethanol should be administered intravenously (the oral route is less reliable) to produce a blood ethanol concentration of 100 to 150 mg/dL. The loading dose is 10 mL/kg of 10% ethanol intravenously, administered concomitantly with a maintenance dose of 10% ethanol of 1.0 mL/kg/h. This dose may need to be increased to 2 mL/kg/h in patients who are heavy drinkers. The blood ethanol concentration should be measured hourly and the infusion rate should be adjusted to maintain a blood ethanol concentration of 100 to 150 mg/dL.

Fomepizole (Antizol, 4-methylpyrazole) inhibits alcohol dehydrogenase more reliability than ethanol and it does not require constant monitoring of ethanol levels and adjustment of infusion rates. Fomepizole is available in 1 g/mL vials of 1.5 mL. The loading dose is 15 mg/kg (0.015 mL/kg) IV; maintenance dose is 10 mg/kg (0.01 mL/kg) every 12 hours for four doses, then 15 mg/kg every 12 hours until the ethylene glycol levels are less than 20 mg/dL. The solution is prepared by being mixed with 100 mL of 0.9% saline or D_5W. Fomepizole can be given to patients requiring hemodialysis but should be dosed as follows:

Dose at the beginning of hemodialysis:

- If <6 hours since last Antizol dose, do not administer dose
- If >6 hours since last dose, administer next scheduled dose

Dosing during hemodialysis:

- Dose every 4 hours

Dosing at the time hemodialysis is completed:

- If <1 hour between last dose and end of dialysis, do not administer dose at end of dialysis
- If 1 to 3 hours between last dose and end of dialysis, administer one half of next scheduled dose
- If >3 hours between last dose and end of dialysis, administer next scheduled dose

Maintenance dosing off hemodialysis:

- Give the next scheduled dose 12 hours from the last dose administered

Hemodialysis is indicated if the ingestion was potentially fatal; if the serum ethylene glycol concentration is greater than 50 mg/dL (some recommend at levels of >25 mg/dL); if severe acidosis or electrolyte abnormalities occur despite conventional therapy; or if congestive heart failure or renal failure is present. Hemodialysis reduces the ethylene glycol half-life from 17 hours on ethanol therapy to 3 hours. Therapy (fomepizole and hemodialysis) should be continued until the serum ethylene glycol concentration is less than 10 mg/dL, the glycolate level is nondetectable (not readily available), the acidosis has cleared, there are no mental disturbances, the creatinine level is normal, and the urinary output is adequate. This may require 2 to 5 days.

Adjunct therapy involving thiamine, 100 mg/d (in children, 50 mg), slowly over 5 minutes intravenously or intramuscularly and repeated every 6 hours and pyridoxine, 50 mg IV or IM every 6 hours, has been recommended until intoxication is resolved, but these agents have not been extensively studied. Folate, 50 mg IV (child 1 mg/kg), can be given every 4 hours for 6 doses.

Disposition

All patients who have ingested significant amounts of ethylene glycol (calculated level above 20 mg/dL), have a history of a toxic dose, or are symptomatic should be referred to the emergency department and admitted. If the serum ethylene glycol concentration cannot be obtained, the patient should be followed for 12 hours, with monitoring of the osmolal gap, acid-base parameters, and electrolytes to exclude development of metabolic acidosis with an anion gap. Transfer should be considered for fomepizole therapy or hemodialysis.

Hydrocarbons

The lower the viscosity and surface tension of hydrocarbons or the greater the volatility, the greater the risk of aspiration. Volatile substance abuse has produced the "Sudden Sniffing's Death Syndrome," most likely caused by dysrhythmias.

Toxicologic Classification and Toxic Mechanism

All systemically absorbed hydrocarbons can lower the threshold of the myocardium to dysrhythmias produced by endogenous and exogenous catecholamines.

Aliphatic hydrocarbons are branched straight chain hydrocarbons. A few aspirated drops produce chemical pneumonitis, but they are poorly absorbed from the gastrointestinal tract and produce no systemic toxicity by this route. However, aspiration of very small amounts can produce chemical pneumonitis. Examples of aliphatic hydrocarbons are gasoline, kerosene, charcoal lighter fluid, mineral spirits (Stoddard's solvent), and petroleum naphtha. Mineral seal oil (signal oil), found in furniture polishes, is a low-viscosity and low-volatility oil with minimum absorption that never warrants gastric decontamination. It can produce severe pneumonia if aspirated.

Aromatic hydrocarbons are six carbon ring structures that are absorbed through the gastrointestinal tract. Systemic toxicity includes CNS depression and, in cases of chronic abuse, multiple organ effects such as leukemia (benzene) and renal toxicity (toluene). Examples are benzene, toluene, styrene, and xylene. The seriously toxic ingested dose is 20 to 50 mL in adults.

Halogenated hydrocarbons are aliphatic or aromatic hydrocarbons with one or more halogen substitutions (Cl, Br, Fl, or I). They are highly volatile and are abused as inhalants. They are well absorbed from the gastrointestinal tract, produce CNS depression, and have metabolites that can damage the liver and kidneys. Examples include methylene chloride (may be converted into carbon monoxide in the body), dichloroethylene (also causes a disulfiram [Antabuse] reaction known as "degreaser's flush" when associated with consumption of ethanol), and 1,1,1-trichloroethane (Glamorene Spot Remover, Scotchgard, typewriter correction fluid). An acute lethal oral dose is 0.5 to 5 mL/kg.

Dangerous additives to the hydrocarbons can be summed up with the mnemonic CHAMP: C, camphor (demothing agent); H, halogenated hydrocarbons; A, aromatic hydrocarbons; M, metals (heavy); and P, pesticides. Ingestion of these substances may warrant gastric emptying with a small-bore nasogastric tube.

Heavy hydrocarbons have high viscosity, low volatility, and minimal gastrointestinal absorption, so gastric decontamination is not necessary. Examples are asphalt (tar), machine oil, motor oil (lubricating oil, engine oil), home heating oil, and petroleum jelly (mineral oil).

Laboratory Investigations

The ECG, ABG, pulmonary function, serum electrolytes, and serial chest radiographs should be continuously monitored. Liver and renal function should be monitored in cases of inhalation of aromatic hydrocarbons.

Management

Asymptomatic patients who ingested small amounts of aliphatic petroleum distillates can be followed at home by telephone for development of signs of aspiration (cough, wheezing, tachypnea, and dyspnea) for 4 to 6 hours. Inhalation of any hydrocarbon vapors in a closed space can produce intoxication. The victim must be removed from the environment, have oxygen administered, and receive respiratory support.

Gastrointestinal decontamination is not advised in cases of hydrocarbon ingestion that usually do not cause systemic toxicity (aliphatic petroleum distillates, heavy hydrocarbons). In cases of ingestion of hydrocarbons that cause systemic toxicity in small amounts (aromatic hydrocarbons, halogenated hydrocarbons), the clinician should pass a small-bore nasogastric tube and aspirate if the ingestion was within 2 hours and if spontaneous vomiting has not occurred. Some toxicologists advocate ipecac-induced emesis under medical supervision instead of small-bore nasogastric gastric lavage; we do not.

Patients with altered mental status should have their airway protected because of concern about aspiration. The use of activated charcoal has been suggested, but there are no scientific data as to effectiveness and it may produce vomiting. Activated charcoal may, however, be useful in adsorbing toxic additives such as pesticides or co-ingestants.

The symptomatic patient who is coughing, gagging, choking, or wheezing on arrival has probably aspirated. The clinician should provide supportive respiratory care and supplemental oxygen, while monitoring pulse oximetry, ABG, chest radiograph, and ECG. The patient should be admitted to the intensive care unit. A chest radiograph for aspiration may be positive as early as 30 minutes after ingestion, and almost all are positive within 6 hours. Negative chest radiographs within 4 hours do not rule out aspiration.

Bronchospasm is treated with a nebulized β-adrenergic agonist and intravenous aminophylline if necessary. Epinephrine should be avoided because of susceptibility to dysrhythmias. Cyanosis in the presence of a normal arterial Pa_{O_2} may be due to methemoglobinemia that requires therapy with methylene blue. Corticosteroids and prophylactic antimicrobial agents have not been shown to be beneficial. (Fever or leukocytosis may be produced by the chemical pneumonitis itself.)

Most infiltrations resolve spontaneously in 1 week; lipoid pneumonia may last up to 6 weeks. It is not necessary to surgically treat pneumatoceles that develop because they usually resolve. Dysrhythmias may require α- and β-adrenergic antagonists or cardioversion.

There is no role for enhanced elimination procedures.

Methylene chloride is metabolized over several hours to carbon monoxide. See treatment of carbon monoxide poisoning. Halogenated hydrocarbons are hepatorenal toxins; therefore, hepatorenal function should be monitored. *N*-acetylcysteine therapy may be useful if there is evidence of hepatic damage.

Extracorporal membrane oxygenation (ECMO) has been used successfully for a few patients with life threatening respiratory failure. Surfactant used for hydrocarbon aspiration was found to be detrimental.

Disposition

Asymptomatic patients with small ingestions of petroleum distillates can be managed at home. Symptomatic patients with abnormal chest radiographic, oxygen saturation, or ABG findings should be admitted. Patients who become asymptomatic and have normal oxygenation and a normal repeat radiograph can be discharged.

Iron

There are more than 100 iron over-the-counter preparations for supplementation and treatment of iron deficiency anemia.

Toxic Mechanism

Toxicity depends on the amount of elemental iron available in various salts (gluconate 12%, sulfate 20%, fumarate 33%, lactate 19%, chloride 21% of elemental iron), not the amount of the salt. Locally, iron is corrosive and may cause fluid loss, hypovolemic shock, and perforation. Excessive free unbound iron in the blood is directly toxic to the vasculature and leads to the release of vasoactive substances, which produces vasodilation. In cases of overdose, iron deposits injure mitochondria in the liver, the kidneys, and the myocardium. The exact mechanism of cellular damage is not clear but is thought to be related to free radical formation.

Toxic Dose

The therapeutic dose is 6 mg/kg/day of elemental iron. An elemental iron dose of 20 to 40 mg/kg may produce mild self-limited gastrointestinal symptoms, 40 to 60 mg/kg produces moderate toxicity, more than 60 mg/kg produces severe toxicity and is potentially lethal, and more than 180 mg/kg is usually fatal without treatment. Children's chewable vitamins with iron have between 12 and 18 mg of elemental iron per tablet or 0.6 mL of liquid drops. These preparations rarely produce toxicity unless very large quantities are ingested and have never caused death.

Kinetics

Absorption occurs chiefly in the upper small intestine. Ferrous (+2) iron is absorbed into the mucosal cells, where it is oxidized to the ferric (+3) state and bound to ferritin. Iron is slowly released from ferritin into the plasma, where it binds to transferrin and is transported to specific tissues for production of hemoglobin (70%), myoglobin (5%), and cytochrome. About 25% of iron is stored in the liver and spleen. In cases of overdose, larger amounts of iron are absorbed because of direct mucosal corrosion. There is no mechanism for the elimination of iron (elimination is 1 to 2 mg/d) except through bile, sweat, and blood loss.

Manifestations

Serious toxicity is unlikely if the patient remains asymptomatic for 6 hours and has a negative abdominal radiograph. Iron intoxication can produce five phases of toxicity. The phases may not be distinct from one another.

Phase I. Gastrointestinal mucosal injury occurs 30 minutes to 12 hours postingestion. Vomiting starts within 30 minutes to 1 hour of ingestion and is persistent; hematemesis and bloody diarrhea may occur; abdominal cramps, fever, hyperglycemia, and leukocytosis may occur. Enteric-coated tablets may pass through the stomach without causing symptoms. Acidosis and shock can occur within 6 to 12 hours.

Phase II. A latent period of apparent improvement occurs over 8 to 12 hours postingestion.

Phase III. Systemic toxicity phase occurs 12 to 48 hours postingestion with cardiovascular collapse and severe metabolic acidosis.

Phase IV. Two to 4 days postingestion, hepatic injury associated with jaundice, elevated liver enzymes, and prolonged prothrombin time occur. Kidney injury with proteinuria and hematuria occur. Pulmonary edema, disseminated intravascular coagulation, and *Yersinia enterocolitica* sepsis can occur.

Phase V. Four to 8 weeks postingestion, pyloric outlet or intestinal stricture may cause obstruction or anemia secondary to blood loss.

Laboratory Investigations

Iron poisoning produces anion gap metabolic acidosis. Monitoring should include complete blood cell counts, blood glucose level, serum iron, stools and vomitus for occult blood, electrolytes, acid-base balance, urinalysis and urinary output, liver function tests, and BUN and creatinine levels. Blood type and match should be obtained.

Serum iron measurements taken at the proper time correlate with the clinical findings. The lavender top Vacutainer tube contains EDTA, which falsely lowers serum iron. One must obtain the serum iron measurement before administering deferoxamine. Serum iron levels of less than 350 μg/dL at 2 to 6 hours predict an asymptomatic course; levels of 350 to 500 μg/dL are usually associated with mild gastrointestinal symptoms; those greater than 500 μg/dL have a 20% risk of shock and serious iron toxicity. A follow-up serum iron measurement after 6 hours may not be elevated even in cases of severe poisoning, but a serum iron measurement taken at 8 to 12 hours is useful to exclude delayed absorption from a bezoar or sustained-release preparation. The total iron-binding capacity is not necessary.

Adult iron tablet preparations are radiopaque before they dissolve by 4 hours postingestion. A "negative" abdominal radiograph more than 4 hours postingestion does not exclude iron poisoning.

Patients who develop high fevers and signs of sepsis following iron overdose should have blood and stool cultures checked for *Yersinia enterocolitica*.

Management

Gastrointestinal decontamination should involve immediate induction of emesis in cases of ingestions of elemental iron of greater than 40 mg/kg if vomiting has not already occurred. Activated charcoal is ineffective. An abdominal radiograph should be obtained after emesis to determine the success of gastric emptying. Children's chewable vitamins and liquid iron preparations are not radiopaque. If radiopaque iron is still present, whole-bowel irrigation with polyethylene glycol solution should be considered. In extreme cases, removal by endoscopy or surgery may be necessary because coalesced iron tablets produce hemorrhagic infarction in the bowel and perforation peritonitis.

Deferoxamine (Desferal) in a dose of about 100 mg binds 8.5 to 9.35 mg of free iron in the serum. The deferoxamine infusion should not exceed 15 mg/kg/h or 6 g daily, but faster rates (up to 45 mg/kg) and larger daily amounts have been administered and tolerated in extreme cases of iron poisoning (>1000 mg/dL). The deferoxamine-iron complex is hemodialyzable if renal failure develops.

Indications for chelation therapy are any of the following:

- Very large, symptomatic ingestions
- Serious clinical intoxication (severe vomiting and diarrhea [often bloody], severe abdominal pain, metabolic acidosis, hypotension, or shock)
- Symptoms that persist or progress to more serious toxicity
- Serum iron level greater than 500 μg/dL

Chelation should be performed as early as possible within 12 to 18 hours to be effective. One should start the infusion slowly and gradually increase to avoid hypotension.

Adult respiratory distress syndrome has developed in patients with high doses of deferoxamine for several days; infusions longer than 24 hours should be avoided.

The endpoint of treatment is when the patient is asymptomatic and the urine clears if it was originally a positive "vin rose" color.

For supportive therapy, intravenous bicarbonate may be needed to correct the metabolic acidosis. Hypotension and shock treatment may require volume expansion, vasopressors, and blood transfusions. The physician should attempt to keep the urinary output at greater than 2 mL/kg/hour. Coagulation abnormalities and overt bleeding require blood products or vitamin K. Pregnant patients are treated in a fashion similar to any other patient with iron poisoning.

Hemodialysis and hemoperfusion are not effective. Exchange transfusion has been used in single cases of massive poisonings in children.

Disposition

The asymptomatic or minimally symptomatic patient should be observed for persistence and progression of symptoms or development of toxicity signs (gastrointestinal bleeding, acidosis, shock, altered mental state). Patients with mild self-limited gastrointestinal symptoms who become asymptomatic or have no signs of toxicity for 6 hours are unlikely to have a serious intoxication and can be discharged after psychiatric clearance, if needed. Patients with moderate or severe toxicity should be admitted to the intensive care unit.

Isoniazid

Isoniazid is a hydrazide derivative of vitamin B_3 (nicotinamide) and is used as an antituberculosis drug.

Toxic Mechanism

Isoniazid produces pyridoxine deficiency by increasing the excretion of pyridoxine (vitamin B_6) and by inhibiting pyridoxal 5-phosphate (the active form of pyridoxine) from acting with L-glutamic acid decarboxylase to form γ-aminobutyric acid (GABA), the major CNS neurotransmitter inhibitor, resulting in seizures. Isoniazid also blocks the conversion of lactate to pyruvate, resulting in profound and prolonged lactic acidosis.

Toxic Dose

The therapeutic dose is 5 to 10 mg/kg (maximum 300 mg) daily. A single acute dose of 15 mg/kg lowers the seizure threshold; 35 to 40 mg/kg produces spontaneous convulsions; more than 80 mg/kg produces severe toxicity. A fatal dose in adults is 4.5 to 15 g. The malnourished patients, those with a previous seizure disorder, alcoholic patients, and slow acetylators are more susceptible to isoniazid toxicity. In cases of chronic intoxication, 10 mg/kg/day produces hepatitis in 10% to 20% of patients but less than 2% at doses of 3 to 5 mg/kg/day.

Kinetics

Absorption from intestine occurs in 30 to 60 minutes, and onset is in 30 to 120 minutes, with peak levels of 5 to 8 μg/mL within 1 to 2 hours. Volume distribution is 0.6 L/kg, with minimal protein binding.

Elimination is by liver acetylation to a hepatotoxic metabolite, acetyl-isoniazid, which is then hydrolyzed to isonicotinic acid. In slow acetylators, isoniazid has a half-life of 140 to 460 minutes (mean 5 hours), and 10% to 15% is eliminated unchanged in the urine. Most (45% to 75%) whites and 50% of African blacks are slow acetylators, and, with chronic use (without pyridoxine supplements), they may develop peripheral neuropathy. In fast acetylators, isoniazid has a half-life of 35 to 110 minutes (mean 80 minutes), and 25% to 30% is excreted unchanged in the urine. About 90% of Asians and patients with diabetes mellitus are fast acetylators and may develop hepatitis on chronic use.

In patients with overdose and hepatic disease, the serum half-life may increase. Isoniazid inhibits the metabolism of phenytoin (Dilantin), diazepam, phenobarbital, carbamazepine (Tegretol), and prednisone. These drugs also interfere with the metabolism of isoniazid. Ethanol may decrease the half-life of isoniazid but increase its toxicity.

Manifestations

Within 30 to 60 minutes, nausea, vomiting, slurred speech, dizziness, visual disturbances, and ataxia are present. Within 30 to 120 minutes, the major clinical triad of severe overdose includes refractory convulsions (90% of overdose patients have one or more seizures), coma, and resistant severe lactic acidosis (secondary to convulsions), often with a plasma pH of 6.8.

Laboratory Investigations

Isoniazid produces anion gap metabolic acidosis. Therapeutic levels are 5 to 8 μg/mL and acute toxic levels are greater than 20 μg/mL. These levels are not readily available to assist in making decisions in acute overdose situations. One should monitor the blood glucose (often hyperglycemia), electrolytes (often hyperkalemia), bicarbonate, ABGs, liver function tests (elevations occur with chronic exposure), BUN, and creatinine.

Management

Seizures must be controlled. Pyridoxine and diazepam should be administered concomitantly through different IV sites. Pyridoxine (vitamin B_6) is given in a dose of 1 g for each gram of isoniazid ingested. If the dose ingested is unknown, at least 5 g of pyridoxine should be given intravenously. Pyridoxine is administered in 50 mL D_5W or 0.9% saline over 5 minutes intravenously. It must not be administered in the same bottle as sodium bicarbonate. Intravenous pyridoxine is repeated every 5 to 20 minutes until the seizures are controlled. Total doses of pyridoxine up to 52 g have been safely administered; however, patients given 132 and 183 g of pyridoxine have developed a persistent crippling sensory neuropathy.

Diazepam is administered concomitantly with pyridoxine but at a different site. They work synergistically. Diazepam should be administered intravenously slowly, 0.3 mg/kg at a rate of 1 mg/min in children or 10 mg at a rate of 5 mg/min in adults. After the seizures are controlled, the remainder of the pyridoxine is administered (1 g/1 g isoniazid) or a total dose of 5 g.

Phenobarbital or phenytoin are ineffective and should not be used.

In asymptomatic patients or patients without seizures, pyridoxine has been advised by some toxicologists prophylactically in gram-for-gram doses in cases of large overdoses (<80 mg/kg/dose) of isoniazid, although there are no studies to support this recommendation. In comatose patients, pyridoxine administration may result in the patient's rapid regaining of consciousness. Correction of acidosis may occur spontaneously with pyridoxine administration and correction of the seizures. Sodium bicarbonate should be administered if acidosis persists.

Hemodialysis is rarely needed because of antidotal therapy and the short half-life of isoniazid, but it may be used as an adjunct for cases of uncontrollable acidosis and seizures. Hemoperfusion has not been adequately evaluated. Diuresis is ineffective.

Disposition

Asymptomatic or mildly symptomatic patients who become asymptomatic can be observed in emergency department for 4 to 6 hours. Larger amounts of isoniazid may warrant pyridoxine administration and longer periods of observation. Intentional ingestions necessitate psychiatric evaluation before the patient is discharged. Patients with convulsions or coma should be admitted to the intensive care unit.

Isopropanol (Isopropyl Alcohol)

Isopropanol can be found in rubbing alcohol, solvents, and lacquer thinner. Coma has occurred in children sponged for fever with isopropanol. See Table 10 for ethanol features of alcohols and glycols.

Toxic Mechanism

Isopropanol is a gastric irritant. It is metabolized to acetone, a CNS and myocardial depressant. It inhibits gluconeogenesis. Normal propyl alcohol is related to isopropyl alcohol but is more toxic.

Toxic Dose

A toxic dose of 0.5 to 1 mg/kg of 70% isopropanol (1 mL/kg of 70%) produces a blood isopropanol plasma concentration of 70 mg/dL. The CNS depressant potency is twice that of ethanol.

Kinetics

Onset of action is within 30 to 60 minutes, and peak is 1 hour postingestion. Volume distribution is 0.6 kg/L. Isopropyl alcohol metabolizes to acetone. Its excretion is renal.

Note: The serum isopropyl concentration and amount ingested can be estimated using the same equation as is used in ethanol kinetics and substituting the specific gravity of 0.785 for isopropyl alcohol.

Manifestations

Ethanol-like inebriation occurs, with an acetone odor to the breath, gastritis, occasionally with hematemesis, acetonuria, and acetonemia without systemic acidosis.

Depression of the CNS occurs: lethargy at blood isopropyl alcohol levels of 50 to 100 mg/dL, coma at levels of 150 to 200 mg/dL, potentially death in adults at levels greater than 240 mg/dL.

Hypoglycemia and seizures may occur.

Laboratory Investigation

Monitoring of blood isopropyl alcohol levels (not readily available in all institutions), acetone, glucose, and ABG should be maintained. The osmolal gap increases 1 mOsm per 5.9 mg/dL of isopropyl alcohol and 1 mOsm per 5.5 mg/dL of acetone. The absence of excess acetone in the blood (normal is 0.3 to 2 mg/dL) within 30 to 60 minutes or excess acetone in the urine within 3 hours excludes the possibility of significant isopropanol exposure.

Management

The airway must be protected with intubation, and assisted ventilation administered if necessary. If the patient is hypoglycemic, glucose should be administered. Supportive treatment is similar to that for ethanol ingestions.

Gastrointestinal decontamination has no role in the treatment of isopropanol ingestion. Hemodialysis is warranted in cases of life-threatening overdose but is rarely needed. A nephrologist should be consulted if the blood isopropanol plasma concentration is greater than 250 mg/dL.

Disposition

Symptomatic patients with concentrations greater than 100 mg/dL require at least 24 hours of close observation for resolution and should be admitted. If the patient is hypoglycemic, hypotensive, or comatose, he or she should be admitted to the intensive care unit.

Lead

Acute lead intoxication is rare and usually occurs by inhalation of lead, resulting in severe intoxication and often death. Lead fumes can be produced by burning of lead batteries or use of a heat gun to remove lead paint. Acute lead intoxication also occurs from exposure to high concentrations of organic lead (e.g., tetraethyl lead).

Chronic lead poisoning occurs most often in children 6 months to 6 years of age who are exposed in their environment and in adults in certain occupations (Table 17). In the United States, the prevalence in children aged 1 to 5 years with a venous blood lead greater than 10 μg/dL decreased from 88.2% in a 1976–1980 survey to 8.9% in 1988–1991 survey due to measures to reduce lead in the environment, particularly leaded gasoline. However, an estimated 1.7 million children between 1 and 5 years of age and more than 1 million workers in over 100 different occupations still have blood lead levels greater than 10 μg/dL.

TABLE 17. **Occupations Associated with Lead Exposure**

Lead production or smelting	Demolition of ships and bridges
Production of illicit whiskey	Battery manufacturing
Brass, copper, and lead foundries	Machining/grinding lead alloys
Radiator repair	Welding of old painted metals
Scrap handling	Thermal paint stripping of old buildings
Sanding of old paint	Ceramic glaze/pottery mixing
Lead soldering	
Cable stripping	
Worker or janitor at a firing range	

Modified from Rempel D: The lead exposed worker. JAMA 262:533, 1989.

TABLE 18. **CDC Questionnaire: Priority Groups for Lead Screening**

1. Children age 6–72 mos (was 12–36 months) who live in or are frequent visitors to older deteriorated housing built before 1960.
2. Children aged 6–72 months who live in housing built prior to 1960 with recent, ongoing, or planned renovation or remodeling.
3. Children 6–72 months who are siblings, housemates, or playmates of children with known lead poisoning.
4. Children aged 6–72 months whose parents or other household members participate in a lead-related industry or hobby.
5. Children aged 6–72 months who live near active lead smelters, battery recycling plants, or other industries likely to result in atmospheric lead release.

Toxic Dose

In cases of chronic lead poisoning, a daily intake of more than 5 μg/kg/day in children or more than 150 μg/day in adults can give a positive lead balance. In 1991, the Centers for Disease Control and Prevention (CDC) recommended routine screening for all children younger than 6 years of age. In children a venous blood level greater than 10 μg/dL was determined to be a threshold of concern. The average venous blood level in the United States is 4 μg/dL. In cases of occupational exposure (see Table 17), a venous blood level greater than 40 μg/dL is indicative of increased lead absorption in adults.

Toxic Mechanism

Lead affects the sulfhydryl enzyme systems, the immature CNS, the enzymes of heme synthesis, vitamin D conversion, the kidneys, the bones, and growth. Lead alters the tertiary structure of cell proteins by denaturing them and causing cell death. Risk factors are mouthing behavior of infants and children and excessive oral behavior (pica), living in the inner city, a poorly maintained home, and poor nutrition (e.g., low calcium and iron). The CDC questionnaire given in Table 18 is recommended at every pediatric visit. If any answers to the CDC questionnaire are "positive," a blood screening test for lead should be administered. To be more accurate, however, identifying lead exposure studies have suggested that the questionnaire will have to be modified for each individual community because it has had poor sensitivity (40%) and specificity (60%) as it stands.

Table 19 lists sources of lead. The number one source is deteriorating lead-based paint, which forms leaded dust. Lead concentrations in indoor paint were not reduced to safer (0.06%) levels until 1978. Lead can also be produced by improper interior or exterior home renovation (scraping or demolition). It is found in pre-1960 built homes. The use of leaded gasoline (limited in 1973) resulted in residue from leaded motor vehicle emissions. Lead persists in the soil near major highways and in deteriorating homes and buildings. Vegetables grown in contaminated soil may contain lead.

Oil refineries and lead-processing smelters produce lead residue. Food cans produced in Mexico contain lead solder (95% do not in United States). Lead water pipes (until 1950) and lead solder (until 1986) deliver lead-containing drinking water (calcium deposits, however,

TABLE 19. **Sources of Lead**

Product	Lead Content (%) by Dry Weight
Paint	0.06
Solder	0.6
Plastic additives	2.0
Priming inks	2.0
Plumbing fixtures	2.0
Pesticides	0.1
Stained glass came	0.1
Wine bottle foils	0.1
Construction material	0.1
Fertilizers	0.1
Glazes, enamels	0.06
Toys/recreational games	0.1
Curtain weights	0.1
Fishing weights	0.1

may offer some protection). Water at a consumer's tap should be contain less than 15 ppb of lead (Table 20).

For occupational exposure, see Table 17. The Occupational Safety and Health Administration (OSHA) standards require employers to provide showering and clothes changing facilities for personnel working with lead; however, businesses with fewer than 25 employees are exempt from the regulation. The OSHA lead standard of 1978 set a limit of 60 µg/dL for occupational exposure to lead. At a blood lead level of 60 µg/dL, a worker should be removed from lead exposure and not allowed back until his or her lead level is below 40 µg/dL. Many authorities believe that this level should be lower. The lead residue on the clothes of the workers may represent a hazard to the family. Other occupations that are potential sources of lead exposure include plumbers, pipe fitters, lead miners, auto repairers, shipbuilders, printers, steel welders and cutters, construction workers, and rubber product manufacturers.

Leaded pots to make molds for "kusmusha" tea represent lead exposure. Imported pottery lined with ceramic glaze can leach large amounts of lead into acids (e.g., citrus fruit juices).

Hobbies associated with lead exposure are listed in Table 21. Some "traditional" folk remedies or cosmetics that contain lead include the following:

- "Azarcon por empacho" ("Maria Louisa" 90 to 95% lead trioxide): a bright orange powder used in Hispanic culture, especially Mexican, for digestive problems and diarrhea.
- "Greta" (4% to 90% lead): a yellow powder "por empacho" ("empacho" refers to a variety of gastrointestinal symptoms), used in Hispanic cultures, especially Mexican.
- "Pay-loo-ah": an orange-red powder used for rash and fever in Southeast Asian cultures, especially among Northern Laos Hmong immigrants.
- "Alkohl" (Al-kohl, kohl, suma 5% to 92% lead): a black powder used in Middle Eastern, African, and Asian cultures as a cosmetic and an umbilical stump astringent.
- "Farouk": an orange granular powder with lead used in Saudi Arabian culture.
- "Bint Al Zahab": used to treat colic in Saudi Arabian culture.
- "Surma" (23% to 26% lead): a black powder used in India as a cosmetic and to improve eyesight.
- "Bali goli": a round black bean that is dissolved in "grippe water," used by Asian and Indian cultures to aid digestion.

Cases of substance abuse involving lead poisoning have been reported, in which the patient sniffs leaded gasoline or uses improperly synthesized amphetamines.

Kinetics

Absorption of lead is 10% to 15% of the ingested dose in adults; in children, up to 40% is absorbed, especially in cases of iron deficiency anemia. With inhalation of fumes, absorption is rapid and complete. Volume distribution in blood (0.9% of total body burden) is 95% in red blood cells. Lead passes through the placenta to the fetus and is present in breast milk.

Organic lead is metabolized in the liver to inorganic lead. Its half-life is 35 to 40 days in blood; in soft tissue, the half-life is 45 days and in bone (99% of the

TABLE 20. **Agency Regulations and Recommendations Concerning Lead Content**

Agency	Specimen	Level	Comments
CDC	Blood (child)	10 µg/dL	Investigate community
OSHA	Blood (adult)	60 µg/dL	Medical removal from work
OSHA	Air	50 µg/m^3	PEL*
	Air	0.75 µg/m^3	Tetraethyl or tetramethyl
ACGIH	Air	150 µg/m^3	TWA†
EPA	Air	1.5 µg/m^3	Three-month average
EPA	Water	15 µg/L (ppb)	5 ppb circulating
EPA	Food	100 µg/day	Advisory
FDA	Wine	300 ppm	Plan to reduce to 200 ppm
EPA	Soil/dust	50 ppm	
CPSC	Paint	600 ppm (0.06%) by dry weight	

ACGIH = American Conference of Governmental Industrial Hygienists; CDC = Centers for Disease Control and Prevention; CPSC = Consumer Product Safety Commission; EPA = Environmental Protection Agency; FDA = Food and Drug Administration; OSHA = Occupational Safety and Health Administration.

*PEL = permissible exposure limit (highest level over an 8-hour workday).

†TWA= time weighted average (air concentration for 8-hour workday and 40 hour workweek).

TABLE 21. **Hobbies Associated with Lead Exposure**

Casting of ammunition	Print making and other fine arts (when lead white, flake white, chrome yellow pigments are involved)
Collecting antique pewter	Liquor distillation
Collecting/painting lead toys (i.e., soldiers and figures)	Hunting and target shooting
Ceramics or glazed pottery	Painting
Refinishing furniture	Car and boat repair
Making fishing weights	Burning/engraving lead-painted wood
Home renovation	Making stained leaded glass
Jewelry making, lead solder	Copper enameling
Glass blowing, lead glass	
Bronze casting	

lead), the half-life is 28 years. The major elimination route is the stool, 80% to 90%, and then renal 10% (80 g/day) and hair, nails, sweat, and saliva. Nine percent of organic lead is excreted in the urine per day.

Manifestations

Adverse health effects are given in Table 22 and include the following.

Hematologic. Lead inhibits γ-aminolevulinic acid dehydratase (early in the synthesis of heme) and ferrochelatase (transfers iron to ferritin for incorporation of iron into protoporphyrin to produce heme). Anemia is a late finding. Decreased heme synthesis starts at >40 μg/dL. Basophilic stippling occurs in 20% of severe lead poisoning.

Neurologic. Segmental demyelination and peripheral neuropathy, usually of the motor type (wrist and ankle drop) occurs in workers. A venous blood level of lead greater than 70 μg/dL (usually >100 μg/dL), produces encephalopathy in children (symptom mnemonic "PAINT": P, persistent forceful vomiting and papilledema; A, ataxia; I, intermittent stupor and lucidity; N, neurologic coma and refractory convulsions; T, tired and lethargic). Decreased cognitive abilities have been reported with a venous blood level of lead greater than 10 μg/dL, including behavioral problems, decreased attention span, and learning disabilities. IQ scores may begin to decrease at 15 μg/dL. Encephalopathy is rare in adults.

Renal. Nephropathy due to damaged capillaries and glomerulus can occur at a venous blood level of lead greater than 80 μg/dL, but recent studies show renal damage and hypertension with low venous blood levels. A direct correlation between hypertension and venous blood level over 30 μg/dL has been reported. Lead reduces excretion of uric acid, and high-level exposure may be associated with hyperuricemia and "saturnine gout," Fanconi's syndrome (aminoaciduria and renal tubular acidosis), and tubular fibrosis.

Reproductive. Spontaneous abortion, transient delay in the child's development (catch up at age 5 to 6 years), decreased sperm count, and abnormal sperm morphology can occur with lead exposure. Lead crosses the placenta and fetal blood levels reach 75 to 100% of maternal blood levels. Lead is teratogenic.

Metabolic. Decreased cytochrome P-450 activity alters the metabolism of medication and endogenously produced substances. Decreased activation of cortisol and decreased growth due to interference in vitamin conversion (25-hydroxyvitamin D to 1,25 hydroxyvitamin D) at venous blood levels of 20 to 30 μg/dL.

Other Manifestations. Abnormalities of thyroid, cardiac, and hepatic function occur in adults. Abdominal colic is seen in children at doses greater than 50 μg/dL. "Lead gum lines" at the dental border of the gingiva can occur in cases of chronic lead poisoning.

TABLE 22. **Summary of Lead-Induced Health Effects in Adults and Children**

Blood lead level (μg/dL)	Age group	Health Effect
>100	Adult	Encephalopathic signs and symptoms
>80	Adult	Anemia
	Child	Encephalopathy
		Chronic nephropathy (e.g., aminoaciduria)
>70	Adult	Clinically evident peripheral neuropathy
	Child	Colic and other gastrointestinal symptoms
>60	Adult	Female reproductive effects
		CNS disturbance symptoms (i.e., sleep disturbances, mood changes, memory and concentration problems, headaches)
>50	Adult	Decreased hemoglobin production
		Decreased performance on neurobehavioral tests
	Adult	Altered testicular function
		Gastrointestinal symptoms (i.e., abdominal pain, constipation, diarrhea, nausea, anorexia)
	Child	Peripheral neuropathy*
>40	Adult	Decreased peripheral nerve conduction
		Hypertension, aged 40–59 yrs
		Chronic neuropathy*
>25	Adult	Elevated erythrocyte protoporphyrin in males
15–25	Adult	Elevated erythrocyte protoporphyrin in females
	Child	Decreased intelligence and growth
>10		Impaired learning
		Reduced birth weight*
		Impaired mental ability
	Fetus	Preterm delivery*

*Controversial.
From MMWR 41:288, 1992.

Laboratory Investigations

Serial venous blood lead measurements are taken on days 3 and 5 during treatment and 7 days after chelation therapy, then every 1 to 2 weeks for 8 weeks, and then every month for 6 months. Intravenous infusion should be stopped at least 1 hour before blood lead levels are measured. Table 23 gives a classification of blood lead concentrations in children.

One should evaluate CBC, serum ferritin, erythrocyte protoporphyrin (>35 μg/dL indicates lead poisoning as well as iron deficiency and other causes), electrolytes, serum calcium and phosphorus, urinalysis, BUN, and creatinine. Abdominal and long bone radiographs may be useful in certain circumstances to identify radiopaque material in bowel and "lead lines" in proximal tibia

TABLE 23. **Classification of Blood Lead Concentrations in Children**

Blood Lead (μg/dL)	Recommended Interventions
<9	None
10–14	Community intervention Repeat blood lead in 3 months
15–19	Individual case management Environmental counseling Nutritional counseling Repeat blood lead in 3 months
20–44	Medical referral Environmental inspection/abatement Nutritional counseling Repeat blood lead in 3 months
45–69	Environmental inspection/abatement Nutritional counseling Pharmacologic therapy DMSA succimer oral or $CaNa_2EDTA$ parenteral Repeat every 2 weeks for 6–8 weeks, then monthly for 4–6 months
>70	Hospitalization in intensive care unit Environmental inspection/abatement Pharmacologic therapy Dimercaprol (BAL in oil) IM initial alone Dimercaprol IM and $CaNa_2EDTA$ together Repeat every week

IM = intramuscular.

(which occur after prolonged exposure in association with venous blood lead levels greater than 50 μg/dL).

Neuropsychological tests are difficult to perform in young children but should be considered at the end of treatment, especially to determine auditory dysfunction.

Management

The basis of treatment is removal of the source of lead. Cases of poisoning in children should be reported to local health department and cases of occupational poisoning should be reported to OSHA. The source must be identified and abated, and dust controlled by wet mopping. Cold water should be let to run for 2 minutes before being used for drinking. Planting shrubbery (not vegetables) in contaminated soil will keep children away.

Supportive care should be instituted, including measures to deal with refractory seizures (continued antidotal therapy, diazepam, and possibly neuromuscular blockers), with the hepatic and renal failure, and intravascular hemolysis in severe cases. Seizures are treated with diazepam followed by neuromuscular blockers if needed.

Lead does not bind to activated charcoal. One must not delay chelation therapy for complete gastrointestinal decontamination in severe cases. Whole-bowel irrigation has been used prior to treatment. Some authorities recommend abdominal radiographs followed by gastrointestinal decontamination if necessary before switching to oral therapy. Chelation therapy can be used for patients in whom venous blood level of lead is greater than 45 μg/dL in children and greater than 80 μg/dL in adults or in adults with lower levels who are symptomatic or who have a "positive" lead mobilization test result (not routinely performed at most centers) (Table 24).

Succimer (dimercaptosuccinic acid, DMSA, Chemet), a derivative of BAL, is an oral agent for chelation in children with a venous blood level of greater than 45 μg/dL. The recommended dose is 10 mg/kg every 8 hours for 5 days, then every 12 hours for 14 days. DMSA is under investigation to determine its role in children with a venous blood level less than 45 μg/dL. Although not approved for adults, it has been used in the same dosage. Monitoring should be maintained by CBC, liver transaminases, and urinalysis for adverse effects.

D-Penicillamine (Cuprimine) is another oral chelator that is given in doses of 20 to 40 mg/kg/day not to exceed 1 g/day. However, it is not FDA approved and has a 10% adverse reaction rate. Nevertheless, D-penicillamine has been used infrequently in adults and children with elevated venous blood lead levels.

Edetate calcium disodium (ethylene diaminetetraacetic acid or $CaNa_2EDTA$ Versenate) is a water-soluble chelator given intramuscularly (with 0.5% procaine) or intravenously. The calcium in the compound is displaced by divalent and trivalent heavy metals, forming a soluble complex, which is stable at physiologic pH (but not at acid pH) and enhances lead clearance in

TABLE 24. **Pharmacologic Chelation Therapy of Lead Poisoning**

Drug	Route	Dose	Duration	Precautions	Monitor
Dimercaprol (BAL in oil)	IM	3–5 mg/kg q4–6 h	3–5 days	G6PD deficiency Concurrent iron therapy	AST/ALT enzymes
$CaNa_2EDTA$ (calcium disodium. versenate)	IM/IV	50 mg/kg per day	5 days	Inadequate fluid intake Renal impairment Penicillin allergy	Urinalysis, BUN Creatinine Urinalysis, BUN
D-Penicillamine (Cuprimine)	PO	10 mg/kg per day increase 30 mg/kg over 2 wks	6–20 wks	Concurrent iron therapy; lead exposure Renal impairment	Creatinine, CBC
2, 3-Dimercaptosuccinic acid (DMSA; succimer)	PO	10 mg/kg per dose tid, 10 mg/kg per dose bid 14 days	19 days	AST/ALT Concurrent iron therapy G6PD deficiency lead exposure	AST/ALT

ALT = alanine aminotransferase; AST = aspartate transaminase; BAL = British antilewisite; BUN= blood urea nitrogen; G6PD = glucose-6-phosphate dehydrogenase.

the urine. EDTA usually is administered intravenously, especially in severe cases. It must not be administered until adequate urine flow is established. It may redistribute lead to the brain; therefore, BAL may be given first at a venous blood lead level of greater than 55 μg/dL in children and greater than 100 μg/dL in adults. Phlebitis occurs at a concentration greater than 0.5 mg/mL. Alkalinization of the urine may be helpful. $CaNa_2EDTA$ should *not* be confused with sodium EDTA (disodium edetate), which is used to treat hypercalcemia; inadvertent use may produce severe hypocalcemia.

Dimercaprol (BAL, British antilewisite) is a peanut oil–based dithiol (two sulfhydryl molecules) that combines with one atom of lead to form a heterocyclic stable ring complex. It is usually reserved for patients in whom venous blood lead is greater than 70 μg/dL, and it chelates red blood cell lead, enhancing its elimination through the urine and bile. It crosses the blood-brain barrier. About 50% of patients have adverse reactions, including bad metallic taste in the mouth, pain at the injection site, sterile abscesses, and fever.

A venous blood lead level greater than 70 μg/dL or the presence of clinical symptoms suggesting encephalopathy in children is a potentially life-threatening emergency. Management should be accomplished in a medical center with a pediatric intensive care unit by a multidisciplinary team including a critical care specialist, a toxicologist, a neurologist, and a neurosurgeon. Careful monitoring of neurologic status, fluid status, and intracranial pressure should be undertaken if necessary. These patients need close monitoring for hemodynamic instability. Hydration should be maintained to ensure renal excretion of lead. Fluids, renal and hepatic function, and electrolyte levels should be monitored.

While waiting for adequate urine flow, therapy should be initiated with intramuscular dimercaprol (BAL) only (25 mg/kg/day divided into 6 doses). Four hours later, the second dose of BAL should be given intramuscularly, concurrently with $CaNa_2EDTA$ 50 mg/kg/day as a single dose infused over several hours or as a continuous infusion. The double therapy is continued until the venous blood level is less than 40 μg/dL.

As long as the venous blood level is greater than 40 μg/dL, therapy is continued for 72 hours and followed by two alternatives: either parenteral therapy with two drugs ($CaNa_2EDTA$ and BAL) for 5 days or continuation of therapy with $CaNa_2EDTA$ alone if a good response is achieved and the venous blood level of lead is less than 40 μg/dL. If one cannot get the venous blood lead report back, one should continue therapy with both BAL and EDTA for 5 days. In patients with lead encephalopathy, parenteral chelation should be continued with both drugs until the patient is clinically stable before changing therapy. Mannitol and dexamethasone can reduce the cerebral edema, but their role in lead encephalopathy is not clear. Surgical decompression is not recommended to reduce cerebral edema in these cases.

If BAL and $CaNa_2EDTA$ are used together, a minimum of 2 days with no treatment should elapse before another 5 day course of therapy is considered. The 5-day course is repeated with $CaNa_2EDTA$ alone if the blood lead level rebounds to greater than 40 μg/dL or in combination with BAL if the venous blood level is greater than 70 μg/dL. If a third course is required, unless there are compelling reasons, one should wait at least 5 to 7 days before administering the course.

Following chelation therapy, a period of equilibration of 10 to 14 days should be allowed and a repeat venous blood lead concentration should be obtained. If the patient is stable enough for oral intake, oral succimer 30 mg/kg/day in three divided doses for 5 days followed by 20 mg/kg/day in two divided doses for 14 days has been suggested, but there are limited data to support this recommendation. Therapy should be continued until venous blood lead level is less than 20 μg/dL in children or less than 40 μg/dL in adults.

Chelators combined with lead are hemodialyzable in the event of renal failure.

Disposition

All patients with a venous blood lead level of greater than 70 μg/dL or who are symptomatic should be admitted. If a child is hospitalized, all lead hazards must be removed from the home environment before allowing the child to return. The source must be eliminated by environmental and occupational investigations. The local health department should be involved in dealing with children who are lead poisoned, and OSHA should be involved with cases of occupational lead poisoning. Consultation with a poison control center or experienced toxicologist is necessary when chelating patients. Follow-up venous blood lead concentrations should be obtained within 1 to 2 weeks and followed every 2 weeks for 6 to 8 weeks, then monthly for 4 to 6 months if the patient required chelation therapy. All patients with venous blood level greater than 10 μg/dL should be followed at least every 3 months until two venous blood lead concentrations are 10 μg/dL or three are less than 15 μg/dL.

Lithium (Eskalith, Lithane)

Lithium is an alkali metal used primarily in the treatment of bipolar psychiatric disorders. Most intoxications are cases of chronic overdose. One gram of lithium carbonate contains 189 mg (5.1 mEq) of lithium; a regular tablet contains 300 mg (8.12 mEq) and a sustained-release preparation contains 450 mg or 12.18 mEq.

Toxic Mechanism

The brain is the primary target organ of toxicity, but the mechanism is unclear. Lithium may interfere with physiologic functions by acting as a substitute for cellular cations (sodium and potassium), depressing neural excitation and synaptic transmission.

Toxic Dose

A dose of 1 mEq/kg (40 mg/kg) of lithium will give a peak serum lithium concentration about 1.2 mEq/L. The therapeutic serum lithium concentration in cases of acute mania is 0.6 to 1.2 mEq/L, and for maintenance it is 0.5 to 0.8 mEq/L. Serum lithium concentration levels are usually obtained 12 hours after the last dose. The toxic dose is determined by clinical manifestations and serum levels after the distribution phase.

Acute ingestion of 20 300-mg tablets (300 mg increases the serum lithium concentration by 0.2 to 0.4 mEq/L) in adults may produce serious intoxication. Chronic intoxication can be produced by conditions listed below that can decrease the elimination of lithium or increase lithium reabsorption in the kidney.

The risk factors that predispose to chronic lithium toxicity are febrile illness, impaired renal function, hyponatremia, advanced age, lithium-induced diabetes insipidus, dehydration, vomiting and diarrhea, and concomitant use of other drugs, such as thiazide and spironolactone diuretics, nonsteroidal anti-inflammatory drugs, salicylates, angiotensin-converting enzyme inhibitors (e.g., captopril), serotonin reuptake inhibitors (e.g., fluoxetine [Prozac]), and phenothiazines.

Kinetics

Gastrointestinal absorption of regular-release preparations is rapid; serum lithium concentration peaks in 2 to 4 hours and is complete by 6 to 8 hours. The onset of toxicity may occur at 1 to 4 hours after acute overdose but usually is delayed because lithium enters the brain slowly. Absorption of sustained-release preparations and the development of toxicity may be delayed 6 to 12 hours.

Volume distribution is 0.5 to 0.9 L/kg. Lithium is not protein bound. The half-life after a single dose is 9 to 13 hours; at steady state, it may be 30 to 58 hours. The renal handling of lithium is similar to that of sodium: glomerular filtration and reabsorption (80%) by the proximal renal tubule. Adequate sodium must be present to prevent lithium reabsorption. More than 90% of lithium is excreted by the kidney, 30% to 60% within 6 to 12 hours.

Manifestations

The examiner must distinguish between side effects, acute intoxication, acute or chronic toxicity, and chronic intoxications. Chronic is the most common and dangerous type of intoxication.

Side effects include fine tremor, gastrointestinal upset, hypothyroidism, polyuria and frank diabetes insipidus, dermatologic manifestations, and cardiac conduction deficits. Lithium is teratogenic.

Patients with acute poisoning may be asymptomatic, with an early high serum lithium concentration of 9 mEq/L, and deteriorate as the serum lithium concentration falls by 50% and the lithium distributes to the brain and the other tissues. Nausea and vomiting may occur within 1 to 4 hours, but the systemic manifestations are usually delayed several more hours. It may take as long as 3 to 5 days for serious symptoms to develop. Acute toxicity and acute on chronic toxicity are manifested by neurologic findings, including weakness, fasciculations, altered mental state, myoclonus, hyperreflexia, rigidity, coma, and convulsions with limbs in hypertension. Cardiovascular effects are nonspecific and occur at therapeutic doses, flat T or inverted T waves, atrioventricular block, and prolonged QT interval. Lithium is not a primary cardiotoxin. Cardiogenic shock occurs secondary to CNS toxicity. Chronic intoxication is associated with manifestations at lower serum lithium concentrations. There is some correlation with manifestations, especially at higher serum lithium concentrations. Although the levels do not always correlate with the manifestations, they are more predictive in cases of severe intoxication. A serum lithium concentration greater than 3.0 mEq/L with chronic intoxication and altered mental state indicates severe toxicity. Permanent neurologic sequelae can result from lithium intoxication.

Laboratory Investigations

Monitoring should include CBC (lithium causes significant leukocytosis), renal function, thyroid function (chronic intoxication), ECG, and electrolytes. Serum lithium concentrations should be determined every 2 to 4 hours until levels are close to therapeutic range. Cross-reactions with green-top Vacutainer specimen tubes containing heparin will spuriously elevate serum lithium concentration 6 to 8 mEq/L.

Management

Vital function must be established and maintained. Seizure precautions should be instituted and seizures, hypotension, and dysrhythmias treated. Evaluation should include examination for rigidity and hyperreflexia signs, hydration, renal function (BUN, creatinine), and electrolytes, especially sodium. The examiner should inquire about diuretic and other drug use that increase serum lithium concentration, and the patient must discontinue the drugs. If the patient is on chronic therapy, the lithium should be discontinued. Serial serum lithium concentrations should be obtained every 4 hours until serum lithium concentration peaks and there is a downward trend toward almost therapeutic range, especially in sustained-release preparations. Vital signs should be monitored, including temperature, and ECG and serial neurologic examinations should be undertaken, including mental status and urinary output. Nephrology consultation is warranted in case of a chronic and elevated serum lithium concentration (>2.5 mEq/L), a large ingestion, or altered mental state.

An intravenous line should be established and hydration and electrolyte balance restored. Serum sodium level should be determined before 0.9% saline fluid is administered in patients with chronic overdose because hypernatremia may be present from diabetes insipidus. Although current evidence supports an initial 0.9% saline infusion (200 mL/h) to enhance excretion of lithium, once hydration, urine output, and normonatremia are established, one should administer 0.45% saline and slow the infusion (100 mL/h) for all patients.

Gastric lavage is often not recommended in cases of acute ingestion because of the large size of the tablets, and it is not necessary after chronic intoxication. Activated charcoal is ineffective. For sustained-release preparations, whole-bowel irrigation may be useful but is not proven. Sodium polystyrene sulfonate (Kayexalate), an ion exchange resin, is difficult to administer and has been used only in uncontrolled studies. Its use is not recommended.

Hemodialysis is the most efficient method for removing lithium from the vascular compartment. It is the treatment of choice for patients with severe intoxication with an altered mental state, those with seizures, and anuric patients. Long runs are used until the serum lithium concentration is less than 1 mEq/L because of extensive re-equilibration. Serum lithium concentration should be monitored every 4 hours after dialysis for rebound. Repeated and prolonged hemodialysis may be necessary. A lag in neurologic recovery can be expected.

Disposition

An acute asymptomatic lithium overdose cannot be medically cleared on the basis of single lithium level. Patients should be admitted if they have any neurologic manifestations (altered mental status, hyperreflexia, stiffness, or tremor). Patients should be admitted to the intensive care unit if they are dehydrated, have renal impairment, or have a high or rising lithium level.

Methanol (Wood Alcohol, Methyl Alcohol)

The concentration of methanol in Sterno fuel is 4% and it contains ethanol, in windshield washer fluid it is 30 to 60%, and in gas-line antifreeze it is 100%.

Toxic Mechanism

Methanol is metabolized by alcohol dehydrogenase to formaldehyde, which is metabolized to formate. Formate inhibits cytochrome oxidase, producing tissue hypoxia, lactic acidosis, and optic nerve edema. Formate is converted by folate-dependent enzymes to carbon dioxide.

Toxic Dose

The minimal toxic amount is approximately 100 mg/kg. Serious toxicity in a young child can be produced by the ingestion of 2.5 to 5.0 mL of 100% methanol. Ingestion of 5-mL 100% methanol by a 10-kg child produces estimated peak blood methanol of 80 mg/dL. Ingestion of 15 mL 40% methanol was lethal for a 2-year-old child in one report. A fatal adult oral dose is 30 to 240 mL 100% (20 to 150 g). Ingestion of 6 to 10 mL 100% causes blindness in adults. The toxic blood concentration is greater than 20 mg/dL; very serious toxicity and potential fatality occur at levels greater than 50 mg/dL.

Kinetics

Onset of action can start within 1 hour but may be delayed up to 12 to 18 hours by metabolism to toxic metabolites. It may be delayed longer if ethanol is ingested concomitantly or in infants. Peak blood methanol concentration is 1 hour. Volume distribution is 0.6 L/kg (total body water).

For metabolism, see Toxic Mechanism.

Elimination is through metabolism. The half-life of methanol is 8 hours, with ethanol blocking it is 30 to 35 hours, and with hemodialysis 2.5 hours.

Manifestations

Metabolism creates a delay in onset for 12 to 18 hours or longer if ethanol is ingested concomitantly. Initial findings are as follows:

- 0 to 6 hours: Confusion, ataxia, inebriation, formaldehyde odor on breath, and abdominal pain can be present, but the patient may be asymptomatic. Note: Methanol produces an osmolal gap (early), and its metabolite formate produces the anion gap metabolic acidosis (see later). Absence of osmolar or anion gap does not always exclude methanol intoxication.
- 6 to 12 hours: Malaise, headache, abdominal pain, vomiting, visual symptoms, including hyperemia of optic disc, "snow vision," and blindness can be seen.
- More than 12 hours: Worsening acidosis, hyperglycemia, shock, and multiorgan failure develop, with death from complications of intractable acidosis and cerebral edema.

Laboratory Investigation

Methanol can be detected on some chromatography drug screens if specified. Methanol and ethanol levels, electrolytes, glucose, BUN, creatinine, amylase, and ABG should be monitored every 4 hours. Formate levels correlate more closely than blood methanol concentration with severity of intoxication and should be obtained if possible.

Management

One should protect the airway by intubation to prevent aspiration and administer assisted ventilation as needed. If needed, 100% oxygen can be administered. A nephrologist should be consulted early regarding the need for hemodialysis.

Gastrointestinal decontamination procedures have no role.

Metabolic acidosis should be treated vigorously with sodium bicarbonate 2 to 3 mEq/kg intravenously. Large amounts may be needed.

Antidote therapy is initiated to inhibit metabolism if the patient has a history of ingesting more than 0.4 mL/kg of 100% with the following conditions:

- Blood methanol level is greater than 20 mg/dL
- The patient has osmolar gap not accounted for by other factors
- The patient is symptomatic or acidotic with increased anion gap and/or hyperemia of the optic disc.

The ethanol or fomepizole therapy outlined below can be used:

Ethanol Therapy. Ethanol should be initiated immediately if fomepizole is unavailable (see fomepizole therapy). Alcohol dehydrogenase has a greater affinity for ethanol than ethylene glycol. Therefore, ethanol blocks the metabolism of ethylene glycol.

Ethanol should be administered intravenously (oral administration is less reliable) to produce a blood ethanol concentration of 100 to 150 mg/dL. The loading dose is 10 mL/kg of 10% ethanol administered intravenously concomitantly with a maintenance dose of 10% ethanol at 1.0 mL/kg/h. This dose may need to be increased to 2 mL/kg/h in patients who are heavy drinkers. The blood ethanol concentration should be measured hourly and the infusion rate should be adjusted to maintain a concentration of 100 to 150 mg/dL.

Fomepizole Therapy. Fomepizole (Antizol, 4-methylpyrazole) inhibits alcohol dehydrogenase more reliably than ethanol and it does not require constant monitoring of ethanol levels and adjustment of infusion rates. Fomepizole is available in 1 g/mL vials of 1.5 mL. The loading dose is 15 mg/kg (0.015 mL/kg) IV, maintenance dose is 10 mg/kg (0.01 mL/kg) every 12 hours for 4 doses, then 15 mg/kg every 12 hours until the ethylene glycol levels are less than 20 mg/dL. The solution is prepared by being mixed with 100 mL of 0.9% saline or D_5W. Fomepizole can be given to patients requiring hemodialysis but should be dosed as follows:

Dose at the beginning of hemodialysis:

- If less than 6 hours since last Antizol dose, do not administer dose
- If more than 6 hours since last dose, administer next scheduled dose

Dosing during hemodialysis:

- Dose every 4 hours

Dosing at the time hemodialysis is completed:

- If less than 1 hour between last dose and end dialysis, do not administer dose at end of dialysis
- If 1 to 3 hours between last dose and end dialysis, administer one half of next scheduled dose
- If more than 3 hours between last dose and end dialysis, administer next scheduled dose

Maintenance dosing off hemodialysis:

- Give the next scheduled dose 12 hours from the last dose administered

Hemodialysis increases the clearance of both methanol and formate 10-fold over renal clearance. A blood methanol concentration greater than 50 mg/dL has been used as an indication for hemodialysis, but recently some toxicologists from the New York City Poison Center recommended early hemodialysis in patients with blood methanol concentration greater than 25 mg/dL because it may be able to shorten the course of intoxication if started early. One should continue to monitor methanol levels and/or formate levels every 4 hours after the procedure for rebound. Other indications for early hemodialysis are significant metabolic acidosis and electrolyte abnormalities despite conventional therapy and if visual or neurologic signs or symptoms are present.

A serum formate level greater than 20 mg/dL has also been used as a criterion for hemodialysis, although this is often not readily available through many laboratories. If hemodialysis is used, the infusion rate of 10% ethanol should be increased 2.0 to 3.5 mL/kg/hour. The blood ethanol concentration and glucose level should be obtained every 2 hours.

Therapy is continued with both ethanol and hemodialysis until the blood methanol level is undetectable, there is no acidosis, and the patient has no neurologic or visual disturbances. This may require several days.

Hypoglycemia is treated with intravenous glucose. Doses of folinic acid (Leucovorin) and folic acid have been used successfully in animal investigations to enhance formate metabolism to carbon dioxide and water. Leucovorin 1 mg/kg up to 50 mg IV is administered every 4 hours for several days.

An initial ophthalmologic consultation and follow-up are warranted.

Disposition

All patients who have ingested significant amounts of methanol should be referred to the emergency department for evaluation and blood methanol concentration measurement. Ophthalmologic follow-up of all patients with methanol intoxications should be arranged.

Monoamine Oxidase Inhibitors

Nonselective monoamine oxidase inhibitors (MAOIs) include the hydrazines phenelzine (Nardil) and isocarboxazid (Marplan), and the nonhydrazine tranylcypromine (Parnate). Furazolidone (Furoxone) and pargyline (Eutonyl)* are also considered nonselective MAOIs. Moclobemide,* which is available in many countries but not the United States, is a selective MAO-A inhibitor. MAO-B inhibitors include selegiline (Eldepryl), an antiparksonism agent, which does not have similar toxicity to MAO-A and is not discussed. Selectivity is lost in an overdose. MAOIs are used to treat severe depression.

Toxic Mechanism

Monoamine oxidase enzymes are responsible for the oxidative deamination of both endogenous and exogenous catecholamines such as norepinephrine. MAO-A in the intestinal wall also metabolizes tyramine in food. MAOIs permanently inhibit MAO enzymes until a new enzyme is synthesized after 14 days or longer. The toxicity results from the accumulation, potentiation, and prolongation of the catecholamine action followed by profound hypotension and cardiovascular collapse.

Toxic Dose

Toxicity begins at 2 to 3 mg/kg and fatalities occur at 4 to 6 mg/kg. Death has occurred after a single dose of 170 mg of tranylcypromine in an adult.

Kinetics

Structurally, MAOIs are related to amphetamines and catecholamines. The hydrazines peak levels are at 1 to 2 hours; metabolism is hepatic acetylation; and

*Not available in the United States.

inactive metabolites are excreted in the urine. For the nonhydrazines, peak levels occur at 1 to 4 hours, and metabolism is via the liver to active amphetamine-like metabolites.

The onset of symptoms in a case of overdose is delayed 6 to 24 hours after ingestion, peak activity is 8 to 12 hours, and duration is 72 hours or longer. The peak of MAO inhibition is in 5 to 10 days and lasts as long as 5 weeks.

Manifestations

Manifestations of an acute ingestion overdose of MAO-A inhibitors are as follows:

Phase I. An adrenergic crisis occurs, with delayed onset for 6 to 24 hours, and may not reach peak until 24 hours. The crisis starts as hyperthermia, tachycardia, tachypnea, dysarthria, transient hypertension, hyperreflexia, and CNS stimulation.

Phase II. Neuromuscular excitation and sympathetic hyperactivity occur with increased temperature greater than 40° C (104° F), agitation, hyperactivity, confusion, fasciculations, twitching, tremor, masseter spasm, muscle rigidity, acidosis, and electrolyte abnormalities. Seizures and dystonic reactions may occur. The pupils are mydriatic, sometimes nonreactive with "ping-pong gaze."

Phase III. CNS depression and cardiovascular collapse occur in cases of severe overdose as the catecholamines are depleted. Symptoms usually resolve within 5 days but may last 2 weeks.

Phase IV. Secondary complications occur, including rhabdomyolysis, cardiac dysrhythmias, multiorgan failure, and coagulopathies.

Biogenic interactions usually occur while the patient is on therapeutic doses of MAOI or shortly after they are discontinued (30 to 60 minutes), before the new MAO enzyme is synthesized. The following substances have been implicated: indirect acting sympathomimetics such as amphetamines, serotonergic drugs, opioids (e.g., meperidine, dextromethorphan), tricyclic antidepressants, specific serotonin reuptake inhibitors (SSRI; e.g., fluoxetine [Prozac], sertraline [Zoloft], paroxetine [Paxil]), tyramine-containing foods (e.g., wine, beer, avocados, cheese, caviar, chocolate, chicken liver), and L-tryptophan. SSRIs should not be started for at least 5 weeks after MAOIs have been discontinued.

In mild cases, usually caused by foods, headache and hypertension develop and last for several hours. In severe cases, malignant hypertension and severe hyperthermia syndromes consisting of hypertension or hyperthermia, altered mental state, skeletal muscle rigidity, shivering (often beginning in the masseter muscle), and seizures may occur.

The serotonin syndrome, which may be due to inhibition of serotonin metabolism, has similar clinical findings to those of malignant hyperthermia and may occur with or without hyperthermia or hypertension.

Chronic toxicity clinical findings include tremors, hyperhidrosis, agitation, hallucinations, confusion, and seizures and may be confused with withdrawal syndromes.

Laboratory Investigations

Monitoring of the ECG, cardiac monitoring, CPK, ABG, pulse oximeter, electrolytes, blood glucose, and acid-base balance should be maintained.

Management

In the case of MAOI overdose, ipecac-induced emesis should not be used. Only activated charcoal alone should be used.

If the patient is admitted to the hospital and is well enough to eat, a nontyramine diet should be ordered.

Extreme agitation and seizures can be controlled with benzodiazepines and barbiturates. Phenytoin is ineffective. Nondepolarizing neuromuscular blockers (not depolarizing succinylcholine) may be needed in severe cases of hyperthermia and rigidity. If the patient has severe hypertension (catecholamine mediated), phentolamine (Regitine), a parenteral β-blocking agent, 3 to 5 mg intravenously, or labetalol (Normodyne), a combination of an α-blocking agent and a β-blocker, 20 mg intravenous bolus, should be given. If malignant hypertension with rigidity is present, a short-acting nitroprusside and benzodiazepine can be used. Hypertension is often followed by severe hypotension, which should be managed by fluid and vasopressors. Caution: Vasopressor therapy should be administered at lower doses than usual because of exaggerated pharmacologic response. Norepinephrine is preferred to dopamine, which requires release of intracellular amines.

Cardiac dysrhythmias are treated with standard therapy but are often refractory, and cardioversion and pacemakers may be needed.

For malignant hyperthermia, dantrolene (Dantrium), a nonspecific peripheral skeletal relaxing agent, is administered, which inhibits the release of calcium from the sarcoplasm. Dantrolene is reconstituted with 60 mL sterile water without bacteriostatic agents. Glass equipment must not be used, and the drug must be protected from light and used within 6 hours. Loading dose is 2 to 3 mg/kg intravenously as a bolus, and the loading dose is repeated until the signs of malignant hyperthermia (tachycardia, rigidity, increased end-tidal CO_2, and temperature) are controlled. Maximum total dose is 10 mg/kg to avoid hepatotoxicity.

When malignant hyperthermia has subsided, 1 mg/kg IV is given every 6 hours for 24 to 48 hours, then orally 1 mg/kg every 6 hours for 24 hours to prevent recurrence. There is a danger of thrombophlebitis following peripheral dantrolene, and it should be administered through a central line if possible. In addition one should administer external cooling and correct metabolic acidosis and electrolyte disturbances. Benzodiazepine can be used for sedation. Dantrolene does not reverse central dopamine blockade; therefore, bromocriptine mesylate (Parlodel) 2.5 to 10 mg should be given orally or through a nasogastric tube three times a day.

Rhabdomyolysis and myoglobinuria are treated with fluids. Urine alkalinization should also be treated.

Hemodialysis and hemoperfusion are of no proven value.

Biogenic amine interactions are managed symptomatically, similar to cases of overdose. For the serotonin syndrome cyproheptadine (Periactin), a serotonin blocker, 4 mg orally every hour for three doses, or methysergide (Sansert), 2 mg orally every 6 hours for three doses, should be considered. The effectiveness of these drugs has not been proven.

Disposition

All patients who have ingested more than 2 mg/kg of an MAOI should be admitted to the hospital for 24 hours of observation and monitoring in the intensive care unit because the life-threatening manifestations may be delayed. Patients with drug or dietary interactions that are mild may not require admission if symptoms subside within 4 to 6 hours and the patients remain asymptomatic. Patients with symptoms that persist or require active intervention should be admitted to the intensive care unit.

Opioids (Narcotic Opiates)

Opioids are used for analgesia, as antitussives, and as antidiarrheal agents and are illicit agents (heroin, opium) used in substance abuse. Tolerance, physical dependency, and withdrawal may develop.

Toxic Mechanism

At least four main opioid receptors have been identified. The μ receptor is considered the most important for central analgesia and CNS depression. The κ and δ receptors predominate in spinal analgesia. The σ receptors may mediate dysphoria. Death is due to dose-dependent CNS respiratory depression or secondary to pulmonary aspiration or noncardiac pulmonary edema. The mechanism of noncardiac pulmonary edema is unknown.

Dextromethorphan can interact with MAOIs, causing severe hyperthermia, and may cause the serotonin syndrome (see SSRI section). Dextromethorphan inhibits the metabolism of norepinephrine and serotonin and blocks the reuptake of serotonin. It is found as a component of a large number of nonprescription cough and cold remedies.

Toxic Dose

The toxic dose depends on the specific drug, route of administration, and degree of tolerance. For therapeutic and toxic doses, see Table 25. In children, respiratory depression has been produced by 10 mg of morphine or methadone, 75 mg of meperidine, and 12.5 mg of diphenoxylate. Infants younger than 3 months of age are more susceptible to respiratory depression. The dose should be reduced by 50%.

Kinetics

Oral onset of analgesic effect of morphine is 10 to 15 minutes; the action peaks in 1 hour and lasts 4 to 6 hours. With sustained-release preparations, the duration is 8 to 12 hours. Opioids are 90% metabolized in the liver by hepatic conjugation and 90% excreted in the urine as inactive compounds. Volume distribution is 1 to 4 L/kg. Protein binding is 35% to 75%. The typical plasma half-life of opiates is 2 to 5 hours, but that of methadone is 24 to 36 hours. Morphine metabolites include morphine-3-glucuronide (inactive) and morphine-6-glucuronide (active) and normorphine (active). Meperidine (Demerol) is rapidly hydrolyzed by tissue esterases into the active metabolite normeperidine, which has twice the convulsant activity of meperidine. Heroin (diacetylmorphine) is deacetylated within minutes to 6-monacetylmorphine and morphine. Propoxyphene (Darvon) has a rapid onset of action, and death has occurred within 15 to

TABLE 25. **Doses and Onset and Duration of Action of Common Opioids**

Drug	Adult Oral Dose	Child Oral Dose	Onset of Action	Duration of Action	Adult Fatal Dose
Camphored tincture of opium	25 mL	0.25–0.50 mL/kg (0.4 mg/mL)	15–30 minutes	4–5 hrs	NA
Codeine	30–180 mg	0.5–1 mg/kg	15–30 minutes	4–6 hrs	800 mg
	>1 mg/kg is toxic in a child, above 200 mg in adult >5 mg/kg fatal in a child				
Dextromethorphan	15 mg 10 mg/kg is toxic	0.25 mg/kg	15–30 minutes	3–6 hrs	NA
Diacetyl-morphine; street heroin is less than 10% pure	60 mg	NA	15–30 minutes	3–4 hrs	100 mg
Diphenoxylate natiopine (Lomotil)	5–10 mg;	NA	120–240 minutes	14 hrs	300 mg
	7.5 mg is toxic in a child, 300 mg is toxic in adult				
Fentanyl (Duragesic)	0.1–0.2 mg	0.001–0.002 mg/kg	7–8 minutes	IM; 1/2–2 hrs;	1.0 mg
Hydrocodone with APAP (Lortab)	5–30 mg	0.15 mg/kg	30 minutes	3–4 hrs	100 mg
Hydromorphone (Dilaudid)	4 mg	0.1 mg/kg	15–30 minutes	3–4 hrs	100 mg
Meperidine (Demerol)	100 mg	1–1.5 mg/kg	10–45 minutes	3–4 hrs	350 mg
Methadone (Dolophine)	10 mg	0.1 mg/kg	30–60 minutes	4–12 hrs	120 mg
Morphine	10–60 mg	0.1–0.2 mg/kg	<20 minutes	4–6 hrs	200 mg
	Oral dose is 6 times parenteral dose, MS Contin sustained release prep				
Oxycodone APAP (Percocet)	5 mg	NA	15–30 minutes	4–5 hrs	NA
Pentazocine (Talwin)	50–100 mg	NA	15–30 minutes	3–4 hrs	NA
Propoxyphene (Darvon)	65–100 mg	NA	30–60 minutes	2–4 hrs	700 mg

30 minutes after a massive overdose. Propoxyphene is metabolized to norpropoxyphene, an active metabolite with convulsive, cardiac dysrhythmic, and heart block properties. Symptoms of diphenoxylate overdose appear within 1 to 4 hours. It is metabolized into the active metabolite difenoxin, which is five times more active as a regular respiratory depressant agent. Death has been reported in children after ingestion of a single tablet.

Manifestations

Initially, mild intoxication produces miosis, dull face, drowsiness, partial ptosis, and "nodding" (head drops to chest then bobs up). Larger amounts produce the classic triad of miotic pupils (exceptions below), respiratory depression, and depressed level of consciousness (flaccid coma). The blood pressure, pulse, and bowel activity are decreased.

Dilated pupils do not exclude opioid intoxication. Some exceptions to the miosis effect include dextromethorphan (paralyzes iris), fentanyl, meperidine, and diphenoxylate (rarely). Physiologic disturbances including acidosis, hypoglycemia, hypoxia, and postictal state, or a co-ingestant may also produce mydriasis.

Usually, the muscles are flaccid, but increased muscle tone can be produced by meperidine and fentanyl (chest rigidity). Seizures are rare but can occur with ingestion of codeine, meperidine, propoxyphene, and dextromethorphan. Hallucinations and agitation have been reported.

Pruritus and urticaria are due to histamine release by some opioids or due to sulfite additives.

Noncardiac pulmonary edema may occur after an overdose, especially with intravenous heroin abuse. Cardiac effects include vasodilation and hypotension. A heart murmur in an intravenous addict suggests endocarditis. Propoxyphene can produce delayed cardiac dysrhythmias.

Fentanyl is 100 times more potent than morphine and can cause chest wall muscle rigidity. Some of its derivatives are 2000 times more potent than morphine.

Laboratory Investigations

For patients with overdose, one should obtain and monitor ABG, blood glucose, and electrolyte levels; chest radiographs; and ECG. For drug abusers, one should consider testing for hepatitis B, syphilis, and HIV antibody (HIV testing usually requires consent). Blood opioid concentrations are not useful. They confirm diagnosis (morphine therapeutic dose, 65 to 80 ng/mL; toxic, <200 ng/mL), but are not useful for making a therapeutic decision. Cross-reactions can occur with Vick's Formula 44, poppy seeds, and other opioids (codeine and heroin are metabolized to morphine). Naloxone 4 mg IV was not associated with a positive enzyme multiplied immunoassay technique urine screen at 60 minutes, 6 hours, or 48 hours.

Management

Supportive care should be instituted, particularly an endotracheal tube and assisted ventilation. Temporary ventilation can be provided by a bag-valve mask with 100% oxygen. The patient should be placed on a cardiac monitor, have intravenous access established, and have specimens for ABG, glucose, electrolytes, BUN, and creatinine levels, CBC, coagulation profile, liver function, toxicology screen, and urinalysis taken.

For gastrointestinal decontamination, emesis should not be induced, but activated charcoal can be administered if bowel sounds are present.

If it is suspected that the patient is an addict, he or she should be restrained first and then 0.1 mg of naloxone (Narcan) should be administered. The dose should be doubled every 2 minutes until the patient responds or 10 to 20 mg has been given. If the patient is not suspected to be an addict, then 2 mg every 2 to 3 minutes to total of 10 to 20 mg is administered.

It is essential to determine whether there is a complete response to naloxone (mydriasis, improvement in ventilation), since it is a diagnostic therapeutic test. A continuous naloxone infusion may be appropriate, using the "response dose" every hour. Repeat doses of naloxone may be necessary because the effects of many opioids can last much longer than naloxone does (30 to 60 minutes). Methadone ingestions may require a naloxone infusion for 24 to 48 hours. Half of the response dose may need to be repeated in 15 to 20 minutes, after the infusion has been started.

Acute iatrogenic withdrawal precipitated by the administration of naloxone to a dependent patient should not be treated with morphine or other opioids. Naloxone's effects are limited to 30 to 60 minutes (shorter than most opioids) and withdrawal will subside in a short time.

Nalmefene (Revex), an FDA-approved long-acting (4 to 8 hours) pure opioid antagonist, is being investigated, but its role in cases of acute intoxication is unclear and it could produce prolonged withdrawal. It may have a role in place of naloxone infusion.

Noncardiac pulmonary edema does not respond to naloxone, and the patient needs intubation, assisted ventilation, positive end-expiratory pressure, and hemodynamic monitoring. Fluids should be given cautiously in patients with opioid overdose because opioids stimulate the antidiuretic hormone.

If the patient is comatose, 50% glucose (3% to 4% of comatose opioid overdose patients have hypoglycemia) and thiamine should be given prior to naloxone. If the patient has seizures that are unresponsive to naloxone, one administers diazepam and examines for metabolic (hypoglycemia, electrolyte disturbances) causes and structural disturbances.

Hypotension is rare and should direct a search for another etiology. If the patient is agitated, hypoxia and hypoglycemia must be excluded before opioid withdrawal is considered as a cause. Complications to consider include urinary retention, constipation, rhabdomyolysis, myoglobinuria, hypoglycemia, and withdrawal.

Disposition

If a patient responds to intravenous naloxone, careful observation for relapse and the development of pulmonary edema is required, with cardiac and respiratory monitoring for 6 to 12 hours. Patients requiring repeated doses of naloxone or an infusion, or those who develop pulmonary edema, require intensive care unit admission and cannot be discharged from the intensive care unit until they are symptom free for 12 hours. Intravenous overdose complications are expected to be present within 20 minutes after injection, and discharge after 4 symptom-free hours has been recommended. Adults with oral overdose have delayed onset of toxicity and require 6 hours of observation. Children with oral opioid overdose should be admitted to the hospital for observation because of delayed toxicity. Some toxicologists advise restraining a patient who attempts to sign out against medical advice after treatment with naloxone, at least until the patient receives psychiatric evaluation.

Organophosphates and Carbamates

Cholinergic intoxication sources are insecticides (organophosphates or carbamates), some medications, and some mushrooms. Examples of organophosphate insecticides are malathion (low toxicity, median lethal dose [LD_{50}] 2800 mg/kg), chlorpyrifos, which has been removed from market (moderate toxicity), and parathion (high toxicity, LD_{50} 2 mg/kg). Carbamate insecticides include carbaryl (low toxicity, LD_{50} 500 mg/kg), propoxpur (moderate toxicity, LD_{50} 95 mg/kg), and aldicarb (high toxicity, LD_{50} 0.9 mg/kg). Pharmaceuticals with carbamate properties include neostigmine (Prostigmin) and physostigmine (Antilirium). Cholinergic compounds also include the "G" nerve war weapons Tubun (GA), Sarin (GB), Soman (GB), and Venom X (VX).

Toxic Mechanism

Organophosphates phosphorylate the active site on red cell acetylcholinesterase and pseudocholinesterase in the serum, neuromuscular and parasympathetic neuroeffector junctions, and in the major synapses of the autonomic ganglia, causing irreversible inhibition. There are two types of organophosphate intoxication: (1) direct action by the parent compound (e.g., tetraethylpyophosphate, or (2) indirect action by the toxic metabolite (e.g., parathoxon or malathoxon).

Carbamates (esters of carbonic acid) cause reversible carbamylation of the active site of the enzymes. When a critical amount, greater than 50%, of cholinesterase is inhibited, acetylcholine accumulates and causes transient stimulation at cholinergic synapses and sympathetic terminals (muscarinic effect), the somatic nerves, the autonomic ganglia (nicotinic effect), and CNS synapses. Stimulation of conduction is followed by inhibition of conduction.

The major differences between the carbamates and the organophosphates are as follows: (1) carbamate toxicity is less and the duration is shorter; (2) carbamates rarely produce overt CNS effects (poor CNS penetration); (3) carbamate inhibition of the acetylcholinesterase enzyme is reversible and activity returns to normal rapidly; (4) pralidoxime, the enzyme regenerator, may not be necessary in the management of mild carbamate intoxication (e.g., carbaryl).

Toxic Dose

Parathion's minimum lethal dose is 2 mg in children and 10 to 20 mg in adults. The lethal dose of malathion is greater than 1375 mg/kg and that of chlorpyrifos is 25 grams; the latter compound is unlikely to cause death.

Kinetics

Absorption is by all routes. The onset of acute ingestion toxicity occurs as early as 3 hours, usually before 12 hours and always before 24 hours. Lipid-soluble agents absorbed by the dermal route (e.g., fenthion), may have a delayed onset of more than 24 hours. Inhalation toxicity occurs immediately after exposure. Massive ingestion can produce intoxication within minutes.

Metabolism is via the liver. With some pesticides (e.g., parathion, malathion), the effects are delayed because they undergo hepatic microsomal oxidative metabolism to their toxic metabolites, the -oxons (e.g., paroxon, malaoxon).

The half-life of malathion is 2.89 hours and that of parathion is 2.1 days. The metabolites are eliminated in the urine and the presence of p-nitrophenol in the urine is a clue up to 48 hours after exposure.

Manifestations

Many organophosphates produce a garlic odor on the breath, in the gastric contents, or in the container. Diaphoresis, excessive salivation, miosis, and muscle twitching are helpful clues to diagnosis.

Early, a cholinergic (muscarinic) crisis develops that consists of parasympathetic nervous system activity. DUMBELS is the mnemonic for *d*efecation, cramps, and increased bowel motility; *u*rinary incontinence; *m*iosis (mydriasis may occur in 20%); *b*ronchospasm and bronchorrhea; *e*xcess secretion; *l*acrimation; and *s*eizures. Bradycardia, pulmonary edema, and hypotension may be present.

Later, sympathetic and nicotinic effects occur, consisting of MATCH: *m*uscle weakness and fasciculation (eyelid twitching is often present), *a*drenal stimulation and hyperglycemia, *t*achycardia, *c*ramps in muscles, and *h*ypertension. Finally, paralysis of the skeletal muscles ensues.

The CNS effects are headache, blurred vision, anxiety, ataxia, delirium and toxic psychosis, convulsions, coma, and respiratory depression. Cranial nerve palsies have been noted. Delayed hallucinations may occur.

Delayed respiratory paralysis and neurologic and neurobehavioral disorders have been described following certain organophosphate ingestions or dermal exposure. The "intermediate syndrome" is paralysis of proximal and respiratory muscles developing 24 to 96 hours after the successful treatment of organophosphate poisoning. A delayed distal polyneuropathy has been described with ingestion of certain organophosphates, such as triorthocresyl phosphate, bromoleptophos, and methomidophos.

Complications include aspiration, pulmonary edema, and acute respiratory distress syndrome.

Laboratory Investigations

Monitoring should include chest radiograph, blood glucose (nonketotic hyperglycemia is frequent), ABG, pulse oximetry, ECG, blood coagulation status, liver function, hyperamylasemia (pancreatitis reported), and urinalysis for the metabolite alkyl phosphate paranitrophenol. Blood should be drawn for red blood cell cholinesterase determination before pralidoxime is given. The red blood cell cholinesterase activity roughly correlates with clinical severity. Mild poisoning is 20% to 50% of normal, moderate poisoning is 10% to 20% of normal, and severe poisoning is 10% of normal (>90% depressed). A postexposure rise of 10% to 15% in the cholinesterase level determined at least 10 to 14 days after the exposure confirms the diagnosis.

Management

Protection of health care personnel with clothing (masks, gloves, gowns, goggles) and respiratory equipment or hazardous material suits, as necessary, is called for. General decontamination consists of isolation, bagging, and disposal of contaminated clothing and other articles. Vital functions should be established and maintained. Cardiac and oxygen saturation monitoring are needed. Intubation and assisted ventilation may be needed. Secretions should be suctioned until atropinization drying is achieved.

Dermal decontamination involves prompt removal of clothing and cleansing of all affected areas of skin, hair, and eyes. Ocular decontamination involves irrigation with copious amounts of tepid water or 0.9% saline for at least 15 minutes. Gastrointestinal decontamination, if the ingestion was recent, involves the administration of activated charcoal.

Atropine sulfate can be given as an antidote. It is both a diagnostic and a therapeutic agent. Atropine counteracts the muscarinic effects but is only partially effective for the CNS effects (seizures and coma). Preservative-free atropine (no benzyl alcohol) should be used. If the patient is symptomatic (bradycardia or bronchorrhea), a test dose should be administered, 0.02 mg/kg in children or 1 mg in adults, intravenously. If no signs of atropinization are present (tachycardia, drying of secretions, and mydriasis), atropine should be administered immediately, 0.05 mg/kg in children or 2 mg in adults, every 5 to 10 minutes as needed to dry the secretions and clear the lungs. Beneficial effects are seen within 1 to 4 minutes and maximum effect in 8 minutes. The average dose in the first 24 hours is 40 mg, but 1000 mg or more has been required in severe cases. Glycopyrrolate (Robinul) can be used if atropine is not available. The maximum dose should be maintained for 12 to 24 hours, then tapered and the patient observed for relapse. Poisoning, especially with lipophilic agents (e.g., fenthion, chlorfenthion), may require weeks of atropine therapy. An alternative is a continuous infusion of atropine 8 mg in 100 mL 0.9% saline at rate of 0.02 to 0.08 mg/kg/hour (0.25 to 1.0 mL/kg/hour) with additional 1 to 5 mg boluses as needed to dry the secretions.

Pralidoxime chloride (Protopam) has both antinicotinic and antimuscarinic effects and possibly also CNS effects. Successful treatment with pralidoxime chloride may result in a reduction in the dose of atropine. Pralidoxime acts to reactivate the phosphorylated cholinesterases by binding the phosphate moiety on the esteritic site and displacing it. It should be given early before "aging" of phosphate bond produces tighter binding. However, recent reports indicate that pralidoxime chloride is beneficial even several days after the poisoning. Improvement is seen within 10 to 40 minutes. The initial dose of pralidoxime chloride is 1 to 2 g in 250 mL 0.89% saline over 5 to 10 minutes, maximum 200 mg/minute, in adults or 25 to 50 mg/kg, maximum 4 mg/kg/minute, in children younger than 12 years of age. The dose can be repeated every 6 to 12 hours for several days. An alternative is a continuous infusion of 1 g in 100 mL 0.89% saline at 5 to 20 mg/kg/hour (0.5 to 12 mL/g/hour) up to 500 mg/hour and titrated to desired response. Maximum adult daily dose is 12 g. Cardiac and blood pressure monitoring are advised during and for several hours after the infusion. The end point is absence of fasciculations and return of muscle strength.

Contraindicated drugs include morphine, aminophylline, barbiturates, opioids, phenothiazine, reserpine-like drugs, parasympathomimetics, and succinylcholine.

Noncardiac pulmonary edema may require respiratory support. Seizures may respond to atropine and pralidoxime chloride but often require anticonvulsants. Cardiac dysrhythmias may require electrical cardioversion or antidysrhythmic therapy if the patient is hemodynamically unstable.

Extracorporeal procedures are of no proven value.

Disposition

Asymptomatic patients with normal examination findings after 6 to 8 hours of observation may be discharged. In cases of intentional poisoning, the patients require psychiatric clearance for discharge. Symptomatic patients should be admitted to the intensive care unit. Observation of milder cases of carbamate poisoning, even those requiring atropine, for 6 to 8 hours symptom-free may be sufficient to exclude significant toxicity. In cases of workplace exposure, OSHA should be notified.

Phencyclidine (Angel Dust)

Phencyclidine is an aryicyclohexylamine related to ketamine and chemically related to the phenothiazines. Originally a "dissociative" anesthetic banned in United States since 1979, it is now an illicit substance, with at least 38 analogues. It is inexpensively manufactured by "kitchen chemists" and is mislabelled as other hallucinogens. Improper phencyclidine synthesis may release cyanide when heated or smoked and can cause explosions.

Toxic Mechanism

The mechanism of phencyclidine is complex and not completely understood. It inhibits some neurotransmitters and causes a loss of pain sensation without depressing the CNS respiratory status. It stimulates α-adrenergic receptors and may act as a "false neurotransmitter." The effects are sympathomimetic, cholinergic, and cerebellar.

Toxic Dose

The usual dose of phencyclidine mixed with marijuana joints is 100 to 400 mg of phencyclidine. Joints or leaf mixtures contain 0.24% to 7.9% of PCP, 1 mg of PCP/150 leaves. Tablets contain 5 mg (the usual street dose). CNS effects at doses of 1 to 6 mg include hallucinations and euphoria, 6 to 10 mg produces toxic psychosis and sympathetic stimulation, 10 to 25 mg produces severe toxicity, and more than 100 mg has resulted in fatalities.

Kinetics

Phencyclidine is a lipophilic weak base, with a pKa of 8.5 to 9.5. It is rapidly absorbed when smoked and snorted, poorly absorbed from the acid stomach, and rapidly absorbed from the alkaline middle small intestine. It has an enterogastric secretion and is reabsorbed in the small intestine. The onset of action when smoked is 2 to 5 minutes, with a peak in 15 to 30 minutes. With oral ingestion, the onset is in 30 to 60 minutes and when taken intravenously it is immediate. Most adverse reactions in cases of overdose begin within 1 to 2 hours. Its duration of action at low doses is 4 to 6 hours and normality returns in 24 hours; in large overdoses, fluctuating coma may last 6 to 10 days.

Volume distribution is 6.2 L/kg. Phencyclidine concentrates in brain and adipose tissue. Protein binding is 70%. The route of elimination is by gastric secretion, liver metabolism, and 10% urinary excretion of conjugates and free phencyclidine. Renal excretion may be increased 50% with urinary acidification. The half-life is 1 hour (in cases of overdose, it is 11 to 89 hours).

Manifestations

The classic picture is bursts of horizontal, vertical, and rotary nystagmus, which is a clue to diagnosis (occurs in 50% of cases), miosis, hypertension, and fluctuating altered mental state. There is a wide spectrum of clinical presentations.

Mild intoxication with 1 to 6 mg produces drunken and bizarre behavior, agitation, rotary nystagmus, and blank stare. Violent behavior and sensory anesthesia make these patients insensitive to pain, self-destructive, and dangerous. Most are communicative within 1 to 2 hours, are alert and oriented in 6 to 8 hours, and recover completely in 24 to 48 hours.

Moderate intoxication with 6 to 10 mg produces excess salivation, hypertension, hyperthermia, muscle rigidity, myoclonus, and catatonia. Recovery of consciousness occurs in 24 to 48 hours and complete recovery in 1 week.

Severe intoxication with 10 to 25 mg results in opisthotonus, decerebrate rigidity, convulsions, prolonged fluctuating coma, and respiratory failure. Patients in this category have a high rate of medical complications. Recovery of consciousness occurs in 24 to 48 hours, with complete normality in a month. Medical complications include apnea, aspiration pneumonia, cardiac arrest, hypertensive encephalopathy, hyperthermia, intracerebral hemorrhage, psychosis, rhabdomyolysis and myoglobinuria, and seizures. Loss of memory and "flashbacks" last for months. Phencyclidine-induced depression and suicide have been reported.

Fatalities occur with ingestions of greater than 100 mg and with serum levels greater than 100 to 250 ng/mL.

Laboratory Investigations

Marked elevation of creatine kinase level may occur. Values greater than 20,000 units have been reported. Urinalysis should be monitored and urine tested for myoglobin. One should monitor the blood for creatine kinase, uric acid (an early clue to rhabdomyolysis), BUN, creatinine, electrolytes (hyperkalemia), blood glucose (20% of patients have hypoglycemia), urinary output, liver function tests, ECG, and ABG if the patient has any respiratory manifestations. Measurement of phencyclidine in the gastric juice is called for because concentrations are 10 to 50 times higher than in blood or urine. Phencyclidine blood concentrations are not helpful. Phencyclidine may be detected in the urine of the average user for 10 days to 3 weeks after the last dose. In chronic users, it can be detected for over 1 month. The analogues of phencyclidine may not produce positive test results for phencyclidine in the urine. Cross-reactions with bleach and dextromethorphan may cause false-positive urine test results on immunoassay, and cross-reaction with doxylamine may produce a false-positive finding on gas chromatography.

Management

The patient should be observed for violent, self-destructive, bizarre behavior and paranoid schizophrenia. Patients should be placed in a low sensory environment and dangerous objects should be removed from the area.

Gastrointestinal decontamination is not effective because phencyclidine is rapidly absorbed from intestines. Overtreating the mild intoxication should be avoided. There is insufficient evidence to support the use of MDAC. In cases of severe toxicity (stupor or coma), continuous gastric suction can be tried (with protection of the airway) because the drug is secreted into the gastric juice. The value of this procedure is controversial because of limited data.

The patient must be protected from harming himself or herself or others. Physical restraints may be necessary, but they should be used sparingly and for the shortest time possible because they increase risk of rhabdomyolysis. Metal restraints such as handcuffs should be avoided. For behavioral disorders and toxic psychosis, diazepam is the agent of choice. Pharmacologic intervention includes diazepam (Valium) 10 to 30 mg orally or 2 to 5 mg intravenously initially and titrated upward to 10 mg; however, up to 30 mg may be required. "Talk down" technique is usually ineffective and dangerous. Phenothiazines and butyrophenones should be avoided in the acute phase because they lower the convulsive threshold; however, they may be needed later for psychosis. Haloperidol (Haldol) administration has been reported to produce catatonia.

Seizures and muscle spasm are managed with diazepam, from 2.5 mg up to 10 mg. Hyperthermia (>38.5°C) is treated with external cooling measures. Hypertension is usually transient and does not require treatment. In the case of emergent hypertensive crisis (blood pressure >200/115 mm Hg) nitroprusside can be used in a dose of 0.3 to 2 μg/kg/min. Maximum infusion rate is 10 μg/kg/min for only 10 minutes.

Acid ion trapping diuresis is not recommended because of the danger of myoglobin precipitation in the renal tubules. Rhabdomyolysis and myoglobinuria are treated by correcting volume depletion and insuring a urinary output of greater than 2 mL/kg/hour. Alkalinization is controversial because of reabsorption of phencyclidine.

Hemodialysis is beneficial if renal failure occurs; otherwise, the extracorporeal procedures are not beneficial.

Disposition

All patients with coma, delirium, catatonia, violent behavior, aspiration pneumonia, sustained hypertension greater than 200/115, and significant rhabdomyolysis should be admitted to the intensive care unit until asymptomatic for at least 24 hours. If patients with mild intoxication are mentally and neurologically stable and become asymptomatic (except for nystagmus) for 4 hours, they may be discharged in the company of a responsible adult. All patients must be assessed for suicide risk before discharge. Drug counseling and psychiatric follow-up should be arranged. Patients should be warned that episodes of disorientation and depression may continue intermittently for 4 weeks or more.

Phenothiazines and Nonphenothiazines (Neuroleptics)

Toxic Mechanism

Neuroleptics have complex mechanisms of toxicity, including (1) block of the postsynaptic dopamine receptors; (2) block of peripheral and central α-adrenergic receptors; (3) block of cholinergic muscarinic receptors; (4) quinidine-like antidysrhythmic and myocardial depressant effect in cases of large overdose; (5) lowering of the convulsive threshold; (6) effect on hypothalamic temperature regulation (Table 26).

Toxic Dose

Extrapyramidal reactions, anticholinergic effects, and orthostatic hypotension may occur at therapeutic doses. The toxic amount is not established, but the maximum daily therapeutic dose may result in significant side effects, and twice this amount may be potentially fatal. Chlorpromazine (Thorazine), the prototype, may produce serious hypotension and CNS depression at doses greater than 200 mg (17 mg/kg) in children and 3 to 5 grams in an adult. Fatalities have been reported after 2.5 grams of loxapine (Loxitane) and mesoridazine (Serentil) and 1.5 grams of thioridazine (Mellaril).

TABLE 26. **Neuroleptics and Properties**

Compound	Antipsychotic	Anticholinergic	Extrapyramidal	Hypotensive and Cardiotoxic	Sedative
Phenothiazine					
Aliphatic Chlorpromazine (Thorazine) Promethazine (Phenergan)	1+	3+	2+	2+	3+
Piperazine Fluphenazine (Prolixin) Perphenazine (Trilafon) Prochlorperazine (Compazine) Trifluoperazine (Stelazine)	3+	1+	3+	1+	1+
Piperidine Mesoridazine (Serentil) Thioridazine (Mellaril)	1+	2+	1+	3+	3+
Nonphenothiazine					
Butyrophenone Haloperidol (Haldol)	3+	1+	3+	1+	1+
Dibenzoxazepine Loxapine (Loxitane)	3+	1+	3+	1+	2+
Dihydroindolone Molindone (Moban)	3+	1+	3+	1+	1+
Thioxanthenes Thiothixene (Navane) Chlorprothixene (Taractan)	3+	1+	3+	3+	1+

1+ = very low activity; 2+ = moderate activity; 3+ = very high activity.

Kinetics

These agents are lipophilic and have unpredictable gastrointestinal absorption. Peak levels occur 2 to 6 hours postingestion and have enterohepatic recirculation.

The mean serum half-life in phase 1 is 1 to 2 hours and the biphasic half-life is 20 to 40 hours. Volume distribution is 10 to 40 L/kg; protein binding is 92% to 98%. Chlorpromazine taken orally has an onset of action in 30 to 60 minutes, peak in 2 to 4 hours, and duration of 4 to 6 hours. With sustained-release preparations, the onset is in 30 to 60 minutes and duration is 6 to 12 hours.

Elimination is by hepatic metabolism, which results in multiple metabolites (some are active). Metabolites can be detected in urine months after chronic therapy. Only 1% to 3% is excreted unchanged in the urine.

Manifestations

In cases of phenothiazine overdose, anticholinergic symptoms may be present early but are not life-threatening. Miosis is usually present (80%) if the phenothiazine has strong α-adrenergic blocking effect (e.g., chlorpromazine), but anticholinergic activity mydriasis may occur. Agitation and delirium rapidly progress into coma. Major problems are cardiac toxicity and hypotension. The cardiotoxic effects are seen more commonly with thioridazine and its metabolite mesoridazine. These agents have produced the largest number of fatalities in patients with phenothiazine overdose. Cardiac conduction disturbances include prolonged PR, QRS, and QTc intervals, U and T wave abnormalities, and ventricular dysrhythmias including torsades de pointes. Seizures occur mainly in patients with convulsive disorders or with administration of loxapine. Sudden death in children and adults has been reported.

Idiosyncratic dystonic reactions are most common with the piperidine group. Reactions are not dose-dependent and consist of opisthotonos, torticollis, orolingual dyskinesia, or oculogyric crisis (painful upward gaze). These reactions are more frequent in children and women. Neuroleptic malignant syndrome occurs in patients on chronic therapy and is characterized by hyperthermia, muscle rigidity, autonomic dysfunction, and altered mental state. There is one case reported with acute overdose. The loxapine syndrome consists of seizures, rhabdomyolysis, and renal failure.

Laboratory Investigations

Monitoring should include arterial blood gases, renal and hepatic function, electrolytes, blood glucose, and creatine kinase and myoglobinemia in neuroleptic malignant syndrome. Most of these agents are detected on routine screening. Quantitative serum levels are not useful in management. Cross-reactions with enzyme multiplied immunoassay technique tests occur with cyclic antidepressants. Phenothiazines give false-negative results on pregnancy urine tests using human chorionic gonadotropin as an indicator, and give false-positive results for urine porphyrins, indirect Coombs test, urobilinogen, and amylase.

Management

Vital functions must be established and maintained. All overdose patients require venous access, 12-lead ECG (to measure intervals), cardiac and respiratory monitoring, and seizure precautions. One should monitor core temperature to detect poikilothermic effect. If the patient is comatose, intubation and assisted ventilation may be required, as well as 100% oxygen, intravenous glucose, naloxone (Narcan), and thiamine.

Emesis is not recommended. Activated charcoal can be administered if ingestion was within 1 hour. MDAC has not been proven beneficial. A radiograph of the abdomen may be useful, if the phenothiazine is radiopaque. Haloperidol (Haldol) and trifluoperazine (Stelazine) are most likely to be radiopaque. Whole-bowel irrigation may be useful when a large number of pills are visualized on radiograph or if sustained-release preparations were taken, but whole-bowel irrigation has not been evaluated in patients with phenothiazine overdose.

Convulsions are treated with diazepam or lorazepam (Ativan). Loxapine (Loxitane) overdose may result in status epilepticus. If nondepolarizing neuromuscular blockade is required, pancuronium (Pavulon) or vecuronium (Norcuron) should be used (not succinylcholine [Anectine], which may cause malignant hyperthermia), and EEG should be monitored during paralysis.

Patients with dysrhythmias should be monitored with serial ECGs. Unstable rhythms can be treated with electrical cardioversion. Class 1a antidysrhythmics (procainamide, quinidine, and disopyramide [Norpace]) must be avoided.

Hypokalemia predisposes to dysrhythmias and should be corrected aggressively. Supraventricular tachycardia with hemodynamic instability is treated with electrical cardioversion. The role of adenosine has not been defined. Calcium channel and β-blockers should be avoided.

Prolongation of the QRS interval is treated with sodium bicarbonate 1 to 2 mEq/kg by intravenous bolus over a few minutes. Torsades de pointes is treated with magnesium sulfate IV 20% solution 2 g over 2 to 3 minutes. If there is no response in 10 minutes, the dose is repeated and followed by a continuous infusion of 5 to 10 mg/min or given as an infusion of 50 mg/minute for 2 hours followed by 30 mg/minute for 90 minutes twice a day for several days, as needed. The dose in children is 25 to 50 mg/kg initially and maintenance dose is 30 to 60 mg/kg/24 hours (0.25 to 0.50 mEq/Kg/24 h) up to 1000 mg/24 hours. Serum magnesium levels should be monitored.

To treat ventricular tachydysrhythmias in a stable patient, lidocaine is used. If the patient is unstable, electrical cardioversion is used. Patients with heart block with hemodynamic instability should be managed with temporary cardiac pacing.

Hypotension is treated with the Trendelenburg position and 0.9% saline. If the condition is refractory to treatment or there is a danger of fluid overload, vasopressors are administered. The vasopressor of choice is α-adrenergic agonist norepinephrine (Levophed), titrated to response. Epinephrine and dopamine should not be used because β-receptor stimulation in the presence of α-receptor blockade may provoke dysrhythmias and phenothiazines are antidopaminogenic.

Hypothermia and hyperthermia are treated with external warming and cooling measures, respectively. Antipyretic drugs must *not* be used.

Management of the neuroleptic malignant syndrome includes the following actions:

- Immediately discontinuing the offending agent
- Hyperventilating the patient, using 100% humidified, cooled oxygen at high gas flows (at least 10 L/min) because of rapid breathing
- Administering a benzodiazepine to control convulsions and facilitate cooling measures
- Initiating appropriate mechanical cooling measures, which may include intravenous cold saline (*not* lactated Ringer's), ice baths, cold lavage of the stomach, bladder, and rectum, and a hypothermic blanket
- Correcting acid-base and electrolyte disturbances and treating significant hyperkalemia with hyperventilation, calcium, sodium bicarbonate, intravenous glucose, and insulin; hemodialysis may be necessary

In addition, dysrhythmias usually respond to correction of the underlying acid-base disturbances and hyperkalemia. If antidysrhythmic agents are required, calcium channel blockers must be avoided because they may precipitate hyperkalemia and cardiovascular collapse. Dantrolene sodium (Dantrium), which is a phenytoin derivative, inhibits calcium release from the sarcoplasmic reticulum and results in decreased muscle contraction. Dantrolene acts peripherally and does not reverse the rigidity or psychomotor disturbances resulting from the central dopamine blockade; it therefore is often used in combination with bromocriptine. Bromocriptine mesylate (Parlodel) acts centrally as a dopamine agonist, as does amantadine hydrochloride (Symmetrel). Bromocriptine and dantrolene have been reported to be successful in combination with cooling and good supportive measures in malignant hyperthermia.

Dosing for these agents is as follows: dantrolene sodium at 2 to 3 mg/kg IV as a bolus, then 1 mg/kg/minute to a maximum of 10 mg/kg or until the tachycardia, rigidity, increased end-tidal CO_2, and temperature elevation are controlled. Note: Hepatotoxicity occurs with doses greater than 10 mg/kg. To prevent symptom recurrence, 1 mg/kg should be administered every 6 hours for 24 to 48 hours after the episode. After that time, oral dantrolene can be used at a dose of 1 mg/kg every 6 hours for 24 hours as necessary. The patient should be observed for thrombophlebitis following intravenous dantrolene. It is best administered via a central line. Bromocriptine mesylate at 2.5 to 10 mg orally or via a nasogastric tube, three times a day, should be used in combination with dantrolene.

Idiosyncratic dystonic reaction can be treated with diphenhydramine (Benadryl) 1 to 2 mg/kg/dose intravenously over 5 minutes up to maximum of 50 mg intravenously; a response is noted within 2 to 5 minutes. This can be followed with oral doses for 4 to 6 days to prevent recurrence.

Extracorporeal measures (hemodialysis, hemoperfusion) are not effective in removing these agents.

Disposition

Asymptomatic patients should be observed for at least 6 hours after gastric decontamination. Symptomatic patients with cardiotoxicity, hypotension, and convulsions should be admitted to the intensive care unit and monitored for 48 hours.

Salicylates (Acetylsalicylic Acid, Salicylic Acid)

Toxic Mechanism

The primary toxic mechanisms include (1) direct stimulation of the medullary chemoreceptor trigger zone and respiratory center; (2) uncoupling oxidative phosphorylation; (3) inhibition of the Krebs' cycle enzymes; (4) inhibition of vitamin K dependent and independent clotting factors; (5) alteration of platelet function; and (6) inhibition of prostaglandin synthesis.

Toxic Dose

Acute mild intoxication occurs at a dose of 150 to 200 mg/kg, moderate intoxication at 200 to 300 mg/kg, and severe intoxication at 300 to 500 mg/kg. Acute salicylate plasma concentration greater than 30 mg/dL (usually >40 mg/dL) may be associated with clinical toxicity. Chronic intoxication occurs at ingestions greater than 100 mg/kg/day for more than 2 days because of accumulation kinetics. Methyl salicylate (oil of wintergreen) is the most toxic form of salicylate. A dose of 1 mL of 98% contains 1.4 g of salicylate. Fatalities have occurred with ingestion of 1 teaspoonful in children and 1 ounce in adults. It is found in topical ointments and liniments (18% to 30%).

Kinetics

Acetylsalicylic acid and salicylic acid are weak acids with a pKa of 3.5 and 3.0, respectively. Acetylsalicylic acid is absorbed from the stomach, from the small bowel, and dermally. Onset of action is within 30 minutes. Methyl salicylate and effervescent tablets are absorbed more rapidly. Salicylate plasma concentration is detectable within 15 minutes after ingestion and peaks in 30 to 120 minutes. The peak may be delayed 6 to 12 hours in cases of large overdose, overdose with enteric-coated or sustained-release preparations, and development of concretions. The therapeutic duration of action is 3 to 4 hours but is markedly prolonged in cases of overdose.

Volume distribution is 0.13 L/kg for salicylic acid but increases as the salicylate plasma concentration increases. Protein binding is greater than 90% for salicylic acid at pH 7.4 and a salicylate plasma concentration of 20 to 30 mg/dL, 75% at a salicylate plasma concentration greater than 40 mg/dL, 50% at a salicylate plasma concentration of 70 mg/dL, and 30% at a salicylate plasma concentration of 120 mg/dL.

The half-life for salicylic acid is 3 hours after a 300 mg dose, 6 hours after a 1 g overdose, and greater than 10 hours after a 10-g overdose. Elimination includes Michaelis-Menten hepatic metabolism by three saturable pathways: (1) glycine conjugation to salicyluric acid (75%); (2) glucuronyl transferase to salicyl phenol glucuronide (10%); and (3) salicyl aryl glucuronide (4%). Nonsaturable pathways are hydrolysis to gentisic acid (<1%). Ten percent is excreted unchanged.

Acidosis increases the severity of the intoxication by increasing the non-ionized salicylate that can cross membranes and enter the brain cells. In kidneys, the un-ionized salicylic acid undergoes glomerular filtration, and the ionized portion undergoes tubular secretion in proximal tubules and passive reabsorption in the distal tubules. Renal excretion of salicylate is enhanced by alkaline urine.

Manifestations

The ingestion of concentrated topical salicylic acid preparations (e.g., wart remover) can cause mucosal caustic injury to the gastrointestinal tract. Occult salicylate overdose should be considered in any patient with unexplained acid-base disturbance.

The manifestations of acute overdose of salicylates are as follows:

Minimal Symptoms. Tinnitus, dizziness, and deafness may occur at high therapeutic salicylate plasma concentrations of 20 to 30 mg/dL. Nausea and vomiting may occur immediately because of local gastric irritation.

Phase I. Mild manifestations occur at 1 to 12 hours after ingestion with a 6-hour salicylate plasma concentration of 45 to 70 mg/dL. Nausea and vomiting followed by hyperventilation are usually present within 3 to 8 hours after acute overdose. Hyperventilation, an increase in both rate (tachypnea) and depth (hyperpnea), is present but it may be subtle. It results in a mild respiratory alkalosis with a serum pH greater than 7.4 and urine pH greater than 6.0. Some patients may have lethargy, vertigo, headache, and confusion. Diaphoresis may be noted.

Phase II. Moderate manifestations occur at 12 to 24 hours after ingestion with a 6-hour salicylate plasma concentration of 70 to 90 mg/dL. Serious metabolic disturbances, including a marked respiratory alkalosis with anion gap metabolic acidosis, dehydration, and urine pH less than 6.0, may occur. Other metabolic disturbances include hypoglycemia or hyperglycemia, hypokalemia, decreased ionized calcium, and increased BUN, creatinine, and lactate. Mental disturbances (confusion, disorientation, hallucinations) may occur. Hypotension and convulsions have been reported.

Phase III. Severe intoxication occurs more than 24 hours after ingestion with a 6-hour salicylate plasma concentration of 90 to 130 mg/dL. In addition to the above clinical findings, coma and seizures develop and indicate severe intoxication. Pulmonary edema may occur. Metabolic disturbances include metabolic acidemia (pH <7.4) and aciduria (pH <6.0). In adults, alkalosis may persist until terminal respiratory failure.

In children younger than 4 years of age, a mixed metabolic acidosis and respiratory alkalosis develop earlier (within 4 to 6 hours) than in adults because children have less respiratory reserve and accumulate lactate and other organic acids. Hypoglycemia is more common in children.

Fatalities occur at 6-hour salicylate plasma concentrations greater than 130 to 150 mg/dL and result from CNS depression, cardiovascular collapse, electrolyte imbalance, and cerebral edema.

Chronic salicylism is more serious than acute intoxication and the 6-hour salicylate plasma concentration does not correlate well with the manifestations in both acute and chronic cases of intoxication. Chronic intoxication usually occurs with therapeutic errors in young children or the elderly with underlying illness, and the diagnosis is delayed because it is not recognized. Noncardiac pulmonary edema is a frequent complication in the elderly. The mortality rate is about 25%. Chronic salicylate poisoning in children may mimic Reye syndrome. It is associated with exaggerated CNS findings (hallucinations, delirium, dementia, memory loss, papilledema, bizarre behavior, agitation, encephalopathy, seizures, and coma). Hemorrhagic manifestations, renal failure, and pulmonary and cerebral edema may occur. The metabolic picture is hypoglycemia and mixed acid-base derangements. A chronic salicylate plasma concentration greater than 60 mg/dL with metabolic acidosis and an altered mental state is very serious.

Laboratory Investigations

All patients with intentional salicylate overdoses should have acetaminophen plasma level measured after 4 hours.

One should continuously monitor ECG, urine output, urine pH, and specific gravity. Every 2 to 4 hours in cases of severe intoxication, salicylate plasma concentration, glucose (in a case of salicylism, CNS hypoglycemia may be present despite normal serum glucose), electrolytes, ionized calcium, magnesium and phosphorous, anion gap, ABGs, and pulse oximeter should be monitored. Daily monitoring of BUN, creatinine, liver function tests, and prothrombin time should take place.

The therapeutic salicylate plasma concentration is less than 10 mg/dL for analgesia and 15 to 30 mg/dL for anti-inflammatory effect. Cross-reaction with diflunisal (Dolobid) will give a falsely high salicylate plasma concentration. The Done nomogram is not considered accurate in evaluating acute or chronic salicylate intoxications.

Management

Treatment is based on clinical and metabolic findings, not on salicylate levels. Continuous monitoring of the urine pH is essential for successful alkalinization treatment. One should always obtain an acetaminophen plasma level.

Vital functions must be established and maintained. If the patient is in an altered mental state, glucose, naloxone, and thiamine are administered in standard doses. Depending on the severity, the initial studies include an immediate and a 6-hour postingestion salicylate plasma concentration, ECG and cardiac monitoring, pulse oximeter, urine (analysis, pH, and specific gravity), chest radiograph, ABGs, blood glucose, electrolytes and anion gap calculation, calcium (ionized), magnesium, renal and liver profiles, and prothrombin time. Gastric contents and stool should be tested for occult blood. Bismuth and magnesium salicylate preparations may be radiopaque on radiographs. Consultation with a nephrologist is warranted in cases of moderate, severe, or chronic intoxication.

For gastrointestinal decontamination, activated charcoal is useful (each gram of activated charcoal binds 550 mg of salicylic acid) if a toxic dose was ingested up to 4 hours postingestion. MDAC is not recommended for salicylate intoxication.

Concretions may occur with massive (usually >300 mg/kg) ingestions. If blood levels fail to decline, prompt contrast radiography of the stomach may reveal concretions that have to be removed by repeated lavage, whole-bowel irrigation, endoscopy, or gastrostomy.

Fluids and electrolyte treatment of salicylate poisonings is given in Table 27. For shock, perfusion and vascular volume should be established with 5% dextrose in 0.9% saline, then the treatment can proceed with correction of dehydration and alkalinization.

For cases of acute moderate or severe salicylism (see Table 27), adults should receive a bolus of 1 to 2 mEq/kg of sodium bicarbonate ($NaHCO_3$) followed by an infusion of 100 to 150 mEq $NaHCO_3$ added to 500 to 1000 mL of 5% dextrose and administered over 60 minutes. Children should receive a bolus of 1 to 2 mEq/kg of $NaHCO_3$ followed by an infusion of 1 to 2 mEq/kg added to 20 mL/kg of 5% dextrose administered over 60 minutes. Potassium is added after the patient voids. The goal is to achieve a urine output of greater than 2 mL/kg/hr and a urine pH of greater than 8. The initial infusion is followed by subsequent infusions (two to three times normal maintenance) of 200 to 300 mL/hour in adults or 10 mL/kg/hour in children. If the patient is acidotic and has a serum pH of less than 7.15, an additional 1 to 2 mEq/kg of $NaHCO_3$ is given over 1 to 2 hours; persistent acidosis may require 1 to 2 mEq/kg of bicarbonate every 2 hours. The infusion rate, the amount of bicarbonate, and the electrolytes should be adjusted to correct serum abnormalities and to maintain the targeted urine output and urinary pH. Diuresis is not as important as the alkalinization. Careful monitoring for fluid overload should take place for patients at risk of pulmonary and cerebral edema (e.g., the elderly) and because of inappropriate secretion of the antidiuretic hormone.

In patients with mild intoxication who are not acidotic and have a urine pH greater than 6, 5% dextrose in 0.45% saline should be administered as maintenance to replace ongoing fluid loss. Some toxicologists may consider adding sodium bicarbonate 50 mEq/L or 1 mEq/kg in some cases.

To achieve alkalinization, sodium bicarbonate is administered to produce a serum pH 7.4 to 7.5 and a urine pH greater than 8. Carbonic anhydrase inhibitors (acetazolamide [Diamox]) should not be used. If the patient is acidotic, additional bicarbonate may be required. About 2 mEq/kg raises the blood pH 0.1. In children, alkalinization may be a difficult problem because of the organic acid production and hypokalemia. Hypokalemic and fluid-depleted patients cannot be adequately alkalinized. Alkalinization is usually discontinued in asymptomatic patients with a salicylate plasma concentration less than 30 to 40 mg/dL but is continued in symptomatic patients regardless of the salicylate plasma concentration. A decreased serum bicarbonate but normal or high blood pH indicates respiratory alkalosis predominating over metabolic acidosis, and the bicarbonate should be administered cautiously. An alkalemic pH of 7.40 to 7.50 is not a contraindication to bicarbonate therapy because these patients have a significant base deficit in spite of elevated blood pH.

Potassium is added, 20 to 40 mEq/L, to the infusion after the patient voids. In cases of severe, late, and chronic salicylism, 60 mEq/L of potassium may be

TABLE 27. **Fluid and Electrolyte Treatment of Salicylate Poisoning**

Type of Salicylism	Metabolic Disturbance	Blood pH	Urine pH	Hydrating Solution	Amount of $NaHCO_3$ (mEq/L)	Amount of Potassium (mEq/L)
Mild	Respiratory alkalosis	>7.4	>6.0	5% dextrose, 0.45% saline	50 (adult) 1 mEq/kg (child)	20
Moderate Chronic Child <4 yrs	Respiratory alkalosis Metabolic acidosis	>7.4 or <7.4	<6.0	5% dextrose in water	100 (adult) 1–2 mEq/kg (child)	40
Severe	Metabolic acidosis	<7.4	<6.0	5% dextrose in water	150 (adult) 2 mEq/kg (child)	60
Chronic Child <4 yrs	Respiratory alkalosis					
CNS depressant co-ingestant	Respiratory acidosis	<7.4	<6.0	5% dextrose in water	100–150*	60

*Correct hypoventilation.

Modified from Linden CH, Rumack BH: The legitimate analgesics, aspirin and acetaminophen. In Hansen W Jr (ed): Toxic Emergencies. New York, Churchill Livingstone, 1984.

needed. When the serum potassium is below 4.0 mEq/L, 10 mEq/L should be added over the first hour. If the patient has hypokalemia less than 3 mEq/L and flat T waves and U waves, 0.25 to 0.5 mEq/kg up to 10 mEq/hour is administered. Potassium should be administered under ECG monitoring. Serum potassium is rechecked after each rapidly administered dose. A paradoxical urine acidosis (alkaline serum pH and acid urine pH) indicates that potassium is probably needed.

Convulsions are treated with diazepam or lorazepam, but hypoglycemia, low ionized calcium, cerebral edema, and hemorrhage should first be excluded with a CT scan. If tetany develops, the $NaHCO_3$ therapy is discontinued and calcium gluconate 0.1 to 0.2 mL/kg 10% administered.

Pulmonary edema management consists of fluid restriction, high FIO_2, mechanical ventilation, and positive end-expiratory pressure.

Cerebral edema management consists of fluid restriction, elevation of the head, hyperventilation, osmotic diuresis, and administration of dexamethasone. Vitamin K_1 is administered parenterally to correct an increased prothrombin time (>20 seconds) and coagulation abnormalities. If the patient has active bleeding, fresh plasma and platelets are administered as needed. Hyperpyrexia is managed by external cooling measures, not antipyretics.

Hemodialysis is the choice for removal of salicylates because it corrects the acid-base, electrolyte, and fluid disturbances as well. The indications for hemodialysis include the following:

- Acute poisoning with salicylate plasma concentration greater than 100 mg/dL without improvement after 6 hours of appropriate therapy
- Chronic poisoning with cardiopulmonary disease and a salicylate plasma concentration as low as 40 mg/dL with refractory acidosis, severe CNS manifestations (coma and seizures), and progressive deterioration, especially in elderly patients
- Impairment of vital organs of elimination
- Clinical deterioration in spite of good supportive care and alkalinization
- Severe refractory acid-base or electrolyte disturbances despite appropriate corrective measures

Disposition

There are limitations of salicylate plasma levels and patients are treated on the basis of clinical and laboratory findings. Patients who are asymptomatic should be monitored for a minimum of 6 hours, and longer if enteric-coated tablets or massive overdose was taken or if there is suspicion of concretions. Those who remain asymptomatic with a salicylate plasma concentration less than 35 mg/dL may be discharged following psychiatric evaluation, if indicated. Chronic salicylate-intoxicated patients with acidosis and an altered mental state should be admitted to the intensive care unit. Patients with acute ingestion and a salicylate plasma concentration less than 60 mg/dL and mild symptoms may be able to be treated in the emergency department. Patients with moderate and severe intoxications should be admitted to the intensive care unit.

Selective Serotonin Reuptake Inhibitors

Selective serotonin reuptake inhibitors (SSRIs) are primarily prescribed as antidepressants. SSRIs include fluoxetine (Prozac), paroxetine (Paxil), and sertraline (Zoloft).

Toxic Mechanism

The SSRIs interfere with the neuron reuptake of serotonin (5-hydroxytryptamine) at the presynaptic ganglia sites in the brain, increasing the activity of serotonin. SSRIs should not be used within 5 weeks of when a MAOI is given, nor should MAOI therapy be initiated or discontinued within 5 weeks of SSRI therapy.

Toxic Dose

The therapeutic oral dose of fluoxetine is 20 to 80 mg/d. No toxicity is seen in children with up to 3.5 mg/kg/dose orally. A fatal dose for adults is 6 g. The therapeutic dose for paroxetine is 20 to 50 mg/d. In 35 adult patients, none developed serious side effects after the ingestion of 10 to 1000 mg, and a study involving 35 children failed to demonstrate serious adverse effects at doses less than 180 mg. The therapeutic dose for sertraline is 50 mg to 200 mg/d. Patients have ingested up to 2.6 g without serious side effects. Overdose involving children who ingested less than 100 mg failed to cause adverse events.

Kinetics

Fluoxetine is well absorbed from the gastrointestinal tract, and has a peak plasma concentration at 6 to 8 hours. Volume distribution is 20 to 42 L/kg; 95% is protein bound. The half-life is 4 days (for the demethylated active metabolite norfluoxetine, the half-life is 7 to 15 days). Elimination is 80% renal. Fluoxetine and other serotonin inhibitors are inhibitors of the cytochrome P450, CYP 2D6 enzyme. Therefore interactions may occur with many other medications, such as antidysrhythmic class IC drugs (quinidine), phenytoin (Dilantin), haloperidol, lithium, TCAs, beta-blockers, codeine, and carbamazepine (Tegretol).

Paroxetine is almost completely absorbed from the gastrointestinal tract, with a peak in 2 to 8 hours. Protein binding is greater than 90%; volume distribution is 13 L/kg. Paroxetine undergoes extensive first-pass liver metabolism by oxidation and methylation to inactive metabolites. It inhibits the P450 system (see fluoxetine metabolism). The average half-life is 21 hours.

Sertraline peaks in 8 to 12 hours. Its volume distribution is 20 L/kg and protein binding is 98%. The average half-life of sertraline is 26 hours. It is metabolized to form a less active metabolite, *N*-desmethylsertraline (half-life of 62 to 104 hours).

Manifestations

All SSRIs may cause serotonin syndrome, a potentially life-threatening reaction, if they are administered concurrently with an MAOI. Serotonin syndrome is due to cerebral serotonergic stimulation and can cause severe hyperthermia, myoclonus, rhabdomyolysis, confusion, tremors, and a variety of psychological disturbances. In addition, cardiovascular complications and extrapyramidal side effects, including akathisia, dyskinesia, and parkinson-like syndromes may occur. Also, increased suicidal ideation, seizures, sexual disorders, and hematologic disorders (platelet serotonin activity blockade leading to prolonged bleeding times) may develop. Inappropriate secretion of antidiuretic hormone resulting in hyponatremia may occur when SSRIs are administered to the elderly. This effect is usually seen within the first week of therapy.

Overdose effects are similar to the serotonin syndrome.

Laboratory Investigations

One should obtain a complete blood count (CBC), electrolytes, glucose levels, a coagulation profile, liver function tests, creatine kinase level, and an ECG.

Management

There is no specific antidote to SSRI intoxication.

Initial management consists of stabilizing vital functions, including thermoregulation. Supportive therapy and anticipation of potential life-threatening manifestations (hypotension, hyperthermia, seizures, coma, disseminated intravascular coagulation, ventricular tachycardia, and metabolic acidosis), are essential. Vital signs, EEG, creatine kinase, and blood chemistry should be monitored.

Benzodiazepines are administered to prevent and control muscle hyperactivity (diazepam [Valium] for seizures, clonazepam [Klonopin] for myoclonus). If benzodiazepine therapy fails to control muscle activity or seizures, anesthesia or nondepolarizing neuromuscular blockade may be necessary.

Electrolyte abnormalities and acid-base balance should be corrected. Fluids are used to maintain a urine output of greater than 2 mL/kg/hour if there is a risk of myoglobinuria.

There are no data to support the use of gastrointestinal decontamination, although activated charcoal may be used if an ingestion has occurred within 1 hour. Hemodialysis and charcoal hemoperfusion are unlikely to be beneficial. Haloperidol (Haldol), phenothiazines, and other highly protein-bound drugs are to be avoided.

Benzodiazepine and cooling therapy can be used for hyperthermia. Serotonin antagonists, such as cyproheptadine (Periactin), may be useful in treating serotonin syndrome, although there are no controlled data. Dantrolene (Dantrium) and bromocriptine (Parlodel) are not recommended and may actually precipitate serotonin syndrome.

Disposition

Cases of ingestions in children up to 5 years of age of less than 180 mg of paroxetine (Paxil), less than 3.5 mg/kg of fluoxetine (Prozac), or less than 100 mg of sertraline (Zoloft) can be observed at home. Symptomatic patients should be admitted to the intensive care unit until asymptomatic for 24 hours. Asymptomatic patients should be observed for 6 hours. All patients should be assessed for risk of suicide before discharge. When taken chronically, SSRIs may increase cholesterol and triglycerides and decrease uric acid, so these test results should be followed.

Theophylline

Theophylline (Slo-Phyllin) is a methylxanthine alkaloid similar to caffeine and theobromine. Aminophylline is 80% theophylline. Theophylline is used in the acute treatment of asthma, pulmonary edema, chronic obstructive pulmonary disease, and neonatal apnea.

Toxic Mechanism

The proposed mechanisms of action include phosphodiesterase inhibition, adenosine receptor antagonism, inhibition of prostaglandins, and increase in serum catecholamines. Theophylline stimulates the central nervous, respiratory, and emetic centers and reduces the seizure threshold. It has positive cardiac inotropic and chronotropic effects, acts as a diuretic, relaxes smooth muscle, and causes peripheral vasodilation but cerebral vasoconstriction. Gastric secretions, gastrointestinal motility, lipolysis, glycogenolysis, and gluconeogenesis are all increased.

Toxic Dose

A single dose of 1 mg/kg produces a theophylline plasma concentration of approximately 2 μg/mL. The therapeutic range usually is 10 to 20 μg/mL. An acute, single dose greater than 10 mg/kg causes mild toxicity, a dose greater than 20 mg/kg causes moderate toxicity, and a dose greater than 50 mg/kg causes serious, possibly fatal toxicity. Fatalities occur at lower doses in patients with chronic toxicity, especially those with risk factors (see Kinetics).

Kinetics

The pKa is 9.5. Absorption from the stomach and upper small intestine is complete and rapid, with onset in 30 to 60 minutes. Peak theophylline plasma concentration occurs within 1 to 2 hours after ingestion of liquid preparations, 2 to 4 hours after ingestion of regular tablets, and 7 to 24 hours after ingestion of slow-release formulations. Volume distribution is 0.3 to 0.7 L/kg. Protein binding is 40% to 60% in adults, mainly to albumin (low albumin increases free active theophylline).

Elimination is 90% by hepatic metabolism to an active metabolite, 2-methyl xanthine. The half-life is 3.5 hours in a child and 4 to 6 hours in an adult. The half-life is shorter in smokers and patients taking enzyme-inducing drugs. Only 8% to 10% of the drug is excreted unchanged in the urine.

Risk factors that produce a longer half-life include age younger than 6 months or older than 60 years, use of enzyme-inhibitor drugs (calcium channel blockers, oral contraceptives, cimetidine [Tagamet], ciprofloxacin [Cipro], erythromycin, macrolide antibiotics, isoniazid), illness (persistent fever >38.9°C [>102°F]), viral illness, liver impairment, heart failure, chronic obstructive pulmonary disease, and influenza vaccination.

Manifestations

Acute toxicity generally correlates with blood levels; chronic toxicity does not (Table 28).

In the case of an acute, single, regular-release overdose, vomiting and occasionally hematemesis occur at low theophylline plasma concentrations. CNS stimulation includes restlessness, muscle tremors, and protracted tonic-clonic seizures, but coma is rare. Convulsions are a sign of severe toxicity and usually are preceded by gastrointestinal symptoms (except with sustained-release and chronic intoxications). Cardiovascular disturbances include cardiac dysrhythmias (supraventricular tachycardia) and transient hypertension with mild overdoses, but hypotension and ventricular dysrhythmias with severe intoxications. Rhabdomyolysis and renal failure are occasionally seen. Children tolerate higher serum levels, and cardiac dysrhythmias and seizures occur at theophylline plasma concentrations greater than 100 μg/mL. Possible metabolic disturbances include hyperglycemia, pronounced hypokalemia, hypocalcemia, hypomagnesemia, hypophosphatemia, increased serum amylase, and elevation of uric acid.

Chronic intoxication, defined as multiple doses of theophylline over 24 hours, or cases in which interacting drugs or illness interfere with theophylline metabolism are more serious and difficult to treat. Cardiac dysrhythmias and convulsions may occur at theophylline plasma concentrations of 40 to 60 μg/mL and there is no correlation with TPC. The seizures occur without warning and are protracted and repetitive and may produce status epilepticus. Vomiting and typical metabolic disturbances do not occur.

Differences with slow-release preparations are that few or no gastrointestinal symptoms occur, peak concentrations and convulsions may be delayed 12 to 24 hours postingestion, and convulsions occur without warning.

TABLE 28. **Theophylline Blood Concentrations and Acute Toxicity**

Plasma Concentration (μg/mL)	Toxicity Degree	Manifestations
8–10	None	Bronchodilation
10–20	Mild	Therapeutic range: nausea, vomiting, nervousness, respiratory alkalosis, tachycardia
15–25		35% have mild manifestations of toxicity
20–40	Moderate	Gastrointestinal complaints and central nervous system stimulation
		Transient hypertension, tachypnea, tachycardia; 80% will have some manifestations of toxicity
60	Severe	Convulsions, dysrhythmias
100		Hypokalemia, hyperglycemia
		Ventricular dysrhythmias, protracted convulsions, hypotension, acid-base abnormalities

Laboratory Investigations

Monitoring includes vital signs, pulse oximeter, ABG, hemoglobin, hematocrit (for gastrointestinal hemorrhage), ECG and cardiac monitor, renal and hepatic function, electrolytes, blood glucose, acid-base balance, and serum albumin. Gastric contents and stools should be tested for occult blood. Samples for theophylline plasma concentration measurement should be drawn within 1 to 2 hours after ingestion of liquid preparations, 2 to 4 hours after ingestion of regular-release formulations, and 4 hours after ingestion of slow-release formulations. One should check the serum albumin level because a decrease in albumin levels may cause manifestations of toxicity despite normal theophylline plasma concentration. A single theophylline plasma concentration reading may be misleading; therefore, theophylline plasma concentration measurement should be repeated every 2 to 4 hours to determine the trend until a declining trend is reached and then monitored every 4 to 6 hours until it is below 20 μg/mL.

Management

Vital functions must be established and maintained. If the patient is in a coma or has convulsions or vomiting, he or she should be intubated immediately. The theophylline plasma concentration is obtained and repeated every 2 to 4 hours to determine peak absorption, and a theophylline bezoar should be considered if the theophylline plasma concentration fails to decline. Consultation with a nephrologist about charcoal hemoperfusion is recommended.

Gastrointestinal decontamination is warranted in the case of an acute overdose, but emesis must not be induced. Activated charcoal is the choice decontamination procedure in a dose of 1 g/kg to all patients, followed with MDAC 0.5 g/kg every 2 to 4 hours until the theophylline plasma concentration is less than 20 μg/mL. MDAC is effective in treating acute, chronic, and intravenous overdoses. Activated charcoal shortens the half-life of theophylline by about 50% and may be indicated up to 24 hours following ingestion.

Whole-bowel irrigation with polyethylene-electrolyte solution has been recommended for cases of massive overdose, possible concretions, and ingestion of sustained-release preparations. If intractable vomiting occurs, the antiemetic metoclopramide (Reglan) (0.1 mg/kg adult dose), droperidol (Inapsine) (2.5 to 10 mg IV), or ondansetron (Zofran) (8 to 32 mg IV) is administered. Ondansetron, however, inhibits metabolism of theophylline after a few doses.

Convulsions are controlled with lorazepam (Ativan) or diazepam (Valium) and phenobarbital. Phenytoin (Dilantin) is ineffective. The convulsions in patients with chronic intoxication are often refractory and may require, in addition to anticonvulsants, neuromuscular paralyzing agents, sedation, assisted ventilation, and EEG monitoring.

Hypotension is treated with fluids and vasopressors, if necessary. Norepinephrine (Levophed) 0.05 μg/kg/min is preferred as the vasopressor over dopamine.

Supraventricular tachycardia with hemodynamic instability requires cardioversion. Low-dose β-blockers may be used but should not be used in patients with reactive airway disease or hypotension. Adenosine (Adenocard) is ineffective. For ventricular dysrhythmias, electrolyte disturbances should be corrected. Lidocaine is the treatment of choice but has the potential to cause seizures at toxic concentrations. Cardioversion may be needed.

Hematemesis is managed with sucralfate (Carafate) 1 g four times daily and/or Maalox TC 30 mL every 2 hours and blood replacement, if necessary. H_2 antihistamine blockers that are enzyme inhibitors are not used.

Fluid and metabolic disturbances should be corrected. Hyperglycemia does not require insulin therapy. Hypokalemia should be corrected cautiously, as it may be largely an intracellular shift and not total body loss. Usually adding 40 mEq potassium to a liter of fluid will suffice. The serum potassium level must be monitored closely.

Charcoal hemoperfusion is the management of choice for patients with serious intoxications. Hemoperfusion can increase the clearance twofold to threefold over hemodialysis, but hemodialysis can be used if hemoperfusion is not available. Criteria for charcoal hemoperfusion are as follows:

- Life-threatening events such as convulsions or dysrhythmias
- Intractable vomiting refractory to antiemetics
- Acute intoxications with a theophylline plasma concentration greater than 80 μg/mL or greater than 70 μg/mL 4 hours after overdose with a sustained-release formulation and greater than 40 μg/mL in the case of chronic intoxication
- Acute or chronic overdoses with a theophylline plasma concentration greater than 40 μg/mL, especially if the patient has risk factors that lengthen the half-life of the drug (see Kinetics).

Disposition

Patients with mild symptoms and a theophylline plasma concentration less than 20 μg/mL can be treated in emergency department and discharged when asymptomatic for a few hours. Any patient with acute ingestion and a theophylline plasma concentration greater than 35 μg/mL should be admitted to a monitored bed with seizure precautions and suicide precautions, if needed. If neurologic or cardiotoxic effects or a theophylline plasma concentration greater than 50 μg/mL is present, the patient should be admitted to the intensive care unit. A patient with an overdose of a sustained-release preparation, regardless of symptoms or initial theophylline plasma concentration, requires admission, monitoring, activated charcoal, and MDAC. In patients on chronic therapy, toxicity may occur at a lower theophylline plasma concentration, and these patients should not be discharged until they are asymptomatic for several hours.

Tricyclic and Cyclic Antidepressants

Historically, tricyclic antidepressants are an important cause of pharmaceutical overdose fatalities. The mortality rate has been reduced from 15% in the 1970s to less than 1% in the 1990s due to better understanding of the pathophysiology of these agents and improvements in management (Table 29).

Toxic Mechanism

The major mechanisms of toxicity of the tricyclic antidepressants are (1) central and peripheral anticholinergic effects; (2) peripheral α-adrenergic blockade; (3) quinidine-like cardiac membrane stabilizing action blockade of the fast inward sodium channels; and (4) inhibition of synaptic neurotransmitter reuptake in the CNS presynaptic neurons. The tetracyclics, monocyclic aminoketones, and dibenzoxazepines possess convulsive activity and less cardiac toxicity in overdose than the older tricyclic antidepressants. Triazolopyridine has less serious cardiac and CNS toxicity.

Toxic Dose

The therapeutic dose of imipramine (Tofranil) is 1.5 to 5 mg/kg; a dose greater than 5 mg/kg may be mildly toxic; 10 to 20 mg/kg may be life threatening, although less than 20 mg/kg has produced few fatalities; greater than 30 mg/kg carries a 30% mortality rate; and at a dose greater than 70 mg/kg, patients rarely survive. In children 375 mg and in adults as little as 500 mg have been fatal. In adults, five times the maximum daily dose is toxic and 10 times is potentially fatal. Although major overdose symptoms are associated with plasma concentrations greater than 1 μg/mL (>1000 ng/mL), plasma tricyclic levels do not correlate well with toxicity; clinical signs and symptoms should guide therapy.

The relative dosage or potency equivalents are as follows: amitriptyline (Elavil) 100 mg = amoxapine (Asendin) 125 mg = desipramine (Norpramin) 75 mg = doxepin (Sinequan) 100 mg = imipramine (Tofranil) 75 mg = maprotiline (Ludiomil) 75 mg = nortriptyline (Pamelor) 50 mg = trazodone (Desyrel) 200 mg. This allows one to determine an equivalent dosage of an agent compared with another (see Table 29).

Kinetics

The tricyclic and cyclic antidepressants are lipophilic. They are rapidly absorbed from the alkaline small intestine, but absorption may be prolonged and delayed in cases of massive overdose owing to anticholinergic action. Onset varies from less than 1 hour (30 to 40 minutes) to, rarely, 12 hours. The peak serum levels are reached in 2 to 8 hours and the peak effect is in 6 hours but may be delayed 12 hours due to erratic absorption. The clinical effects correlate poorly with plasma levels.

Cyclic antidepressants are highly protein-bound to plasma glycoproteins, 98% at a pH 7.5 and 90% at 7.0. Volume distribution is 10 to 50 L/kg. The elimination route is by hepatic metabolism. The tertiary amines are metabolized into active demethylated secondary

TABLE 29. **Cyclic Antidepressants, Daily Dose and Their Major Properties**

Generic Name	Adult Daily Dose (mg)	Therapeutic Range (ng/mL)	Half-Life (hours)	Toxicity		
				*Antichol**	*CNS*	*Cardiac*
Tertiary amines						
Amitriptyline (Elavil)	75–300	120–250	31–46	3+	3+	3+
Imipramine (Tofranil)	75–300	125–250	9–24	3+	3+	2+
Doxepin (Sinequan)	75–300	30–150	8–24	3+	3+	2+
Trimipramine (Surmantil)	75–200	10–240	16–18	3+	3+	2+
Secondary amines						
Nortriptyline (Pamelor)	75–150	50–150	18–93	2+	3+	3+
Desipramine (Norpramin)	75–200	75–160	14–62	1+	3+	3+
Protriptyline (Vivactil)	20–60	70–250	54–198	2+	3+	3+
Newer cyclic antidepressants						
Tetracyclic						
Maprotiline (Ludiomil)	75–300	—	30–60	1+	2+	3+
Trizolopyridine, a noncyclic, produces less serious cardiac and CNS toxicity						
Trazodone (Desyrel)	50–600	700	4–7	1+	1+	1+
Monocyclic aminoketone						
Bupropion (Wellbutin)	200–400	—	8–24	1+	3+	1+
Dibenzazepine						
Clomipramine (Anafranil)	100–250	200–500	21–32	2+	2+	2+
Dibenoxazepine						
Amoxapine (Ascendin)	150–300	200–500	6–10	1+	3+	2+

*Antichol, anticholinergic effect; CNS, Central nervous system effect primarily seizures; Cardiac, cardiac effect.

Other drugs with similar structures are cyclobenzaprine, a muscle relaxant (similar to amitriptyline) and carbamazepine, an anticonvulsant (similar to imipramine); however, they cause less cardiac toxicity.

amine metabolites. The active secondary amine metabolites undergo a 15% enterohepatic recirculation and are metabolized over a period of days into nonactive metabolites. The intestinal bacterial flora may reconstitute the metabolites, which are active.

The half-life varies from 10 hours for imipramine to 81 hours for amitriptyline and 100 hours for nortriptyline. The active metabolites have longer half-lives.

Only 3% of the ingested dose is excreted in the urine unchanged.

Manifestations

There are reports of asymptomatic patients who, upon arrival to an emergency department, suddenly have a seizure, develop hemodynamically unstable dysrhythmias, and die shortly thereafter from ingestion of a tricyclic antidepressant. Most patients with severe toxicity develop symptoms within 1 to 2 hours, but symptoms may be delayed 6 hours after overdose.

Small overdoses produce early anticholinergic effects, agitation, and transient hypertension, which are not life-threatening. Large overdoses produce depression of the CNS and myocardium, convulsions, and hypotension. Death can occur within the first 2 to 6 hours following ingestion.

Some ECG screening tools for predicting cardiac or neurologic toxicity from ingestion of a tricyclic antidepressant have been developed: (1) A QRS greater than 0.10 second may produce seizures, and if greater than 0.16 second, 50% of patients may develop ventricular dysrhythmias (20% of these may be life-threatening) and seizures; (2) a terminal 40 msec of the QRS axis greater than 120 degrees in the right frontal plane may be associated with toxicity; or (3) a large R wave greater than 3 mm in ECG lead aVR may predispose the patient to toxicity. The quinidine cardiac membrane stabilizing effect produces depression of myocardium, conduction, and ECG changes. The peripheral α-adrenergic blockade produces hypotension.

The secondary amines are metabolized to inactive metabolites. The tetracyclics produce a high incidence of cardiovascular disturbances and seizures. Moncyclic aminoketones produce seizures in doses greater than 600 mg. Dibenoxazepines produce a syndrome of convulsions, rhabdomyolysis, and renal failure.

Laboratory Investigations

If the patient has altered mental status or ECG abnormalities, ABG, ECG, chest radiograph, blood glucose, serum electrolytes, calcium, magnesium, blood urea nitrogen, and creatinine levels, liver profile, creatine kinase level, urine output, and, in severe cases, hemodynamic monitoring are indicated. Levels of the tricyclic and cyclic antidepressants less than 300 ng/mL are therapeutic; levels greater than 500 ng/mL indicate toxicity, and levels greater than 1000 ng/mL indicate serious poisoning and are associated with QRS widening.

Management

Vital functions must be established and maintained. Even if the patient is asymptomatic, intravenous access should be established, vital signs and neurologic status monitored, and baseline 12-lead ECG and continuous cardiac monitoring obtained for at least 6 hours from admission or 8 to 12 hours postingestion. QRS interval should be measured on a limb lead ECG every 15 minutes for 6 hours postingestion.

For gastrointestinal decontamination, emesis should not be induced and gastric lavage should not be used. Activated charcoal is preferable. If the patient is in an altered mental state, the airway must be protected. Activated charcoal 1 g/kg is recommended up to 1 hour postingestion. Benefit from MDAC has not been demonstrated.

Alkalinization does not control seizures; diazepam or lorazepam should be used. Status epilepticus may require high-dose barbiturates or neuromuscular blockers with intravenous diazepam. If not successful, the patient can be paralyzed with short-term nondepolarizing neuromuscular blockers such as vecuronium (Norcuron), intubation, and assisted ventilation. A bolus of sodium bicarbonate is recommended as an adjunct to correct the acidosis produced by the seizures.

Sodium bicarbonate is administered in a dose of 1 to 2 mEq/kg undiluted as a bolus and repeated twice a few minutes apart, if needed, for "sodium loading" and alkalinization, which may increase protein binding from 90% to 98%. The sodium loading overcomes the sodium channel blockage and is more important than the alkalinization. Indications include (1) a QRS complex greater than 0.12 second, (2) ventricular tachycardia, (3) severe conduction disturbances, (4) metabolic acidosis, (5) coma, and (6) seizures. A continuous infusion of sodium bicarbonate is of limited usefulness for controlling dysrhythmias. Bolus therapy should be used as needed.

Hyperventilation alone has been recommended, but the pH elevation is not as instantaneous and there is compensatory renal excretion of bicarbonate; therefore, we do not recommend it. The combination of hyperventilation and sodium bicarbonate has produced fatal alkalemia and is not recommended. One should monitor serum potassium level (the sudden increase in blood pH can aggravate or precipitate hypokalemia), serum sodium, and ionized calcium levels (hypocalcemia may occur with alkalinization) and blood pH.

Specific cardiovascular complications should be treated as follows: Hypotension is treated with norepinephrine, a predominantly α-adrenergic drug, which is preferred over dopamine. Hypertension that occurs early rarely requires treatment. Sinus tachycardia usually does not require treatment. Supraventricular tachycardia in a patient who is hemodynamically unstable requires synchronized electrical cardioversion, starting at 0.25 to 1.0 watt-second per kg, after sedation. Ventricular tachycardia that persists after alkalinization requires intravenous lidocaine or countershock if the patient is hemodynamically unstable. Ventricular fibrillation should be treated with defibrillation. Torsades de pointes is treated with magnesium sulfate IV 20% solution, 2 g over 2 to 3 minutes, followed by a continuous infusion of 1.5 mL 10% solution or 5 to 10 mg per minute. For the treatment of bradydysrhythmias, atropine is contraindicated because of the anticholinergic activity. Isoproterenol 0.1 μg/kg/minute, used with caution, may produce hypotension. If the patient is hemodynamically unstable, a pacemaker is used.

Extraordinary measures, such as aortic balloon pump and cardiopulmonary bypass, have been successful.

Investigational treatments include FAB fragments specific for tricyclic antidepressant, which have been successful in animals. Prophylactic $NaHCO_3$ to prevent dysrhythmias is also being investigated.

Physostigmine has produced asystole, and flumazenil has produced seizures. Both are contraindicated.

Disposition

A patient with an antidepressant overdose who meets any of the following criteria should be admitted to the intensive care unit for 12 to 24 hours: (1) ECG abnormalities except sinus tachycardia, (2) altered mental state, (3) seizures, (4) respiratory depression, and (5) hypotension. Low-risk patients include those in whom the above symptoms are absent at 6 hours postingestion, those who present with minor transient manifestations such as sinus tachycardia who subsequently become and remain asymptomatic for a 6-hour period, and asymptomatic patients who remain asymptomatic for 6 hours. These patients may be discharged if the ECG remains normal, they have normal bowel sounds, and they undergo psychiatric disposition.

Even if the patient is asymptomatic upon presentation to the health care facility, intravenous access should be established, vital signs and neurologic status monitored, a baseline 12-lead ECG obtained, and cardiac monitoring continued for at least 6 hours. Caution: in 25% of fatal cases, the patients were initially alert and awake at presentation. However, in most cases of fatality initially deemed as sudden cardiac death, the patient, upon reexamination, actually had symptoms that were missed.

Children younger than 6 years of age with nonintentional (accidental) exposures to amitriptyline (Elavil), desipramine (Norpramin), doxepin (Sinequan), imipramine (Tofranil), or nortriptyline (Aventyl) in a dose less than 5 mg/kg, who are asymptomatic and have what are deemed reliable caregivers, can be observed at home, with close poison control follow-up for 6 hours. Parents or caregivers should be given instructions regarding signs and symptoms to be alert for. Children who are symptomatic, or who ingested greater than 5 mg/kg, should be referred to the emergency department for monitoring, observation, and activated charcoal treatment.

Section 19
Appendices and Index

REFERENCE INTERVALS FOR THE INTERPRETATION OF LABORATORY TESTS

method of
WILLIAM Z. BORER, M.D.
Thomas Jefferson University Hospital
Philadelphia, Pennsylvania

Most of the tests performed in a clinical laboratory are quantitative; that is, the amount of a substance present in blood or serum is measured and reported in terms of concentration, activity (e.g., enzyme activity), or counts (e.g., blood cell counts). The laboratory must provide reference intervals to assist the clinician in the interpretation of laboratory results. These reference intervals represent the physiologic quantities of a substance (concentrations, activities, or counts) to be expected in healthy persons. Deviation above or below the reference range may be associated with a disease process, and the severity of the disease process may be associated with the magnitude of the deviation. Unfortunately, a sharp demarcation rarely exists to distinguish between physiologic and pathologic values, and the time of transition between the two is often gradual as the disease process progresses.

The terms *normal* and *abnormal* have been used to describe laboratory values that fall inside and outside the reference range, respectively. Use of these terms is inappropriate because no good definition of normality exists in the clinical sense and the term *normal* may be confused with the statistical term *gaussian*. Reference ranges are established from statistical studies in groups of healthy volunteers. These study subjects must be free of disease, but they may have lifestyles or habits that result in variations in certain laboratory values. Examples of these variables include diet, body mass, exercise, and geographic location. Age and gender may also affect reference values.

When the data from a large cohort of healthy subjects fit a gaussian distribution, the usual statistical approach is to define the reference limits as 2 SD above and below the mean. By definition, the reference range excludes the 2.5% of the population with the lowest values and the 2.5% with the highest values. Nongaussian distributions are handled by different statistical methods, but the result is similar in that the reference range is defined by the central 95% of the population. In other words, the probability that a healthy person will have a laboratory result that falls outside the reference range is 1 in 20. If 12 laboratory tests are performed, the probability that at least one of the results will be outside the reference range increases to about 50%, which means that all healthy persons are likely to have a few laboratory results that are unexpected. The clinician must then integrate these data with other clinical information, such as the history and physical examination, to arrive at an appropriate clinical decision.

The reference intervals for many tests (especially enzyme and immunochemical measurements) vary with the method used. Accordingly, each laboratory must establish reference intervals that are appropriate for the methods used.

SI UNITS

During the 1980s, a concerted effort was made to introduce SI units (le Système International d'Unités). The rationale for conversion to SI units is sound. Laboratory data are scientifically more informative when the units are based on molar concentration rather than on mass concentration. For example, the conversion of glucose to lactate and pyruvate or the binding of a drug to albumin is more easily understood in units of molar concentration. Another example is illustrated as follows:

Conventional Units

1.0 g of hemoglobin:

- Combines with 1.37 mL of oxygen
- Contains 3.4 mg of iron
- Forms 34.9 mg of bilirubin

SI Units

4.0 mmol of hemoglobin:

- Combines with 4.0 mmol of oxygen
- Contains 4.0 mmol of iron
- Forms 4.0 mmol of bilirubin

The use of SI units would also enhance the standardization of nomenclature to facilitate global communication of medical and scientific information.

TABLE 1. **Base SI Units**

Property	Base Unit	Symbol
Length	Meter	m
Mass	Kilogram	kg
Amount of substance	Mole	mol
Time	Second	s
Thermodynamic temperature	Kelvin	K
Electrical current	Ampere	A
Luminous intensity	Candela	cd
Catalytic amount	Katal	kat

The units, symbols, and prefixes used in the international system are shown in Tables 1, 2, and 3.

Unfortunately, problems have arisen with the implementation of SI units in the United States. The introduction of this system in 1987 prompted many medical journals to report laboratory values in both SI and conventional units in anticipation of complete conversion to SI units in the early 1990s. The lack of a coordinated effort toward this goal forced a retrenchment on the issue. Physicians continue to think and practice with laboratory results expressed in conventional units, and few, if any, hospitals or clinical laboratories in the United States use SI units exclusively. Complete conversion to SI units is not likely to occur in the foreseeable future, but most medical journals will probably continue to publish both sets of units. For this reason, the values in the tables of reference ranges in this appendix are given in both conventional units and SI units.

TABLES OF REFERENCE INTERVALS

Some of the values included in the tables that follow have been established by the Clinical Laboratories at Thomas Jefferson University Hospital in Philadelphia and have not been published elsewhere. Other values have been compiled from the sources cited in the suggested readings. These tables are provided for information and educational purposes only. Laboratory values must always be interpreted in the context of clinical data derived from other sources, including the medical history and physical examination. One must exercise individual judgment when using the information provided in this appendix.

TABLE 2. **Derived SI Units and Non-SI Units Retained for Use With SI Units**

Property	Unit	Symbol
Area	Square meter	m^2
Volume	Cubic meter	m^3
	Liter	L
Mass concentration	Kilogram/cubic meter	kg/m^3
	Gram/liter	g/L
Substance concentration	Mole/cubic meter	mol/m^3
	Mole/liter	mol/L
Temperature	Degree Celsius	C = K – 273.15

TABLE 3. **Standard Prefixes**

Prefix	Multiplication Factor	Symbol
yocto	10^{-24}	y
zepto	10^{-21}	z
atto	10^{-18}	a
femto	10^{-15}	f
pico	10^{-12}	p
nano	10^{-9}	n
micro	10^{-6}	μ
milli	10^{-3}	m
centi	10^{-2}	c
deci	10^{-1}	d
deca	10^{1}	da
hecto	10^{2}	h
kilo	10^{3}	k
mega	10^{6}	M
giga	10^{9}	G
tera	10^{12}	T

SUGGESTED READINGS

Bick RL (ed): Hematology: Clinical and Laboratory Practice. St Louis, Mosby-Year Book, 1993.

Borer WZ: Selection and use of laboratory tests. In Tietz NW, Conn RB, Pruden EL (eds): Applied Laboratory Medicine. Philadelphia, WB Saunders, 1992, pp 1-5.

Campion EW: A retreat from SI units. N Engl J Med 327:49, 1992.

Drug Evaluations Annual. Chicago, American Medical Association, 1994.

Friedman RB, Young DS: Effects of Disease on Clinical Laboratory Tests, 3rd ed. Washington, DC, AACC Press, 1997.

Henry JB: Clinical Diagnosis and Management by Laboratory Methods, 19th ed. Philadelphia, WB Saunders, 1996.

Hicks JM, Young DS: DORA 97-99: Directory of Rare Analyses. Washington, DC, AACC Press, 1997.

Jacob DS, Demott WR, Grady HJ, et al (eds): Laboratory Test Handbook, 4th ed. Baltimore, Williams & Wilkins, 1996.

Kaplan LA, Pesce AJ: Clinical Chemistry: Theory, Analysis, and Correlation, 3rd ed. St Louis, Mosby-Year Book, 1996.

Kjeldsberg CR, Knight JA: Body Fluids: Laboratory Examination of Amniotic, Cerebrospinal, Seminal, Serous and Synovial Fluids, 3rd ed. Chicago, ASCP Press, 1993.

Laposata M: SI Unit Conversion Guide. Boston, NEJM Books, 1992.

Scully RE, McNeely WF, Mark EJ, McNeely BU: Normal reference laboratory values. N Engl J Med 327:718-724, 1992.

Speicher CE: The Right Test: A Physician's Guide to Laboratory Medicine, 3rd ed. Philadelphia, WB Saunders, 1998.

Tietz NW (ed): Clinical Guide to Laboratory Tests, 3rd ed. Philadelphia, WB Saunders, 1995.

Wallach J: Interpretation of Diagnostic Tests: A Synopsis of Laboratory Medicine, 6th ed. Boston, Little, Brown, 1996.

Young DS: Effects of Preanalytical Variables on Clinical Laboratory Tests, 2nd ed. Washington, DC, AACC Press, 1997.

Young DS: Effects of Drugs on Clinical Laboratory Tests, 4th ed. Washington, DC, AACC Press, 1995.

Young DS: Determination and validation of reference intervals. Arch Pathol Lab Med 116:704-709, 1992.

Young DS: Implementation of SI units for clinical laboratory data. Ann Intern Med 106:114-129, 1987.

Reference Intervals for Hematology

Test	Conventional Units	SI Units
Acid hemolysis (Ham test)	No hemolysis	No hemolysis
Alkaline phosphatase, leukocyte	Total score, 14-100	Total score, 14-100
Cell counts		
Erythrocytes		
Males	4.6-6.2 million/mm^3	4.6-6.2 × 10^{12}/L
Females	4.2-5.4 million/mm^3	4.2-5.4 × 10^{12}/L
Children (varies with age)	4.5-5.1 million/mm^3	4.5-5.1 × 10^{12}/L
Leukocytes, total	4500-11,000/mm^3	4.5-11.0 × 10^9/L
Leukocytes, differential counts*		
Myelocytes	0%	0/L
Band neutrophils	3-5%	150-400 × 10^6/L
Segmented neutrophils	54-62%	3000-5800 × 10^6/L
Lymphocytes	25-33%	1500-3000 × 10^6/L
Monocytes	3-7%	300-500 × 10^6/L
Eosinophils	1-3%	50-250 × 10^6/L
Basophils	0-1%	15-50 × 10^6/L
Platelets	150,000-400,000/mm^3	150-400 × 10^9/L
Reticulocytes	25,000-75,000/mm^3 (0.5-1.5% of erythrocytes)	25-75 × 10^9/L
Coagulation tests		
Bleeding time (template)	2.75-8.0 min	2.75-8.0 min
Coagulation time (glass tube)	5-15 min	5-15 min
D Dimer	<0.5 μg/mL	<0.5 mg/L
Factor VIII and other coagulation factors	50-150% of normal	0.5-1.5 of normal
Fibrin split products (Thrombo-Welco test)	<10 μg/mL	<10 mg/L
Fibrinogen	200-400 mg/dL	2.0-4.0 g/L
Partial thromboplastin time, activated (aPTT)	20-25 s	20-35 s
Prothrombin time (PT)	12.0-14.0 s	12.0-14.0 s
Coombs' test		
Direct	Negative	Negative
Indirect	Negative	Negative
Corpuscular values of erythrocytes		
Mean corpuscular hemoglobin (MCH)	26-34 pg/cell	26-34 pg/cell
Mean corpuscular volume (MCV)	80-96 μm^3	80-96 fL
Mean corpuscular hemoglobin concentration (MCHC)	32-36 g/dL	320-360 g/L
Haptoglobin	20-165 mg/dL	0.20-1.65 g/L
Hematocrit		
Males	40-54 mL/dL	0.40-0.54
Females	37-47 mL/dL	0.37-0.47
Newborns	49-54 mL/dL	0.49-0.54
Children (varies with age)	35-49 mL/dL	0.35-0.49
Hemaglobin		
Males	13.0-18.0 g/dL	8.1-11.2 mmol/L
Females	12.0-16.0 g/dL	7.4-9.9 mmol/L
Newborns	16.5-19.5 g/dL	10.2-12.1 mmol/L
Children (varies with age)	11.2-16.5 g/dL	7.0-10.2 mmol/L
Hemoglobin, fetal	<1.0% of total	<0.01 of total
Hemoglobin A_{1C}	3-5% of total	0.03-0.05 of total
Hemoglobin A_2	1.5-3.0% of total	0.015-0.03 of total
Hemoglobin, plasma	0.0-5.0 mg/dL	0.0-3.2 μmol/L
Methemoglobin	30-130 mg/dL	19-80 μmol/L
Erythrocyte sedimentation rate (ESR)		
Wintrobe:		
Males	0-5 mm/h	0-5 mm/h
Females	0-15 mm/h	0-15 mm/h
Westergren:		
Males	0-15 mm/h	0-15 mm/h
Females	0-20 mm/h	0-20 mm/h

*Conventional units are percentages; SI units are absolute cell counts.

Reference Intervals* for Clinical Chemistry (Blood, Serum, and Plasma)

Analyte	Conventional Units	SI Units
Acetoacetate plus acetone		
Qualitative	Negative	Negative
Quantitative	0.3-2.0 mg/dL	30-200 μmol/L
Acid phosphatase, serum (thymolphthalein monophosphate substrate)	0.1-0.6 U/L	0.1-0.6 U/L
ACTH (see Corticotropin)		
Alanine aminotransferase (ALT), serum (SGPT)	1-45 U/L	1-45 U/L
Albumin, serum	3.3-5.2 g/dL	33-52 g/L
Aldolase, serum	0.0-7.0 U/L	0.0-7.0 U/L
Aldosterone, plasma		
Standing	5-30 ng/dL	140-830 pmol/L
Recumbent	3-10 ng/dL	80-275 pmol/L
Alkaline, phosphatase (ALP), serum		
Adult	35-150 U/L	35-150 U/L
Adolescent	100-500 U/L	100-500 U/L
Child	100-350 U/L	100-350 U/L
Ammonia nitrogen, plasma	10-50 μmol/L	10-50 μmol/L
Amylase, serum	25-125 U/L	25-125 U/L
Anion gap, serum, calculated	8-16 mEq/L	8-16 mmol/L
Ascorbic acid, blood	0.4-1.5 mg/dL	23-85 μmol/L
Aspartate aminotransferase (AST), serum (SGOT)	1-36 U/L	1-36 U/L
Base excess, arterial blood, calculated	0±2 mEq/L	0±2 mmol/L
Bicarbonate		
Venous plasma	23-29 mEq/L	23-29 mmol/L
Arterial blood	21-27 mEq/L	21-27 mmol/L
Bile acids, serum	0.3-3.0 mg/dL	0.8-7.6 μmol/L
Bilirubin, serum		
Conjugated	0.1-0.4 mg/dL	1.7-6.8 μmol/L
Total	0.3-1.1 mg/dL	5.1-19.0 μmol/L
Calcium, serum	8.4-10.6 mg/dL	2.10-2.65 mmol/L
Calcium, ionized, serum	4.25-5.25 mg/dL	1.05-1.30 mmol/L
Carbon dioxide, total, serum or plasma	24-31 mEq/L	24-31 mmol/L
Carbon dioxide tension (Pco_2), blood	35-45 mm Hg	35-45 mm Hg
β-Carotene, serum	60-260 μg/dL	1.1-8.6 μmol/L
Ceruloplasmin, serum	23-44 mg/dL	230-440 mg/L
Chloride, serum or plasma	96-106 mEq/L	96-106 mmol/L
Cholesterol, serum or EDTA plasma		
Desirable range	<200 mg/dL	<5.20 mmol/L
Low-density lipoprotein (LDL) cholesterol	60-180 mg/dL	1.55-4.65 mmol/L
High-density lipoprotein (HDL) cholesterol	30-80 mg/dL	0.80-2.05 mmol/L
Copper	70-140 μg/dL	11-22 μmol/L
Corticotropin (ACTH), plasma, 8 AM	10-80 pg/mL	2-18 pmol/L
Cortisol, plasma		
8:00 AM	6-23 μg/dL	170-630 nmol/L
4:00 PM	3-15 μg/dL	80-410 nmol/L
10:00 PM	<50% of 8:00 AM value	<50% of 8:00 AM value
Creatine, serum		
Males	0.2-0.5 mg/dL	15-40 μmol/L
Females	0.3-0.9 mg/dL	25-70 μmol/L
Creatine kinase (CK), serum		
Males	55-170 U/L	55-170 U/L
Females	30-135 U/L	30-135 U/L
Creatinine kinase MB isoenzyme, serum	<5% of total CK activity <5% of ng/mL by immunoassay	<5% of total CK activity <5% ng/mL by immunoassay
Creatinine, serum	0.6-1.2 mg/dL	50-110 μmol/L
Estradiol-17β, adult		
Males	10-65 pg/mL	35-240 pmol/L
Females		
Follicular	30-100 pg/mL	110-370 pmol/L
Ovulatory	200-400 pg/mL	730-1470 pmol/L
Luteal	50-140 pg/mL	180-510 pmol/L
Ferritin, serum	20-200 ng/mL	20-200 μg/L
Fibrinogen, plasma	200-400 mg/dL	2.0-4.0 g/L
Folate, serum	3-18 ng/mL	6.8-41 nmol/L
Erythrocytes	145-540 ng/mL	330-1220 nmol/L
Follicle-stimulating hormone (FSH), plasma		
Males	4-25 mU/mL	4-25 U/L
Females, premenopausal	4-30 mU/mL	4-30 U/L
Females, postmenopausal	40-250 mU/mL	40-250 U/L
Gastrin, fasting, serum	0-100 pg/mL	0-100 mg/L
Glucose, fasting, plasma or serum	70-115 mg/dL	3.9-6.4 nmol/L
γ-Glutamyltransferase (GGT), serum	5-40 U/L	5-40 U/L
Growth hormone (hGH), plasma, adult, fasting	0-6 ng/mL	0-6 μg/L

Continued

Reference Intervals* for Clinical Chemistry (Blood, Serum, and Plasma)—cont'd

Analyte	Conventional Units	SI Units
Haptoglobin, serum	20-165 mg/dL	0.20-1.65 g/L
Immunoglobulins, serum (see table of Reference Intervals for Tests of Immunologic Function)		
Iron, serum	75-175 μg/dL	13-31 μmol/L
Iron-binding capacity, serum		
Total	250-410 μg/dL	45-73 μmol/L
Saturation	20-55%	0.20-0.55
Lactate		
Venous whole blood	5.0-20.0 mg/dL	0.6-2.2 mmol/L
Arterial whole blood	5.0-15.0 mg/dL	0.6-1.7 mmol/L
Lactate dehydrogenase (LD), serum	110-220 U/L	110-220 U/L
Lipase, serum	10-140 U/L	10-140 U/L
Lutropin (LH), serum		
Males	1-9 U/L	1-9 U/L
Females		
Follicular phase	2-10 U/L	2-10 U/L
Midcycle peak	15-65 U/L	15-65 U/L
Luteal phase	1-12 U/L	1-12 U/L
Postmenopausal	12-65 U/L	12-65 U/L
Magnesium, serum	1.3-2.1 mg/dL	0.65-1.05 mmol/L
Osmolality	275-295 mOsm/kg water	275-295 mOsm/kg water
Oxygen, blood, arterial, room air		
Partial pressure (Pao_2)	80-100 mm Hg	80-100 mm Hg
Saturation (Sao_2)	95-98%	95-98%
pH, arterial blood	7.35-7.45	7.35-7.45
Phosphate, inorganic, serum		
Adult	3.0-4.5 mg/dL	1.0-1.5 mmol/L
Child	4.0-7.0 mg/dL	1.3-2.3 mmol/L
Potassium		
Serum	3.5-5.0 mEq/L	3.5-5.0 mmol/L
Plasma	3.5-4.5 mEq/L	3.5-4.5 mmol/L
Progesterone, serum, adult		
Males	0.0-0.4 ng/mL	0.0-1.3 mmol/L
Females		
Follicular phase	0.1-1.5 ng/mL	0.3-4.8 mmol/L
Luteal phase	2.5-28.0 ng/mL	8.0-89.0 mmol/L
Prolactin, serum		
Males	1.0-15.0 ng/mL	1.0-15.0 μg/L
Females	1.0-20.0 ng/mL	1.0-20.0 μg/L
Protein, serum, electrophoresis		
Total	6.0-8.0 g/dL	60-80 g/L
Albumin	3.5-5.5 g/dL	35-55 g/L
Globulins		
α_1	0.2-0.4 g/dL	2.0-4.0 g/L
α_2	0.5-0.9 g/dL	5.0-9.0 g/L
β	0.6-1.1 g/dL	6.0-11.0g/L
γ	0.7-1.7 g/dL	7.0-17.0 g/L
Pyruvate, blood	0.3-0.9 mg/dL	0.03-0.10 mmol/L
Rheumatoid factor	0.0-30.0 IU/mL	0.0-30.0 kIU/L
Sodium, serum or plasma	135-145 mEq/L	135-145 mmol/L
Testosterone, plasma		
Males, adult	300-1200 ng/dL	10.4-41.6 nmol/L
Females, adult	20-75 ng/dL	0.7-2.6 nmol/L
Pregnant females	40-200 ng/dL	1.4-6.9 nmol/L
Thyroglobulin	3-42 ng/mL	3-42 μg/L
Thyrotropin (hTSH), serum	0.4-4.8 μIU/mL	0.4-4.8 mIU/L
Thyrotropin-releasing hormone (TRH)	5-60 pg/mL	5-60 ng/L
Thyroxine (FT_4), free, serum	0.9-2.1 ng/dL	12-27 pmol/L
Thyroxine (T_4), serum	4.5-12.0 μg/dL	58-154 nmol/L
Thyroxine-binding globulin (TBG)	15.0-34.0 μg/mL	15.0-34.0 mg/L
Transferrin	250-430 mg/dL	2.5-4.3 g/L
Triglycerides, serum, after 12-h fast	40-150 mg/dL	0.4-1.5 g/L
Triiodothyronine (T_3), serum	70-190 ng/dL	1.1-2.9 nmol/L
Triiodothyronine uptake, resin (T_3RU)	25-38%	0.25-0.38
Urate		
Males	2.5-8.0 mg/dL	150-480 μmol/L
Females	2.2-7.0 mg/dL	130-420 μmol/L
Urea, serum or plasma	24-49 mg/dL	4.0-8.2 nmol/L
Urea, nitrogen, serum or plasma	11-23 mg/dL	8.0-16.4 nmol/L
Viscosity, serum	1.4-1.8 × water	1.4-1.8 × water
Vitamin A, serum	20-80 μg/dL	0.70-2.80 μmol/L
Vitamin B_{12}, serum	180-900 pg/mL	133-664 pmol/L

*Reference values may vary, depending on the method and sample source used.

Reference Intervals for Therapeutic Drug Monitoring (Serum or Plasma)*

Analyte	Therapeutic Range	Toxic Concentrations	Proprietary Name(s)
Analgesics			
Acetaminophen	10-40 μg/mL	>150 μg/mL	Tylenol Datril
Salicylate	100-250 μg/mL	>300 μg/mL	Aspirin Bufferin
Antibiotics			
Amikacin	20-30 μg/mL	Peak >35 μg/mL Trough >10 μg/mL	Amikin
Gentamicin	5-10 μg/mL	Peak >10 μg/mL Trough >2 μg/mL	Garamycin
Tobramycin	5-10 μg/mL	Peak >10 μg/mL Trough >2 μg/mL	Nebcin
Vancomycin	5-35 μg/mL	Peak >40 μg/mL Trough >10 μg/mL	Vancocin
Anticonvulsants			
Carbamazepine	5-12 μg/mL	>15 μg/mL	Tegretol
Ethosuximide	40-100 μg/mL	>250 μg/mL	Zarontin
Phenobarbital	15-40 μg/mL	40-100 ng/mL (varies widely)	Luminal
Phenytoin	10-20 μg/mL	>20 μg/mL	Dilantin
Primidone	5-12 μg/mL	>15 μg/mL	Mysoline
Valproic acid	50-100 μg/mL	>100 μg/mL	Depakene
Antineoplastics and Immunosuppressives			
Cyclosporine	100-300 ng/mL	>400 ng/mL	Sandimmune
Methotrexate, high-dose, 48-h	Variable	>1 μmol/L, 48 h after dose	
Tacrolimus (FK-506), whole blood	3-20 μg/L	>15 μg/L	Prograf
Bronchodilators and Respiratory Stimulants			
Caffeine	3-15 ng/mL	>30 ng/mL	
Theophylline (aminophylline)	10-20 μg/mL	>30 μg/mL	Elixophyllin Quibron
Cardiovascular Drugs			
Amiodarone (obtain specimen more than 8 h after last dose)	1.0-2.0 μg/mL	>2.0 μg/mL	Cordarone
Digoxin (obtain specimen more than 6 h after last dose)	0.8-2.0 ng/mL	>2.4 ng/mL	Lanoxin
Disopyramide	2-5 μg/mL	>7 μg/mL	Norpace
Flecainide	0.2-1.0 μg/mL	>1 μg/mL	Tambocor
Lidocaine	1.5-5.0 μg/mL	>6 μg/mL	Xylocaine
Mexiletine	0.7-2.0 μg/mL	>2 μg/mL	Mexitil
Procainamide	4-10 μg/mL	>12 μg/mL	Pronestyl
Procainamide plus NAPA	8-30 μg/mL	>30 μg/mL	
Propranolol	50-100 ng/mL	Variable	Inderal
Quinidine	2-5 μg/mL	>6 μg/mL	Cardioquin Quinaglute
Tocainide	4-10 ng/mL	>10 ng/mL	Tonocard
Psychopharmacologic Drugs			
Amitriptyline	120-150 ng/mL	>500 ng/mL	Elavil Triavil
Bupropion	25-100 ng/mL	Not applicable	Wellbutrin
Desipramine	150-300 ng/mL	>500 ng/mL	Norpramin
Imipramine	125-250 ng/mL	>400 ng/mL	Tofranil
Lithium (obtain specimen 12 h after last dose)	0.6-1.5 mEq/L	>1.5 mEq/L	Lithobid
Nortriptyline	50-150 ng/mL	>500 ng/mL	Aventyl Pamelor

*Values may vary depending on the method and sample collection device used. Always consult the reference values provided by the laboratory performing the analysis.

Reference Intervals* for Clinical Chemistry (Urine)

Analyte	Conventional Units	SI Units
Acetone and acetoacetate, qualitative	Negative	Negative
Albumin		
Qualitative	Negative	Negative
Quantitative	10-100 mg/24 h	0.15-1.5 μmol/d
Aldosterone	3-20 μg/24 h	8.3-55 nmol/d
δ-Aminolevulinic acid (δ-ALA)	1.3-7.0 mg/24 h	10-53 μmol/d
Amylase	<17 U/h	<17 U/h
Amylase/creatinine clearance ratio	0.01-0.04	0.01-0.04
Bilirubin, qualitative	Negative	Negative
Calcium (regular diet)	<250 mg/24 h	<6.3 nmol/d
Catecholamines		
Epinephine	<10 μg/24 h	<55 nmol/d
Norepinephine	<100 μg/24 h	<590 nmol/d
Total free catecholamines	4-126 μg/24 h	24-745 nmol/d
Total metanephrines	0.1-1.6 mg/24 h	0.5-8.1 μmol/d
Chloride (varies with intake)	110-250 mEq/24 h	110-250 mmol/d
Copper	0-50 μg/24 h	0.0-0.80 μmol/d
Cortisol, free	10-100 μg/24 h	27.6-276 nmol/d
Creatine		
Males	0-40 mg/24 h	0.0-0.30 mmol/d
Females	0-80 mg/24 h	0.0-0.60 mmol/d
Creatinine	15-25 mg/kg/24 h	0.13-0.22 mmol/kg/d
Creatinine clearance (endogenous)		
Males	110-150 mL/min/1.73 m^2	110-150 mL/min/1.73 m^2
Females	105-132 mL/min/1.73 m^2	105-132 mL/min/1.73 m^2
Cystine or cysteine	Negative	Negative
Dehydroepiandrosterone		
Males	0.2-2.0 mg/24 h	0.7-6.9 μmol/d
Females	0.2-1.8 mg/24 h	0.7-6.2 μmol/d
Estrogens, total		
Males	4-25 μg/24 h	14-90 nmol/d
Females	5-100 μg/24 h	18-360 nmol/d
Glucose (as reducing substance)	<250 mg/24 h	<250 mg/d
Hemoglobin and myoglobin, qualitative	Negative	Negative
Homogentisic acid, qualitative	Negative	Negative
17-Hydroxycorticosteroids		
Males	3-9 mg/24 h	8.3-25 μmol/d
Females	2-8 mg/24 h	5.5-22 μmol/d
5-Hydroxyindoleacetic acid		
Qualitative	Negative	Negative
Quantitative	2-6 mg/24 h	10-31 μmol/d
17-Ketogenic steroids		
Males	5-23 mg/24 h	17-80 μmol/d
Females	3-15 mg/24 h	10-52 μmol/d
17-Ketosteroids		
Males	8-22 mg/24 h	28-76 μmol/d
Females	6-15 mg/24 h	21-52 μmol/d
Magnesium	6-10 mEq/24 h	3-5 mmol/d
Metanephrines	0.05-1.2 ng/mg creatinine	0.03-0.70 mmol/mmol creatinine
Osmolality	38-1400 mOsm/kg water	38-1400 mOsm/kg water
pH	4.6-8.0	4.6-8.0
Phenylpyruvic acid, qualitative	Negative	Negative
Phosphate	0.4-1.3 g/24 h	13-42 mmol/d
Porphobilinogen		
Qualitative	Negative	Negative
Quantitative	<2 mg/24 h	<9 μmol/d
Porphyrins		
Coproporphyrin	50-250 μg/24 h	77-380 nmol/d
Uroporphyrin	10-30 μg/24 h	12-36 nmol/d
Potassium	25-125 mEq/24 h	25-125 mmol/d
Pregnanediol		
Males	0.0-1.9 mg/24 h	0.0-6.0 μmol/d
Females		
Proliferative phase	0.0-2.6 mg/24 h	0.0-8.0 μmol/d
Luteal phase	2.6-10.6 mg/24 h	8-33 μmol/d
Postmenopausal	0.2-1.0 mg/24 h	0.6-3.1 μmol/d
Pregnanetriol	0.0-2.5 mg/24 h	0.0-7.4 μmol/d

*Values may vary, depending on the method used.

Continued

Reference Intervals* for Clinical Chemistry (Urine)—cont'd

Analyte	Conventional Units	SI Units
Protein, total		
Qualitative	Negative	Negative
Quantitative	10-150 mg/24 h	10-150 mg/d
Protein/creatinine ratio	<0.2	<0.2
Sodium (regular diet)	60-260 mEq/24 h	60-260 mmol/d
Specific gravity		
Random specimen	1.003-1.030	1.003-1.030
24-h collection	1.015-1.025	1.015-1.025
Urate (regular diet)	250-750 mg/24 h	1.5-4.4 mmol/d
Urobilinogen	0.5-4.0 mg/24 h	0.6-6.8 μmol/d
Vanillylmandelic acid (VMA)	1.0-8.0 mg/24 h	5-40 μmol/d

Reference Intervals for Toxic Substances

Analyte	Conventional Units	SI Units
Arsenic, urine	<130 μg/24 h	<1.7 μmol/d
Bromides, serum, inorganic	<100 mg/dL	<10 mmol/L
Toxic symptoms	140-1000 mg/dL	14-100 mmol/L
Carboxyhemoglobin, blood	Saturation, percent	
Urban environment	<5%	<0.05
Smokers	<12%	<0.12
Symptoms		
Headache	>15%	>0.15
Nausea and vomiting	>25%	>0.25
Potentially lethal	>50%	>0.50
Ethanol, blood	<0.05 mg/dL <0.005%	<1.0 mmol/L
Intoxication	>100 mg/dL >0.1%	>22 mmol/L
Marked intoxication	300-400 mg/dL 0.3%-0.4%	65-87 mmol/L
Alcoholic stupor	400-500 mg/dL 0.4%-0.5%	87-109 mmol/L
Coma	>500 mg/dL >0.5%	>109 mmol/L
Lead, blood		
Adults	<20 μg/dL	<1.0 μmol/L
Children	<10 μg/dL	<0.5 μmol/L
Lead, urine	<80 μg/24 h	<0.4 μmol/d
Mercury, urine	<10 μg/24 h	<150 nmol/d

Reference Intervals for Tests Performed on Cerebrospinal Fluid

Test	Conventional Units	SI Units
Cells	<5/mm^3; all mononuclear	<5 × 10^6/L, all mononuclear
Protein electrophoresis	Albumin predominant	Albumin predominant
Glucose	50–75 mg/dL (20 mg/dL less than in serum)	2.8–4.2 mmol/L (1.1 mmol/L less than in serum)
IgG		
Children <14 y	<8% of total protein	<0.08 of total protein
Adults	<14% of total protein	<0.14 of total protein
IgG index		
$\left(\frac{\text{CSF/serum IgG ratio}}{\text{CSF/serum albumin ratio}}\right)$	0.3–0.6	0.3–0.6
Oligoclonal banding on electrophoresis	Absent	Absent
Pressure, opening	70–180 mm H_2O	70–180 mm H_2O
Protein, total	15–45 mg/dL	150–450 mg/L

Reference Intervals for Tests of Gastrointestinal Function

Test	Conventional Units
Bentiromide	6-h urinary arylamine excretion >57% excludes pancreatic insufficiency
β-Carotene, serum	60-250 ng/dL
Fecal fat estimation	
Qualitative	No fat globules seen by high-power microscope
Quantitative	<6 g/24 h (>95% coefficient of fat absorption)
Gastric acid output	
Basal	
Males	0.0-10.5 mmol/h
Females	0.0-5.6 mmol/h
Maximum (after histamine or pentagastrin)	
Males	9.0-48.0 mmol/h
Females	6.0-31.0 mmol/h
Ratio: basal/maximum	
Males	0.0-0.31
Females	0.0-0.29
Secretin test, pancreatic fluid	
Volume	>1.8 mL/kg/h
Bicarbonate	>80 mEq/L
D-Xylose absorption test, urine	>20% of ingested dose excreted in 5 h

Reference Intervals for Tests of Immunologic Function

Test	Conventional Units	SI Units
Complement, serum		
C3	85-175 mg/dL	0.85-1.75 g/L
C4	15-45 mg/dL	150-450 mg/L
Total hemolytic (CH_{50})	150-250 U/mL	150-250 U/mL
Immunoglobulins, serum, adult		
IgG	640-1350 mg/dL	6.4-13.5 g/L
IgA	70-310 mg/dL	0.70-3.1 g/L
IgM	90-350 mg/dL	0.90-3.5 g/L
IgD	0.0-6.0 mg/dL	0.0-60 mg/L
IgE	0.0-430 ng/dL	0.0-430 μg/L

Lymphocytes Subsets, Whole Blood, Heparinized

Antigen(s) Expressed	Cell Type	Percentage	Absolute Cell Count
CD3	Total T cells	56-77	860-1880
CD19	Total B cells	7-17	140-370
CD3 and CD4	Helper-inducer cells	32-54	550-1190
CD3 and CD8	Suppressor-cytotoxic cells	24-37	430-1060
CD3 and DR	Activated T cells	5-14	70-310
CD2	E rosette T cells	73-87	1040-2160
CD16 and CD56	Natural killer (NK) cells	8-22	130-500
Helper/Suppressor ratio: 0.8-1.8			

Reference Values for Semen Analysis

Test	Conventional Units	SI Units
Volume	2-5 mL	2-5 mL
Liquefaction	Complete in 15 min	Complete in 15 min
pH	7.2-8.0	7.2-8.0
Leukocytes	Occasional or absent	Occasional or absent
Spermatozoa		
Count	$60\text{-}150 \times 10^6$ mL	$60\text{-}150 \times 10^6$ mL
Motility	>80% motile	>0.80 motile
Morphology	80-90% normal forms,	>0.80-0.90 normal forms
Fructose	>150 mg/dL	>8.33 mmol/L

TOXIC CHEMICAL AGENTS REFERENCE CHART: CLINICAL CONSIDERATIONS

method of
JAMES J. JAMES, M.D., DR.P.H., M.H.A., and
JAMES M. LYZNICKI, M.S., M.P.H.
Center for Disaster Preparedness and Emergency Response
American Medical Association
Chicago, Illinois

Chemical weapon agents are poisonous vapors, aerosols, gases, liquids, or solids that have toxic effects on people, animals, or plants. Most of these agents are liquid at room temperature and are disseminated as vapors and aerosols. They may be released as bombs, sprayed from aircraft and boats, or disseminated by other means intentionally to create a hazard to people and the environment. Some of these agents are highly toxic and persistent, features that can render a site uninhabitable and can require costly and potentially hazardous decontamination and remediation. Health effects range from irritation and burning of skin and mucous membranes to rapid cardiopulmonary collapse and death.

Efficient deployment of hazardous materials (HazMat) teams is critical to control a chemical agent attack. Although all major cities and emergency medical systems in the United States have plans and equipment in place to address this situation, physicians and other health professionals must be aware of principles involved in managing a patient or multiple patients exposed to these agents. Chemical weapon agents have a high potential for secondary contamination from victims to responders. This requires that medical treatment facilities have clearly defined procedures for handling contaminated casualties, many of whom will transport themselves to the facility. Precautions must be used until thorough decontamination has been performed or the specific chemical agent is identified. Health care professionals must first protect themselves (e.g., by using protective suits and chemical-resistant gloves) because secondary contamination with even small amounts of these substances (particularly nerve agents such as VX) may be lethal.

Primary detection of exposure to chemical agents will be based on the signs and symptoms of the potential victim (Table 1). Confirmation of a chemical agent, using detection equipment or laboratory analyses, will take considerable time and will not likely contribute to the early management of mass casualties. Several patients presenting with the same symptoms should alert physicians and hospital staff to the possibility of a chemical attack. If a chemical attack occurs, most victims will likely arrive within a short time. This situation differentiates a chemical attack from a biologic attack involving infectious microorganisms. Additional diagnostic clues include:

- Unusual temporal or geographic clustering of illness.
- Any sudden increase in illness in previously healthy persons.
- Sudden increase in nonspecific syndromes (e.g., sudden unexplained weakness in previously healthy persons; dimmed or blurred vision; and hypersecretion, inhalation, or burnlike syndromes).

A coordinated communication network is critical for transmitting reliable information from the incident scene to treatment facilities. Any suspicious or confirmed exposure to a chemical weapons agent should be reported to the local health department, the local Federal Bureau of Investigation office, and the Centers for Disease Control and Prevention (1-770-488-7100).

TABLE 1. **Quick Reference Chart on Chemical Weapon Agents**

Chemical Agent	Diagnostic Considerations	Treatment Considerations*
Cyanides Cyanogen chloride (CK) Hydrogen cyanide (AC)	Symptom onset: rapid, seconds to minutes Odor: bitter almonds Nonspecific hypoxic and hypoxemic symptoms Binds cellular cytochrome oxidase, causing chemical asphyxia Respiratory: shortness of breath, chest tightness, hyperventilation, respiratory arrest Gastrointestinal: nausea, vomiting Cardiovascular: ventricular arrhythmias, hypotension, cardiac arrest, shock CNS: anxiety, headache, drowsiness, weakness, apnea, convulsions, seizure, coma CNS effects may be confused with carbon monoxide and hydrogen sulfide poisoning Metabolic acidosis and increased concentration of venous oxygen ("bright-red" venous blood) Laboratory testing: cyanide, thiocyanate, serum lactate levels; venous and arterial partial oxygen pressure	Antidote: sodium nitrite and sodium thiosulfate; repeat one-half of initial doses of both agents in 30 minutes if there is inadequate clinical response Amyl nitrate capsules are available for first aid until intravenous access is achieved "Cyanide antidote kits" are commercially available Investigational in the United States, available in Europe: hydroxycobalamin (vitamin B_{12a}) administered with thiosulfate Activated charcoal for oral exposure Mechanical ventilation as needed Circulatory support with crystalloids and vasopressors Metabolic acidosis corrected with IV sodium bicarbonate Seizures controlled with benzodiazepines

Continued

TABLE 1. **Quick Reference Chart on Chemical Weapon Agents—cont'd**

Chemical Agent	Diagnostic Considerations	Treatment Considerations*
Incapacitating Agents Agent 15 3-Quinuclidinyl benzilate (BZ)	Symptom onset: hours 0-4 h: parasympathetic blockade and mild CNS effects 4-20 h: stupor with ataxia and hyperthermia 20-96 h: full-blown delirium Resolution phase: paranoia, deep sleep, reawakening, crawling, climbing automatisms, eventual reorientation Odorless Competitive inhibitor of acetylcholine muscarinic receptor Mydriasis, blurred vision, dry mouth, dry skin, possible atropine-like flush, initial rise in heart rate, decreased level of consciousness, confusion, disorientation, visual hallucinations, impaired memory	Antidote: physostigmine salicylate (Antilirium) Support, intravenous fluids
Nerve Agents Cyclohexyl sarin (GF) Sarin (GB) Soman (GD) Tabun (GA) VX	Symptom onset: vapor (seconds), liquid (minutes to hours) Odor: none (GB, VX), fruity (GA), camphor-like (GD) Most toxic of known chemical agents Irreversible acetylcholinesterase inhibitors Eyes: lacrimation, miosis Respiratory: rhinorrhea, bronchospasm, respiratory failure Gastrointestinal: hypersalivation, nausea, vomiting, diarrhea Skin: localized sweating Cardiac: sinus bradycardia Skeletal muscles: fasciculations followed by weakness, flaccid paralysis CNS: loss of consciousness, convulsions, apnea, seizures May be confused with organophosphate and carbamate pesticide poisoning Laboratory testing: erythrocyte or serum cholinesterase activity to confirm exposure	Antidote: Atropine and pralidoxime chloride (Protopam Chloride, 2-PAM); additional doses until bronchial secretions are cleared and ventilation improved Early administration of 2-PAM is critical to minimize permanent agent inactivation of acetylcholinesterase (i.e., "aging") Benzodiazepines to control nerve agent–induced seizures Airway and ventilatory support as needed Atropine, pralidoxime, and diazepam are available in autoinjector kits through the U.S. military
Pulmonary or Choking Agents Acrolein Ammonia (NH_3) Chlorine (Cl) Choloropicrin (PS) Diphosgene (DP) Nitrogen oxides (NO_x) Perflouroisobutylene (PFIB) Phosgene (CG) Sulfur dioxide (SO_2)	Symptom onset: rapid or delayed; 1-24 h (rarely ≤72 h) Odor (CG): freshly mown hay or grass Easily absorbed by mucous membranes of eyes, nose, oropharynx; degree of water solubility of the agent influences onset and severity of respiratory injury Eye and airway irritation, dyspnea, chest tightness, rhinorrhea, hypersalivation, cough, wheezing High-dose inhalation may produce laryngospasm, pneumonitis, and acute lung injury with delayed onset (≤48 h) of acute respiratory distress syndrome Chest radiograph: hyperinflation, noncardiogenic pulmonary edema May be confused with inhalation exposure to industrial chemicals (e.g., HCl, Cl_2, NH_3)	Supportive measures; specific treatment depends on the agent IV fluids for hypotension; no diuretics Ventilation with or without positive airway pressure Bronchodilators for bronchospasm Methylprednisone may be effective in preventing noncardiogenic pulmonary edema No antidotes
Riot-Control Agents Mace (CN) Tear gas (CS)	Symptom onset: immediate Odor: apple blossom (CN); pepper (CS) Metallic taste SN_2 alkylating agents Burning and pain on mucosal membranes and skin Eyes: irritation, pain, tearing, blepharospasm Airways: burning in nose and mouth, respiratory discomfort, bronchospasm (may be delayed 36 h) Skin: tingling, erythema Nausea and vomiting common CN can cause corneal opacification No specific laboratory tests	Supportive Irrigation as necessary Persons with asthma or emphysema may need oxygen, inhaled bronchodilators, steroids, assisted ventilation Calamine for erythema

Continued

TABLE 1. **Quick Reference Chart on Chemical Weapon Agents—cont'd**

Chemical Agent	Diagnostic Considerations	Treatment Considerations*
Vesicant or Blister Agents	Symptom onset: immediate (L, CX); delayed 2-48 h (H, HD) Primary liquid hazard May be confused with skin exposure to caustic irritants (e.g., sodium hydroxide, ammonia)	Thermal burn–type treatment; supportive care Symptomatic management of lesions Immediate decontamination
Sulfur mustard (H) Distilled mustard (HD)	Intracellular enzyme and DNA alkylating agents Odor: garlic, horseradish, or mustard Skin: erythema and blisters (may be delayed ≤8 h), pruritus Eye: irritation, conjunctivitis, corneal damage, lacrimation, pain, blepharospasm Respiratory: mild to marked acute airway damage, pneumonitis within 1-3 d, respiratory failure Gastrointestinal effects (nausea, vomiting, diarrhea) may be present Bone marrow stem cell suppression leading to pancytopenia and increased susceptibility to infection Fever, sputum production Combination Lewisite (called mustard-Lewisite or HL) results in rapid effects of Lewisite and delayed effects of mustard agents	No antidote Skin: silver sulfadiazine Eye: homatropine ophthalmic ointment Pulmonary: antibiotics, bronchodilators, steroids Colony-stimulating factor may be helpful for leukopenia Systemic analgesic and antipruritics Early use of positive end-expiratory pressure or continuous positive airway pressure Maintain fluid and electrolyte balance (do not excessively fluid resuscitate as in thermal burns)
Lewisite (L)	Odor: fruity or geranium More volatile than mustard Damages eyes, skin, and airways by direct contact Skin: gray area of dead skin within 5 min, erythema within 30 min, blistering 2-3 h, immediate irritation or burning pain, severe tissue necrosis	Antidote: British antilewisite (BAL or dimercaprol)
Phosgene Oxime (CX)	Eyes: pain, blepharospasm, conjunctival and lid edema Airway: pseudomembrane formation, nasal irritation Intravascular fluid loss, hypovolemia, shock, organ congestion, leukocytosis, miosis, immediate pain on contact Odor: freshly mown hay Urticant, nonvesicant agent Vapor extremely irritating; vapor and liquid cause tissue damage on contact Immediate burning, irritation, wheal-like skin lesions, eye and airway damage, conjunctivitis, lacrimation, lid edema, blepharospasm No distinctive laboratory findings	No antidote Parenteral methylprednisone may be effective in preventing noncardiogenic pulmonary edema Experimental: aerosolized dexamethasone and theophylline for pulmonary involvement
Vomiting (Arsine-Based) Agents Adamsite (DM) Diphenylchlorarsine (DA) Diphenylcyanoarsine (DC)	Symptom onset: all rapidly acting within minutes Odor: none (DA), garlic (DC), burning fireworks (DM) Primary route of absorption is through respiratory system Arsine gas depletes erythrocyte glutathione and causes hemolysis Eyes: conjunctival irritation, tearing, and blepharospasm Airways: sneezing, mucosal lung irritation, edema, progressive cough, wheezing Cardiac: tachypnea, tachycardia Gastrointestinal: intestinal cramps, emesis, diarrhea Skin: erythema, edema at the site of dermal contact CNS depression, syncope Chest radiograph to rule out chemical pneumonitis	Supportive care Monitor for hemolysis Wheezing or dyspnea may need albuterol inhalation Eye irrigation (water, normal saline, lactated Ringer's solution) in patients sustaining ocular exposure Treat repetitive emesis with IV hydration and antiemetics Blood transfusion may be required Exchange transfusion may be required Hemodialysis may be useful in decreasing arsenic level and treating renal failure

*Different situations may require different treatment and dosage regimens. Please consult other references as well as a regional poison control center (1-800-222-1222), medical toxicologist, clinical pharmacologist, or other drug information specialist for definitive dosage information, especially dosages for pregnant women and children.

CNS, central nervous system.

BIOLOGIC AGENTS REFERENCE CHART: CLINICAL CONSIDERATIONS

method of
JAMES J. JAMES, M.D., Dr.P.H., M.H.A., AND JAMES M. LYZNICKI, M.S., M.P.H.
Center for Disaster Preparedness and Emergency Response
American Medical Association
Chicago, Illinois

Biologic weapons are devices used intentionally to cause disease or death through dissemination of microorganisms or toxins in food and water, by insect vectors, or by aerosols. Potential targets include human beings, food crops, livestock, and other resources essential for national security, economy, and defense. Unlike nuclear, chemical, and conventional weapons, the onset of a biologic attack will probably be insidious. Its impact may continue with secondary and tertiary transmission of the agent and sequelae, weeks or months after the initial attack.

Initial detection of an unannounced biologic attack will likely occur when an astute health professional notices an unusual case or disease cluster and reports his or her concerns to local public health authorities. Physicians and other health professionals should be alert to:

- Unusual temporal or geographic clustering of illnesses.
- Sudden increase of illness in previously healthy persons.
- Sudden increase in nonspecific illnesses (e.g., pneumonia, flulike illness; bleeding disorders; unexplained rashes, particularly in adults; neuromuscular illness; and diarrhea).

To enhance detection and treatment capabilities, physicians in acute care settings should be familiar with the clinical manifestations, diagnostic techniques, isolation precautions, treatment, and prophylaxis for likely causative agents (e.g., smallpox, pneumonic plague, anthrax, viral hemorrhagic fevers). Table 1 provides a quick summary of diagnostic and treatment considerations for various infectious and toxic biologic agents. For some of these agents, delay in medical response could result in a potentially devastating number of casualties. To mitigate such consequences, early identification and intervention are imperative. Front-line physicians must have an increased level of suspicion regarding the possible intentional use of biologic agents as well as an increased sensitivity to reporting those suspicions to public health authorities, who, in turn, must be willing to evaluate a predictable increase in false-positive reports.

Medical response efforts require coordination and planning with emergency management agencies, law enforcement, health care facilities, and social services agencies. Health care agencies should ensure that physicians know whom to call with reports of suspicious cases and clusters of infectious diseases and should work to build a good relationship with the local medical community. Resource integration is necessary to establish adequate surge capacity to initiate rapid investigation of an outbreak, to educate the public, to begin mass distribution of antibiotics and vaccines, to ensure mass medical care, and to control public anger and fear. In an epidemic, catastrophic numbers of critically ill patients will require acute and follow-up medical care. Both infected persons and the "worried well" would seek medical attention, with a corresponding need for medical supplies, diagnostic tests, and hospital beds. The impact—or even the threat—of an attack can elicit widespread panic and civil disorder, can overwhelm hospital resources, and can disrupt social services.

Any suspicious or confirmed exposure to a biologic weapons agent should be immediately reported to the local health department, the local Federal Bureau of Investigation office, and the Centers for Disease Control and Prevention (1-770 488-7100).

TABLE 1. **Quick Reference Chart on Biologic Weapon Agents**

Disease/Agent	Diagnostic Considerations	Treatment Considerations[1]	Prophylaxis
Bacteria			
Anthrax *Bacillus anthracis*	Incubation period: 1-5 d (perhaps ≤60 d)[2] *Cutaneous:* Evolving skin lesion (face, neck, arms), progresses to vesicle, depressed ulcer, and black necrotic lesion Lethality: 20% if untreated, otherwise rarely fatal *Gastrointestinal:* Nausea, vomiting, abdominal pain, bloody diarrhea, sepsis Lethality: approaches 100% if untreated but data are limited; rapid, aggressive treatment may reduce mortality *Inhalational:* Abrupt onset of flulike symptoms, fever with or without chills, sweats, fatigue	Combination therapy of ciprofloxacin (Cipro) or doxycycline (Vibramycin) plus one or two other antimicrobials should be considered with inhalational anthrax[6] Penicillin should be considered if strain is susceptible and does not possess inducible β-lactamases If meningitis is suspected, doxycycline (Vibramycin) may be less optimal because of poor central nervous system penetration	Ciprofloxacin (Cipro) or doxycycline (Vibramycin) with or without vaccination; if strain is susceptible, penicillin or amoxicillin (Amoxil) should be considered Inactivated vaccine (licensed but not readily available); six injections and annual booster

Continued

TABLE 1. **Quick Reference Chart on Biologic Weapon Agents—cont'd**

Disease/Agent	Diagnostic Considerations	Treatment Considerations[1]	Prophylaxis
	or malaise, nonproductive or minimally productive cough, nausea, vomiting, dyspnea, headache, chest pain, followed in 2-5 d by severe respiratory distress, mediastinitis, hemorrhagic meningitis, sepsis, shock[3] Widened mediastinum on chest radiograph is characteristic of inhalational and occasionally gastrointestinal anthrax[4] Lethality: Once respiratory distress develops, mortality rates may approach 90%; begin treatment when inhalational anthrax is suspected; do not wait for confirmatory testing[5] Gram stain and culture of blood, pleural fluid, cerebrospinal fluid, ascitic fluid, vesicular fluid or lesion exudate; sputum rarely positive; confirmatory serologic and PCR tests available through public health laboratory network	Steroids may be considered for severe edema and for meningitis	
Brucellosis *Brucella abortus* *Brucella canis* *Brucella mellitensis* *Brucella suis*	Incubation period: 5-60 d (usually 1-2 mo) Nonspecific flulike symptoms, fever, headache, profound weakness and fatigue, gastrointestinal symptoms such as anorexia, nausea, vomiting, diarrhea, or constipation Osteoarticular complications common Lethality: less than 5% even if untreated; tends to incapacitate rather than kill Blood and bone marrow culture (may require 6 wk to grow *Brucella*); confirmatory culture and serologic testing available through public health laboratory network.	Doxycycline (Vibramycin) plus streptomycin or rifampin (Rifadin) Alternative therapies: Ofloxacin (Floxin) plus rifampin (Rifadin) Doxycycline (Vibramycin) plus gentamicin (Garamycin) Trimethoprim-sulfamethoxazole (Bactrim, Septra) plus gentamicin (Garamycin)	Doxycycline (Vibramycin) plus streptomycin or rifampin (Rifadin) No approved human vaccine
Inhalational (pneumonic) tularemia *Francisella tularensis*	Incubation period: 3-5 d (range, 1-21 d) Sudden onset of acute febrile illness, weakness, chills, headache, generalized body aches, elevated white blood cells Pulmonary symptoms such as dry cough, chest pain, or tightness with or without objective signs of pneumonia Progressive weakness, malaise, anorexia, and weight loss, potentially leading to sepsis and organ failure Largely clinical diagnosis Lethality: ~30-60% fatal if untreated Culture of blood, sputum, biopsies, pleural fluid, bronchial washings. (culture is difficult and potentially dangerous); confirmatory testing available through public health laboratory network	Streptomycin or gentamicin (Garamycin) Alternatives: Ciprofloxacin (Cipro) Doxycycline (Vibramycin) Chloramphenicol (Chloromycetin)	Tetracycline Doxycycline (Vibramycin) Ciprofloxacin (Cipro) Live attenuated vaccine (USAMRIID, IND) given by scarification; currently under FDA review; limited availability
Pneumonic plague *Yersinia pestis*	Incubation period: 1-10 d (typically 2-3 d) Acute onset of flulike prodrome: fever, myalgia, weakness, headache; within 24 h of prodrome, chest discomfort, cough, and dyspnea; by day 2 to 4 of illness, symptoms progressing to cyanosis, respiratory distress, and hemodynamic instability Lethality: almost 100% if untreated; 20-60% if appropriately treated within 18-24 h of symptoms; begin treatment when diagnosis of plague is suspected; do not wait for confirmatory testing. Gram stain and culture of blood, cerebrospinal fluid, sputum, lymph node aspirates, bronchial washings;	Streptomycin; gentamicin (Garamycin) Alternatives: Doxycycline (Vibramycin) Tetracycline Ciprofloxacin (Cipro) Chloramphenicol (Chloromycetin) is first choice for meningitis except for pregnant women	Tetracycline Doxycycline (Vibramycin) Ciprofloxacin (Cipro) Inactivated whole cell vaccine licensed but not readily available; injection with boosters Vaccine not effective against aerosol exposure

Continued

TABLE 1. **Quick Reference Chart on Biologic Weapon Agents—cont'd**

Disease/Agent	Diagnostic Considerations	Treatment Considerations[1]	Prophylaxis
	confirmatory serologic and bacteriologic tests available through public health laboratory network		
Rickettsia			
Q fever *Coxiella burnetii*	Incubation period: 2-14 d (may be ≤40 d) Nonspecific febrile disease, chills, cough, weakness and fatigue, pleuritic chest pain, possible pneumonia Lethality: 1-3%; fatalities uncommon even if untreated, but relapsing symptoms possible Isolation of organism may be difficult; confirmatory testing by serology or PCR available through public health laboratory network	Tetracycline Doxycycline (Vibramycin)	Tetracycline Doxycycline (Vibramycin) Inactivated whole cell vaccine (IND) Skin test to determine prior exposure to *C. burnetii* recommended before vaccination
Viruses			
Smallpox Variola viruses	Incubation period: 7-17 d Prodrome of high fever, malaise, prostration, headache, vomiting, delirium followed in 2-3 d by maculopapular rash uniformly progressing to pustules and scabs, mostly on extremities and face Requires astute clinical evaluation; may be confused with chickenpox, erythema multiforme with bullae, or allergic contact dermatitis Lethality: 30% in unvaccinated persons Pharyngeal swab, vesicular fluid, biopsies, scab material for electron microscopy and PCR testing through public health laboratory network Notify CDC Poxvirus Section at 1-404 639-2184	Supportive care Cidofovir (Vistide) shown to be effective in vitro and in experimental animals infected with surrogate orthopox virus	Attenuated-strain vaccinia vaccine derived from calf lymph; given by scarification (licensed, limited supply) Vaccination given within 3-4 d of exposure can prevent or decrease the severity of disease
Viral Encephalitis Eastern (EEE) Western (WEE) Venezuelan (VEE)	Incubation period: 2-6 d (VEE); 7-14 d (EEE, WEE) Systemic febrile illness, with encephalitis developing in some populations Generalized malaise, spiking fevers, headache, myalgia Incidence of seizures and/or focal neurologic deficits may be higher after biologic attack White blood cell count may show striking leukopenia and lymphopenia Clinical and epidemiologic diagnosis Lethality: <10% (VEE); 10% (WEE); 50-75% (EEE) Confirmatory test and viral isolation available through public health laboratory network	Supportive care Analgesics, anticonvulsants as needed	Several IND vaccines, poorly immunogenic, highly reactogenic
Viral hemorrhagic fevers (VHFs) Arenaviruses (Lassa, Junin, and related viruses) Bunyaviruses (Hanta, Congo-Crimean, Rift Valley) Filoviruses (Ebola, Marburg) Flaviviruses (yellow fever, dengue, various tick-borne disease viruses)	Incubation period: 4-21 d Fever with mucous membrane bleeding, petechiae, thrombocytopenia, and hypotension in patients without underlying malignancies Malaise, myalgias, headache, vomiting, diarrhea possible Lethality: variable depending on viral strain; 15-25% with Lassa fever to ≤90% with Ebola Confirmatory testing and viral isolation available through public health laboratory network Call CDC Special Pathogens Office at 1-404 639-1115	Supportive therapy Ribavirin (Virazole may be effective for Lassa fever, Argentine hemorrhagic fever, and Congo-Crimean hemorrhagic fever	Ribavarin (Virazole) is suggested for Congo-Crimean hemorrhagic fever and Lassa fever Yellow fever vaccine is the only licensed vaccine available Vaccines for some of the other VHFs exist but are for investigational use only

Continued

TABLE 1. **Quick Reference Chart on Biologic Weapon Agents—cont'd**

Disease/Agent	Diagnostic Considerations	Treatment Considerations[1]	Prophylaxis
Biologic Toxins			
Botulism *Clostridium botulinum* toxin	Symptom onset: 1-5 d (typically 12-36 h) Blurred vision, diplopia, dry mouth, ptosis, fatigue As disease progresses, acute bilateral descending flaccid paralysis, respiratory paralysis resulting in death Clinical diagnosis Lethality: 60% without ventilatory support Serum and stool should be assayed for toxin by mouse neutralization bioassay, which may require several days	Intensive and prolonged supportive care; ventilation may be necessary Trivalent equine antitoxin (serotypes A,B,E licensed, available from the CDC) should be administered immediately after clinical diagnosis Anaphylaxis and serum sickness are potential complications of antitoxin Aminoglycosides and clindamycin (Cleocin) must not be used	Pentavalent toxoid (A-E), yearly booster (IND, CDC) Not available to the public Antitoxin may be sufficient to prevent illness after exposure but is not recommended until patient is showing symptoms
Enterotoxin B *Staphylococcus aureus*	Symptom onset: 3-12 h Acute onset of fever, chills headache, nonproductive cough Normal chest radiograph Clinical diagnosis Lethality: probably low (few data available for respiratory exposure) Serology on acute and convalescent serum can confirm diagnosis	Supportive care	No vaccine available
Ricin toxin *Ricinus communis*	Symptom onset: 18-24 h Weakness, nausea, chest tightness, fever, cough, pulmonary edema, respiratory failure, circulatory collapse, hypoxemia resulting in death (usually within 36-72 h) Clinical and epidemiologic diagnosis Lethality: mortality data not available but is likely to be high with extensive exposure Confirmatory serologic testing available through public health laboratory network	Supportive care Treatment for pulmonary edema Gastric decontamination if toxin ingested	No vaccine available
T-2 Mycotoxins *Fusarium* *Myrothecium* *Trichoderma* *Stachbotrys* Other filamentous fungi	Symptom onset: minutes to hours Abrupt onset of mucocutaneous and airway irritation and pain May include skin, eyes, and gastrointestinal tract; systemic toxicity may follow Lethality: severe exposure can cause death in hours to days Consult with local health department regarding specimen collection and diagnostic testing procedures; confirmation requires testing blood, tissue, and environmental samples	Clinical support Soap and water washing within 4-6 h reduces dermal toxicity; washing within 1 h may eliminate toxicity entirely No effective medications or antidotes	No vaccine available

[1]Different situations may require different dosage and treatment regimens. Please consult other references and an infectious disease specialist for definitive dosage information, especially dosages for pregnant women and children.

[2]Data from 22 patients infected with anthrax in October and November 2001 indicate a median incubation period of 4 d (range, 4-7 d) for inhalational anthrax and a mean incubation of 5 d (range, 1-10 d) for cutaneous anthrax.

[3]Limited data from the October/November 2001 anthrax infections indicate hemorrhagic pleural effusions to be strongly associated with inhalational anthrax; rhinorrhea was present in only 1/10 patients.

[4]Chest radiograph abnormalities include paratracheal and hilar fullness and may be subtle. Consider chest computed tomography if diagnosis is uncertain.

[5]Limited data from the 2001 terrorist-related anthrax infections indicate that early treatment significantly decreased the mortality rate.

[6]Other agents with in vitro activity suggested for use in conjunction with ciprofloxacin (Cipro) or doxycycline (Vibramycin) for treatment of inhalational anthrax include rifampin (Rifadin), vancomycin (Vancocin), imipenem (Primaxin), chloramphenicol (Chloromycetin), penicillin and ampicillin, clindamycin (Cleocin), and clarithromycin (Biaxin).

CDC, Centers for Disease Control and Prevention; IND, investigational new drug; PCR, polymerase chain reaction; USAMRIID, U.S. Army Medical Research Institute of Infectious Diseases.

Adapted from American Medical Association: Biological Weapons: Quick Reference Guide. Chicago, American Medical Association, 2002. Available at http://www.ama-assn.org/ama1/pub/upload/mm/415/quickreference0902.pdf.

SOME POPULAR HERBS AND NUTRITIONAL SUPPLEMENTS

method of
MIRIAM M. CHAN, R.PH., PHARM.D.
Riverside Family Practice Residency Program
Columbus, Ohio

Herb/Nutritional Supplement	Common Uses	Reasonable Adult Oral Dosage*	Precautions and Drug Interactions
Black cohosh root	Commonly used to relieve menopausal symptoms, such as hot flashes Also used to treat premenstrual discomfort and dysmenorrhea	20 mg bid of the rhizome extract standardized to triterpene glycosides The German guidelines do not recommend its use for >6 mo	Black cohosh has an estrogen-like effect and has been shown to decrease luteinizing hormone Large doses may induce miscarriage, and it is contraindicated during pregnancy It may cause GI disturbances, headache, and hypotension
Chamomile flower	Used orally to calm nerves and treat GI spasms and inflammatory diseases of the GI tract Used topically to treat wounds, skin infections, and skin or mucous membrane inflammation	1 cup of freshly made tea three to four times daily (1 tbsp or 3 g of dried flower in 150 mL boiling water for 5-10 min)	Chamomile may cause an allergic reaction, especially in people with severe allergies to ragweed or other members of the daisy family (e.g., echinacea, feverfew, and milk thistle) It should not be taken concurrently with other sedatives, such as alcohol or benzodiazepines
Chromium	For diabetes For hypercholesterolemia Commonly found in weight-loss products Also promoted for body building	For diabetes, 100 μg bid for ≤4 mo or 500 μg bid for 2 mo For hypercholesterolemia, 200 μg tid or 500 μg bid for 2-4 mo For body building, 200-400 μg/d Chromium picolinate has been been used in most studies, even though the chloride form is also available	Adverse effects are rare, but they may include headaches, insomnia, sleep disturbances, irritability and mood changes. Some patients may also experience cognitive, perceptual, and motor dysfunction Long-term use of high doses (600-2400 μg/d) can cause anemia, thrombocytopenia, hemolysis, hepatic dysfunction, and renal failure There have been two case reports of interstitial nephritis A few studies suggest that chromium may cause DNA damage Chromium competes with iron for binding to transferrin and can cause iron deficiency Antacids, H_2 blockers, and proton pump inhibitors can decrease the absorption of chromium
Chondroitin	For osteoarthritis, commonly used in combination with glucosamine	400 mg tid; chondroitin derived from bovine cartilage may carry a potential risk of contamination with diseased animals	Occasional mild side effects include nausea, indigestion, and allergic reactions
Coenzyme Q10	As adjunctive treatment for congestive heart failure, angina, and hypertension Also used for reducing cardiotoxicity associated with doxorubicin	For heart failure, 100 mg/d in two or three divided doses For angina, 50 mg tid For hypertension, 60 mg bid	Mild adverse events include gastric distress, nausea, vomiting, and hypotension Doses >300 mg/d may cause elevated liver enzymes Coenzyme Q10 may reduce the anticoagulation effects of warfarin Oral hypoglycemic agents and HMG-CoA reductase inhibitors may reduce serum coenzyme Q10 levels
Creatine	To enhance muscle performance, especially during short-duration, high-intensity exercise	A loading dose of 20 g/d for 5-7 d followed by a maintenance dose of ≥2 g/d An alternative regimen of of 3 g/d for 28 d has been suggested	Creatine can cause gastroenteritis, diarrhea, heat intolerance, muscle cramps, and elevated serum creatinine levels Creatine is contraindicated in patients taking diuretics

Continued

Herb/Nutritional Supplement	Common Uses	Reasonable Adult Oral Dosage*	Precautions and Drug Interactions
			Concurrent use with cimetidine, probenecid, or nonsteroidal anti-inflammatory drugs increase the risk of adverse renal effects Caffeine may decrease creatine's ergogenic effects
Echinacea	As an immune stimulant, particularly for the prevention and treatment of the common cold and influenza Supportive therapy for lower urinary tract infections Used topically to treat skin disorders and promote wound healing	300 mg tid of *Echinacea pallida* root or 2-3 mL tid of expressed juice of *Echinacea purpurea* herb Do not use for >8 wk because echinacea may suppress immunity if used long term	Echinacea should not be used in transplant recipients and those with autoimmune disease or liver dysfunction Allergic reactions have been reported Adverse events are rare and may include mild GI effects It should be discontinued as far in advance of surgery as possible Echinacea may decrease effectiveness of immunosuppressants
Ephedra (ma huang)	For diseases of the respiratory tract with mild bronchospasm Commonly found in weight-loss products Also marketed as a stimulant for performance enhancement	1 tsp or 2 g of dried herb (15-30 mg of ephedrine) in 240 mL boiling water for 10 min The FDA recommends that ephedra products contain no more than 8 mg ephedrine/dose or 24 mg/d and the duration of use be <7 d	Ephedra contains ephedrine, which has sympathomimetic activities; consequently, it should not be used in patients who have cardiovascular disease, diabetes, glaucoma, hypertension, hyperthyroidism, prostate enlargement, psychiatric disorders, or seizures Serious adverse effects, including seizures, arrhythmias, heart attack, stroke, and death, have been associated with the use of ephedra Because of the cardiovascular effects of ephedrine, patients taking ephedra should discontinue use at least 24 h before surgery Concurrent use of ephedra and digitalis, guanethidine, monoamine oxidase inhibitors, or other stimulants, including caffeine, is not recommended
Evening primrose oil	For premenstrual syndrome, especially if mastalgia is present Licensed in the United Kingdom for the treatment of atopic eczema Also used for other medical conditions, including rheumatoid arthritis, Raynaud's phenomenon, Sjögren's syndrome, and diabetic neuropathy	For premenstrual syndrome, 2-4 g/d For atopic eczema, 6-8 g/d For rheumatoid arthritis, 2.8 g/d These doses are based on products standardized to 9% γ-linolenic acid The daily dose can be given in divided doses	Evening primrose oil may increase the risk of pregnancy complications Side effects may include indigestion, nausea, soft stools, and headache Seizures have been reported in patients with schizophrenia who were taking phenothiazines and evening primrose oil concomitantly Evening primrose oil may interact with anesthesia and cause seizures
Feverfew	For migraine headache prophylaxis For treatment of fever, menstrual problems, and arthritis	50-125 mg qd of the encapsulated dried leaf extract standardized to at least 0.2% parthenolide	Feverfew may induce menstrual bleeding and is contraindicated in pregnancy Fresh leaves may cause oral ulcers and GI irritation Sudden discontinuation of feverfew can precipitate rebound headache Feverfew may interact with anticoagulants and potentiate the antiplatelet effect of aspirin
Garlic	To lower blood pressure and serum cholesterol To prevent artherosclerosis	Fresh clove: 1 (4 g)/d Tablet: 300 mg bid to tid standardized to 0.6-1.3% allicin	Intake of large quantities can lead to stomach complaints Garlic has antiplatelet effects, so patients should discontinue use of garlic at least 7 d before surgery Concomitant use of garlic and anticoagulants may increase the risk of bleeding
Ginger root	As an antiemetic For prevention of motion sickness	Fresh rhizome: 2-4 g /d Powdered ginger: 250 mg three to four times daily	Ginger should not be used in patients with gallstones because of its cholagogic effect

Continued

Herb/Nutritional Supplement	Common Uses	Reasonable Adult Oral Dosage*	Precautions and Drug Interactions
		Tea: 1 cup tea tid (0.5-1 g dried root in 150 mL boiling water for 5-10 min)	It may inhibit platelet aggregation; cases of postoperative bleeding have been reported Large doses of ginger may increase bleeding time in patients taking antiplatelet agents
Ginkgo biloba leaf	To slow cognitive deterioration in dementia To increase peripheral blood flow in claudication To treat sexual dysfunction associated with the use of SSRIs	60-120 mg bid of extract Egb761 standardized to 24% flavonoids and 6% terpenoids	Adverse effects are rare and may include mild stomach or intestinal upset, headache, or allergic skin reaction Ginkgo can inhibit platelet aggregation; reports of spontaneous bleeding have been published Patients should discontinue ginkgo at least 36 h before surgery Concurrent use of ginkgo and anticoagulants, antiplatelet agents, vitamin E, or garlic may increase the risk of bleeding
Ginseng root	As a tonic during times of stress, fatigue, disability, and convalescence To improve physical performance and stamina	Root: 1-2 g/d Tablet: 100 mg bid of extract standardized to 4-7% ginsenosides A 2-3-wk period of using ginseng followed by a 1-2-wk "rest" period is generally recommended Ginseng is commonly adulterated, especially Siberian ginseng products	Ginseng has a mild stimulant effect and should be avoided in patients with cardiovascular disease Tachycardia and hypertension can occur Overdosages can lead to "ginseng abuse syndrome," characterized by insomnia, hypotonia, and edema Ginseng has estrogenic effects and may cause vaginal bleeding and breast tenderness Ginseng has been shown to inhibit platelets, so patients should discontinue ginseng use at least 7 d before surgery Ginseng should not be used with other stimulants Patients taking antidiabetic agents and ginseng should be monitored to avoid the hypoglycemic effects of ginseng Ginseng may interact with warfarin and cause a decreased international normalized ratio Siberian ginseng may increase digoxin levels There have been reports of a drug interaction between ginseng and phenelzine (a monoamine oxidase inhibitor) resulting in insomnia, headache, tremulousness, and manic-like symptoms
Glucosamine	For osteoarthritis	500 mg tid with meals Glucosamine is available in the form of sulfate, hydrochloride, or n-acetyl salt Glucosamine sulfate is the form that has been used in most clinical studies	Side effects are generally limited to mild GI symptoms, including stomach upset, heartburn, diarrhea, nausea, and indigestion Glucosamine derived from marine exoskeletons may cause reactions in people allergic to shellfish Glucosamine may raise blood glucose levels in patients with diabetes
Hawthorn leaf with flower	Commonly used in Germany to increase cardiac output in patients with New York Heart Association class I and II heart failure	160-900 mg water-ethanol extract (30-160 mg procyanidins or 3.5-19.8 mg flavonoids) divided into two to three doses	Side effects include GI upset, palpitations, hypotension, headache, dizziness, and insomnia Concomitant use with CNS depressants may have additive CNS effects Hawthorn may potentiate effects of digoxin and vasodilators

Continued

Herb/Nutritional Supplement	Common Uses	Reasonable Adult Oral Dosage*	Precautions and Drug Interactions
Horse chestnut seed	To relieve symptoms of chronic venous insufficiency	250 mg bid of extract standardized to 50 mg aescin in delayed-release form It is unsafe to ingest the raw seed, which contains significant amounts of the most toxic constituent, esculin	Mild GI symptoms, headache, dizziness, and pruritus have been reported Ingestion of high doses may cause renal, hepatic, and hematologic toxicity Concomitant use with anticoagulants may increase the risk of bleeding Horse chestnut may potentiate the effects of hypoglycemic drugs
Kava kava	As an anxiolytic for nervous anxiety, stress, and restlessness As a sedative to induce sleep	Herb and preparations equivalent to 60-120 mg kava pyrones/d Most clinical trials have used 100 mg tid of extract standardized to 70% kava pyrones for anxiety disorders	Kava should not be used by patients with depression or by pregnant or nursing women Kava may affect motor reflexes and judgment, so it should not be taken while driving and/or operating heavy machinery Accommodative disturbances have been reported; kava may exacerbate Parkinson's disease Extended use can cause a temporary yellow discoloration of skin, hair, and nails Reports have linked kava use to at least 25 cases of severe liver toxicity Kava has been shown to have additive CNS depressant effects with benzodiazepines, alcohol, and herbal tranquilizers Kava may also potentiate the sedative effects of anesthetics, so kava should be discontinued at least 24 h before surgery
Melatonin	For jet lag, insomnia, shift-work disorder, and circadian rhythm disorders Also for other medical conditions, including depression, multiple sclerosis, tinnitus, headache, and cancer	For jet lag, 5 mg at bedtime for 2-5 d beginning the day of return For sleep disorders, 0.3-5 mg taken 2 h before bedtime Avoid melatonin from animal pineal gland because of the possibility of contamination	Avoid use in pregnancy because melatonin decreases serum luteinizing hormone concentrations and increases serum prolactin levels Common adverse reactions include headache, transient depressive symptoms, daytime fatigue and drowsiness, dizziness, abdominal cramps, irritability, and reduced alertness Concomitant use of melatonin with alcohol, benzodiazepines, or other CNS depressants may cause additive sedation Melatonin can affect immune function and may interfere with immunosuppressive therapy Concomitant use with other herbs that have sedative properties (e.g., chamomile, goldenseal, hops, kava, valerian) may produce additive CNS-impairing effects
Milk thistle fruit	As a hepatoprotectant and antioxidant, particularly for the treatment of hepatitis, cirrhosis, and toxic liver damage Used in Europe for the treatment of hepatotoxic mushroom poisoning from *Amanita phalloides*	Average daily dose is 12-15 g of crude drug or formulations equivalent to 200-400 mg of silymarin	Adverse effects are rare but may include diarrhea and allergic reactions Milk thistle may potentiate the hypoglycemic effect of antidiabetic agents
SAMe (S-adenosyl-L-methionine)	For treatment of osteoarthritis, depression, fibromyalgia, and liver disease	For osteoarthritis, 200 mg tid For depression and fibromyalgia, 800 mg bid For liver disease, 600-800 mg bid	Common side effects include flatulence, nausea, vomiting, and diarrhea SAMe can cause anxiety in people with depression and hypomania in people with bipolar disorder Concurrent use of SAMe and other antidepressant may cause serotonin syndrome

Continued

Herb/Nutritional Supplement	Common Uses	Reasonable Adult Oral Dosage*	Precautions and Drug Interactions
Saw palmetto berry	To treat symptomatic benign prostatic hyperplasia and irritable bladder	160 mg bid of extract standardized to 85-95% fatty acids and sterols	Adverse effects are rare but may include headache, nausea, and upset stomach High doses can cause diarrhea
St. John's wort	Effective for the treatment of mild to moderate depression May have anti-inflammatory and anti-infective activities	300 mg tid of hypericum extract standardized to 0.3% hypericin	St. John's wort should not be used in pregnancy Side effects include dry mouth, GI upset, dizziness, fatigue, and constipation St. John's wort may induce photosensitivity, especially in fair-skinned individuals It may cause serotonin syndrome if used with other antidepressants, including SSRIs, or other serotonergic drugs It has been shown to induce the cytochrome P-450 isoenzymes and decrease blood levels of many drugs such as indinavir, cyclosporine, digoxin, theophylline, oral contraceptive pills, and warfarin St. John's wort should be discontinued at least 5 d before surgery to avoid any potential drug interactions
Soy	Commonly used for cholesterol reduction in combination with a low-fat diet Also used for menopausal symptoms and for preventing osteoporosis and cardiovascular disease in postmenopausal women	For lowering cholesterol, 25-50 g/d of soy protein For hot flashes, 20-60 g/d of soy protein For osteoporosis, 40 g/d of soy protein containing 90 mg isoflavones	Soy may cause GI side effects such as constipation, bloating, and nausea Allergic reactions such as rash and itching have been reported Soy may inhibit the effects of estrogen replacement therapy Soy may reduce the absorption of zinc, iron, or calcium supplements
Valerian root	Used as a mild sedative for insomnia and anxiety	2-3 g of dried root or 1-3 mL of tincture, qd to several times/d Two clinical trials have found 400-450 mg of the root extract effective for insomnia	Valerian has a bad odor and can cause morning drowsiness Long-term administration may lead to paradoxical stimulation including restlessness and palpitations Because of the risk of benzodiazepine-like withdrawal, valerian should be tapered over a period of several weeks before surgery It may potentiate the sedative effect of CNS depressants (e.g., benzodiazepines, alcohol) and other herbal tranquilizers

*Doses presented in the table are adapted from the German Commission E Monographs and/or data from clinical trials. Products from different manufacturers vary considerably. A reliable product should have a label clearly stating the botanical name of the herb and the milligram amount contained in the product. Standardized extracts should be used whenever possible and are often disclosed on the label of high-quality products.

CNS, central nervous system; GI, gastrointestinal; HMG-CoA, 3-hydroxy-3-methylglutaryl coenzyme A; SSRIs, selective serotonin reuptake inhibitors.

NEW DRUGS IN 2002 AND AGENTS PENDING FDA APPROVAL

method of
MIRIAM CHAN, PHARM.D.
Riverside Family Practice Residency Program
Columbus, Ohio

and

BELLA MEHTA, PHARM.D.
The Ohio State University College of Pharmacy
Columbus, Ohio

TABLE 1. **New Drugs Approved in 2002**

Generic Name	Trade Name (Manufacturer)	Strength	Dosage form	Normal Dosage Range	Pregnancy Rating*	FDA Approval Date	Indication	Classification
Adalimumab	Humira (Abbott)	40 mg/0.8 mL in 1-mL prefilled syringes or 2-mL vials	Injection	40 mg SC every other week	B	12/02	Treatment of moderately to severely active rheumatoid arthritis	Immuno-modulator
Adefovir dipivoxil	Hepsera (Gilead)	10 mg	Tablet	10 mg qd	C	09/02	Treatment of patients with chronic hepatitis B, including treatment-naive and treatment-experienced patients	Antiretroviral agent (prodrug nucleotide analogue)
Alosetron	Lotronex (GlaxoSmithKline)	1.124 mg (1 mg as alosetron base)	Tablet	1 mg qd	B	06/02	Reintroduction with restrictions (prescriber program and informed consent) and narrowed indication; indicated only in treatment of severe diarrhea-prominent irritable bowel syndrome in women who have chronic irritable bowel syndrome symptoms, who have failed to respond to conventional therapy, and in whom anatomic and biochemical abnormalities of the gastrointestinal tract have been excluded	Selective 5-HT_3 receptor antagonist
Anastrozole	Arimidex (AstraZeneca)	1 mg	Tablet	1 mg qd	D	09/02	First-line treatment for post-menopausal women with hormone receptor positive or hormone receptor unknown localized metastatic or advanced breast cancer	Antineoplastic agent
Aripiprazole	Abilify (Bristol Myers Squibb/Otsuka)	10, 15, 20, 30 mg	Tablet	10-15 mg qd (maximum 30 mg/d)	C	11/02	Treatment of schizophrenia	Antipsychotic

Atomoxetine	Strattera (Eli Lilly)	10, 18, 25, 40, 60 mg	Capsule	Children ≤70 kg: Initially 0.5 mg/kg/d for minimum 3 d, increase to target dose of 1.2 mg/kg/d; Adults and children >70 kg: initially 40 mg for a minimum of 3 d then increase to target dose of 80 mg/d (maximum 80 mg/d in children >70 kg and 100 mg/d in adults)	C	11/02	Treatment of attention deficit/hyperactivity syndrome	Selective norepinephrine reuptake inhibitor
Buprenorphine	Subutex (Reckitt Benckiser)	2, 8 mg	Sublingual tablet	12-16 mg/d	C	10/02	Treatment of opioid dependence	Narcotic agonist/ antagonist
Buprenorphine/ naloxone	Suboxone (Reckitt Benckiser)	2 mg/0.5 mg, 8 mg/2 mg	Sublingual tablet	12-16 mg/d	C	10/02	Treatment of opioid dependence	Narcotic agonist/ antagonist
Dimyristoyl-phosphatidyl-choline/ perflexane lipid micro-spheres	Imagent (Alliance)	200 mg	Injection	0.125 mg/kg as a single IV bolus dose	C	05/02	For imaging studies in subjects with suboptimal echocardiograms to opacify the left ventricular chamber and to improve the delineation of the left ventricular endocardial border	Diagnostic imaging agent
Dutasteride	Avodart (GlaxoSmithKline)	0.5 mg	Capsule	0.5 mg qd	X	10/02	Treatment of symptomatic benign prostatic hyperplasia in men with an enlarged prostate to improve symptoms and reduce the risk of acute urinary retention and need for surgery related to benign prostatic hyperplasia	Androgen hormone inhibtor
Eletriptan	Relpax (Pfizer)	20, 40 mg	Tablet	40 mg initially, may repeat dose in 2 h (maximum 80 mg/d)	C	12/02	Treatment of acute migraine headache	Serotonin 5-HT 1b/1d receptor agonist
Eplerenone	Inspra (Pharmacia)	25, 50, 100 mg	Tablet	50 mg qd	B	09/02	Treatment of hypertension	Antihypertensive (selective aldosterone blocker)
Escitalopram oxalate	Lexapro (Forest Laboratories)	10, 20 mg tablet; 5 mg/5 mL solution	Tablet, solution	10 mg qd	C	08/02	Treatment of major depressive disorder	Antidepressant (selective serotonin

Continued

TABLE 1. **New Drugs Approved in 2002—cont'd**

Generic Name	Trade Name (Manufacturer)	Strength	Dosage form	Normal Dosage Range	Pregnancy Rating*	FDA Approval Date	Indication	Classification
								reuptake inhibitor)
Ezetimibe	Zetia (Schering)	10 mg	Tablet	10 mg qd	C	10/02	Treatment of primary hypercholesterolemia as monotherpay or as adjunct in combination with an HMG-coenzyme A reductase inhibitor	Antihyper-lipidemic (cholesterol absorption inhibitor)
Fulvestrant	Faslodex (AstraZeneca)	50 mg/mL in 5-mL or two 2.5-mL prefilled syringes	Injection	250 mg IM/mo	D	04/02	Treatment of hormone receptor–positive metastatic breast cancer in postmenopausal women with disease progression after antiestrogen therapy	Antineoplastic (estrogen receptor antagonist)
Glatiramer acetate	Copaxone (Teva)	20-mg premixed syringe or 2-mL vial with 1-mL diluent	Injection	20 mg/d SC	B	02/02	For reduction in the frequency of relapses in patients with relapsing-remitting multiple sclerosis	Immuno-suppressant
Glipizide and metformin	Metaglip (Bristol Myers Squibb)	2.5 mg/250 mg, 2.5 mg/500 mg, 5 mg/500 mg	Tablet	Initial therapy 2.5 mg/ 250 mg qd with a meal (maximum 20 mg/2000 mg)	C	10/02	As initial therapy to improve glycemic control in type 2 diabetes or as a second-line agent in nonresponders to sulfonylurea or metformin alone	Antidiabetic
Hydroxy-amphetamine hydrobromide/ tropicamide	Paremyd (Akorn)	1%/0.25% combination	Ophthalmic solution	Instill 1-2 drops into the conjuctival sac(s)	C	01/02	Pupil dilation in routine ophthalmic diagnostic procedures and eye examinations	Ophthalmic-mydriatric combination
Ibritumomab tiuxetan	Zevalin (IDEC Pharmaceuticals)	3.2 mg/2 mL	Injection	Two-step regimen given after rituximab infusion	D	02/02	Treatment of relapsed or refractory low-grade, follicular, or transformed B-cell non-Hodgkin's lymphoma, including rituximab-refractory follicular non-Hodgkin's lymphoma	Monoclonal antibody/radio-pharmaceutical

Icodextrin	Extraneal (Baxter)	7.5%	Solution	Use qd for the long-dwell (8-16 h) dialysis exchange	C	12/02	For use in a single daily exchange for the long dwell during continuous ambulatory peritoneal dialysis or automated peritoneal dialysis for the management of chronic renal failure	Peritoneal dialysis solution (glucose polymer osmotic agent)
Interferon β-1a	Rebif (Serono)	22-, 44-μg prefilled syringes	Injection	44 μg SC three times/wk	C	03/02	Treatment of patients with relapsing forms of multiple sclerosis to decrease the frequency of clinical exacerbations and delay the accumulation of physical disability	Immuno-modulator
Nitazoxanide	Alinia (Romark)	100 mg/5 mL in 60-mL bottle	Oral suspension	Age 12-47 mo: 100 mg q12h × 3 d; age 4-11 y: 200 mg q12h × 3 d	B	12/02	Treatment of diarrhea caused by *Cryptosporidium parvum* and *Giardia lamblia* in pediatric patients 1-11 y old	Antiparasitic
Nitisinone	Orfadin (Swedish Orphan AB)	2, 5, 10 mg	Capsule	1 mg/kg/d divided into two doses, then titrate to individual patient response	C	01/02	As an adjunct to dietary restriction of tyrosine and phenylalanine in the treatment of hereditary tyrosinemia type 1	Enzyme inhibitor of hydroxy-phenyl pyruvate dioxygenase
Olmesartan medoxomil	Benicar (Sankyo Pharma)	5, 20, 40 mg	Tablet	20-40 mg qd	C (first trimester)/ D (second and third trimesters)	04/02	Treatment of hypertension	Angiotension II receptor blocker
Oxaliplatin	Eloxatin (Sanofi-Synthelabo)	50, 100 mg	Injection	85 mg/m^2 IV infusion with leucovorin followed by 5-fluorouracil q2wk	D	08/02	For patients with metastatic carcinoma of the colon or rectum whose disease has recurred or progressed during or within 6 months of completion of first-line therapy with the combination of bolus 5-fluorouracil/ leucovorin and irinotecan	Antineoplastic agent (alkylating agent)
Oxybate sodium	Xyrem (Orphan Medical)	500 mg/mL in 180-mL bottle	Oral solution	Start at 4.5 g/d divided into two equal doses (first dose at	B	07/02	Treatment of cataplexy related to narcolepsy (access restricted by the	Central nervous system depressant

Continued

TABLE 1. **New Drugs Approved in 2002—cont'd**

Generic Name	Trade Name (Manufacturer)	Strength	Dosage form	Normal Dosage Range	Pregnancy Rating*	FDA Approval Date	Indication	Classification
				bedtime then second dose 2.5-4 h later)			FDA and manufacturer)	
Pegfilgrastim	Neulasta (Amgen)	6 mg/0.6-mL prefilled syringe	Injection	6 mg SC once per chemotherapy cycle (do not administer the drug in the period 14 d before to 24 h after chemotherapy)	C	01/02	To decrease the incidence of infection in patients with nonmyeloid malignancies who are receiving myelosuppressive anticancer drugs associated with a clinically significant incidence of febrile neutropenia	Colony-stimulating factor
Peginterferon alfa-2a	Pegasys (Roche)	180 μg/mL	Injection	180 μg SC once/wk for 48 weeks	C	10/02	Treatment of adults with chronic hepatitis C who have compensated liver disease and who have not been previously treated with interferon-α	Immuno-modulator
Rasburicase	Elitek (Sanofi-Synthelabo)	1.5 mg	Injection	0.15 or 0.20 mg/kg as a single daily dose × 5d (chemotherapy should be initiated 4-24 h after the first dose of the drug)	C	07/02	For the initial management of hyperuricemia in pediatric patients with leukemia, lymphoma, and solid tumor malignancies who are receiving chemotherapy	Recombinant urate-oxidase enzyme
Rosiglitazone/ metformin	Avandamet (GlaxoSmithKline)	1 mg/500 mg, 2 mg/500 mg, 4 mg/500 mg	Tablet	Dose is based on the patient's current doses of rosiglitzaone and/or metformin (maximum 8 mg/2000 mg/d)	C	10/02	Improvement of glycemic control in patients with type 2 diabetes mellitus who are already treated with combination rosiglitazone and metformin or whose disease is not adequately controlled on metformin alone	Antidiabetic
Secretin	SecreFlo (RepliGen)	16 μg	Injection	0.2 or 0.4 μg/kg, depending on type of testing	C	04/02	To aid in the diagnosis of pancreatic exocrine dysfunction and gastrinoma; and also to facilitate the identification of	Diagnostic agent (peptide hormone)

							ampulla of Vater and accessory papilla during endoscopic retrograde cholangio-pancreatography	
Tegaserod maleate	Zelnorm (Novartis)	2, 6 mg	Tablet	6 mg bid before meals for 4-6 wk (an additional 4-6-wk course for those who respond)	B	07/02	Short-term treatment of women with constipation-predominant irritable bowel syndrome	Serotonin (5-HT_4) receptor partial agonist
Teriparatide	Forteo (Eli Lilly)	750 µg/3 mL prefilled pen delivery device	Injection	20 µg SC once daily	C	12/02	Treatment of postmenopausal women with osteoporosis who are at high risk of fractures and men with primary or hypogonadal osteoporosis who are at high risk of fractures	Recombinant human parathyroid hormone
Treprostinil sodium	Remodulin (United Therapeutics)	1, 2.5, 5, 10 mg/mL in 20-mL vial	Injection	Continuous subcutaneous infusion at initial rate of 1.25 ng/kg/min, then titrate	B	05/02	Treatment of pulmonary arterial hypertension in patients with New York Heart Association class II-IV symptoms to diminish symptoms associated with exercise	Vasodilator
Urofollitropin	Bravelle (Ferring)	75 IU follicle-stimulating hormone activity	Injection	Initiate at 150 IU/d × 5 d, adjust subsequent dose according to response	X	05/02	In conjunction with human chorionic gonadotropin for ovulation induction in patients who previously received pituitary suppression	Gonadotropin-ovulation stimulants
Voriconazole	Vfend (Pfizer)	200-mg injection; 50-, 200-mg tablet	Injection, tablet	Loading dose of 6 mg/kg q12h × two doses, followed by a maintenance dose of 4 mg/kg IV q12h; oral maintenance dose of 200 mg q12h for >40 kg and 100 mg q12h for <40 kg	D	05/02	Treatment of invasive aspergillosis and serious fungal infections caused by *Scedosporium apiospermum* and *Fusarium* sp. including *Fusarium solani,* in patients intolerant of, or refractory to, other therapy	Triazole antifungal agents

*FDA Pregnancy Categories:

A: Adequate studies in pregnant women have not demonstrated a risk to the fetus in the first trimester of pregnancy, and there is no evidence of risk in later trimesters.

B: Animal studies have shown an adverse effect, but adequate studies in pregnant women have not demonstrated a risk to the fetus during the first trimester of pregnancy, and there is no evidence of risk in later trimesters.

C: Animal studies have shown an adverse effect on the fetus but there are no adequate studies in human patients; the benefit from the use of the drug in pregnant women may be acceptable despite its potential risks.

D: There is evidence of human fetal risk, but the potential benefit from the use of the drug in pregnant women may be acceptable despite its potential risks.

X: Adverse reaction reports indicate evidence of fetal risks; the risk of use in a pregnant women clearly outweighs any possible benefit. No drug should be administered during pregnancy unless it is clearly needed and the potential benefit outweighs the potential hazard to the fetus, regardless of the pregnancy category.

TABLE 2. **Agents Pending FDA Approval**

Generic Name	Trade Name (Manufacturer)	Indication
Alefacept	Amevive (Biogen)	Treatment of patients with chronic plaque psoriasis
Alfuzosin	Xatral (Skepharma)	Treatment of prostatic hyperplasia
Apomorphine	Uprima (TAP Holdings)	Treatment of erectile dysfunction
Artesunate	No current trade name (World Health Organization)	Treatment of malaria
Duloxetine	Cymbalta (Eli Lilly)	Treatment of depression
Etoricoxib	Arcoxia (Merck)	Treatment of arthritis pain
Gefitinib	Iressa (AstraZeneca)	Treatment of patients with advanced nonsmall cell lung cancer
Influenza vaccine	FluMist vaccine (Anron)	Nasal spray flu vaccine
Latanoprost and timolol	Xalcom (Pharmacia)	Reduction of intraocular pressure in open-angle glaucoma or ocular hypertension unresponsive to other treatments
Lercanidipine	Zanidip (Forest Laboratories)	Treatment of hypertension
Leuprolide	One-Month Leuprogel (Atrix Laboratories)	Treatment of advanced prostate cancer
Norastemizole	Soltara (Sepracor)	Treatment of allergic rhinitis
Parecoxib sodium	No current trade name (Pharmacia)	Management of acute pain
Pleconaril	Picovir (VioPharma)	Treatment of viral respiratory infection in adults
Pramlintide acetate	Symlin (Amylin Pharmaceuticals)	Treatment of patients with diabetes mellitus using insulin
Prasterone (dehydroepiandrosterone)	Aslera (Genelabs Technologies)	Treatment of systemic lupus erythematosus
Rifaximin	Lumenax (Salix Pharmaceuticals)	Treatment of traveler's diarrhea
Ropivacaine	Naropin (AstraZeneca)	Regional anesthesia in pediatric patients
Rosuvastatin calcium	Crestor (AstraZeneca)	Treatment of high cholesterol
Tadalafil	Cialis (Eli Lilly)	Treatment of erectile dysfunction
Telithromycin	Ketek (Aventis)	Treatment of community-acquired pneumonia in patients 18 yrs and older
Tibolone	Xyvion (Akzo Nobel)	Treatment of osteoporosis
Tiotropium	Spiriva (Boehringer Ingelheim)	Treatment of patients with chronic obstructive pulmonary disease
Vardenafil	Levitra (Bayer and GlaxoSmithKline)	Treatment of erectile dysfunction
Verteporfin	Visudyne (Novartis/QLT Inc.)	Treatment of pathologic myopia and ocular histoplasmosis syndrome
Ziconotide	Prialt (Elan)	Treatment of chronic pain

Body Mass Index Table

	Normal						Overweight					Obese										Extreme Obesity														
BMI	**19**	**20**	**21**	**22**	**23**	**24**	**25**	**26**	**27**	**28**	**29**	**30**	**31**	**32**	**33**	**34**	**35**	**36**	**37**	**38**	**39**	**40**	**41**	**42**	**43**	**44**	**45**	**46**	**47**	**48**	**49**	**50**	**51**	**52**	**53**	**54**
Height (inches)	**Body Weight (pounds)**																																			
58	91	96	100	105	110	115	119	124	129	134	138	143	148	153	158	162	167	172	177	181	186	191	196	201	205	210	215	220	224	229	234	239	244	248	253	258
59	94	99	104	109	114	119	124	128	133	138	143	148	153	158	163	168	173	178	183	188	193	198	203	208	212	217	222	227	232	237	242	247	252	257	262	267
60	97	102	107	112	118	123	128	133	138	143	148	153	158	163	168	174	179	184	189	194	199	204	209	215	220	225	230	235	240	245	250	255	261	266	271	276
61	100	106	111	116	122	127	132	137	143	148	153	158	164	169	174	180	185	190	195	201	206	211	217	222	227	232	238	243	248	254	259	264	269	275	280	285
62	104	109	115	120	126	131	136	142	147	153	158	164	169	175	180	186	191	196	202	207	213	218	224	229	235	240	246	251	256	262	267	273	278	284	289	295
63	107	113	118	124	130	135	141	146	152	158	163	169	175	180	186	191	197	203	208	214	220	225	231	237	242	248	254	259	265	270	278	282	287	293	299	304
64	110	116	122	128	134	140	145	151	157	163	169	174	180	186	192	197	204	209	215	221	227	232	238	244	250	256	262	267	273	279	285	291	296	302	308	314
65	114	120	126	132	138	144	150	156	162	168	174	180	186	192	198	204	210	216	222	228	234	240	246	252	258	264	270	276	282	288	294	300	306	312	318	324
66	118	124	130	136	142	148	155	161	167	173	179	186	192	198	204	210	216	223	229	235	241	247	253	260	266	272	278	284	291	297	303	309	315	322	328	334
67	121	127	134	140	146	153	159	166	172	178	185	191	198	204	211	217	223	230	236	242	249	255	261	268	274	280	287	293	299	306	312	319	325	331	338	344
68	125	131	138	144	151	158	164	171	177	184	190	197	203	210	216	223	230	236	243	249	256	262	269	276	282	289	295	302	308	315	322	328	335	341	348	354
69	128	135	142	149	155	162	169	176	182	189	196	203	209	216	223	230	236	243	250	257	263	270	277	284	291	297	304	311	318	324	331	338	345	351	358	365
70	132	139	146	153	160	167	174	181	188	195	202	209	216	222	229	236	243	250	257	264	271	278	285	292	299	306	313	320	327	334	341	348	355	362	369	376
71	136	143	150	157	165	172	179	186	193	200	208	215	222	229	236	243	250	257	265	272	279	286	293	301	308	315	322	329	338	343	351	358	365	372	379	386
72	140	147	154	162	169	177	184	191	199	206	213	221	228	235	242	250	258	265	272	279	287	294	302	309	316	324	331	338	346	353	361	368	375	383	390	397
73	144	151	159	166	174	182	189	197	204	212	219	227	235	242	250	257	265	272	280	288	295	302	310	318	325	333	340	348	355	363	371	378	386	393	401	408
74	148	155	163	171	179	186	194	202	210	218	225	233	241	249	256	264	272	280	287	295	303	311	319	326	334	342	350	358	365	373	381	389	396	404	412	420
75	152	160	168	176	184	192	200	208	216	224	232	240	248	256	264	272	279	287	295	303	311	319	327	335	343	351	359	367	375	383	391	399	407	415	423	431
76	156	164	172	180	189	197	205	213	221	230	238	246	254	263	271	279	287	295	304	312	320	328	336	344	353	361	369	377	385	394	402	410	418	426	435	443

Source: Adapted from National Heart, Lung, and Blood Institute: Clinical Guidelines on the Identification, Evaluation, and Treatment of Overweight and Obesity in Adults: The Evidence Report. See http://www.nhlbi.nih.gov/guidelines/obesity/bmi_tbl.pdf

NOMOGRAM FOR THE DETERMINATION OF BODY SURFACE AREA OF CHILDREN AND ADULTS

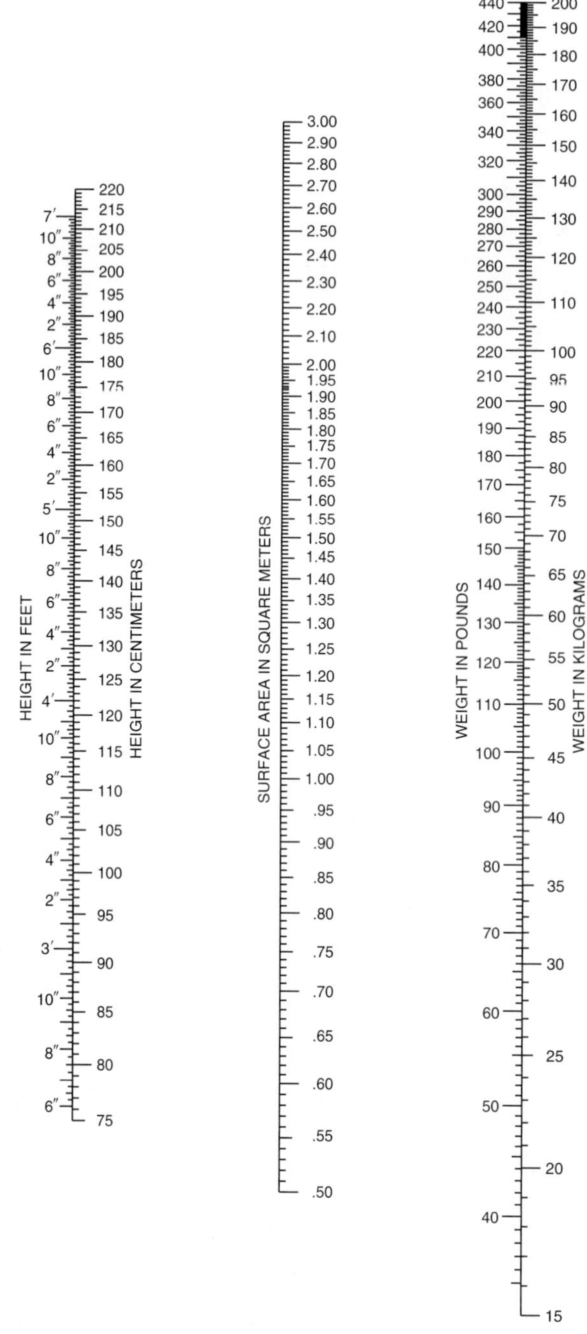

From Boathy WM, Sandiford RB: Boston Med Surg J 185:337, 1921.

Index

Note: Page numbers followed by f indicate figures; those followed by t indicate tables. Drugs are listed under the generic name.

B

C

J

K

L

O

Q

R

W

X

Y

Z

ISBN 0-7216-0401-3

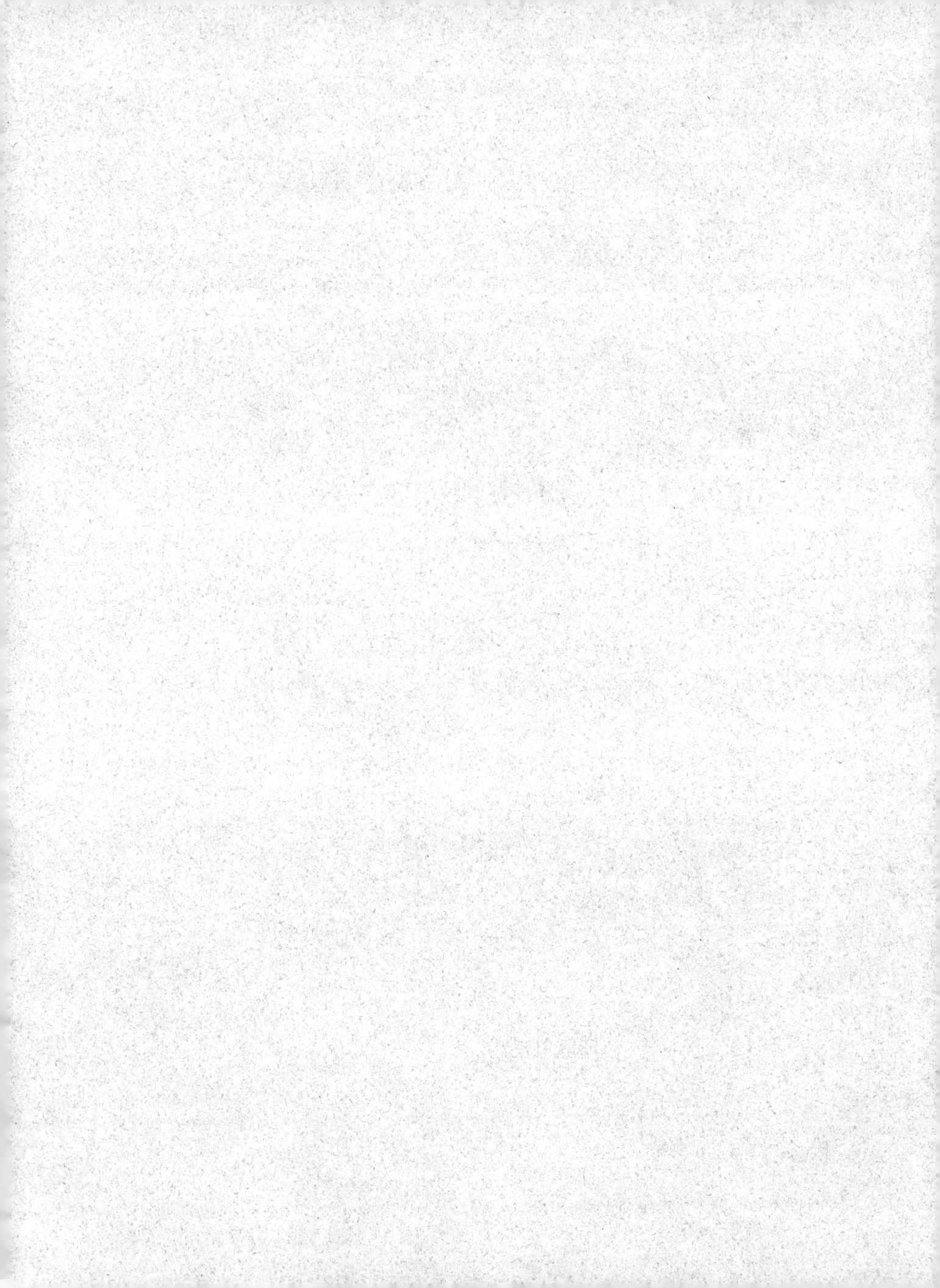